Evidence-based Nephrology

Evidence-based Nephrology

EDITED BY

DONALD A. MOLONY
Division of Renal Disease and Hypertension
University of Texas
Houston Medical School
Houston, Texas, USA

JONATHAN C. CRAIG
School of Public Health
University of Sydney
Department of Nephrology
The Children's Hospital at Westmead
Sydney, Australia

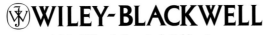

WILEY-BLACKWELL

A John Wiley & Sons, Ltd., Publication

This edition first published 2009, ©2009 by Blackwell Publishing Ltd

BMJ Books is an imprint of BMJ Publishing Group Limited, used under licence by Blackwell Publishing which was acquired by John Wiley & Sons in February 2007. Blackwell's publishing programme has been merged with Wiley's global Scientific, Technical and Medical business to form Wiley-Blackwell.

Registered office
John Wiley & Sons Ltd, The Atrium, Southern Gate, Chichester, West Sussex,
PO19 8SQ, UK

Editorial office
9600 Garsington Road, Oxford, OX4 2DQ, UK
The Atrium, Southern Gate, Chichester, West Sussex, PO19 8SQ, UK
111 River Street, Hoboken, NJ 07030-5774, USA

For details of our global editorial offices, for customer services and for information about how to apply for permission to reuse the copyright material in this book please see our website at www.wiley.com/wiley-blackwell

The right of the author to be identified as the author of this work has been asserted in accordance with the Copyright, Designs and Patents Act 1988.

Wiley also publishes its books in a variety of electronic formats. Some content that appears in print may not be available in electronic books.

Designations used by companies to distinguish their products are often claimed as trademarks. All brand names and product names used in this book are trade names, service marks, trademarks or registered trademarks of their respective owners. The publisher is not associated with any product or vendor mentioned in this book. This publication is designed to provide accurate and authoritative information in regard to the subject matter covered. It is sold on the understanding that the publisher is not engaged in rendering professional services. If professional advice or other expert assistance is required, the services of a competent professional should be sought.

The contents of this work are intended to further general scientific research, understanding, and discussion only and are not intended and should not be relied upon as recommending or promoting a specific method, diagnosis, or treatment by physicians for any particular patient. The publisher and the author make no representations or warranties with respect to the accuracy or completeness of the contents of this work and specifically disclaim all warranties, including without limitation any implied warranties of fitness for a particular purpose. In view of ongoing research, equipment modifications, changes in governmental regulations, and the constant flow of information relating to the use of medicines, equipment, and devices, the reader is urged to review and evaluate the information provided in the package insert or instructions for each medicine, equipment, or device for, among other things, any changes in the instructions or indication of usage and for added warnings and precautions. Readers should consult with a specialist where appropriate. The fact that an organization or Website is referred to in this work as a citation and/or a potential source of further information does not mean that the author or the publisher endorses the information the organization or Website may provide or recommendations it may make. Further, readers should be aware that Internet Websites listed in this work may have changed or disappeared between when this work was written and when it is read. No warranty may be created or extended by any promotional statements for this work. Neither the publisher nor the author shall be liable for any damages arising herefrom.

Library of Congress Cataloging-in-Publication Data

Data available
ISBN: 978-1-4051-3975-5

A catalogue record for this book is available from the British Library

Set in 9.25/12pt Minion by Aptara® Inc., New Delhi, India
Printed in Singapore by Ho Printing, Singapore Pte Ltd

3   2010

Contents

Contents

A companion website for this book with updates, a chance to send us your feedback, and links to other useful Evidence Based resources is provided at:

www.blackwellpublishing.com/medicine/bmj/nephrology

List of contributors

Kevin C. Abbott MD, MPH
Walter Reed Army Medical Center
Washington, DC, USA

Marcin Adamczak MD
Department of Nephrology
Endocrinology and Metabolic Diseases
Medical University of Silesia
Katowice, Poland

Dwomoa Adu MD, FRCP
Department of Nephrology
Queen Elizabeth Hospital
Birmingham, United Kingdom

Behdad Afzali MD
Department of Nephrology and Transplantation
Guy's Hospital
London, United Kingdom

Anil K. Agarwal MD
Department of Internal Medicine
The Ohio State University Medical Center
Columbus, Ohio, USA

Rajiv Agarwal MD
Division of Nephrology
Department of Medicine
Indiana University School of Medicine,
Indianapolis, Indiana, USA

Aimun Ahmed MD
Sheffield Kidney Institute
Sheffield, United Kingdom

M. Aamir Ali MD
Division of Renal Diseases and Hypertension
Department of Medicine
George Washington University Medical Center
Washington, DC, USA

Sandra Amaral MD, MHS
Division of Pediatric Nephrology
Emory Healthcare & Children's Healthcare of
Atlanta, Atlanta, Georgia, USA

Sharon Phillips Andreoli MD
Bryon P. and Frances D. Hollett Professor of
Pediatrics
Director of the Division of Pediatric Nephrology
James Whitcomb Riley Hospital for Children
Indianapolis, Indiana, USA

Phyllis August MD, MPH
Weill Medical College of Cornell University
Ithaca, New York, USA

Justine Bacchetta MD
Département de Pédiatrie & Inserm
Hôpital Edouard-Herriot
Hospices Civils de Lyon & Université Lyon
Lyon, France

Joanne M. Bargman MD
Department of Medicine
Division of Nephrology
University of Toronto
Toronto, Canada

Jonathan Barratt MD
Department of Infection
John Walls Renal Unit
Leicester General Hospital
Leicester, United Kingdom

Brendan J. Barrett MBBS, PhD
Division of Nephrology and Clinical Epidemiology
Faculty of Medicine
Memorial University of Newfoundland
St. John's, Newfoundland, Canada

Patrina Caldwell MBBS, PhD
Centre for Kidney Research
The Children's Hospital at Westmead
Westmead, Australia

Giovanni Cancarini MD
Section and Division of Nephrology
Department of Experimental and Applied
Medicine
University and Spedali Civili
Brescia, Italy

Andrés Cárdenas MD, MMSc
Liver Unit
Institut de Malalties Digestives i Metaboliques
Hospital Clinic
University of Barcelona
Barcelona, Spain

Daniel C. Cattran MD, FRCP
University of Toronto
Toronto, Ontario, Canada

Monique E. Cho MD
Kidney Disease Section
National Institute of Diabetes and Digestive and
Kidney Diseases
National Institutes of Health
US Department of Health and Human Services
Bethesda, Maryland, USA

Annabelle Chua MD
Section of Pediatric Nephrology
Texas Children's Hospital
Baylor College of Medicine
Houston, Texas, USA

Pierre Cochat MD
Département de Pédiatrie
Hôpital Edouard-Herriot
Lyon, France

Scott D. Cohen MD
Division of Renal Diseases and Hypertension
Department of Medicine
George Washington University Medical Center
Washington, DC, USA

Jonathan C. Craig MD, PhD
School of Public Health
University of Sydney
Deptartment of Nephrology
The Children's Hospital at Westmead
Sydney, Australia

Erica Daina MD
Mario Negri Institute for Pharmacological
Research
Negri Bergamo Laboratories
Bergamo, Italy

Connie L. Davis MD
Division of Nephrology
Department of Medicine
University of Washington School of Medicine
Seattle, Washington, USA

Allison Eddy MD
Children's Hospital & Regional Medical Center
Seattle, Washington, USA

Meguid El Nahas PhD, FRCP
Sheffield Kidney Institute
Northern General Hospital
Sheffield, United Kingdom

Chukwuma Eze MD
Good Samaritan Hospital
Dayton, Ohio, USA

John Feehally MD
University of Leicester
The John Walls Renal Unit
Leicester General Hospital
Leicester, United Kingdom

Bengt C. Fellström MD, PhD
Department of Medical Sciences
Nephrology Unit
University Hospital
Uppsala, Sweden

Fernando C. Fervenza MD, PhD
Division of Nephrology and Hypertension
Mayo Clinic College of Medicine
Rochester, Minnesota, USA

Kevin W. Finkel MD
Division of Renal Diseases and Hypertension
University of Texas Medical
School at Houston
Houston, Texas, USA

Danilo Fliser MD
Department of Internal Medicine
Division of Nephrology
Medical School Hannover
Hannover, Germany

Robert N. Foley MB, MSc
Chronic Disease Research Group
University of Minnesota
Minneapolis, Minnesota, USA

John R. Foringer MD
Division of Renal Diseases and Hypertension
University of Texas Medical School at Houston
Houston, Texas, USA

Diane L. Frankenfield MD
Centers for Medicare & Medicaid Services
Office of Clinical Standards and Quality
Baltimore, Maryland, USA

Marc Froissart MD, PhD
Paris-Descartes University School of Medicine
Georges Pompidou European Hospital
INSERM U652
Paris, France

Susan Furth MD, PhD
Pediatrics and Epidemiology Welch Center for
Prevention
Epidemiology and Clinical Research
Johns Hopkins Medical Institutions
Baltimore, Maryland, USA

Pere Ginès MD
Liver Unit
Institut de Malalties Digestives i Metaboliques
Hospital Clinic
University of Barcelona
Barcelona, Spain

Fabrizio Ginevri MD
Pediatric Nephrology Unit
Istituto G. Gaslini
Genova, Italy

Richard J. Glassock MD
David Geffen School of Medicine
University of California Los Angeles
Los Angeles, California, USA

David S. Goldfarb MD
Nephrology Division
NYU Medical Center
Professor of Medicine and Physiology
NYU School of Medicine
New York, USA

David J. A. Goldsmith MD
Department of Nephrology and Transplantation
Guy's Hospital
London, United Kingdom

Stuart L. Goldstein MD
Baylor College of Medicine
Medical Director
Renal Dialysis Unit and Pheresis Service
Houston, Texas, USA

Frank Gotch MD
University of California San Francisco
San Francisco, California, USA

Jaap W. Groothoff MD, PhD
Department of Pediatric Nephrology
Emma Children's Hospital
Academic Medical Center
Amsterdam, The Netherlands

Nabil Haddad MD
Department of Internal Medicine
The Ohio State University Medical Center
Columbus, Ohio, USA

Michael Haderlie MD
Department of Medicine
Tulane University School of Medicine
New Orleans, Louisiana, USA

L. Lee Hamm MD
Department of Medicine
Tulane University School of Medicine
New Orleans, Louisiana, USA

Lee A. Hebert MD
Department of Internal Medicine
The Ohio State University Medical Center
Columbus, Ohio, USA

Jonathan Himmelfarb MD
Kidney Research Institute
Division of Nephrology
University of Washington Medical School
Seattle, Washington, USA

List of contributors

Hans H. Hirsch MD, MS
Transplantation Virology & Molecular Diagnostics
Institute for Medical Microbiology
University of Basel
Basel, Switzerland

Elisabeth M, Hodson MD
Cochrane Renal Group
Centre for Kidney Research
The Children's Hospital at Westmead
Westmead, Australia

Ronald Hogg MD
Division of Pediatric Nephrology
Children's Health Center
St. Joseph's Hospital and Medical Center
Phoenix, Arizona, USA

Hallvard Holdaas MD
Department of Nephrology
Rikshospitalet
Oslo, Norway

Byron P. Hollett MD
Department of Pediatrics
James Whitcomb Riley Hospital for Children
Indiana University Medical Center
Indianapolis, Indiana, USA

Frances D. Hollett MD
Department of Pediatrics
James Whitcomb Riley Hospital for Children
Indiana University Medical Center
Indianapolis, Indiana, USA

Eric AJ Hoste MD, PhD
The Clinical Research, Investigation and Systems
Modeling of Acute Illness (CRISMA)
Laboratory, Department of Critical Care Medicine
University of Pittsburgh School of Medicine
Pittsburgh, PA
Intensive Care Unit
Ghent University Hospital
Ghent, Belgium

Fairol H. Ibrahim MD
Sheffield Kidney Institute
Northern General Hospital
Sheffield, United Kingdom

Alan Jardine MD
Nephrology & Transplantation
BHF Cardiovascular Research Centre
University of Glasgow
Glasgow, United Kingdom

David W. Johnson MD
Department of Renal Medicine
University of Queensland at Princess Alexandra
Hospital
Brisbane, Australia

Bertram L. Kasiske MD
University of Minnesota
Department of Medicine
Hennepin County Medical Center
Minneapolis, Minnesota, USA

John A Kellum MD
The Clinical Research, Investigation, and Systems
Modeling of Acute Illness (CRISMA)
Laboratory, Department of Critical Care Medicine
University of Pittsburgh School of Medicine
Pittsburgh, Pennsylvania, USA

Paul A. Keown MD
Departments of Medicine and Pathology and
Laboratory Medicine
University of British Columbia
Vancouver, BC, Canada

Byrce Kiberd MD
Department of Medicine
Dalhousie University
Halifax, Nova Scotia, Canada

Paul L. Kimmel MD, FACP, FASN
Division of Renal Diseases and Hypertension
Department of Medicine
George Washington University
Medical Center
Washington, DC, USA

Jeffrey B. Kopp MD
Kidney Disease Section
National Institute of Diabetes and Digestive and
Kidney Diseases
National Institutes of Health
US Department of Health and Human Services
Bethesda, Maryland, USA

Peter Kotanko MD
Krankenhaus der Barmherzigen Brüder
Department of Internal Medicine
Graz, Austria

Jay L. Koyner MD
Section of Nephrology
University of Chicago
Chicago, Illinois, USA

Vera Krane MD
Department of Medicine
Division of Nephrology
University of Würzburg
Würzburg, Germany

Raymond T. Krediet MD, PhD
Academic Medical Center
Amsterdam, The Netherlands

Dirk R. J. Kuypers MD, PhD
Department of Nephrology and Renal
Transplantation
University Hospitals Leuven
University of Leuven
Leuven, Belgium

Norbert Lameire MD
Renal Division
Department of Internal Medicine
University Hospital Ghent
Ghent, Belgium

Krista L. Lentine MD, MS
Center for Outcomes Research and Division of
Nephrology
Saint Louis University School of Medicine
St. Louis, Missouri, USA

Mary B. Leonard MD, MSCE
Department of Pediatrics
The Children's Hospital of Philadelphia
Department of Biostatistics and Epidemiology
University of Pennsylvania School of Medicine
Philadelphia, Pennsylvania, USA

Nathan W. Levin MD
Renal Research Institute
New York, USA

Philip Kam-Tao Li MD, FRCP, FACP
Honorary Professor of Medicine
Chief of Nephrology and Consultant
Department of Medicine & Therapeutics
Prince of Wales Hospital
The Chinese University of Hong Kong
Hong Kong, China

Alison Macleod BMedBiol, MB, ChB, MD,
FRCP
Department of Medicine and Therapeutics
University of Aberdeen
Aberdeen, United Kingdom

Robert Mactier MD
Glasgow Royal Infirmary
Scotland, United Kingdom

Crispín Marin Villalobos MD
Nephrology Section
Hospital Universitario and Universidad del Zulia
School of Medicine
Maracaibo, Venezuela

William M. McClellan MD
Renal Division
Emory University School of Medicine
Atlanta, Georgia, USA

Maruschka P. Merkus PhD
Department of Pediatric Nephrology
Emma Children's Hospital
Academic Medical Center
Amsterdam, The Netherlands

Alain Meyrier MD
Service de Nephrologie
Hôpital Georges Pompidou
Paris, France

Malot G. Minnick-Belarmino PhD
Chronic Kidney Disease in Children
Study Welch Center for Prevention
Baltimore, Maryland, USA

Donald A. Molony MD
Division of Renal Disease and Hypertension
University of Texas
Houston Medical School
Houston, Texas, USA

Norman Muirhead MD
Division of Nephrology
University of Western Ontario
London, Ontario, Canada

Patrick T. Murray MD
Section of Nephrology
University of Chicago
Chicago, Illinois, USA

Sankar Navaneethan MD, MPH
Department of Medicine
Unity Health System
Rochester, New York, USA

Sharon J. Nessim MD
Department of Medicine
Division of Nephrology
University of Toronto
Toronto, Canada

Christopher Norris MD
Division of Renal Diseases and Hypertension
University of Texas Medical School at Houston
Houston, Texas, USA

Paul M. Palevsky MD
Renal-Electrolyte Division
Department of Medicine
University of Pittsburgh School of Medicine
Pittsburgh, Pennsylvania, USA

Patrick S. Parfrey MD
Division of Nephrology and Clinical Epidemiology
Faculty of Medicine, Memorial University of Newfoundland
St. John's, Newfoundland, Canada

Mark G. Parker MD
Maine Medical Center
Portland, Maine, USA

Robert M. Perkins MD
Department of Medicine/Nephrology Service
Medigan Army Medical Center
Ft. Lewis, Washington, USA

Tiina Podymow MD
McGill University
Montreal, Quebec, Canada

Kevan R. Polkinghorne MD
Department of Nephrology
Monash Medical Centre
Melbourne, Australia

Friedrich K. Port MD
Arbor Research Collaborative for Health
Ann Arbor, Michigan, USA

Kannaiyan S. Rabindranath MD
Renal Unit
Churchill Hospital
Oxford, United Kingdom

Jörg Radermacher MD
Department of Nephrology
Klinikum Minden
Minden, Germany

Sylvia Paz B. Ramirez MD, MPH, MBA
Arbor Research Collaborative for Health
Ann Arbor, USA

Lesley Rees MD, FRCP, FRCPCH
Consultant Paediatric Nephrologist
Great Ormond St Hospital for Children NHS Trust
London, United Kingdom

Giuseppe Remuzzi MD, FRCP
Clinical Research Center for Rare Diseases
Mario Negri Institute for Pharmacological Research
Bergamo, Italy

Eberhard Ritz MD
Department of Internal Medicine
Division Nephrology
Ruperto Carola University
Heidelberg, Germany

Michael V. Rocco MD
Wake Forest University School of Medicine
Department of Internal Medicine
Section on Nephrology,
Winston-Salem, North Carolina, USA

Bernardo Rodriguez-Iturbe MD
Nephrology Section
Hospital Universitario and
Universidad del Zulia
School of Medicine
Maracaibo, Venezuela

Jerome Rossert MD
Paris-Descartes University School of Medicine
Georges Pompidou European Hospital
INSERM U872
Paris, France

Richard L. Roudebush MD
Division of Nephrology
Department of Medicine
Indiana University School of Medicine
Indianapolis, Indiana, USA

Piero Ruggenenti MD
Unit of Nephrology
Azienda Ospedaliera Ospedali Riuniti di Bergamo
Bergamo, Italy

Kamalanathan K. Sambandam MD
Renal Division
Washington University School of Medicine
St. Louis, Missouri, USA

Sangeetha Satyan MD
Division of Nephrology
Department of Medicine
Indiana University School of Medicine
Indianapolis, Indiana, USA

Franz Schaefer MD
Division of Pediatric Nephrology
Center for Pediatric and Adolescent Medicine
University of Heidelberg
Heidelberg, Germany

Arrigo Schieppati MD
Division of Nephrology and Dialysis
Mario Negri Institute for Pharmacological Research
Negri Bergamo Laboratories
Bergamo, Italy

Eric E. Simon MD
Department of Medicine
Tulane University School of Medicine
New Orleans, Louisiana, USA

Benedicte Stengel MD
Université Paris-Sud
INSERM U780
Villejuif, France

Brett W. Stephens MD
Division of Renal Disease and Hypertension
University of Texas
Houston Medical School
Houston, Texas, USA

Giovanni F. M. Strippoli MD
Centre for Kidney Research
The Children's Hospital at Westmead
Westmead, Australia
Cochrane Renal Group
University of Sydney
School of Public Health
Sydney, Australia

Premala Sureshkumar MD
Centre for Kidney Research
The Children's Hospital at Westmead
Westmead, Australia

Cheuk-Chun Szeto MD, FRCP
Department of Medicine & Therapeutics,
Prince of Wales Hospital
The Chinese University of Hong Kong
Hong Kong, China

Robert Daniel Toto MD
Nephrology Division
University of Texas Southwestern Medical Center
Dallas, Texas, USA

Wai Y. Tse BSc, FRCP, PhD
Department of Neprology
Derriford Hospital
Plymouth, United Kingdom

Wim van Biesen MD
Renal Division
Department of Internal Medicine
University Hospital Ghent
Ghent, Belgium

Raymond Vanholder MD
University of Ghent
Associate Head of the Nephrology
Division of the Ghent University Hospital
Ghent, Belgium

Yves Vanrenterghem MD
Department of Nephrology
University Hospital Gasthuisberg
Leuven, Belgium

William G. van't Hoff BSc, MD,
FRCPCH, FRCP
Nephro-Urology Unit
Great Ormond Street Hospital for Children
London, United Kingdom

Ramesh Venkataraman MD
The Clinical Research, Investigation, and Systems
Modeling of Acute Illness (CRISMA)
Department of Critical Care Medicine
University of Pittsburgh School of Medicine
Pittsburgh Pennsylvania, USA

Anitha Vijayan MD
Renal Division
Washington University School of Medicine
St. Louis, Missouri, USA

Christoph Wanner MD, PhD
Department of Medicine
Division of Nephrology
University of Würzburg
Würzburg, Germany

Nicholas J. A. Webb DM, FRCP, FRCPCH
Department of Nephrology
Royal Manchester Children's Hospital
Manchester, United Kingdom

Richard P. Wedeen MD
Universily of Medicine and Dentistry of New Jersey
The New Jersey Medical School
New Jersey, New Jersey, USA

Steven D. Weisbord MD, MSc
Renal-Electrolyte Division
Department of Medicine
University of Pittsburgh School of Medicine
Pittsburgh, Pennsylvania, USA

David C. Wheeler MD
Royal Free and University College Medical School
London, United Kingdom

Kathryn J. Wiggins MD
The University of Melbourne
Department of Medicine at St. Vincent's Hospital
Melbourne, Australia

Gabrielle Williams MPH, PhD
Centre for Kidney Research
The Children's Hospital at Westmead
Westmead, Australia
University of Sydney
Sydney, Australia

John D. Williams MD
Department of Nephrology
Cardiff University
Cardiff, United Kingdom

Narelle S. Willis
Centre for Kidney Research
Cochrane Renal Group
The Children's Hospital at Westmead
Westmead, Australia

Elke Wühl MD
Division of Pediatric Nephrology
Center for Pediatric and Adolescent Medicine
University of Heidelberg
Heidelberg, Germany

Peter Yorgin MD
Section of Pediatric Nephrology
Loma Linda University Children's Hospital
Loma Linda, California, USA

Foreword

The evidence-based approach to health care is assuming a greater role in informing patient care worldwide. This approach arises from a convergence of factors, including the easy availability of evidence-based resources that synthesize the evidence, as exemplified by the Cochrane database, the desire of practitioners to attain best practices in the face of an almost overwhelming volume of new biomedical information, and the realization that, in an environment of limited health care resources, the best evidence of effectiveness should be central to the determination of which specific treatments warrant full investment. On the most immediate level, best evidence should inform the rational care of individual patients by the practitioner. On a broader level, best evidence should also influence specific decisions by society on the provision of specific health care services. In each case, evidence forms one of the two main components of a medical decision, as described by David Eddy [1,2].

Because the term evidence-based medicine was first coined by Sackett and colleagues more than 15 years ago, the emphasis in evidence-based medicine has been on evidence as it informs the choices of individual patients and of practitioners caring for these individuals, where the choices are determined by the evidence and by the individual preferences of the patients but not, strictly speaking, by the relative value or cost-effectiveness of these interventions [3,4]. Although cost-effectiveness determinations naturally evolve from a consideration of the evidence, we have chosen in this first evidence-based medicine-centered textbook in nephrology to address the evidence principally from the perspectives of the patient and the individual practitioner, not the policy maker. It is our hope that this evidence-based nephrology textbook will provide a resource for practitioners, and therefore we have focused on the primary clinical evidence and, where available, systematic reviews of this evidence. Health economic assessments are considered in this text only insofar as such analyses and the policy choices they have engendered may influence the various current national and international management guidelines, such as the National Kidney Foundation's Kidney Disease Outcomes Quality Initiative and the European Best Practice Guidelines.

What then is the potential for an evidence-based approach to nephrology for the individual practitioner and patient? As noted by Eddy [1], "different value judgments are unavoidable. Yet, a thorough and judicious assessment of the best evidence will promote treatment decisions that are: less arbitrary, better informed, more individualized, more transparent, and more broadly acceptable. The first contribution of evidence-based medicine is to change the anchor for the decision from the beliefs of experts to evidence of effectiveness." An important consequence of a comprehensive examination of the evidence broadly covering all clinical topics in nephrology as necessitated by this textbook is the exposure of the scope of evidence that informs the diagnosis and management of patients in our field, the laying bare, so to speak, of what is known and what is not known. Recently, Strippoli and coworkers evaluated the number of randomized controlled trials in nephrology compared to other fields in internal medicine [5]. They found that the number of randomized trials in nephrology was substantially lower than for other internal medicine subspecialties. In this evidence-based nephrology textbook, evidence from high-quality observational studies is considered in many cases in conjunction with the randomized controlled trials evidence, a reflection of the current state of the best available evidence that informs the practice of nephrology.

The examination of the totality of evidence should have the following principal outcomes. An explicit acknowledgment of the limited scope of the evidence, specifically, that it is rather incomplete in many areas, should permit a responsible challenge of opinion-based (even expert opinion) practice recommendations and should, thus, reduce the reliance on dogma. Identifying those areas of disease management for which there is only poor-grade evidence should suggest a research agenda. Because evidence-based medicine has traditionally emphasized patient-centered research, it is anticipated that an evidence-based approach will be more robustly patient centered.

In the spirit of evidence-based medicine, we have embarked on this book with the following goals in mind. First, we wish to provide the student of nephrology with a single convenient source of clinical evidence that has been passed through an evidence-based filter. Second, we wish to provide a forum for the reasonable inclusion of data of multiple types as these determine best practice in nephrology, including high-quality observational and

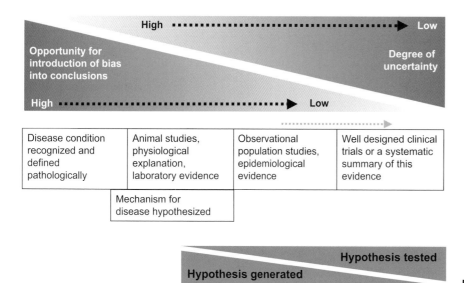

Figure 1 The spectrum of clinical uncertainty.

epidemiological data, in particular where high-quality experimental data are lacking. Third, by uncovering the areas where evidence is lacking, we hope to help inform the hierarchy of need for clinical trials. We hope that this textbook reflects current best evidence and that it is sufficiently comprehensive to cover the major clinical questions encountered by nephrologists, including those caring for the transplant patient and the pediatric patient. In compiling a textbook we have had to make some editing choices for clarity and organization. There may be areas, we hope very few, that have not been covered as comprehensively as the majority of topics in this text. We have included very little discussion of some topics that are covered extensively in traditional nephrology textbooks, including discussions of the mechanisms of disease and/or pathophysiology that emerge from *in vitro* studies, unless a discussion of these is likely required to understand clinical evidence on treatment of the relevant renal disorder. Thus, the treatment of electrolyte disorders that typically occupies one-third of most textbooks in nephrology is confined to one rather brief section, as clinical trials evidence is entirely lacking for much of the dogma on this topic.

By definition a textbook is likely to be less up to date than an evidence-based medicine website that can undergo comprehensive updating in real time. The latter type of resource, as exemplified by the Cochrane database, requires a large investment of intellectual resources, and for this reason the promise of a truly comprehensive constantly updated review of all topics in nephrology has not been fully achieved to date. In the absence of such resources, we hope that this textbook, *Evidence-Based Nephrology*, will fill a substantial portion of this void. Furthermore, unlike the Cochrane database, which is almost exclusively focused on questions of therapy, we have also included comparisons of many of the current evidence-based guidelines and we have included a discussion of the evidence as it relates to diagnosis, prognosis, and risk identification. We begin with a discussion of the sources of this evidence and the qualities that differentiate high-quality evidence from that of lower quality. We acknowledge that inclusion of nonexperi-

mental evidence does not permit robust conclusions in the absence of a significant degree of clinical uncertainty. This general concept of a spectrum of clinical uncertainty, in which all clinical decisions are made along a continuum from higher degrees of uncertainty to lower degrees of uncertainty, is illustrated in Figure 1.

It is our hope that this evidence-based nephrology textbook will, by moving the practice of nephrology toward the right-hand end of this spectrum, result in better clinical decisions. In the true spirit of evidence-based medicine, we hope that this text will thus push the specialty toward greater reliance on less biased evidence and make explicit the fact that we will never be able to manage patients without some uncertainty.

We also wish to acknowledge, along with the benefits we have enumerated above, some of the risks of an evidence-based approach in developing a textbook. In sum, we do believe the practice of nephrology is far better off with an evidence-based approach based on the principles that we have tried to exemplify in compiling this text as the starting point of an understanding of our field. To the material detailed in the various chapters, we hope or rather expect that our evidence-based medicine-centered learners and readers will add, through their own judicious application of evidence-based medicine principles, their own new knowledge as it emerges from the medical literature. Additionally, we acknowledge that an evidence-based medicine text might be most up to date when first published but that new information will always emerge between editions; hence, a textbook like this can at best be only one of several resources for the evidence-based medicine practitioner. We hope this effort will provide a core resource for the evidence-based nephrology practitioner who is otherwise limited by time constraints from researching every question that may arise daily in the care of patients.

Donald A. Molony, MD
Jonathan C. Craig, MD

References

1 Eddy DM. Clinical decision making: from theory to practice—anatomy of a decision. *JAMA* 1990; **263:** 441–443.

2 Tunis SR, Eddy D. Reflections on science, judgment and value in evidence-based decision making: a conversation with David Eddy. *Health Affairs* 2007; **26:** 500–515.

3 Sackett DL, Haynes RB, Guyatt GH, Tugwell P. *Clinical Epidemiology: a Basic Science for Clinical Medicine*, 2nd edn. Little Brown & Co., Boston, 1992; 173–186.

4 Guyatt G, EBM Working Group. Evidence based medicine. A new approach to teaching the practice of medicine. *JAMA* 1992; **268:** 2420–2425.

5 Strippoli GF, Craig JC, Schena FP. The number, quality, and coverage of randomized controlled trials in nephrology. *J Am Soc Nephrol* 2004; **15(2):** 411–419.

Introduction: Trials, Systematic Reviews, Grading Evidence, and Implications for Nephrology Research

Jonathan C. Craig

Why a trial (evidence)-based book

Readers of this book will be very familiar with the usual rationale for why randomized controlled trials (RCTs) should be central to routine clinical care [1]. Fundamentally, health care is about improving health outcomes, and an RCT is the study design which best estimates the true effects of interventions. Clearly, to practice good health care, other types of questions need to be addressed, diagnostic and prognostic questions in particular, and for these questions other study designs are needed. Inevitably in a book like this, some prioritization is needed, and because treatment questions are critical, results of relevant RCTs have been highlighted in all chapters.

The recent history of RCTs is interesting and was begun not in health care but in agricultural science by R. A. Fisher in 1935 [2]. Like many advances in biomedical science, innovators and leaders are always needed, and this came in the form of two eminent English scientists, Major Greenwood and Bradford Hill. Major Greenwood, as head of the Medical Research Council's (MRC) Statistical Committee, was able to convince the Therapeutic Trials Committee of the MRC in the 1930s to 1940s of the importance of RCTs. Bradford Hill took over Major Greenwood's position in 1945, and under his supervision the MRC's randomized trial of streptomycin was conducted in 1946 and published in 1948 [3]. Richard Doll, another major figure in the development of clinical trials during the 20th century, reflected upon the impact of this landmark study. The expert judgment of the Professor in deciding whether an intervention worked or not was rejected in favor of am explicit, quantitative, methodologically robust study design, the randomized trial [4].

The history of RCTs has also been marked by critics who typically suggest that observational studies are more "real world," and because they are larger, follow patients for longer time periods, are more inclusive, they are at least as valid as RCTs for evaluating whether interventions work, and they are probably more valid [5–10]. This debate occurred during the so-called outcomes research movement in the 1980s, but it was comprehensively decided in favor of trial-based evaluation of interventions, given that for the past 20 years major research funders, guidelines groups, regulators, and purchasers of health care had almost universally accepted the trial as the most valid study design to evaluate the effects of interventions, with observational studies a clear second [11]. Recently, this debate has been reignited, largely it would seem, to lower the barrier for new drugs and devices for the purposes of approval and subsidization [12].

The fundamental flaw of observational studies is that the allocation of interventions to patients is not random [13–16]. Consequently, any difference in outcomes between the patients who did and those who did not receive the intervention may be due to differences in patient characteristics, and unfortunately these differences can never be reliably and completely adjusted for, despite regression analysis, propensity scores, and the other statistical methods. A large-scale empirical comparison of the results of trials and observational studies was commissioned by the National Health Service and published as a Health Technology Assessment report [17]. The conclusion was clear. Most of the time, the results of observational studies and trials are concordant, but sometimes they are not, and the results of trials cannot be predicted with certainty based upon observational studies. There are many examples, tightness of glucose control in type 2 diabetics being a recent one. Contrary to observational studies, which have consistently shown tight glucose control improves macrovascular and microvascular outcomes, the ACCORD [18] and ADVANCE [19] studies showed no improvement in macrovascular outcomes, and in ACCORD, an increased all-cause mortality was reported. Studies like these reaffirm the importance of proper evaluation of interventions in RCTs, even though they are expensive and take time. The conduct of trials will become increasingly important when the marginal gains in health care become smaller and the potential harms and costs, greater.

Why a systematic review-based book

Decisions on treatment should be based upon all, and not just some, relevant RCTs. Currently, the Cochrane Renal Group has a register of RCTs in kidney disease that contains the records of about 10,000 trials and 12,000 publications arising out of those trials. The registry steadily increases at about 2000 trials/year. A simple Medline search would find only about two-thirds of these trials, because of problems in classification of the disease category and study design in the Medline coding. Also, about one-fourth of all trials in the registry come from handsearching, mainly from abstract compilations from the major nephrology and transplantation meetings. These studies may never be published (publication bias) or may be published relatively late (publication delay bias). Why systematic reviews of RCTs should form the basis of treatment recommendations and not just narrative reviews or a single trial chosen by an expert is beyond the scope of this introduction, but I will summarize the key points.

For clinicians it is easier to look at one systematic review than the many trials that are summarized in that review. Second, many trials are relatively underpowered, and a formal quantitative synthesis of the results may find a statistically significant benefit (or harm) that none of the component studies found. Meta-analysis provides a summary estimator of treatment effects, where appropriate, and this is necessary to inform practice, to ensure that benefits numerically exceed harms. Third, the variabilities in populations and interventions in a systematic review may increase the applicability of the findings. For example, interleukin 2 receptor antagonists have a remarkably homogeneous effect in reducing acute rejection despite the variability in baseline immunosuppression used [20]. Critics of meta-analyses argue that like should only be kept with like, and that "apples and oranges" should never be combined. Actually, it is often only in a context of a meta-analysis that there can be formal testing of whether treatment effects vary according to prior beliefs. Fourth, systematic reviews may minimize and/or highlight the various publication biases that might occur. One publication bias, the tendency for so-called "negative studies" not to be published, can be minimized if a comprehensive search of the "grey literature" (meeting abstract compilations, etc.) is conducted. The opposite bias, duplication bias, is where one study, typically one that is favorable to an intervention, is published multiple times and this is not disclosed to readers. Some "salami slicing" is reasonable, when studies are extremely large and report many outcomes. Many is not, particularly when the net effect is to mislead clinicians into thinking an intervention is more effective than it really is because of multiple, undisclosed publications. Finally, systematic reviews can highlight an outcomes reporting bias. It has been shown that trialists frequently change their primary outcomes during the trial, and this tends to favor the intervention under evaluation [21,22]. Trialists may only report what is improved with an intervention and not what is most important to a patient or what they said they would do at the inception of a study. These observations have led to calls for public disclosure of trial protocols. Systematic reviews can highlight these potential biases by demonstrating discrepancies in the number of trials reporting important outcomes. For example, many trials of calcineurin inhibitors did not report diabetes, acute rejection, or graft survival [23].

Why a book which "GRADEs" evidence

Most evidence-based textbooks and guidelines only evaluate the study design. Randomized trials become the proxy for evidence, when the reality is much more complex. What about when the trials are poorly done? What about when the wrong outcomes are measured? What about when the benefits are evaluated but the harms are not? Recently, the GRADE group, an open, multidisciplinary, international group of researchers and policy makers, developed a comprehensive approach to evidence, which forms the basis of this book [24–26]. Many of the chapters in this book have one or more evidence profile tables, with the simple two-tier (strong or recommend, weak or suggest) recommendations developed by GRADE. Full details of the process are provided elsewhere, but in short, GRADE begins with a systematic review of the available evidence. The overall evidence supporting an intervention, against the comparator intervention, is assessed. Domains considered are the study design (RCTs, observational studies, etc.), study quality (for RCTs this would include allocation concealment, blinding, intention to treat, loss to follow-up), consistency (are all the studies reporting the same results or are they different, and are the differences unexplained), and directness. Directness concerns whether the results of the trials can be generalized to the patient group being considered for the intervention and whether the outcomes being assessed are relevant or of a surrogate or unimportant nature. These four domains are considered in evaluating the overall strength of the evidence for the intervention being evaluated. Importantly, both benefits and harms are given equal consideration, and so even if there was high-quality evidence of the benefits of an intervention, if the quality of data for the adverse effects was very low, then the overall quality of evidence would also be rated as very low. Conceptually, evidence is rated as high quality when the evidence is so robust that no new studies could be justified because the benefits and harms are clear. The GRADE framework is a net clinical benefit, a benefit–harm framework, informed by the quality of the evidence. The evidence profile is then converted into a treatment recommendation after considering the quality of the evidence, values and preferences, local applicability considerations, and the benefit–harm trade-off in the patient group being considered for treatment. Conceptually, a strong recommendation would be equivalent to a recommendation that most clinicians and patients would follow if well-informed.

Clearly, judgment is required, but GRADE requires that such judgments be explicit and incorporate all of the relevant domains. GRADE reinforces the notion that, although trials are essential for evidence-based health care, they are insufficient. Observational studies are often needed to quantify the baseline risk values of individuals for outcomes that are averted by an intervention and to quantify the harms of rare events. GRADE also reinforces the importance of systematic reviews as the first step in the recommendation process.

Why evidence-based nephrology is a work in progress

More and better trials are needed

It has been shown that the number of trials in kidney disease lags behind all other specialties, and the standard quality reporting domains of allocation concealment, blinding, and intention to treat analysis are low and not improving [27]. Nephrology patients deserve the same quality of evidence-based care as patients with cancer. This can only occur when the standard of clinical care is for participation in a trial of a new promising intervention versus the current standard of care that is large enough to answer the question and in which simple outcomes that matter to patients are measured in all participants, both benefits and harms. This model of a large, simple trial, which has been adopted so successfully in cardiology and oncology, is a long way from the current model in nephrology [28]. The typical current model is a small trial (presumably because of large per-patient recruitment costs or a lack of a cohesive recruiting network) and one that sometimes compares a new intervention against a nonstandard, clinically inferior intervention [29]. Superiority is typically demonstrated, but such trials have questionable ethics and give results with uncertain policy relevance where the best standard care is expected to be the comparator. Trials may also be short term (months), and not all patient-relevant outcomes are reported, suggesting outcomes reporting bias in which only favorable outcomes are reported. In nephrology trials, the generic call for mandatory registration of trials and study protocols, and for complete reporting of all outcomes, both harmful and beneficial, should be heeded [21,22]. The nephrology community needs to follow the example of other disciplines and develop a consensus on what outcomes should be reported in trials and what definitions should be used [30].

More and better systematic reviews are needed

To date, the nephrology community has summarized in systematic reviews only about 1000 of the available 10,000 trials. In short, we are only about 10% of the way towards the goal of up-to-date systematic reviews of all RCTs. Readers of this book will notice that not all chapters have tabulated evidence summaries based on the GRADE methods. Reasons for this are many but include the absence of existing systematic reviews in areas of high clinical importance.

Although the focus on interventions is justifiable, ideally we need systematic reviews of all diagnostic tests used in nephrology and, some would argue, we equally need systematic reviews of prognosis studies. This can only be achieved with much larger-scale cooperation across the peak nephrology bodies and among researchers and clinicians than has occurred to date. Until this

occurs, and the relevant reviews are done, unnecessarily duplicative and unethical studies will continue, and needed studies will go undone. Research will be dominated by commercial interests and not patient needs.

More and better recommendations are needed

Not all authors in this book have used the GRADE system. This is to be expected, given the absence of existing systematic reviews and lack of familiarity with the GRADE process, which is still in development.

One critical lack is an almost complete absence of evidence about the values and preferences of patients with chronic kidney disease, which is needed to inform and assign weights to recommendations. Researchers tend to assume that they can correctly assign priorities to outcomes that reflect the values held by patients but, when evaluated, this has not been the case for other chronic diseases. A qualitative research agenda needs to be developed around patient perspectives of research and health care in nephrology.

In conclusion, this book has been deliberately ambitious. If readers are better informed by better evidence compared to their pre-reading state, then the goal of the book will have been achieved. A bonus will be if this book prompts a better evidence base that will make whatever subsequent editions of this book that appear more comprehensive, valid, and useful to clinical decision makers [31].

References

1 Collins R, Peto R, Gray R, Parish S. Large-scale randomised evidence: trials and overviews. *In*: Maynard A, Chalmers I, editors. *Non-Random Reflections on Health Services Research*. BMJ Books, London, 1998; 197–230

2 Mathews JR. *Quantification and the Quest for Medical Certainty*. Princeton University Press, Princeton, 1995.

3 MRC Streptomycin in Tuberculosis Trials Committee. Streptomycin treatment for pulmonary tuberculosis. *BMJ* 1948; **ii**: 769–782.

4 Doll R. Controlled trials: the 1948 watershed. *BMJ* 1998; **317**: 1217–1220.

5 Greenfield S. The state of outcome research: are we on target? *N Engl J Med* 1989; **320**: 1142–1143.

6 Clinton JJ. Outcomes research: a way to improve medical practice. *JAMA* 1991; **266**: 2057.

7 Cross design synthesis: a new strategy for studying medical outcomes (editorial). *Lancet* 1992; **340**: 944–946.

8 Wennberg JE, Barry MJ, Fowler FJ, Mulley A. Outcomes research, PORTs, and health care reform. *Ann N Y Acad Sci* 1993; **703**: 52–62.

9 Lu-Yao GL, McLerran D, Wasson J, Wennberg JE. An assessment of radical prostatectomy. Time trends, geographic variation, and outcomes. The Prostate Patient Outcomes Research Team. *JAMA* 1993; **269**: 2633–2636.

10 Welch WP, Miller ME, Welch HG, Fisher ES, Wennberg JE. Geographic variation in expenditures for physicians' services in the United States. *N Engl J Med* 1993; **328**: 621–627.

11 Hill SR, Mitchell AS, Henry DA. Problems with the interpretation of pharmacoeconomic analyses: a review of submissions to the Australian

Pharmaceutical Benefits Scheme. *JAMA* 2000; **283**: 2116–2121.

12 Vandenbroucke JP. Observational research, randomised trials, and two views of medical science. *PLoS Med* 2008; **5**:e67.

13 Miettinen OS. The need for randomization in the study of intended effects. *Stat Med* 1983; **2**: 267–271.

14 Colditz GA, Miller JN, Mosteller F. How study design affects outcomes in comparisons of therapy. II. Medical. *Stat Med* 1989; **8**: 441–454.

15 Miller JN, Colditz GA, Mosteller F. How study design affects outcomes in comparisons of therapy. II. Surgical. *Stat Med* 1989; **8**: 455–466.

16 Davey Smith G, Phillips AN, Neaton JD. Smoking as "independent" risk factor for suicide: illustration of an artifact from observational epidemiology. *Lancet* 1992; **340**: 709–712.

17 Deeks JJ, Dinnes J, D'Amico R, Sowden AJ, Sakarovitch C, Song F *et al*. Evaluating non-randomised intervention studies. *Health Technol Assess* 2003; **7**: 1–173.

18 Effects of intensive glucose lowering in type 2 diabetes. The action to control cardiovascular risk in diabetes study group. *N Engl J Med* 2008; **358**: 2545–2559.

19 Intensive blood glucose control and vascular outcomes in patients with type 2 diabetes. The ADVANCE collaborative group. *N Engl J Med* 2008; **358**: 2560–2572.

20 Webster AC, Playford EG, Higgins G, Chapman JR, Craig J. Interleukin 2 receptor antagonists for kidney transplant recipients. *Cochrane Database Syst Rev* 2004; **1**: CD003897.

21 Chan AW, Hrobjartsson A, Haahr MT, Gotzsche PC, Altman DG. Empirical evidence for selective reporting of outcomes in randomized trials: comparison of protocols to published articles. *JAMA* 2004; **291**: 2457–2465.

22 Zarin DA, Ide NC, Tse T, Harlan WR, West JC, Lindberg DAB. Issues in the registration of clinical trials. *JAMA* 2007; **297**: 2112–2120.

23 Webster A, Woodroffe RC, Taylor RS, Chapman JR, Craig JC. Tacrolimus versus cyclosporin as primary immunosuppression for kidney transplant recipients. *Cochrane Database Syst Rev* 2005; **4**: CD003961.

24 Guyatt GH, Oxman AD, Kunz R, Falck-Ytter Y, Vist GE, Liberati A *et al*. GRADE Working Group. Going from evidence to recommendations. *BMJ* 2008; **336**: 1049–1051.

25 Guyatt GH, Oxman AD, Kunz R, Vist GE, Falck-Ytter Y, Schunemann HJ. GRADE Working Group. What is "quality of evidence" and why is it important to clinicians? *BMJ* 2008; **336**: 995–998.

26 Guyatt GH, Oxman AD, Vist GE, Kunz R, Falck-Ytter Y, Alonso-Coello P *et al*. GRADE Working Group. GRADE: an emerging consensus on rating quality of evidence and strength of recommendations. *BMJ* 2008; **336**: 924–926.

27 Strippoli GF, Craig JC, Schena FP. The number, quality, and coverage of randomized controlled trials in nephrology. *J Am Soc Nephrol* 2004; **15**: 411–419.

28 Peto R, Baigent C. Trials: the next 50 years. *BMJ* 1998; **317**: 1170–1171.

29 Johansen HK, Gotzsche PC. Problems in the design and reporting of trials of antifungal agents encountered during meta-analysis. *JAMA* 1999; **282**: 1752–1759.

30 Boers M, Brooks P, Simon LS, Strand V, Tugwell P. OMERACT: an international initiative to improve outcome measurement in rheumatology. *Clin Exp Rheumatol* 2005; **23**: S10–S13.

31 Glasziou PP, Irwig LM. An evidence based approach to individualising treatment. *BMJ* 1995; **311**: 1356–1359.

1 Epidemiology of Kidney Disease

1 Epidemiology of Chronic Kidney Disease

William M. McClellan[1] & Friedrich K. Port[2]

[1] Emory University School of Medicine, Atlanta, USA
[2] Arbor Research Collaborative for Health, Ann Arbor, USA

Introduction

End-stage renal disease (ESRD) is defined by the cessation of effective kidney function and the substitution of renal replacement therapy (RRT), such as hemodialysis, peritoneal dialysis, or kidney transplantation, for native kidney function to sustain life. During the last 3 decades, an epidemic of ESRD has occurred in both industrialized and developing countries [1,2]. The epidemic increase in ESRD was initially attributed to the dissemination and adoption of RRT with the attendant extension of productive life. Although there is evidence that the rate of increase in ESRD incidence has abated in the USA, continuing increases in ESRD incidence rates after access to RRT becomes available to an entire population of a particular country have been documented by registries throughout the world [3].

The public health impact of the epidemic of ESRD is substantial. In the USA, it is estimated that the lifetime risk of being treated for ESRD is 2.5% for white men, 1.8% for white women, 7.3% for black men, and 7.8% for black women [4]. Life expectancy among individuals treated for ESRD is substantially shortened, and treatment is punctuated by frequent hospitalizations and progressive disability [3]. The economic costs of the epidemic are substantial as well, and the per-patient cost of care can exceed by severalfold the costs incurred by age-, gender-, and ethnicity-matched individuals in the general population. Furthermore, these costs only partially capture the full economic burden of ESRD, which includes the costs of chronic disability, premature mortality, and diminished quality of life.

Given the population cost burden of this epidemic of ESRD, it is increasingly recognized that strategies must be designed to increase the early detection and care of the antecedent diseases that contribute to this epidemic of end-organ failure [5,6]. There are multiple causes of kidney injury that result in ESRD, and the

evidence-based diagnosis and management of these conditions are discussed in detail in subsequent chapters of this textbook. Common to each, however, is a continuum of progressive decline in kidney function that leads to a syndrome of chronic kidney disease (CKD), which is characterized by hypertension, anemia, renal/metabolic bone disease, nutritional impairment, neuropathy, impaired quality of life, and reduced life expectancy and which culminates in ESRD. The purpose of this chapter is to describe the definition of CKD and the measurement of the population-based health burden of CKD across the continuum of disease, from mild impairment to ESRD, as an essential foundation for the evidence-based management of kidney disease. Problems inherent in using biomarkers and prediction equations to define kidney function and detect CKD are discussed in chapter 2. The epidemiology of CKD is discussed in chapter 4, and risk factors associated with progressive loss of kidney function can be found in chapter 3. Chapter 2 examines how surveillance systems have been used to measure and improve the care of patients receiving RRT.

Definition of chronic kidney disease

CKD can be defined as the persistence for 3 or more months of structural and/or functional abnormalities of the kidney [7]. This definition replaces previous case definitions that described variable degrees of impaired kidney function [8,9]. The rationale for adopting a uniform case definition of CKD includes the need for 1) improved comparability across observational and clinical studies, 2) an improved capability for uniform comparisons of kidney disease incidence and prevalence, and 3) improved communications about diagnosis and treatment of kidney disease. The most important anticipated benefit of a common terminology is more effective communication with patients and the public.

The "structural" abnormalities used to define CKD are 1) microalbuminuria or overt proteinuria; 2) an abnormal urinary sediment as evidenced by the presence of red blood cells (RBCs), RBC casts, white blood cells (WBCs), WBC casts, tubular cells, cellular casts, granular casts, oval fat bodies, fatty casts, or free

Evidence-based Nephrology. Edited by Donald Molony and Jonathan Craig
© 2009 Blackwell Publishing, ISBN: 978-1-4051-3975-5.

Table 1.1 Prevalence of decreased kidney function and CKD in the noninstitutionalized US population

Kidney function				Albuminuria Within Each Level of GFR (%)				CKD			
Estimated GFR (mL/min/1.73 m²)	n	Prevalence (%)	N (1,000s)	None	Micro-albuminuria	Macro-albuminuria	Persistence of Micro-albuminuria (%)	Stage	Prevalence (%)	N* (1,000s)	N† (1,000s)
>90	10,183	64.3	114,000	90.8	8.7	0.5	53.9	1	3.3	5,900	10,500
60–89	4,404	31.2	55,300	87.2	11.7	1.2	72.7	2	3.0	5,300	7,100
30–59	961	4.3	7,600	61.3	31.5	7.2	‡	3	4.3	7,600	7,600
15–29	52	0.2	400	‡	‡	‡	‡	4	0.2	400	400
<15	‡	‡	300§	‡	‡	‡	‡	5	0.2	300§	300§
Total	15,600	100	177,300	88.4	10.5	1.1	63.2	Total	11.0	19,200	25,600

NOTE: Dark shading indicates individuals with CDK, and light shading indicates CKD in a subgroup with persistent microalbuminuria. Estimates based on repeated visit of individuals with microalbuminuria ($n = 102$ for GFR > 90 mL/min/1.73 m², $n = 44$ for GFR of 60 to 89 mL/min/1.73 m²). Microalbuminuria defined as albumin-creatnine ratio (ACR) of $17 \leq ACR \leq 250$ for men and $25 \leq ACR \leq 355$ for women; macroalbuminuria defined as ACR > 250 for men and ACR > 355 for women (persistence assumed to be 100%).

Abbreviations: n, number of NHANES III participants; N, estimated number of individuals in the United States.

* Estimates based on persistent microalbuminuria at two visits for CKD stages 1 and 2.

† Estimates based on albuminuria in a single spot urine sample.

‡ Denotes cells with fewer than 30 NHANES III participants.

§ Estimated from the US Renal Data System.[1]

Source: Coresh *et al.* 2003 [105].

fat; and 3) abnormal findings on imaging tests, including ultrasound, intravenous pyelogram, computer tomography, magnetic resonance imaging, and nuclear scans. Overt proteinuria is defined as an increased urinary concentration of albumin and other proteins detected by routine laboratory measures (e.g. urine dipstick test for protein), and microalbuminuria is an increased albumin excretion that can be detected only by laboratory methods more sensitive than the standard protein assay that uses the urine dipstick.

The functional component of the definition of CKD uses creatinine-based estimates of clearance derived from the Modification of Diet in Renal Disease (MDRD) glomerular filtration rate (GFR) estimating equation or the Cockcroft–Gault creatinine clearance equation [10]. The derivation and use of these multivariate prediction equations are discussed in chapter 5. At present, no single method of GFR estimation is strongly recommended. Clinicians should choose a method that is appropriate for their population to determine the estimated GFR (eGFR) and assign a stage of kidney disease, always cognizant that failing to account for the modification of the complex association between serum creatinine and GFR by age, gender, and race is likely to lead to misclassification of kidney function and attendant errors in clinical decision making.

The available estimating equations are imprecise at higher levels of GFR, and there is great interest in revising them or identifying better filtration markers that will improve our ability to measure kidney function across the continuum of kidney performance from normal to ESRD [10]. The inherent imprecision of all methods of estimating GFR led to the decision to rank the degree of impaired kidney function into more global stages (levels) by the eGFR in the following manner:

Stage 1: eGFR >90 mL/min/1.73 m² (with structural abnormalities)
Stage 2: 60–90 mL/min/1.73 m² (with structural abnormalities)
Stage 3: 30–59 mL/min/1.73 m²
Stage 4: 15–29 mL/min/1.73 m²
Stage 5: <15 mL/min/1.73 m²

In addition to these eGFR ranges, the persistence of structural abnormalities for at least 3 months is necessary to assigning CKD stages 1 and 2, and stages 3–5 of CKD are defined by persistent impairments for greater than 3 months in the eGFR alone.

This staging algorithm is illustrated by using data from the US population aged 20 years and older (Table 1.1). The prevalence of CKD based on eGFR and presence and degree of proteinuria CKD is estimated to be 11% of the US population [7]. Over 50% of the prevalent disease is due to the presence of proteinuria among individuals with stage 1 (3.3%) and stage 2 (3.0%) CKD, and this proteinuria is largely due to microalbuminuria. Among individuals with stages 3–5 CKD, which are defined by eGFR alone, 85% of individuals have stage 3 disease (4.3%).

Kidney disease: improving global outcomes

The definition of CKD was reviewed at the 2004 "Kidney Disease: Improving Global Outcomes (KDIGO)" Controversies Conference [11]. Two further modifications were proposed to better

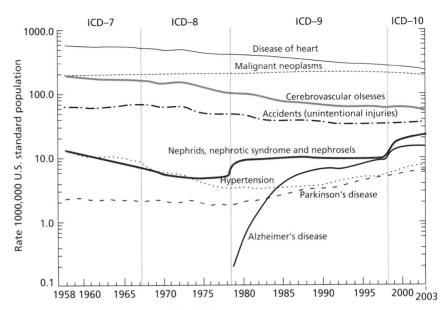

Figure 1.1 Secular trends in mortality attributed to various causes illustrating discontinuities in trends with changes in ICD classification of cause of death. (Reprinted with permission [13].)

Note : Age-adjusted rates per 100,000 U.S. standard populattion, area "Technical Notes" "Essential" (primary) hyperien aion and Hypertension renal disease.

adapt the staging algorithm for international use: 1) clinical judgment should be used to decide the relevance of nonproteinuric markers of kidney damage prior to diagnosing CKD in individuals without either proteinuria or reduced GFR; 2) individuals with a transplanted kidney should be considered as having CKD irrespective of other structural or functional markers. The KDIGO modified the CKD risk stratification by adding the letter T to denote CKD in a transplanted kidney and recommended that stage 5 CKD be modified by the letter D to denote RRT by dialysis [11].

International Classification of Diseases and kidney diseases

The *International Classification of Diseases* (ICD) classifies each condition that has given rise to the chain of events leading to death (underlying cause of death) as recorded on death certificates. The ICD is used by national vital statistics registries. At present, it provides the only uniform population-based case definition for international comparisons of the burden of disease attributable to earlier stages of CKD and, as such, is an important actuarial tool in defining the health burden of CKD across populations and, with certain limitations described below, temporally. The Ninth Revision of the ICD (ICD-9), used between January 1, 1979 and December 31, 1998, was replaced by ICD-10 on January 1, 1999 [12].

Revisions of the ICD reflect the evolution of disease classification and emergence of new diseases, and they resolve administrative issues that have stemmed from a particular version of the codes. Clinicians should be aware that ICD revisions often introduce changes in the classification of an underlying cause of death. Comparisons of death rates due to specific causes, such as kidney disease, across different ICD revisions can be facilitated by using comparability ratios that relate rates from different time periods. The comparability ratio relating rate computed from ICD-9 (ICD-9 codes 580–589) and ICD-10 (ICD-10 codes N00–N07, N17–N19, and N25–N27) data is estimated to be 1.23, indicating that the new ICD-10 coding will result in a 23% increase in classification of deaths due to kidney disease compared with the ICD-9 codes [12]. This version-to-version difference is due, in part, to a change in the classification of ESRD from an unspecified disorder of the kidney in ICD-9 to ESRD (N18.0), a subcategory of kidney failure (N17–N19) in ICD-10.

Secular trends in kidney disease as an underlying cause of death need to be interpreted with these changes in mind. This can be illustrated by trends in kidney disease as a cause of death in the USA (Figure 1.1), which declined between 1958 and 1978 and then increased substantially until the end of the century [13]. The transition from ICD-9 to ICD-10 in 1998 is represented by the discontinuity in the trend line for deaths due to nephritis, nephrotic syndrome, and nephrosis.

The Clinical Modification of ICD-9 (ICD-9-CM) is used administratively in the USA and was modified in 2005 to reflect the new nomenclature for CKD. ICD-9-CM code 585, "Chronic renal failure," was dropped, and seven new four-digit codes were introduced to code for the presence of CKD [14]. These new codes reflect the National Kidney Foundation (NKF) CKD staging definitions:

585.1: Chronic kidney disease, stage 1
585.2: Chronic kidney disease, stage 2 (mild)
585.3: Chronic kidney disease, stage 3 (moderate)
585.4: Chronic kidney disease, stage 4 (severe)
585.5: Chronic kidney disease, stage 5
585.6: End-stage renal disease
585.9: Chronic kidney disease, unspecified

Furthermore, in 2006, the ICD-9-CM nomenclature for codes 403 and 404, denoting kidney complications of hypertension, were changed from "renal disease" to "kidney disease" and from "renal failure" to "chronic kidney disease." A revision of the clinical modification of ICD-9 to reflect the ICD-10 coding conventions is currently being developed.

The standardized ICD nomenclature provides some uniformity of data that allows descriptions of population-to-population differences in death rates attributed to kidney disease. This standard nomenclature stands in contrast to the information reported by national ESRD registries that collect and report information on the occurrence of stage 5D CKD (see chapter 2). A report by Maisonneuve *et al.* found substantial variability in the definition and classification of primary causes of ESRD throughout the world [15]. Comparisons of the burden of CKD based on ICD-related mortality statistics also avoid the skewing of prevalence rates based on ESRD rates that would be introduced by the variable coverage of ESRD registries in economically developing countries.

The use of international comparisons of kidney disease burden can be illustrated by considering the proportionate mortality attributed to kidney disease throughout the world. Kidney disease is the 9th leading cause of death in the USA [6] and the 12th leading cause of death worldwide [16]. The burden of mortality due to kidney disease in different world regions was recently reported by the Global Burden of Disease Report [17]. Age- and gender-adjusted proportionate death rates for genito-urinary diseases, which include nephritis and nephrosis, benign prostatic hypertrophy, and other genito-urinary system diseases, vary from less than half of to 50% greater than those observed in high-income regions of the world (Figure 1.2) [17].

There are multiple potential explanations for this region-to-region variability in the overall mortality burden due to kidney disease. Regional differences in the prevalence of risk factors for

kidney injury and progressive loss of kidney function, access to health care, detection and treatment of kidney disease, and diagnostic convention could contribute to the observed variability. The main point of international comparisons is that a better understanding of the source of variation is essential for better control of CKD and its risk factors through public health measures and may lead to important generalizable insights into the reasons for the occurrence and progression of CKD.

Functional and etiologic diagnoses for CKD

CKD is a nonspecific diagnosis that describes the presence and degree of structural and functional abnormalities of the kidney. CKD does not identify the cause for the injury and/or impaired kidney function. Thus, the stage of CKD is an incomplete clinical description of the underlying disease process, and identification of CKD should also lead to a clinical diagnosis that includes a cause (etiology) for the kidney disease and the stage of CKD. For example, a diagnosis for CKD might be stated as "stage 3 CKD due to diabetes," "immunoglobulin A nephropathy with stage 4 CKD," or "stage 2 CKD of unknown etiology."

At present, the best estimates for the relative contributions of specific etiologies to the total burden of CKD within populations are derived from the proportionate, cause-specific incidence of ESRD within a population (see below). These estimates, however, have a number of limitations. Most important is the possibility that variations in survival and progression to stage 5 CKD among individuals with kidney disease due to different causes might alter the patterns of disease and the proportionate health burden over the course of CKD. It is also likely that there are substantial regional and ethnic variations within and between groups with respect to specific causes of initial kidney injury. It is likely that many individuals with prevalent kidney disease will have a number of competing risk factors associated with the initiation and progression of kidney disease, and the precise temporal relationship between these and the etiology of the initial kidney injury remains obscure. Finally, systematic studies to estimate the risk of kidney injury among individuals with less common forms of stage 5 CKD remain to be conducted.

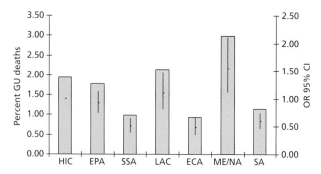

Figure 1.2 Proportion of all deaths attributed to genito-urinary causes (ICD-9 codes 580–611 and 617–629 or ICD-10 codes N00–N64 and N75–N98). These codes include nephritis and nephrosis, benign prostatic hypertrophy, and other genito-urinary system diseases. Regions in the Global Burden of Disease study were defined as high-income countries (HIC), East Asia and Pacific (EPA), sub-Saharan Africa (SSA), Latin America and the Caribbean (LAC), Europe and Central Asia (ECA), Middle East and North Africa (ME/NA), and South Asia (SA). Data were derived from regional tables for deaths by cause, sex, and age. (Reprinted with permission [17].)

Prognostic importance of the stage of CKD

As discussed in chapter 2, the classification of CKD using the NKF stages provides substantial prognostic and diagnostic information concerning 1) outcomes (progression to ESRD and mortality) [18,19] and 2) ocurrence of intercurrent morbidity (ischemic heart disease, stroke, and peripheral vascular disease) [20–28]. Further, the stage of CKD is predictive of the prevalence of complications associated with impaired kidney function (anemia, bone disease, and nutritional and functional status) (Table 1.2).

Table 1.2 CKD stage characterizations and risk factors associated with progressive kidney disease

Characteristic or risk factor	Stages 1 and 2	Stage 3	Stage 4	Stage 5
CKD stage characterization				
Description	Chronic kidney damage with normal to mildly decreased GFR	Moderate GFR loss	Severe GFR loss	Kidney failure
GFR (mL/min/1.73 m^2) [2]	$\geq$60	30–59	15–29	<15 or dialysis
Prevalence [7]	6.6%	4.3%	0.2%	0.2%
Proteinuria [45]	8.1%	23.3%	63.4%	–
Cardiovascular risk factors				
Hypertension [7]	40%	55%	77%	75%
Diabetes [45]	3.1–6.5%	16.8%	22.8%	–
C-reactive protein >0.21 mg/dL [44]	25–30%	48.7%	57.7%	–
Nutritional risk factors	–	2%	20%	50%
Albumin <3.5 g/dL [44]	1.7–2.2%	6.2%	8.2%	–
Bicarbonate <22 mmol/L [44]	1.3–1.6%	2.3%	19.1%	–
Risk factors for bone disease				
PO$_4$ >4.5 mg/dL [7,32]	–	<5%	20%	50%
Ca <8.5 mg/dL [7,32]	–	<5%	8%	28%
25(OH)-vitamin D $\leq$75 nmol/L [32]	–	71%	83%	–
iPTH (pg/mL) (<70 CKD-3 or <110 CKD-4) [32]	–	35.4%	31%	–
Quality of life				
Difficulty walking [7]	5%	8%	22%	30%
Hemoglobin <13 g/dL [38]	4%	7%	29%	69%
Outcomes				
5-year ESRD rate [18]	1.1%	1.3%	19.9%	–
5-year mortality rate [18]	19.5%	24.3	45.7%	–
3-year CVD rate [18]	2.1%	4.8%	11.4%	14.1%

Abbreviations: iPTH, intact parathyroid hormone; CVD, cardiovascular disease.

Complications of CKD and CKD stages

Complications that develop in CKD are listed in Table 1.2. The diagnosis and management of these complications are discussed in greater detail in the sections Prognostic importance of the stage of CKD and Complications of CKD and CKD stage of this text. Some of the important CKD-specific associations between the development of comorbidities and CKD stage that have emerged from epidemiologic studies are described in brief below.

Disordered metabolism of 25(OH)-vitamin D, phosphorous and calcium balance, and serum parathyroid hormone levels are well-documented for stage 5 CKD [1] and are noted to begin at or before stage 3 CKD. LaClair *et al.* studied patients with stage 3–5 CKD and found that 25(OH)-vitamin D deficiency was present in 71% and 83% of these patients, and parathyroid hormone levels outside of the recommended normal range were present in 64.6% and 69% of individuals with stages 3 and 4 of CKD [32]. Interestingly, geographic locations characterized by lower latitudes were inversely associated with an intact parathyroid hormone level. A recent study by Binkley *et al.* questioned the role of sun exposure on 25(OH)-vitamin D deficiency because deficiency remains relatively common even in sun-exposed individuals [33]. The prevalence of elevated serum phosphorous levels and low albumin-adjusted serum calcium levels increases with increasing stage of CKD. Analyses of data from a cohort study of left ventricular hypertrophy and anemia by Levin *et al.* estimated that the prevalence of a serum phosphorous level greater than 4.5 mg/dL increased from less than 5% among individuals with stage 3 CKD to 20% of those with stage 4 CKD; comparable prevalence estimates for a serum calcium level of less than 8.5 mg/dL were less than 5% and 8% [34]. In contrast to these observations, Hsu *et al.* found that age-, gender-, and race-adjusted femoral bone density among National Health and Nutrition Survey III (NHANES III) participants was unchanged among individuals with mild and moderate kidney disease [35].

Abnormalities of calcium and phosphorous metabolism are associated with increased risks of death and cardiovascular disease. Kestenbaum *et al.* reported that patients with CKD in the Veterans Affairs medical system with an elevated serum phosphorous level were at increased risk for all-cause mortality (hazard ratio [HR] per 1 mg/dL increase, 1.33; 95% confidence interval [CI],

1.15–1.54) [36]. Menton *et al.* reported that, after adjusting for other risk factors, cardiovascular disease but not all-cause mortality rates were marginally associated with increased serum phosphorous among participants in the MDRD study (adjusted HR per 1 mg/dL increase, 1.27; 95% CI, 0.94–1.73) [37]. Similarly, the calcium–phosphorus product was marginally associated with cardiovascular disease, but not all-cause mortality (HR, 1.22; 95% CI, 0.89–1.66; $P = 0.23$) in the MDRD participants. Among individuals with stage 5 CKD, the association between disorders of mineral metabolism, including elevated serum phosphorus and calcium levels and hyperparathyroidism, are well-documented and are estimated to account for 17.5% of the population attributable risk for proportionate mortality.

Astor *et al.* used the NHANES III data to determine the association between GFR and the prevalence of anemia, defined as hemoglobin less than 12 g/dL for men and less than 11 g/dL for women [38]. The prevalence of anemia increased from 1% among individuals with no CKD to 5.2% of individuals with stage 3 CKD and 44.1% of those with stage 4 CKD.

As the stage of CKD increases, functional impairment and magnitude of diminished quality of life reported by patients increase as well [39,40]. A recent report from the Chronic Renal Insufficiency Cohort study compared standard disease-specific measures of quality of life, the Kidney Disease Quality of Life Short Form 36, and general measures, including the SF-12 Physical and Mental Health Short Form, the Health Utilities Index 3, and the Time Trade-Off score among individuals with CKD [39]. The Chronic Renal Insufficiency Cohort study investigators observed a strong inverse association between stage of CKD and baseline measures of disease-specific and general quality of life. Furthermore, among individuals with CKD of stage 4 or greater who were tested sequentially over 2 years, progression of CKD was associated with further impairment of quality of life [40].

There is also evidence that the prevalence of cognitive impairment increases with increasing stage of CKD and that individuals with impaired kidney function at any level are at increased risk of developing cognitive impairment [41–43]. A report from the Health, Aging, and Body Composition study found that baseline cognitive function measured by the Modified Mini-Mental State Exam was inversely associated with degree of impaired kidney function, which declined from a total score of 87.5 among individuals without CKD to 86.9 among those with a GFR between 45 and 59 mL/min/1.73 m^2 and to 84.7 for those with a GFR less than 45 mL/min/1.73 m^2, with a score of less than 80 indicative of cognitive impairment [42]. After controlling for other risk factors, both individuals with a GFR between 45 and 59 mL/min/1.73 m^2 (odds ratio [OR], 1.32; 95% CI, 1.03–1.69) and those with a GFR of less than 45 mL/min/1.73 m^2 (OR, 2.43; 95% CI, 1.38–4.29) were at an increased risk of developing dementia during follow-up.

Individuals in the Cardiovascular Health Cognition Study underwent a three-stage evaluation for dementia that included an assessment of dementia risk, neuropsychological testing on high-risk patients (and a sample of other study subjects), and neurological and psychiatric evaluation for those classified as abnormal on the neuropsychological tests [42]. Subjects with an increased serum creatinine of ≥1.3 mg/dL for women and ≥1.5 mg/dL for men were found to be at increased risk of developing incident dementia during follow-up (OR, 1.37; 95% CI, 1.06–1.78). Of interest from this study, these associations were observed only among individuals who were healthy at baseline and were observed for vascular-type but not Alzheimer's-type dementia.

Descriptive epidemiology of CKD

Prevalence of Stage 1–4 CKD

The epidemiology of CKD is not well understood. NHANES is an ongoing series of surveys of representative samples of the US population conducted by the National Center for Health Statistics of the Centers for Disease Control and Prevention. These surveys are cross-sectional, complex, random samples of the US population, and they have been analyzed to provide CKD prevalence estimates. The prevalence of CKD among adults aged 20 years and older in the USA based on NHANES III data is estimated as 11%, with 6.3% of the population in the combined stages 1 and 2 CKD, 4.3% in stage 3 CKD, and 0.2% of the population in each of stage 4 and stage 5 CKD (Table 1.1).

Microalbuminuria, defined as an albumin–creatinine ratio of 17–250 mg/g in men and 25–355 mg/g in women, is present in 10.5% of the population on initial screening and persists over time on repeated measures in the same individual in 63.2%, whereas overt proteinuria (albumin–creatinine ratio of >250 mg/g for men and >355 mg/g for women) is present in 1.1% of the population [45]. Proteinuria increases in prevalence with decreasing GFR and is found in 0.5% of individuals with an estimated GFR greater than 90 mL/min/1.73 m^2, 1.2% of those with stage 3 CKD, and 7.2% of those with stage 4 CKD.

There is substantial heterogeneity in the prevalence of stage 3 and 4 CKD across subgroups of the US population. CKD stages 3 and 4 are more prevalent among women (5.3%) than men (3.6%), and prevalence increases from 0.2% among individuals age 20–39 years to 7.5% of individuals age 60–69 years. The non-Hispanic white population has the highest prevalence of stage 3 and 4 CKD in the US population (5.0%), compared with the non-Hispanic black population (3.3%) and Mexican–Americans (1.0%). CKD stage 3 and 4 prevalence is higher among individuals with diabetes (15.1%) and those with treated (17.5%) and untreated (7.9%) hypertension.

Comparisons of CKD estimates between the US population and other countries are difficult to make for several reasons. The measure of kidney function needs to be based on a standardized measure of kidney function that has been validated within each population. A standard classification needs to be applied to each population. Estimates need to be adjusted for differences in the underlying demographic characteristics (age, gender, and ethnicity) of the respective populations.

CKD prevalence estimates currently available in the literature are shown in Table 1.3 [46–57]. There is substantial variability

Table 1.3 Prevalence estimates for Stage 3 and 4 CKD by world region

Region [reference]	N	Ages (yrs)	Sample	Prevalence (%) with indicated stage(s)		
				Stage 3	Stage 4	Total, stages 3 and 4
North America						
USA [105]		≥18	Random, stratified national	4.3	0.2	4.5
Morelia, Mexico [46]	3564	≥18	Random sample clinic patients	8.1	0.3	8.4
Mexico City (diabetes) [47]	1586	35–64	Random, stratified Mexico City	23.8	0.7	41.2
Europe						
Norway [48]	65,181	≥20	Total population, Nord-Trondelag County	4.5	0.2	4.7
Groningen, Netherlands [49]				5.7	0.1	5.8
Galicia, Spain [50]	237	≥20	Random community	5.3	0.4	5.7
Reykjavik, Iceland [51]	19,381	≥30	Total population, Reykjavik area	3.7 (M)		
				11.0 (F)	0.0–0.3	–
Switzerland [52]	1778	55–65	Random national	7.1 (M)		
				23.5 (F)	–	–
East Asia/Pacific						
China [53]	15,540	35–74	Random, stratified national	2.4	0.1	2.5
Australia (diabetes) [54]	11,247	≥25	Random, stratified national	10.9	0.3	22.4
Hisayama, Japan [55]	2634	≥40	Community survey	10.2	–	10.2
South Asia				–		
Karachi, Pakistan [56]	262	≥40	Random, stratified community	29.4	–	29.4
India* [57]	4972	≥30	Random, stratified, regional (Delhi)	–	0.8	0.8

* Serum creatinine > 1.8 mg/dL.

across the studies in the age strata studied, classification methods, and methods of estimating GFR. Despite these variations, it is possible to discern the substantial drop-off in prevalence between stage 3 and stage 4 CKD across these varied populations; the estimated prevalence of CKD stage 4 is consistently less than 0.5% among nondiabetic populations. It is also evident that stage 3 and 4 CKD is a substantial public health problem across the world, exceeding 4% prevalence in all but one population. Finally, the population-to-population variability in prevalence suggests that, similar to the risk for cardiovascular disease, population-specific risk factors for CKD may exist.

CKD and race

The lifetime risks of incidence of ESRD, based on 1993–1995 US Renal Data System (USRDS) data, for 20-year-old white men has been estimated to be 1.98%, 1.67% for white women, 5.49% for black men, and 6.31% for black women, and these cumulative incidences increased further during the 1990s [4]. The racial disparity is reflected in age-adjusted ESRD rates, which are 3.8- to 4-fold higher among black people compared with white people [3]. The excess ESRD incidence for the black population stands in stark contrast to the prevalence data of stage 3 and 4 CKD estimated from the NHANES III population-based sample of the US population [58]. These studies report that CKD among adults age 20 years and older is found in 5.0% of the white population and 3.4% of the black population [58]. These racial disparities persisted after controlling for age, hypertension, and diabetes. Analyses of

the REGARDS cohort study showed that these disparities are particularly evident in stage 3 CKD. As GFR declines, the black–white prevalence gap diminishes and crosses in stage 4 CKD such that the prevalence among Black people with advanced stages of CKD becomes consistent with the observed ESRD incidence rate disparities [59].

The disparity in black and white population ESRD incidence rates persists after accounting for differences in the prevalence of hypertension [60] and diabetes [61] in the at-risk population. Factors associated with these racial disparities in ESRD incidence include access to health care, poverty, and community poverty [62–64]. Tarver-Carr and her associates used follow-up data from NHANES II to examine risk factors associated with racial differences in the incidence of all-cause ESRD [65]. They reported a 2.7-fold-higher ESRD incidence for black people compared with white people. Adjustment for a number of sociodemographic factors (poverty status, educational attainment, and marital status) explained 12% of the excess ESRD risk among black people, and adjusting for life-style factors (smoking status, physical activity, alcohol use, and body mass index) explained an additional 24% of the excess risk. Models that adjusted for prevalent diabetes mellitus, hypertension, and cardiovascular disease and baseline values of systolic blood pressure and serum cholesterol levels explained 32% of the excess risk. When all of these factors were controlled, the adjusted relative risk was 1.95 (95% CI, 1.05–3.63), accounting for 44% of the excess risk. Furthermore, the excess risk among black people for ESRD reported by Tarver-Carr and her colleagues was much greater among middle-aged than among older adults [65].

The unexpected reversal of prevalence of CKD among black individuals compared with the white population and the failure of multiple risk factors to explain the observed disparities in ESRD incidence are consistent with observations that black people with the same degree of impaired kidney function are at increased risk of progressive kidney failure [62–69]. Hsu *et al.* recently examined this possibility in an ecologic analysis of NHANES III and USRDS data [70,71]. They estimated that, despite a comparable prevalence of CKD, 5% of black people and 1% of white people in the US population will develop ESRD over a 5-year period, which is consistent with the progression hypothesis.

Incidence and prevalence of stage 5 CKD

Stage 5 CKD is defined by a GFR of <15 mL/min/1.73 m^2 and has two phases. The first phase is treated conservatively without dialysis, and the second, slightly later phase involves the initiation of RRT—either dialysis or kidney transplantation. The latter has been called stage 5D, or ESRD, which is defined by its treatment [11]. Whereas there is ample information available about patients treated with RRT, epidemiological information about stage 5 prior to starting dialysis is quite limited.

During the earlier phase of stage 5 CKD, conservative therapy includes the same factors discussed in chapter 3 for stage 4 but requires much closer monitoring of laboratory data and clinical symptoms of uremia. Symptoms or laboratory abnormalities are the main indications for starting dialysis. The optimal time for initiation of dialysis therapy has been a focus of many debates, as reports appear to be conflicting. Collins *et al.* showed that late stages of CKD are associated with a high risk of mortality even before starting dialysis [72]. Therefore, it appears reasonable that early initiation of dialysis will save lives. Retrospective analyses of mortality risk after initiation of dialysis, by level of kidney function at the start of dialysis, suffer from a major bias: patients who are started on dialysis with relatively higher levels of kidney function tend to be older and frailer, whereas those who start with poorer kidney function tend to be otherwise healthier with relatively few comorbidities. Thus, due to selection bias, retrospective data may falsely suggest that a later start is associated with better survival on dialysis. Prospective studies that randomize patients to early versus late start are scarce, but they appear to suggest that earlier start of dialysis is associated with better outcomes after dialysis [73]. Such studies must consider the lead time bias, which can be avoided by studying survival not from the start of dialysis but from the time of randomization to early versus late start. This takes into account mortality risk while being treated without dialysis for those randomized to a later start. As with stage 4, various causes of CKD have different rates of loss of kidney function, which needs to be considered in such studies, for example, by stratified randomization. The contributors to the recent NKF Kidney Disease Outcomes Quality Initiative (K/DOQI) guidelines reviewed the available evidence on optimal RRT start time in great detail [7]. These guidelines do not offer a specific level of GFR to indicate the need for starting dialysis but suggest that impairment of nutritional status is one of several key indications for the initiation of

dialysis therapy. The evidence regarding when to initiate dialysis therapy and what dialysis modality results in the best outcomes is reviewed in detail in chapters 7 and 8 of this textbook.

There is a wealth of epidemiologic information available about the later stage 5D of CKD (i.e. for patients who have started RRT, usually with dialysis). Numerous national and regional registries have relatively complete information on patients undergoing RRT. Patients initiating dialysis should be viewed as survivors of stage 4 CKD and the earlier phase of stage 5 CKD. This applies to numerous retrospective studies on patient management during the months prior to the start of dialysis.

The Dialysis Outcomes and Practice Patterns Study (DOPPS) inquired from patients how long they had seen a nephrologist prior to starting dialysis and found (among those surviving to dialysis) that, for each of the 12 DOPPS countries, about 66.8–82% had seen a nephrologist for more than 4 months and 8.4–20.6% had seen one for less than 1 month prior to starting dialysis. Patients who received longer pre-ESRD nephrology care were sixfold more likely to have a permanent vascular access rather than a catheter in use, and they were more likely to have an arteriovenous fistula rather than a graft [74].

Incidence

The number of patients starting RRT per year has been increasing steadily since maintenance dialysis became available in 1960, with roughly a doubling in the annual number of new patients during each decade in the 1970s, 1980s, and 1990s [75]. Thus, the incidence has been growing at an exponential rate. Each registry has shown clearly that this rate of growth has been substantially lower for younger patients and highest for the oldest age group. This epidemic of dialysis-requiring CKD may have several causes, although it may be difficult to quantify the role of each contributor. Causes may be categorized into three major groups: 1) patient selection, 2) competing risk, and 3) increased incidence of advanced CKD.

Selection of patients to RRT

The steep increase in incidence for older age groups suggests that very elderly patients and those with particularly severe comorbid conditions were likely not offered dialysis therapy in earlier years and have been increasingly offered RRT in each subsequent decade. In fact, in the early 1970s, a common exclusion for dialysis was age over 60 or 65 years and presence of any systemic disease, such as diabetes or lupus erythematosus. Such patients did have stage 5 CKD but were not counted in registries because registries dealt only with patients who actually received dialysis therapy. The "epidemic" of ESRD was defined only by its treatment.

Competing risks

There is clearly a high mortality risk among patients with earlier stages of CKD, and most individuals with stage 3 and 4 CKD die before starting RRT [18,19]. In fact, impaired kidney function is now recognized as one of the most important risk factors for coronary artery disease, and these risks persist into stage 5 CKD [20].

Substantial improvements in the treatment of heart disease and in survival have occurred in recent decades, which may have allowed such patients to survive to advanced stages of CKD and to the need for dialysis, whereas in earlier eras, these same patients would have died from heart disease during an earlier stage of CKD. A recent analysis by Muntner *et al.* investigated the possibility that the increase in ESRD between 1978 and 1991 could be attributed to increased survival among individuals with diabetes, myocardial infarction, and stroke [76]. They estimated that changes in the numbers of persons in the US population with these conditions could account for slightly over 40% of the increased ESRD incidence (diabetes, 27.6%; myocardial infarction, 4.8%; stroke, 7.9%). These results suggest that some, but not all, of the increase in ESRD in the USA is due to improved care and survival among high-risk groups.

True increase in incidence of CKD

It is also possible that the increased incidence of ESRD reflects increases in the underlying prevalence of CKD. There are potential reasons for more CKD to occur, but these are somewhat speculative. The incidence of type 2 diabetes mellitus has doubled from the 1970s to the 1990s, according to the Framingham study [77]. The availability of nonsteroidal anti-inflammatory drugs without prescription has likely increased their widespread use and the potential for nephrotoxic injury. Greater intensity of medical care may have led to greater exposure to potentially nephrotoxic agents, such as antibiotics and chemotherapeutic agents. Specifically, the growth in nonrenal organ transplantation has been associated with a substantial incidence of CKD and ESRD [78].

Influence of race on incidence of ESRD

Incidence rates for newly treated ESRD differ markedly by race and ethnic group. Incidence is highest among African Americans and among indigenous populations of North America, Australia, and New Zealand [7,78]. Diabetes as the cause of ESRD is also particularly high in these populations. Low incidence rates are recorded in developing countries, but this may reflect more limited availability of dialysis therapy, rather than less CKD. Japan and the USA have relatively high overall incidence rates. The USA also has a particularly high fraction of incident patients with diabetes as the cause of their kidney failure. It is surprising that incidence rates of RRT and of the fraction with diabetes are substantially lower among Europeans than among white Americans, since the latter are mostly of European descent [7,79]. As ESRD incidence rates continue to rise everywhere, European rates have been similar to those observed in the USA nearly a decade earlier. As the rates of increase gradually level off in the USA, one may speculate that rates in Europe and the USA will eventually become more similar.

Trends in incidence

The first indication of a significant slowing of the rate of rise in the incidence of stage 5D CKD was noted by Wolfe and Port for nondiabetic patients, according to USRDS data for the year 1997 [80]. More recent USRDS data confirm the earlier change in trend for nondiabetic patients and show that, for patients with diabetic ESRD, the annual rise in incidence rates has also significantly slowed in more recent years. This is shown in Figure 1.3 by the evidence that, since 2001, annual incidence rates for diabetic patients have been below the projected 95% CI of prior years. USRDS data

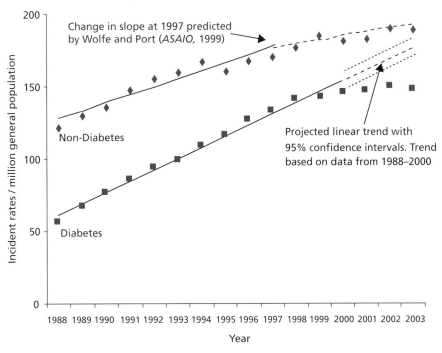

Figure 1.3 USRDS data showing trends for non-diabetic and diabetic patients.

Table 1.4 Comorbid conditions for representative samples of prevalent and incident hemodialysis patients by geographic region in 2002–2003 based on DOPPS-II

Comorbid condition	Prevalent cross-section (%)			Incident prevalent cross-section (%)[a]		
	Europe (n = 3938)	Japan (n = 1805)	US (n = 2260)	Europe (n = 230)	Japan (n = 75)	US (n = 162)
CAD	44.3	25.2	61.1	40.8	14.9	60.7
Cancer	12.9	6.0	11.9	18.9	10.4	15.8
Cardiac (other than CAD or CHF)	40.1	31.7	31.7	31.1	17.5	29.7
Cerebrovascular	16.5	14.6	19.1	13.8	14.3	15.4
CHF	24.5	16.4	40.1	24.7	25.6	44.0
Diabetes	25.6	26.8	51.4	34.8	33.8	52.5
GI bleed	5.6	4.1	6.5	8.6	0.8	3.7
HIV/AIDS	0.5	0.1	1.0	1.5	0.0	0.6
HTN	74.2	63.9	87.8	75.6	67.5	87.0
Lung disease	11.3	2.2	12.9	15.4	0.0	15.3
Neurological	11.7	6.8	14.2	11.3	9.5	13.2
Psychiatric	20.2	3.4	25.5	15.4	1.9	33.0
PVD	28.5	11.7	29.3	26.7	10.7	26.9
Recurrent cellulitis, gangrene	7.2	3.1	10.2	5.0	4.3	9.5

Abbreviations: CAD, coronary artery disease; CHF, congestive heart failure
[a] Defined as entering the DOPPS study within 90 days of their first-ever hemodialysis treatment.
Note: Analyses are weighted for dialysis facility size.

also show that the age group of patients that shows essentially no increase in incidence now extends beyond childhood and adolescence to also include young adults [80]. Despite these encouraging trends, it is important to note that there continues to be an increase in the incidence rate overall, even in the USA. The epidemic may have slowed in the USA, but it continues to be a major concern. Recent reports from non-US ESRD registries indicate that similar trends may be emerging throughout the world [81].

Prevalence

Data on the true prevalence of stage 5 CKD are lacking, except for the detailed registry data on those treated with dialysis or transplant. The number of patients undergoing RRT at the end of a year (point prevalence) and the number at any time during a year (period prevalence) are much higher than the number starting RRT during the year (incidence). Prevalence rates have been rising steeply over time. Prevalence of a disease increases if patient survival increases at a constant incidence rate or if the incidence rises at a constant survival rate. Thus, the prevalence rate corresponds to the product of the incidence and survival rates. For RRT, both a rise in the incidence (Figure 1.1) and an improvement in survival have been well-documented in the USA [82]. The issues described above related to incidence also apply to prevalence of treated ESRD, except where modified by differences in survival for certain groups. Because of the lower survival rates for the oldest age groups, their relative rate of rise in prevalence is not as steep as that observed for incidence. Worldwide, more than a million patients were undergoing ESRD therapy at the beginning of the millennium, and this number continues to grow.

Comorbidity in stage 5D CKD patients

Patients starting RRT usually have numerous comorbid conditions. International data from the DOPPS indicate that, at the initiation of hemodialysis, the vast majority of patients carry a diagnosis of hypertension. Heart disease, particularly coronary artery disease and congestive heart failure, lead the list of serious conditions. Other major factors are noted in Table 1.4 both for incident and for a cross-section of prevalent hemodialysis patients. With diabetes as a leading cause of ESRD, it is noteworthy that the prevalence of comorbidities is even higher in diabetic patients than in nondiabetic patients. Compared with patients on dialysis for over 1 year, incident hemodialysis patients (<30 days) are more markedly anemic [82], and almost half of them have phosphorous levels above the guideline level of <5.5 mg/dL (DOPPS unpublished information). Patients starting ESRD with peritoneal dialysis may have a positive selection because greater independence and ability to learn self-care may select healthier patients. On the other hand, difficulties with vascular access or lack of prior nephrologic care may select higher-risk patients to peritoneal dialysis [84]. Transplant recipients have substantially less comorbidity, largely due to patient selection. This has been documented by the finding that the mortality risk for wait-listed transplant candidates on dialysis is substantially lower than for all dialysis patients who are not (yet) wait-listed [85].

Comparisons of treatment modalities for ESRD and for patient groups need to consider differences in case mix (i.e. comorbidities and demographics). This can be accomplished in part through statistical adjustment for those factors that are recorded. The DOPPS and other studies showed that a long list of factors needs to be considered to allow meaningful comparisons between treatments, patient groups, regions, or centers. Some factors, such as age, cancer, and diabetes, may be considered as givens, whereas others, such as control of anemia, phosphorus, and malnutrition, may be modifiable. Studies of the latter factors, while adjusting for the former, have the potential to identify ways to improve patient care and longevity. This has been the focus of observational studies, such as the DOPPS, and of panels that review evidence to develop practice guidelines, such as the K/DOQI.

Survival after initiation of RRT

Morbidity and mortality are high in late stages of CKD and remain high among those who survive to the start of dialysis therapy. After initiation of dialysis, mortality depends largely on patient characteristics and comorbid conditions, particularly age and diabetes. Comparative studies of treatment modalities have clearly identified that kidney transplantation provides superior outcomes [85], and even more so when from a living donor [86]. Studies of the mortality risk for peritoneal dialysis versus hemodialysis have been somewhat inconclusive, as no large randomized studies of these dialytic treatment options have been performed and patient selection may influence the outcomes. Age may serve as an example for important differences in patient selection; compared with patients treated with hemodialysis, those treated with peritoneal dialysis are on average younger in the USA and older in Italy [87]. Thus, selection practice may explain some of the conflicting comparative survival results of peritoneal dialysis versus hemodialysis from different countries. In the USA, peritoneal dialysis appears to be associated with lower mortality risk in the first 1 or 2 years of dialysis, followed by a higher mortality risk. This early benefit of peritoneal dialysis, particularly among nondiabetic patients, may be related to greater preservation of residual kidney function with peritoneal dialysis [88]. These issues are reviewed in detail in the chapters in part 6 (hemodialysis) and in part 7 (peritoneal dialysis) of this textbook.

Differences in ESRD patient survival for Europe, Japan, and the USA have been found to be based largely on registry data, after adjusting for age and diabetes [89]. Subsequent study of hemodialysis patients, based on the DOPPS, confirmed these significant differences, albeit of a lesser magnitude, when allowing for greater adjustments for case mix and achieving better death ascertainment [90]. A more recent analysis of the DOPPS II data indicated that the mortality difference between the USA and Europe was confirmed but suggested that it could be largely explained by differences in vascular access [91].

Further studies of hemodialysis patients have indicated that several treatment factors are associated with mortality risk. The DOPPS pointed to a large number of factors that may be modifiable. Specifically, significantly lower mortality risk was associated with less catheter use and greater arteriovenous fistula use [92] as well as greater compliance with guidelines for Kt/V, hemoglobin, albumin, phosphorus, and calcium and avoiding large interdialytic fluid weight gains [93]. Additionally, the DOPPS analyses suggest

that better quality of life indicators [94], less depression [95], and better nutrition [96] are strongly associated with longer survival.

The mortality risk has been shown to be relatively high in the early phase after initiation of dialysis. According to the DOPPS, this risk is elevated for the first 4 months and then appears to level off [97]. Among survivors to subsequent years, the mortality risk appears to show a gradual increasing trend by the fifth year compared with the second year [98].

Among causes of death, those related to atherosclerotic heart disease and congestive heart failure are dominant. Infection deaths are strongly associated with catheter use for vascular access. Withdrawal from dialysis precedes death in about 20% of deaths in the USA, about half of them due to failure to thrive and half following acute complications [99]. Withdrawal from dialysis is practiced differently in different countries; for example, much lower rates have been reported in Japan and Italy and much higher rates have been reported in the USA [100].

Hospitalization may serve as a proxy for morbidity. On average, dialysis patients are hospitalized nearly twice yearly [7]. Modifiable factors associated with higher case mix-adjusted hospital admissions include more severe anemia and hyperphosphatemia [83,101]. Cardiac problems account for most admissions, and these same laboratory abnormalities are associated more prominently with cardiac admissions. Catheter use for vascular access is strongly associated with greater risks of hospitalization for infections [102].

Dialysis therapy is successful overall in prolonging life. However, survival of patients on dialysis is similar to survival of patients with serious malignancies, such as colon or prostate cancer [103]. A greater focus on modifiable practices may influence better outcomes. A recent study strongly suggested a causal relationship between practice and outcomes by showing that dialysis facilities that improved their compliance with guidelines for dialysis dose and anemia control had improvements in their patients' survival during the same time period compared with those with little change in treatment, where outcomes did not improve [82]. Transplantation clearly provides a better quality of life [104] and longer survival than dialysis in virtually all patient groups [85].

References

1 Gilbertson DT, Liu J, Xue JL, Louis TA, Solid CA, Ebben JP *et al.* Projecting the number of patients with end-stage renal disease in the United States to the year 2015. *J Am Soc Nephrol* 2005; **16**: 3736–3741.

2 Atkins RC. The epidemiology of chronic kidney disease. *Kidney Int Suppl* 2005; **94**: S14–S18.

3 U.S. Renal Data System (USRDS). *USRDS 2005 Annual Data Report: Atlas of End-Stage Renal Disease in the United States.* National Institutes of Health, National Institute of Diabetes and Digestive and Kidney Diseases, Bethesda, MD, 2005.

4 Kiberd BA, Clase CM. Cumulative risk for developing end-stage renal disease in the US population. *J Am Soc Nephrol* 2002; **13**: 1635–1644.

5 Dirks JH, de Zeeuw D, Agarwal SK, Atkins RC, Correa-Rotter R, D'Amico G *et al.* Prevention of chronic kidney and vascular disease:

toward global health equity: the Bellagio 2004 Declaration. *Kidney Int Suppl* 2005; **98**: S1–S6.

6 Schoolwerth AC, Engelgau MM, Hostetter TH, Rufo KH, Chianchiano D, McClellan WM et al. Chronic kidney disease: a public health problem that needs a public health action plan. *Prev Chronic Dis* 2006; **3**: A57.

7 National Kidney Foundation. K/DOQI clinical practice guidelines for chronic kidney disease: evaluation, classification and stratification. *Am J Kidney Dis* 2002; **39(Suppl 1)**: S1–S266.

8 Hsu CY, Chertow GM. Chronic renal confusion: insufficiency, failure, dysfunction, or disease. *Am J Kidney Dis* 2000; **36**: 415–418.

9 Levin A. The advantage of a uniform terminology and staging system for chronic kidney disease (CKD). *Nephrol Dial Transplant* 2003; **18**: 1446–1451.

10 Stevens LA, Coresh J, Greene T, Levey AS. Assessing kidney function—measured and estimated glomerular filtration rate. *N Engl J Med* 2006; **354**: 2473–2483.

11 Levey AS, Eckardt KU, Tsukamoto Y, Levin A, Coresh J, Rossert J et al. Definition and classification of chronic kidney disease: a position statement from Kidney Disease: Improving Global Outcomes (KDIGO). *Kidney Int* 2005; **67**: 2089–2100.

12 Anderson RN, Minino AM, Hoyert DL, Rosenberg HM. Comparability of cause of death between ICD-9 and ICD-10: preliminary estimates. *Natl Vital Stat Rep* 2001; **49**: 1–32.

13 Hoyert DL, Heron MP, Murphy SL, Kung HC. Deaths: final data for 2003. *Natl Vital Stat Rep* 2006; **54**: 1–120.

14 New ICD-9-CM Code for Beneficiaries with Chronic Kidney Disease. *Trans. 737, CR #4108, Pub. 100-04, Medlearn Matters Number: MM4108 Published Online: 11/4/2005* (http://www.cms.hhs.gov/MLNMattersArticles/downloads/MM4108.pdf.)

15 Maisonneuve P, Agodoa L, Gellert R, Stewart JH, Buccianti G, Lowenfels AB et al. Distribution of primary renal diseases leading to end-stage renal failure in the United States, Europe, and Australia/New Zealand: results from an international comparative study. *Am J Kidney Dis* 2000; **35**: 157–165.

16 Dirks J, Remuzzi G, Horton S, Schieppati A, Hasan Rizvi SA. Diseases of the kidney and the urinary system. *Disease Control Priorities in Developing Countries*, 2nd edn. Oxford University Press, New York, 2006; 695–706.

17 Ezzati M, Jamison DT, Murray CJL, Lopez AD, Mathers CD. *Global Burden of Disease and Risk Factors*. World Bank Publications, Washington DC, 2006.

18 Keith DS, Nichols GA, Guillion CM, Brown JB, Smith DH. Longitudinal follow-up and outcomes among a population with chronic kidney disease in a large managed care organization. *Arch Intern Med* 2004; **164**: 659–663.

19 Go AS, Chertow GM, Fan D, McCulloch CE, Hsu CY. Chronic kidney disease and the risks of death, cardiovascular events, and hospitalization. *N Engl J Med* 2004; **351**: 1296–1305.

20 Sarnak MJ, Levey AS, Schoolwerth AC, Coresh J, Culleton B, Hamm LL et al. Kidney disease as a risk factor for development of cardiovascular disease: a statement from the American Heart Association Councils on Kidney in Cardiovascular Disease, High Blood Pressure Research, Clinical Cardiology, and Epidemiology and Prevention. *Hypertension* 2003; **42**: 1050–1065.

21 Vanholder R, Massy Z, Argiles A, Spasovski G, Verbeke F, Lameire N. European Uremic Toxin Work Group. Chronic kidney disease as cause of cardiovascular morbidity and mortality. *Nephrol Dial Transplant* 2005; **20**: 1048–1056.

22 Foley RN, Murray AM, Li S, Herzog CA, McBean AM, Eggers PW et al. Chronic kidney disease and the risk for cardiovascular disease, renal replacement, and death in the United States Medicare population, 1998 to 1999. *J Am Soc Nephrol* 2005; **16**: 489–495.

23 Weiner DE, Tighiouart H, Amin MG, Stark PC, MacLeod B, Griffith JL et al. Chronic kidney disease as a risk factor for cardiovascular disease and all-cause mortality: a pooled analysis of community-based studies. *J Am Soc Nephrol* 2004; **15**: 1307–1315.

24 Manjunath G, Tighiouart H, Ibrahim H, MacLeod B, Salem DN, Griffith JL et al. Level of kidney function as a risk factor for atherosclerotic cardiovascular outcomes in the community. *J Am Coll Cardiol* 2003; **41**: 47–55.

25 O'Hare AM, Glidden DV, Fox CS, Hsu CY. High prevalence of peripheral arterial disease in persons with renal insufficiency: results from the National Health and Nutrition Examination Survey 1999–2000. *Circulation* 2004; **109**: 320–323.

26 O'Hare AM, Vittinghoff E, Hsia J, Shlipak MG. Renal insufficiency and the risk of lower extremity peripheral arterial disease: results from the Heart and Estrogen/Progestin Replacement Study (HERS). *J Am Soc Nephrol* 2004; **15**: 1046–1051.

27 Jaar BG, Astor BC, Berns JS, Powe NR. Predictors of amputation and survival following lower extremity revascularization in hemodialysis patients. *Kidney Int* 2004; **65**: 613–620.

28 O'Hare AM, Feinglass J, Reiber GE, Rodriguez RA, Daley J, Khuri S et al. Postoperative mortality after nontraumatic lower extremity amputation in patients with renal insufficiency. *J Am Soc Nephrol* 2004; **15**: 427–434.

29 Foley RN, Wang C, Collins AJ. Cardiovascular risk factor profiles and kidney function stage in the US general population: the NHANES III study. *Mayo Clin Proc* 2005; **80**: 1270–1277.

30 Muntner P, He J, Astor BC, Folsom AR, Coresh J. Traditional and non-traditional risk factors predict coronary heart disease in chronic kidney disease: results from the atherosclerosis risk in communities study. *J Am Soc Nephrol* 2005; **16**: 529–538.

31 Verhave JC, Hillege HL, Burgerhof JG, Gansevoort RT, de Zeeuw D, de Jong PE. PREVEND Study Group. The association between atherosclerotic risk factors and renal functio 6n in the general population. *Kidney Int* 2005; **67**: 1967–1973.

32 LaClair RE, Hellman RN, Karp SL, Kraus M, Ofner S, Li Q et al. Prevalence of calcidiol deficiency in CKD: a cross-sectional study across latitudes in the United States. *Am J Kidney Dis* 2005; **45**: 1026–1033.

33 Binkley N, Novotny R, Krueger D, Kawahara T, Daida YG, Lensmeyer G et al. Low vitamin D status despite abundant sun exposure. *J Clin Endocrinol Metab* 2007; **92**: 2130–2135.

34 Levin A, Thompson CR, Ethier J, Carlisle EJ, Tobe S, Mendelssohn D et al. Left ventricular mass index increase in early renal disease: impact of decline in hemoglobin. *Am J Kidney Dis* 1999; **34**: 125–134.

35 Hsu CY, Cummings SR, McCulloch CE, Chertow GM. Bone mineral density is not diminished by mild to moderate chronic renal insufficiency. *Kidney Int* 2002; **61**: 1814–1820.

36 Kestenbaum B, Sampson JN, Rudser KD, Patterson DJ, Seliger SL, Young B et al. Serum phosphate levels and mortality risk among people with chronic kidney disease. *J Am Soc Nephrol* 2005; **16**: 520–528.

37 Menon V, Greene T, Pereira AA, Wang X, Beck GJ, Kusek JW et al. Relationship of phosphorus and calcium-phosphorus product with mortality in CKD. *Am J Kidney Dis* 2005; **46**: 455–463.

38 Astor BC, Muntner P, Levin A, Eustace JA, Coresh J. Association of kidney function with anemia: the Third National Health and Nutrition

Examination Survey (1988–1994). *Arch Intern Med* 2002; **162:** 1401–1408.

39 Gorodetskaya I, Zenios S, McCulloch CE, Bostrom A, Hsu CY, Bindman AB *et al.* Health-related quality of life and estimates of utility in chronic kidney disease. *Kidney Int* 2005; **68:** 2801–2808.

40 Perlman RL, Finkelstein FO, Liu L, Roys E, Kiser M, Eisele G *et al.* Quality of life in chronic kidney disease (CKD): a cross-sectional analysis in the Renal Research Institute-CKD study. *Am J Kidney Dis* 2005; **45:** 658–666.

41 Sehgal AR, Grey SF, DeOreo PB, Whitehouse PJ. Prevalence, recognition, and implications of mental impairment among hemodialysis patients. *Am J Kidney Dis* 1997; **30:** 41–49.

42 Seliger SL, Siscovick DS, Stehman-Breen CO, Gillen DL, Fitzpatrick A, Bleyer A *et al.* Moderate renal impairment and risk of dementia among older adults: The Cardiovascular Health Cognition Study. *J Am Soc Nephrol* 2000; **15:** 1904–1911.

43 Kurella M, Chertow GM, Fried LF, Cummings SR, Harris T, Simonsick E *et al.* Chronic kidney disease and cognitive impairment in the elderly: the health, aging, and body composition study. *J Am Soc Nephrol* 2005; **16:** 2127–2133.

44 Eustace JA, Astor B, Muntner PM, Ikizler TA, Coresh J. Prevalence of acidosis and inflammation and their association with low serum albumin in chronic kidney disease. *Kidney Int* 2004; **65:** 1031–1040.

45 Garg AX, Kiberd BA, Clark WF, Haynes RB, Clase CM. Albuminuria and renal insufficiency prevalence guides population screening: results from the NHANES III. *Kidney Int* 2002; **61:** 2165–2175.

46 Amato D, Alvarez-Aguilar C, Castaneda-Limones R, Rodriguez E, Avila-Diaz M, Arreola F *et al.* Prevalence of chronic kidney disease in an urban Mexican population. *Kidney Int Suppl* 2005; **97:** S11–S17.

47 Cueto-Manzano AM, Cortes-Sanabria L, Martinez-Ramirez HR, Rojas-Campos E, Barragan G, Alfaro G *et al.* Detection of early nephropathy in Mexican patients with type 2 diabetes mellitus. *Kidney Int Suppl* 2005; **97:** S40–S45.

48 Hallan SI, Coresh J, Astor BC, Astor BC, Asberg A, Romundstad S *et al.* International comparison of the relationship of chronic kidney disease prevalence and ESRD risk. *J Am Soc Nephrol* 2006; 17; 2275–2284.

49 de Zeeuw D, Hillege HL, de Jong PE. The kidney, a cardiovascular risk marker, and a new target for therapy. *Kidney Int Suppl* 2005; **98:** S25–S29.

50 Otero A, Gayoso P, Garcia F, de Francisco AL, on behalf of the EPIRCE study group. Epidemiology of chronic renal disease in the Galician population: results of the pilot Spanish EPIRCE study. *Kidney Int Suppl* 2005; **99:** S16–S19.

51 Viktorsdottir O, Palsson R, Andresdottir MB, Aspelund T, Gudnason V, Indridason OS. Prevalence of chronic kidney disease based on estimated glomerular filtration rate and proteinuria in Icelandic adults. *Nephrol Dial Transplant* 2005; **20:** 1799–1807.

52 Nitsch D, Dietrich DF, von Eckardstein A, Gaspoz JM, Downs SH, Leuenberger P *et al.* Prevalence of renal impairment and its association with cardiovascular risk factors in a general population: results of the Swiss SAPALDIA study. *Nephrol Dial Transplant* 2006; **21:** 935–944.

53 Chen J, Wildman RP, Gu D, Kusek JW, Spruill M, Reynolds K *et al.* Prevalence of decreased kidney function in Chinese adults aged 35 to 74 years. *Kidney Int* 2005; **68:** 2837–2845.

54 Chadban SJ, Briganti EM, Kerr PG, Dunstan DW, Welborn TA, Zimmet PZ *et al.* Prevalence of kidney damage in Australian adults: The AusDiab kidney study. *J Am Soc Nephrol* 2003; **14(Suppl 2):** S131–S138.

55 Ninomiya T, Kiyohara Y, Kubo M, Tanizaki Y, Doi Y, Okubo K *et al.* Chronic kidney disease and cardiovascular disease in a general Japanese population: the Hisayama Study. *Kidney Int* 2005; **68:** 228–236.

56 Jafar TH, Schmid CH, Levey AS. Serum creatinine as marker of kidney function in South Asians: a study of reduced GFR in adults in Pakistan. *J Am Soc Nephrol* 2005; **16:** 1413–1419.

57 Agarwal SK, Dash SC, Irshad M, Raju S, Singh R, Pandey RM. Prevalence of chronic renal failure in adults in Delhi, India. *Nephrol Dial Transplant* 2005; **20:** 1638–1642.

58 Clase CM, Garg AX, Kiberd BA. Prevalence of low glomerular filtration rate in nondiabetic Americans: Third National Health and Nutrition Examination Survey (NHANES III). *J Am Soc Nephrol* 2002; **13:** 1338–1349.

59 McClellan W, Warnock DG, McClure L, Campbell RC, Newsome BB, Howard V *et al.* Racial differences in the prevalence of chronic kidney disease among participants in the Reasons for Geographic and Racial Differences in Stroke (REGARDS) Cohort Study. *J Am Soc Nephrol* 2006; **17:** 1710–1715.

60 McClellan W, Tuttle E, Issa A. Racial differences in the incidence of hypertensive end-stage renal disease (ESRD) are not entirely explained by differences in the prevalence of hypertension. *Am J Kidney Dis* 1988; **12:** 285–290.

61 Lopes AA, Port FK. Differences in the patterns of age-specific black/white comparisons between end-stage renal disease attributed and not attributed to diabetes. *Am J Kidney Dis* 1995; **25:** 714–721.

62 Whittle JC, Whelton PK, Seidler AJ, Klag MJ. Does racial variation in risk factors explain black-white differences in the incidence of hypertensive end-stage renal disease? *Arch Intern Med* 1991; **151:** 1359–1364.

63 Brancati FL, Whittle JC, Whelton PK, Seidler AJ, Klag MJ. The excess incidence of diabetic end-stage renal disease among blacks. A population-based study of potential explanatory factors. *JAMA* 1992; **268:** 3079–3084.

64 Perneger TV, Whelton PK, Klag MJ. Race and end-stage renal disease. Socioeconomic status and access to health care as mediating factors. *Arch Intern Med* 1995; **155:** 1201–1208.

65 Tarver-Carr ME, Powe NR, Eberhardt MS, LaVeist TA, Kington RS, Coresh J *et al.* Excess risk of chronic kidney disease among African-American versus white subjects in the United States: a population-based study of potential explanatory factors. *J Am Soc Nephrol* 2002; **13:** 2363–2370.

66 Rostand S, Kirk K, Rutsky E, Pate B. Racial differences in the incidence of treatment for end-stage renal disease. *N Engl J Med* 1982; **306:** 1276–1279.

67 Shulman NB, Ford CE, Hall WD, Blaufox MD, Simon D, Langford HG *et al.* Prognostic value of serum creatinine and effect of treatment of hypertension on renal function. Results from the hypertension detection and follow-up program. The Hypertension Detection and Follow-up Program Cooperative Group. *Hypertension* 1989; **13(Suppl):** I80–I93.

68 Walker WG, Neaton JD, Cutler JA, Neuwirth R, Cohen JD. Renal function change in hypertensive members of the Multiple Risk Factor Intervention Trial. Racial and treatment effects. The MRFIT Research Group. *JAMA* 1992; **268:** 3085–3091.

69 Hunsicker LG, Adler S, Caggiula A, England BK, Greene T, Kusek JW *et al.* Predictors of the progression of renal disease in the Modification of Diet in Renal Disease Study. *Kidney Int* 1997; **51:** 1908–1919.

70 Hsu CY, Lin F, Vittinghoff E, Shlipak MG. Racial differences in the progression from chronic renal insufficiency to end-stage renal disease in the United States. *J Am Soc Nephrol* 2003; **14:** 2902–2907.

71 Hsu CY, Vittinghoff E, Lin F, Shlipak MG. The incidence of end-stage renal disease is increasing faster than the prevalence of chronic renal insufficiency. *Ann Intern Med* 2004; **141:** 95–101.

72 Foley RN, Murray AM, Li S, Herzog CA, McBean AM, Eggers PW *et al.* Chronic kidney disease and the risk for cardiovascular disease, renal replacement, and death in the United States Medicare population, 1998 to 1999. *J Am Soc Nephrol* 2005; **16:** 489–495.

73 Khan SS, Xue JL, Kazmi WH, Gilbertson DT, Obrador GT, Pereira BJ *et al.* Does predialysis nephrology care influence patient survival after initiation of dialysis? *Kidney Int* 2005; **67:** 1038–1046.

74 Pisoni RL, Young EW, Dykstra DM, Greenwood RN, Hecking E, Gillespie B *et al.* Vascular access use in Europe and the United States: Results from the DOPPS. *Kidney Int* 2002; **61:** 305–316.

75 Port FK. End-stage renal disease: magnitude of the problem, prognosis of future trends and possible solutions. *Kidney Int Suppl* 1995; **50:** S3–S6.

76 Muntner P, Coresh J, Powe NR, Klag MJ. The contribution of increased diabetes prevalence and improved myocardial infarction and stroke survival to the increase in treated end-stage renal disease. *J Am Soc Nephrol* 2003; **14:** 1568–1577.

77 Fox CS, Pencina MJ, Meigs JB, Vasan RS, Levitzky YS, D'Agostino RB. Trends in the incidence of type 2 diabetes mellitus from the 1970s to the 1990s: The Framingham Heart Study. *Circulation* 2006; **113:** 2914–2918.

78 Ojo AO, Held PJ, Port FK, Wolfe RA, Leichtman, AB, Young EW *et al.* Chronic renal failure after transplantation of a nonrenal organ. *N Engl J Med* 2003; **349:** 931–940.

79 Bottalico D, Schena FP, Port FK. Outcomes in dialysis: a global assessment. In: Hoerl WH, Koch KM, Lindsay RM, Ronco C, Winchester J, editors. *Replacement of Renal Function by Dialysis*, 5th edn. Kluwer Academic Publishers, Dordrecht, 2004; 1411–1453.

80 Wolfe RA, Port FK. Good news, bad news for diabetic versus non-diabetic ESRD: Incidence and mortality. *ASAIO J* 1999; **45:** 117–118.

81 ESRD Incidence Group. Geographic, ethnic, age-related and temporal variation in the incidence of end-stage renal disease in Europe, Canada and the Asia-Pacific region, 1998–2002. *Nephrol Dial Transplant* 2006; **21:** 2178–2183.

82 Wolfe RA, Hulbert-Shearon TE, Ashby VB, Mahadevan S, Port FK. Improvements in dialysis patient mortality are associated with improvements in urea reduction ratio and hematocrit, 1999 to 2002. *Am J Kidney Dis* 2005; **45:** 127–135.

83 Pisoni RL, Bragg-Gresham JL, Young EW, Akizawa T, Asano Y, Locatelli F *et al.* Anemia management outcomes from 12 countries in the Dialysis Outcomes and Practice Patterns Study (DOPPS). *Am J Kidney Dis* 2004; **44:** 94–111.

84 Port FK, Wolfe RA, Bloembergen WE, Held PJ, Young EW. The study of outcomes for CAPD versus hemodialysis patients. *Perit Dial Int* 1996; **16:** 628–633.

85 Wolfe RA, Ashby VB, Milford EL, Ojo AO, Ettenger RE, Agodoa LYC *et al.* Comparison of mortality in all patient on dialysis, patients awaiting transplantation, and recipients of a first cadaveric transplant. *N Engl J Med* 1999; **341:** 1725–1730.

86 Cohen DJ, St. Martin L, Christensen LL, Bloom RD, Sung RS. Kidney and pancreas transplantation in the United States, 1995-2004. *Am J Transplant* 2006; **6:** 1153–1169.

87 Port FK, Wolfe RA, Bloembergen WE, Held PJ, Young EW. The study of outcomes for CAPD versus hemodialysis patients. *Perit Dial Int* 1996; **16:** 628–633.

88 Moist LM, Port FK, Orzol SM, Young EW, Ostbye T, Wolfe RA *et al.* Predictors of loss of residual renal function among new dialysis patients. *J Am Soc Nephrol* 2000; **11:** 556–564.

89 Held PJ, Brunner F, Odaka M, Garcia J, Port FK, Gaylin DS. Five-year survival for end stage renal disease patients in the U.S., Europe, and Japan 1982-87. *Am J Kidney Dis* 1990; **15:** 451–457.

90 Goodkin DA, Bragg-Gresham JL, Koenig KG, Wolfe RA, Akiba T, Andreucci VE *et al.* Association of comorbid conditions and mortality in hemodialysis patients in Europe, Japan, and the United States in the Dialysis Outcomes and Practice Patterns Study (DOPPS). *J Am Soc Nephrol* 2003; **14:** 3270–3277.

91 Pisoni RL, Young EW, Mapes DL, Keen ML, Port FK. Vascular access use and outcome in the U.S., Europe, and Japan: results from the Dialysis Outcomes and Practice Patterns Study. *Nephrol News Issues* 2003; **17:** 38–43.

92 Ethier J, Mendelssohn DC, Elder SJ, Hasegawa T, Akizawa T, Akiba T, Canaud BJ, Pisoni RL. Vascular access use and outcomes: an international perspective from the dialysis outcomes and practice patterns study. *Nephrol Dial Transplant* 2008 May 29.

93 Port FK, Pisoni RL, Bragg-Gresham JL, Satayathum S, Young EW, Wolfe RA *et al.* DOPPS estimates of patient life years attributable to modifiable hemodialysis treatment practices in the United States. *Blood Purif* 2004; **22:** 175–180.

94 Mapes DL, Lopes AA, Satayathum S, McCullough KP, Goodkin D, Locatelli F *et al.* Health-related quality of life as a predictor of mortality and hospitalization: the Dialysis Outcomes and Practice Patterns Study (DOPPS). *Kidney Int* 2003; **64:** 339–349.

95 Lopes AA, Albert JM, Young EW, Satayathum S, Pisoni RL, Andreucci VE *et al.* Screening for depression in hemodialysis patients: Associations with diagnosis, treatment, and outcomes in the DOPPS. *Kidney Int* 2004; **66:** 2047–2053.

96 Pifer TB, McCullough KP, Port FK, Goodkin DA, Maroni BJ, Held PJ *et al.* Mortality risk and changes in nutritional indicators among hemodialysis patients in the DOPPS. *Kidney Int* 2002; **62:** 2238–2245.

97 Bradbury B, Fissell RB, Albert JM, Anthony MS, Critchlow CW, Pisoni RL *et al.* Predictors of early mortality among incident US hemodialysis patients in the Dialysis Outcomes and Practices Patterns Study (DOPPS). *Clin J Am Soc Nephrol* 2007; **2:** 89–99.

98 Okechukwu CN, Lopes AA, Stack A, Feng S, Wolfe RA, Port FK. The impact of years of dialysis therapy on mortality risk and the characteristics of long-term dialysis survivors. *Am J Kidney Dis* 2002; **39:** 533–538.

99 Leggat JE, Bloembergen WE, Levine G, Hulbert-Shearon T, Port FK. An analysis of risk factors for withdrawal from dialysis prior to death. *J Am Soc Nephrol* 1997; **8:** 1755–1763.

100 Fissell RB, Bragg-Gresham JL, Lopes AA, Cruz JM, Fukuhara S, Asano Y *et al.* Factors associated with "Do not resuscitate" orders and rates of withdrawal from hemodialysis in the international DOPPS. *Kidney Int* 2005; **68:** 1282–1288.

101 Saran R, Bragg-Gresham JL, Rayner HC, Goodkin DA, Keen ML, van Dijk PC *et al.* Nonadherence in hemodialysis: associations with mortality, hospitalization, and practice patterns in the DOPPS. *Kidney Int* 2003; **64:** 254–262.

102 Pisoni RL, Young EW, Combe C, Leavey SF, Greenwood RN, Hecking E *et al.* Higher catheter use within facilities is associated with increased

mortality and hospitalization: results from the DOPPS. *J Am Soc Nephrol* 2005; **12:** 299A.

103 US Renal Data System. Patient mortality and survival. *Am J Kidney Dis* 1995; **26(Suppl 2):** S69–S84.

104 Evans RW, Manninen DL, Garrison LP, Hart LG, Blagg CR, Gutman RA *et al.* The quality of life of patients with end-stage renal disease. *N Engl J Med* 1985; **312:** 553–559.

105 Coresh J, Astor BC, Greene T, Eknoyan G, Levey AS. Prevalence of chronic kidney disease and decreased kidney function in the adult US population: Third National Health and Nutrition Examination Survey. *Am J Kidney Dis* 2003; **41:** 1–12.

2 Chronic Disease Surveillance and Chronic Kidney Disease

Information for evidence-based practice

Diane L. Frankenfield[1] & Michael V. Rocco[2]

[1]Centers for Medicare & Medicaid Services, Office of Clinical Standards and Quality, Baltimore, USA
[2]Wake Forest University School of Medicine, Winston-Salem, USA

Definition of surveillance

The US Centers for Disease Control and Prevention (CDC) defines surveillance as "the ongoing, systematic collection, analysis, interpretation, and dissemination of data regarding a health-related event for use in public health action to reduce morbidity and mortality and to improve health" [1]. Data obtained through surveillance may be used for public health action, program planning and evaluation, measuring the burden of disease in specified populations, monitoring the quality of care patients receive, and evaluating trends in outcomes of care [1–4].

Chronic kidney disease (CKD) patients have a unique set of medical comorbidities that can affect morbidity and mortality rates, including anemia, renal osteodystrophy, and blood pressure. In addition, several process measures, such as dose of dialysis, type of vascular access, and markers of nutritional status, are associated with morbidity and mortality. Data from a number of surveillance systems have demonstrated that there is marked variation in the care of patients with CKD. This variation in care offers opportunities for the improvement in the care of patients, and surveillance systems provide an excellent mechanism to identify these variations in care [5–7]. In this chapter, we describe several sentinel surveillance systems in place for these medically complex patients, including governmental systems, such as the US Renal Data System (USRDS) and the End-Stage Renal Disease Clinical Performance Measures (ESRD-CPM) Project Database in the USA, and private systems, such as the Dialysis Outcomes and Practice Patterns Study (DOPPS) and the National Kidney Foundation (NKF) Kidney Early Evaluation Program (KEEP).

US ESRD surveillance systems

There are two national surveillance systems in the USA for patients with ESRD. These are the USRDS and the ESRD-CPM Project Database.

USRDS

The USRDS, a national registry of ESRD patients in the USA, was created in 1988 with funding from the National Institute of Diabetes and Digestive and Kidney Diseases. Patient-level data are supplied by the Centers for Medicare & Medicaid Services (CMS), the Organ Procurement and Transplant Network (OPTN), and proprietary databases. Until 2002, when their program was terminated, the CDC also provided the USRDS with facility-level data on reuse practices, water treatment, antibiotic use, hepatitis levels, and rates of human immunodeficiency virus infection and AIDS. Data from these sources have been integrated and compiled in a format suitable for biomedical and economic research analyses.

From the USRDS, an Annual Data Report is produced each year that provides information on the characterization of the total kidney disease patient population and the distribution of patients by sociodemographic characteristics across treatment modalities, the incidence and prevalence of ESRD, hospitalization, transplantation, and mortality rates, and economic analyses.

The USRDS database (more information may be obtained at http://www.usrds.org) contains the following information:
- Demographic, diagnosis, and treatment history for all Medicare beneficiaries with ESRD
- Medicare enrollment and entitlement data, including historical information on Medicare secondary payor status and employee group health plan status

Evidence-based Nephrology. Edited by Donald Molony and Jonathan Craig
© 2009 Blackwell Publishing, ISBN: 978-1-4051-3975-5.

- CMS paid claims records
- CMS Standard Information Management System data maintained by the ESRD Networks and used for patient tracking
- CMS ESRD Annual Facility Survey data
- Dialysis facility ownership status
- CMS ESRD CPM data
- CMS minimum data set to determine which ESRD beneficiaries are nursing home residents
- Medicare 5% enrollment and utilization data, used to estimate numbers of persons with CKD, diabetes, and/or heart disease in the general Medicare population
- OPTN wait list information, transplant events, and posttransplant follow-up
- MEDSTAT Marketscan databases
- CDC surveillance data (historical; data collection was terminated in 2002).

Researchers interested in obtaining data from the USRDS may complete a study request form online, following the processes outlined on the USRDS website (http://www.usrds.org/request.asp).

The ESRD-CPM Project Database

CMS's Health Care Quality Improvement Program is a national surveillance system designed to monitor the quality of care provided to beneficiaries. Since 1994, CMS, in collaboration with the 18 ESRD Networks (regional organizations contracted by CMS to perform quality oversight activities to ensure the appropriateness of services and protection for dialysis patients), has conducted an annual data collection to assess the quality of care of US dialysis patients. The data collection effort was known as the ESRD Core Indicators Project from 1994 to 1999. In response to the Balanced Budget Act of 1997, CMS sought the broad participation of the nephrology community in the development of CPMs based on NKF's Dialysis Outcome Quality Initiative (DOQI) clinical practice guidelines [8–11]. In 1999, the ESRD Core Indicators Project was merged with the ESRD-CPM development effort. Since 1999, the ESRD-CPM Project has collected quality-of-care information in the areas of anemia management, hemodialysis adequacy, peritoneal dialysis adequacy, and vascular access for hemodialysis patients. Although not an official CPM, information is also collected on serum albumin. (Reports and data collection forms may be found at http://www.cms.hhs.gov/CPMProject.)

Annually, each ESRD Network validates the census of ESRD patients within their geographic region. The following groups of patients have been included in the project:
- A nationally representative 5% sample of adult ($\geq$ or 18 years or older) in-center hemodialysis patients, stratified by the 18 ESRD Networks (1994 to present)
- A nationally representative 5% sample of adult peritoneal dialysis patients (1995 to present)
- The identified universe of pediatric in-center hemodialysis patients, ages 12 to under 18 years (2000–2001)
- The identified universe of pediatric in-center hemodialysis patients, ages 0 to under 18 years (2002 to present)
- The identified universe of pediatric peritoneal dialysis patients, ages 0 to under 18 years (2005 to present).

Data are collected on in-center hemodialysis patients from October to December of the year prior to the study year (i.e. October–December 2004 for the 2005 study year) and for the peritoneal dialysis patients from October of the year prior to the study year to March of the study year (i.e. October 2004–March 2005 for the 2005 study year). The data are aggregated, analyzed, and reported annually in the ESRD-CPM Annual Report. Every facility in the country receives the Annual Report and is able to compare their performance against regional and national findings for their adult hemodialysis patients. For adult peritoneal dialysis patients and for all pediatric patients (hemodialysis and peritoneal dialysis patients), national comparison findings are provided.

ESRD Network and treatment center quality improvement activities

A primary function of the ESRD surveillance system is to promote practice-based quality improvement activities designed to remedy less-than-adequate care [5]. These activities facilitate the translation of information about facility-specific, guideline-based performance measures into activities to improve care. Although each Network designs its own intervention activities, these interventions are typically directed at treatment centers needing improvement, rather than the system of treatment centers, and include dissemination of relevant guidelines (national, Network, and facility feedback reports on quality of care; distribution of management algorithms; workshops on methods to improve the quality of care in the treatment center) and continued supervision of poorly performing treatment centers [6]. Network-specific interventions that were subsequently found to be independently associated with an increased rate of improvement in care included workshop participation and continuing Network supervision of facilities selected for intervention [12]. Additional data suggest that changes in care documented by this surveillance system were associated with improved survival among ESRD patients [13].

Improvement has been noted in the areas of hemodialysis adequacy and in anemia management for adult hemodialysis and peritoneal dialysis patients. The percentage of in-center hemodialysis patients with a mean single-pool Kt/V of 1.2 increased from 74% in late 1996 to 91% in late 2004 (Figure 2.1). From 1997 to 2004, the percentage of adult in-center hemodialysis patients with a mean hemoglobin of 11 g/dL increased from 43% to 83%; for adult peritoneal dialysis patients, the increase was from 55% to 82% (Figure 2.2). Similar improvement has been noted for pediatric in-center hemodialysis patients. The percentage of pediatric patients with a mean single-pool Kt/V of 1.2 increased from 87% in late 2001 to 89% in late 2004. Sixty-two percent of pediatric patients had a mean hemoglobin of 11 g/dL in late 2001 compared with 67% in late 2004.

The NKF's Kidney Disease Outcomes Quality Initiative (K/DOQI) clinical practice guidelines for vascular access in 2001

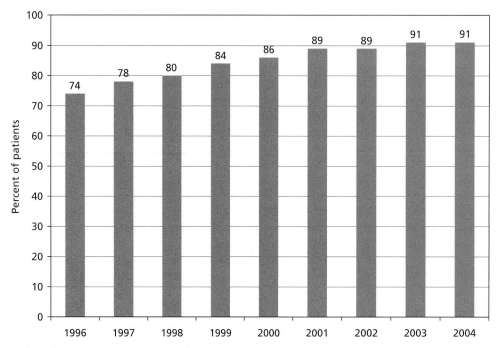

Figure 2.1 Percentage of adult hemodialysis patients in the USA with mean single-pool Kt/V of ≥1.2, 1996–2004. Data are from the ESRD-CPM Project.

recommended that primary arteriovenous (AV) fistulae be constructed in at least 50% of all new kidney failure patients and that 40% of prevalent patients have a native AV fistula [14]. Trend data from the ESRD-CPM Project indicate only modest improvement toward attaining these goals. For the last quarter of 2004, 37% of incident and 39% of prevalent adult in-center hemodialysis patients were dialyzed with an AV fistula as their access (Figure 2.3).

Thus far, there have been 52 publications and 123 abstracts describing findings from the ESRD-CPM Project data. One of the

goals of *Healthy People 2010* [15] is to eliminate disparity for all groups. Data from the ESRD-CPM Project have been examined to determine whether disparity exists for groups of ESRD patients in regard to both processes of care and outcomes, such as subsequent hospitalization, transplantation, and mortality [16–20]. Other analyses linking the ESRD-CPM Project data with CMS administrative and claims data have examined the association of intermediate outcomes with hospitalization and mortality [7,21–24].

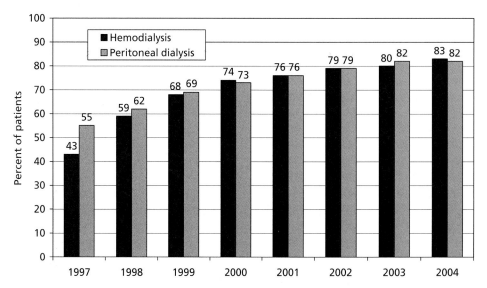

Figure 2.2 Percentage of adult ESRD patients in the USA with mean hemoglobin of ≥11 g/dL by modality, 1997–2004. Data are from the ESRD-CPM Project.

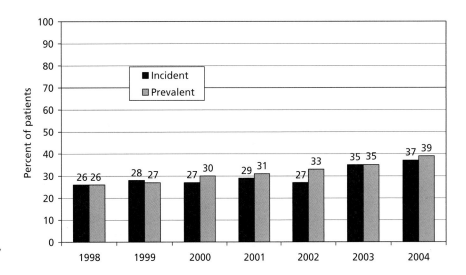

Figure 2.3 Percentage of adult hemodialysis patients in the USA with an AV fistula as their access, 1998–2004. Data are from the ESRD-CPM Project.

Other national ESRD surveillance systems

A number of other national or international registries for ESRD patients have been developed by either governmental or private agencies. The defining characteristic of these registries is that they have been voluntary and capture a variable fraction of the ESRD population. Some of the larger registries are presented below. The reader is referred to the websites of these organizations for additional information.

European Renal Association–European Dialysis and Transplant Association Registry

The European Renal Association–European Dialysis and Transplant Association (ERA-EDTA) Registry collects data on renal replacement therapy (RRT) via the national and regional renal registries in Europe. The 2003 annual report included information based on 55 registries from 27 countries. Section A of this report contains data on incidence and prevalence from 32 national and regional registries from 12 countries whose individual patient data are included in the ERA-EDTA Registry database (shown in dark gray in Figure 2.4) as well as data on patient survival, graft survival, and expected remaining lifetimes. Section B of the report provides aggregated data from 24 national and regional registries from 17 countries that were obtained via individual patient data, center questionnaire data, or information from health authorities (shown in light gray in Figure 2.4). Data in Section B are not included in the ERA-EDTA Registry database. These registries complete the tables themselves and return them to the ERA-EDTA Registry office for inclusion in the annual report(http://www.era-edta-reg.org/index.jsp) [25].

Canadian Organ Replacement Register

The Canadian Organ Replacement Register (CORR) is the national information system on renal and extrarenal organ failure and transplantation in Canada. The first Renal Failure Register was started in 1972. CORR collects data from hospital dialysis programs, regional transplant programs, organ procurement organizations, and kidney dialysis services offered at independent health facilities. The registry includes information on both renal and extrarenal transplantation. The most recent annual report provides data for a 10-year period (http://secure.cihi.ca/cihiweb/dispPage.jsp?cw_page=AR_5_E) [26].

Australia and New Zealand Dialysis and Transplant Registry

The Australia and New Zealand Dialysis and Transplant Registry (ANZDATA) is an organization set up by Kidney Health Australia and the Australia and New Zealand Society of Nephrology to monitor dialysis and transplant treatments. ANZDATA is funded by the Australian and New Zealand governments and Kidney Health Australia. All kidney specialists throughout Australia and New Zealand report patient information every 12 months to ANZDATA. The most recent annual report includes data from the calendar year 2004 (http://www.anzdata.org.au/) [27].

Other ESRD surveillance systems

DOPPS

DOPPS is a prospective, observational study that was initiated in 1996 (DOPPS I) with data from 308 hemodialysis units in seven countries (17,000 patients), including 145 facilities from the USA, followed by additional data from 62 facilities from Japan and 101 facilities from five European countries (France, Germany, Italy, Spain, and the UK). More than 12,800 patients were added in DOPPS II from 322 hemodialysis units from the seven DOPPS I countries as well as Australia, Belgium, Canada, New Zealand, and Sweden (Figure 2.5). DOPPS III was initiated in 2005, and the data collection effort includes parameters that allow for a better

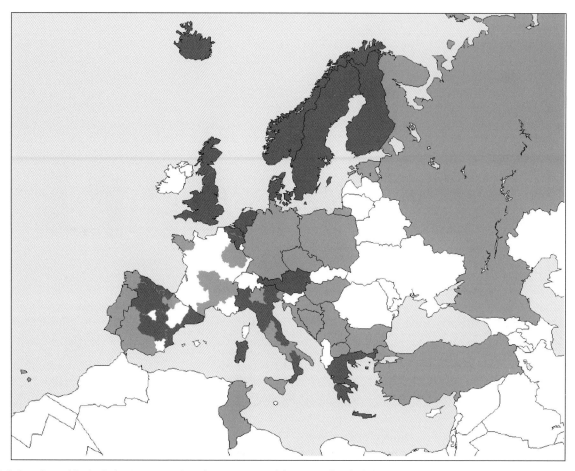

Figure 2.4 Countries participating in the ERA-EDTA Registry. The 12 countries in dark grey provide individual patient data. The 17 countries in medium grey provide aggregated patient data from 24 national and regional registries [25].

understanding on how some dialysis facilities accomplish better adherence and achievement of K/DOQI targets than others.

For DOPPS I and II, the study design focused on five key elements: 1) within each country, random selection of dialysis units stratified by type of facility and geographic region, with facility sampling proportional to size within each stratum; 2) collection of demographic data, diabetes as the cause of ESRD, and mortality data for all chronic maintenance hemodialysis patients in each study dialysis unit (cumulative hemodialysis census); 3) collection of additional detailed patient data from a random selection of 20–40 patients within each dialysis unit at study entry (medical questionnaire) and at 4-month intervals throughout the study (interval summary); 4) collection of kidney disease quality-of-life information from this random sample as well as other data regarding a patient's medical care as indicated in a questionnaire completed by the patient at study entry and annually thereafter (patient questionnaire); and 5) collection of detailed facility practice information, assessed from patient data and from questionnaires completed annually by the dialysis unit's medical director (medical directors survey) and by the unit's nurse manager or designee

(unit practices survey) [28]. In DOPPS II, data were collected for both a cross-section of chronic hemodialysis patients and sequentially on 5354 new patients within 30 days of initiating dialysis. The latter cohort allowed for the determination of the practices, characteristics, and outcomes of patients since the initiation of chronic hemodialysis therapy.

Facilities chosen for participation in DOPPS were required to treat more than 25 hemodialysis patients to ensure that the facility was of sufficient size to obtain accurate estimates of facility practices and outcomes. Patients from each dialysis unit were chosen randomly. In addition, facilities were chosen so that there was a representative sample of dialysis units in each country. The implementation of these criteria allowed for the investigators to provide nationally representative results for in-center hemodialysis therapy.

The data collected in DOPPS II provide detailed information on sampled patients, including patient demographics and more than 70 other variables, including medical comorbidity, socioeconomic status, insurance coverage, laboratory values, medication use, hospitalization and outpatient events, vascular access use and

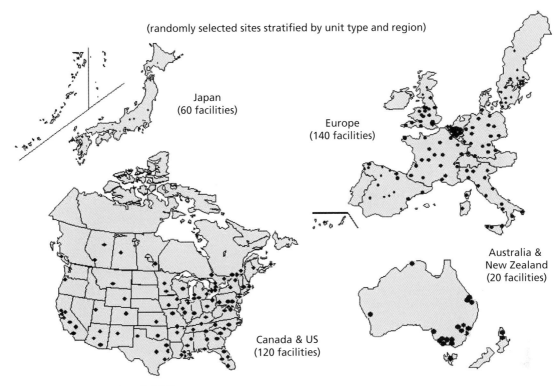

(randomly selected sites stratified by unit type and region)

Japan
(60 facilities)

Europe
(140 facilities)

Australia &
New Zealand
(20 facilities)

Canada & US
(120 facilities)

Figure 2.5 Countries participating in the DOPPS [28].

vascular access procedures, dialysis prescription, delivered dialysis dose, residual kidney function, nutritional measures, aspects of medical care before ESRD, kidney transplant wait-listing, patient quality of life, physician-diagnosed and patient-reported measures of depression, date and cause(s) of death for patients who died during the study, and transfer to or from peritoneal dialysis or kidney transplantation.

This extensive database allows DOPPS investigators to analyze information on patient demographics, comorbidities, laboratory measures, and practice patterns for characterization of these data elements, as well as to determine cross-sectional associations and prospective associations with outcomes of interest. The database includes mortality data for more than 100,000 patients and detailed longitudinal data from almost 30,000 hemodialysis patients. This large database also allows for analyses of practice pattern variations in hemodialysis patients. Thus far, more than 70 publications have described findings from the DOPPS data [29].

Surveillance systems for CKD stages 1–4

There are few surveillance systems for stage 1–4 CKD that are available in the public domain. Difficulties with identifying patients with CKD have hampered efforts to develop surveillance systems. The October 2005 ninth revision of the *International Classification of Disease* (ICD-9) coding now includes specific codes for each of the five stages of CKD (ICD-9 codes 585.1–585.5). In addition, legislation in both British Columbia (Canada) and New Jersey (USA) now mandate that laboratories provide an estimate of glomeru-

lar filtration rate (GFR) based on serum creatinine levels. More widespread use of these specific CKD codes, in conjunction with more widespread use of automated estimates of GFR based on serum creatinine levels, will facilitate the development of additional surveillance systems. In the absence of these systems, mass screenings have substituted for surveillance systems in identifying patients with CKD.

KEEP

In the USA, the NKF developed the KEEP program to 1) evaluate the feasibility of detecting large numbers of previously unidentified persons with CKD or at high risk for CKD in communities with at-risk populations, and 2) determine the prevalence of selected risk factors and level of kidney function within that group.

The pilot study, KEEP 1, was conducted from 1997 to 1999 in 21 cities, and data from this study demonstrated that 71.4% of 889 individuals screened had at least one abnormal test value [30]. Since then, KEEP screening programs conducted by NKF affiliates had enrolled more than 37,000 individuals at the time of publication of the 3rd Annual Data Report from KEEP in 2005 [31]. Screenings are advertised through local media (radio and television stations and newspapers), announcements by clergy from the pulpit, flyers, posters, and information provided to dialysis patients, with an emphasis on minority communities [32]. Screening sites include churches, hospitals, health centers, schools, community centers, and dialysis units.

Consenting individuals completed a screening questionnaire, a self-report instrument that collects information regarding sociodemographic status (e.g. race and ethnicity, age, education), personal and family health history, and life-style behavior (e.g. smoking). Those persons with hypertension or diabetes or a first-order relative with hypertension, diabetes, or kidney disease were screened for kidney disease risk factors. Blood pressure, blood glucose, serum creatinine, hemoglobin, microalbuminuria, hematuria, pyuria, body mass index, and estimated GFR (eGFR) were obtained for these eligible persons. Those persons who did not meet eligibility criteria were given educational material and encouraged to maintain a healthy life-style [30].

At the completion of data collection, participants were given a copy of their test results that had been reviewed by a KEEP physician, educational materials and, if needed, a list of health care providers who could provide follow-up care. Approximately 2 months after the screening, participants who had been encouraged to see their physician were contacted to determine whether follow-up had occurred and whether abnormal test results had been corroborated.

Although less than 10% of KEEP participants reported that they had kidney disease or kidney stones, more than 50% of participants had CKD as defined by NKF K/DOQI guidelines, compared with 13% of National Health and Nutrition Survey (NHANES) participants. CKD of stages 1, 2, and 3 was found in 16%, 22%, and 15% of KEEP participants, respectively, compared with <5% in each stage for NHANES participants (Figure 2.6). Among those patients with CKD (Figure 2.7), stage 2 CKD was noted in 41% of KEEP participants, with a range of 39–42% among different race and ethnic groups. Stage 3 CKD was found in 42% of the White population compared with 17–21% in other racial and ethnic groups [31].

Fifty-seven percent of KEEP participants returned the study follow-up form. Of these 14,441 participants, a total of 8244 saw a doctor, of which 51% were seen for hypertension and 48% for abnormal urine testing. A total of 3449 participants learned that they had anemia, 1605 participants learned that they had hypertension, and 741 participants learned that they had diabetes mellitus; all were started on a medical intervention [31].

The KEEP study demonstrates the high yield of a high-risk screening program in detecting previously unknown disease as well as the benefit of a screening program in tracking individuals with known clinical conditions to evaluate the control and progress of management of hypertension and diabetes, conditions that are well-recognized as risk factors for CKD.

Province of British Columbia

The British Columbia Renal Agency (BCPRA) and the British Columbia Ministry of Health Services have jointly developed a patient register to help identify and track the quality of care and status of patients at all stages of CKD, including at-risk populations. The register is supported by existing Ministry administrative data and the BCPRA's Patient Registration and Outcome Management Information System. This registry includes data from more than 30 nephrology (CKD and ESRD) units in British Columbia to provide information on individual patient management, nephrology unit management, continuous quality improvement and research, and outcomes-based planning.

As of October 2002, more than 2000 dialysis patients and 2600 CKD patients were registered in this database, which captures data on all patients seen by nephrologists. Once registered, patients are tracked over their entire clinical course; thus complete data, including medication lists, dialysis start dates, and death, are accessible. Demographic variables such as age, gender, and diagnosis of kidney disease are entered into the database as part of essential information. Diabetic status (either insulin-requiring or non-insulin-requiring) is entered as a comorbid condition, and the level of kidney function at the time of registration is also entered. Laboratory values including hemoglobin, transferrin saturation, and serum chemistries are all either manually entered or automatically uploaded from laboratory systems in the province. Changes in treatment status (from CKD to dialysis or transplant or death) are captured within the database, as it forms the basis of funding of kidney services. Any patient requiring erythropoietin therapy must have hemoglobin and transferrin saturation values entered into the database before the prescription for the drug can be processed. Other prescribed medications are also entered into the database [33]. Additional information about the British Columbia Renal Agency may be found on their website (http://www.bcrenalagency.ca/).

Okinawa (Japan) Screening Program

The Okinawa Screening program is a unique demonstration of a longitudinal cohort study of a community-based screening program that was first conducted in 1983. The study has provided

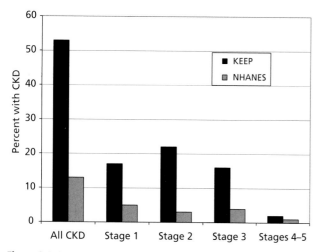

Figure 2.6 CKD in KEEP and NHANES participants by CKD stage. CKD stages 1, 2, and 3 were found in 16%, 22%, and 15% of KEEP participants, respectively; occurrence of each stage was 5% or less in the NHANES population. Adapted from KEEP 2005 Annual Report, Figure 5.3.

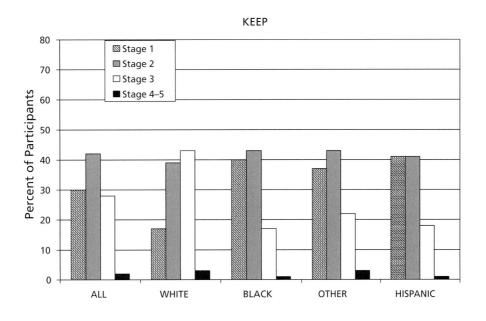

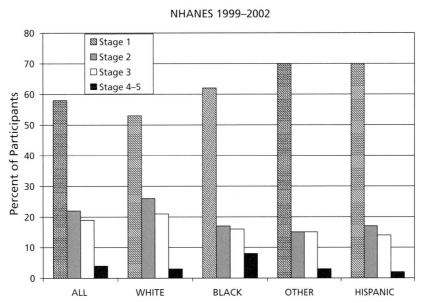

Figure 2.7 CKD in KEEP and NHANES participants by CKD stage and race and ethnicity. The percentage of KEEP participants with stage 2 CKD was similar across race and ethnicity groups, at 39–42%. Stage 3 CKD, however, was found in 42% of the white population but only 17–21% of other racial and ethnic groups. From KEEP 2005 Annual Report, Figure 3.35.

insights on the natural history of risk factors and longitudinal outcomes of the thousands of individuals who participated in the screening program. Over 10% of the adult population in Okinawa participated in the 1983 screening survey [34]. This program identified several key findings, including the following: 1) the strong association between dipstick proteinuria at baseline and increased risk of ESRD after 17 years of follow-up, even at levels of proteinuria of 1+ (odds ratio of 1.93 for ESRD) [34]; 2) a continuous increase in risk of ESRD with increasing body mass index, primar-

ily in men [35]; 3) uric acid as an independent risk factor for ESRD [36] and other.

National Kidney Foundation of Singapore Screening Program

Similarly, the National Kidney Foundation of Singapore Screening Program is unique in its goal of developing a comprehensive multilevel strategy for the prevention of ESRD in the population. The design of the Singapore model includes 1) screening populations at risk for CKD, 2) monitoring of standards of care for chronic diseases associated with CKD, 3) institution of a disease management program to facilitate management of patients with diabetes and hypertension, which are among the leading causes of ESRD in the country, and 4) longitudinal tracking of individuals who participated in the screening program [37]. Given Singapore's multi-ethnic population and high burden of chronic diseases that are associated with CKD, the Singapore program suggests that differences in risk for kidney disease exist across racial and ethnic subgroups. In particular, the program demonstrates that 1) the relationship between body mass index and proteinuria in this multi-ethnic population is J-shaped, 2) the association between blood pressure and proteinuria is continuous and begins to occur even at levels considered within the normal range for Western populations, 3) a family history of kidney disease is a risk factor for proteinuria, and 4) among its pediatric population, a low body weight was found to be predictive of proteinuria [37,38].

Altogether, these population-based studies suggest the possible use of a surveillance and screening program, not merely in identifying persons at increased risk for CKD but also to determine unique population-specific risk factors that may be modifiable. Longitudinal analyses of these populations should be performed in order to evaluate whether interventions aimed at these risk factors are effective in reducing the burden of CKD in the population.

Practice-based screening and quality management for CKD

Practice-based screening for CKD is a relatively undeveloped field. This is due to the difficulties in identifying patients with CKD based on ICD-9 codes (as discussed above) and the slow acceptance of the provision of automated estimates of GFR by local and national laboratories.

Quality management of both dialysis and nondialysis CKD patients has been facilitated by guideline development in key areas of CKD. In 1995, the NKF launched the DOQI to develop clinical practice guidelines for dialysis patients and health care providers. The goal of this project was to improve the quality of care delivered to all patients with kidney disease. The first set of guidelines for dialysis patients, in the areas of hemodialysis, peritoneal dialysis, anemia management, and vascular access, was published in 1997 [8–11]. These guidelines were updated in 2001 [14,39–41] and again in 2006 [42–45].

In 1999, the NKF developed guidelines for CKD patients who were not on dialysis. The rationale for this change was that early intervention and appropriate measures can prevent the loss of kidney function in some patients, slow the progression of the disease in many other patients, and ameliorate organ dysfunction and comorbid conditions in those patients who progress to kidney failure and ESRD. To reflect these expanded goals, the reference to "dialysis" in DOQI was changed to "disease," and the new initiative was termed the Kidney Disease Outcomes Quality Initiative (K/DOQI). The first of these K/DOQI guidelines, on the evalua-

tion, classification, and stratification of CKD, was released in 2002 [46].

CKD is defined in five stages, based on the estimated level of kidney function and the presence of other signs of kidney disease, such as proteinuria, as detailed in chapter 1 of this text. The GFR is estimated from equations using serum creatinine, patient demographics, and in some cases, other serum and laboratory data. This classification of CKD provides a framework for additional guidelines in CKD, where evaluation and management are linked to the level of kidney function. There are now K/DOQI guidelines for anemia (in 2006 for dialysis and nondialysis patients) [42], nutrition [47], hypertension [48], hyperlipidemia [49], bone and mineral metabolism [50], and cardiovascular disease [51]. Guidelines for the care of the CKD patient with diabetes mellitus published in 2007.

The process of guideline development follows several principles. First, guideline development is scientifically rigorous and based on a critical appraisal of the available evidence. This process is carried out by both an evidence review team and the workgroup members. Second, participants involved in developing the guidelines are from multiple disciplines. These participants include not only nephrologists, but also other internists, surgeons, nurses, dietitians, social workers, and other content experts as deemed appropriate by the workgroup. Third, the workgroups charged with developing the guidelines are the final authority on their content and evidence rating. The guidelines are evidence based whenever possible, and the rationale and evidentiary basis of each guideline are explicit. Each of the draft guidelines undergoes a peer review process where nephrologists and other content experts worldwide are asked to provide comments that are reviewed by the workgroup. Modifications to the guidelines are made by the workgroup prior to the publication of the guidelines.

These guidelines have been widely adopted. They were used as a template for national clinical performance measures in the USA that were developed and implemented by the Health Care Financing Administration (now named the Centers for Medicare & Medicaid Services). They have been translated into more than a dozen languages, and selected components of these guidelines have been adopted in various countries across the world. The new classification of CKD into five stages has been widely adopted in research and was adopted in a revision of the ICD-9 codes released in October 2005. Implementation tools for each of the guidelines are available from Kidney Learning System (http://www.kidney.org/professionals/KLS/). This NKF organization develops implementation tools by using information provided by workgroup members, other content experts, and Kidney Learning System staff.

Other guideline development organizations

A number of other national and international organizations have developed guidelines, and many of these guidelines are summarized at the website http://www.kdigo.org/welcome.htm. Although in general these guideline statements are similar to those developed by K/DOQI, there are differences not only in the targets recommended for particular parameters but also in the evidence review and evidence-grading processes. It thus became evident that there would be benefits both in terms of a standard approach to guideline development worldwide; also, the potential duplication of effort among these many organizations led to the formation of an international guideline development group called Kidney Disease Improving Global Outcomes, or KDIGO. The stated goal of KDIGO, launched in 2003, is "to improve the care and outcomes of kidney disease patients worldwide through promoting coordination, collaboration and integration of initiatives to develop and implement clinical practice guidelines" [52]. The KDIGO website has a list of guideline statements from a number of national and international organizations that allows for the direct comparison of recommended targets among different guidelines.

Summary

A number of surveillance systems have been developed for patients with CKD. ESRD surveillance systems are well-established in many countries, and documentation of improvement in intermediate outcomes over time has been demonstrated. CKD surveillance systems are of more recent origin and are not prevalent in most developed countries. Additional efforts are needed to expand CKD surveillance programs. The development of guidelines in a number of areas of CKD should help to facilitate the choice of intermediate outcomes for these surveillance systems.

References

1 Updated guidelines for evaluating public health surveillance systems. *MMWR Recomm Rep* 2001; **50(RR-13):** 1–35.

2 Thacker SB. *Principles and Practice of Public Health Surveillance.* New York, 2000. Oxford University Press, Second edition, p. 1–16.

3 Buehler JW. *Modern Epidemiology.* Philadelphia, 1998. Lippincott Williams & Wilkins, p. 435–458.

4 Teutsch SC, Thacker SB. Planning a public health surveillance system. *Epidemiol Bull* 1995; **16:** 1–6.

5 McClellan WM, Frankenfield DL, Frederick PR, Helgerson SD, Wish JB, Sugarman JR. Improving the care of ESRD patients: a success story. *Health Care Financ Rev* 2003; **24:** 89–100.

6 McClellan WM, Frankenfield DL, Frederick PR, Flanders WD, Alfaro-Correa A, Rocco MV *et al.* Can dialysis therapy be improved? A report from the ESRD Core Indicators Project. *Am J Kidney Dis* 1999; **34:** 1075–1082.

7 Rocco MV, Frankenfield DL, Hopson SD, McClellan WM. Relationship between clinical performance measures and outcomes among chronic hemodialysis patients. *Ann Intern Med* 2006; **145:** 512–519.

8 Hemodialysis Adequacy Work Group. NKF-DOQI clinical practice guidelines for hemodialysis. *Am J Kidney Dis* 1997; **30 (Suppl 2):** S15–S66.

9 National Kidney Foundation. NKF-DOQI clinical practice guidelines for peritoneal dialysis adequacy. *Am J Kidney Dis* 1997; **30 (Suppl 2):** S67—S136.

10 National Kidney Foundation. NKF-DOQI clinical practice guidelines for vascular access. *Am J Kidney Dis* 1997; **30 (Suppl 3):** S150–S191.

11 National Kidney Foundation. NKF-DOQI clinical practice guidelines for the treatment of anemia of chronic renal failure. *Am J Kidney Dis* 1997; **30 (Suppl 3):** S192–S240.

12 McClellan WM, Hodgin E, Pastan S, McAdams L, Soucie M. A randomized evaluation of two health care quality improvement program (HCQIP) interventions to improve the adequacy of hemodialysis care of ESRD patients: feedback alone versus intensive intervention. *J Am Soc Nephrol* 2004; **15:** 754–760.

13 Wolfe RA, Hulbert-Shearon T, Ashby VB, Mahadevan S, Port FK. Improvements in dialysis patient mortality are associated with improvements in urea reduction ratio and hematocrit, 1999 to 2002. *Am J Kidney Dis* 2005; **45:** 127–135.

14 National Kidney Foundation. K/DOQI clinical practice guidelines for vascular access. *Am J Kidney Dis* 2001; **37 (Suppl 1):** S137–S181.

15 U.S. Department of Health and Human Services. With Understanding and Improving Health and Objectives for Improving Health, 2nd edn. U.S. Government Printing Office, Washington DC, 2000.

16 Frankenfield DL, Rocco MV, Frederick PR, Pugh J, McClellan WM, Owen W Jr. Racial/ethnic analysis of selected intermediate outcomes for hemodialysis patients: results from the 1997 ESRD Core Indicators Project. *Am J Kidney Dis* 1999; **34:** 721–730.

17 Rocco MV, Frankenfield DL, Frederick PR, Pugh J, McClellan WM, Owen WF. Intermediate outcomes by race and ethnicity in peritoneal dialysis patients: results from the 1997 ESRD Core Indicators Project. National ESRD Core Indicators Workgroup. *Perit Dial Int* 2000; **20:** 328–335.

18 Frankenfield DL, Ramirez SP, McClellan WM, Frederick PR, Rocco MV. Differences in intermediate outcomes for Asian and non-Asian adult hemodialysis patients in the United States. *Kidney Int* 2003; **64:** 623–631.

19 Frankenfield DL, Roman SH, Rocco MV, Bedinger MR, McClellan WM. Disparity in outcomes for adult Native American hemodialysis patients? Findings from the ESRD Clinical Performance Measures Project. *Kidney Int* 1999; **65:** 1426–1434.

20 Frankenfield DL, Atkinson MA, Fivush BA, Neu AM. Outcomes for adolescent Hispanic hemodialysis patients: findings from the ESRD Clinical Performance Measures Project. *Am J Kidney Dis* 2006; **47:** 870–878.

21 Rocco MV, Frankenfield DL, Prowant B, Frederick PR, Flanigan MJ. Risk factors for early mortality in U.S. peritoneal dialysis patients: impact of residual renal function. *Perit Dial Int* 2002; **22:** 371–379.

22 Speckman RA, Frankenfield DL, Roman SH, Eggers PW, Bedinger MR, Rocco MV *et al.* Diabetes is the strongest risk factor for lower extremity amputation in new hemodialysis patients. *Diabetes Care* 2004; **27:** 2198–2203.

23 Gorman G, Furth S, Hwang W, Parekh R, Astor B, Fivush B *et al.* Clinical outcomes and dialysis adequacy in adolescent hemodialysis patients. *Am J Kidney Dis* 2006; **47:** 285–293.

24 Fadrowski JJ, Hwang W, Frankenfield DL, Fivush BA, Neu AM, Furth SL. Clinical course associated with vascular access type in a national cohort of adolescents receiving hemodialysis: findings from the ESRD CPM Project. *Clin J Am Soc Nephrol* 2006; **1:** 987–992.

25 ERA-EDTA Registry. ERA-EDTA Registry 2003 Annual Report. Academic Medical Center, Amsterdam, 2005.

26 Treatment of End-Stage Organ Failure in Canada 2002 and 2003 Report. Canadian Institute for Health Information, Ottawa, 2005.

27 McDonald S, Excell L. ANZDATA Registry Report 2005 Australia and New Zealand Dialysis and Transplant Registry. Adelaide, 2006.

28 Pisoni RL, Gillespie BW, Dickinson DM, Chen K, Kutner MH, Wolfe RA. The Dialysis Outcomes and Practice Patterns Study (DOPPS): design,

data elements and methodology. *Am J Kidney Dis* 2004; **44 (Suppl 2):** S7–S15.

29 Pisoni RL, Greenwood RN. Selected lessons learned from the Dialysis Outcomes and Practice Patterns Study (DOPPS). *Contrib Nephrol* 2005; **149:** 58–68.

30 Brown WW, Collins A, Chen SC, King K, Molony DA, Gannon M. Identification of persons at high risk for kidney disease via targeted screening: The NKF Kidney Early Evaluation Program. *Kidney Int* 2003; **63:** S50–S55.

31 National Kidney Foundation. KEEP Annual Data Report. *Am J Kidney Dis* 2005; **46 (Suppl 3):** S1–S158.

32 Brown WW, Peters RM, Ohmit SE, Keane WF, Collins A, Chen SC *et al.* Early detection of kidney disease in community settings: The Kidney Early Evaluation Program (KEEP). *Am J Kidney Dis* 2003; **42:** 22–35.

33 Levin A, Djurdjev O, Duncan J, Rosenbaum D, Werb R. Haemoglobin at time of referral prior to dialysis predicts survival: an association of haemoglobin with long-term outcomes. *Nephrol Dial Transplant* 2005; **21:** 370–377.

34 Iseki K, Ikemiya Y, Iseki C, Takishita S. Proteinuria and the risk of developing end-stage renal disease. *Kidney Int* 2003; **63:** 1468–1474.

35 Iseki K, Ikemiya Y, Kinjo K, Inoue T, Iseki C, Takishita S. Body mass index and the risk of development of end-stage renal disease in a screened cohort. *Kidney Int* 2004; **65:** 1870–1876.

36 Iseki K, Ikemiya Y, Inoue T, Iseki C, Kinjo K, Takishita S. Significance of hyperuricemia as a risk factor for developing ESRD in a screened cohort. *Am J Kidney Dis* 2004; **44:** 642–650.

37 Ramirez SPB, McClellan W, Port FK, Hsu SIH. Risk factors for proteinuria in a large, multiracial, Southeast Asian population. *J Am Soc Nephrol* 2002; **13:** 1907–1917.

38 Ramirez SPB, Hsu SIH, McClellan W. Low body weight is a risk factor for proteinuria in a multiracial Southeast Asian population. *Am J Kidney Dis* 2001; **38:** 1045–1054.

39 National Kidney Foundation. NKF-K/DOQI clinical practice guidelines for hemodialysis adequacy, 2000. *Am J Kidney Dis* 2001; **37(Suppl 1):** S7–S64.

40 National Kidney Foundation. NKF-K/DOQI clinical practice guidelines for peritoneal dialysis adequacy, 2000. *Am J Kidney Dis* 2001; **37 (Suppl 1):** S65–S136.

41 National Kidney Foundation. NKF-K/DOQI clinical practice guidelines for anemia of chronic kidney disease, 2000. *Am J Kidney Dis* 2001; **37(Suppl 1):** S182–S238.

42 National Kidney Foundation. NKF-K/DOQI clinical practice guidelines and clinical practice recommendations for anemia in chronic kidney disease. *Am J Kidney Dis* 2006; **47(Suppl 3):** S11–S145.

43 K/DOQI Workgroup for Hemodialysis. K/DOQI clinical practice guidelines and clinical practice recommendations for hemodialysis. *Am J Kidney Dis* 2006; **48(Suppl 1):** S2–S90.

44 K/DOQI Workgroup for Peritoneal Dialysis. K/DOQI clinical practice guidelines and clinical practice recommendations for peritoneal dialysis. *Am J Kidney Dis* 2006; **48(Suppl 1):** S91–S175.

45 K/DOQI Workgroup for Vascular Access. K/DOQI clinical practice guidelines and clinical practice recommendations for vascular access. *Am J Kidney Dis* 2006; **48(Suppl 1):** S176–S306.

46 National Kidney Foundation. NKF-K/DOQI clinical practice guidelines for chronic kidney disease: evaluation, classification and stratification. *Am J Kidney Dis* 2002; **39(Suppl 1):** S1–S266.

47 K/DOQI NKF. Clinical practice guidelines for nutrition in chronic renal failure. *Am J Kidney Dis* 2000; **35:** S1–S40.

48 Kidney Disease Quality Initiative (K/DOQI). K/DOQI clinical practice guidelines on hypertension and antihypertensive agents in chronic kidney disease. *Am J Kidney Dis* 2004; **43(Suppl 1):** S1–S290.

49 Kidney Disease Outcomes Quality Initative (K/DOQI). K/DOQI clinical practice guidelines for management of dyslipidemias in patients with kidney disease. *Am J Kidney Dis* 2003; **41(Suppl 3):** S1–S91.

50 National Kidney Foundation. K/DOQI clinical practice guidelines for bone metabolism and disease in chronic kidney disease. *Am J Kidney Dis* 2003; **42(Suppl 3):** S1–S201.

51 K/DOQI Workgroup. K/DOQI clinical practice guidelines for cardiovascular disease in dialysis patients. *Am J Kidney Dis* 2005; **45(Suppl 3):** S1–S153.

52 National Kidney Foundation. K/DOQI clinical practice guidelines and clinical practice recommendations for diabetes and CKD. *Am J Kidney Dis* 2007; **49:** 51–5180.

53 Eknoyan G, Lameire N, Barsoum R, Eckardt KU, Levin A, Locatelli F *et al.* The burden of kidney disease: improving global outcomes. *Kidney Int* 2004; **66:** 1310–1314.

3 Risk Factors for Progression of Chronic Kidney Disease

Eberhard Ritz,[1] Danilo Fliser,[2] & Marcin Adamczak[3]

[1] Department of Internal Medicine, Nierenzentrum, Ruperto Carola University, Heidelberg, Germany
[2] Department of Internal Medicine, Division of Nephrology, Medical School Hannover, Hannover, Germany
[3] Department of Nephrology, Endocrinology and Metabolic Diseases, Medical University of Silesia, Katowice, Poland

Evidence for progression of primary and secondary chronic kidney diseases

Etiology as a determinant of progression

In experimental studies, progressive loss of kidney function is consistently observed in many different animal models of chronic kidney diseases (CKD) [1]. In contrast, observational clinical data and available data from the recruitment phase prior to enrollment in controlled prospective studies have revealed that a considerable proportion of patients with CKD progress at a slow rate, and we know from our clinical observations that a substantial proportion of patients do not progress at all. One of the factors determining the rate of progression (i.e. the natural course of CKD) is the underlying renal disease. For example, progression is rather slow in membranous glomerulonephritis (GN) and immunoglobulin A (IgA) GN and more rapid in focal segmental glomerulosclerosis, autosomal-dominant polycystic kidney disease (ADPKD), and diabetic nephropathy, whereas in malignant hypertension and scleroderma fulminant progression is usually observed in the short term. Because controlled clinical trials with placebo treatment are ethically no longer permissible in patients with progressive CKD, historical data on spontaneous rates of progression are still of considerable interest [2–10].

Risk factors of progression

It is clinically useful to distinguish between modifiable and non-modifiable risk factors for progression of CKD (Table 3.1). Some modifiable risk factors of progression can be eliminated simply by avoidance, for example, smoking, nonsteroidal anti-inflammatory drugs (NSAIDs), or herbal medicines, whereas elimination of others, such as elevated blood pressure and proteinuria, necessitates aggressive treatment and strict control. The list of modifiable risk factors also includes recently discovered potential risk factors, such

Evidence-based Nephrology. Edited by Donald Molony and Jonathan Craig
© 2009 Blackwell Publishing, ISBN: 978-1-4051-3975-5.

as the endogenous nitric synthase inhibitor asymmetric dimethylarginine [11,12]. In diabetic patients glycemic control (as reflected by the level of HbA_{1C}) determines long-term cardiovascular (CV) risk [13,14] and also renal risk, particularly in the first years of the disease.

Although there is no controlled prospective evidence available on this point, it is plausible to assume that the earlier intervention starts, the greater the effect on retardation of progression. In support of this view are the observations in several studies that low baseline glomerular filtration rate (GFR) is a strong predictor of progression and the comparison of outcomes for diabetic nephropathy, hypertension, and renin–angiotensin–aldosterone system (RAAS) blockade between studies with early [15] versus late [16,17] interventions.

Confounding effect of cardiovascular prognosis on progression

It is of note that even in early diabetic or nondiabetic renal disease, the risk of death (mainly from cardiovascular causes) is greater than the risk of progress to end-stage renal disease (ESRD) [18] (Table 3.2), and results from several recent large clinical trials have revealed that even incipient renal failure is an important independent CV risk factor [19–28].

Assessment of CKD progression

Measurement of GFR

GFR can be assessed using different methods. The gold standard for measurement of true GFR is still inulin clearance, but iohexol, Cr-EDTA, or iothalamate clearances are valuable alternatives. These clearance measurements are cumbersome, however, and too expensive for use in clinical routine or epidemiological studies. Thus, estimates of GFR based on the measurement of serum creatinine are widely accepted, for example, the MDRD or Cockroft-Gault equation, but in the interpretation of literature one has to keep in mind that these estimates of GFR are not very accurate, particularly in the near-normal range [29,30]. Furthermore, the equations

Table 3.1 Some modifiable and nonmodifiable risk factors for progression of CKD.

Risk factor for CKD progression
Modifiable risk factors
Blood pressure
Albuminuria, proteinuria
Obesity, metabolic syndrome
Smoking
Glycemic control in diabetic patients
Use of NSAIDs
Herbal medicine (e.g. Chinese herbs)
Lead
Radiocontrast media
Some antibiotics and antiviral drugs (e.g. amino glycoside antibiotics)
Dyslipidemia?
Nonmodifiable risk factors
Age
Gender
Etiology of renal disease
Family history
Ethnicity

have not been validated for specific populations and ethnicities, for example, the very old, patients with a renal allograft, or African Americans or Asians. A major problem remains, because the results of the MDRD equation depend on the accuracy of serum creatinine measurement, which can vary considerably between laboratories, and this again has to be considered when evaluating the literature. Alternative possibilities are new indicators of GFR, such as serum cystatin C, that are not confounded by muscle mass or tubular transport of creatinine, etc. [29,31].

Quantification of albuminuria and proteinuria

Albuminuria is usually categorized as micro- or macroalbuminuria, but several important questions concerning the measurement of urinary albumin excretion rate have not been resolved: in which sample should albumin be measured, that is, in spot urine (with or without creatinine correction), morning urine, or 24-h urine, and which method should be used for the measurement, that is, immune detection or high-performance liquid chromatography [32].

Despite these unresolved methodological problems albuminuria, as a continuous variable, is an impressively powerful predictor of both renal and cardiovascular outcomes in nondiabetic [33] as well as in diabetic [34] individuals (Table 3.3).

The urinary protein excretion is measured as total urinary protein (Biuret); the upper limit is 150 mg/24 h. Confounders of proteinuria (and also of albuminuria) are physical exercise, fever, and orthostasis (particularly in lordotic young individuals). In patients with CKD proteinuria is an independent treatment target, in addition to blood pressure lowering, to prevent progression, and reduction of proteinuria is predictive for lower rate of progression and renal function (GFR) loss (see below).

Renal resistance index

Studies in kidney transplant recipients have indicated that an increased renal segmental arterial resistance index (RI) measured by Doppler ultrasound is associated with worse renal outcome [35]. In patients with type 2 diabetes mellitus, an increased RI is associated with the presence of established diabetic nephropathy, that is, a higher-grade albumin excretion rate accompanied by reduced creatinine clearance [36,37]. It has been speculated that assessment of RI in patients with CKD is an easy-to-assess indicator of progression [38]. Because biopsy studies are lacking, it is not clear whether a high renal RI in diabetic patients is merely the result of structural changes of renal vessels or changes of the elastic properties of larger vessels (e.g. aortic stiffness) also modify RI. As a result, studies using this index will not be considered in the following discussion of the clinical measures of progression in CKD.

Perspectives

The assessment of GFR is not an optimal index of renal function loss, because the remaining glomeruli compensate by increasing single-nephron GFR so that up to 40% of renal parenchyma may be lost without a change in whole-kidney GFR (Table 3.4). This may explain metabolic abnormalities in patients with primary renal disease compared to healthy controls despite normal or near-normal whole-kidney GFR, for example, elevated asymmetric dimethylarginine levels [39], insulin resistance [40], or dyslipidemia [41]. Thus, there is a need for novel indicators of kidney function, perhaps those assessing processes beyond perfusion and filtration. Moreover, apart from assessing steady-state renal function, there is

Table 3.2 Estimated GFR reductions and relative risks of death and of progression to ESRD.[a]

Patient group GFR (mL/min/1.73 m^2) and CKD stage	No. of patients	% on renal replacement therapy	% Mortality
60–89 without proteinuria	14,202	0.07	14.9
60–89 with proteinuria, CKD stage 2	1741	1.1	19.5
30–59, CKD stage 3	11,278	1.3	24.3
15–29, CKD stage 4	777	19.9	45.7

[a] The risk of death was greater than risk of progression to ESRD during the 5-year observation period of 27,998 patients who had estimated GFRs of less than 90 mL/min/1.73 m^2 (data are from reference 18). CKD stages 2, 3, and 4 are the stages of CKD according to the National Kidney Foundation K/DOQI) criteria.

Table 3.3 Studies suggesting that albuminuria predicts CV events and diabetes.

Event that albuminuria predicts and study(s)
Cardiovascular death
Klausen *et al.* 2004
Hillege *et al.* 2002
Romundstad *et al.* 2003
Cardiovascular events
Gerstein *et al.* 2001
Wachtell *et al.* 2003
Cardiac ischemic events
Borch-Johsen *et al.* 1999
Coronary artery disease
Tuttle *et al.* 1999
Survival after myocardial infarction
Berton *et al.* 2004
Stroke
Yuyun *et al.* 2004
Onset of type 2 diabetes
Brantsma *et al.* 2005

also a need to monitor the activity of the kidney-specific processes underlying renal damage. Promising approaches are the measurement of podocyte excretion rates, urinary angiotensinogen excretion, and proteomic analysis of the urine [42–44]. Some of the more promising alternatives to GFR are listed in Table 3.4.

Prevention of progression of CKD

Prevention or delay of progression

Measures designed to reduce or prevent chronic kidney injury and the risk factors known to mediate this injury have been shown to reduce progression in controlled studies. However, to date, we do

Table 3.4 Limitations of GFR and potential alternative approaches to assess renal dysfunction beyond GFR.

Limitation or alternative approach
Limitations of GFR
• Whole-kidney GFR does not take into account partial compensation by single-nephron hyperfiltration
• GFR does not capture processes initiating and maintaining progressive loss of renal function
• GFR does not capture injury to tubular cells
Selected examples of parameters beyond GFR
• Podocyte count in urine
• Podocyte protein in urine
• Exosomes in urine
• Proteomic analysis of urine
• Tubular marker proteins in urine

not know whether any of these measures will completely abrogate the risk of progression to the hard end point of ESRD or merely delay its onset, valuable though this might be. If the evolution of the incidence of ESRD in type 1 and recently also type 2 diabetes is any indication, however, the observation of a progressive reduction of the incidence of ESRD in type 1 diabetes and its stabilization in type 2 diabetes is cause for cautious optimism. Recent evidence emerging from experimental models of kidney damage indicates that to a limited extent glomeruli with focal segmental glomerulosclerosis are capable of undergoing self-repair with reversal of glomerulosclerosis, presumably as long as the number of podocytes is not too seriously depleted [45,46]. Additionally, progressive loss of renal function after an episode of acute renal failure, particularly in the elderly, is now recognized as a potential cause for CKD. Thus, optimal management to prevent acute renal failure [47,48], including that from nephrotoxic injury, should reduce the burden of CKD [49]. These conditions and management options are detailed in section 3 of this book. Evidence from observational studies and from controlled clinical trials supports the efficacy of a number of therapeutic interventions that may ameliorate the development and progression of CKD. These measures are summarized in Table 3.5. These are discussed in the context of the CKD burden in populations and are detailed further in section 6 of this book.

Treatment strategies
Blood pressure lowering
In patients with CKD an important unresolved issue is which aspect of blood pressure should be targeted for control. Observational studies and post hoc analyses of intervention trials have documented that systolic blood pressure is more predictive of renal function loss than diastolic blood pressure or pulse pressure (the latter of which is also highly predictive for cardiovascular events) [50,51]. Currently poorly documented in kidney disease patients are the relative roles of casual blood pressure, home blood pressure, ambulatory 24-h blood pressure, night-time blood pressure, or blood pressure variability as predictors of renal outcome. Observational data indicate that, independent of time-averaged 24-h blood pressure, high nocturnal blood pressure is associated with more rapid loss of renal function in nondiabetic [52] and diabetic [53] patients.

Published guidelines propose a target blood pressure of below 130/80 mmHg for patients with CKD and diabetes [54–56]. The prospective controlled evidence for this recommendation is problematic, however. In the Modification of Diet in Renal Disease (MDRD) trial, which examined 840 patients with predominantly nondiabetic kidney disease, a nonsignificant trend was observed for the primary end point of less GFR loss during a mean observation period of 2.2 years in patients randomized to intensified blood pressure control (i.e. a target mean arterial blood pressure of 92 mmHg) compared to those randomized to usual blood pressure control (i.e. a target mean arterial blood pressure of 107 mmHg), or -2.8 versus -3.9 ml/min/1.73 m^2/year in patients with baseline GFR between 25 and 55 mL [57]. Closer inspection of the

Table 3.5 Interventions proposed to halt progression of CKD

Intervention	Strength of evidence[a]	Strength of recommendations[b]	Reference(s)
Blood pressure lowering	A	Is recommended	57–59, 62, 63
Reduction of proteinuria	A	Is recommended	16, 17, 58, 73–76
Blockade of RAAS			
With ACEi or ARB in conventional doses	A	Is recommended	15–17, 74, 88, 158, 159
Dose escalation and/or combination ACEI or ARBs if response unsatisfactory	Indirect	May be considered	91–93
Mineralocorticoid receptor blocker (spironolactone, eplerenone)	Indirect	May be considered[c]	98
Renin inhibitors	No evidence	Cannot yet be recommended	
Cessation of smoking	B	Is recommended	102, 104–107
Weight reduction in obese subjects	Indirect	Is recommended[d]	113, 116–120
Avoidance of NSAIDs and other nephrotoxic drugs	C	Is recommended	160–164
Reduction of salt intake	C	Should be considered	135
Low-protein diet	B	May be considered[c]	57, 141–157

Source: Based on ADA 2005 [158].

[a] Strength level A, randomized controlled clinical trials, may be assigned based on results of a single trial; level B, cohort and case–control studies, post hoc, subgroup analysis, or meta-analysis, prospective observational studies and registries; level C, expert opinion, observational studies, epidemiological findings, safety reporting from large-scale use in practice.

[b] "Is recommended," part of routine care, exception to therapy should be minimized; "Should be considered," majority of patients should receive the intervention; some discretion in application to individual patients should be allowed; "May be considered," individualization of therapy is indicated; "Is not recommended" (or cannot yet be recommended), therapeutic intervention should not be used.

[c] Until safety data are available, considered only if estimated GFR is normal and no hyperkalemia is present.

[d] Note of caution: because of the risk of malnutrition and the potential adverse impact on later outcome of dialysis, this is no longer advisable in advanced kidney failure.

[e] Is recommended particularly if protein intake is very high, as assessed by urinary urea excretion.

data revealed, however, that initially GFR decreased more in the group randomized to intensified blood pressure control (i.e. 3.4 ml/min/1.73 m² vs. 1.9 mL/min/1.73 m² for 4 months), an effect that was thought to be hemodynamically mediated. The subsequent decline in GFR in the intensified blood pressure control group, however, was less than in the control group. Further post hoc analysis has indicated that the benefit of blood pressure lowering was restricted mainly to patients with proteinuria of >1 g/24 h [58]. Patients with proteinuria of <1 g/24 h were mostly patients with ADPKD; it remains unclear whether they were less responsive to the intervention because of their underlying renal disease rather than because of the absence of significant proteinuria. The evidence from the MDRD study has become more solid with the results of a longer-term observation of these patients for a median observation period of 5.9 years. A significant and persisting, but not progressively widening, difference in the slowing of the decline in GFR has been observed in patients randomized to intensified blood pressure control versus usual care [59].

In contrast to the positive results from the MDRD long-term follow-up study, two large prospective studies, the African American Study of Kidney Disease and Hypertension (AASK) and the REIN 2 study [60,61], have found no significant difference overall between patients randomized to ordinary and lower blood pressure targets. It may not be appropriate, however, to consider all patients with advanced CKD as one homogenous group. In the AASK trial there was a tendency in patients with proteinuria above 300 mg/24 h to have a slower rate of loss of GFR at the lower blood pressure target, and this was most evident in the few patients with proteinuria above 1 g/24 h. This observation raises the issue as to whether one identical blood pressure target is appropriate for all patients with kidney disease irrespective of their rate of protein excretion. Post hoc analyses of two recent major clinical trials in patients with advanced diabetic nephropathy, the Irbesartan Diabetic Nephropathy Trial (IDNT) study [62] and the Reduction of Endpoints in Non-Insulin-Dependent Diabetes Mellitus with the Angiotensin II Antagonist Losartan (RENAAL) study [63], clearly show that at any given level of systolic blood pressure, renal end points, defined as a doubling of serum creatinine or ESRD, were progressively lower with lower achieved seated systolic blood pressure at 12 months (Figure 3.1) However, at systolic blood pressures below 120 mmHg all-cause mortality was higher by a factor of 3. It is unclear whether this higher observed mortality at the lowest treated blood pressures was caused by preexisting cardiac or other diseases or whether it was the result of too-aggressive antihypertensive treatment. This observation is reminiscent of the J-curve phenomenon, specifically, a paradoxical increase of mortality with aggressive lowering of diastolic blood pressure in hypertensive patients in general, presumably because of cardiac events. This finding was recently reiterated in the International Verapamil-Trandolapril Study (INVEST) in patients with known coronary

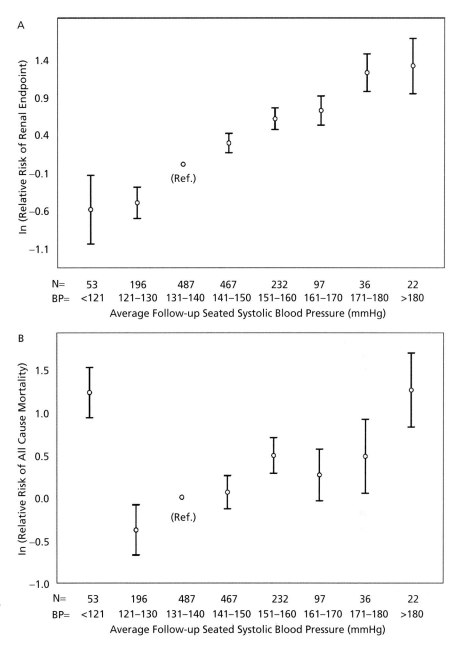

Figure 3.1 Achieved systolic blood pressure and progression of diabetic nephropathy (A) and all cause mortality (B) in patients with type 2 diabetes. From the IDNT study, post hoc analysis [63].

heart disease [64]. From these observations, it may be prudent not to lower systolic blood pressure below 120 mmHg or diastolic blood pressure below approximately 70 mmHg in kidney disease patients with known coronary heart disease.

Reduction of proteinuria

It has been known for a long time that proteinuria is a predictor of more rapid loss of renal function in patients with CKD [65]. Quite unexpectedly it has also been shown that the change in proteinuria during treatment is a powerful predictor of progression beyond that predicted because of any concomitant change in blood pressure [66,67]. This observation lends support to the hypothesis of

Remuzzi *et al.* [68] that proteinuria is a potent CKD progression promoter. Furthermore, the change in proteinuria predicts not only renal but also cardiovascular events, and this holds true both for patients with frank proteinuria and also in patients with microalbuminuria [69,70]. The conclusion of Khosla and Bakris [71] therefore seems justified, that proteinuria per se is an important therapeutic target apart from and independent of blood pressure. This recommendation has been integrated into the recent National Kidney Foundation Kidney Disease Outcomes Quality Initiative (K/DOQI) guidelines [56]. Specifically, the K/DOQI guidelines recommend reduction of proteinuria to less than 1 g/24 h [56], and some authors have even recommended 0.3 g/24 h [72].

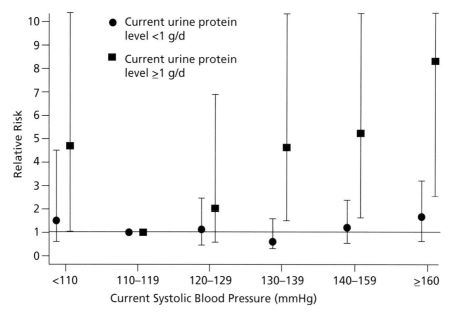

Figure 3.2 Progression: effects of current level of systolic blood pressure and current urine protein excretion. From reference 73 with permission of the publisher. Data show the relative risks for patients with a current urine protein excretion of 1.0 g/day or greater (223 events) and in patients with a current urine protein excretion of less than 1.0 g/day (88 events). Patients with a systolic blood pressure of 110–119 mmHg as the reference group. Single multivariable model including two levels for urine protein excretion, six levels for systolic blood pressure, and the interaction of current systolic blood pressure and current urine protein excretion. Covariates include assignment to angiotensin-converting enzyme inhibitor versus control group, sex, age, baseline systolic blood pressure, baseline diastolic blood pressure, baseline urine protein excretion, baseline serum creatinine concentration (<2.0 or 2.0 mg/dL [<177 or 177 μmol/L]), interaction of baseline serum creatinine and baseline urine protein excretion, interaction of baseline serum creatinine and current urine protein excretion, and study terms.

The evidence for this guideline recommendation in nondiabetic patients comes from clinical trials summarized by Jafar *et al.* [73] (Figure 3.2), including particularly the REIN [74,75] and AIPRI [76] studies for angiotensin converting enzyme inhibitors (ACEi), but also from the results of the RENAAL [16] and IDNT [17] studies for angiotensin receptor blockers (ARBs). As with MDRD trial, the attenuation of GFR loss in these trials was greater in CKD patients with proteinuria of >1 g/day [58]. In the REIN study mostly nondiabetic patients with advanced CKD were randomized to treatment groups after stratification according to baseline proteinuria (below 1 g/day, between 1 and 3 g/day, and above 3 g/day). The rate of progression in placebo-treated patients was greatest in patients with proteinuria above 3 g/day. They were also the ones who benefited most from RAAS blockade with ramipril, with the greatest attenuation of the rate of loss of GFR [74].

The validity of the assumption that, independent of blood pressure control, the combination of ACEi and ARBs can reduce proteinuria further compared to the monotherapies was supported by several recent studies [77,78]. Furthermore, in diabetic [79] as well as in nondiabetic patients [80], it has been noted that an inverse correlation exists between the initial reduction of proteinuria and the subsequent decline in GFR. For ARBs, post hoc analyses of two recent studies (RENAAL for losartan and IDNT for irbesartan) provided evidence that reduction of proteinuria predicts the occurrence of fewer renal end points, independent of the antihypertensive agent used (in the IDNT study irbesartan, amlodipine, or alternative antihypertensive medication was used) [62,63].

In nondiabetic individuals, an increased albumin excretion rate is a predictor of a future decrease in estimated GFR [80]. However, there is no controlled clinical trial evidence to date that a reduction of albumin excretion in the microalbuminuric range at baseline reduces the renal risk in nondiabetic patients. Such evidence is, however, available with respect to reduction of CV events [69]. In contrast, there is abundant evidence in diabetic patients that reduction of microalbuminuria is associated with less progression of diabetic nephropathy; the evidence initially arose from observational studies on patients with type 1 diabetes [82] and later from controlled clinical trials in patients with type 1 [83,84] and type 2 [85] diabetes. Additionally, the Bergamo Nephrologic Diabetes Complications Trial (BENEDICT) by Ruggenenti *et al.* [86] documented that it is not only possible to attenuate microalbuminuria but also to prevent its development in a large proportion of patients. In this study, administration to nonmicroalbuminuric patients with type 2 diabetes of trandolapril, but not verapamil, with attainment with both of equally intense lowering of blood pressure, reduced the onset of albuminuria over a median of 3.6 years of observation significantly from 10.0% for patients on placebo combined with control antihypertensive treatment compared to 6.0% for those on trandolapril. This question is currently

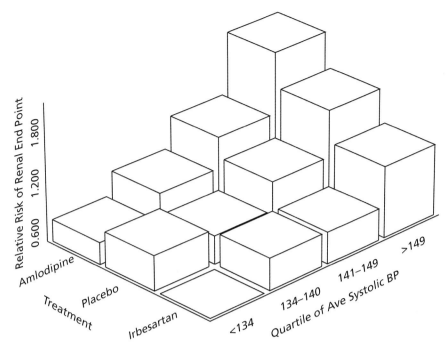

Figure 3.3 Progression of nephropathy in type 2 diabetes: influence of achieved systolic blood pressure, RAAS blockade with irbesartan, and their interaction. Data are from a post hoc analysis of the IDNT results (reference 62).

being investigated further in the ROADMAP study using the ARB olmesartan [87].

RAAS blockade

The US National Kidney Foundation recommends either ARBs or ACEi as first-line antihypertensive agents for the treatment of diabetic renal disease [56]. This recommendation is based largely on the findings from clinical studies demonstrating their renoprotective effects in patients with type 1 and type 2 diabetes and nephropathy (Figure 3.3) [15,16,17,88]. In addition to lowering blood pressure and reducing proteinuria, these clinical trials data support the view that blockade of renin, angiotensin, or aldosterone, the RAAS, might have direct and specific renoprotective effects. In normotensive patients with type 2 diabetes and microalbuminuria, treatment with enalapril for 5 years stabilized the decline in renal function (and reduced proteinuria) compared to placebo [85]. Similarly, in normoalbuminuric patients with type 2 diabetes and hypertension, treatment with enalapril for 6 years stabilized creatinine clearance and prevented the development of albuminuria [89]. These study results highlight the potential clinical impact of initiating RAAS blockade even before the onset of overt albuminuria in patients with type 2 diabetes.

One important question has yet to be resolved in large-scale clinical trials, specifically, whether increasing the dose of ACEi and/or ARBs above the level of maximal blood pressure lowering offers additional renoprotection through a direct RAAS inhibition in patients with nondiabetic or diabetic kidney disease. Studies in experimental models of kidney disease have documented increased intrarenal RAAS activity, and treatment with RAAS inhibitors

resulted in significant attenuation of progression independent of the effect on systemic blood pressure [90]. Clinical evidence for a blood pressure-independent effect by RAAS inhibition on proteinuria as an accepted surrogate marker of progression comes from two recent small studies in patients with nondiabetic [91] and diabetic [92] CKD and from the much larger IRMA 2 study (Irbesartan in Patients with Type 2 Diabetes and Microalbuminuria) [93]. In the IRMA 2 study, 590 hypertensive patients with type 2 diabetes and microalbuminuria were randomized to the addition of either placebo to conventional antihypertensive treatment or the ARB irbesartan, at a dose of either 150 mg or 300 mg daily, and were followed for 2 years. The primary outcome was the time to the onset of diabetic nephropathy, defined by persistent albuminuria of >200 μg/min. In the 300-mg irbesartan treatment group 5.2% of patients reached the primary end point, whereas in the 150-mg Irbesartan group 9.7% developed persistent albuminuria, and in the placebo group 14.9% developed persistent albuminuria (hazard ratios: 0.30 [95% confidence interval 0.14–0.61] [$P < 0.001$] and 0.61 [95% confidence interval 0.34–1.08] [$P = 0.08$] for the two irbesartan groups compared to control, respectively). Because the average blood pressure during the course of the study was similar in both ARB treatment groups, the authors concluded that irbesartan has renoprotective effects independent of its clinical blood pressure effects. Importantly, serious adverse events were less frequent among the patients treated with irbesartan ($P = 0.02$) [93]. In the two smaller studies with ultra-high-dose ARB therapy no adverse effects were observed, including, notably, no effects on measured GFR [91,92].

When considering the role of each of the components of the RAAS in mediating the progression of nondiabetic and diabetic CKD, one must take into account recent data that support the view that aldosterone may be of importance as well. This is somewhat reminiscent of what has been shown for chronic congestive heart failure. There is experimental [94] as well as indirect clinical [95–98] evidence that aldosterone inhibition may be beneficial in arresting progression of CKD. Schjoedt *et al.* [98] evaluated the short-term effect of spironolactone on albuminuria in 20 diabetic patients with nephrotic-range albuminuria (>2500 mg/24 h) in a double-blind, crossover trial. Patients were randomly assigned initial treatment with either 25 mg of spironolactone once a day or placebo added to their baseline antihypertensive regimen, which included an ACEi or an ARB at maximally recommended doses. They found that spironolactone treatment significantly reduced proteinuria and concluded that inhibition of aldosterone may offer further renoprotection when added to recommended renoprotective strategies, including maximal RAAS blockade. Concerns remain with respect to the risk of hyperkalemia, particularly in patients with advanced CKD. Large prospective trials are necessary to evaluate the efficacy and safety of this approach. The preliminary clinical trials data described above indicate, however, that complete RAAS inhibition may not be accomplished even with high-dose ACEi and ARB monotherapy [91,92] or combination therapy [99], raising expectations for direct renin inhibitors. It remains to be proven whether this new class of antihypertensive agents that act by blocking "completely" the RAAS will confer renoprotection of greater magnitude than that observed with the ACEi and ARBs.

Smoking

In the general population cigarette smoking is associated with an increased risk of albuminuria and renal disease [100,101]. Smoking is also associated with an increased renal risk in nondiabetic and diabetic patients with CKD. Among patients with IgA GN (as a model of immunological renal disease) or ADPKD (as a model of nonimmunological disease) in a retrospective case–control study, Orth *et al.* [102] found that the risk of progressing to ESRD was significantly higher in smokers compared to nonsmokers, but the risk was markedly attenuated in patients on ACEi therapy. In diabetic patients it has been known for a long time that smokers have a higher risk of developing microalbuminuria and also progress more rapidly to overt nephropathy and renal failure [103–107]. According to Biesenbach *et al.* [106], smokers progress twice as fast to ESRD as nonsmokers. Although ACEi obviously attenuate GFR loss in smokers, they do not completely prevent it, even when target blood pressure values are reached [107]. Because no difference of proteinuria was observed in smoking compared to nonsmoking diabetic persons with renal disease, it has been concluded that vascular lesions are more important promoters of the excess CKD progression among smokers than the glomerular lesions of classical Kimmelstiel-Wilson glomerulosclerosis [108]. Regalado, Yang, and Wesson demonstrated in a prospective cohort an association of smoking with more rapid progression of CKD in hypertensive patients in the absence of diabetes [109]. This risk appeared to be particularly important for African Americans in their cohort study. These data further support the notion that the risk of CKD from smoking is mediated through the effects of smoking on renal microvascular disease.

Is there evidence that cessation of smoking improves renal prognosis? Controlled studies to address this question would be unethical. In an observational study Sawicki *et al.* [104] compared progression in type 1 diabetic patients according to smoking habits. Progression was loosely defined as an increase in proteinuria or serum creatinine or a decrease in GFR. Progression was observed in 53% of the smokers ($n = 34$) but significantly less in exsmokers ($n = 24$; 33%) and nonsmokers ($n = 35$; 11%). Chuahirun *et al.* also demonstrated that markers of kidney injury in diabetic patients without overt nephropathy but with controlled hypertension on ACEi improved in a cohort of individuals who were successful in quitting smoking [110].

Obesity

In patients with morbid obesity a unique form of focal segmental glomerulosclerosis may be found with nephrotic proteinuria [111] and rapid progression to kidney failure [112]. In patients with various types of kidney disease, body mass index (BMI) is an independent predictor of proteinuria and loss of kidney function, particularly in IgA GN [113], in kidney transplant recipients [114,115], and in patients with unilateral renal agenesis or a remnant kidney [116]. In uninephrectomized individuals, for example, live kidney donors [117], the risks of proteinuria and loss of kidney function are higher if the individual is obese.

The question arises whether weight reduction improves indices of kidney damage. In severely obese patients without overt kidney disease but with hyperfiltration, Chagnac *et al.* observed normalization of GFR and reduction of albuminuria after gastroplasty following a decrease of BMI from 48 to 32.1 kg/m^2 [118]. In morbidly obese patients with chronic proteinuric nephropathy (including diabetic nephropathy and chronic glomerulonephritis), weight loss after caloric restriction with a decrease of BMI from 37.1 to 32.6 kg/m^2 reduced urinary protein excretion from 2.9 to 0.4 g/day [119]. The reduction of proteinuria was similar in magnitude to what is achieved with ACEi treatment [119]. The effect of weight reduction has also been studied in proteinuric patients with moderate obesity [120]. In such obese patients with chronic proteinuric nephropathies, a loss of 4.1% of body weight (BMI reduction from 33.0 to 31.6 kg/m^2) decreased proteinuria by 31.2% (from 2.8 to 1.9 g/day) [120]. However, in patients with advanced kidney failure on hemodialysis, a low BMI predicts poor CV survival, and the survival advantage progressively improves with higher BMI values extending into the range of morbid obesity [121]. It is therefore likely prudent to advise against weight reduction in patients with advanced stages of CKD, possibly CKD stage 3 or higher; however, the exact threshold of CKD where the risks of weight reduction outweigh the benefits cannot be determined from the clinical trial evidence currently available.

Salt intake

In the early decades of the past century low salt intake was a standard feature of the treatment of patients with renal disease [122]. With the advent of diuretics this aspect of management of renal patients was largely abandoned. However, in addition to the large body of clinical evidence that low dietary salt intake reduces blood pressure [123] and oxidative stress [124], low dietary salt has been demonstrated to attenuate proteinuria, renal function loss, glomerulosclerosis, and interstitial fibrosis in various experimental models of renal damage [125–131]. It is important to emphasize that the benefits of low salt intake could not be reproduced in the experimental model of uninephrectomized SHR rats by the administration of a diuretic [127]. This observation could have potential clinical importance.

In humans, evidence pointing to the renal benefit of dietary salt restriction comes from short-term studies on renal function that suggest a transient increase of filtration fraction as a surrogate marker of glomerular capillary pressure [132], which could be reversed by RAAS blockade and presumably represents evanescent counterregulation [133]. Reduction of proteinuria was seen in Black patients during short-term intervention [134]. Both a slowing of loss of GFR and cessation of further increases of proteinuria after reduction of sodium intake were reported from a retrospective analysis of an Italian series [135]. In particular because of its potential multiple health benefits, salt restriction as a public health measure directed towards individuals at risk for CKD and CKD progression is in great need of further well-designed human studies and constitutes a promising area of renal research.

Water intake

As Koranyi observed in the 19th century, reduced urinary osmolality (and hence the capacity to concentrate urine) is one of the first functional signs of renal dysfunction and primary kidney disease [136]. Both the capacity to concentrate urine and the capacity to excrete excess water are reduced in advanced renal disease. Because of the limited urine-concentrating capacity, and uncontrolled clinical observations that volume depletion may cause acute deterioration of renal function, it had been recommended conventionally that in patients with impaired renal function, the daily water intake should be above 1500 mL. As a safeguard against hyponatremia in these patients with limited excretory capacity for water, the daily water intake has usually been restricted to 3000 mL. Fishberg suggested that "if renal function is poor as revealed by the concentration test one should not restrict the fluid intake, because the elimination of a large volume of urine is the only safeguard of the patient with impaired concentrating power" [137]. Experimental studies by Bankir et al. [138,139] have provided evidence that water intake might attenuate progression. They reported that increased water intake in the animal renal ablation model attenuated progression in parallel with reduced vasopressin concentrations and less O_2-demanding solute transport in the ascending limb of Henle's loop. Until recently, no further human clinical trial

evidence was available to inform this question beyond the above recommendations, which are based largely on biological plausibility and customary practice. However, recent evidence from clinical trials in humans has seriously challenged the validity of these prior recommendations. Thus, in a retrospective analysis of data from the MDRD study, higher urine volumes and, by implication, higher water intakes in the steady state were associated with more adverse renal outcome, even when adjusted for a number of relevant confounders [140]. This has led to the competing recommendation that CKD patients should not be encouraged to ingest high water loads. The issue has remained controversial and is in need of controlled studies.

Protein intake

A recent observational study found that the risk of a progressive decline of renal function increases with increasing protein intake in women with moderate CKD [141]. A large randomized trial, however, failed to demonstrate that low-protein diets improved renal survival (MDRD), although several small studies with less rigorous end points showed better renal outcomes in those on low-protein diets among nondiabetic [142,143,144] as well as diabetic patients [145,146]. This finding was not consistent across all studies, however [147,148,149]. Several meta-analyses came to the conclusion that dietary protein restriction had a positive effect on renal outcomes despite significant heterogeneity between the studies [150,151,152]. The data are difficult to interpret, however, because observation periods and end points differed between the studies. The one study to address this issue which is regarded as definitive because of its size and study design was the MDRD study [57]. A total of 585 patients with moderate CKD (GFR, 25–55 mL/min) were randomized to a typical protein (1.3 g/kg/day) or low-protein (0.58 g/kg/day) diet (study A). In addition 255 patients with severe CKD (GFR, 13–24 mL/min) were randomized to a low (0.58 g/kg/day) or very low (0.28 g/kg/day) protein diet plus a mixture of ketoacids (study B). After an average of 2.2 years the intention-to-treat analysis showed no significant difference between the diets, although there was a trend toward a slower rate of GFR decline in the very low protein group in patients with advanced CKD [57]. A secondary analysis of the data from study B of the MDRD trial evaluating the achieved dietary protein intake found an inverse correlation between achieved total protein intake and GFR loss [153]. An achieved total protein intake lower by 0.2 g/kg/day was associated with a 1.15-mL/min/year reduced loss of GFR, equivalent to 29% of the mean GFR decline [153].

Although under properly supervision very low protein diets have been claimed to be nutritionally safe [154,155] and do not adversely affect function and structure of skeletal muscle [156], follow-up observations of the MDRD study have documented a nutritional decline in patients on protein restriction, which is a matter of considerable concern in view of the high mortality associated with reduced body weight observed in incident dialysis patients [157].

References

1 Zoja C, Abbate M, Remuzzi G. Progression of chronic kidney disease: insights from animal models. *Curr Opin Nephrol Hypertens* 2006; **15**: 250–257.

2 Davison AM, Cameron JS, Kerr DN, Ogg CS, Wilkinson RW. The natural history of renal function in untreated idiopathic membranous glomerulonephritis in adults. *Clin Nephrol* 1984; **22**: 61–67.

3 D'Amico G, Minetti L, Ponticelli C, Fellin G, Ferrario F, Barbiano di Belgioioso G *et al.* Prognostic indicators in idiopathic IgA mesangial nephropathy. *Q J Med* 1986; **228**: 363–378.

4 D'Amico G. Natural history of idiopathic IgA nephropathy and factors predictive of disease outcome. *Semin Nephrol* 2004; **24**: 179–196.

5 Habib R, Kleinknecht C, Gubler MC, Maiz HB. Idiopathic membranoproliferative glomerulonephritis. Morphology and natural history. *Perspect Nephrol Hypertens* 1973; **1**: 491–514.

6 Habib R, Kleinknecht C. Idiopathic extramembranous glomerulonephritis in children. Morphology and natural history. *Perspect Nephrol Hypertens* 1973; **1**: 449–459.

7 Jungers P, Hannedouche T, Itakura Y, Albouze G, Descamps-Latscha B, Man NK. Progression rate to end-stage renal failure in non-diabetic kidney diseases: a multivariate analysis of determinant factors. *Nephrol Dial Transplant* 1995; **10**: 1353–1360.

8 Wight JP, Salzano S, Brown CB, el Nahas AM. Natural history of chronic renal failure: a reappraisal. *Nephrol Dial Transplant* 1992; **7**: 379–383.

9 Gabow PA, Johnson AM, Kaehny WD, Kimberling WJ, Lezotte DC, Duley IT *et al.* Factors affecting the progression of renal disease in autosomal-dominant polycystic kidney disease. *Kidney Int* 1992; **41**: 1311–1319.

10 Gretz N, Zeier M, Geberth S, Strauch M, Ritz E. Is gender a determinant for evolution of renal failure? A study in autosomal dominant polycystic kidney disease. *Am J Kidney Dis* 1989; **14**: 178–183.

11 Ravani P, Tripepi G, Malberti F, Testa S, Mallamaci F, Zoccali C. Asymmetrical dimethylarginine predicts progression to dialysis and death in patients with chronic kidney disease: a competing risks modeling approach. *J Am Soc Nephrol* 2005; **16**: 2449–2455.

12 Fliser D, Kronenberg F, Kielstein JT, Morath C, Bode-Boger SM, Haller H *et al.* Asymmetric dimethylarginine (ADMA) and progression of chronic kidney disease: the Mild to Moderate Kidney Disease (MMKD) study. *J Am Soc Nephrol* 2005;**16**: 2456–2461.

13 Diabetes Control and Complications Trial/Epidemiology of Diabetes Interventions and Complications Research Group. Retinopathy and nephropathy in patients with type 1 diabetes four years after a trial of intensive therapy. *N Engl J Med* 2000; **342**: 381–389.

14 Nathan DM, Cleary PA, Backlund JY, Genuth SM, Lachin JM, Orchard TJ *et al.* Intensive diabetes treatment and cardiovascular disease in patients with type 1 diabetes. *N Engl J Med* 2005; **353**: 2643–2653.

15 Barnett AH, Bain SC, Bouter P, Karlberg B, Madsbad S, Jervell J *et al.* Angiotensin-receptor blockade versus converting-enzyme inhibition in type 2 diabetes and nephropathy. *N Engl J Med* 2004; **351**: 1952–1961.

16 Maschio G, Alberti D, Janin G, Locatelli F, Mann JF, Motolese M *et al.* Effect of the angiotensin-converting-enzyme inhibitor benazepril on the progression of chronic renal insufficiency. The Angiotensin-Converting-Enzyme Inhibition in Progressive Renal Insufficiency Study Group. *N Engl J Med* 1996; **334**: 939–945.

17 Brenner BM, Cooper ME, de Zeeuw D, Keane WF, Mitch WE, Parving HH *et al.* Effects of losartan on renal and cardiovascular outcomes in patients with type 2 diabetes and nephropathy. *N Engl J Med* 2001; **345**: 861–869.

18 Keith DS, Nichols GA, Gullion CM, Brown JB, Smith DH. Longitudinal follow-up and outcomes among a population with chronic kidney disease in a large managed care organization. *Arch Intern Med* 2004; **164**: 659–663.

19 Mann JF, Gerstein HC, Pogue J, Bosch J, Yusuf S. Renal insufficiency as a predictor of cardiovascular outcomes and the impact of ramipril: the HOPE randomized trial. *Ann Intern Med* 2001; **134**: 629–636.

20 Go AS, Chertow GM, Fan D, McCulloch CE, Hsu CY. Chronic kidney disease and the risks of death, cardiovascular events, and hospitalization. *N Engl J Med* 2004; **351**: 1296–1305.

21 Manjunath G, Tighiouart H, Ibrahim H, MacLeod B, Salem DN, Griffith JL *et al.* Level of kidney function as a risk factor for atherosclerotic cardiovascular outcomes in the community. *J Am Coll Cardiol* 2003; **41**: 47–55.

22 Weiner DE, Tighiouart H, Amin MG, Stark PC, MacLeod B, Griffith JL *et al.* Chronic kidney disease as a risk factor for cardiovascular disease and all-cause mortality: a pooled analysis of community-based studies. *J Am Soc Nephrol* 2004, **15**: 1307–1315.

23 Fried LF, Shlipak MG, Crump C, Bleyer AJ, Gottdiener JS, Kronmal RA *et al.* Renal insufficiency as a predictor of cardiovascular outcomes and mortality in elderly individuals. *J Am Coll Cardiol* 2003; **41**: 1364–1372.

24 Henry RM, Kostense PJ, Bos G, Dekker JM, Nijpels G, Heine RJ *et al.* Mild renal insufficiency is associated with increased cardiovascular mortality: the Hoorn study. *Kidney Int* 2002; **62**: 1402–1407.

25 Muntner P, He J, Hamm L, Loria C, Whelton PK. Renal insufficiency and subsequent death resulting from cardiovascular disease in the United States. *J Am Soc Nephrol* 2002; **13**: 745–753.

26 Ruilope LM, Salvetti A, Jamerson K, Hansson L, Warnold I, Wedel H *et al.* Renal function and intensive lowering of blood pressure in hypertensive participants of the hypertension optimal treatment (HOT) study. *J Am Soc Nephrol* 2001; **12**: 218–225.

27 Hillege HL, Girbes AR, de Kam PJ, Boomsma F, de Zeeuw D, Charlesworth A *et al.* Renal function, neurohormonal activation, and survival in patients with chronic heart failure. *Circulation* 2000; **102**: 203–210.

28 Tonelli M, Wiebe N, Culleton B, House A, Rabbat C, Fok M *et al.* Chronic kidney disease and mortality risk: a systematic review. *J Am Soc Nephrol* 2006; **17**: 2034–2047.

29 Stevens LA, Coresh J, Greene T, Levey AS. Assessing kidney function—measured and estimated glomerular filtration rate. *N Engl J Med* 2006; **354**: 2473–2483.

30 Levey AS, Bosch JP, Lewis JB, Greene T, Rogers N, Roth D. A more accurate method to estimate glomerular filtration rate from serum creatinine: a new prediction equation. Modification of Diet in Renal Disease Study Group. *Ann Intern Med* 1999; **130**: 461–470.

31 Fliser D, Ritz E. Serum cystatin C concentration as a marker of renal dysfunction in the elderly. *Am J Kidney Dis* 2001; **37**: 79–83.

32 Brinkman JW, Bakker SJ, Gansevoort RT, Hillege HL, Kema IP, Gans RO *et al.* Which method for quantifying urinary albumin excretion gives what outcome? A comparison of immunonephelometry with HPLC. *Kidney Int Suppl* 2004; **92**: S69–S75.

33 Hillege HL, Fidler V, Diercks GF, van Gilst WH, de Zeeuw D, van Veldhuisen DJ *et al.* Urinary albumin excretion predicts cardiovascular and non-cardiovascular mortality in general population. *Circulation* 2002; **106**: 1777–1782.

34 Rachmani R, Levi Z, Lidar M, Slavachevski I, Half-Onn E, Ravid M. Considerations about the threshold value of microalbuminuria in patients with diabetes mellitus: lessons from an 8-year follow-up study of 599 patients. *Diabetes Res Clin Pract* 2000; **49:** 187–194.

35 Radermacher J, Mengel M, Ellis S, Stuht S, Hiss M, Schwarz A *et al.* The renal arterial resistance index and renal allograft survival. *N Engl J Med* 2003; **349:** 115–124.

36 Boeri D, Derchi LE, Martinoli C, Simoni G, Sampietro L, Storace D *et al.* Intrarenal arteriosclerosis and impairment of kidney function in NIDDM subjects. *Diabetologia* 1998; **41:** 121–124.

37 Ishimura E, Nishizawa Y, Kawagishi T, Okuno Y, Kogawa K, Fukumoto S *et al.* Intrarenal hemodynamic abnormalities in diabetic nephropathy measured by duplex Doppler sonography. *Kidney Int* 1997; **51:** 1920–1927.

38 Petersen LJ, Petersen JR, Talleruphuus U, Ladefoged SD, Mehlsen J, Jensen HA. The pulsatility index and the resistive index in renal arteries. Associations with long-term progression in chronic renal failure. *Nephrol Dial Transplant* 1997; **12:** 1376–1380.

39 Kielstein JT, Boger RH, Bode-Boger SM, Frolich JC, Haller H, Ritz E *et al.* Marked increase of asymmetric dimethylarginine in patients with incipient primary chronic renal disease. *J Am Soc Nephrol* 2002; **13:** 170–176.

40 Becker B, Kronenberg F, Kielstein JT, Haller H, Morath C, Ritz E *et al.* Renal insulin resistance syndrome, adiponectin and cardiovascular events in patients with kidney diseases: the Mild to Moderate Kidney Disease (MMKD) study. *J Am Soc Nephrol* 2005; **16:** 1091–1098.

41 Kronenberg F, Kuen E, Ritz E, Junker R, Konig P, Kraatz G *et al.* Lipoprotein(a) serum concentrations and apolipoprotein(a) phenotypes in mild and moderate renal failure. *J Am Soc Nephrol* 2000; **11:** 105–115.

42 Yu D, Petermann A, Kunter U, Rong S, Shankland SJ, Floege J. Urinary podocyte loss is a more specific marker of ongoing glomerular damage than proteinuria. *J Am Soc Nephrol* 2005; **16:** 1733–1741.

43 Fliser D, Wittke S, Mischak H. Capillary electrophoresis coupled to mass spectrometry (CE/MS) for clinical diagnostic purposes. *Electrophoresis* 2005; **26:** 2708–2716.

44 Vidal BC, Bonventre JV, I-Hong Hsu S. Towards the application of proteomics in renal disease diagnosis. *Clin Sci* 2005; **109:** 421–430.

45 Adamczak M, Gross M-L, Krtil J, Kodi A, Tyralla K, Amann K *et al.* Reversal of glomerulosclerosis after high dose enalapril treatment in subtotally nephrectomised rats. *J Am Soc Nephrol* 2003; **14:** 2833.

46 Aldrigier JC, Kanjanbuch T, Ma L-J, Brown NJ, Fogo AB. Regression of existing glomerulosclerosis by inhibition of aldosterone. *J Am Soc Nephrol* 2005; **16:** 3306–3314.

47 Kellum JA, Leblanc M, Gibney RT, Tumlin J, Lieberthal W, Ronco C. Primary prevention of acute renal failure in the critically ill. *Curr Opin Crit Care* 2005; **11:** 537–541.

48 Van den Berghe G, Wouters P, Weekers F, Verwaest C, Bruyninckx F, Schetz M *et al.* Intensive insulin therapy in critically ill patients. *N Engl J Med* 2001; **345:** 1359–1367.

49 Pannu N, Wiebe N, Tonelli M, Alberta Kidney Disease Network. Prophylaxis strategies for contrast-induced nephropathy. *JAMA* 2006; **295:** 2765–2779.

50 Opelz G, Wujciak T, Ritz E. Association of chronic kidney graft failure with recipient blood pressure. Collaborative Transplant Study. *Kidney Int* 1998; **53:** 217–222.

51 Bakris GL, Weir MR, Shanifar S, Zhang Z, Douglas J, van Dijk DJ *et al.* Effects of blood pressure level on progression of diabetic nephropathy: results from the RENAAL study. *Arch Intern Med* 2003; **163:** 1555–1565.

52 Timio M, Venanzi S, Lolli S, Lippi G, Verdura C, Monarca C *et al.* "Non-dipper" hypertensive patients and progressive renal insufficiency: a 3-year longitudinal study. *Clin Nephrol* 1995; **43:** 382–387.

53 Nakano S, Ishii T, Kitazawa M, Kigoshi T, Uchida K, Morimoto S. Altered circadian blood pressure rhythm and progression of diabetic nephropathy in non-insulin dependent diabetes mellitus subjects: an average three year follow-up study. *J Investig Med* 1996; **44:** 247–253.

54 Cifkova R, Erdine S, Fagard R, Farsang C, Heagerty AM, Kiowski W *et al.* Practice guidelines for primary care physicians: 2003 ESH/ESC hypertension guidelines. *J Hypertens* 2003; **21:** 1779–1786.

55 Chobanian AV, Bakris GL, Black HR, Cushman WC, Green LA, Izzo JL. Jr., *et al.* The Seventh Report of the Joint National Committee on Prevention, Detection, Evaluation, and Treatment of High Blood Pressure: the JNC 7 report. *JAMA* 2003; **289:** 2560–2572.

56 Kidney Disease Outcomes Quality Initiative. K/DOQI clinical practice guidelines on hypertension and antihypertensive agents in chronic kidney disease. *Am J Kidney Dis* 2004; **43 (Suppl 1):** S1–S290.

57 Klahr S, Levey AS, Beck GJ, Caggiula AW, Hunsicker L, Kusek JW, Striker G. The effects of dietary protein restriction and blood-pressure control on the progression of chronic renal disease. Modification of Diet in Renal Disease Study Group. *N Engl J Med* 1994; **330:** 877–884.

58 Peterson JC, Adler S, Burkart JM, Greene T, Hebert LA, Hunsicker LG *et al.* Blood pressure control, proteinuria, and the progression of renal disease. The Modification of Diet in Renal Disease Study. *Ann Intern Med* 1995; **123:** 754–762.

59 Sarnak MJ, Greene T, Wang X, Beck G, Kusek JW, Collins AJ *et al.* The effect of a lower target blood pressure on the progression of kidney disease: long-term follow-up of the modification of diet in renal disease study. *Ann Intern Med* 2005; **142:** 342–351.

60 Wright JT, Jr., Bakris G, Greene T, Agodoa LY, Appel LJ, Charleston J *et al.* Effect of blood pressure lowering and antihypertensive drug class on progression of hypertensive kidney disease: results from the AASK trial. *JAMA* 2002; **288:** 2421–2431.

61 Ruggenenti P, Perna A, Loriga G, Ganeva M, Ene-Iordache B, Turturro M *et al.* Blood-pressure control for renoprotection in patients with non-diabetic chronic renal disease (REIN-2): multicentre, randomised controlled trial. *Lancet* 2005; **365:** 939–946.

62 Pohl MA, Blumenthal S, Cordonnier DJ, De Alvaro F, Deferrari G, Eisner G *et al.* Independent and additive impact of blood pressure control and angiotensin II receptor blockade on renal outcomes in the irbesartan diabetic nephropathy trial: clinical implications and limitations. *J Am Soc Nephrol* 2005; **16:** 3027–3037.

63 Bakris GL, Weir MR, Shanifar S, Zhang Z, Douglas J, van Dijk DJ *et al.* Effects of blood pressure level on progression of diabetic nephropathy: results from the RENAAL study. *Arch Intern Med* 2003; **163:** 1555–1565.

64 Messerli FH, Mancia G, Conti CR, Hewkin AC, Kupfer S, Champion A *et al.* Dogma disputed: can aggressively lowering blood pressure in hypertensive patients with coronary artery disease be dangerous? *Ann Intern Med* 2006; **144:** 884–893.

65 Cameron JS, Glassock RJ, editors. *The Nephrotic Syndrome.* Marcel Dekker, Inc., New York, 1988.

66 de Zeeuw D, Remuzzi G, Parving HH, Keane WF, Zhang Z, Shahinfar S *et al.* Proteinuria, a target for renoprotection in patients with type 2 diabetic nephropathy: lessons from RENAAL. *Kidney Int* 2004; **65:** 2309–2320.

67 Atkins RC, Briganti EM, Lewis JB, Hunsicker LG, Braden G, Champion de Crespigny PJ *et al.* Proteinuria reduction and progression to renal

failure in patients with type 2 diabetes mellitus and overt nephropathy. *Am J Kidney Dis* 2005; **45**: 281–287.

68 Remuzzi G, Bertani T. Pathophysiology of progressive nephropathies. *N Engl J Med* 1998; **339**: 1448–1456.

69 Ibsen H, Olsen MH, Wachtell K. Reduction in albuminuria translates to reduction in cardiovascular events in hypertensive patients: losartan intervention for endpoint reduction in hypertension study. *Hypertension* 2005; **45**: 198–202.

70 Asselbergs FW, Diercks GF, Hillege HL. Effects of fosinopril and pravastatin on cardiovascular events in subjects with microalbuminuria. *Circulation* 2004; **110**: 2809–2816.

71 Khosla N, Bakris G. Lessons learned from recent hypertension trials about kidney disease. *C J Am Soc Nephrol* 2006; **1**: 229–235.

72 Ruggenenti P, Schieppati A, Remuzzi G. Progression, remission, regression of chronic renal diseases. *Lancet* 2001; **357**: 1601–1608.

73 Jafar TH, Stark PC, Schmid CH, Landa M, Maschio G, de Jong PE *et al*. Progression of chronic kidney disease: the role of blood pressure control, proteinuria, and angiotensin-converting enzyme inhibition. A patient-level meta-analysis. *Ann Intern Med* 2003; **139**: 244–225.

74 Ruggenenti P, Perna A, Gherardi G, Gaspari F, Benini R, Remuzzi G. Renal function and requirement for dialysis in chronic nephropathy patients on long-term ramipril: REIN follow-up trial. Gruppo Italiano di Studi Epidemiologici in Nefrologia (GISEN). Ramipril Efficacy in Nephropathy. *Lancet* 1998; **352**: 1252–1256.

75 Ruggenenti P, Perna A, Mosconi L, Pisoni R, Remuzzi G. Urinary protein excretion rate is the best independent predictor of ESRF in non-diabetic proteinuric chronic nephropathies. "Gruppo Italiano di Studi Epidemiologici in Nefrologia" (GISEN). *Kidney Int* 1998; **53**: 1209–1216.

76 Lewis EJ, Hunsicker LG, Clarke WR, Berl T, Pohl MA, Lewis JB *et al*. Renoprotective effect of the angiotensin-receptor antagonist irbesartan in patients with nephropathy due to type 2 diabetes. *N Engl J Med* 2001; **345**: 851–860.

77 Rossing K, Jacobsen P, Pietraszek L, Parving HH. Renoprotective effects of adding angiotensin II receptor blocker to maximal recommended doses of ACE inhibitor in diabetic nephropathy: a randomized double-blind crossover trial. *Diabetes Care* 2003; **26**: 2268–2274.

78 Schjoedt KJ, Jacobsen P, Rossing K, Boomsma F, Parving HH. Dual blockade of the renin-angiotensin-aldosterone system in diabetic nephropathy: the role of aldosterone. *Horm Metab Res* 2005; **37**: 4–8.

79 Rossing P, Hommel E, Smidt UM, Parving HH. Reduction in albuminuria predicts a beneficial effect on diminishing the progression of human diabetic nephropathy during antihypertensive treatment. *Diabetologia* 1994; **37**: 511–516.

80 Appperloo AJ, de Zeeuw D, de Jong PE. Short-term antiproteinuric response to antihypertensive treatment predicts long-term GFR decline in patients with non-diabetic renal disease. *Kidney Int* 1994; **45**: S174–S178.

81 Verhave JC, Gansevoort RT, Hillege HL, Bakker SJ, De Zeeuw D, de Jong PE *et al*. An elevated urinary albumin excretion predicts de novo development of renal function impairment in the general population. *Kidney Int Suppl* 2004; **92**: S18–S21.

82 Mogensen CE. Long-term antihypertensive treatment inhibiting progression of diabetic nephropathy. *BMJ* 1982; **285**: 685–688.

83 Parving H-H, Andersen AR, Smidt UM, Hommel E, Mathiesen ER, Svendsen PA. Effect of antihypertensive treatment on kidney function in diabetic nephropathy. *BMJ* 1987; **294**: 1443–1447.

84 Parving H-H, Smidt UM, Hommel E, Mathiesen ER, Rossing P, Nielsen F *et al*. Effective antihypertensive treatment postpones renal insuf-

ficiency in diabetic nephropathy. *Am J Kidney Dis* 1993; **22**: 188–195.

85 Ravid M, Savin H, Jutrin I, Bental T, Katz B, Lishner M. Long-term stabilizing effect of angiotensin-converting enzyme inhibition on plasma creatinine and on proteinuria in normotensive type II diabetic patients. *Ann Intern Med* 1993; **118**: 577–581.

86 Ruggenenti P, Fassi A, Ilieva AP, Bruno S, Iliev IP, Brusegan V *et al*. Preventing microalbuminuria in type 2 diabetes. *N Engl J Med* 2004; **351**: 1941–1951.

87 Haller H, Viberti GC, Mimran A, Remuzzi G, Rabelink AJ, Ritz E *et al*. Preventing microalbuminuria in patients with diabetes: rationale and design of the Randomised Olmesartan and Diabetes Microalbuminuria Prevention (ROADMAP) study. *J Hypertens* 2006; **24**: 403–408.

88 Lewis EJ, Hunsicker LG, Bain RP, Rohde RD. The effect of angiotensin-converting-enzyme inhibition on diabetic nephropathy. *N Engl J Med* 1993; **329**: 1456–1462.

89 Ravid M, Brosh D, Levi Z, Bar-Dayan Y, Ravid D, Rachmani R. Use of enalapril to attenuate decline in renal function in normotensive, normoalbuminuric patients with type 2 diabetes mellitus. A randomized, controlled trial. *Ann Intern Med* 1998; **128**: 982–988.

90 Taal MW, Brenner BM. Renoprotective benefits of RAS inhibition: from ACEI to angiotensin II antagonists. *Kidney Int* 2000; **57**: 1803–1817.

91 Schmieder RE, Klingbeil AU, Fleischmann EH, Veelken R, Delles C. Additional antiproteinuric effect of ultrahigh dose candesartan: a double-blind, randomized, prospective study. *J Am Soc Nephrol* 2005; **16**: 3038–3045.

92 Rossing K, Schjoedt KJ, Jensen BR, Boomsma F, Parving HH. Enhanced renoprotective effects of ultrahigh doses of irbesartan in patients with type 2 diabetes and microalbuminuria. *Kidney Int* 2005; **68**: 1190–1198.

93 Parving HH, Lehnert H, Bröchner-Mortensen J, Gomis R, Andersen S, Arner P. Irbesartan in Patients with Type 2 Diabetes and Microalbuminuria Study Group. The effect of irbesartan on the development of diabetic nephropathy in patients with type 2 diabetes. *N Engl J Med* 2001; **345**: 870–878.

94 Fiebeler A, Nussberger J, Shagdarsuren E, Rong S, Hilfenhaus G, Al-Saadi N *et al*. Aldosterone synthase inhibitor ameliorates angiotensin II-induced organ damage. *Circulation* 2005; **111**: 3087–3094.

95 Schjoedt KJ, Andersen S, Rossing P, Tarnow L, Parving HH. Aldosterone escape during blockade of the renin-angiotensin-aldosterone system in diabetic nephropathy is associated with enhanced decline in glomerular filtration rate. *Diabetologia* 2004; **47**: 1936–1939.

96 Bianchi S, Bigazzi R, Campese VM. Antagonists of aldosterone and proteinuria in patients with CKD: an uncontrolled pilot study. *Am J Kidney Dis* 2005; **46**: 45–51.

97 Schjoedt KJ, Rossing K, Juhl TR, Boomsma F, Rossing P, Tarnow L *et al*. Beneficial impact of spironolactone in diabetic nephropathy. *Kidney Int* 2005; **68**: 2829–2836.

98 Schjoedt KJ, Rossing K, Juhl TR, Boomsma F, Tarnow L, Rossing P *et al*. Beneficial impact of spironolactone on nephrotic range albuminuria in diabetic nephropathy. *Kidney Int* 2006; **70**: 536–542.

99 Wolf G, Ritz E. Combination therapy with ACE inhibitors and angiotensin II receptor blockers to halt progression of chronic renal disease: pathophysiology and indications. *Kidney Int* 2005; **67**: 799–812.

100 Pinto-Sietsma SJ, Mulder J, Janssen WM, Hillege HL, de Zeeuw D, de Jong PE. Smoking is related to albuminuria and abnormal renal function in non-diabetic persons. *Ann Intern Med* 2000; **133**: 585–591.

101 Haroun MK, Jaar BG, Hoffman SC, Comstock GW, Klag MJ, Coresh J. Risk factors for chronic kidney disease: a prospective study of 23534 men and women in Washington County, Maryland. *J Am Soc Nephrol* 2003; **14:** 2934–2941.

102 Orth SR, Stockmann A, Conradt C, Ritz E, Ferro M, Kreusser W *et al.* Smoking as a risk factor for end-stage renal failure in men with primary renal disease. *Kidney Int* 1998; **54:** 926–931.

103 Christiansen JS. Cigarette smoking and prevalence of microangiopathy in juvenile-onset insulin-dependent diabetes mellitus. *Diabetes Care* 1978; **1:** 146–149.

104 Sawicki PT, Didjurgeit U, Muhlhauser I, Bender R, Heinemann L, Berger M. Smoking is associated with progression of diabetic nephropathy. *Diabetes Care* 1994; **17:** 126–131.

105 Orth SR, Schroeder T, Ritz E, Ferrari P. Effects of smoking on renal function in patients with type 1 and type 2 diabetes mellitus. *Nephrol Dial Transplant* 2005; **20:** 2414–2419.

106 Biesenbach G, Grafinger P, Janko O, Zazgornik J. Influence of cigarette-smoking on the progression of clinical diabetic nephropathy in type 2 diabetic patients. *Clin Nephrol* 1997; **48:** 146–150.

107 Chuahirun T, Wesson DE. Cigarette smoking predicts faster progression of type 2 established diabetic nephropathy despite ACE inhibition. *Am J Kidney Dis* 2002; **39:** 376–382.

108 Lhotta K, Rumpelt HJ, Konig P, Mayer G, Kronenberg F. Cigarette smoking and vascular pathology in renal biopsies. *Kidney Int* 2002; **61:** 648–654.

109 Regalado M, Yang S, Wesson DE. Cigarette smoking is associated with augmented progression of renal insufficiency in severe essential hypertension. *Am J Kidney Dis* 2000; **35:** 687–694.

110 Chuahirun T, Simoni J, Hudson C, Seipel T, Khanna A, Harrist RB *et al.* Cigarette smoking exacerbates and its cessation ameliorates renal injury in type 2 diabetes. *Am J Med Sci* 2004; **327:** 57–67.

111 Weisinger JR, Kempson RL, Eldridge FL, Swenson RS. The nephrotic syndrome: a complication of massive obesity. *Ann Intern Med* 1974; **81:** 440–447.

112 Kambham N, Markowitz GS, Valeri AM, Lin J, D'Agati VD. Obesity-related glomerulopathy: an emerging epidemic. *Kidney Int* 2001; **59:** 1498–1509.

113 Bonnet F, Deprele C, Sassolas A, Moulin P, Alamartine E, Berthezene F *et al.* Excessive body weight as a new independent risk factor for clinical and pathological progression in primary IgA nephritis. *Am J Kidney Dis* 2001; **37:** 720–727.

114 Modlin CS, Flechner SM, Goormastic M, Goldfarb DA, Papajcik D, Mastroianni B *et al.* Should obese patients lose weight before receiving a kidney transplant? *Transplantation* 1997; **64:** 599–604.

115 Meier-Kriesche HU, Arndorfer JA, Kaplan B. The impact of body mass index on renal transplant outcomes: a significant independent risk factor for graft failure and patient death. *Transplantation* 2002; **73:** 70–74.

116 Gonzalez E, Gutierrez E, Morales E, Hernandez E, Andres A, Bello I *et al.* Factors influencing the progression of renal damage in patients with unilateral renal agenesia and remnant kidney. *Kidney Int* 2005; **68:** 263–270.

117 Praga M, Hernandez E, Herrero JC, Morales E, Revilla Y, Diaz-Gonzalez R *et al.* Influence of obesity on the appearance of proteinuria and renal insufficiency after unilateral nephrectomy. *Kidney Int* 2000; **58:** 2111–2118.

118 Chagnac A, Weinstein T, Herman M, Hirsh J, Gafter U, Ori Y. The effects of weight loss on renal function in patients with severe obesity. *J Am Soc Nephrol* 2003; **14:** 1480–1486.

119 Praga M, Hernández E, Andres A, Leon M, Ruilope LM, Rodicio JL. Effects of body-weight loss and captopril treatment on proteinuria associated with obesity. *Nephron* 1995; **70:** 35–41.

120 Morales E, Valero MA, Leon M, Hernandez E, Praga M. Beneficial effects of weight loss in overweight patients with chronic proteinuric nephropathies. *Am J Kidney Dis* 2003; **41:** 319–327.

121 Leavey SF, McCullough K, Hecking E, Goodkin D, Port FK, Young EW. Body mass index and mortality in 'healthier' as compared with 'sicker' haemodialysis patients: results from the Dialysis Outcomes and Practice Patterns Study (DOPPS). *Nephrol Dial Transplant* 2001; **16:** 2386–2394.

122 Volhard F, Fahr T. *Die Brightsche Nierenkrankheit.* Julius Springer Verlag, Berlin; 1914.

123 Denton D, Weisinger R, Mundy NI, Wickings EJ, Dixson A, Moisson P *et al.* The effect of increased salt intake on blood pressure of chimpanzees. *Nat Med* 1995; **1:** 1009–1016.

124 Kitiyakara C, Chabrashvili T, Chen Y, Blau J, Karber A, Aslam S *et al.* Salt intake, oxidative stress, and renal expression of NADPH oxidase and superoxide dismutase. *J Am Soc Nephrol* 2003; **14:** 2775–2782.

125 Dworkin LD, Benstein JA, Tolbert E, Feiner HD. Salt restriction inhibits renal growth and stabilizes injury in rats with established renal disease. *J Am Soc Nephrol* 1996; **7:** 437–442.

126 Lax DS, Benstein JA, Tolbert E, Dworkin LD. Effects of salt restriction on renal growth and glomerular injury in rats with remnant kidneys. *Kidney Int* 1992; 41: 1527–1534.

127 Benstein JA, Feiner HD, Parker M, Dworkin LD. Superiority of salt restriction over diuretics in reducing renal hypertrophy and injury in uninephrectomized SHR. *Am J Physiol* 1990; **258:** F1675–F1681.

128 Suzuki H, Yamamoto T, Ikegaya N, Hishida A. Dietary salt intake modulates progression of antithymocyte serum nephritis through alteration of glomerular angiotensin II receptor expression. *Am J Physiol Renal Physiol* 2004; **286:** F267–F277.

129 Sanders PW, Gibbs CL, Akhi KM, MacMillan-Crow LA, Zinn KR, Chen YF *et al.* Increased dietary salt accelerates chronic allograft nephropathy in rats. *Kidney Int* 2001; **59:** 1149–1157.

130 Sanders MW, Fazzi GE, Janssen GM, Blanco CE, De Mey JG. High sodium intake increases blood pressure and alters renal function in intrauterine growth-retarded rats. *Hypertension* 2005; **46:** 71–75.

131 Allen TJ, Waldron MJ, Casley D, Jerums G, Cooper ME. Salt restriction reduces hyperfiltration, renal enlargement, and albuminuria in experimental diabetes. *Diabetes* 1997; **46:** 19–24.

132 Luik PT, Hoogenberg K, van der Kleij FGH, Beusekamp BJ, Kerstens MN, Jong PE *et al.* Short-term moderate sodium restriction induces relative hyperfiltration in normotensive normoalbuminuric type I diabetes mellitus. *Diabetologia* 2002; **454:** 535–541.

133 Fliser D, Nowack R, Wolf G, Ritz E. Differential effects of ACE inhibitors and vasodilators on renal function curve in patients with primary hypertension. *Blood Press* 1993; **2:** 296–300.

134 Swift PA, Markandu ND, Sagnella GA, He FJ, MacGregor GA. Modest salt reduction reduces blood pressure and urine protein excretion in black hypertensives: a randomized control trial. *Hypertension* 2005; **46:** 308–312.

135 Cianciaruso B, Bellizzi V, Minutolo R, Tavera A, Capuano A, Conte G *et al.* Salt intake and renal outcome in patients with progressive renal disease. *Miner Electrolyte Metab* 1998; **24:** 296–301.

136 Koranyi A. Physikalisch-chemische Methoden und Gesichtspunkte in ihrer Anwendung auf die pathologische Physiologie der Nieren. In: Korányi A, Richter P, editors. *Physikalische Chemie und Medizin.* Thieme Verlag, Berlin, 1907; 133–190.

137 Fishberg AM. *Hypertension and Nephritis*. Lea and Febiger, Philadelphia, 1939.

138 Bouby N, Bachmann S, Bichet D, Bankir L. Effect of water intake on the progression of chronic renal failure in the 5/6 nephrectomized rat. *Am J Physiol* 1990; **258:** F973–F979.

139 Bankir L, Bouby N, Trinh-Trang-Tan MM. Vasopressin-dependent kidney hypertrophy: role of urinary concentration in protein-induced hypertrophy and in the progression of chronic renal failure. *Am J Kidney Dis* 1991; **17:** 661–665.

140 Hebert LA, Greene T, Levey A, Falkenhain ME, Klahr S. High urine volume and low urine osmolality are risk factors for faster progression of renal disease. *Am J Kidney Dis* 2003; **41:** 962–971.

141 Knight EL, Stampfer MJ, Hankinson SE, Spiegelman D, Curhan GC. The impact of protein intake on renal function decline in women with normal renal function or mild renal insufficiency. *Ann Intern Med* 2003; **138:** 460–467.

142 Ihle BU, Becker GJ, Whitworth JA, Charlwood RA, Kincaid-Smith PS. The effect of protein restriction on the progression of renal insufficiency. *N Engl J Med* 1989; **321:** 1773–1777.

143 D'Amico G, Gentile MG, Fellin G, Manna G, Cofano F. Effect of dietary protein restriction on the progression of renal failure: a prospective randomized trial. *Nephrol Dial Transplant* 1994; **9:** 1590–1594.

144 Rosman JB, ter Wee PM, Meijer S, Piers-Becht TP, Sluiter WJ, Donker AJ. Prospective randomised trial of early dietary protein restriction in chronic renal failure. *Lancet* 1984; **ii:** 1291–1296.

145 Zeller K, Whittaker E, Sullivan L, Raskin P, Jacobson HR. Effect of restricting dietary protein on the progression of renal failure in patients with insulin-dependent diabetes mellitus. *N Engl J Med* 1991; **324:** 78–84.

146 Walker JD, Bending JJ, Dodds RA, Mattock MB, Murrells TJ, Keen H *et al.* Restriction of dietary protein and progression of renal failure in diabetic nephropathy. *Lancet* 1989; **ii:** 1411–1415.

147 Williams PS, Stevens ME, Fass G, Irons L, Bone JM. Failure of dietary protein and phosphate restriction to retard the rate of progression of chronic renal failure: a prospective, randomized, controlled trial. *Q J Med* 1991; **81:** 837–855.

148 Locatelli F, Alberti D, Graziani G, Buccianti G, Redaelli B, Giangrande A. Prospective, randomised, multicentre trial of effect of protein restriction on progression of chronic renal insufficiency. Northern Italian Cooperative Study Group. *Lancet* 1991; **337:** 1299–1304.

149 Wingen AM, Fabian-Bach C, Schaefer F, Mehls O. Randomised multicentre study of a low-protein diet on the progression of chronic renal failure in children. European Study Group of Nutritional Treatment of Chronic Renal Failure in Childhood. *Lancet* 1997; **349:** 1117–1123.

150 Pedrini MT, Levey AS, Lau J, Chalmers TC, Wang PH. The effect of dietary protein restriction on the progression of diabetic and nondiabetic renal diseases: a meta-analysis. *Ann Intern Med* 1996; **124:** 627–632.

151 Fouque D, Laville M, Boissel JP, Chifflet R, Labeeuw M, Zech PY. Controlled low protein diets in chronic renal insufficiency: meta-analysis. *BMJ* 1992; **304:** 216–220.

152 Fouque D, Wang P, Laville M, Boissel JP. Low protein diets delay end-stage renal disease in non diabetic adults with chronic renal failure. *Cochrane Database Syst Rev* 2000; **2:** CD001892.

153 Levey AS, Adler S, Caggiula AW, England BK, Greene T, Hunsicker LG *et al.* Effects of dietary protein restriction on the progression of advanced renal disease in the Modification of Diet in Renal Disease Study. *Am J Kidney Dis* 1996; **27:** 652–663.

154 Aparicio M, Chauveau P, De Precigout V, Bouchet JL, Lasseur C, Combe C. Nutrition and outcome on renal replacement therapy of patients with chronic renal failure treated by a supplemented very low protein diet. *J Am Soc Nephrol* 2000; **11:** 708–716.

155 Vendrely B, Chauveau P, Barthe N, El Haggan W, Castaing F, de Precigout V *et al.* Nutrition in hemodialysis patients previously on a supplemented very low protein diet. *Kidney Int* 2003; **63:** 1491–1498.

156 Cupisti A, Licitra R, Chisari C, Stampacchia G, D'Alessandro C, Galetta F *et al.* Skeletal muscle and nutritional assessment in chronic renal failure in patients on a protein-restricted diet. *J Intern Med* 2004; **255:** 115–124.

157 Kopple JD, Levey AS, Greene T, Chumlea WC, Gassman JJ, Hollinger DL *et al.* Effect of dietary protein restriction on nutritional status in the Modification of Diet in Renal Disease Study. *Kidney Int* 1997; **52:** 778–791.

158 American Diabetes Association. Standard of medical care in diabetes. *Diabetes Care* 2005; **38:** S4–S36.

159 Randomised placebo-controlled trial of effect of ramipril on decline in glomerular filtration rate and risk of terminal renal failure in proteinuric, non-diabetic nephropathy. The GISEN Group (Gruppo Italiano di Studi Epidemiologici in Nefrologia) *Lancet* 1997; **349:** 1857–1863.

160 Curhan GC, Knight EL, Rosner B, Hankinson SE, Stampfer MJ, Lifetime nonnarcotic analgesic use and decline in renal function in women. *Arch Intern Med.* 2004; **164:** 1519–1524.

161 Perneger TV, Whelton PK, Klag MJ. Risk of kidney failure associated with the use of acetaminophen, aspirin, and nonsteroidal anti-inflammatory drugs. *N Engl J Med.* 1994; **331:** 1675–1679.

162 Sandler DP, Smith JC, Weinberg CR, Buckalew VM Jr, Dennis VW, Blythe WB, Burgess WP. Analgesic use and chronic renal disease. *N Engl J Med.* 1989; **320:** 1238–1243.

163 Pommer W, Bronder E, Greiser E, Helmert U, Jesdinsky HJ, Klimpel A, Borner K, Molzahn M. Regular analgesic intake and the risk of end-stage renal failure. *Am J Nephrol* 1989; **9:** 403–412.

164 Muntner P, Coresh J, Klag MJ, Whelton PK, Perneger TV. Exposure to radiologic contrast media and an increased risk of treated end-stage renal disease. *Am J Med Sci.* 2003; **326:** 353–359.

4 Epidemiology and Screening for Chronic Kidney Disease

Sylvia Paz B. Ramirez

Arbor Research Collaborative for Health, Ann Arbor, USA

Epidemiology of chronic kidney disease as a basis for a population-based system for surveillance and screening for kidney disease

Applying a standard system for the definition and classification of chronic kidney disease (CKD) is essential. Only through an established system that is consistently utilized can disease trends be tracked over time. To achieve this, the National Kidney Foundation in its Kidney Disease Outcomes Quality Initiative (K/DOQI) guidelines has proposed a staging classification for CKD, and these guidelines have been extensively described elsewhere [1]. The guidelines also provide an extensive review of the test characteristics of the various screening tests for CKD, and this is further discussed in chapter 2 of this textbook.

Screening for CKD serves two general goals. The first is to diagnosis and intervene early in the chronic phase of kidney disease in order to modify renal outcomes, particularly in high-risk populations. The second is to intervene in order to improve nonrenal outcomes, including cardiovascular outcomes and mortality. Numerous studies of a wide spectrum of populations have shown that low glomerular filtration rate (GFR) is clearly associated with cardiovascular disease and cardiovascular disease risk factors. For instance, systolic blood pressure, cholesterol levels, and the percentage of patients with low levels of high-density lipoproteins are more prevalent in patients with reduced GFR, as shown in the Heart Outcomes and Prevention Evaluation (HOPE) study and the Cardiovascular Health Study [2,3], the Hypertension Optimal Treatment Study [4], the Framingham and Framingham Offspring studies [5,6], and the Atherosclerosis Risk in Communities study [7]. Similarly, the prevalence of cardiovascular disease is higher in those with a decreased GFR [4,5,8,9]. The implications of CKD and proteinuria as risk markers for cardiovascular disease are not within the scope of this discussion; a more extensive analysis of

the cardiovascular implications of CKD is presented in chapter 5 of this textbook.

For screening and surveillance to be feasible, it is important to consider the following factors:
- The natural history of CKD, including the likelihood of disease progression based on the stage of CKD detected. Screening and surveillance become relevant only if it is clear that the associated abnormality increases the risk of disease progression. The natural history of disease is also relevant in determining the optimal interval of screening for a particular population.
- The target population for screening, as this determines the screening tool's success at identifying a true increase in risk for CKD and CKD progression (positive predictive value)
- Screening frequency or the interval between two successive screening tests.
- Ability of a screening program to impact clinical outcomes, including mortality, progression to end-stage renal disease (ESRD), and development of other comorbidities.

These factors will be described in detail in the following sections.

Impact of natural history of CKD on screening

Tables 4.1 and 4.2 present a summary of the published literature on the natural history of CKD in general and proteinuria in particular. As is evident from the literature, there is clear variability in the progression of CKD, particularly in the presence of clinical factors such as diabetes, hypertension, or proteinuria.

Table 4.1 reflects the annual decline in GFR, whereas Table 4.2 presents the likelihood of disease progression by degree of proteinuria. An extensive body of literature shows that the presence of elevated levels of albumin in the urine is associated with a significantly greater risk of development of progressive renal insufficiency and should be a component of surveillance and screening programs for CKD.

As shown in Table 4.1, the annual decline of GFR differs markedly by clinical history and presence of proteinuria. Based on the National Health and Nutrition Evaluation Survey (NHANES),

Evidence-based Nephrology. Edited by Donald Molony and Jonathan Craig
© 2009 Blackwell Publishing, ISBN: 978-1-4051-3975-5.

Table 4.1 Annual decline in GFR by clinical history.

Clinical history and GFR	References	Annual decline in GFR (mL/min/1.73 m^2)
No diabetes or hypertension No proteinuria, normal GFR	Coresh *et al.* 2003 [10] NKF Clinical Practice Guidelines 2000 (http://www.kidney.org/professionals/doqi/kdoqi/-4_class_g1.htm)	Mean decrease, 1.0
Proteinuria Progression from stages 2–4 CKD to ESRD	Ruggenenti *et al.* 1998 [12] Jones *et al.* 2006 [91]	4.2 5.3
Hypertension No proteinuria, progression from stages 2–4 CKD to ESRD	Agodoa *et al.* 2001 [11]	1.4
Proteinuria, progression from stages 2–4 CKD to stage 5	Agodoa *et al.* 2001 [11] Ruggenenti *et al.* 1998 [12] Klahr *et al.* 1994 [13] Toto *et al.* 1995 [102] Wright *et al.* 2002 [104]	3.9
Diabetes No proteinuria, normal GFR to K/DOQI stages 2–4	Nelson *et al.* 1996 [14] Nosadini *et al.* 2000 [15] Rachmani *et al.* 2000 [16]	1.1
Stages 2–4 to 5 Proteinuria, normal GFR to K/DOQI stages 2–4	Lebovitz *et al.* 1994 [105] Gaede *et al.* 1999 [106] Gaede *et al.* 2003 [107] Nosadini *et al.* 2000 [15]	2.8 4.1
Stages 2–4 to 5	Lewis *et al.* 2001 [17] Brenner *et al.* 2001 [18] Ruggenenti *et al.* 2000 [19]	5.2

in the absence of diabetes or hypertension, the average member of the adult US population is estimated to have an approximate annual decline in GFR of 1 mL/min/1.73 m^2 in the presence of normal renal function at baseline [10]. The degree to which renal function continues to decline beyond a certain GFR in the absence of hypertension, diabetes, or proteinuria is not known.

In the presence of hypertension, but without proteinuria, Agodoa and others [11] showed a GFR decline of 1.4 mL/min/1.73 m^2, and this deterioration increased significantly to approximately 3.9 mL/min/1.73 m^2 in the presence of proteinuria [12,13]. In the presence of diabetes, multiple studies have demonstrated an annual decline in GFR that increases from 1.1 mL/min/1.73 m^2 in

Table 4.2 Disease progression by degree of proteinuria.

Clinical history and [reference]	Predictor	Outcome	Population
No hypertension or diabetes			
Verhave *et al.* 2004 [20]	Elevated urinary albumin excretion	4.2% developed GFR <60 mL/min/1.73 m^2 after 4-year follow-up	The Netherlands, excluded those with GFR <60 mL/min/1.73 m^2 at baseline
Iseki *et al.* 2003 [21]	No proteinuria to trace 1+ proteinuria ≥ 2+ proteinuria	18-yr ESRD incidence 0.2% 18-yr ESRD incidence 1.4% 9.2%	Japanese
Tozawa *et al.* 2003 [109]	Proteinuria 1+ or greater	RR of ESRD, 11.29 in men, 12.5 in women	Japanese
High risk for CVD Ishani *et al.* 2006 [22]	Proteinuria 1+ Proteinuria ≥2+	OR 3.1 (CI, 1.8–5.4) OR 15.7 (CI, 10.3–23.9)	12,866 men at high risk for CVD

Abbreviation: RR, relative risk.

the absence of baseline proteinuria and renal insufficiency [14–16] to 5.2 mL/min/1.73 m^2 among patients with proteinuria and renal insufficiency at baseline [17–19]. What these studies demonstrate is the following: 1) there is a background rate of deterioration of renal function, 2) this decline in renal function is dramatically hastened by the presence of diabetes and hypertension, and 3) the presence of proteinuria is an important marker for progression of CKD.

Table 4.2 is another representation of the clinical importance and natural history of proteinuria, as it presents the likelihood of progression to significant chronic renal insufficiency and ESRD based on clinical history and presence of proteinuria. As shown in Table 4.2, numerous studies support that albuminuria in and of itself, regardless of the level of GFR, is an important predictor of renal function decline. In the absence of hypertension or diabetes, the PREVEND study (Prevention of Renal and Vascular End-Stage Renal Disease), a longitudinal study initiated in 1997 that looked at the impact of albuminuria in the development of renal and cardiovascular disease in the general population, showed that the presence of an elevated urinary albumin excretion was associated with development of renal insufficiency 4 years after follow-up [20]. The study identified older age, higher blood pressure, serum cholesterol and serum glucose, degree of albuminuria, and relatively lower GFR as predictors of significant renal insufficiency in a population without known risk factors for CKD. Similarly, Iseki and colleagues in an 18-year longitudinal study of the general population of Okinawa revealed a significant stepwise increase in the incidence of future ESRD based on a screening dipstick proteinuria [21]. As shown in Table 4.2, the presence of dipstick-positive proteinuria of 2+ or greater is associated with a 9.2% incidence of ESRD, and even with lower degrees of proteinuria (1+), there was an increased risk of ESRD compared to patients with dipstick-negative proteinuria. The increased risk of ESRD associated with proteinuria was even higher in a population at high risk for cardiovascular disease [22]. As shown in the MRFIT study (Multiple Risk Factor Intervention Trial), which included 12,866 men who were at high risk for heart disease, the presence of a single dipstick proteinuria of 1+ was associated with an odds ratio (OR) of 3.1 (confidence interval, 1.8–5.4) for development of ESRD in over 25 years of follow-up. When dipstick proteinuria was 2+ or greater, the associated OR was 15.7 (confidence interval, 10.3–23.9). A similar predictive power of proteinuria in the development of ESRD in other populations considered at high risk for development of ESRD will be discussed extensively below. These studies unequivocally show the relationship between proteinuria and subsequent development of ESRD.

Less clear is the relationship between normal levels of albuminuria and microalbuminuria on the development of CKD. Indeed, although there are numerous studies that show that microalbuminuria is associated with an increase in both all-cause and cardiovascular mortality in apparently healthy populations [23–25], as well as in those with existing cardiovascular risk factors in the HOPE trial [26] or hypertension in the LIFE and AASK trials [27], studies that show an association between lower levels of albuminuria and renal outcomes have only been recently published. In the PREVEND study, for instance, high-normal levels of urinary albumin were found to be associated with an increased risk of chronic kidney disease in the general population [20].

Thus, published evidence on the natural history of CKD unequivocally demonstrates the relationship between high levels of albuminuria and progression to CKD, supporting the use of this measure in a surveillance and screening system. Whether this is of value in the general population or only in high-risk populations is further discussed below. Finally, because there is no evidence on the use of normoalbuminuria or microalbuminuria for screening in the general population, this does not appear to be justified at present.

Impact of other factors on development of a surveillance and screening system

A second consideration in developing a surveillance and screening system is to define the target population. If CKD were extremely infrequent in a population, then screening would not be productive. A screening test's likelihood of truly detecting an individual at increased risk for CKD, or the positive predictive value, depends on the proportion of the screened population with CKD [28,29]. Indeed, a screening program's positive predictive value can be improved by focusing on the population at increased risk, that is, the group of individuals with a higher prevalence of CKD. A summary of the published literature identifying the populations at increased risk for CKD is presented in the next section.

Another important factor to consider is the screening frequency, or the interval between two successive screening tests. This, too, depends primarily on the incidence rate of CKD in the target population. For a low-risk population with a low incidence of CKD, high frequencies of screening will yield a lower number of identified cases and, as a consequence, the potential for a reduction in the number of cases of ESRD will be low.

Finally, evaluating a screening program for CKD in terms of its ability to impact on the number of ESRD cases, or the development of cardiovascular and all-cause morbidity and mortality, is complex. Even a randomized study that evaluates the effects of a screening program is difficult for a variety of reasons, as summarized by McClellan and others [30], including the feasibility and cost of the study and the unique biases associated with screening programs. In particular, when comparing survival curves between screened and unscreened populations, it is certain that longer survival will be observed in the screened population [28,29]. This is due to three factors: 1) lead time bias, with which patients are detected earlier than they would have been based on clinical symptoms; 2) length time bias, with which patients with a longer preclinical, and likely less-aggressive, kidney disease course are more likely to be detected by screening programs; and 3) selection bias, with which patients who are relatively healthy have a greater tendency to participate in screening programs. Indeed, the improved outcomes that may be attributed to early detection and early intervention with screening

Table 4.3 Older age and risk of CKD.

Data source [reference]	Study population	Exposure	End point	Results
Patel *et al.* 2005 [32]	VA, retrospective longitudinal cohort, 48% with CKD at baseline	GFR (stage of CKD)	Mortality rate, 3-yr follow-up	Mortality in those without CKD, 4.7 deaths/100 person-yrs; increased w/ progressive CKD to 20.1 deaths/100 person-yrs if GFR 15–29 mL/min/1.73 m^2
Shlipak *et al.* 2006 [35]	The Cardiovascular Health Study, population-based study of adults $\geq$65 yrs in 4 US communities	GFR and cystatin C conc	Death, cardiovascular outcomes, CKD, and others	High prevalence of "preclinical disease," those at greater risk for progression to CKD in this elderly population

programs are difficult to separate from these inherent biases of screening programs.

High-risk populations for CKD

Elderly

Older age is significantly associated with mortality regardless of the presence of preexisting disease [31]. Several studies have demonstrated an increased risk of CKD progression in older populations. Working with the Veterans Administration (VA) population, Patel and others evaluated the 3-year mortality rate of older patients with or without CKD [32]. As shown in Table 4.3, the mortality rate increased with worsening degree of baseline GFR. Furthermore, the authors noted that the risk in the VA population, previously reported to have a greater illness burden than the general population [33], is greater than that observed using a community-based population, with a sevenfold-greater risk of death among those with relatively higher GFR levels in the VA population [34]. Similarly, the Cardiovascular Health Study, a longitudinal cohort study of elderly persons in four communities in the USA demonstrated the high prevalence of a condition that the authors identified as "preclinical disease" in the elderly community. The term preclinical disease was likened to prediabetes by those authors, in that the constellation of clinical characteristics is associated with a high rate of progression to CKD [35]. The study further noted that in this older population, there was a value in the use of cystatin C as a predictor for future CKD. In the absence of any other evidence of CKD, those elderly patients with elevated cystatin C concentrations were found to have a fourfold-increased risk for developing CKD on follow-up. These studies demonstrate the elevated risk of CKD associated with older age.

Hypertension

Hypertension as a risk factor for CKD has been clearly established. As shown in Table 4.4, CKD is highly prevalent in patients with treated essential hypertension. An analysis of the NHANES data showed that reduced GFR was present in 51.4% of screened adults with hypertension and on no medications and in 64.4% of screened adults with hypertension and receiving medications [10]. An analysis of the SHEP study (Systolic Hypertension in the Elderly Program) demonstrated a relative risk of 2.4 for a decline in kidney function among SHEP participants (placebo group) in the highest quartile of systolic blood pressure compared to those in the lowest quartile [36]. Perneger and colleagues, by integrating several population studies, estimated a rate of 14.6/100 patients for the development of CKD in hypertensive patients with normal baseline renal function [37]. Similarly, Segura and colleagues observed a deterioration in creatinine clearance (CrCl) to less than 60 mL/min/1.73 m^2 in 14.6% of a hypertensive population with baseline normal renal function [38]. Indeed, more recent studies have demonstrated an increased risk of CKD among patients with essential hypertension, in contrast to the earlier thought that the prevalence of CKD in the presence of essential hypertension is quite low [39].

Cardiovascular disease

Innumerable studies have documented the increased risk of cardiovascular disease in the presence of CKD [40,41]. This is discussed in chapter 5. Similarly, in addition to the strong relationship between hypertension and ESRD, cardiovascular disease in and of itself is also known to increase the risk for CKD, resulting in a vicious cycle given that CKD is known to amplify cardiovascular disease [42]. Using the HOPE study findings, which was a randomized trial designed to test the use of an angiotensin converting enzyme inhibitor (ACEi) and vitamin E in patients at high risk of cardiovascular events (Heart Outcomes and Prevention Evaluation Study), Mann and colleagues evaluated the predictive value of low levels of albuminuria that were below the cutoff used to define microalbuminuria for the development of clinical proteinuria and several cardiovascular outcomes [26]. Their analysis showed that in the individuals with established risk factors for cardiovascular disease, even low levels of albuminuria were significantly associated with development of clinical proteinuria. The relative risk for developing higher-grade proteinuria was 17.5 in both diabetic and nondiabetic patients. In fact, other findings of the HOPE study included that one of every three patients with diabetes developed microalbuminuria, and of these, one of five developed nephropathy

Table 4.4 Hypertension and cardiovascular disease as risk factors for CKD.

Data source [reference]	Study population	Exposure	End point	Results
Coresh et al. 2003 [10]	NHANES III cross-sectional survey	Hypertension (among others)	Presence of CKD	51.4% of those with hypertension on no medication and 64.4% of those with hypertension and on medication had reduced GFR
Young et al. 2002 [36]	Placebo arm of the Systolic Hypertension in the Elderly Program	Elderly men and women; blood pressure	Risk of decline of kidney function	2.4 adjusted RR for decline in kidney function in the highest quartile of SBP compared to lowest quartile
Perneger et al. 1993 [37]	Integrated analysis of several population studies	Four national databases (US Census, NHANES, Hypertension Detection and Follow-up Program trial, USRDS)	Abnormal serum creatinine	14.6/100 patients (over 13 yrs follow-up)
Segura et al. 2004 [38]	Patients with essential hypertension and normal renal function at baseline	Observational cohort study looking at relationship between blood pressure and CKD	CrCl <60 mL/min/1.73 m^2	Mean follow-up of 13.2 yrs, 14.6% developed renal insufficiency
Mann et al. 2004 [26]	Heart Outcomes and Prevention Evaluation (HOPE) study, a randomized trial designed to test use of an ACEi and vitamin E in patients at high risk of cardiovascular events	Normoalbuminuria (below microalbuminuria cutoff, >2 mg/mmol)	Clinical proteinuria	Baseline microalbuminuria predicted clinical proteinuria with RR of 17.5 in both diabetic and nondiabetic patients over 4.5-year follow-up; baseline microalbuminuria also increased RR of primary outcome of MI, stroke, or CV death (RR, 1.83)
McClellan et al. 2004 [44]	Medicare fee-for-service patients with primary diagnosis of AMI and a primary diagnosis of CHF	Presence of preexisting cardiovascular disease as defined by AMI and CHF diagnoses	Presence of CKD (defined as MDRD eGFR <60 mL/min/1.73 m^2	CKD in 51.7% of AMI and 60.4% of CHF patients; CKD increased risk of death in yr 1 for CHF patients (OR 1.6) and AMI (OR 3.1); increased risk of progression to ESRD among those with CKD

Abbreviations: ACEi, angioteusin converting enzyme inhibitor; AMI, acute myocardial infarction; CHF, congestive heart failure; RR, relative risk.

[43]. McClellan and others also demonstrated the increased risk of progressive CKD among patients with cardiovascular disease [44]. Using the Medicare database, those authors evaluated the relationship between CKD as defined by a reduced estimated GFR of <60 mL/min/1.73 m^2 in Medicare patients with a discharge diagnosis of either acute myocardial infarction or congestive heart failure. The study revealed that not only was there a high prevalence of previously undetected CKD in these two patient groups, but also there was an increased risk of ESRD among patients with CKD in addition to their cardiovascular disease, and they had an increased risk of death within 1 year after discharge.

That the presence of cardiovascular disease is a risk factor for CKD is most clearly apparent with the inclusion of kidney disease screening in the guidelines for the management of cardiovascular disease [45]. This advisory acknowledges the strong correlation between the risk factors and the occurrence of cardiovascular disease and CKD, and strongly recommends the routine screening of patients with cardiovascular disease for evidence of kidney disease.

Table 4.5 Diabetes and risk of CKD.

Data source	Study population	Exposure	End point	Results
Kramer et al. 2003 [48]	Type 2 diabetes mellitus in NHANES	Albuminuria	Low GFR	In 30% of adults with type 2 diabetes and normoalbuminuria, GFR was low
MacIsaac et al. 2004 [49]	Type 2 diabetes mellitus, cross-sectional survey of outpatients of a hospital	Albuminuria	Low GFR	In 39% of adults with type 2 diabetes and normoalbuminuria, GFR was <60 mL/min/1.73 m^2

Table 4.6 Family history and risk of CKD.

Data source [reference]	Study population	Exposure	End point	Results
Jurkovitz et al. 2002 [50]	Voluntary screening of family members of patients with ESRD	Family history	CrCl <60 mL/min, proteinuria	13.9% of family members had a CrCl <60 mL/min; 9.9% had proteinuria of ≥1+
Freedman et al. 2001 [51]	4365 incident dialysis patients treated in a single year	Incident dialysis patients	Family history of ESRD	20% of patients reported having a first- or second-degree relative with ESRD
Ferguson et al. 1988 [52]	Matched case–control study of dialysis patients matched to controls residing in area surrounding dialysis centers	History of CKD in a first- or second-degree relative	Risk of ESRD	History of CKD in first- or second-degree relative was associated with increased risk for being a prevalent ESRD patient
Bergman et al. 1996 [108]	First-degree relatives of patients with hypertensive ESRD	Relative of ESRD patient	Renal abnormality	Evidence for CKD was seen in 65% of participating families
O'Dea et al. 1998 [53]	Patients with ESRD	ESRD	Family history of ESRD	28% of patients had a first-, second-, or third-degree relative with CKD, compared with 15% of comparison spouses
Lei et al. 1998 [54]	First-degree relatives of new ESRD patients	Family member of ESRD patient	ESRD	OR of ESRD was 1.33 (CI, 0.7–2.6) for one first-degree relative with CKD, 10.4 (2.7–40.2) for two or more first-degree relatives

Diabetes

Diabetes is well-recognized to have reached epidemic proportions worldwide. In fact, an analysis by Jones and others suggested that the increase in incident ESRD over recent years is directly attributable to the combination of the rise in the incidence and prevalence of diabetes, as well as an increased risk in developing ESRD among patients with diabetes [46]. That there is a clear and established relationship between diabetes and CKD is well-documented, and this has been the subject of extensive review elsewhere [47]. Rather than providing a review of the overwhelmingly convincing data documenting the increased risk for nephropathy in diabetes, it is important to point out a novel finding presented by Kramer and others (Table 4.5). In their analysis of adults in their study with type 2 diabetes mellitus, 30% were found to have a low GFR in the absence of proteinuria [48]. That a reduced GFR can exist in diabetic patients in the absence of albuminuria was also shown in a study in Australia in which 39% of adults with type 2 diabetes had a GFR of <60 mL/min/1.73 m^2 despite having a normal albumin excretion level [49]. These studies provide evidence that for patients with diabetes, screening for nephropathy requires testing for both albuminuria and reduced GFR. Whether those diabetic patients who present only with reduced GFR in the absence of albuminuria follow a different clinical course and require different interventions deserves further study.

Family history

Several studies have demonstrated that individuals with a family history of CKD are at greater risk for kidney disease compared to those without any family history (Table 4.6). Among family members of patients with ESRD, it was shown that 13.9% had reduced CrCl (below 60 mL/min) and 9.9% had proteinuria of 1+ or greater on voluntary screening [50]. In another study, 20% of incident dialysis patients were reported to have a first- or second-degree relative with ESRD [51]. In a case–control study of dialysis patients matched to controls residing in areas surrounding dialysis centers, it was also shown that compared to controls, those with a family history of CKD was a significant predictor for being a prevalent ESRD patient [52]. That a family history of CKD is associated with CKD has been shown in both black and white patients [53]. Finally, the association between family history and CKD appears to be dose dependent. Lei et al. showed that the OR for ESRD was 1.3 for those with a single first-degree relative with CKD but that the odds dramatically increased to 10.4 in the presence of two or more first-degree relatives [54]. These studies demonstrate the association between CKD and a positive family history, arguing for targeted screening for CKD among individuals with such a family history.

Race and ethnicity

Evidence for race and ethnicity as risk factors for CKD is extensive (Table 4.7). To begin with, the US Renal Data System (USRDS) has shown that certain racial and ethnic groups have a higher age- and gender-adjusted risk of ESRD compared to the white population [55]. Factors that potentially account for the racial disparity in CKD include true biologic differences in risk and disease progression [56], a higher prevalence of low birth weight in certain racial and ethnic groups, which evidence reveals is a risk factor not only for CKD but also for hypertension and diabetes [57], and socio-economic factors leading to differential quality of and access to health care [58]. Low birth weight as a partial explanation of the observed racial difference is of interest [59]. As discussed in a separate section below, evidence exists that suggests an association between low birth weight and risk of CKD. Furthermore, the prevalence of low birth weight is up to twofold higher among African Americans compared to white and Hispanic groups [60]. Together, these suggest the potential contribution of prenatal and postnatal characteristics in the subsequent development of CKD.

Another contributing factor to the excess burden of CKD in certain racial and ethnic groups is the higher rates of predisposing factors to kidney disease development and progression, including higher rates of diabetes mellitus, hypertension, and glomerulonephritis [61]. With diabetes, for instance, African Americans, Hispanics, and Native Americans are recognized to have markedly higher rates of diabetes mellitus compared to white people. Similarly, as shown by the NHANES data, 34% of African Americans have hypertension, compared to 29% in the white population and 21% in Hispanic populations [62], and more African Americans develop hypertension-related ESRD compared to white people [63]. Socio-economic factors that lead to disparities in access to care have also been documented, with 31% of the African American population living below the federal poverty level compared to 11% of the white population [64].

As shown in Table 4.7, racial differences in the prevalence and risk for CKD are striking. Using the NHANES data, Jones and colleagues showed that the prevalence of albuminuria in African Americans is 50% higher compared to other racial and ethnic groups [65]. Interestingly, clear differences in various Asian ethnic groups have also been demonstrated in Hong Kong and Singapore [66,67]. The NHANES data were also used in an analysis that showed that the higher incidence of ESRD in African Americans is partly attributable to a faster rate of progression of CKD compared to that in other racial groups [56].

Racial differences in the rate of ESRD were also demonstrated in the health screening of the integrated health care system of Kaiser Permanente, in which Blacks and Asians were found to have significantly higher age-adjusted rates of ESRD compared to Whites [68]. The differences between black and white populations were similarly demonstrated in the MRFIT study, although the racial difference identified by this study was significantly attenuated by adjustments for multiple confounding factors [63]. Even the risk of developing ESRD secondary to diabetes appeared to have racial differences, as shown by Karter *et al.*, who found that Asians had an adjusted risk of 1.85 for developing diabetic ESRD compared to white people [69].

Analyses from the REGARDS cohort study, which aims to identify risk factors that lead to an increased mortality rate from stroke among black patients, has provided additional insight into the question of race and CKD risk. In this analysis of racial differences in the prevalence of CKD among participants in this cohort, there was a clear shift in the black/white OR with advancing degrees of renal insufficiency. In particular, the OR for a GFR between 50 and 59 mL/min/1.73 m^2 was 0.51, with fewer blacks than whites

having this degree of renal insufficiency, whereas at a GFR of <10 mL/min/1.73 m^2, the OR had flipped to 4.19, with a significantly greater odds for Black patients to have a more advanced degree of renal insufficiency compared to White patients [70].

Thus, for numerous reasons, it is evident that certain racial subgroups are at markedly greater risk for the development or more aggressive progression of CKD. Screening programs aimed to identify those at increased risk can potentially lead to earlier and more aggressive intervention. Although such an approach is theoretically appropriate, no published studies exist that demonstrate the clinical benefit gained from taking part in a screening program. Even if a randomized controlled trial for screening were performed, as stated in the earlier section of this chapter, unique screening-specific biases would need to be teased out from the true benefit gained from taking part in a screening program.

Other risk factors for CKD

Data exist on several other clinical features that may place individuals at increased risk for CKD. As summarized in Table 4.8, these factors include obesity, low birth weight, and the presence of metabolic syndrome. In Sweden for instance, Ejerblad and colleagues demonstrated that a body mass index (BMI) of 25 kg/m^2 or greater at the age of 29 years was associated with a threefold-increased risk of having an elevated serum creatinine [71]. Indeed as shown in Table 4.8, obesity as a risk factor for CKD was seen whether CKD was defined as a decline in GFR or as the presence of microalbuminuria and whether this was evaluated in a cohort study or in a cross-sectional study.

There is also significant evidence that low birth weight is associated with CKD. In nondiabetic populations, Yudkin and others showed an association between low ponderal index (weight for height) and an increased OR for microalbuminuria [72]. Among Pima Indians with type 2 diabetes, it was also shown that both extremes of BMI were significantly associated with albuminuria, with an OR of 2.3 for albuminuria among those with low birth weight compared to those with normal birth weight [73]. A similar increased risk for nephropathy in low birth weight women with type 1 diabetes was also reported by Rossing and colleagues [74]. Finally, low birth weight was also shown to be associated with ESRD, with an OR of 1.4 for developing ESRD among those with a birth weight of <2.5 kg compared to those with normal birth weight [75]. These studies potentially show that obesity and low birth weight should be increasingly recognized as risk factors for CKD, and these factors should be considered in developing screening and surveillance programs.

Patterns of awareness and treatment of stage 1–4 CKD in the general population

There is growing evidence that the detection and treatment of earlier stages of diabetic [47] and nondiabetic kidney disease [76,77] can delay, if not prevent, further progression of kidney injury, and this evidence has been incorporated into clinical practice

Table 4.7 Race and ethnicity and risk of CKD.

Data source [reference]	Study population	Exposure	End point	Results
Jones *et al.* 2005 [46]	National Health and Nutrition Evaluation Survey (US, multiethnic)	Race	Albuminuria	Prevalence of albuminuria 50% higher in African Americans than in non-African Americans
Li *et al.* 2005 [66]	Population-based screening program (Hong Kong, Chinese)	Predictors of urinary abnormalities	Urinary abnormalities	Prevalence of 5% for proteinuria
Chadban *et al.* 2003 [110]	Cross-sectional study, Australians of European descent and Asians	Predictors of urinary abnormalities	Urinary abnormalities	Prevalence of 2.4% for proteinuria, 16% with either proteinuria, hematuria, or reduced GFR
Ramirez *et al.* 2003 [67]	Cross-sectional study, multiethnic	Clinical and demographic factors	Urinary abnormalities	Prevalence of 1.1% for proteinuria
Hsu *et al.* 2003 [56]	National Health and Nutrition Evaluation Survey and US Renal Data System (US, multiethnic)	Race	Development of ESRD	More aggressive disease and increased rate of progression of CKD contributes to higher incidence of ESRD in African Americans
Hall *et al.* 2005 [68]	299,168 adult members of an integrated health care delivery system who underwent screening in 1964 and 1985 (Kaiser Permanente) (US, multiethnic)	Race and ethnicity	Incidence of ESRD	Age-adjusted rate of ESRD 14.0/100,000 PY in Asians (10.5–18.5); 7.9/100,000 PY in whites (6.5–9.6); 43.4/100,000 PY in blacks (36.6–51.4)
Klag *et al.* 1997 [63]	Men screened for entry into MRFIT study	Race and ethnicity	Incidence of ESRD	Age-adjusted ESRD incidence 13.9 and 44.2/100,000 yrs for white and black populations, respectively, after adjustments RR reduced to 1.9 in blacks vs whites
Karter *et al.* 2002 [69]	Prospective cohort study of 62,432 diabetic members of a health insurance plan (US, multiethnic)	Race	Risk of ESRD and other diabetic complications	Adjusted risk of 1.85 (1.4–2.4) for diabetic ESRD among Asians compared to whites
McClellan *et al.* 2006 [70]	Nationally representative, population-based cohort of individuals ≥45 yrs old	Race	GFR	Distribution of GFR significantly different between black and white participants, whereas CKD more prevalent among white than black participants at relatively lower grades of CKD; odds of lower GFR for blacks vs whites increased with more advanced degrees of CKD
Toto 2004 [103]	AASK, prospective randomized controlled trial of use of antihypertensive regimens in 1100 nondiabetic African American adults (US)	Effect of aggressive blood pressure vs usual blood pressure lowering in African Americans with hypertensive nephrosclerosis using three different regimens	Rate of decline of GFR	No difference in rate of decline and renal outcomes between blood pressure groups or between antihypertensive regimens; those assigned to ramipril had significantly lower ESRD and composite renal outcome

Abbreviation: PY, person-years.

guidelines [50,78,79], and the contemporary management of CKD is discussed in section 6 of this textbook.

Despite the well-documented benefits of early detection and treatment of CKD, population-based studies have found that awareness of impaired kidney function among individuals with CKD is minimal, and this lack of awareness should be considered a potential risk factor for progressive CKD. Analyses of the NHANES data found that 8% of participants with stage 3 CKD responded that they had been told by a health care provider that they had "weak or failing kidneys" (excluding kidney stones, bladder

Table 4.8 Other potential risk factors for CKD.

Risk factor and data source [reference]	Study population	Exposure	End point	Results
Obesity				
Ejerblad *et al.* 2006 [71]	Population-based case–control study of incident moderately severe CKF in Sweden	BMI at age 25 and highest lifetime BMI	Creatinine >3.4 in men, >2.8 in women	BMI ≥25 kg/m² at age 29 associated with 3-fold increased risk of CKD; BMI ≥30 among men and ≥35 in women anytime during lifetime had a 3- to 4-fold increased risk. High BMI increased risk of GFR in 5th or lower percentile; each unit increase in BMI SD was associated with 1.2-fold increased risk for new-onset kidney disease
Fox *et al.* 2004 [111]	Framingham Offspring cohort	BMI	GFR	A continuous increase in risk of ESRD with increasing BMI primarily in men; higher BMI associated with higher degrees of albumin excretion, primarily in men
Iseki *et al.* 2004 [21]	Okinawa longitudinal cohort study	BMI	CKD	BMI ≥30 associated with RR of 1.77 for CKD; after adjusting for diabetes and other predictors, remained significant at 1.57
Cirillo *et al.* 1998 [112]	Population-based cohort study	Predictors of albuminuria	Microalbuminuria	Higher baseline BMI associated with increased risk for CKD, OR of 1.45 in those with BMI >26.6 vs those with BMI <22.7
Hallan *et al.* 2006 [113]	Cross-sectional survey of Nord-Trondelag County (HUNT Study); 30,485 men and 34,708 women	BMI	CKD	Each 1 unit increase in BMI was associated with 5% increase in CKD risk
Gelber *et al.* 2005 [114]	Physicians Health Study, cohort study of 11,104 healthy men	BMI	GFR	Those with weight gain >10% had increase in CKD risk to 1.27 compared to those with weight that remained within 5% of their baseline
Low birth weight				
Yudkin *et al.* 2001 [72]	Community-based populations	BW, length, and ponderal index	Albuminuria	Those in the lowest third for ponderal index had an OR of 3.1 for microalbuminuria compared to those in highest third for ponderal index
Nelson *et al.* 1998 [73]	Pima Indians with type 2 diabetes	BW	Albuminuria	As compared to those with normal BW, those with low BW had an OR of 2.3 and those with high BW had an OR of 3.2
Rossing *et al.* 1995 [74]	Type 1 diabetes	BW percentile	Nephropathy	Among women with IDDM, 75% had evidence of nephropathy among those whose BW was ≤2.7 kg (10th percentile) compared to 35% in those with BW ≥4 kg (90th percentile)
Lackland *et al.* 2002 [75]	Medicaid beneficiaries in a US region	BW	ESRD	Among those with BW <2.5 kg, OR for developing ESRD was 1.4 compared to those with normal birth weight

Abbreviations: CRF, chronic kidney failure; BW, birth weight; IDDM, insulin-dependent diabetes mellitus.

infections, or incontinence) [78]. Awareness of CKD increased as the stage of CKD increased and was higher among individuals with albuminuria and among women [78]. Similar low levels of awareness of impaired kidney function and proteinuria have been reported for other high-risk populations [50].

The lack of reported awareness among individuals with stage 3–4 CKD is consistent with reports that clinicians frequently fail to recognize evidence of injury and impaired kidney function among their patients [79,80] and that patients in North America and Europe with CKD may not be referred early for specialist care [81,82], which may be associated with less than optimal care of CKD [83]. There is evidence that the care of CKD patients by both primary care physicians and kidney specialists is characterized by inadequately managed hypertension [84] and anemia [85] and under prescription of cardiovascular medications [86,87] as well as routine preventive care [88]. Recently there has been interest both in Europe and North America in the role of clinics dedicated to the management of CKD [89] with growing evidence that such care is better in quality [84,90,91] and may be associated with improved outcomes, including delayed progression of CKD [92–94].

Cost-effectiveness analyses for CKD screening

Another important consideration in determining the appropriateness of a screening program is its cost-effectiveness [30]. Because of the lack of studies that evaluate the effectiveness of screening programs in improving clinical and economic outcomes, the limited number of publications that have addressed the issue of cost-effectiveness of screening have largely been based on computer simulation models. Furthermore, the focus of the literature is on cost-effectiveness of screening for nephropathy in the context of diabetes mellitus.

Diabetic nephropathy

Without exception, all studies on the cost-effectiveness of screening for nephropathy in patients with diabetes, whether type 1 or type 2, have been based on simulation models as summarized in Table 4.9. Simulation models are subject to a number of limitations, including dependence on key assumptions, such as the rate of progression of various stages of CKD as well as the efficacy of treatment in reducing the risk of progression. Nevertheless, the findings of the cost-effectiveness analyses for screening for diabetic nephropathy are overwhelmingly in favor of either one of two strategies: routine screening for microalbuminuria followed by treatment, or routine treatment with an ACEi or angiotensin receptor blocker (ARB) upon diagnosis of diabetes mellitus. Clearly dominated, that is, not deemed to be cost-effective, is screening for gross proteinuria.

Studies that have evaluated the cost-effectiveness of screening for diabetic nephropathy are shown in Table 4.9. Of further importance for study is the routine treatment of patients with diabetes with antiproteinuric therapy. Golan and others, modeling patients with newly diagnosed type 2 diabetes mellitus, demonstrated that routine treatment had the lowest progression to ESRD or death and had a marginal cost-effectiveness of only $7500 for every quality-adjusted life year (QALY) compared to the strategy of screening for microalbuminuria followed by treatment [95]. Similarly, Kiberd and Jindal showed that routine treatment with ACE inhibitors 5 years after diagnosis of type 1 diabetes produced the longest life expectancy, more quality-adjusted life years, and had the lowest cost of care if ACE treatment were assumed to reduce microalbuminuria development by 26% [96]. These analyses raise the question of whether there is a potential value in designing a clinical trial that compares routine treatment with ACEI or ARB on diagnosis of type 2 diabetes, or after several years of having type 1 diabetes, with the current standard of care that includes annual screening for microalbuminuria.

Nondiabetic nephropathy

In contrast to screening for type 1 and 2 diabetic nephropathy, cost-effectiveness studies for the screening for proteinuria in a nondiabetic population are extremely limited. Boulware and colleagues examined the cost-effectiveness of annual screening for proteinuria in the absence of diabetes mellitus [97]. In this study, routine screening with a urine dipstick test during annual physical examination tests was compared with incidental testing or testing during symptom development. The authors demonstrated that in the absence of diabetes or hypertension, routine screening for proteinuria was not within the range considered cost-effective, with an estimated cost of $282,818/QALY gained. Only in patients

60 years or older did screening in the absence of hypertension or diabetes approach a cost-effectiveness range, with $53,372/QALY gained. In contrast, routine screening in the presence of hypertension was highly favorable, with a cost of $18,621/QALY gained, and this was cost-effective even with screening at 30 years of age. Screening in patients with diabetes was cost-saving, with a savings of $217 and gain of 0.1 QALY/person. Indeed, this analysis suggests the value of screening high-risk populations, in that screening for proteinuria only in the presence of hypertension, diabetes, or older age is cost-effective. This is in marked contrast to the findings of Craig *et al.* who showed that a single opportunistic dipstick screening results in significant cost savings [98]. The differences in the conclusions of these two analyses demonstrate the limitations of simulation models given that analyses are sensitive to model assumptions, including reliability and reproducibility of screening tools and the natural history of disease progression [99]. Another important shortcoming of existing cost-effectiveness studies is the failure to account for the benefit gained from preventing the cardiovascular outcomes of proteinuria. Thus, these evaluations of the cost-effectiveness of screening using simulation models only highlight the lack of appropriately designed studies to evaluate the outcomes of screening for CKD.

Discussion and recommendations for future research

Evidence for improving population outcomes through the implementation of population-based CKD screening programs is not convincing. However, the value of surveillance systems in tracking trends of disease and overall disease burden should be considered. In addition, though definitive randomized clinical trials evaluating the effectiveness of screening programs in reducing ESRD rates may not be feasible, review of the extensive literature on the outcomes of CKD in populations at high risk, such as those in certain clinical and demographic subgroups, warrants the consideration of targeted screening and intervention among high-risk populations.

Other important questions on the value of screening for CKD in the population remain, including 1) determining the optimal time to initiate screening in high-risk populations, 2) identifying an appropriate screening frequency that balances cost and utility of screening, 3) determining whether it is truly clinically feasible and appropriate to treat all diabetic patients upon diagnosis with an ACEi or ARB rather than to perform screening for evidence of early or overt nephropathy, 4) performing follow-up of programs that focus on screening high-risk populations, and 5) defining the harms and costs of screening.

In evaluating the true increase in risk for CKD in certain demographic and clinical populations, additional studies on the following aspects should be considered, as summarized by Ramirez [99]: 1) continued evaluation and examination of clinical biomarkers and genetic markers for the occurrence and progression of CKD, 2) development of race- and ethnicity-specific prediction

Table 4.9 Cost-effectiveness analysis of screening for diabetic nephropathy.

Data source [reference]	Comparison groups	Diabetes type and population	Outcome
Kiberd et al. 1999 [115]	Annual screening for microalbuminuria 1 yr after diagnosis of diabetes and then treatment with ACEi, vs treat all with ACEi 1 yr after diagnosis	Type 2, Pima Indians	If routine ACEi treatment reduced development of microalbuminuria by 9% and reduced progression of microalbuminuria to macroalbuminuria by 50%, cost per life year gained was $15,000
Herman et al. 2003 [117]	Treatment with losartan for hypertension and nephropathy, vs conventional antihypertensive treatment (non-ACEi, non-ARB)	Type 2 diabetes with nephropathy and hypertenison; analysis of the RENAAL clinical trial	Treatment with losartan resulted in reduction in ESRD days by 33.6 over 3.5 yrs, translating to net cost savings per patient of $3522 over 3.5 yrs
Palmer et al. 2004 [118]	Early treatment with irbesartan (microalbuminuria only), late treatment with irbesartan (overt diabetic nephropathy) vs standard antihypertensive treatment (non-ACEi, non-ARB)	Type 2 diabetes with nephropathy and hypertension; analysis of the IDNT data	Compared to standard therapy, early irbesartan treatment resulted in savings of $11.9 million; late irbesartan resulted in savings of $3.3 million for every 1000 patients
Golan et al. 2000 [95]	Routine treatment with ACEi, screening for microalbuminuria or screening for gross proteinuria	Patients with newly diagnosed type 2 diabetes	Routine treatment of newly diagnosed diabetes had lowest progression to ESRD or death, screening for gross proteinuria had lowest benefit and highest cost; marginal cost-effectiveness of routine treatment was $7500 per QALY compared with screening for microalbuminuria
Kiberd & Jindal 1998 [96]	Screening for microalbuminuria then treatment, routine ACEi treatment 5 yrs after diagnosis, vs a risk-based strategy in which high-risk patients received routine treatment and low-risk patients received treatment only upon abnormalities	Type 1 diabetes	Routine treatment with ACEi 5 yrs after diagnosis produced longest life expectancy, more QALYs, and had lowest associated cost if routine drug therapy reduced microalbuminuria development by 26%.
Siegel et al. 1992 [120]	Screening for microalbuminuria then treatment vs screening for gross proteinuria and treatment	Type 1 diabetes	Screening for microalbuminuria and treatment cost $7900 to $16,500 per QALY, within range considered cost-effective
Borch-Johnsen et al. 1993 [121]	Screening and intervention program vs no screening	Type 1 diabetes	Increase in life expectancy by 4–14 yrs depending on effectiveness of ACEi treatment, estimated 33–67% effectiveness
Kiberd et al. 1999 [116]	Screening for microalbuminuria vs screening for gross proteinuria and hypertension	Type 1 diabetes	Screening for microalbuminuria would produce an additionally QALY at an incremental cost of $27,042 compared to screening for gross proteinuria and hypertension
Palmer et al. 2000 [119]	Modeled seven different complications of diabetes; evaluated nephropathy management including screening for microalbuminuria and then treatment	Type 1 diabetes	Screening for microalbuminuria and treatment dominate altenatives, as this was both cost-saving and life-saving
Dong et al. 2004 [122]	Treatment with ACEi immediately following diagnosis of type 1 diabetes vs treatment after onset of microalbuminuria	Type 1 diabetes	Routine treatment with ACEi following diagnosis is cost-effective; estimated cost per QALY gained is $13,814 if onset of diabetes is 20 yrs and HbA1c is 9%; cost is $39,350 per QALY gained if onset is at 25 yrs and HbA1c is 7%
Rodby et al. 1996 [123]	Compared treatment of diabetic nephropathy with captopril vs placebo	Types 1 and 2 diabetes, reanalysis of clinical trial (Collaborative Study Group)	Treatment with captopril was cost-savings with benefit of $32,550 direct costs saved for IDDM and $9900 direct costs saved for NIDDM per patient

Abbreviations: IDDM, insulin-dependent diabetes mellitus; NIDDM, non-insulin-dependent diabetes mellitus.

equations for the occurrence and progression of CKD, 3) an evaluation of the generalizability of intervention strategies across populations, 4) development of a CKD surveillance model (and not just an ESRD registry), among others. Both the KDIGO position statement and the ISN Consensus Workshops on Prevention have also released similar position statements on additional studies required in the field of kidney disease surveillance, screening, and prevention [100,101].

References

1 National Kidney Foundation. K/DOQI clinical practice guidelines for chronic kidney disease: evaluation, classification and stratification. *Am J Kidney Dis* 2002; **39(Suppl 1):** S1–S266.

2 Gerstein HC, Mann JF, Yi Q, Zinman B, Dinneen SF, Hoogwerf B *et al.* Albuminuria and risk of cardiovascular events, death and heart failure in diabetic and nondaibetic individuals. *JAMA* 2001; **186:** 421–426.

3 Manjunath G, Tighiouart H, Coresh J, Macleod B, Salem DN, Griffith JL *et al.* Level of kidney function as a risk factor for cardiovascular outcomes in the elderly. *Kidney Int* 2003; **63:** 1121–1129.

4 Ruilope LM, Salvetti A, Jamerson K, Hansson L, Warnold I, Wedel H *et al.* Renal function and intensive lowering of blood pressure in hypertensive participants of the Hypertension Optimal Treatment (HOT) study. *J Am Soc Nephrol* 2001; **12:** 218–225.

5 Culleton BF, Larson MG, Wilson PW, Evans JC, Parfrey PS, Levy D. Cardiovacular disease and mortality in a community-based cohort with mild renal insufficiency. *Kidney Int* 1999; **56:** 2214–2219.

6 Jacques PF, Bostom AM, Wilson PW, Rich S, Rosenberg IH, Selhub J. Determinants of plasma total homocysteine concentration in the Framingham Offspring Cohort. *Am J Clin Nutr* 2001; **73:** 613–621.

7 Shillaci G, Reboldi G, Verdecchia P. High normal serum creatinine concentration is a predictor of cardiovascular risk in essential hypertension. *Arch Intern Med* 2001; **161:** 886–891.

8 Mann JF, Berstein HC, Pogue J, Bosch J, Yusuf S. Renal insufficiency as a predictor of cardiovascular outcomes and the impact of ramipril. The HOPE randomized trial. *Ann Intern Med* 2001; **134:** 629–636.

9 Manjunath G, Tighiouart H, Ibrahim H, MacLeod B, Salem DN, Griffith JL *et al.* Level of kidney function as a risk factor for atherosclerotic cardiovascular disease in the community. *J Am Coll Cardiol* 2003; **41:** 47–55.

10 Coresh J, Astor BC, Greene T, Eknoyan G, Levey AS. Prevalence of chronic kidney disease and decreased kidney function in the adult US population. *Am J Kidney Dis* 2003; **41:** 1–12.

11 Agodoa LY, Appel L, Bakris G, Beck G, Bourgoignie J, Briggs JP *et al.* Effect of ramipril vs amlodipine on renal outcomes in hypertensive nephrosclerosis a randomized controlled trial. *JAMA* 2001; **285:** 2719–2728.

12 Ruggenenti P, Gaspari F, Perna A, Remuzzi G. Cross-sectional longitudinal study of spot morning urine protein. *BMJ* 1998; **316:** 504–509.

13 Klahr S, Levey AS, Beck GJ, Caggiula AW, Hunsicker L, Kusek JW *et al.* The effects of dietary protein restriction and blood-pressure control on the progression of chronic renal disease. *N Engl J Med* 1994; **330:** 877–884.

14 Nelson RG, Benett RH, Beck GJ, Tan M, Knowler WC, Mitch WE *et al.* Development and progression of renal disease in Pima Indians with non-insulin dependent diabetes mellitus. *N Engl J Med* 1996; **335:** 1636–1642.

15 Nosadini R, Velussi M, Brocco E, Bruseghin M, Abaterusso C, Saller A *et al.* Course of renal function in type 2 diabetic patients with abnormalities of albumin excretion rate. *Diabetes* 2000; **49:** 476–484.

16 Rachmani R, Levi Z, Lidar M, Slavachevski J, Half-Onn E, Ravid M. Considerations about the threshold vale of microalbuminuria in patients with diabetes mellitus: lessons from an 8-year follow-up study of 599 patients. *Diabetes Res Clin Pract* 2000; **49:** 187–194.

17 Lewis EJ, Hunsicker LG, Clarke WR, Berl T, Pohl MA, Lewis JB *et al.* Renoprotective effect of the angiotensin-receptor antagonist irbesartan in patients with nephropathy due to type 2 diabetes. *N Engl J Med* 2001; **345:** 851–860.

18 Brenner BM, Cooper ME, de Zeeuw D, Keane WF, Mitch WE, Parving HH *et al.* Effects of losartan on renal and cardiovascular outcomes in patients with type 2 diabetes and nephropathy. *N Engl J Med* 2001; **345:** 861–869.

19 Ruggenenti P, Perna A, Gherardi G, Benini R, Remuzzi G. Chronic proteinuric nephropathies. *Am J Kidney Dis* 2000; **35:** 1155–1165.

20 Verhave JC, Gansevoort RT, Hillege HL, Bakker SJL, De Zeeuw D, De Jong PE *et al.* An elevated urinary albumin excretion predicts de novo development of renal function impairment in the general population. *Kidney Int* 2004; **66(Suppl 92):** S18–S21.

21 Iseki K, Ikemiya Y, Iseki C, Takishita S. Proteinuria and the risk of developing end-stage renal disease. *Kidney Int* 2003; **63:** 1468–1474.

22 Ishani A, Grandits GA, Grimm RH *et al.* Association of dipstick proteinuria, estimated glomerular filtration rate, and hematocrit with 25-year incidence of end-stage renal disease in the Multiple Risk Factor Intervention Trial. *J Am Soc Nephrol* 2006; **17:** 1444–1452.

23 Hillege HL, Janssen WM, Bak AA, Diercks GF, Grobbee DE, Crijns HJ *et al.* Microalbuminuria is common, also in an nondiabetic, nonhypertensive population, and an independent indicator of cardiovascular risk factors and cardiovascular morbidity. *J Intern Med* 2001; **249:** 519–526.

24 Romundstad S, Holmen J, Kvenild K, Hallan H, Ellekjaer H. Microalbuminuria and all-cause mortality in 2089 apparently healthy individuals: a 4.4-year follow-up study. The Nord-Trundelag Health Study (HUNT), Norway. *Am J Kidney Dis* 2003; **42:** 466–473.

25 Yuyun MF, Khaw KET, Luben R, Welch A, Bingham S, Day NE *et al.* Microalbuminuria independently predicts all-cause and cardiovascular mortality in a British population. The European Prospective Investigation into Cancer in Norfolk (EPIC-Norfolk) population study. *Int J Epidemiol* 2004; **33:** 189–198.

26 Mann JFE, Yi QL, Gerstein HC. Albuminuria as a predictor of cardiovascular and renal outcomes in people with known atherosclerotic cardiovascular disease. *Kidney Int* 2004; **66(Suppl 92):** S59–S62.

27 Wachtell K, Ibsen H, Olsen MH, Borch-Johnsen K, Lindholm LH, Mogensen CE *et al.* Albuminuria and cardiovascular risk in hypertensive patients with left ventricular hypertrophy. The LIFE study. *Ann Intern Med* 2003; **139:** 902–906.

28 Rothman KJ, Greenland S, editors. *Modern Epidemiology*, 2nd edn. Lippincott-Raven, Philadelphia, 1998; 435–438.

29 Morrison AS. Screening. In: Rothman KJ, Greenland S, editors, *Modern Epidemiology*, 2nd edn. Lippincott-Raven, Philadelphia, 1998; 499–518.

30 McClellan WM, Ramirez SPB, Jurkovitz C. Screening for kidney disease: unresolved issues. *J Am Soc Nephrol* 2003; **14:** S81–S87.

31 Kochanek KD, Smith BL. Deaths: preliminary data for 2002. *Nat Vital Stat Rep* 2004; **52:** 1–47.

32 Patel UD, Young EW, Ojo AO, Hayward RA. CKD progression and mortality among older patients with diabetes. *Am J Kidney Dis* 2005; **46(3):** 406–414.

33 Petersen LA, Normand S-L, Daley J, McNeil BJ. Outcome of myocardial infarction in Veterans Health Administration patients as compared with Medicare patients. *N Engl J Med* 2000; **343**: 1934–1941.

34 Go AS, Chertow GM, Fan D, McCulloch CE, Hsu CY. Chronic kidney disease and the risks of death, cardiovascular events and hospitalization. *N Engl J Med* 2004; **351**: 1296–1305.

35 Shlipak MG, Katz R, Sarnak MJ, Fried LF, Newman AB, Stehman-Breen C *et al.* Cystatin C and prognosis for cardiovascular and kidney outcomes in elderly persons without chronic kidney disease. *Ann Intern Med* 2006; **145**: 237–246.

36 Young JH, Klag MJ, Muntner P, Whyte JL, Pahor M, Coresh J. Blood pressure and decline in kidney function: findings from the Systolic Hypertension n the Elderly Program (SHEP). *J Am Soc Nephrol* 2002; **13**: 2776–2782.

37 Perneger TV, Klag MJ, Feldman HI, Whelton PK. Projections of hypertension-related renal disease in middle-aged residents of the United States. *JAMA* 1993; **269**: 1272–1277.

38 Segura J, Campo C, Gil P, Roldan C, Visil L, Rodicio JL *et al.* Development of chronic kidney disease and cardiovascular prognosis in essential hypertensive patients. *J Am Soc Nephrol* 2004; **15**: 1616–1622.

39 Wesstuch JM, Dowrkin LD. Does essential hypertension cause end-stage renal disease? *Kidney Int* 1992; **41(Suppl 36)**: S33–S37.

40 Sarnak MJ, Levey AS, Schoolwerth AC *et al.* Kidney disease as a risk factor for development of cardiovascular disease: a statement from the American Heart Association Councils on Kidney in Cardiovascular Disease, High Blood Pressure Research, Clinical Cardiology and Epidemiology and Prevention. *Circulation* 2003; **108**: 2154–2169.

41 Foley RN, Murray AM, Li S, Herzog CA, McBean AM, Eggers PW *et al.* Chronic kidney disease and the risk for cardiovascular disease, renal replacement, and death in the United States Medicare population, 1998 to 1999. *J Am Soc Nephrol* 2005; **16**: 489–495.

42 Roberts MA, Hare DL, Ratnaike S, Ierino FL. Cardiovascular biomarkers in CKD: pathophysiology and implications for clinical management of cardiac disease. *Am J Kid Dis* 2006; **48**: 341–360.

43 Mann JF, Gerstein HC, Yi Q, Lonn EM, Hoogwerf BJ, Rashkow A *et al.* Development of renal disease in people at high cardiovascular risk: results of the HOPE randomized study. *J Am Soc Nephrol* 2003; **14**: 641–647.

44 McClellan WM, Langston RD, Presley R. Medicare patients with cardiovascular disease have a high prevalence of chronic kidney disease and a high rate of progression to end-stage renal disease. *J Am Soc Nephrol* 2004; **15**: 1912–1919.

45 Brosius FC, III, Hostetter TH, Kelepouris E, Mitsnefes MM, Moe SM, Moore MA *et al.* Detection of chronic kidney disease in patients with or at increased risk of cardiovascular disease. A science advisory from the American Heart Association Kidney and Cardiovascular Disease Council; the Councils on High Blood Pressure Research, Cardiovascular Disease in the Young, and Epidemiology and Prevention; and the Quality of Care and Outcomes Research Interdisciplinary Working Group developed in collaboration with the National Kidney Foundation. *Circulation* 2006; **114**: 1083–1087.

46 Jones CA, Krolewski AS, Rogus J, Xue JL, Collins A, Warram JH. Epidemic of end-stage renal disease in people with diabetes in the United States population: do we know the cause? *Kidney Int* 2005; **67**: 1684–1691.

47 American Diabetes Association. Nephropathy in diabetes. *Diabetes Care* 2004; **27(Suppl 1)**: S79–S83.

48 Kramer HJ, Nguyen OD, Curhan G, Hsu CY. Renal insufficiency in the absence of albuminuria and retinopathy among adults with type 2 diabetes mellitus. *JAMA* 2003; **289**: 3273–3277.

49 MacIsaac RJ, Tsalamandria C, Pangiotopoulos S, Smith TJ, McNeil KJ, Jerums G. Nonalbuminuric renal insufficiency in type 2 diabetes. *Diabetes Care* 2004; **27**: 195–200.

50 Jurkovitz C, Franch H, Shoham D, Bellenger J, McClellan W. Family members of patients treated for ESRD have high rates of undetected kidney disease. *Am J Kidney Dis* 2002; **40**: 1173–1178.

51 Freedman BI, Soucie JM, Kenderees B, Krisher J, Garrett LE, Caruana RJ *et al.* Family history of end-stage renal disease does not predict dialytic survival. *Am J Kidney Dis* 2001; **38**: 547–552.

52 Ferguson R, Grim CE, Opgenorth TJ. A familial risk of chronic renal failure among blacks on dialysis? *J Clin Epidemiol* 1988; **41**: 1189–1196.

53 O'Dea DF, Murphy SW, Hefferton D, Parfrey PS. Higher risk for renal failure in first-degree relatives of white patients with end-stage renal disease: a population-based study. *Am J Kidney Dis* 1998; **32**: 794–801.

54 Lei HH, Perneger TV, Klag MJ, Whelton PK, Coresh J. Familial aggregation of renal disease in a population-based case-control study. *J Am Soc Nephrol* 1998; **9**: 1270–1276.

55 United States Renal Data System: 2004 Annual Data Report. *Am J Kidney Dis* 2005; **45(Suppl 1)**: 8–2880.

56 Hsu CY, Lin F, Vittinghoff E, Shlipak MG. Racial differences in the progression from chronic renal insufficiency to end-stage renal disease in the United States. *J Am Soc Nephrol* 2003; **14**: 2902–2907.

57 Lopes AA, Port FK. The low birth weight hypothesis as a plausible explanation for the black/white differences in hypertension, non-insulin dependent diabetes, and end-stage renal disease. *Am J Kidney Dis* 1995; **25**: 350–356.

58 Perneger TV, Whelton PK, Klag MJ. Race and end-stage renal disease. Socioeconomic status and access to health care as mediating factors. *Arch Intern Med* 1995; **155**: 1201–1208.

59 Luyckx VA, Brenner BM. Low birth weight, nephron number and kidney disease. *Kidney Int* 2005; **68(Suppl 97)**: S68–S77.

60 Fang J, Madhavan S, Alderman MH. The influence of maternal hypertension on low birth weight: differences among ethnic populations. *Ethn Dis* 1999; **9**: 369–376.

61 Norris KC, Agodoa LY. Unraveling the racial disparities associated with kidney disease. *Kidney Int* 2005; **68**: 914–924.

62 Hajjar I, Kotchen TA. Trends in prevalence, awareness, treatment and control of hypertension in the United States, 1988–2000. *JAMA* 2003; **290**: 199–206.

63 Klag MJ, Whelton PK, Randall BL, Neaton JD, Brancati FL, Stamler J. End-stage renal disease in African-American and white men. 16 year-MRFIT findings. *JAMA* 1997; **277**: 1293–1298.

64 Henry J. Kaiser Family Foundation. *Key Facts: Race, Ethnicity and Medical Care.* Kaiser Family Foundation, Menlo Park, CA, 2003.

65 Jones CA, Francis M, Eberhardt MS, *et al.* Microalbuminuria in the US population. Third National Health and Nutrition Examination Survey. *Am J Kidney Dis* 2005; **29**: 445–459.

66 Li PKT, Kwan BCH, Leung CB, *et al.* Prevalence of silent kidney disease in Hong Kong: the Screening for Hong Kong Asymptomatic Renal Population and Evaluation (SHARE) program. *Kidney Int Suppl* 2005; **96**: S36–S40.

67 Ramirez SP, McClellan W, Port FK, Hsu SI. Risk factors for proteinuria in a large, multiracial southeast Asian population. *J Am Soc Nephrol* 2003; **13**: 1907–1917.

68 Hall YN, Hsu CY, Iribarren C, Darbinian J, McCulloch CE, Go AS. The conundrum of increased burden of end-stage renal disease in Asians. *Kidney Int* 2005; **68:** 2310–2316.

69 Karter AJ, Ferrara A, Liu JY, Moffett HH, Ackerson LM, Selby JV. Ethnic disparities in diabetic complications in an insured population. *JAMA* 2002; **287:** 2519–2527.

70 McClellan W, Warnock DG, McClure L, Campbell RC, Newsome BB, Howard V *et al.* Racial differences in the prevalence of chronic kidney disease among participants in the Reasons for Geographic and Racial Differences in Stroke (REGARDS) cohort study. *J Am Soc Nephrol* 2006; **17:** 1710–1715.

71 Ejerblad E, Fored CM, Lindblad P, Fryzek J, McLaughlin JK, Nyren O. Obesity and risk for chronic renal failure. *J Am Soc Nephrol* 2006; **17:** 195–1702.

72 Yudkin JS, Martyn CN, Phillips DI, Gale CR. Association of microalbuminuria with intra-uterine growth retardation. *Nephron* 2001; **89:** 309–314.

73 Nelson RG, Morgenstern H, Bennett PH. Birth weight and renal disease in Pima Indians with type 2 diabetes mellitus. *Am J Epidemiol* 1998; **148:** 650–656.

74 Rossing P, Tarnow L, Nielsen FS, Hansen BV, Brenner BM, Parving HH. Low birth weight: a risk factor for development of diabetic nephropathy? *Diabetes* 1995; **44:** 1405–1407.

75 Lackland DT, Egan BM, Syddall HE, Barker DJ. Association between birth weight and antihypertensive medication in black and white Medicaid recipients. *Hypertension* 2002; **39:** 179–183.

76 Chobanian AV, Bakris GL, Black HR, Cushman WC, Green LA, Izzo JL, Jr., *et al.* Seventh Report of the Joint National Committee on Prevention, Detection, Evaluation, and Treatment of High Blood Pressure. *Hypertension* 2003; **42:** 1206–1252.

77 Levey AS, Coresh J, Balk E, Kausz AT, Levin A, Steffes MW *et al.* National Kidney Foundation practice guidelines for chronic kidney disease: evaluation, classification, and stratification. *Ann Intern Med* 2003; **139:** 137–147.

78 Coresh J, Byrd-Holt D, Astor BC, Briggs JP, Eggers PW, Lacher DA *et al.* Chronic kidney disease awareness, prevalence, and trends among U.S. adults, 1999 to 2000. *J Am Soc Nephrol* 2005; **16:** 180–188.

79 Stevens LA, Fares G, Fleming J, Martin D, Murthy K, Qiu J *et al.* Low rates of testing and diagnostic codes usage in a commercial clinical laboratory: evidence for lack of physician awareness of chronic kidney disease. *J Am Soc Nephrol* 2005; **16:** 2439–2348.

80 Akbari A, Swedko PJ, Clark HD, Hogg W, Lemelin J, Magner P *et al.* Detection of chronic kidney disease with laboratory reporting of estimated glomerular filtration rate and an educational program. *Arch Intern Med* 2004; **164:** 1788–1792.

81 John R, Webb M, Young A, Stevens PE. Unreferred chronic kidney disease: a longitudinal study. *Am J Kidney Dis* 2004; **43:** 825–835.

82 Roderick P, Jones C, Tomson C, Mason J. Late referral for dialysis: improving the management of chronic renal disease. *QJM* 2002; **95:** 363–370.

83 Cleveland DR, Jindal KK, Hirsch DJ, Kiberd BA. Quality of prereferral care in patients with chronic renal insufficiency. *Am J Kidney Dis* 2002; **40:** 30–36.

84 Minutolo R, De Nicola L, Zamboli P, Chiodini P, Signoriello G, Toderico C *et al.* Management of hypertension in patients with CKD: differences between primary and tertiary care settings. *Am J Kidney Dis* 2005; **46:** 18–25.

85 Horl WH, Macdougall IC, Rossert J, Rutkowski B, Wauters JP, Valderrabano F *et al.* Predialysis survey on anemia management: patient referral. *Am J Kidney Dis* 2003; **41:** 49–61.

86 Bailie GR, Eisele G, Liu L, Roys E, Kiser M, Finkelstein F *et al.* Patterns of medication use in the RRI-CKD study: focus on medications with cardiovascular effects. *Nephrol Dial Transplant* 2005; **20:** 1110–1115.

87 Reddan DN, Szczech L, Bhapkar MV, Moliterno DJ, Califf RM, Ohman EM *et al.* Renal function, concomitant medication use and outcomes following acute coronary syndromes. *Nephrol Dial Transplant* 2005; **20:** 2105–2112.

88 Kausz AT, Guo H, Pereira BJ, Collins AJ, Gilbertson DT. General medical care among patients with chronic kidney disease: opportunities for improving outcomes. *J Am Soc Nephrol* 2005; **16:** 3092–3101.

89 St. Peter WL, Schoolwerth AC, McGowan T, McClellan WM. Chronic kidney disease: issues and establishing programs and clinics for improved patient outcomes. *Am J Kidney Dis* 2003; **41:** 903–924.

90 Herget-Rosenthal S, Quellmann T, Linden C, Reinhardt W, Philipp T, Kribben A. Management of advanced chronic kidney disease in primary care: current data from Germany. *Int J Clin Pract* 2006; **60:** 941–948.

91 Jones C, Roderick P, Harris S, Rogerson M. An evaluation of a shared primary and secondary care nephrology service for managing patients with moderate to advanced CKD. *Am J Kidney Dis* 2006; **47:** 103–114.

92 Curtis BM, Ravani P, Malberti F, Kennett F, Taylor PA, Djurdjev O *et al.* The short- and long-term impact of multi-disciplinary clinics in addition to standard nephrology care on patient outcomes. *Nephrol Dial Transplant* 2005; **20:** 147–154.

93 Jones C, Roderick P, Harris S, Rogerson M. Decline in kidney function before and after nephrology referral and the effect on survival in moderate to advanced chronic kidney disease. *Nephrol Dial Transplant* 2006; **21:** 2133–2143.

94 Martinez-Ramirez HR, Jalomo-Martinez B, Cortes-Sanabria L, Rojas-Campos E, Barragan G, Alfaro G *et al.* Renal function preservation in type 2 diabetes mellitus patients with early nephropathy: a comparative prospective cohort study between primary health care doctors and a nephrologist. *Am J Kidney Dis* 2006; **47:** 78–87.

95 Golan L, Birkmeyer JD, Welch HG. The cost-effectiveness of treating all patients with type 2 diabetes with angiotensin-conveting enzyme inhibitors. *Ann Intern Med* 2000; **131:** 660–667.

96 Kiberd BA, Jindal K. Routine treatment of insulin-dependent diabetic patients with ACE inhibitors to prevent renal failure: an economic evaluation. *Am J Kid Dis* 1998; **31:** 49–54.

97 Boulware LE, Jaar BG, Tarver-Carr ME, Brancati FL, Powe NR. Screening for proteinuria in US adults: a cost-effectiveness analysis. *JAMA* 2003; **290:** 3101–3114.

98 Craig JC, Barratt A, Cumming R, Irwig L, Salkeld G. Feasibility of the early detection and treatment of renal disease by mass screening. *Intern Med J* 2002; **32:** 6–14.

99 Ramirez SPB *et al.* First International Summit on Kidney Disease Prevention, 25–27 July 2002: consensus document. *J Am Soc Nephrol* 2003; **14:** S205–S207.

100 Levey AS, Eckardt KU, Tsukamoto Y, *et al.* Definition and classification of chronic kidney disease: a position statement from Kidney Disease: Improving Global Outcomes (KDIGO). *Kidney Int* 2003; **67:** 2089–2100.

101 Li PKT, Weenin JJ, Dirks J, *et al.* A report with consensus statements of the International Society of Nephrology 2004 Consensus Workshop on Prevention of Progression of Renal Disese, Hong Kong, June 29, 2004. *Kidney Int* 2005; **67(Suppl 94):** S2–S7.

102 Toto R, Mitchell H, Smith R, Lee HC, McIntire D, Pettinger WA. Strict blood pressure control and progression of renal disease in hypertensive nephrosclerosis. *Kidney Int* 1995; **48:** 851–859.

103 Toto RD. Proteinuria and hypertensive nephrosclerosis in African Americans. *Kidney Int* 2004; **66(Suppl 92):** S102–S104.

104 Wright JJ, Bakris G, Greene T, Agodoa LY, Appel LJ, Charleston J *et al.* Effect of blood pressure lowering and anti-hypertensive drug class on progression of hypertensive kidney disease: results from AASK trial. *JAMA* 2002; **288:** 2421–2431.

105 Lebovitz HE, Wiegmann TB, Cnaan A, Shahinfar S, Sica DA, Broadstone V *et al.* Renal protective effects of enalapril in hypertensive NIDDM. *Kidney Int Suppl* 1994; **45:** S150–S155.

106 Gaede P, Vedel P, Parving HH, Pederson O. Intensified mutifactorial intervention in patients with type 2 diabetes mellitus and microalbuminuria: the Steno type 2 randomised study. *Lancet* 1999; **353:** 617–622

107 Gaede P, Vedel P, Larsen N, Jensen GV, Parving HH, Pedersen O. Multifactorial intervention and cardiovascular disease in patients with type 2 diabetes. *N Engl J Med* 2003; **348:** 383–393.

108 Bergman S, Key BO, Kirk KA, Warnock DG, Rostant SG. Kidney disease in the first-degree relatives of African-Americans with hypertensive end-stage renal disease. *Am J Kidney Dis* 1996; **27:** 341–346.

109 Tozawa M, Iseki K, Iseki C, Kinjo K, Ikemiya Y, Takashita S. Blood pressure predicts risk of developing end-stage renal disease in men and women. *Hypertension* 2003; **41:** 1341–1345.

110 Chadban SJ, Briganti EM, Kerr PG, Dunstan DW, Welborn TA, Zimmet PA *et al.* Prevalence of kidney damage in Australian adults: the AusDiab Kidney Study. *J Am Soc Nephrol* 2003; **14:** S131–S138.

111 Fox CS, Larson MG, Leip EP, Culleton B, Wilson PW, Levy D. Predictors of new-onset kidney disease in a community-based population. *JAMA* 2004; **291:** 844–850.

112 Cirillo M, Senigalliesi L, Laurenzi M, Alfieri R, Stamler J, Stamler R *et al.* Microalbuminuria in nondiabetic adults: relation of blood pressure, body mass index, plasma cholesterol levels and smoking. The Gubbio Population Study. *Arch Intern Med* 1998; **158:** 1933–1939.

113 Hallan S, de Mutsert R, Carlsen S, Dekker FW, Aasarod K, Holmen J. Obesity, smoking, and physical inactivity as risk factors for CKD: are men more vulnerable? *Am J Kid Dis* 2006; **47(3):** 396–405.

114 Gelber RP, Kurth T, Kausz AT, Manson JE, Buring JE, Levey AS *et al.* Association between body mass index and CKD in apparently healthy men. *Am J Kidney Dis* 2005; **46(5):** 871–880.

115 Kiberd BA, Jindal K. Should all Pima Indians with type 2 diabetes mellitus be prescribed routine angiotensin converting enzyme inhibition therapy to prevent renal failure. *Mayo Clin Proc* 1999; **74(6):** 559–564.

116 Kiberd BA, Jindal K. Screening to prevent renal failure in insulin dependent diabetic patients: an economic analysis. *BMJ* 1995; **311:** 1595–1599.

117 Herman WH, Shahinfar S, Carides GW, Dasbach EJ, Gerth WC, Alexander CM *et al.* Losartan reduces the costs associated with diabetic end-stage renal disease: the RENAAL study economic evaluation. *Diabetes Care* 2003; **26:** 683–687.

118 Palmer AJ, Annemans L, Roze S, Lamotte M, Lapuerta P, Chen R *et al.* Cost-effectiveness of early irbesartan treatment versus control or late irbesartan treatment in patients with type 2 diabetes, hypertension and renal disease. *Diabetes Care* 2004; **27:** 1897–1903.

119 Palmer AJ, Weiss S, Sendi PP, Neeser K, Brandt A, Singh G *et al.* The cost-effectiveness of different management strategies for type 1 diabetes: a Swiss perspective. *Diabetologia* 2000; **43:** 13–26.

120 Siegel JE, Krolewski AS, Warram JH, Weinstein MC. Cost-effectiveness of screening and early treatment of nephropathy in patients with insulin dependent diabetes mellitus. *J Am Soc Nephrol* 1992; **3:** S111–S119.

121 Borch-Johnsen K, Wenzel H, Viberti GC, Mogensen CE. Is screening and intervention for microalbuminuria worthwhile in patients with insulin-dependent diabetes? *BMJ* 1993; **306:** 1722–1725.

122 Dong FB, Sorensen SW, Manninen DL, Thompson TJ, Narayan V, Orians CE *et al.* Cost effectiveness of ACE inhibitor treatment for patients with type 1 diabetes mellitus. *Pharmacoeconomics* 2004; **22(15):** 1015–1027.

123 Rodby RA, Firth LM, Lewis EJ. An economic analysis of captopril in the treatment of diabetic nephropathy. The Collaborative Study Group. *Diabetes Care* 1996; **19(10):** 1051–1061.

5

Prediction of Risk and Prognosis: Decision Support for Diagnosis and Management of Chronic Kidney Disease

Benedicte Stengel,[1,2] **Marc Froissart,**[3,4,5] **& Jerome Rossert**[3,4,5]

[1] INSERM U780, Villejuif, France
[2] Université Paris-Sud, UMR, Villejuif, France
[3] Paris-Descartes University School of Medicine, Paris, France
[4] AP-HP, Georges Pompidou European Hospital, Paris, France
[5] INSERM U872, Paris, France

In establishing a severity stage classification for chronic kidney disease (CKD), the goal of the National Kidney Foundation Kidney Disease Outcomes Quality Initiative (K/DOQI) was to develop a public health approach to the disease aimed at facilitating epidemiological studies and clinical trials as well as the application of clinical practice guidelines [1]. Although this classification did not aim at predicting renal risk, albuminuria and glomerular filtration rate (GFR) cutoff levels set to define CKD stages reflect a graded increase in the risk of major renal and cardiovascular outcomes, including progression to end-stage renal disease (ESRD) and premature death [1,2].

Recommendations for evaluating individuals at risk mainly rely on urine albumin measurement and equation-estimated GFR. In this chapter, we will first very briefly describe the reference methods for these two measures as well as issues related to their use in specific subgroups. In the second part, we will review the main studies providing risk estimates of ESRD as well as of all-cause mortality and cardiovascular events associated with CKD, with special emphasis on variations by age, gender, and race.

Estimation of GFR

GFR has been considered the best indicator of global kidney function for many years [3–6]. It can be measured using slightly different methods, each of which has advantages and limitations. All of these are based on measurement of renal or plasma clearance of an exogenous tracer, such as inulin, which is historically the gold standard, radiolabeled molecules ([51Cr]EDTA, [125I]iothalamate, and 99mTc-DTPA), or radiocontrast agents (iohexol and iothalamate). However, these GFR measurements can only be performed in specialized centers, and they are much too time-consuming and costly for routine use in monitoring kidney function. Thus, in clinical practice, GFR has to be estimated using endogenous filtration markers. Creatinine, which is an amino acid derivative with a molecular mass of 113.12 Da, is by far the most widely used one, although it does not fulfill all the criteria of an ideal filtration marker. In particular, creatinine production depends on muscle mass and to a lesser extent on protein intake. As a consequence, serum creatinine concentration is thus influenced by factors such as gender, age, ethnicity, and diet. In addition, although creatinine is principally eliminated by glomerular filtration, urinary excretion is in part mediated by tubular secretion, especially in subjects with reduced renal function. Different equations have been developed that provide an estimation of GFR based on serum creatinine concentration and on subject characteristics, such as age, gender, ethnicity, or body weight. They have been derived by using regression techniques to model the observed relationship between serum creatinine concentration and measured GFR in study populations. Up to now, two creatinine-based equations have been extensively studied and are widely used: the historical Cockcroft-Gault formula [7] and the abbreviated Modification of Diet in Renal Disease (MDRD) study equation [8,9]. The results of the main studies that assessed the performance of these formulas have been recently reviewed by Coresh *et al.* [10] and are summarized in Table 5.1.

The Cockcroft-Gault equation, which was developed to be an estimation of creatinine clearance rather than measured GFR, has several limitations. It tends to systematically overestimate GFR in subjects with low GFR and in subjects with high body mass index, while it tends to underestimate GFR in the elderly [11–14]. For example, in a cohort of subjects with GFR higher than 60 mL/min/1.73 m^2 and older than 65 years, on average the Cockcroft-Gault formula underestimated GFR by 14.5 mL/min/1.73 m^2 in men and by 10.7 mL/min/1.73 m^2 in women [12]. By contrast, the MDRD formula tends to perform better than

Evidence-based Nephrology. Edited by Donald Molony and Jonathan Craig
© 2009 Blackwell Publishing, ISBN: 978-1-4051-3975-5.

Table 5.1 The main studies that have analyzed the performance of the Cockcroft-Gault and MDRD formulas adapted from [10].

Author [reference]	Year	Type	Population	Subgroup (n)	Marker	Mean GFR (range) (mL/min/1.73 m²)	Creatinine calibration	MDRD vs. Cockcroft-Gault	Bias (%)ᵃ	R^2	P₃₀
Lewis et al. [82]	2001	RS	African Americans with hypertensive nephrosclerosis	Total (1703)	[¹²⁵I]iothalamate (U)	57 (10–140)	Yes	MDRD better	−3	0.82	88
Poggio et al. [11]	2005	CP	Cleveland Clinic Foundation GFRs	CKD overall (828) w/ diabetes (249) w/o diabetes (579) kidney donors (457)	[¹²⁵I]iothalamate (U)	32 (10–74) 24 (9–52) 36 (10–81) 106 (85–130)	Indirect	MDRD better	−3 m 1 m −4 m −9 m	0.81 0.13	71 63 74 86
Rule et al. [15,83]	2004	CP	Mayo Clinic GFRs	CKD (320) kidney donors (580)	Cold iothalamate	48 (5–133) 101 (63–177)	No	MDRD better Neither	−6.2 −29	0.79 0.19	75 54
Gonwa et al. [84]	2004	CP	iver Tx patients	Pre-Tx (1447) 3 mos post-Tx (887) 1 yr post-Tx (1297) 5 yrs post-Tx (521)	[¹²⁵I]iothalamate (U)	91 (2–260) 59 (2–240) 53 (2–150) 55 (2–140)	No	Neither (MDRD better)	−4 7 −15 −18	0.45 0.38 0.52 0.56	67 62 68 66
Froissart et al. [12,18]	2005	CP	HEGP GFRs (French clinical site)	Overall (2095) mGFR <60 (1051) mGFR >60 (1044) age <65 (1500) age >65 (595) kidney donors (162)	[⁵¹Cr]EDTA (U)	61 (2–166) 67 (2–166) 45 (3–127) 98 (68–153)	Yes	MDRD	−1.0 1.3 −3.3 −1.2 −0.6 −5.5	0.83 0.74 0.44 0.80 0.86 0.29	87 83 92 87 87 64
Ibrahim et al. [17]	2005	RS	Type 1 diabetics in DCCT	Total (1286)	[¹²⁵I]iothalamate (U)	122 (75–140)	Indirect	Neither	−22	0.13	78
Verhave et al. [16]	2005	CP	CVD risk screening	SCr <1.5 mg/dL (850)	⁹⁹ᵐTc-DTPA (U)	99 (33–201)	No	Similar	−12.4	0.34	89
Stevens et al. [23]	2007	CP-RS	CKD-EPI collaborative study	Total (5504) eGFR < 60 (2874) eGFR > 60 (2630)	[¹²⁵I]iothalamate	68	Yes, IDMS	ND	5.8 m 3.0 m 8.7 m		83 82 84

Abbreviations: RS, research study; CP, clinical practice; Tx, transplant; CVD, cardiovascular disease; mGFR, mean GFR (in mL/min/1.73 m²); SCr, serum creatinine.
ᵃ An "m" following the bias value indicates the value is the median.

the Cockcroft-Gault equation in these subgroups of patients, and it appears to be reasonably accurate in most CKD patients. The major limitation of the MDRD formula seems to be an underestimation of GFR in subjects with high GFR. This has been shown by analysis of different cohorts, including potential kidney donors [15,16], diabetic patients without CKD [17], or subjects with and without CKD [11,18]. However, it should be stressed that, at high levels of GFR, a small relative error in serum creatinine measurement will induce a large error in estimated GFR and that the uncertainty of the estimate increases with the absolute value of the GFR. This can be depicted by plotting the interquartile range of measured GFR as a function of estimated GFR (Figure 5.1). It emphasizes the fact that variability of serum creatinine measurements among clinical laboratories can lead to very significant differences in GFR estimation, particularly in subjects with high GFR, and the necessity to calibrate creatinine assays [19,20]. Recently, initiatives have been developed to standardize serum creatinine measurements and im-

prove their accuracy through the preparation of high-level certified reference materials set by isotope–dilution mass spectrometry (IDMS) [21]. A slightly modified IDMS-MDRD formula is now available that should be used with calibrated serum creatinine assays [22], since the formula has been validated on a large external set of data collected through the CKD-EPI collaborative study [23].

Cystatin C, a 13-kDa protein, is an alternative endogenous filtration marker. Its main advantage is the relative stability of its production, which is mainly independent of muscular mass variations. During the past few years, some predictive equations to estimate GFR have been developed. Two sets of equations issued from the CKD-EPI collaborative study have been proposed: one using cystatin alone as a GFR marker, and a second using both creatinine and cystatin [24]. This combined approach slightly improves the predictive performance of the formula. The main recent GFR predictive equations are summarized in Table 5.2.

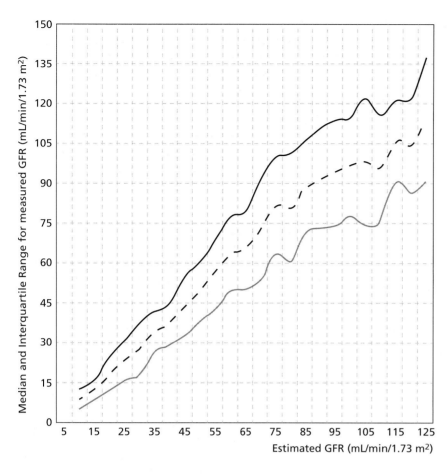

Figure 5.1 Predicted values of the measured GFR as a function of the estimated GFR value using the MDRD formula. Solid lines represent the upper and lower boundaries of the 95% confidence interval of the measured GFR values for each value of eGFR. The dotted line represents the mean measured GFR value for each value of eGFR [12].

Table 5.2 GFR prediction formulas recently developed based on large data sets of patients (900–3400 independent patients).

GFR marker, method (reference lab or reference material)	eGFR formula [reference]
Creatinine, Jaffe colorimetric (Cleveland Clinic Foundation)	Abbreviated MDRD (four variables) [9] SCr (mg/dL): eGFR = 186 × (SCr)$^{-1.154}$ × (age)$^{-0.203}$ × (0.742 if female) × (1.212 if Black) SCr (μmol/L): eGFR = 32,789 × (SCr)$^{-1.154}$ × (age)$^{-0.203}$ × (0.742 if female) × (1.212 if Black)
Creatinine, Jaffe colorimetric (Mayo Clinic Clinical Lab)	Mayo quadratic [15] SCr (in mg/dL; SCr with a constant value of 0.8 mg/dL if measured creatinine < 0.8 mg/dL): eGFR = exp[1.911 + (5.249/SCr) − (2.114/SCr^2) − (0.00686 × age) − (0.205 if female)]
Creatinine, Jaffe colorimetric calibrated to IDMS-standardized Roche enzymatic assay (IDMS, NIST 914a)	Abbreviated MDRD refitted for IDMS standardization [22] Scr (mg/dL): eGFR = 175 × (SCr)$^{-1.154}$ × (age)$^{-0.203}$ × (0.742 if female) × (1.212 if Black) SCr (μmol/L): eGFR = 30,850 × (SCr)$^{-1.154}$ × (age)$^{-0.203}$ × (0.742 if female) × (1.212 if Black)
Cystatin C, nephelometry (Dade-Behring/Siemens)	CKD-EPI cystatin alone [24] SCys (mg/L): eGFR = 127.7 × (SCr)$^{-1.17}$ × (age)$^{-0.13}$ × (0.91 if female) × (1.06 if Black)
Creatinine and cystatin C, nephelometry for SCys (Dade-Behring/Siemens) and Jaffe colorimetric calibrated to IDMS-standardized Roche enzymatic assay (IDMS, NIST 914a) for SCr	CKD-EPI combined SCr and SCys formula [24] SCr (mg/dL) and SCys (mg/L): eGFR = 177.6 × (SCr)$^{-0.65}$ × (SCys)$^{-0.57}$ × (age)$^{-0.20}$ × (0.82 if female) × (1.11 if Black) SCr (μmol/L) and SCys (mg/L): eGFR = 3271 × (SCr)$^{-0.65}$ × (SCys)$^{-0.57}$ × (age)$^{-0.20}$ × (0.82 if female) × (1.11 if Black)

Abbreviations: BSA, body surface area; SCr, serum creatinine; SCys, serum cystatin; NIST, National Institute of Standards and Technology.

It is worth noting that although similar in structure to risk prediction equations, such as the Framingham risk function [25], currently utilized GFR equations do not provide an estimate of risk directly; that is, calculated GFR is not expressed as a risk estimate for future events. However, the combined cystatin and creatinine equation may be a first step in integrating relative risk in GFR prediction formulas, because cystatin on its own has been recognized as an independent risk marker for cardiovascular morbidity and overall mortality [26].

Assessment of proteinuria

Timed versus untimed urine sample

Measurement of proteins in a 24-h urine collection has long been considered the gold standard for quantitative assessment of proteinuria. However, collecting urine over such a long period of time is quite burdensome, and reliable 24-h urine collections are quite difficult to obtain. This has prompted the National Kidney Foundation and KDIGO to recommend using protein/creatinine or albumin/creatinine ratios obtained in untimed urine samples to quantitatively assess proteinuria or albuminuria. Although the excretion rate of creatinine in the urine varies according to age, gender, ethnicity, and body size, and although protein and albumin excretion rates may vary throughout the day, different studies have shown a strong correlation between protein and albumin excretion rates and protein/creatinine and albumin/creatinine ratios in a spot urine sample. In 2005, Price *et al.* performed a systematic review of studies comparing 24-h protein excretion and protein/creatinine ratios assessed in a random spot urine sample [27]. Their analysis of 20 studies showed that the correlation coefficient between the two values was above 0.90 in 14 studies of 20 and above 0.80 in 16 studies of 20.

Albuminuria versus proteinuria

In adults, the National Kidney Foundation K/DOQI guidelines recommend measurement of albuminuria rather than proteinuria, because it is a more sensitive marker of CKD due to diabetes, hypertension, or glomerular disease [1]. In addition, it seems logical to measure a well-defined protein that is filtered in increased amounts even when glomerular lesions are minimal rather than a mixture of proteins that include albumin but also proteins that are normally filtered by the glomerulus and reabsorbed by tubular cells, such as low-molecular-weight proteins, and proteins that are normally produced by tubular cells and excreted in the urine, such as uromodulin. However, the usefulness of albuminuria for diagnosis of CKD has been mostly demonstrated in patients with diabetes and kidney disease. In these patients, albuminuria provides the earliest clinical evidence of nephropathy and is an early predictor of patients at higher risk of progressive loss of renal function, both in type 1 and type 2 diabetic patients [28–31]. In the general population, the PREVEND study has provided evidence that at low level albuminuria are also a risk factor for subsequent impairment of renal function. In this large epidemiological study that included more than 80,000 subjects with a mean follow-up of 4 years, an albumin/creatinine ratio above 30 mg/g at inclusion was an independent risk factor for an estimated GFR (eGFR) of <60 mL/min/1.73 m² at 4 years [32].

Threshold values

The threshold used to define proteinuria is usually 300 mg/day or 200 mg/g of creatinine [1], which roughly correspond to protein concentrations that are detected by dipstick analyses. Although this threshold appears not to be grossly flawed on clinical grounds, one can question the fact that it is not higher than the limit used to define "clinical albuminuria" or "macroalbuminuria" [1].

Regarding albuminuria, the Third National Health and Nutrition Evaluation Survey showed that, in a very large cohort of subjects, about 95% of those less than 50 years of age had an albumin/creatinine ratio of less than 3 mg/g [33]. Because creatinine excretion rate varies according to gender and ethnicity, it may seem necessary, for the sake of precision, to define gender-specific cutoff values for albuminuria as defined by this ratio. However, due to the greater complexity that such modifications would introduce, the inherent uncertainty in assay precision, and the existence of other factors influencing importantly creatinine excretion rate besides gender, a KDIGO position paper did not advocate using gender-specific cutoff values for diagnosis of CKD and considered 30 mg/g as the threshold level [34]. Furthermore, this threshold is consistent with the recommendations of JNC-7 and recommendations from the American Diabetes Association [35]. However, when assessing albuminuria, it is important to remember that verification of increased albumin excretion requires at least two out of three positive tests on independent determinations.

Mortality and ESRD risk associated with CKD

There are numerous studies that have linked CKD to all-cause mortality and cardiovascular events in various populations, including cohort studies and cohort analyses of randomized trials, but those linking CKD to the risk of ESRD are scarce [36,37]. With a few exceptions, risks associated with GFR level or albuminuria have been analyzed separately.

GFR level and risk for progression to ESRD

In most studies, renal replacement therapy (RRT) is used as a surrogate outcome for ESRD. Therefore, ESRD risk estimates are influenced by geographic variations and trends over time in access to treatment. Based on data from the US Renal Data System 2000 annual report, the cumulative lifetime risk of developing ESRD requiring RRT was estimated by gender and race in 20-year-old Americans as follows: 7.3% and 7.8% in African American men and women and 2.5% and 1.8% in white men and women [38]. Because RRT incidence rates are 2 to 3 times lower in Europe and Australia than in the USA [39,40], cumulative risks are likely to be reduced proportionally in these countries.

Table 5.3 Cumulative 5- and 10-year incidence rates of competing risks for kidney failure and death in patients with CKD stage 3 (n = 3047)

Patient age and incidence data category	No. of cases (%) or incidence (95% CI)		
	Men	Women	Total
Age <69 yrs			
No. (%)	279 (28)	704 (72)	983
Renal failure[a]			
5 yrs	0.05 (0.03–0.09)	0.02 (0.01–0.03)	0.03 (0.02–0.04)
10 yrs	0.12 (0.08–0.20)	0.04 (0.02–0.08)	0.07 (0.05–0.11)
Death			
5 yrs	0.20 (0.16–0.27)	0.08 (0.06–0.11)	0.12 (0.10–0.15)
10 yrs	0.26 (0.20–0.35)	0.13 (0.09–0.17)	0.17 (0.14–0.21)
Age 70–79 yrs			
No. (%)	404 (35)	759 (65)	1163
Renal failure			
5 yrs	0.02 (0.01–0.04)	0.01 (0.01–0.02)	0.01 (0.01–0.02)
10 yrs	0.06 (0.03–0.11)	0.03 (0.01–0.07)	0.04 (0.02–0.07)
Death			
5 yrs	0.41 (0.35–0.46)	0.21 (0.18–0.25)	0.28 (0.25–0.31)
10 yrs	0.65 (0.58–0.73)	0.40 (0.35–0.46)	0.49 (0.45–0.54)
Age >79 yrs			
No. (%)	245 (27)	656 (73)	901
Renal failure			
5 yrs	0.02 (0.01–0.05)	0.01 (0.00–0.02)	0.01 (0.00–0.02)
10 yrs	0.05 (0.03–0.11)	0.01 (0.00–0.03)	0.03 (0.01–0.05)
Death			
5 yrs	0.64 (0.57–0.71)	0.53 (0.49–0.57)	0.56 (0.52–0.60)
10 yrs	0.88 (0.81–0.95)	0.83 (0.77–0.89)	0.84 (0.80–0.89)
Total			
No. (%)	928 (30)	2119 (70)	3047
Renal failure			
5 yrs	0.03 (0.02–0.04)	0.01 (0.01–0.02)	0.02 (0.01–0.02)
10 yrs	0.08 (0.05–0.11)	0.03 (0.02–0.04)	0.04 (0.03–0.06)
Death			
5 yrs	0.41 (0.38–0.45)	0.28 (0.26–0.30)	0.32 (0.30–0.34)
10 yrs	0.61 (0.56–0.67)	0.47 (0.43–0.50)	0.51 (0.48–0.55)

Source: Reference 43.
[a] Kidney failure was defined as irreversible CKD stage 5 or initiation of RRT.

Available studies have consistently shown that at any stage of CKD the risk of death is greater than the risk of progression to ESRD. Some studies have also shown that the magnitude of both risks, i.e. death or ESRD, stratified by CKD stage varies importantly with age, gender, and race.

In a large cohort of 28,000 health maintenance organization members (>17 years old; mean age, 66 years), Keith *et al.* [41] showed that the percentages of patients reaching RRT, either transplant or dialysis, over a 5-year observation period versus those dying were 1.1 versus 19.5%, 1.3 versus 24.3%, and 19.9 versus 45.7% for those patients at baseline with CKD stages 2, 3, and 4, respectively. Moreover, among patients with comparable levels of eGFR, older patients have higher rates of death and lower rates of treated ESRD than younger patients [42].

Table 5.3, adapted from Eriksen and Ingebretsen [43], displays the 5- and 10-year competing risks of true ESRD and death in a population-based cohort of 3047 Norwegian patients (>20 years old; median age, 75 years) with persistent CKD stage 3 at baseline, identified from all serum creatinine levels measured in a geographically defined population. The 10-year risk of ESRD, defined as

CKD stage 5, that is, either an eGFR of less than 15 mL/min/1.73 m² or RRT, was 4%, 13 times lower than the risk of death in this cohort. The risk of ESRD was 3 times higher in men than in women and twice as high in patients less than 69 years old than in older patients. As expected, the relative risk of death versus ESRD increased strongly with age, from 2.4 (17% vs. 7%) among the youngest age group to 28 (84% vs. 3%) in the oldest group. Compared with the general population, the standardized incidence rate ratios of ESRD and death for CKD patients in this Norwegian population were 36.6 and 3.1, respectively, among those younger than 69 years but only 3.7 and 2.2, respectively, in the oldest age group. Similar results with regard to the risk of progression to ESRD versus mortality according to age were observed in a retrospective cohort from England [44].

The competing risks of death versus ESRD were examined in advanced CKD stages in a population-based inception cohort of 920 Swedish adults aged 18–74 years with CKD stage 4 or stage 5 not on dialysis. Of this cohort, 8% started RRT within 6 years, only 10% died before initiating RRT, but 42% were dead by 6 years [45]. These findings taken together favor the conclusion that premature death rather than denial of RRT explains the higher risk of death versus ESRD for patients with earlier stages of CKD.

Finally, ecologic studies linking data on the CKD prevalence derived from nationally representative population-based surveys with the RRT incidence derived from national renal registries have shown that the 5-year risk of treated ESRD is 5 times higher in African Americans with stage 3 plus CKD (5%) than in their white counterparts (1%) [46] and 2.5 times higher in US whites than in Norwegians [40]. Causal interpretation of these results should nevertheless be made with caution, as ecologic associations based on aggregate measures may not accurately reflect true associations at the individual level [47].

GFR level and risk for all-cause mortality and cardiovascular events

Studies linking GFR level with mortality have been extensively reviewed by Tonelli *et al.* and Vanholder *et al.* [36,48]. Despite variations in design, study populations, event rates in controls, and definitions of CKD, more than 90% of the studies found an increased risk of all-cause and cardiovascular mortality with decreasing GFR, both before and after adjustment for potential confounders [36]. An independent graded association between a reduced eGFR and the risk of death and *de novo* or recurrent cardiovascular events was consistently observed in cohorts of patients with heart failure [49,50], cardiovascular disease or high cardiovascular risk [51,52], and hypertension [53], as well as in the general population [54–63].

In a cohort of 1,120,000 health plan members, Go *et al.* [57] showed that the age-standardized rates for death from any cause and for cardiovascular events, defined as any hospitalization for coronary heart disease, heart failure, ischemic stroke, or peripheral arterial disease, increased substantially with progressively lower GFR. Taking patients with an eGFR of ≥60 mL/min/1.73 m² as the reference, and after adjustment for demographics and several

comorbidities, the risk of death strongly increased as GFR declined, from a 17% increase in risk with an eGFR of 45–59 mL/min/1.73 m² to 80%, 220%, and nearly 500% increases for GFRs of 30–44, 15–29, and <15, respectively. The adjusted risk of any cardiovascular events followed a similar pattern, with a 43% increase in risk for a GFR of 45–59 mL/min/1.73 m² and 100%, 180%, and 240% increases for GFRs of 30–44, 15–29, and <15, respectively. However, O'Hare *et al.* [62] demonstrated using a different study population that whereas severe reductions in eGFR were associated with an increased risk for death in all age groups, very moderate reductions in GFR (50–59 ml/min/1.73 m²) were not associated with significantly increased risk among those older than 65 years.

In a pooled analysis of data from four large US community-based longitudinal studies including 22,634 individuals, Weiner *et al.* [60] found that CKD was an independent risk factor for all-cause mortality but not for myocardial infarction or stroke. However, there was a significant interaction between kidney function and race. In African Americans, CKD defined as an eGFR of <60 mL/min/1.73 m² was associated with a more than a 100% increase in risk of myocardial infarction and 83% increase of all-cause mortality, whereas in whites the risk of all-cause mortality only was significantly increased by 31%. Reduced kidney function was also associated with increased risk for incident heart failure [64]. Finally, in a large cohort of participants in the MONICA Augsburg survey, the authors investigated the gender-specific association of CKD with cardiovascular mortality and incident myocardial infarction. After adjusting for common cardiovascular disease risk factors, they found similar hazard ratios for both events in men and women [63].

Proteinuria and risk for ESRD and cardiovascular outcomes

Urinary protein (or albumin) excretion of 300 mg/24 h (300 mg/g urinary creatinine) or greater is a major and well-established determinant of progressive kidney failure in patients with glomerular, diabetic, and hypertensive nephropathies. Numerous clinical studies have shown a strong graded relationship between proteinuria level and the risk of either 50% decrease in GFR, ESRD, or death. Moreover, there is evidence that treating proteinuria in these patients improves renal outcome [65–67]. These studies are reviewed and discussed in detail by Ritz in chapter 3.

In contrast, studies investigating the link between the presence of proteinuria at screening and the risk for poor renal outcomes in the general population are scarce. In a 17-year follow-up of 106,177 participants in a community-based mass screening in Japan, Iseki *et al.* [68] showed that a positive dipstick proteinuria (1+ or greater) was associated with a relative risk for developing ESRD of 1.9 in men and 2.4 in women, compared with participants with no or trace proteinuria. Similarly, in the PREVEND study, which was a large population-based cohort of 6894 adults aged 20–75 years from the city of Groningen, the Netherlands, participants with baseline screened macroalbuminuria (>300 mg/24 h), which was present in 0.6% of the general population, had faster annual declines in GFR (7.2 mL/min/1.73 m^2/year) than controls without albuminuria (2.3 mL/min/1.73 m^2/year) [69]. The 4-year follow-up of this study was not long enough, however, to evaluate the risk of the progression to ESRD.

The significance of microalbuminuria, in the range of 30–300 mg/24 h (30–300 mg/g urinary creatinine), as an early marker of renal injury and a predictor of progressive CKD is less clear [70]. Microalbuminuria was initially defined as a range of dipstick-negative albuminuria predicting future overt nephropathy in patients with type 1 diabetes mellitus [71]. Its predictive value was later extended to patients with type 2 diabetes mellitus. In the UK Prospective Diabetes Study (UKPDS), a randomized clinical trial including 5097 patients with newly diagnosed type 2 diabetes and a median follow-up of 10.4 years, the annual probability of progression from stage to stage of kidney injury (incidence) was estimated as follows: 2%/year from no nephropathy to microalbuminuria, 2.8% from microalbuminuria to macroalbuminuria, and 2.3% from macroalbuminuria to elevated serum creatinine or RRT [72]. The annual probability of not progressing to a more advanced stage of nephropathy or death was 93.8% for patients with microalbuminuria, and the estimated median duration in this stage was 10.9 years. For patients with microalbuminuria, the annual death rate, 3%/year, was similar to that of progressing to macroalbuminuria, but for those with macroalbuminuria, the annual death rate of 4.6% was twice as high as that of progressing to worse nephropathy. Relative to patients with no nephropathy, those with microalbuminuria, macroalbuminuria, or an elevated serum creatinine or RRT had a 2.2-fold, 3.4-fold, and 13.9-fold increased risk of death, respectively.

Although similarly robust evidence of progression from microalbuminuria to overt nephropathy and ESRD are lacking in other segments of the population, there is increasing evidence that microalbuminuria is associated with GFR decline in the general population as in patients with hypertension [70]. Data from the PREVEND study showed that an elevated urinary albumin excretion predicted *de novo* development of chronic kidney failure defined as an eGFR of <60 mL/min/1.73 m^2 [32]. In the African American Study of Kidney Disease and Hypertension (AASK), there was a graded relationship between continuous level of albuminuria and the risk of either a 50% decrease of GFR, ESRD, or death, starting in the microalbuminuric range [67].

Both micro- and macroalbuminuria are well-established risk factors for cardiovascular outcomes, including fatal and nonfatal coronary heart disease, chronic heart failure, and stroke. Multiple studies and secondary analyses of large databases have shown strong independent associations of albuminuria with an increased risk for these events, as reviewed by Basi *et al.* [70]. This association is well-documented in patients with diabetes or hypertension [39-41], as well as in nondiabetic, nonhypertensive individuals from either selected or unselected populations [56,73–78].

It is evident from all these studies that microalbuminuria is definitely a major predictor of cardiovascular risk in all individuals and of progressive renal disease in diabetic patients. Whether it also predicts poor renal outcomes in nondiabetic populations is likely, albeit not yet proven. These results are important from a public health perspective of primary prevention of both cardiovascular disease and ESRD, as albuminuria is a potentially modifiable risk factor. Lowering of albuminuria by either an angiotensin converting enzyme inhibitor or an angiotensin II receptor blocker is indeed associated with a better renal and cardiovascular outcome in patients with overt proteinuric nephropathy as well as in diabetic patients with microalbuminuria [65,66,81]. However, robust clinical trials evidence that similar treatment of nondiabetic individuals with microalbuminuria [75], a condition that can affect from 6 to 20% of all adults depending on the population, is beneficial, safe, and cost-effective to prevent cardiovascular and renal diseases is currently not available.

References

1 Definition and classification of stages of chronic kidney disease. *Am J Kidney Dis* 2002;**39(2)**: S46–S75.

2 Stevens LA, Coresh J, Greene T, Levey AS. Assessing kidney function: measured and estimated glomerular filtration rate. *N Engl J Med* 2006; **354(23)**: 2473–2483.

3 Smith HW. Comparative physiology of the kidney. In: Smith HW, editor, *The Kidney: Structure and Function in Health and Disease.* Oxford University Press, New York, 1951; 520–574.

4 Smith HW. Measurement of the rate of glomerular filtration. In: Smith HW, editor, *Principles of Renal Physiology.* Oxford University Press, New York, 1957; 25–35.

5 Wesson LG. Renal hemodynamics in physiological states. In: Wesson LG, editor, *Physiology of the Human Kidney.* Grune & Stratton, New York, 1969; 96–108.

6 Wesson LG. Renal hemodynamics in pathological states. In: Wesson LG, editor, *Physiology of the Human Kidney.* Grune & Stratton, New York, 1969; 109–154.

7 Cockcroft DW, Gault MH. Prediction of creatinine clearance from serum creatinine. *Nephron* 1976; **16:** 31–41.

8 Levey AS, Bosch JP, Lewis JB, Greene T, Rogers N, Roth D. A more accurate method to estimate glomerular filtration rate from serum creatinine: a new prediction equation. Modification of Diet in Renal Disease Study Group. *Ann Intern Med* 1999; **130(6):** 461–470.

9 Levey AS, Greene T, Kusek JW, *et al.* A simplified equation to predict glomerular filtration rate from serum creatinine. *J Am Soc Nephrol* 2000; **11:** 155A.

10 Coresh J, Stevens LA. Kidney function estimating equations: where do we stand? *Curr Opin Nephrol Hypertens* 2006; **15(3):** 276–284.

11 Poggio ED, Wang X, Greene T, Van Lente F, Hall PM. Performance of the Modification of Diet in Renal Disease and Cockcroft-Gault equations in the estimation of GFR in health and in chronic kidney disease. *J Am Soc Nephrol* 2005; **16(2):** 459–466.

12 Froissart M, Rossert J, Jacquot C, Paillard M, Houillier P. Predictive performance of the Modification of Diet in Renal Disease and Cockcroft-Gault equations for estimating renal function. *J Am Soc Nephrol* 2005; **16(3):** 763–773.

13 Cirillo M, Anastasio P, De Santo NG. Relationship of gender, age, and body mass index to errors in predicted kidney function. *Nephrol Dial Transplant* 2005; **20(9):** 1791–1798.

14 Rigalleau V, Lasseur C, Perlemoine C, Barthe N, Raffaitin C, Chauveau P *et al*. Cockcroft-Gault formula is biased by body weight in diabetic patients with renal impairment. *Metabolism* 2006; **55(1):** 108–112.

15 Rule AD, Larson TS, Bergstralh EJ, Slezak JM, Jacobsen SJ, Cosio FG. Using serum creatinine to estimate glomerular filtration rate: accuracy in good health and in chronic kidney disease. *Ann Intern Med* 2004; **141(12):** 929–937.

16 Verhave JC, Fesler P, Ribstein J, du Cailar G, Mimran A. Estimation of renal function in subjects with normal serum creatinine levels: influence of age and body mass index. *Am J Kidney Dis* 2005; **46(2):** 233–241.

17 Ibrahim H, Mondress M, Tello A, Fan Y, Koopmeiners J, Thomas W. An alternative formula to the Cockcroft-Gault and the Modification of Diet in Renal Diseases formulas in predicting GFR in individuals with type 1 diabetes. *J Am Soc Nephrol* 2005; **16(4):** 1051–1060.

18 Froissart MC, Rossert J, Houillier P. The new Mayo Clinic equation for estimating glomerular filtration rate. *Ann Intern Med* 2005; **142(8):** 679. [Author reply, **142:** 681.]

19 Coresh J, Astor BC, McQuillan G, Kusek J, Greene T, Van Lente F *et al*. Calibration and random variation of the serum creatinine assay as critical elements of using equations to estimate glomerular filtration rate. *Am J Kidney Dis* 2002; **39:** 920–929.

20 Murthy K, Stevens LA, Stark PC, Levey AS. Variation in the serum creatinine assay calibration: a practical application to glomerular filtration rate estimation. *Kidney Int* 2005; **68(4):** 1884–1887.

21 Myers GL, Miller WG, Coresh J, Fleming J, Greenberg N, Greene T *et al*. Recommendations for improving serum creatinine measurement: a report from the Laboratory Working Group of the National Kidney Disease Education Program. *Clin Chem* 2006; **52(1):** 5–18.

22 Levey AS, Coresh J, Greene T, Stevens LA, Zhang YL, Hendriksen S *et al*. Using standardized serum creatinine values in the modification of diet in renal disease study equation for estimating glomerular filtration rate. *Ann Intern Med* 2006; **145(4):** 247–254.

23 Stevens LA, Coresh J, Feldman HI *et al*. Evaluation of the Modification of Diet in Renal Disease study equation in a large diverse population. *J Am Soc Nephrol* 2007; **18(10):** 2749–2757.

24 Stevens LA, Coresh J, Schmid C *et al*. Estimation glomerular filtration rate using serum cystatin C alone and in combination with serum creatinine: a pooled analysis of 3418 individuals. *Am J Kidney Di*s 2008; **51(3):** 395–406.

25 Anderson KM, Wilson PW, Odell PM, Kannel WB. An updated coronary risk profile. A statement for health professionals. *Circulation* 1991; **82(1):** 356–362.

26 Menon V, Shlipak MG, Wang X *et al*. Cystatin C as a risk factor for outcomes in chronic kidney disease. *Ann Intern Med* 2007; **147(1):** 19–27.

27 Price CP, Newall RG, Boyd JC. Use of protein:creatinine ratio measurements on random urine samples for prediction of significant proteinuria: a systematic review. *Clin Chem* 2005; **51(9):** 1577–1586.

28 Viberti GC, Hill RD, Jarrett RJ, Argyropoulos A, Mahmud U, Keen H. Microalbuminuria as a predictor of clinical nephropathy in insulin-dependent diabetes mellitus. *Lancet* 1982; **i(8287):** 1430–1432.

29 Parving HH, Oxenboll B, Svendsen PA, Christiansen JS, Andersen AR. Early detection of patients at risk of developing diabetic nephropathy. A longitudinal study of urinary albumin excretion. *Acta Endocrinol* (Copenhagen) 1982; **100(4):** 550–555.

30 Mogensen CE. Microalbuminuria predicts clinical proteinuria and early mortality in maturity-onset diabetes. *N Engl J Med* 1984; **310(6):** 356–360.

31 Nelson RG, Bennett PH, Beck GJ, Tan M, Knowler WC, Mitch WE *et al*. Development and progression of renal disease in Pima Indians with non-insulin-dependent diabetes mellitus. Diabetic Renal Disease Study Group. *N Engl J Med* 1996; **335(22):** 1636–1642.

32 Verhave JC, Gansevoort RT, Hillege HL, Bakker SJ, De Zeeuw D, de Jong PE *et al*. An elevated urinary albumin excretion predicts de novo development of renal function impairment in the general population. *Kidney Int Suppl* 2004; **66(S92):** S18–S21.

33 Garg AX, Kiberd BA, Clark WF, Haynes RB, Clase CM. Albuminuria and renal insufficiency prevalence guides population screening: results from the NHANES III. *Kidney Int* 2002; **61(6):** 2165–2175.

34 Levey AS, Eckardt KU, Tsukamoto Y, Levin A, Coresh J, Rossert J *et al*. Definition and classification of chronic kidney disease: a position statement from Kidney Disease: Improving Global Outcomes (KDIGO). *Kidney Int* 2005; **67(6):** 2089–2100.

35 Diabetic Nephropathy. *Diabetes Care* 2002; **25:** 85S–89S.

36 Tonelli M, Wiebe N, Culleton B, House A, Rabbat C, Fok M *et al*. Chronic kidney disease and mortality risk: a systematic review. *J Am Soc Nephrol* 2006; **17(7):** 2034–2047.

37 Sarnak MJ, Levey AS, Schoolwerth AC, Coresh J, Culleton B, Hamm LL *et al*. Kidney disease as a risk factor for development of cardiovascular disease: a statement from the American Heart Association Councils on Kidney in Cardiovascular Disease, High Blood Pressure Research, Clinical Cardiology, and Epidemiology and Prevention. *Circulation* 2003; **108(17):** 2154–2169.

38 Kiberd BA, Clase CM. Cumulative risk for developing end-stage renal disease in the US population. *J Am Soc Nephrol* 2002; **13(6):** 1635–1644.

39 McCredie M. Geographic, ethnic, age-related and temporal variation in the incidence of end-stage renal disease in Europe, Canada and the Asia-Pacific region, 1998-2002. *Nephrol Dial Transplant* 2006; **21(8):** 2178–2183.

40 Hallan SI, Coresh J, Astor BC, Asberg A, Powe NR, Romundstad S *et al*. International comparison of the relationship of chronic kidney disease prevalence and ESRD risk. *J Am Soc Nephrol* 2006; **17(8):** 2275–2284.

41 Keith DS, Nichols GA, Gullion CM, Brown JB, Smith DH. Longitudinal follow-up and outcomes among a population with chronic kidney disease in a large managed care organization. *Arch Intern Med* 2004; **164(6):** 659–663.

42 O'Hare AM, Choi AI, Bertenthal D *et al*. Age affects outcomes in chronic kidney disease. *J Am Soc Nephrol* 2007; **18(10):** 2758–2765.

43 Eriksen BO, Ingebretsen OC. The progression of chronic kidney disease: a 10-year population-based study of the effects of gender and age. *Kidney Int* 2006; **69(2):** 375–382.

44 Drey N, Roderick P, Mullee M, Rogerson M. A population-based study of the incidence and outcomes of diagnosed chronic kidney disease. *Am J Kidney Dis* 2003; **42(4):** 677–684.

45 Evans M, Fryzek JP, Elinder CG, Cohen SS, McLaughlin JK, Nyren O *et al*. The natural history of chronic renal failure: results from an unselected, population-based, inception cohort in Sweden. *Am J Kidney Dis* 2005; **46(5):** 863–870.

46 Hsu CY, Lin F, Vittinghoff E, Shlipak MG. Racial differences in the progression from chronic renal insufficiency to end-stage renal disease in the United States. *J Am Soc Nephrol* 2003; **14(11):** 2902–2907.

47 Stengel B, Couchoud C. Chronic kidney disease prevalence and treated end-stage renal disease incidence: a complex relationship. *J Am Soc Nephrol* 2006; **17(8):** 2094–2096.

48 Vanholder R, Massy Z, Argiles A, Spasovski G, Verbeke F, Lameire N *et al.* Chronic kidney disease as cause of cardiovascular morbidity and mortality. *Nephrol Dial Transplant* 2005; **20(6):** 1048–1056.

49 McAlister FA, Ezekowitz J, Tonelli M, Armstrong PW. Renal insufficiency and heart failure: prognostic and therapeutic implications from a prospective cohort study. *Circulation* 2004; **109(8):** 1004–1009.

50 Smith GL, Lichtman JH, Bracken MB, Shlipak MG, Phillips CO, Di-Caupa P *et al.* Renal impairment and outcomes in heart failure: systematic review and meta-analysis. *J Am Coll Cardiol* 2006; **47(10):** 1987–1996.

51 Mann JF, Gerstein HC, Pogue J, Bosch J, Yusuf S. Renal insufficiency as a predictor of cardiovascular outcomes and the impact of ramipril: the HOPE randomized trial. *Ann Intern Med* 2001; **134(8):** 629–636.

52 Weiner DE, Tighiouart H, Stark PC, Amin MG, MacLeod B, Griffith JL *et al.* Kidney disease as a risk factor for recurrent cardiovascular disease and mortality. *Am J Kidney Dis* 2004; **44(2):** 198–206.

53 Hailpern SM, Cohen HW, Alderman MH. Renal dysfunction and ischemic heart disease mortality in a hypertensive population. *J Hypertens* 2005; **23(10):** 1809–1816.

54 Manjunath G, Tighiouart H, Coresh J, Macleod B, Salem DN, Griffith JL *et al.* Level of kidney function as a risk factor for cardiovascular outcomes in the elderly. *Kidney Int* 2003; **63(3):** 1121–1129.

55 Manjunath G, Tighiouart H, Ibrahim H, MacLeod B, Salem DN, Griffith JL *et al.* Level of kidney function as a risk factor for atherosclerotic cardiovascular outcomes in the community. *J Am Coll Cardiol* 2003; **41(1):** 47–55.

56 Muntner P, He J, Hamm L, Loria C, Whelton PK. Renal insufficiency and subsequent death resulting from cardiovascular disease in the United States. *J Am Soc Nephrol* 2002; **13(3):** 745–753.

57 Go AS, Chertow GM, Fan D, McCulloch CE, Hsu CY. Chronic kidney disease and the risks of death, cardiovascular events, and hospitalization. *N Engl J Med* 2004; **351(13):** 1296–1305.

58 Fried LF, Shlipak MG, Crump C, Bleyer AJ, Gottdiener J, Kronmal RA *et al.* Renal insufficiency as a predictor of cardiovascular outcomes and mortality in elderly individuals. *J Am Coll Cardiol* 2003; **41(8):** 1364–1372.

59 Fried LF, Katz R, Sarnak MJ, Shlipak MG, Chaves PH, Jenny NC *et al.* Kidney function as a predictor of noncardiovascular mortality. *J Am Soc Nephrol* 2005; **16(12):** 3728–3735.

60 Weiner DE, Tighiouart H, Amin MG, Stark PC, MacLeod B, Griffith JL *et al.* Chronic kidney disease as a risk factor for cardiovascular disease and all-cause mortality: a pooled analysis of community-based studies. *J Am Soc Nephrol* 2004; **15(5):** 1307–1315.

61 Mazza A, Pessina AC, Tikhonoff V, Montemurro D, Casiglia E. Serum creatinine and coronary mortality in the elderly with normal renal function: the CArdiovascular STudy in the ELderly (CASTEL). *J Nephrol* 2005; **18(5):** 606–612.

62 O'Hare AM, Bertenthal D, Covinsky KE, Landefeld CS, Sen S, Mehta K *et al.* Mortality risk stratification in chronic kidney disease: one size for all ages? *J Am Soc Nephrol* 2006; **17(3):** 846–853.

63 Meisinger C, Doring A, Lowel H. Chronic kidney disease and risk of incident myocardial infarction and all-cause and cardiovascular disease mortality in middle-aged men and women from the general population. *Eur Heart J* 2006; **27(10):** 1245–1250.

64 Kottgen A, Russell SD, Loehr LR *et al.* Reduced kidney function as a risk factor for incident heart failure: the Atherosclerosis Risk in Communities (ARIC) study. *J Am Soc Nephrol* 2007; **18(4):** 1307–1315.

65 Jafar TH, Stark PC, Schmid CH, Landa M, Maschio G, de Jong PE *et al.* Progression of chronic kidney disease: the role of blood pressure control, proteinuria, and angiotensin-converting enzyme inhibition: a patient-level meta-analysis. *Ann Intern Med* 2003; **139(4):** 244–252.

66 de Zeeuw D, Remuzzi G, Parving HH, Keane WF, Zhang Z, Shahinfar S *et al.* Proteinuria, a target for renoprotection in patients with type 2 diabetic nephropathy: lessons from RENAAL. *Kidney Int* 2004; **65(6):** 2309–2320.

67 Agodoa LY, Appel L, Bakris GL, Beck G, Bourgoigne J, Briggs JP *et al.* Effect of ramipril vs amlodipine on renal outcomes in hypertensive nephrosclerosis: a randomized controlled trial. *JAMA* 2001; **285(21):** 2719–2728.

68 Iseki K, Kinjo K, Iseki C, Takishita S. Relationship between predicted creatinine clearance and proteinuria and the risk of developing ESRD in Okinawa, Japan. *Am J Kidney Dis* 2004; **44(5):** 806–814.

69 Halbesma N, Kuiken DS, Brantsma AH, Bakker SJ, Wetzels JF, De Zeeuw D *et al.* Macroalbuminuria is a better risk marker than low estimated GFR to identify individuals at risk for accelerated GFR loss in population screening. *J Am Soc Nephrol* 2006; **17(9):** 2582–2590.

70 Basi S, Lewis JB. Microalbuminuria as a target to improve cardiovascular and renal outcomes. *Am J Kidney Dis* 2006; **47(6):** 927–946.

71 Mogensen CE, Keane WF, Bennett PH, Jerums G, Parving HH, Passa P *et al.* Prevention of diabetic renal disease with special reference to microalbuminuria. *Lancet* 1995; **346(8982):** 1080–1084.

72 Adler AI, Stevens RJ, Manley SE, Bilous RW, Cull CA, Holman RR *et al.* Development and progression of nephropathy in type 2 diabetes: the United Kingdom Prospective Diabetes Study (UKPDS 64). *Kidney Int* 2003; **63(1):** 225–232.

73 Culleton BF, Larson MG, Parfrey PS, Kannel WB, Levy D. Proteinuria as a risk factor for cardiovascular disease and mortality in older people: a prospective study. *Am J Med* 2000; **109(1):** 1–8.

74 Miettinen H, Haffner SM, Lehto S, Ronnemaa T, Pyorala K, Laakso M. Proteinuria predicts stroke and other atherosclerotic vascular disease events in nondiabetic and non-insulin-dependent diabetic subjects. *Stroke* 1996; **27(11):** 2033–2039.

75 Hillege HL, Fidler V, Diercks GF, van Gilst WH, de Zeeuw D, van Veldhuisen DJ *et al.* Urinary albumin excretion predicts cardiovascular and noncardiovascular mortality in general population. *Circulation* 2002; **106(14):** 1777–1782.

76 Yuyun MF, Khaw KT, Luben R, Welch A, Bingham S, Day NE *et al.* A prospective study of microalbuminuria and incident coronary heart disease and its prognostic significance in a British population: the EPIC-Norfolk study. *Am J Epidemiol* 2004; **159(3):** 284–293.

77 Arnlov J, Evans JC, Meigs JB, Wang TJ, Fox CS, Levy D *et al.* Low-grade albuminuria and incidence of cardiovascular disease events in nonhypertensive and nondiabetic individuals: the Framingham Heart Study. *Circulation* 2005; **112(7):** 969–975.

78 Tillin T, Forouhi N, McKeigue P, Chaturvedi N. Microalbuminuria and coronary heart disease risk in an ethnically diverse UK population: a prospective cohort study. *J Am Soc Nephrol* 2005; **16(12):** 3702–3710.

79 Astor BC, Hallan SI, Millere ER, III, Yeung E, Coresh J. Glomerular filtration rate, albuminuria, and risk of cardiovascular and all-cause mortality in the US population. *Am J Epidemiol* 2008; **167(10):** 1226–1234.

80 Hallan S, Astor B, Romundstad S, Aasarod K, Kvenild K, Coresh J. Association of kidney function and albuminuria with cardiovascular

mortality in older vs younger individuals: the HUNT II study. *Arch Intern Med* 2007; **167(22):** 2490–2496.

81 Andersen S, Brochner-Mortensen J, Parving HH. Kidney function during and after withdrawal of long-term irbesartan treatment in patients with type 2 diabetes and microalbuminuria. *Diabetes Care* 2003; **26(12):** 3296–3302.

82 Lewis J, Agodoa L, Cheek D, Greene T, Middleton J, O'Connor D *et al.* Comparison of cross-sectional renal function measurements in African Americans with hypertensivenephrosclerosis and of primary formulas to estimate glomerular filtration rate. *Am J Kidney Dis* 2001; **38(4):** 744–753.

83 Rule AD, Gussak HM, Pond GR, Bergstrath EJ, Stegall MD, Cosio FG *et al.* Measured and estimated GFR in healthy potential kidney donors. *Am J Kidney Dis* 2004; **43(1):** 112–119.

84 Gonwa TA, Jennings L, Mai ML, Stark PC, Levey AS, Klintmaim GB. Estimation of glomerular filtration rates before and after orthotopic liver transplantation: evaluation of current equations. *Liver Transplant* 2004; **10(2):** 301–309.

2 Acute Kidney Injury

6 Definition, Classification, and Epidemiology of Acute Kidney Disease

Eric A. J. Hoste,[1,2] Ramesh Venkataraman,[1] & John A. Kellum[1]

[1]The Clinical Research, Investigation, and Systems Modeling of Acute Illness Laboratory, Department of Critical Care Medicine, University of Pittsburgh, School of Medicine, Pittsburgh, USA

[2]Intensive Care Unit, Ghent University Hospital, De Pintelaan 185, Belgium

Introduction

The concept of acute renal failure (ARF) has undergone significant reexamination in recent years. Mounting evidence suggests that acute, relatively mild dysfunction of the kidney, manifest by changes in urine output and blood chemistries, portends serious clinical consequences [1]. Although the term acute renal failure is relatively new, its first description as *ischuria renalis* was by William Heberden in 1802 [2]; it has nonetheless become entrenched in our medical lexicon. During the first World War the syndrome was named "War Nephritis" [3] and was reported in several publications. The syndrome was then largely forgotten until the second World War, when Bywaters and Beall published their classical paper on crush syndrome [4]. It is Homer W. Smith who is credited for the introduction of the term acute renal failure, in a chapter on "Acute renal failure related to traumatic injuries" in his textbook *The Kidney—Structure and Function in Health and Disease* (1951). The same year, an entire issue of the *Journal of Clinical Investigation* was dedicated to ARF [5].

Thus, it should come as little surprise that in most reviews and textbook chapters [6,7], the concept of acute kidney dysfunction still emphasizes the most severe forms, with severe azotemia and often with oliguria or anuria. It has only been in the past few years that moderate decreases of kidney function have been recognized as potentially important, e.g. by the SOFA score [8] and in studies on radiocontrast-induced nephropathy [9].

However, not only has there been a lack of consensus regarding the concept of ARF, but also there has been, until very recently, no consensus on the diagnostic criteria or clinical definition of ARF. Distressingly, this has resulted in multiple different definitions being used. For example, a recent survey revealed the use of at least 35 different definitions of ARF in the literature

[10]. Along with differences in patient characteristics, this lack of uniformity in the diagnosis has probably contributed to the wide variation in the reported incidence and outcome of ARF (incidence ranges between 1 and 31% [11,12], and mortality is between 28 and 82% [12,13]). Obviously if one study defines ARF as a 25% or greater rise in serum creatinine while another study defines ARF based on the need for renal replacement therapy (RRT), the two studies will not describe the same cohort of patients. A linear correlation between the degree of kidney dysfunction and the outcome of acute kidney dysfunction has been described; the more strict the definition of ARF, the greater the mortality [10].

Another element that has emerged in recent years is the observation that small decrements in kidney function are important. For example, Levy *et al.* [9] found that a 25% increase in serum creatinine after administration of radiocontrast was associated with a worse outcome in those patients experiencing the decrement in function compared to those patients who did not experience a 25% or greater increase in serum creatinine. Chertow *et al.* [14] defined hospital-acquired acute kidney dysfunction as an increase of serum creatinine of >0.3 mg/dL and found that this was independently associated with mortality.

Similarly, Lassnigg *et al.* [15] saw, in a cohort of patients who underwent cardiac surgery, that acute kidney dysfunction, defined as an increase of serum creatinine of ≥ 0.5 mg/dL or a decrease greater than 0.3 mg/dL, was associated with decreased survival.

The reasons why small alterations in kidney function lead to increases in hospital mortality are unclear. Possible explanations include the untoward effects of acute kidney dysfunction, such as volume overload, retention of uremic compounds, acidosis, electrolyte disorders, increased risk for infection, and anemia [16]. Although, acute kidney dysfunction could simply be colinear with unmeasured variables that lead to increased mortality, multiple attempts to control for known clinical variables have led to the consistent conclusion that kidney dysfunction is independently associated with adverse outcome. Furthermore, more severe kidney dysfunction tends to be associated with even worse outcome compared to milder abnormalities.

Evidence-based Nephrology. Edited by Donald Molony and Jonathan Craig
© 2009 Blackwell Publishing, ISBN: 978-1-4051-3975-5.

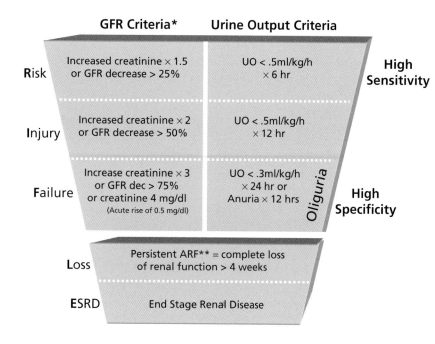

GFR Criteria* **Urine Output Criteria**

Risk — Increased creatinine × 1.5 or GFR decrease > 25% | UO < .5ml/kg/h × 6 hr — **High Sensitivity**

Injury — Increased creatinine × 2 or GFR decrease > 50% | UO < .5ml/kg/h × 12 hr

Failure — Increase creatinine × 3 or GFR dec > 75% or creatinine 4 mg/dl (Acute rise of 0.5 mg/dl) | UO < .3ml/kg/h × 24 hr or Anuria × 12 hrs — Oliguria — **High Specificity**

Loss — Persistent ARF** = complete loss of renal function > 4 weeks

ESRD — End Stage Renal Disease

Figure 6.1 RIFLE classification scheme for AKI. The classification system includes separate criteria for serum creatinine (SCreat) and urine output (UO). The criterion that leads to the worst possible classification should be used. Note that RIFLE-F is present even if the increase in SCreat is <3-fold, as long as the new SCreat is ≥4.0 mg/dL (350 μmol/L) in the setting of an acute increase of at least 0.5 mg/dL (44 μmol/L). The shape of the figure denotes the fact that more patients (high sensitivity) will be included in the mild category, including some without actually having kidney failure (less specificity). In contrast, at the bottom, the criteria are strict and therefore specific, but some patients will be missed. From Bellomo *et al.* [17]; used with permission.

From acute kidney failure to acute kidney injury

As with many conditions in acute medicine, early detection affords a better opportunity to intervene. Furthermore, milder forms of renal dysfunction have clinical importance and therefore staging (mild to severe) is desirable in order to better describe the syndrome. For these reasons, the Acute Dialysis Quality Initiative (ADQI), an international consensus group comprised of nephrologists and intensivists with expertise in acute kidney dysfunction, proposed the RIFLE criteria to define and stage acute kidney dysfunction (www.ccm.upmc.edu/adqi/ADQI2) [17]. The acronym RIFLE stands for the three severity stages of *r*isk, *i*njury, and *f*ailure (in order of increasing severity) and the two outcome stages of *l*oss and *e*nd-stage kidney disease. The three severity stages are defined on the basis of either increases in serum creatinine or decreases in urine output (Figure 6.1), where the more severe of either criterion is used. The two outcome criteria, loss and end-stage kidney disease, are defined by the duration of loss of kidney function.

The RIFLE criteria were published as a workgroup document on the ADQI website in June 2003 and published online May 2004 and in print August 2004 [17]. Since then multiple studies have been published using the RIFLE criteria [18–29] (Table 6.1), with the majority published within the past 12 months. In addition, the Acute Kidney Injury Network (AKIN) organized two conferences endorsed by critical care and nephrology societies from around the world with the aim of developing a broader consensus on the definitions and terminology for ARF. In particular, this group has proposed the term acute kidney injury (AKI) to define the entire spectrum of acute kidney dysfunction from its earliest and mildest forms to the need for RRT. We will therefore adopt this term for new

studies, as we have previously [1,24], although we will continue to use ARF when describing older studies.

Epidemiology of AKI

In one Spanish multicenter study, Liaño *et al.* defined ARF as a sudden rise in serum creatinine concentration to >177 μmol/L in patients with normal kidney function, or a ≥50% rise in serum creatinine in patients with previous mild to moderate chronic kidney failure (serum creatinine <264 μmol/L) [30]. In this study, a collaborative prospective protocol with 98 variables was developed to assess all ARF episodes encountered in the 13 tertiary care hospitals in Madrid, Spain. An overall incidence of ARF of 209 cases per million population (pmp)/year; (95% confidence interval [CI], 195–223) was reported. The incidence of acute tubular necrosis (ATN) was 88 cases pmp (95% CI, 79–97), prerenal ARF was 46 pmp (95% CI, 40–52), acute onset chronic kidney failure presenting as ARF was 29 pmp (95% CI, 24–34), and obstructive ARF was 23 pmp (95% CI, 19–27). In 187 cases, mortality was attributed to underlying disease, and thus corrected mortality due to ARF was 26.7%. Dialysis was required in 36% of patients and was associated with a significantly higher mortality (65.9 vs. 33.2%; P < 0.001). More recently, in a prospective study of adult patients admitted in 43 Spanish intensive care units (ICUs), ARF was defined as a creatinine level of ≥2 mg/dL or oliguria and a urine volume of <400 mL/24 h in patients with normal baseline function, and in patients with chronic kidney disease, ARF was defined as a 100% increase in serum creatinine, excluding patients with a baseline creatinine of ≥4 mg/dL [31]. This study found an incidence of ARF of 5.7%, with 55% of cases occurring on admission. Mortality was 42.3% during the ARF episode, and recovery

Table 6.1 Studies in which the RIFLE criteria for AKI were used.

Study [reference]	Cohort	Aim of study	AKI defined by GFR (1) or by UO and GFR (2)	Outcome criteria	Occurrence of AKI	No. patients with max RIFLE score/total patients in subgroup
Herget-Rosenthal [18]	85 ICU patients, initial normal GFR	Evaluate cystatin C vs creatinine	1	No	44/85 (51.8%)	R: 3/85 (3.5%) I: 13/85 (15.3%) F: 28/85 (32.9%)
Hoste [19]	704 AKI patients treated with RRT	Impact of BSI	NA	Yes	NA	L: 9.2% (no BSI), 43.5%(BSI) E: 0.5% (no BSI), 8.1% (BSI)
Bell [20][a]	207 CRRT patients	Long-term outcome	2	Yes	NA	R: 17/207 (8.2%) I: 50/207 (24.2%) F: 121/207 (58.5%) L: 3/207 (1.4%) E: 16/207 (7.7%)
Abosaif [21][a]	183 ICU patients with AKI on admission	Outcome	2	No	NA	R: 60/159 (37.7%) I: 56/159 (35.2%) F: 43/159 (27.0%)
Kuitunen [22]	813 cardiac surgery patients	Incidence and outcome of AKI	2	No	156/813 (19.2%)	R: 88/813 (10.8%) I: 28/813 (3.4%) F: 40/813 (4.9%)
Guitard [23]	94 liver transplant patients	Incidence and outcome of AKI	1	No	60/94 (63.8%)	I: 39/94 (41.5%) F: 21/94 (22.3%)
Hoste [24]	5383 ICU patients	Incidence and outcome of AKI	2	No	3,617/5,383 (67.2%)	R: 670/5383 (12.4%) I: 1436/5383 (26.5%) F: 1511/5383 (28.1%)
Uchino [25]	20,126 patients admitted to the hospital	Incidence and outcome of AKI	1	No	18%	R: 9.1% I: 5.2% F: 3.7%
Lin [26]	46 ECMO patients	Incidence and outcome of AKI	2	No	36/46 (78.3%)	R: 7/46 (15.2%) I: 18/46 (39.1%) 11/46 (23.9%)
Heringlake [27]	29,623 cardiac surgery patients	Incidence and outcome of AKI	1	No	15.4% (range, 3.1–75%)	R: 9% (2–40%) I: 5% (0.8–30%) F: 2% (0.6–33%)
Lopes [28][b]	126 burn patients	Incidence and outcome of AKI	2	No	35.7%	R: 14.3% I: 8.7% F:: 12.7%
Ahlstrom [29]	658 ICU patients, classified w/in 3 days of ICU admission	Evaluation of different scoring systems, including RIFLE criteria, for hospital mortality	2	Yes	52.0%	R: 168/658 (25.5%) I: 100/658 (15.2%) F: 74/658 (11.2%) L: 1/658 (0.2%)

Abbreviations: NA, not applicable or not available; BSI, bloodstream infection; ECMO, extracorporeal membrane oxygenation.
[a] Patients were classified at inclusion in the study (on admission to the ICU or at the start of CRRT).
[b] Patients were classified on occurrence of maximum RIFLE class during the first 10 days of hospital admission.

of kidney function occurred in 85.6% of the survivors. Four other large epidemiological surveys, in which a less sensitive but more specific definition of ARF was used, i.e. ARF defined by the need for RRT, found an incidence of approximately 100 pmp/year. The incidence in Australia ranged from 80 to 134 pmp/year [32,33], in Finland an incidence of 80 pmp/year was found [34], and recently,

Bagshaw *et al.* reported an incidence of severe ARF defined as needing new RRT of 110 pmp/year in a Canadian population [35].

Recent retrospective data suggest that there is a rise in the incidence of ARF in the USA, while mortality rates are declining [36,37]. Different definitions or coding of ARF may hamper correct interpretation of these findings. However, this limitation seems unlikely based on the study by Waikar *et al.* [37]. Those authors evaluated the accuracy of administrative codes for ARF for applications in clinical epidemiology and health services research by comparing codes of the *International Classification of Diseases,* 9th Revision, Clinical Modification (ICD-9-CM) from hospital discharge records against serum creatinine-based definitions of ARF [38]. The study revealed that 4.2% of discharges received a code for ARF. In comparison to a diagnostic standard of a 100% change in serum creatinine, ICD-9-CM codes for ARF had a sensitivity of 35.4%, specificity of 97.7%, positive predictive value of 47.9%, and negative predictive value of 96.1%. Compared with reviews of medical records, ICD-9-CM codes for ARF had a positive predictive value of 94.0% and negative predictive value of 90.0%.

AKI defined by the RIFLE criteria

An overview of studies using the RIFLE criteria for AKI is presented in Table 6.1.

All studies used the severity grading criteria of risk, injury, and failure, but only three studies [19,20,29] also used the outcome criteria loss and end-stage kidney disease. Two of these studies were in a cohort of AKI patients defined by the need for RRT. Ahlstrom *et al.* [29] and Bell *et al.* [20] classified both severity grades and outcome classes. However, all patients included in the study by Bell and colleagues were treated with chronic RRT for AKI. These subjects therefore had severe AKI, and thus represent only a subgroup of the overall population.

Severity grading was performed according to the RIFLE criteria on creatinine and urine output criteria in 8 of the 11 studies that reported on severity grading [20–24,26,28]. However, Lin *et al.* [26] used different urine output criteria cutoffs than those of RIFLE. The three remaining studies defined severity of AKI based only on change of serum creatinine level and not on urine output [18,25,27]. The reasons for this were diverse. Herget-Rosenthal compared assessment of glomerular filtration rate (GFR) by serum creatinine and cystatin C levels. Uchino retrospectively evaluated hospital-wide cases, which prevented assessment of urine output [25]. In addition, the study by Heringlake was a large prospective study on practice patterns in cardiac surgery in German cardiovascular centers [27], and urine output was not collected. Interestingly, one group chose to use the Cockcroft-Gault equation for assessment of creatinine clearance, rather than use a change in serum creatinine levels, as all other authors did [21]. When the baseline serum creatinine level is unknown in a patient without a history of chronic kidney insufficiency, ADQI proposed backcalculation of the "baseline" serum creatinine concentration using the four-variable Modification of Diet in Renal Disease (MDRD) study equation, assuming a GFR of >75 mL/min/1.73 m^2 [17]. This was done in only four studies [24–26,29]. Kuitunen also used the MDRD formula, however not for assessment of a baseline creatinine level but for assessment of GFR [22].

Most studies used the RIFLE criteria to assess the occurrence of AKI in specific cohorts. However, two studies used the RIFLE criteria for other specific purposes. Herget-Rosenthal evaluated whether a serum level of cystatin C is a better marker for GFR than

a serum creatinine level [18], and Hoste used the RIFLE outcome criteria as a secondary outcome parameter in a study on the impact of bloodstream infection in AKI patients treated with RRT [19].

The occurrence of AKI defined by RIFLE criteria in various different cohorts ranged from 15.4 to 78.3% (Table 6.1). This is higher than is generally accepted when the classic terminology of ARF is used. The large study by Uchino demonstrated that almost 18% of hospitalized patients in a large tertiary care hospital had an episode of AKI as defined by RIFLE using serum creatinine criteria [25]. This is much higher than the incidence of 4.9% reported in a hallmark study using data from 1979 [39] or 7.2% in a follow-up study that used data from 1996 [40]. Although the definition of AKI used in these earlier studies differs from the RIFLE criteria, the sensitivity seems comparable. Hou and Nash defined AKI as a rise in serum creatinine of >0.5mg/dL for patients with a baseline of <1.9 mg/dL, >1.0 mg/dL for patients with a baseline between 2 and 4.9 mg/dL, and >1.5 mg/dL for patients with a serum creatinine level of >5.0 mg/dL [39]. An explanation for the higher rates of AKI could be that the RIFLE criteria are more sensitive, especially for patients with acute or chronic disease. Alternatively, the three cohorts may have had different baseline characteristics and/or different comorbidities. The trend of increasing incidence for the same definition suggests that the latter explanation seems more plausible. Increasingly, patients are now older, suffer from more comorbidities, such as diabetes or cardiovascular disease, and are more frequently exposed to diagnostic and therapeutic procedures with potential to harm the kidneys.

Two large studies in cardiac surgery patients using the RIFLE criteria indicated that the incidence of AKI after cardiac surgery is about 15–20% [22,27]. This is a considerably higher incidence than the incidence of AKI of <8% that is generally accepted in this specific cohort of patients [11,41–44]. In a single-center, tertiary care, general ICU setting, two out of three patients experienced an episode of AKI [24]. This was comparable to the 52% incidence found by another group in a study that included two different ICUs from the same hospital [29] and considerably higher than the incidence of renal dysfunction generally reported (generally ranging from about 5% [45] up to 31% in specific patient subgroups [12,46]). Finally, small studies in specific groups of patients, such as patients with cardiogenic shock on extracorporeal membrane oxygenation, liver transplantation, or burns, also demonstrated high ICU period prevalence rates for AKI, with rates of 78, 64, and 35.7%, respectively [23,26,28].

In summary, the RIFLE criteria for AKI are more sensitive than more traditional definitions of ARF. The incidence of AKI defined by the RIFLE criteria is much higher (2–10 times higher) than the incidence of more traditionally defined ARF, but the incidence for both appears to be increasing.

Outcomes in AKI

Most studies, with few exceptions, have reported a stepwise increase of mortality for increasing RIFLE class. One exception is

Table 6.2 Mortality outcome of AKI defined by RIFLE criteria and by individual RIFLE severity grades after correction for other comorbidities.

Study [reference]	Statistical test used	RIFLE criterion	OR (for LR) or HR (for CPH) (95% CI)	P value
Kuitunen [22]	LR	AKI	2.616	<0.001
Hoste [24]	CPH	AKI	1.7 (1.28–2.13)	<0.001
	CPH	Risk	1.0 (0.68–1.56)	0.896
		Injury	1.4 (1.02–1.88)	0.037
		Failure	2.7 (2.03–3.55)	<0.001
Uchino [25]	LR	Risk	2.536 (2.152–2.988)	<0.0001
		Injury	5.412 (4.547–6.442)	<0.0001
		Failure	10.124 (8.318–12.32)	<0.0001
Lopes [28]	LR	Risk	5.6 (1.2–26.8)	<0.001
		Injury	6.2 (1.1–47.8)	0.008

Abbreviations: LR, logistic regression analysis; CPH, Cox proportional hazard analysis; OR, odds ratio; HR, hazard ratio.

the study by Bell *et al.* [20], who included only patients who were treated with CRRT, suggesting that these patients already had severe AKI. In all other studies, increasing severity classes of AKI indeed had worse outcomes. In four studies, multivariate analyses were performed to assess the impact of AKI defined by RIFLE after correction for other comorbidities (Table 6.2). AKI defined by RIFLE criteria was associated with increased mortality in all four studies.

Limitations of the RIFLE criteria

Use of the urine output criterion of the RIFLE criteria has been more controversial and less widely used compared to the creatinine criterion. Although decreased urine output has a high specificity and sensitivity for acute kidney dysfunction, the urine output criteria have significant limitations. First, sensitivity and specificity may be lost when diuretics are used. The use of diuretics is not explicitly addressed in the RIFLE criteria, although their use is common practice with AKI patients worldwide (with reported utilization rates ranging between 59 and 70%) [47,48]. The urine output criterion can only be accurately assessed in patients with urinary catheters. Thus, the use of urine output criterion may be limited to an ICU cohort. However, these data should also prompt reconsideration of the need for monitoring urine output and improved rigor in this monitoring in most hospital settings outside of the ICU or operating room. Another limitation of the urine output criterion is that there are many reasons that might interfere with exact measurement of urine output, such as mechanical issues, including obstruction of the urinary bladder catheter by debris or blood clots and kinking of the catheter. Finally, the sensitivity of the urine output criterion for risk, injury, and failure may not be well-calibrated with the respective creatinine criteria. In other words, at-risk patients defined by the creatinine criterion may be more severely ill compared to at-risk patients defined by the urine output criterion. This could be one explanation for the different impact of increasing RIFLE class on mortality in the two large studies by Hoste (creatinine and urine output criteria) [24] and Uchino (creatinine criterion only) [25]. Baseline mortality in non-AKI patients was comparable. However, mortality for patients in the risk, injury, and failure groups was much higher in the cohort studied by Uchino compared to the cohort studies by Hoste, despite the fact that the latter was derived from a hospital-wide population and the former a general ICU population.

Another limitation of the RIFLE criteria is the need for a baseline creatinine level in order to calculate the proportional decrease of kidney function. A proportional increase in serum creatinine better represents changes in kidney function compared to a severity gradation based completely on specific cutoffs, as in the SOFA score [8]. A patient who has an increase of serum creatinine from 0.5 to 1.1 mg/dL has a 120% decrease of kidney function and this would be classified as RIFLE injury; however, this same patient would have a renal SOFA score of 0. Baseline serum creatinine levels are, however, not always known in patients who are admitted to the emergency department or ICU. And if there are data, what is the correct baseline? For example, a serum creatinine level after a 1.5-week hospitalization period in an elderly patient with pneumonia may be falsely low due to loss of muscle mass and decreased creatinine production [49]. Creatinine at admission is probably less biased by loss of muscle mass; however, it may be elevated already due to early kidney dysfunction. In patients without a history of chronic kidney disease, back-calculation of a "baseline" creatinine level using the MDRD equation has been proposed; however, this can only provide an approximate value, and the validity of this equation across all populations has been questioned. The MDRD equation was validated in a large data set of US patients with moderate to severe chronic kidney insufficiency and was not validated in patients with near-normal kidney function, in patients with underlying diabetes mellitus, or in the very elderly. However, recent reports from different parts of the world suggest general validity in other groups of patients and ethnicities [50–52].

Another issue was raised by Herget-Rosenthal *et al.* [18]. These authors demonstrated that serum cystatin C levels allow for an earlier determination of AKI than serum creatinine. Although serum creatinine has its limitations, it has been the biomarker of choice for evaluation of kidney function for many years. Recently, other biomarkers for detection of AKI have emerged.

Biomarkers of renal tubular injury

Several serum and urinary markers, such as neutrophil gelatinase-associated lipocalin (NGAL) [53,54], kidney injury molecule-1 (KIM-1) [55], cysteine-rich protein 61 (also called CCN1) [56], spermidine/spermine $N(1)$-acetyltransferase [57], cystatin C [18,58], and urine interleukin-18 (IL-18) [59–61], have been identified as potential markers of early tubular injury (see Table 6.3).

Table 6.3 Potential biomarkers in early detection and surveillance of AKI.

Biomarker	Study	Patients	Results	Comments
Cystatin C	Villa *et al.* [62]	50 critically ill patients	Serum cystatin C correlated better with GFR than did serum creatinine	1/cystatin C versus C_{Cr}: $r = 0.832$, $P < 0.001$ 1/creatinine versus C_{Cr}: $r = 0.426$, $P = 0.002$
	Herget-Rosenthal *et al.* [18]	85 patients at high risk to develop AKI	Increase in blood level of cystatin C significantly preceded that of creatinine	Serum cystatin C increased by ≥50%, 1.5 ± 0.6 days earlier than creatinine
	Ahlstrom *et al.* [58]	202 consecutive adult ICU patients	Serum cystatin C was as good as plasma creatinine in detecting AKI in intensive care patients	Cystatin C had poor predictive value for hospital mortality
NGAL	Mishra *et al.* [53]	71 children undergoing cardiopulmonary bypass	NGAL in urine at 2 h after cardiopulmonary bypass was the most powerful independent predictor of acute renal injury	NGAL conc in urine at 2 h had area under ROC curve of 0.998; sensitivity was 1.00 and specificity was 0.98 for a cutoff value of 50 μg/L
KIM-1	Han *et al.* [55]	6 patients with biopsy-proven ATN	For each unit increase in normalized KIM-1 there was a >12-fold-higher risk for the presence of ATN (odds ratio, 12.4; 95% CI, 1.2–119)	Small study with questionable statistical and clinical relevance
IL-18	Parikh *et al.* [59]	Nested case–control study within Acute Respiratory Distress Syndrome Network trial (400 urine specimens from 52 patients and 86 controls)	Urine IL-18 levels of >100 pg/mL are associated with increased odds of AKI of 6.5 (95% CI, 2.1–20.4) in the next 24 h	On multivariable analysis, urine IL-18 on day 0 was independent predictor of mortality

Of these markers, cystatin C has been evaluated most extensively. Cystatin C is a nonglycosylated protein that is produced at a constant rate by nucleated cells. Its low molecular mass (13.3 kDa) and positive charge at physiological pH levels facilitate its glomerular filtration. Following filtration, it is reabsorbed and almost completely catabolized in the proximal renal tubule. Because of its constant rate of production, its serum concentration is determined by glomerular filtration. For these reasons, cystatin C has the potential to be a useful marker in detecting AKI. Villa *et al.* conducted an evaluation of serum cystatin C concentration as a real-time marker of AKI in critically ill patients and demonstrated that cystatin C correlated better with GFR than did creatinine and was diagnostically superior to creatinine (receiver-operating characteristic [ROC] area under the curve for cystatin C, 0.927; 95% confidence interval, 86.1–99.4; ROC area under the curve for creatinine, 0.694; 95% confidence interval, 54.1–84.6) [62]. Subsequently, Herget-Rosenthal and coworkers evaluated early detection of AKI by cystatin C and showed that the increase in blood levels of this marker significantly preceded that of creatinine [18]. Moreover, according to the R, I, and F criteria of RIFLE, cystatin C detected renal dysfunction 2 days earlier than did creatinine. It also predicted the long-term need for RRT in patients with AKI moderately well. A subsequent study evaluated serum cystatin C as a marker of kidney function in ARF and its power in predicting survival of ARF patients [58]. Serum cystatin C, plasma creatinine, and plasma urea were measured in 202 patients upon admission to the ICU, daily during the first 3 days, and 5–7 times a week during the rest of the ICU stay. In this study, serum cystatin C showed excellent positive predictive value for ARF in critical illness. However, it was not clinically useful in predicting mortality.

Using a genome-wide interrogation strategy, investigators have identified NGAL as one of the most strikingly up-regulated genes and overexpressed proteins in the kidney after ischemia [54,63]. The clinical applicability of NGAL in AKI was demonstrated by Mishra *et al.*, who studied 71 children undergoing cardiopulmonary bypass [53]. Serial urine and blood samples were analyzed by Western blotting and enzyme-linked immunosorbent assay for NGAL expression. Using multivariate analysis, the investigators found that the urinary NGAL 2 h after cardiopulmonary bypass was the most powerful independent predictor of acute renal injury. The study also revealed that for the concentration of NGAL in the urine at 2 h, the area under the receiver-operating characteristic curve was 0.998, sensitivity was 1.00, and specificity was 0.98, using a cutoff value of 50 μg/L.

KIM-1 is a type 1 transmembrane protein whose expression is markedly up-regulated in the proximal tubule in the postischemic kidney in rat models. In a pilot study, Han *et al.* evaluated the appearance of KIM-1 in the urine of 40 patients with acute (23 patients) or chronic (9 patients) kidney failure and normal kidney function (8 patients) and the tissue expression of KIM-1 in kidney biopsy specimens from 6 patients with biopsy-proven ATN [55]. The investigators found that there was extensive expression of KIM-1 in proximal tubule cells in biopsies from the six patients with confirmed ATN. Moreover, when adjusted for age, gender,

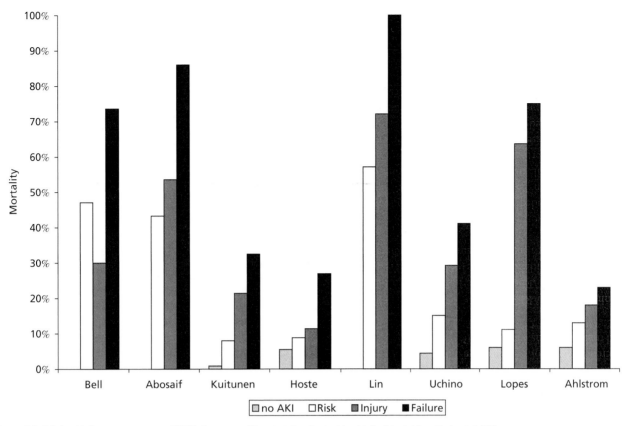

Figure 6.2 Relationship between outcome and RIFLE class across different studies. See text for details. Adapted from Hoste *et al.* [64].

and length of time between the initial insult and sampling of the urine, these investigators found that for subjects in this small cohort, a 1-unit increase in normalized KIM-1 was associated with a 12-fold risk (odds ratio, 12.4; 95% CI, 1.2–119) for the presence of ATN.

IL-18 has been shown to be an important mediator of inflammation. Urine IL-18 levels have been shown to increase in patients with ATN, both in animal models and human studies [59–61]. In humans, IL-18 was shown to have a sensitivity and specificity of >90% for diagnosis of established kidney injury [59]. In this study, on multivariable analysis, the urine IL-18 concentration was an independent predictor of mortality.

Large human trials evaluating the usefulness of various biomarkers for early detection of AKI are lacking. However, theoretically such biomarkers could play an important role in the diagnosis and management of AKI. Currently available serum markers for other disease processes, such as troponin-I and brain natriuretic peptide, have correlated fairly well with the degree of the underlying disease. Serum brain natriuretic peptide levels also decline with adequate response to therapy. Theoretically, serial measurement of a biomarker could potentially help clinicians identify early disease and/or follow the response to treatment once disease is advanced. With ongoing research, an analogous biomarker for AKI is perhaps not too far in the future. In addition, further research exploring

the value of biomarkers in terms of prognosticating for patients with AKI (both survival and renal recovery) will be necessary.

Conclusions

Small changes in kidney function in hospitalized patients are important and impact outcomes, hence the shift of terminology from ARF to AKI. RIFLE criteria provide a uniform definition of AKI and are increasingly used in the literature. RIFLE severity grades represent patient groups with increasing severity of illness, as illustrated by the increasing proportion of patients who die or require treatment with RRT.

References

1 Hoste EA, Kellum JA. RIFLE criteria provide robust assessment of kidney dysfunction and correlate with hospital mortality. *Crit Care Med* 2006; **34**: 2016–2017.
2 Eknoyan G. Emergence of the concept of acute renal failure. *Am J Nephrol* 2002; **22**: 225–230.
3 Davies F, Weldon R. A contribution to the study of "war nephritis." *Lancet* 1917; **ii**: 118–120.

4 Bywaters EG, Beall D. Crush injuries with impairment of renal function. *Br Med J* 1941; **1**: 427–432.

5 Oliver J, Mac DM, Tracy A. The pathogenesis of acute renal failure associated with traumatic and toxic injury; renal ischemia, nephrotoxic damage, and the ischemic episode. *J Clin Invest* 1951; **30**: 1307–1439.

6 Gill N, Nally JV, Jr., Fatica RA. Renal failure secondary to acute tubular necrosis: epidemiology, diagnosis, and management. *Chest* 2005; **128**: 2847–2863.

7 Kumar P, Clark M (editors). *Clinical Medicine*, 6th edn. Elsevier Saunders, Philadelphia, PA, USA; 2005.

8 Vincent JL, Moreno R, Takala J, Willats S, De Mendonca A, Bruining H *et al*. The SOFA (sepsis-related organ failure assessment) score to describe organ dysfunction/failure. *Intensive Care Med* 1996; **22**: 707–710.

9 Levy EM, Viscoli CM, Horwitz RI. The effect of acute renal failure on mortality. A cohort analysis. *JAMA* 1996; **275**: 1489–1494.

10 Kellum JA, Levin N, Bouman C, Lameire N. Developing a consensus classification system for acute renal failure. *Curr Opin Crit Care* 2002; **8**: 509–514.

11 Chertow G, Lazarus J, Christiansen C, Cook EF, Hammermeister KE, Grover F *et al*. Preoperative renal risk stratification. *Circulation* 1997; **95**: 878–884.

12 Vivino G, Antonelli M, Moro M, Cottini F, Conti G, Bufi M *et al*. Risk factors for acute renal failure in trauma patients. *Intensive Care Med* 1998; **24**: 808–814.

13 Schiffl H, Lang SM, Fischer R. Daily hemodialysis and the outcome of acute renal failure. *N Engl J Med* 2002; **346**: 305–310.

14 Chertow GM, Burdick E, Honour M, Bonventre JV, Bates DW. Acute kidney injury, mortality, length of stay, and costs in hospitalized patients. *J Am Soc Nephrol* 2005; **16**: 3365–3370.

15 Lassnigg A, Schmidlin D, Mouhieddine M, Bachmann LM, Druml W, Bauer P *et al*. Minimal changes of serum creatinine predict prognosis in patients after cardiothoracic surgery: a prospective cohort study. *J Am Soc Nephrol* 2004; **15**: 1597–1605.

16 Hoste EA, Kellum JA. ARF in the critically ill: Impact on morbidity and mortality. *Contrib Nephrol* 2004; **144**: 1–11.

17 Bellomo R, Ronco C, Kellum JA, Mehta RL, Palevsky P. Acute renal failure: definition, outcome measures, animal models, fluid therapy, and information technology needs: the Second International Consensus Conference of the Acute Dialysis Quality Initiative (ADQI) Group. *Crit Care* 2004; **8**: R204–R212.

18 Herget-Rosenthal S, Marggraf G, Husing J, Goring F, Pietruck F, Janssen O *et al*. Early detection of acute renal failure by serum cystatin C. *Kidney Int* 2004; **66**: 1115–1122.

19 Hoste EA, Blot SI, Lameire NH, Vanholder RC, De Bacquer D, Colardyn FA. Effect of nosocomial bloodstream infection on the outcome of critically ill patients with acute renal failure treated with renal replacement therapy. *J Am Soc Nephrol* 2004; **15**: 454–462.

20 Bell M, Liljestam E, Granath F, Fryckstedt J, Ekbom A, Martling CR. Optimal follow-up time after continuous renal replacement therapy in actual renal failure patients stratified with the RIFLE criteria. *Nephrol Dial Transplant* 2005; **20**: 354–360.

21 Abosaif NY, Tolba YA, Heap M, Russell J, El Nahas AM. The outcome of acute renal failure in the intensive care unit according to RIFLE: model application, sensitivity, and predictability. *Am J Kidney Dis* 2005; **46**: 1038–1048.

22 Kuitunen A, Vento A, Suojaranta-Ylinen R, Pettila V. Acute renal failure after cardiac surgery: evaluation of the RIFLE classification. *Ann Thorac Surg* 2006; **81**: 542–546.

23 Guitard J, Cointault O, Kamar N, Muscari F, Lavayssiere L, Suc B *et al*. Acute renal failure following liver transplantation with induction therapy. *Clin Nephrol* 2006; **65**: 103–112.

24 Hoste EA, Clermont G, Kersten A, Venkataraman R, Angus DC, De Bacquer D *et al*. RIFLE criteria for acute kidney injury are associated with hospital mortality in critically ill patients: a cohort analysis. *Crit Care* 2006; **10**: R73.

25 Uchino S, Bellomo R, Goldsmith D, Bates S, Ronco C. An assessment of the RIFLE criteria for acute renal failure in hospitalized patients. *Crit Care Med* 2006; **34**: 1913–1917.

26 Lin C-Y, Chen Y-C, Tsai F-C, Tian YC, Jeng CC, Fang JT *et al*. RIFLE classification is predictive of short-term prognosis in critically ill patients with acute renal failure supported by extracorporeal membrane oxygenation. *Nephrol Dial Transplant* 2006; **21**: 2867–2873.

27 Heringlake M, Knappe M, Vargas Hein O, Lufft H, Kindgen-Milles D, Bottiger BW *et al*. Renal dysfunction according to the ADQI-RIFLE system and clinical practice patterns after cardiac surgery in Germany. *Minerva Anestesiol* 2006; **72**: 645–654.

28 Lopes JA, Jorge S, Neves FC, Caneira M, da Costa AG, Ferriera AC *et al*. An assessment of the RIFLE criteria for acute renal failure in the severely burned patients. *Nephrol Dial Transplant* 2007; **22**: 285

29 Ahlstrom A, Kuitunen A, Peltonen S, Hynninen M, Tallgren M, Aaltonen *et al*. Comparison of 2 acute renal failure severity scores to general scoring systems in the critically ill. *Am J Kidney Dis* 2006; **48**: 262–268.

30 Liaño F, Pascual J, the Madrid Acute Renal Failure Study Group. Epidemiology of acute renal failure: a prospective, multicenter, community-based study. *Kidney Int* 1996; **50**: 811–818.

31 Herrera-Gutierrez ME, Seller-Perez G, Maynar-Moliner J, Sanchez-Izquierdo-Riera JA. Epidemiology of acute kidney failure in Spanish ICU. Multicenter prospective study FRAMI. *Med Intensiva* 2006; **30**: 260–267.

32 Cole L, Bellomo R, Silvester W, Reeves JH. A prospective, multicenter study of the epidemiology, management, and outcome of severe acute renal failure in a "closed" ICU system. *Am J Respir Crit Care Med* 2000; **162**: 191–196.

33 Silvester W, Bellomo R, Cole L. Epidemiology, management, and outcome of severe acute renal failure of critical illness in Australia. *Crit Care Med* 2001; **29**: 1910–1915.

34 Korkeila M, Ruokonen E, Takala J. Costs of care, long-term prognosis and quality of life in patients requiring renal replacement therapy during intensive care. *Intensive Care Med* 2000; **26**: 1824–1831.

35 Bagshaw SM, Laupland KB, Doig CJ, Mortis G, Fick GH, Mucenski M *et al*. Prognosis for long-term survival and renal recovery in critically ill patients with severe acute renal failure: a population-based study. *Crit Care* 2005; **9**: R700–R709.

36 Xue JL, Daniels F, Star RA, Kimmel PL, Eggers PW, Molitoris BA *et al*. Incidence and mortality of acute renal failure in Medicare beneficiaries, 1992 to 2001. *J Am Soc Nephrol* 2006; **17**: 1135–1142.

37 Waikar SS, Curhan GC, Wald R, McCarthy EP, Chertow GM. Declining mortality in patients with acute renal failure, 1988 to 2002. *J Am Soc Nephrol* 2006; **17**: 1143–1150.

38 Waikar SS, Wald R, Chertow GM, Curhan GG, Winkelmayer WC, Liangos O *et al*. Validity of *International Classification of Diseases*, Ninth Revision, clinical modification codes for acute renal failure. *J Am Soc Nephrol* 2006; **17**: 1688–1694.

39 Hou S, Bushinsky D, Wish J, Cohen JJ, Harrington HT. Hospital-acquired renal insuffciency: a prospective study. *Am J Med* 1983; **74**: 243–248.

40 Nash K, Hafeez A, Hou S. Hospital-acquired renal insufficiency. *Am J Kidney Dis* 2002; **39**: 930–936.

41 Mangano CM, Diamondstone LS, Ramsay JG, Aggarwal A, Herkowitz A, Mangano DT. Renal dysfunction after myocardial revascularization: risk factors, adverse outcomes, and hospital resource utilization. *Ann Intern Med* 1998; **128**: 194–203.

42 Conlon P, Stafford-Smith M, White W, Newman MF, King S, Winn MP *et al.* Acute renal failure following cardiac surgery. *Nephrol Dial Transplant* 1999; **14**: 1158–1162.

43 Stallwood MI, Grayson AD, Mills K, Scawn ND. Acute renal failure in coronary artery bypass surgery: independent effect of cardiopulmonary bypass. *Ann Thorac Surg* 2004; **77**: 968–972.

44 Thakar CV, Liangos O, Yared JP, Nelson D, Piedmonte MR, Hariachar S *et al.* ARF after open-heart surgery: Influence of gender and race. *Am J Kidney Dis* 2003; **41**:742-751.

45 Uchino S, Kellum JA, Bellomo R, Doig GS, Morimatsu H, Morgera S *et al.* Acute renal failure in critically ill patients: a multinational, multicenter study. *JAMA* 2005; **294**: 813–818.

46 de Mendonca A, Vincent JL, Suter PM, Moreno R, Dearden NM, Antonelli M *et al.* Acute renal failure in the ICU: risk factors and outcome evaluated by the SOFA score. *Intensive Care Med* 2000; **26**: 915–921.

47 Mehta RL, Pascual MT, Soroko S, Chertow GM. Diuretics, mortality, and nonrecovery of renal function in acute renal failure. *JAMA* 2002; **288**: 2547–2553.

48 Uchino S, Doig GS, Bellomo R, Morimatsu H, Morgera S, Schetz M *et al.* Diuretics and mortality in acute renal failure. *Crit Care Med* 2004; **32**: 1669–1677.

49 Hoste EA, Damen J, Vanholder RC, Lameire NH, Delanghe JR, Van den Hauwe K *et al.* Assessment of renal function in recently admitted critically ill patients with normal serum creatinine. *Nephrol Dial Transplant* 2005; **20**: 747–753.

50 Hallan S, Asberg A, Lindberg M, Johnsen H. Validation of the Modification of Diet in Renal Disease formula for estimating GFR with special emphasis on calibration of the serum creatinine assay. *Am J Kidney Dis* 2004; **44**: 84–93.

51 Nobrega AM, Gomes CP, Lemos CC, Bregman R. Is it possible to use modification of diet in renal disease (MDRD) equation in a Brazilian population? *J Nephrol* 2006; **19**: 196–199.

52 Aizawa M, Hayashi K, Shimaoka T, Yamaji K, Horikoshi S, Tomino Y. Comparison of prediction equations of glomerular filtration rate in Japanese adults. *Nippon Jinzo Gakkai Shi* 2006; **48**: 62–665.

53 Mishra J, Dent C, Tarabishi R, Mitsnefes MM, Ma Q, Kelly C *et al.* Neutrophil gelatinase-associated lipocalin (NGAL) as a biomarker for acute renal injury after cardiac surgery. *Lancet* 2005; **365**: 1231–1238.

54 Mishra J, Ma Q, Prada A, Mitsnefes M, Zahedi K, Yang J *et al.* Identification of neutrophil gelatinase-associated lipocalin as a novel early urinary biomarker for ischemic renal injury. *J Am Soc Nephrol* 2003; **14**: 2534–2543.

55 Han WK, Bailly V, Abichandani R, Thadhani R, Bonventre JV. Kidney injury molecule-1 (KIM-1): a novel biomarker for human renal proximal tubule injury. *Kidney Int* 2002; **62**: 237–244.

56 Muramatsu Y, Tsujie M, Kohda Y, Pham B, Perantoni AO, Zhao H *et al.* Early detection of cysteine rich protein 61 (CYR61, CCN1) in urine following renal ischemic reperfusion injury. *Kidney Int* 2002; **62**: 1601–1610.

57 Zahedi K, Wang Z, Barone S, Prada AE, Kelly CN, Casero RA *et al.* Expression of SSAT, a novel biomarker of tubular cell damage, increases in kidney ischemia-reperfusion injury. *Am J Physiol Renal Physiol* 2003; **284**: F1046–F1055.

58 Ahlstrom A, Tallgren M, Peltonen S, Pettila V. Evolution and predictive power of serum cystatin C in acute renal failure. *Clin Nephrol* 2004; **62**: 344–350.

59 Parikh CR, Abraham E, Ancukiewicz M, Edelstein CL. Urine IL-18 is an early diagnostic marker for acute kidney injury and predicts mortality in the intensive care unit. *J Am Soc Nephrol* 2005; **16**: 3046–3052.

60 Parikh CR, Jani A, Melnikov VY, Faubel S, Edelstein CL. Urinary interleukin-18 is a marker of human acute tubular necrosis. *Am J Kidney Dis* 2004; **43**: 405–414.

61 Parikh CR, Mishra J, Thiessen-Philbrook H, Dursun B, Ma Q, Kelly C *et al.* Urinary IL-18 is an early predictive biomarker of acute kidney injury after cardiac surgery. *Kidney Int* 2006; **70**: 199–203.

62 Villa P, Jimenez M, Soriano MC, Manzanares J, Casasnovas P. Serum cystatin C concentration as a marker of acute renal dysfunction in critically ill patients. *Crit Care* 2005; **9**: R139–R143.

63 Devarajan P, Mishra J, Supavekin S, Patterson LT, Potter S. Gene expression in early ischemic renal injury: clues towards pathogenesis, biomarker discovery, and novel therapeutics. *Mol Genet Metab* 2003; **80**: 365–376.

64 Hoste E, Kellum JA. Acute kidney injury: epidemiology and diagnostic criteria. *Curr Opin Crit Care* 2006; **12**: 531–537.

7 Pre-Renal Failure and Obstructive Disease

Kevin W. Finkel

Division of Renal Diseases & Hypertension, University of Texas Medical School, Houston, USA

Introduction

Pre-renal azotemia is the most common form of acute renal failure (ARF) in hospitalized patients and, if uncorrected, can lead to ischemic parenchymal damage and acute tubular necrosis (ATN) [1,2]. The clinical syndrome of pre-renal failure is characterized by intact tubular function with impaired filtration function because of renal hypoperfusion and usually manifests as low urine volume, reduced urinary concentration of sodium (UNa) and fractional excretion of sodium (FeNa%), and an elevated ratio of blood urea nitrogen to serum creatinine (Cr).

Pre-renal failure is the result of either true volume depletion, as occurs with hemorrhage or excessive diuresis, or "effective" volume depletion in circumstances such as congestive heart failure (cardiorenal syndrome), liver failure with ascites (hepatorenal syndrome), and sepsis. The etiologies for pre-renal failure are outlined in Table 7.1. In both instances decreased intravascular volume causes baroreceptor stimulation and enhanced adrenergic output, leading to systemic and local regulatory mechanisms aimed at restoring normal perfusion pressure.

At the level of the kidney, a complex interplay between neuroendocrine and vasoactive agents initially compensates for decreased perfusion pressure. Specifically, angiotensin II causes preferential vasoconstriction of the efferent arteriole, increased proximal tubular reabsorption, elevation of glomerular hydrostatic pressure, and a reduced glomerular ultrafiltration coefficient. Because of angiotensin II preferential constriction of the efferent arteriole, with mild to moderate volume depletion, the glomerular filtration rate (GFR) is maintained. With severe volume depletion, frank ischemic ATN may ensue. Since the GFR in such situations is dependent on relative efferent arteriolar vasoconstriction, the use of angiotensin II antagonists, such as angiotensin converting enzyme (ACE) inhibitors and angiotensin receptor blockers (ARBs),

can precipitate ATN. The vasoconstrictor effects of angiotensin II are opposed by endogenously produced prostaglandins and nitric oxide. When used acutely in pre-renal failure, nonsteroidal anti-inflammatory drugs lead to unopposed vasoconstriction and worsening of renal function.

In response to decreased renal perfusion, activation of the renin–aldosterone axis and release of antidiuretic hormone also occur, increasing sodium and water retention in an attempt to restore intravascular volume. These temporizing physiologic measures are necessary to maintain perfusion pressures in the face of frank volume depletion but are ineffective in sepsis and clearly deleterious in conditions such as heart failure with pulmonary edema.

Given this background, pre-renal failure is not a simple case of hypovolemia that can be corrected by administration of intravascular crystalloid or colloid. Treatment must, by necessity, be directed at the underlying pathophysiology that has triggered the compensatory physiologic response common to all etiologies. Therefore, an evidence-based approach to the treatment of pre-renal azotemia requires a review of the available data in several subgroups of patients and cannot take a "one size fits all" approach.

Diagnosis

Many causes of pre-renal failure are clinically obvious. With reliance on history, physical examination, and certain laboratory findings, patients with true volume depletion are often easily identified and can be treated with aggressive volume repletion. Such patients demonstrate orthostatic hypotension, tachycardia, dry mucous membranes, low urinary output, and poor skin turgor. Although much has been made of the utility of urinary indices in ARF (*vide infra*), they are unnecessary in such situations, and patients promptly respond to volume resuscitation. Likewise, the argument over using colloid or crystalloid in these patients is moot, as simple crystalloid solutions have proven very effective. It is only in the complex patient, usually in an intensive care unit (ICU), that such controversies are more germane. In essence, one is trying to differentiate the patient with pre-renal failure physiology

Evidence-based Nephrology. Edited by Donald Molony and Jonathan Craig
© 2009 Blackwell Publishing, ISBN: 978-1-4051-3975-5.

Table 7.1 Causes of pre-renal failure.

Decreased Cardiac Output	Redistribution/Vasodilation
Myocardial infarction	Cirrhosis
Congestive heart failure	Nephrotic syndrome
Pericardial tamponade	Pancreatitis
Positive pressure ventilation	Sepsis
Pulmonary embolism	Crush injuries
	Intestinal obstruction
Hypovolemia	**Vascular Disease**
Hemorrhage	Renal artery stenosis
Diuresis	Atheroembolism
Diarrhea	Vasculitis
Excessive sweating	Aortic aneurysm dissection

who will not benefit (or be frankly harmed) by fluid resuscitation from one who will quickly recover with crystalloid or colloid infusion. For example, a patient with cirrhosis of the liver and ARF has clinical and laboratory findings consistent with pre-renal failure. Will volume repletion reverse the renal failure because true volume depletion is present, or is it hepatorenal syndrome? In both scenarios the kidneys are underperfused, but administration of fluid will only help in the former and be deleterious in the latter. In the liver failure patient measurement of the central venous pressure (CVP) or pulmonary artery occlusion pressure (PAOP) could be used as a guide to therapy, or the clinical response to an infusion of saline, as recommended by the Second International Ascites Club [3]. Yet, none of these diagnostic methods has been subjected to rigorous scientific analysis. Similarly, in the patient with septic shock, on multiple vasopressors and positive pressure ventilation, early ARF may be pre-renal failure in nature but aggressive fluid resuscitation may only serve to aggravate hypoxemia by worsening acute respiratory distress syndrome (ARDS). Indeed, in the recently published Fluids and Catheter Treatment Trial by the ARDS Network group, a fluid-conservative treatment strategy targeting a CVP of 3 or a PAOP of 7 decreased the number of ventilator days and ICU length of stay without any increase in the incidence of ARF or need for dialysis [4].

CVP and PAOP

Although physicians often rely on CVP and PAOP to guide fluid administration and determine whether or not a patient has true volume depletion, there is little evidence that such measurements are clinically useful. Although there are no trials that have assessed the utility of these measurements specifically for determining the reversibility of pre-renal failure, one can reasonably extrapolate from available data regarding their ability to predict improvement in stroke volume, cardiac output, and urine output.

The CVP and PAOP are frequently used as means of determining cardiac preload and volume status. However, their use has been criticized because of poor ability to predict which patients will have improvement in their hemodynamic status when given fluid resuscitation [5]. As reviewed by Michard and Teboul, in three of five

trials assessing the ability of CVP to predict fluid responsiveness in critically ill patients, defined as an improvement in either stroke volume or cardiac output, there was no significant difference in the baseline CVP measurements between responders and nonresponders. The two remaining studies reported lower baseline values of CVP in responders; however, the marked overlap of individual CVP levels did not allow for the identification of a discriminatory cutoff value. Likewise, baseline PAOP was not significantly lower in responders versus nonresponders in seven of nine studies. Three studies reported a significant difference in the baseline PAOP between the groups, being higher in responders in a single study and lower in responders in two studies. However, in none of the studies could a cutoff PAOP value be found that predicted the hemodynamic response to volume expansion. In normal subjects, Kumar and associates demonstrated a lack of correlation between initial CVP and PAOP values and both end diastolic volume and stroke volume [6]. Furthermore, changes in both parameters following 3-L saline infusion did not correlate with changes in end diastolic volume and cardiac performance.

In addition, numerous randomized controlled trials (RCTs) and meta-analyses assessing the benefit of pulmonary artery catheters (PAC) in a variety of clinical circumstances have been reported [7–9]. In a meta-analysis of 13 RCTs, the use of PAC neither increased overall mortality and hospital days nor conferred any benefit [10]. Likewise, in an RCT of 676 patients with shock mainly from sepsis, ARDS, or both, early use of PAC did not significantly affect mortality or morbidity, including the need for dialysis [11]. Therefore, in critically ill patients with multiple reasons for pre-renal failure (sepsis, capillary leak with third spacing, positive pressure ventilation, hypoalbuminemia, cardiac dysfunction, and liver disease), measurement of CVP and/or PAOP does not improve outcome and has poor predictive value for improvement in renal function.

Urine output

The development of oliguria (urine output of less than 400 mL/day) does not assure the presence of pre-renal failure. It occurs in both pre-renal failure states and numerous other causes of ARF, including ATN, obstructive nephropathy, glomerulonephritis, and atheroembolic disease. Despite the compensatory mechanisms invoked in response to decreased renal perfusion that increase salt and water retention by the kidneys in pre-renal failure states, higher urine outputs can ensue in the face of underlying chronic kidney disease, salt wasting states such as adrenal insufficiency and cerebral salt wasting, concomitant use of diuretics, osmotic diuresis, and the presence of nonreabsorbed anions, such as ketones and bicarbonate in the urine.

Urinalysis

Urinalysis is often used to differentiate various causes of ARF. In pre-renal failure, the urine is concentrated and the urinary sediment is bland. Bland urinary sediment, however, does not allow for discrimination between true and effective volume depletion. Furthermore, patients with pre-renal failure can have abnormal sediment if they have a pre-existing renal disorder, bilirubin in the

Table 7.2 Urinary indices in ARF.

Index and range	No. of patients with condition/total no. of patients		
	Pre-renal failure	Oliguric ATN	Nonoliguric ATN
Urine Na (mEq/L)			
<20	18/30 (60%)	0/24 (0%)	2/13 (6%)
20–40	12/30 (40%)	14/24 (59%)	11/31 (35%)
>40	0/30 (0%)	10/24 (41%)	18/31 (59%)
FeNa%			
<1	27/30 (90%)	1/24 (4%)	4/31 (12%)

Source: Adapted from reference 14.

urine (causing granular casts), or microscopic hematuria and bacteriuria from an indwelling bladder catheter. The utility of the urinalysis in differentiating pre-renal failure from acute kidney injury (AKI) has been called further into question by the results of two recent systematic reviews on the urinary findings in sepsis-related AKI (human and experimental animal studies). These systematic reviews demonstrated substantial heterogeneity between studies and suggested that the scientific basis for the use of urinary microscopy in septic AKI and, by extension, to differentiating ATN from pre-renal failure is weak [12,13].

Urinary indices

The measurement of UNa and calculation of the FeNa% has been routinely recommended as a means to differentiate oliguric pre-renal failure from oliguric ATN, as shown in Table 7.2. In the sentinel study reported by Miller *et al.* a UNa concentration of less than 20 mEq/L had an 80% sensitivity and specificity for differentiating pre-renal failure from ATN in the face of oliguria [14]. The FeNa% performed even better, with a sensitivity and specificity of 98 and 95%, respectively. The utility of either measurement was significantly less in the absence of oliguria. However, there are numerous exceptions to the general rule [15–17]. Both UNa and FeNa% can be low, suggestive of pre-renal failure with ARF from rhabdomyolysis, radiocontrast nephropathy, acute glomerulonephritis, multiple myeloma, amphotericin B toxicity, and early obstructive nephropathy. More to the point, the finding of renal sodium avidity does not allow one to discriminate between true and effective volume depletion nor reliably predict reversibility with volume administration.

It is also important to point out that in the study by Miller *et al.* patients were excluded if they had an elevated baseline creatinine (>1.6 mg/dL), received any diuretic within the preceding 24 h, had evidence of underlying adrenal or liver disease, or had glucosuria or bicarbonaturia [14]. Also, the percentage of patients with sepsis was not described, nor was the actual cause of ATN provided. With only 85 patients included in the study, it is probable that in the medically complex patient these indices have lower sensitivity and specificity or predictive powers than the paper actually suggests.

The use of diuretics can increase urinary sodium loss even in the face of pre-renal failure, thus negating the utility of the FeNa%. Since the fractional excretion of urea (FeUN%) is primarily dependent on passive forces, it is less influenced by the administration of diuretics and may be useful in the evaluation of ARF. A group of 102 patients with ARF was divided into three subgroups: pre-renal failure, pre-renal failure treated with diuretics, and ATN. The FeNa% was low in 92% of prerenal failure patients and 48% of pre-renal failure patients receiving diuretics. Both groups had similar and significantly lower FeUN% values than the ATN patients [18].

Treatment

In the patient with clinically obvious volume depletion, adequate fluid resuscitation can be achieved by the administration of crystalloids, such as normal saline or lactated Ringers solution. Such patients often show remarkable improvement in their renal function over a short period of time.

In the complex or critically ill patient, the situation is more challenging. In this population, it is difficult to accurately determine intravascular volume and whether the pre-renal failure is due to true or effective volume depletion, while concern is great for the potential harm of indiscriminant fluid administration in the face of acute lung injury or frank ARDS. There is also debate on what type of fluid, colloid versus crystalloid, is best for volume resuscitation in such patients. Although not specifically done to address pre-renal failure, review of recent clinical trials in these areas can provide some type of general guideline.

Goal-directed hemodynamic management and fluid therapy

Previous observational nonrandomized studies had shown that patients who survived critical illness had higher values for cardiac index and oxygen delivery than those who died and that those values were higher than normal physiologic levels [19,20]. Two studies of surgical patients showed significant decreases in mortality associated with therapy directed at increasing hemodynamic parameters to supraphysiologic values, whereas no benefit was seen in patients with sepsis and mixed groups of critically ill patients [21–24]. Subsequently, two RCTs assessed the benefit of goal-directed hemodynamic therapy in critically ill patients. In one trial of 100 patients randomized to dobutamine or placebo, there were no differences in mean arterial pressure or oxygen consumption despite higher cardiac index and oxygen delivery in the treatment group [25]. In fact, the treatment group had a significantly higher mortality rate than the placebo group. In another trial of 762 patients randomized into one of three intervention groups, hemodynamic therapy aimed at achieving supranormal values for cardiac index or normal values for mixed venous oxygenation saturation did not reduce morbidity or mortality [26].

More recently, Rivers and colleagues reported their experience with early goal-directed therapy in the treatment of severe sepsis and septic shock [27]. Patients with severe sepsis or septic shock were randomly assigned upon arrival to the emergency center to either 6 h of early goal-directed therapy or standard therapy prior to admission to the ICU. Active intervention aimed at achieving a central venous oxygen saturation of 70% included saline boluses targeted to a CVP level of 8–12 mmHg, vasopressor agents to maintain a mean arterial pressure greater than 65 mmHg, transfusion to a hematocrit of 30%, and dobutamine. Although the patients assigned to active intervention received more fluid and blood products in the initial 24-h period, they experienced a significantly reduced rate of organ failure and death.

Finally, the ARDS Clinical Trials Network assessed optimal fluid management in patients in the ICU with acute lung injury [4]. In this RCT, 1000 patients were assigned to either a conservative or liberal strategy of fluid management using explicit protocols applied for 7 days. The mean cumulative fluid balances in the conservative versus liberal groups were −136 ml and 6992 mL, respectively. Although there was no difference in mortality, the conservative group had significantly reduced ventilator and ICU days and improved oxygenation. Importantly, conservative fluid management did not increase the need for RRT.

Crystalloid versus colloid fluids

The putative superiority of colloid over crystalloid fluids in the resuscitation of the critically ill patient has been a source of considerable controversy. Aggressive hydration with crystalloid solutions such as normal saline can worsen interstitial edema and pulmonary function. Colloidal solutions, such as various starches and human albumin, might appear to be attractive alternatives, but there is little solid evidence of their superiority in clinical trials. Systematic reviews of randomized controlled trials comparing crystalloids with colloids have yielded conflicting results. Some trials have found an increased mortality rate associated with the administration of human albumin and hydroxyethyl-starch, while others have not [28–31]. More recently, a large, randomized, controlled prospective trial of albumin versus saline in almost 7000 critically ill patients found no benefit of one over the other [32]. Specifically, there was no demonstrable effect on mortality, renal function, or the frequency of renal replacement therapy. Of note, patients with cirrhosis were excluded from this trial, and limited data suggest that albumin is useful to prevent ARF in cirrhotic patients with spontaneous bacterial peritonitis [33].

Summary

In the complex medical patient, pre-renal failure can occur from either true or effective volume depletion. Since both circumstances share the same physiologic derangements, clinical parameters such as urine output and urinary electrolytes do not have any discriminatory power between the two. It is also difficult to predict which patients will benefit from volume resuscitation based on measurement of the CVP or PAOP. Often, the only way to determine if the renal failure is reversible is to provide an empiric "fluid challenge" and assess the clinical response. With regard to approaching the critically ill patient who may be functionally pre-renal failure, fluid management is dependent on timing. Early intervention with goal-directed therapy, resulting in a positive fluid balance in the first 24 h, is associated with reduced organ failure. In patients already in the ICU with lung injury, a conservative fluid approach improves pulmonary function without adverse renal effects.

Cardiorenal syndrome

Cardiorenal syndrome is a recently recognized constellation of findings in patients with combined cardiac and renal dysfunction. Such patients have pulmonary edema refractory to diuretics, recurrent hospitalizations, progressive renal failure, and markedly reduced quality of life. However, no explicit diagnostic criteria have been adopted, as yet, for cardiorenal syndrome. It is nonetheless a common medical condition. The prevalence of chronic kidney disease (GFR of ≤ 60 mL/min) in the US population is estimated to be 16 million adults. In these patients, cardiac failure is frequently present and a major cause of mortality [34,35]. Likewise, the development of renal dysfunction in heart failure patients has a significantly negative impact on prognosis. In the Evaluation of Losartan in the Elderly (ELITE) study, comparing an ACE inhibitor to an ARB in the treatment of heart failure, nearly 30% of patients experienced worsening renal function [36]. In the Studies of Left Ventricular Dysfunction trial, risk factors for renal failure included older age, low ejection fraction, use of diuretics, low systolic blood pressure, and diabetes mellitus [37]. Patients who develop worsening renal function have increased hospital length of stay, higher costs, and higher mortality rates [38].

The pathophysiology of cardiorenal syndrome is incompletely understood. It is not simply a "low cardiac output" syndrome, since up to as many as one-half of patients have cardiac ejection fractions greater than 40%, and several studies could not find a correlation between worsening renal function and ejection fraction [38,39]. More than likely, cardiorenal syndrome is the result of a complex interplay between local and systemic neurohumoral systems, such as the renin–angiotensin–aldosterone system, sympathetic nervous system, natriuretic peptides, nitric oxide, prostaglandins, endothelin, and inflammatory mediators. It is not surprising, therefore, that traditional methods for treating heart failure prove either ineffective or exacerbate renal dysfunction and have prompted interest in novel therapies, such as isolated ultrafiltration.

Treatment of cardiorenal syndrome

Determining the best evidence-based treatment of cardiorenal syndrome is a challenging clinical problem, since most heart failure trials have excluded patients with impaired renal function. Furthermore, as mentioned, cardiorenal syndrome is not simply a low-flow problem that corrects with traditional therapies used in congestive heart failure. Each organ dysfunction appears to interact in such a way that traditional measures may be rendered ineffective.

Diuretics

The role of diuretics in cardiorenal syndrome is controversial. Often, they are not effective in achieving the desired fluid removal and weight loss. In heart failure trials, 20% of patients treated with intravenous diuretics fail to lose weight or actually gain weight during their hospitalization [40]. This diuretic resistance has been shown to be an independent marker of poor outcome. Aggressive attempts to overcome the resistance with higher diuretic doses, continuous infusion, or addition of a second diuretic agent acting distally to a loop diuretic often are associated with worsening renal function, an independent risk factor for mortality [41].

Loop-diuretic resistance results from the interplay of several factors, including poor intestinal absorption, decreased delivery to the kidney, increased sodium absorption proximal and distal to the loop of Henle, and excess sodium intake. Strategies to overcome resistance include adding an additional diuretic agent that acts at another site, increasing the dose and frequency of the diuretic, and changing from intermittent to continuous infusion. However, a Cochrane review comparing continuous to intermittent bolus diuretic for congestive heart failure was unable to confirm any superiority from this maneuver [42]. Addition of hyperoncotic (>5%) albumin has also been advocated as a means of increasing diuresis. In analbuminemic animals, addition of albumin increases salt excretion [43]. However, albumin did not improve diuresis in a small trial of humans with nephrotic syndrome [44].

ACE inhibitors and ARBs

ACE inhibitors and ARBs have clearly been shown to improve survival in patients with heart failure [45]. Most studies, however, excluded patients with significant chronic kidney disease (Cr $\geq$ 2.0 mg/dL).

The Cooperative North Scandinavian Enalapril Survival Study (CONSENSUS) included severe heart failure patients with creatinine values less than 3.5 mg/dL [46]. In the subgroup with Cr greater than 2.0 mg/dL, use of an ACE inhibitor significantly improved outcome. Nevertheless, in CONSENSUS 30% of all patients experienced an increase in their serum Cr, although few patients needed to stop the medication.

In order to avoid precipitating acute renal dysfunction, ACE inhibitors and ARBs should be started at low doses in patients who are considered not to be volume depleted and who are off of any nonsteroidal anti-inflammatory agents.

Natriuretic peptides

B-type natriuretic peptide (BNP) is produced by the myocardial ventricles in response to increased stress. BNP results in arterial and venous vasodilation, increased sodium excretion, and suppression of the renin–angiotensin–aldosterone system.

Nesiritide, a synthetic BNP, was assessed in heart failure patients in the Vasodilation in the Management of Acute Congestive Heart Failure trial [47]. Compared to intravenous nitroglycerine, nesiritide significantly lowered PAOP at 1 h, although there was no difference in the degree of dyspnea. Nesiritide was equally effective in patients with or without renal dysfunction (Cr > 2.0 mg/dL) [48].

In another trial nesiritide was given to patients with recent increases in baseline Cr associated with congestive heart failure exacerbation (mean Cr increase from 1.5 to 1.8 mg/dL) [49]. Compared to placebo, there were no changes in urine output, sodium excretion, glomerular filtration rate, or effective renal plasma flow. This finding suggests that nesiritide is ineffective in cardiorenal syndrome.

More concerning are recent reports that the use of nesiritide in congestive heart failure may be associated with an increased risk of acute renal dysfunction and mortality. In a meta-analysis of five randomized trials including 1,269 patients, the use of nesiritide was significantly associated with the development of acute renal dysfunction (an increase of Cr of ≥ 0.5 mg/dL) [50]. Furthermore, in three RCTs that reported mortality rates, the use of nesiritide was associated with a hazard ratio for death of 1.8 ($P = 0.057$) [51].

Ultrafiltration

Ultrafiltration (UF) for therapy-resistant chronic volume overload is an increasingly utilized treatment modality. With the advent of technology that allows for low blood flow and ultrafiltration rates, and also venous access through a peripheral location, the use of isolated UF will likely become commonplace in the treatment of cardiorenal syndrome.

The Ultrafiltration Versus IV Diuretics for Patients Hospitalized for Acute Decompensated Congestive Heart Failure trial compared UF and intravenous diuretics in 200 patients [52]. Compared to patients who received diuretics, patients randomized to UF lost more weight and, at 90 days, had less rehospitalization and unscheduled clinic and emergency center visits. However, overall mortality rates were equal in both groups. In addition, there is justified concern if isolated UF becomes more prevalent outside the research environment that excessive UF rates may result in hypotension and worsening renal function.

Obstructive nephropathy

Urinary tract obstruction should always be considered in the differential diagnosis of ARF. Regardless of cause, obstruction of urinary flow leads to renal impairment, which early in the course of the condition is reversible if the obstruction is alleviated. Tubular function is initially affected; however, prolonged obstruction leads to tubular damage and parenchymal atrophy.

Clinical manifestations of urinary tract obstruction vary depending on the location, duration, and degree of obstruction. In patients with complete bilateral obstruction or with an obstructed solitary kidney, anuria (<50 mL urine output in 24 h) can be the presenting feature, whereas in patients with partial obstruction, the urinary output can vary from oliguria to polyuria. Although pain is more likely to be associated with acute blockage, obstruction may be totally asymptomatic and occur without overt clinical manifestations or suggestive laboratory findings. Therefore, obstructive nephropathy should always be considered as a cause of renal failure when an obvious pre-renal failure or intrinsic renal cause is not identified. The location of obstruction is anatomically divided into upper and lower urinary tract at or below the level of the bladder. Common causes of lower urinary tract obstruction include urethral strictures, prostatic hypertrophy, and neurogenic bladder.

Diagnosis of urinary tract obstruction can be difficult. Anuria, flank pain with a palpable mass, or a palpable bladder are obvious clues. The laboratory evaluation can be helpful. Hyperkalemia with a nonanion gap metabolic acidosis is suggestive of a renal tubular acidosis associated with obstruction [53]. The urinary sediment may be bland or demonstrate crystals or hematuria, depending on the etiology of the obstruction. Patients may have very dilute urine due to the presence of an acquired form of nephrogenic diabetes insipidus [54].

Ultrasonography is the most useful test for the presence of obstruction. Although hydronephrosis is usually demonstrated, there are circumstances when hydronephrosis is not seen despite urinary tract obstruction: 1) early in the course of obstruction (12–24 h) when the collecting system is relatively noncompliant; 2) in the face of severe volume depletion when glomerular filtration is severely depressed; and 3) when the collecting system is encased by retroperitoneal lymphadenopathy or fibrosis [55,56].

Conversely, the finding of hydronephrosis on ultrasound does not prove the presence of obstruction, since it is also seen in high urinary flow states such as diuretic use and diabetes insipidus, pregnancy, previous obstruction, and congenital megaureter. In a series of 192 patients with ARF, hydronephrosis unrelated to obstruction was noted in 11% of patients [57].

Although ultrasound is the preferred imagining modality for initial assessment of obstruction, its use has been supplanted by noncontrast helical computed tomography (CT) scan in the evaluation of flank pain and nephrolithiasis. In a single-center study of 864 patients evaluated for flank pain, 34 underwent both helical CT scan and ultrasound [58]. Compared to helical CT, ultrasound was found to have a sensitivity and specificity for renal stones of 81 and 100%, respectively, although the sensitivity for ureteric stones was only 46%. In the same study, the sensitivity and specificity for the detection of hydronephrosis were 93 and 100%, respectively.

In another study, 181 consecutive patients with acute flank pain underwent a combination of helical CT, ultrasound, and unenhanced radiography [59]. When compared with the diagnostic accuracy for ureterolithiasis of combined ultrasound and unenhanced radiography, helical CT had greater sensitivity (92% vs. 77%) and negative predictive value (87% vs. 68%).

Treatment of obstruction and its timing is dependent on the etiology. Patients with small stones (>5 mm) can be managed conservatively with aggressive hydration and pain control in the absence of infection. Bladder catheterization should be performed if there is reason to suspect that bladder outlet obstruction is present; possible clues to this diagnosis include suprapubic pain, a palpable bladder, or an older man with unexplained renal failure. Measurement of a urinary postvoid residual is often advocated in the detection of outlet obstruction but has not been subjected to any rigorous evaluation. Nor is there a standard method of measurement or definition. Up to one-third of patients with bladder outlet obstruction demonstrated by urodynamic testing do not have an elevated postvoid residual [60]. Upper tract obstruction is relieved with either percutaneous nephrostomy tubes or ureteral stenting, depending on cause, availability, and local expertise.

The duration and severity of obstruction are the major determinants for the recovery of renal function after its correction. The longer the duration of obstruction, the less likely are the chances for complete renal recovery. There are few published data on the relationship between duration and obstruction and renal recovery rates. The variability is likely related to the severity and cause of obstruction, the presence of underlying chronic kidney disease, and concurrent infection. Case reports, however, have documented renal recovery after correction of obstruction lasting 12 months [59].

Postobstructive diuresis

Postobstructive diuresis occurs when there is correction of complete bilateral obstruction or complete obstruction of a solitary kidney. It involves the production of a large volume of urine that results from a defect in urine-concentrating ability, impaired reabsorption of urinary sodium, and solute diuresis from the retained urea and intravenous administration of sodium-containing solutions [62]. Although numerous textbooks discuss the proposed pathogenesis and treatment of postobstructive diuresis, there is very little information in the medical literature that describes its clinical course or outcome other than case reports and case series. There certainly are no RCTs. Patients with relief of complete obstruction are considered at risk for developing postobstructive diuresis and should be carefully monitored. It has been recommended for patients without pulmonary edema, congestive heart failure, or altered consciousness from uremia that urine losses be replaced by oral intake. Intravenous replacement fluids are given only if the patients develop orthostatic hypotension, tachycardia, hyponatremia, or a urine output of more than 200 mL/h [63]. On the other hand, in high-risk patients with altered sensorium, congestive heart failure, or pulmonary edema, replacement of half the hourly urine output with half-normal saline has been recommended. If the patient is hyponatremic, normal saline should be used instead. None of these recommendations has been subjected to any rigorous clinical trial. Nonetheless, they do appear to be prudent and reasonable based on clinical experience.

References

1 Liano F, Pascual J. Epidemiology of acute renal failure: a prospective, multicenter, community-based study. Madrid Acute Renal Failure Study Group. *Kidney Int* 1996; **50**: 811–818.

2 Thadhani R, Pascual M, Bonventre JV. Acute renal failure. *N Engl J Med* 1996; **334**: 1448–1460.

3 Arroyo V, Gines P, Gerbes AL, Dudley EJ, Gentillini P, Laffi G *et al*. Definition and diagnostic criteria of refractory ascites and hepatorenal

syndrome in cirrhosis. International Ascites Club. *Hepatology* 1996; **23**: 164–176.

4 Wiedemann HP, Wheeler AP, Bernard GR, Thompson BT, Hayden D, deBloisblanc B *et al.* Comparison of two fluid-management strategies in acute lung injury. *N Engl J Med* 2006; **354**: 2564–2575.

5 Michard F, Teboul JL. Predicting fluid responsiveness in ICU patients: a critical analysis of the evidence. *Chest* 2002; **121**: 2000–2008.

6 Kumar A, Anel R, Bunnell E, Habet K, Zanotti S, Marshall S *et al.* Pulmonary artery occlusion pressure and central venous pressure fail to predict ventricular filling volume, cardiac performance, or the response to volume infusion in normal subjects. *Crit Care Med* 2004; **32**: 691–699.

7 Sandham JD, Hull RD, Brant RF, Knox L, Pineo GF, Doig CJ *et al.* A randomized, controlled trial of the use of pulmonary-artery catheters in high-risk surgical patients. *N Engl J Med* 2003; **348**: 5–14.

8 Harvey S, Harrison DA, Singer M, Ashcroft J, Jones CM, Elbourne D *et al.* Assessment of the clinical effectiveness of pulmonary artery catheters in management of patients in intensive care (PAC-Man): a randomised controlled trial. *Lancet* 2005; **366**: 472–477.

9 Binanay C, Califf RM, Hasselblad V, O'Connor CM, Shah MR, Sopko G *et al.* Evaluation study of congestive heart failure and pulmonary artery catheterization effectiveness: the ESCAPE trial. *JAMA* 2005; **294**: 1625–1633.

10 Shah MR, Hasselblad V, Stevenson LW, Binanay C, O'Connor CM, Sopko G *et al.* Impact of the pulmonary artery catheter in critically ill patients: meta-analysis of randomized clinical trials. *JAMA* 2005; **294**: 1664–1670.

11 Richard C, Warszawski J, Anguel N, Deye N, Combes A, Barnoud D *et al.* Early use of the pulmonary artery catheter and outcomes in patients with shock and acute respiratory distress syndrome: a randomized controlled trial. *JAMA* 2003; **290**: 2713–2720.

12 Bagshaw SM, Langenberg C, Bellomo R. Urinary biochemistry and microscopy in septic acute renal failure: a systematic review. *Am J Kidney Dis* 2006; **48**: 695–705.

13 Bagshaw SM, Langenberg C, Wan L, May CN, Bellomo R. A systematic review of urinary findings in experimental septic acute renal failure. *Crit Care Med* 2007; **35**: 1592–1598.

14 Miller TR, Anderson RJ, Linas SL, Henrich WL, Berns AS, Gabow PA *et al.* Urinary diagnostic indices in acute renal failure: a prospective study. *Ann Intern Med* 1978; **89**: 47–50.

15 Corwin HL, Schreiber MJ, Fang LS. Low fractional excretion of sodium. Occurrence with hemoglobinuric- and myoglobinuric-induced acute renal failure. *Arch Intern Med* 1984; **144**: 981–982.

16 Vaz AJ. Low fractional excretion of urine sodium in acute renal failure due to sepsis. *Arch Intern Med* 1983; **143**: 738–739.

17 Zarich S, Fang LS, Diamond JR. Fractional excretion of sodium. Exceptions to its diagnostic value. *Arch Intern Med* 1985; **145**: 108–112.

18 Carvounis CP, Nisar S, Guro-Razuman S. Significance of the fractional excretion of urea in the differential diagnosis of acute renal failure. *Kidney Int* 2002; **62**: 2223–2229.

19 Bland RD, Shoemaker WC, Abraham E, Cobo JC. Hemodynamic and oxygen transport patterns in surviving and nonsurviving postoperative patients. *Crit Care Med* 1985; **13**: 85–90.

20 Shoemaker WC, Montgomery ES, Kaplan E, Elwyn DH. Physiologic patterns in surviving and nonsurviving shock patients. Use of sequential cardiorespiratory variables in defining criteria for therapeutic goals and early warning of death. *Arch Surg* 1973; **106**: 630–636.

21 Shoemaker WC, Appel PL, Kram HB, Waxman K, Lee TS. Prospective trial of supranormal values of survivors as therapeutic goals in high-risk surgical patients. *Chest* 1988; **94**: 1176–1186.

22 Boyd O, Grounds RM, Bennett ED. A randomized clinical trial of the effect of deliberate perioperative increase of oxygen delivery on mortality in high-risk surgical patients. *JAMA* 1993; **270**: 2699–2707.

23 Tuchschmidt J, Fried J, Astiz M, Rackow E. Elevation of cardiac output and oxygen delivery improves outcome in septic shock. *Chest* 1992; **102**: 216–220.

24 Yu M, Levy MM, Smith P, Takiguchi SA, Miyasaki A, Myers SA. Effect of maximizing oxygen delivery on morbidity and mortality rates in critically ill patients: a prospective, randomized, controlled study. *Crit Care Med* 1993; **21**: 830–838.

25 Hayes MA, Timmins AC, Yau EH, Palazzo M, Hinds CJ, Watson D. Elevation of systemic oxygen delivery in the treatment of critically ill patients. *N Engl J Med* 1994; **330**: 1717–1722.

26 Gattinoni L, Brazzi L, Pelosi P, Latini R, Tognoni G, Pesenti A *et al.* A trial of goal-oriented hemodynamic therapy in critically ill patients. SvO2 Collaborative Group. *N Engl J Med* 1995; **333**: 1025–1032.

27 Rivers E, Nguyen B, Havstad S, Ressler J, Muzzin A, Knoblich B *et al.* Early goal-directed therapy in the treatment of severe sepsis and septic shock. *N Engl J Med* 2001; **345**: 1368–1377.

28 Schierhout G, Roberts I. Fluid resuscitation with colloid or crystalloid solutions in critically ill patients: a systematic review of randomised trials. *BMJ* 1998; **316**: 961–964.

29 Choi PT, Yip G, Quinonez LG, Cook DJ. Crystalloids vs. colloids in fluid resuscitation: a systematic review. *Crit Care Med* 1999; **27**: 200–210.

30 Ragaller MJ, Theilen H, Koch T. Volume replacement in critically ill patients with acute renal failure. *J Am Soc Nephrol* 2001; **12(Suppl 17)**: S33–S39.

31 Reviewers CIGA. Human albumin administration in critically ill patients: systematic review of randomised controlled trials. Cochrane Injuries Group Albumin Reviewers. *BMJ* 1998; **317**: 235–240.

32 Finfer S, Bellomo R, Boyce N, French J, Myburgh J, Norton R *et al.* A comparison of albumin and saline for fluid resuscitation in the intensive care unit. *N Engl J Med* 2004; **350**: 2247–2256.

33 Sort P, Navasa M, Arroyo V, Aldequer X, Planas R, Ruiz-del-Arbol L *et al.* Effect of intravenous albumin on renal impairment and mortality in patients with cirrhosis and spontaneous bacterial peritonitis. *N Engl J Med* 1999; **341**: 403–409.

34 Shlipak MG. Pharmacotherapy for heart failure in patients with renal insufficiency. *Ann Intern Med* 2003; **138**: 917–924.

35 Initiative KDOQ. K/DOQI clinical practice guidelines for chronic kidney disease: evaluation, classification, and stratification. *Am J Kidney Dis* 2002; **39**: S1–S266.

36 Pitt B, Segal R, Martinez FA, Meurers G, Cowley AJ, Thomas I *et al.* Randomised trial of losartan versus captopril in patients over 65 with heart failure (Evaluation of Losartan in the Elderly Study, ELITE). *Lancet* 1997; **349**: 747–752.

37 Dries DL, Exner DV, Domanski MJ, Greenberg B, Stevenson LW. The prognostic implications of renal insufficiency in asymptomatic and symptomatic patients with left ventricular systolic dysfunction. *J Am Coll Cardiol* 2000; **35**: 681–689.

38 Forman DE, Butler J, Wang Y, Abraham WT, O'Connor CM, Gottlieb SS *et al.* Incidence, predictors at admission, and impact of worsening renal function among patients hospitalized with heart failure. *J Am Coll Cardiol* 2004; **43**: 61–67.

39 Butler J, Forman DE, Abraham WT, Gottlieb SS, Loh E, Massie BM *et al.* Relationship between heart failure treatment and development of worsening renal function among hospitalized patients. *Am Heart J* 2004; **147**: 331–338.

40 Registry AADHFN. ADHERE (Acute Decompensated Heart Failure National Registry) www.adhereregistry.com/nat.html 2004.

41 Gottlieb SS. Renal effects of adenosine A1-receptor antagonists in congestive heart failure. *Drugs* 2001; **61**: 1387–1393.

42 Salvador DR, Rey NR, Ramos GC, Punzalan FE. Continuous infusion versus bolus injection of loop diuretics in congestive heart failure. *Cochrane Database Syst Rev* 2004; **3**: CD003178.

43 Inoue M, Okajima K, Itoh K, Ando Y, Watanabe N, Yasaka T *et al*. Mechanism of furosemide resistance in analbuminemic rats and hypoalbuminemic patients. *Kidney Int* 1987; **32**: 198–203.

44 Fliser D, Zurbruggen I, Mutschler E, Bischoff I, Nussberger J, Franek E *et al*. Coadministration of albumin and furosemide in patients with the nephrotic syndrome. *Kidney Int* 1999; **55**: 629–634.

45 Investigators TS. Effect of enalapril on survival in patients with reduced left ventricular ejection fractions and congestive heart failure. The SOLVD Investigators. *N Engl J Med* 1991; **325**: 293–302.

46 Ljungman S, Kjekshus J, Swedberg K. Renal function in severe congestive heart failure during treatment with enalapril (the Cooperative North Scandinavian Enalapril Survival Study [CONSENSUS] Trial). *Am J Cardiol* 1992; **70**: 479–487.

47 Investigators PCftV. Intravenous nesiritide vs nitroglycerin for treatment of decompensated congestive heart failure: a randomized controlled trial. *JAMA* 2002; **287**: 1531–1540.

48 Butler J, Emerman C, Peacock WF, Mathur VS, Young JB. The efficacy and safety of B-type natriuretic peptide (nesiritide) in patients with renal insufficiency and acutely decompensated congestive heart failure. *Nephrol Dial Transplant* 2004; **19**: 391–399.

49 Wang DJ, Dowling TC, Meadows D, Ayala T, Marshall J, Minshall S *et al*. Nesiritide does not improve renal function in patients with chronic heart failure and worsening serum creatinine. *Circulation* 2004; **110**: 1620–1625.

50 Sackner-Bernstein JD, Skopicki HA, Aaronson KD. Risk of worsening renal function with nesiritide in patients with acutely decompensated heart failure. *Circulation* 2005; **111**: 1487–1491.

51 Sackner-Bernstein JD, Kowalski M, Fox M, Aaronson K. Short-term risk of death after treatment with nesiritide for decompensated heart failure: a pooled analysis of randomized controlled trials. *JAMA* 2005; **293**: 1900–1905.

52 Costanza M. Ultrafiltration versus IV diuretics for patients hospitalized for acute decompensated heart failure. 55th Annual Scientific Session of the American College of Cardiology, Atlanta, GA, 2006.

53 Batlle DC, Arruda JA, Kurtzman NA. Hyperkalemic distal renal tubular acidosis associated with obstructive uropathy. *N Engl J Med* 1981; **304**: 373–380.

54 Kato A, Hishida A, Ishibashi R, Nakajima T, Ohura M, Furuya R *et al*. Nephrogenic diabetes insipidus associated with bilateral ureteral obstruction. *Intern Med* 1994; **33**: 231–233.

55 Webb JA. Ultrasonography in the diagnosis of renal obstruction. *BMJ* 1990; **301**: 944–946.

56 Rascoff JH, Golden RA, Spinowitz BS, Charytan C. Nondilated obstructive nephropathy. *Arch Intern Med* 1983; **143**: 696–698.

57 Amis ES, Jr., Cronan JJ, Pfister RC, Yoder IC. Ultrasonic inaccuracies in diagnosing renal obstruction. *Urology* 1982; **19**: 101–105.

58 Ather MH, Jafri AH, Sulaiman MN. Diagnostic accuracy of ultrasonography compared to unenhanced CT for stone and obstruction in patients with renal failure. *BMC Med Imag* 2004; **4**: 2.

59 Catalano O, Nunziata A, Altei F, Siani A. Suspected ureteral colic: primary helical CT versus selective helical CT after unenhanced radiography and sonography. *Am J Roentgenol* 2002; **178**: 379–387.

60 Turner-Warwick R, Whiteside CG, Worth PH, Milroy EJ, Bates CP. A urodynamic view of the clinical problems associated with bladder neck dysfunction and its treatment by endoscopic incision and trans-trigonal posterior prostatectomy. *Br J Urol* 1973; **45**: 44–59.

61 Cohen EP, Sobrero M, Roxe DM, Levin ML. Reversibility of long-standing urinary tract obstruction requiring long-term dialysis. *Arch Intern Med* 1992; **152**: 177–179.

62 Schlossberg SM, Vaughan ED, Jr. The mechanism of unilateral postobstructive diuresis. *J Urol* 1984; **131**: 534–536.

63 Narins RG. Post-obstructive diuresis: a review. *J Am Geriatr Soc* 1970; **18**: 925–936.

8 Hepatorenal Syndrome

Andrés Cárdenas & Pere Ginès

Liver Unit, Institut de Malalties Digestives i Metaboliques, Hospital Clinic, University of Barcelona, Barcelona, Spain.

Renal failure in the setting of cirrhosis is a common complication that accounts for major morbidity and mortality. A frequent cause of kidney dysfunction in patients with advanced cirrhosis is hepatorenal syndrome (HRS), which occurs in the absence of parenchymal kidney disease. HRS is defined as functional renal failure characterized by renal vasoconstriction and a low glomerular filtration rate (GFR) that develops in patients with advanced cirrhosis and ascites; however, it occasionally occurs in patients with alcoholic hepatitis or acute liver failure [1–4]. There are two types of HRS, as previously defined by the International Ascites Club: type 1 HRS is the acute form and is associated with very poor prognosis, and type 2 HRS is a chronic form that develops slowly over weeks with a better survival rate [1]. Although advances in medical therapy are very promising, liver transplantation remains the treatment of choice in suitable candidates. Uncontrolled studies demonstrate that the use of splanchnic vasoconstrictors, such as terlipressin, midodrine, and norepinephrine, in combination with albumin as a plasma expander or the use of a transjugular intrahepatic portosystemic shunts (TIPS) are effective in improving renal function in cirrhosis. HRS can be prevented in the setting of spontaneous bacterial peritonitis (SBP) with intravenous albumin and in alcoholic hepatitis with oral pentoxifylline [3,5]. This chapter will review the pathogenesis, clinical features, therapy, and prevention of HRS.

Pathogenesis

The main characteristic of HRS is the presence of renal vasoconstriction [6,7]. This vasoconstriction occurs late in the natural history of patients with cirrhosis and ascites and is a consequence of a continuous process where several underlying mechanisms, including changes in systemic arterial circulation, increased portal pressure, impaired cardiac function, and activation of systemic

and renal vasoconstrictor factors, act on the renal circulation and lead to functional renal failure without histological damage of the kidneys.

Arterial vasodilation

Portal hypertension due to an abnormal liver architecture and increased intrahepatic resistance of blood flow is the main factor responsible for the development of splanchnic arterial vasodilation. This vasodilation occurs mainly due to the production of nitric oxide and other vasodilators (calcitonin gene-related peptide, substance P, carbon monoxide, and endogenous cannibinoids) as a consequence of endothelial stretching and possibly bacterial translocation [8]. Plasma volume accumulates in the splanchnic bed, causing a compensatory response due to a fall in central blood volume with activation of systemic vasoconstrictor and antinatriuretic systems, such as the renin–angiotensin–aldosterone system (RAAS), the sympathetic nervous system (SNS), and arginine vasopressin (AVP), accounting for sodium and water retention and in advanced stages, renal vasoconstriction as the kidney senses a relative hypovolemic state (Figure 8.1) [9–11]. The ongoing action of such vasoconstrictor factors acting on the kidney eventually leads to HRS. This occurs because although in the early stages of cirrhosis renal blood flow may be kept within normal limits due to the effect of local renal vasodilators, with time circulating vasoconstrictors overcome the effect of renal vasodilators, leading to severe renal vasoconstriction and reduction in GFR [7,12]. In some patients precipitating factors such as bacterial infections worsen circulatory dysfunction and may trigger renal vasoconstriction [5,13]. At this stage, the stimulation of the RAAS, SNS, and AVP is so intense that their vasoconstrictor effects cannot be overcome, and HRS develops.

Reduced cardiac output

Circulatory dysfunction in cirrhosis has been the classic defining pathophysiological alteration that leads to HRS; however, recent evidence suggests that a reduction in cardiac output may play a role as well [14]. As discussed above, a complex interplay between the splanchnic, systemic, and renal circulation takes place once

Evidence-based Nephrology. Edited by Donald Molony and Jonathan Craig
© 2009 Blackwell Publishing, ISBN: 978-1-4051-3975-5.

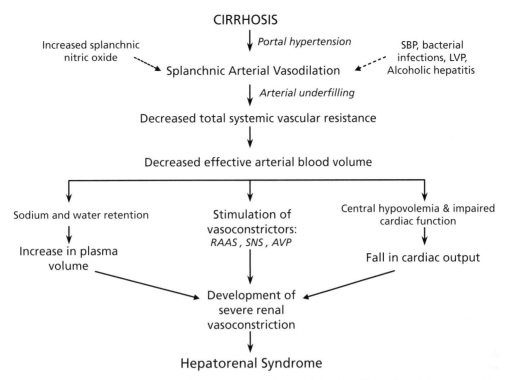

Figure 8.1 Pathogenesis of HRS in cirrhosis. Extrahepatic nitric oxide production is secondary to endothelial stretching and bacterial translocation. The main precipitating factors are SBP, other bacterial infections, large volume paracentesis (LVP) without plasma expanders, and alcoholic hepatitis. Splanchnic vasodilation arising from portal hypertension, an increased plasma volume, and a decreased cardiac output seem to play an equally important role in the decreased renal perfusion leading to HRS.

portal hypertension is established. In the initial stages of cirrhosis in the process of progressive vasodilation, both intravascular volume and cardiac output increase to maintain systemic hemodynamic homeostasis. However, with progression to decompensated cirrhosis a patient's clinical status may worsen, for instance, due to a bacterial infection. A consequent decrease in cardiac output and effective arterial blood volume may occur, thereby reducing renal perfusion and possibly contributing to the development of HRS. Two studies suggested that the development of HRS occurs in the setting of a reduction in cardiac output and that the progression of circulatory and renal dysfunction in cirrhosis is not only due to splanchnic vasodilation but also to a fall in cardiac output [15,16]. In the first study of 23 patients with SBP, the 8 patients who developed renal failure had a significantly reduced cardiac output compared to those that did not develop renal failure [15]. In the second study, 66 patients with cirrhosis and ascites were longitudinally followed. Twenty-seven patients (41%) developed HRS, and in all cases cardiac output at the time of HRS was significantly decreased compared to the cardiac output in the same patients measured before the occurrence of HRS [16]. These studies support the concept that HRS occurs in the setting of worsening circulatory function with a significant decrease in cardiac output in the setting of marked splanchnic vasodilation [15,16] (Figure 8.1). The exact pathogenic mechanisms that cause this decrease in cardiac output are not completely understood and therefore deserve further investigation.

Clinical features

HRS occurs in about 10% of hospitalized patients with cirrhosis and ascites [17]. The probability of developing HRS in patients with cirrhosis and ascites is 18% at 1 year and 39% at 5 years of follow-up [17]. Individuals who have HRS for the most part exhibit clinical features of advanced cirrhosis, and most have high model for end-stage liver disease (MELD) and Child-Pugh scores, along with low arterial blood pressure and severe urinary sodium retention (urine sodium, ≤10 meq/L) [17,18]. The MELD score is a mathematically derived score calculated from serum bilirubin, serum creatinine, and the international normalized ratio for prothrombin time used for organ allocation by liver transplant centers in the USA [19]. Spontaneous dilutional hyponatremia (serum sodium, ≤130 meq/L) is commonly present in patients with HRS due to an increased solute-free water retention because of elevated levels of AVP [20]. Serum creatinine levels are elevated and in fact define HRS; however, they are usually lower than those seen in noncirrhotic patients with acute renal failure, due to a reduced muscle mass and low endogenous production of creatinine in cirrhosis [21–23]. The two types of HRS as previously defined by the International Ascites Club [1] are shown in Table 8.1. In type 1 HRS renal function deteriorates with an increase in serum creatinine to a level higher than 2.5 mg/dL in less than 2 weeks. This type of HRS, if not treated, is associated with a very poor

Table 8.1 Clinical types of HRS.

Type 1: Rapid and progressive impairment of renal function, defined by a doubling of initial serum creatinine to a level higher than 2.5 mg/dL or a 50% reduction of the initial 24-h creatinine clearance to a level lower than 20 mL/min in less than 2 weeks.

Type 2: Impairment in renal function with serum creatinine of >1.5 mg/dL that does not meet criteria for type 1.

Table 8.2 Diagnostic criteria of HRS.

Major criteria[a]
- Chronic or acute liver disease with advanced hepatic failure and portal hypertension
- Low GFR, as indicated by a serum creatinine concentration greater than 1.5 mg/dL or 24-h creatinine clearance of <40 mL/min
- Exclusion of shock, ongoing bacterial infection, volume depletion, or use of nephrotoxic drugs
- No sustained improvement in renal function (decrease in serum creatinine to 1.5 mg/dL or less) despite stopping diuretics and volume repletion with 1.5 L of isotonic saline
- No proteinuria or ultrasonographic evidence of obstructive uropathy or parenchymal renal disease

Minor Criteria
- Urine volume lower than 500 mL/day
- Urine sodium lower than 10 mEq/L
- Urine osmolality greater than plasma osmolality
- Urine red blood cells less than 50 per high power field
- Serum sodium concentration lower than 130 mEq/L

Source: Adapted from reference 1.
[a]Only major criteria are necessary for the diagnosis of hepatorenal syndrome.

prognosis, with a median survival time of 2 weeks (Figure 8.2) [16,17]. In type 2 HRS there is a steady decline in renal function, and serum creatinine levels usually range between 1.5 and 2.5 mg/dL [1]. Most patients with type 2 HRS have a median survival time of 6 months if they do not receive a transplant (Figure 8.2) [17,18,23].

Type 1 HRS may develop spontaneously, but in many cases it is precipitated by bacterial infections, such as SBP or sepsis, acute alcoholic hepatitis, and large-volume paracentesis without albumin expansion [3,5,13,24]. Bacterial infections and SBP precipitate type 1 HRS in 10–30% of patients with advanced cirrhosis and ascites despite resolution of the infection [5,13,25]. Therapeutic paracentesis (≥5 L) without albumin expansion may precipitate type 1 HRS in nearly 15–20% of cases [24]. Renal failure may occur in up to 10% of cirrhotic patients with gastrointestinal bleeding, but in most cases it is due to acute tubular necrosis (ATN) and not HRS [26]. Contrast medium for radiological procedures does not seem to be associated with an increased risk of kidney failure in patients with cirrhosis and ascites [27].

Clinical diagnosis

The diagnosis of HRS is based on specific clinical criteria that aim to exclude other causes of kidney failure that are not functional. The diagnostic criteria proposed by the International Ascites Club for the diagnosis of HRS are outlined in Table 8.2 [1]. Unfortunately, it seems that in clinical practice HRS is not accurately diagnosed, as evidenced by two retrospective studies. In one study, 59% of patients with cirrhosis and kidney failure labeled as having HRS fulfilled the proposed criteria [28]. Another report from a large tertiary care center indicated that out of 140 patients diagnosed as having HRS only 29% met the diagnostic criteria and the majority of misdiagnosed cases were due to ATN and sepsis-related renal failure [29].

Common causes of renal failure in cirrhosis that should be excluded before the diagnosis of HRS is made include pre-renal failure secondary to volume depletion, ATN secondary to shock, drug-induced renal failure (mainly from nonsteroidal anti-inflammatory agents or aminoglycosides), and glomerulopathies in patients with viral hepatitis [30,31]. In cases of pre-renal failure, renal function usually improves after plasma volume expansion with an intravenous dose of 20–40 g of albumin. Proteinuria (>500 mg/day) and/or ultrasonographic abnormalities of the kidneys indicate parenchymal renal disease and preclude the diagnosis of HRS.

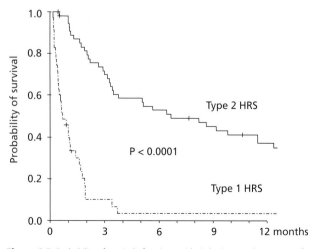

Figure 8.2 Probability of survival of patients with cirrhosis according to type of HRS. (From Alessandria *et al.*, 2005 [18], with permission.)

Management

When considering treatment, the type of HRS must always be taken into account, as the two types differ in time course and prognosis. In type 1 HRS patients, current practice supports their hospitalization in a closely monitored acute care unit. A central line may be helpful in assessing volume status after patients receive plasma expansion when ruling out other causes of renal failure, but the utility of central pressure monitoring has yet to be established with

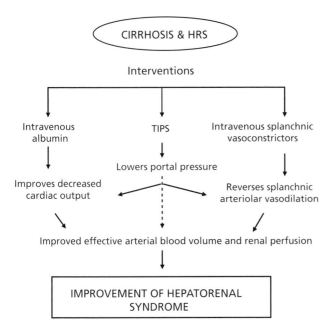

Figure 8.3 Possible mechanism of action of the different therapies for HRS. Therapies that improve renal function are vasoconstrictors, such as terlipressin, midodrine, or norepinephrine (which act by ameliorating arterial vasodilation) combined with albumin (which improves circulatory function). TIPS may reverse HRS by reducing portal pressure as well as increasing effective arterial blood volume.

an randomized, controlled trial (RCT) in this specific patient population. Patients with type 2 HRS can be managed as outpatients.

Given that patients are frequently malnourished and require a sodium-restricted diet, a nutritionist should be a part of the team taking care of the patient. In patients with dilutional hyponatremia, fluid restriction of 1 L/day is recommended, as pharmacological therapy is not yet available for this condition [20]. Apart from routine hematological and biochemistry blood tests, all patients must undergo a diagnostic paracentesis to rule out SBP and have blood cultures performed to rule out other bacterial infections, as prompt treatment of infections may result in improvements in renal function. Diuretics need to be stopped, because they can worsen renal failure and may cause electrolyte disturbances. Finally, probably the most important aspect of providing care to patients with HRS is assessment of candidacy for orthotopic liver transplantation (OLT).

In patients that are candidates for OLT, all efforts should be made to improve renal function in order to obtain a better outcome after transplantation. Current available therapies for type 1 HRS include the use of splanchnic vasoconstrictors, albumin, and TIPS. A summary of the therapeutic interventions available for HRS is outlined in Figure 8.3.

Pharmacological therapy

Systemic vasoconstrictors given with plasma expansion are currently the most-used form of pharmacologic therapy for HRS [2,12,32–50]. Splanchnic vasoconstrictors are used in conjunc-

tion with albumin because they counteract the intense vasodilation of the splanchnic circulation and improve effective arterial blood volume, which in turn supresses the endogenous vasoconstrictor factors responsible for HRS (Figure 8.3). Vasoconstrictor therapies used in HRS include vasopressin analogues (ornipressin and terlipressin) and α-adrenergic agonists (midodrine and norepinephrine). Albumin has been used concomitantly with these vasoconstrictors as a means of improving effective arterial blood volume and therefore further suppressing endogenous vasoconstrictor factors (RAAS and SNS) responsible for the intense renal vasoconstriction in HRS [35,39,40,42,43,47–50]. In addition, albumin administration by expanding circulating blood volume may increase cardiac preload and cardiac output, which may improve effective arterial blood volume leading to improved GFR [51] (Figure 8.3).

Terlipressin

Vasopressin analogs have a marked vasoconstrictor effect in the splanchnic circulation and therefore have been used for treating patients with portal hypertension-related complications, such as bleeding gastroesophageal varices. Ornipressin, although effective in HRS, caused significant ischemic side effects in about one-third of patients and was abandoned [32,33,52]. Terlipressin, a safer synthetic analog of vasopressin with fewer side effects (approximately <10% of cases) has been succesfully used in the past decade, and one randomized and several nonrandomized studies indicate that it reverses renal failure in type 1 HRS [35–37,39–46,50]. The administration of terlipressin and intravenous albumin improves renal function, with a reduction of serum creatinine and improvement in GFR in aproximately 60% of patients with type 1 HRS (range, 42–92% initial response rates in the reported clinical trial) [35–37,39,46,50] (Table 8.3). The dose of terlipressin ranged from 0.5 to 1 mg every 6–12 h in two studies [42,43]. In other studies, the administered dose was an intravenous bolus of 0.5 mg every 4 h, and it was increased in a stepwise fashion to 1 mg every 4 h and 2 mg every 4 h every 3 days if a significant reduction in serum creatinine level (≥1 mg/dL) was not observed during each 3-day period [35,39]. Also in another study terlipressin, administered as a continuous intravenous infusion starting at 2 mg/day with an increase every 2 days (in a stepwise manner to 4, 6, 8, and 12 mg/day if no significant reduction in serum creatinine [≥30%] was observed), was found to be efficacious when given in combination with albumin [50].

The dose of albumin administered in most studies was 20–40 g/day [35,39,40,42,43,50]. In most cases renal function starts to improve within 48–72 hours. The end point of treatment is a reduction in serum creatinine to a value less than 1.5 mg/dL, and in general this takes between 1 and 2 weeks. In four studies of patients with type 1 HRS, the recurrence of HRS among initial responders after stopping treatment ranged between 17 and 64% [36,39,42,50]. In the study with the highest rate of recurrence (64%), albumin was not administered with terlipressin [36]. In the other studies with lower recurrence rates (17–55%), albumin was administered at the doses described above, and in most cases

Table 8.3 Treatment of type 1 HRS patients with terlipressin.

Study [reference]	Response[a] (%)	Recurrence[b] (%)	Response in control group	Severe side effects[c] (%)	Median survival (days)	Median survival, control group
Uriz 2000 [35][d]	7/9 (77)	0/7 (0)		1/9	39	
Mulkay 2001 [36]	11/12 (92)	6/11 (55)		0/12	42	
Moreau 2002 [37]	53/91 (58)	NR[e]		18/99	43	
Colle 2002 [42][d]	11/18 (61)	7/11 (64)		0/18	24	
Halimi 2002 [41]	13/18 (72)	NR		4/18	NR	
Ortega 2002 [39][d]	14/21 (66)	2/12 (17)		1/21	40	
Solanki 2003 [43][d,f]	5/12 (42)	NR	0/12	3/12	NR	0/12
Danalioglu 2003 [40][d]	3/7 (42)	NR		NR	NR	
Angeli 2006 [50][d]	12/19 (63%)	3/12 (25)		NR	230[g]	

[a]The definition of response varied between studies; however, in all studies it was defined as a marked decrease in serum creatinine.

[b]Recurrence of HRS after treatment withdrawal in responder patients; the definition of recurrence also varied between studies.

[c]Many patients presented with self-limited abdominal cramps and/or diarrhea during the administration of the first doses of terlipressin, which were not counted as severe side effects.

[d]Received concomitant albumin as plasma expander.

[e]NR, not reported.

[f]An RCT.

[g]Mean transplant-free survival in complete responders.

a repeat course of terlipressin with albumin was effective in decreasing serum creatinine [39,42,50] if HRS recurred after completion of the first course. Short-term (15 days to 1 month) survival among patients responding to terlipressin has ranged from 40% to 80% [35–37,39,42,50] (Table 8.3). In the one RCT that compared terlipressin-based therapy to customary care, survival at 15 days was 40% in the terlipressin group and zero in the control [42]. Survival was seen only in those who demonstrated improvement in renal function. Although the data on this therapeutic approach are encouraging, there is undoubtedly a need for additional prospective RCTs assessing the role of terlipressin and albumin in improving renal function in HRS.

Midodrine, octreotide, and norepinephrine

The use of midodrine (an α-adrenergic agonist) in association with octreotide, an inhibitor of the release of glucagon, and albumin also may improve renal function in cirrhotic patients with HRS. However, available data are so far limited to only two nonrandomized observational cohort studies with a total of 19 patients [47,48]. In these two studies there was improvement in renal function and GFR with suppression of renin, aldosterone, norepinephrine, and AVP to normal or near-normal levels in 73% of cases (15/19 patients). Overall survival in these two cohorts was 58% at 3 months. In the second, larger study, long-term survival was seen only in patients who had undergone either a TIPS procedure or a liver transplant [48]. In the earlier of these cohort studies, the administered dose of midodrine was between 7.5 mg orally three times daily with an increase to 12.5 mg three times daily if needed and octreotide at 100 μg subcutaneously three times daily with an increase to 200 μg three times daily if needed [47]. In addition, 20–40 g of in-

travenous albumin was given daily [47]. In contrast, in the second study the investigators used midodrine at 2.5 mg daily combined with a continuous intravenous infusion of octreotide of 25 μg/h (previous bolus injection of 25 μg/h) and 50 g/day of intravenous albumin [48]. Interestingly, another study showed that octreotide was ineffective when administered alone [53]. The administration of a continuous infusion of norepinephrine (0.5–3 mg/h) for 5 days combined with intravenous albumin resulted in a significant improvement of renal function in a cohort of 12 cirrhotic patients with type 1 HRS [49]. Improvement in renal function was observed in 10 patients in association with an increase in mean arterial pressure and a marked reduction in renin and aldosterone levels [49]. Unfortunately, there is scarce rigorous clinical trials' evidence on these therapeutic regimens for HRS; only two of these trials are formal RCTs and both are of very small size. Despite the fact that the available data from observational and cohort studies are promising, more rigorous randomized controlled studies are needed in order to determine if any of these interventions have a beneficial role in HRS (Table 8.4) in terms of long-term renal function preservation, overall survival, and/or transition to OLT.

Aim of pharmacological therapy

The most important objective when treating HRS is to reverse renal failure in order to provide a successful bridge to OLT, so that suitable candidates can undergo transplantation with less morbidity and side effects to posttransplant medications and have similar survival as patients without HRS. Patients with HRS treated sucessfully with terlipressin and albumin before OLT have a similar posttransplantation outcome and survival as patients transplanted without HRS [54]. In four cohort studies, patients that responded

Table 8.4 Treatment of type 1 HRS patients with oral midodrine (Mido) and subcutaneous or intravenous octreotide (oct), octreotide intravenous infusion alone, intravenous norepinephrine, and TIPS.

Treatment [reference]	Response[a] (%)	Recurrence[b] (%)	Response control group	Side effects[c]	1-month survival (%)	1-month survival in control group (%)
Mido + Oct [47][d]	5/5 (100)	0/5 (0)	1/8	3/5	80	15
Mido + Oct, TIPS [48]	10/14 (71)	4/14 (29)		NR	50	
Norepinephrine [49]	10/12 (83)	NR		2/12	50	
Oct [53][d,e]	2/7 (61)	NR	2/9	NR	28.5	55

Abbreviations: Mido, midodrine; Oct, octreotide; NR, not reported.

[a] The definition of response varied between studies; however, in all studies it was defined as a marked decrease in serum creatinine.

[b] Recurrence of HRS after treatment withdrawal in responder patients; definition of recurrence also varied between studies.

[c] Patients presented with self-limited tingling, abdominal cramps, and/or diarrhea during the administration of the first doses of midodrone–octreotide.

[d] Patients received concomitant albumin as plasma expander.

[e] Crossover study of placebo and octreotide.

to therapy of HRS with terlipressin plus albumin or octretide, midodrine, and albumin had an increased survival compared to those who did not respond [37,39,48,50]. Whether this observed increase in survival after transplant in responders is a direct effect specific to a particular pharmacological therapy or rather simply a result of the identification of a less-ill patient group cannot be determined from these studies.

Nonpharmacological therapy
Liver transplantation
In the past OLT was the only available effective therapy for patients with HRS, and it continues to be the treatment of choice for HRS in candidate patients. The survival of cirrhotic patients with HRS treated by OLT is 85% at 1 year and 73% at 3 years, although the presence of HRS is associated with increased morbidity and early mortality after transplantation [55]. In fact, patients with HRS who undergo transplantation have more complications, spend more days in the intensive care unit, and have a higher in-hospital mortality rate than transplanted patients without antecedent HRS. Transplantation for type 1 HRS is limited by the fact that many patients die before the operation because of their advanced liver disease, a short average survival time after onset of HRS, and a prolonged waiting time for transplantation in most liver transplant centers [56]. Therefore, since patients with type 1 HRS have a very poor prognosis, this group of patients should be given higher priority for transplantation [56]. In fact, the implementation of the MELD score in the USA has placed patients with HRS at a higher priority level for liver transplantation due to the fact that creatinine is a strong variable in the mathematical model [19]. In addition, the MELD score provides a good estimate of prognosis in patients with type 2 HRS [18].

TIPS
TIPS is a nonsurgical intervention performed percutaneously that creates a connection (by means of a prosthetic shunt) within the liver between the portal and hepatic vein, thereby reducing portal pressure. This method has been used as an alternative therapy to surgical shunts for cirrhotic patients bleeding from esophageal or gastric varices who are refractory to endoscopic and medical treatment. The rationale for using TIPS in HRS is based on the fact that reduction of portal pressure improves circulatory function and supresses RAAS and SNS activity (Figure 8.3).

There are scarce data regarding the use of TIPS in HRS. Four uncontrolled studies indicate that TIPS may improve renal function and GFR as well as reduce the activity of RAAS and SNS in patients with cirrhosis and HRS [48,57–59]. Improvement in renal function observed in these uncontrolled studies after TIPS placement alone was slow and successful in approximately 60–70% of patients [48,57–59]. Studies assesing TIPS for type 1 HRS have only included patients with preserved liver function and excluded those with a history of hepatic encephalopathy, Child-Pugh scores of $\geq$12 or serum bilirubin of >5 mg/dL. A combined approach using the combination of vasoconstrictors with TIPS in 14 patients for the treatment of type 1 HRS revealed that those with preserved liver function (Child score, <12) who responded to oral midodrine plus intravenous octreotide and albumin and then had a TIPS performed had an excellent outcome, with renal function that continued to improve and completely normalize [48]. Nonetheless, this study included a limited number of patients, was uncontrolled for either aspect of the intervention, and was associated with an overall mortality of 50% at 2 months. Thus, larger studies using this approach are required in patients with type 1 HRS before the efficacy of this combined approach can be accepted.

Dialysis
The use of hemodialysis and peritoneal dialysis is ineffective in HRS because patients are prone to develop significant side effects, including arterial hypotension, coagulopathy, and gastrointestinal

bleeding [60,61]. Although dialysis is not routinely recommended in HRS, it may be a temporary option in patients who have exhibited no response to vasoconstrictors or TIPS or in those who develop severe volume overload, metabolic acidosis, or refractory hyperkalemia. Data on the extracorporeal albumin dialysis (MARS) system seem to be promising. This system uses a cell-free albumin-containing dialysate that is recirculated and perfused through charcoal and anion exchange columns connected to a hemodialysis machine, enabling the removal of albumin-bound substances, such as bilirubin, bile acids, and cytokines [62]. In a prospective RCT of 19 patients with Child C cirrhosis and type 1 HRS, there was a decrease in serum bilirubin and serum creatinine levels and an improvement in serum sodium, urine volume, mean arterial blood pressure, and mortality when the data were analyzed using parametric statistical tests for the 13 patients who underwent MARS versus the 5 patients who received hemofiltration and customary care [62]. In a recent systematic review of MARS compared to conventional therapy in patients with severe liver failure, a meta-analysis of the four RCTs identified and that included the only RCT in patients with HRS failed to demonstrate a survival benefit from MARS in liver patients in general [63]. A survival advantage was demonstrated only when nonrandomized trials were included in the review. MARS should, therefore, still be considered an experimental treatment, and further controlled studies are clearly needed before advocating its use in the management of patients with type 1 HRS. An alternative approach to MARS, Prometheus, is currently undergoing clinical evaluation and comparison to MARS [64].

Prevention

The two clinical scenarios in which prevention of HRS has been successful are SBP and alcoholic hepatitis. In SBP, intravenous albumin (1.5 g/kg at diagnosis of infection and 1 g/kg 48 h later) prevents the development of HRS because it counteracts an enhanced arterial splanchnic vasodilation triggered by the infection, causing an even more reduced effective arterial blood volume with additional activation of vasoconstrictor systems [5]. In one study, the incidence of HRS in patients with SBP not administered albumin was 33% and only 10% in those that received albumin [5]. In addition, there was less in-hospital mortality in those receiving albumin (10%) than in those not receiving albumin (29%) [5]. However, it seems that other plasma expanders, such as intravenous hydroxyethyl starch, are not effective in preventing renal failure in the setting of SBP [65]. In patients with acute alcoholic hepatitis, oral pentoxifylline (400 mg three times daily for 1 month) also reduces the incidence of (8% in pentoxiphylline vs. 35% in placebo) and mortality (24% in pentoxiphylline vs. 46% in placebo) of HRS [3]. There have been no follow-up studies confirming these results nor studies to evaluate their generalizability to other clinical settings; however, these two methods of prevention are widely accepted in the clinical setting.

References

1 Arroyo V, Ginès P, Gerbes A, Dudley FJ, Gentilini P, Laffi G et al. Definition and diagnostic criteria of refractory ascites and hepatorenal syndrome in cirrhosis. *Hepatology* 1996; **23**: 164–176.

2 Ginès P, Guevara M, Arroyo V, Rodés J. Hepatorenal syndrome. *Lancet* 2003; **362**: 1819–1827.

3 Akriviadis E, Botla R, Briggs W, Han S, Reynolds T, Shakil O. Pentoxifylline improves short-term survival in severe acute alcoholic hepatitis: a double-blind, placebo-controlled trial. *Gastroenterology* 2000; **119**: 1637–1648.

4 Moore K. Renal failure in acute liver failure. *Eur J Gastroenterol Hepatol* 1999; **11**: 967–75.

5 Sort P, Navasa M, Arroyo V, Aldeguer X, Planas R, Ruiz-del-Arbol L et al. Effect of intravenous albumin on renal impairment and mortality in patients with cirrhosis and spontaneous bacterial peritonitis. *N Engl J Med* 1999; **341**: 403–409.

6 Bataller R, Ginés P, Guevara M, Arroyo V. Hepatorenal syndrome. *Semin Liver Dis* 1997; **17**: 233–247

7 Schrier RW, Arroyo V, Bernardi M, Epstein M, Henriksen JH, Rodes J et al. Peripheral arterial vasodilation hypothesis: a proposal for the initiation of renal sodium and water retention in cirrhosis. *Hepatology* 1988; **8**: 1151–1157.

8 Iwakiri Y, Groszmann R. The hyperdynamic circulation of chronic liver diseases: from the patient to the molecule. *Hepatology* 2006; **43**: S121–S131.

9 Bernardi M, Domenicali M. The renin-angiotensin-aldosterone system in cirrhosis. In: Ginès P, Arroyo V, Rodés J, Schrier RW, editors. *Ascites and Renal Dysfunction in Liver Disease*. Blackwell Publishing, Oxford, 2005; 43–53.

10 Dudley F, Esler M. The sympathetic nervous system in cirrhosis. In: Ginès P, Arroyo V, Rodés J, Schrier RW, editors. *Ascites and Renal Dysfunction in Liver Disease*. Blackwell Publishing, Oxford, 2005; 54–72.

11 Schrier RW. Water and sodium retention in edematous disorders: role of vasopressin and aldosterone. *Am J Med* 2006; **119**: S47–S53.

12 Arroyo V, Terra C, Gines P. New treatments of hepatorenal syndrome. *Semin Liver Dis* 2006; **26**: 254–64.

13 Terra C, Guevara M, Torre A, Gilabert R, Fernandez J, Martin-Llahi M et al. Renal failure in patients with cirrhosis and sepsis unrelated to spontaneous bacterial peritonitis. Value of MELD score. *Gastroenterology* 2005; **129**: 1944–1953.

14 Gines P, Guevara M, Perez-Villa F. Management of hepatorenal syndrome: another piece of the puzzle. *Hepatology* 2004; **40**: 16–18.

15 Ruiz-del-Arbol W, Urman J, Fernandez J, Gonzalez M, Navasa M, Monescillo A et al. Systemic, renal, and hepatic hemodynamic derangement in cirrhotic patients with spontaneous bacterial peritonitis. *Hepatology* 2003; **38**: 1210–1218.

16 Ruiz del Arbol L, Monescillo A, Arocena C, Valer P, Gines P, Moreira V et al. Circulatory function and hepatorenal syndrome in cirrhosis. *Hepatology* 2005; **42**: 439–447.

17 Ginès A, Escorsell A, Ginès P, Salo J, Jimenez W, Inglada L et al. Incidence, predictive factors, and prognosis of hepatorenal syndrome in cirrhosis. *Gastroenterology* 1993; **105**: 229–236.

18 Alessandria C, Ozdogan O, Guevara M, Restuccia T, Jimenez W, Arroyo V et al. MELD score and clinical type predict prognosis in hepatorenal syndrome: relevance to liver transplantation. *Hepatology* 2005; **41**: 1282–1289.

19 Kamath PS, Wiesner RH, Malinchoc M, Kremers W, Therneau TM, Kosberg CL *et al.* A model to predict survival in patients with end-stage liver disease. *Hepatology* 2001; **33**: 464–470.

20 Cárdenas A, Ginès P. Management of hyponatremia in cirrhosis. In: Ginès P, Arroyo V, Rodés J, Schrier RW, editors. *Ascites and Renal Dysfunction in Liver Disease.* Blackwell Publishing, Oxford, 2005; 305–314.

21 Caregaro L, Menon F, Angeli P, Amodio P, Merkel C, Bortoluzzi A *et al.* Limitations of serum creatinine level and creatinine clearance as filtration markers in cirrhosis. *Arch Intern Med* 1994; **154**: 201–205.

22 Sherman D, Fish DN, Teitelbaum I. Assessing renal function in cirrhotic patients: problems and pitfalls. *Am J Kidney Dis* 2003; **41**: 269–278.

23 Cárdenas A, Gines P. Therapy insight: hepatorenal syndrome. *Nat Clin Gastroenterol Hepatol* 2006; **3**: 862–865.

24 Ginès P, Titó L, Arroyo V, Planas R, Panes J, Viver J *et al.* Randomized comparative study of therapeutic paracentesis with and without intravenous albumin in cirrhosis. *Gastroenterology* 1988; **94**: 1493–1502.

25 Follo A, Llovet JM, Navasa M, Planas R, Forns X, Francitorra A *et al.* Renal impairment after spontaneous bacterial peritonitis in cirrhosis: incidence, clinical course, predictive factors and prognosis. *Hepatology* 1994; **20**: 1495–1501.

26 Cárdenas A, Ginès P, Uriz J, Bessa X, Salmeron JM, Mas A *et al.* Renal failure after upper gastrointestinal bleeding in cirrhosis. Incidence, clinical course, predictive factors and short-term prognosis. *Hepatology* 2001; **34**: 671–676.

27 Guevara M, Fernandez-Esparrach G, Alessandria C, Torre A, Terra C, Montana X *et al.* Effects of contrast media on renal function in patients with cirrhosis: a prospective study. *Hepatology* 2004; **40**: 646–651.

28 Watt K, Uhanova J, Minuk GY. Hepatorenal syndrome: diagnostic accuracy, clinical features, and outcome in a tertiary care center. *Am J Gastroenterol* 2002; **97**: 2046–2050.

29 Servin-Abad L, Regev A, Contreras G, *et al.* Retrospective analysis of 140 patients labeled as hepatorenal syndrome in a referral center. *Hepatology* 2005; **42**: 543A.

30 Meyers CM, Seeff LB, Stehman-Breen CO, Hoofnagle JH. Hepatitis C and renal disease: an update. *Am J Kidney Dis* 2003; **42**: 631–657.

31 McGuire BM, Julian BA, Bynon JS, Jr., Cook WJ, King SJ, Curtis JJ *et al.* Brief communication: glomerulonephritis in patients with hepatitis C cirrhosis undergoing liver transplantation. *Ann Intern Med* 2006; **144**: 735–741.

32 Guevara M, Ginès P, Fernandez-Esparrach G, Sort P, Salmeron JM, Jimenez W *et al.* Reversibility of hepatorenal syndrome by prolonged administration of ornipressin and plasma volume expansion. *Hepatology* 1998; **27**: 35–41.

33 Gulberg V, Bilzer M, Gerbes AL. Long-term therapy and retreatment of hepatorenal syndrome type 1 with ornipressin and dopamine. *Hepatology* 1999; **30**: 870–875.

34 Hadengue A, Gadano A, Moreau R, Giostra E, Durand F, Valla D *et al.* Beneficial effects of the 2-day administration of terlipressin in patients with cirrhosis and hepatorenal syndrome. *J Hepatol* 1998; **29**: 565–570.

35 Uriz J, Ginès P, Cárdenas A, Sort P, Jimenez W, Salmeron JM *et al.* Terlipressin plus albumin infusion: an effective and safe therapy of hepatorenal syndrome. *J Hepatol* 2000; **33**: 43–48.

36 Mulkay JP, Louis H, Donckier V, Bourgeois N, Adler M, Deviere J *et al.* Long-term terlipressin administration improves renal function in cirrhotic patients with type 1 hepatorenal syndrome: a pilot study. *Acta Gastroenterol Belg* 2001; **64**: 15–19.

37 Moreau R, Durand F, Poynard T, Duhamel C, Cervoni JP, Ichai P *et al.* Terlipressin in patients with cirrhosis and type 1 hepatorenal syndrome: a retrospective multicenter study. *Gastroenterology* 2002; **122**: 923–930.

38 Alessandria C, Venon WD, Marzano A, Barletti C, Fadda M, Rizzetto M. Renal failure in cirrhotic patients: role of terlipressin in clinical approach to hepatorenal syndrome type 2. *Eur J Gastroenterol Hepatol* 2002; **14**: 1363–1368.

39 Ortega R, Ginès P, Uriz J, Cardenas A, Calahorra B, De Las Heras D *et al.* Terlipressin therapy with and without albumin for patients with hepatorenal syndrome. Results of a prospective, non-randomized study. *Hepatology* 2002; **36**: 941–948.

40 Danalioglu A, Cakaloglu Y, Karaca C, Aksoy N, Akyuz F, Ozdil S *et al.* Terlipressin and albumin combination in hepatorenal syndrome. *Hepatogastroenterology* 2003; **50 Suppl 2**: ccciii–cccv.

41 Halimi C, Bonnard P, Bernard B, Mathurin P, Mofredj A, di Martino V *et al.* Effect of terlipressin (Glypressin) on hepatorenal syndrome in cirrhotic patients: results of a multicentre pilot study. *Eur J Gastroenterol Hepatol* 2002; **14**: 153–158.

42 Colle I, Durand F, Pessione F, Rassiat E, Bernuau J, Barriere E *et al.* Clinical course, predictive factors and prognosis in patients with cirrhosis and type 1 hepatorenal syndrome treated with terlipressin: a retrospective analysis. *J Gastroenterol Hepatol* 2002; **17**: 882–888.

43 Solanki P, Chawla A, Garg R, Gupta R, Jain M, Sarin SK *et al.* Beneficial effects of terlipressin in hepatorenal syndrome: a prospective, randomized placebo-controlled clinical trial. *J Gastroenterol Hepatol* 2003; **18**: 152–156.

44 Saner F, Kavuk I, Lang H, Biglarnia R, Fruhauf NR, Schafers RF *et al.* Terlipressin and gelafundin: safe therapy of hepatorenal syndrome. *Eur J Med Res* 2004; **9**: 78–82.

45 Saner FH, Fruhauf NR, Schafers RF, Lang H, Malago M, Broelsch CE *et al.* Terlipressin plus hydroxyethyl starch infusion: an effective treatment for hepatorenal syndrome. *Eur J Gastroenterol Hepatol* 2003; **15**: 925–927.

46 Gluud LL, Kjaer M, Taastroem, Christensen E. Terlipressin for hepatorenal syndrome: a Cochrane systematic review. *J Hepatol* 2005; **42**: 206A.

47 Angeli P, Volpin R, Gerunda G, Craighero R, Roner P, Merenda R *et al.* Reversal of type 1 hepatorenal syndrome with the administration of midodrine and octreotide. *Hepatology* 1999; **29**: 1690–1697.

48 Wong F, Pantea L, Sniderman K. Midodrine, octreotide, albumin, and TIPS in selected patients with cirrhosis and type 1 hepatorenal syndrome. *Hepatology* 2004; **40**: 55–64.

49 Duvoux C, Zanditenas D, Hezode C, Chauvat A, Monin JL, Roudot-Thoroval F *et al.* Effects of noradrenaline and albumin in patients with type 1 hepatorenal syndrome: a pilot study. *Hepatology* 2002; **36**: 374–380.

50 Angeli P, Guarda S, Fasolato S, Miolo E, Craighero R, Piccolo F *et al.* Switch therapy with ciprofloxacin vs. intravenous ceftazidime in the treatment of spontaneous bacterial peritonitis in patients with cirrhosis: similar efficacy at lower cost. *Aliment Pharmacol Ther* 2006; **23**: 75–84.

51 Arroyo V, Ruiz del Arbol, Ginés P. Circulatory dysfunction in cirrhosis. In: Arroyo V, Navasa M, Forns X, Bataller R, Sanchez-Fueyo A, Rodes J, editors. *Update in Treatment of Liver Disease.* Ars Medica, Barcelona, 2005; 19–28.

52 Arroyo V, Terra C, Torre A, Gines P. Hepatorenal syndrome in cirrhosis: clinical features, diagnosis, and management. In: Ginès P, Arroyo V, Rodés J, Schrier RW, editors. *Ascites and Renal Dysfunction in Liver Disease.* Blackwell Publishing, Oxford, 2005; 341–359.

53 Pomier-Layrargues G, Paquin SC, Hassoun Z, Lafortune M, Tran A. Octreotide in hepatorenal syndrome: a randomized, double-blind, placebo-controlled, crossover study. *Hepatology* 2003; **38**: 238–243.

54 Restuccia T, Ortega R, Guevara M, Gines P, Alessandria C, Ozdogan O et al. Effects of treatment of hepatorenal syndrome before transplantation on posttransplantation outcome. A case-control study. *J Hepatol* 2004; **40:** 140–146.

55 Rimola A, Navasa M, Grande L, Garcia-Valdecasas JC. Liver transplantation for patients with cirrhosis and ascites. In: Ginès P, Arroyo V, Rodés J, Schrier RW, editors. *Ascites and Renal Dysfunction in Liver Disease.* Blackwell Publishing, Oxford, 2005; 271–285.

56 Cárdenas A, Ginès P. Management of complications of cirrhosis in patients awaiting liver transplantation. *J Hepatol* 2005; **42:** S124–S133.

57 Testino G, Ferro C, Sumberaz A, Messa P, Morelli N, Guadagni B et al. Type-2 hepatorenal syndrome and refractory ascites: role of transjugular intrahepatic portosystemic stent-shunt in eighteen patients with advanced cirrhosis awaiting orthotopic liver transplantation. *Hepatogastroenterology* 2003; **50:** 1753–1755.

58 Brensing KA, Textor J, Perz J, Schiedermaier P, Raab P, Strunk H et al. Long-term outcome after transjugular intrahepatic portosystemic stent-shunt in non-transplant cirrhotics with hepatorenal syndrome: a phase II study. *Gut* 2000; **47:** 288–295.

59 Guevara M, Ginès P, Bandi JC, Gilabert R, Sort P, Jimenez W et al. Transjugular intrahepatic portosystemic shunt in hepatorenal syndrome: effects on renal function and vasoactive systems. *Hepatology* 1998; **28:** 416–422.

60 Kapling RK, Bastani B. The clinical course of patients with type 1 hepatorenal syndrome maintained on hemodialysis. *Ren Fail* 2004; **26:** 563–568.

61 Keller F, Heinze H, Jochimsen F, Passfall J, Schuppan D, Buttner P et al. Risk factors and outcome of 107 patients with decompensated liver disease and acute renal failure (including 26 patients with hepatorenal syndrome): the role of hemodialysis. *Ren Fail* 1995; **17:** 135–146.

62 Mitzer SR, Stange J, Klammt S, Risler T, Erley CM, Bader BM et al. Improvement of hepatorenal syndrome with extracorporeal albumin dialysis MARS: results of a prospective, randomized, controlled clinical trial. *Liver Transpl* 2000; **6:** 277–286.

63 Khuroo MS, Khuroo MS, Farahat KLC. Molecular adsorbent recirculating system for acute and acute-on-chronic liver failure: a meta-analysis. *Liver Transpl* 2004; **10:** 1099–1106.

64 Krisper P, Stauber RE. Technology insight: artificial extracorporeal liver support- how does Prometheus® compare with MARS®? *Nat Clin Practice Nephrol* 2007; **3:** 267–276.

65 Fernandez J, Monteagudo J, Bargallo X, Jimenez W, Bosch J, Arroyo V et al. A randomized unblinded pilot study comparing albumin versus hydroxyethyl starch in spontaneous bacterial peritonitis. *Hepatology* 2005; **42:** 627–634.

9 Acute Tubular Necrosis

Jay L. Koyner & Patrick T. Murray

Section of Nephrology, University of Chicago, Chicago, USA.

Introduction

The incidence, etiology, and outcomes of acute kidney injury (AKI) vary greatly, depending on the chosen definition and specific population being studied. In the majority of hospitalized patients, AKI is usually the result of prerenal azotemia (reversible renal insufficiency caused by renal hypoperfusion) or acute tubular necrosis (ATN) [1,2]. ATN is a form of AKI that results from injury (ischemic or toxic) to the tubular epithelial cells. In recent case series ATN has accounted for 45–63% of AKI cases hospitalized [3,4]. Furthermore, a study based upon the Program to Improve Care in Acute Renal Disease found ischemic (nonnephrotoxic) ATN to be the most common cause of AKI, occurring in over 40% of all patients [5]. It should be noted that sustained prerenal azotemia has been shown to be a major predisposing factor towards the development of ischemic ATN [6]. In hospitalized patients, ATN commonly results from a variety of ischemic (hypotension, sepsis, etc.) and nephrotoxic (pharmacologic, radiocontrast, rhabdomyolysis, etc.) insults, often in additive or synergistic combinations [7]. ATN results in intrinsic renal parenchymal injury characterized by tubular cell apoptosis and necrosis, which leads to impairment of renal function.

Diagnosis

The diagnosis of ATN (nephrotoxic or ischemic) may be distinguished from that of prerenal azotemia via serum markers (plasma electrolytes, blood urea nitrogen, and creatinine) and evaluation of urine electrolytes, osmolality, and sediment [8,9]. The tubular dysfunction of ATN may be associated with an elevated urine sodium concentration and a fractional excretion of sodium (FeNa) $\{[(\text{urine sodium/plasma sodium})/(\text{urine creatinine/plasma creatinine})] \times 100\}$ greater than 1%. Additionally, owing to tubular

damage that results in the impaired ability to concentrate and dilute urine, isosthenuria is present [10]. Of course there are exceptions to these findings; in the setting of chronic kidney disease or following recent diuretic use, the diagnostic accuracy of urine chemistries to distinguish prerenal azotemia versus ATN decreases. Additionally, ATN in the setting of rhabdomyolysis, hemolysis, sepsis, or heart failure has been shown to be associated with urine sodium of less than 10 mEq/L and a fractional excretion of sodium of less than 1% [11–13]. As such, one must use caution when attempting to make a diagnosis of ATN based solely on laboratory data. Fortunately, ATN does have characteristic urinary sediment that includes renal tubular epithelial cells and granular and muddy brown casts, but these findings may be transient or unrecognized by an inexperienced observer. Despite years of investigation, no "gold standard" for the diagnosis of ATN exists. Thus, the diagnosis must rely on a combination of data from the patient's history, physical examination, and laboratory studies, including urine sediment. The utility of various diagnostic strategies to differentiate pre-renal azotemia from ATN are discussed in further detail in chapter 3.

Pathophysiology

Although there is still much to be discovered in the complex biology of ATN, there are increasingly sophisticated experimental data characterizing the pathophysiology of this syndrome (Figure 9.1). Current evidence suggests that the course of ischemic ATN has several phases: prerenal, initiation, extension, maintenance, and repair. Tubular cell structure and function are severely impaired during the renal hypoperfusion of the initiation phase. Eventually, the tubular basement membrane is denuded by the sloughing of tubular cells. This sloughing leads to cast formation and intratubular obstruction, which results in a decrease in glomerular filtration rate (GFR) [12,13]. Additionally, this permits glomerular filtrate back-leak, which leads to a further decrease in GFR [14]. In the extension and maintenance phases of ATN, several inflammatory cytokines and chemokines promote vasoconstriction, contributing

Evidence-based Nephrology. Edited by Donald Molony and Jonathan Craig
© 2009 Blackwell Publishing, ISBN: 978-1-4051-3975-5.

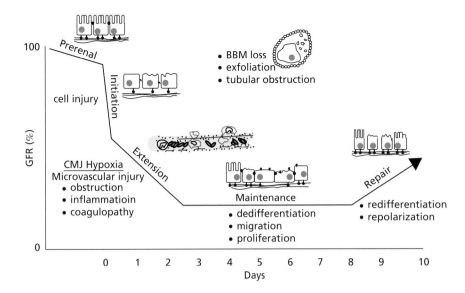

Figure 9.1 The serial phases of ischemic ATN. (Reprinted from Sutton *et al.* [16] with permission of the publisher.)

to a milieu that promotes renal hypoperfusion, medullary congestion, and generalized tissue injury [14,15]. Lastly, when successful, the repair phase (which is an area of extremely active investigation) consists of death and exfoliation of the proximal tubular cells. These cells are then repopulated and eventually mature and regain their differentiated character [1]. Although ATN is a complex and poorly understood syndrome, a broad spectrum of research initiatives are currently in progress to further our understanding of its pathogenesis and pathophysiology to inform the timing and targeting of prophylactic and therapeutic efforts to improve patient outcomes.

Outcomes

In the early stages of ATN there is an opportunity to correct insults (ischemic or nephrotoxic) that have caused the initial damage. Provided this adjustment is made, renal function will generally improve, although it may not return to preinsult level. It should be noted, however, that severe and acutely irreversible loss of renal function may occur in the setting of ATN. When such a loss of function does occur, it often requires initiation of renal replacement therapy (RRT) and is associated with much higher morbidity and mortality. Severe acute irreversible loss of function with ATN is most likely in the setting of preexisting renal disease and/or repeated ischemic or nephrotoxic insults [16].

Several studies have attempted to gain a clinical understanding of factors that contribute to patient mortality in ATN. Chertow *et al.* [17] performed a multicenter prospective study that followed over 250 patients with "early ATN." They documented a 60-day mortality rate of 36%. Additionally, multivariate analysis identified the following independent predictors of death in acute renal failure (ARF) (with relative risks in parentheses): mechanical ventilation (1.86), male gender (2.01), oliguria (<0.4 L/day) (2.25),

chronic immunosuppression (2.37), acute stroke or seizure (3.08), and acute myocardial infarction (3.14). Similarly, in a multicenter, prospective, controlled trial that evaluated the use of biocompatible hemodialysis membranes, Parker and colleagues showed that the severity-of-illness scores (APACHE) within 24 h of the initiation of RRT for ATN can predict patient survival and recovery of renal function [18]. Despite several recent advances in critical care and renal replacement therapy, recent studies show that AKI from ATN still carries a 35–70% mortality rate, depending on the center and patient population studied [19,20]. Given the severe adverse impact from ATN, it is imperative that clinicians employ as many clinically effective preventative strategies as possible in patients known to be at increased risk for development of ATN by virtue of their demographic characteristics or their risk of exposure to ischemia or nephrotoxicants.

Preventive strategies

Ischemic events (vascular and cardiothoracic surgeries, sepsis, and hypotension) and exposure to several known potential nephrotoxicants (aminoglycosides, amphotericin B, and rhabdomyolysis) are part of the everyday experience of modern medicine. As such, several trials have been performed to determine if any preventative strategies are successful when the clinician is faced with the potential of an ATN-inciting agent or event. This section seeks to describe the studies currently available that inform best practices with regards to preventive strategies and that provide guidance for our current evidence-based recommendations.

Prevention of ATN from aminoglycosides

Despite their severe toxicities, aminoglycosides are still a mainstay of the treatment of life-threatening gram-negative bacterial infections. Nephrotoxicity occurs in 10–20% of patients, whereas ototoxicity occurs in 3–10% [21–22]. Briefly, the nephrotoxicity stems from the proximal tubular damage the drugs induce after being freely filtered at the glomerulus and absorbed into the proximal tubular cell from the tubular lumen. The potential for tubular damage persists as long as 4 weeks after a single dose because of prolonged intracellular aminoglycoside accumulation; this may account for the observations of nephrotoxicity several days after the drug has been discontinued. It should be noted that aminoglycosides may also affect the distal nephron. This damage normally manifests itself as a defect in the concentrating ability of the kidney (polyuria) as well as severe magnesium wasting [24]. Despite the elucidation of several risk factors for developing aminoglycoside nephrotoxicity (duration of treatment, concurrent diuretics or nephrotoxins, elevated plasma drug trough levels, and liver dysfunction) [24–23], severe nephrotoxicity still occurs. Accordingly, several studies have been performed to evaluate strategies to minimize this potentially devastating side effect.

Over 60 trials have been conducted that have explored the benefit of altering the dosing schedule for aminoglycoside antibiotics. Traditionally, these drugs were dosed three times daily, but concerns over the dose exposure led to trials investigating the utility of once-a-day dosing. Due to the inherent differences in both the protocols and results of the clinical trials, no fewer than four meta-analyses have been performed in the hopes of clarifying some of the contradicting aspects of these studies [24–30]. Each of these works analyzed 20–42 randomized clinical trials; it should be noted that 10 studies were included in all four of these meta-analyses. Blaser *et al.* [27] reported improved clinical efficacy (89.5% vs. 84.7%; $P < 0.001$) as well as improved bacteriological efficacy (88.6% vs. 83.4%; $P < 0.01$) with once-a-day dosing but found no statistical improvement based on toxicity rates. Barza *et al.* [29] found a reduced incidence of nephrotoxicity (from 7.7% to 5.5%) with daily dosing but no significant change in the patient's clinical course. The largest of these studies, Hatala *et al.* [30] reported equivalence with regard to bacteriologic cure and a statistical "trend" toward reduced mortality and toxicity with once-daily dosing (risk ratio for nephrotoxicity, 0.87; 95% confidence interval [CI], 0.60–1.26). Lastly, Munckhof *et al.* [28] compared 20 trials involving 2881 patients and concluded that clinical efficacy improved 3.5% ($P = 0.027$) with once-daily dosing but that there were no differences in terms of the bacteriologic efficacy or toxicity rates. Taken together, these data have led to the commonplace use of daily aminoglycoside dosing in clinical practice, even though none of these meta-analyses reported a statistically robust renal advantage with daily dosing regimens. A recent systematic review in the Cochrane Database comparing aminoglycoside-based treatment regimens in patients with cystic fibrosis demonstrated a reduced renal toxicity benefit to once-daily dosing in children but not in adults with cystic fibrosis [31].

Unfortunately, there are still several grey areas where the safety and efficacy of aminoglycoside dosing remains unclear, including in the elderly, the morbidly obese, and those with chronic kidney disease (CKD). Additionally, in the face of the ever-growing threat of antibiotic resistance, several studies have also sought to facilitate further reductions in drug exposure by evaluating regimens that entail dosing less frequently than once daily. Although no large randomized trials or meta-analyses exist, studies like the prospective controlled trial by Bartal *et al.* raise the question of whether all patients should receive aminoglycosides doses on an individual pharmacokinetic basis (according to personalized trough levels drawn in response to daily drug administration) [32].

Prevention of ATN from amphotericin B

Amphotericin B, an effective therapeutic agent in treating systemic and invasive mycoses, induces nephrotoxicity in 20–80% of patients, depending on a variety of factors, including the dose, total drug exposure, and the population being investigated, as well as the definition of AKI that is used [33,34]. Despite recent advances and new agents to treat fungal infections, amphotericin B still remains an often-used agent for hospital-acquired ATN. All too often ATN arises with concomitant use of amphotericin B and another nephrotoxic agent (aminoglycosides, calcineurin inhibitors, etc.) [35]. It should be noted that amphotericin B nephrotoxicity can take on several forms besides ATN (as measured by increased serum creatinine); these other symptoms include hypokalemia with urinary potassium wasting and hypomagnesemia with urinary magnesium wasting (due to increased distal tubular membrane permeability), as well as nephrogenic diabetes insipidus or type 1 (distal) renal tubular acidosis [36]. In addition to decreasing some of the concomitant risk factors (drug dosage and avoidance of concomitant nephrotoxins), several other preventative measures have been investigated.

Prevention of ATN from amphotericin B by saline (volume expansion)

Animal models have suggested that, in part, the nephrotoxicity of amphotericin B stems from its ability to enhance tubuloglomerular feedback [37]. Because volume expansion (salt loading) has been shown to decrease the sensitivity of tubuloglomerular feedback, it has been used in an attempt to lower the rates of amphotericin B nephrotoxicity. Several studies have attempted to evaluate the utility of volume expansion prior to amphotericin B administration. A review by Anderson [38] compiled the results from five studies (120 total patients) that investigated the use of volume expansion. Anderson concluded that supplementing dietary intake of sodium chloride before amphotericin B therapy is initiated "will likely" prevent nephrotoxicity. This statement is based in large part on the results from the only prospective, double-blind placebo-controlled trial among the five studies included in the Anderson review. In that study, Llanos *et al.* looked at 20 individuals in Peru being treated with thrice-weekly amphotericin B for mucocutaneous leishmaniasis [39]. They found that serum creatinine rose and creatinine clearance decreased in those individuals who received the usual care compared to those who received intravenous saline prior to amphotericin administration ($P < 0.05$). Overall it is difficult to enthusiastically endorse volume expansion, as adequate trials have not been performed, but based on current data there appears to be minimal harm in giving patients a saline load prior to amphotericin B administration.

Prevention of ATN from amphotericin B: lipid-based formulations

Because of the dose-limiting nephrotoxicity of conventional amphotericin B, several other formulations have been tried. Additionally, co-administration of a wide variety of therapeutic agents, including dopamine [40], has been investigated in the hopes of reducing amphotericin B nephrotoxicity, but these efforts have generally been disappointing.

The results of studies with lipid-based formulations of amphotericin B are more promising. Human studies have shown that there is likely an equal or decreased incidence and severity of AKI with the administration of lipid-based formulations of amphotericin B [41–44]. To date there have been few randomized trials demonstrating unequivocal superior efficacy and safety of lipid-based formulations compared to standard amphotericin B when the latter is given under optimal conditions. Walsh *et al.* [44] conducted a randomized double-blind multicenter trial in 687 patients that compared liposomal amphotericin B with conventional amphotericin B as empiric antifungal therapy. They showed that liposomal amphotericin B was as effective as conventional amphotericin B when used as empirical antifungal therapy and that it was associated with fewer breakthrough fungal infections, less infusion-related toxicity, and less nephrotoxicity (16.6% had a threefold increase in baseline serum creatinine with convention amphotericin B compared with 8.2% with liposomal). Wingard *et al.* performed a double-blind randomized controlled trial (RCT) that compared two doses of liposomal amphotericin B (3 and 5 mg/kg/day) with amphotericin B lipid complex in 244 neutropenic patients [45]. They found significantly lower rates of nephrotoxicity in those who received liposomal amphotericin B compared to amphotericin B lipid complex. In a systematic Cochrane review of this topic that included literature through April 2000, Jonhansen and Gotzche [46] noted that all lipid-based preparations appeared to decrease the occurrence of nephrotoxicity, but conventional amphotericin was rarely administered under optimal conditions and, therefore, they concluded that it was not clear that lipid-based formulations conferred any benefit. Moreover, it should be noted that under optimal clinical conditions, as achieved in the clinical trials, AKI still occurs with the lipid-based formulations and is more likely to occur in the setting of concurrent patient exposure to other nephrotoxic agents [42,44]. Overall, although large-scale and long-term outcome trials comparing lipid formulations of amphotericin B to the conventional formulation have not been performed, it appears that the former may cause less nephrotoxicity.

Prevention of ATN from rhabdomyolysis

Rhabdomyolysis and its associated myonecrosis often results in ATN and oliguric AKI. The ATN associated with rhabdomyolysis is often multifactorial. Volume depletion (renal ischemia), renal tubular obstruction from heme pigment casts, and tubular injury

from the free iron (released from dying muscle) all contribute to the development of ATN. As many as 50% of all patients with traumatic rhabdomyolysis develop ATN [47], but this number can vary greatly depending on the clinical cause of the rhabdomyolysis as well as the definition used to indentify cases of rhabdomyolysis and of AKI. Current standard therapy for treating rhabdomyolysis, regardless of its cause (which can be quite varied), involves aggressive fluid resuscitation with saline and then, once volume repletion is achieved, urinary alkalinization. The vast majority of studies on prevention of rhabdomyolysis-induced ATN involve trauma patients (natural disaster or accidental). Due to the nature of this type of injury, large-scale RCTs in humans have not been performed to evaluate the recommended therapeutic interventions.

Prevention of ATN from rhabdomyolysis with saline resuscitation

Saline resuscitation is the first step in interrupting the pathophysiology of rhabdomyolysis-induced ATN. The damaged and dying muscles sequester large volumes of water and sodium, which results in rapid intravascular hypovolemia if aggressive fluid resuscitation is not initiated [48]. Although mostly retrospective, human studies have indicated that in order to maintain adequate intravascular volume in traumatized patients at risk for rhabdomyolysis, it is important to start the fluid resuscitative effort prior to the extraction of the patient from the scene of the crush injury [49]. The rationale behind this is to restore intravascular volume prior to the release of heme pigment from injured muscle into the circulation and thus help to prepare the kidneys in advance of the crush relief. In a small retrospective study, this technique was shown to decrease the rate of ATN requiring RRT [50]. The ultimate goal of fluid administration is to initiate a volume diuresis, thereby washing out any obstructing heme pigment casts in the setting of massive fluid sequestration into injured muscle tissue. Overall, the observational trials data support the conclusion that the benefits of attempting saline resuscitation outweigh the risks for fluid overload and pulmonary edema, and as a result it should be attempted in patients presenting with rhabdomyolysis.

Prevention of ATN from rhabdomyolysis with mannitol and bicarbonate

In the setting of a successful saline resuscitation, several studies have attempted to show an additional benefit from initiating a forced alkalinization of the urine. This is often performed through the administration of a combination of mannitol and bicarbonate in intravenous solutions. The rationale behind this treatment is that urine alkalinization prevents the precipitation of the heme pigment casts and thus prevents tubular obstruction and AKI. Additionally, it is thought that it helps to prevent the dissociation of free iron from myoglobin [51]. Animal models have shown that in the setting of experimental traumatic rhabdomyolysis a combination of 0.9% saline, sodium bicarbonate, and mannitol reduces tissue injury (via oxidant stress) and restores renal blood flow, better than either 0.9% saline alone or hypertonic saline [48]. Unfortunately, these animal data have not been replicated in human studies. The literature supporting the use of urinary alkalinization in patients suffers from the same deficiencies as the saline resuscitation studies. It is limited to retrospective, nonrandomized studies. Furthermore, these observational studies offer conflicting results with regards to the utility and effectiveness of urinary alkalinization in preventing ATN from rhabdomyolysis [50,52–54]. These studies vary in size from 15 patients to 382 patients, the largest of which (Brown *et al.*) did not demonstrate any improvement in the ATN or mortality rates in those individuals with rhabdomyolysis (creatine kinase level greater than 5000 U/L) treated with bicarbonate and mannitol [53]. The use of these agents cannot be recommended on the basis of any proven effectiveness reported in the current body of literature. Additionally, multiple toxicities and complications can occur with the administration of these agents (e.g. worsening of hypocalcemia, hypokalemia, hyperosmolality, mannitol-induced proximal tubular damage, systemic alkalosis) necessitating close monitoring of electrolytes, intravascular volume status, and serum and urine pH whenever this intervention is used.

Prevention of ischemic and postoperative ATN

Patients exposed to hypotension, regardless of the etiology (surgery, sepsis, hypovolemia, drug induced, etc.) are at risk for developing ischemic ATN. As mentioned above, the pathophysiology of ATN is complex, but much of what we know is based on animal and clinical models of ischemic ATN. Combining insights obtained from animal models with the availability of well-defined patient cohorts that are at high risk for postoperative ATN, several studies have been conducted to investigate the prevention (and therapy) of ATN in the perioperative setting. However, the majority of these controlled investigations have focused on patients with established ATN rather than those in the early initiation phase prior to clinically overt renal failure. Additionally, it should be noted that although several interventions evaluated in the aforementioned animal models showed dramatic effects in their ability to minimize injury and dysfunction, their translation to human studies and clinical practice has been negligible. These interventions include the use of loop diuretics, dopamine, and fenoldopam. The evidence supporting the role of these interventions in human ischemic ATN prevention and treatment is outlined below. A recent systematic review of loop diuretics, dopamine, calcium channel blockers, angiotensin converting enzyme inhibitors, and fluid therapy as renoprotective strategies for patients undergoing surgery has been published by the Cochrane Library [55].

Loop diuretics

In animal models of ATN, loop diuretics minimize the extent of renal damage and dysfunction [56]. As a result they have been extensively investigated as a means of preventing ATN in patients at risk. Randomized controlled trials comparing diuretic infusion to placebo and other agents (e.g. dopamine) have been performed, and the results have been varied. In 1996, Hager *et al.* [57] randomized 121 patients to receive low-dose infusions of furosemide (1 mg/h) or placebo throughout their intensive care

unit (ICU) stay following major thoraco-abdominal or vascular surgery. They found that there was no difference in serum creatinine or creatinine clearances nor incidence of AKI. It should be noted that no patient in this study (regardless of study arm) developed AKI requiring RRT. Subsequent studies have demonstrated a potential deleterious effect of loop diuretics. In a double-blind, placebo-controlled trial, Lassnigg *et al.* randomized 123 patients to furosemide, dopamine, or saline during and after cardiac surgery [58]. They described an increased rate of AKI (defined as a 0.5-mg/dL increase in serum creatinine) in those patients receiving the diuretic infusion (6 of 41) compared to those receiving saline (0 of 40) ($P < 0.01$). In light of the data reviewed, indicating that loop diuretic administration in patients with established acute renal failure might result in poorer outcomes [59–61] and the finding that loop diuretic administration does not reduce the incidence or duration of AKI and RRT, their routine use in patients at risk of ATN cannot be recommended.

Dopamine

Dopamine, when infused at low doses, has the ability to dilate both the afferent and efferent arterioles in experimental models and has been investigated extensively as a preventative tool in ATN. In the best study of low-dose dopamine therapy for ATN, the ANZICS group performed a randomized, double-blind, controlled trial in 328 critically ill patients with early signs of renal dysfunction (not specifically ATN), comparing dopamine (2 μg/kg/min) with placebo [62]. They found no difference between the groups in the primary end point (peak serum creatinine during study drug infusion) ($P = 0.93$) or with a variety of secondary end points, including development of RRT-requiring ATN ($P = 0.55$), length of ICU stay ($P = 0.67$), or hospital-based mortality ($P = 0.66$). Although this study may not have been a "pure prevention" trial, other more conventional prophylaxis trials have been performed with dopamine therapy. Marik [63] performed a meta-analysis of the kidney-protective effects of low-dose dopamine and found 21 RCTs that had compared low-dose dopamine to placebo and, after a quality review, Marik included 15 studies in the final analysis. Nine of these 15 studies involved postoperative or ischemia-related ATN; none of these demonstrated a significant beneficial effect of low-dose dopamine in preventing renal injury. Two additional meta-analyses [64,65] have been conducted that have included but were not limited to studies investigating dopamine on postoperative or ischemic ATN. Both of these meta-analyses failed to find a benefit from low-dose dopamine. The recent analysis by Friedrich *et al.* [66] included 61 trials (more than 40 of which involved postoperative or ischemic insults) encompassing over 3300 patients. Their analysis demonstrated that dopamine may offer "transient improvement in renal physiology" (as measured by urine output during the first 24 h of infusion) but no improvement in survival, need for RRT, or incidence of AKI (Figures 9.2 and 9.3).

Despite the robust clinical trials literature, use of dopamine persists in clinical practice because of the perceived beneficial effects of dopamine on renal perfusion in patients with AKI. The basic premise of this physiological argument has not been tested

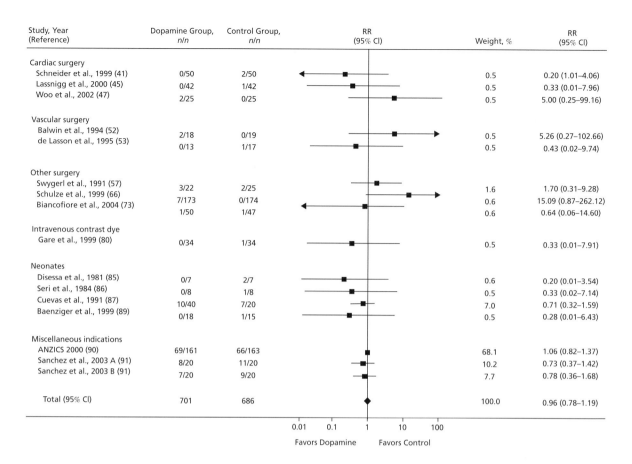

Study, Year (Reference)	Dopamine Group, n/n	Control Group, n/n	RR (95% CI)	Weight, %	RR (95% CI)
Cardiac surgery					
Schneider et al., 1999 (41)	0/50	2/50		0.5	0.20 (1.01–4.06)
Lassnigg et al., 2000 (45)	0/42	1/42		0.5	0.33 (0.01–7.96)
Woo et al., 2002 (47)	2/25	0/25		0.5	5.00 (0.25–99.16)
Vascular surgery					
Balwin et al., 1994 (52)	2/18	0/19		0.5	5.26 (0.27–102.66)
de Lasson et al., 1995 (53)	0/13	1/17		0.5	0.43 (0.02–9.74)
Other surgery					
Swygerl et al., 1991 (57)	3/22	2/25		1.6	1.70 (0.31–9.28)
Schulze et al., 1999 (66)	7/173	0/174		0.6	15.09 (0.87–262.12)
Biancofiore et al., 2004 (73)	1/50	1/47		0.6	0.64 (0.06–14.60)
Intravenous contrast dye					
Gare et al., 1999 (80)	0/34	1/34		0.5	0.33 (0.01–7.91)
Neonates					
Disessa et al., 1981 (85)	0/7	2/7		0.6	0.20 (0.01–3.54)
Seri et al., 1984 (86)	0/8	1/8		0.5	0.33 (0.02–7.14)
Cuevas et al., 1991 (87)	10/40	7/20		7.0	0.71 (0.32–1.59)
Baenziger et al., 1999 (89)	0/18	1/15		0.5	0.28 (0.01–6.43)
Miscellaneous indications					
ANZICS 2000 (90)	69/161	66/163		68.1	1.06 (0.82–1.37)
Sanchez et al., 2003 A (91)	8/20	11/20		10.2	0.73 (0.37–1.42)
Sanchez et al., 2003 B (91)	7/20	9/20		7.7	0.78 (0.36–1.68)
Total (95% CI)	701	686		100.0	0.96 (0.78–1.19)

0.01   0.1   1   10   100

Favors Dopamine   Favors Control

Weight refers to the contribution of each study to the overall estimate of treatment effect. The pooled estimate is calculated by using a random-effects model. The summary relative risk is calculated on the natural logarithm scale. The weight of each study is calculated as the inverse of the variance of the natural logarithm of its relative risk. The size of the symbol denoting the point estimate does not represent the weighting of the study. See the Methods section for a discussion of the weighting. ANZICS = Australian and New Zealand Intensive Care Society; n/n = numbers of deaths/patients randomly assigned; RR = relative risk.

Figure 9.2 Effect of low-dose dopamine on mortality. (Reprinted from Friedrich et al. [65] with permission of the publisher.)

in humans until recently. Recently, Lauschke et al. demonstrated that "low-dose" dopamine may have a deleterious effect on renal perfusion, specifically in those patients with AKI [66]. They conducted a prospective, double-blind, randomized controlled crossover trial in 40 patients (30 with AKI and 10 without). The patients received, in randomly assigned sequence, alternating doses of dopamine (2 μg/kg/min) or placebo and had renal resistive and pulsatility indices measured during four 60-min study periods. Patients with AKI (doubling of baseline serum creatinine or a value above 2.0 mg/dL) demonstrated an increase in resistance indices from baseline ($P < 0.01$) in response to dopamine. This study was the first to demonstrate that dopamine adversely affects renal perfusion and hemodynamics in patients with AKI and that this response differs from that observed in patients without AKI. Robust RCTs and meta-analyses of these RCTs demonstrate no renal or survival benefit from the administration of dopamine to prevent AKI in patients at risk. On the basis of these clinical trials data, dopamine cannot be recommended as an intervention to prevent ischemia-related ATN in the medical or surgical ICU patient.

Fenoldopam

Fenoldopam, a selective dopamine 1 receptor agonist, has been investigated for renoprotective uses because, like dopamine, it has been shown in low doses to increase renal blood flow in animal models without significant systemic adverse hemodynamic effects [67]. Several RCTs have evaluated the potential prophylactic effects of fenoldopam in preventing ATN in the settings of radio-contrast exposure [68,69], sepsis [70], liver transplantation [71], and cardio-aortic surgery [73–75].

In a prospective randomized placebo-controlled trial, Halpenny et al. studied 31 hemodynamically stable post-cardiovascular surgery patients administered either fenoldopam or placebo immediately postoperatively. They assessed renal function in patients who were sufficiently stable to remain on fenoldopam or placebo at 0–4 and 4–8 h and then on days 1, 2, 3, and 5 postoperatively. They reported their findings for the first three time periods only, during which they observed improved renal function in the fenoldopam group [73]. The long-term benefits and clinical importance of these data are unclear. In a second prospective randomized double-blind controlled study, Halpenny et al. [74] studied 28 individuals

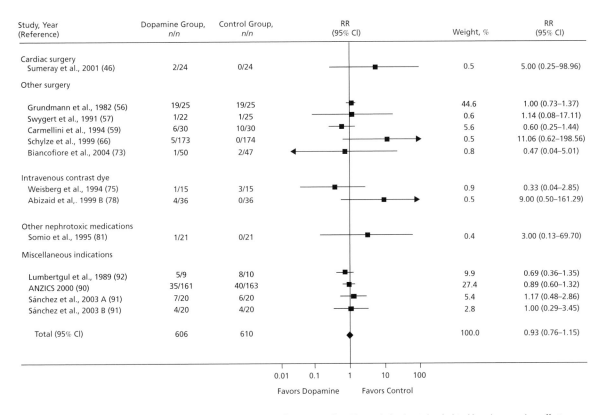

Study, Year (Reference)	Dopamine Group, n/n	Control Group, n/n	RR (95% CI)	Weight, %	RR (95% CI)
Cardiac surgery					
Sumeray et al., 2001 (46)	2/24	0/24		0.5	5.00 (0.25–98.96)
Other surgery					
Grundmann et al., 1982 (56)	19/25	19/25		44.6	1.00 (0.73–1.37)
Swygert et al., 1991 (57)	1/22	1/25		0.6	1.14 (0.08–17.11)
Carmellini et al., 1994 (59)	6/30	10/30		5.6	0.60 (0.25–1.44)
Schylze et al., 1999 (66)	5/173	0/174		0.5	11.06 (0.62–198.56)
Biancofiore et al., 2004 (73)	1/50	2/47		0.8	0.47 (0.04–5.01)
Intravenous contrast dye					
Weisberg et al., 1994 (75)	1/15	3/15		0.9	0.33 (0.04–2.85)
Abizaid et al,. 1999 B (78)	4/36	0/36		0.5	9.00 (0.50–161.29)
Other nephrotoxic medications					
Somio et al., 1995 (81)	1/21	0/21		0.4	3.00 (0.13–69.70)
Miscellaneous indications					
Lumbertgul et al., 1989 (92)	5/9	8/10		9.9	0.69 (0.36–1.35)
ANZICS 2000 (90)	35/161	40/163		27.4	0.89 (0.60–1.32)
Sánchez et al., 2003 A (91)	7/20	6/20		5.4	1.17 (0.48–2.86)
Sánchez et al., 2003 B (91)	4/20	4/20		2.8	1.00 (0.29–3.45)
Total (95% CI)	606	610		100.0	0.93 (0.76–1.15)

0.01   0.1   1   10   100

Favors Dopamine   Favors Control

Weight refers to the contribution of each study to the overall estimate of treatment effect. The pooled estimate is calculated by using a random-effects model. The summary relative risk is calculated on the natural logarithm scale. The weight of each study is calculated as the inverse of the variance of the natural logarithm of its relative risk. The size of the symbol denoting the point estimate does not represent the weighting of the study. See the Methods section for a discussion of the weighting. ANZICS = Australian and New Zealand Intensive Care Society; n/n = numbers of patients requiring renal replacement therapy/patients randomly assigned; RR = relative risk.

Figure 9.3 Effect of low-dose dopamine on need for RRT. (Reprinted from Friedrich *et al.* [65] with permission of the publisher.)

undergoing aortic cross-clamping and the effects of intraoperative administration of fenoldopam. Plasma creatinine concentration increased significantly from baseline on the first postoperative day in the placebo group ($P < 0.01$) and not in the fenoldopam group, but no subsequent data were reported, and the utility of this small pilot study in informing care is, therefore, limited. Caimmi *et al.* [75] randomized 160 patients with CKD (serum creatinine > 1.5 mg/dL) undergoing hypothermic cardiopulmonary bypass to receive intraoperative and postoperative fenoldopam (0.1–0.3 µg/kg/min) or conventional care. They found that fenoldopam was correlated with a shorter duration of mechanical ventilation, shorter ICU stays, and a lower immediately postoperative serum creatinine. Unfortunately, once again there was no report of effects on long-term postoperative renal function compared to placebo. In the last of these studies, Bove *et al.* [76] randomized 80 patients undergoing cardiac surgery to receive an infusion of either fenoldopam or dopamine for the 24 h following the induction of anesthesia. The merits of using dopamine as a control aside, this study failed to show any incremental improvement or benefit on renal outcomes from the fenoldopam infusion compared to dopamine.

Morelli *et al.* [71] conducted a randomized, double-blind, placebo-controlled trial of 300 patients with sepsis in which pa-

tients received fenoldopam (0.09 µg/kg/min) or placebo for the entire length of their ICU stay. They found that prophylactic fenoldopam decreased the rate of renal failure (serum creatinine > 300 µmol/L) compared to placebo (29 vs. 51 patients; $P = 0.006$). Additionally, they noted a decrease in the length of ICU stay with fenoldopam (10.6 ± 9.3 days vs. 13.4 ± 14.0 days; $P < 0.001$). These promising data for sepsis suggest that a larger trial should be conducted for this indication.

Although some of these studies report benefits from the use of fenoldopam for prevention of ATN, the data do not support the clinical use of fenoldopam for this purpose at this time, particularly given the potential risk of fenoldopam-induced hypotension, pending further confirmatory prospective studies.

N-Acetylcysteine

N-acetyl-cysteine (NAC) is thought to potentially protect patients from contrast-associated nephropathy because of its anti-inflammatory properties and through modulation of oxidative stress as an oxygen free radical scavenger [77]. NAC has therefore been tested in the setting of increased oxidative stress and renal ischemia associated with either cardiopulmonary bypass (CPB) or cross-clamping of the aorta for abdominal surgery where NAC has been administered prior to the onset of overt renal injury in order to reduce postoperative AKI. Seven RCTs have evaluated the renoprotective effects of intra- and/or postoperative NAC infusion in patients at risk for ischemic and oxidative stress-related ATN from cardiac or aorta surgery [78–84]. No systematic review of the literature has been performed to date that summarizes this literature. Fisher *et al.* in a post hoc analysis of an RCT of NAC in cardiac surgery reported a significantly greater decline in calculated creatinine clearance in patients receiving placebo compared to those who received NAC [78]. In an RCT of 295 high renal risk coronary artery bypass graft patients that compared high-dose NAC (2400 mg/24 h) versus placebo, Burns and colleagues were unable to demonstrate kidney-protective effects from NAC [79]. They conducted a post hoc analysis of those patients with baseline renal dysfunction (Cr > 1.4 mg/dL) and reported a non-significant trend toward less renal dysfunction in this subset of patients when they received NAC. Ristikankare *et al.* randomized 80 subjects with CKD undergoing elective cardiac surgery and CPB to receive either NAC intra- and postoperatively or placebo [80]. They evaluated biomarkers of tubular damage (*N*-acetyl-beta-D-glucosaminidase) and serum cystatin C and creatinine clearance during the first 5 days postoperatively and observed no protective effect on renal function with NAC [80]. In a second study from the same institution, Hynninen *et al.* evaluated whether NAC administered intraoperatively afforded renoprotection from ischemic ATN for patients with normal baseline renal function undergoing abdominal aortic surgery and aortic cross-clamping [81]. They measured serum creatinine and cystatin C and urinary NAG levels. They were unable to demonstrate any renoprotective effect with NAC administration. In a small study of Brazilian patients, Macedo also was unable to demonstrate renoprotective effects from NAC during abdominal aortic surgery [82]. In the most recent studies, Haase *et al.* investigated the effects of high doses of NAC (300 mg/kg over 24 h by continuous infusion) on renal function in a high-risk group of patients undergoing cardiac surgery with CPB. In this RCT there was no difference in the two groups in terms of serum creatinine or cystatin C level or urinary NAG during the 5-day postoperative follow-up period [83]. Thus, only one RCT demonstrated a small potential benefit from prophylactic NAC administration, one reported a trend toward a benefit in individuals with CKD, and the remainder of studies reported to date have demonstrated no benefit in patients at risk for ischemic ATN associated with cardiac or abdominal surgery. These studies are mostly small and, therefore, not sufficiently powered to preclude a small beneficial effect. At this time, however, routine use of NAC in cardiac and aortic surgery as a renoprotective strategy cannot be recommended.

Modulation of mechanical ventilation settings

Positive-pressure mechanical ventilation alters renal perfusion and function through a variety of mechanisms [76,85]. In patients with decreased effective circulating blood volume, increased intrathoracic pressure promotes a decrease in venous return from the periphery and may cause hypovolemic shock. Positive pressure ventilation, even in the absence of hypovolemia, alters neuro-hormonal

systems (stimulates increased sympathetic outflow, activates the renin–angiotensin–aldosterone axis, increases nonosmotic vasopressin release, and decreases atrial natriuretic peptide release). Overall these effects promote systemic and renal vasoconstriction, decreased renal blood flow, and lower GFR. Hypercapnia and severe hypoxemia ($PaO_2 < 40$ mmHg) have similarly been shown to result in renal vasoconstriction and decreased blood flow [85]. Overall, in critically ill patients with compromised circulatory function, it is well-documented that diminished systemic and renal perfusion (ATN) are common adverse outcomes of respiratory failure requiring mechanical ventilation.

Several studies have shown that fluid administration and the use of vasoactive drugs (dopamine, fenoldopam) can improve the renal hypoperfusion and decreased GFR associated with positive pressure ventilation [86–88]. Recently, ventilator-induced pulmonary and systemic inflammation have been identified as risk factors for ARF, in addition to known hemodynamic and neuro-hormonal mechanisms of ventilator-induced renal injury. Evidence from large-scale randomized trials suggests that the proinflammatory effects of positive pressure ventilation, specifically those of lung-injurious ventilatory strategies, may be a source of AKI [85,89–91]. The ARDSNet Tidal Volume Trial demonstrated that patients assigned to the lower tidal volume group experience an increased number of ventilator-free days, improved survival, and less AKI (defined as serum creatinine > 2.0 mg/dL) (20 ± 11 vs. 18 ± 11 days; $P = 0.005$) [90]. Additionally, in an RCT, Ranieri *et al.* [91] demonstrated that lower tidal volumes and higher PEEP (lung protective strategy) caused less systemic inflammation compared to standard care, and this correlated with fewer patients with organ system failures, including less AKI at 72 h postadmission. Overall, recent developments have shown that combinations of hemodynamic and lung-protective ventilatory strategies are the best current approach to minimizing ventilator-induced AKI. Hopefully, the widespread adoption of these guidelines will result in a decrease in AKI in critically ill patients.

Other agents

Over the years several additional agents have been investigated as potential preventative measures. The adenosine agonist theophylline has been studied in the setting of radiocontrast nephropathy [92] as well as following cardiovascular surgery [93]. In RCTs of 80 and 56 patients, respectively, theophylline was shown to be ineffective at preventing ATN. Similarly, mannitol has been compared to standard hydration in a wide variety of settings for ATN prophylaxis. Although some data support its use in the perioperative kidney transplant setting (discussed in chapter 51), in several small RCTs mannitol failed to prevent ATN following cardiovascular surgery [94], vascular surgery [95], and biliary tract surgery [96].

Pharmacologic therapy of established ATN

Several classes of agents have been investigated as potential therapeutic options for established ATN, but the results have been disappointing.

Therapy of established ATN with loop diuretics

Loop diuretics are often used during the management of ATN in the hopes of "converting" oliguric ATN to a nonoliguric state. Several decades ago, two small RCTs (with 58 and 66 patients) showed no benefit from increasing urine output with loop diuretics on the duration or severity of AKI [62,97]. Recently, there has been a renewed interest in this phenomenon, and several new investigations have sought to redefine the role of loop diuretics in the setting of established ATN. Cantarovich et al. found that high-dose furosemide (25 mg/kg/day), in the setting of established AKI, showed no impact on patient survival or renal recovery rate, despite increasing total urine output [98]. In this prospective, randomized, double-blind, placebo-controlled multicenter trial of 338 patients with AKI requiring RRT, there was no between-groups difference in the total time on RRT (11.4 ± 8.6 vs. 12.4 ± 8.7 days; not significant) despite achieving 2.0 L of urine output with furosemide administration. Furthermore, Mehta et al. evaluated a multicenter retrospective cohort of 552 patients with AKI in the intensive care unit setting. They found that diuretic use in critically ill patients was associated with an increased risk of death and nonrecovery of renal function [60]. In contrast, Uchino et al. examined diuretic use in 1743 patients with AKI at 54 centers [99]. Overall, 64% of that cohort received diuretic therapy, and extensive multivariate analysis found that diuretic use was not associated with any increase in mortality. Regrettably, due to lack of randomization and other confounders, the latter cohort studies are not definitive. In summary, the current literature does not support the use of loop diuretics as therapy for ATN to hasten renal recovery or improve mortality, but when clinically indicated it appears that their use to control fluid balance remains justified.

Therapy of established ATN with dopamine

As previously mentioned, although several meta-analyses have examined the role of dopamine in the setting of ATN, many of these results have combined prevention and therapeutic trials. For instance, in the Friedrich et al. meta-analysis of 61 randomized trials, only 6 trials studied dopamine as a treatment option for those with established renal dysfunction [66]. Of these six, only four investigated dopamine use in the setting of potential ATN (critical illness and congestive heart failure). The remaining two studies measured dopamine's performance in the settings of preeclampsia and contrast nephropathy [66]. The largest of the included trials was the ANZICS trial [63], which as previously mentioned examined 328 patients with two or more manifestations of systemic inflammatory syndrome in a 24-h period and at least one indicator of early renal dysfunction (decreased urine output or changes in serum creatinine). Patients received dopamine (at 2 μg/kg/min) or placebo until one of the study end points was met (death, RRT, 24 h postresolution of systemic inflammatory syndrome or adverse event). In the end, low-dose dopamine did not confer any clinically significant protection from renal dysfunction; there was no observed difference in the primary outcome of peak serum creatinine during the study ($P = 0.93$), RRT rate ($P = 0.55$), length of ICU stay ($P = 0.67$), or in-hospital mortality ($P = 0.66$). Similarly, a systematic review by Kellum and Decker [100] looked at dopamine use in a total of 17 RCTs. They concluded from their systematic review that "the use of low-dose dopamine for treatment or prevention of acute renal failure cannot be justified...and should be eliminated from routine clinical use." It should be noted that this meta-analysis did not formally distinguish between prevention and therapeutic trials. Based on these findings as well as those from the prevention trials discussed above, the use of dopamine as a therapeutic option in the setting of ATN cannot be endorsed.

Therapy of established ATN with fenoldopam

In addition to investigation as a prophylactic agent for radio-contrast nephropathy [101] and sepsis-induced renal dysfunction, fenoldopam has been studied as therapy for established ATN [102,103]. Tumlin et al. studied 155 ICU patients with early ATN and randomized them in a double-blind fashion to receive fenoldopam or 0.45% saline. They demonstrated that fenoldopam patients tended to have lower mortality ($P = 0.068$) and a decreased need for RRT. Unfortunately, the study was underpowered, and the 11% difference in RRT-free survival did not reach statistical significance. A secondary post hoc analysis of the trial data by these authors supported the view that in the subsets of patients without diabetes and those recently undergoing CV surgery improved outcomes might have been achieved with fenoldopam. The authors recommended that a larger multicenter trial with stratification for diabetes mellitus be performed to further explore the potential therapeutic utility of fenoldopam in the setting of early ATN [104].

Similarly, Brienza et al. [105] recently published their study of 110 ICU patients with AKI, comparing therapy with 4 days of fenoldopam with low-dose dopamine. Although this study was randomized, the investigators were not blinded, and the use of low-dose dopamine as a control arm was less than ideal. Nevertheless, the study showed that the mean serum creatinine as in the fenoldopam group was lower than that of the dopamine group after the 4-day infusion period (1.56 vs. 1.81 mg/dl). There was, however, no difference observed in the rate of RRT in either group. The clinical significance of this slightly lower serum creatinine after the 4-day infusion period remains unclear. Based upon the results of these two studies, a larger, multicenter, randomized, double-blind, placebo-controlled trial of fenoldopam therapy for ATN, stratified for subpopulations such as diabetic status, seems warranted.

Therapy of established ATN with natriuretic peptides

The natriuretic peptides (NP) are a family of hormones and pro-hormones that work in concert with the renin–angiotensin–aldosterone axis to maintain salt and water homeostasis. Atrial natriuretic peptide (ANP), which promotes afferent arteriolar vasodilation and efferent arteriolar vasoconstriction, leading to an increase in GFR [104], is the best-studied in this family. ANP and its analogs have been studied as treatment for ATN in several settings, including radiocontrast nephropathy [105], post-cardiac surgery [106], and generalized ATN (sepsis, nephrotoxin reaction, etc.) [107].

In a multicenter randomized, double-blind, placebo-controlled trial, Allgren et al. looked at anaritide (a synthetic analog of ANP) in 504 patients with preexisting ATN [108]. They concluded that anaritide did not improve the overall rate of RRT-free survival; however, they reported some possible benefit for the subset of individuals with oliguric ATN. Only 73% of those with oliguric ATN required RRT in the anaritide arm compared to 92% receiving placebo. To evaluate this possibility, Lewis et al. conducted a randomized, double-blind, placebo-controlled trial of 222 patients with oliguric ATN and found no improvement in the dialysis-free survival time after a 24-h infusion of ANP (200 ng/kg/min) [108]. It should be noted that 36% of those studied by Lewis et al. received radiocontrast agent as the precipitating source of their ATN and that hypotension was more common in the ANP-treated subjects.

Looking at ANP exclusively in the post-cardiac surgery setting, Sward et al. found that administering 50 ng/kg/min of ANP to patients with early postoperative renal dysfunction decreased the requirement of RRT and improved dialysis-free survival [106]. In this prospective, double-blind, randomized placebo-controlled trial of 61 patients, only 8 patients (28%) receiving anaritide required RRT or died in the first 21 postoperative days, compared to 17 (57%) in the placebo arm (hazard ratio, 0.35; $P = 0.017$).

However, these studies have dosing discrepancies; the Allgren and Lewis studies that failed to show a benefit in RRT-free survival dosed ANP at 200 ng/kg/min (resulting in more hypotension in the experimental arm), compared to 50 ng/kg/min in the Sward et al. study. The duration of ANP treatment was also different. Thus, the possibility exists that the negative results from the former, high-dose studies might be the result of ANP-induced hypotension or some other confounder. As such, more trials investigating the use of "low-dose" anaritide are needed in order to fully evaluate the utility of these agents as ATN therapy.

Recent meta-analyses of brain natriuretic peptide (BNP; nesiritide) trials in the setting of congestive heart failure have generated some controversy. Sackner-Bernstein et al. in a meta-analysis of five trials with 1269 patients found nesiritide doses of 0.03 μg/kg/min significantly increased the risk of renal dysfunction (serum creatinine increase > 0.5 mg/dL) compared to non-inotrope-based controls or compared to all control groups (including inotropes) [109]. This association with renal dysfunction was noted at doses as low as 0.015 μg/kg/min compared to controls; however, there was no noted difference in dialysis rates. In a separate meta-analysis by the same authors, nesiritide showed a trend toward increased 30-day mortality [110]. Although none of the studies analyzed was performed with renal function as a primary end point, the use of nesiritide for the prevention or treatment of AKI in patients with CHF is not supported by the current literature.

Therapy of established ATN: other modalities

As previously mentioned, the pathophysiology of AKI is an active area of investigation, and several potential therapeutic agents have been identified in experimental models of AKI. Unfortunately, their role in clinical practice remains unclear [111]. Insulin-like growth factor 1 (IGF-1) showed a great degree of promise in early basic science studies and animal models. Yet, despite this early promise, several clinical trials have failed to demonstrate an appreciable beneficial effect. Among these studies is the multicenter, randomized, double-blind, placebo-controlled trial conducted by Hirschberg et al. [112]. In this trial, 72 patients were randomized to receive either recombinant human IGF-1 (rhIGF-1) or placebo. In this RCT, rhIGF-1 did not hasten recovery from AKI. Among the other negative studies, Hladunewich et al. performed a randomized placebo-controlled trial in 44 patients with delayed graft function immediately following cadaveric kidney allografts (a commonly used model for postischemic ATN) and compared the use of IGF-1 to placebo [113]. Patients receiving twice-daily infusions of IGF-1 for the first six postoperative days achieved no significant improvement in their renal function, as measured by day 7 inulin clearance ($P = 0.67$). IGF-1 is one agent on a long list of potential therapeutic agents that have shown promise in animal models, but to date none has demonstrated a clear benefit in clinical practice.

Summary

ATN is an all-too-common and serious complication for hospitalized patients. Its course is extremely variable, often necessitates that patients undergo RRT, and carries a very high mortality rate. Despite countless trials to investigate potential preventative and therapeutic agents, to date there exist few proven effective interventions for ATN.

References

1 Lameire N, Van Biesen W, Vanholder R. Acute renal failure. *Lancet* 2005; **365(9457)**: 417–430.

2 Blantz RC. Pathophysiology of prerenal azotemia. *Kidney Int* 1998; **53(2)**: 512–523.

3 Prakash J, Sen D, Kumar NS, Kumar H, Tripathi LK, Saxena RK. Acute renal failure due to intrinsic renal disease: review of 1122 cases. *Ren Fail* 2003; **25(2)**: 225–233.

4 Liano F, Pascual J, and the Madrid Acute Renal Failure Study Group. Epidemiology of acute renal failure: a prospective, multicenter, community-based study. *Kidney Int* 1996; **50(3)**: 811–818.

5 Mehta RL, Pascual MT, Soroko S, Savage BR, Himmelfarb J, Ikizler TA *et al.* Spectrum of acute renal failure in the intensive care unit: the PICARD experience. *Kidney Int* 2004; **66(4)**: 1613–1621.

6 Liano F, Junco E, Pascual J, Madero R, Verde E. The spectrum of acute renal failure in the intensive care unit compared with that seen in other settings. The Madrid Acute Renal Failure Study Group. *Kidney Int Suppl* 1998; **66**: S16–S24.

7 Zager RA. Endotoxemia, renal hypoperfusion, and fever: interactive risk factors for aminogylcoside and sepsis-induced acute renal failure. *Am J Kidney Dis* 1992; **20(3)**: 223–230.

8 Gill N, Nally JV, Fatica RA. Renal failure secondary to acute tubular necrosis: epidemiology, diagnosis and management. *Chest* 2005; **128(4)**: 2847–2863.

9 Esson ML, Schrier RW. Diagnosis and treatment of acute tubular necrosis. *Ann Intern Med* 2002; **137(9)**: 744–752.

10 Miller TR, Anderson RJ, Linas SL, Henrich WL, Berns AS, Gabow PA et al. Urinary diagnostic indices in acute renal failure: a prospective study. Ann Intern Med 1978; **89**(1): 47–50.

11 Corwin HL, Schreiber MJ, Fang LS. Low fractional excretion of sodium. Occurence with hemoglobinuric- and myoglobinuric-induced acute renal failure. Arch Intern Med 1980; **144**: 981–982.

12 Zarich S, Fang LS, Diamond TR. Fractional excretion of sodium: exceptions to its diagnostic value. Arch Intern Med 1985; **145**(1): 108–112.

13 Vaz AJ. Low fraction excretion of sodium in acute renal failure due to sepsis. Arch Intern Med 1985; **143**: 738–739.

14 Lameire N, Vanholder R. Pathophysiologic features and prevention of human and experimental acute tubular necrosis. J Am Soc Nephrol 2001; **12**(Suppl 1): S20–S32.

15 Bonventre JV, Weinberg JM. Recent advances in the pathophysiology of ischemic acute renal failure. J Am Soc Nephrol 2003; **14**(8): 2199–2210.

16 Sutton TA, Fisher CJ, Molitoris BA. Microvascular endothelial injury and dysfunction during ischemic acute renal failure. Kidney Int 2002; **62**(5): 1539–1549.

17 Molitoris BA, Sutton TA. Endothelial injury and dysfunction: role in the extension phase of acute renal failure. Kidney Int 2004; **66**(2): 496–499.

18 Spurney RF, Fulkerson WJ, Schwab SJ. Acute renal failure in critically ill patients: prognosis for recovery of kidney function after prolonged dialysis support. Crit Care Med 1991; **19**(10): 8–11.

19 Chertow GM, Lazarus JM, Paganini EP, Allgren RL, Lafayette RA, Sayegh MH. Predictors of mortality and the provision of dialysis in patients with acute tubular necrosis. The Auriculin Anaritide Acute Renal Failure Study Group. J Am Soc Nephrol 1998; **9**(4): 692–698.

20 Parker RA, Himmelfarb J, Tolkoff-Rubin N, Chandran P, Wingard RL, Hakim RM. Prognosis of patients with acute renal failure requiring dialysis: results of a multicenter study. Am J Kid Dis 1998; **32**(3): 432–443.

21 Schrier RW, Wang W. Acute renal failure and sepsis. N Engl J Med 2004; **351**(2): 159–169.

22 Bagshaw SM, Laupland KB, Doig CJ, Mortis G, Fick GH, Mucenski M et al. Prognosis for long-term survival and renal recovery in critically ill patients with severe acute renal failure: a population-based study. Crit Care 2005; **9**(6): R700–R709.

23 Prins JM, Buller HR, Kuijer EJ, Tange RA, Speelman P. Once versus thrice daily gentamicin in patients with serious infections. Lancet 1993; **341**(8841): 335–339.

24 Humes HD. Aminoglycoside nephtoxicity. Kidney Int 1988; **33**(4): 900–911.

25 Meyer RD. Risk factors and comparisons of clinical nephrotoxicity of aminoglycosides. Am J Med 1986; **80**(6B): 119–125.

26 Moore SD, Smith CR, Lietman PS. Increased risk of renal dysfunction due to interaction of liver disease and aminoglycosides. Am J Med 1986; **80**(6): 1093–1097.

27 Blaser J, Konig C. Once daily dosing of aminoglycosides. Eur J Clin Microbiol Infect Dis 1995; **14**(12): 1029–1038.

28 Munckhof WJ, Grayson ML, Turnidge JD. A metanalyisis of studies on the safety and efficacy of aminglycosides given either once daily or as divided doses. J Antimicrob Chemother 1996; **37**(4): 645–663.

29 Barza M, Ioannidis JPA, Cappelleri JC, Lau J. Single or multiple daily doses of aminoglycosides: a meta analysis. BMJ 1996; **312**(7027): 338–345.

30 Hatala R, Dinh T, Cook DJ. Once-daily aminoglycoside dosing in immunocompetent adults: a meta analysis. Ann Intern Med 1996; **124**(8): 717–725.

31 Smyth AR, Tan KH. Once-daily versus multiple-daily dosing with intravenous aminoglycosides for cystic fibrosis. Cochrane Database Syst Rev 2006; **3**: CD002009.

32 Bartal C, Danon A, Sclaaeffer F, Reisenberg K, Alkan M, Smoliakov R et al. Pharmacokinetic dosing of aminoglycosides: a controlled trial. Am J Med 2003; **114**(4): 194–198.

33 Butler WT, Bennett JE, Ailing DW, Wertlake PT, Utz JP, Hill GJ. Nephrotoxicity of amphotericin B—early and late events in 81 patients. Ann Intern Med 1964; **61**: 175–187.

34 Arning M, Scharf RE. Prevention of amphotericin B-induced nephrotoxicity with sodium chloride: a report of 1291 days of treatment with amphotericin B with renal failure. Klin Wochenschr 1989; **67**: 1020–1028.

35 Harbarth S, Pestotnik SL, Lloyd JF, Burke JP, Samore MH. The epidemiology of nephrotoxicity associated with conventional amphotericin B therapy. Am J Med 2001; **111**(7): 528–534.

36 Sawaya BP, Briggs JP, Schnermann J. Amphotericin B nephrotoxicity: the adverse consequences of altered membrane properties. J Am Soc Nephrol 1995; **6**(2): 154–164.

37 Gerkens JF, Branch RA. The influence of sodium status and furesomide on canine acute amphotericin B nephrotoxicity. J Pharmacol Exp Ther 1980; **214**: 306–311.

38 Anderson CM. Sodium chloride treatment of amphotericin B nephrotoxicity: Standard of care? West J Med 1995; **162**(4): 313–317.

39 Llanos A, Cieza J, Bernado J, Echevarria J, Biaggioni I, Sabra R et al. Effect of salt supplementation on amphotericin B nephrotoxicity. Kidney Int 1991; **40**(2): 302–308.

40 Camp MJ, Wingard JR, Gilmore CE, Lin LS, Dix SP, Davidson TG et al. Efficacy of low-dose dopamine in preventing amphotericin B nephrotoxicity in bone marrow transplant patients and leukemia patients. Antimicrob Agents Chemother 1998; **42**(12): 3103–3106.

41 Walsh TJ, Hiemenz JW, Seibel NL, Perfect JR, Horwith G, Lee L et al. Amphotericin B lipid complex for invasive fungal infections: analysis of safety and efficacy in 556 cases. Clin Infect Dis 1998; **26**(6): 1383–1396.

42 Alexander BD, Wingard JR. Study of renal safety in amphotericin B lipid complex-treated patients. Clin Infect Dis 2005; **40**(Suppl 6): S414–S421.

43 Aguado JM, Lumbreras C, Gonzalez-Vidal D. Assessment of nephrotoxicity in patients receiving amphotericin B lipid complex: a pharmaco-surveillance study in Spain. Clin Microbiol Infect 2004; **10**(9): 785–790.

44 Walsh TJ, Finberg RW, Arndt C, Hiemenz J, Schwartz C, Bodensteiner D et al. Liposomal amphotericin B for empirical therapy in patients with persistent fever and neutropenia. N Engl J Med 1999; **340**(10): 764–771.

45 Wingard JR, White MH, Anaissie E, Raffalli J, Goodman J, Arrieta A et al. A randomized, double-blind comparative trial evaluating the safety of liposomal amphotericin B versus amphotericin B lipid complex in the empirical treatment of febrile neutropenia. Clin Infect Dis 2000; **31**: 1155–1163.

46 Johansen HK, Gotzsche PC. Amphotericin B lipid soluble formulations vs amphotericin B in cancer patients with neutropenia. Cochrane Database Syst Rev 2000; **3**: CD000969.

47 Ozguc H, Kahveci N, Akkose S, Serdar Z, Balci V, Ocak O. Effect of different resuscitation fluid on tissue blood flow and oxidant injury in experimental rhabdomyolysis. Crit Care Med 2005; **33**(11): 2579–2586.

48 Better OS, Stein JH. Early management of shock and prophylaxis of acute renal failure in traumatic rhabdomyolysis. N Engl J Med 1990; **322**(12): 825–829.

49 Ron D, Taitelman U, Michealson M, Bar-Joseph G, Bursztein S, Better OS. Prevention of acute renal failure in traumatic rhabdomyolysis. Arch Intern Med 1984; **144**(2): 277–280.

50 Gunal AI, Celiker H, Dogukan A, Ozalp G, Kirciman E, Simsekli H *et al.* Early and vigorous fluid resuscitation prevents acute renal failure in the crush victims of catastrophic earthquakes. *J Am Soc Nephrol* 2004; **15**(7): 1862–1867.

51 Zager RA. Rhabdomyolysis and myohemoglobinuric acute renal failure. *Kidney Int* 1996; **49**(2): 314–26.

52 Brown CVR, Rhee P, Chan L, Evans K, Demetriades D, Velmahos GC. Preventing renal failure in patients with rhabdomyolysis: do bicarbonate and mannitol make a difference? *J Trauma* 2004; **56**(6): 1191–1196.

53 Homsi E, Barreiro MF, Orlando JM, Higa EM. Prophylaxis of acute renal failure in patients with rhabdomyolysis. *Ren Fail* 1997; **19**(2): 283–288.

54 Eneas JF, Schoenfeld PY, Humphreys MH. The effect of infusion of mannitol-sodium bicarbonate on the clinical course of myoglobinuria. *Arch Intern Med* 1979; **139**(7): 801–805.

55 Zacharias M, Gilmore ICS, Herbison GP, Sivalingam P, Walker RJ. Interventions for protecting renal function in the perioperative period. *Cochrane Database Syst Rev* 2005; **3**: CD003590.

56 Hanley MJ, Davidson, K. Prior mannitol and furosemide infusion in a model of ischemic acute renal failure. *Am J Physiol* 1981; **241**(5): F556–F564.

57 Hager B, Betschart M, Krapf R. Effect of postoperative intravenous loop diuretic on renal function after major surgery. *Schweiz Med Wochenschr* 1996; **126**(16): 666–673.

58 Lassnigg A, Donner E, Grubhofer G, Presterl E, Druml W, Hiesmayr M. Lack of renoprotective effect of dopamine and furosemide during cardiac surgery. *J Am Soc Nephrol* 2000; **11**(1): 97–104.

59 Brown CB, Ogg CS, Cameron JS. High dose frusemide in acute renal failure: a controlled study. *Clin Nephrol* 1981; **15**(2): 90–96.

60 Mehta RL, Pascual MT, Soroko S, Chertow GM. Diuretics, mortality and nonrecovery of renal function in acute renal failure. *JAMA* 2002; **288**(20): 2547–2553.

61 Sirivella, S, Gielchinsky I, Parsonnet V. Mannitol, furosemide, and dopamine infusion in postoperative renal failure complicating cardiac surgery. *Ann Thorac Surg* 2000; **69**(2): 501–506.

62 Bellomo R, Chapman M, Finfer S, Hicking K, Myburgh J. Low-dose dopamine in patients with early renal dysfunction: a placebo-controlled randomized trial. *Lancet* 2000; **356**(9248): 2139–2143.

63 Marik PE. Low-dose dopamine: a systemic review. *Intensive Care Med* 2002; **28**: 877–883.

64 Kellum JA, Decker JM. Use of dopamine in acute renal failure: a meta-analysis. *Crit Care Med* 2001; **29**: 1526–1531.

65 Friedrich JO, Adhikari N, Herridge MS, Beyene J. Meta-analysis: low-dose dopamine increases urine output but does not prevent renal dysfunction or death. *Ann Intern Med* 2005; **142**(7): 510–524.

66 Lauschke A, Teichgräber UKM, Frei U, Eckardt K-U. 'Low-dose' dopamine worsens renal perfusion in patients with acute renal failure. *Kidney Int* 2006; **69**: 1669–1674.

67 Mathur VS, Swan SK, Lambrecht LJ, Anjum S, Fellmann J, McGuire D *et al.* The effect of fenoldopam, a selective dopamine receptor agonist, on systemic and renal hemodynamics in normotensive patients. *Crit Care Med* 1999; **27**(9): 1832–1837.

68 Tumlin JA, Wang A, Murray PT, Mathur VS. Fenoldopam mesylate blocks reductions in renal plasma flow after radiocontrast dye infusion: a pilot trial in the prevention of contrast nephropathy. *Am Heart J* 2002; **143**(5): 894–903.

69 Stone GW, McCullough PA, Tumlin JA, Lepor NE, Madyoon H, Murray P *et al.* Fenoldopam mesylate for the prevention of contrast-induced nephropathy: a randomized controlled trial. *JAMA* 2003; **290**(17): 2284–2291.

70 Morelli A, Ricci Z, Bellomo R, Ronco C, Conti G, De Gaetano A *et al.* Prophylatic fenoldopam for renal protection in sepsis: a randomized, placebo controlled pilot trial. *Crit Care Med* 2005; **33**(11): 2451–2456.

71 Biancofiore G, Della Rocca G, Bindi L, Romanelli A, Esposito M, Meacci L *et al.* Use of fenoldopam to control renal dysfunction early after liver transplantation. *Liver Transpl* 2004; **10**(8): 986–992.

72 Halpenny M, Lakshmi S, O'Donnell A, O'Callaghan-Enright S, Shorten GD. Fenoldopam: renal and splanchnic effects in patients undergoing coronary artery bypass grafting. *Anaesthesia* 2001; **56**(10): 953–960.

73 Halpenny M, Rushe C, Breen P, Cunningham AJ, Boucher-Hayes D, Shorten GD. The effects of fenoldopam on renal function in patients undergoing elective aortic surgery. *Eur J Anaesthesiol* 2002; **19**(1): 32–39.

74 Caimmi PP, Pagani L, Micalizzi E, Fiume C, Guani S, Bernardi M *et al.* Fenoldopam for renal protection in patients undergoing cardiopulmonary bypass. *J Cardiothorac Vasc Anesth* 2003; **17**(4): 491–494.

75 Bove T, Landoni G, Calabro MG, Aletti G, Marino G, Cerchierini E *et al.* Renoprotective action of fenoldopam in high-risk patients undergoing cardiac surgery: a prospective, double-blind, randomized clinical trial. *Circulation* 2005; **111**(24): 3230–3235.

76 Kuiper JW, Groeneveld AB, Slutsky AS, Plotz FB. Mechanical ventilation and acute renal failure. *Crit Care Med* 2005; **33**: 1460–1461.

77 Tossios P, Bloch W, Huebner A, Raji MR, Dodos F, Klass O *et al.* N-acetylcysteine prevents reactive oxygen species-mediated myocardial stress in patients undergoing cardiac surgery: results of a randomized, double blind, placebo controlled clinical trial. *J Thorac Cardiovasc Surg* 2003; **126**: 1513–1520.

78 Fischer UM, Tossios P, Mehlhorn U. Renal protection by radical scavenging in cardiac surgery patients. *Curr Med Res Opin* 2005; **21**: 1161–1164.

79 Burns KEA, Chu MWA, Novick RJ, Fox SA, Gallo K, Martin CM *et al.* Perioperative N-acetylcysteine to prevent renal dysfunction in high-risk patients undergoing CABG surgery. *JAMA* 2005; **294**: 342–350.

80 Ristikankare A, Kuitunen T, Kuitunen A, Uotila L, Vento A, Suojaranta-Ylinen R *et al.* Lack of renoprotective effect of iv N-acetylcysteine in patients with chronic renal failure undergoing cardiac surgery. *Br J Anaesth* 2006; **97**: 611–616.

81 Hynninen MS, Nieni TT, Poyhia R, Raininko EI, Salmenera MT, Lepantalo MJ *et al.* N-acetylcysteine for the prevention of kidney injury in abdominal aortic surgery: a randomized, double-blind, placebo-controlled trial. *Anesth Analg* 2006; **102**: 1638–1645.

82 Macedo E, Abdulkader R, Castro I, Sobrinho ACC, Yu L, Vieira JM. Lack of protection of N-acetylcysteine (NAC) in acute renal failure related to elective aortic aneurysm repair; a randomized controlled trial. *Nephrol Dial Transplant* 2006; **21**: 1863–1869.

83 Haase M, Haase-Fielitz A, Bagshaw SM, Reade MC, Morgera S, Seevenayagam S *et al.* Phase II, randomized, controlled trial of high-dose N-acetylcysteine in high-risk cardiac surgery patients. *Crit Care Med* 2007; **35**: 1324–1331.

84 El-Hamamsy IE, Stevens LM, Carrier M, Pellerin M, Bouchard D, Demers P *et al.* Effects of intravenous N-acetylcysteine on outcomes after coronary artery bypass surgery: a randomized, double-blind, placebo controlled clinical trial. *J Thorac Cardiovasc Surg* 2007; **133**: 7–12.

85 Pannu, N, Mehta RL. Mechanical ventilation and renal function: an area for concern? *Am J Kidney Dis* 2002; **39**: 616–624.

86 Ramamoorthy C, Rooney M, Dries DJ, Mathru M. Aggressive hydration during continuous positive pressure ventilation restores atrial

transmural pressure, plasma atrial natriuretic peptide concentrations, and renal function. *Crit Care Med* 1992; **20**: 1014–1019.

87 Schuster HP, Suter PM, Hemmer M, *et al.* Fenoldopam improves renal dysfunction secondary to ventilation with PEEP. *Intensivmedizin* 1991; **28**: 348–355.

88 Poinsot O, Romand JA, Favre H, Suter PM. Fenoldopam improves renal hemodynamics impaired by positive pressure. *Anesthesiology* 1993; **79**: 680–684.

89 ARDSNet: ventilation with lower tidal volumes as compared with traditional tidal volumes for acute lung injury and the acute respiratory distress syndrome. *N Engl J Med* 2000; **342**: 1301–1308.

90 Ranieri VM, Suter P, Tortoerlla C, De Tullio R, Dayer JM, Brienza A *et al.* Effect of mechanical ventilation on inflammatory mediators in patients with acute respiratory distress syndrome: a randomized controlled trial. *JAMA* 1999; **282**: 54–61.

91 Ranieri VM, Suter PM, Slutsky AS. Mechanical ventilation as a mediator of multisystem organ failure in acute respiratory distress syndrome. *JAMA* 2000; **284**: 43–44.

92 Erley CM. Does hydration prevent radiocontrast-induced acute renal failure? *Nephrol Dial Transplant* 1999; **14**: 1064–1066.

93 Kramer BK, Preuner J, Ebenburger A, Kaiser M, Bergner U, Eilles C *et al.* Lack of renal protective effect of theophylline during aortocoronary bypass surgery. *Nephrol Dial Transplant* 2002; **17**: 910–915.

94 Io-Yam PC, Murphy S, Baines M. Renal function and proteinuria after cardiopulmonary bypass; the effects of temperature and mannitol. *Anesth Analg* 1994; **78**: 842–847.

95 Beall AC, Holman MR, Morris GC. Mannitol-induced osmotic diuresis during vascular surgery. *Arch Surg* 1963; **86**: 34–42.

96 Gubern JM, Sancho JJ, Simo J. A randomized trial on the effect of mannitol on postoperative renal function in patients with obstructive jaundice. *Surgery* 1988; **103**: 39–44.

97 Kleinknecht D, Ganeval D, Gonzalez-Duque LA, Fermanian J. Furosemide in acute oliguric renal failure. A controlled trial. *Nephron* 1976; **17(1)**: 51–58.

98 Cantorivch F, Rangoonwala B, Lorenz H, Verho M, Esnault VLM. High dose furesomide for established ARF: a prospective, randomized, double-blind, placebo controlled, multicenter trial. *Am J Kidney Dis* 2004; **44(3)**: 402–409.

99 Uchino S, Doig GS, Bellomo R, Morimatsu H, Morgera S, Schetz M *et al.* Diuretics and mortality in acute renal failure. *Crit Care Med* 2004; **32(8)**: 1669–1677.

100 Kellum JA, Decker JM. Use of dopamine in acute renal failure: a meta-analysis. *Crit Care Med* 2001; **29(8)**: 1526–1531.

101 Stone GW, McCullough PA, Tumlin JA, Lepor NE, Madyoon H, Wang A *et al.* Fenoldopam mesylate for the prevention of contrast-induced nephropathy: a randomized controlled trial. *JAMA* 2003; **290**: 2284–2291.

102 Brienza N, Malcangi V, Dalfino L, Trerotoli P, Guagliardi C, Bortone D *et al.* A comparison between fenoldopam and low-dose dopamine in early renal dysfunction in critically ill patients. *Crit Care Med* 2006; **34(3)**: 707–714.

103 Tumlin JA, Finkel KW, Murray PT, Samuels J, Cotsonis G, Shaw AD. Fenoldopam mesylate in early acute tubular necrosis: a randomized, double-blind, placebo-controlled clinical trial. *Am J Kidney Dis* 2005; **46(1)**: 26–34.

104 Weidmann P, Hasler L, Gnadinger MP, Lang RE, Uehlinger DE, Shaw S *et al.* Blood levels and renal effects of atrial natriuretic peptide in normal man. *J Clin Invest* 1986; **77(3)**: 734–742.

105 Kurnik BRC, Allgren RL, Genter FC, Solomon RJ, Bates ER, Weisberg LS. Prospective study of atrial natriuretic peptide for the prevention of radiocontrast-induced nephropathy. *Am J Kidney Dis* 1998; **31(4)**: 674–680.

106 Sward K, Valsson F, Odencrants P, Samuelsson O, Ricksten SE. Recombinant human atrial natriuretic peptide in ischemic acute renal failure: a randomized placebo-controlled trial. *Crit Care Med* 2004; **32(6)**: 1310–1315.

107 Allgren RL, Marbury TC, Rahman SN, Weisberg LS, Fenves AZ, Lafayette RA *et al.* Anaritide in acute tubular necrosis. *N Engl J Med* 1997; **336(12)**: 828–834.

108 Lewis J, Salem MM, Chertow GM, Weisberg LS, McGrew F, Marbury TC *et al.* Atrial natriuretic factor in oliguric acute renal failure. *Am J Kidney Dis* 2000; **36(4)**: 767–774.

109 Sackner-Bernstein JD, Skopicki HA, Aaronson KD. Risk of worsening renal function with nesiritide in patients with acutely decompensated heart failure. *Circulation* 2005; **111**: 1487–1491.

110 Sackner-Bernstein JD, Kowalski M, Fox M, Aaronson K. Short-term risk of death after treatment with nesiritide for decompensated heart failure. A pooled analysis of randomized controlled trials. *JAMA* 2005; **293**: 1900–1905.

111 Nigam S, Lieberthal W. Acute renal failure. III. The role of growth factors in the process of renal regeneration and repair. *Am J Physiol Renal Physiol* 2000; **279**: F3–F11.

112 Hirschberg R, Kopple J, Lipsett P, Benjamin E, Minei J, Albertson T *et al.* Multicenter clinical trial of recombinant human insulin-like growth factor I in patients with acute renal failure. *Kidney Int* 1999; **55**: 2423–2432.

113 Hladunewich MA, Corrigan G, Derby GC, Ramaswamy D, Kambham N, Scandling JD *et al.* A randomized, placebo controlled trial of IGF-1 for delayed graft function: a human model to study postischemic ARF. *Kidney Int* 2003; **64**: 593–602.

10 Radiocontrast Nephropathy

Brendan J. Barrett & Patrick S. Parfrey

Division of Nephrology and Clinical Epidemiology Unit, Faculty of Medicine, Memorial University of Newfoundland, St. John's, Newfoundland, Canada.

Introduction

Iodinated contrast media are commonly employed to enhance aspects of radiographic images during diagnostic or interventional radiological procedures. The contrast media are injected intravascularly, into either an artery or vein. As discussed below, the route of administration and population studied may be important determinants in the potential for kidney injury and its prevention. Most of the recent literature on contrast-induced nephropathy has been in the setting of cardiac angiography and percutaneous coronary intervention. Estimates of risk, the mechanism of kidney injury, and the impact of preventive therapies may differ according to the population studied.

Definition of contrast-induced nephropathy

After exposure to intravascular iodinated contrast medium, sensitive tests of kidney function have identified mild, transient changes in most cases [1]. Clinically important injury, or contrast-induced nephropathy (CIN), is less common. There is no single satisfactory definition of CIN. CIN is often defined as an acute change in kidney function, occurring after contrast injection and in the absence of other potential causes of acute renal failure. Change in kidney function is usually recognized as a rise in serum creatinine in terms of either a fixed (e.g. 0.5 mg/dL [44 µmol/L]) or relative (e.g. 25%) change following contrast. Despite the prevailing definition, contrast solution may be a contributory rather than a sole cause of acute kidney failure. Concomitant insults may include low blood volume, surgery, atheroembolic disease, and other nephrotoxins. There is no specific diagnostic marker for CIN in humans, and these concomitant insults to the kidney may contribute indepen-

dently to a portion of the higher rate of acute renal failure seen after cardiac angiography.

The clinical importance of minor, usually transient, changes in serum creatinine is debatable. Although a 25% increase in serum creatinine following contrast exposure has been associated with prolonged hospital stay, adverse cardiac events, and higher mortality both in hospital and in the long term [2–7], these associations may be explained at least in part by comorbidities, acuity of illness, or by alternate causes of acute kidney failure, such as atheroembolism. However, the fact that interventions, such as prophylactic hemofiltration and N-acetylcysteine (NAC), have been found to reduce both the occurrence of CIN and premature death in some studies leaves open the possibility that minor acute changes in kidney function may in some way contribute to the other adverse outcomes [8–10].

Burden of disease

CIN was reported in one recent cohort study to be the third most common cause of acute renal failure in hospitalized patients [11]. In this study, contrast was assumed to be the cause of the renal failure if administered within the prior 24 h and no other major kidney insult was identified. The reported incidence of contrast nephropathy, however, varies among studies due to differences in definition, background risk, type and dose of contrast, imaging procedure, and the frequency of other potential causes of acute renal failure.

The presence or absence of background risk factors and the type of imaging procedure are the most relevant factors influencing the incidence of CIN. Preexisting renal function is a major determinant of risk for CIN [2]. In one study of patients undergoing coronary angiography, serum creatinine rose by more than 25% in 14.5% of cases (95% confidence interval [CI], 12.9–16.1), while 0.77% required dialysis [2]. Baseline estimated creatinine clearance was below 47 mL/min (0.78 mL/s) in all cases requiring dialysis, many of whom were close to end-stage kidney disease prior to angiography [2]. Registry data suggest an incidence of

Evidence-based Nephrology. Edited by Donald Molony and Jonathan Craig
© 2009 Blackwell Publishing, ISBN: 978-1-4051-3975-5.

nephropathy requiring dialysis after percutaneous intervention of 0.44% [12]. In the absence of preexisting renal disease, the incidence is much lower. In a large clinical trial, only 8% of patients whose baseline serum creatinine was below 1.5 mg/dL (135 μmol/L) had an increase in serum creatinine of more than 0.5 mg/dL, and none had a rise of more than 1 mg/dL [13]. All of the above incidence rates were derived from studies of cardiac angiography. The literature on risk following intravenous injection of modern contrast agents for routine diagnostic computed tomography, for example, is more sparse. The frequency of minor changes in serum creatinine after intravenous contrast would appear to be much lower than the frequency reported after cardiac angiography. The importance of the background level of kidney function on the incidence rate of acute change in kidney function has recently been reemphasized [14].

Risk stratification of patients

The first steps in reducing the risk for kidney injury are to identify modifiable risk factors, to estimate the magnitude of risk, and to review the indications for contrast. Table 10.1 lists the major factors that have been associated with an increased risk for CIN. Most risk factors can be detected with a routine history and physical examination. Some risk factors, like hypovolemia, can be at least partially corrected prior to administration of contrast agent. The risk for decline in kidney function after contrast rises exponentially with the number of risk factors present [4,5,22]. Validated risk prediction models, such as the one shown in Table 10.2 and

Table 10.1 Risk factors for the development of radiocontrast nephropathy.

Risk factor	Comment [references]
Preexisting kidney disease	Risk inversely related to level of kidney function [2,12]
Diabetes mellitus	Less of a factor on its own but interacts with presence of kidney disease [2,15,16]
Heart failure or reduced systolic function	Seen with NYHA class III/IV pulmonary edema or LVEF <40% [10,16,17]
Hypotension	[16,17]
Low hematocrit	[17,18]
Older age	[16,17]
High dose of contrast	"Tolerable" dose may depend on level of kidney function [12,19,20]
High-osmolality contrast	Risk only clearly shown in presence of preexisting kidney disease [13,21]
Route of administration, cardiac angiography	Higher rates of CIN reported after cardiac angiography than after i.v. exposure [13,14]

Abbreviations: NYHA, New York Heart Association; LVEF, left ventricular ejection fraction.

Table 10.2 Risk prediction scores for acute decline in kidney function following percutaneous coronary intervention.

Risk factor	Score
Systolic pressure <80 mmHg for >1 h and requiring inotropic of intra-aortic balloon pump support within 24 h of procedure	5
Use of intra-aortic balloon pump	5
Heart failure, New York Heart Association class III/IV and/or history of pulmonary edema	5
Age >75 yrs	4
Hematocrit <39% for men, <36% for women	3
Diabetes	3
Contrast media volume	1 (for each 100 ml)
Serum creatinine >1.5 mg/dL or eGFR[a] <60 mL/min/1.73m^2	4 or 2 (for eGFR 40–60) 4 (for 20–40) 6 (for <20)

Source: adapted from Mehran *et al.* [16].
[a]Formula for eGFR: $186 \times$ (serum creatinine [mg/dL])$^{-1.154} \times$ (age)$^{-0.203} \times$ (0.742 [for women]) $\times$ (1.21 [for African Americans]).

illustrated in Table 10.3, have been developed for those undergoing percutaneous coronary intervention [16].

It is not necessary to measure serum creatinine for every patient prior to contrast, but this should be done prior to intra-arterial use and in patients with a history of kidney disease, proteinuria, kidney surgery, diabetes, hypertension, or gout [23]. Patients with reduced kidney function may be more easily recognized if estimated creatinine clearance or estimated glomerular filtration rate (eGFR) is determined from the serum creatinine, using either the Cockroft-Gault [24] or MDRD [25] formula [eGFR = $186 \times$ (serum creatinine, in mg/dL)$^{-1.154} \times$ (age)$^{-0.203} \times$ (factor of 0.742 if female) $\times$ (factor of 1.21 if African American). It should be noted that the

Table 10.3 Association of total risk prediction score with specific risks related to acute decline in kidney function.

Total risk score[a]	% of patients with indicated total risk score who will:	
	Have a serum creatinine rise >25% or 0.5 mg/dL	Require dialysis
≤5	7.5	0.04
6–10	14.0	0.12
11–16	26.1	1.09
≥16	57.3	12.6

[a]The total risk score is determined by addition of the scores for each element (illustrated in Table 10.2).

Cockroft-Gault formula progressively overestimates GFR as GFR reaches lower levels whereas the MDRD formula yields an estimate corrected to a body surface area of 1.73 m^2, which may not be appropriate in judging the impact of drug exposure (e.g. contrast agent) for an individual. Alternate imaging modalities not requiring contrast should be considered in those patients with any risk factors. High-dose gadolinium chelates should not be substituted for iodinated radiocontrast medium in patients at risk for CIN, as the former have been shown to be at least as nephrotoxic as the latter medium when used in this fashion and recently have been associated with the occurrence of nephrogenic systemic fibrosis [26]. Serum creatinine should be measured again at 24–72 h postcontrast in patients at risk for CIN, but estimates of GFR should not be calculated at that time, as the estimating equations rely on kidney function being stable and are not valid when kidney function is changing acutely. Because of the risk of lactic acidosis when CIN occurs in a patient with diabetes mellitus who receives metformin, it is recommended that metformin be stopped at the time of contrast injection and held until CIN has been excluded [27,28]. The balance of risks and benefits associated with interrupting a patient's ongoing therapy with diuretics, angiotensin converting enzyme inhibitors, or angiotensin receptor blockers in patients at risk for CIN has not been thoroughly studied [29]. It is generally recommended that nonsteroidal anti-inflammatory drug therapy be interrupted, but empirical data on which to base this recommendation are lacking.

Preventive interventions

No full Cochrane reviews have been published for preventive interventions for CIN. Meta-analyses of the impact of *N*-acetylcysteine and theophylline have been published and are discussed below. A general systematic overview of the prevention of CIN has recently been published [30]. The preventive approaches discussed below generally have been evaluated in randomized clinical trials as discussed in the relevant sections.

Contrast agent
Contrast media can be classified in a number of ways, including by osmolality, viscosity, and ionicity. High-osmolality agents, such as sodium diatrizoate, have largely been abandoned because of their greater general toxicities. Studies comparing the nephrotoxicities of contrast agents are presented in Table 10.4. In a meta-analysis of comparative trials, an increase in serum creatinine of more than 0.5 mg/dL (44 µmol/L) following administration of contrast in patients with reduced kidney function was less frequent with low- as opposed to high-osmolality medium (odds ratio, 0.61; 95% CI, 0.48–0.77) [21]. In that analysis, the results for subgroups in trials examining the intervention in particular patient populations were qualitatively similar but statistically significant only for intraarterial injection of contrast and in those patients with preexisting renal impairment. Due to the small number of events, no conclusion could be reached about the need for dialysis.

More recently, trials have compared the nephrotoxicity of low-osmolal media, such as iohexol or iopamidol, to the iso-osmolal agent iodixanol. The results have not been consistent. Only one trial of patients with diabetes with renal impairment and undergoing cardiac angiography suggested a benefit with iodixanol [31]. Results of further trials are awaited. Thus, either low- or iso-osmolal medium could be used at this time for patients at risk for CIN.

The nephrotoxicity of iodinated radiocontrast agents seems to be dose related. This feature of contrast solution was not always clear from the early observational studies, because exposure to contrast was based on the volume injected (in milliliters). However, different contrast agents have different concentrations of iodine, and iodinated media are largely excreted through the kidney. It has been shown that the area under the curve as a measure of contrast exposure is closely estimated by dividing the amount (in grams) of iodine injected by the creatinine clearance [20]. The related measure, the maximum radiographic contrast dose, in milliliters, can be determined from the following formula: [(5 ml) × body weight in kilograms]/(serum creatinine in mg/dL). A value of >1.0 for the ratio of volume of contrast actually received to the calculated maximum radiographic contrast dose strongly predicts nephropathy requiring dialysis [12]. These studies support the recommendation that limiting the volume of iodinated contrast injected to the minimum required to complete the diagnostic or therapeutic procedure reduces the risk for CIN.

Fluid administration
Administration of fluids is recommended to reduce the risk of CIN. However, data to support a specific fluid regimen are lacking, and the optimal fluid regimen remains unclear. Studies evaluating prophylactic fluid therapy are summarized in Table 10.5. Three small trials compared prolonged intravenous (i.v.) fluid prophylaxis to regimens involving oral fluid with or without brief supplemental i.v. fluids administration [36,38,39]. The results were not entirely consistent, but the trend favors prolonged i.v. therapies. Isotonic saline was slightly better than 0.45% saline in a large trial of patients with well-preserved kidney function [37]. Almost all participants in these trials had received intra-arterial contrast. Based on this evidence the best recommendations at present are to ensure that patients receiving contrast are in a state of optimal volume and hydration as determined by clinical assessment. Fluid restriction prior to exposure to i.v. contrast should be limited to those cases where this is truly necessary. For cases at risk for CIN, particularly those undergoing cardiac angiography, it is recommended that fluids such as 0.9% saline be continued intravenously for at least 6 h after contrast, in the absence of data showing that a shorter duration or oral fluid supplementation is comparable.

Bicarbonate
Alkalinization of tubular fluid has been proposed to reduce the rate of CIN. The mechanism of any benefit might include reduction of pH-dependent free radical generation in the kidney. In the only reported trial to date, which involved 119 patients, 81%

Table 10.4 Trials comparing risk of CIN following exposure to contrast agents of various osmolalities.

Study [reference]	Route of contrast	Contrast agent #1	Contrast agent #2	No. of participants	Mean baseline kidney function	Outcome measure	Results, contrast #1 vs. contrast #2	95% CI or P value
Barrett 1992 [21]	i.a.	Various LOCM	Various HOCM	3000	NA	SCr increase =0.5 mg/dL at 24–72 h	OR 0.62	CI 0.0–1.3
Barrett 1992 [21]	i.v.	Various LOCM	Various HOCM	1187	NA	SCr increase =0.5 mg/dL at 24–72 h	OR 0.64	CI 0.48–0.8
Aspelin 2003 [31]	i.a.	Iodixanol	Iohexol	129	CrCl 50 mL/min	SCr increase =0.5 mg/dL by 3 days	3.1% vs. 26.1%	P = 0.002
Barrett 2006 [32]	i.v.	Iodixanol	Iopamidol	153	SCr 1.6	SCr increase =25% by 42–78 h	4% vs. 3.9%	P = NS
Cararo 1998 [33]	i.v.	Iodixanol	Iopromide	64	SCr 1.68	SCr increase =50% by 24 h	3.1% vs. 0%	P = NS
Chalmers 1999 [34]	i.a.	Iodixanol	Iohexol	102	SCr 3.1	SCr increase =25% w/in 7 days	3.7% vs. 10%	P = NS
Davidson 2000 [35]	i.a.	Iodixanol	Ioxaglate	856	NA	Nondefined renal failure requiring medication	0.5% vs. 0.5%	P = NS

Abbreviations: i.a., intra-arterial; LOCM, low-osmolality contrast medium; HOCM, high-osmolality contrast medium; NA, not available; NS, not significant.

Table 10.5 Trials of prophylactic fluid therapy for prevention of CIN.

Study [reference]	Contrast osmolality, route	Intervention regimen	Control regimen	No. of participants	Mean baseline kidney function	Outcome measure	Results, intervention vs. control	P value
Bader 2004 [36]	Low, i.v.	300 ml i.v. fluid during, 1.5–2.0 L fluid p.o. (12 h post)	2 L i.v. fluid (12 h pre/12 h post)	39	GFR 110 mL/min	Mean change in GFR by contrast clearance at 48 h	−34.6 vs. −18.3 mL/min/1.73 m²	<0.05
Mueller 2002 [37]	Low, i.a.	1 mL/kg/h i.v. 0.9% saline (24 h pre)	1 mL/kg/h i.v. 0.45% saline (24 h pre)	1383	CrCl 84 mL/min/50 kg lean mass	SCr increase =0.5 mg/dL w/in 48 h	5 pts (0.7%) vs. 14 (2%)	0.04
Taylor 1998 [38]	Multiple, i.a.	75 mL/h i.v. 0.45% saline (12 h pre/12 h post)	1 L water p.o. (>10 h pre), 300 mL/h i.v. 0.45% saline (6 h from call to lab)	36	CrCl 48 mL/min	Mean max change in SCr w/in 48 h	0.21 vs. 0.12 mg/dL	NS
Trivedi 2003 [39]	Low, i.a.	1 mL/kg/h i.v. 0.9% saline (24 h)	Unrestricted oral fluids	53	CrCl 79.6 mL/min	SCr increase =0.5 mg/dL w/in 48 h	1 pts (3.7%) vs. 9 (34.6%)	0.005
Merten 2004 [40]	Low, multiple	3 mL/kg/h (1 h pre), 1 mL/kg/h (6 h post), i.v. sodium bicarbonate 154 mmol/L	3 mL/kg/h (1 h pre), 1 mL/kg/h (6 h post) i.v. 0.9% saline	119	GFR 41–45 mL/min/1.73 m²	SCr increase =25% w/in 48 h	1 pts (1.7%) vs. 8 (13.6%)	0.02

Abbreviations: i.a., intra-arterial; p.o., per os; CrCl, creatinine clearance; NS, not significant.

of whom were undergoing cardiac angiography, isotonic sodium bicarbonate resulted in a lower frequency of a 25% increase in serum creatinine within 2 days compared to that following 0.9% saline infusion [40]. However, the trial was terminated early due to a lower than expected rate of "events" in the bicarbonate group, but the timing of the interim analysis and the stopping rules were not prespecified, and the P value for the difference in event rates was higher than generally used to prematurely terminate a trial. Additionally, visual inspection of Figure 3 from the study report raises the concern that the apparent, albeit small, benefit from bicarbonate versus saline might be due, at least in part, to a loss of one tail of the distribution of patients in the bicarbonate arm of this study. Although it may be reasonable to use a bicarbonate infusion judiciously in an effort to reduce the rate of CIN, the results of this trial require replication before bicarbonate-containing solutions can be recommended as the fluid of choice.

N-Acetylcysteine

NAC might reduce the nephrotoxicity of contrast through antioxidant and vasodilatory effects [41]. Data from trials evaluating the impact of prophylactic NAC on CIN risk are presented in Table 10.6. The results of an initial trial were dramatic, but the event rate, defined as a rise in serum creatinine of >05. mg/dL in the controls, was unexpectedly high for patients given low-dose intravenous low-osmolality contrast [62]. Subsequent trials have largely involved patients with reduced kidney function undergoing cardiac angiography. Some have shown benefit and others not; many are limited by low power and a lack of blinding. The dose of NAC employed in most trials has not been chosen based on pharmacologic principles. Two trials comparing doses of NAC suggested that higher doses may be required, especially if higher doses of contrast are being employed [10,45]. Several meta-analyses of trials of NAC have been reported. The trials included in these analyses vary, but more recent and comprehensive meta-analyses suggest some benefit with NAC (pooled odds ratio range, 0.54–0.73 for contrast nephropathy, defined variably as elevations of serum creatinine) [64–68]. However, this estimate must be interpreted with caution, given the heterogeneous results of the individual trials and the possibility of publication bias, with small negative studies underrepresented. Also, the effect of NAC on outcomes other than minor changes in serum creatinine is largely unknown. Indeed, studies in healthy volunteers have suggested that NAC might have an effect on creatinine levels unrelated to an effect on GFR [69]. However, in a recent trial involving patients undergoing primary angioplasty following myocardial infarction, NAC showed a dose-related improvement in CIN (defined as a serum creatinine rise), and there was a parallel beneficial effect on the in-hospital death rate [10].

Theophylline

Theophylline and aminophylline have the potential to reduce CIN through antagonizing adenosine-mediated vasoconstriction. These drugs have been tested in several small trials. Recent meta-analyses found that the mean rise in serum creatinine was sig-

nificantly but slightly lower at 48 h after contrast administration among those receiving active therapy than among the placebo group, but the clinical importance of this finding is not clear, and there was significant heterogeneity among studies with regard to changes in serum creatinine [70,71]. There is potential for adverse effects with theophylline, and the optimal dose for prevention of CIN has not been established. Further studies are warranted.

Other pharmacological agents

Several other interventions have been proposed to reduce the risk of CIN, but data are limited to support them. Forced diuresis with furosemide, mannitol, dopamine, or a combination of these compounds given at the time of the contrast exposure has been associated with similar or higher rates of CIN compared to prophylactic fluids alone [72–75]. Negative fluid balance might underlie some of the observed detrimental outcomes from these pharmacological interventions.

Generally small randomized trials of vasodilation with dopamine, fenoldopam, ANP, calcium channel blockers, prostaglandin E_1, or a nonselective endothelin receptor antagonist failed to show a reduction in rate of CIN compared to fluid therapy alone [75–80].

Two small studies of captopril as a prophylactic agent yielded opposite results. In the first trial serum creatinine rose by more than 0.5 mg/dL (44 μmol/L) in two (6%) patients given captopril for 3 days versus 10 (29%) given placebo ($P < 0.02$) [81]. In the second study CIN was reported to occur in five (8.3%) patients given captopril versus one (3.1%) given placebo ($P = 0.02$) [82].

Ascorbic acid as an antioxidant has been tested in a single randomized trial with patients undergoing cardiac angiography [83]. Serum creatinine rose by 25% or more than 0.5 mg/dL (44 μmol/L) within 2–5 days in 11 (9%) cases given ascorbic acid versus 23 (20%) given placebo ($P = 0.02$) [83]. However, these results are difficult to interpret, as the baseline serum creatinine level was lower in the placebo group and both groups reached a similar creatinine level postcontrast [83].

Prophylactic renal replacement therapy

Hemodialysis during or shortly after contrast has not been shown to prevent CIN [84–86]. However, in an initial trial involving patients with advanced kidney disease (mean creatinine clearance, 26 mL/min) undergoing cardiac procedures, those randomized to prophylactic hemofiltration in an intensive care unit before and after contrast had a 25% increase in serum creatinine in three (5%) cases versus 28 (50%) cases given fluid alone ($P < 0.001$) [8]. Death in hospital was also less frequent in the hemofiltration group (2 versus 14%; $P = 0.02$) [8]. These results were replicated in another trial by the same investigators, in which they further demonstrated that the effects of hemofiltration limited to the postcontrast period were not significantly different from those with saline alone [9]. The change in serum creatinine during and soon after hemofiltration is affected by creatinine removal. This biases the primary outcome of the proportion suffering a 25% increase in serum creatinine within a time unspecified by the investigators.

Table 10.6 Trials of NAC for prevention of CIN.

Study [reference]	Contrast osmolality, route	Intervention regimen (NAC dose)	Control regimen	Co-intervention(s)	No. of participants	Mean baseline SCr (mg/dL)	Definition of CIN	Results	P value
Azmus 2005 [42]	Multiple, i.a.	600 mg p.o. b.i.d. (1 day pre/1.5 days post)	Placebo	1 L 0.9% saline i.v. (pre/post)	414	1.3	Increased SCr ≥25% or 0.5 mg/dL by 48 h	7.1% vs. 8.4%	NS
Baker 2003 [43]	Iso, i.a.	150 mg/kg i.v. pre + 50 mg/kg in 0.9% saline 4 h post	1 ml/kg/h 0.9% saline (12 h pre/12 h post)	None	80	1.8	Increased SCr ≥25% at 2–4 days	5% vs. 21%	0.045
Briguori 2002 [44]	Low, i.a.	600 mg p.o. b.i.d. (1 day pre/1 day post)	0.9% saline	1 ml/kg/h 0.45% saline (12 h pre/12 h post)	183	1.5	Increased SCr ≥25% at 48 h or dialysis	6.5% vs. 11%	NS
Briguori 2004 [45]	Iso, i.a.	1200 mg p.o. b.i.d. (1 day pre/1 day post)	NAC 600 mg p.o. b.i.d. (1 day pre/1 day post)	1 ml/kg/h 0.45% saline (12 h pre/12 h post)	223	1.6	Increased SCr ≥0.5 mg/dL at 48 h or dialysis	3.5% vs. 11%	0.038
Diaz-Sandoval 2002 [46]	Low, i.a.	600 mg p.o. b.i.d. (1 dose pre/3 doses post)	Placebo	1 ml/kg/h 0.45% saline (2–12 h pre/12 h post)	54	1.6	Increased SCr ≥25% or 0.5 mg/dL at 48 h	8% vs. 45%	0.005
Drager 2004 [47]	Low, i.a.	600 mg p.o. b.i.d. (2 days pre/2 days post)	Placebo	2 ml/kg/h saline (4 h pre/4 h post)	30	1.8	None	Mean CrCl change +12.5 vs. 0.3 mL/min	0.02
Durham 2002 [48]	Low, i.a.	1200 mg p.o. (1 h pre/3 h post)	Placebo	1 ml/kg/h 0.45% saline (12 h pre/12 h post)	81	2.3	Increased SCr ≥0.5 mg/dL at 48 h	26.3% vs. 22%	NS
Efrati 2003 [49]	Low, i.a.	1 g p.o. b.i.d. (1 day pre/1 day post)	Placebo	1 ml/kg/h 0.45% saline (12 h pre/12 h post)	55	1.5	Increased SCr ≥25% w/in 1–4 days	0% vs. 6.9%	NS
Fung 2004 [50]	Low, i.a.	400 mg p.o. t.i.d. (1 day pre/1 day post)	None	10 ml/h 0.9% saline (12 h pre/12 h post) unless heart failure	91	2.3	Increased SCr ≥0.5 mg/dL or decreased eGFR at 48 h	17.4% vs. 13.3%	NS
Goldenberg 2004 [51]	Low, i.a.	600 mg p.o. t.i.d. (1 day pre/1 day post)	Placebo	1 ml/kg/h 0.45% saline (12 h pre/12 h post)	80	2.0	Increased SCr ≥0.5 mg/dL at 48 h	10% vs. 8%	NS
Gomes 2005 [52]	Low, i.a.	600 mg p.o. b.i.d. (1 day pre/1 day post)	Placebo	1 ml/kg/h 0.9% saline (12 h pre/12 h post)	156	1.3	Increased SCr ≥0.5 mg/dL at 48 h	10.4% vs. 10.1%	NS
Gulel 2005 [53]	Low, i.a.	600 mg p.o. t.i.d. (1 day pre/1 day post)	None	1 ml/kg/h 0.9% saline (12 h pre/12 h post)	50	1.7	Increased SCr ≥0.5 mg/dL at 48 h	12% vs. 8%	NS
Kay 2003 [54]	Low, i.a.	600 mg p.o. b.i.d. (1 day pre/1 day post)	Placebo	1 ml/kg/h 0.9% saline (12 h pre/6 h post)	200	1.3	Increased SCr ≥25% at 48 h	4% vs. 12%	0.03
Kotlyar 2005 [55]	Low, i.a.	300 mg i.v. (1–2 h pre and 2–4 h post) or 600 mg i.v. (1–2 h pre and 2–4 h post)	Placebo	200 mL/h 0.9% saline (2 h pre/5 h post)	65	1.8	Increased SCr ≥0.5 mg/dL at 48 h	No cases in any group	NS

Study	Contrast	NAC regimen	Control	Hydration	N	SCr	Outcome definition	Result	p
MacNeill 2003 [56]	Low, i.a.	600 mg p.o. b.i.d. (1 dose pre/1 dose 4 h post/3 doses every 12 h post)	Placebo	Inpatients: 1 ml/kg/h 0.45% saline (12 h pre); Outpatients: 2 ml/kg/h (4 h pre) + 75 mL/h 0.45% saline (12 h post)	57	1.9	Increased SCr =25%	5% vs. 32%	0.046
Marenzi 2006 [10]	Low, i.a.	600 mg i.v. + 600 mg p.o. b.i.d. (4 doses post) or 1200 mg i.v. + 1200 mg p.o. b.i.d. (4 doses post)	Placebo	1 ml/kg/h 0.9% saline (12 h post)	354	1.02 (median)	Increased SCr ≥25% w/in 72 h	15% vs. 8% vs. 33%	<0.001
Miner 2004 [57]	Low, i.a.	2000 mg p.o. b.i.d. (4000–6000 mg total)	Placebo	75 mL/h 0.45% saline (24 h from enrollment)	180	1.4	Increased SCr by ≥25% at 48–72 h	9.6% vs. 22.2%	0.04
Ochoa 2004 [58]	Multiple, i.a.	1000 mg p.o. (1 h pre/4 h post)	Placebo	150 mL/h 0.9% saline (4 h pre/6 h post)	105	2.0	Increased SCr ≥25% at 48 h	8% vs. 25%	0.051
Oldemeyer 2003 [59]	Low, i.a.	1500 mg p.o. b.i.d. for 48 h beginning evening before	Placebo	1 ml/kg/h 0.45% saline (12 h pre/12 h post)	96	1.6	Increased SCr ≥0.5 mg/dL or 25% at 24 or 48 h	8.2% vs. 6.4%	NS
Rashid 2004 [60]	Low, i.a.	1 g i.v.	Placebo	500 ml 0.9% saline (4–6 h pre/ 4–6 h post)	103	1.3	Increased SCr ≥0.5 mg/dL or 25% at 48 h	6.5% vs. 6.2%	NS
Shyu 2002 [61]	Low, i.a.	400 mg p.o. b.i.d. (1 day pre/1 day post)	Placebo	1 ml/kg/h 0.45% saline (12 h pre/23 h post)	121	2.8	Increased SCr ≥0.5 mg/dL at 48 h	3.3% vs. 24.6%	<0.001
Tepel 2000 [62]	Low, i.v.	600 mg p.o. b.i.d. (1 d aypre/1 day post)	Placebo	1 ml/kg/h 0.45% saline (12 h pre/12 h post)	104	2.5	Increased SCr ≥0.5 mg/dL at 48 h	2% vs. 21%	0.01
Webb 2004 [63]	Low, i.a.	500 mg i.v. (1 h pre)	Placebo	1.5 ml/kg/h 0.9% saline (6 h post)	487	1.6	Decreased estimated CrCl >5 mL/min	23.3% vs. 20.7%	NS

Abbreviations: i.a., intra-arterial; p.o., per os; b.i.d., two times/day; t.i.d., three times/day; NS, not significant.

Table 10.7 Recommendations to reduce risks for CIN.

1. Assess overall risk–benefit balance for the proposed contrast-requiring procedure

2. Assess kidney function prior to contrast injection by eGFR or creatinine clearance from serum creatinine in those due to have intra-arterial contrast and in those at increased risk of either preexisting reduced kidney function or with other risk factors for CIN

3. Consider whether a non-contrast-requiring procedure would provide the necessary diagnostic or therapeutic result(s)

4. Attempt to correct any modifiable risk factors prior to administration of contrast, including optimization of fluid volume status

5. Avoid use of high-osmolality contrast agents in those at risk for CIN

6. Use the lowest dose of contrast compatible with adequate completion of the diagnostic or therapeutic procedure

7. In patients at risk for CIN, where possible administer i.v. fluids, either 0.9% saline or isotonic sodium bicarbonate, beginning at least 1 h preoperative and continuing for at least 6 h post-contrast injection. The usual rate of administration is at least 1 mL/kg/h, but care is required in those at risk for fluid overload or pulmonary edema, and fluid status and balance must be clinically monitored during fluid administration.

8. Consider the use of NAC in patients at risk for CIN. The optimal dose is unclear, but doses of 1200 mg twice a day for 48 h, beginning prior to contrast injection, may be appropriate, especially if higher doses of contrast are likely to be required.

9. Consider prophylactic hemofiltration before and after contrast in patients with advanced preexisting kidney disease

10. Reassess kidney function by measurement of serum creatinine between 24 and 72 h post-contrast injection in those at risk for CIN

The mechanism of benefit, if any, to the kidney remains speculative. Marenzi *et al.* [9] suggest controlled high-volume administration as one possibility, but their protocol for hemofiltration should leave the patient in neutral, not positive, fluid balance. Alkalinization by bicarbonate in the hemofiltration replacement fluid is another possible mechanism. In both trials, hemofiltration, especially pre- and postcontrast together, was associated with reduced in-hospital cardiovascular mortality, but the mechanism by which this might occur is unclear. Given the resource implications, prophylactic hemofiltration should be considered a preventive option only for those at highest risk due to advanced kidney disease. Further studies are indicated to best define the group of patients who might benefit and the magnitude of this benefit.

Conclusions and recommendations

CIN remains a concern for patients with risk factors, including those with preexisting kidney disease, who must undergo cardiac procedures with iodinated radiocontrast. It is not clear that the same magnitude of risk applies to patients undergoing other radiocontrast-requiring procedures, particularly computer tomography with i.v. contrast. Data on risk from other contrast agents, such as gadolinium, in this patient population have not been as robustly assembled, and therefore evidence-based recommendations for prevention of nephrotoxicity from this second class of agents are not possible at this time.

Many different measures have been suggested to reduce the risk for CIN from iodinated contrast. Many of the trials of prophylaxis suffer from methodologic flaws. In most instances the dramatic apparent efficacy of preventive interventions was observed in initial trials with very small sample sizes and was not replicated in subsequent larger studies. Despite the limitations in the evidence base, some recommendations can be made to prevent kidney injury associated with radiocontrast agents. These are summarized in Table 10.7.

References

1 Katholi RE, Taylor GJ, McCann WP, Woods, WT, Jr., Womack KA, McCoy CD *et al.* Nephrotoxicity from contrast media: attenuation with theophylline. *Radiology* 1995; **195**: 17–22.

2 McCullough PA, Wolyn R, Rocher LL, Levin RN, O'Neill WW. Acute renal failure after coronary intervention: incidence, risk factors, and relationship to mortality. *Am J Med* 1997; **103**: 368–375.

3 Rihal CS, Textor SC, Grill DE, Berger PB, Ting HH, Best PJ *et al.* Incidence and prognostic importance of acute renal failure after percutaneous coronary intervention. *Circulation* 2002; **105**: 2259–2264.

4 Marenzi G, Lauri G, Assanelli E, Campodonico J, De Metrio M, Marana I *et al.* Contrast-induced nephropathy in patients undergoing primary angioplasty for acute myocardial infarction. *J Am Coll Cardiol* 2004; **44**: 1780–1785.

5 Bartholomew BA, Harjai KJ, Dukkipati S, Boura JA, Yerkey MW, Glazier S *et al.* Impact of nephropathy after percutaneous coronary intervention and a method for risk stratification. *Am J Cardiol* 2004; **93**: 1515–1519.

6 Dangas G, Iakovou I, Nikolsky E, Aymong ED, Mintz GS, Kipshidze NN *et al.* Contrast-induced nephropathy after percutaneous coronary interventions in relation to chronic kidney disease and hemodynamic variables. *Am J Cardiol* 2005; **95**: 13–19.

7 Abizaid AS, Clark CE, Mintz GS, Dosa S, Popma JJ, Pichard AD *et al.* Effects of dopamine and aminophylline on contrast-induced acute renal failure after coronary angioplasty in patients with preexisting renal insufficiency. *Am J Cardiol* 1999; **83**: 260–263.

8 Marenzi G, Marana I, Lauri G, Assanelli E, Grazi M, Campodonico J *et al.* The prevention of radio-contrast-agent-induced nephropathy by hemofitration. *N Engl J Med* 2003; **349**: 1333–1340.

9 Marenzi G, Lauri G, Campodonico J, Marana I, Assanelli E, De Metrio M *et al.* Comparison of two hemofiltration protocols for prevention of contrast-induced nephropathy in high-risk patients. *Am J Med* 2006; **119**(2): 155–162.

10 Marenzi G, Assanelli E, Marana I, Lauri G, Campodonico J, Grazi M et al. N-acetylcysteine and contrast-induced nephropathy in primary angioplasty. *N Engl J Med* 2006 Jun 29; **354(26)**: 2773–2782.

11 Nash K, Hafeez A, Hou S. Hospital-acquired renal insufficiency. *Am J Kidney Dis* 2002; **39**: 930–936.

12 Freeman RV, O'Donnell MO, Share D, Meengs WL, Kline-Rogers E, Clark VL et al. Nephropathy requiring dialysis after percutaneous coronary intervention and the critical role of an adjusted contrast dose. *Am J Cardiol* 2002; **90**: 1068–1073.

13 Rudnick MR, Goldfarb S, Wexler L, Ludbrook PA, Murphy MJ, Halpern EF et al. Nephrotoxicity of ionic and non-ionic contrast in 1196 patients: a randomized trial. *Kidney Int* 1995; **47**: 254–261.

14 Rao QA, Newhouse JH. Risk of nephropathy after intravenous administration of contrast material: a critical literature analysis. *Radiology* 2006; **239(2)**: 392–397.

15 Parfrey PS, Griffiths SM, Barrett BJ, Paul MD, Genge M, Withers J et al. Contrast material-induced renal failure in patients with diabetes mellitus, renal insufficiency, or both. A prospective controlled study. *N Engl J Med* 1989; **320(3)**: 143–149.

16 Mehran R, Aymong ED, Nikolsky E, Lasic Z, Iakovou I, Fahy M et al. A simple risk score for prediction of contrast-induced nephropathy after percutaneous coronary intervention. *J Am Coll Cardiol* 2004; **44**: 1393–1399.

17 Dangas G, Iakovou I, Nikolsky E, Aymong ED, Mintz GS, Kipshidze NN et al. Contrast-induced nephropathy after percutaneous coronary interventions in relation to chronic kidney disease and hemodynamic variables. *Am J Cardiol* 2005; **95(1)**: 13–19.

18 Nikolsky E, Mehran R, Lasic Z, Mintz GS, Lansky AJ, Na Y et al. Low hematocrit predicts contrast-induced nephropathy after percutaneous coronary interventions. *Kidney Int* 2005; **67(2)**: 706–713.

19 Cigarroa RG, Lange RA, Williams RH, Hillis LD. Dosing of contrast material to prevent contrast nephropathy in patients with renal disease. *Am J Med* 1989; **86**: 649–652.

20 Sherwin PF, Cambron R, Johnson JA, Pierro JA. Contrast dose-to-creatinine clearance ratio as a potential indicator of risk for radiocontrast-induced nephropathy: correlation of D/CrCL with area under the contrast concentration-time curve using iodixanol. *Invest Radiol* 2005; **40**: 598–603.

21 Barrett BJ, Carlisle EJ. Metaanalysis of the relative nephrotoxicity of high- and low-osmolality iodinated contrast media. *Radiology* 1993; **188**: 171–178.

22 Rich MW, Crecelius CA. Incidence, risk factors, and clinical course of acute renal insufficiency after cardiac catheterization in patients 70 years of age or older. *Arch Intern Med* 1995; **150**: 1237–1242.

23 Thomsen HS, Morcos SK, Contrast Media Safety Committee of European Society of Urogenital Radiology (ESUR). In which patients should serum creatinine be measured before iodinated contrast medium injection? *Eur Radiol* 2005; **15**: 749–754.

24 Cockroft DW, Gault MH. Prediction of creatinine clearance from serum creatinine. *Nephron* 1976; **16**: 31–41.

25 Levey AS, Bosch JP, Lewis JB, Greene T, Rogers N, Roth D. A more accurate method to estimate glomerular filtration rate from serum creatinine: a new prediction equation. Modification of Diet in Renal Disease Study Group. *Ann Intern Med* 1999; **130**: 461–470.

26 Thomsen HS, Almen T, Morcos SK, Contrast Media Safety Committee Of The European Society Of Urogenital Radiology (ESUR). Gadolinium-containing contrast media for radiographic examinations: a position paper. *Eur Radiol* 2002; **12(10)**: 2600–2605.

27 Thomsen HS. Guidelines for contrast media from the European Society of Urogenital Radiology. *Am J Roentgenol* 2003; **181**: 1463–1471.

28 RANZCR Guidelines for metformin hydrochloride and intravascular contrast media. http://www.ranzcr.edu.au/collegegroups/reference/EBM /mhicm_guidelines.cfm. Accessed 29 June 2006.

29 Erley C. Concomitant drugs with exposure to contrast media. *Kidney Int Suppl* 2006; **(100)**: S20–S24.

30 Pannu N, Wiebe N, Tonelli M, Alberta Kidney Disease Network. Prophylaxis strategies for contrast-induced nephropathy. *JAMA* 2006; **295(23)**: 2765–2779.

31 Aspelin P, Aubry P, Fransson SG, Strasser R, Willenbrock R, Berg KJ et al. Nephrotoxic effects in high-risk patients undergoing angiography. *N Engl J Med* 2003; **348**: 491–499.

32 Barrett BJ, Katzberg RW, Thomsen HS, Chen N, Sahani D, Soulez G et al. Contrast-induced nephropathy in patients with chronic kidney disease undergoing computed tomography: a double blind comparison of iodixanol and iopamidol. *Invest Radiol* 2006; **41**: 815–821.

33 Carraro M, Malalan F, Antonine R, Stacul F, Cova M, Petz S et al. Effects of a dimeric vs a monomeric non-ionic contrast medium on renal function in patients with mild to moderate real insufficiency: a double-blind, randomized clinical trial. *Eur Radiol* 1998; **8**: 144–147.

34 Chalmers N, Jackson RW. Comparison of iodixanol and iohexol in renal impairment. *Br J Radiol* 1999; **72**: 701–703.

35 Davidson CJ, Laskey WK, Hermiller JB, Harrison JK, Matthai W, Jr., Vlietstra RW et al. Randomized trial of contrast media utilization for high risk PTCA. *Circulation* 2000; **101**: 2172–2177.

36 Bader BD, Berger ED, Heede MB, Silberbauer I, Duda S, Risler T et al. What is the best hydration regimen to prevent contrast media-induced nephrotoxicity? *Clin Nephrol* 2004; **62**: 1–7.

37 Mueller C, Buettner HJ, Petersen J, Perruchoud AP, Eriksson U, Marsch S et al. Prevention of contrast media-associated nephropathy. Randomized comparison of 2 hydration regimens in 1620 patients undergoing coronary angioplasty. *Arch Intern Med* 2002; **162**: 329–336.

38 Taylor AJ, Hotchkiss D, Morse RW, McCabe J. PREPARED: preparation for angiography in renal dysfunction, a randomized trial of inpatient vs outpatient hydration protocols for cardiac catheterization in mild-to-moderate renal dysfunction. *Chest* 1998; **114**: 1570–1574.

39 Trivedi HS, Moore H, Nasr S, Aggarwal A, Agrawal A, Goel P et al. A randomized prospective trial to assess the role of saline hydration on the development of contrast nephrotoxicity. *Nephron Clin Pract* 2003; **93**: c29–c34.

40 Merten GJ, Burgess WP, Gray LV, Holleman JH, Roush TS, Kowalchuk GJ et al. Prevention of contrast-induced nephropathy with sodium bicarbonate: a randomized controlled trial. *JAMA* 2004; **291**: 2328–2334.

41 Fishbane S, Durham JH, Marzo K, Rudnick M. N-acetylcysteine in the prevention of radio-contrast-induced nephropathy. *J Am Soc Nephrol* 2004; **15**: 251–260.

42 Azmus AD, Gottschall C, Manica A, Manica J, Duro K, Frey M et al. Effectiveness of acetylcysteine in prevention of contrast nephropathy. *J Invasive Cardiol* 2005; **17(2)**: 80–84.

43 Baker CS, Wragg A, Kumar S, De Palma R, Baker LR, Knight CJ. A rapid protocol for the prevention of contrast-induced renal dysfunction: the RAPPID study. *J Am Coll Cardiol* 2003; **41**: 2114–2118.

44 Briguori C, Manganelli F, Scarpato P, Elia PP, Golia B, Riviezzo G et al. Acetylcysteine and contrast agent-associated nephrotoxicity. *J Am Coll Cardiol* 2002; **40**: 298–303.

45 Briguori C, Colombo A, Violante A, Balestrieri P, Manganelli F, Paolo Elia P et al. Standard vs double dose of N-acetylcysteine to prevent

contrast agent associated nephrotoxicity. *Eur Heart J* 2004; **25**: 206–211.

46 Diaz-Sandoval LJ, Kosowsky BD, Losordo DW. Acetylcysteine to prevent angiography-related renal tissue injury (the APART trial). *Am J Cardiol* 2002; **89**: 356–358.

47 Drager LF, Andrade L, Barros de Toledo JF, Laurindo FR, Machado Cesar LA, Seguro AC. Renal effects of N-acetylcysteine in patients at risk for contrast nephropathy: decrease in oxidant stress-mediated renal tubular injury. *Nephrol Dial Transplant* 2004; **19**: 1803–1807.

48 Durham JD, Caputo C, Dokko J, Zaharakis T, Pahlavan M, Keltz J *et al.* A randomized controlled trial of N-acetylcysteine to prevent contrast nephropathy in cardiac angiography. *Kidney Int* 2002; **62**: 2202–2207.

49 Efrati S, Dishy V, Averbukh M, Blatt A, Krakover R, Weisgarten J *et al.* The effect of N-acetylcysteine on renal function, nitric oxide, and oxidative stress after angiography. *Kidney Int* 2003; **64**: 2182–2187.

50 Fung JW, Szeto CC, Chan WW, Kum LC, Chan AK, Wong JT *et al.* Effect of N-acetylcysteine for prevention of contrast nephropathy in patients with moderate to severe renal insufficiency: a randomized trial. *Am J Kidney Dis* 2004; **43**: 801–808.

51 Goldenberg I, Shechter M, Matetzky S, Jonas M, Adam M, Pres H *et al.* Oral acetylcysteine as an adjunct to saline hydration for the prevention of contrast-induced nephropathy following coronary angiography. A randomized controlled trial and review of the current literature. *Eur Heart J* 2004; **25**: 212–218.

52 Gomes VO, Poli de Figueredo CE, Caramori P, Lasevitch R, Bodanese LC, Araujo A *et al.* N-acetylcysteine does not prevent contrast induced nephropathy after cardiac catheterisation with an ionic low osmolality contrast medium: a multicentre clinical trial. *Heart* 2005; **91**: 774–778.

53 Gulel O, Keles T, Eraslan H, Aydogdu S, Diker E, Ulusoy V. Prophylactic acetylcysteine usage for prevention of contrast nephropathy after coronary angiography. *J Cardiovasc Pharmacol* 2005; **46**: 464–467.

54 Kay J, Chow WH, Chan TM, Lo SK, Kwok OH, Yip A *et al.* Acetylcysteine for prevention of acute deterioration of renal function following elective coronary angiography and intervention: a randomized controlled trial. *JAMA* 2003; **289**: 553–558.

55 Kotlyar E, Keogh AM, Thavapalachandran S, Allada CS, Sharp J, Dias L *et al.* Prehydration alone is sufficient to prevent contrast-induced nephropathy after day-only angiography procedures—a randomised controlled trial. *Heart Lung Circ* 2005; **14**: 245–251.

56 MacNeill BD, Harding SA, Bazari H, Patton KK, Colon-Hernandez P, DeJoseph D *et al.* Prophylaxis of contrast-induced nephropathy in patients undergoing coronary angiography. *Catheter Cardiovasc Interv* 2003; **60**: 458–461.

57 Miner SE, Dzavik V, Nguyen-Ho P, Richardson R, Mitchell J, Atchison D *et al.* N-acetylcysteine reduces contrast-associated nephropathy but not clinical events during long-term follow-up. *Am Heart J* 2004; **148**: 690–695.

58 Ochoa A, Pellizzon G, Addala S, Grines C, Isayenko Y, Boura J *et al.* Abbreviated dosing of N-acetylcysteine prevents contrast-induced nephropathy after elective and urgent coronary angiography and intervention. *J Interv Cardiol* 2004; **17**: 159–165.

59 Oldemeyer JB, Biddle WP, Wurdeman RL, Mooss AN, Cichowski E, Hilleman DE. Acetylcysteine in the prevention of contrast-induced nephropathy after coronary angiography. *Am Heart J* 2003; **146**: E23.

60 Rashid ST, Salman M, Myint F, Baker DM, Agarwal S, Sweny P *et al.* Prevention of contrast-induced nephropathy in vascular patients un-

dergoing angiography: a randomized controlled trial of intravenous N-acetylcysteine. *J Vasc Surg* 2004; **40**: 1136–1141.

61 Shyu KG, Cheng JJ, Kuan P. Acetylcysteine protects against acute renal damage in patients with abnormal renal function undergoing a coronary procedure. *J Am Coll Cardiol* 2002; **40**: 1383–1388.

62 Tepel M, van der Giet M, Schwarzfeld C, Laufer U, Liermann D, Zidek W. Prevention of radiographic contrast-agent-induced reductions in renal function by acetylcysteine. *N Engl J Med* 2000; **343**: 180–184.

63 Webb JG, Pate GE, Humphries KH, Buller CE, Shalansky S, Al Shamari A *et al.* A randomized controlled trial of intravenous N-acetylcysteine for the prevention of contrast-induced nephropathy after cardiac catheterization: lack of effect. *Am Heart J* 2004; **148**: 422–429.

64 Kshirsagar AV, Poole C, Mottl A, Shoham D, Franceschini N, Tudor G *et al.* N-acetylcysteine for the prevention of radio-contrast induced nephropathy: a meta-analysis of prospective controlled trials. *J Am Soc Nephrol* 2004; **15**: 761–769.

65 Pannu N, Manns B, Lee H, Tonelli M. Systematic review of the impact of N-acetylcysteine on contrast nephropathy. *Kidney Int* 2004; **65**: 1266–1274.

66 Bagshaw SM, Ghali WA. Acetylcysteine for prevention of contrast-induced nephropathy after intravascular angiography: a systematic review and meta-analysis. *BMC Med* 2004; **2**: 38.

67 Nallamothu BK, Shojania KG, Saint S, Hofer TP, Humes HD, Moscucci M *et al.* Is acetylcysteine effective in preventing contrast-related nephropathy? A meta-analysis. *Am J Med* 2004; **117**: 938–947.

68 Duong MH, MacKenzie TA, Malenka DJ. N-acetylcysteine prophylaxis significantly reduces the risk of radio-contrast-induced nephropathy: comprehensive meta-analysis. *Catheter Cardiovasc Interv* 2005; **64(4)**: 471–479.

69 Hoffmann U, Fischereder M, Kruger B, Drobnik W, Kramer BK. The value of *N*-acetylcysteine in the prevention of radio-contrast agent-induced nephropathy seems questionable. *J Am Soc Nephrol* 2004; **15**: 407–410.

70 Bagshaw SM, Ghali WA. Theophylline for prevention of contrast-induced nephropathy. *Arch Int Med* 2005; **165**: 1087–1093.

71 Ix JH, McCulloch CE, Chertow GM. Theophylline for the prevention of radiocontrast nephropathy: a meta-analysis. *Nephrol Dial Transplant* 2004; **19(11)**: 2747–2753.

72 Weinstein J-M, Heyman S, Brezis M. Potential deleterious effect of furosemide in radiocontrast nephropathy. *Nephron* 1992; **62**: 413–415.

73 Solomon R, Werner C, Mann D, D'Elia J, Silva P. Effects of saline, mannitol, and furosemide on acute decreases in renal function induced by radiocontrast agents. *N Engl J Med* 1994; **331**: 1416–1420.

74 Stevens MA, McCullough PA, Tobin KJ, Speck JP, Westveer DC, Guido-Allen DA *et al.* A prospective randomized trial of prevention measures in patients at high risk for contrast nephropathy. *J Am Coll Cardiol* 1999; **33**: 403–411.

75 Weisberg LS, Kurnik PB, Kurnik BRC. Risk of radiocontrast nephropathy in patients with and without diabetes mellitus. *Kidney Int* 1994; **45**: 259–265.

76 Kurnik BR, Allgren RL, Genter FC, Solomon RJ, Bates ER, Weisberg LS. Prospective study of atrial natriuretic peptide for the prevention of radio-contrast-induced nephropathy. *Am J Kidney Dis* 1998; **31**: 674–680.

77 Stone GW, McCullough PA, Tumlin JA, Lepor NE, Madyoon H, Murray P *et al.* Fenoldopam mesylate for the prevention of contrast-induced nephropathy: a randomized controlled trial. *JAMA* 2003; **290**: 2284–2291.

78 Wang A, Holcslaw T, Bashore TM, Freed MI, Miller D, Rudnick MR *et al.* Exacerbation of radiocontrast nephrotoxicity by endothelin receptor antagonism. *Kidney Int* 2000; **57**: 1675–1680.

79 Sketch MH, Whelton A, Schollmayer E, Koch JA, Bernink PJ, Woltering F *et al.* Prevention of contrast media-induced renal dysfunction with prostaglandin E_1: a randomized, double-blind, placebo-controlled study. *Am J Ther* 2001; **8**: 155–162.

80 Khoury Z, Schlicht JR, Como J, Karschner JK, Shapiro AP, Mook WJ *et al.* The effect of prophylactic nifedipine on renal function in patients administered contrast media. *Pharmacotherapy* 1995; **15**: 59–65.

81 Gupta RK, Kapoor A, Tewari S, Sinha N, Sharma RK. Captopril for prevention of contrast-induced nephropathy in diabetic patients: a randomised study. *Indian Heart J* 1999; **51**: 521–526.

82 Toprak O, Cirit M, Bayata S, Yesil M, Aslan SL. The effect of pre-procedural captopril on contrast-induced nephropathy in patients who underwent coronary angiography. *Anadolu Kardiyol Derg* 2003; **3(2)**: 98–103. (Article in Turkish.)

83 Spargias K, Alexopoulos E, Kyrzopoulos S, Iokovis P, Greenwood DC, Manginas A *et al.* Ascorbic acid prevents contrast-mediated nephropathy in patients with renal dysfunction undergoing coronary angiography or intervention. *Circulation* 2004; **110**: 2837–2842.

84 Frank H, Werner D, Lorusso V, Klinghammer L, Daniel WG, Kunzendorf U *et al.* Simultaneous hemodialysis during coronary angiography fails to prevent radio-contrast-induced nephropathy in chronic renal failure. *Clin Nephrol* 2003; **60**: 176–182.

85 Vogt B, Ferrari P, Schonholzer C, Marti HP, Mohaupt M, Wiederkehr M *et al.* Prophylactic hemodialysis after radiocontrast media in patients with renal insufficiency is potentially harmful. *Am J Med* 2001; **111**: 692–698.

86 Sterner G, Frennby B, Kurkus J, Nyman U. Does post-angiographic hemodialysis reduce the risk of contrast-medium nephropathy? *Scand J Urol Nephrol* 2000; **34**: 323–326.

Miscellaneous Etiologies of Acute Kidney Injury

Kamalanathan K. Sambandam & Anitha Vijayan

Washington University School of Medicine, Renal Division, St. Louis, USA

Introduction

This chapter will review some of the less frequent causes of acute kidney injury (AKI): acute interstitial nephritis, atheroembolic renal disease, renal myeloma, crystalline nephropathies, and renovascular syndromes. Due to the relative rarity of these conditions, there are few randomized controlled trials to guide management. However, several observational and retrospective studies provide some insight into the clinical features, natural histories, and therapeutic responses.

Acute interstitial nephritis

Definition, etiology, and pathogenesis

Acute interstitial nephritis (AIN) represents a hypersensitivity reaction that causes AKI by immune-mediated tubular injury with interstitial infiltration and glomerular sparing. In one large case series, AIN was the predominant finding in 2.4% of all native kidney biopsies and in 10.3% of those biopsies performed in cases of AKI. There has been a documented increase in the incidence over a 12-year period, perhaps as a result of more liberal prescribing practices and the expanding drug armamentarium [1].

The localization of inflammatory injury to the renal tubules may occur through diverse mechanisms, including molecular mimicry with tubular epitopes or deposition of immunogenic portions of the inciting agent at the renal interstitium, either alone or as a hapten [2]. Similar to other hypersensitivity reactions, it is not dose dependent, there is recrudescence in disease activity upon re-exposure to compounds with similar biochemical structure, and there is often multiorgan involvement. Cell-mediated immunity plays a major pathogenic role, as evidenced by large numbers of T cells found in the interstitial infiltrates as well as occasional gran-

uloma formation. Immune complexes or anti-tubular basement membrane antibodies are infrequently noted [3,4], suggesting that humoral immunity may also be involved.

The major causes of AIN are drugs, infections, and systemic diseases (Table 11.1). When AIN was first described by Councilman in 1898, it reportedly occurred in the context of scarlet fever and diphtheria [6], and prior to the advent of antibiotics, infections were the most common cause of AIN. However, in a recent analysis of three series totaling 128 cases from 1968 to 2001, drugs were the leading etiology (71%). Other causes included infections (16%), idiopathic (8%), tubulointerstitial nephritis with uveitis syndrome (TINU) (5%), and sarcoidosis (1%) [7]. Among drug-induced AIN, nonsteroidal anti-inflammatory drugs (NSAIDs; including salicylates and cyclooxygenase-2 [COX-2] inhibitors) and antibiotics were responsible for 44% and 33% of the cases, respectively [1,7].

Clinical features

In the 1960s, methicillin was a leading cause of AIN, with up to 17% of patients that received prolonged courses of the drug developing the disease [8]. Methicillin-induced AIN was thus considered the prototype for this disease, and AIN was viewed as having a relatively monomorphic presentation. Multiple etiologies have since been recognized with quite variable clinical features (Table 11.2). The combination of AKI, urinary symptoms (e.g. flank pain, macroscopic hematuria, or oliguria), and symptoms of hypersensitivity (e.g. rash, fever, or arthralgias) should alert the clinician to the possibility of AIN. However, signs and symptoms of hypersensitivity may not be present in up to 45% of patients with AIN (especially in cases attributable to NSAIDs), and in one series they were present in 19% of patients with drug-induced, biopsy-proven acute tubular necrosis (ATN) [17]. The temporal relationship between the initiation of a new drug and the development of renal injury may also aid in making the diagnosis. Disease manifestations develop within 3 weeks of initiation of the inciting drug in about 80% of patients, with an average latency of onset of 10 days (range, 1 day to >1 year) [2]. The duration of onset may be longer with NSAIDs, with a mean latent period of 2–3 months [9, 10]. In

Evidence-based Nephrology. Edited by Donald Molony and Jonathan Craig
© 2009 Blackwell Publishing, ISBN: 978-1-4051-3975-5.

Table 11.1 Causes of AIN.

<u>Drugs[a]</u>

Antimicrobial agents

Penicillins[b] (especially penicillin, ampicillin, and methicillin), cephalosporins, ciprofloxacin,[b] indinavir, rifampin,[b] and sulfonamides[b] (including cotrimoxazole[b])

NSAIDs, COX-2 inhibitors, salicylates

fenoprofen,[b] ibuprofen,[b] indomethacin,[b] naproxen, phenylbutazone, piroxicam,[b] tolmentin, zomepirac

Anticonvulsants

Phenytoin[b]

Diuretics

Furosemide,[b] thiazides

Gastric antisecretory drugs

Cimetidine,[b] omeprazole

Other drugs

Allopurinol,[b] phenindione[b]

<u>Infections</u>

Bacteria

Brucella spp.,[b] *Campylobacter jejuni, Corynebacterium diphtheriae, Chlamydia* spp., *Escherichia coli, Legionella* spp., *L. interrogans, Mycobacterium tuberculosis,*[b] *Mycoplasma pneumoniae, Rickettsia* spp., *Salmonella* spp.,[b] *Staphylococcus* spp., *Streptococcus* spp., *Yersinia pseudotuberculosis*

Viruses

Cytomegalovirus, Epstein-Barr virus,[b] hantaviruses, hepatitis B virus, human immunodefficiency virus, herpes simplex virus, measles virus, polyomaviruses

Parasites

Leishmania donovani, Toxoplasma gondii[b]

<u>Systemic diseases</u>

Light chain gammopathy, sarcoidosis,[b] Sjogren's syndrome,[b] systemic lupus erythematosus, tubulointerstitial nephritis and uveitis sydrome,[b] Wegener's and other vasculitides

<u>Other causes</u>

Wasp sting, Chinese herbs, idiopathic[b]

Source: Johnson & Feehally [5].
[a] Due to the fact that a very large number of drugs have been associated with AIN, only drug classes and the most common individual offending medicines are listed here.
[b] Agent that may be associated with granulomatous interstitial nephritis

AIN related to infection or systemic diseases, the clinical features of the inciting disease usually predominate.

Laboratory findings

Hematuria and/or sterile pyuria are often present but are non-specific findings. The presence of white blood cell (WBC) casts is more specific, although they can also be seen in pyelonephritis and certain proliferative glomerulonephritides. Eosinophiluria (urine eosinophils numbering >1% of the urine WBC count) can be seen, usually detected more reliably with Hansel's stain than with Wright's stain [18,19]. However, by combining the data from three series, the presence of eosinophiluria using Hansel's stain has a positive predictive value of only 62% and sensitivity of 62%, even when considering only cases with AKI [18,19,20]. Though the negative predictive value is high (92%), this is not much greater than the combined prevalence of the other non-AIN causes of AKI in these studies (82%). The diagnostic value of eosinophiluria might be improved if other causes of eosinophiluria, such as urinary tract infection (28% prevalence of eosinophiluria) and atheroembolic disease (up to 88% prevalence), are excluded [2,21].

Other laboratory abnormalities that may be present in AIN include renal tubular acidosis, a concentrating defect, or elements of a Fanconi's syndrome. Mild proteinuria is common, but sometimes it may be in the nephrotic range. Though heavy proteinuria has been reported with AIN from various drugs, it is classically associated with NSAIDs. Minimal change glomerulopathy with nephrotic syndrome is present in approximately 38% of AIN cases from NSAIDs [9]. Signs of multiorgan dysfunction, such as elevated transaminases and hemolysis, are occasionally seen. Lymphocyte stimulation testing can confirm hypersensitivity to the culprit medication if several drug exposures, each with a potential for causing AIN, have occurred [22]. Renal imaging often reveals normal to large kidneys with increased echogenicity.

Renal biopsy is the gold standard for the definitive diagnosis of AIN. A cellular infiltrate consisting mostly of T cells and macrophages with edema increases the separation of tubules from

Table 11.2 Causes of AIN and characteristic clinical and laboratory features.

Inciting agent [reference(s)]	Clinical features	Laboratory findings	Clinical course
All drugs other than methicillin [2,5,9]	• Fever (45%) • Rash (42%) • Arthralgia (12%) • Flank pain (45%) • Oliguria (40%) • Macroscopic hematuria (17%) • New or worsened hypertension (20%)	• Hematuria (53%) • Pyuria (50%) • Mild proteinuria (58%) • Eosinophilia (40%)	• Mean 10-day exposure prior to onset • Temporary dialysis required in 32–50% • CKD remains in 36–40%

Methicillin [2,5]	• **Hypersensitivity symptoms common:**
	  • **Fever** (85%)
	  • Rash (25%)
	  • Arthralgias (10%)
	• Oliguria (25%)
	• **Macroscopic hematuria** (80%)
		• Hematuria (90%)
		• Pyuria (95%, often w/ WBC casts)
		• Mild proteinuria (80%)
		• **Eosinophilia** (80%)
		• **Eosinophiluria** (almost all patients)
			• Mean duration of impaired renal function, 1.5 mos
			• Temporary dialysis required in 17%
			• **CKD remains in only 10%**

NSAIDs [2,5,9,10]	• **Hypersensitivity symptoms uncommon:** • Fever, rash, or arthralgias (10%) • Macroscopic hematuria (7%) • New or worsened hypertension (17%)	• **Nephrotic-range proteinuria** (38%) • Hematuria (38%) • Pyuria (40%) • Eosinophilia (40%) • Renal biopsy may also show **minimal change disease**	• **Mean exposure 2–3 mos before presentation** • Temporary dialysis required in 20–38% • **CKD remains in 56%**
Allopurinol [11]	• **Hypersensitivity symptoms very common & robust** • Signs of vasculitis possible • **Often occurs in setting of renal insufficiency** from accumulation of the inciting metabolite, oxypurinol	• **Eosinophilia** fairly common • **Hepatitis** common • Renal biopsy may reveal **immune complex deposition at TBM**	• **Mortality may be as high as 25%** • Rate of renal recovery unknown

Rifampin [12]	• **Hypersensitivity symptoms common & robust:**
	  • Fever (45%)
	  • **Nausea or vomiting** (72%)
	  • **Abdominal pain** (40%)
	  • Rash uncommon
	• Flank pain (17%)
	• **Oligoanuria** (96%)
		• Eosinophilia (7%)
		• Coombs-positive **hemolysis** (25%)
		• **Thrombocytopenia** (50%)
		• **Hemoglobinuria** (17%)
		• Hepatitis (25%)
		• **Antirifampin antibodies** (almost all patients)
		• Renal biopsy rarely shows immune complex deposition at TBM
			• **Usually occurs 24 h after dose** with current intermittent dosing or after previous continuous exposure (up to 1 yr prior)
			• Dialysis required in almost all cases
			• **CKD remains in only 3%**

Leptospiral nephropathy [13]	• Preceding **exposure to animal excrement** • Fever (93%) • **Jaundice** (93%) • Hepatomegaly (76%) • Gingival/GI **bleeding**, purpura (79%) • Macroscopic hematuria (26%) • **Conjunctival suffusion** (12%) • Altered mental status (50%) • Hypotension (62%) • **Oligoanuria** (95%) • Rhabdomyolysis (62%)	• **Cholestatic hepatitis** (93%) • **Hemolytic anemia** (72%) • **Thrombocytopenia** (81%) • **Hypokalemia** (renal wasting) (38%) • **Hyponatremia** (79%) • Rhabdomyolysis (62%) • **Positive blood/urine cultures or serology** • Renal biopsy reveals inflammation predominating at proximal tubules early; interstitial hemorrhage possible	• Nephropathy occurs in 40% of cases of leptospirosis • **Mortality of 26%** • Temporary dialysis required in 74% • **Persistent tubular transport defects may remain in 29%** • CKD remains in only 10.3%

(continued)

Table 11.2 (*cont.*)

Inciting agent [reference(s)]	Clinical features	Laboratory findings	Clinical course
BK nephropathy [14]	• Usually occurs in renal allografts 1 yr after transplant in setting of **aggressive immunosuppression** • May occur in other immunosuppressed states also (e.g. HIV) • Fever uncommon • Macroscopic hematuria rare	• **"Decoy cells"** (tubular cells with enlarged nucleus, intranuclear inclusions) in urine sediment, 100% sensitivity/71% specificity • **Viremia by PCR** 100% sensitive/88% specific • Renal biopsy reveals **SV40 stain positive intranuclear inclusion bodies**	• Acute or gradual deterioration in renal function • Decreases 5-year renal allograft survival from 76 to 46% • Often **resolves with decrease in immunosuppression**
Sarcoidosis [15]	• Extrarenal symptoms of sarcoidosis predominate with **pulmonary, ocular, and skin symptoms** most common • Renal limited disease is very rare • Most often occurs in young adults • Higher incidence in black population	• Eosinophilia (25%) • **Hypercalcemia** or normocalcemia despite advanced kidney failure • **Chest radiography with hilar adenopathy** and/or infiltrates (90%) • Elevated ACE level not reliable with renal involvement • Renal biopsy reveals **noncaseating granulomas** and giant cells	• Often a remitting/relapsing course responsive to pulse increase in steroids • **CKD remains in 90%**
TINU [16]	• 3:1 female predominance • **Median age of onset, 15 yrs** • **Eye pain or redness** (32%) • Fever (53%) • Weight loss (47%) • Abdominal or flank pain (28%) • Arthralgias or myalgias (17%) • Rash (1%)	• Eosinophilia (17%) • **Elevated serum IgG** (83%) • Renal biopsy shows granulomas in 13%; unlike sarcoidosis, uveitis is not granulomatous	• Uveitis precedes renal disease in 21%, is concurrent in 15%, and follows it in 65% • **Complete renal recovery often occurs spontaneously within 1 yr** • Uveitis recurs in 54%, but recurrence of AIN is rare • CKD is rare

Abbreviations: GI, gastrointestinal; TBM, tubular basement membrane; SV40, simian virus 40; IgG, immunoglobulin G; CKD, chronic kidney disease.
Note: Particularly distinctive features are noted in bold. The percentages are estimates of the prevalence of the associated finding for each etiology.

one another, and there may be tubulitis or frank tubular necrosis in severe AIN (Figure 11.1). Neutrophils, eosinophils, and plasma cells can often also be found. Occasionally there is granulomatous inflammation, which might provide clues as to the offending agent, since this is associated with a limited list of causes (Table 11.1). Immunofluorescence and electron microscopy usually reveal no immune complexes, but tubular basement membrane deposition can rarely be seen. Glomeruli are usually normal, but electron microscopy may reveal foot process effacement in NSAID-associated AIN. A summary of the relevant laboratory findings is given in Table 11.2.

Course and treatment
Given the polymorphic nature of the disease and the multiple potential causative agents, AIN does not have a uniform course or response to treatment. In the prototype, methicillin-induced AIN, the prognosis was excellent, with complete recovery of renal function noted in 90% of patients after a mean period of 1.5 months after cessation of the drug exposure [2]. In nonmethicillin, drug-induced AIN, chronic kidney disease (CKD) is an expected

sequela in 36–40% of cases [2,9]. The prevalence of CKD is even higher (56%) with NSAID-induced AIN [9]. In one series consisting of seven cases of infection-associated AIN, all had complete renal recovery. However, in this case series the inciting infections were readily treatable or self-limited [9]. Indeed, the prognosis for AIN may depend on the promptness of elimination of the inciting agent, with those etiologies associated with milder symptoms and therefore delayed diagnosis (e.g. NSAIDs, chronic infections, sarcoidosis) having worse prognosis than those with more acute and dramatic presentations (e.g. methicillin, rifampin, acute bacterial or viral infections) (Table 11.2).

The heterogeneity of AIN and the lack of randomized, controlled trials have made it difficult to formulate evidence-based therapeutic strategies. Clearly, the most important therapeutic maneuver is prompt removal of the inciting agent. Although it is tempting to combat the hypersensitivity response with adjunctive corticosteroids, the usefulness of this intervention remains uncertain. Retrospective studies, including a series of 100 cases pooled from seven reports [5] and a recent series of 42 cases [1], suggest no reduction in the incidence of CKD with corticosteroids. However, it can

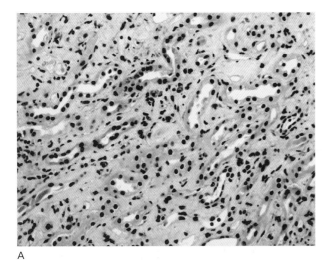

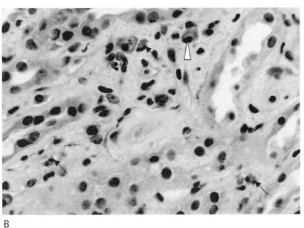

Figure 11.1 AIN, drug induced, with hematoxylin and eosin stain. Note the presence of interstitial edema and predominantly mononuclear inflammatory cells separating the normally adjacent tubules (A). A few eosinophils (arrows) and a plasma cell (arrowhead) can be seen on higher power (B). (Courtesy of Dr. Rosa Davila, Washington University School of Medicine.)

be argued that a beneficial effect is less evident because patients with more severe disease are more likely to receive corticosteroids. Indeed, in the two large negative analyses just mentioned, the patients who received corticosteroids had a tendency toward a higher peak creatinine (Cr) than the untreated group (mean peak Cr, 9.3 vs. 6.5 mg/dL [reference 5] and 8.0 vs. 6.2 mg/dL [reference 1]). Although peak serum creatinine has not been shown to correlate with prognosis [9,23,24], it is still possible that other markers of worse disease bias clinicians towards corticosteroid treatment.

The best data supporting the use of corticosteroids come from a series of 14 patients, all with methicillin-induced AIN. Corticosteroids were associated with complete renal recovery in six of eight treated patients, compared to only two of six untreated patients, and the treated group recovered more quickly (9.3 vs. 54 days) [25]. Positive observational data with corticosteroids in AIN from other etiologies exist but are limited to small case series [25,27,28]. In many reports, the most apparent effect of corticosteroids was

an association with a more rapid recovery of renal function. As for the use of other immunosuppressants, the literature is limited to rare case reports, mostly involving the more unusual causes of AIN. One recent retrospective series described the use of mycophenolate mofetil in eight cases of steroid-dependent AIN (renal function worsened with attempts at steroid withdrawal, and all patients received at least 6 months of corticosteroids). Only two of the eight cases were thought to be drug induced, with the remaining cases being idiopathic or associated with systemic diseases such as sarcoidosis or collagen vascular disease. Treatment with mycophenolate mofetil resulted in a stabilization or slight improvement in renal function (mean creatinine decreased from 2.3 to 1.6 mg/dL); however, an average of 2 years of therapy were required [29].

Given these data, a reasonable treatment strategy would be to reserve corticosteroids for patients with idiopathic AIN, systemic diseases for which corticosteroids have a proven role (e.g. sarcoidosis, Sjogren's, vasculitides), or cases with characteristics associated with worse renal prognosis. The latter includes delayed onset of renal recovery after removal of the inciting agent (>1 week), prolonged exposure to the offending agent (>2–3 weeks), preexisting CKD, and histology with intense and diffuse interstitial infiltrate, granuloma formation, or significant fibrosis and tubular atrophy [9,23,24]. A frequently used regimen is oral prednisone, 1 mg/kg, for a duration of therapy guided by the improvement in renal function, usually 3 weeks. The presence of conditions that can be exacerbated by corticosteroid therapy (e.g. slow-healing wounds, brittle diabetes, or active infection) should dissuade the clinician from this option. Furthermore, studies have suggested that corticosteroids do not alter the course of NSAID-induced AIN [1,30], but if poor prognostic factors are present, treatment can still be considered. Other immunosuppressants should be reserved for cases that are not responsive to withdrawal of the inciting agent alone when corticosteroid resistance or dependence occurs.

AKI associated with multiple myeloma

Definitions and etiology

Multiple myeloma (MM) is a malignancy of plasma cells, with an incidence of about 2–4/100,000 people. AKI has been reported as the presenting feature in 12–20% of patients with MM [31,32]. The major causes of AKI associated with MM or plasma cell dyscrasias include prerenal AKI secondary to hypercalcemia and volume depletion, AKI from glomerular disease (light chain deposition disease and amyloidosis), cast nephropathy (myeloma kidney), and drug-induced AKI (e.g. intravenous bisphosphonates). Only the latter two will be discussed in this chapter.

Cast nephropathy
Clinical features and laboratory findings

The diagnosis of cast nephropathy is suspected when patients present with rapidly declining renal function associated with the presence of free light chains detected by plasma or urine electrophoresis. There is a paucity of data regarding characteristic

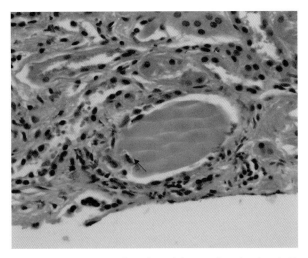

Figure 11.2 Myeloma cast nephropathy, with hematoxylin and eosin stain. Note the characteristic eosinophilic, "corrugated paper" appearance of this cast that is adherent to the wall of the tubule. There is resulting tubular cell toxicity and inflammation, with an interstitial infiltrate and cells engulfing the cast at its point of adherence (arrow). (Courtesy of Dr. Helen Liapis, Washington University School of Medicine.)

diagnostic studies, such as the fractional excretion of sodium, urinalysis, and proteinuria that distinguish cast nephropathy from other causes of AKI in patients with myeloma. The definitive diagnosis is made by kidney biopsy, but this is not routinely performed unless there are confounding factors that make the diagnosis uncertain or if the treating physician feels that it is necessary to guide therapy. On light microscopy, cast nephropathy is manifested by the presence of large lamellated eosinophilic casts in the distal convoluted and collecting tubules. Leakage of tubular contents into the interstitium can elicit an inflammatory response similar in appearance to interstitial nephritis [33] (Figure 11.2). The casts are comprised primarily of monoclonal light chains but also contain albumin, Tamm-Horsfall protein, fibrin, and polyclonal light chains.

Course and treatment

Treatment of cast nephropathy should include hydration, correction of hypercalcemia, and discontinuation of nephrotoxic medications, such as NSAIDs and angiotensin converting enzyme inhibitors (ACEi). A retrospective study revealed that patients with MM and AKI have decreased survival compared to MM patients without renal impairment (median survival of 22 vs. 47 months) [34]. However, there was no difference in survival between those with AKI requiring dialysis versus those with AKI that did not require dialysis. Thus, there are no data to suggest that dialysis should be withheld from patients with MM. Three prospective controlled trials have evaluated the role of therapeutic plasma exchange (TPE) in the treatment of cast nephropathy. The first study evaluated 29 patients with Bence-Jones proteinuria in the setting of MM and AKI [35]. All patients received corticosteroids and cytotoxic therapy, with 15 patients undergoing TPE with hemodialysis as required (group 1) and the other 14 patients all undergoing peritoneal dialysis regardless of need (group 2). Renal recovery

was noted in 13 patients in group 1, compared to only 2 patients in group 2. One-year survival was also significantly higher in group 1 (66% vs. 28%; $P < 0.01$).

The second study reported no difference in patient survival or in renal recovery in those assigned to chemotherapy plus TPE versus chemotherapy alone [36]. The third and largest study evaluated 104 patients with AKI and MM and randomized them to conventional therapy plus TPE versus conventional therapy alone [32]. There was no difference in the primary composite end point of death, dialysis, or GFR of <30 ml/min. There was a 52% reduction in dialysis dependency among survivors at 6 months in the TPE arm, but this was not statistically significant. Given the conflicting data, TPE cannot be generally recommended in the treatment of cast nephropathy, but it can be considered in patients with cast nephropathy and rapidly deteriorating renal function in order to improve renal function and decrease the risk of dialysis dependency.

AKI secondary to bisphosphonate therapy

Intravenous bisphosphonates are widely used in the treatment of hypercalcemia of malignancy. Several case reports have documented AKI and severe symptomatic hypocalcemia associated with intravenous bisphosphonate (zoledronate and pamidronate) use in MM. In a series of six patients with AKI associated with zolendronate, kidney biopsy revealed evidence of tubular injury with luminal ectasia, cytoplasmic vacuolization, hypereosinophilia, loss of brush border, and apoptosis along with interstitial inflammation and fibrosis [37]. The 2003 MM Guidelines recommend that serum creatinine should be measured prior to administration of intravenous bisphosphonates [38]. An elevation of serum creatinine by 0.5 mg/dL from baseline should trigger either a dose or schedule adjustment in the administration of bisphosphonates. Zoledronate is not recommended if serum creatinine is greater than 3 mg/dL. A recent case report also suggests that evaluation for and correction of vitamin D deficiency should be done before administration of bisphosphonates, to reduce the risk for life-threatening hypocalcemia [39].

Crystalline nephropathies

Definition, etiology, and pathogenesis

Crystalline nephropathies describe the AKI that results from the intratubular precipitation of substances. The most common cause of crystalline nephropathy is tumor lysis syndrome (TLS), which consists of acute uric acid nephropathy and acute phosphate nephropathy. Less common causes of crystalline nephropathy include calcium oxalate, acyclovir, sulfonamides, methotrexate, indinavir, and triamterene. There are also case reports associated with ciprofloxacin, foscarnet, ampicillin, and plasma cell dyscrasias.

Intratubular crystal formation and deposition of a substance is promoted by three mechanisms: high concentrations in the tubular fluid, prolonged intratubular transit time, and decreased solubility [40]. The first two mechanisms occur in the setting of decreased effective circulating volume, which is a major risk factor for all of the crystalline nephropathies. Decreased effective circulating volume results in increased proximal tubular sodium and fluid re-absorption, resulting in both a high concentration of the offending compound in the distal tubule and decreased distal flow rates. This allows the substance a longer time to precipitate out of the saturated tubular fluid and to accumulate. Underlying CKD is also a major risk factor for the crystalline nephropathies, because a larger amount of the compound is excreted per functioning nephron and drug overdosing for the level of renal function is frequent. The third mechanism, decreased solubility, is often dependent on the distal tubular fluid pH. Compounds with a pKa <7, such as uric acid, calcium oxalate, sulfonamides, methotrexate, and triamterene, tend to precipitate in acidic urine, whereas compounds with a pKa >7, such as indinavir and calcium phosphate, tend to precipitate in alkaline urine. The clinical contexts in which the more common crystalline nephropathies occur are summarized in Table 11.3. Crystalline AKI from TLS and ethylene glycol intoxication are discussed separately due to their unique pathogenic mechanisms and treatment strategies.

Clinical features

Extensive crystal deposition results in pain from distention of the renal capsule and is similar in nature to the pain due to nephrolithiasis. In certain cases (especially with indinavir and sulfonamides), macroscopic lithiasis and its characteristic presenting symptoms can exist alone or concomitantly with intratubular crystal nephropathy [47,48]. Hypocalcemia due to coprecipitation of calcium in acute phosphate nephropathy and oxalate nephropathy may result in paresthesias, lethargy, or tetany. High levels of acyclovir seen in AKI can lead to hallucinations, delirium, and myoclonus. Methotrexate can cause stroke-like symptoms (not dose related) as well as nausea, rash, and mucositis (usually dose related).

Laboratory findings

Urine sediment findings are nonspecific and will often reveal hematuria, pyuria, and mild proteinuria. Although the offending substances have unique crystal morphologies on urine microscopy, examining the sediment is not independently diagnostic. Obstructed tubules may not empty urine into the collecting system, and therefore the absence of crystals dose not exclude crystalline nephropathy. The presence of crystals does not prove their pathogenic role, because calcium oxalate, calcium phosphate, and uric acid crystalluria can very often be seen in normal individuals. Furthermore, crystalluria has been found in patients without AKI in frequencies varying from 100% of healthy individuals receiving a single 100-mg dose of triamterene and ascorbic acid (for urinary acidification) to 17% of all patients taking indinavir [47,52].

Renal ultrasound may reveal bilaterally enlarged and echogenic kidneys and can identify concomitant macroscopic lithiasis. Renal biopsy is required to make a definitive diagnosis. Light microscopy can reveal crystalline deposits (usually in the distal tubules), with a surrounding interstitial infiltrate that may contain giant cells as part of a foreign body reaction. Evidence of ATN can also be present, as many of the inciting agents display direct tubular cell toxicity. Polarized microscopy may demonstrate birefringence, depending on the offending agent (Figure 11.3). A summary of the characteristic laboratory findings is outlined in Table 3.

Course and management

In most cases of crystalline nephropathy, the renal prognosis is excellent if further exposure to the precipitating substance can be avoided. In drug-related crystalline nephropathies, recovery of renal function is expected to occur within days to weeks after cessation or even just dose reduction of the drug. An exception is the underrecognized phosphate nephropathy that may occur after the use of phosphate-containing laxatives prior to colonoscopy. Although there was likely selection bias for more severe cases, the largest series characterizing this disease found that none of 21 affected patients returned to their previous level of renal function and 4 progressed to require chronic dialysis [41].

The mainstay of prevention is avoidance of the two most frequent predisposing factors: volume depletion and drug overdosing by failing to adjust for renal dysfunction. Establishing a brisk urine output (e.g.100–150 mL/h or greater) in high-risk patients is extremely important. For substances with pKa <7 (e.g. uric acid, calcium oxalate, sulfonamides, methotrexate, triamterene) urinary alkalinization by administering intravenous isotonic bicarbonate solutions or oral citrate can be considered. Urine pH should be periodically followed to ensure an appropriate level of alkalinization. Acetazolamide may be added if a metabolic alkalosis ensues. Attempting to acidify the urine to increase the solubility of weakly basic compounds is dangerous and not recommended. These preventive strategies are based on underlying pathophysiologic mechanisms, and evidence proving reduced renal complications with these measures is lacking, except perhaps with high-dose methotrexate administration.

Treatment of established AKI consists of discontinuing the culprit agent and, if nonoliguric and not volume overloaded, applying many of the same principles used in prevention: forced diuresis (aggressive volume expansion with judicious use of diuretics) and, for weak acids, urinary alkalinization. In the setting of AKI, moderate to large doses of diuretics may be required to establish adequate urine flow, and care must be taken with bicarbonate loading to avoid profound alkalosis. Additionally, early initiation of renal replacement therapy (RRT) can rapidly decrease the concentration of some inciting agents (e.g. phosphate, oxalate, and methotrexate). Again, evidence for improvement in renal outcome with these maneuvers is lacking. See Table 11.3 for details on specific management strategies.

Tumor lysis syndrome
Pathophysiology
TLS results from the sudden release of several intracellular constituents to the extracellular space from massive tumor cell death.

Table 11.3 Causes of crystalline nephropathy, their distinctive clinical and laboratory features, and strategies for prevention and treatment.

Inciting agent [reference]	Clinical context	Laboratory findings	Prevention and treatment	Disease course
Phosphate [41]	• TLS, especially posttreatment form • Phosphasoda bowel prep with risk increased by ACEi/diuretic use, advanced age, CKD, and/or female gender • Rhabdomyolysis (rare) • Severe hemolysis (rare)	• Crystalluria with weakly birefringent, long prisms, often in rosettes • Hyperphosphatemia (peaking 1–2 days after initiation of treatment in TLS) out of proportion to renal insufficiency • Hypocalcemia • Hyperkalemia out of proportion to renal insufficiency • High LDH in TLS, rhabdomyolysis, & hemolysis • Renal biopsy: von Kossa-positive crystals	*Prevention* • Forced diuresis[b] • Non-calcium-based phosphate binders *Treatment* • Forced diuresis[b] • Non-calcium-based phosphate binders • Avoid treatment of hypocalcemia unless symptomatic or ECG changes present • Consider early initiation of RRT, especially CRRT	Incidence of CKD higher in cases caused by phosphasoda
Uric acid [42,43]	• TLS, especially spontaneous form • Rhabdomyolysis (rare) • HGPRT deficiency (rare)	• Crystalluria with brownish, strongly birefringent, rhomboid plates, rosettes, or needles • UA >15 mg/dL (peaking 2–3 days after initiation of treatment in TLS) • Urine UA/urine Cr >1 (<0.75 suggests alternative diagnosis) • Hyperkalemia out of proportion to renal insufficiency • Elevated LDH in TLS & rhabdomyolysis	*Prevention* • Forced diuresis[b] • Allopurinol or rasburicase *Treatment* • Rasburicase • RRT (if rasburicase not available)	Full renal recovery expected in the absence of other insults; higher mortality in spontaneous TLS
Oxalate [44]	• EG poisoning (9/19 in largest series developed AKI) • High-dose i.v. ascorbic acid–xylitol–sorbitol infusions (rare) • Primary hyperoxaluria (rare)	• Crystalluria with birefringent monohydrate needles or dihydrate envelope shapes appearing >4 h after EG ingestion • Hypocalcemia • In EG poisoning, osmolal gap >10 mOsm/L & detectable serum and urine EG early with subsequent development of severe anion gap acidosis • Renal biopsy: silver nitrate/rubeanic acid stain-positive crystals	*Prevention* • Forced diuresis[b] • Consider urine alkalinization • Fomepizole for high-risk EG ingestion[a] (ethanol is 2nd line) • i.v. thiamine, magnesium, and pyridoxine in alcoholic patients *Treatment* • Forced diuresis[b] • Consider urine alkalinization • Avoid treatment of hypocalcemia unless symptomatic or ECG changes present • Fomepizole (ethanol is 2nd line) if EG level >20 mg/dL • Early initiation of RRT, esp. if EG >50 mg/dL and renal insufficiency or acidosis present	• Full renal recovery occurred in 6/9 patients; dration & severity of AKI is predicted by severity of acidosis at presentation
Acyclovir [46]	• 11% develop AKI with high-dose rapid i.v. bolus • Very rare with oral acyclovir or valacyclovir	• Crystalluria with birefringent needles with occasional engulfment by WBC	*Prevention* • Forced diuresis[b] • Increase time of i.v. infusion to 1 h *Treatment* • Forced diuresis[b] • Decreasing the dose is sufficient in 40–50% of patients	Full renal recovery expected

(continued)

Table 11.3 (cont).

Inciting agent [reference]	Clinical context	Laboratory findings	Prevention and treatment	Disease course
Indinavir [47]	• 18.6% develop AKI, especially with longer treatment, smaller body size, & concurrent TMP-SMX	• Crystalluria with birefringent plates, fans, or starbursts • Isosthenuria common • CT with i.v. contrast shows wedge-shaped perfusion defects in up to 50%	*Treatment* • Forced diuresis[b] • Urologic consultation if concomitant macroscopic obstruction present (not uncommon)	AKI is easily reversible as opposed to the slowly progressive injury seen in indinavir-induced AIN
Methotrexate [48,49]	• 2–4% develop AKI with high-dose i.v. therapy; increased risk in older patients and with concomitant use of NSAID or other highly protein-bound drugs which increase free methotrexate levels	• Crystalluria with amorphous yellow casts • High serum methotrexate level • Anemia, leukopenia, or thrombocytopenia possible	*Prevention* • Forced diuresis[b] • Urinary alkalinization to pH $\geq$8 *Treatment* • Forced diuresis[b] • Urinary alkalinization to pH $\geq$8 • Leucovorin rescue $\pm$ thymidine for extrarenal toxicity until methotrexate level <0.05 μmol/L • Consider carboxypeptidase G2 (>98% fall in levels by 15 min) vs. daily 6-h high-flux hemodialysis (clears drug in 5.5 days)	Median time to renal recovery to 2–3 wks
Sulfonamides [50]	• Usually with high-dose therapy • More common with sulfadiazine (1.9–7.5% incidence in AIDS patients) • Low serum albumin may increase risk from higher free drug levels	• Crystalluria with variable shapes from shocks of wheat to spheres • Positive lignin test (orange urine upon mixing with 10% hydrochloric acid) • Densities in parenchyma and in collection system on ultrasound are common	*Treatment* • Forced diuresis[b] • Urine alkalinization to pH >7.1 • Dose reduction usually sufficient • Urologic consultation if macroscopic obstruction present (not uncommon)	Full renal recovery is prompt, sometimes within hours, but median 6 days
Triamterene [40]	• Rare; must distinguish from the much more common AIN, or AKI with concomitant NSAID use	• Crystalluria with birefringent orange casts & spheres • Hyperkalemia out of proportion to renal insufficiency	*Treatment* • Forced diuresis[b] • Urine alkalinization to pH >7.5 • May require urologic consultation for the more common triamterene stone if obstructed	Full renal recovery is expected

Abbreviations: HGPRT, hypoxanthine-guanine phosphoribosyl transferase; EG, ethylene glycol; i.v., intravenous; TMP-SMX, trimethoprim-sulfamethoxazole; LDH, lactate dehydrogenase; UA, uric acid; CT, computerized tomography; ECG, electrocardiogram; CRRT, continuous renal replacement therapy; TLS, tumor lysis syndrome.
[a]Patients at high risk for organ dysfunction in EG poisoning are those with serum EG of >20 mg/dL, or with known recent ingestion of EG with osmolal gap >10mOsm/L, OR strong suspicion of recent ingestion and 2 of the following: pH <7.3, HCO3 <20mEq/L, osmolal gap >10mOsm/L, and urinary oxalate crystals [45].
[b]Forced diuresis refers to aggressive hydration with judicious use of diuretics to achieve and maintain brisk urine flow rate.

The main risk factor is the presence of a large tumor burden with a rapid doubling time and thus exquisite response to cytolytic therapy. Most cancers associated with TLS are high-grade lymphoproliferative malignancies, with up to 6% of these patients developing this complication [51]. It has also been reported with several aggressive solid tumors, including lung and breast carcinoma. Although the disease usually arises in the setting of traditional potent chemotherapy directed against nucleic acid processing, it has also

been observed with interferon therapy, endocrine therapies such as corticosteroids or tamoxifen, and radiation therapy. Furthermore, spontaneous TLS can occur when aggressive cancers rapidly outstrip their nutrient supply.

The AKI due to TLS has historically been thought of as an acute uric acid nephropathy. Purine nucleosides are released by dying cells and are metabolized to hypoxanthine and xanthine. Xanthine oxidase converts both intermediates to uric acid. At normal

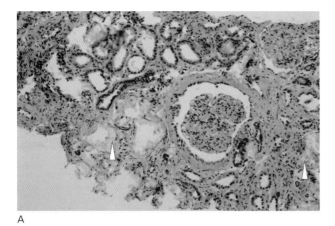

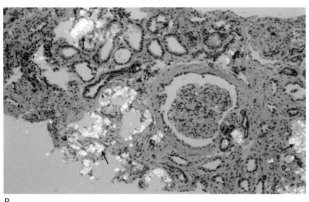

Figure 11.3 Oxalate nephropathy, shown with hematoxylin and eosin stain. This patient developed kidney failure in the setting of primary hyperoxaluria. (A) Note the distortion of the tubular architecture associated with intratubular deposits of calcium oxalate (arrowheads). There is an interstitial infiltrate along with interstitial fibrosis consistent with disease chronicity. (B) Under polarized light the deposits exhibit birefringence (black arrows). (Courtesy of Dr. Rosa Davila, Washington University School of Medicine.)

plasma pH, 98% of uric acid exists as the more-soluble ionized salt, urate (pKa 5.5). In the normally acidic tubular fluid, it exists primarily as the less-soluble, nonionized uric acid and may precipitate. Recently, it has become apparent that acute phosphate nephropathy is also an important cause of AKI in TLS, now that hypouricemic therapy is commonly employed for prophylaxis in patients at risk for TLS [51]. Significant amounts of phosphate complexed with adenosine exist in the intracellular compartment, especially in metabolically active cancer cells. Once released by cell death, phosphate precipitates in the renal tubules and other tissues as calcium phosphate. In spontaneous TLS, severe hyperphosphatemia is less likely, since the surviving tumor cells, with their high metabolic rate, rapidly recycle released phosphate.

Management

Patients at high risk for TLS, such as those with high-grade lymphoproliferative malignancies and large tumor burdens about to receive aggressive cytoreductive chemotherapy, or those with high pretreatment lactate dehydrogenase, WBC count and serum uric acid values or patients with urine uric acid/urine creatinine ratio of >1, preexisting renal insufficiency or leukemic kidney infiltration [42] should receive preventive therapy. Patients with "laboratory TLS" (modest perturbations in serum electrolytes but no symptoms or evidence of organ dysfunction) should also receive preventive measures. Volume expansion to achieve brisk urine flow and hypouricemic therapy should be initiated 2 days prior to the start of chemotherapy. Urine alkalinization is *not* recommended given the potential risk of calcium phosphate precipitation in alkaline urine. Alkalemia can also worsen hypocalcemia by increasing protein binding of free calcium. Furthermore, data from animal studies revealed no reduction in the occurrence of uric acid nephropathy with urine alkalinization [53].

Two options for hypouricemic therapy exist: allopurinol and rasburicase. Allopurinol (400–800 mg, total daily dose) competitively inhibits xanthine oxidase, thus preventing the *further* production of uric acid. Uric acid levels decrease over the subsequent 2 days with continued excretion of preformed uric acid. Rasburicase is a recombinant uricase enzyme and can convert *existing* uric acid to allantoin, which is 5–10 times more soluble in urine than uric acid. After intravenous administration (0.05–0.20 mg/kg over 30 min), uric acid levels decrease by 86% at 4 h compared to the 12% reduction with allopurinol [54]. However, comparative data between allopurinol and rasburicase regarding meaningful clinical end points, such as reductions in AKI, dialysis requirement, or death do not exist. Therefore, the extremely high cost of rasburicase deters its use in prevention unless an allopurinol allergy is present. Nevertheless, one analysis, albeit with serious limitations, estimated that the prophylactic use of rasburicase over allopurinol might be cost-effective in children with high-grade lymphoproliferative malignancies [55].

Patients with evidence of organ system dysfunction have "clinical TLS" and require therapeutic rather than preventive interventions. Most patients with resulting AKI will not require dialysis and will recover to their previous renal function, although patient and renal prognosis may be worse with spontaneous TLS. Similar to preventive methods, maintaining adequate urine flow and suppressing further rises in the serum concentration of uric acid and phosphate is essential. Previously, hemodialysis was sometimes initiated early in order to rapidly reduce uric acid levels, with a 50% reduction occurring after 6 h of hemodialysis (clearance of 70–145 mL/min) [56]. Rasburicase results in more prompt reduction of uric acid and eliminates this indication for RRT. However, when significant hyperphosphatemia is present, early RRT may still be required along with non-calcium-based phosphate binders to prevent further phosphate precipitation and/or hypocalcemia. Indeed, hypocalcemia should not be treated with intravenous calcium without first lowering the phosphorus, unless the patient is symptomatic or there is evidence of electrocardiographic changes. With intermittent hemodialysis, phosphorus clearance is fairly inefficient (50–90 mL/min) and daily or twice-daily treatments are needed to achieve negative phosphorus balance. Continuous RRT (up to 40-mL/min clearance) may be more effective at reducing phosphorus levels [57].

Ethylene glycol poisoning

Ethylene glycol is metabolized by hepatic alcohol dehydrogenase to four toxic organic compounds: glycoaldehyde, glycolic acid, glyoxylic acid, and oxalic acid. Accumulation of organic anions (glycolate, glyoxylate, and oxalate) leads to severe anion gap metabolic acidosis. These compounds, especially glycolic acid, are direct cell toxins and cause multiorgan dysfunction leading to cardiotoxicity, ATN, and nervous system depression. Oxalate precipitates with calcium in several tissues, including the renal tubules, causing crystalline nephropathy.

The clinical manifestations of ethylene glycol intoxication evolve over time as the alcohol is metabolized. During the first 30 min to 12 h, ethylene glycol causes inebriation, with progression to seizures or coma. Twelve to 36 h postingestion, peak concentrations of organic acid intermediates lead to profound acidosis, with Kussmaul's respirations and cardiopulmonary failure. Twenty-four to 72 h postingestion, the oxalate end product accumulates in tissues, resulting in AKI. This time course is prolonged in cases of ethanol co-ingestion, due to its competitive inhibition of alcohol dehydrogenase.

Treatment of ethylene glycol toxicity should be focused on decreasing the concentration of toxic metabolites. This can be achieved by 1) reducing organic acid formation through the use of competitive alcohol dehydrogenase inhibitors, such as fomepizole or ethanol, 2) increasing metabolite clearance through early initiation of RRT, and 3) conversion to less toxic metabolites by cofactor supplementation (Table 11.3).

Atheroembolic renal disease

Definition, prevalence, and pathogenesis

Atheroembolic renal disease refers to the progressive AKI that arises from occlusion of the renal microvasculature by lipid debris and subsequent inflammation. It is an underrecognized cause of renal insufficiency in the older patient population, with 4.2% of renal biopsies from patients over 65 years revealing this significant finding [58]. Clinically significant renal atheroemboli occur in <0.2% of cardiac catheterizations [59] but are more common with aortography and aortic surgeries. With the progress of invasive endovascular procedures, the incidence is likely to increase.

Most patients who develop atheroembolic renal disease have significant aortic atherosclerosis, with more severe vascular disease correlating with a higher incidence of cholesterol embolism [60]. There is usually an inciting event leading to plaque destabilization and distal showering of lipid debris, although spontaneous atheroemboli may occur in up to 21% of cases. Plaque destabilization may occur either from vascular wall trauma from vascular surgery or percutaneous endovascular procedures (which accounts for 65% of cases with an inciting event) or from anticoagulation (21% of provoked cases) [61]. Anticoagulation is thought to cause hemorrhage into plaques or prevent protective thrombus formation over ulcerated plaques. The administration of thrombolytics also can cause lipid release. The cholesterol lodges in the small arterioles and incites thrombus formation, causing distal ischemia and infarction. Within 5 days there may be recanalization of the thrombus, but an inflammatory foreign body arteritis ensues. Because the cholesterol is not soluble and it is never successfully cleared by phagocytes, inflammation persists and leads to progressive fibrosis and later obliteration of the lumen of the small vessel. With involvement of multiple arterioles, the result is persistent, patchy ischemia of several nephrons, instigating progressive renal insufficiency.

Clinical features and laboratory findings

Atheroembolic renal disease is a disease of the elderly (mean age, 66–70 years) with a male (4:1) and Caucasian (30:1 vs. African Americans) predominance. Because a significant embolic shower can occur after an unpredictable period following plaque disturbance, the time of disease onset can be quite variable: from 3 days up to 3 months after the initiating event. Other organ systems, such as the skin, gastrointestinal tract, and central nervous system, are commonly involved as well (Table 11.4). In fact, the reliance on characteristic skin findings for diagnosis (reported in 80% of cases) may contribute to the underrepresentation of this disease among the dark-skinned African American population [65]. The multisystem involvement along with the frequent occurrence of eosinophilia (48% of cases) and an elevated erythrocyte sedimentation rate mimics vasculitis. Depressed complement levels can also be seen, with reported rates varying from <15% to 66% [69,71].

Renal biopsy reveals empty clefts in arcuate and interlobular arteries and, less commonly, afferent arterioles. These result from the dissolution of lipid from these sites by the fixation process. Depending on the age of the lesion, varying degrees of arteritis and intimal fibrosis can be seen (Figure 4). In severe, acute cases there may be signs of ATN. Late in evolution, patchy glomerular sclerosis and tubular atrophy may be visualized in areas supplied by the affected vessels. Similar arteriolar inflammation or fibrosis can be found in other tissues, especially the muscle, gastrointestinal tract, and skin. Biopsy of skin lesions may have the most diagnostic yield, with a reported sensitivity of 92% [66].

Course and management

Three patterns of disease evolution are apparent in atheroembolic renal disease [61]. An acute course (35% of cases) resulting from a massive embolic load is characterized by an abrupt deterioration in renal function and multiorgan involvement 3–7 days after the inciting event. The more common, subacute course (56%) occurs after repeated smaller embolic showers or through progression

Table 11.4 Clinical findings in patients with renal atheroembolic disease and frequency of occurrence.

Clinical finding	Frequency of occurrence (%)
Signs and symptoms	
New-onset, accelerated, or labile hypertension	78
Skin findings (cyanotic or ulcerated digits or scrotum, livedo reticularis on back or lower extremities, nodules, less commonly purpura)	80
GI symptoms (nausea, abdominal pain, GI bleeding)	24
CNS symptoms (focal neurologic deficits, progressive dementia)	11
Retinal emboli (Hollenhorst plaque on fundoscopy)	19
Fevers	Uncommon
Laboratory findings [reference]	
Microscopic hematuria [62,63]	53
Mild proteinuria (rarely nephrotic associated with a secondary collapsing FSGS or accelerated hypertension) [63,64]	63
Eosinophiluria (by Hansel's stain) [21]	88
Peripheral blood eosinophilia [69]	48–88%
Hypocomplementemia [69,71]	<15–66
Various markers of ischemic organ injury (elevated creatinine kinase, amylase/lipase, transaminases)	Not uncommon
Elevated erythrocyte sedimentation rate and/or C-reactive protein	Very common
Renal artery stenosis by Doppler or angiography [61,62]	44

Abbreviations: GI, gastrointestinal; CNS, central nervous system; FSGS, focal and segmental glomerulosclerosis.

Unless otherwise indicated, frequency data come from combining 3 case series of *clinically significant* renal disease totaling 171 patients [61, 62, 63]. CK, creatine kinase; CNS, central nervous system; FSGS, focal segmental glomerular sclerosis; GI, gastrointestinal.

of the obliterative arteritis in previously involved vessels. There is a stepwise deterioration in renal function, with stabilization by 3–8 weeks. The least common chronic course (9% of cases) manifests as a slowly progressive renal insufficiency that is hard to discriminate from worsening hypertensive nephrosclerosis or ischemic renovascular disease.

Progression to dialysis dependence occurs in one-third of the patients who survive the initial insult. Preexisting CKD and a history of significant claudication confers greater risk for this outcome [62,67]. Some mild improvement in renal function can occur with time, from progressive hyperfiltration by the remaining nephrons. As a result, 21–32% of patients on chronic dialysis from

atheroembolic renal disease can recover enough renal function to stop dialysis [62,68,69].

Early studies revealed a grim outcome for patients with acute, multivisceral atheroembolic disease, with 1-year survival rates of 13–36% [63,70]. Death usually occurs from cardiac ischemia, heart failure, stroke, or gastrointestinal ischemia with malnutrition [61,63,68]. An aggressive supportive regimen specifically targeting these mechanisms of mortality was prospectively evaluated in a population with acute multivisceral atheroembolic disease [62]. Principles of therapy included the following: 1) a proscription against further anticoagulation or intravascular manipulations, even in the setting of recurrent cardiac ischemia or vascular

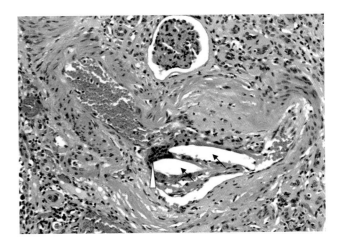

Figure 11.4 Renal atheroembolic disease, H and E stain. Cholesterol clefts remaining in an intralobular artery where lipid had been prior to the fixation process are indicated by arrows. The early inflammatory arteritis composed of eosinophils, neutrophils, and macrophages is later replaced by a giant cell foreign body reaction (arrow head), intimal proliferation, and fibrosis. (Courtesy of Dr. Helen Liapis, Washington University School of Medicine)

stents (if dialysis was required, it was performed without antico-agulation); 2) aggressive management of heart failure and blood pressure reduction to <140/80 mmHg with the stepwise use of va-sodilators (preferentially ACEi), diuretics, and then ultrafiltration; 3) aggressive nutritional support, parenterally if needed. This in-tensive support strategy resulted in a 1-year survival of 77%, a vast improvement from previous series. Interestingly, the aggressive use of ACEi in the setting of AKI was not associated with an increase in the need for dialysis and allowed eventual dialysis cessation in sev-eral patients. A similar result (1-year survival of 69%) was noted in a second uncontrolled study employing the same basic princi-ples, although there was no mention of preferential ACEi therapy [61]. Although limited, these studies represent the best data re-garding treatment, and these principles should be incorporated in the management of this disease. If the relative contraindica-tion for anticoagulation makes hemodialysis difficult, peritoneal dialysis should be considered.

Several adjunctive therapies to improve renal outcome have been attempted in cases of atheroembolic renal disease. Corticos-teroids have not been proven to affect renal outcome, but low doses (0.3 mg of prednisone/kg) might improve anorexia and abdominal pain from mesenteric involvement [62]. Statins have theoretical benefits in decreasing inflammation and stabilizing atheroscle-rotic plaques, thus potentially reducing risks of further embolic events. An observational analysis found a lower rate of statin ther-apy among those patients who eventually progressed to end-stage renal disease (4.3 vs. 30.6% in those not requiring chronic dialy-sis) [67]. Given the cardiovascular risk factors in this population, it is prudent to include statin therapy in the treatment regimen. A few case reports have shown encouraging results with vasodila-tory prostaglandins (iloprost); however, larger studies are required [72]. Regarding prevention, one study evaluated the brachial artery approach during cardiac catheterization in those with extensive aortic atherosclerotic disease. Although this did not reveal a lower incidence of cholesterol emboli, the incidence of atheroembolic disease in this analysis was likely too small to detect an effect [73]. This approach is a reasonable consideration in high-risk patients undergoing cardiac catheterization.

Renal artery and vein thromboses

Renal artery thrombosis

Acute renal artery thrombosis (RAT) is extremely rare, with only about 300 cases reported in the literature. Most of the cases are uni-lateral, and only a few cases of bilateral RAT leading to AKI have been described. The leading causes of acute RAT are blunt ab-dominal trauma (acceleration–deceleration injury) and the anti-phospholipid antibody syndrome [74,75]. Other hypercoagulable diseases, such as nephrotic syndrome (NS), have also been as-sociated with RAT. Computerized tomography with intravenous contrast of the abdomen is the diagnostic modality of choice. Treat-ment of traumatic RAT is dependent on the duration of ischemia. In one case series, surgical revascularization had a success rate (de-

fined as independence from dialysis) of 56% if the ischemia time was less than 12 h. The median ischemic time in the unsuccessful revascularizations was 48 h, and the mortality in these patients was 29% [76]. At present, there are insufficient data to recommend an evidence-based treatment plan for RAT.

Renal vein thrombosis

Renal vein thrombosis (RVT), either unilateral or bilateral, is also a rare cause of AKI. The common etiologies are NS and other hyper-coagulable states, such as anti-phospholipid antibody syndrome. Of all the causes of NS, patients with membranous glomeru-lonephritis have the highest prevalence of RVT (37%) [77]. Se-lective renal venogram is considered the gold standard for diag-nosis, but it is not routinely performed due to a high risk for contrast-induced AKI as well as vascular complications. In one se-ries, computerized tomography had a sensitivity of 92% and speci-ficity of 100%. A series investigating Doppler ultrasonography re-vealed a sensitivity of 85% and specificity of 56%, but this modality is heavily operator dependent [77]. Magnetic resonance imaging can also be used, although adequate studies have not evaluated this modality.

Treatment of RVT involves conventional anticoagulation with intravenous heparin and warfarin sodium. Use of thrombolytics in RVT has been reported, but given the risk for bleeding, their use should be considered only in patients with severe bilateral RVT with rapidly declining renal function [78]. There are insufficient data to support the use of primary prophylactic anticoagulation in patients with NS. At this time, the decision to use prophylactic anticoagulation should be made on a case-by-case basis, keeping in mind that membranous glomerulonephritis and patients with profound hypoalbuminemia (albumin less than 2 mg/dL) proba-bly have the highest risk of thromboembolism. However, once a patient has developed a thrombotic event, anticoagulation should be continued until the resolution of the NS, since the risk of recur-rence is extremely high [79]. Given these data, it would be prudent to restart anticoagulation in this select group of patients if the NS recurs.

References

1 Clarkson MR, Giblin L, O'Connell FP, O'Kelly P, Walshe JJ, Conlon P et al. Acute interstitial nephritis: clinical features and response to corti-costeroid therapy. *Nephrol Dial Transplant* 2004; **19**: 2778–2783.

2 Rossert J. Drug-induced acute interstitial nephritis. *Kidney Int* 2001; **60**: 804–817.

3 Arellano F, Sacristan JA. Allopurinol hypersensitivity syndrome: a review. *Ann Pharmacother* 1993; **27**: 337–343.

4 Mori Y, Kishimoto N, Yamahara H, Kijima Y, Nose A, Uchiyama-Tanaka Y et al. Predominant tubulointerstitial nephritis in a patient with systemic lupus nephritis. *Clin Exp Nephrol* 2005; **9**: 79–84.

5 Johnson R, Feehally J. Acute interstitial nephritis. In: *Comprehensive Clin-ical Nephrology*, 2nd edn. Mosby, Philadelphia, 2003; 769–776.

6 Councilman WT. Acute interstitial nephritis. *J Exp Med* 1898; **3**: 393.

7 Baker RJ, Pusey CD. The changing profile of acute tubulointerstitial nephritis. *Nephrol Dial Transplant* 2004; **19:** 8–11.

8 Nolan CM, Abernathy RS. Nephropathy associated with methicillin therapy: prevalence and determinants in patients with staphylococcal bacteremia. *Arch Intern Med* 1977; **137:** 997–1000.

9 Schwarz A, Krause PH, Kunzendorf U, Keller F, Distler A. The outcome of acute interstitial nephritis: risk factors for the transition from acute to chronic interstitial nephritis. *Clin Nephrol* 2000; **54:** 179–90.

10 Kleinknecht D, Landais P, Goldfarb B. Analgesic and non-steroidal anti-inflammatory drug-associated acute renal failure: a prospective collaborative study. *Clin Nephrol* 1986; **25:** 275–281.

11 Arellano F, Sacristan JA. Allopurinol hypersensitivity syndrome: a review. *Ann Pharmacother* 1993; **27:** 337–343.

12 Covic A, Goldsmith DJ, Segall L, Stoicescu C, Lungu S, Volovat C *et al.* Rifampicin-induced acute renal failure: a series of 60 patients. *Nephrol Dial Transplant* 1998; **13:** 924–929.

13 Covic A, Goldsmith DJ, Gusbeth-Tatomir P, Seica A, Covic M. A retrospective 5-year study in Moldova of acute renal failure due to leptospirosis: 58 cases and a review of the literature. *Nephrol Dial Transplant* 2003; **18:**1128–1134.

14 Hirsch HH, Knowles W, Dickenmann M, Passweg J, Klimkait T, Mihatsch MG *et al.* Prospective study of polyomavirus type BK replication and nephropathy in renal-transplant recipients. *N Engl J Med* 2002; **347:** 488–496.

15 Hannedouche T, Grateau G, Noel LH. Renal granulomatous sarcoidosis: report of six cases. *Nephrol Dial Transplant* 1990; **5:** 18–24.

16 Mandeville JT, Levinson RD, Holland GN. The tubulointerstitial nephritis and uveitis syndrome. *Surv Ophthalmol* 2001; **46:** 195–208.

17 Kleinknecht D, Landais P, Goldfarb B. Drug-associated acute renal failure. A prospective collaborative study of 81 biopsied patients. *Adv Exp Med Biol* 1987; **212:** 125–128.

18 Corwin HL, Bray RA, Haber MH. The detection and interpretation of urinary eosinophils. *Arch Pathol Lab Med* 1989; **113:** 1256–1258.

19 Nolan CR, Anger MS, Kelleher SP. Eosinophiluria: a new method of detection and definition of the clinical spectrum. *N Engl J Med* 1986; **315:** 1516–1519.

20 Ruffing KA, Hoppes P, Blend D, Cugino A, Jarjoura D, Whittier FC. Eosinophils in urine revisited. *Clin Nephrol* 1994; **41:** 163–166.

21 Wilson DM, Salazer TL, Farkouh ME. Eosinophiluria in atheroembolic renal disease. *Am J Med* 1991; **91:** 186–189.

22 Joh K, Aizawa S, Yamaguchi Y, Inomata I, Shibasaki T, Sakai O *et al.* Drug-induced hypersensitivity nephritis: lymphocyte stimulation testing and renal biopsy in 10 cases. *Am J Nephrol* 1990; **10:** 212–230.

23 Kida H, Abe T, Tomosugi N, Koshino Y, Yokoyama H, Hattori N. Prediction of the long-term outcome in acute interstitial nephritis. *Clin Nephrol* 1984; **22:** 55–60.

24 Laberke HG, Bohle A. Acute interstitial nephritis: correlation between clinical and morphological findings. *Clin Nephrol* 1980; **14:** 263–273.

25 Galpin JE, Shinaberger JH, Stanley TM, Blumenkrantz MJ, Bayer AS, Friedman GS *et al.* Acute interstitial nephritis due to methicillin. *Am J Med* 1978; **65:** 756–764.

26 Buysen JGM, Houtlhoff HJ, Krediet RT, Arisz L. Acute interstitial nephritis: a clinical and morphologic study in 27 patients. *Nephrol Dial Transplant* 1990; **5:** 94–9.

27 Handa SP. Drug-induced acute interstitial nephritis: report of 10 cases. *CMAJ* 1986; **135:** 1278–1281.

28 Laberke HG. Treatment of acute interstitial nephritis. *Klin Wochenschr* 1980; **58:** 531–532.

29 Preddie DC, Markowitz GS, Radhakrishnan J, Nickolas TL, D'Agati VD, Schwimmer JA *et al.* Mycophenolate mofetil for the treatment of interstitial nephritis. *Clin J Am Soc Nephrol* 2006; **1:** 718–722.

30 Porile JL, Bakris GL, Garella S. Acute interstitial nephritis with glomerulopathy due to nonsteroidal anti-inflammatory agents: a review of its clinical spectrum and effects of steroid therapy. *J Clin Pharmacol* 1990; **30:** 468–475.

31 Blade J, Fernandez-Llama P, Bosch F, Montoliu J, Lens XM, Montoto S *et al.* Renal failure in multiple myeloma. *Arch Intern Med* 1998; **158:** 1889–1893.

32 Clark WF, Stewart AK, Rock GA, Sternbach M, Sutton DM, Barrett BJ *et al.* Plasma exchange when myeloma presents as acute renal failure. *Ann Intern Med* 2005; **143:** 777–784.

33 Iggo N, Winearls CG, Davies DR. The development of cast nephropathy in multiple myeloma. *QJM* 1997; **90:** 635–636.

34 Sharland A, Snowdon L, Douglas EJ, Gibson J, Tiller DJ. Hemodialysis: an appropriate therapy in myeloma-induced renal failure. *Am J Kidney Dis* 1997; **30:** 786–792.

35 Zucchelli P, Pasquali S, Cagnoli L, Ferrari G. Controlled plasma exchange trial in acute renal failure due to multiple myeloma. *Kidney Int* 1988; **33:** 1175–1180.

36 Johnson WJ, Kyle RA, Pineda AA, O'Brien PC, Holley KE. Treatment of renal failure associated with multiple myeloma. Plasmapheresis, hemodialysis and chemotherapy. *Arch Intern Med* 1990; **150:** 863–869.

37 Markowitz GS, Fine PL, Stack JI, Kunis CL, Radhakrishnan J *et al.* Toxic acute tubular necrosis following treatment with zolendronate. *Kidney Int* 2003; **64:** 281–289.

38 Durie BG, Kyle RA, Belch A, Bensinger W, Blade J, Boccadoro M *et al.* Myeloma management guidelines. *Hematol J* 2003; **4:** 379–398.

39 Henley D, Kaye J, Walsh J, Cull G. Symptomatic hypocalcemia and renal impairment associated with bisphosphonates treatment in patients with multiple myeloma. *Intern Med J* 2005; **35:** 726–728.

40 Perazella MA. Crystal-induced acute renal failure. *Am J Med* 1999; **106:** 459–465.

41 Markowitz GS, Stokes MB, Rhadhakrishnan J, D'Agati VD. Acute phosphate nephropathy following oral sodium phosphate bowel purgative: and under-recognized cause of chronic renal failure. *J Am Soc Nephrol* 2005; **16:** 3389–3396.

42 Oldfield V, Perry CM. Rasburicase: a review of its use in the management of anticancer therapy-induced hyperuricaemia. *Drugs* 2006; **66:** 529–545.

43 Kelton J, Kelley WN, Holmes EW. A rapid method for the diagnosis of acute uric acid nephropathy. *Arch Intern Med* 1978; **138:** 612–615.

44 Brent J, McMartin K, Philips S, Burkhart KK, Donovan JW, Wells M *et al.* Fomepizole for the treatment of ethylene glycol poisoning. *N Engl J Med* 1999; **340:** 832–838.

45 Barceloux DG, Krenzelok EP, Olson K, Watson W. American Academy of Clinical Toxicology Practice Guidelines on the Treatment of Ethylene Glycol Poisoning. *J Toxicol Clin Toxicol* 1999; **37:** 537–560.

46 Keeney RE, Kirk LE, Bridgen D. Acyclovir tolerance in humans. *Am J Med* 1982; **73:** 176–181.

47 Boubaker K, Sudre P, Bally F, Vogel G, Meuwly JY, Glauser MP *et al.* Changes in renal function associated with indinavir. *AIDS* 1998; **12:** F249–F254.

48 Wall SM, Johansen MJ, Molony DA, DuBose TD, Jr., Jaffe N, Madden T. Effective clearance of methotrexate using high-flux hemodialysis membranes. *Am J Kidney Dis* 1996; **28:** 846–854.

49 Widemann BC, Balis FM, Kempf-Bielack B, Bielack S, Pratt CB, Ferrari S *et al.* High-dose methotrexate-induced nephrotoxicity in patients with osteosarcoma. *Cancer* 2004; **100:** 2222–2232.

50 Becker K, Jablonowski H, Haussinger D. Sulfadiazine-associated nephrotoxicity in patients with the acquired immunodeficiency syndrome. *Medicine* 1996; **75:** 185–194.

51 Hande KR. Garrow GC. Acute tumor lysis syndrome in patients with high-grade non-Hodgkin's lymphoma. *Am J Med* 1993; **94:** 133–139

52 Fairley KF, Woo KT, Birch DF, Leaker BR, Ratnaike S. Triamterene-induced crystalluria and cylinduria: clinical and experimental studies. *Clin Nephrol* 1986; **26:** 169–173.

53 Conger JD, Falk SA. Intrarenal dynamics in the pathogenesis and prevention of acute urate nephropathy. *J Clin Invest* 1977; **59:** 786–793.

54 Goldman SC, Holcenberg JS, Finkelstein JZ, Hutchinson R, Kreissman S, Johnson S *et al.* A randomized comparison between rasburicase and allopurinol in children with lymphoma or leukemia at high risk for tumor lysis. *Blood* 2001; **97:** 2998–3003.

55 Annemans L, Moeremans K, Lamotte M, Garcia Conde J, van den Berg H, Myint H *et al.* Pan-European multicentre economic evaluation of recombinant urate oxidase (rasburicase) in prevention and treatment of hyperuricaemia and tumour lysis syndrome in haematological cancer patients. *Support Care Cancer* 2003; **11:** 249–257.

56 Kjellstrand CM, Campbell DC, von Hartitzsch B,Buselmeier TJ. Hyperuricemic acute renal failure. *Arch Intern Med* 1974; **133:** 349–359.

57 Pichette V, Leblanc M, Bonnardeaux A, Ouimet D, Geadah D, Cardinal J. High dialysate flow rate continuous arteriovenous hemodialysis: a new approach for the treatment of acute renal failure and tumor lysis syndrome. *Am J Kidney Dis* 1994; **23:** 591–596.

58 Preston RA, Stemmer CL, Materson BJ, Perez-Stable E, Pardo V. Renal biopsy in patients 65 years of age or older: an analysis of the results of 334 biopsies. *J Am Geriatr Soc* 1990; **38:** 669–674.

59 Drost H, Buis B, Haan D, Hillers JA. Cholesterol embolism as a complication of left heart catheterisation. Report of seven cases. *Br Heart J* 1984; **52:** 339–342.

60 Flory CM. Arterial occlusion produced by emboli from eroded aortic atheromatous plaques. *Am J Pathol* 1945; **21:** 549–565.

61 Scolari F, Tardanico R, Zani R, Pola A, Viola BF, Movilli E *et al.* Cholesterol crystal embolism: a recognizable cause of renal disease. *Am J Kidney Dis* 2000; **36:** 1089–1109.

62 Belenfant X, Meyrier A, Jacquot C. Supportive treatment improves survival in multivisceral cholesterol crystal embolism. *Am J Kidney Dis* 1999; **33:** 840–850.

63 Thadhani RI, Camargo CA Jr, Xavier RJ, Fang LS, Bazari H. Atheroembolic renal failure after invasive procedures. Natural history based on 52 histologically proven cases. *Medicine* 1995; **74:** 350–358.

64 Greenberg A, Bastacky SI, Iqbal A, Borochovitz D, Johnson JP. Focal segmental glomerulosclerosis associated with nephrotic syndrome in cholesterol atheroembolism: clinicopathological correlations. *Am J Kidney Dis* 1997; **29:** 334–344.

65 Saklayen MG. Atheroembolic renal disease. Preferential occurrence in whites only. *Am J Nephrol* 1989; **9:** 87–88.

66 Falanga V, Fine MJ, Kapoor WN. The cutaneous manifestations of cholesterol crystal embolization. *Arch Dermatol* 1986; **122:** 1194–1198.

67 Scolari F, Ravani P, Pola P, Guerini S, Zubani R, Movilli E *et al.* Predictors of renal and patient outcomes in atheroembolic renal disease: a prospective study. *J Am Soc Nephrol* 2003; **14:** 1584–1590.

68 Lye WC, Cheah JS, Sinniah R. Renal cholesterol embolic disease: case report and review of the literature. *Am J Nephrol* 1993; **13:** 489–493.

69 Theriault J, Agharazzi M, Dumont M, Pichette V, Ouimet D, Leblanc M. Atheroembolic renal failure requiring dialysis: potential for renal recovery. *Nephron* 2003; **94:** c11–c18.

70 Dahlberg P, Frecentese D, Cogbill T. Cholesterol embolism: experience with 22 histologically proven cases. *Surgery* 1989; **105:** 737–746.

71 Cosio FG, Zager RA, Sharma HM. Atheroembolic renal disease causes hypocomplementemia. *Lancet* 1985; **ii:** 118–121.

72 Elinav E, Chajek-Shaul T, Stern M. Improvement in cholesterol emboli syndrome after iloprost therapy. *BMJ* 2002; **324:** 268–269.

73 Johnson LW, Esente P, Giambartolomei A, Grant WD, Loin M, Reger MJ *et al.* Peripheral vascular complications of coronary angioplasty by the femoral and brachial techniques. *Cathet Cardiovasc Diagn* 1996; **31:** 165–172.

74 Van der Wal MA, Wisselink W, Rauwerda JA. Traumatic bilateral renal artery thrombosis: case report and review of the literature. *Cardiovasc Surg* 2003; **11:** 537–539.

75 Rysava R, Zabka J, Peregrin JH, Tesar V, Merta M, Rychlik I. Acute renal failure due to bilateral renal artery thrombosis associated with primary antiphospholipid syndrome. *Nephrol Dial Transplant* 1998; **3:** 2645–2647.

76 Haas CA, Spirnak JP. Traumatic renal artery occlusion: a review of the literature. *Techniques Urol* 1998; **4:** 1–11.

77 Singhal R, Brimble KS. Thromboembolic complications in the nephritic syndrome: pathophysiology and clinical management. *Thromb Res* 2006; **118:** 397–407.

78 Markowitz GS, Brignol F, Burns ER, Koenigsberg M, Folkert VW. RVT treated with thrombolytic therapy: case report and brief review. *Am J Kidney Dis* 1995; **25:** 801–806.

79 Briefel GR, Manis T, Gordon DH, Nicastri AD, Friedman EA. Recurrent RVT consequent to membranous glomerulonephritis. *Clin Nephrol* 1978; **10:** 32–37.

12 Renal Replacement Therapy in Acute Kidney Injury

Steven D. Weisbord & Paul M. Palevsky

Renal Section, VA Pittsburgh Healthcare System, and Renal-Electrolyte Division, Department of Medicine, University of Pittsburgh School of Medicine, Pittsburgh, USA.

Introduction

Acute kidney injury (AKI) is a common condition in hospitalized patients and is an independent risk factor for mortality [1–6]. Interventions to prevent the development of AKI are limited to a small number of clinical settings, including pre-renal azotemia, radiocontrast nephropathy, and pigment-induced AKI. In addition, there are no effective pharmacologic interventions for the treatment of most forms of intrinsic AKI. As a result, renal replacement therapy (RRT) is the cornerstone of care in patients with severe AKI. Over the past 2 decades there has been a proliferation of modalities of RRT available for the management of AKI. Whereas the options for therapy were previously limited to intermittent hemodialysis (IHD) and peritoneal dialysis (PD), the current armamentarium also includes various modalities of continuous RRT (CRRT) and newer "hybrid" therapies, such as extended duration dialysis and sustained low-efficiency dialysis (SLED). Despite the increasing technological sophistication of RRT, key management issues, such as the optimal timing of initiation, selection of modality, and dosing of RRT, remain controversial. The clinical complexity of patients with severe AKI has made clinical trials addressing these questions particularly challenging.

This chapter focuses on the role of RRT in the treatment of AKI and summarizes the current evidence basis for the optimal timing of initiation of treatment and effects of selection of modality and dose of therapy on patient outcomes. We also address several management issues related to the delivery of specific modalities of RRT for patients with AKI.

Prescription and delivery of RRT

Timing of initiation of RRT

In patients with AKI complicated by intractable hyperkalemia, severe metabolic acidosis, volume overload, or overt uremic symptoms, the decision to initiate RRT is straightforward. However, in the absence of these overt manifestations, there is uncertainty regarding the optimal time to initiate renal support. Whether the initiation of RRT before the development of absolute indications, including overt uremia, volume overload, or metabolic complications, improves patient outcome has been a matter of some debate. Those who favor early initiation argue that RRT should be instituted as soon as a significant and persistent reduction in the glomerular filtration rate develops, prior to the development of potentially deleterious metabolic abnormalities or volume overload. The counterargument is that early initiation of RRT will expose some patients to risks of treatment, such as the insertion and prolonged placement of intravenous catheters, the need for anticoagulation, and the potential for hypotension and other treatment-related complications; these patients, if managed conservatively, might recover renal function without ever developing an "absolute" indication for RRT.

Nearly 50 years ago, the prophylactic benefits of dialysis were initially proposed by Teschan and colleagues and by Easterling and Forland in uncontrolled case series [7,8]. Several subsequent retrospective studies aimed to substantiate this hypothesis [9–11] (Table 12.1). The first prospective study evaluating timing of initiation of RRT was published in 1975 by Conger [12]. In that study, 18 consecutive patients were assigned in an alternating fashion to early (intensive) or late (nonintensive) IHD [12]. Patients receiving the intensive regimen exhibited lower mortality (20% vs. 64%; $P < 0.01$) and less frequent infectious and gastrointestinal complications. In the only subsequent prospective study on the timing of initiation of IHD, Gillum et al. randomized 34 patients to initiate dialysis with even smaller elevations of blood urea nitrogen (BUN) and serum creatinine, and they found lower mortality (47% vs. 59%) but more frequent hemorrhagic and septic complications with the nonintensive management strategy [13]. These differences, however, failed to reach statistical significance. Collectively, these early studies formed the basis for conventional teaching that dialytic support should be initiated when the BUN approaches 100 mg/dL and that there is no added benefit from earlier initiation in the absence of other specific indications. The

Evidence-based Nephrology. Edited by Donald Molony and Jonathan Craig
© 2009 Blackwell Publishing, ISBN: 978-1-4051-3975-5.

Table 12.1 Timing of initiation of RRT.

Study	Study method	Early RRT	Late RRT	No. of patients	Effect(s) of early initiation
IHD studies					
Parsons et al. 1961 [10]	Prospective/ observational	BUN 120–150 mg/dL	BUN >200 mg/dL, clinical deterioration	33	↓mortality, ↓ infection
Fisher 1966 [9]	Prospective/ observational	BUN <150 mg/dL, clinical deterioration	BUN >200 mg/dL	235	↓ mortality
Kleinknecht et al. 1972 [11]	Prospective/ observational	Maintenance of BUN <200 mg/dL	BUN >350 mg/dL, electrolyte disturbance	500	↓ mortality, ↓ GI hemorrhage
Conger 1975 [12]	Prospective/ randomized	Maintenance of pre-HD BUN <70 mg/dL, Scr <5 mg/dL	BUN ~150 mg/dL, Scr ~10 mg/dL, clinical indications	18	↓ mortality, ↓ infectious and GI complications
Gillum et al. 1986 [13]	Prospective/ randomized	Maintenance of pre-HD BUN <60 mg/dL, Scr <5 mg/dL	Maintenance of pre-HD BUN <100 mg/dL, Scr <9 mg/dL	34	↓ mortality, ↑ hemorrhagic and septic complications
CRRT studies					
Gettings et al. 1999 [14]	Retrospective	BUN <60 mg/dL	BUN >60 mg/dL	100	↓ mortality
Bouman et al. 2002 [17]	Prospective/ randomized	12 h after meeting inclusion criteria	BUN >112 mg/dL, K >6.5 mEq/L, severe pulmonary edema	106	No effect on mortality
Elahi et al. 2004 [16]	Retrospective	0.78 ± 0.2 days between surgery and RRT	2.55 ± 2.2 days between surgery and RRT	64	↓ mortality
Demirkilic et al. 2004 [15]	Prospective/ observational	Urine output <100 mL within 8 h after surgery	Scr >5 mg/dL or serum K >5.5 mEq/L	61	↓ mortality
Multiple modality studies					
Liu et al. 2006 [18]	Retrospective	BUN ≤ 76 mg/dL	BUN >76 mg/dL	243	↓ mortality

Abbreviations: Scr, serum creatinine.

inherent methodological limitations of these studies, including the retrospective design of the earlier studies and the small number of subjects in the two prospective studies, as well as the differences in technology between the eras when these studies were performed and current practice, must be taken into consideration in interpreting these results.

More recent studies have focused on the timing of initiation of CRRT. Gettings and colleagues retrospectively assessed outcomes among 100 consecutive adults with posttraumatic AKI treated with continuous venovenous hemofiltration (CVVH), stratifying timing of initiation based on the pretreatment BUN [14]. The early group (BUN < 60 mg/dL) started CRRT an average of 9 days sooner than the late group (BUN ≥ 60 mg/dL) (10 ± 15 days vs. 19 ± 27 days; $P < 0.0001$) and had substantially lower preinitiation BUN (43 ± 13 mg/dL vs. 94 ± 28 mg/dL; $P < 0.0001$). Survival was found to be nearly twofold greater in the early group (39% vs. 20%; $P = 0.041$). Although acuity of illness was comparable in the two groups, the retrospective study design precluded a comprehensive assessment of whether the outcomes were related to unrecognized differences in the clinical characteristics of the two groups. Similarly, two retrospective analyses in post-cardiac surgery patients

revealed lower mortality rates in patients in whom CVVH was initiated based on a urine output of less than 100 mL/8 h, independent of metabolic parameters, compared to patients in whom CVVH was not begun until overt metabolic thresholds were met [15,16]. The only prospective randomized study evaluating the timing of initiation of CRRT to date, reported by Bouman and colleagues, failed to observe superior outcomes with early initiation of renal support, although the sample size was small and the overall patient survival of 70–75% suggested a lower acuity of illness than most studies of critically ill patients with AKI [17].

Recently, Liu and colleagues analyzed prospectively collected data from the Program to Improve Care in Acute Renal Disease, a multicenter observational study of AKI, and assessed risk of death in patients requiring RRT as a function of BUN prior to initiation of therapy [18]. Patients were stratified based on the median BUN, 76 mg/dL. Crude survival rates were slightly lower for the patients who started RRT at higher BUN concentrations, despite a lower burden of organ system failure. After adjustment for covariates, stratification by study site and by initial modality of RRT, and utilization of a propensity score model, the relative risk for death associated with initiation of renal support at a higher BUN was 2.0

Table 12.2 Studies comparing modalities of RRT.

Study	No. of IHD patients	IHD mortality (%)	No. of CRRT patients	CRRT mortality (%)	Unadjusted odds of death with IHD (95% CI)	Risk-adjusted odds or risk of death with IHD[a]
Observational studies of IHD vs. CRRT						
Mauritz *et al.* 1986 [64]	22	91	36	75	3.3	NR
Paganini *et al.* 1988 [65]	47	81	27	82	1.0	NR
Bastien *et al.* 1991 [66]	32	75	34	50	3.0	NR
McDonald *et al.* 1991 [67]	10	70	22	82	0.5	NR
Kierdorf *et al.* 1991 [68]	73	93	73	78	3.8	NR
Kruczynski *et al.* 1993 [69]	23	83	12	33	9.5	NR
Bellomo *et al.* 1995 [70][b]	84	70	150	61	1.5	NR
van-Bommel *et al.* 1995 [71]	34	41	60	57	0.5	NR
Neveu *et al.* 1996 [55]	141	58	28	89	0.2	NR
Rialp *et al.* 1996 [72][c]	21	67	43	76	0.6	NR
Swartz *et al.* 1999 [19]	137	41	90	68	0.3	NS
Bellomo *et al.* 1999 [73]	47	57	47	53	1.2	NR
Ji *et al.* 2002 [74]	92	36	101	41	0.8	NR
Guérin *et al.* 2002 [20]	233	59	354	79	0.4	NS
Chang *et al.* 2004 [75]	95	54	53	79	0.3	NR
Gangji *et al.* 2005 [76]	66	58	36	64	0.8	NS
Swartz *et al.* 2005 [77]	183	40	200	65	0.4	NS
Randomized studies of IHD vs. CRRT						
Mehta *et al.* 2001 [22]	82	48	84	66	0.63[d] (0.3–1.4)	
John *et al.* 2001 [21]	20	70	10	70	1.0 (0.1–6.6)	
Augustine *et al.* 2004 [23]	40	70	40	68	1.12 (0.4–3.2)	
Uehlinger *et al.* 2006 [25]	55	51	70	47	1.16 (0.5–2.5)	
Vinsonneau *et al.* 2006 [24]	184	68	175	67	1.05 (0.6–1.7)	
Studies of PD vs. CRRT						
Phu *et al.* 2002 [36] (PD patients)[e]	36	47	34	15	5.1	

[a] NR, not reported; NS, not statistically significant.
[b] Conventional dialysis predominantly IHD with small number of patients treated with PD and combination of PD and IHD.
[c] Included some patients who received PD.
[d] Adjusted for clinical differences in study groups.
[e] Patients received PD, not IHD.

(95% confidence interval, 1.2–3.2). Thus, although there are data suggesting that "early" initiation of renal support in AKI is associated with improved survival, the evidence base is not sufficiently robust to draw firm conclusions. Resolution of this question will require adequately powered, prospective, randomized trials.

Modality of RRT

Although previously limited to IHD or PD, the current armamentarium of available RRT modalities includes the multiple forms of CRRT and the recently introduced hybrid treatments (e.g. SLED and extended duration dialysis). Unfortunately, objective and sound data to guide the selection of modality remain limited (Table 12.2).

Although clinical practices suggest that it is commonly believed that CRRT is superior to IHD in hemodynamically unstable patients, clinical trials have failed to demonstrate that this is the case. However, the propensity for seriously ill and more hemodynamically tenuous patients to receive CRRT rather than IHD, along with the inherent limitations of retrospective and nonrandomized study designs, confounded many of the early studies that compared continuous and intermittent therapies. Several studies have applied multivariable analyses to adjust for these issues. In a single-center retrospective study, Swarz and colleagues compared patients treated with either CVVH or IHD and found an unadjusted twofold-greater mortality in patients treated with CVVH [19]. After adjusting for the greater severity of illness in the CVVH group, no differences in mortality were observed. Similarly, in a prospective, multicenter, observational study published by Guérin and colleagues, mortality was 79% in patients managed with CRRT compared to 59% in patients who received IHD [20]. However, after adjustment for comorbidities, modality of RRT was not independently associated with outcome.

Four randomized controlled trials comparing CRRT and IHD have been published in peer-reviewed journals. In a small randomized controlled trial designed to compare the effects of CVVH and IHD on systemic hemodynamics and splanchnic perfusion in patients with septic shock, mortality was 70% in 20 patients randomized to CVVH and in 10 patients who received IHD [21]. In a multicenter randomized controlled trial of 166 patients with AKI, Mehta and colleagues observed intensive care unit and hospital mortality rates of 59.5% and 65.5%, respectively, in patients randomized to CRRT, compared to 41.5% and 47.6%, respectively, in patients randomized to IHD ($P < 0.02$) [22]. However, imbalanced randomization resulted in patients in the CRRT arm having greater severity of illness as measured by APACHE III score and a higher rate of liver failure, both of which were independently associated with increased mortality. After covariate adjustment, the investigators found no difference in mortality attributable to modality of RRT. In addition to the issues related to imbalanced randomization, interpretation of this study is also confounded by a very high rate of crossover between treatment modalities in both study arms. In a single-center randomized trial involving 80 patients, Augustine and colleagues reported more effective fluid removal and greater hemodynamic stability associated with continuous venovenous hemodialysis (CVVHD) compared to IHD but observed no difference in survival [23]. Similarly, in another single-center randomized controlled trial from Switzerland, Uehlinger and colleagues observed no difference in survival in 70 patients randomized to continuous venovenous hemodiafiltration (CVVHDF) compared to 55 patients assigned to IHD [25]. Most recently, the Hemodiafe study, a multicenter randomized controlled trial conducted in 21 intensive care units in France, demonstrated no difference in mortality in 184 patients randomized to IHD compared to 175 patients randomized to (CVVHDF) [24]. This study is particularly notable for the fact that IHD was delivered to patients despite marked hemodynamic instability, with very little crossover between treatment groups.

Multiple meta-analyses comparing outcomes between these modalities of RRT have been published [26–30]. The first two of these meta-analyses were published prior to the most recent randomized controlled trials [26,27]. One included both randomized and nonrandomized studies and concluded that weaknesses in the quality of the studies significantly limited meaningful comparisons between modalities [26]. However, based on weighting of the studies using an *a priori* assessment of study quality and comparability of severity of illness between treatment arms, the authors suggested that CRRT might be associated with a lower relative mortality risk. The second of these early meta-analyses was limited to six randomized trials, of which only one, the trial reported by Mehta and colleagues, was designed to evaluate mortality as an outcome and had been published in a peer-reviewed journal [27]. The authors found no differences in survival associated with modality of RRT. The three subsequent meta-analyses [28–30], which included the more recent randomized controlled trials of Uehlinger *et al.* [24] and the Hemodiafe study [25], differed in their criteria for including studies, resulting in minor differences

in their calculated odds ratios (ORs) for mortality, but all three found no differences in mortality associated with use of IHD or CRRT.

The propensity for hemodynamic instability and intradialytic hypotension during IHD has led to the suggestion that CRRT may be associated with an increased likelihood for recovery of renal function [22,31,32]. Although this benefit has been observed in surviving patients, to conclude that this is attributable to the modality would fail to account for the competing risk of mortality. Reanalyzing the data from these studies using the combined end point of death or nonrecovery of renal function, no difference in outcome between modalities is observed [33]. In addition, no differences in recovery of renal function were observed in either the single-center randomized controlled trial published by Augustine *et al.* or by Uehlinger *et al.*, or in the Hemodiafe study [23–25].

The initial modalities of CRRT utilized an arteriovenous circuit. Blood flow through the extracorporeal circuit was driven by the gradient between mean arterial pressure and central venous pressure. Although these modalities required little technology, they have been largely supplanted by pump-driven venovenous therapies. Several factors favor the use of venovenous therapies. The intrinsic resistance of the extracorporeal circuit coupled with the limited arteriovenous pressure gradient limits blood flow and ultimately the maximal achievable solute clearance with arteriovenous therapies. In addition, the arteriovenous circuit is associated with a significantly greater risk of vascular-related complications [34]. For this reason, the arteriovenous therapies should generally be restricted to situations where equipment for venovenous therapy is not available.

Solute removal during RRT may occur by diffusion (HD), convection (hemofiltration), or a combination of both (hemodiafiltration). Theoretically, convective clearance provides greater removal of middle- and higher-molecular-weight solutes. It has been postulated that this may be clinically relevant, particularly in patients with sepsis-associated AKI, because proinflammatory cytokines are in this molecular size range. In one study, lower tumor necrosis factor alpha levels were demonstrated using CVVH compared to continuous venovenous HD; however, no clinical outcome benefit was reported [35]. No studies comparing the relative benefits of convective and diffusive therapies on mortality have been reported.

Studies comparing other forms of RRT have been limited. One randomized controlled trial found that CVVH was superior to PD in infection-associated AKI, although the predominance of malaria as the cause of AKI limited the study's generalizability for Western populations [36]. No studies have directly compared "hybrid" treatments to either IHD or CRRT, although hybrid therapies have been shown to provide similar hemodynamic stability and solute control compared to CRRT [37].

In summary, methodological limitations in the observational studies to date and negative results of randomized trials preclude the development of evidence-based guidelines for the selection of RRT modality for the treatment of AKI. Choice of modality should therefore be guided by the individual patient's clinical status, provider expertise, and the availability of equipment and personnel.

Dose of RRT

Although there are extensive data guiding the dosing of dialysis for patients with end-stage renal disease, the body of evidence informing prescription of RRT dose in AKI is much more limited. When evaluating the dosing of IHD, both the dose per treatment and the treatment frequency need to be considered.

There is a paucity of data regarding the "adequate" per-treatment dose of IHD in AKI. Paganini and colleagues retrospectively evaluated survival as a function of the delivered dose of dialysis in critically ill patients with AKI [38]. Among patients at either the low or high extremes of severity of illness, dialysis dose had no impact on patient outcome. However, in patients with an intermediate severity of illness, the delivery of dialysis dose in excess of the 50th percentile (Kt/V, ~1) was associated with lower mortality risk than the delivery of lower doses of dialysis. It should be noted that this median delivered dialysis dose was substantially lower than what would be deemed appropriate in the setting of end-stage renal disease. No prospective studies addressing this issue have been published. As a result, given the lack of specific data for AKI, a consensus panel convened by the multinational Acute Dialysis Quality Initiative recommended that patients with AKI receive at least the minimum dose that is considered appropriate for patients with end-stage renal disease [39]. It is important to note that several studies have established that there is a significant discrepancy between prescribed and delivered dose for IHD; however, routine monitoring of the delivered dose of dialysis is not common [40–42].

Only one study has evaluated the effects of treatment frequency of IHD on outcomes among patients with AKI. Schiffl and colleagues assigned 160 critically ill patients with acute tubular necrosis to daily or alternate-day dialysis on an alternating basis and found that patients who received daily dialysis had both lower mortality 14 days after discontinuation of RRT (28% vs. 46%; $P = 0.01$) and shorter duration of AKI (9 ± 2 vs. 16 ± 6 days; $P = 0.001$) [40]. However, it is important to note that the dose of dialysis delivered to the alternate-day treatment group was exceptionally low (mean delivered Kt/V, 0.94 ± 0.11). This resulted in a markedly elevated time-averaged BUN concentration, which may have been the reason that this treatment group had a high incidence of complications, including gastrointestinal bleeding, mental status alterations, and infections, complications that may have resulted from inadequate dialysis [40]. Therefore, although this study demonstrates that increasing the delivered dose of dialysis from a very low level by increasing the frequency of treatment improves survival, it is not possible to conclude that increasing the frequency of "adequate" alternate-day or a thrice-weekly schedule versus daily therapy would improve outcome.

There are more data regarding the appropriate dosing of CRRT. Ronco and colleagues randomized 435 patients to one of three CVVH doses, defined by ultrafiltration rates of 20, 35, and 45 mL/kg/h [6]. Mortality was markedly lower in the intermediate- and high-dose arms (43% and 42%, respectively) compared to the low-dose arm (59%; $P < 0.001$). The absence of a survival benefit of high-dose therapy compared to the intermediate dose argued against a linear relationship between dose and outcome. Similarly, Saudan and colleagues reported overall improved mortality when dialysate flow (CVVHDF) was added to a fixed dose of CVVH [43]. A total of 102 patients were randomized to receive CVVH with a mean ultrafiltration rate of 25 ± 5 mL/kg/h, and 104 patients were randomized to CVVHDF with a mean ultrafiltration rate of 24 ± 6 mL/kg h and a mean dialysate flow rate of 18 ± 5 mL/kg/h. The addition of diffusive clearance was associated with an increase in 28-day survival from 39% to 59% ($P = 0.03$) and increased 90-day survival from 34% to 59% ($P = 0.0005$). In contrast, Bouman and colleagues did not observe this advantage with higher doses of CRRT [17]. However, the overall study mortality of less than 30% suggests that the enrolled patients were poorly representative of most critically ill patients with AKI. More recently, Tolwani and colleagues reported no difference in outcomes in 200 patients randomized to CVVHDF at either 20 to 35 mL/kg/h [44]. Survival to ICU discharge or 30 days, whichever was earlier, was 49% in the patients randomized to the higher dose group, compared to 56% of patients randomized to the lower dose of therapy.

The largest study evaluating intensity of RRT in AKI, the VA/NIH Acute Renal Failure Trial Network (ATN) study, utilized a strategy that included both IHD in hemodynamically stable patients and either CVVHDF or SLED in hemodynamically unstable patients [45]. In the intensive management strategy, IHD and SLED were provided daily (except Sunday), and CVVHDF was provided with an effluent flow of 35 mL/kg/h; in the less-intensive strategy, IHD and SLED were provided every other day (except Sunday), and CVVHDF was dosed at 20 mL/kg/h. In both treatment arms the target delivered single-pool Kt/V$_{urea}$ for IHD and SLED was 1.2–1.4/treatment, with an actual delivered dose during IHD of 1.32 ± 0.36. Sixty-day all-cause mortality was 53.6% in the 563 patients randomized to intensive therapy, compared to 51.5% in the 561 patients randomized to the less-intensive therapy (OR, 1.09; 95% CI, 0.86–1.40; $P = 0.47$). There was also no difference in the duration of RRT, recovery of kidney function, or course of nonrenal organ system failure.

Thus, although several smaller single-center studies have suggested that increased intensity of RRT is associated with improved outcomes, this approach is not supported across studies. Differences between study results most likely reflect differences among study designs and populations. For example, the delivered dose of IHD in the ATN study [45] was substantially higher than in the earlier study of Schifl and colleagues [40]. Similarly, only 12% of the patients in the study of Ronco and colleagues had sepsis [6], compared to 63% in the ATN study [45].

In summary, current evidence suggests that in the absence of specific medical indications (e.g. control of hyperkalemia) in patients with AKI, there is no additional benefit to providing IHD more frequently than every other day, with a delivered single-pool Kt/V$_{urea}$ of at least 1.2/treatment. Similarly, current evidence

Table 12.3 Randomized studies of dialysis membranes.

Study [reference]	Biocompatible membrane	Bioincompatible membrane	No. of patients	Biocompatible membrane mortality (%)	Bioincompatible membrane mortality (%)	P value for mortality difference
Schiffl et al. 1995 [46]	Polyacrylonitrile	Cuprophane	76	37	66	<0.05
Schiffl et al. 1994 [78][a]	Polyacrylonitrile	Cuprophane	52	38	65	<0.05
Kurtal et al. 1995 [52]	Polyamide	Cuprophane	57	36	28	NS[b]
Himmelfarb et al. 1998 [48]	Polymethylmethacrylate/polysulfone	Cellulosic based	153	43	54	0.03
Hakim et al. 1995 [47][c]	Polymethylmethacrylate/polysulfone	Cellulosic based	72	43	63	0.11
Jorres et al. 1999 [49]	Polymethylmethacrylate	Cuprophane	180	40	42	0.87
Gastaldello et al. 2000 [50]	Polysulfone[d]	Cellulose diacetate	159	60	55	0.57
Albright et al. 2000 [51]	Polysulfone	Cellulose acetate	66	27	24	0.61

[a] Patients in this study were included in the 1995 Schiffl et al. study.

[b] No P value reported. NS, not statistically significant.

[c] A subgroup of patients that were included in the 1998 Himmelfarb et al. study.

[d] Included both high-flux and low-flux membranes.

suggests that there is no additional benefit associated with provision of CRRT at an effluent flow rate of more than 20 mL/kg/h.

Mechanistic considerations in RRT

There are multiple technical considerations that need to be considered when prescribing RRT. We present data on the choice of hemodialyzer and hemofilter, use and type of anticoagulation, and selection of dialysate buffer.

Choice of hemodialyzer and hemofilter

As the result of animal studies suggesting that the activation of cellular and humoral processes by exposure of blood to bioincompatible dialysis membranes delays recovery from experimental AKI, a series of studies evaluated the effects of membrane biocompatibility on outcomes in patients with AKI (Table 12.3). More than a decade ago, Shiffl and colleagues randomized 76 patients with AKI to receive RRT with either cuprophane or polyacrylonitrile membranes [46]. Among patients dialyzed with cuprophane, there was a higher overall mortality (66% vs. 37%) and increased death from sepsis (55% vs. 16%). A subsequent single-center trial by Hakim et al., which was later extended to include additional study sites, demonstrated improved survival and recovery of renal function with the use of polymethylmethacrylate or polysulfone membranes compared to cellulosic membranes [47,48]. The benefit in this study was more substantial in nonoliguric than oliguric patients. However, a subsequent trial by Jorres et al. did not replicate these results [49]. Subsequent studies have compared various unsubstituted and substituted cellulosic membranes to more biocompatible synthetic dialyzers and have reported conflicting results as to the benefit of biocompatible membranes on survival and renal recovery [48,50–52].

Three meta-analyses have been conducted to help resolve these conflicting data. Jaber and colleagues examined seven studies, including both randomized and nonrandomized trials, encompassing a total of 722 patients [53]. Overall mortality rates were similar in those dialyzed with bioincompatible versus biocompatible membranes (46% vs. 45%). A subsequent meta-analysis broadened the study sample by including an additional observational study by Neveu et al. [54,55]. Overall survival was greater with synthetic membranes than cellulose-based membranes (62% vs. 55%; OR, 1.37; $P = 0.03$), although there were no differences in recovery of renal function. Using sensitivity analyses, the authors also found a survival benefit when synthetic membranes were compared to cuprophane membranes (OR, 1.64; $P = 0.013$), yet no overall survival advantage could be demonstrated with the use of synthetic membranes (OR, 1.2; not statistically significant). A more recent Cochrane analysis included nine studies with a total of 1062 patients and concluded that there is no demonstrable clinical advantage to the use of biocompatible membranes [56].

Thus, the current body of knowledge suggests that synthetic membranes provide a survival advantage(s) over cuprophane membranes for patients with AKI. Data comparing synthetic and substituted cellulose dialysis membranes are conflicting, and no firm conclusions can be drawn on the impact of membrane composition on recovery of renal function. Since the major advantage of cellulosic membranes compared to synthetic membranes is their low cost, these issues may have become moot with the recent reductions in the costs of synthetic membranes.

Use of anticoagulation

The most widely used anticoagulant for RRT in patients with AKI is unfractionated heparin [57]. Although an effective anticoagulant, heparin is associated with a risk of bleeding and with the

Table 12.4 Trials comparing lactate-buffered to bicarbonate-buffered fluid in CRRT.

Study [reference]	No. of patients	Study method	Effects of bicarbonate
Kierdorf [60]	20	Randomized, crossover	↑ chloride,[a] ↓ lactate, ↓ calcium and magnesium,[b,c] ↓ nitrogen excretion[b]
Thomas et al. [61]	40	Randomized trial	↑sodium and chloride, ↓ lactate
Barenbrock et al. [62]	117	Randomized trial	↑HCO₃, ↓ lactate, ↓ hypotensive crises, ↓cardiovascular events, ↓ mortality[d]
McLean [63]	54	Nonrandomized crossover cohort	↑mean arterial pressure, ↓ inotrope requirement, ↑ sodium, ↑ correction of acidosis, ↓ lactate

[a] Within-group effect.
[b] Variable effect by time period of therapy.
[c] Within- and between-group differences.
[d] Among patients with cardiac failure.

development of heparin-induced thrombocytopenia (HIT). Regional heparinization protocols, with reversal of heparin by infusion of protamine into the return line, have been developed to prevent systemic anticoagulation and minimize bleeding risk. Unfortunately, these protocols are cumbersome, may be associated with paradoxical increased risk of bleeding if excess protamine is infused, and do not alter the risk of HIT. Other anticoagulants that are safe in patients with a history of HIT include prostacylin (prostaglandin I_2), hirudin, and argatroban.

Regional citrate anticoagulation has also emerged as a viable alternative to standard approaches to anticoagulant therapy, particularly for patients managed with CRRT. Citrate is infused into the prefilter line and exerts its effect in the extracorporeal circuit by chelating calcium, which is an essential component in the coagulation cascade. A normal systemic ionized calcium concentration is maintained through the concomitant infusion of calcium into the return line or a peripheral vein. Multiple protocols for regional citrate anticoagulation have been developed, but until recently there were few direct comparisons with standard heparin therapy. In a study of patients with AKI receiving CVVH, Monchi and colleagues randomized patients to heparin or regional citrate anticoagulation [58]. Patients who required the use of more than one dialysis filter were administered the alternate anticoagulant for subsequent circuits. Median filter patency was greater (70 h vs. 40 h; $P = 0.0007$), and transfusion requirements were lower with citrate anticoagulation, whereas adverse events were comparable between study arms. In a trial of 30 critically ill patients receiving CRRT that was published by Kutsogiannis and colleagues, hemofilter survival was nearly three times longer with citrate therapy than heparin (124.5 h vs. 38.3 h; $P < 0.001$), whereas risk of hemorrhage was lower in patients anticoagulated with citrate (relative risk, 0.14; $P = 0.05$) [59]. Although unfractionated heparin remains the most commonly employed strategy for anticoagulation in patients with AKI who require RRT, these emerging data support the safety and potential superiority of regional citrate anticoagulation.

Choice of dialysate buffer for CRRT

Historically, lactate and acetate have been the primary buffers used in replacement fluid and dialysate for CRRT. Both are rapidly metabolized by the liver and skeletal muscle to bicarbonate, providing their basis for use as effective buffers. Elevations in blood lactate levels can occur during lactate-buffered CRRT, particularly among patients with underlying lactic acidosis and/or impaired hepatic function, potentially contributing to increased protein catabolism and impaired myocardial contractility. Until relatively recently, commercially available bicarbonate-based fluids for CRRT were unavailable due to the instability of bicarbonate solutions stored in gas-permeable containers. The recent introduction of commercially available bicarbonate-buffered fluids for CRRT coupled with the findings of studies over the past decade that have compared the effects of lactate-buffered and bicarbonate-buffered fluids forms the basis for recommendations for the use of bicarbonate-buffered fluids for CRRT (Table 12.4).

In 1995, Kierdorf and colleagues randomized 20 patients treated with CVVH to receive lactate-buffered or bicarbonate-buffered replacement fluids using a crossover study design [60]. No substantive differences in metabolic parameters, pH, control of azotemia, or hemodynamic status were seen between the two groups. Subsequently, Thomas et al. randomized 40 patients receiving hemofiltration to receive replacement fluids with either bicarbonate or lactate as the primary buffer and found no differences in correction of acidosis, hemodynamic parameters, or oxygen transport variables [61].

More recently, Barenbrock and colleagues demonstrated that bicarbonate-buffered replacement fluid was associated with fewer hypotensive episodes (0.26 ± 0.9 episodes/24 h vs. 0.60 ± 0.31 episodes/24 h; $P < 0.05$) and a lower rate of cardiovascular events (15% vs. 38%; $P < 0.01$) than lactate-buffered replacement fluid [62]. Although overall mortality rates and rates of death in patients with sepsis were comparable, there was a trend toward decreased mortality with the use of bicarbonate among those with cardiac failure (29% vs. 57%; $P = 0.058$). A crossover cohort study by McLean *et al.* revealed more rapid control of systemic acidosis with bicarbonate-buffered fluids than with lactate-buffered fluids in patients treated with continuous venovenous hemodiafiltration [63]. Mean arterial pressure rose by 5.76 mmHg with bicarbonate-buffered fluids and fell by 2.66 mmHg during the use of lactate-containing fluids.

Thus, despite the paucity of data demonstrating a survival benefit with bicarbonate-buffered dialysate and/or replacement fluid, the preponderance of evidence to date suggests a benefit on hemodynamic and cardiovascular parameters.

Summary

1) RRT remains the mainstay of supportive care for patients with established AKI. Unfortunately, there is insufficient evidence to make firm recommendations on the optimal timing of initiation of RRT.

2) Current data do not suggest superiority of any specific modality of renal support in patients with AKI, although outcomes with PD may be inferior. Clinical characteristics of patients, provider expertise, and locally available technology may all need to be considered when addressing these issues.

3) In the absence of specific medical indications (e.g. control of hyperkalemia), there is no additional benefit to providing IHD more frequently than every other day, so long as the delivered single-pool Kt/V_{urea} is at least 1.2/treatment. Although some studies have observed improved survival with higher doses of CRRT, current data suggest that there is no additional benefit associated with effluent flow rates exceeding 20 mL/kg/h.

4) The benefit associated with biocompatible dialysis membranes is uncertain, although there may be survival advantages relative to cuprophane membranes. The importance of resolving this issue, however, may be moot, given the marked reductions in costs for synthetic membranes over the past decade.

5) Heparin continues to be the primary means of anticoagulation, yet citrate may offer certain advantages and should be considered an effective alternative.

6) Bicarbonate-buffered fluids for CRRT are now commercially available. Although it remains unclear whether bicarbonate-buffered fluids are associated with a survival advantage over lactate- or acetate-buffered fluids, cardiovascular events may be less pronounced and hemodynamic stability improved with the use of bicarbonate-buffered fluid.

Ongoing studies should help resolve many of these unanswered questions related to the delivery of RRT and the overall goal of improving outcomes among patients with AKI.

Acknowledgment

Dr. Weisbord is supported by a VA Health Services Research and Development Career Development Award.

References

1 Metnitz PG, Krenn CG, Steltzer H, Lang T, Ploder J, Lenz K *et al.* Effect of acute renal failure requiring renal replacement therapy on outcome in critically ill patients. *Crit Care Med* 2002; **30**: 2051–2058.

2 Clermont G, Acker CG, Angus DC, Sirio CA, Pinsky MR, Johnson JP. Renal failure in the ICU: comparison of the impact of acute renal failure and end-stage renal disease on ICU outcomes. *Kidney Int* 2002; **62**: 986–996.

3 Chertow GM, Christiansen CL, Cleary PD, Munro C, Lazarus JM. Prognostic stratification in critically ill patients with acute renal failure requiring dialysis. *Arch Intern Med* 1995; **155**: 1505–1511.

4 Guerin C, Girard R, Selli JM, Perdrix JP, Avzac L.Initial versus delayed acute renal failure in the intensive care unit. A multicenter prospective epidemiological study. Rhone-Alpes Area Study Group on Acute Renal Failure. *Am J Respir Crit Care Med* 2000; **161**: 872–879.

5 Maher ER, Robinson KN, Scoble JE, Farrimond JG, Browne DR, Sweny P *et al.* Prognosis of critically ill patients with acute renal failure: APACHE II score and other predictive factors. *Q J Med* 1989; **72**: 857–866.

6 Ronco C, Bellomo R, Homel P, Brendolan A, Dan M, Piccinni P *et al.* Effects of different doses in continuous veno-venous haemofiltration on outcomes of acute renal failure: a prospective randomised trial. *Lancet* 2000; **356**: 26–30.

7 Teschan PE, Baxter CR, O'Brien TF, Freyhof JN, Hall WH. Prophylactic hemodialysis in the treatment of acute renal failure. *Ann Intern Med* 1960; **53**: 992–1016.

8 Easterling RE, Forland M. A five year experience with prophylactic dialysis for acute renal failure. *Trans Am Soc Artif Intern Organs* 1964; **10**: 200–208.

9 Fischer RP, Griffen WO, Jr., Reiser M, Clark DS. Early dialysis in the treatment of acute renal failure. *Surg Gynecol Obstet* 1966; **123**: 1019–1023.

10 Parsons FM, Hobson SM, Blagg CR, McCracken BH. Optimum time for dialysis in acute reversible renal failure. Description and value of an improved dialyser with large surface area. *Lancet* 1961; **i**: 129–134.

11 Kleinknecht D, Jungers P, Chanard J, Barbanel C, Ganeval D. Uremic and non-uremic complications in acute renal failure: evaluation of early and frequent dialysis on prognosis. *Kidney Int* 1972; **1**: 190–196.

12 Conger JD. A controlled evaluation of prophylactic dialysis in post-traumatic acute renal failure. *J Trauma* 1975; **15**: 1056–1063.

13 Gillum DM, Dixon BS, Yanover MJ, Kelleher SP, Shapiro MD, Benedetti RG *et al.* The role of intensive dialysis in acute renal failure. *Clin Nephrol* 1986; **25**: 249–255.

14 Gettings LG, Reynolds HN, Scalea T. Outcome in post-traumatic acute renal failure when continuous renal replacement therapy is applied early vs. late. *Intensive Care Med* 1999; **25**: 805–813.

15 Demirkilic U, Kuralay E, Yenicesu M, Caglar K, Oz BS, Cingoz F *et al.* Timing of replacement therapy for acute renal failure after cardiac surgery. *J Card Surg* 2004; **19**: 17–20.

16 Elahi MM, Lim MY, Joseph RN, Dhannapnuneni RR, Spyt TJ. Early hemofiltration improves survival in post-cardiotomy patients with acute renal failure. *Eur J Cardiothorac Surg* 2004; **26**: 1027–1031.

17 Bouman CS, Oudemans-Van Straaten HM, Tijssen JG, Zandstra DF, Kesecioglu J. Effects of early high-volume continuous venovenous hemofiltration on survival and recovery of renal function in intensive care patients with acute renal failure: a prospective, randomized trial. *Crit Care Med* 2002; **30**: 2205–2211.

18 Liu KD HJ, Paganini E, Ikizler TA, Soroko SH, Mehta RL, Chertow GM. Timing of initiation of dialysis in critically ill patients with acute kidney injury. *Clin J Am Soc Nephrol* 2006;**1:** 915–919.

19 Swartz RD, Messana JM, Orzol S, Port FK. Comparing continuous hemofiltration with hemodialysis in patients with severe acute renal failure. *Am J Kidney Dis* 1999; **34:** 424–432.

20 Guerin C, Girard R, Selli JM, Ayzac L. Intermittent versus continuous renal replacement therapy for acute renal failure in intensive care units: results from a multicenter prospective epidemiological survey. *Intensive Care Med* 2002; **28:** 1411–1418.

21 John S, Griesbach D, Baumgartel M, Weihprecht H, Schmieder RE, Geiger H. Effects of continuous haemofiltration vs intermittent haemodialysis on systemic haemodynamics and splanchnic regional perfusion in septic shock patients: a prospective, randomized clinical trial. *Nephrol Dial Transplant* 2001; **16:** 320–327.

22 Mehta RL, McDonald B, Gabbai FB, Pahl M, Pascual MT, Farkas A *et al.* A randomized clinical trial of continuous versus intermittent dialysis for acute renal failure. *Kidney Int* 2001; **60:** 1154–1163.

23 Augustine JJ, Sandy D, Seifert TH, Paganini EP. A randomized controlled trial comparing intermittent with continuous dialysis in patients with ARF. *Am J Kidney Dis* 2004; **44:** 1000–1007.

24 Uehlinger DE, Jakob SM, Ferrari P *et al.* Comparison of continuous and intermittent renal replacement therapy for acute renal failure. *Nephrol Dial Transplant* 2005; **20:** 1630–1637.

25 Vinsonneau C, Camus C, Combes A, Costa de Beauregard MA, Klouche K, Boulain T *et al.* Continuous venovenous haemodiafiltration versus intermittent haemodialysis for acute renal failure in patients with multiple-organ dysfunction syndrome: a multicentre randomised trial. *Lancet* 2006; **368:** 379–385.

26 Kellum JA, Angus DC, Johnson JP, Leblanc M, Griffin M, Ramakrishnan N *et al.* Continuous versus intermittent renal replacement therapy: a meta-analysis. *Intensive Care Med* 2002; **28:** 29–37.

27 Tonelli M, Manns B, Feller-Kopman D. Acute renal failure in the intensive care unit: a systematic review of the impact of dialytic modality on mortality and renal recovery. *Am J Kidney Dis* 2002; **40:** 875–885.

28 Rabindranath K, Adams J, Macleod AM, Muirhead N. Intermittent versus continuous renal replacement therapy for acute renal failure in adults. Cochrane Database Syst Rev 2007; **3:** CD003773.

29 Pannu N, Klarenbach S, Wiebe N *et al.* Renal replacement therapy in patients with acute renal failure: a systematic review. *JAMA* 2008; **299:** 793–805.

30 Bagshaw SM, Berthiaume LR, Delaney A, Bellomo R. Continuous versus intermittent renal replacement therapy for critically ill patients with acute kidney injury: a meta-analysis. *Crit Care Med* 2008; **36:** 610–617.

31 Manns B, Doig CJ, Lee H, Dean S, Tonelli M, Johnson D *et al.* Cost of acute renal failure requiring dialysis in the intensive care unit: clinical and resource implications of renal recovery. *Crit Care Med* 2003; **31:** 449–455.

32 Jacka MJ, Ivancinova X, Gibney RT. Continuous renal replacement therapy improves renal recovery from acute renal failure. *Can J Anaesth* 2005; **52:** 327–332.

33 Palevsky PM, Baldwin I, Davenport A, Goldstein S, Paganini E. Renal replacement therapy and the kidney: minimizing the impact of renal replacement therapy on recovery of acute renal failure. *Curr Opin Crit Care* 2005; **11:** 548–554.

34 Bellomo R, Parkin G, Love J, Boyce N. A prospective comparative study of continuous arteriovenous hemodiafiltration and continuous venovenous hemodiafiltration in critically ill patients. *Am J Kidney Dis* 1993; **21:** 400–404.

35 Kellum JA, Johnson JP, Kramer D, Palevsky P, Brady JJ, Pinsky MR. Diffusive vs. convective therapy: effects on mediators of inflammation in patient with severe systemic inflammatory response syndrome. *Crit Care Med* 1998; **26:** 1995–2000.

36 Phu NH, Hien TT, Mai NT, Chau TT, Chuong LV, Loc PP *et al.* Hemofiltration and peritoneal dialysis in infection-associated acute renal failure in Vietnam. *N Engl J Med* 2002; **347:** 895–902.

37 Kielstein JT, Kretschmer U, Ernst T, Hafer C, Bahr MJ, Haller H *et al.* Efficacy and cardiovascular tolerability of extended dialysis in critically ill patients: a randomized controlled study. *Am J Kidney Dis* 2004; **43:** 342–349.

38 Paganini EP, Taployai M, Goormastic M, Halstenberg W, Kozlowski L, *et al.* Establishing a dialysis therapy/patient outcome link in intensive care unit acute dialysis for patients with acute renal failure. *Am J Kidney Dis* 1996; **28:** s81–s89.

39 Kellum JA, Mehta RL, Angus DC, Palevsky P, Ronco C, ADQI Workgroup. The first international consensus conference on continuous renal replacement therapy. *Kidney Int* 2002; **62:** 1855–1863.

40 Schiffl H, Lang SM, Fischer R. Daily hemodialysis and the outcome of acute renal failure. *N Engl J Med* 2002; **346:** 305–310.

41 Pesacreta MOP, Palevsky PM, and the VA/NIH Acute Renal Failure Trial Network. Management of renal replacement therapy in acute renal failure: a survey of practitioner prescribing practices. *J Am Soc Nephrol* 2004; **15:** 350A.

42 Evanson JA, Himmelfarb J, Wingard R, Knights S, Shyr Y, Schulman G *et al.* Prescribed versus delivered dialysis in acute renal failure patients. *Am J Kidney Dis* 1998; **32:** 731–738.

43 Saudan P, Niederberger, De Seigneux S *et al.* Adding a dialysis dose to continuous hemofiltration increases survival in patients with acute renal failure. *Kidney Int* 2006; **70:** 1312–1317.

44 Tolwani AJ, Campbell RC, Stofan BS *et al.* Standard versus high-dose CVVHDF for ICU-related acute renal failure. *J Am Soc Nephrol* 2008; **19:** 1233–1238.

45 Palevsky PM, Zhang JH, O'Connor TZ *et al.* Intensity of renal support in critically ill patients with acute kidney injury. *N Engl J Med* 2008; **359:** 7–20.

46 Schiffl H, Sitter T, Lang S, Konig A, Haider M, Held E. Bioincompatible membranes place patients with acute renal failure at increased risk of infection. *ASAIO J* 1995; **41:** M709–M712.

47 Hakim RM, Wingard RL, Parker RA. Effect of the dialysis membrane in the treatment of patients with acute renal failure. *N Engl J Med* 1994; **331:** 1338–1342.

48 Himmelfarb J, Tolkoff Rubin N, Chandran P, Parker RA, Wingard RL, Hakim R. A multicenter comparison of dialysis membranes in the treatment of acute renal failure requiring dialysis. *J Am Soc Nephrol* 1998; **9:** 257–266.

49 Jorres A, Gahl GM, Dobis C, Polenakovic MH, Cakalaroski K, Rutkowski B *et al.* Haemodialysis-membrane biocompatibility and mortality of patients with dialysis-dependent acute renal failure: a prospective randomised multicentre trial. International Multicentre Study Group. *Lancet* 1999; **354:** 1337–1341.

50 Gastaldello K, Melot C, Kahn RJ, Vanherweghem JL, Vincent JL, Tielemans C. Comparison of cellulose diacetate and polysulfone membranes in the outcome of acute renal failure. A prospective randomized study. *Nephrol Dial Transplant* 2000; **15:** 224–230.

51 Albright RC, Jr., Smelser JM, McCarthy JT, Homburger HA, Bergstrath EJ, Larson TS. Patient survival and renal recovery in acute renal failure:

randomized comparison of cellulose acetate and polysulfone membrane dialyzers. *Mayo Clin Proc* 2000; **75**: 1141–1147.

52 Kurtal H, von Herrath D, Schaefer K. Is the choice of membrane important for patients with acute renal failure requiring hemodialysis? *Artif Organs* 1995; **19**: 391–394.

53 Jaber BL, Lau J, Schmid CH, Karsou SA, Levey AS, Pereira BJ. Effect of biocompatibility of hemodialysis membranes on mortality in acute renal failure: a meta-analysis. *Clin Nephrol* 2002; **57**: 274–282.

54 Subramanian S, Venkataraman R, Kellum JA. Influence of dialysis membranes on outcomes in acute renal failure: a meta-analysis. *Kidney Int* 2002; **62**: 1819–1823.

55 Neveu H, Kleinknecht D, Brivet F, Loirat P, Landais P. Prognostic factors in acute renal failure due to sepsis. Results of a prospective multicentre study. The French Study Group on Acute Renal Failure. *Nephrol Dial Transplant* 1996; **11**: 293–299.

56 Alonso ALJ, Jaber BL. Biocompatible hemodialysis membranes for acute renal failure (Cochrane Review). In: *The Renal Health Library*, Update Software Ltd., Oxford, UK, 2005.

57 Davenport A, Mehta S. The Acute Dialysis Quality Initiative, part VI: access and anticoagulation in CRRT. *Adv Ren Replace Ther* 2002; **9**: 273–281.

58 Monchi M, Berghmans D, Ledoux D, Canivet JL, Dubois B, Damas P. Citrate vs. heparin for anticoagulation in continuous venovenous hemofiltration: a prospective randomized study. *Intensive Care Med* 2004; **30**: 260–265.

59 Kutsogiannis DJ, Gibney RT, Stollery D, Gao J. Regional citrate versus systemic heparin anticoagulation for continuous renal replacement in critically ill patients. *Kidney Int* 2005; **67**: 2361–2367.

60 Kierdorf H, Leue C, Heintz B, Riehl J, Melzer H, Sieberth HG. Continuous venovenous hemofiltration in acute renal failure: is a bicarbonate- or lactate-buffered substitution better? *Contrib Nephrol* 1995; **116**: 38–47.

61 Thomas AN, Guy JM, Kishen R, Geraghty IF, Bowles BJ, Vadgama P. Comparison of lactate and bicarbonate buffered haemofiltration fluids: use in critically ill patients. *Nephrol Dial Transplant* 1997; **12**: 1212–1217.

62 Barenbrock M, Hausberg M, Matzkies F, de la Motte S, Schaefer RM. Effects of bicarbonate- and lactate-buffered replacement fluids on cardiovascular outcome in CVVH patients. *Kidney Int* 2000; **58**: 1751–1757.

63 McLean AG, Davenport A, Cox D, Sweny P. Effects of lactate-buffered and lactate-free dialysate in CAVHD patients with and without liver dysfunction. *Kidney Int* 2000; **58**: 1765–1772.

64 Mauritz W, Sporn P, Schindler I, Zadrobilek E, Roth E, Appel W. [Acute renal failure in abdominal infection. Comparison of hemodialysis and continuous arteriovenous hemofiltration]. *Anasth Intensivther Notfallmed* 1986; **21**: 212–217.

65 Paganini EP. Slow continuous hemofiltration and slow continuous ultrafiltration. *ASAIO Trans* 1988; **34**: 63–66.

66 Bastien O, Saroul C, Hercule C, George M, Estanove S. Continuous venovenous hemodialysis after cardiac surgery. *Contrib Nephrol* 1991; **93**: 76–78.

67 McDonald BR, Mehta RL. Decreased mortality in patients with acute renal failure undergoing continuous arteriovenous hemodialysis. *Contrib Nephrol* 1991; **93**: 51–56.

68 Kierdorf H. Continuous versus intermittent treatment: clinical results in acute renal failure. *Contrib Nephrol* 1991; **93**: 1–12.

69 Kruczynski K, Irvine-Bird K, Toffelmire EB, Morton AR. A comparison of continuous arteriovenous hemofiltration and intermittent hemodialysis in acute renal failure patients in the intensive care unit. *ASAIO J* 1993; **39**: M778–M781.

70 Bellomo R, Farmer M, Parkin G, Wright C, Boyce N. Severe acute renal failure: a comparison of acute continuous hemodiafiltration and conventional dialytic therapy. *Nephron* 1995; **71**: 59–64.

71 van Bommel E, Bouvy ND, So KL, Zietse R, Vincent HH, Bruining HA *et al.* Acute dialytic support for the critically ill: intermittent hemodialysis versus continuous arteriovenous hemodiafiltration. *Am J Nephrol* 1995; **15**: 192–200.

72 Rialp G, Roglan A, Betbese AJ, Perez-Marquez M, Ballus J, Lopez-Velarde G *et al.* Prognostic indexes and mortality in critically ill patients with acute renal failure treated with different dialytic techniques. *Ren Fail* 1996; **18**: 667–675.

73 Bellomo R, Farmer M, Bhonagiri S, Porceddu S, Ariens M, M'Pisi D *et al.* Changing acute renal failure treatment from intermittent hemodialysis to continuous hemofiltration: impact on azotemic control. *Int J Artif Organs* 1999; **22**: 145–150.

74 Ji D, Gong D, Xie H, Xu B, Liu Y, Li L. A retrospective study of continuous renal replacement therapy versus intermittent hemodialysis in severe acute renal failure. *Chin Med J* (Engl) 2001; **114**: 1157–1161.

75 Chang JW, Yang WS, Seo JW, Lee JS, Lee SK, Park SK. Continuous venovenous hemodiafiltration versus hemodialysis as renal replacement therapy in patients with acute renal failure in the intensive care unit. *Scand J Urol Nephrol* 2004; **38**: 417–421.

76 Gangji AS, Rabbat CG, Margetts PJ. Benefit of continuous renal replacement therapy in subgroups of acutely ill patients: a retrospective analysis. *Clin Nephrol* 2005; **63**: 267–275.

77 Swartz RD, Bustami RT, Daley JM, Gillespie BW, Port FK. Estimating the impact of renal replacement therapy choice on outcome in severe acute renal failure. *Clin Nephrol* 2005; **63**: 335–345.

78 Schiffl H, Lang SM, Konig A, Strasser T, Haider MC, Held E. Biocompatible membranes in acute renal failure: prospective case-controlled study. *Lancet* 1994; **344**: 570–572.

3   Primary Glomerulonephritis

13 Management of Idiopathic Nephrotic Syndrome in Adults: Minimal Change Disease and Focal Segmental Glomerulosclerosis

Alain Meyrier

Hôpital Georges Pompidou and Faculté de Médecine René Descartes, Paris, France.

In 1999, evidence-based recommendations for treating adult idiopathic nephrotic syndrome (INS) were published in *Kidney International* [1,2]. One could assume that little has changed regarding minimal change disease (MCD) and focal segmental glomerulonephritis (FSGS) since then, but a review of the literature shows that new treatment-related concepts have been developed. First, not all recommendations presented in the 1999 compendium meet the second millennium nephrologist's experience. Second, some patients with genetic mutations affecting podocin, ACTN-4, or CD2AP, may develop their first episode of nephrosis as an adult when it does not respond to immunosuppressive treatment [3–12]. In a series of 139 cases Ghiggheri *et al.* [13] excluded 18 patients with mutations, 11% of the entire group. This indicates that some patients with mutations and who fail immunosuppression may explain some of the variability in observed treatment effects in trials. In addition, a number of publications suggest that cases of FSGS might stem from viral or toxic factors that were not considered in 1999 but could lead to a response to immunosuppressive therapy different from that of cases with an immunologic background [14–17].

Other research has led to the notion that MCD and FSGS might be distinct entities rather than two subsets of INS [18–24]. Finally, a number of new immunosuppressive agents, marketed in the field of organ transplantation, have now been tried in the treatment of INS, and the evidence supporting their use merits discussion.

Definitions

MCD

The definition of MCD has not changed. It presents as nephrotic syndrome of sudden onset. In adults proteinuria is less selective than in children. Hypertension may be present. A functional impaired glomerular filtration rate is common at onset and normal-

izes with remission. Light microscopy and immunofluorescence show normal glomeruli. Electron microscopy discloses foot process flattening and no immune deposits.

FSGS

In contrast with MCD, our current clinical and histologic knowledge of FSGS has evolved. The onset of nephrotic syndrome can be more insidious than in MCD, except in the so-called glomerular tip lesion, a variant whose response to treatment is comparable to that of MCD [26–28]. In other forms, an explosive onset also seems to entail a response to treatment closer to MCD than in more progressive forms, although considerable overlap exists [29]. Hypertension and renal insufficiency are not unusual from the onset. Proteinuria is not selective. A detailed discussion of the histopathology of FSGS is beyond the scope of this chapter but is available elsewhere [30–34]; it is not covered further here because there are no implications for specific treatment [33,34].

Remission

Complete remission

There is general agreement regarding the definition of complete remission (CR): 24-h proteinuria of ≤ 0.3 g and serum albumin of ≥ 3.5 g/dL, persisting for at least 1 month.

Partial remission

Partial remission (PR) has been variably defined among publications. An acceptable definition is 24-h proteinuria of > 0.3 g and < 3 g, along with a rise of serum albumin of ≥ 3 g/dL and stable renal function. A 50% reduction from peak proteinuria has prognostic relevance and has recently been suggested as an added component to the definition.

Relapse

The definition of relapse also varies among publications. In fact, clinicians' experiences suggest that some patients in whom treatment has achieved remission may occasionally experience short spells of minimal and spontaneously decreasing proteinuria without hypoalbuminemia or clinical manifestations justifying

Evidence-based Nephrology. Edited by Donald Molony and Jonathan Craig
© 2009 Blackwell Publishing, ISBN: 978-1-4051-3975-5.

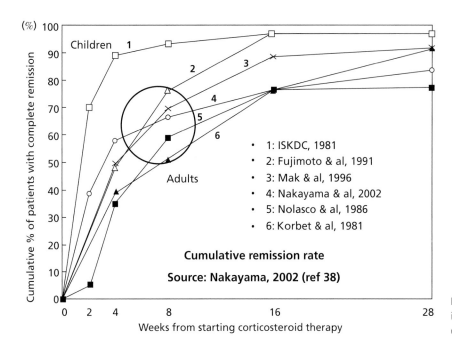

Cumulative remission rate

Source: Nakayama, 2002 (ref 38)

- 1: ISKDC, 1981
- 2: Fujimoto & al, 1991
- 3: Mak & al, 1996
- 4: Nakayama & al, 2002
- 5: Nolasco & al, 1986
- 6: Korbet & al, 1981

Figure 13.1 Time to remission in children (ISKDC) and in adults treated with corticosteroids for minimal change disease. (Adapted from ref 38).

treatment. From this experience, 24-h proteinuria of ≥3 g/day for more than 3 days with incipient decline in serum albumin levels appears to be an acceptable definition of relapse.

Steroid dependency

Two relapses occurring during steroid therapy or within 14 days of completing steroid therapy can be accepted as defining steroid dependency. More than 3 relapses/year may be considered to meet the definition of "multiple relapses."

Spontaneous remission

Spontaneous remission may occur in 10–20% of MCD [38]. It is considered rare in FSGS (3/81 [reference 46] or 1/42 [reference 47]). Yet, it is worth noting that in the most severe variant of FSGS, that is, collapsing glomerulopathy, Valeri *et al.* [48] observed three cases of spontaneous remission.

Renal function: progression to chronic kidney disease

Aside from functional renal insufficiency, which is not rare in case of severe proteinuria [49], renal function remains normal in MCD and tends to decline in FSGS, especially in cases with proteinuria of >14 g/day and in steroid-resistant patients, in whom end-stage renal disease (ESRD) is reached within an average time course of 5.5 years [50]. The risk of persistent renal insufficiency in MCD is extremely low, the only exceptions being concurrent acute tubular necrosis, seen in the elderly and in people with preexisting severe hypertension and compromised cortical blood flow [1]. Conversely, the risk for adult patients with nephrotic FSGS who

progress to ESRD following a CR is very low (2/119; 1.7%), somewhat higher following a PR (9/67; 13%), and occurs in over half of the steroid-resistant group (94/175; 54%) [33]. On a whole, decline in renal function is the rule in FSGS resistant to treatment. A partial remission portends a significantly better prognosis than in the treatment-resistant nephrotic patient [29].

MCD

Natural history
MCD presenting in adulthood

In contrast with about 95% of cases of INS, which occur in children and are due to MCD, this histologic variant makes up less than 50% of such cases in adults [49]. Although most patients experience a single attack, a multirelapsing course may occur, especially if the onset is before 30 years of age.

MCD presenting in the elderly

More than 20% of adult MCD cases affect persons older than 70 years [49]. The precise pathologic diagnosis can be ambiguous, as some glomerular lesions of focal sclerosis may be secondary to aging. Elderly nephrotic patients are prone to present with functional renal insufficiency and in some cases acute tubular necrosis.

A first attack of MCD-related NS in adults is usually corticosteroid sensitive. Relapses are distinctly less frequent in adults than in children. Corticosteroid response is slower in adults than in children [38,52–54] (Figure 13.1), and 4 months of continuous steroid treatment is required before one can conclude steroid resistance. Because of the risks of long-term steroid use, including diabetes and osteonecrosis, 6 months of full-dose corticosteroid treatment before considering alternate therapy, as suggested by the earlier literature [1], does not seem the proper balance between risk and benefit today.

Management

Recommendations

Recommendation 1: corticosteroids

Corticosteroids remain the mainstay of first-line treatment of MCD in adults. The drug of choice is prednisone. Prednisolone is commonly prescribed, but the pharmacokinetics of this form of steroid may vary with its intestinal absorption. This is true, for instance, in patients taking aluminum gels. Prednisone should be used instead of prednisolone (opinion), with a recommended dose of 1 mg/kg/day, not exceeding 80 mg. In the elderly some clinicians use a dosage of 2 mg/kg given on an alternate-day basis, although no specific study has addressed the issue of similar efficacy and better tolerability. The issue of steroid toxicity is well-recognized, but although weight gain, diabetes, and osteonecrosis are constantly cited regarding prolonged treatment with steroids in adult MCD, very few published studies have provided specific long-term data on the rates of these complications. In adults there are no randomized controlled trials (RCTs) that provide evidence on the dose of corticosteroids that should be given or the frequency or duration.

Only one paper has addressed the option of cyclosporine A (CsA) as first-line treatment in high-risk patients with adult MCD [41]. In that study, high-risk patients were those with a history of psychosis, a history of bleeding duodenal ulcer, or morbid obesity.

Recommendation 2: alkylating agents

Alkylating agents (cyclophosphamide or chlorambucil) are indicated in multirelapsing cases more than for steroid-resistant forms (opinion), although true steroid resistance is rare in true MCD, that is, cases in which a repeat renal biopsy carried out after 4 months of unsuccessful corticosteroid therapy still shows MCD. In most cases the second histopathologic examination discloses lesions of FSGS that had been overlooked or not sampled on the first biopsy, or had not yet appeared at the onset of the nephrotic syndrome, which explains the initial failure of steroids [38,51–54].

Despite the lack of studies specifically related to adult multirelapsers, it is likely that cytotoxic agents result in prolonged remissions, as shown in RCTs in children. Cyclophosphamide, at 2–3 mg/kg/day, is more commonly used than chlorambucil, without clear evidence of the superiority of one over the other. It should be administered orally and not in the form of intravenous pulses, and presumably, considering the experience acquired with childhood onset cases, for 8 weeks. Alkylating agents entail known hazards of hematologic, infectious, and oncologic side effects, but quantifying these risks is not possible given the available data. In men and women the risk of sterility is significant if the course is prolonged, and the risk increases with increasing age at the time of onset of the therapy.

Recommendation 3: CsA

CsA has been used in adults with MCD since 1986 [1]. Its side effects include hypertension, tremor, gingival hyperplasia, and hypertrichosis. Conversely, CsA has the advantage of not being cytotoxic, does not induce sterility, and entails fewer metabolic disturbances. These reasons may justify its use as first-line treatment in patients at risk of diabetes, osteonecrosis, or infertility.

One of the main safety concerns of CsA therapy in INS is the potential for nephrotoxicity. This is a class effect common to all calcineurin inhibitors, including tacrolimus [55,56]. Previous studies indicated that the dosage and type of primary renal disease are two elements to keep in mind when interpreting a decline in renal function [45].

A problem that has appeared since 1999 is that of formulation. Most publications mention "cyclosporine" and do not specify whether they are discussing Sandimmune or Neoral or a generic form of the drug, which may be important because it is known that the better pharmacokinetic profile of Neoral may lead to better efficacy and hence a distinct reduction of dosage [55,56] below the maximum of 5 mg/kg/day recommended for Sandimmune [45].

Evidence

Aside from clinical scenarios in which steroids are contraindicated [41], CsA first-line monotherapy has been used in many case series (level IV studies) with very low dosages [57]. One such study [41] included 86 adult patients with MCD and nephrotic syndrome that were resistant to conventional therapy or were steroid dependent or multirelapsers. They were treated with the Sandimmune formulation at a dose of 5.18 ± 0.94 mg/kg/day. Superior efficacy was reported in steroid-dependent patients (CR in 73% of cases and PR in 14%) compared to those who were steroid resistant (30% and 26%, respectively). Serum creatinine levels remained stable during CsA treatment. These patients were not all CsA dependent, as $\sim$20–25% were progressively tapered off after 2 years without relapsing [45].

Recommendation 4: mycophenolate mofetil

Studies of mycophenolate mofetil (MMF) in the treatment of MCD in adults are few and are limited to case series and reports [58–60]. Considering the encouraging results obtained in childhood nephrosis (see chapter 66–68), MMF may have a place in the treatment of adult MCD, but so far evidence either supporting or refuting its use is absent.

Summary

MCD is not uncommon in adults and may assume a multirelapsing course. The majority of patients respond to corticosteroids with complete remission, although this may require 4 months of treatment, compared with 6–8 weeks in children, with the attendant hazards of steroid toxicity. Steroid resistance may be due to an initially missed diagnosis of FSGS, and resistance should be considered an indication to verify the diagnosis by a repeat kidney biopsy. The frequency of relapses diminishes with age: after 30 years of age a single attack of NS is the most common variant

Table 13.1 Treatment of adult MCD[a].

Study author [reference]	Study design	No. of patients	Treatment outcomes	Comments and recommendations
Nakayama [38]	Retrospective study Prednisolone 60–80 mg/day in 57 pts + Cyc for 6 + CsA for 2	57 (originally 62, −5 with spontaneous remissions)	CR: 53/57 (38 within 8 wks, 15 later) PR: 3/57 F: 1/57 Age of Early relapsers: 24.4 ± 3.2 yrs Late relapsers: 42.5 ± 4.4 yrs Nonrelapsers: 41.9 ± 4.1 yrs	The study suggests that remission requires 4 mos of treatment before pronouncing failure
Meyrier [41]	Open collaborative prospective multicenter study (1986–1996) of CsA (Sandimmune) ~ 5mg/kg/day	82	CR: 60 (74%) PR: 11 (13%) F: 11 (13%)	High predictive value of previous response to steroids No decline in renal function
Tse [39]	Retrospective study based on age at onset	50 (35 18–50 yrs old, 15 >50 yrs)	18–50 yrs, CR at wks 2, 4, 6, and 8: 15.6, 62.5, 87.5, and 93.75% >50 yrs, CR: 9, 45.5, 91, and 100%	The response to steroids is similar, irrrespective of age The study confirms that remission requires 4 mos of treatment before admitting failure
Matsumoto [57]	CsA monotherapy, 2–3 mg/kg/day, after pulse MP or oral prednisone	36 (26 first attack, 10 relapses)	CR: 75% CsA alone, 100% CsA + MP, 92% prednisone alone	Too few patients to determine the superiority of CsA over steroids

Abbreviations: Cyc, cyclophosphamide; F, failure; Rx, treatment; MP, methylprednisolone.
[a] All studies are case series, level IV.

of MCD. In selected cases, low-dose CsA can be considered an alternative to steroids, with very little nephrotoxicity. The place of MMF in the treatment of adult MCD remains to be determined. The strength of evidence supporting these statements is very low, being largely based on case series (Table 13.1).

FSGS

Natural history

The incidence and the prevalence of nephrotic FSGS are steadily rising [61,62]. Patients of black African ancestry are twice as likely to develop FSGS than patients of white European origin [50]. This is true of most histological variants, especially the cellular variants [33,47]. The exception is the glomerular tip lesion [26–28]. The response to corticosteroid treatment in black people is distinctly worse than in white people [63], although the overall outcome of the disease in each race follows the same trend.

Management

All forms of FSGS require treatment, irrespective of the histopathologic variant [27,28,33,34]. The goal of therapy is to reduce, if not eliminate, proteinuria. Inducing even a partial remission reduces the rate of deterioration in renal function [29]. Corticosteroids remain the first-line treatment. Response to steroids is also the best indicator of a better long-term prognosis. In case of failure, a panoply of immunosuppressive drugs have been tried, including

new immunosuppressive agents used in solid organ transplantation. Unfortunately, the majority of these studies have included few patients and are case series (level IV studies). A few recent publications on rituximab (reviewed in reference 64) indicate that the anti-CD20 monoclonal antibody may inconstantly obtain a remission in cases of FSGS, especially when the NS relapses after renal transplantation.

Recommendations
Recommendation 1: corticosteroids
The initial response to treatment in adults with FSGS was analyzed by Korbet et al. [33,66,67]. The trend before 1980 was to treat for a short time and with low doses of steroids. The highest CR rates, >30%, were observed in cases treated for >5 months, and the lowest, ≤20%, were seen in patients treated for ≤2 months. Thus, corticosteroid treatment must be sufficiently long. Full-dose (1 mg/kg/day) prednisone is given for 8–12 weeks, followed in case of remission, even partial, by slow tapering over months to avoid a "rebound" relapse [68]. CR portends a favorable outcome, comparable to that of steroid-responsive MCD [50]. In fact, a minority of patients with nephrotic FSGS achieve stable remission after tapering steroids to complete withdrawal. Most cases are steroid dependent, usually to a high threshold dose. This poses a serious problem, as pursuing indefinite treatment with a high-maintenance dose leads to steroid side effects. Steroid dependency or resistance leads to the need to consider other treatment options, with the aim of

reducing proteinuria. In the case of steroid dependency, this may mean trading steroid toxicity for other complications.

In steroid-responsive cases, the rates of CR, PR, and failure are, respectively, on the order of 50%, 25%, and 25% of cases [33]. The response to steroids is significantly lower in black patients. Crook *et al.* analyzed the response to steroids in a retrospective case series comprised of 65 African Americans [63] and concluded that in this group of patients, steroids were in general ineffective and that the rate of complications was high.

Evidence

Few studies have addressed specifically the effect of steroids on nephrotic FSGS, with the exception of Crook *et al.* [63]. A single case series [64] included a surprisingly high proportion of patients doing well without treatment. Four case series [36,37,47,69] included 151 patients and showed that steroids were credited with about a 30% complete or partial remission. Troyanov *et al.* [29] estimated by multivariate analysis the significance of PR in nephrotic FSGS. They showed that even PR portends a significantly better prognosis than steroid resistance. A special case is that of glomerular tip lesion, classified by the Columbia group as a variant of FSGS. A majority of this subset responds to steroids as in MCD, as shown by Stokes *et al.* [28] and by Chun *et al.* [34].

In summary, in the absence of any RCT data, current consensus remains that corticosteroids are the first line of therapy. Full doses must be applied for an extended period of time before determining failure. CR portends a very favorable outcome. PR is also a goal pursued with steroid therapy. A minority of patients with nephrotic FSGS achieve stable remission after tapering steroids to a stop. Most cases are steroid dependent. Steroid dependency or resistance leads to the need to consider other treatment options aimed at reducing proteinuria, but which trade steroid toxicity for other complications.

Recommendation 2: alkylating agents

The best indication for use of an alkylating agent is the case of a steroid-dependent or multirelapsing patient, which is rare in nephrotic FSGS. Some studies included patients treated with a combination of cyclophosphamide or chlorambucil and steroids.

Evidence

The best study was a randomized trial in 57 patients by Heering *et al.* [70], which included 23 patients treated for 6 months with steroids and chlorambucil. They achieved 17% CR and 48% PR. Five of 23 progressed to ESRD. The contributions of other studies to treatment recommendations about alkylating agents are uncertain, such as Martinelli *et al.*'s case series [71]. In short, there is no strong evidence to recommend alkylating agents in the treatment of FSGS.

Recommendation 3: CsA

CsA has been used for 2 decades in the treatment of FSGS. It has been shown that its efficacy is greatly increased by a combination with low-dose steroids [41]. A comparison was made in 226 patients treated for steroid-resistant nephrotic syndrome (the majority were FSGS with some cases of MCD), with 127 receiving CsA alone and 103 receiving CsA plus steroids. The proportions of patients with CR, PR, and failure were, respectively, 14% versus 24%, 12% versus 24%, and 74% versus 52%. CsA combined with low-dose steroids can therefore be considered both an immunosuppressive drug and a steroid-sparing agent to treat resistant forms of FSGS.

Evidence

In Cattran's study [35], patients were randomized to a 26-week regimen of low-dose CsA (3.5 mg/kg/day) or placebo in 49 patients with steroid-resistant FSGS. CsA was tapered over the next 4 weeks and then stopped. Both groups also received low-dose prednisone (0.15 mg/kg/day), which was then tapered over the subsequent 8 weeks. Patients were followed up for an average of 200 weeks. CR was rare. By week 26, CR or PR had occurred in 70% of the treatment group versus only 4% of the placebo group ($P < 0.001$). Relapse off of CsA occurred in 40% of patients achieving remission by 52 weeks and in a further 20% by week 78, with the remainder continuing in remission to the end of the observation period. Long-term renal function was significantly better preserved in the CsA group. This trial was the first to demonstrate that low-dose CsA-induced partial remission reduces the rate of progression of nephrotic FSGS patients to renal insufficiency.

Another case series [41] was based on 68 patients treated with 5.18 ± 0.94 mg/kg/day of cyclosporine (Sandimmune formulation). The results on nephrotic syndrome were 14 CR (21%), 19 PR (28%), and 35 failures (51%). Other case series have comprised patients treated with CsA (among other immunosuppressants) and support the beneficial effect of CsA for inducing at least PR in nephrotic FSGS.

Recommendation 4: tacrolimus (FK-506)

Tacrolimus, like CsA, is a calcineurin inhibitor that inhibits T-cell-driven elaboration of cytokines [18,41]. The results with this medication are roughly comparable to those obtained with CsA in clinical practice, but there are no RCTs for this indication. So far, the experience acquired is too scarce to lead to specific recommendations regarding its use in FSGS.

Recommendation 5: sirolimus

Sirolimus (Rapamycin) inhibits the response to cytokines. The current experience with this drug is controversial and inadequate to allow recommendations on its use in FSGS [74,75].

Recommendation 6: MMF

The current experience regarding MMF in the treatment of FSGS seems more or less encouraging [76–78], but the lack of RCTs precludes firm recommendations regarding this new immunosuppressive drug.

Table 13.2 Treatment of FSGS.

Study author [reference]	Study design	n	Treatment outcomes	Comments and recommendations
Cattran [35]	RCT, 26 weeks CsA (3.5 mg/kg/day) + low-dose prednisone	49 (26 CsA, 23 placebo)	70% of treated group CR or PR by 26 wks, vs 4% in placebo group Relapse: 60% by wk 78; remainder remained in remission; renal function decline was less in treatment group than in placebo group	This RCT showed the efficacy for inducing CR + PR in nephrotic FSGS without affecting renal function
Ponticelli [36]	Retrospective multicenter study; included pts with serum creatinine up to 3 mg/dL Various regimens applied (steroids, combination or succession of steroids, and alkylating agents or CsA)	80 (initially 53 steroids, 27 immunosuppressive drugs)	First treatment Steroids (n = 53) Cytotoxic drugs (n = 27) CR: 21 CR: 8 PR: 10 PR: 3 F: 22 F: 16 Second treatment Steroids (n = 6) Cytotoxic Rx CsA CR: 1 CR: 1 CR: 0 PR: 1 PR: 5 PR: 7	1) Major side effects in 11 2) 70% of patients may maintain stable renal function with prolonged Rx 3) Inclusion of pts with renal insufficiency and variability of treatment courses make analysis of data and recommendations difficult
Alexopoulos [37]	17 nephrotic pts with FSGS, 6 not treated and 11 treated w/ prednisolone 4 PR and 4 F treated with add-on Cyc (n = 2) ⟶ or CsA (n = 6), 2–3 mg/kg/day for 6–12 mos ⟶	11 treated	CR 3 (28 %) PR 4 (36 %) F 4 (36 %) PR: 1 PR: 1	Renal survival at 5 yrs: 86% in treated, 65% untreated pts (P < 0.03) Nephrotic FSGS responding to treatment had better renal survival than in case of F. Age and serum creatinine at biopsy independent risk factors leading to ESRD Analysis of data quite difficult
Ghiggheri [13]	Retrospective open nonrandomized study, children and adults; 84 not treated and 55 treated	139 (18 [11%] who had mutations were excluded)	20 pts (36%) responsive to CsA	No signs of renal toxicity on repeat biopsy Note significant percentage of genetic mutations
Chun 2004 [34]	Retrospective study based on histology Prednisone at 1 mg/kg/day for 3–4 mos (up to 80 mg/day) tapered progressively Elderly pts: alternate-day Rx 4–5 mos	51	Classic FSGS Cell FSGS Tip lesion 17 25 9 CR 6 16 7 PR 3 10 2 NB: Pts in this series could be the same as those described in Schwartz 1999 (same numbers except for tip lesion type)	The authors consider cellular FSGS and collapsing glomerulopathy the same entity Results of steroid Rx are the same irrespective of histology Pts with FSGS benefit from prolonged steroid Rx irrespective of histology
Stirling [69]	Retrospective record review in 5 UK renal units (1975–1999)	136 (76 on steroids; 45 alone, 31 with additional immunosuppression: 26 Cyc, 26 CsA, 20 Aza)	CR + PR: 67% Remission with 5-yr survival off dialysis in 94%; F with 5-yr survival off dialysis in 53%	Pts treated with steroids are more likely to enter remission than those left untreated Remission rate of up to 80% can be achieved with prolonged treatment Pts who do not achieve remission have a poor prognosis
Crook [63]	Retrospective review of charts, selection of majority of African Americans with nephrotic FSGS	72 (65 African Americans, 43 treated with steroids) Follow-up: 48.3 mos	17/43 reached ESRD 26/43 doubled their initial serum creatinine conc 1/3 treated with steroids developed complications	A beneficial effect of steroids was not observed in this series of predominantly African American adults with nephrotic FSGS
Deegens [65]	Retrospective study of initially untreated patients with normal renal function and negative family history; median follow-up 9.4 yrs (2.1–18.6)	20	13 pts in remission without any treatment Renal function deterioration in 7, among which 4 were treated 10-year renal survival, 89%	This series has an unusual percentage of patients with spontaneous remission
Segarra [72]	Prospective open study; switch to FK-506 + full-dose steroids for 25 patients who did not attain remission with CsA + full-dose steroids	25	At 6 mos, 10 CR + 2 PR + 5 with "diminution of proteinuria" Time to remission: 112 ± 24 days Reversible nephrotoxicity in 40% FK-506 dependency in 76%	Preliminary results might indicate some superiority of FK-506 + steroids over CsA + steroids in treatment of FSGS
Voehringer [74]	Prospective open trial of sirolimus in FSGS (5 primary) following failure of CsA–FK-506, prednisone + MMF, and in 3 on Cyc	7	No effect at 6 mos	Sirolimus did not prove to a beneficial effect on nephrotic syndrome or renal function
Segarra [78]	Prospective open trial of MMF in FSGS resistant to other treatment options	22	Slow remission (150 ± 68 days), CR in 2, PR in 10, F in 10	MMF Rx causes a moderate decrease in proteinuria in 50% of pts who do not have other treatment options; the response to therapy is largely influenced by preserved renal function and requires sustained MMF treatment

Abbreviations: FSGS: focal segmental glomerulosclerosis. RCT: randomized controlled trial. CR: complete remission. PR: partial remission. F: failure (no remission). ESRD: end-stage renal disease. Rx: treatment. CsA: cyclosporine Cyc: cyclophosphamide. Aza: azathioprine MMF: mycophenolate mofetil Pts: patients.

Summary

Nephrotic FSGS, irrespective of its histopathologic variant, is always an indication for a course of full-dose steroids, preferably prednisone (opinion) and for a minimum of 4 months prior to labeling the patient steroid resistant (opinion). CR portends an excellent prognosis. PR is beneficial, both clinically and in terms of preservation of renal function. In the case of steroid resistance, the use of a combination of CsA and low-dose steroids obtains partial or, more rarely, complete remission in about 50–70% of patients, with a definite advantage regarding long-term preservation of renal function. Among the various other immunosuppressants tried in the treatment of FSGS, MMF has the advantage of no nephrotoxicity, but the studies to date, although positive, have been small and pilot in nature (Table 13.2).

Plasmapheresis

The rationale for treating nephrotic FSGS with plasma exchange is based on the concept of a glomerular permeability factor, postulated by Shalhoub in 1974 [79], and despite this factor being the subject of numerous publications, much remains uncertain about this factor [18]. There is no evidence that plasma exchange modifies the course of FSGS, outside of the particular case of relapse of nephrotic syndrome in a kidney transplant recipient [33]. Based on the concept of a "circulating factor," plasmapheresis has been advocated to remove it, reduce proteinuria, and avoid the progression to renal insufficiency, but there is little evidence for or against its use [80–86]. In 2001 Bosch and Wendler [87] concluded, in a review of extracorporeal plasma treatment in primary and recurrent FSGS, that there was only poor evidence to support its use, and no significant additional data have been added since that time.

Similarly, plasma protein adsorption on columns coated with staphylococcal protein A [88] does not seem to remove specifically the elusive circulating factor responsible for the proteinuria, as this experimental protocol also reduces proteinuria in other glomerulopathies [89].

Pregnancy

INS occurring during pregnancy poses a unique situation. The majority of the data relative to the effects of immunosuppressive treatment in pregnancy are based on post-kidney transplantation reports. High-dose corticosteroids entail a risk to the fetus [90]. Alkylating agents are contraindicated. In the CsA era, case reports, center reports, and registry data have supported the concept that successful pregnancy outcomes are possible for mother and newborn in the presence of stable graft function and well-controlled maternal comorbidities, such as hypertension. While the risks of prematurity and low birth weight are greater than those seen in the general population, there has been no increase in the malformation rate of newborns. Successful pregnancy outcomes have been reported in non-renal CsA recipients as well [91–93]. The available

experience with MMF has been limited to organ transplantation [91–93]. Two newborns with malformations were noted in a limited case series with MMF exposure, but other factors may have also been at play. The use of MMF during pregnancy continues to be an unresolved issue. In summary, CsA seems to be the less toxic agent to treat a case of INS during pregnancy, but the data are weak.

References

1 Bargman JM. Management of minimal lesions glomerulonephritis: evidence-based recommendations. *Kidney Int* 1999; **55 (Suppl 70)**: S3–S16.

2 Burgess E. Management of focal segmental glomerulosclerosis: evidence-based recommendations. *Kidney Int* 1999; **55(Suppl 70)**: S26–S32.

3 Conlon PJ, Lynn K, Winn MP, Quarles LD, Bembe ML, Pericak-Vance M *et al.* Spectrum of disease in familial focal and segmental glomerulosclerosis. *Kidney Int* 1999; **56**: 1863–1871.

4 Ruf RG, Lichtenberger A, Karle SM, Haas JP, Anacleto FE, Schultheiss M *et al.* Patients with mutations in NPHS2 (podocin) do not respond to standard steroid treatment of nephrotic syndrome. *J Am Soc Nephrol* 2004; **15**: 722–732.

5 Winn MP. Approach to the evaluation of heritable diseases and update on familial focal segmental glomerulosclerosis. *Nephrol Dial Transplant* 2003; **18(Suppl 6)**: vi14–vi20.

6 Boute N, Gribouval O, Roselli S, Benessy F, Lee H, Fuchshuber A *et al.* NPHS2, encoding the glomerular protein podocin, is mutated in autosomal recessive steroid-resistant nephrotic syndrome. *Nat Genet* 2000; **24**: 349–354.

7 Huber TB, Simons M, Hartleben B, Sernetz L, Schmidts M, Gundlach E *et al.* Molecular basis of the functional podocin–nephrin complex: mutations in the NPHS2 gene disrupt nephrin targeting to lipid raft microdomains. *Hum Mol Genet* 2003; **12**: 3397–3405.

8 Caridi G, Bertelli R, Di Duca M, Dagnino M, Emma F, Onetti Muda A *et al.* Broadening the spectrum of diseases related to podocin mutations. *J Am Soc Nephrol* 2003; **14**: 1278–1286.

9 Kaplan JM, Kim SH, North KN, Rennke H, Correia LA, Tong HQ *et al.* Mutations in ACTN4, encoding alpha-actinin-4, causes familial focal segmental glomerulosclerosis. *Nat Genet* 2000; **24**: 251–256.

10 Komatsuda A, Wakui H, Maki N, Kigawa A, Goto H, Ohtani H *et al.* Analysis of mutations in alpha-actinin 4 and podocin genes of patients with chronic renal failure due to sporadic focal segmental glomerulosclerosis. *Ren Fail* 2003; **25**: 87–93.

11 Niaudet P. Podocin and nephrotic syndrome: implications for the clinician. *J Am Soc Nephrol* 2004; **15**: 832–834.

12 Ghiggeri GM, Carraro M, Vicenti F. Recurrent focal glomerulosclerosis in the era of genetics of podocyte proteins: theory and therapy. *Nephrol Dial Transpl* 2004; **19**: 1036–1040.

13 Ghiggeri GM, Catarsi P, Scolari F, Caridi G, Bertelli R, Carrea A *et al.* Cyclosporine in patients with steroid-resistant nephrotic syndrome: an open-label carried out genetic profiling. *Clin Ther* 2004; **26**: 1411–1418.

14 Tanawattanacharoen S, Falk RJ, Jennette JC, Kopp JB. Parvovirus B19 DNA in kidney tissue of patients with focal segmental glomerulosclerosis. *Am J Kidney Dis* 2000; **35**: 1166–1174.

15 Moudgil A, Nast CC, Bagga A, Wei L, Nurmamet A, Cohen AH *et al.* Association of parvovirus B19 infection with idiopathic collapsing glomerulopathy. *Kidney Int* 2001; **59**: 2126–2133.

16 Li RM, Branton M, Tanawattanacharoen S, Falk RJ, Jennette JC, Kopp JB. Molecular identification of SV 40 infection in human subjects and possible association with kidney disease. *J Am Soc Nephrol* 2002; **13**: 2320–2330.

17 Barri YM, Munshi NC, Sukumalchantra S, Abulezz SR, Bonsib SM, Wallach J *et al.* Podocyte injury associated glomerulopathies induced by pamidronate. *Kidney Int* 2004; **65**: 634–641.

18 Meyrier A. Mechanisms of disease: focal segmental glomerulosclerosis. *Nat Clin Pract Nephrol* 2005; **1**: 44–54.

19 Kerjaschki D. Caught flat-footed: podocyte damage and the molecular bases of focal glomerulosclerosis. *J Clin Invest* 2001; **8**: 1583–1587.

20 Pavenstädt H, Kriz W, Kretzler M. Cell biology of the glomerular podocyte. *Physiol Rev* 2003; **83**: 253–307.

21 Shankland SJ, Eitner F, Hudkins KL, Goodpaster T, d'Agati V, Alpers CE. Differential expression of cyclin-dependent kinase inhibitors in human glomerular disease: role in podocyte proliferation and maturation. *Kidney Int* 2000; **58**: 674–683.

22 Bariety J, Nochy D, Mandet C, Jacquot C, Glotz D, Meyrier A. Podocytes undergo phenotypic changes and express macrophagic-associated markers in idiopathic collapsing glomerulopathy. *Kidney Int* 1998; **53**: 918–928.

23 Barisoni L, Kriz W, Mundel P, d'Agati V. The dysregulated podocyte phenotype; a novel concept in the pathogenesis of collapsing idiopathic focal segmental glomerulosclerosis and HIV-associated nephropathy. *J Am Soc Nephrol* 1999; **10**: 51–61.

24 Bariety J, Bruneval P, Hill G, Irinopoulou T, Mandet C, Meyrier A. Post-transplantation relapse of FSGS is characterized by glomerular epithelial cell transdifferentiation. *J Am Soc Nephrol* 2001; **12**: 261–274.

25 Feldman RD, Campbell N, Larochelle P, Bolli P, Burgess ED, Carruthers SG *et al.* Development of the 1999 Canadian recommendations for the management of hypertension. Task Force for the Development of the 1999 Canadian Recommendations for the Management of Hypertension. *CMAJ* 1999; **161(Suppl 12)**: S1–S17.

26 Howie AJ, Pankhurst T, Sarioglou S, Turhan N, Adu D. Evolution of nephrotic-associated focal segmental glomerulosclerosis and relation to the glomerular tip lesion. *Kidney Int* 2005; **67**: 987–1001.

27 Haas M. The glomerular tip lesion: what does it really mean? *Kidney Int* 2005; **67**: 1188–1189.

28 Stokes BM, Markowitz GS, Lin J, Valeri AM, D'Agati VD. Glomerular tip lesion. A distinct entity within the minimal change disease/focal segmental glomerulosclerosis spectrum. *Kidney Int* 2004; **65**: 1690–1702.

29 Troyanov S, Wall CA, Miller JA, Scholey JW, Cattran DC, Toronto Glomerulonephritis Registry Group. Focal and segmental glomerulosclerosis: definition and relevance of a partial remission. *J Am Soc Nephrol* 2005; **16**:1061–1068.

30 d'Agati VD, Fogo AB, Bruijn JA, Jennette JC. Pathologic classification of focal segmental glomerulosclerosis: a working proposal. *Am J Kidney Dis* 2004; **43**: 368–382.

31 Meyrier AY. Collapsing glomerulopathy: expanding interest in a shrinking tuft. *Am J Kidney Dis* 1999; **33**: 801–803.

32 Meyrier A. E pluribus unum: the riddle of focal-segmental glomerulosclerosis. *Semin Nephrol* 2003; **23**: 135–140.

33 Korbet SM. Treatment of primary focal segmental glomerulosclerosis. *J Am Soc Nephrol* 2002; **62**: 2301–2310.

34 Chun MJ, Korbet SM, Schwartz MM, Lewis EJ. Focal segmental glomerulosclerosis in nephrotic adults: presentation, prognosis, and response to therapy of the histologic variants. *J Am Soc Nephrol* 2004; **8**:2169–2177.

35 Cattran DC, Appel GB, Hebert LA, Hunsicker LG, Pohl MA, Hoy WE *et al.* A randomized trial of cyclosporine in patients with steroid-resistant focal segmental glomerulosclerosis. North America Nephrotic Syndrome Study Group. *Kidney Int* 1999; **56**: 2220–2226.

36 Ponticelli C, Villa M, Banfi G, Cesana B, Pozzi C, Pani A *et al.* Can prolonged treatment improve the prognosis in adults with focal segmental glomerulosclerosis? *Am J Kidney Dis* 1999; **34**: 618–625.

37 Alexopoulos E, Stangou M, Papagianni A, Pantzaki A, Papadimitriou M. Factors influencing the course and the response to treatment in primary focal segmental glomerulosclerosis. *Nephrol Dial Transplant* 2000; **15**: 1348–1356.

38 Nakayama M, Katafuchi R, Yanase T, Ikeda K, Tanaka H, Fujimi S. Steroid responsiveness and frequency of relapse in adult-onset minimal change nephrotic syndrome. *Am J Kidney Dis* 2002; **39**: 503–512.

39 Tse KC, Lam MF, Yip PS, Li FK, Choy BY, Lai KN *et al.* Idiopathic minimal change nephrotic syndrome in older adults: steroid responsiveness and pattern of relapses. *Nephrol Dial Transplant* 2003; **18**: 1316–1320.

40 Huang JJ, Hsu SC, Chen FF, Sung JM, Tseng CC, Wang MC. Adult onset minimal change disease among Taiwanese: clinical features, therapeutic response, and prognosis. *Am J Nephrol* 2001; **21**: 28–34.

41 Meyrier A. Treatment of idiopathic nephrosis by immunophillin modulation. *Nephrol Dial Transplant* 2003; **18(Suppl 6)**: vi79–vi86.

42 Tumlin JA, Miller D, Near M, Selvaraj S, Hennigar R, Guasch A. A prospective, open-label trial of sirolimus in the treatment of focal segmental glomerulonephritis. *Clin J Am Soc Nephrol* 2006; **1**: 109–116.

43 Sandoz Pharma. Sanimmun use in nephrotic syndrome, part IV B, clinical experience. Study OL-9507, vol. 5, p. 7.

44 Meyrier A, Condamin MC, Broneer D. Treatment of adult idiopathic nephrotic syndrome with cyclosporine A: minimal change disease and focal-segmental glomerulosclerosis. *Clin Nephrol* 1991; **35**: 37–42.

45 Meyrier A, Noël LH, Auriche P, Callard P. Long-term renal tolerance of cyclosporin A treatment in adult idiopathic nephrotic syndrome. *Kidney Int* 1994; **45**: 1446–1456.

46 Pokhariyal S, Gulati S, Prasad N, Sharma RK, Singh U, Gupta RK. Duration of therapy for idiopathic focal segmental glomerulosclerosis. *J Nephrol* 2003; **16**: 691–696.

47 Schwartz MM, Evans J, Bain R, Korbet SM. Focal segmental glomerulosclerosis: prognostic implication of the cellular lesion. *J Am Soc Nephrol* 1999; **10**: 1900–1907.

48 Valeri A, Barisoni L, Appel GB, Seigle R, D'Agati V. Idiopathic collapsing focal segmental glomerulosclerosis. *Kidney Int* 1996; **50** :1734–1746.

49 Cameron SJ. The nephrotic syndrome and its complications. *Am J Kidney Dis* 1987; **10**: 157–171.

50 Korbet SM. Clinical picture and outcome of primary focal segmental glomerulosclerosis. *Nephrol Dial Transpl* 1999; **14(Suppl 3)**: 68–73.

51 Nolasco F, Cameron JS, Heywood EF, Hicks J, Ogg C, Williams DG. Adult-onset minimal change nephrotic syndrome: a long-term follow-up. *Kidney Int* 1986; **29**: 1215–1223.

52 Korbet SM, Schwartz MM, Lewis EJ. Minimal-change glomerulopathy of adulthood. *Am J Nephrol* 1988; **8**: 291–297.

53 Fujimoto S, Yamamoto Y, Hisanaga S, Morita S, Eto T, Tanaka K. Minimal change nephrotic syndrome in adults: response to corticosteroid therapy and frequency of relapse. *Am J Kidney Dis* 1991; **17**: 687–692.

54 Mak SK, Short CD, Mallick NP. Long term outcome of adult-onset minimal change nephropathy. *Nephrol Dialysis Transplant* 1996; **11**: 2192–2201.

55 Serkova N, Christians U. Transplantation: toxicokinetics and mechanisms of toxicity of cyclosporine and macrolides. *Curr Opin Invest Drugs* 2003; **4**: 1287–1296.

56 Filler G. How should microemulsified cyclosporine A (Neoral®) therapy in patients with nephrotic syndrome be monitored? *Nephrol Dial Transplant* 2005; **20**:1032–1034.

57 Matsumoto H, Nakao T, Okada T, Nagaoka Y, Shino T, Yoshino M et al. Initial remission-inducing effect of very low-dose cyclosporine monotherapy for minimal-change nephrotic syndrome in Japanese adults. *Clin Nephrol* 2001; **55** :143–148.

58 Day CJ, Cockwell P, Lipkin GW, Savage CO, Howie AJ, Adu D. Mycophenolate mofetil in the treatment of resistant idiopathic nephrotic syndrome. *Nephrol Dial Transplant* 2002; **17**: 2011–2013.

59 Choi MJ, Eustace JA, Gimenez LF, Atta MG, Scheel PJ, Sothinathan R et al. Mycophenolate mofetil for primary glomerular diseases. *Kidney Int* 2002; **61**: 1098–1114.

60 Norona B, Valentin M, Gutierrez E, Praga M. Treatment of steroid-dependent minimal change nephrotic syndrome with mycophenolate mofetil. *Nefrologia* 2004; **24**: 79–82. (In Spanish.)

61 Braden GL, Mulhern JG, O'Shea MH, Nash SV, Ucci AA, Germain MJ. Changing incidence of glomerular diseases in adults. *Am J Kidney Dis* 2000; **35**: 878–883.

62 Dragovic D, Rosenstock JL, Wahl SJ, Panagopoulos G, DeVita MV, Michelis MF. Increasing incidence of focal segmental glomerulosclerosis and an examination of demographic patterns. *Clin Nephrol* 2005; **63**: 1–7.

63 Crook ED, Habeeb D, Gowdy O, Nimmagadda S, Salem M. Effects of steroids in focal segmental glomerulosclerosis in a predominantly African-American population. *Am J Med Sci* 2005; **330**: 19–24.

64 Ahmed MS, Wong CF. Rituximab and nephrotic syndrome: a new therapeutic hope? *Nephrol Dial Transplant* 2008; **23**: 11–17.

65 Deegens JK, Assmann KJ, Steenbergen EJ, Hilbrands LB, Gerlag PG, Jansen H et al. Idiopathic focal segmental glomerulosclerosis: a favourable prognosis in untreated patients? *Neth J Med* 2005; **63**: 393–398.

66 Korbet S, Schwartz M, Lewis E. Primary focal segmental glomerulosclerosis: clinical course and response to therapy. *Am J Kidney Dis* 1994; **23**: 773–783.

67 Korbet SM. Management of idiopathic nephrosis in adults, including steroid-resistant nephrosis. *Curr Opin Nephrol Hypertens* 1995; **4**: 169–176.

68 Meyrier A. Treatment of focal segmental glomerulosclerosis. *Expert Opin Pharmacother* 2005; **6**: 1539–1549.

69 Stirling CM, Mathieson P, Boulton-Jones JM, Feehally J, Jayne D, Murray HM et al. Treatment and outcome of adult patients with primary focal segmental glomerulosclerosis in five UK units. *Q J Med* 2005; **98**: 443–449.

70 Heering P, Braun N, Mullejans R, Ivens K, Zauner J, Funfstuck R et al. Cyclosporine A and chlorambucil in the treatment of idiopathic focal segmental glomerulosclerosis. *Am J Kidney Dis* 2004; **43**: 10–18.

71 Martinelli R, Pereira LJ, Silva OMM, Okumura AS, Rocha H. Cyclophosphamide in the treatment of focal segmental glomerulosclerosis. *Braz J Med Biol Res* 2004; **37**: 1365–1372.

72 Segarra A, Vila J, Pou L, Majo J, Arbos A, Quiles T et al. Combined therapy of tacrolimus and corticosteroids in cyclosporin-resistant or -dependent idiopathic focal glomerulosclerosis: a preliminary uncontrolled study with prospective follow-up. *Nephrol Dial Transplant* 2002; **17**: 655–662.

73 Duncan N, Dhaygude A, Owen J, Cairns TD, Griffith M, LcLean AG et al. Treatment of focal and segmental glomerulosclerosis in adults with tacrolimus monotherapy. *Nephrol Dial Transplant* 2004; **19**: 3062–3067.

74 Voehringer M, Keller F. Effect of sirolimus on nephrotic syndrome and renal function in 7 patients with focal sclerosing glomerulonephritis. *J Am Soc Nephrol* 2004; **15**: 555A.

75 Tumlin JA, Miller D, Near M, Selvaraj S, Hennigar R, Guasch A. A prospective, open-label trial of sirolimus in the treatment of focal segmental glomerulonephritis. *Clin J Am Soc Nephrol* 2006; **1**: 109–116.

76 Choi MJ, Eustace JA, Gimenez LF, Atta MG, Scheel PJ, Sothinathan R et al. Mycophenolate mofetil for primary glomerular diseases. *Kidney Int* 2002; **61**: 1098–1114.

77 Cattran DC, Wang MM, Appel G, Matalon A, Briggs W. Mycophenolate mofetil in the treatment of focal segmental glomerulosclerosis. *Clin Nephrol* 2004; **62** :405–411.

78 Segarra A, Amoedo ML, Martinez Garcia JM, Pons S, Praga M, Garcia EI et al. Efficacy and safety of 'rescue therapy' with MMF in resistant primary glomerulonephritis: a multicentre study. *Nephrol Dial Transpl* 2007; **22**: 1351–1360.

79 Shalhoub RJ. Pathogenesis of lipoid nephrosis: a disorder of T cell function. *Lancet* 1974; **ii**: 556–559.

80 Matalon A, Markowitz GS, Joseph RE, Cohen DJ, Saal SD, Kaplan B et al. Plasmapheresis treatment of recurrent FSGS in adult renal transplant recipients. *Clin Nephrol* 2001; **56**: 271–278.

81 Davenport RD. Apheresis treatment of recurrent focal segmental glomerulosclerosis after kidney transplantation: re-analysis of published case-reports and case-series. *J Clin Apher* 2001; **16**: 175–178.

82 Shariatmadar S, Noto TA. Therapeutic plasma exchange in recurrent focal segmental glomerulosclerosis following transplantation. *J Clin Apher* 2002; **17** :78–83.

83 Otsubo S, Tanabe K, Shinmura H, Ishikawa N, Tokumoto T, Hattori M et al. Effect of post-transplant double filtration plasmapheresis on recurrent focal and segmental glomerulosclerosis in renal transplant recipients. *Ther Apher Dial* 2004; **8**: 299–304.

84 Valdivia P, Gonzalez Roncero F, Gentil MA et al. Plasmapheresis for the prophylaxis and treatment of recurrent focal segmental glomerulosclerosis following renal transplant. *Transplant Proc* 2005; **37**: 1473–1474.

85 Gohh RY, Yango AF, Morrissey PE, Monaco AP, Gautam A, Sharma M et al. Preemptive plasmapheresis and recurrence of FSGS in high-risk renal transplant recipients. *Am J Transplant* 2005; **5**: 2907–2912.

86 Pardon A, Audard V, Caillard S, Moulin B, Desvaux D, Bentaari B et al. Risk factors and outcome of focal and segmental glomerulosclerosis recurrence in adult renal transplant recipients. *Nephrol Dial Transplant* 2006; **21**:1053–1059.

87 Bosch T, Wendler T. Extracorporeal plasma treatment in primary and recurrent focal segmental glomerular sclerosis: a review. *Ther Apher* 2001; **5** :155–160.

88 Dantal J, Bigot E, Bogers W, Testa A, Kriaa F, Jacques Y et al. Effect of plasma protein adsorption in kidney-transplant recipients with recurrent nephrotic syndrome. *N Engl J Med* 1994; **330**: 7–14.

89 Esnault VL, Besnier D, Testa A, Coville P, Simon P, Subra JF et al. Effect of protein A immunoadsorption in nephrotic syndrome of various etiologies. *J Am Soc Nephrol* 1999; **10**: 2014–2017.

90 Nijland MJM. Fetal exposure to corticosteroids: how low can we go? *J Physiol* 2003; **549(1)**: 1.

91 Bar Oz B, Hackman R, Einarson T, Koren G. Pregnancy outcome after cyclosporine therapy during pregnancy: a meta-analysis. *Transplantation* 2002; **71** :1051–1055.

92 Armenti GT. Immunosuppression and teratology: evolving guidelines. *J Am Soc Nephrol* 2004; **15**: 2759–2760.

93 Armenti VT, Radomski JS, Moritz MJ, Gaughan WJ, McGrory CH, Coscia LA. Report from the National Transplantation Pregnancy Registry (NTPR): outcomes of pregnancy after transplantation. *Clin Transpl* 2003; **2003**: 131–141.

14 Membranous Nephropathy

Fernando C. Fervenza[1] & Daniel C. Cattran[2]

[1]Division of Nephrology and Hypertension, Mayo Clinic College of Medicine, Rochester, USA
[2]Department of Medicine, University of Toronto, Toronto, Ontario, Canada

Introduction

Idiopathic membranous nephropathy (MN) is a relatively common immune-mediated glomerular disease and remains the leading cause of nephrotic syndrome (NS) in Caucasian adults. Its incidence rate has remained constant over the past 3 decades, in contrast to other primary glomerular diseases, such as immunoglobulin A (IgA) nephropathy and focal segmental glomerulosclerosis [1,2]. In the majority of cases, the etiological agent is unknown, and the disorder is termed idiopathic. Secondary MN forms may account for up to one-third of cases and are associated with autoimmune diseases (e.g. systemic lupus erythematosus [SLE]), infections (e.g. hepatitis B and C), medications (e.g. nonsteroidal anti-inflammatory drugs [NSAIDs], D-penicillamine, gold), and neoplasias (e.g. carcinomas) [3]. The association with malignancy increases with age of the patient, reaching up to 20% in patients over the age of 60. Because idiopathic and secondary forms have similar clinical presentations, the designation of idiopathic is made only after ruling out secondary causes by a careful history, physical examination, and laboratory evaluation of the patient. It is crucial to rule out secondary causes of MN, because the management of these cases is directed towards removing or correcting the underlying cause. The disease is rare in children, and when it does occur, it is commonly associated with an immunologically mediated disorder such as SLE.

Natural history

MN is a chronic disease, with spontaneous remission and relapses. There is great variability in the rate of disease progression, and the natural course is difficult to assess in part due to the different criteria the nephrologist uses to select patients for biopsy, as well as geographic variability and genetic characteristics of the subjects

that have been presented in the different studies [4–6]. Much of the data comes from studies that included patients with both idiopathic MN and secondary MN as well as treated and untreated patients [7]. In addition, the majority of studies were conducted prior to the availability of agents that could potentially modify the natural course of the disease, such as angiotensin converting enzyme inhibitors (ACEi). Spontaneous remissions are said to occur in up to 30% of cases, usually in the first 2 years after presentation, but this may happen at any time over the course of the illness. The proportion of patients going into spontaneous remission is much lower when patients are selected who have higher grades of proteinuria at presentation, for example, proteinuria of >8 g/24 h. The remaining two-thirds of patients who do not undergo spontaneous remission generally divide equally into either those with persistent proteinuria who will maintain renal function long term or those patients who will progress to kidney failure. In Caucasian patients with NS, 10-year kidney survival of <70% has been reported [4,8–11]. Because of its high incidence rate, MN remains the second or third leading cause of end-stage renal disease (ESRD) among the primary glomerulonephritis types [12]. Even patients who do not progress but remain nephrotic are at an increased risk for life-threatening thromboembolic and cardiovascular events. A rapid change in either the degree of proteinuria or in the rate of loss of renal function, especially in a previously stable patient, should raise the possibility of a superimposed condition, for example, interstitial nephritis, anti-glomerular basement membrane disease, or renal vein thrombosis.

Clinical manifestations

The disease affects patients of all ages and races, but it is more common in men than women by a 2:1 to 3:1 ratio. Idiopathic MN is most often diagnosed in middle-aged patients, with the peak incidence during the fourth and fifth decades of life, and is relatively uncommon in patients under 20 years. At presentation, 60–70% of patients will have NS. The remaining 30–40% of cases present with proteinuria of <3.5 g/24 h and are most commonly found at

Evidence-based Nephrology. Edited by Donald Molony and Jonathan Craig
© 2009 Blackwell Publishing, ISBN: 978-1-4051-3975-5.

the time of a routine examination in an otherwise-asymptomatic patient. The presence of microscopic hematuria is common (30–40%), but macroscopic hematuria and red cell casts are rare and suggest a different histopathology. In patients with idiopathic MN, serum C3 and C4 complement levels are always normal. At presentation, the great majority of patients are normotensive, with only 10–20% having hypertension, and only a small fraction of patients (<10%) having significant renal insufficiency. Patients with MN have significant abnormalities in their lipid profile and are at increased risk for thromboembolic events.

Predicting factors

Evaluating the prognosis is critical in making decisions regarding when and what to use in terms of treatment, for example, conservative versus immunosuppressive treatment in patients with MN [13–15]. An accurate predictor of outcome of patients with idiopathic MN would allow separation of those patients who are likely to have a long-term renal survival without treatment from those who are likely to progress. This would allow us to target immunosuppressive treatment to patients at high risk of renal disease progression. However, finding useful markers that predict this last group has been difficult. Many individual factors, such as advanced age, male gender, and selected biopsy findings (e.g. degree of interstitial fibrosis, glomerulosclerosis, vascular damage, or glomeruli with focal segmental glomerulosclerosis) have all been found to be predictors of prognosis and/or response to immunosuppressive therapy in patients with MN [16]. In addition, the degree of proteinuria may also predict those who are most likely to progress. Pei *et al.* observed a 47% risk for progression in patients with proteinuria of >4 g/24 h for longer than 18 months and a 66% risk in patients with proteinuria of >8 g/24 h for more than 6 months [17]. Urinary excretion ratios of α_1-microglobulin, β_2-microglobulin, IgM, and IgG have also been found to be strong predictors of outcome in MN [18–21]. Determining these ratios has been helpful in assessing the severity of overall renal injury and to predict those who are most likely to respond to immunosuppressive therapy [22]. Unfortunately, methods for quantification of urinary α_1-microglobulin, β_2-microglobulin, IgM, and IgG are not widely available and this limits their clinical use. There is also concern with the establishment of cutoff values for these ratios because they may reflect activity only at certain times during the course of the disease and under certain conditions, which may vary widely over time and be independent of the activity of the primary disease. The degree of renal impairment at presentation has also been found to correlate with long-term renal survival. However, renal function at presentation is widely variable and may be independent of disease severity. A recent study by Hladunewich *et al.* that used glomerular filtration rate (GFR) determinations based on inulin clearance indicated that, among patients with MN, for those with nephrotic-range proteinuria the presenting GFR may be artificially low [23]. Estimating renal function by using a serum creatinine value is also problematic in these patients because in NS

there is an increase in the tubular secretion of creatinine which may result in a marked overestimation of the GFR [24]. Thus, the use of immunosuppressive treatment limited only to those patients who exhibit deterioration in renal function, based on reaching a determined serum creatinine threshold, e.g. ≥1.5 mg/dL, may result in delaying treatment beyond the point at which the kidney damage may still be reversible.

Thus far, the best model for the identification of patients at risk was developed with data derived from the Toronto Glomerulonephritis Registry [17,25]. This model takes into consideration the initial creatinine clearance (CrCl), the slope of the CrCl curve, and the lowest level of proteinuria during a 6-month observation period. This risk score assessment has good performance characteristics and to date is the only one that has been validated in two geographically diverse MN populations, one from Italy and the other from Finland [25]. Based on data using this model, patients who present with a normal CrCl, proteinuria of ≤4 g/24 h, and stable renal function over a 6-month observation period have an excellent long-term prognosis. Patients whose CrCl remains unchanged during 6 months of observation but who continue to have proteinuria of >4 g but <8 g/24 h have a 55% probability of developing chronic renal insufficiency, and patients with persistent proteinuria of >8 g/24 h, independent of the degree of renal dysfunction, have a 66–80% probability of progression to chronic kidney failure within 10 years. On the other hand, patients with MN who were never nephrotic have an excellent long-term renal survival. A review of this algorithm has recently been published [12].

Response measurements

The best-accepted responses are improved renal survival and complete remission (CR) of proteinuria. About 30% of MN cases will relapse subsequent to a CR [26]. The great majority who do, however, will relapse to sub-nephrotic-range proteinuria and will have stable long-term function. More recently, partial remission (PR) has been also recognized as a positive outcome. A recent review of 350 nephrotic patients with MN found that the 10-year renal survival was 100% in the CR group, 90% in the PR group, and 45% in the no-remission group [27]. Patients with CR or PR have a similar rate of decline: −1.5 mL/min/year in the CR group and −2 mL/min/year in the PR group. In contrast, the no-remission group lost GFR at a rate of −10 mL/min/year. Thus, both CR and PR appear to be excellent predictors of long-term renal survival. In the two largest studies of patients with MN who achieved CR, only a few developed mild renal insufficiency, over a long observation period, and none progressed to ESRD.

Treatment

Using the algorithm for predicting outcome described above, we can rationally assign patients to conservative, nonimmunosuppressive therapy or to immunosuppressive therapy according to their risk for renal disease progression.

Conservative therapy

Conservative therapy is based on controlling edema, dietary protein intake, blood pressure, and hyperlipidemia. Dietary protein intake should be restricted to 0.8 g of high-quality protein/kg ideal body weight/day, as protein restriction may reduce proteinuria (15–25%) and slow renal disease progression. Blood pressure control is important both as protection against cardiovascular events and to reduce proteinuria and slow the progression of the renal disease. In the Modification of Diet in Renal Disease study, patients with proteinuria of >1 g/day had a significantly better outcome if their blood pressure was reduced to 125/75 mmHg [28]. Thus, in patients with proteinuric renal disease, including MN, the current target for blood pressure is ≤125/75 mmHg. ACEi and/or angiotensin receptor blockers (ARBs) are effective antihypertensive agents that can reduce proteinuria and slow progression of renal disease in both diabetic and nondiabetic chronic nephropathy patients, and for these reasons they are the preferred agents to treat hypertension in proteinuric renal diseases. However, the following issues need to be considered when using an ACEi and/or an ARB in patients with MN: 1) The degree of renal protection is related to the degree of proteinuria reduction, and if proteinuria is not lowered, the benefit is substantially attenuated. 2) In patients with MN, the antiproteinuric effect is modest (<30% decrease) and is more significant in patients with lower levels of proteinuria [29–31]. 3) In contrast to other proteinuric renal diseases, for example, diabetes mellitus, ACEi may not offer the same degree of renal protection to patients with MN [31]. In studies by du Buf-Vereijken *et al.* [11] and in a review by Troyanov *et al.* [26], the use of ACEi or ARBs when subjected to multivariate analysis did not have independent value in determining the prognosis for patients with MN. Furthermore, Praga *et al.* showed that in patients with NS, the majority of which had MN, ACEi were ineffective in reducing proteinuria, and this poor antiproteinuric response in MN patients was associated with a poor renal function outcome [33,34]. In those patients with a significant antiproteinuric response, the effect is usually seen within 2 months of initiation of therapy [29]. Thus, for patients with lower levels of proteinuria (<4 g/24 h), treatment with and ACEi and/or an ARB may be enough to reduce proteinuria to subnephrotic levels with little chance of significant adverse effect. However, in patients with higher degrees of proteinuria, the use of these medications alone is unlikely to result in a substantial reduction in proteinuria or preservation of renal function. Patients need to be instructed to follow a low-salt diet, because high salt intake (e.g. 200 mg Na or 4.6 g sodium/day) can significantly impair the beneficial effects of angiotensin II blockade.

Lipid abnormalities associated with proteinuria are likely important players in the high cardiovascular risk seen in these patients and provide an important target for treatment. Statins may have a synergistic antiproteinuric effect when combined with ACEi, but this effect is small and mainly observed in patients with proteinuria of <3 g/24 h. When used in combination with high-dose cyclosporine (CsA), statins may increase the risk of rhabdomyolysis.

Patients with severe NS are at increased risk for thromboembolic complications. Mahmoodi *et al.* recently reported on the incidence of thromboembolism in a cohort of 298 patients with NS [35]. During a mean follow-up of 10 years, 29 patients had at least one episode of venous thromboembolism (VTE) and 43 had at least one episode of arterial thromboembolism (ATE). The resulting annual incidence rates for VTE and ATE were 1.02% and 1.48%, respectively. However, the incidence of VTE and ATE was considerably higher in the first 6 months following the diagnosis of NS (9.85% and 5.52% for VTE and ATE, respectively) [35]. Prophylactic anticoagulation has been shown in retrospective reviews to be beneficial in reducing fatal thromboembolic episodes in nephrotic patients with MN without a concomitant increase in the risk of bleeding [36]. In general, MN patients who are severely nephrotic (proteinuria of >10 g/day and serum albumin of <2.5 g/day) are candidates for anticoagulation.

In severe untreatable NS, NSAIDs can reduce proteinuria by 30–50%, are additive to the effects of ACEi, and can provide symptomatic relief [37,38]. The combined use of NSAIDs and ACEi or ARBs should be conducted under careful monitoring, especially in elderly patients and in those with hypertension and renal insufficiency, because acute and nonreversible renal failure may ensue.

Immunosuppressive therapy

Several treatment strategies, including a variety of immunosuppressive agents, have been shown to be at least partially successful in reducing proteinuria in MN [39]. The available evidence is presented according to the risk group (e.g. low, medium, and high) that the patients in the studies most closely represent.

Treatment of low-risk patients

Patients in the low-risk group are categorized by a <5% risk for progression over 5 years of observation. They are defined by normal renal function and proteinuria of ≤4 g/24 h over a 6-month observation period. Evidence to support this approach comes from published validation studies and from recent data on the clinical relevance of PR [25,27]. Treatment should be conservative only, given the excellent prognosis of this group of patients when untreated.

Treatment of medium-risk patients

Patients in the medium-risk group are defined by normal renal function and persistent proteinuria between 4 and 8 g/24 h over 6 months of observation despite the institution of maximum conservative therapy.

Corticosteroids

The early US collaborative study of adult idiopathic NS reported that a 2- to 3-month course of high-dose alternate-day prednisone resulted in a significant reduction, compared to placebo, in progression to renal failure, although there was no effect on the degree of proteinuria [40]. Subsequently, the Toronto Glomerulonephritis Study Group conducted a prospective randomized study in which patients were assigned to receive either a 6-month course of prednisone given on alternate days ($n = 81$) or no specific

Table 14.1 Corticosteroids treatment in idiopathic membranous nephropathy

Author	Year	Level of Evidence	Risk group	N	Treatment regimens	Follow-up (months)	Outcomes/comments
CSAINS [40]	1979	1	Medium	72	Prednisone 100–150 mg p.o. on alternate days × 8–12 weeks vs. placebo	23	10 of 38 controls, but only 1 of 34 given prednisone had SCr > 5mg/dl or died. Rapid decline of renal function in controls considered unexpected.
Cattran [41]	1989	1	Medium	158	Prednisone 125–150 mg p.o. on alternate days × 6 mos vs. placebo	48	Proportion of patients with CR similar in the 2 groups. No differences in annual change in CrCl between the 2 groups. No sustained difference in proteinuria
Cameron [42]	1990	1	High	107	Prednisolone 45 mg/m² on alternate days × 8 weeks vs placebo	52	No difference in remission rates for NS in either short (6 and 12 months) or long (48 months) term. No differences in rates of renal function decline
Short [43]	1987	5	High	15	MTP 1g I.v. × 5 days followed by prednisolone 100 mg, 75 mg 50 mg, then 25 mg on alternate days for 4 weeks; then dose decreasing by a further 5 mg each month	32	Serum creatinine fell by a mean of 46%. In 10 patients the beneficial effect was sustained, but in 3 it had reversed by six months. In the other 2 patients the progressive decline of renal function was not influenced

Abbreviations are: p.o., oral; NS, nephrotic syndrome; MTP, methylprednisolone; SCr, serum creatinine; CrCl, creatinine clearance

treatment ($n = 77$) [41]. Patients in the prednisone group entered the study with a median CrCl of 72 mL/min/1.73 m² (range, 15–156) and a median rate of urinary protein excretion of 6.8 g/24 h (range, 0.3–26). The study showed no significant benefit of corticosteroid treatment alone in either induction of remission or preservation of renal function, even after the data were adjusted to include only patients with proteinuria at entry of >3.5 g/24 h [41]. Whether greater and more prolonged courses of prednisone, as in patients with idiopathic focal segmental glomerulosclerosis, may prove more effective in MN is unknown, but this approach is likely to be associated with significant steroid toxicity. These studies are summarized in Table 14.1 [40–43].

Cytotoxic agents combined with corticosteroids
In patients with a moderate risk of progression, a number of randomized trials have suggested that monthly cycling of steroids and cytotoxic agents is four to five times more likely to induce CR of NS, and halt disease progression, compared to no therapy or corticosteroids alone. The largest studies and with the longest follow-up were conducted by Ponticelli's group. The first study compared the effects of 6-month cycles of methylprednisolone (MTP) administered intravenously and oral steroids alternating monthly with chlorambucil, compared to conservative treatment [44]. CR was achieved in 50%, and PR was found in 31% of the cases. Among the controls, CR was achieved in 7% and PR in 24% of the patients. After up to 10 years of follow-up, patients treated with combination therapy had a 92% probability of renal survival compared with 60% in the control group, and only 8% of treated patients versus 40% of untreated ones had reached ESRD [45]. Women and patients with mild glomerular lesions (stages 1 and 2) were more likely to enter remission after therapy in this study. A second study

compared 6 months of alternating monthly pulses of MTP plus oral steroids and chlorambucil cycled as described above versus MTP pulses plus steroids alone, and the investigators found at 3 years that 66% of the patients given steroids and chlorambucil versus 42% of patients given steroids alone were in remission; this differences was significant [46]. At 4 years this difference was no longer statistically significant, although a seemingly large 20% difference favoring the combined treatment persisted. In a third study from the same investigators, patients were enrolled in a 6-month study comparing MTP pulses on months 1, 3, and 5 followed by oral prednisone alternating monthly with either chlorambucil (same doses as in prior studies) or oral cyclophosphamide [47]. The study showed that 82% of patients assigned to MTP and chlorambucil versus 93% of patients assigned to MTP and cyclophosphamide entered a complete or partial remission of the NS ($P = 0.116$, not significant). The use of cyclophosphamide was associated with fewer side effects, but renal function was equally preserved in both groups for up to 3 years.

These observations have been recently confirmed by Jha et al., who reported the 10-year follow-up of a randomized controlled trial on 93 patients allocated to either conservative therapy or to receive a 6-month course of alternating predisolone [48]. Proteinuria was 5.9 ± 2.2 and 6.1 ± 2.5 g/24 h in the conservative and immunosuppressive therapy groups, respectively. Renal function was well-preserved, with estimated GFRs above 80 mL/min in both groups. Of the 47 patients treated with immunosuppressive therapy, 34 achieved remission (15 CR and 19 PR), compared with 16 (5 CR and 11 PR) of 46 in the control group ($P < 0.0001$). The 10-year dialysis-free survival was 89 and 65% ($P = 0.016$), and the likelihood of survival without death, dialysis, or doubling of serum creatinine was 79% in the treated group versus 44% in the control group ($P = 0.0006$). The incidence of infections was similar in the two groups [48].

Thus, in a number of studies, both cyclophosphamide and chlorambucil in combination with corticosteroids appear to be effective in the treatment of patients with idiopathic MN and preserved renal function, with benefits maintained well beyond the 1-year treatment period, although relapse rates approached 35% at 2 years. The long-term adverse effects of these cytotoxic agents, in particular, effects on fertility and also malignancy are the major drawbacks to the universal application of this form of therapy. A recent publication suggests that the risk of malignancy is not increased for patients treated with cumulative cyclophosphamide doses of ≤ 36 g but increases significantly in patients with cumulative cyclophosphamide doses of ≥ 36 g [49]. These studies are summarized in Table 14.2 [45–48,50–61].

Cyclosporine A

Early uncontrolled studies of CsA suggested an initial benefit but a high relapse rate [31,62]. In the first single-blind randomized controlled study, 51 patients with steroid-resistant MN were treated with low-dose prednisone plus CsA and compared to patients treated with placebo plus prednisone [63]. At the end of 26 weeks of treatment, 75% of patients (21 of 28) in the CsA group versus only 22% of patients (5 of 23) in the controls had achieved a PR or CR ($P < 0.001$) (CR in two patients in the CsA group versus one in the placebo group). CsA was well-tolerated, and no subjects had to discontinue treatment because of adverse effects. Relapses occurred in about 40% of patients within 1 year of discontinuation of CsA treatment; this is a very similar relapse rate to that seen with combined cytotoxic agent–corticosteroid regimens. Relapses should not be considered failure of therapy, because reintroduction of CsA or its alternative, that is, the cytotoxic agent–corticosteroid regimen, are usually capable of inducing another remission. Data from the German Cyclosporine in NS Study Group suggest that prolonging CsA treatment (>1 year) results in a higher (34% CR at 1 year) and more sustained rate of remission [64]. Taken together, these data suggest that CsA can induce a remission (CR or PR) of NS in 50–60% of patients. Prolonged low-dose CsA (~ 1.5 mg/kg/day) could be considered for long-term maintenance of patients who achieve CR or PR, especially in patients at high risk for relapse [65]. It is important to emphasize that although reduction of proteinuria usually occurs within a few weeks, the majority of CR occurred after more than 6 months of treatment. On the other hand, if after 3–4 months of CsA therapy at adequate doses proteinuria is not significantly reduced, it is unlikely that the therapy will be effective. Significant adverse effects, including hypertension and nephrotoxicity, can accompany prolonged CsA treatment. The latter is dose and duration dependent as well as age dependent. These studies are summarized in Table 14.3 [31,66–69].

Tacrolimus

An alternative to CsA was reported in a recent study by Praga *et al.* which evaluated tacrolimus (TAC) monotherapy in idiopathic MN [70]. In this study, 25 patients with normal renal function (mean proteinuria, ~ 8 g/24 h) received TAC (0.05 mg/kg day) over 12 months with a 6-month taper, whereas 23 patients served as controls. After 18 months, the probability of remission was 94% in the TAC group but only 35% in the control group. Six patients in the control group and only one in the TAC group reached the secondary end point of a 50% increase in serum creatinine [70]. Unfortunately, almost half of the patients relapsed after TAC was withdrawn, and similar to patients treated with CsA, maintenance of remission may require prolonged use of TAC at a low dose.

Treatment of high-risk patients

Patients in the high-risk group are characterized by progressive loss of renal function and/or by persistent high-grade proteinuria of ≥ 8 g/24 h during the 6 months of observation.

Corticosteroids

The UK Medical Research Council study, a randomized, prospective, double-blind, controlled trial, assessed the medium-term effect of an 8-week course of high-dose prednisolone in this patient population [42]. A total of 103 patients with preserved renal function (average CrCl, 88 ± 30 mL/min) were randomized to the treatment group ($n = 52$) or to the control group ($n = 51$). Entry 24-h urinary protein excretion was 10.8 ± 6 in the treated group versus 10.4 ± 5 in the control group. At 36 months, there was no significant difference regarding the degree of proteinuria between the control and the treatment group. Similarly, there were no differences with regard to loss of renal function between the treatment and control groups (Table 14.1) [40–43]. Renal function did deteriorate equally in both groups, confirming that this study population was indeed high risk.

Cytotoxic agents combined with corticosteroids

There has not been a randomized, controlled trial of cytotoxic agents plus corticosteroids in this high-risk group. A summary of the studies conducted in this group of patients is presented in Table 14.2 [45–47,50–61].

Cyclosporine

There has been only one controlled trial with CsA in patients with high-grade proteinuria and progressive renal failure. In this study, 17 patients of the initial 64 MN patients who had a loss in CrCl of ≥ 8 mL/min during the 12-month observation period were randomly assigned to either CsA treatment (9 patients) or placebo (8 patients) for 12 months (phase 2) [69]. At the time of initiation of treatment, the average CrCl of these patients was in the mid-50s, and they had an average proteinuria of 11 g/day. After 12 months, there was a significant reduction in proteinuria, and the rate of loss (slope) of renal function in the CsA group was reduced from -2.4 to -0.7 mL/min/month, whereas in the placebo group the change was insignificant, -2.2 to -2.1 mL/min/month ($P < 0.02$). This improvement was sustained in $\sim 50\%$ of the patients for up to 2 years after CsA was stopped (Table 14.3) [33,66–69].

Table 14.2 Cytotoxic treatment in idiopathic membranous nephropathy

Author	Year	Level of Evidence	Risk group	N	Treatment regimens	Mean Follow-up (months)	Outcomes/comments
Ponticelli [51]	1984	1	Medium	67	MTP 1g i.v. × 3 days followed by MTP 0.4 mg/kg p.o. × 27 days, on months 1, 3 and 5 and CHL (0.2 mg/kg/d) on months 2, 4 and 6, vs. symptomatic therapy.	31	At the end of follow-up 23 of 32 treated patients (72%) were in CR or PR, as compared with 9 out of 30 controls (30%).
Ponticelli [46]	1992	1	Medium	92	MTP 1g, i.v. × 3 days; followed by MTP 0.4 mg/kg p.o. × 27 days, on months 1, 3 and 5 and CHL (0.2 mg/kg/d) on months 2, 4 and 6, vs MTP alone	48	At 3 years, 66% remission in MTP/CHL group vs 40% in MTP group. At 4 years, the difference was no longer statistically significant.
Ponticelli [45]	1995	1	Medium	67	MTP 1g i.v. × 3 days followed by prednisone 0.5 mg/kg/d × 27 days on months 1, 3 and 5 and CHL (0.2 mg/kg/d) on months 2, 4 and 6, vs symptomatic therapy	120	92% probability of renal survival in treated compared with 60% in the control group. 8% of treated patients vs. 40% of the untreated group reached ESRD.
Ponticelli [47]	1998	1	Medium	87	MTP 1g i.v. × 3 days followed by MTP 0.4 mg/kg/d p.o. × 27 days on months 1, 3 and 5 alternating with either CHL 0.2 mg/kg/d or CYC 2.5 mg/kg/d on months 2, 4 and 6	36	CR/PR in 82% of patients on MTP/CHL vs 93% on MTP/CYC ($P = $ NS). Side effects lower in the MTP/CYC group
Jha [48]	2007	1	Medium	93	MTP 1 g i.v. × 3 days followed by prednisolone 0.5 mg/kg/d p.o. × 27 days on months 1, 3 and 5 and CYC 2 mg/kg/d on months 2, 4, and 6, vs. conservative therapy	120	CR/PR in 72% of patients on MTP/CYC vs 35% in control group
Murphy [52]	1992	2	Medium	40	CYC 1.5 mg/kg × 6 months + DIP/W24 X 2 years vs symptomatic therapy		Treatment group had less proteinuria. No differences in renal function at 2 years
Donadio [50]	1974	2	Medium	22	CYC 1.5 to 2.5 mg/kg p.o. × 1 year vs. symptomatic therapy	12	No benefit of CYC on proteinuria, renal function, or histology
Falk [56]	1992	2	High	26	Prednisone 2 mg/kg on alternate days × 8 weeks, tapered over 4 weeks, vs. CYC 0.5–1 g/m² i.v. monthly × 6 months, + MTP (7 mg/kg) × 3 followed by prednisone (2 mg/kg/alternate days) for 8 weeks, then tapered over next 4 weeks.	29	No impact of CYC on renal function, level of proteinuria, or progression to ESRD
West [53]	1987	4	High	26	CYC 2 mg/kg × 20 ± 4 months ± prednisone vs. prednisone or symptomatic therapy	49	CYC associated with an increased rate of remission of NS and better preservation of renal function. Adverse effects were significant.
Jindal [57]	1992	4	High	9	CYC (1–2 mg/kg/d) for a mean of 23. ± 4 months (8 to 54) ± prednisone (6/9 patients; dose 33 ± 9 mg/d) compared to 17 controls receiving prednisone, max. dose 50–125 mg alternate days in 9/17 and 40–80 mg in 6/17, for a mean of 20 ± 4 months.	64–83	CR in 4/9 and PR in 5/9 in CYC group. One patient in the CYC group and 10 patients in control group reached ESRD. Four relapses in 3 treated patients, and 3 of 4 responded to repeat therapy. Of the 7 controls who did not reach ESRD, only 2 had persistent NS.
Torres [60]	2002	4	High	19	Prednisone (1 mg/kg/d month 1 0.5 mg/kg/d month 2, 0.5 mg/kg/d months 3 to 6) together with CHL 0.15 mg/kg/d for the first 14 weeks, vs. historic control group on symptomatic therapy	48	At the end of follow-up, 65% of patients in the control group had reached ESRD, 10% had advanced renal failure, and 25% had died. Majority of treated patients showed stabilization or improvement of renal function.

(continued)

Table 14.2 (cont.)

Author	Year	Level of Evidence	Risk group	N	Treatment regimens	Mean Follow-up (months)	Outcomes/comments
Bruns [55]	1991	5	High	11	CYC, 100 mg/d in all patients + prednisone (60–100 mg alternate days) in 10/11 patients, for 1 year	24–25	Serum creatinine decreased in 10 patients on combined therapy by 6 months and remained stable in 7/8 followed long-term. Proteinuria decreased from 11.9 to 2.3 g/d. Similar course observed in the 1 patient on CYC alone.
Warwick [58]	1994	5	High	21	Prednisolone 125 mg alternate days on months 1, 3 and 5 and CHL 10 mg/d on months 2, 4 and 6. Later patients received MTP 1g i.v. × 3 at the start first cycle of treatment. Four patients were retreated.	39	Renal function stable or improved in 11/21 patients (52%). Of these 11, PR in 4 and CR in 2. Serum creatinine >5.7 mg/dl or ESRD in 6 patients (29%). 3 patients died. Side effects + significant complications related to therapy in >50% of patients.
Branten [59]	1998	5	High	32	MTP 1g i.v. × 3 days, followed by prednisone (0.5 mg/kg/d months 1, 3 and 5), and CHL (0.15 mg/kg/d months 2, 4 and 6); or CYC (1.5–2 mg/kg/d for 1 year) + steroids in a comparable dose.	26–38	Renal function improved in both groups but the improvement was short-lived in the CHL group. Remissions of proteinuria more frequent after CYC treatment (15/17 vs. 5/15). CHL associated with more side effects.
Du Buf-Vereijken [61]	2004	5	High	65	MTP 1g i.v. × 3 days at months 1, 3 and 5, and prednisone 0.5 mg/kg/48h for 6 months + CYC (1.5–2 mg/kg/d) × 12 months	51	Renal function improved or stabilized in all patients. At the end of follow-up, CR in 16, PR in 31, 4 progressed to ESRD, and 5 patients had died. Overall survival 86% after 5 years.
Mathieson [54]	1988	6	High	8	MTP 1g i.v. × 3 days; 0.5 mg/kg/d p.o. × 27 days, then CHL 0.15–0.2 mg/kg × 28 days × 3 cycles	8	Renal function improved in 6, stabilized in 1, and deteriorated in 1 patient. Proteinuria fell from 15 to 2 g/d. Side effects were severe.

Abbreviations are: MTP, methylprednisolone; CYC, cyclophosphamide; CHL, chlorambucil; DIP/W, dipyridamole/warfarin; CR, complete remission; PR, partial remission.

New therapies

A number of uncontrolled studies have evaluated the effects of new immunosuppressive agents in the treatment of patients with MN.

Mycophenolate mofetil

There has been a paucity of studies using mycophenolate mofetil (MMF) for MN. In a pilot study, Miller *et al.* treated 16 patients with 1.5–2 g/day of MMF for a mean of 8 months [71]. These patients would be categorized as either medium or high risk for progression given the severity of their proteinuria and the fact that they had previously failed a variety of other immunosuppressive drugs. The results were modest: six patients had a ≥50% reduction in their proteinuria, two had a minor reduction in proteinuria, four had no change, three were withdrawn because of significant adverse effects, and one stopped treatment on his own. There were no significant changes in mean serum creatinine, or serum albumin levels, over the course of the study. In patients who responded, the lowest degree of proteinuria was reached within 6 months, suggesting that patients who are likely to respond would do so in this time frame. This was a pilot study and is somewhat difficult to interpret as negative or positive, given the setting of resistance to all other agents. Similar results were reported in a retrospective analysis of 17 patients with MN who were treated by Choi *et al.*

(15 patients had nephrotic-range proteinuria and 6 had renal insufficiency) [72]. Patients were either steroid dependent, steroid resistant, or steroid intolerant, with or without CsA, or they had been resistant or had a suboptimal response to CsA, or they had signs of progressive renal failure. Overall, treatment with MMF (0.5–1.0 g twice daily for a mean of 12 months) combined with steroids in most patients resulted in a 61% reduction of proteinuria (7.8 to 2.3 g/24 h; $P = 0.001$), with eight patients having PR and two patients CR. Renal function improved in three of six patients with kidney failure.

More recently, Branten *et al.* reported on 32 patients with MN and renal insufficiency (serum creatinine of >1.5 mg/dL) treated with MMF (1 g, twice daily) for 12 months and compared the results with those obtained for 32 patients from a historic control group treated for the same period of time with oral cyclophosphamide (1.5 mg/kg/day) [73]. Both groups received high-dose steroid treatment (methylpredisone, intravenously, 1 g three times at months 1, 3, and 5, followed by oral predisone at 0.5 mg/kg every other day for 6 months, with subsequent tapering). Overall, 21 MMF-treated patients developed PR of proteinuria, in 6 patients proteinuria decreased by at least 50%, and no response was observed in 5 patients. Cumulative incidences of remission of proteinuria at 12 months were 66% in the MMF group versus 72% in the cyclophosphamide group ($P = 0.3$). Side effects occurred

Table 14.3 Cyclosporin A treatment in idiopathic membranous nephropathy

Author	Year	Level of Evidence	Risk group	N	Treatment regimens	Follow-up (months)	Outcomes/comments
Cattran [63]	2001	1	Medium	51	Prednisone (0.15 mg/kg/d) plus CsA (3–4 mg/kg/d) vs. placebo plus prednisone × 26 weeks.	19.5	75% of patients in CsA group vs. 22% in control group achieved PR or CR. Relapse rate 43% in CsA group vs. 40% in placebo by week 52.
Cattran [69]	1995	2	High	17	CsA 3.5 mg/kg/d × 12 months vs. placebo	21	CsA associated with slower rate of decline in renal function. Sustained remission of proteinuria in 6/8 CsA patients.
Alexopoulos [65]	2006	3	Medium	51	CsA 2–3 mg/kg/day and prednisone vs CsA (same dose) alone for 12 mo. responders were placed on long-term low dose CsA 1–1.5 mg/kg/d and prednisone vs CsA alone	26	After 12 months of treatment, 26 patients in the combination group and 17 patients in the CsA alone group had a CR or PR of proteinuria. Daily CsA dose was higher in non-relapsers in both groups while relapsers in both groups had lower CsA trough levels
Ambalavanan [31]	1996	5	Medium	41	CsA 4–5 mg/kg/d for 3–6 months. Lupus serology (+) in 12 patients Retreatment in 20 of 31 patients who relapsed after stopping CsA	18	CsA lowered median proteinuria by 56%, from 7.3 to 3.2 g/24h. In 6 patients with declining GFR during prolonged CsA therapy, a repeat biopsy showed more prominent immune deposits and thicker GBM.
Rostoker [68]	1993	5	High	15	CsA 4–5 mg/kg × 12–30 months Prednisone 1–2 mg/kg/d × 2 months	40	CR or PR in 11/15 (73%) patients. Relapse in 3/9 on CsA withdrawal, but the relapse remain sensitive to CsA. All patients had received corticosteroids (1 mg/kg/d × 2 months) prior to enrollment.
DeSanto [66]	1987	6	Medium-Low	5	CsA 7 mg/kg/d for 6 months plus MTP 1–0.3 mg/kg/d for one month, reduced to 0.3–0.15 mg/kg on the second month, and then down to 0.15 mg/kg for 4 months	8	All had failed prior cytotoxic therapy. Prompt remission of proteinuria in 4/5 patients. No renal failure.

Abbreviations are: MTP, methylprednisolone; CsA, cyclosporin A; CR, complete remission; PR, partial remission; GBM, glomerular basement membrane

at a similar rate between the two groups, but relapses were much more common in the MMF-treated group [73].

Rituximab

Evidence from both experimental and human studies has indicated that MN is mediated by the deposition of IgG antibodies in the subepithelial aspect of the glomerular basement membrane. Thus, it is reasonable to postulate that suppression of antibody production by depleting B cells and/or plasma cells may improve or even resolve the glomerular pathology in MN. Rituximab is a genetically engineered, chimeric, murine/human IgG1κ monoclonal antibody against the CD20 antigen that is found on the surface of normal and malignant pre-B and mature B cells but is not expressed on hematopoietic stem cells, normal plasma cells, or other normal tissues. In a pilot study of rituximab in idiopathic MN, Ruggenenti *et al.* prospectively treated eight nephrotic patients with MN with four weekly courses of rituxan (375 mg/m^2) and followed them for 1 year [74,75]. All patients had complete depletion of circulating B cells lasting up to 1 year. Proteinuria significantly decreased from a mean (±standard deviation [SD]) of 8.6 ± 4.2 g at baseline to 3.0 ± 2.5 g at 12 months; −66%; *P* <0.005). This included two patients with <0.5 g/24 h and <3.5

g/24 h in three other patients. Proteinuria decreased in the three remaining patients by 74, 44, and 41%. Renal function remained stable in all patients. Adverse effects were reported as mild and included chills and fever in one patient and an anaphylactic reaction in another patient. A recent publication from these investigators suggests that rituximab is likely to be most effective in patients with a minimal degree of tubulo-interstitial injury [76].

We recently conducted a prospective open-label pilot trial in 15 newly biopsied patients (<3 years) with idiopathic MN and proteinuria of >4 g/24 h despite ACEi or ARB use for >3 months and systolic BP of <130 mmHg [71]. Thirteen men and 2 women, median age 47 years (range, 33–63) and with a mean serum creatinine of 1.4 ± 0.5 mg/dL, were treated with rituximab (1 g) on days 1 and 15. At 6 months, patients who still had proteinuria of >3 g/24 h and in whom the total CD19$^+$ B-cell count was >15 cells/μl received a second identical course of rituximab. All patients tolerated rituximab well and achieved swift B-lymphocyte depletion by day 28. Baseline proteinuria of 13.0 ± 5.7 g/24 h (range, 8.4–23.5) decreased to 9.1 ± 7.4, 9.3 ± 7.9, 7.2 ± 6.2, and 6.0 ± 7.0 g/24 h (range, 0.2–20) at 3, 6, 9, and 12 months, respectively (means ± SD). Fourteen patients completed a 12-month follow-up: CR (proteinuria <0.3 g/24 h) was achieved in two patients, PR (<3 g/24 h)

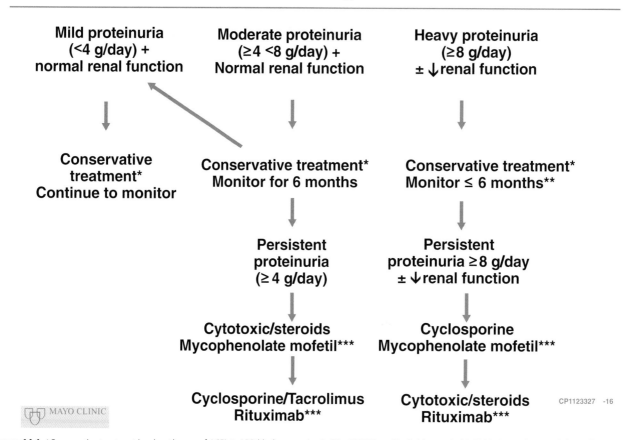

MN Treatment Algorithm

Figure 14.1 *Conservative treatment involves the use of ACEi ± ARB blocker to maintain BP<125/75 mmHg, lipid control with HMG-CoA reductase inhibitor, dietary protein restriction (0.6–0.8g/kg ideal body weight/day), dietary NaCl intake (goal is 2 to 3 g Na) to optimize antiproteinuric effects of ACEi and ARBs, smoking cessation, and attempt to reduce obesity, if present.
**Decreasing function or complication: start treatment early
***Data from non randomized control studies.

was achieved in six patients, and five patients did not respond. Two patients progressed to ESRD. The mean drop in proteinuria from baseline to 12 months was 6.2 ± 5.1 g and was statistically significant ($P = 0.002$, paired t test). Rituximab was well-tolerated and was effective in reducing proteinuria in patients with idiopathic MN. However, the responses varied widely among patients, and further research is needed in order to identify *a priori* which of the patients would be likely to benefit from rituximab treatment. These pilot studies, although encouraging, need to be confirmed by larger randomized controlled studies before recommendations can be made regarding rituximab.

Eculizumab

Eculizumab is a new, humanized anti-C5 monoclonal antibody designed to prevent the cleavage of C5 into its proinflammatory by-products. In a recent randomized controlled trial (currently reported in abstract form only), 200 patients with MN were treated

every 2 weeks with two different intravenous dose regimens and compared to a placebo group, over a total of 16 weeks [78]. Neither of the active drug regimens of eculizumab showed any significant effect on proteinuria or renal function compared to placebo. It was later determined that adequate inhibition of C5 was seen in only a small proportion of patients, suggesting that the doses given were inadequate. More encouraging results were seen in a continuation of the original study, in which eculizumab was used for up to 1 year, with a significant reduction in proteinuria in some patients (including two patients who went into CR). Whether complement inhibition with higher doses of eculizumab will prove to be more effective, as well as safe, in the treatment of MN remains a question.

Adrenocorticotropic hormone

In a study by Berg and colleagues, synthetic adrenocorticotropic hormone (ACTH) administered for 1 year decreased proteinuria in patients with idiopathic MN [79,80]. More recently, Ponticelli *et al.* conducted a randomized pilot study comparing methyl-prednisolone plus a cytotoxic agent versus synthetic ACTH in 32 patients with idiopathic MN [81]. Of these, 16 were randomly assigned to receive methylprednisolone plus chlorambucil or cyclophosphamide (group A), and 16 were assigned to receive ACTH (group B). ACTH was administered by one intramuscular injection (1 mg) every other week, with the frequency increased to two injections per week for a total treatment period of 1 year. Data were reported according to intention-to-treat analysis. CR or PR as a first event was attained by 93% of patients in group A (5 CR and 10 PR) and 87% in group B (10 CR and 4 PR), and the difference between the two groups was not significant. Side effects associated with the use of ACTH included dizziness, glucose intolerance, diarrhea, and the development of bronze-colored skin, which resolved after the end of therapy. Whereas these studies suggest that prolonged synthetic ACTH therapy may represent an effective therapy in patients with idiopathic MN, more extensive randomized studies with longer follow-up are needed before therapeutic recommendations can be made. At the present time, the synthetic formulation of ACTH used in the above studies is not available in the USA.

Disease and treatment summary

In conclusion, control of NS, specifically with CR or PR, is clearly associated with prolonged renal survival and a slower rate of renal disease progression. There are no standard or universal first-line specific therapeutic options for idiopathic MN. Supportive or conservative care should be given in all cases and should include the use of potentially renal protective agents such as ACEi and ARBs and lipid-lowering agents. In patients who are at low risk of progression, conservative therapy should suffice, given their excellent prognosis, although long-term follow-up is needed to ensure that there is no disease progression or worsening of proteinuria. Patients at medium or high risk are candidates for immunosuppressive therapy. Patients with persistent nephrotic-range proteinuria are at increased risk for cardiovascular and thromboembolic complications. Proteinuria is an inducer of kidney injury and plays a major role in the development of progressive tubular injury, interstitial fibrosis, and subsequent loss in GFR. The higher the sustained level of proteinuria, the more likely the development of ESRD. Therefore, even if the main benefit of immunosuppressive therapy is to accelerate the induction of a remission, it may still have value in the long term. A treatment algorithm that combines the predictive factors and best evidence for immunosuppressive therapy is presented in Figure 14.1. In following this algorithm, physicians must also take into account the individual patient and their wishes in order to make the best decision regarding which therapy should be initiated. These routines are not mutually exclusive and may follow one after the other (with a drug holiday) if the first one chosen does not succeed in reducing the proteinuria to the desired range and/or adverse side effects make completion of a course of therapy untenable. Patients who do not respond well or relapse after a first course of immunosuppression therapy may benefit from a second course of immunosuppression [82].

Preliminary evidence on the use of anti-CD20 antibodies suggests this is another agent that may be as effective, and safer, than our current regimens, but it needs further assessment before being widely recommended. Patients with severe renal insufficiency (serum creatinine of ≥ 3 mg/dL) are less likely to benefit from immunosuppression therapy, and the risk of treatment is significantly higher, and so these patients should be considered for conservative therapy only and with plans made for transplantation in the future.

References

1 Swaminathan SLD, Melton LJ, III, Bergstralh EJ, Leung N, Fervenza FC. Changing incidence of glomerular disease in the Olmstead County: a 30-year renal biopsy study. *Clin J Am Soc Nephrol* 2006; **1**: 483–487.

2 Haas M, Meehan SM, Karrison TG, Spargo BH. Changing etiologies of unexplained adult nephrotic syndrome: a comparison of renal biopsy findings from 1976–1979 and 1995–1997. *Am J Kidney Dis* 1997; **30**: 621–631.

3 Glassock RJ. Secondary membranous glomerulonephritis. *Nephrol Dial Transplant* 1992; **7(Suppl 1)**: 64–71.

4 Donadio JV, Jr., Torres VE, Velosa JA, Wagoner RD, Holley KE, Okamura M *et al.* Idiopathic membranous nephropathy: the natural history of untreated patients. *Kidney Int* 1988; **33**: 708–715.

5 Erwin DT, Donadio JV, Jr., Holley KE. The clinical course of idiopathic membranous nephropathy. *Mayo Clin Proc* 1973; **48**: 697–712.

6 Glassock RJ. Diagnosis and natural course of membranous nephropathy. *Semin Nephrol* 2003; **23**: 324–332.

7 Gluck MC, Gallo G, Lowenstein J, Baldwin DS. Membranous glomerulonephritis. Evolution of clinical and pathologic features. *Ann Intern Med* 1973; **78**: 1–12.

8 Troyanov SWC, Cattran DC. Natural history of patients with idiopathic membranous nephropathy (IMGN) who never become nephrotic. *J Am Soc Nephrol* 2003; **14**: 287A.

9 Zucchelli P, Ponticelli C, Cagnoli L, Passerini P. Long-term outcome of idiopathic membranous nephropathy with nephrotic syndrome. *Nephrol Dial Transplant* 1987; **2**: 73–78.

10 Schieppati A, Mosconi L, Perna A, Mecca G, Bertani T, Garattini S *et al.* Prognosis of untreated patients with idiopathic membranous nephropathy. *N Engl J Med* 1993; **329**: 85–89.

11 Maisonneuve P, Agodoa L, Gellert R, Stewart JJH, Buccianti G, Lowenfels AB *et al.* Distribution of primary renal diseases leading to end-stage renal failure in the United States, Europe, and Australia/New Zealand: results from an international comparative study. *Am J Kidney Dis* 2000; **35**: 157–165.

12 du Buf-Vereijken PW, Branten AJ, Wetzels JF, Idiopathic membranous nephropathy: outline and rationale of a treatment strategy. *Am J Kidney Dis* 2005; **46**: 1012–1029.

13 Cattran D. Management of membranous nephropathy: when and what for treatment. *J Am Soc Nephrol* 2005; **16**: 1188–1194.

14 Glassock RJ. The treatment of idiopathic membranous nephropathy: a dilemma or a conundrum? *Am J Kidney Dis* 2004; **44**: 562–566.

15 Marx BE, Marx M. Prediction in idiopathic membranous nephropathy. *Kidney Int* 1999; **56**: 666–673.

16 Wehrmann M, Bohle A, Bogenschutz O, Eissele R, Freislederer A, Ohlschlegel C *et al.* Long-term prognosis of chronic idiopathic

membranous glomerulonephritis. An analysis of 334 cases with particular regard to tubulo-interstitial changes. *Clin Nephrol* 1989; **31:** 67–76.

17 Pei Y, Cattran D, Greenwood C. Predicting chronic renal insufficiency in idiopathic membranous glomerulonephritis. *Kidney Int* 1992; **42:** 960–966.

18 Reichert LJ, Koene RA, Wetzels JF. Urinary IgG excretion as a prognostic factor in idiopathic membranous nephropathy. *Clin Nephrol* 1997; **48:** 79–84.

19 Reichert LJ, Koene RA, Wetzels JF. Urinary excretion of β2-microglobulin predicts renal outcome in patients with idiopathic membranous nephropathy. *J Am Soc Nephrol* 1995; **6:** 1666–1669.

20 Branten AJ, du Buf-Vereijken PW, Klasen IS, Bosch FH, Feith GW, Hollander DA *et al.* Urinary excretion of β2-microglobulin and IgG predict prognosis in idiopathic membranous nephropathy: a validation study. *J Am Soc Nephrol* 2005; **16:** 169–174.

21 Bakoush O, Torffvit O, Rippe B, Tencer J. Renal function in proteinuric glomerular diseases correlates to the changes in urine IgM excretion but not to the changes in the degree of albuminuria. *Clin Nephrol* 2003; **59:** 345–352.

22 Bazzi C, Petrini C, Rizza V, Arrigo G, Beltrame A, Pisano L *et al.* Urinary excretion of IgG and α1-microglobulin predicts clinical course better than extent of proteinuria in membranous nephropathy. *Am J Kidney Dis* 2001; **38:** 240–248.

23 Hladunewich MA, Lemley KV, Blouch KL, Myers BD. Determinants of GFR depression in early membranous nephropathy. *Am J Physiol Ren Fluid Electrolyte Physiol* 2003; **284:** F1014–F1022.

24 Branten AJ, Vervoort G, Wetzels JF. Serum creatinine is a poor marker of GFR in nephrotic syndrome. *Nephrol Dial Transplant* 2005; **20:** 707–711.

25 Cattran DC, Pei Y, Greenwood CM, Ponticelli C, Passerini P, Honkanen E. Validation of a predictive model of idiopathic membranous nephropathy: its clinical and research implications. *Kidney Int* 1997; **51:** 901–907.

26 Ponticelli C, Passerini P, Altieri P, Locatelli F, Pappalettera M. Remissions and relapses in idiopathic membranous nephropathy. *Nephrol Dial Transplant* 1992; **7(Suppl 1):** 85–90.

27 Troyanov SWC, Miller JA, Scholey JW, Cattran DC. Idiopathic membranous nephropathy: definition and relevance of a partial remission. *Kidney Int* 2004; **66:** 1199–1205.

28 Klahr S, Levey AS, Beck GJ, Caggiula AW, Hunsicker L, Kusek JW *et al.* The effects of dietary protein restriction and blood-pressure control on the progression of chronic renal disease. Modification of Diet in Renal Disease Study Group. *N Engl J Med* 1994; **330:** 877–884.

29 Gansevoort RT, Heeg JE, Vriesendorp R, de Zeeuw D, de Jong PE. Antiproteinuric drugs in patients with idiopathic membranous glomerulopathy. *Nephrol Dial Transplant* 1992; **7(Suppl 1):** 91–96.

30 Ruggenenti P, Mosconi L, Vendramin G, Moriggi M, Remuzzi A, Sangalli F *et al.* ACE inhibition improves glomerular size selectivity in patients with idiopathic membranous nephropathy and persistent nephrotic syndrome. *Am J Kidney Dis* 2000; **35:** 381–391.

31 Ambalavanan S, Fauvel JP, Sibley RK, Myers BD. Mechanism of the antiproteinuric effect of cyclosporine in membranous nephropathy. *J Am Soc Nephrol* 1996; **7:** 290–298.

32 Rostoker G, Ben Maadi A, Remy P, Lang P, Lagrue G, Weil B. Low-dose angiotensin-converting-enzyme inhibitor captopril to reduce proteinuria in adult idiopathic membranous nephropathy: a prospective study of long-term treatment. *Nephrol Dial Transplant* 1995; **10:** 25–29.

33 Praga M, Hernandez E, Montoyo C, Andres A, Ruilope LM, Rodicio JL. Long-term beneficial effects of angiotensin-converting enzyme inhibition in patients with nephrotic proteinuria. *Am J Kidney Dis* 1992; **20:** 240–248.

34 Praga M, Borstein B, Andres A, Arenas J, Oliet A, Montoyo C *et al.* Nephrotic proteinuria without hypoalbuminemia: clinical characteristics and response to angiotensin-converting enzyme inhibition. *Am J Kidney Dis* 1991; **17:** 330–338.

35 Manood BK, ten Kate MK, Waanders F, Veeger NJ, Brouwer JL, Vogt L *et al.* High absolute risks and predictors of venous and arterial thromboembolic events in patients with nephrotic syndrome: results from a large retrospective cohort study. *Circulation* 2008; **117:** 224–230.

36 Sarasin FP, Schifferli JA. Prophylactic oral anticoagulation in nephrotic patients with idiopathic membranous nephropathy. *Kidney Int* 1994; **45:** 578–585.

37 Velosa JA, Torres VE. Benefits and risks of nonsteroidal antiinflammatory drugs in steroid-resistant nephrotic syndrome. *Am J Kidney Dis* 1986; **8:** 345–350.

38 Velosa JA, Torres VE, Donadio JV, Jr., Wagoner RD, Holley KE, Offord KP. Treatment of severe nephrotic syndrome with meclofenamate: an uncontrolled pilot study. *Mayo Clin Proc* 1985; **60:** 586–592.

39 Perna A, Schieppati A, Zamora J, Giuliano GA, Braun N, Remuzzi G. Immunosuppressive treatment for idiopathic membranous nephropathy: a systematic review. *Am J Kidney Dis* 2004; **44:** 385–401.

40 A controlled study of short-term prednisone treatment in adults with membranous nephropathy. Collaborative Study of the Adult Idiopathic Nephrotic Syndrome. *N Engl J Med* 1979; **301:** 1301–1306.

41 Cattran DC, Delmore T, Roscoe J, Cole E, Cardella C, Charron R *et al.* A randomized controlled trial of prednisone in patients with idiopathic membranous nephropathy. *N Engl J Med* 1989; **320:** 210–215.

42 Cameron JS, Healy MJ, Adu D. The Medical Research Council trial of short-term high-dose alternate day prednisolone in idiopathic membranous nephropathy with nephrotic syndrome in adults. The MRC Glomerulonephritis Working Party. *Q J Med* 1990; **74:** 133–156.

43 Short CD, Solomon LR, Gokal R, Mallick NP. Methylprednisolone in patients with membranous nephropathy and declining renal function. *Q J Med* 1987; **65:** 929–940.

44 Ponticelli C, Zucchelli P, Passerini P, Cagnoli L, Cesana B, Pozzi C *et al.* A randomized trial of methylprednisolone and chlorambucil in idiopathic membranous nephropathy. *N Engl J Med* 1989; **320:** 8–13.

45 Ponticelli C, Zucchelli P, Passerini P, Cesana B, Locatelli F, Pasquali S *et al.* A 10-year follow-up of a randomized study with methylprednisolone and chlorambucil in membranous nephropathy. *Kidney Int* 1995; **48:** 1600–1604.

46 Ponticelli C, Zucchelli P, Passerini P, Cesana B. Methylprednisolone plus chlorambucil as compared with methylprednisolone alone for the treatment of idiopathic membranous nephropathy. The Italian Idiopathic Membranous Nephropathy Treatment Study Group. *N Engl J Med* 1992; **327:** 599–603.

47 Ponticelli C, Altieri P, Scolari F, Passerini P, Roccatello D, Cesana B *et al.* A randomized study comparing methylprednisolone plus chlorambucil versus methylprednisolone plus cyclophosphamide in idiopathic membranous nephropathy. *J Am Soc Nephrol* 1998; **9:** 444–450.

48 Jha V, Ganguli A, Saha TK, Kohli HS, Sud K, Gupta KL *et al.* A randomized, controlled trial of steroids and cyclophosphamide in adults with nephrotic syndrome caused by idiopathic membranous nephropathy. *J Am Soc Nephrol* 2007; **18:** 1899–1904.

49 Faurschou M, Sorensen IJ, Mellemkjaer L, Loft AG, Thomsen BS, Tvede N *et al.* Malignancies in Wegener's granulomatosis: incidence and relation to cyclophosphamide therapy in a cohort of 293 patients. *J Rheumatol* 2008; **35:** 100–105.

50 Donadio JV, Jr., Holley KE, Anderson CF, Taylor WF. Controlled trial of cyclophosphamide in idiopathic membranous nephropathy. *Kidney Int* 1974; **6:** 431–439.

51 Ponticelli C, Zucchelli P, Imbasciati E, Cagnoli L, Pozzi C, Passerini P *et al.* Controlled trial of methylprednisolone and chlorambucil in idiopathic membranous nephropathy. *N Engl J Med* 1984; **310:** 946–950.

52 Murphy BF, McDonald I, Fairley KF, Kincaid-Smith PS. Randomized controlled trial of cyclophosphamide, warfarin and dipyridamole in idiopathic membranous glomerulonephritis. *Clin Nephrol* 1992; **37:** 229–234.

53 West ML, Jindal KK, Bear RA, Goldstein MB. A controlled trial of cyclophosphamide in patients with membranous glomerulonephritis. *Kidney Int* 1987; **32:** 579–584.

54 Mathieson PW, Turner AN, Maidment CG, Evans DJ, Rees AJ. Prednisolone and chlorambucil treatment in idiopathic membranous nephropathy with deteriorating renal function. *Lancet* 1988; **ii:** 869–872.

55 Bruns FJ, Adler S, Fraley DS, Segel DP. Sustained remission of membranous glomerulonephritis after cyclophosphamide and prednisone. *Ann Intern Med* 1991; **114:** 725–730.

56 Falk RJ, Hogan SL, Muller KE, Jennette JC. Treatment of progressive membranous glomerulopathy. A randomized trial comparing cyclophosphamide and corticosteroids with corticosteroids alone. The Glomerular Disease Collaborative Network. *Ann Intern Med* 1992; **116:** 438–445.

57 Jindal K, West M, Bear R, Goldstein M. Long-term benefits of therapy with cyclophosphamide and prednisone in patients with membranous glomerulonephritis and impaired renal function. *Am J Kidney Dis* 1992; **19:** 61–67.

58 Warwick GL, Geddes CG, Boulton-Jones JM. Prednisolone and chlorambucil therapy for idiopathic membranous nephropathy with progressive renal failure. *Q J Med* 1994; **87:** 223–229.

59 Branten AJ, Reichert LJ, Koene RA, Wetzels JF. Oral cyclophosphamide versus chlorambucil in the treatment of patients with membranous nephropathy and renal insufficiency. *Q J Med* 1998; **91:** 359–366.

60 Torres A, Dominguez-Gil B, Carreno A, Hernandez E, Morales E, Segura J *et al.* Conservative versus immunosuppressive treatment of patients with idiopathic membranous nephropathy. *Kidney Int* 2002; **61:** 219–227.

61 du Buf-Vereijken PW, Branten AJ, Wetzels JF. Cytotoxic therapy for membranous nephropathy and renal insufficiency: improved renal survival but high relapse rate. *Nephrol Dial Transplant* 2004; **19:** 1142–1148.

62 Guasch A, Suranyi M, Newton L, Hall BM, Myers BD. Short-term responsiveness of membranous glomerulopathy to cyclosporine. *Am J Kidney Dis* 1992; **20:** 472–481.

63 Cattran DC, Appel GB, Hebert LA, Hunsicker LG, Pohl MA, Hoy WE *et al.* Cyclosporine in patients with steroid-resistant membranous nephropathy: a randomized trial. *Kidney Int* 2001; **59:** 1484–1490.

64 Meyrier A, Noel LH, Auriche P, Callard P. Long-term renal tolerance of cyclosporin A treatment in adult idiopathic nephrotic syndrome. Collaborative Group of the Societe de Nephrologie. *Kidney Int* 1994; **45:** 1446–1456.

65 Alexopoulos E, Papagianni A, Tsamelashvili M, Leontsini M, Memmos D. Induction and long-term treatment with cyclospirin A in membranous glomerulonephritis with the nephrotic syndrome. *J Am Soc Nephrol* 2005; **16:** 780A.

66 DeSanto NG, Capodicasa G, Giordano C. Treatment of idiopathic membranous nephropathy unresponsive to methylprednisolone and chlorambucil with cyclosporin. *Am J Nephrol* 1987; **7:** 74–76.

67 Cattran DC. Idiopathic membranous glomerulonephritis. *Kidney Int* 2001; **59:** 1983–1994.

68 Rostoker G, Belghiti D, Ben Maadi A, Remy P, Lang P, Weil B *et al.* Long-term cyclosporin A therapy for severe idiopathic membranous nephropathy. *Nephron* 1993; **63:** 335–341.

69 Cattran DC, Greenwood C, Ritchie S, Bernstein K, Churchill DN, Clark WF *et al.* A controlled trial of cyclosporine in patients with progressive membranous nephropathy. Canadian Glomerulonephritis Study Group. *Kidney Int* 1995; **47:** 1130–1135.

70 Praga M, Barrio V, Juarez GF, Luno J. Tacrolimus monotherapy in membranous nephropathy: a randomized controlled trial. *Kidney Int* 2007; **71:** 924–930.

71 Miller G, Zimmerman R, III, Radhakrishnan J, Appel G. Use of mycophenolate mofetil in resistant membranous nephropathy. *Am J Kidney Dis* 2000; **36:** 250–256.

72 Choi MJ, Eustace JA, Gimenez LF, Atta MG, Scheel PJ, Sothinathan R *et al.* Mycophenolate mofetil treatment for primary glomerular diseases. *Kidney Int* 2002; **61:** 1098–1114.

73 Branten AJ, du Buf-Veriejken PW, Vervloet M, Wetzels JF. Mycophenolate mofetil in idiopathic membranous nephropathy: a clinical trial with comparison to a historic control group treated with cyclophosphamide. *Am J Kidney Dis* 2007; **50:** 248–256.

74 Remuzzi G, Chiurchiu C, Abbate M, Brusegan V, Bontempelli M, Ruggenenti P. Rituximab for idiopathic membranous nephropathy. *Lancet* 2002; **360:** 923–924.

75 Ruggenenti P, Chiurchiu C, Brusegan V, Abbate M, Perna A, Filippi C *et al.* Rituximab in idiopathic membranous nephropathy: a one-year prospective study. *J Am Soc Nephrol* 2003; **14:** 1851–1857.

76 Ruggenenti P, Chiurchiu C, Abbate M, Perna A, Cradevi P, Bontempelli M *et al.* Rituximab for idiopathic membranous nephropathy: who can benefit? *Clin J Am Soc Nephrol* 2006; **1:** 738–748.

77 Fervenza FC, Cossio FG, Leung N, Wasiluk A, Cohen I, Wochos D *et al.* A pilot study on the use of rituximab for the treatment of idiopathic membranous nephropathy: preliminary results. *J Am Soc Nephrol* 2005; **16:** 555A.

78 Appel G NP, Hogan S, Radhakrishnan J, Old C, Hebert L, Fervenza F *et al.* Eculizumab (C5 complement inhibitor) in the treatment of idiopathic membranous nephropathy (abstract). *J Am Soc Nephrol* 2002; **13:** 668A.

79 Berg AL, Arnadottir M. ACTH-induced improvement in the nephrotic syndrome in patients with a variety of diagnoses. *Nephrol Dial Transplant* 2004; **19:** 1305–1307.

80 Berg AL, Nilsson-Ehle P, Arnadottir M. Beneficial effects of ACTH on the serum lipoprotein profile and glomerular function in patients with membranous nephropathy. *Kidney Int* 1999; **56:** 1534–1543.

81 Ponticelli C, Passerini P, Salvadori M, Manno C, Viola BF, Pasquali S et al. A randomized pilot trial comparing methylprednisolone plus a cytotoxic agent versus synthetic adrenocorticotropic hormone in idiopathic membranous nephropathy. *Am J Kidney Dis* 2006; **47:** 233–240.

82 du Buf-Vereijken PW, Wetzels JF. Efficacy of a second course of immunosuppressive therapy in patients with membranous nephropathy and persistent or relapsing disease activity. *Nephrol Dial Transplant* 2004; **19:** 2036–2043.

15 IgA Nephropathy in Adults and Children

Jonathan Barratt,[1] John Feehally,[1] & Ronald Hogg[2]

[1]The John Walls Renal Unit, Leicester General Hospital, and Department of Infection, Immunity & Inflammation, University of Leicester, Leicester, United Kingdom
[2]Division of Pediatric Nephrology, Children's Health Center, St. Joseph's Hospital and Medical Center, Phoenix, USA

Introduction

Immunoglobulin A nephropathy (IgAN) is the most common pattern of glomerulonephritis in all countries where renal biopsy is widely practiced and is an important cause of end-stage renal disease (ESRD) at all ages [1]. IgAN is a mesangial proliferative glomerulonephritis characterized by the predominant deposition of IgA in the glomerular mesangium. The degree of histopathologic injury is extremely variable, and this is reflected in the varied tempo and severity of clinical presentation seen in this disease [2]. Closely associated with IgAN is Henoch-Schönlein purpura (HSP), a small vessel systemic vasculitis characterized by small blood vessel deposition of IgA predominantly affecting the skin, joints, gut, and kidney. The nephritis of HSP is also characterized by mesangial IgA deposition and may be histologically indistinguishable from IgAN [3].

No clinical presentation is pathognomonic of IgAN, not even the archetypal young male with episodic macroscopic hematuria following an upper respiratory tract infection. Also, although a number of abnormalities in circulating IgA and its production have been reported in IgAN patients, cohorts are heterogeneous with respect to these abnormalities, making their diagnostic utility poor [4]. Therefore, a diagnosis of IgAN currently requires a renal biopsy.

Recurrence of IgAN after transplantation, and also the rare cases of resolution of IgA deposits in transplanted kidneys from donors with IgAN, supports the hypothesis that mesangial IgA is derived from a pathogenic IgA fraction within the circulating pool of serum IgA [4–6]. What defines this pathogenic IgA fraction is incompletely understood, but there is evidence for the importance of low-affinity, undergalactosylated polymeric IgA1 molecules forming circulating IgA immune complexes with a propensity for both mesangial deposition and mesangial cell activation [7]. The lack of a complete understanding of the pathogenesis of IgAN has resulted in there still being no treatment known to modify mesangial deposition of IgA. Available treatment options are mostly directed at downstream immune and inflammatory events in the glomerulus and the tubulo-interstitium that may lead to renal scarring. It is therefore likely that these are generic treatments with potential benefit in other chronic glomerular diseases.

In this chapter, we summarize the published studies according to their level of evidence and provide recommendations for the common clinical situations that confront the nephrologist treating patients with idiopathic IgAN (Figure 15.1). In each section, we will describe the results of therapeutic approaches to these clinical situations in adults with IgA nephropathy, followed by a pediatric perspective for which we review the results of similar therapeutic trials in children and adolescents. Some of these reports have been reviewed previously [8]. Whenever possible, the pediatric experience with each treatment will be compared with evidence-based conclusions drawn from adult studies. In this way, we will attempt to facilitate comparison between pediatric and adult recommendations for the management of patients with IgAN. Discussions of the treatment of HSP or secondary forms of IgAN are not included in this chapter.

Natural history

Adult IgAN

The natural history of IgAN has now been well-defined in a number of large series with prolonged follow-up [9]. Fewer than 10% of all patients with IgAN have complete resolution of urinary abnormalities [10] and episodes of macroscopic hematuria become less frequent with time after diagnosis, although the majority of patients will still have persistent microscopic hematuria. All patients have the potential for slowly progressive chronic kidney disease leading eventually to ESRD. Approximately 25–30% of any cohort will require renal replacement therapy within 20–25 years of presentation. From the first renal symptom, on average, 1.5% of patients with IgAN have been calculated to reach ESRD per year [11], but the observed risk varies with the diagnostic approach. Centers

Evidence-based Nephrology. Edited by Donald Molony and Jonathan Craig
© 2009 Blackwell Publishing, ISBN: 978-1-4051-3975-5.

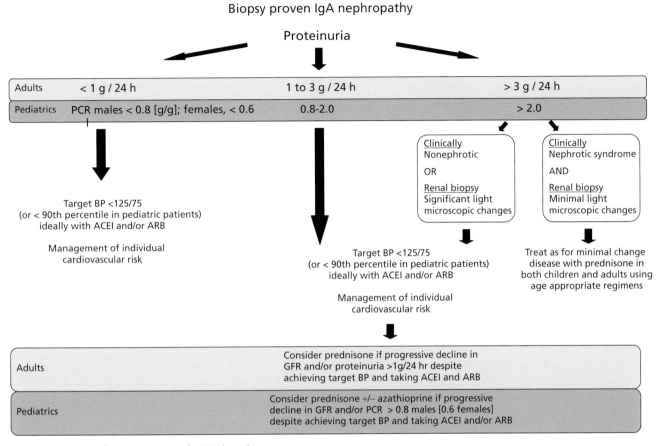

Biopsy proven IgA nephropathy

Proteinuria

Adults	< 1 g / 24 h	1 to 3 g / 24 h	> 3 g / 24 h
Pediatrics	PCR males < 0.8 [g/g]; females, < 0.6	0.8-2.0	> 2.0

Clinically
Nonephrotic

OR

Renal biopsy
Significant light
microscopic changes

Clinically
Nephrotic syndrome

AND

Renal biopsy
Minimal light
microscopic changes

Target BP <125/75
(or < 90th percentile in pediatric patients)
ideally with ACEI and/or ARB

Management of individual
cardiovascular risk

Target BP <125/75
(or < 90th percentile in pediatric patients)
ideally with ACEI and/or ARB

Management of individual
cardiovascular risk

Treat as for minimal change
disease with prednisone in
both children and adults using
age appropriate regimens

Adults	Consider prednisone if progressive decline in GFR and/or proteinuria >1g/24 hr despite achieving target BP and taking ACEI and ARB
Pediatrics	Consider prednisone +/– azathioprine if progressive decline in GFR and/or PCR > 0.8 males [0.6 females] despite achieving target BP and taking ACEI and/or ARB

Figure 15.1 Flowchart for the management of IgA Nephropathy.

with a low threshold for renal biopsy for patients with mild urine abnormalities, particularly those in countries where urine screening programs are established, will likely diagnose IgAN in a larger number of patients with mild disease and good prognosis (length bias) and at an earlier stage in their disease (lead-time bias), thus favorably influencing the overall outcome of the cohort.

Rarely, acute kidney injury can complicate preexisting IgAN, and evaluation should include a further renal biopsy unless renal function improves rapidly with supportive measures. Acute kidney injury develops by two distinct mechanisms (Figure 15.2). There may be acute, severe immune and inflammatory injury producing crescent formation, or crescentic IgA nephropathy, which may be amenable to intensive immunosuppression. Alternatively, acute kidney injury can occasionally occur with mild glomerular injury when heavy glomerular hematuria leads to tubular occlusion and/or damage by red blood cells. This is a reversible phenomenon, and recovery of renal function occurs with supportive measures.

Pediatric IgAN

Children with progressive forms of IgAN will often not develop ESRD until they are adults [12,13]. Thus, most pediatric trials must rely on surrogate measures, as discussed in the next sec-

tion. Some reports of childhood IgAN have concluded that the risk of progressive renal failure is very low [14–16], whereas others have shown that a significant number of pediatric patients with IgAN will progress to ESRD [12,13,17]. It has been estimated that as many as 30% will progress to ESRD in the USA [13], but for Japanese children only 11–20% are expected to progress to ESRD [12,16,17]. However, similar to many adult studies, predictions are based on different selection criteria for renal biopsy candidates [16,18]. In addition, when progressive disease occurs, it is often insidious, resulting in considerable difficulty in assessing outcomes over the short term. This also presents a significant obstacle when designing clinical trials to evaluate the effect of therapeutic interventions within a feasible time period (i.e. 3–5 years).

Prognostic factors

Many studies have identified features at presentation that mark a poor prognosis (Table 15.1) [9]: proteinuria more than 1 g/24 h, raised serum creatinine, and hypertension. The severity of proteinuria has been shown to correlate with extent of glomerular lesions [19]. In one study 98% of patients presenting with proteinuria of <1 g/24 h had at least a 15-year renal survival [20].

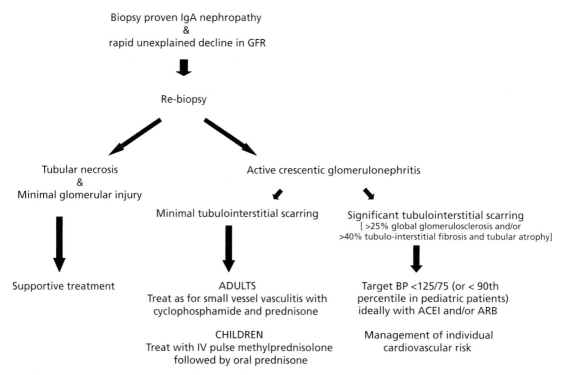

Biopsy proven IgA nephropathy
&
rapid unexplained decline in GFR

Re-biopsy

Tubular necrosis
&
Minimal glomerular injury

Active crescentic glomerulonephritis

Minimal tubulointerstitial scarring

Significant tubulointerstitial scarring
[>25% global glomerulosclerosis and/or
>40% tubulo-interstitial fibrosis and tubular atrophy]

Supportive treatment

ADULTS
Treat as for small vessel vasculitis with
cyclophosphamide and prednisone

Target BP <125/75 (or < 90th
percentile in pediatric patients)
ideally with ACEI and/or ARB

CHILDREN
Treat with IV pulse methylprednisolone
followed by oral prednisone

Management of individual
cardiovascular risk

Figure 15.2 Flowchart for the evaluation and management of patients with previously diagnosed IgA Nephropathy who present with a rapid unexplained decline in renal function.

Another analysis identified those with proteinuria of more than 1 g/24 h and serum creatinine more than 1.7 mg/dL. The 7-year renal survival was 99% if both values were below this threshold, 87% if either one was above the cutoff, and 21% if both were above the cutoff [21]. More recently, serum uric acid levels have been found to correlate with a poor prognosis (and severity of tubulo-interstitial injury) [22]. Episodic macroscopic hematuria does not entail a poor prognosis. It is likely that this observation reflects the variation in time between clinical presentation and diagnosis, which can hinder the accurate interpretation of the natural history. Histopathologic features marking a poor prognosis include glomerulosclerosis, tubular atrophy, and interstitial fibrosis. Clearly, none of these features is specific to IgAN, and they would all mark a poor prognosis in any chronic glomerular disease. Capillary wall IgA deposits are the only histologic feature specific to IgAN which has prognostic significance [11].

The various prognostic factors described may be informative for groups of patients but do not have sufficient accuracy to predict the prognosis of an individual patient with complete confidence. More refined methods of assessing disease activity are required to define those patients in whom IgA deposition will lead to substantial and sustained glomerular injury. An approach incorporating sequential information on blood pressure (BP) and proteinuria can further refine the prediction of risk of progression [23–25], although this will still only account for 30% of overall risk. In milder disease, one study suggested that proteinuria may in fact be a less powerful predictive factor than expected [26]. Although prognostic formulae using simple clinical and laboratory data have been proposed [24,26], there is not yet sufficient consensus to recommend their use in clinical practice for the prediction of individual progression risk.

Methods

We have reviewed the English literature published on the treatment of IgAN since 1976. Despite the prevalence of IgAN, published randomized controlled trials (RCTs) are few in number, and even recent RCTs are not always sufficiently powered to provide definitive information on tested interventions. In part, this is because IgAN is a slowly progressive disease, making it necessary to study large numbers of patients for prolonged periods of time to determine the efficacy of any therapeutic intervention. Another consequence of the slowly progressive nature of IgAN is that for many of the trials now published, patient recruitment occurred at a time when the management of progressive glomerular disease was less clearly defined than it is now. These caveats are even more relevant for reports dealing with therapeutic interventions in children with IgAN. Although the most important outcome indicator for all patients with IgAN is based on deterioration of the glomerular filtration rate (GFR), the period from diagnosis to ESRD in patients with onset in childhood may be decades. Thus, most studies of therapy for pediatric IgAN have relied on surrogate markers, such as deterioration in renal biopsy findings [27,28] and/or decline in the amount of proteinuria or hematuria [28–30]. Significant deterioration in renal function (i.e. 40–50% reduction of GFR or

Table 15.1 Prognostic markers at presentation.

Prognosis category	Clinical finding(s)	Histopathological findings
Worse prognosis	Increasing age Duration of preceding symptoms Severity of proteinuria Hypertension Renal impairment Increased body mass index Serum uric acid	*Light microscopy* Capsular adhesions and crescents Glomerular sclerosis Tubule atrophy Interstitial fibrosis Vascular wall thickening *Immunofluorescence* Capillary loop IgA deposits *Ultrastructure* Capillary wall electron-dense deposits Mesangiolysis GBM abnormalities
Good prognosis	Recurrent macroscopic hematuria	Minimal light microscopic abnormalities
No effect on prognosis	Gender Ethnicity Serum IgA level	Intensity of IgA deposits Codeposition of mesangial IgG, IgM, or C3

Abbreviation: GBM, glomerular basement membrane.

doubling of serum creatinine concentration) is the surrogate end point most associated with progression to ESRD, although this occurs infrequently in patients participating in pediatric trials of IgAN [31].

Recommendations

All patients with IgAN
Recommendations for adults
All adult patients with IgAN should have a BP of <125/75 to 130/80 mmHg (level I recommendation). The antihypertensive agents of choice should be angiotensin converting enzyme inhibitors (ACEi) and angiotensin II receptor blockers (ARB) (level I recommendation). Combination therapy with an ACEi and ARB may provide additional benefit compared to either single agent alone (level II recommendation). Furthermore, all patients should have an individual assessment of their cardiovascular risk, particularly those with progressive chronic kidney disease, hypertension, and dyslipidemia, and treated accordingly (reviewed in Chapter 6).

Recommendations for children
It is also important to maintain pediatric patients with IgAN in a normotensive range, utilizing age-, gender-, and height-appropriate norms for BP [32] (grade I recommendation). ACEi and ARB are the first choice for treatment of hypertension and/or proteinuria (grade I recommendation).

Evidence in adults
In common with virtually all kidney diseases, hypertension is a risk factor for progression in IgAN and should be treated early in the course of the disease [9,33]. There is, however, limited RCT evidence devoted specifically to IgAN concerning a target BP required to preserve renal function. In one 3-year RCT of 49 patients with IgAN, the achieved mean BP of 129/70 mmHg stabilized GFR over 3 years, whereas patients with an achieved mean BP of 136/76 mmHg showed an average decline in GFR of 13 mL/min over 3 years [34]. As with other proteinuric glomerular diseases, the antiproteinuric effect of antihypertensive treatment appears to predict renoprotection, and so therapy should be titrated not only to target BP values but also to maximize reduction of proteinuria. There is increasing evidence that the antihypertensive strategy of choice should be maximal renin–angiotensin system (RAS) blockade, to both achieve a target BP of <125/75 to 130/80 mmHg and to minimize proteinuria [35] (Table 15.2). Retrospective data from the Toronto GN registry have shown that patients with IgAN treated with an ACEi to control BP had a lower rate of annual loss of renal function than similar patients treated with alternative antihypertensives [36]. This is supported by an RCT of 44 patients that demonstrated an additional benefit of an ACEi (enalapril) on progressive kidney disease in IgAN despite equivalent BP control [37]. This benefit was believed to have arisen from the additional reduction in proteinuria seen in the ACEi-treated group. Similarly, a more recent and larger RCT of 109 Asian patients showed benefit with an ARB (valsartan) both in proteinuria reduction and in retarding the rate of renal deterioration, although the investigators were unable to demonstrate a significant improvement in their

Table 15.2 Evidence for use of RAS blockade in IgAN.[a]

Author [reference]	Design	N	Treatment	Follow-up (mos)	Results
Cattran [36]	NRCT	115	ACEi	29	↑ GFR, ↓ proteinuria
Coppo [83]	NRCT	27	Captopril	26	↑ GFR, ↓ proteinuria
Maschio [84]	RCT	39	Fosinopril	9	↓ proteinuria
Kanno [34]	RCT	49	Benazapril and amlodipine	36	≈ GFR
Praga [37]	RCT	44	Enalapril	74	slower ↓ GFR, ↓ proteinuria
Li [38]	RCT	109	Valsartan	24	slower ↓ GFR, ↓ proteinuria
Russo [39]	NRCT	8	ACEi and losartan	3	↓ proteinuria
Song [40]	NRCT	14	Ramipril and candersartan	6	↓ proteinuria
Nakao [41]	RCT	336[b]	Trandolapril and losartan	36	slower ↓ GFR, ↓ proteinuria
Coppo [42]	RCT	66	Benazepril	38	slower ↓ GFR, ↓ proteinuria

Abbreviation: NRCT, nonrandomized controlled trial.

[a] Overall quality of evidence is moderate: consistent effects, variable quality of design and reporting, moderate-sized and small studies, surrogate outcomes.

[b] Of the 336 patients in the COOPERATE study, 131 had IgAN.

primary end points of doubling of serum creatinine or ESRD at 2 years [38].

A number of studies have demonstrated the potential for additive renoprotection when an ACEi is given in combination with an ARB in IgAN, but no studies have long-term outcome data [39,40]. The COOPERATE study, in which 131 of 301 patients had IgAN, demonstrated superior renoprotection with an ACEi (trandolapril)–ARB (losartan) combination than an ACEi or ARB alone, with no further lowering of BP in nonnephrotic proteinuric renal diseases [41]. No formal subgroup analysis of those with IgAN in this study has been reported, however.

Evidence in children

A recent placebo-controlled RCT conducted in 23 centers in five European countries that evaluated benazepril (0.2 mg/kg/day) in 66 children and young adults <35 years of age provided evidence to support the use of ACEi in pediatric patients [42]. The patient cohort included 29 patients ≤18 years of age. Seventy-four percent of the patients had their initial renal abnormalities when they were ≤18 years old. The overall allocation of patients was 32 in the benazepril arm and 34 in the placebo arm. There was a significant benefit with benazepril in preventing progression of renal disease in these patients (defined as a reduction in GFR by 30% versus baseline, or worsening of proteinuria to ≤3.5 g/L/1.73 m^2/day). Such progression was seen in 9/34 (26%) of the placebo group but only 1/32 (3%) of the benazepril group. Furthermore, at the end of the trial, the number of patients with proteinuria of <0.5 g/L/1.73 m^2/day in the benazepril group was significantly higher than the number in the placebo group (13/32 [40%] vs. 3/34 [9%]; $P = 0.0002$). This was evident in both the groups of children (6/10 [60%] vs. 2/19 [10%]) and adults (7/12 [58%] vs. 1/15 [7%]) in this trial.

Patients with recurrent macroscopic hematuria
Recommendation for adults and children
Patients with recurrent macroscopic hematuria require no specific additional intervention (level II recommendation).

Evidence in adults
Episodes of macroscopic hematuria are self-limiting and can be provoked by a range of mucosal, most commonly respiratory, infections. There is no evidence supporting prophylactic use of antibiotics, even in the minority of patients in whom recurrent episodes are provoked by bacterial tonsillitis. Tonsillectomy is still favored as therapy in some regions of the world, notably Japan. Although several retrospective studies of the effectiveness of tonsillectomy have been published, most contain small numbers of patients, are nonrandomized, uncontrolled trials, and have generated conflicting data. In one Japanese study tonsillectomy was shown to be an independent factor in predicting remission in 329 patients followed for a minimum of 3 years [43]. A second retrospective study from Japan looked at the outcome in 118 patients followed over 20 years, of which 48 underwent tonsillectomy [44]. Benefit from the tonsillectomy only became apparent 10 years after initial diagnosis. The concomitant use of other treatment modalities and changing therapeutic goals during the follow-up period make these data difficult to interpret. A retrospective study from Germany of 55 patients in whom 16 had had a tonsillectomy suggested no benefit of tonsillectomy at 10 years [45]. A retrospective study of 112 Chinese patients, of whom 54 underwent tonsillectomy, similarly showed no difference in renal survival at 130 months [46]. Preliminary data from a prospective Japanese RCT of tonsillectomy combined with steroids versus steroids alone reported improvement in hematuria and proteinuria in the tonsillectomy group but no difference in the proportion of patients doubling their serum creatinine at 24 months [47].

Evidence in children

As for adults, there are no prospective clinical trials evaluating the role of tonsillectomy in children with IgAN. In 1985, Lozano *et al.* reported on eight Spanish patients of mean age 18.7 years with a history of frequent episodes of gross hematuria following upper respiratory tract infections and who had had a tonsillectomy. These patients, over the subsequent 2 years, had significantly fewer episodes of gross hematuria, and the percentage of their blood lymphocytes producing polymeric IgA also fell [48]. In 1996, Tomioka *et al.* reported that 13 of 15 children with IgAN who underwent tonsillectomy had improved urinalyses, with 6 of them going into remission [49]. More recently, changes in the levels of hematuria and proteinuria were assessed by Sanai *et al.* in eight children treated with "medication" combined with tonsillectomy compared to 7 "control" children treated with "medication" [50]. These patients were a small subset of a larger patient cohort (ages 3–13 years) that included five children with HSP nephritis and eight with "other" types of glomerulonephritis. No details were given regarding the "medication" that was employed. The authors reported that both proteinuria and hematuria improved in five of eight patients in the tonsillectomy group compared to only one of the seven children with IgAN who received "medication only." However, it is of interest that significant improvement also followed tonsillectomy in five of the eight children with "other glomerulonephritis."

These limited data on the effect of tonsillectomy in children with IgAN are similar to the reports in adults. Most of the studies that have been reported in both groups are retrospective in nature, are based on unvalidated surrogate markers for outcome, and are confounded by co-interventions. There is no convincing evidence that tonsillectomy will prevent progressive renal disease in children or adults, and so this procedure should not be done (level II recommendation).

Patients with isolated microscopic hematuria and proteinuria of <1 g/24 h

Recommendation for adults and children

Adult patients with isolated microscopic hematuria and proteinuria of <1 g/24 h require no specific additional intervention (level II recommendation). There are insufficient data to establish a specific evidence-based recommendation for children in this category, but we suggest that such patients require no additional therapy if their urinary protein (grams)/creatinine (grams) ratio is <0.6 (boys) or <0.8 (girls) (grade II recommendation).

Evidence

Available data suggest that most patients presenting with proteinuria of <1 g/24 h have at least a 15-year renal survival [20]. It is generally accepted that these patients require no additional treatment, although they should receive regular follow-up. It is, however, important to note that while a threshold for proteinuria of 1 g/24 h is commonly used to identify those at increased risk of progression (and therefore warranting treatment), this is an arbitrary value, and the risk attributable to proteinuria is almost certainly a continuum. Interventions that may lower proteinuria further, and are therefore likely renoprotective, for example RAS blockade, have not been tested in this setting in either adults or children.

Patients with rapidly declining GFR

Recommendations for adults

Unexplained acute kidney injury complicating preexistent IgAN requires evaluation with a kidney biopsy (Figure 15.2). Crescentic IgAN associated with active glomerular inflammation and deteriorating renal function in the absence of significant chronic damage should be treated with induction therapy comprising cyclophosphamide and corticosteroids followed by maintenance therapy of azathioprine and corticosteroids at doses similar to those used for the treatment of ANCA-positive small vessel vasculitis (level II recommendation).

Recommendation for children

Although there are no controlled trials of treatment regimens for children with crescentic IgAN, we recommend that pediatric patients with rapidly progressive disease and crescents in ≥50% of their glomeruli be treated with a 2-week course of intravenous (i.v.) methylprednisone pulses (six doses of $1 \text{ g}/1.73 \text{ m}^2$ every other day), followed by 1 month of daily prednisone (1 mg/kg/day) and then alternate-day prednisone for 2–3 months (level II recommendation). Additional therapy with cyclophosphamide should be considered in patients who fail to respond to the pulse therapy (level II recommendation).

Evidence in adults

Acute kidney injury may occur as the first presentation of IgAN with little preceding renal insult or, alternatively, may be superimposed on a background of preexistent disease with variable degrees of chronic glomerular and tubulo-interstitial scarring. Even if the diagnosis of IgAN has previously been established, evaluation should include renal biopsy to distinguish between acute kidney injury due to acute tubular necrosis, which should be self-limiting with supportive treatment, and crescentic IgAN, which may be amenable to intensive immunosuppression.

Crescentic IgAN has a less favorable prognosis, even with immunosuppressive therapy, than other forms of crescentic glomerulonephritis, such as ANCA-associated small vessel vasculitis; cumulative published cases suggest that renal survival in crescentic IgAN is only 50% at 1 year and 20% at 5 years [9,51]. Evidence of chronic glomerular and tubulo-interstitial injury with scarring usually predicts a poor response to intensive immunosuppression. There is no published systematic definition of the degree of chronicity that predicts poor response to immunosuppressive treatment, but we do not recommend such an approach if a representative renal biopsy shows >40% tubulo-interstitial fibrosis and/or >25% global glomerulosclerosis.

A number of case series have recently been published that indicate good preservation of renal function when using treatment regimens similar to those recommended for renal vasculitis, usually with high-dose corticosteroids and cyclophosphamide, and

Table 15.3 Evidence for management of crescentic IgAN with acute kidney injury.[a]

Author [reference]	Design	N	Treatment	Follow-up (mos)	Results
Lai [85]	NRCT	2	Plasma exchange	12	Unsustained slower ↓ GFR
Nicholls [86]	NRCT	13	Plasma exchange		Unsustained slower ↓ GFR
Roccatello [87]	NRCT	9	Plasma exchange, CP and steroids	60	Unsustained slower ↓ GFR
Roccatello [88]	NRCT	20	CP and steroids	60	Slower ↓ GFR
McIntyre [89]	NRCT	9	CP and steroids	17	↑ GFR, ↓ proteinuria
Tumlin [90]	NRCT	24	CP and steroids	36	Stabilized GFR, ↓ proteinuria

Abbreviations: NRCT, nonrandomized controlled trial; CP, cyclophosphamide.

[a] Overall quality very low: inconsistent effects, nonrandomized, very small studies, surrogate outcomes.

in some cases plasma exchange (Table 15.3). However, all of these series are small nonrandomized studies, most using historical controls. There has still been no RCT of these treatments in crescentic IgAN, and response to treatment is not uniform. In addition, comparisons across studies are difficult because published reports use varying definitions of crescentic IgAN. Some include cases where crescents are seen, but others include acute injury where the glomerular tuft is not intense and renal function is not deteriorating. One report indicated that there is a subset of crescentic IgAN with circulating ANCA antibodies which respond well to immunosuppression [52].

Evidence in children

As in adults, the prognosis for children with crescentic IgAN is also poor according to most reports [53]. However, in the largest pediatric experience reported to date, Niaudet *et al.* described a very aggressive and successful approach to 12 children aged 8–14 years with crescentic IgAN, 10 of whom had crescents in ≥50% of their glomeruli [54]. The patients received i.v. methylprednisone in a dose of 1 gm/1.73 m² every other day, followed by 1 month of daily prednisone (1 mg/kg/day) and then alternate-day prednisone for 2–3 months. Three of the patients received a second course of pulse methylprednisone, whereas three others received cyclophosphamide. Although uncontrolled, the authors described very good results after a follow-up period of 1–9 years, because none of the children progressed to ESRD, nine had improved histology on repeat biopsy, and six had recovered clinically, although one patient was still hypertensive.

Patients with nephrotic syndrome
Recommendation for adults and children

In patients presenting with nephrotic syndrome, preserved renal function, and minimal glomerular injury evident on light microscopy, a trial of high-dose corticosteroids using a regimen appropriate for minimal change disease in IgAN should be considered (level I recommendation). However, there is no evidence to support prolonged exposure to corticosteroids if there is not a prompt

response, nor for their use in nephrotic syndrome in the presence of structural glomerular damage.

Evidence in adults

In many patients with IgAN, nephrotic syndrome-range proteinuria is a manifestation of significant structural glomerular damage and progressive renal dysfunction. However, a small minority of both adults and children have nephrosis with minimal glomerular change on renal biopsy, although there are also IgA deposits, and proteinuria remits promptly in response to corticosteroids. In these patients, two common glomerular diseases may coincide: minimal change nephrotic syndrome and IgAN [55,56]. The only RCT of corticosteroids in nephrotic IgAN confirmed this approach, since there was remission of proteinuria only in patients with minimal glomerular change on light microscopy [57]. More recent RCTs of corticosteroids in IgAN have excluded those with nephrotic-range proteinuria, so there is little evidence to inform treatment choices for nephrotic IgAN with significant histologic glomerular injury.

Evidence in children

A number of reports have also described the association of mesangial IgA deposition in association with steroid-responsive nephrotic syndrome in children [58–60]. In at least two of the patients described in the SPNSG report, there was a temporal dissociation between the onset and course of nephrotic syndrome and the later development of clinical features of IgAN [58].

Patients with slowly progressive renal impairment
Recommendations for adults

Tight BP control to a target of <125/75 mmHg and evaluation of individual cardiovascular risk are essential in this group of patients. In patients with persistent proteinuria (>1 g/24 h) despite tight BP control (<125/75 mmHg) and maximal RAS blockade, a 6-month treatment course of corticosteroids may reduce proteinuria (level II recommendation) and stabilize kidney function (level II recommendation). Available evidence does not support a role for mycophenolate mofetil (MMF) (level I recommendation), although additional evidence from appropriately designed studies may soon be available. We cannot recommend the use of cyclophosphamide (grade I recommendation), fish oil (level I recommendation), and other agents at the present time.

Recommendations for children

Based upon the limited evidence currently available, we are unable to make a specific recommendation regarding the use of fish oil supplements for treatment of IgAN in the pediatric patient, although preliminary data from the North American IgA Nephropathy Trials indicate that such therapy may be efficacious in reducing proteinuria in such patients (77). We recommend that a trial of alternate-day prednisone be considered in pediatric patients who have deterioration of GFR or persistent proteinuria (level II recommendation). If prednisone alone is unhelpful, we recommend therapy combining corticosteroids with azathioprine (level II recommendation)

Evidence in adults and children

Patients at risk of progressive renal dysfunction are typically those with hypertension, proteinuria of >1 g/24 h, or reduced GFR at the time of diagnosis. Specific treatment strategies in this group of patients remain contentious. Progression is usually slow, and therefore large studies with prolonged follow-up are necessary to evaluate new treatment strategies in these patients. Recently reported RCTs have tested interventions intended to slow immune and inflammatory events implicated in progressive IgAN, including corticosteroids, cyclophosphamide, and MMF. Because of the long duration required to identify with confidence the benefit of interventions, it is inevitable that recruitment into a number of these studies goes back 10 years or more, to a time when the generic approach to progressive glomerular disease was less well defined, so that BP targets and the use of RAS blockade are variable in these studies.

Immunosuppressive treatments

Corticosteroids in adults

The recent review of immunosuppressive treatments for IgAN by the Cochrane Renal Group identified six RCTs of sufficient quality to be included in their meta-analysis of corticosteroid treatment in IgAN (Table 15.4) [61]. This analysis suggests that corticosteroid therapy may be effective in reducing proteinuria (six trials, 263 patients) and reducing risk of ESRD (six trials, 341 patients), although the meta-analysis was unable to evaluate the influence of RAS blockade or achieved BP in the analysis. Follow-up in a large Italian study of corticosteroid treatment has now reached 10 years. and the investigators report impressive benefit of treatment in reducing proteinuria and preventing ESRD [62]. However, the high-dose corticosteroid regimen, with pulse methylprednisone (1 g daily for 3 days at induction and beginning of months 2 and 4) and alternate-day oral prednisone (0.5 mg/kg) for 6 months, is

regarded by many physicians as likely to carry considerable toxicity, even though none was reported by the investigators. Notably, RAS blockade was only used in a minority of patients in this study, although equally distributed among the participants, and achieved BP was not in line with current recommendations. Another recent RCT of corticosteroids (20-mg/day induction and 5-mg/day maintenance) from Japan in which BP control was tight even though RAS blockade was not used showed only a modest reduction in proteinuria with no protection of GFR [63]. It is unclear whether this lack of renoprotection was due to the lower dose of corticosteroid or a genuine lack of effect in patients managed to current BP targets.

Corticosteroids in children

The short-term effects of prednisone on proteinuria and hematuria were examined by Welch *et al.* in a group of children with IgAN. Twenty patients were randomized to either placebo or prednisone (2 mg/kg/day, maximum 80 mg) for 2 weeks, followed by the same dose on alternate days for 10 weeks [30]. After a 12-week washout period, the treatments were reversed in each subject. No difference in the severity of hematuria was reported after treatment with prednisone compared to placebo. However, most of the subjects had only mild histologic changes, and the subjects in this study would not be expected to have progressive disease.

Waldo and Wyatt *et al.* compared the outcomes of 13 children with IgAN in Alabama followed for 4–10 years after they received alternate-day prednisone for 2 years with 15 children in Tennessee who received no steroid therapy [29]. All of the patients had either proteinuria of >1 g/m^2/day or renal biopsies showing more than a minimal degree of interstitial fibrosis, tubular atrophy, or glomerular sclerosis. None of the 13 treated patients progressed to ESRD, compared to 5 of 15 of the untreated patients ($P = 0.04$). At last follow-up, 12 of 13 treated patients had no hematuria and normal protein excretion ($P < 0.001$ compared with nontreated historic control patients).

Cyclophosphamide with/without azathioprine in adults

The use of cyclophosphamide in patients at very high risk of progression (ESRD predicted in all cases within 5 years) is supported by a single study. Patients received cyclophosphamide (1.5 mg/kg/day for 3 months) followed by azathioprine (1.5 mg/kg/day) in conjunction with high-dose prednisone (40-mg/day induction, 10-mg/day maintenance) and were followed for at least 2 years [64]. Notably, BP control and use of RAS blockade in this trial fell outside current recommendations. Previous RCTs of cyclophosphamide in less severe, slowly progressive IgAN have shown no consistent benefit (reviewed by Feehally [65]), and this is supported by the Cochrane Renal Group meta-analysis, which failed to show any significant renal survival benefit from those RCTs incorporating cyclophosphamide, cyclosporine, or other cytotoxic agents, although there was a significant reduction in daily proteinuria [61]. These studies were, however, insufficiently powered to exclude any effect on progression with certainty.

Table 15.4 RCTs included in the Cochrane Renal Group meta-analysis evaluating the benefit of corticosteroids in IgAN.[a]

Author [reference]	N	Treatment	Follow-up (mos)	Results
Julian [91]	35	Pred, 60 mg/alt day (3/12)	6–24	Stabilized GFR, ↓ proteinuria
		Controls: no treatment		
Kobayashi [92]	46	Pred, 40 mg/day (tapering over 7/12)	120	Stabilized GFR, ↓ proteinuria
		Controls: no treatment		
Katafuchi [63]	90	Pred, 20 mg/day (tapering to 5 mg/day over 24/12)	60	No effect on GFR decline, ↓ proteinuria
		Controls: dipyridamole 150–300 mg/day		
Lai [57]	34	Pred, 40–60 mg/day (halved at 2/12 for further 2/12)	38	Stabilized GFR, ↓ proteinuria
		Controls: no treatment		
Pozzi [93]	86	MP, 1 g i.v. 3 times then 0.5 mg/kg/day for 6/12	60	Stabilized GFR, ↓ proteinuria
		Controls: no treatment		
Shoji [94]	21	Pred, 0.8 mg/kg/day (tapering to 10 mg alt day for 12/12)	13	Stabilized GFR, ↓ proteinuria
		Controls: dipyridamole 300 mg/dy (12/12)		

Abbreviations: Pred, prednisone; MP, methylprednisone.

[a] Overall quality low: inconsistent effects, variable quality of RCT design and reporting, small studies, surrogate outcomes.

Cyclophosphamide with/without azathioprine in children

The efficacy of a 1-year course of prednisone and azathioprine in combination was evaluated in 10 children with IgAN by Andreoli *et al.* [66]. Outcome measures included proteinuria and changes in acute and chronic scores on pre- and posttreatment renal biopsies. Prednisone at 60 mg/m^2 (maximum, 60 mg) once daily for 8 weeks was followed by the same dose every other day for 10 months. Azathioprine at 2–3 mg/kg/day was given for 12 months. Proteinuria fell from 4.1 to 1.6 g/day after treatment ($P < 0.01$). Serial renal biopsies showed that the activity score improved ($P > 0.01$), but the chronicity score was unchanged. The level of microscopic hematuria (red blood cells per high-power field) also improved in each of the 10 patients.

In 1994, Murakami *et al.*, in a retrospective study, evaluated the efficacy of a 6-month course of prednisolone at 10–15 mg on alternate days, cyclophosphamide at 1 mg/kg once daily, and dipyridamole at 5 mg/kg once daily in 17 pediatric patients (age 10.4 ± 3.4 years) who had proteinuria of >1 g/m^2/day plus histologic risk factors for progressive disease, and they compared the results to 21 patients (age 10.1 ± 3.0 years) with similar features who received the same regimen plus warfarin for 3 months in a dose that was adjusted to maintain the thrombotest in the anticoagulant range (as stated by the authors) [67]. The dipyridamole therapy was subsequently continued in all patients until the patient had ≤1 proteinuria. The patients were then followed for 2–10 years (mean, 4.8 years). The authors reported that both groups of patients showed significant improvement in proteinuria but noted that chronic histology indices on posttherapy biopsies (performed in 14 patients) were similar to those reported by Andreoli *et al.* [66], in that they showed persistent signs of chronic disease. Subsequent follow-up studies showed rebound deterioration of proteinuria 5–6 years after the therapy was given. These authors speculated

that their protocol was effective in delaying the progression of renal disease in their patients and that more sustained benefit might be achieved with longer courses of therapy, and with agents having less risk of toxicity.

In 1999, Yoshikawa *et al.* reported an RCT evaluating 2 years of therapy in two groups of children: group 1 received prednisone, azathioprine, heparin, warfarin, and dipyridamole; group 2 received heparin, warfarin, and didyridamole [28]. The prednisone dose was 2 mg/kg/day (maximum, 80 mg) for 4 weeks, followed by 2 mg/kg every other day for 4 weeks, 1.5 mg/kg every other day for 4 weeks, and 1 mg/kg every other day for 21 months. The azathioprine dose was 2 mg/kg/day. Although there was no significant change in GFR in either group, group 1 patients had a significant reduction of proteinuria following therapy (1.35 to 0.22 g/day), whereas group 2 patients did not (0.98 to 0.88 g/day). There was also a significant decrease in glomerular IgA staining in follow-up biopsies in group 1 patients but not in group 2. These follow-up biopsies showed progression of glomerular sclerosis in control patients but not in those receiving prednisone and azathioprine.

In a more recent report in 2006, Yoshikawa *et al.* described the results of a second RCT that compared the effects of combination therapy using prednisone, azathioprine, warfarin, and dipyridanole in 40 children versus prednisone alone in 40 children [68]. Both regimens were given for 24 months. The authors did not incorporate any clinical or laboratory entry requirements in their study design, but all patients were required to have diffuse mesangial hypercellularity on initial renal biopsy. Both treatment regimens were associated with remarkable improvement: proteinuria was less than 100 mg/m^2/day at the end of therapy in 92% of the combination therapy group and in 74% of the prednisone group ($P = 0.007$). In addition, whereas the percentage of glomeruli showing sclerotic changes was unchanged from baseline

Table 15.5 Evidence for the use of MMF in IgAN.[a]

Author [reference]	Design	N	MMR treatment	Follow-up (mos)	Results
Maes [69]	RCT	34	2 g/day for 36/12	36	No effect on GFR decline, no effect on proteinuria
Chen [71]	RCT	93	1–1.5g/day for 6/12 1 g/day for 6/12 0.75 g/day for 6/12	18	No effect on GFR decline, ↓ proteinuria
Tang [72]	RCT	40	2 g/day for 6/12	18	No effect on GFR decline, ↓ proteinuria
Frisch [70]	RCT	32	2 g/day for 12/12	24	No effect on GFR decline, no effect on proteinuria

[a] Overall quality low: inconsistent effects, variable quality of RCT design and reporting, small studies, surrogate outcomes.

in the patients receiving combination therapy (5.0% at baseline and 4.6% at follow-up), it was significantly higher at follow-up in those receiving only prednisone (3.1% and 14.6%, respectively; $P = 0.0003$). However, it should be noted the use of ACEi and ARB was prohibited in all of the patients in this trial; hence, it is not clear whether such aggressive immunosuppressive therapy would be the first choice of therapy in clinical practice for patients with laboratory and biopsy features comparable to those of the patients described.

MMF and mizoribine in adults and children

MMF has been used in four major trials for IgAN (Table 15.5). Two studies reported no benefit from MMF (2 g/day) in patients either at risk of progression (hypertensive and/or proteinuria of >1 g/24 h and/or reduced GFR within 5 years of diagnosis) [69] or with more advanced disease (mean serum creatinine at entry, 2.6 mg/dL) [70]. Both of these studies achieved rigorous BP control with use of an ACEi. In two separate studies on patients with less advanced renal impairment, MMF (1–2 g/day) did reduce proteinuria over an 18-month follow-up period, but neither study demonstrated a change in rate of renal decline [71,72]. Again, both studies achieved tight BP control with ACE inhibition.

A recent retrospective study in Japan showed that mizoribine, which blocks purine synthesis in a manner similar to MMF, resulted in a significant reduction in proteinuria when given to 20 pediatric patients in combination with prednisone, warfarin, and dipyridamole [73]. This was significantly better than the reduction in proteinuria seen in 21 historic control patients who were given only prednisone, warfarin, and dipyridamole, or in 20 historic control patients who also received i.v. pulses of methylprednisone. Follow-up renal biopsies in the mizoribine-treated patients showed no progression of chronic lesions, whereas the other two sets of patients had a significant increase in the chronicity index. A recent pilot study using mizoribine, again in combination with prednisone, warfarin, and dipyridamole, confirmed the efficacy and safety of this regimen in treating children with IgAN [74].

The relatively small size and short duration of the studies to date justify further evaluation of MMF and related compounds, and other studies are in progress [75].

Fish oil in adults

A number of studies have evaluated the role of fish oils (eicosapentanoic acid and docosahexanoic acid in IgAN (Table 15.6). An RCT of 106 patients with proteinuria of >1 g/24 h and impaired renal function at enrollment (60% also hypertensive) found those treated with fish oil had a slower rate of decline in GFR at both 2 and 5 years [76,77]. This effect appeared independent of the dose used [78]. These results have not been replicated in other RCTs studying similar patient cohorts [79–81]. A recent meta-analysis (three trials, 175 patients [76,79,81]) failed to detect a benefit of fish oils on renal outcome in IgAN [82]. Furthermore, a recent RCT showed no benefit following 2 years of treatment with fish oil

Table 15.6 Evidence for the use of fish oil in IgAN.[a]

Author [reference]	Design	N	EPA + DHA daily doses (g)	Follow-up (mos)	Results
Bennett [79]	RCT	37	1.8 + 1.2	24	No effect on GFR decline
Pettersson [81]	RCT	32	3.3 + 1.8	6	↓ GFR, no effect on proteinuria
Donadio [76, 77]	RCT	106	1.8 + 1.2	24 and 60	Slower ↓ GFR
Donadio [78]	RCT	73	3.8 + 2.9 1.9 + 1.5	24	No difference between high- and low-dose EPA–DHA
Hogg [80]	RCT	96	1.88 + 1.48	24	No effect on GFR decline, ↓ proteinuria

Abbreviations: EPA, eicosapentanoic acid; DHA, docosahexanoic acid.
[a] Overall quality low: inconsistent effects, variable quality of RCT design and reporting, small studies, surrogate outcomes.

compared to placebo [80], although a subsequent post hoc analysis of the data in the study revealed a dose-dependent decrease in proteinuria in the fish oil group [77].

Other therapies

Warfarin, urokinase, antiplatelet agents, phenytoin, sodium cromoglycate, dietary gluten restriction, and a low-antigen content diet have all been assessed for the treatment of IgAN and have not been shown to affect renal outcomes [65].

The use of newer immunosuppressive agents, such as leflunomide, rituximab, and sirolimus, while of potential interest for this group of patients, should be considered experimental therapies at this point.

References

1 Barratt J, Feehally J. IgA nephropathy. *J Am Soc Nephrol* 2005; **16:** 2088–2097.

2 Berthoux FC, Mohey H, Afiani A. Natural history of primary IgA nephropathy. *Semin Nephrol* 2008; **28:** 4–9.

3 Davin JC, Ten Berge IJ, Weening JJ. What is the difference between IgA nephropathy and Henoch-Schonlein purpura nephritis? *Kidney Int* 2001; **59:** 823–834.

4 Barratt J, Smith AC, Molyneux K, Feehally J. Immunopathogenesis of IgAN. *Semin Immunopathol* 2007; **29:** 427–443.

5 Floege J. Recurrent IgA nephropathy after renal transplantation. *Semin Nephrol* 2004; **24:** 287–291.

6 Silva FG, Chander P, Pirani CL, Hardy MA. Disappearance of glomerular mesangial IgA deposits after renal allograft transplantation. *Transplantation* 1982; **33:** 241–246.

7 Novak J, Julian BA, Tomana M, Mestecky J. IgA glycosylation and IgA immune complexes in the pathogenesis of IgA nephropathy. *Semin Nephrol* 2008; **28:** 78–87.

8 Wyatt RJ, Hogg RJ. Evidence-based assessment of treatment options for children with IgA nephropathies. *Pediatr Nephrol* 2001; **16:** 156–167.

9 D'Amico G. Natural history of idiopathic IgA nephropathy and factors predictive of disease outcome. *Semin Nephrol* 2004; **24:** 179–196.

10 Costa RS, Droz D, Noel LH. Long-standing spontaneous clinical remission and glomerular improvement in primary IgA nephropathy (Berger's disease). *Am J Nephrol* 1987; **7:** 440–444.

11 Ibels LS, Gyory AZ. IgA nephropathy: analysis of the natural history, important factors in the progression of renal disease, and a review of the literature. *Medicine* (Baltimore) 1994; **73:** 79–102.

12 Kusumoto Y, Takebayashi S, Taguchi T, Harada T, Naito S. Long-term prognosis and prognostic indices of IgA nephropathy in juvenile and in adult Japanese. *Clin Nephrol* 1987; **28:** 118–124.

13 Wyatt RJ, Kritchevsky SB, Woodford SY, Miller PM, Roy S, III, Holland NH *et al.* IgA nephropathy: long-term prognosis for pediatric patients. *J Pediatr* 1995; **127:** 913–919.

14 Kher KK, Makker SP, Moorthy B. IgA nephropathy (Berger's disease): a clinicopathologic study in children. *Int J Pediatr Nephrol* 1983; **4:** 11–18.

15 Michalk D, Waldherr R, Seelig HP, Weber HP, Scharer K. Idiopathic mesangial IgA-glomerulonephritis in childhood. Description of 19 pediatric cases and review of the literature. *Eur J Pediatr* 1980; **134:** 13–22.

16 Nozawa R, Suzuki J, Takahashi A, Isome M, Kawasaki Y, Suzuki S *et al.* Clinicopathological features and the prognosis of IgA nephropathy in Japanese children on long-term observation. *Clin Nephrol* 2005; **64:** 171–179.

17 Yoshikawa N, Ito H, Yoshiara S, Nakahara C, Yoshiya K, Hasegawa O *et al.* Clinical course of immunoglobulin A nephropathy in children. *J Pediatr* 1987; **110:** 555–560.

18 Hogg RJ, Silva FG, Wyatt RJ, Reisch JS, Argyle JC, Savino DA. Prognostic indicators in children with IgA nephropathy. Report of the Southwest Pediatric Nephrology Study Group. *Pediatr Nephrol* 1994; **8:** 15–20.

19 Neelakantappa K, Gallo GR, Baldwin DS. Proteinuria in IgA nephropathy. *Kidney Int* 1988; **33:** 716–721.

20 Bailey RR, Lynn KL, Robson RA, Smith AH, Wells JE. Long term follow up of patients with IgA nephropathy. *N Z Med J* 1994; **107:** 142–144.

21 Frimat L, Briancon S, Hestin D, Aymard B, Renoult E, Huu TC *et al.* IgA nephropathy: prognostic classification of end-stage renal failure. L'Association des Nephrologues de l'Est. *Nephrol Dial Transplant* 1997; **12:** 2569–2575.

22 Myllymaki J, Honkanen T, Syrjanen J, Helin H, Rantala I, Pasternack A *et al.* Uric acid correlates with the severity of histopathological parameters in IgA nephropathy. *Nephrol Dial Transplant* 2005; **20:** 89–95.

23 Feehally J. Predicting prognosis in IgA nephropathy. *Am J Kidney Dis* 2001; **38:** 881–883.

24 Bartosik LP, Lajoie G, Sugar L, Cattran DC. Predicting progression in IgA nephropathy. *Am J Kidney Dis* 2001; **38:** 728–735.

25 Donadio JV, Bergstralh EJ, Grande JP, Rademcher DM. Proteinuria patterns and their association with subsequent end-stage renal disease in IgA nephropathy. *Nephrol Dial Transplant* 2002; **17:** 1197–1203.

26 Rauta V, Finne P, Fagerudd J, Rosenlof K, Tornroth T, Gronhagen-Riska C. Factors associated with progression of IgA nephropathy are related to renal function: a model for estimating risk of progression in mild disease. *Clin Nephrol* 2002; **58:** 85–94.

27 Tanaka H, Waga S, Yokoyama M. Age-related histologic alterations after prednisolone therapy in children with IgA nephropathy. *Tohoku J Exp Med* 1998; **185:** 247–252.

28 Yoshikawa N, Ito H, Sakai T, Takekoshi Y, Honda M, Awazu M *et al.* A controlled trial of combined therapy for newly diagnosed severe childhood IgA nephropathy. The Japanese Pediatric IgA Nephropathy Treatment Study Group. *J Am Soc Nephrol* 1999; **10:** 101–109.

29 Waldo FB, Wyatt RJ, Kelly DR, Herrera GA, Benfield MR, Kohaut EC. Treatment of IgA nephropathy in children: efficacy of alternate-day oral prednisone. *Pediatr Nephrol* 1993; **7:** 529–532.

30 Welch TR, Fryer C, Shely E, Witte DP, Quinlan M. Double-blind, controlled trial of short-term prednisone therapy in immunoglobulin A glomerulonephritis. *J Pediatr* 1992; **121:** 474–477.

31 Hogg RJ, Lee J, Nardelli N, Julian BA, Cattran D, Waldo B *et al.* Clinical trial to evaluate omega-3 fatty acids and alternate day prednisone in patients with IgA nephropathy: report from the Southwest Pediatric Nephrology Study Group. *Clin J Am Soc Nephrol* 2006; **1:** 467–474.

32 The fourth report on the diagnosis, evaluation, and treatment of high blood pressure in children and adolescents. *Pediatrics* 2004; **114:** 555–576.

33 Katafuchi R, Takebayashi S, Taguchi T. Hypertension-related aggravation of Iga nephropathy: a statistical approach. *Clin Nephrol* 1988; **30:** 261–269.

34 Kanno Y, Okada H, Saruta T, Suzuki H. Blood pressure reduction associated with preservation of renal function in hypertensive patients with IgA nephropathy: a 3-year follow-up. *Clin Nephrol* 2000; **54:** 360–365.

35 Jafar TH, Stark PC, Schmid CH, Landa M, Maschio G, de Jong PE *et al.* Progression of chronic kidney disease: the role of blood pressure control,

proteinuria, and angiotensin-converting enzyme inhibition. A patient-level meta-analysis. *Ann Intern Med* 2003; **139:** 244–252.

36 Cattran DC, Greenwood C, Ritchie S. Long-term benefits of angiotensin-converting enzyme inhibitor therapy in patients with severe immunoglobulin A nephropathy: a comparison to patients receiving treatment with other antihypertensive agents and to patients receiving no therapy. *Am J Kidney Dis* 1994; **23:** 247–254.

37 Praga M, Gutierrez E, Gonzalez E, Morales E, Hernandez E. Treatment of IgA nephropathy with ACE inhibitors: a randomized and controlled trial. *J Am Soc Nephrol* 2003; **14:** 1578–1583.

38 Li PK, Leung CB, Chow KM, Cheng YL, Fung SK, Mak SK *et al.* Hong Kong study using valsartan in IgA nephropathy (HKVIN): a double-blind, randomized, placebo-controlled study. *Am J Kidney Dis* 2006; **47:** 751–760.

39 Russo D, Pisani A, Balletta MM, De Nicola L, Savino FA, Andreucci M *et al.* Additive antiproteinuric effect of converting enzyme inhibitor and losartan in normotensive patients with IgA nephropathy. *Am J Kidney Dis* 1999; **33:** 851–856.

40 Song JH, Lee SW, Suh JH, Kim ES, Hong SB, Kim KA *et al.* The effects of dual blockade of the renin-angiotensin system on urinary protein and transforming growth factor-beta excretion in 2 groups of patients with IgA and diabetic nephropathy. *Clin Nephrol* 2003; **60:** 318–326.

41 Nakao N, Yoshimura A, Morita H, Takada M, Kayano T, Ideura T. Combination treatment of angiotensin-II receptor blocker and angiotensin-converting-enzyme inhibitor in non-diabetic renal disease (COOPERATE): a randomised controlled trial. *Lancet* 2003; **361:** 117–124.

42 Coppo R, Peruzzi L, Amore A, Piccoli A, Cochat P, Stone R *et al.* IgACE: a placebo-controlled, randomized trial of angiotensin-converting enzyme inhibitors in children and young people with IgA nephropathy and moderate proteinuria. *J Am Soc Nephrol* 2007; **18:** 1880–1888.

43 Hotta O, Miyazaki M, Furuta T, Tomioka S, Chiba S, Horigome I *et al.* Tonsillectomy and steroid pulse therapy significantly impact on clinical remission in patients with IgA nephropathy. *Am J Kidney Dis* 2001; **38:** 736–743.

44 Xie Y, Nishi S, Ueno M, Imai N, Sakatsume M, Narita I *et al.* The efficacy of tonsillectomy on long-term renal survival in patients with IgA nephropathy. *Kidney Int* 2003; **63:** 1861–1867.

45 Rasche FM, Schwarz A, Keller F. Tonsillectomy does not prevent a progressive course in IgA nephropathy. *Clin Nephrol* 1999; **51:** 147–152.

46 Chen Y, Tang Z, Wang Q, Yu Y, Zeng C, Chen H *et al.* Long-term efficacy of tonsillectomy in Chinese patients with IgA nephropathy. *Am J Nephrol* 2007; **27:** 170–175.

47 Komatsu H, Fujimoto S, Hara S, Sato Y, Yamada K, Eto T. A prospective cohort study on the effect of tonsillectomy combined with steroid pulse on IgA nephropathy [abstract]. *J Am Soc Nephrol* 2005; **16:** 523A.

48 Lozano L, Garcia-Hoya R, Egido J, Blasco R, Sancho J. Tonsillectomy decreases the synthesis of polymeric IgA by blood lymphocytes and clinical activity in patients with IgA nephropathy. *Proc EDTA-ERA* 1985; **22:** 33–37.

49 Tomioka S, Miyoshi K, Tabata K, Hotta O, Taguma Y. Clinical study of chronic tonsillitis with IgA nephropathy treated by tonsillectomy. *Acta Otolaryngol Suppl* 1996; **523:** 175–177.

50 Sanai A, Kudoh F. Effects of tonsillectomy in children with IgA nephropathy, purpura nephritis, or other chronic glomerulonephritides. *Acta Otolaryngol Suppl* 1996; **523:** 172–174.

51 Tumlin JA, Hennigar RA. Clinical presentation, natural history, and treatment of crescentic proliferative IgA nephropathy. *Semin Nephrol* 2004; **24:** 256–268.

52 Haas M, Jafri J, Bartosh SM, Karp SL, Adler SG, Meehan SM. ANCA-associated crescentic glomerulonephritis with mesangial IgA deposits. *Am J Kidney Dis* 2000; **36:** 709–718.

53 Welch TR, McAdams AJ, Berry A. Rapidly progressive IgA nephropathy. *Am J Dis Child* 1988; **142:** 789–793.

54 Niaudet P, Murcia I, Beaufils H, Broyer M, Habib R. Primary IgA nephropathies in children: prognosis and treatment. *Adv Nephrol Necker Hosp* 1993; **22:** 121–140.

55 Clive DM, Galvanek EG, Silva FG. Mesangial immunoglobulin A deposits in minimal change nephrotic syndrome: a report of an older patient and review of the literature. *Am J Nephrol* 1990; **10:** 31–36.

56 Furuse A, Hiramatsu M, Adachi N, Karashima S, Hattori S, Matsuda I. Dramatic response to corticosteroid therapy of nephrotic syndrome associated with IgA nephropathy. *Int J Pediatr Nephrol* 1985; **6:** 205–208.

57 Lai KN, Lai FM, Ho CP, Chan KW. Corticosteroid therapy in IgA nephropathy with nephrotic syndrome: a long-term controlled trial. *Clin Nephrol* 1986; **26:** 174–180.

58 Association of IgA nephropathy with steroid-responsive nephrotic syndrome. A report of the Southwest Pediatric Nephrology Study Group. *Am J Kidney Dis* 1985; **5:** 157–164.

59 Saint-Andre JP, Simard C, Spiesser R, Houssin A. [Nephrotic syndrome in a child, with minimal glomerular lesions and mesangial IgA deposits]. *Nouv Presse Med* 1980; **9:** 531–532.

60 Sinnassamy P, O'Regan S. Mesangial IgA deposits with steroid responsive nephrotic syndrome: probable minimal lesion nephrosis. *Am J Kidney Dis* 1985; **5:** 267–269.

61 Samuels JA, Strippoli GF, Craig JC, Schena FP, Molony DA. Immunosuppressive treatments for immunoglobulin A nephropathy: a meta-analysis of randomized controlled trials. *Nephrology* (Carlton) 2004; **9:** 177–185.

62 Pozzi C, Andrulli S, Del Vecchio L, Melis P, Fogazzi GB, Altieri P *et al.* Corticosteroid effectiveness in IgA nephropathy: long-term results of a randomized, controlled trial. *J Am Soc Nephrol* 2004; **15:** 157–163.

63 Katafuchi R, Ikeda K, Mizumasa T, Tanaka H, Ando T, Yanase T *et al.* Controlled, prospective trial of steroid treatment in IgA nephropathy: a limitation of low-dose prednisolone therapy. *Am J Kidney Dis* 2003; **41:** 972–983.

64 Ballardie FW, Roberts IS. Controlled prospective trial of prednisolone and cytotoxics in progressive IgA nephropathy. *J Am Soc Nephrol* 2002; **13:** 142–148.

65 Feehally J. IgA nephropathy and Henoch-Schonlein purpura. In: Brady HR, Wilcox CS, editors, *Therapy in Nephrology and Hypertension*, 2nd edn. WB Saunders, Philadelphia, 2002.

66 Andreoli SP, Bergstein JM. Treatment of severe IgA nephropathy in children. *Pediatr Nephrol* 1989; **3:** 248–253.

67 Murakami K, Yoshioka K, Akano N, Takemura T, Okada M, Aya N *et al.* Combined therapy in children and adolescents with IgA nephropathy. *Nippon Jinzo Gakkai Shi* 1994; **36:** 38–43.

68 Yoshikawa N, Honda M, Iijima K, Awazu M, Hattori S, Nakanishi K *et al.* Steroid treatment for severe childhood IgA nephropathy: a randomized, controlled trial. *Clin J Am Soc Nephrol* 2006; **1:** 511–517.

69 Maes BD, Oyen R, Claes K, Evenepoel P, Kuypers D, Vanwalleghem J *et al.* Mycophenolate mofetil in IgA nephropathy: results of a 3-year prospective placebo-controlled randomized study. *Kidney Int* 2004; **65:** 1842–1849.

70 Frisch G, Lin J, Rosenstock J, Markowitz G, D'Agati V, Radhakrishnan J *et al.* Mycophenolate mofetil (MMF) vs placebo in patients with moderately advanced IgA nephropathy: a double-blind randomized controlled trial. *Nephrol Dial Transplant* 2005; **20:** 2139–2145.

71 Chen X, Chen P, Cai G, Wu J, Cui Y, Zhang Y *et al.* [A randomized control trial of mycophenolate mofeil treatment in severe IgA nephropathy]. *Zhonghua Yi Xue Za Zhi* 2002; **82:** 796–801.

72 Tang S, Leung JC, Chan LY, Lui YH, Tang CS, Kan CH *et al.* Mycophenolate mofetil alleviates persistent proteinuria in IgA nephropathy. *Kidney Int* 2005; **68:** 802–812.

73 Kawasaki Y, Hosoya M, Suzuki J, Onishi N, Takahashi A, Isome M *et al.* Efficacy of multidrug therapy combined with mizoribine in children with diffuse IgA nephropathy in comparison with multidrug therapy without mizoribine and with methylprednisolone pulse therapy. *Am J Nephrol* 2004; **24:** 576–581.

74 Yoshikawa N, Nakanishi K, Ishikura K, Hataya H, Iijima K, Honda M. Combination therapy with mizoribine for severe childhood IgA nephropathy: a pilot study. *Pediatr Nephrol* 2008; **23:** 757–763.

75 Hogg RJ, Wyatt RJ. A randomized controlled trial of mycophenolate mofetil in patients with IgA nephropathy [ISRCTN6257616]. *BMC Nephrol* 2004; **5:** 3.

76 Donadio JV, Jr., Bergstralh EJ, Offord KP, Spencer DC, Holley KE. A controlled trial of fish oil in IgA nephropathy. Mayo Nephrology Collaborative Group. *N Engl J Med* 1994; **331:** 1194–1199.

77 Donadio JV, Jr., Grande JP, Bergstralh EJ, Dart RA, Larson TS, Spencer DC. The long-term outcome of patients with IgA nephropathy treated with fish oil in a controlled trial. Mayo Nephrology Collaborative Group. *J Am Soc Nephrol* 1999; **10:** 1772–1777.

78 Donadio JV, Jr., Larson TS, Bergstralh EJ, Grande JP. A randomized trial of high-dose compared with low-dose omega-3 fatty acids in severe IgA nephropathy. *J Am Soc Nephrol* 2001; **12:** 791–799.

79 Bennett WM, Walker RG, Kincaid-Smith P. Treatment of IgA nephropathy with eicosapentanoic acid (EPA): a two-year prospective trial. *Clin Nephrol* 1989; **31:** 128–131.

80 Hogg RJ, Lee J, Narelli N, Cattran DC, Hirschman G, Julian BA. Multicenter placebo-controlled trial of alternate day prednisolone or daily omega-3 fatty acids in children and young adults with IgA nephropathy. Report from the Southwest Pediatric Nephrology Study Group. *J Am Soc Nephrol* 2003; **14:** 751A.

81 Pettersson EE, Rekola S, Berglund L, Sundqvist KG, Angelin B, Diczfalusy U *et al.* Treatment of IgA nephropathy with omega-3-polyunsaturated fatty acids: a prospective, double-blind, randomized study. *Clin Nephrol* 1994; **41:** 183–190.

82 Strippoli GF, Manno C, Schena FP. An "evidence-based" survey of therapeutic options for IgA nephropathy: assessment and criticism. *Am J Kidney Dis* 2003; **41:** 1129–1139.

83 Coppo R, Amore A, Gianoglio B, Cacace G, Picciotto G, Roccatello D *et al.* Angiotensin II local hyperreactivity in the progression of IgA nephropathy. *Am J Kidney Dis* 1993; **21:** 593–602.

84 Maschio G, Cagnoli L, Claroni F, Fusaroli M, Rugiu C, Sanna G *et al.* ACE inhibition reduces proteinuria in normotensive patients with IgA nephropathy: a multicentre, randomized, placebo-controlled study. *Nephrol Dial Transplant* 1994; **9:** 265–269.

85 Lai KN, Lai FM, Leung AC, Ho CP, Vallance-Owen J. Plasma exchange in patients with rapidly progressive idiopathic IgA nephropathy: a report of two cases and review of literature. *Am J Kidney Dis* 1987; **10:** 66–70.

86 Nicholls K, Becker G, Walker R, Wright C, Kincaid-Smith P. Plasma exchange in progressive IgA nephropathy. *J Clin Apher* 1990; **5:** 128–132.

87 Roccatello D, Ferro M, Coppo R, Giraudo G, Quattrocchio G, Piccoli G. Report on intensive treatment of extracapillary glomerulonephritis with focus on crescentic IgA nephropathy. *Nephrol Dial Transplant* 1995; **10:** 2054–2059.

88 Roccatello D, Ferro M, Cesano G, Rossi D, Berutti S, Salomone M *et al.* Steroid and cyclophosphamide in IgA nephropathy. *Nephrol Dial Transplant* 2000; **15:** 833–835.

89 McIntyre CW, Fluck RJ, Lambie SH. Steroid and cyclophosphamide therapy for IgA nephropathy associated with crescenteric change: an effective treatment. *Clin Nephrol* 2001; **56:** 193–198.

90 Tumlin JA, Lohavichan V, Hennigar R. Crescentic, proliferative IgA nephropathy: clinical and histological response to methylprednisolone and intravenous cyclophosphamide. *Nephrol Dial Transplant* 2003; **18:** 1321–1329.

91 Julian BA, Barker C. Alternate-day prednisone therapy in IgA nephropathy. Preliminary analysis of a prospective, randomized, controlled trial. *Contrib Nephrol* 1993; **104:** 198–206.

92 Kobayashi Y, Hiki Y, Kokubo T, Horii A, Tateno S. Steroid therapy during the early stage of progressive IgA nephropathy. A 10-year follow-up study. *Nephron* 1996;**72:** 237–242.

93 Pozzi C, Bolasco PG, Fogazzi GB, Andrulli S, Altieri P, Ponticelli C *et al.* Corticosteroids in IgA nephropathy: a randomised controlled trial. *Lancet* 1999; **353:** 883–887.

94 Shoji T, Nakanishi I, Suzuki A, Hayashi T, Togawa M, Okada N *et al.* Early treatment with corticosteroids ameliorates proteinuria, proliferative lesions, and mesangial phenotypic modulation in adult diffuse proliferative IgA nephropathy. *Am J Kidney Dis* 2000; **35:** 194–201.

16 Membranoproliferative Glomerulonephritis

Richard J. Glassock

The David Geffen School of Medicine, UCLA, Los Angeles, USA

Introduction

The term membranoproliferative glomerulonephritis (MPGN) has been used for many decades to describe a group of glomerular diseases that have in common (by light microscopic examination) a pathologic increase in the cellularity of the mesangium, accompanied by an increase in mesangial matrix, and in which the peripheral capillary walls are thickened and distorted. This capillary wall alteration is the consequence of a disturbance of the glomerular basement membrane structure and/or a layering effect of the capillary wall (double contour) caused by interposition of mesangial cells or trapping of circulating cells between old and newly synthesized layers of basement membrane [1,2]. These abnormalities are most often diffuse and generalized and lead to a simplification of the architecture of the glomeruli and an accentuation of the lobulation of the glomerular capillaries. Extracapillary crescent formation can complicate the pathological picture. The terms mesangiocapillary glomerulonephritis and lobular glomerulonephritis have also been used to describe this group of entities. The strong association of MPGN with hypocomplementemia, discovered by West and coworkers in 1965, also led to the use of "hypocomplementemic persistent (chronic) glomerulonephritis" as an early term for this group of disorders [3].

The light microscopic lesions of MPGN are extremely heterogeneous with respect to underlying immunopathology, ultrastructure, presumed etiology, and pathogenesis. This extraordinary diversity complicates attempts to evaluate the therapeutic responsiveness of the lesions of MPGN. It is not the intent of this chapter to review the origins of this diversity in detail but to provide a brief analysis is in order to help make some sense of the confusing literature on treatment of MPGN.

Classification

The ultrastructural appearance of the light microscopic pattern of MPGN gives rise to several subtypes [1,2]. The most common subtype, accounting for about 60–80% of cases of MPGN, is MPGN type I, which is characterized by subendothelial electron-dense deposits (often presumed to be immune complexes) and regularly contains immunoglobulin G (IgG) and/or C3. The intensity of the C3 deposits tend to predominate over the intensity of the IgG deposits. These deposits may acquire an organized substructure when associated with cryoglobulinemia (such as that associated with chronic hepatitis C viral infection) [4] or a nonamyloid monoclonal immunoglobulin deposition disease (MIDD). A form of type I MPGN due to disturbances in complement dysregulation in which only C3 is deposited in glomeruli has also recently been defined [5,6]. The nephritis associated with systemic lupus erythematosus (SLE) also commonly presents with a membranoproliferative pattern by light microscopy. Chronic thrombotic microangiopathies (such as thrombotic thrombocytopenic purpura [TTP] and hemolytic uremia syndrome [HUS]) can also lead to a pattern superficially resembling MPGN type I by light microscopy but usually without any subendothelial dense deposits by electron microscopy. Amorphous, non-electron-dense, flocculent subendothelial deposits may be seen in this circumstance. Fibrillary or immunotactoid glomerulonephritis can also evoke a pattern of MPGN.

The form of MPGN type I in which deposits of both IgG and C3 are common has been traced to a chronic infection with hepatitis C virus in many cases (80% in Europe, 50–70% in the USA, and rarely in parts of Africa and some developing developing countries) [4,7–9]. Systemic hypocomplementemia (lowered levels of C3 and or C4) are found in 50–70% of patients with MPGN type I. Low C4 and normal or low C3 levels are characteristic of hepatitis C virus-associated MPGN [4,7], especially when mixed IgG/IgM cryoglobulinemia (type II cryoglobulinemia) is concomitantly present [4]. Numerous other chronic infections may also produce a

Evidence-based Nephrology. Edited by Donald Molony and Jonathan Craig
© 2009 Blackwell Publishing, ISBN: 978-1-4051-3975-5.

pattern of MPGN type I, but some cases remain to be explained by an unknown underlying disease (idiopathic MPGN type I). The infection-related glomerulopathies are covered in chapter 23 of this textbook.

In recent years the idiopathic forms of MPGN type I have become increasingly uncommon in developed countries, but they remain a frequent cause of glomerular disease in developing nations [8,9]. Although unproven, it seems likely that many cases of so-called idiopathic MPGN type I, unassociated with any regulatory abnormality of complement metabolism, thrombotic microangiopathy, MIDD, fibrillary glomerulonephritis, or SLE, are in fact examples of chronic infections with as-yet-unidentified organisms (possibly lentiviruses). The disparity in the frequency of MPGN type I in developed compared to developing nations has given rise to the "Hygiene Hypothesis" of Johnson and coworkers [10]. This hypothesis suggests that the high prevalence of MPGN observed in developing countries and its steady decline in prevalence in developed countries is due to poor hygienic conditions in the developing countries and an imbalance of the Th1/Th2 functional subsets of lymphocytes, favoring vigorous humoral and cellular responses to infectious organisms.

The MPGN type II pattern is very distinctive by electron microscopic analysis, accounts for about 10–20% of all cases of MPGN [1,2,11], and is seen more often in children and young adults. In this form of MPGN the glomerular basement membrane is transformed into a thickened layer due to the presence of an electron-dense material in what was previously recognized as the lamina densa. The findings gave rise to the name dense deposit disease as a synonym for MPGN type II [11]. Subepithelial deposits can also be seen, particularly early in the course of the disease or during acute exacerbations associated with hypocomplementemia. Subendothelial deposits are typically absent, in contradistinction to MPGN type I. Variable degrees of mesangial and extraglomerular capillary hypercellularity, including crescents, are also present, and the capillary wall may be thickened due to the presence of the dense intramembranous deposits. MPGN type II is also characterized by extensive deposits of C3 (usually C3c fragment) in the mesangium and in the capillary wall (and can include subepithelial deposits) [12]. IgG and IgM deposits are usually absent or scanty. Similar deposits can be found in extrarenal tissue, including the spleen and Bruch's membrane of the eye, leading to "drusen" in the retina, suggesting that they arise from the circulation [11].

Abnormalities in complement metabolism are very common in MPGN type II, and 80% or more of patients will exhibit a decrease in serum C3 (but not C4) concentration [11]. Acquired and genetic forms of factor H deficiency (a complement regulatory protein) are also particularly common in MPGN type II. An IgG autoantibody to the C3 convertase (C3 nephritic factor, or C3Nef) of the alternative pathway of complement activation is commonly found in hypocomplementemic subjects. MPGN type II is also associated with partial lipodystrophy (Dunnigan-Koeberling syndrome)

[11]. Thus, MPGN type II is very different from MPGN type I in regard to appearance and underlying pathogenesis. Rarely, MPGN type II can evolve as a sequela of postinfectious GN, but most cases are idiopathic. The morphology and pathogenesis of MPGN type II are distinctly different from MPGN type I, and some believe that MPGN type II should not be classified as a form of MPGN at all [13,14]. The light microscopic findings in MPGN type II are quite varied, with only about 25% showing the typical membranoproliferative pattern [13,14].

MPGN type III is very heterogeneous, and some studies have divided this group even further into types IIIA and IIIB, depending on the appearance of the glomerular basement membrane and the deposits [1,2]. MPGN type IIIA, also known as the Strife and Anders variant, is characterized by electron-dense deposits and a disruption of the glomerular basement membrane with fragmentation and multilayering [1,2]. MPGN type IIIB, also known as the Burkholder variant, is characterized by subendothelial, intramembranous, and subepithelial electron-dense deposits, often resembling class IV and class V lupus nephritis [1,2]. Together, MPGN types IIIA and IIIB account for less than 10% of all cases of MPGN. Complement abnormalities, including persistently reduced levels of C3, are very common, occurring in 50–80% of cases.

All three major forms of MPGN can recur in the transplanted kidney, and the frequency of recurrence is more related to the severity of the disease than to the underlying subtype [15]. Because MPGN type II is more commonly associated with crescents and a more progressive course, it is more frequently associated with a recurrence in the allografted kidney. Such recurrence rates for MPGN type II have approached 100% in some series, with at least 50% leading to graft failure [11].

A light microscopic pattern resembling MPGN can also be observed in MIDD (kappa light chain nephropathy), complement regulatory protein deficiencies (factor H and I deficiency), fibrillary glomerulonephritis, lupus nephritis (class IV and class V), chronic thrombotic microangiopathy (TTP and HUS), chronic allograft nephropathy, some cases of diabetic nephropathy (nodular diabetic glomerulosclerosis), and in idiopathic lobular glomerulopathy. These disorders can generally be distinguished from MPGN secondary to hepatitis C virus infection or idiopathic forms by careful immunohistological and electron microscopic analysis [1,2,4] supplemented by serological analysis. Genetic analysis may be required in some cases of complement regulatory disturbances [11].

In summary, the light microscopic lesions of MPGN encompass an extremely diverse group of disorders. It is not surprising that the results of treatment have been so varied, since each therapeutic study may have examined a collection of subjects with different underlying pathogenetic alterations. Failure to recognize important etiologic factors, particularly concomitant hepatitis C viral infection (4), but also monoclonal immunoglobulin deposition diseases, thrombotic microangiopathies, or complement regulatory abnormalities, may have also contributed to the varying results of treatments as reported in the literature, particularly those appearing before 1990.

Clinical features and natural history

Despite the morphologic and pathogenetic heterogeneity of the subtypes, the clinical presentation of MPGN is rather uniform and quite independent of subtype [1,2]. Proteinuria, commonly evoking the nephrotic syndrome, hematuria (gross and microscopic), hypertension, and impaired glomerular filtration rate (GFR) are frequent presenting findings. The discovery of hypocomplementemia (reduced levels of C3 and/or C4 or lowered C/H50) is the feature which distinguishes MPGN from the other forms of primary idiopathic glomerular disease (minimal change disease, focal and segmental glomerulosclerosis, membranous nephropathy, and IgA nephropathy seldom, if ever, display hypocomplementemia). Once a renal biopsy diagnosis of MPGN is made,

additional studies are always indicated to properly assign the patient to an etio-pathogenetic category, if possible (Figure 16.1).

If MPGN type I is found, then a search for an underlying infection (particularly hepatitis C viral infection), a monoclonal immunoglobulin deposition disease, an autoimmune disease (such as SLE), a complement regulatory abnormality, or another systemic disease should be sought. If MPGN type II is found, then a complement regulatory abnormality (particularly factor H deficiency and mutations in the *CFH* gene) should be investigated and a search made for extrarenal deposits (in the eye with an ophthalmologic search for retinal drusen) as well as an examination for lipodystrophy [11,16]. If MPGN type IIIA or IIIB is found, then a search for autoimmune disease (particularly SLE) or a chronic infection is in order. If an "organized" substructure of the electron-dense deposits is observed by electron microscopy, then an evaluation for cryoglobulinemia or an MIDD is in order. Only after all of these searches prove negative can one reasonably assign the label "idiopathic" to a case of MPGN identified by light microscopy of a renal biopsy.

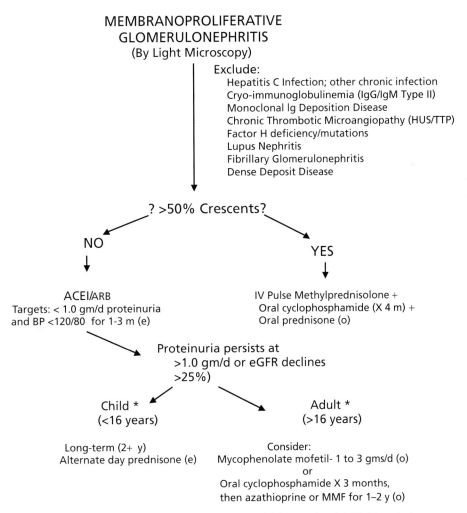

Figure 16.1 Suggested algorithm for evaluation and treatment of MPGN. (e), evidence based; (o), opinion based; *, MPGN type I only.

A contemporary analysis of the natural history of MPGN (unmodified by any specific therapy), and all of its varieties, is extraordinarily difficult. The reasons for this are multiple. Older studies did not take into account the possible influence of concomitant infection with hepatitis C virus or the presence of complement regulatory protein abnormalities [4,16]. Many observational studies included patients treated with various regimens; direct comparisons of outcomes among such studies are not possible. Many studies did not take into account the impact of length and lead-time bias when cases were identified through screening efforts [17]. Changes in conservative therapy, particularly the more extensive use of antihypertensive agents (including angiotensin II inhibitors) may have changed outcomes in those subjects with more severe levels of proteinuria and/or hypertension.

Despite these limitations, general statements can be made regarding factors that appear to be associated with a progressive course leading to end-stage renal disease (ESRD) and factors which are associated with a more benign outcome, even including spontaneous clinical remission. Broad agreement exists that persistence of nephrotic-range proteinuria (>3.0 g/g of creatinine in a spot urine sample in an adult or >40 mg/h/m^2 in a child) is associated with a poor prognosis. Elevation of serum creatinine into the abnormal range at the time of discovery and the presence of hypertension (blood pressure >140/90 mmHg) are also signs portending an unfavorable outcome [1,2]. By contrast, the presence of hematuria and its severity have variable effects on outcome. Marked hematuria (>500,000 erythrocytes/mL of uncentrifuged urine) is strongly associated with the presence of crescents, which usually confers a less favorable prognosis. The presence and magnitude of hypocomplementemia in MPGN is generally of little consequence from the standpoint of prognosis. Concomitant infection with hepatitis C virus often confers a worse prognosis, although this may be altered by successful eradication of the infection (see below) [4]. Patients with MPGN who have normal renal function at discovery and have persistent nonnephrotic proteinuria seldom progress to ESRD [18].

Pathological features of the renal biopsy at the time of diagnosis also impact on determination of likely outcomes. Extensive crescentic disease (>50% involvement of glomeruli) is associated with a highly unfavorable course (in the absence of treatment) [1,2]. Extensive glomerulosclerosis, tubulo-interstitial fibrosis, and tubular atrophy signify an established chronic process and indicate a future likelihood of further progression. Such findings often are strongly associated with an elevation of serum creatinine levels. Whether the subvarieties of MPGN (types I, II, and III) really have differing prognoses, independent of the severity of the disease (e.g. presence of nephrotic syndrome, superimposed crescentic disease, glomerulosclerosis, interstitial fibrosis) remains uncertain [15,19–24]. Claims have been made that MPGN type III has a more benign evolution than either MPGN type I or type II [23,24]. Whatever the true state of affairs may be, it is reasonable to assume that the majority of patients with MPGN and persistence of nephrotic syndrome will show progression toward ESRD, but at variable rates. Overall renal survival (free of the need for renal replacement therapy) is in the vicinity of 60–80% at 10 years from the time of diagnosis, with a mean renal survival of about 8 years for those patients with MPGN who have persisting nephrotic syndrome [1,19].

Characterization of the overall long-term renal survival (5 and 10 years after diagnosis) for untreated idiopathic MPGN can be in part reconstructed from reports in the literature. Some factors that limit the accuracy of these predictions have been mentioned previously and include the following: 1) lead-time bias for patients discovered during screening; 2) lack of stratification of patients into hepatitis C virus-positive and -negative cases; 3) inclusion of treated patients in observational studies of prognosis; 4) lack of information regarding the degree of blood pressure control and the use of agents affecting angiotensin II action; 5) lack of detailed information regarding concomitant renal lesions affecting outcome (e.g. crescentic involvement); 6) failure to stratify patients according to the presence and persistence of complement regulatory dysfunction, thrombotic microangiopathy, or monoclonal immunoglobulin deposition disease.

Despite these caveats, approximate values for the anticipated renal survival in groups (but not individuals) not receiving any specific therapy for MPGN can be gleaned from the placebo or untreated arms of the reported randomized controlled trials of specific therapies (see also below).

For example, in the open-label, randomized controlled trial of therapy for MPGN in children and adults reported by Cattran *et al.* in 1985, the control group (*n*= 32) who received no specific therapy displayed a 2-year renal survival of 85% in MPGN type I and 90% in MPGN type II [25]. All of these patients had an initial creatinine clearance of <80 mL/min/1.73 m^2 and proteinuria of >2.0 g/day at entry. It is also noteworthy that in this study 8 of 32 control patients achieved a spontaneous clinical remission. In the randomized, placebo-controlled trial of treatment of MPGN reported by Tarshish *et al.* in 1992 (completed in 1980), the actuarial renal survival (stable renal function) in the placebo group (*n*= 40) was only 12% at 130 months, and a progressive decline of renal function was noted in about 60% of the placebo group [26]. In this study 52% had MPGN type I, 17% had MPGN type II, and 30% had MPGN type III or other types of MPGN. The hepatitis C virus status of these patients was not known.

In the randomized, double-blind placebo-controlled trial of therapy for MPGN type I (hepatitis C status unknown) reported by Donadio*et al.* in 1984, the average decline in GFR was 19.6 mL/min/year/1.73 m^2 in the placebo group [27]. A total of 9 of 19 patients in the placebo group developed ESRD after 33 months. However, a later reappraisal of this study suggested that the poor prognosis observed in the placebo group could be accounted for by the long duration of disease prior to entry into the randomized trial [17].

Observational studies involving untreated patients can also give some insight into the natural history of MPGN, but these studies are also confounded by lack of information concerning control of blood pressure, use of angiotensin II inhibition, and stratification of underlying disease (e.g. hepatitis C viral infection). In

2004, Cansick *et al.* studied the long-term outcome of 53 children with MPGN (58% type I, 26% type II, and 16% type III and others) [19]. The median follow-up was 3.5 years (range, 0–17 years). Twenty-nine of the 53 children were treated with steroids in an uncontrolled manner. Overall renal survival (including the treated patients and patients without nephrotic syndrome) was 92% at 5 years and 83% at 10 years. In the group of patients with nephrotic syndrome at discovery, the mean renal survival was 8.9 years compared to 13.6 years when nephrotic syndrome was absent. In the study by Chan *et al.* in 1989, 27 of 46 (59%) patients with MPGN (including 20% with hepatitis B virus infection) developed or died of ESRD within a follow-up period averaging 60 months, with no differences in outcome between a treated group (*n*= 19) and an untreated group (*n*= 27) [21]. In a recent report by Fujita *et al.*, the prognosis for untreated "atypical" (unclassifiable) forms of MPGN has been quite favorable (five of six underwent a spontaneous clinical remission after a 10-year follow-up) [28].

In summary, it is a challenging task to reconstruct a consistent pattern of long-term outcome for untreated MPGN from an inspection of the contemporary literature. Very clearly, the presence of nephrotic syndrome connotes an unfavorable prognosis, with a 50% actuarial renal survival being reached at somewhere between 5 and 9 years after discovery. Impaired renal function in addition to nephrotic syndrome would likely indicate an even more unfavorable prognosis, but the outcome would also depend on the severity of hypertension and its treatment with angiotensin II inhibition. Spontaneous clinical recovery appears to be more likely when patients are discovered during screening surveys in childhood and perhaps in those with atypical forms of MPGN. Concomitant hepatitis C virus infection likely confers a worse prognosis, but this has not been well-studied [4]. Overall renal survival of MPGN type I patients among treated and untreated adults and

children averages about 60% at 10 years (range, 50–80%), with children having a somewhat more favorable outcome than adults [21,24].

Evidence base for treatment decisions

Randomized controlled trials

Given the extraordinary diversity of the group of disorders covered under the generic heading of MPGN, it is not surprising that the evaluation of the evidence for treatment of MPGN leads down a controversial and generally confusing path. Unfortunately, much of the evidence bearing on the question of treatment is observational and uncontrolled, and even the limited number of controlled trials that have been conducted thus far have had serious flaws (in design or execution) or limitations in light of contemporary knowledge regarding MPGN. Only six randomized, controlled trials (involving fewer than 270 patients with MPGN) have been conducted, completed, and reported for MPGN to date (Table 16.1).

One study by Cattran and colleagues [25] evaluated the effects of combinations of cyclophosphamide, dipyridamole, and anticoagulants. This study failed to show any difference between control and treated groups but may have been underpowered to show a difference even if one existed. Two studies of alternate-day glucocorticoids alone (Tarshish *et al.* [26] and Mota-Hernandez [24]) and two studies of dipyridamole and aspirin (Donadio *et al.* [27] and Zauner *et al.* [30]) have been conducted. One of the two dipyridamole–aspirin trials failed to show any difference between treatment and control groups upon reappraisal (Donadio *et al.* [17]). One additional nonrandomized crossover trial of warfarin and dipyridamole was reported in 1983 by Zimmerman *et al.* [31]. A randomized trial of cyclophosphamide, anticoagulants,

Table 16.1 Key characteristics of randomized and controlled or cross-over trials of therapy in MPGN (in order of year of publication)

Study	No. of patients	MPGN type	Design	Results
Tiller *et al.*(1981)	39 (A)	I/II	Open-label, CP/Wa/S vs. no therapy	Inconclusive; underpowered
Mota-Hernandez *et al.* (1982)	18 (C)	I	Placebo vs. alt-day steroids	Reduced ESRD
Zimmerman *et al.* (1983)	18 (A)	I	Cross-over, open label Wa/DiP vs. no therapy	Better renal function in unpaired analysis but not with paired analysis
Donadio *et al.* (1984)	40 (A)	I	Double-blind, placebo vs. aspirin/DiP	Better GFR (not confirmed in later analysis)
Cattran *et al.* (1985)	59 (A/C)	I/II	Open-label, CP/Wa/DiP vs. no therapy	No benefit for renal function or proteinuria (25% remission in control)
Tarshish *et al.* (1992)	80 (C)	I/II/III	Double-blind, placebo vs. alt-day steroids	Nonsignificant ($P = 0.07$) trend for better renal function
Zauner *et al.* (1994)	18 (A)	I/II	Open-label, nonplacebo vs. aspirin/DiP	Reduced proteinuria, no GFR change
Giri *et al.* (2002)	30 (A)	I	ACEi vs. non-ACEi	Improved renal function and proteinuria in ACEi group

Abbreviations: A, adults; c, children; S, steroids; CP, cyclophosphamide; Wa, warfarin; DiP, dipyridamole; ACEi, angiotensin converting enzyme inhibitor.

and steroids was interrupted after randomization of 39 subjects due to difficulty in recruiting subjects [32]. No differences in the outcomes for treated and control groups were observed in this study, but the power to detect differences in outcomes was very low. An additional study of angiotensin II inhibition has also been reported (Giri *et al.* [33]). Due to the paucity of trials and the heterogeneity of the studies, no meta-analyses specifically directed to MPGN have been conducted to date; however, Schena has conducted a meta-analysis of immunosuppressive therapy of nephrotic syndrome due to primary glomerulonephritis in adults, which included an analysis of MPGN [34]. Schena concluded that no benefits of immunosuppression in MPGN could be determined because of the substantial imprecision around the point estimates of effect due to sparse data (wide confidence limits). It is important to point out that the entire randomized trial evidence base for treatment of MPGN comes from trials conducted 12–26 years ago. One might legitimately ask how relevant these studies are for the "modern" approach to management of MPGN. Nevertheless, it is appropriate to describe these studies in some detail, especially to point out their strengths and weaknesses.

The study by Cattran *et al.* was an open-label, nonblinded, randomized prospective trial (untreated patients served as controls) [25]. A total of 59 patients (adults and children) with MPGN were randomized to receive cyclophosphamide, warfarin, and dipyridamole for 18 months or no specific therapy. At entry, all patients had an endogenous creatinine clearance of <80 mL/min and >2.0 g of protein in the urine/day. Both MPGN type I and type II were included. The actuarial renal survival rate was not different between the treated and nontreated groups at 2 years, and there was no difference in the outcome of MPGN type I and type II. No differences in protein excretion rates were noted in either group at any time. There was no influence of the initial level of renal function on the subsequent rate of decline in creatinine clearance, as assessed by the slope of 1/serum creatinine. This negative study was underpowered to show a difference even if it existed, and too few patients with MPGN type II were randomized to make any statement regarding efficacy of therapy in this variant of MPGN.

The study by Tarshish *et al.* was actually completed 12 years earlier than it was published, and it was conducted as part of the International Study of Kidney Disease in Children (26). This study was a randomized, double-blind, placebo-controlled study of long-term alternate-day prednisone therapy (40 mg/m^2 every other day) in MPGN. A total of 80 patients (all children) were randomized, including 42 with type I, 14 with type II, 17 with type III, and 7 with nonclassified MPGN. Only patients with nephrotic syndrome and an initial GFR of >70mL/min/1.73 m^2 were included. The mean duration of therapy was 41 months. Treatment failure was the main prespecified end point of the study, and it was defined as achieving an increase in serum creatinine from baseline of 30% or more or an absolute rise of serum creatinine of >35 μmol/L from baseline. It is noteworthy that the mean duration of disease prior to randomization was only 8.9 months in the prednisone-treated group

and 18.1 months in the placebo-treated group ($P < 0.05$). This baseline difference is likely to have biased the results of the study. Actuarial renal survival showed a nonsignificant ($P = 0.07$) trend to better survival in the treated group (61% in treated vs. 12% in the placebo group at 130 months of follow-up). Overall treatment failure occurred in 40% of the prednisone-treated group versus 55% in the placebo-treated group (not significant). In a secondary analysis which excluded MPGN type II and the unclassified forms of MPGN, the prednisone-treated group had only 33% treatment failures while the placebo-treated group had 58% treatment failures. These differences in outcome were not noted until after 90 months of observation, when only 11 prednisone-treated and 7 placebo-treated patients were still under observation. The power of the study to detect differences was small (0.35). In general, treatment was well-tolerated except for a tendency of prednisone to aggravate hypertension (which could have biased the study in favor of the placebo treatment). Overall, one would have to regard this study as negative (or at best, inconclusive) and underpowered, despite the presence of trends favoring treatments. The differences in the time between discovery and randomization between the treated and placebo groups and the differences in blood pressure between the groups could easily have confounded the results.

Mota-Hernandez *et al.* conducted a placebo-controlled study in children with MPGN [29]. In this study 18 patients were randomized to receive prednisone or a placebo and were followed for up to 5 years. One of nine patients in the prednisone group developed ESRD compared to four of nine patients in the placebo group. Repeat kidney biopsies at 3 and 5 years showed improvement in mesangial hypercellularity and resolution of deposits. Tubulo-interstitial lesions did not improve, except in those whose proteinuria remitted. The small number of patients enrolled in this study precludes any definite conclusions, but the trend toward improvement was noticeable. Thus, the evidence for efficacy of alternate-day prednisone treatment of MPGN must remain suggestive but inconclusive.

Two studies have examined the efficacy of combined aspirin and dipyridamole therapy in MPGN. Donadio *et al.* conducted a randomized, double-blind, placebo-controlled trial of dipyridamole (225 mg/day) and aspirin (975 mg/day) for 1 year in 40 adult patients with MPGN type I [27]. Abnormal platelet survival at baseline was corrected by this treatment. Three of 21 patients receiving active therapy developed ESRD after 62 months of follow-up, compared to 9 of 19 after 33 months of follow-up in the placebo group. The main end point of the study was the change in measured GFR over time. The analysis was not by intention-to-treat. The GFR declined by 1.3 mL/min/1.73 m^2/year in the active drug-treated group and declined by 19.6 mL/min/1.73 m^2/year in the placebo group ($P < 0.01$). Mild bleeding complications, requiring discontinuance of treatment (but no transfusions), were noted in about 15% of patients. The initial interpretation of this study was that dipyridamole and aspirin therapy slows progression of renal disease in MPGN type I. However, 5 years later the same authors reanalyzed the data from this trial [17]. When the results were examined in a fashion enabling comparisons of the two groups from the time of onset of therapy (from randomization) rather than from the time of onset of disease, no differences in patient survival or survival free of renal failure were demonstrated. The previously suggested benefits of dipyridamole and aspirin were an artifact of differential lengths of observation from clinical onset of disease. Similar biases are likely to be present in observational studies utilizing historical controls for comparison purposes (see below).

Zauner *et al.* and the German Collaborative Glomerulonephritis Study Group conducted a further randomized, open-label, non-placebo-controlled trial of dipyridamole (75 mg/day) and aspirin (500 mg/day) for 36 months in 18 adult patients with MPGN (type I in 15 and type II in 3) [30]. All patients had impaired renal function and heavy proteinuria at randomization. Proteinuria declined significantly in both groups, but to a greater extent in the active drug-treated group ($P < 0.05$). A total of 7 of 10 patients reached a partial remission in the treated group, while only 2 of 8 reached a similar level of remission in the control group ($P < 0.05$). There was no difference in serum creatinine values in either group postrandomization, but the observation period was probably too short to show any difference in progression of renal disease between the two groups. The decline in proteinuria also might have been due to better blood pressure control in the treated group.

Thus, there is no consistent evidence of efficacy for a combination of dipyridamole and aspirin in slowing the rate of progression of renal disease in MPGN, but all studies so far reported have been underpowered to show such an effect even if it were present. No controlled studies of this form of therapy have been conducted in children.

A prospective, open-label trial with a crossover design utilizing warfarin and dipyridamole was reported by Zimmerman *et al.* in 1983 [31]. Eighteen patients with MPGN, primarily type I, completed either a control or an active treatment year, whereas 13 patients completed both a control and an active treatment year. The analysis involved both unpaired (10 patients in an initial control year compared to 8 patients receiving treatment first) and paired comparisons (13 patients). In the unpaired comparisons, renal function (as assessed by the slope of 1/serum creatinine) was preserved in the treated group but deteriorated in the control group ($P < 0.025$). Proteinuria also fell in the treated group. Doubling of the serum creatinine occurred in 40% of the control group but in 0% of the treated group. Paired analysis of the crossover patients tended to support the findings in the unpaired analysis, but the overall differences were insignificant. Bleeding complications were frequent (cerebral, gastrointestinal, menorrhagia, and hematuria) and were the primary cause for dropping out from the study. Although this small study was encouraging, the findings have never been confirmed in a separate randomized controlled study analyzed using intention-to-treat principles, and the side effects of anticoagulation were sufficient to dampen enthusiasm for this approach to treat MPGN, despite the well-known involvement

of coagulation and platelet aggregation in the disorder. There is good reason to suggest that this study needs to be repeated in a randomized, double-blind, placebo-controlled fashion using modern anticoagulant drugs that have a more favorable profile of bleeding complications in order to evaluate its status as an approach to treatment of MPGN.

Finally, inhibition of angiotensin II action has been clearly demonstrated in randomized, controlled clinical trials to have beneficial effects on the course of many forms of proteinuric renal disease [35]. The effects are mediated both by better control of blood pressure and by a reduction in proteinuria. Many of these trials have included small numbers of patients with MPGN, with too few to justify a specific independent evaluation of angiotensin II inhibition on MPGN. Only one randomized controlled trial examined the specific effects of angiotensin II inhibition in MPGN. Giri *et al.* conducted a small, randomized, controlled trial of angiotensin II inhibition in patients with MPGN and mild to moderate renal insufficiency (serum creatinine of >1.4 mg/dL) [33]. All patients were controlled to the same level of blood pressure ($<140/90$ mmHg). Three groups were studied: group I, a control group with BP controlled to $<140/90$ mmHg with non-angiotensin II inhibition or calcium channel blockers; group II, a group treated with nifedipine at 30 mg/day; and group III, a group treated with nifedipine at 30 mg/day and enalapril at 10 mg/day. Each group consisted of only 10 patients. After 9 months of observation, serum creatinine and albuminuria increased in the control group, whereas serum creatinine and albuminuria decreased in the enalapril-treated group. There was no change in serum creatinine in the nifedipine-treated group, but albuminuria did increase. All patients had adequate blood pressure control during the observation period. Even though they are of a short-term nature, these findings are quite consistent with those of other larger and longer-term studies of other forms of glomerular disease and proteinuria. They add to the evidence base, which suggests that all patients with MPGN (regardless of type) and abnormal blood pressure or proteinuria should be treated with angiotensin II inhibitors with a goal of blood pressure control (to values of <130 mmHg systolic) and reduction of proteinuria to values of <500 mg/day.

In summary, the evidence base concerning efficacy of treatment strategies from randomized controlled trials in MPGN is weak and inconsistent (a very low to low level). Moderate evidence of efficacy for long-term alternate steroids is available for children only. Combinations of dipyridamole and aspirin do not appear to be consistently effective over long-term periods of observation in adults with MPGN, even though they are remarkably safe and may produce a reduction in proteinuria over the short term. Multidrug immunosuppressive–anticoagulant–antithrombotic therapy using cyclophosphamide, warfarin, and dipyridamole did not appear to be effective in MPGN, but studies were underpowered to show such an effect and the entry criteria for the studies may have diminished the likelihood of observing any benefit. Combinations of anticoagulants and antithrombotics (warfarin and dipyridamole) may be effective in MPGN but have an undesirable profile of side effects (bleeding). The best-studied and probably most effective measure is to employ inhibitors of angiotensin II in patients with proteinuria with the goal of reducing blood pressure and proteinuria.

Observational, uncontrolled studies

The majority of published data on the natural history and treatment of MPGN are in the form of observational, uncontrolled studies. The weaknesses of such studies are readily apparent and have been emphasized by Donadio and Offord [17]. At best they are hypothesis-generating rather than proof of efficacy. They are also subject to publication bias (positive studies are selected for reporting), so that compilation of the results of multiple studies cannot be relied upon to give a true reflection of overall efficacy. Despite these caveats, observational studies can give clues to the existence of therapies that might have beneficial effects. Due to the uncommon occurrence of MPGN (at least in developed countries), such reports may be the only data which can be generated, as randomized trials with adequate power are extraordinarily difficult to execute for MPGN.

The use of long-term (6–8 years), high-dose, alternate-day glucocorticoid (prednisone) therapy of MPGN has attracted the most attention in observational studies. Beginning with the pioneering efforts of the Cincinnati group (West, McEnery, McAdams, Strife, and Braun), benefits of long-term, alternate-day steroids have been suggested to modify the course of MPGN in children [36–38]. Renal survival was improved in treated patients compared to historical controls (particularly when diffuse mesangial cell proliferation was seen on initial renal biopsy). Cumulative renal survival of 82% at 10 years and 56% at 20 years has been reported. These renal survival values are superior to those reported in untreated patients, but direct comparison is hazardous because of differences in baseline conditions in the different groups (e.g. presence of impaired renal function at baseline, nephrotic syndrome, etc.). Serial biopsies in treated patients have shown improvements in histopathology [36–40]. A return of urinalysis values to normal has been observed in about 30% of treated patients [41], whereas spontaneous remissions are thought to be uncommon in MPGN. Hematuria, proteinuria, and hypoalbuminemia also improve with steroid therapy. Stable or normal renal function is seen in about 75% of patients, while 25% deteriorate under treatment. These findings have been supported by other independent observational studies. Differences in "responsiveness" to treatment among the various subtypes have also been reported. Braun et al. found that MPGN type I was most responsive to alternate-day steroid therapy, whereas MPGN type III was unresponsive, progressive, and showed a tendency for more relapses [38]. Hypocomplementemia was also more persistent in MPGN type III than in MPGN type I.

Early therapy with steroids, before renal function is impaired, may be more effective than delayed therapy, but this has not been well-established [42]. Limited courses of steroids may also be effective, at least over the short term [40–44]. Patients with MPGN who do not have nephrotic syndrome tend to have a more favorable

course, and the purported benefits of steroids seen in nephrotic children have not been replicated in nonnephrotic children with MPGN [18]. Rarely, clinical remission may occur after steroid therapy is discontinued [45].

Pulses of high-dose methylprednisolone followed by short-term daily oral prednisone have been studied in small observational trials [40,43,44,46]. Bahat et al. recently reported on a small, uncontrolled observational trial of intravenous pulse steroid therapy ($n = 11$) compared to oral steroid therapy ($n = 8$) in children with MPGN. After a follow-up period of about 6 years, 1 of 11 in the pulse steroid therapy group and 4 of 8 in the oral steroid therapy group had developed ESRD [47]. About 60% of patients "improved," but follow-up was short (averaging 27 months) in most studies, so long-term benefits of this approach to therapy are unknown, although the observational studies are encouraging. The combination of pulse methyl prednisolone, short-term oral steroids, and dipyridamole may allow for earlier discontinuance of steroid therapy without sacrificing putative benefits. No comparison of this regimen and the high-dose alternate-day regimen has been reported, so it cannot be claimed that one is better than the other. The benefits of steroids in MPGN type II are much less well understood. No evidence of efficacy has been noted in very limited analyses. Other, atypical (nonclassifiable) forms of MPGN may have a more favorable course, even without therapy [28].

Thus, observational and uncontrolled studies have rather consistently demonstrated beneficial effects of steroid therapy (using a variety of regimens) in children with MPGN type I. Publication bias may have been involved in these studies, however. Side effects are important considerations, since long-term steroids can produce growth retardation, osteopenia, cataracts, diabetes, psychiatric abnormalities, and obesity. Hypertension may be aggravated by this therapeutic approach and requires very careful observation and aggressive therapy. Observational studies of steroid therapy alone, either alternate day, daily, or pulse, in adults with MPGN are very limited and inconclusive.

Observational studies of aspirin and dipyridamole combinations for MPGN are very limited. In general, reduction in proteinuria and stabilization of renal function have been seen [46,48], especially when combined with steroid therapy [46].

Combinations of cyclophosphamide, warfarin, and dipyridamole were among the first therapies examined for MPGN. Very impressive and favorable results were reported by Kincaid-Smith as early as 1972 [49]. Many patients treated in this manner also had "malignant hypertension," and some of the benefits observed may have been due to better control of blood pressure rather than a specific effect of the combination therapy. Patients with an initial creatinine clearance of <31 mL/min nearly always deteriorated, whereas six of eight patients with creatinine clearances of >31 mL/min improved with this therapy. The overall 3-year survival was 85% in the treated group ($n = 16$) versus 0% 3-year survival in a historical control group of 13 untreated patients [49]. Similar results were reported 8 years later by Chapman et al., who employed a regimen of azathioprine, warfarin, dipyridamole, and steroids in a small group of 10 patients with MPGN, including

4 with MPGN type II [50]. In 1994, Faedda and coworkers reported an uncontrolled trial of pulse methylprednisolone, oral prednisone, and cyclophosphamide in 19 patients with MPGN (4 of whom had MPGN type II) [51]. After 10 months, 15 of 19 entered remission, 3 of 19 improved, and 1 of 19 progressed. Relapses occurred in 6 of the 15 patients who remitted, and those who were retreated for a relapse all improved. As a whole group, serum creatinine changed from 165 μmol/L (1.9 mg/dL) before treatment to 156 μmol/L (1.8 mg/dL) during therapy and to 224 μmol/L (2.5 mg/dL) at the end of follow-up. Urine protein excretion declined. No data were given on blood pressure control. These very impressive results of combined steroid and cyclophosphamide therapy of MPGN have not yet been replicated in a controlled, randomized trial.

Thus, combinations of immunosuppressive agents and steroids (orally or as intravenous pulses) or anticoagulants or antithrombotics have shown beneficial effects in observational, uncontrolled studies. The lack of controls and the possibility that other concomitant measures (such as better blood pressure control) contributed to the positive findings must be mentioned as mitigating factors. Obviously, a controlled randomized trial is needed to confirm these very suggestive observations.

Other agents have also been used to treat MPGN. Published studies are generally small, are of short duration, and lack controls. The use of nonsteroidal anti-inflammatory drugs (NSAIDs) was advocated based on longitudinal, uncontrolled studies conducted in the 1970s and 1980s [52–54]. Results equivalent to those claimed by advocates of the alternate-day steroid regimens were observed. This form of therapy fell into disuse as the potential renal-damaging and gastrointestinal effects of NSAIDs became recognized. No controlled studies were ever performed. Cyclosporine or tacrolimus have also been suggested as effective agents for MPGN, but the basis for these claims are a few case reports, and publication bias needs to be considered [55–58]. Buckley's syndrome (hyper-IgE syndrome) associated with MPGN apparently responds to cyclosporine [57].

Mycophenolate mofetil (MMF) has emerged as a promising new agent for the treatment of MPGN [59–63]. Approximately a dozen patients have been treated with MMF combined with steroids in various dosages (usually 2.0 g/day or less of MMF for 6 months to 1 year) with substantial decline in proteinuria and stabilization or improvement in renal function in the majority of reports. Side effects have been mild, usually consisting of leukopenia and/or diarrhea at higher doses. These adverse effects are self-limited and improve with reductions in dose. Improvement in renal function and/or proteinuria is not seen in all cases, and the follow-up has been very short in most reports. A randomized controlled trial is needed to evaluate the significance of these anecdotal reports and to separate the effects of the concomitant use of steroids from the effects of MMF. A single case report of MPGN arising in a patient with X-linked agammaglobulinemia during intravenous immunoglobulin therapy reported that the patient responded with a complete remission following pulse methylprednisolone therapy alone [64].

Plasma replacement and/or plasma exchange could theoretically be of benefit in patients with MPGN types I or II due to deficiencies in factor H or I, but this has not yet been rigorously tested (see below).

MPGN can frequently recur in a transplanted kidney, especially when the disease is severe and progressive or associated with crescentic involvement [15, 65]. All types of MPGN can recur, but this event is most common in MPGN type II, largely due to the greater severity of this variant and its more common association with crescentic disease [15,65,66]. Recurrent MPGN often leads to loss of graft function. Treatment of recurrent disease is quite uncertain, but recent studies suggest a possible role for intensive plasma exchange, cyclophosphamide, or high-dose MMF (3.0 g/day) [66–68].

The therapy of hepatitis C virus infection-associated MPGN type I [4] is discussed in chapter 25 and will not be reviewed here. It is likely that some of the studies quoted and analyzed in prior sections of this report included patients with unrecognized hepatitis C virus infections [1,4,7]. Many of these patients also have mixed essential cryoglobulinemia (type II cryoglobulinemia), and they may also have overt chronic liver disease. All patients presenting with MPGN type I are now routinely tested for antibodies to hepatitis C virus and often are also examined for circulating hepatitis C virions by reverse polymerase chain reaction. Thus, it should not be difficult to separate MPGN type I due to hepatitis C from the idiopathic forms of MPGN type I. The former predominate in Western cultures, but the latter are seen more frequently in developing countries, such as in Africa [7–9].

The management of MPGN type II (dense deposit disease) requires special consideration, as detailed in a recent special communication based on the Hixton Retreat of the Dense Deposit Disease Focus Group [16]. According to an analysis from the Hixton Retreat group, if MPGN type II is diagnosed by renal biopsy and ultrastructural examination, serologic assays for C3 nephritic factor (C3Nef) and factor H gene (*CFH*) mutations should be performed. If assays for C3Nef are positive (expected in about 75% of cases), then a trial of plasma exchange–plasma infusion and/or rituximab should be attempted. No prospective trials have been conducted to evaluate the safety or efficacy of this approach. If a *CFH* mutation is found (expected in about 15–25% of cases and presumably associated with a functional deficiency of the complement regulator factor H), then therapy with plasma infusion is indicated. Anecdotal and experimental evidence is available to support such a recommendation [16,69]. If neither C3Nef nor a *CFH* mutation is found, then empirical therapy with eculizumab (Soliris; Alexion Pharmaceuticals, Inc., Cheshire, CT), a monoclonal antibody directed to the C5 component of the complement cascade that inhibits complement-mediated cell injury, could be initiated. Eculizumab is approved by the US Food and Drug Administration for treatment of paroxysmal nocturnal hemoglobinuria but has not yet been studied for MPGN type II. Sulodexide, a proprietary mixture of sulfated glycoso-aminoglycans, has also been suggested for therapy, but no trials have been conducted as yet [16]. It is apparent that steroids administered in conventional dosages are ineffective for MPGN type II, and immunosuppressive agents would not likely be effective either [16]. High-dose pulse steroid therapy combined with cyclophosphamide and plasma exchange may be tried for MPGN type II associated with extensive crescents and rapidly progressive glomerulonephritis, but there is no clear evidence for efficacy and safety for this approach. Very rarely, steroid therapy may be effective in acute nonproliferative glomerulonephritis, which can be confused with MPGN type II in children [70]. The role of mutations in the factor H gene in the production of both MPGN types I and II and glomerulonephritis with isolated C3 deposition [5,6] and HUS is gradually becoming better understood, especially because of the availability of animal models of disease [71–74].

Treatment of the underlying plasma cell dyscrasia in MPGN type I associated with MIDD is nearly always indicated.

Management of thrombotic microangiopathy (TTP and HUS) in those patients with concomitant MPGN is difficult, but if a deficiency of ADAMTS-13 or factor H (or I) can be documented, plasma infusions and/or plasma exchange may be indicated [16,69,74]. The treatment of lupus nephritis and a lesion of MPGN and fibrillary glomerulonephritis is also covered elsewhere (see chapters 22).

Summary and recommendations

It should be abundantly clear that the evidence base for treatment decisions in MPGN is weak and inconsistent, with a paucity of rigorously designed and executed controlled trials that would conform to modern-day standards of excellence (see references 1 and 75 for reviews). Thus, treatment decisions in MPGN are often made on the basis of less-convincing evidence from observational studies, many of which were short term and used only historical controls. A summary of an evidence- and opinion-based approach to evaluation and therapeutic decision making in MPGN is given in Figure 16.1. MPGN presenting with persistent nephrotic-range proteinuria is a progressive disease which can and frequently does lead to loss of renal function and ESRD. All patients with the lesion of MPGN type I should be thoroughly and systematically evaluated for secondary causes, particularly hepatitis C viral infection, with or without concomitant cryoglobulinemia, monoclonal immunoglobulin deposition diseases, chronic thrombotic microangiopathy, fibrillary or immunotactoid glomerulonephritis, autoimmune diseases (such as atypical SLE), and complement regulatory dysfunction (e.g. factor H deficiency) before commencing a trial of therapy. MPGN type II is equally heterogeneous, with some cases reflecting an abnormality in regulation of complement metabolism (factor H deficiency), which would not be expected to respond simply to steroids or immunosuppressive agents but might respond to plasma infusions or plasma exchange [16,69]. MPGN type III is relatively uncommon but may have a greater resistance to any form of therapy. Other atypical, nonclassifiable forms of MPGN may have a more benign outcome, even if left untreated. Recurrences of MPGN in allografts are common and

often result in graft loss. Treatment of recurrent disease is difficult and problematical.

At the present time the cumulative evidence from controlled and randomized trials and observational data suggests that a trial of high-dose alternate-day steroid therapy *may* be indicated in children with otherwise-idiopathic MPGN type I (low evidence; level II recommendation). Long-term therapy may be required with the attendant risks of steroid toxicity. Children with MPGN types II and III respond less favorably to this regimen, and there is no evidence of efficacy of steroids in any form or dosage in these subvariants of MPGN. Initiation of steroid therapy with high-dose intravenous pulses of methylprednisolone and shorter-term therapy with daily steroids may achieve equivalent effects, but no head-to-head comparisons of the two steroid-based regimens are available. Exacerbations of hypertension can develop with steroid treatment and must be aggressively managed. There are no data to support this steroid-based approach in adults with idiopathic MPGN type I.

Combinations of dipyridamole and aspirin may result in short-term beneficial effects (reduced proteinuria), but there is no evidence to support any long-term benefits or prevention of ESRD in adults with MPGN types I, II, or III. Insufficient data for the efficacy of these regimens in children are available to make any recommendations. Use of this combination of agents in adults is optional (very low evidence; level II recommendation).

Combinations of cyclophosphamide, warfarin, and dipyridamole (without concomitant steroids) are probably not effective in MPGN of any type (low evidence; level I recommendation). Whether combinations of cyclophosphamide, intravenous methylprednisolone pulses, and oral steroids are beneficial needs to be evaluated in a randomized controlled trial, but observational data suggest benefits, at least over the short term, in a subset of patients treated before irreversible renal disease has developed (e.g. estimated GFR of >30 mL/min/1.73 m^2). Such an approach might be especially helpful in patients with extensive crescentic glomerular disease and rapidly progressive glomerulonephritis (low evidence; level II recommendation). Before embarking on this unproven and potentially risky regimen, the presence of an occult infection with hepatitis C or hepatitis B virus, a complement regulatory abnormality (e.g. factor H deficiency), chronic thrombotic microangiopathy, or MIDD should be rigorously excluded (see figure 16.1). The benefits of an anticoagulant or antithrombotic approach (using warfarin and dipyridamole without steroids or immunosuppressive agents) has been validated in a limited crossover trial, but bleeding complications are worrisome and no confirmation of the putative benefits has appeared in the several decades since a trial with this combination was first reported. Little enthusiasm can be generated for use of this regimen (very low evidence; level I recommendation).

The most widely used and evidence-based regimen is strict control of blood pressure (to values below 130/80 mmHg), preferably with the use of inhibitors of angiotensin II action (angiotensin converting enzyme inhibitors alone or in combination with angiotensin II receptor antagonists), often in combination with a low-salt diet and diuretics (high evidence; level I recommendation). This approach is strongly supported from multiple randomized controlled trials, though not specifically for MPGN. The goal of this therapy should be to reduce proteinuria to the lowest possible value consistent with side effects and symptoms as well as to lower blood pressure. This regimen is indicated in all patients with MPGN (regardless of type) who have proteinuria (>500 mg/day) and/or hypertension (blood pressure of >130 mmHg systolic). Patients with MPGN who have stable renal function and who have nonnephrotic levels of proteinuria probably do not need any therapy other than maintenance of normal blood pressure through use of angiotensin II inhibition (moderate evidence; level I recommendation).

The roles of other agents in therapy remain uncertain, largely due to the lack of controlled randomized trials. Cyclosporine or tacrolimus are generally ineffective but may reduce proteinura in the short term (low evidence; level II recommendation). NSAIDs may reduce proteinuria but have no proven benefit for the long-term course and may be associated with side effects (gastrointestinal), aggravate hypertension, and may be potentially nephrotoxic (very low evidence; level I recommendation). MMF is a promising new agent with preliminary favorable effects reported in very limited observational studies. A controlled trial is needed before this agent can be routinely recommended for MPGN type I. Its use should be limited to patients with an adverse prognosis until more information regarding effectiveness is available (low evidence; level I recommendation).

Patients with very severe MPGN associated with extensive crescents may benefit from aggressive use of cyclophosphamide, pulse methylprednisolone, and plasma exchange, but no controlled trials are available and none are unlikely to be conducted due to the rarity of this complication of MPGN (low evidence; level I recommendation).

Patients with MPGN type II require an approach tailored to the underlying abnormality. If a *CFH* mutation can be identified, then therapy with plasma infusions are probably indicated (moderate evidence, level II recommendation). The therapy for patients with MPGN type II not associated with a *CFH* mutation is very uncertain. Rituximab, eculizumab, or plasma exchange or plasma infusion could be tried, but no data are available to evaluate the safety or efficacy of this highly experimental approach.

Patients with recurrent MPGN in a renal allograft would possibly best be managed by a trial of plasma exchange or plasma infusion (possibly for MPGN type II only), oral cyclophosphamide, or high-dose MMF plus prednisone (MPGN type I only; very low evidence; level I recommendation).

References

1 Glassock RJ. Membranoproliferative glomerulonephritis. In: Ponticelli C, Glassock R, editors. *Treatment of Primary Glomerulonephritis*, Oxford Medical Publications, Oxford, 1997; 218–233.

2 Holley KE, Donadio JV. Membranoproliferative glomerulonephritis. In: Tisher CC, Brenner BM, editors, *Renal Pathology (with Clinical and Functional Correlations)*, 2nd edn. Lippincott and Co., Philadelphia, 1994; 294–329.

3 West CD, McAdams AJ, McConville JM, Davis NC, Holland NH. Hypocomplementemic and normocomplementemic persistent (chronic) glomerulonephritis: clinical and pathologic characteristics. *J Pediatr* 1965; **67:** 1089–1112.

4 Roccatello D, Fornasieri A, Giachino O, Rossi D, Beltrame A, Banfi G et al. Multi-center study of hepatitis C virus-related cryoglobulinemic glomerulonephritis. *Am J Kidney Dis* 2007; **49:** 69–82.

5 Servais A, Fremeaux-Bacchi V, Salomon R, Lequintrec M, Noel L-H, Knebelman B et al. Mutations in complement regulatory genes, factor H, I and CD46 and C3 nephritic factor predispose to membranoproliferative glomerulonephritis with isolated mesangial C3 deposits. *J Am Soc Nephrol* 2005; **16:** 51A.

6 Servais A, Fremeaux-Bacchi V, Lequintrec M, Salomon R, Blouin J, Knebelmann B et al. Primary glomerulonephritis with isolated C3 deposits: a new entity which shares common genetic risk factors with hemolytic uremic syndrome. *J Med Genet* 2007; **44:** 193–199.

7 Johnson RJ, Gretch DR, Yamabe H, Hart J, Bacchi CE, Hartwell P et al. Membranoproliferative glomerulonephritis associated with hepatitis C infection. *N Engl J Med* 1993; **328:** 465–470.

8 Madala ND, Naicker S, Singh B, Naidoo M, Smith AN, Rughubar K. The pathogenesis of membranoproliferative glomerulonephritis in KwaZulu-Natal, South Africa is unrelated to hepatitis C virus infection. *Clin Nephrol* 2003; **60:** 69–73.

9 Asinobi AO, Gbadegesin RA, Adeyemo AA, Akang EE, Arowolo FA, Abiola OA et al. The predominance of membranoproliferative glomerulonephritis in childhood nephrotic syndrome in Ibadan, Nigeria. *West Afr J Med* 1999; **18:** 203–206.

10 Johnson RJ, Hurtado A, Merszei J, Rodriguez-Iturbe B, Feng L. Hypothesis: dysregulation of immunologic balance resulting from hygiene and socio-economic factors may influence the epidemiology and cause of glomerulonephritis worldwide. *Am J Kidney Dis* 2003; **42:** 575–581.

11 Appel GB, Cook HT, Hageman G, Jennette JC, Kashgarian M, Kirschfink M et al. Membranoproliferative glomerulonephritis type II (dense deposit disease): an update. *J Am Soc Nephrol* 2005; **16:** 1392–1403.

12 West CD, Witte DP, McAdams AJ. Composition of nephritic-factor generated glomerular deposits in membranoproliferative glomerulonephritis type 2. *Am J Kidney Dis* 2001; **37:** 1120–1130.

13 Walker PD, Ferrario F, Joh K, Bonsib SM. Dense deposit disease is not a membranoproliferative glomerulonephritis. *Mod Pathol* 2007; **20:** 605–616.

14 Walker PD. Dense deposit disease: new insights. *Curr Opin Nephrol Hypertens* 2007; **16:** 204–212.

15 Little MA, Dupont P, Campbell E, Dorman A, Walshe JJ. Severity of primary MPGN, rather than MPGN type determines renal survival and post-transplant recurrence risk. *Kidney Int* 2006; **69:** 504–511.

16 Smith RJH, Alexander J, Barlow PN, Botto M, Cassavant TL, Cook HT et al. New approaches to the treatment of dense deposit disease. *J Am Soc Nephrol* 2007; **18:** 2447–2456.

17 Donadio JV, Offord KP. Reassessment of treatment results in membranoproliferative glomerulonephritis, with emphasis on life-table analysis. *Am J Kidney Dis* 1989; **14:** 445–451.

18 Somers M, Kertesz S, Rosen S, Herrin J, Colvin R, Palaciaos de Carreta N et al. Non-nephrotic children with membranoproliferative glomerulonephritis: are steroids needed? *Pediatr Nephrol* 1995; **9:** 140–144.

19 Cansick JC, Lennon R, Cummins CL, Howie AJ, McGraw ME, Saleem MA *et al.* Prognosis, treatment and outcome of childhood mesangiocapillary (membranoproliferative) glomerulonephritis. *Nephrol Dial Transplant* 2004; **19**: 2769–2777.

20 Wu MJ, Shu KH, Chan LP, Lu YS, Cheng CH, Sheu SS *et al.* Long-term clinical and morphological evaluation of primary membranoproliferative glomerulonephritis. *Zhonghua Yi Xue Za Zhi* (Taipei) 1996; **57**: 34–41.

21 Chan MK, Chan KW, Chan PC, Fang GX, Cheng IK. Adult-onset mesangiocapillary glomerulonephritis: a disease with a poor prognosis. *Q J Med* 1989; **72**: 599–607.

22 Arslan S, Saatci U, Ozen S, Bakkaloglu A, Besbas N, Tinaztepe K *et al.* Membranoproliferative glomerulonephritis in childhood: factors affecting prognosis. *Int Urol Nephrol* 1997; **29**: 711–716.

23 Abreo K, Moorthy AV. Type 3 membranoproliferative glomerulonephritis: clinicopathologic correlations and long-term follow-up in nine patients. *Arch Pathol Lab Med* 1982; **106**: 413–417.

24 Iitaka K, Moriya S, Nakamura S, Tomonaga K, Sakai T. Long-term follow-up of type III membranoproliferative glomerulonephritis in children. *Pediatr Nephrol* 2002; **17**: 373–378.

25 Cattran DC, Cardella CJ, Roscoe JM, Charron, RC, Rance PC, Ritchie SM *et al.* Results of a controlled drug trial in membranoproliferative glomerulonephritis. *Kidney Int* 1985; **27**: 436–441.

26 Tarshish P, Bernstein J, Tobin JN, Edelmann CM. Treatment of mesangiocapillary glomerulonephritis with alternate-day prednisone—a report of the International Study of Kidney Disease in Children. *Pediatr Nephrol* 1992; **6**: 123–130.

27 Donadio JV, Anderson CF, Mitchell JC, Holley CE, Ilstrup DM, Fuster V *et al.* Membranoproliferative glomerulonephritis. A prospective clinical trial of platelet-inhibitor therapy. *N Engl J Med* 1984; **310**: 1421–1426.

28 Fujita T, Nozu K, Iijima L, Kamioka I, Yoshiya K, Tanaka R. Long-term follow-up of atypical membranoproliferative glomerulonephritis: are steroids indicated? *Pediatr Nephrol* 2006; **21**: 194–200.

29 Mota-Hernandez F, Gordillo-Paniagua G, Munoz-Aripe R. Prednisone vs placebo in membranoproliferative glomerulonephritis: long-term clinico-pathologic correlation. *Int J Pediatr Nephrol* 1985; **6**: 25–28.

30 Zauner I, Bohler J, Braun N, Grupp C, Herring P, Schollmeyer P. Effect of aspirin and dipyridamole on proteinuria in idiopathic membranoproliferative glomerulonephritis. *Nephrol Dial Transplant* 1994; **9**: 619–622.

31 Zimmerman SW, Moorthy AV, Dreher WH, Friedman A, Varanasi U. Prospective trial of warfarin and dipyridamole in patients with membranoproliferative glomerulonephritis. *Am J Med* 1983; **75**: 920–927.

32 Tiller D, Clarkson A, Mathew T. A prospective randomized trial of the use of cyclophosphamide, dipyridamole and warfarin in membranous and membranoproliferative glomerulonephritis. In: Robinson R, Glassock R, Tisher C, Andreoli T, Kokko J. *Proceedings of the 8th International Congress of nephrology.* Karger, Basel, 1981; 345–351.

33 Giri S, Mahajan SK, Sen R, Sharma A. Effects of angiotensin converting enzyme inhibitors on renal function in patients with membranoproliferative glomerulonephritis with mild to moderate renal insufficiency. *J Assoc Physicians India* 2002; **50**: 1245–1249.

34 Schena FP. Primary glomerulonephritides with nephrotic syndrome. Limitations of therapy in adult patients. *J Nephrol* 1999; **12**(**Suppl 2**): S125–S130.

35 Remuzzi G, Chiurchiu C, Ruggenenti P. Proteinuria predicting outcome in renal disease: nondiabetic nephropathies (REIN). *Kidney Int Suppl* 2004; **92**: S90–S96.

36 McEnery PT, McAdams AJ, West CD. The effect of prednisone in a high-dose, alternate day regimen on the natural history of idiopathic membranoproliferative glomerulonephritis. *Medicine* (Baltimore) 1985; **64**: 401–424.

37 McEnery PT. Membranoproliferative glomerulonephritis: the Cincinnati experience, cumulative renal survival from 1957–1989. *J Pediatr* 1990; **116**: S109–S114.

38 Braun MC, West CD, Strife CF. Difference between membranoproliferative glomerulonephritis type I and III in long-term response to an alternate-day prednisone regimen. *Am J Kidney Dis* 1999; **34**: 1022–1032.

39 Warady BA, Guggenheim SJ, Sedman A, Lum GM. Prednisone therapy of membranoproliferative glomerulonephritis in children. *J Pediatr* 1985; **107**: 702–707.

40 Ford DM, Briscoe DM, Shanley PF, Lum GM. Childhood membranoproliferative glomerulonephritis type I: limited steroid therapy. *Kidney Int* 1992; **41**: 1606–1612.

41 Bergstein JM, Andreoli SP. Response of type I membranoproliferative glomerulonephritis to pulse methyl prednisolone and alternate day prednisone therapy. *Pediatr Nephrol* 1995; **9**: 268–271.

42 Yanagihara T, Hayakawa M, Yoshida J, Tsuchiya M, Morita T, Murakami M *et al.* Long-term follow-up of diffuse membranoproliferative glomerulonephritis type I. *Pediatr Nephrol* 2005; **20**: 585–590.

43 Emre S, Sirin A, Alpay H, Tanman F, Uysal V, Nayir A *et al.* Pulse methylprednisolone therapy in children with membranoproliferative glomerulonephritis. *Acta Paediatr Jpn* 1995; **37**: 626–629.

44 Iitaka K, Ishidate T, Hojo M, Kuwao S, Kasai N, Sakai T. Idiopathic membranoproliferative glomerulonephritis in Japanese children. *Pediatr Nephrol* 1995; **9**: 272–277.

45 Kazama I, Matsubara M, Ejima Y, Michimata M, Suzuki M, Miyama N *et al.* Steroid resistance in prolonged type I membranoproliferative glomerulonephritis and accelerated disease remission after steroid withdrawal. *Clin Exp Nephrol* 2005; **9**: 62–68.

46 Takeda A, Niimura F, Matsutani H. Long-term corticosteroid and dipyridamole treatment of membranoproliferative glomerulonephritis type I in children. *Nippon Jinzo Gakkai Shi* 1995; **37**: 330–335.

47 Bahat E, Akkaya BK, Akman S, Karpuzoglu G, Guven AG. Comparison of pulse and oral steroid in childhood membranoproliferative glomerulonephritis. *J Nephrol* 2007; **20**: 234–245.

48 Harmankaya O, Basturk T, Ozturk Y, Karabiber N, Obek A. Effect of acetylsalicylic acid and dipyridamole in primary membranoproliferative glomerulonephritis type I. *Int Urol Nephrol* 2001; **33**: 583–587.

49 Kincaid-Smith P. The treatment of chronic mesangiocapillary (membranoproliferative) glomerulonephritis with impaired renal function. *Med J Aust* 1972; **2**: 587–592.

50 Chapman SJ, Cameron JS, Chantler C, Turner D. Treatment of mesangiocapillary glomerulonephritis in children with combined immunosuppression and anti-coagulation. *Arch Dis Child* 1980; **55**: 446–451.

51 Faedda R, Satta A, Tanda F, Pirisi M, Bartole E. Immunosuppressive treatment of membranoproliferative glomerulonephritis. *Nephron* 1994; **67**: 59–65.

52 Lagrue G, Laurent J, Beighiti D. Renal survival in membranoproliferative glomerulonephritis (MPGN): role of long-term treatment with non-steroidal anti-inflammatory drugs (NSAID). *Int Urol Nephrol* 1988; **20**: 669–677.

53 Vanrenterghem Y, Roels L, Verberckmoes R. Treatment of chronic glomerulonephritis with a combination of indomethacin and cyclophosphamide. *Clin Nephrol* 1975; **4**: 218–222.

54 Michielsen P, van Damme B, Dotremont G, Verberckmoes R, Oei LS, Vermylen J. Indomethacin treatment of membranoproliferative and lobular glomerulonephritis. In: Kincaid-Smith P, T Mathew T, Becker E, editors, *Glomerulonephritis*. John Wiley and Sons, New York, 1973; 611–620.

55 Kiyomasu T, Shibata M, Kurosu H, Shiraishi K, Hashimoto H, Hayashidera T *et al.* Cyclosporin A treatment for membranoproliferative glomerulonephritis type II. *Nephron* 2002; **91:** 509–511.

56 Matsumoto H, Shibasaki T, Ohno I, Sakai O, Kuriyama S, Tomohari H *et al.* Effect of cyclosporin monotherapy on proteinuria in patients with membranoproliferative glomerulonephritis. *Nippon Jinzo Gakkai Shi* 1995; **37:** 258–262.

57 Lagrue G, Laurent J, Robeva R. Membranoproliferative glomerulonephritis associated with Buckley's syndrome treated with cyclosporin. *Nephron* 1986; **44:** 382–383.

58 Haddad M, Lau K, Butani L. Remission of membranoproliferative glomerulonephritis type 1 with the use of Tacrolimus. *Pediatr Nephrol* 2007; **22:** 1787–1791.

59 Choi MJ, Eustace JA, Giminez LF, Atta MG, Scheel PJ, Sothinathan R *et al.* Mycophenolate mofetil treatment for primary glomerular diseases. *Kidney Int* 2002; **61:** 1098–1114.

60 Jones G, Juszczak M, Kingdon E, Harber M, Sweny P, Burns A. Treatment of idiopathic membranoproliferative glomerulonephritis with mycophenolate mofetil and steroids. *Nephrol Dial Transplant* 2004; **19:** 3160–3164.

61 Levin ML. Mycophenolate mofetil for primary glomerular diseases (editorial). *Kidney Int* 2002; **62:** 1475.

62 Karim MY, Abbas IC. Mycophenoalte mofetil in non-lupus glomerulonephropathy. *Lupus* 2005; **14(Suppl 1):** S39–S41.

63 Bayazit AK, Noyan A, Cengiz N, Anarat A. Mycophenolate mofetil in children with multi-drug resistant nephrotic syndrome. *Clin Nephrol* 2004; **61:** 25–29.

64 Yoshino A, Honda M, Kanegane H, Obata K, Matsukura H, Sakazume S *et al.* Membranoproliferative glomerulonephritis in a patient with X-linked agammaglobulinemia. *Pediatr Nephrol* 2006; **21:** 36–38.

65 Braun MC, Stablein DM, Hamiwka LA, Bell L, Bartosh SM, Strife CF. Recurrence of membranoproliferative glomerulonephritis type II in renal allografts. The North American Pediatric Renal Transplant Cooperative Study experience. *J Am Soc Nephrol* 2005; **16:** 2225–2233.

66 Kurtz KA, Schlueter AJ. Management of membranoproliferative glomerulonephritis type II with plasmapheresis. *J Cin Apher* 2002; **17:** 135–137.

67 Lien YH, Scott K. Long-term cyclophosphamide treatment for recurrent type I membranoproliferative glomerulonephritis after transplantation. *Am J Kidney Dis* 2000; **35:** 539–543.

68 Wu J, Jaar BG, Briggs WA, Choi MJ, Kraus ES, Racusen LC *et al.* High-dose mycophenolate mofetil in the treatment of post-transplant glomerular disease in the allograft: a case series. *Nephron Clin Pract* 2004; **98:** c61–c66.

69 Licht C, Weyersberg A, Heinen S, Stapenhorst C, Devenge J, Beck B *et al.* Successful plasma therapy for atypical hemolytic uremia syndrome caused by factor H deficiency owing to a novel mutation in the complement cofactor protein domain 15. *Am J Kidney Dis* 2005; **45:** 515–424.

70 West CD, McAdams AJ, Witte DP. Acute non-proliferative glomerulonephritis: a cause of renal failure unique to children. *Pediatr Nephrol* 2000; **14:** 786–793.

71 Licht C, Schlotzer-Schrehardt U, Kirschfink M, Zipfel PF, Hoppe B. MPGN-II-genetically determined by defective complement regulation? *Pediatr Nephrol* 2007; **22:** 2–9.

72 de Cordoba SR, de Jorge EG. Translational mini-review series on complement factor H. Genetics and disease associations of human complement factor H. *Clin Exp Immunol* 2008; **151:** 1–13.

73 Pickering MC, Cook HT. Translational mini-review series on complement factor H. Renal diseases associated with complement factor H: novel insights from human and animals. *Clin Exp Immunol* 2008; **151:** 210–230.

74 Noris M, Remuzzi G. Translational mini-review series on complement factor H. Therapies of renal diseases associated with complement factor H abnormalities: atypical hemolytic uremic syndrome and membranoproliferative glomerulonephritis. *Clin Exp Immunol* 2008; **151:** 199–209.

75 Levin A. Management of membranoproliferative glomerulonephritis: evidence-based recommendations. *Kidney Int* 1999; **46(Suppl 70):** S41–S46.

4 Secondary Diseases of the Kidney

Hypertensive Renal Disease

17 Hypertension: Classification and Diagnosis

Bernardo Rodriguez-Iturbe & Crispín Marin Villalobos

Nephrology Section, Hospital Universitario, and Universidad del Zulia, School of Medicine, Maracaibo, Venezuela

Introduction

A high level of arterial blood pressure, or hypertension, is a mortality and morbidity risk factor for cardiovascular and kidney disease and is responsible for 7.1 million deaths and 64 million disease adjusted life-years lost worldwide [1]. It is estimated that 25–35% of the world's population older than 18 years and more than 60% of individuals older than 70 years have blood pressure levels of $\geq$140/90 mmHg [2].

Because blood pressure levels are on a continuum, separation of normal and high values is somewhat arbitrary, with excess cardiovascular risk found with blood pressure values higher than 115 mmHg systolic and 75 mmHg diastolic blood pressure [3]. Guidelines from the *Seventh Report of the Joint National Committee on Prevention, Detection, Evaluation and Treatment of High Blood Pressure* [4] (Table 17.1) define hypertension in adults as a systolic blood pressure of $\geq$140 mmHg or diastolic blood pressure of $\geq$90 mmHg (average of two or more blood pressure determinations at two or more clinic visits). The category of prehypertension (systolic blood pressure of 120–139 mmHg or diastolic blood pressure of 80–89 mmHg) is also included, as this group of patients usually develop hypertension, and prehypertension is present in about 25% of the general population. Target levels for antihypertensive treatment have recently been lowered in patients with diabetes or kidney disease who are at increased risk for cardiovascular disease. In growing children, the blood pressure increases at about 1.5 mmHg systolic and 0.7 mmHg diastolic per year, and hypertension is defined as blood pressure levels equal to or greater than the 95th percentile of the distribution for age, sex, and height. Blood pressure levels between the 90th and 95th percentiles are considered high-normal [5].

A similar classification was essentially agreed upon by the World Health Organization, International Society of Hypertension, European Society of Hypertension, and the European Society of Cardiology (Table 17.1) [6].

Isolated systolic hypertension, isolated diastolic hypertension, "white coat" hypertension, isolated ambulatory hypertension, pseudohypertension, and orthostatic hypotension are defined in Table 17.2.

Auscultatory determination of Korotkoff sounds by trained personnel using a mercury sphygmomanometer is the traditionally accepted reference standard for blood pressure measurement. The systolic blood pressure corresponds to the beginning (phase I) and diastolic blood pressure to the cessation (phase V) of Korotkoff sounds. In older individuals with a wide pulse pressure there may be an auscultatory gap, when the sound disappears between systolic and diastolic pressure and reappears as cuff deflation continues. This can be avoided if the arm is elevated for 30 s before inflating the cuff.

Determination of blood pressure in different settings

Blood pressure in a clinic

Determination of blood pressure in a clinic is assumed to be a surrogate marker for the average blood pressure over time in a given patient, but it should be recognized that errors may result from misclassification of individuals as hypertensive when they are not (false positives) as well as from failure to recognize hypertension in some patients who have normal clinic readings (false negatives). Furthermore, clinic blood pressure does not disclose patients whose blood pressure remains high at night ("nondippers") and who have higher cardiovascular morbidity [7]. The mercury sphygmomanometer is the reference equipment for blood pressure determination but, like all technical items, regular maintenance is essential. It should be routinely checked for leaks and other problems, which affect as many as 25% of the devices currently in use [8]. Recently, aneroid and oscillometric automated devices have been used more commonly and, while generally accurate [9,10], they should be calibrated periodically with a mercury manometer

Evidence-based Nephrology. Edited by Donald Molony and Jonathan Craig
© 2009 Blackwell Publishing, ISBN: 978-1-4051-3975-5.

Table 17.1 Classification and definition of hypertension.

Classification system and hypertension category	Systolic BP (mmHg)	Diastolic BP (mmHg)
JNC-7		
Normal	<120	<80
Prehypertensive	120–139	80–89
Stage 1 hypertension	140–159	90–99
Stage 2 hypertension	≥160	≥100
WHO/ISH/ESH/ESC		
Optimal	<120	<80
Normal	120–129	80–84
High-normal	130–139	85–89
Stage 1 hypertension	140–159	90–99
Stage 2 hypertension	160–179	100–109
Stage 3 hypertension	≥180	≥110

Abbreviations: JNC-7, Joint National Committee on Prevention, Detection, Evaluation and Treatment of High Blood Pressure, 7th report (National Heart, Lung, and Blood Institute); WHO/ISH/ESH/ESC, a joint committee of the World Health Organization, International Society of Hypertension, European Society of Hypertension, and European Society of Cardiology.

[11]. In small children and neonates, Doppler ultrasound (systolic blood pressure) and oscillometric equipment (systolic, diastolic, and mean blood pressure) are commonly used.

There are several details that need to be considered when measuring blood pressure in the clinic. The patient should be seated with back support, without crossing the legs, and relaxed for more

Table 17.2 Hypertension definitions, from the AHA scientific statement.

Category	Definition
Isolated systolic hypertension	SBP ≥140, DBP <90
Isolated diastolic hypertension	SBP <140, DBP ≥90
White coat hypertension	Clinic BP >140/90 Ambulatory BP (avg) <135/85
Isolated ambulatory hypertension	Clinic BP <135/85 Ambulatory BP (avg) >140/90
Ambulatory hypertension	24-h avg >135/85
Ambulatory daytime hypertension	Avg daytime values >140/90
Ambulatory nighttime hypertension	Avg nighttime values >125/75
Pseudohypertension	Advanced or calcified arteries require high cuff pressure to compress them
Accelerated or malignant hypertension	DBP usually >120 in association with grade III (arteriolar narrowing and "nicking," flame-shaped hemorrhages, and exudates) or grade IV retinopathy (papilledema); treat as medical emergency

Source: American Heart Association [11].
Abbreviations: SBP, systolic blood pressure; DBP, diastolic blood pressure (all BP values are in mmHg).

than 5 min before measurements are taken. The cuff should have a length and width that are about 80% and 40%, respectively, of the arm circumference and should be placed on the upper arm at about the level of the right atrium. These conditions are important because, if not followed, they could result in an overestimation by as much as 20–25 mmHg (5 mmHg higher for undercuffing large arms, 8 mmHg higher in the supine position, 5 mmHg for crossing the legs, 5 mmHg for having the arm 2–3 in. above the right atrium) [12–14]. Ideally, three readings should be taken to reduce measurement error, and additional readings are required when differences between readings exceed 5 mmHg [11].

Specific problems may be present in elderly individuals (frequency of orthostatic hypotension), children (inappropriately small cuff size, anxiety), patients with arrhythmias (variability), and pulseless syndromes (Takayasu's arteritis, occlusive arterial disease, atherosclerosis) that may result in interarm blood pressure differences of greater than 10 mmHg [15].

Home monitoring of blood pressure

Home monitoring is convenient, cheap, and probably a better predictor of cardiovascular morbidity than clinic measurements [16]. Also, home monitoring of blood pressure is associated with increased compliance with recommended treatment [17]. Home blood pressure is usually determined by electronic oscillometric equipment rather than aneroid sphygmomanometers. A list of validated equipment for this purpose is available elsewhere (http://www.dableducational.org). The preferred devices measure blood pressure in the arm. It is recommended that these devices have annual checks for accuracy. Devices that give printed records are recommended, to avoid erroneous verbal reports to the physician [18]. In addition it is recommended that the patient follow the same guidelines discussed earlier and take three readings, usually in the morning and at night. The accepted upper limit of normal for ambulatory blood pressure is 135/85 mmHg [19].

Ambulatory blood pressure

Ambulatory blood pressure is measured with automated noninvasive equipment that takes blood pressure readings every 30 min over a 24-h period and, after computerized analysis, reports summary data of specific determinations, average 24-h values, and average day and night values. Although ambulatory blood pressure probably provides the most valid prognostic information [20], it is cumbersome, costly, uncomfortable, and not universally available. Ambulatory blood pressure measurement is usually done to identify individuals with "white coat" hypertension and those who do not have a nighttime reduction (nondippers). It may also prove useful in evaluating patients in whom episodes of hypertension or hypotension are suspected, in patients whose blood pressure is found intermittently to be above 140/90 mmHg (borderline hypertension), and in patients whose blood pressure varies widely during clinic visits.

Abnormally high ambulatory blood pressure is defined by 24-h average values of >135/85 mmHg, average daytime values of

Table 17.3 Frequencies of hypertension conditions.

Clinical condition[a] and etiology	Frequency
Essential hypertension Unknown cause	90–95%
Isolated systolic hypertension Reduced aortic compliance	>60% of hypertension after age 65 yrs
Increased systolic load (aortic insufficiency, patent ductus arteriosus, arteriovenous fistula, thyrotoxicosis, anemia, Paget's bone disease	<1%
Renal parenchymal diseases Glomerulonephritis (acute or chronic), pyelonephritis, polycystic disease, tubulo-interstitial disease, diabetic nephropathy, obstructive uropathy	4–6%
Pregnancy Eclampsia, preeclampsia	5% of all pregnancies
Renal vascular disorders Renal artery stenosis (atherosclerosis, fibromuscular hyperplasia)	1–4%
Endocrine diseases Primary aldosteronism, Cushing's disease, congenital adrenogenital syndromes (17α- or 11β-hydroxylase deficiency), pheochromocytoma, hypo- or hyperthyroidism, hyperparathyroidism (hypercalcemia), acromegaly	1%
Medications or toxic exposure Glucorticoids, mineralocorticoids, sympatho-mimetics, oral contraceptives, cyclosporine, nonsteroidal anti-infammatory drugs, erythropoietin, cocaine, amphetamines	1%
Coarctation of aorta	0.1–1%
Increased vascular volume or viscosity Polycythemia (vera, high altitude, or overtransfusion)	
Neurogenic disorders Familiar dysautonomia, acute spinal cord section, increased intracranial pressure	
Miscellaneous Acute porphyria, acute withdrawal from clonidine	

[a] Conditions are listed in order of decreasing frequency.

>140/90 mmHg, and average nighttime values of >125/75 mmHg (Table 17.2) [11].

Other settings

Determination of blood pressure in public places with automated devices does not meet accuracy requirements [21], and their usefulness rests primarily in increasing public awareness of the need for evaluation and treatment of hypertension.

Classification of hypertension

The etiologic classification of hypertension is traditionally made by separating the known (secondary) causes of increased blood pressure from the vast majority of cases without a discernible cause, which are designated as primary, idiopathic, or more commonly, essential hypertension (Table 17.3). The pathogenic mechanisms responsible for essential hypertension are discussed in chapter 18.

As indicated in Table 17.3, the vast majority of patients have essential hypertension, and the most common cause of secondary hypertension is parenchymal renal disease.

In children the prevalence of hypertension is about 1% [22]. The prevalence of persistent secondary hypertension is less than 0.1%, and 70–80% of these patients have parenchymal renal disease (acute glomerulonephritis, Henoch-Schönlein nephritis, hemolytic uremic syndrome, reflux nephropathy, etc.) and 5–10% have renovascular disease (fibromuscular dysplasia or arteritis). Coarctation of the aorta is reported in 0–29% of pediatric patients [23,24], and endocrine causes of hypertension (pheochromocytoma, congenital adrenal hyperplasia, apparent mineralocorticoid excess, and glucocorticoid remediable aldosteronism) are found in 1–8%. Renal tumors (Wilms' tumor, hamartoma, and hemangiopericytoma) rarely cause hypertension. Hypertension occurs in 60–90% of children who have received transplants, which is a higher percentage than in adults with functioning renal grafts [25].

Hypertension as a cause and consequence of kidney disease

For many years, malignant hypertension has been known to cause end-stage renal disease, but it was debated for some time whether

Does hypertension require immediate treatment (≥180/110)?

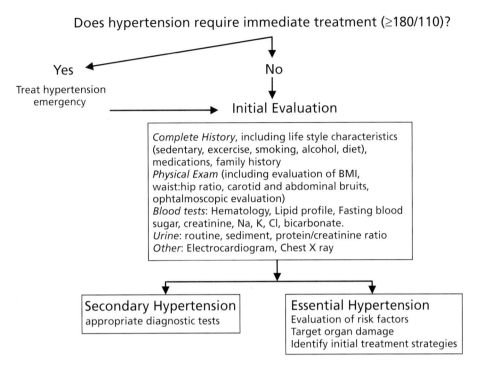

Figure 17.1 Initial evaluation of the patient with hypertension.

uncomplicated hypertension was the cause of nephrosclerosis [26]. This question was answered by the Multiple Risk Factor Intervention Trial, which demonstrated that both systolic and diastolic hypertension were strong independent risk factors of end-stage renal disease [27], and other studies have shown that reducing blood pressure with angiotensin converting enzyme inhibitors reduces the risk of end-stage renal disease or death by as much as 55% in 3–5 years if the systolic blood pressure is controlled to levels of 139 mmHg or lower [28,29]. There is considerable variation in reports of the incidence of hypertension as a cause of end-stage renal disease, ranging from 27% in the USA [30] to 13% in Europe and 6% in Japan [31]. In Latin America there is considerable variation between countries and within countries, but the reported mean value is 28% [32].

Hypertension is also a consequence of renal disease. Reduction in nephron number of any cause, intrarenal inflammation, and increased intrarenal angiotensin II and oxidative stress result in a tendency to sodium retention, leading to hypertension [33]. Diabetic nephropathy occurs in about 40% of type 2 diabetics and is the most common cause of end-stage renal disease worldwide, and hypertension is present in almost all patients with type 2 diabetes.

Unilateral renal disease is also a cause of hypertension. Unilateral segmental renal hypoplasia (associated with vesicourethral reflux), unilateral renal agenesis, hydronephrosis, and renal trauma may occasionally result in hypertension. Hypertension associated with perirenal hematoma has been considered to be renin-induced due to parenchymal compression, in a manner similar to the hypertension resulting from the perinephritic hull resulting from cellophane wrapping of the kidney (Page kidney). Recently, evi-

dence has been advanced indicating that in the Page kidney model, hypertension is caused by interstitial inflammation and increased intrarenal (rather than plasma) angiotensin II activity [34], and it is likely that similar mechanisms may be operating in subcapsular renal hematoma because nephrectomy, but not the relief of the compression, is frequently associated with normalization of blood pressure [35].

Evaluation of the hypertensive patient

When a patient with hypertension is initially evaluated, the severity of the hypertension may warrant immediate treatment. A cost-effective initial evaluation of the patient is shown in Figure 17.1, and this evaluation should be directed to 1) examine the possibility of secondary causes of hypertension, 2) determine the existence of risk factors and target organ damage, and 3) define initial treatment strategies. If secondary causes of hypertension are suspected (Table 17.3), specific diagnostic tests are indicated (Table 17.4).

In the patient history, information on diet, habits, ingestion of medications such as oral contraceptives and nonsteroidal anti-inflammatory agents, family history of hypertension or kidney disease, and past history of edema, proteinuria, or hematuria, among other factors, is important. Recent onset of hypertension before the age of 20 years or after the age of 60 years should raise suspicion of renal artery stenosis in addition to the findings listed in Table 17.4.

Physical examination may disclose palpable kidneys (polycystic kidney disease), abdominal murmurs (renal artery stenosis),

Table 17.4 Diagnostic evaluation of the most common causes of secondary hypertension.

Condition	Clinical finding(s)	Abnormal laboratory tests	Sensitivity/specificity (%)[a]	Reference(s)
Renal parenchymal disease	History of renal disease, edema, flank pain, urinary symptoms, hematuria	Serum creatinine, proteinuria, blood glucose, urine sediment		
Renal artery stenosis	Recent development or sudden worsening of hypertension, abdominal bruit, azotemia induced by ACE inhibitor, flash pulmonary edema, hypokalemia, azotemia with normal urine sediment	Captopril-enhanced Doppler ultrasound scan	60–65/NR	[38,39]
		MRA	62–94/85 (for transplant artery stenosis, 100/75) 64/92	[40,41,42]
		Gadolinium-enhanced MRA	88–100/71–100	[40]
		Angio-CT		
		Digital subtraction renal artery angiography	Gold standard	[41]
Hyperaldosteronism	Hypokalemia	Serum aldosterone/plasma renin ratio	89 /96	[43]
		CT scan	62/77	[44]
		MRI	100/64	[44]
Pheochromocytoma	Episodes of headache, palpitation, and sweating	Urinary metanephrines	100/NR	[45]
		Plasma cathecholamines	85/NR	[45]
		Urinary VMA	89/NR	[45]
		CT scan (localization)	85–95	[45,46]
		MRI (localization)	>95	[45,46]

Abbreviations: MRI, magnetic resonance imaging; MRA, magnetic resonance angiography; CT, computer tomography (CAT scan); ACE, angiotensin converting enzyme; NR, not reported; VMA, vanillyl madelic acid.

deafness (Alport's disease), neurofibromatosis (pheochromocytoma), or adenoma sebaceum (tuberous sclerosis).

Laboratory investigations should always include urine sediment analysis and, if proteinuria is detected, 24-h urinary protein excretion or a spot creatinine/protein concentration ratio should be determined. A test for albuminuria (micral test or albumin/creatinine ratio in spot morning urine, followed by quantified excretion in timed urine samples if the data are in the microalbuminuric range) may help detect kidney damage before the appearance of clinical proteinuria. In addition, for all patients the levels of plasma creatinine (used to calculate the glomerular filtration rate by standard formulas), electrolytes (hypokalemia would suggest diuretic therapy, renal artery stenosis, or hyperaldosteronism), and fasting glucose (if abnormal, evaluate for diabetes), lipid profile, and body mass index (to determine risk factors) should be determined. An electrocardiogram and echocardiogram are indicated to detect and monitor left ventricular hypertrophy.

Radiological and image analyses are not routinely indicated. Depending on the suspected diagnosis, renal ultrasonography (for obstruction, stone disease, and polycystic kidneys), intravenous urography (for obstruction, stone disease, and to determine whether macroscopic hematuria is present), computerized tomography, magnetic resonance angiography, and renal angiography (as the reference standard for renal artery stenosis, prior to correction) may all be useful. Renography with isotopes that are eliminated by glomerular filtration (e.g. ^{99}Tc-diethylenetriaminepenta acetic acid) are markers of renal blood flow, and evaluation with [^{123}I]iodohippurate may occasionally also be useful. Magnetic resonance angiography is useful in the study of renal artery stenosis (Table 17.4) but only when the stenosis is in the main renal artery.

In children, hypertension is usually asymptomatic or presents with nonspecific symptoms: failure to thrive, irritability, and convulsions in infants, and headache, visual disturbances, vomiting, epistaxis, growth retardation, and facial palsy in older children [36]. If hypertension is severe, the initial evaluation in children should include not only hematology, blood chemistries, and urinary sediment but also abdominal ultrasound studies and ^{99}mTc-dimercaptosuccinic acid scans (for detecting segmental scars resulting from pyelonephritis) and determinations of end-organ damage (echocardiography, electrocardiography) [37]. Intravenous urography and voiding cystourethrography are only indicated if vesicouretheral reflux or obstruction is suspected.

References

1 WHO. *The World Health Report 2002: Reducing Risks, Promoting Healthy Life*, chapter 4. http://www.who.int/whr/2002/chapter4/en/.

2 Staessen JA, Wang J, Bianchi G, Birkenhager WH. Essential hypertension. *Lancet* 2003; **361**: 1629–1641.

3 Lewington S, Clarke R, Qizilbash N, Peto R, Collins R, Prospective Studies Collaboration. Age-specific relevance of usual blood pressure to vascular mortality: a meta-analysis of individual data for one million adults in 61 prospective studies. *Lancet* 2002; **360**: 1903–1913.

4 Chobanian AV, Bakris GL, Black HR, Cushman WC, Green LA, Izzo JL *et al.* Joint National Committee on Prevention, Detection, Evaluation and Treatment of High Blood Pressure; National Heart, Lung, and Blood Institute. Seventh report. *Hypertension* 2003; **42**: 1206–1252.

5 National High Blood Pressure Education Program Working Group on Hypertension Control in Children and Adolescents. Update on the 1987 Task Force report on high blood pressure in children and adolescents: a working group report. *Pediatrics* 1996; **98**: 649–658.

6 Cifkova R, Erdine S, Fagard C, Heagerty AM, Kiowski W, Kjeldsen S *et al.* 2003 ESH/ESC Hypertension Guidelines Committee: practice guidelines. *J Hypertens* 2003; **21**: 1779–1786.

7 Verdecchia P, Schillaci G, Borgioni C, Ciucci A, Gattobigio R, Porcellatti C. Nocturnal pressure is the true pressure. *Blood Press Monit* 1966; **1(Suppl 2)**: S81–S85.

8 Mion D, Pierin AM. How accurate are sphygmomanometers? *J Hum Hypertens* 1998; **12**: 245–248.

9 Canzanello VJ, Jensen PL, Schwartz GL. Are aneroid sphygmomanometers accurate in hospital and clinical settings? *Arch Intern Med* 2001; **161**: 729–773.

10 Cates EM, Sclussel YR, James GD, Pickering TG. A validation study of the Spacelabs 90207 ambulatory blood pressure monitor. *J Ambul Monitor* 1990; **3**: 149–154.

11 Pickering TG, Hall JE, Appel LJ, Falkner BE, Graves J, Hill MN *et al.* Recommendations for blood pressure measurement in humans and experimental animals. Part 1: blood pressure measurement in humans. *Hypertension* 2005; **45**: 142–161.

12 Terent A, Breig-Asberg E. Epidemiological perspective of body position and arm level in blood pressure measurements. *Blood Press* 1994; **3**: 156–163.

13 Peters GL, Binder SK, Campbell NR. The effect of crossing legs on blood pressure: a randomized single-blind cross-over study. *Blood Press Monit* 1999; **4**: 97–101.

14 Netea RT, Lenders JW, Smits P, Thien T. Arm position is important for blood pressure measurement. *J Hum Hypertens* 1999; **3**: 471–474.

15 Materson BJ. Inter-arm blood pressure differences. *J Hypertens* 2004; **22**: 2267–2268.

16 Tsuji I, Imai Y, Nagai K, Ohkubo T, Watanabe N, Minami N *et al.* Proposal of reference values for home blood pressure measurement: prognostic criteria based on prospective observations of the general population in Ohasama, Japan. *Am J Hypertens* 1997; **10**: 409–418.

17 Stahl SM, Kelley CR, Neil PJ, Grim CE, Mamlin J. Effects of home blood pressure measurement on long-term BP control. *Am J Public Health* 1984; **74**: 704–709.

18 Mengden T, Hernandez-Medina RM, Beltran B, Alvarez E, Kraft K. Vetter H. Reliability of reporting self-measured blood pressure values by hypertensive patients. *Am J Hypertens* 1998; **11**: 1413–1417.

19 Pickering T. Recommendations for the use of home, self and ambulatory blood pressure monitoring. American Society of Hypertension Ad Hoc Panel. *Am J Hypertens* 196; **9**: 1–11.

20 Staesseb JA, Asmar R, De Buyzere M, Imai Y, Parati G, Shimada K *et al.* Consensus conference on ambulatory blood pressure measurement and cardiovascular outcome. *Blood Press Monit* 2001; **6**: 355–370.

21 Lewis JE, Boyle E, Magharious L, Myers MG. Evaluation of a community-based automated blood pressure measuring device. *CMAJ* 2002; **166**: 1145–1148.

22 Adrogue HE, Sinaiko AR. Prevalence of hypertension in junior high school-aged children: effect of new recommendations in the 1996 Updated Task Force Report. *Am J Hypertens* 2001; **14**: 412–414.

23 Loirat C, Azancot-Benisty A, Bossu C, Durant I. Value of ambulatory blood pressure monitoring in borderline hypertension in the child. *Ann Pediatr* (Paris) 1991; **38**: 381–386.

24 Uhari M, Koskimies O. A survey of 164 Finnish children and adolescent with hypertension. *Acta Paediatr Scand* 1979; **68**: 193–198.

25 Baluarte HJ, Gruskin AB, Ingelfinger JR, Stablein D, Tejani DA. Analysis of hypertension in children post-renal transplantation. A report of the North American Pediatric Renal Transplant Cooperative Study (NAPRTCS). *Pediatr Nephrol* 1994; **8**: 570–573.

26 Zucchelli P, Zuccala A. Recent data on hypertension and progressive renal disease. *J Hum Hyperten* 1996; **10**: 679–682.

27 Klag MJ, Whelton PK, Randall BL, Neaton JD, Brancata FL, Ford CE *et al.* Blood pressure and end-stage renal disease in men. *N Engl J Med* 1996; **334**: 13–18.

28 Agoda LY, Appel L, Bakris GL, Beck G, Bourgoignie J, Briggs, JP *et al.* Effect of ramipril vs amlodipine on renal outcomes in hypertensive nephrosclerosis: a randomized controlled trial. *JAMA* 2001; **285**: 2719–2728.

29 Jafar TH, Schmid CH, Landa M, Giatras I, Toto R, Ramuzzi G *et al.* Angiotensin-converting enzyme inhibitors and progression of nondiabetic renal disease. A meta-analysis of patient-level data. *Ann Intern Med* 2001; **135**: 73–87.

30 US Renal Data System. *Annual Data Report: Atlas of ESRD in the United States.* National Institute of Diabetes and Digestive and Kidney Diseases, National Institutes of Health, Bethesda, 2001.

31 Vaderrabano F, Gomez-Campdera F, Jones EM. Hypertension as a cause of end-sate renal disease: lessons from international registries. *Kidney Int Suppl* 1998; **68**: S60–S66.

32 Rodriguez-Iturbe B, Bellorin-Font E. End-stage renal disease prevention strategies in Latin America. *Kidney Int Suppl* 2005; **68(Suppl 98)**: S30–S36.

33 Rodriguez-Iturbe B, Vaziri ND, Herrera-Acosta J, Johnson RJ. Oxidative stress, renal infiltration of immune cells and salt-sensitive hypertension: all for one and one for all. *Am J Physiol Renal Physiol* 2004; **286**: F606–F616.

34 Vanegas V, Ferrebuz A, Quiroz Y, Rodriguez-Iturbe B. Hypertension in Page (cellophane wrapped) kidney is due to interstitial nephritis. *Kidney Int* 2005; **68**: 1161–1170.

35 Sterns RH, Rabonovitz R, Segal AJ, Spitzer EM. Page kidney: hypertension caused by subcapsular hematoma. *Arch Intern Med* 1985; **145**: 1609–1701.

36 Tirodker UH, Dabbagh F. Facial paralysis in childhood hypertension. *J Paediatr Health* 2001; **37**: 193–194.

37 Recommendations for Management of Hypertension in Children and Adolescents. *Clin Exp Hypertens* 1986; **A8**: 901–918.

38 Postma CT, van Aalen J, de Boo T, Rosenbusch G, Thien T. Doppler ultrasound scanning in the detection of renal artery stenosis in hypertensive patients. *Br J Radiol* 1992; **65**: 857–860.

39 Qanadli SD, Soulez G, Therasse E, Nicolet V, Turpin S, Froment D *et al.* Detection of renal artery stenosis: prospective comparison of captopril-enhanced Doppler sonography, captopril-enhanced sonography, and MR angiography. *Am J Roentgenol* 2001; **177**: 1123–1129.

40 Tan KT, van Beek EJ, Brown PW, van Delden OM, Tijssen J, Ramsay LE. Magnetic resonance angiography for the diagnosis of renal artery stenosis: a meta-analysis. *Clin Radiol* 2002; **57**: 617–624.

41 Vasbinder GB, Nelemans PJ, Kessels AG, Kroon AA, Maki JH, Leiner T *et al.* Accuracy of computed tomographic angiography and magnetic

resonance angiography for diagnosis of renal artery stenosis. *Ann Intern Med* 2004; **141**: 674–682.

42 Chan YL, Leung CB, Yu SC, Yeung DK, Li PK. Comparison of non-breath-hold high resolution gadolimium-enhanced MRA with digital subtraction angiography in the evaluation of allograft renal artery stenosis. *Clin Radiol* 2001; **56**: 127–132.

43 Trenkel S, Seifarth C, Schobel H, Hahn EG, Hensen J. Ratio of serum aldosterone to plasma renin concentration in essential hypertension and primary aldosteronism. *Exp Clin Endocrinol Diabetes* 2002; **110**: 80–85.

44 Rossi GP, Chiesura-Corona M, Tregnanhi A, Zanin L, Perale R, Saottin S *et al.* Imaging of aldosterone-secreting adenomas: a prospective comparison of computed tomography and magnetic resonance imaging in 27 patients with suspected primary aldosteronism. *J Hum Hypertens* 1993; **7**: 357–363.

45 Witteles RM, Kaplan EL, Roizen MF. Sensitivity of diagnostic and localization tests for pheochromocytoma in clinical practice. *Arch Intern Med* 2000; **160**: 2521–2525.

46 Plouin PF, Chatellier G, Delahousse M, Rougeot MA, Duclos JM, Pagny JY *et al.* Detection, diagnosis and localization of pheochromocytoma. 77 cases in a population of 21,420 hypertensive patients. *Presse Med* 1987; **16**: 2211–2215.

18 Management of Essential Hypertension

Eberhard Ritz,[1] Danilo Fliser,[2] & Marcin Adamczak[3]

[1] Department of Internal Medicine, Nierenzentrum, Ruperto Carola University, Heidelberg, Germany.
[2] Department of Internal Medicine, Division of Nephrology, Medical School Hannover, Hannover, Germany.
[3] Department of Nephrology, Endocrinology and Metabolic Diseases, Medical University of Silesia, Katowice, Poland.

Evidence for hypertensive renal damage

Historically, renal failure in patients with hypertension occurred mainly as the result of malignant hypertension [1]. However, with the introduction of potent antihypertensive drugs, malignant hypertension and kidney failure caused by malignant hypertension have become rare [2]. Because virtually no renal end points were observed in individuals with primary hypertension in relatively short-term studies, it had been widely assumed that primary hypertension caused few, if any, renal sequelae in individuals without primary kidney disease. More recent observational data over longer periods of time suggested that this view needed modification. The failure to observe renal sequelae may be explained primarily by the insufficient duration of trials designed to observe cardiovascular end points. Today, evidence from long-term observational studies has shown that, in individuals without primary chronic kidney disease (CKD), a relationship exists between the level of blood pressure (BP) and impaired renal function. These studies also show that the evolution of kidney failure in patients with nonmalignant hypertension usually takes decades [3–7]. The true frequency of this is unknown, because no series have been reported where the diagnosis of "renal failure from hypertensive nephropathy" was confirmed by renal biopsy. Registry data are unreliable, as shown by large differences in end-stage renal disease incidence data due to hypertension reported from different countries. The most convincing evidence comes from small series where the diagnosis has been established by renal biopsy [8]. These findings support the view that the term "benign nephrosclerosis" (which goes back to Volhard and Fahr [9]) is a misnomer and underestimates the role of primary hypertension in the initiation and progression of CKD. Even more common, the mild impairment of renal function seen in many elderly patients with primary hypertension, although infrequently causing dialysis-dependent kidney failure, is not benign because of the high cardiovascular risk conferred by even minor renal dysfunction, as reflected by diminished estimated glomerular filtration rate (GFR) [10–12] or albuminuria or proteinuria [13–15].

The evidence that essential hypertension may (relatively infrequently) lead even to end-stage renal disease is based on experimental as well as human studies. In animal models of primary hypertension that may result in CKD, for example, Dahl salt-sensitive rats and some strains of spontaneously hypertensive rats, a clear-cut relationship exists between the BP increase and development of kidney failure [16,17], particularly when sensitizing maneuvers such as unilateral nephrectomy are performed [18,19] that are known to cause dilatation of the afferent (preglomerular) artery, thus triggering glomerular hypertension [20–22]. Moreover, in these animals lowering BP retards progression of renal injury [23–25]. The hypothesis of "nephron underdosing," proposed by Brenner [26], potentially provides a link between the genesis of hypertension and the evolution of CKD in these experimental settings and in humans [27–30]. According to this theory, a reduced number of nephrons causes hypertension, which in turn may further accelerate the development of abnormalities in renal structure and function.

What is the evidence in humans? Evidence for an important role of high BP in the development of CKD and progressive loss of renal function has been provided by historical observations of untreated hypertensive patients [31], although these observations are confounded by the occurrence of malignant hypertension. In the tradition of the classical anatomical descriptions of Gull and Suton [32] and Volhard and Fahr [9], additional information has come from the scarce biopsy studies in hypertensive patients with presumed "hypertensive nephropathy" and no evidence of primary kidney disease or diabetes mellitus [8,33–36], autopsy studies [37,38], and long-term observational studies in patients with presumed primary hypertension who have been followed for more than a decade [3–6]. Registry information of patients on hypertensive nephropathy as a cause for renal replacement therapy, for instance, in the US Renal Data System [39], is unreliable because of the absence of biopsy confirmation. Striking differences in the reported frequencies between countries [40] may, in part, be due to varying susceptibilities of some ethnicities, particularly black people, to hypertensive kidney damage [36]. In the general US population, approximately 0.2% developed terminal kidney failure during an average observational period of 16 years, and this risk was clearly related to BP [5]. In patients with primary hypertension this proportion was considerably higher and increased in parallel with the severity of hypertension. In patients with severe hypertension, more than 3% developed end-stage renal disease, that is, their relative risk for the development of kidney failure was 12.4 compared to subjects with "optimal" BP. Progression to kidney failure was a function of the BP value in several studies, systolic BP being more tightly correlated than diastolic BP, with the elderly and Black people having a worse prognosis [3,4]. In individuals without evidence of kidney disease at baseline, as reflected by an absence of proteinuria, a graded increase of the risk to develop end-stage renal disease with time was found even for BP values within the "normal" range according to past WHO definitions [6]. Hypertension may also cause renal failure indirectly, by promoting atherosclerosis of the abdominal aorta with ischemic nephropathy resulting from renal artery stenosis, cholesterol embolism, or arteriolosclerosis, or a combination of these conditions [38].

One interesting observation is the finding that BP goes with the transplanted kidney in humans [42] as it does in experimental animals [43], suggesting that in humans a functional defect in the kidneys plays a causal role in the development of primary hypertension. It has been argued that the kidney is the culprit as well as the victim of high BP [44]. This argument is not invalidated by the evidence, from cross-kidney transplantation experiments in AT_1 receptor knockout animals, that extrarenal vascular territories make nonredundant contributions to BP regulation [45].

Diagnosis of hypertensive renal damage

Classically, it has been postulated that the typical finding in primary hypertension is ischemic kidney disease leading to the constellation of small kidneys with impaired renal function but without significant proteinuria. This assumption was disproved by findings in biopsy studies showing that even nephrotic proteinuria may be found in patients with ischemic kidney disease [34].

Measurement of GFR

The GFR can be measured using different methods. The gold standard for the measurement of true GFR is still inulin clearance, but iohexol, Cr-EDTA, or iothalamate clearances are valuable alternatives. However, these clearance measurements are cumbersome and too expensive for routine clinical use or use in epidemiological studies. Thus, estimates of GFR based on the measurement of serum creatinine, such as with the MDRD [46] and Cockcroft-Gault equation [47], are widely accepted, but these estimates are not very accurate, particularly in the near-normal range [46]. Also, they have not been validated in specific populations and

ethnicities, such as the very old, patients with a renal allograft, African Americans, or Asians. The newer MDRD formula, which was derived from data of the Modification of Diet in Renal Disease trial, is more accurate for advanced rather than early-stage CKD [46]. A major problem with the MDRD equation is that it depends on the accuracy of serum creatinine measurement, which may vary considerably between different laboratories. In addition, interethnic differences may result in different estimates. Newer tests for GFR, such as serum cystatin C, are becoming available that are not confounded by muscle mass or tubular transport of creatinine [46,48].

Quantification of urinary albumin and protein excretion

Albuminuria is usually categorized into micro- and macroalbuminuria, but the method by which urine should be collected is still unresolved: spot urine (with or without creatinine correction), morning urine, or 24-h urine. It is also unclear how urinary albumin should be measured: immune detection or high-performance liquid chromatography [49,50]. Albuminuria also varies physiologically and is reversibly elevated by physical exercise, fever, and heart failure.

Despite these unresolved methodological problems, an increased urinary albumin (and protein) excretion rate has been clearly documented in patients with essential hypertension, although recent epidemiologic studies have shown that the prevalence of albuminuria is rather modest [51–55]. Nevertheless, this parameter is of considerable interest, because it identifies hypertensive individuals at particularly high risk of cardiovascular complications and death [13,56] (see Table 30.3 in chapter 30 for more information on risk factors in CKD progression). In the Göteborg study the proteinuria was even more predictive than total cholesterol for adverse cardiovascular outcomes [56]. The reasons why urinary albumin excretion is predictive of cardiovascular death have not been clarified, but it has been hypothesized that elevated urinary albumin excretion, as a result of glomerular injury, may reflect generalized endothelial dysfunction in nonrenal vascular beds as well [57]. In line with this assumption, an increased transcapillary escape rate of albumin as a potential marker of generalized endothelial dysfunction has been found in patients with essential hypertension [58]. It is also not clear whether albuminuria reflects a functional disturbance of the glomerulus, structural renal damage, or both, and whether albuminuria is fully explained by glomerular leakage or whether abnormalities of tubular albumin reabsorption contribute. Further information from biopsy studies with ultrastructural and gene expression analyses would be highly desirable. It is also uncertain whether in patients with essential hypertension (micro)albuminuria is associated with the long-term risk of progressive renal injury [59] as it is in diabetes mellitus [60]. Despite such gaps in our knowledge, measurement of urinary albumin provides information important for patient management because of the tight relation between urinary albumin excretion (even in the high-normal range) and the risk of cardiovascular complications.

Prevention and treatment

Strategies of prevention and treatment of hypertension-induced CKD are all based on observational studies, because large controlled prospective trials on this issue are completely lacking with the exception of the African American Study of Kidney Disease and Hypertension (AASK) study in the specific population of African American patients. The few relevant observational studies that are available suffer from drawbacks such as insufficient duration and/or inclusion of mostly young individuals in whom renal risk is considerably lower, absence of information on albuminuria and/or proteinuria as a renal risk modifier, and selecting (and validating) cardiovascular events, assuming that factors affecting cardiovascular end points also affect renal outcome (what is good for the heart is good for the kidney). Also, in the studies that did measure a renal end point, this was frequently confounded by comorbidities such as (undetected) chronic heart failure, diabetes, and prediabetes. In the studies where medication has been used which reduces renin–angiotensin–aldosterone system (RAAS) activity it is difficult to evaluate whether, for example, changes in GFR are the result of natural history, RAAS blockade, or BP lowering.

These shortcomings mean there is some uncertainty inherent in the following recommendations concerning BP and the choice of specific antihypertensive drugs.

Target BP

Relatively small studies have suggested that antihypertensive treatment reduces renal damage caused by hypertension [61,62]. This was not confirmed in a meta-analysis of the available literature by Hsu, in which no significant overall effect could be shown [63], with the exception of the AASK study in African Americans.

It is uncertain which BP parameter is the most important treatment target for renoprotection in hypertensive CKD: systolic BP, diastolic BP, or pulse pressure. It is also unclear which measurement is most relevant: clinic BP, home BP, 24-h ambulatory BP monitoring, nighttime BP, monitoring of early morning surge, or BP variability.

In patients with CKD due to diabetes mellitus, observational studies and post hoc analyses of intervention trials have shown that systolic BP is more predictive of renal function loss than diastolic BP or pulse pressure [64]. Further, observational data indicate that high nocturnal BP is associated with a more rapid loss of renal function in nondiabetic patients [65], but such information is lacking for patients with hypertensive renal damage. The authors concluded that general recommendations based on clinic BP do not do justice to the complexity of BP control. Published guidelines define a target BP of below 140/90 mmHg in the absence of renal disease, below 130/85 mmHg for patients with CKD and diabetes, and even values below this threshold in patients with gross proteinuria [66–68].

The only currently available solid evidence to support these recommendations in patients with CKD as a result of hypertension-induced kidney failure is the AASK study [69]. In that study, comprising a total of 1094 African Americans with hypertensive kidney disease (GFR between 20 and 65 mL/min/1.73 m^2), the effects of two levels of BP control and three antihypertensive drug classes on change in GFR (i.e. GFR slope) during a follow-up period of 3–6.4 years were examined. Participants were randomly assigned to either usual BP control, that is, mean arterial BP between 102 and 107 mmHg ($n = 554$), or lower BP, that is, mean arterial BP of ≤92 mmHg ($n = 540$). The initial treatment was either the β-receptor blocker metoprolol ($n = 441$), the angiotensin converting enzyme inhibitor (ACEI) ramipril ($n = 436$), or the dihydropyridine calcium channel blocker amlodipine ($n = 217$). Open-label agents were added if necessary to achieve the assigned BP goals. The GFR slope was determined separately during the first 3 months following randomization (acute slope) and after 3 months (chronic slope), because the acute effects of the interventions on GFR may have differed from their long-term effects on disease progression. They achieved BP on average 128/78 mmHg in the lower BP group and 141/85 mmHg in the usual BP group, but the mean GFR slope from baseline through 4 years did not differ significantly between either intervention (lower BP group, −2.21 mL/min, vs. usual BP group, −1.95 mL/min/1.73 m^2/year) (Figure 18.1) [69]. Moreover, the lower BP goal did not significantly reduce the rate of the clinical composite outcome, including occurrence of end-stage renal failure. None of the drug group comparisons showed consistent significant differences in the GFR slope. However, compared with the metoprolol and amlodipine groups, the ramipril group had a reduced relative risk of 22% ($P = 0.04$) and 38% ($P = 0.004$), respectively. The authors concluded that lower BP control has no additional benefit of slowing progression of hypertensive nephrosclerosis and that an ACEI appears to be more effective than a β-receptor blocker or dihydropyridine calcium channel blockers in slowing GFR decline. However, the increase in proteinuria over time during the observation period was significantly less ($P < 0.001$) with lower target BP (Figure 18.2), and the same was true for the ACEI and β-receptor blocker treatment arms, compared to the amlodipine group ($P < 0.001$). Given the important role of proteinuria as a progression promoter in primary kidney disease and diabetic nephropathy, this finding corroborates the importance of insufficient trial duration for the proper assessment of progression in patients with hypertensive nephrosclerosis. Another limitation of the AASK trial is that the results are restricted to African Americans, so that they must be confirmed for other ethnicities. It should be stressed that to achieve the assigned BP goals in the AASK trial, most patients required more than monotherapy. The average number of antihypertensive drugs was 2.7 in the usual BP group and 3.5 in the lower BP group [69].

All classes of antihypertensive drugs are effective in lowering BP in patients with renal malfunction. However, adverse effects should be considered, particularly for aggressive BP lowering in the elderly with comorbidities, which may increase cardiac events and/or mortality, as recently shown in intervention trials [70,71]. When the systolic BP was reduced below 120 mmHg, all-cause mortality was higher by a factor of 3, a finding that is reminiscent

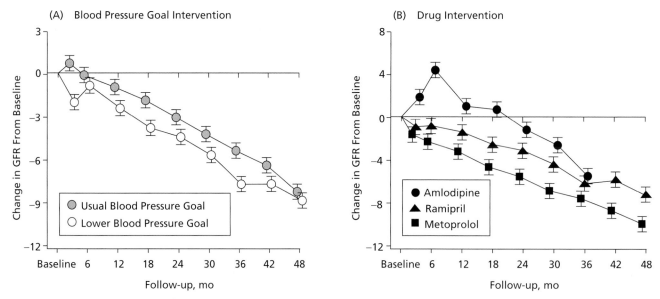

Figure 18.1 Effects of BP goal and selection of antihypertensive agent on GFR (AASK trial [69]). Mean changes in GFR by randomized group are shown. Data are the estimated mean changes (with standard errors of the means) in GFR (in mL/min/1.73 m^2) from baseline through follow-up with the two BP goal interventions (A) and with the three drug interventions (B). The plot is based on a multislope generalization of the two-slope mixed-effects model, in which different mean slopes are estimated within each treatment group for each interval between scheduled GFR measurements. Numbers of patients with GFR data at years 0, 1, 2, 3, 4, and 5 in all treatment groups combined were 1094, 953, 837, 731, 469, and 262, respectively.

of the J-curve phenomenon, that is, a paradoxical increase in mortality. As a consequence, in patients with known coronary heart disease, systolic BP should not be reduced below 120 mmHg and diastolic BP should not be reduced below approximately 70 mmHg (in order to avoid coronary under perfusion). The sensitivity to low diastolic BP is explained by the fact that coronary perfusion occurs during diastole only. Some caution with aggressive BP lowering is also appropriate in patients with disseminated atherosclerosis, particularly of the arteries supplying the central nervous system

(cerebral ischemia) or the kidneys, that is, bilateral or dominant kidney renal artery stenosis (ischemic nephropathy). This is especially true in disease states such as diabetes, when autoregulation is disturbed, exposing the patient to the risk of organ ischemia (e.g. cerebral micro-infarction) when BP is lowered excessively.

Specific benefit of RAAS blockade

Generally, no preference for a specific antihypertensive agent is justified on the basis of currently available data, although results

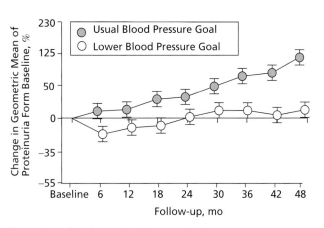

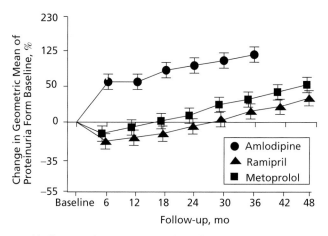

Figure 18.2 Effect of BP goal and selection of antihypertensive agent on proteinuria (AASK trial [69]). Percent changes in proteinuria by randomized group are shown. Data are the estimated percent changes in the urine protein/creatinine ratio from baseline through follow-up by BP goal and drug regimen. Based on the two-slope linear spline model for the log(urinary protein/creatinine) ratio, the percent change in geometric mean proteinuria to 4 years was significantly lower for the lower BP goal than the usual BP goal ($P < 0.001$) and was significantly higher in the amlodipine group than the other two drug groups ($P < 0.001$).

of some studies in patients with primary hypertension show better reduction of albuminuria and perhaps also better renal outcome [72,73] with RAAS blockade. Nevertheless, a specific renoprotective effect has been proven only in primary CKD and patients with diabetic nephropathy. The relevance of these findings for managing patients with primary hypertension and renal dysfunction remains questionable in the absence of prospective controlled data.

References

1 Kincaid-Smith P, McMicheal J, Murphy EA. The clinical course and pathology of hypertension with papilledema (malignant hypertension). *Q J Med* 1958; **27**: 117–152.

2 Gudbrandsson T, Hansson L, Herlitz H, Andren L. Malignant hypertension: improving prognosis in a rare disease. *Acta Med Scand* 1979; **206**: 495–499.

3 Rosansky SJ, Hoower DR, King L, Gibson J. The association of blood pressure levels and change in renal function in hypertensive and non-hypertensive subjects. *Arch Intern Med* 1990; **150**: 2073–2076.

4 Perneger TV, Nieto FJ, Whelton PK, Klag MJ, Comstock GW, Szklo M. A prospective study of blood pressure and serum creatinine. *JAMA* 1993; **269**: 488–493.

5 Klag MJ, Whelton PK, Randall BL, Neaton JD, Brancati FL, Ford CE *et al.* Blood pressure and end-stage renal disease in men. *N Engl J Med* 1996; **334**: 13–18.

6 Hsu CY, McCulloch CE, Darbinian J, Go AS, Iribarren C. Elevated blood pressure and risk of end-stage renal disease in subjects without baseline kidney disease. *Arch Intern Med* 2005; **165**: 923–928.

7 Fox CS, Larson MG, Leip EP, Culleton B, Wilson PW, Levy D. Predictors of new-onset kidney disease in a community-based population. *JAMA* 2004; **291**: 844–850.

8 Vikse BE, Aasarod K, Bostad L, Iversen BM. Clinical prognostic factors in biopsy-proven benign nephrosclerosis. *Nephrol Dial Transplant* 2003; **18**: 517–523.

9 Volhard F, Fahr T. *Die Brightsche Nierenkrankheit.* Julius Springer Verlag, Berlin, 1914.

10 Go AS, Chertow GM, Fan D, McCulloch CE, Hsu CY. Chronic kidney disease and the risks of death, cardiovascular events, and hospitalization. *N Engl J Med* 2004; **351**: 1296–1305.

11 Mann JF, Gerstein HC, Pogue J, Bosch J, Yusuf S. Renal insufficiency as a predictor of cardiovascular outcomes and the impact of ramipril: the HOPE randomized trial. *Ann Intern Med* 2001; **134**: 629–636.

12 Ritz E, McClellan WM. Overview: increased cardiovascular risk in patients with minor renal dysfunction: an emerging issue with far-reaching consequences. *J Am Soc Nephrol* 2004; **15**: 513–516.

13 Hillege HL, Fidler V, Diercks GF, van Gilst WH, de Zeeuw D, van Veldhuisen DJ *et al.* Urinary albumin excretion predicts cardiovascular and non-cardiovascular mortality in general population. *Circulation* 2002; **106**: 1777–1782.

14 Wachtell K, Ibsen H, Olsen MH, Borch-Johnsen K, Lindholm LH, Mogensen CE *et al.* Albuminuria and cardiovascular risk in hypertensive patients with left ventricular hypertrophy: the LIFE study. *Ann Intern Med* 2003; **139**: 901–916.

15 Klausen K, Borch-Johnsen K, Feldt-Rasmussen B, Jensen G, Clausen P, Scharling H *et al.* Very low levels of microalbuminuria are associated with increased risk of coronary heart disease and death independently of renal function, hypertension, and diabetes. *Circulation* 2004; **110**: 32–35.

16 Sterzel RB, Luft FC, Gao Y, Schnermann J, Briggs JP, Ganten D *et al.* Renal disease and the development of hypertension in salt-sensitive Dahl rats. *Kidney Int* 1988; **33**: 1119–1129.

17 Dworkin LD, Feiner HD. Glomerular injury in uninephrectomized spontaneously hypertensive rats. A consequence of glomerular capillary hypertension. *J Clin Invest* 1986; **77**: 797–809.

18 Raij L, Azar S, Keane WF. Role of hypertension in progressive glomerular immune injury *Hypertension* 1985; **7**: 398–404.

19 Feld LG, Van Liew JB, Brentjens JR, Boylan JW. Renal lesions and proteinuria in the spontaneously hypertensive rat made normotensive by treatment. *Kidney Int* 1981; **20**: 606–614.

20 Dworkin LD, Benstein JA. Impact of antihypertensive therapy on progressive kidney damage. *Am J Hypertens* 1989; **2**: 162S–172S.

21 Bidani AK, Griffin KA. Long-term renal consequences of hypertension for normal and diseased kidneys. *Curr Opin Nephrol Hypertens* 2002; **11**: 73–80.

22 Pelayo JC, Westcott JY. Impaired autoregulation of glomerular capillary hydrostatic pressure in the rat remnant nephron. *J Clin Invest* 1991; **88**: 101–105.

23 Feld LG, Cachero S, Van Liew JB, Zamlauski-Tucker M, Noble B. Enalapril and renal injury in spontaneously hypertensive rats. *Hypertension* 1990; **16**: 544–554.

24 Dworkin LD, Feiner HD, Parker M, Tolbert E. Effects of nifedipine and enalapril on glomerular structure and function in uninephrectomized SHR. *Kidney Int* 1991; **39**: 1112–1117.

25 Hayakawa H, Coffee K, Raij L. Endothelial dysfunction and cardiorenal injury in experimental salt-sensitive hypertension: effects of antihypertensive therapy. *Circulation* 1997; **96**: 2407–2413.

26 Brenner BM, Garcia DL, Anderson S. Glomeruli and blood pressure. Less of one, more of the other? *Am J Hypertens* 1988; **1**: 335–347.

27 Keller G, Zimmer G, Mall G, Ritz E, Amann K. Nephron number in patients with primary hypertension. *N Engl J Med* 2003; **348**: 101–108.

28 Hoy WE, Douglas-Denton RN, Hughson MD, Cass A, Johnson K, Bertram JF. A stereological study of glomerular number and volume: preliminary findings in a multiracial study of kidneys at autopsy. *Kidney Int Suppl* 2003; **83**: S31–S37.

29 Hughson MD, Douglas-Denton R, Bertram JF, Hoy WE. Hypertension, glomerular number, and birth weight in African Americans and white subjects in the southeastern United States. *Kidney Int* 2006; **69**: 671–678.

30 Hoy WE, Hughson MD, Bertram JF, Douglas-Denton R, Amann K. Nephron number, hypertension, renal disease, and renal failure. *J Am Soc Nephrol* 2005; **16**: 2557–2564.

31 Perera GA. Hypertensive vascular disease description and natural history. *J Chron Dis* 1955; **1**: 33–42.

32 Gull WW, Suton HG. On the pathology of the morbid state commonly called chronic Bright's disease with contracted kidney ("arterio-capillary fibrosis"). *Medico-Chirurg Trans* 1872; **55**: 273–326.

33 Harvey JM, Howie AJ, Lee SJ, Newbold KM, Adu D, Michael J *et al.* Renal biopsy findings in hypertensive patients with proteinuria. *Lancet* 1992; **340**: 1435–1436.

34 Innes A, Johnston PA, Morgan AG, Davison AM, Burden RP. Clinical features of benign hypertensive nephrosclerosis at time of renal biopsy. *Q J Med* 1993; **86**: 271–275.

35 Caetano ER, Zatz R, Saldanha LB, Praxedes JN. Hypertensive nephrosclerosis as a relevant cause of chronic renal failure. *Hypertension* 2001; **38**: 171–176.

36 Fogo A, Breyer JA, Smith MC, Cleveland WH, Agodoa L, Kirk KA *et al.* Accuracy of the diagnosis of hypertensive nephrosclerosis in African Americans. A report from the African American Study of Kidney Disease (AASK) Trial. *Kidney Int* 1997; **51**: 244–252.

37 Tracy RE, Berenson G, Wattigney W, Barret TJ. The evolution of benign arterio-nephrosclerosis from age 6 to 70 years. *Am J Pathol* 1990; **136**: 429–439.

38 Freedman BI, Iskandar SS, Appel RG. The link between hypertension and nephrosclerosis. *Am J Kidney Dis* 1995; **25**: 207–221.

39 US Renal Data System. *USRDS 2004 Annual Data Report: Atlas of End-Stage Renal Disease in the United States.* NIH publication no. 26-5-2005. National Institute of Diabetes and Digestive and Kidney Diseases, National Institutes of Health, Bethesda, 2004. http://www.usrds.org/adr_2004.htm.

40 Stewart JH, McCredie MR, Williams SM, McDonald SP. Interpreting incidence trends for treated end-stage renal disease: implications for evaluating disease control in Australia. *Nephrology* (Carlton) 2004; **9**: 238–246.

41 Perneger TV, Whelton PK, Klag MJ, Rossiter KA. Diagnosis of hypertensive end-stage renal disease: effect of patient's race. *Am J Epidemiol* 1995; **141**: 10–15.

42 Curtis JJ, Luke RG, Dustan HP, Kashgarian M, Whelchel JD, Jones P *et al.* Remission of essential hypertension after renal transplantation. *N Engl J Med* 1983; **309**: 1009–1015.

43 Rettig R, Folberth C, Stauss H, Kopf D, Waldherr R, Unger T. Role of the kidney in primary hypertension: a renal transplantation study in rats. *Am J Physiol* 1990; **258**: F606–F611.

44 Klahr S. The kidney in hypertension—villain and victim. *N Engl J Med* 1989; **320**: 731–733.

45 Crowley SD, Gurley SB, Oliverio MI, Pazmino AK, Griffiths R, Flannery PJ *et al.* Distinct roles for the kidney and systemic tissues in blood pressure regulation by the renin-angiotensin system. *J Clin Invest* 2005; **115**: 1092–1099.

46 Stevens LA, Coresh J, Greene T, Levey AS. Assessing kidney function: measured and estimated glomerular filtration rate. *N Engl J Med* 2006; **354**: 2473–2483.

47 Cockcroft DW, Gault MH. Prediction of creatinine clearance from serum creatinine. *Nephron* 1976; **16**: 31–41.

48 Fliser D, Ritz E. Serum cystatin C concentration as a marker of renal dysfunction in the elderly. *Am J Kidney Dis* 2001; **37**: 79–83.

49 Brinkman JW, Bakker SJ, Gansevoort RT, Hillege HL, Kema IP, Gans RO *et al.* Which method for quantifying urinary albumin excretion gives what outcome? A comparison of immunonephelometry with HPLC. *Kidney Int Suppl* 2004; **92**: S69–S75.

50 Comper WD, Osicka TM, Clark M, MacIsaac RJ, Jerums G. Earlier detection of microalbuminuria in diabetic patients using a new urinary albumin assay. *Kidney Int* 2004; **65**: 1850–1855.

51 Parving HH, Mogensen CE, Jensen HA, Evrin PE. Increased urinary albumin excretion rate in benign essential hypertension. *Lancet* 1974; **i**: 1190–1192.

52 Bigazzi R, Bianchi S, Campese VM, Baldari G. Prevalence of microalbuminuria in a large population of patients with mild to moderate essential hypertension. *Nephron* 1992; **61**: 94–97.

53 Mimran A, Ribstein J, DuCailar G, Halimi JM. Albuminuria in normals and essential hypertension. *J Diabetes Complications* 1994; **8**: 150–156.

54 Hörner D, Fliser D, Klimm HP, Ritz E. Albuminuria in normotensive and hypertensive individuals attending offices of general practitioners. *J Hypertens* 1996; **14**: 655–660.

55 Agrawal B, Berger A, Wolf K, Luft FC. Microalbuminuria screening by reagent strip predicts cardiovascular risk in hypertension. *J Hypertens* 1996; **14**: 223–228.

56 Samuelsson O, Wilhelmsen L, Elmfeldt D, Pennert K, Wedel H, Widstrand J *et al.* Predictors of cardiovascular morbidity in treated hypertension. Results from the primary preventive trial in Göteborg, Sweden. *J Hypertens* 1985; **3**: 167–176.

57 Deckert T, Feldt-Rasmussen B, Borch-Johnsen K, Jensen T, Kofoed-Enevoldsen A. Albuminuria reflects widespread vascular damage: the Steno hypothesis. *Diabetologia* 1989; **32**: 219–226.

58 Parving HH, Gyntelberg F. Transcapillary escape rate of albumin and plasma volume in essential hypertension. *Circ Res* 1973; **32**: 642–651.

59 Verhave JC, Gansevoort RT, Hillege HL, Bakker SJ, De Zeeuw D, de Jong PE *et al.* An elevated urinary albumin excretion predicts de novo development of renal function impairment in the general population. *Kidney Int Suppl* 2004; **92**: S18–S21.

60 Mogensen CE, Christensen CK. Predicting diabetic nephropathy in insulin-dependent patients. *N Engl J Med* 1984; **311**: 89–93.

61 VA Cooperative Study Group on Antihypertensive Agents. Effects of treatment on morbidity in hypertension. Results in patients with diastolic blood pressures averaging 115 through 129 mm Hg. *JAMA* 1967; **202**: 1028–1034.

62 VA Cooperative Study Group on Antihypertensive Agents. Effects of treatment on morbidity in hypertension. II. Results in patients with diastolic blood pressure averaging 90 through 114 mm Hg. *JAMA* 1970; **213**: 1143–1152.

63 Hsu CY. Does treatment of non-malignant hypertension reduce the incidence of renal dysfunction? A meta-analysis of 10 randomised, controlled trials. *J Hum Hypertens* 2001; **15**: 99–106.

64 Mroczek WJ, Davidov M, Gavrilovich L, Finnerty FA. The value of aggressive therapy in the hypertensive patients with azotemia. *Circulation* 1969; **15**: 893–904.

65 Timio M, Venanzi S, Lolli S, Lippi G, Verdura C, Monarca C *et al.* "Non-dipper" hypertensive patients and progressive renal insufficiency: a 3-year longitudinal study. *Clin Nephrol* 1995; **43**: 382–387.

66 Cifkova R, Erdine S, Fagard R, Farsang C, Heagerty AM, Kiowski W *et al.* Practice guidelines for primary care physicians: 2003 ESH/ESC hypertension guidelines. *J Hypertens* 2003; **21**: 1779–1786.

67 Chobanian AV, Bakris GL, Black HR, Cushman WC, Green LA, Izzo JL, Jr, *et al.* The Seventh Report of the Joint National Committee on Prevention, Detection, Evaluation, and Treatment of High Blood Pressure: the JNC 7 report. *JAMA* 2003; **289**: 2560–2572.

68 Kidney Disease Outcomes Quality Initiative (K/DOQI). K/DOQI clinical practice guidelines on hypertension and antihypertensive agents in chronic kidney disease. *Am J Kidney Dis* 2004; **43(Suppl 1)**: S1–S290.

69 Wright JT, Jr, Bakris G, Greene T, Agodoa LY, Appel LJ, Charleston J *et al.* Effect of blood pressure lowering and antihypertensive drug class on progression of hypertensive kidney disease: results from the AASK trial. *JAMA* 2002; **288**: 2421–2431.

70 Pohl MA, Blumenthal S, Cordonnier DJ, De Alvaro F, Deferrari G, Eisner G *et al.* Independent and additive impact of blood pressure control and angiotensin II receptor blockade on renal outcomes in the irbesartan diabetic nephropathy trial: clinical implications and limitations. *J Am Soc Nephrol* 2005; **16**: 3027–3037.

71 Messerli FH, Mancia G, Conti CR, Hewkin AC, Kupfer S, Champion A *et al.* Dogma disputed: can aggressively lowering blood pressure in hypertensive patients with coronary artery disease be dangerous? *Ann Intern Med* 2006; **144**: 884–893.

72 Asselbergs FW, Diercks GF, Hillege HL, van Boven AJ, Janssen WM, Voors AA *et al.* Effects of fosinopril and pravastatin on cardiovascular events in subjects with microalbuminuria. *Circulation* 2004; **110**: 2809–2816.

73 Schrader J, Luders S, Kulschewski A, Hammersen F, Zuchner C, Venneklaas U *et al.* Microalbuminuria and tubular proteinuria as risk predictors of cardiovascular morbidity and mortality in essential hypertension: final results of a prospective long-term study (MARPLE Study). *J Hypertens* 2006; **24**: 541–548.

19 Management of Hypertension in Chronic Kidney Disease

Aimun Ahmed, Fairol H. Ibrahim, & Meguid El Nahas

Sheffield Kidney Institute, Sheffield, UK.

Hypertension and risk of developing chronic kidney disease

A large number of community-based studies have identified a number of markers and factors known to be associated with increased risk of developing chronic kidney disease (CKD), foremost among them, systemic hypertension and diabetes mellitus, but also dyslipidemia, obesity, and smoking. These markers are identical to those associated with increased risk of cardiovascular disease (CVD), highlighting the close association between CKD and CVD. Of these, systemic hypertension is the single most important factor predicting the onset of CKD; a number of large community-based studies have linked raised blood pressure (BP) levels to the increased incidence of CKD.

In the USA, the Multiple Risk Factor Intervention Trial screened 332,544 men aged 35–57 years between 1973 and 1975 and followed them for an average of 16 years [1]. Of these, 814 subjects either died of end-stage renal disease (ESRD) or were treated for that condition (15.6 cases/100,000 person-years of observation) [1]. A strong, graded relation between both systolic and diastolic BP and ESRD was identified independent of associations with age, race, income, use of medication for diabetes mellitus, history of myocardial infarction, serum cholesterol concentration, and cigarette smoking. Compared with men with an optimal level of BP (<120/80 mmHg), the relative risk of ESRD for those with stage 4 hypertension (systolic pressure of ≥210 mmHg or diastolic pressure of ≥120 mmHg) was 22.1 [1].

Also in the USA, the Washington County, Maryland study [2] showed that the association between hypertension and smoking on the future risk of CKD in 23,534 men and women was proportional to the baseline levels of BP. The adjusted hazard ratio of developing

CKD among women was 2.5 for normal BP, 3.0 for high-normal BP, 3.8 for stage 1 hypertension, 6.3 for stage 2 hypertension, and 8.8 for stage 3 or 4 hypertension compared with individuals with optimal BP. In men, the relationship was similar but somewhat weaker. A large proportion of the attributable risk of CKD in this population was associated with stage 1 hypertension (23%) and cigarette smoking (31%) (Table 19.1) [2].

Data from Kaiser Permanente in northern California that were based on a total of 316,675 US adults showed that the adjusted rate for developing CKD was 1.62 for a BP of 120–129/80–85 mmHg, 1.98 for BP of 130–139/85–89 mmHg, 2.59 for BP of 140–159/90–99 mmHg, and up to 3.86 for BP of 160–179/100–109 mmHg [3].

It could be concluded from these studies that increased risk of incident CKD is observed with BP levels considered in the high-normal or the prehypertensive range (120–139/80–89 mmHg).

Similarly, data from Japan's Okinawa island survey of over 110,000 individuals followed for over 17 years also linked the development of proteinuria and CKD to high baseline levels of BP [4].

Hypertension and risk of progression of CKD

As with the development of CKD, its progression has been associated with a number of factors. They consist of modifiable and nonmodifiable factors. Among the modifiable risk factors, both systemic hypertension and proteinuria are the most significant [5]. They are associated with a faster rate of progression of established disease. A faster rate of progression of CKD has been associated with both high systolic as well as high diastolic BP levels. Some have also linked faster progression with raised pulse pressure [6]. Correlations have also been made between an overall high BP level detected by 24-h ambulatory BP monitoring and a faster rate of decline of glomerular filtration rate (GFR) [7].

Of the 49 studies examining the relationship between raised BP and faster progression of CKD published by the Kidney Disease Outcomes Quality Initiative (K/DOQI) in 2002, 29 studies showed

Evidence-based Nephrology. Edited by Donald Molony and Jonathan Craig
© 2009 Blackwell Publishing, ISBN: 978-1-4051-3975-5.

Table 19.1 Classification of hypertension.[a]

BP classification	Systolic BP (mmHg)	Diastolic BP (mmHg)
Optimal	<120	*and* <80
Prehypertension		
Normal	120–129	80–84
High-normal	130–139	85–89
Stage 1 (mild) hypertension	140–159	*or* 90–99
Stage 2 (moderate) hypertension	160–179	100–109
Stages 3 and 4 (severe) hypertension	≥180	≥110
Isolated systolic (grade 1) hypertension	140–159	<90
Isolated systolic (grade2) hypertension	≥160	<90

[a] This classification is based on that of the British Hypertension Society, ESH, JNC-7, and that of WHO/ISH. If systolic BP and diastolic BP fall into different categories, the higher value should be used for classification purposes.

an association by univariate analysis and 20 remained significant by multivariate analysis evaluation [8].

Mechanisms of hypertension in CKD

The kidney is the key organ involved in the regulation of systemic BP. It is involved in the pathogenesis of hypertension and is one of the organs most severely affected by raised BP. Conventional teaching has implicated fluid and salt overload and the activation of the renin–angiotensin–aldosterone system (RAAS) in the pathogenesis of hypertension in CKD. However, additional data also suggest other mediators. For instance, there is no doubt that the sympathetic nervous system is activated in CKD [9]. This may be a direct effect of kidney injury and scarring with afferent renal signals stimulating the sympathetic nervous system or indirectly via the activation of the RAAS [10]. Experimental data show that renal denervation results in a fall in systemic BP and an attenuation of CKD [11,12]. Endothelin (ET) has also been shown to be raised in CKD, implicating ET1 and ET3 in the pathogenesis of hypertension [13], which may be mediated by the activation of the ET agonist receptor known to cause vascular constriction. ET antagonists have been shown to reduce systemic hypertension and slow the progression of experimental CKD. Other putative mechanisms of raised BP in CKD include the well-known increased arterial stiffness associated with impaired kidney function and reflected in the increased arterial pulse wave velocity observed early in the course of CKD [14]. Arterial stiffness is associated with systolic hypertension and coronary artery disease. Finally, a significant number of elderly and diabetic patients with

CKD suffer from atherosclerotic renovascular disease and renal ischemia.

Guidelines for management of hypertension

When to treat

Global guidelines for the management of essential hypertension agree on a number of points. These include the threshold of initiation of antihypertensive therapy based on risk stratification. In general, it is acceptable to consider those at increased CVD risk for earlier treatment. High CVD risk is defined as a >20% event risk over 10 years, which is equivalent to a congestive heart disease (CHD) risk of approximately 10% over 10 years [15].

The European Best Practice Guidelines (EBPG) for the management of hypertension stipulate that those with a >20% increased CVD risk over 10 years should be treated based on a lower threshold of BP (<130/80 mmHg) to achieve the maximum reduction in the total cardiovascular risk [16]. The EBPG, like most other guidelines [17], consider patients with CKD at high CVD risk, thus warranting early intervention [8,17,18]. In those patients with CKD and high CVD risk, an integrated therapeutic intervention (statin and antiplatelet therapy) frequently should be considered [16,19].

The EBPG recommend that proteinuria should be lowered in patients with CKD to values as near to normal as possible with either an angiotensin converting enzyme inhibitor (ACEi) or an angiotensin receptor blocker (ARB) (or a combination of both). To achieve the BP goal, combination therapy is usually required, with the addition of a diuretic, a calcium antagonist, and other antihypertensive agents [16]. The EBPG also recommend the treatment of all modifiable risk factors associated with hypertension (hyperglycemia, dyslipidemia, and smoking). Nondiabetic CKD patients with minimal proteinuria, however, have no benefit from treatment with an ACEi [20].

The Seventh Report of the Joint National Committee for the Prevention, Detection, Evaluation and Treatment of High Blood Pressure (JNC-7) recommended treating systolic BP and diastolic BP to targets of <140/90 mmHg, aiming to decrease cardiovascular and renal morbidity and mortality in healthy subjects. In patients with hypertension and diabetes or CKD, the BP goal is lower, <130/80 mmHg [21].

Similar recommendations have been made by the British Hypertension Society, with a threshold for intervention of ≥140/90 mmHg in individuals with high CVD risk, including patients with CKD [22]. Target BP for those with CKD are <130/80 mmHg, and reducing BP to <125/75 mmHg may produce additional effects in those with proteinuria of >1 g/24 h (urine protein/creatinine ratio of >100 mg/mmol) [22].

In general, it is acceptable that patients with CKD are considered at the highest CVD risk [17,18], thus warranting a low threshold for initiation of antihypertensive treatment and lower target BP levels.

Table 19.2 Life-style modification recommendations for management of hypertension.

Intervention	Recommendation
Weight reduction	Maintain ideal body mass index (20–25 kg/m^2)
DASH eating plan	Consume diet rich in fruit, vegetables, and low-fat dairy products and with reduced content of saturated and total fat
Dietary sodium restriction	Reduce dietary sodium intake to 100 mmol/day (<2.4 g sodium or <6 g sodium chloride)
Physical activity	Engage in regular aerobic physical activity, e.g. brisk walking for at least 30 min most days
Alcohol moderation	Men: ≤21 units/wk; women: ≤14 units/wk

Guidelines for management of hypertensive CKD

How to treat
Nonpharmacological interventions
A range of nonpharmacological interventions have been advocated for the control of mild hypertension. These include life-style modifications, such as weight loss, regular exercise, and reduction in dietary salt and fat as well as increased intake of fruits and vegetables [23,24]. The Dietary Approaches to Stop Hypertension (DASH) studies showed the beneficial effect of a diet rich in fruits and vegetables and low in fat on blood pressure level. In addition, the DASH-Salt studies showed that dietary salt restriction further reduces BP in those already on a standard DASH diet [25]. Cessation of smoking and reduction of alcohol intake [25,26], weight reduction, and increased physical activity have also been shown to reduce BP [24] (Table 19.2).

Pharmacological interventions
In patients with CKD, pharmacological intervention, often with more than one drug, is required to control hypertension. In general, it is acceptable that the control of systemic BP has to be associated with a reduction in proteinuria to effect maximum protection in slowing the rate of decline of GFR [27]. In fact, recent studies have suggested that the control of proteinuria may be as important as, if not more important than, the control of hypertension per se [28].

Target BP levels
The K/DOQI guidelines on the management of hypertension in patients with CKD have recommended target BP levels of <130/80 mmHg [17]. These guidelines also suggested consideration of lower targets in heavy proteinuric [29] as well as diabetic patients [29,30]. These recommendations are based on observational and intervention studies.

Sources of data for these recommendations include the original report of the Modification of Diet in Renal Disease (MDRD) study, which suggested that lower blood pressure levels (<140/90 mmHg) may be needed in patients with moderate to heavy proteinuria (>1 g/24 h) [29]. These recommendations are also based on a systematic review of the literature that suggests that the lower the mean arterial BP (MAP) level, the slower the progression of CKD [31] for both diabetic and nondiabetic nephropathies. For the latter, reduction of MAP to levels below 92 mmHg has led to a normalization of the rate of decline in GFR (−1 mL/min/year), prompting those study authors to talk of regression of diabetic nephropathy [32].

The updated MDRD data suggested that a low target BP (MAP of <92 mmHg, compared to <107 mmHg) delayed the onset of kidney failure and a composite outcome of kidney failure and all-cause mortality [33]. This beneficial effect was observed in participants with various causes of nondiabetic CKD and extended across a wide range of proteinuria levels [34], although this was not the randomized intervention of this study.

In contrast, neither the Ramipril Efficacy in Nephropathy 2 (REIN-2) nor the African-American Study of Kidney Disease (AASK) studies showed additional advantage from further BP reduction [34].

Among the REIN-2 patients with nondiabetic proteinuric nephropathies receiving background ACEi therapy (134/82 mmHg), no additional benefit from further BP reduction by felodipine (130/80 mmHg) was shown [35]. However, this study was conducted over a relatively short period of time (1.6 years) and added a calcium antagonist for patients already controlled on an ACEi and achieving a 4.8-mmHg difference in systolic BP.

The AASK of African Americans with hypertensive CKD (baseline GFR around 46 mL/min, median baseline proteinuria of 0.81 g/24 h, follow-up of 5 years) failed to show an advantage to further BP reduction; patients with a mean BP of 128/78 mmHg experienced renal deterioration at the same rate as those achieving a mean of 141/85 mmHg [36]. However, subgroup analysis of those with proteinuria of >1 g/day showed a trend towards slower progression in the lower BP group. In this study, there was a therapeutic advantage for the ACEi (ramipril) on progression and proteinuria (−20%) compared to those treated with beta blockers (−14% for proteinuria). CKD patients treated with the calcium antagonist amlodipine showed a 58% increase in proteinuria.

In diabetic nephropathy (type 2 diabetes), the ABCD trial compared the effects of moderate BP control (target diastolic pressure, 80–89 mmHg) with those of intensive control (target diastolic pressure, 75 mmHg) on the incidence and progression of diabetic vascular complications. During a 5-year follow-up period, no difference was observed between intensive versus moderate BP control and between those randomized to nisoldipine versus enalapril for the outcome of change in creatinine clearance. After the first year of antihypertensive treatment, creatinine clearance stabilized in both the intensive and moderate BP control groups in those patients with baseline normo- or microalbuminuria. In

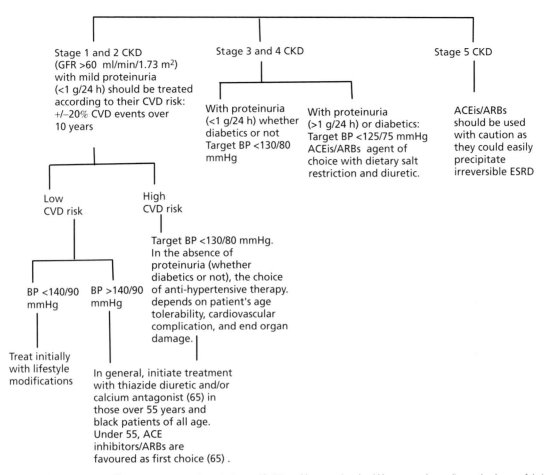

Figure 19.1 Algorithm for management of hypertensive CKD patients. Patients with CKD and hypertension should be managed according to the degree of their hypertension, proteinuria, and the stage of CKD.

contrast, patients starting with overt albuminuria demonstrated a steady decline in creatinine clearance of 5–6 mL/min/1.73 m^2/year throughout the follow-up period whether they were on intensive or moderate therapy. There was also no difference between the interventions for the risk of progression from normoalbuminuria to microalbuminuria (25% intensive therapy vs. 18% moderate therapy) or microalbuminuria to overt albuminuria (16% intensive therapy vs. 23% moderate therapy) [37].

Regarding target BP levels, it is important to consider levels that would minimize CKD complications, including CVD morbidity and mortality. Although there are no data available for the target level needed to reduce CVD in CKD, results from other non-kidney-related studies are informative. For example, in the HOT trial, for each 5 mmHg decrease in diastolic BP, there was a significant reduction in cardiovascular events [38]. In diabetics at high CVD risk, every 2-mmHg reduction in systolic BP was associated with a 7% reduction in CHD and a 10% reduction in stroke. In this trial, a diastolic BP value of 85 mmHg appeared to reduce risk of major CV events by 27% with no further improvement at lower diastolic BP levels (80 mmHg) [38,39]. Of note, a recent study in patients with CKD and estimated GFR of

<60 mL/min suggested that low BP levels (systolic, <133 mmHg; diastolic, <65 mmHg) are associated with increased mortality in moderate to severe CKD as in patients on hemodialysis [40]. However, the increased mortality noted in these patients could not be dissociated from the patients' underlying cardiovascular status (i.e. reverse causality). Furthermore, diastolic values of less than 65 mmHg are seldom achieved in patients with CKD and hypertension. Regarding the type of agents used to reduce CVD, reports are available to suggest that every single antihypertensive agent has some advantage; ACEi is favored by some to minimize cardiac remodeling.

Target proteinuria

Albuminuria and proteinuria are well-known markers associated with diabetic and nondiabetic kidney disease [41]. Recent data suggest a high prevalence of albuminuria (microalbuminuria) in the general population [42,43]. It is elevated in a variety of conditions, including old age, obesity, hypertension, diabetes, CVD, and CKD. It is also increased in a number of chronic inflammatory conditions, including arthritis, chronic hepatitis, and inflammatory bowel disease. A growing body of evidence points to the fact that albuminuria therefore may be more a marker of chronic inflammation and/or endothelial dysfunction rather than progressive CKD. In support of such an assumption is the reversibility of albuminuria with the control of the underlying pathology or predisposing factor. In diabetes, it has been shown that albuminuria does not always progress to proteinuria and is readily reversible with glycemic and hypertension control [44].

In other conditions associated with endothelial dysfunction and/or chronic inflammation, albuminuria reduction often parallels the fall in C-reactive protein (CRP) associated with the control of chronic inflammation. Data from the PREVEND study in the Netherlands highlighted this close association between albuminuria and CRP [45,46] and showed that, for example, weight reduction was associated with a fall in albuminuria and CRP levels [47]. Albuminuria should be considered a marker of endothelial dysfunction and inflammation rather than CKD.

In contrast, proteinuria [29,48], along with hypertension, is a very significant risk marker of progressive CKD. Over the last decade a body of evidence has implicated baseline as well as follow-up proteinuria levels in the progression of CKD [29,48], and the extent of the reduction of baseline proteinuria over a short period, 1–6 months [49], can predict the long-term renal functional response to an intervention. This was shown initially with dietary protein restriction [50] and more recently with hypertension control as well as ACEi [49] and ARBs [51]. In fact, some studies suggested that the beneficial impact of proteinuria reduction is greater and is independent from that of hypertension [52].

Choice of antihypertensive agents

Based on these data, a number of guidelines have favored the use of ACEi and ARBs in the management of hypertensive CKD, and these apply to diabetic and nondiabetic CKD patients. However, a number of observations suggest that the superiority of ACEi and ARBs in the management of hypertensive CKD in slowing the progression of CKD is greater among patients with a higher level of proteinuria [52]. In fact, the pivotal study of the impact of ACEi on the progression of nondiabetic CKD (REIN) failed to show benefit in those with proteinuria of <3 g/24 h [53]. Furthermore, this study also failed to show a therapeutic advantage of ramipril in those with MAP of <101 mmHg, for whom progression was slow, and both conventional agents, including calcium channel blockers (CCBs) and ACEi, had a comparable impact on CKD progression

Other studies that investigated the management of systemic hypertension (ALLHAT, ASCOT, and others) included some patients with CKD, although the degree of functional impairment was variable and often mild (CKD stages 1–3). The ALLHAT study of 33,357 individuals included 5662 patients with CKD (diabetic and nondiabetic, with an estimated GFR of <60 mL/min/1.73 m^2) who were followed for over 4.9 years. They noted that lisinopril was not more effective than chlorthalidone in slowing the progression of CHD or CKD [54]. Consequently, the therapeutic advantage of ACEi or ARBs is uncertain, particularly in patients with early CKD and in those with nondiabetic nephropathy and proteinuria of <1 g/24 h. It is likely that patients included in these trials, including ALLHAT, with mild to moderate hypertensive CKD may not have had severe proteinuria [54].

A meta-analysis of the impact of ACEi on the progression of diabetic and nondiabetic nephropathies showed some advantage on the progression of CKD in the latter but not in diabetics [55]. The data from this meta-analysis have been criticized for the inclusion of data on primary and secondary CKD, including the ALLHAT data, which showed thiazide diuretics to be superior to ACEi. Also, the primary and secondary end points of some of the studies included in the meta-analysis were not directly focused on the impact of treatment on CKD progression. However, the conclusion of the meta-analysis, that the beneficial effect of RAAS inhibition on progression is primarily dependent on better BP control, agrees with a number of observations made for essential hypertension and for diabetic nephropathy. In fact, data from the Steno Institute have shown over the years, in a number of relatively small studies, that progression of diabetic nephropathy can be halted with good BP control and MAP of <92 mmHg regardless of the antihypertensive agent used [56]. The UKPDS confirmed that lower BP led to slower decline in renal function regardless of whether atenolol or captopril was used [57]. Also, the ABCD trial, in a similar population of type 2 diabetic individuals, failed to show an advantage of enalapril over nisoldipine [37]. These observations in diabetic CKD and the implication of the Casas meta-analysis support a large body of literature on the impact of treatment on hypertensive CVD complications, from which the benefit derives primarily from the degree of BP reduction regardless of the antihypertensive agent used [58].

Finally, the indiscriminate use of ACEi and ARBs in CKD patients is not without risks. It is well known that patients with renovascular disease and ischemic nephropathy may be at risk of further renal dysfunction when using these agents. Distinction is also seldom made in the prescribing of RAAS inhibitors to patients with type 2 diabetes mellitus and CKD between those with genuine diabetic nephropathy and significant proteinuria and those with severe atherosclerosis or hypertensive or ischemic nephropathy. This may explain the high incidence of side effects. Also, a recent long-term analysis of the outcome of patients with diabetic nephropathy treated with ACEi suggested that after an initial stabilization, a higher number of patients progressed to ESRD compared to controls [59].

It is generally accepted that an up to 30% acute increase, within a week, in serum creatinine or a fall in GFR of less than 25% is acceptable, and predictable, upon initiation of ACEi and ARBs in patients with CKD [60]. However, close and prolonged monitoring is warranted, as some patients continue to have a rise in serum creatinine within the first 3 months of ACEi or ARB initiation.

Risk stratification of CKD and CVD risk: the CKD-CVD complex

With the above in mind, what recommendations can be made regarding the management of hypertensive CKD? The choice of agents in hypertensive CKD may have to take into consideration the presence of other CKD and CVD risk markers.

Proteinuria

Evidence suggests that ACEi and ARBs are more effective than conventional agents in CKD patients with heavy proteinuria and MAP levels of >110 mmHg (BP >140/90 mmHg) [53]. This would justify their use as the initial treatment of choice under these conditions. In such patients, including those with advanced diabetic nephropathy, it has been suggested that dihydropyridine CCBs may not be effective at reducing proteinuria, as they have been shown to increase, rather than decrease, glomerular filtration and intraglomerular capillary pressure in experimental animals. There may be an advantage for using one of the nondihydropyridine CCBs, such as verapamil or diltiazem, which have been shown, in a small number of studies, to be as effective in reducing proteinuria as ACEi in type2 diabetic nephropathy [61,62]. Beta blockers have a modest, if any, intrinsic antiproteinuric effect.

In such patients, it is generally acceptable that the threshold for initiation of antihypertensive treatment should be 130/80 mmHg and the target BP level should be <125/75 mmHg [17,21].

To control proteinuria, ACEi and ARB treatment is often ineffective unless combined with dietary salt restriction (below 100 mmol/day; <2.4 g sodium or <6 g sodium chloride) and diuretic therapy. This may explain the inferiority of these agents in some large studies, such as ALLHAT, where lisinopril was not combined with a diuretic. The beneficial effect of adding a diuretic to RAAS inhibition has been demonstrated with thiazide and loop diuretics as well as aldosterone antagonists, with all showing synergy with ACEi and ARB in reducing proteinuria.

As the initial (1–6 months) proteinuria-reducing effect determines long-term outcome, it is sensible to aim at maximal suppression of proteinuria with values of <1 g/24 h; for that level of suppression, the combination of an ACEi and an ARB may be justifiable. The COOPERATE study showed that ACEi and ARBs have additive antiproteinuric effects independent of their blood pressure-lowering impacts [63]. The combination led to a beneficial effect on the progression of CKD as a function of the reduction of proteinuria and independently of BP levels [63].

While reduction of albuminuria may impact favorably on CVD outcomes [62], there are suggestions that in diabetic nephropathy the reduction of proteinuria also favorably affects CVD complications [63,64]. Albuminuria may prove to be a useful CVD risk stratification marker in CKD patients, thus affecting the choice of antihypertensive agents.

Stage of CKD

There is little doubt that the initial level of GFR at the initiation of treatment affects prognosis, with patients with CKD stages of 3–5 at higher risk. Most data evaluating the impact of antihypertensives on the progression of CKD have focused on those patients with the highest risk of progression, in whom changes in BP levels and proteinuria have detectable impacts on CKD progression over short observation times.

Patients with CKD stages 3 and 4 and heavy proteinuria would benefit from ACEi and ARBs, as discussed above, with a target BP of <125/75 mmHg. It has also been argued that even those with CKD stage 5 would benefit from such treatment(s) [65,66]; this awaits confirmation and warrants caution, as these agents could easily precipitate irreversible ESRD.

In patients with CKD stages 1 and 2 with mild proteinuria (<1 g/24 h), progression is often slow and there is little evidence that progression is affected by the type of antihypertensive agent used. There is also a paucity of data on their CVD risk in the absence of decreased GFR (<60 mL/min) and/or anemia. In these patients it would therefore be reasonable to apply the risk stratification recommendations drawn for the treatment of essential hypertension:

1 High risk for CVD: 20% chance of an event over a 10-year period: Those aged >55 years, male, smokers, and hyperlipidemic and/or with a family history of CVD should be treated early (BP 140/90 mmHg), and BP levels should be reduced to <130/80 mmHg [16,17,21].
2 Low risk for CVD: target BP levels of 140/90 mmHg would be acceptable, bearing in mind their low CKD and CVD risk.

Recent guidelines issued by the National Institute of Health and Clinical Excellence suggest that the initiation of antihypertensive therapy with a thiazide diuretic and/or a calcium antagonist would be a reasonable and cost-effective first choice in those over the age of 55 years and for Black patients of any age [67]. These agents seem to provide better CVD risk reduction than beta blockers, in particular against stroke, and are marginally more cost-effective than ACEi and ARBs [67]. This choice is based on a meta-analysis of major hypertension clinical trials as well as a formal economic evaluation [67]. They recommend ACEi as first-line treatment in hypertensive patients younger than 55 years. If more than two agents need to be used to control BP, they recommend a combination of a diuretic, calcium antagonist, and ACEi or ARB [67].

At a recent UK CKD consensus meeting, it was suggested that for most patients with early CKD (stages 1–3) without significant proteinuria (<1 g/24 h or urinary protein/creatinine ratio of <100 mg/mmol), the primary objective of treatment should be to reduce the risk of stroke and heart disease with the choice of antihypertensive agents according to national guidelines; for the UK, initial therapy in those <55 years with an ACEi and in those older than 55 years with a calcium antagonist and/or a diuretic [68]. These recommendations agree with those of the National Institute of Health and Clinical Excellence and the British Hypertension Society and take into consideration the absence of evidence of an additional renoprotective effect of angiotensin inhibitors in nonproteinuric CKD.

Type of CKD

Patients with diabetic nephropathy should preferentially be treated by initial inhibition of the RAAS; there is no evidence of difference in efficacy between ACEi and ARBs in these patients. In nondiabetic CKD patients, the stage of CKD and proteinuria should be the major determinants in selecting an antihypertensive agent, rather than the nature of the underlying nephropathy. In a number of chronic glomerulonephritis patients, including those with membranous and immunoglobulin A nephropathy, ACEi have been shown to be effective at reducing proteinuria and slowing the progression of renal insufficiency. In patients with polycystic kidney disease it has been argued that ACEi are both beneficial and detrimental; this may reflect the stage of CKD, with early intervention having a more beneficial effect.

An increasing number of patients are recognized as having renovascular disease. These also include a proportion of type 2 diabetic patients with CKD. It is imperative to have a high index of suspicion of such patients in the face of a disproportionately high systolic BP and a wide pulse pressure in patients with a history of atherosclerotic vascular disease. ACEi and ARBs should be avoided in these patients, as they can precipitate further deterioration in renal function as the ischemic kidney depends to a large extent on angiotensin II-mediated efferent arteriolar vasoconstriction to maintain the capillary pressure and filtration of its hypoperfused glomeruli.

Race and ethnicity

It is generally accepted that black people of African or African-Caribbean origin have higher rates of hypertension and higher BP levels than white individuals. This is associated with higher CKD and CVD risks, with the exception of CHD, which is lower than in white people. Hypertension in the black population is often volume dependent and salt sensitive, reflecting a low renin status, favoring dietary salt restriction and diuretic therapy. Among black patients in the ALLHAT study, ACE inhibition led to a significantly higher rate of CVD events: strokes and CHF [69]. However, the AASK trial of African American patients with CKD showed ramipril to be superior to amlodipine; the amlodipine arm had to be stopped prematurely because of apparent worsening of CKD. The decision was controversial, because it implied that CCB may not be suitable for black individuals with CKD. In general, it is advisable to treat black patients with CKD along similar lines to their white counterparts, including the inhibition of the RAAS along with dietary salt restriction and vigorous diuretic therapy.

In the USA and UK, individuals of Asian origin have a higher prevalence of diabetes mellitus and hypertension as well as renal and cardiovascular complications. British Asians may also have a faster rate of progression of diabetic nephropathy [70]. There is no evidence that these individuals respond differently to antihypertensive agents compared to Caucasians. However, their high susceptibility to glucose intolerance and diabetes, obesity, and dyslipidemia may affect the choice of antihypertensive agents. With that in mind, agents modifying the RAAS may have therapeutic advantages, as they decrease the incidence of diabetes and have beneficial effects on components of metabolic syndrome.

Smoking

Patients with CKD who are heavy smokers are at increased risk of progression of diabetic and nondiabetic CKD [71]. It was shown in one study that ACE inhibition considerably reduced the smoking-associated risk of progression to ESRD [72].

Dyslipidemia

It is of relevance that the initiation and progression of CKD has been linked to serum lipid levels [73], which should be considered when prescribing antihypertensive agents because some, such as diuretics and beta blockers, increase serum lipids.

In conclusion, the management of hypertension in CKD depends on the renal and cardiovascular risk profile of the patient. Patients with low renal and cardiovascular risk, namely, those with CKD stages 1 and 2 and no or mild proteinuria (<1 g/24 h), could be treated according to guidelines set by hypertension societies in the EU and USA. On the other hand, those with more advanced renal insufficiency (CKD stages 3–5) and/or those with proteinuria who are at high renal and CVD risk should be treated according to the K/DOQI guidelines for the management of hypertension with lower treatment and target thresholds (i.e. <130/80 mmHg) [54]. The great majority of these patients will require more than one agent to control their BP to recommended target levels of <130/80 mmHg. Compliance is often a problem, and so the conventional stepped-care approach to the management of hypertension may not be optimal to minimize side effects and improve compliance. Combination therapy of two or three drugs at lower doses may be a better initial option [39].

Acknowledgments

The authors are grateful to Andrew Levey for his constructive comments.

A.A. and F.H.I. contributed equally to the chapter.

References

1 Klag MJ, Whelton PK, Randall BL, Neaton JD, Brancati FL, Ford CE *et al.* Blood pressure and end-stage renal disease in men. *N Engl J Med* 1996; **334**: 13–18.

2 Haroun MK, Jaar BG, Hoffman SC, Comstock GW, Klag MJ, Coresh J. Risk factors for chronic kidney disease: a prospective study of 23,534 men and women in Washington County, Maryland. *J Am Soc Nephrol* 2003; **14**: 2934–2941.

3 Hsu CY, McCulloch CE, Darbinian J, Go AS, Iribarren C. Elevated blood pressure and risk of end-stage renal disease in subjects without baseline kidney disease. *Arch Intern Med* 2005; **165**: 923–928.

4 Tozawa M, Iseki K, Iseki C, Kinjo K, Ikemiya Y, Takishita S. Blood pressure predicts risk of developing end-stage renal disease in men and women. *Hypertension* 2003; **41**: 1341–1345.

5 Yu HT. Progression of chronic renal failure. *Arch Intern Med* 2003; **163**: 1417–1429.

6 Banerjee D, Brincat S, Gregson H, Contreras G, Streather C, Oliveira D *et al.* Pulse pressure and inhibition of renin–angiotensin system in chronic kidney disease. *Nephrol Dial Transplant* 2006; **21**: 975–978.

7 Agarwal R, Andersen MJ. Prognostic importance of ambulatory blood pressure recordings in patients with chronic kidney disease. *Kidney Int* 2006; **69**: 1175–1180.

8 NKF. K/DOQI Clinical practice guidelines for chronic kidney disease: evaluation, classification, and stratification. *Am J Kidney Dis* 2002; **39(Suppl)**: S7–S266.

9 Koomans HA, Blankestijn PJ, Joles JA. Sympathetic hyperactivity in chronic renal failure: a wakeup call. *J Am Soc Nephrol* 2004; **15**: 524–537.

10 Neumann J, Ligtenberg G, Klein II, Koomans HA, Blankestijn PJ. Sympathetic hyperactivity in chronic kidney disease: pathogenesis, clinical relevance, and treatment. *Kidney Int* 2004; **65**: 1568–1576.

11 Campese VM, Kogosov E. Renal afferent denervation prevents hypertension in rats with chronic renal failure. *Hypertension* 1995; **25**: 878–882.

12 Jacob F, Ariza P, Osborn JW. Renal denervation chronically lowers arterial pressure independent of dietary sodium intake in normal rats. *Am J Physiol Heart Circ Physiol* 2003; **284**: H2302–H2310.

13 Dhaun N, Goddard J, Webb DJ. The endothelin system and its antagonism in chronic kidney disease. *J Am Soc Nephrol* 2006; **17**: 943–955.

14 Briet M, Bozec E, Laurent S, Fassot C, London GM, Jacquot C *et al.* Arterial stiffness and enlargement in mild-to-moderate chronic kidney disease. *Kidney Int* 2006; **69**: 350–357.

15 Rosendorff C, Black HR, Cannon CP, Gersh BJ, Gore J, Izzo JL, Jr., *et al.* Treatment of hypertension in the prevention and management of ischemic heart disease: a scientific statement from the American Heart Association Council for High Blood Pressure Research and the Councils on Clinical Cardiology and Epidemiology and Prevention. *Circulation* 2007; **115**: 2761–2788.

16 Guidelines Committee, 2003 European Society of Hypertension–European Society of Cardiology guidelines for the management of arterial hypertension. *J Hypertens* 2003; **21**: 1011–1053.

17 K/DOQI clinical practice guidelines on hypertension and antihypertensive agents in chronic kidney disease. *Am J Kidney Dis* 2004; **43**(Suppl 1): S1–S290.

18 Sarnak MJ, Levey AS, Schoolwerth AC, Coresh J, Culleton B, Hamm LL *et al.* Kidney disease as a risk factor for development of cardiovascular disease: a statement from the American Heart Association Councils on Kidney in Cardiovascular Disease, High Blood Pressure Research, Clinical Cardiology, and Epidemiology and Prevention. *Hypertension* 2003; **108**: 2154–2169.

19 Mancia G, De Backer G, Dominiczak A, Cifkova A, Farard R, Germano G *et al.* 2007 Guidelines for the management of arterial hypertension: The Task Force for the Management of Arterial Hypertension of the European Society of Hypertension (ESH) and of the European Society of Cardiology (ESC). *Eur Heart J* 2007; **28**: 1462–1536.

20 Kent DM, Jafar TH, Hayward RA, Tighiouart H, Landa M, de Jong P *et al.* Progression risk, urinary protein excretion, and treatment effects of angiotensin-converting enzyme inhibitors in nondiabetic kidney disease. *J Am Soc Nephrol* 2007; **18**: 1959–1965.

21 Chobanian AV, Bakris GL, Black HR, Cushman WC, Green LA. Seventh Report of the Joint National Committee on Prevention, Detection, Evaluation, and Treatment of High Blood Pressure. *Hypertension* 2003; **42**: 1206–1252.

22 Williams B, Poulter NR, Brown MJ, Davis M, McInnes GT, Potter JF *et al.* Guidelines for management of hypertension: report of the fourth working party of the British Hypertension Society, 2004—BHS IV. *J Hum Hypertens* 2004; **18**: 139–185.

23 Appel LJ, Brands MW, Daniels SR, Karanja N, Elmer PJ, Sacks FM. Dietary approaches to prevent and treat hypertension: a scientific statement from the American Heart Association. *Hypertension* 2006; **47**: 296–308.

24 Writing Group of the PREMIER Collaborative Research Group. Effects of comprehensive lifestyle modification on blood pressure control. *JAMA* 2003; **289**: 2083–2093.

25 Sacks FM, Svetkey LP, Vollmer WM, Appel LJ, Bray GA. Effects on blood pressure of reduced dietary sodium and the dietary approaches to stop hypertension (DASH) diet. *N Engl J Med* 2001; **344**: 3–10.

26 Xin X, He J, Frontini MG, Ogden LG, Motsamai OI, Whelton PK. Effects of alcohol reduction on blood pressure: a meta-analysis of randomized controlled trials. *Hypertension* 2001; **38**: 1112–1117.

27 Jafar TH, Schmid CH, Landa M, Giatras I, Toto R, Remuzzi G *et al.* Angiotensin-converting enzyme inhibitors and progression of nondiabetic renal disease. *Ann Intern Med* 2001; **135**: 73–87.

28 Vogt L, Navis G, de Zeeuw D. Renoprotection: a matter of blood pressure reduction or agent characteristics? *J Am Soc Nephrol* 2002; **13**: S202–S207.

29 Peterson JC, Adler S, Burkatt J, Greene T, Hebert LA, Hunsicker LG *et al.* Blood pressure control, proteinuria, and the progression of renal disease: the Modification of Diet in Renal Disease Study. *Ann Intern Med* 1995; **123**: 754–762.

30 Lewis JB, Berl T, Bain RP, Rohde RD, Lewis EJ. Effect of intensive blood pressure control on the course of type 1 diabetic nephropathy. *Am J Kidney Dis* 1999; **34**: 809–817.

31 Bakris GL, Williams M, Dworkin L, Elliott WJ, Epstein M, Toto R *et al.* Preserving renal function in adults with hypertension and diabetes: a consensus approach. *Am J Kidney Dis* 2000; **36**: 646–661.

32 Hovind P, Rossing P, Tarnow L, Toft H, Parving J, Parving H-H. Remission of nephrotic-range albuminuria in type 1 diabetic patients. *Diabetes Care* 2001; **24**: 1972–1977.

33 Sarnak MJ, Greene T, Wang X, Beck G, Kusek JW, Collins AJ *et al.* The effect of a lower target blood pressure on the progression of kidney disease: long-term follow-up of the Modification of Diet in Renal Disease study. *Ann Intern Med* 2005; **142**: 342–351.

34 Levey AS. An editorial update: what level of blood pressure control in chronic kidney disease? *Ann Intern Med* 2005; **143**: 79–83.

35 Ruggenenti P, Perna AF, Loriga G, Ganeva M, Ene-Iordache B, Turturro M *et al.* Blood-pressure control for renoprotection in patients with nondiabetic chronic renal disease (REIN-2): multicentre, randomised controlled trial. *Lancet* 2005; **365**: 939–946.

36 Wright JT, Bakris GL, Greene T, Agodoa LY, Appel LJ, Charelston J *et al.* Effect of blood pressure lowering and antihypertensive drug class on progression of hypertensive kidney disease. *JAMA* 2002; **288**: 2421–2431.

37 Estacio RO, Jeffers BW, Hiatt WR, Biggerstaff SL, Gifford N, Schrier RW. The effect of nisoldipine as compared with enalapril on cardiovascular outcomes in patients with non-insulin-dependent diabetes and hypertension. *N Engl J Med* 1998; **338**: 645–652.

38 Hansson L, Zanchetti A, Carruthers SG, Dahlof B, Elmfeldt D, Julius S *et al.* Effects of intensive blood-pressure lowering and low-dose aspirin in patients with hypertension: principal results of the Hypertension Optimal Treatment (HOT) randomised trial. *Lancet* 1998; **351**: 1755–1762.

39 Neutel JM. The role of combination therapy in the management of hypertension. *Nephrol Dial Transplant* 2006; **21**: 1469–1474.

40 Kovesdy CP, Trivedi BK, Kalantar-Zadeh K, Anderson JE. Association of low blood pressure with increased mortality in patients with moderate to severe chronic kidney disease. *Nephrol Dial Transplant* 2006; **21**: 1257–1262.

41 Jafar TH, Stark PC, Schmid CH, Landa M, Maschio G, Marcantoni C *et al.* Proteinuria as a modifiable risk factor for the progression of non-diabetic renal disease. *Kidney Int* 2001; **60**: 1131–1140.

42 Garg AX, Kiberd BA, Clark WF, Haynes RB, Clase CM. Albuminuria and renal insufficiency prevalence guides population screening: results from the NHANES III. *Kidney Int* 2002; **61**: 2165–2175.

43 Hillege HL, Janssen WM, Bak AA, Diercks GF, Grobbee DE, Crijns HJ et al. Microalbuminuria is common, in a nondiabetic, nonhypertensive population, and an independent indicator of cardiovascular risk factors and cardiovascular morbidity. *J Intern Med* 2001; **249**: 519–526.

44 Perkins BA, Ficociello LH, Silva KH, Finkelstein DM, Warram JH, Krolewski AS. Regression of microalbuminuria in type 1 diabetes. *N Engl J Med* 2003; **348**: 2285–2293.

45 Brantsma AH, Bakker SJL, Hillege HL, de Zeeuw D, de Jong PE, Gansevoort RT. Urinary albumin excretion and its relation with C-reactive protein and the metabolic syndrome in the prediction of type 2 diabetes. *Diabetes Care* 2005; **28**: 2525–2530.

46 Stuveling EM, Bakker SJL, Hillege HL, Burgerhof JG, de Jong PE, Gans RO et al. C-reactive protein modifies the relationship between blood pressure and microalbuminuria. *Hypertension* 2004; **43**: 791–796.

47 Bello AK, de Zeeuw D, El Nahas M, Brantsma AH, Bakker SJ, de Jong PE et al. Impact of weight change on albuminuria in the general population. *Nephrol Dial Transplant* 2007; **22**: 1619–1627.

48 Locatelli F, Marcelli D, Comelli M, Alberti D, Graziani G, Buccianti G et al. Proteinuria and blood pressure as causal components of progression to end-stage renal failure. *Nephrol Dial Transplant* 1996; **11**: 461–467.

49 Ruggenenti P, Perna A, Remuzzi G. Retarding progression of chronic renal disease: the neglected issue of residual proteinuria. *Kidney Int* 2003; **63**: 2254–2261.

50 El Nahas AM, Masters-Thomas A, Brady SA, Farrington K, Wilkinson V, Hilson AJ et al. Selective effect of low protein diets in chronic renal diseases. *Br Med J* (Clin Res Ed) 1984; **289**: 1337–1341.

51 Atkins RC, Briganti EM, Lewis JB, Hunsicker LG, Braden G, Champion de Crespigny PJ et al. Proteinuria reduction and progression to renal failure in patients with type 2 diabetes mellitus and overt nephropathy. *Am J Kidney Dis* 2005; **45**: 281–287.

52 Maschio G, Alberti D, Janin G. Effect of the angiotensin-converting-enzyme inhibitor benazepril on the progression of chronic renal insufficiency. The Angiotensin-Converting-Enzyme Inhibition in Progressive Renal Insufficiency Study Group. *N Engl J Med* 1996; **334**: 939–945.

53 Remuzzi G. Randomised placebo-controlled trial of effect of ramipril on decline in glomerular filtration rate and risk of terminal renal failure in proteinuric, non-diabetic nephropathy. *Lancet* 1997; **349**: 1857–1863.

54 Levey AS, Uhlig K. Which antihypertensive agents in chronic kidney disease? *Ann Intern Med* 2006; **144**: 213–215.

55 Casas JP, Chua W, Loukogeorgakis S, Vallance P, Smeeth L, Hingorani AD et al. Effect of inhibitors of the renin-angiotensin system and other antihypertensive drugs on renal outcomes: systematic review and meta-analysis. *Lancet* 2005; **366**: 2026–2033.

56 Gaede P, Vedel P, Parving H-H, Pedersen O. Intensified multifactorial intervention in patients with type 2 diabetes mellitus and microalbuminuria: the Steno type 2 randomised study. *Lancet* 1999; **353**: 617–622.

57 UK Prospective Diabetes Study Group. Efficacy of atenolol and captopril in reducing risk of macrovascular and microvascular complications in type 2 diabetes: UKPDS 39. *BMJ* 1998; **317**: 713–720.

58 Khosla N, Bakris GL. Lessons learned from recent hypertension trials about kidney disease. *Clin J Am Soc Nephrol* 2006; **1**: 229–235.

59 Suissa S, Hutchinson T, Brophy JM, Kezouh A. ACE-inhibitor use and the long-term risk of renal failure in diabetes. *Kidney Int* 2006; **69**: 913–919.

60 Bakris GL, Weir MR. Angiotensin-converting enzyme inhibitor-associated elevations in serum creatinine: is this a cause for concern? *Arch Intern Med* 2000; **160**: 685–693.

61 Bakris GL, Weir MR, Secic M, Campbell B, Weis-McNulty A. Differential effects of calcium antagonist subclasses on markers of nephropathy progression. *Kidney Int* 2004; **65**: 1991–2002.

62 Bakris GL, Copley JB, Vicknair N, Sadler R, Leurgans S. Calcium channel blockers versus other antihypertensive therapies on progression of NIDDM associated nephropathy. *Kidney Int* 1996; **50**: 1641–1650.

63 Nakao N, Yoshimura A, Morita H, Takada M, Kayano T, Ideura T. Combination treatment of angiotensin-II receptor blocker and angiotensin-converting-enzyme inhibitor in non-diabetic renal disease (COOPERATE): a randomised controlled trial. *Lancet* 2003; **361**: 117–124.

64 Berl T, Hunsicker LG, Lewis JB, Pfeffer MA, Porush JG, Rouleau JL et al. Cardiovascular outcomes in the Irbesartan Diabetic Nephropathy Trial of patients with type 2 diabetes and overt nephropathy. *Ann Intern Med* 2003; **138**: 542–549.

65 Hou FF, Zhang X, Zhang GH, Xie D, Chen PY, Zhang WR et al. Efficacy and safety of benazepril for advanced chronic renal insufficiency. *N Engl J Med* 2006; **354**: 131–140.

66 Ruggenenti P, Perna AF, Remuzzi G. ACE inhibitors to prevent end-stage renal disease: when to start and why possibly never to stop: a post hoc analysis of the REIN Trial results. *J Am Soc Nephrol* 2001; **12**: 2832–2837.

67 NICE hypertension guidelines, UK. 2006.

68 Williams B, Rodger SC. Consensus conference on early chronic kidney disease. *Nephrol Dial Transplant* 2007; **22**(Suppl 9): ix1–ix63.

69 Wright JT, Dunn JK, Cutler JA, Davis BR, Cushman WC, Ford CE et al. Outcomes in hypertensive black and nonblack patients treated with chlorthalidone, amlodipine, and lisinopril. *JAMA* 2005; **293**: 1595–1608.

70 Lightstone L, Rees AJ, Tomson C, Walls J, Winearls CG, Feehally J. High incidence of end-stage renal disease in Indo-Asians in the UK. *QJM* 1995; **88**: 191–195.

71 Orth SR. Smoking and the kidney. *J Am Soc Nephrol* 2002; **13**: 1663–1672.

72 Orth SR, Stockmann A, Conradt C, Ritz E. Smoking as a risk factor for end-stage renal failure in men with primary renal disease. *Kidney Int* 1998; **54**: 926–931.

73 Moorhead JF, Chan MK, El Nahas AM, Varghese Z. Lipid nephrotoxicity in chronic progressive glomerular and tubulo-interstitial disease. *Lancet* 1982; **ii**: 1309–1311.

20 Diagnosis and Management of Renovascular Disease

Jörg Radermacher

Department of Nephrology, Klinikum Minden, 32427 Minden, Germany

Introduction

End-stage renal disease requiring renal replacement therapy puts a major economic burden on the health care system. Atherosclerotic renovascular disease has been found in about 12–31% of patients >45 years old with end-stage renal disease [1,2] and constitutes the fastest-growing group of these patients [3]. In unselected patients with hypertension, the prevalence is only about 1–5% [4]. In certain patient populations, such as those with severe hypertension, refractory hypertension, aortic aneurysm [5], or coronary artery disease [6], the prevalence is as high as 20–40% [7].

Patients with renal artery stenosis of >50–70% renal artery diameter are frequently advised to undergo correction of the stenosis. The reason for treatment usually is difficult-to-control hypertension; however, amelioration of kidney failure should also be considered a reason for treatment. Identifying patients whose blood pressure and/or renal function will improve postintervention is difficult. Retrospective studies have shown a lack of improvement in blood pressure and renal function despite correction of the stenosis in 20–46% of patients [8–15]. The term renovascular hypertension is reserved for those patients with improved, or rarely even normalization of, blood pressure after intervention. The term renovascular azotemia is used for those patients who have improved renal function. Frequently, the term ischemic nephropathy is used, but this term does not tell whether a patient is going to be a responder. Renal artery stenosis and renovascular hypertension are frequently used as synonyms in the literature [16]. However, the term renal artery stenosis should be reserved for an anatomical description, whereas renovascular hypertension and renovascular azotemia describe the functional relevance of the stenosis.

Because angioplasty and surgery can lead to complications like cholesterol embolism, persistent acute kidney failure, and even patient death, these procedures should only be performed in patients with a high likelihood of benefit. Possible reasons for a lack of treatment effect are correction of trivial stenoses (<60%), underlying renoparenchymatous disease, technical failure, cholesterol embolism, or radiocontrast toxicity. These aspects will be discussed in this chapter.

Pathophysiology of renal artery stenosis

Renal artery stenosis leads to renal ischemia, causing the release of renin from the juxtaglomerular cells of the kidney and resulting in the conversion of angiotensin I to angiotensin II, subsequent release of aldosterone from the adrenal gland, vasoconstriction, and sodium and water retention. The long-term consequences are the buildup of extracellular matrix and collagen IV via angiotensin II-induced increased expression of transforming growth factor β and interstitial platelet-derived growth factor, resulting in irreversible parenchymal damage [17] also in the nonaffected kidney. The challenge of treatment of atherosclerotic renal artery stenosis is to intervene at a stage before major parenchymal damage has occurred.

Patients who should be screened for renal artery stenosis

Because renal artery stenosis is present in only about 1% of unselected patients with hypertension, general screening is not advisable. The clinical signs suggesting renovascular disease include an abdominal bruit, difficult-to-control hypertension (requiring ≥3 antihypertensive agents), accelerated hypertension or hypertension that was previously well-controlled, worsening of renal function 4–31 days after introduction of angiotensin converting enzyme inhibitor (ACEi) or angiontensin II receptor blocker treatment [18], severe atherosclerosis in other vascular beds, otherwise-unexplained chronic kidney disease, hypertension associated with sudden and repeated left heart failure or pulmonary edema, the onset of hypertension before the age of 30 years (from fibromuscular renal artery disease) or after the age of 55 years (from atherosclerotic renal artery disease), and differences in the sizes of the two kidneys. It is important to identify these clinical clues, because the prevalence of renal artery stenosis rises up to 39% among these patients [19]. Once renal artery stenosis is suspected, a screening test is used to confirm its presence.

Screening methods for renal artery stenosis

Screening tests should be inexpensive, accurate (i.e. with a low rate of technical failure and high sensitivity and specificity), and noninvasive. This excludes angiography, although angiography is still considered the reference standard for detection and quantification of stenosis. A high interobserver variability for stenosis quantification has been shown (kappa < 0.4) [20]. One study found a pressure gradient of ≥ 30 mmHg in 13 of 22 renal arteries in which arteriography had shown only minor degrees of stenoses (<50%) [21], a pressure gradient generally associated with a reduction of the glomerular filtration rate (GFR) [22]. Angiography may also cause atheromatous embolization of the kidneys or renal impairment due to radiocontrast nephrotoxicity.

Spiral computed tomography angiography (CTA) and magnetic resonance angiography are noninvasive imaging techniques that have high sensitivity and specificity (>95%) for detecting renal artery stenosis [23–26], although a more recent study did not find the same level of accuracy when these methods were applied in everyday practice [26]. The latter study reported a sensitivity of 64% and a specificity of 92% for CTA and 62% and 84%, respectively, for magnetic resonance angiography. These techniques are also limited by their high costs and, in the case of spiral CT, the use of contrast agents. Magnetic resonance is not suitable for patients with claustrophobia and certain types of metallic implants. Measurement of the concentrations of renin in the renal veins have been used to predict the potential success of surgical revascularization. False-negative and false-positive results are common with this technique, and it is therefore not recommended as a reliable screening test for renal artery stenosis. In theory, the accuracy of renal vein renins are enhanced by using an ACEi (captopril test), which attenuates the vasoconstrictive effect of angiotensin II on the efferent arteriole and reduces filtration on the side of the stenosis [23]. The reported sensitivity and specificity after 25–50 mg of captopril, however, are also low [27].

Captopril scintigraphy (25–50 mg of oral captopril given 12 h before isotope) can detect renal artery stenosis with high sensitivity and acceptable specificity and has also been shown to be of value in identifying patients whose blood pressure will improve after correcting the stenotic lesion [28]. This test, however, has not been shown to predict an improvement in renal function after correction of renal artery stenosis, and it cannot locate the stenosis or determine its severity [23]. Furthermore, the sensitivity of this test is reduced to 80% in patients with renal insufficiency (GFR of <50 mL/min) or in patients with bilateral stenoses or a stenosis in a single functioning kidney [23,29]. It is particularly important to identify significant stenoses in these patients, because the major rationale for performing surgery or angioplasty is to preserve renal function.

In experienced hands Doppler ultrasonography is highly sensitive and specific for detecting renal artery stenosis, and it is rapid and inexpensive [30]. Two main approaches are used to detect a significant renal artery stenosis of 50–70% [30,31]. The first (direct) approach looks at flow acceleration at the site of the stenosis. This approach has good sensitivity and specificity for detecting stenoses of $\geq 50\%$. Obesity, excessive bowel gas, or poor blood flow in the main renal artery can, however, interfere with direct visualization of the renal arteries [30]. The second (indirect) approach looks at poststenotic flow phenomena (tardus and parvus). This approach can be used in nearly all patients but will only detect severe stenoses of >70%. A combination of both approaches is the most suitable technique for accurate detection of renal artery stenosis in almost all patients. In patients with normal or impaired renal function, we reported no technical failure with this combination method and showed high sensitivity (96.7%) and specificity (98.0%) for detecting renal artery stenosis of $\geq 50\%$ compared with angiography [30,31]. The value of Doppler ultrasonography to reliably detect stenoses of 50% and more has been shown in the majority of more recent studies (Table 20.1).

In summary the best screening test is probably the test performed most frequently at an individual facility. In patients with a GFR of <50 mL/min, CTA (due to radiocontrast toxicity) and captopril scintigraphy (due to low sensitivity) should be avoided.

Quantification of stenosis and estimation of functional relevance

Other than detecting the presence of stenosis, Doppler ultrasonography can also be used to estimate the severity of renal artery stenosis, with reliable estimates for up to 70% diameter reduction. A good correlation compared to intravascular ultrasound has been shown ($R = 0.97$) [44].

There is general agreement [45] that a diameter stenosis of <50% causes neither high blood pressure nor impairment of renal function. For this reason intervention should not be performed for these low-degree stenoses. Stenoses of <60% progress slowly and almost never proceed directly to occlusion [46]. A policy of watchful waiting (e.g. ultrasonographic follow-up of stenoses) is reasonable. Stenoses of >65–80% are considered to be hemodynamically relevant [14,47]. Stenoses in most studies have been graded by angiography. Simon *et al.* found hypersecretion of renin, suggesting functional relevance, in stenoses of >80% diameter reduction [47]. Unfortunately, data on the improvement of blood pressure or renal function after correction of stenosis are lacking. Giroux retrospectively evaluated the degree of stenosis in patients who did or did not have improved blood pressure after correction of renal artery stenosis. They found tighter stenoses in patients that did benefit (79 ± 9% vs. 74 ± 9%; $P < 0.05$), but the differences

Table 20.1 Stenosis criteria and sensitivity and specificity for detection of renal artery stenosis with Doppler ultrasound compared to selective angiography.[a]

Criterion and study [reference]	No. of patients	Criterion	% Technical failure[b]	Degree (%) of stenosis[c]	% Sensitivity/ specificity
Direct stenosis criteria					
Hansen *et al.* 1990 [32]	74	RAR > 3.5	8	≥ 60	93/98
Karasch *et al.* 1993 [33]	53	V_{max} > 180 cm/s	15	≥ 50	92/92
Olin *et al.* 1995 [4]	102	V_{max} > 200 cm/s or RAR > 3.5	10	≥ 60	98/98
Postma *et al.* 1992 [34]	61	Doppler freq. >4 kHz and broadened Doppler spectrum	25	≥ 50	63/86
Schäberle *et al.* 1992 [35]	76	V_{max} > 140 cm/s	NA	≥ 50	86/83
Indirect stenosis criteria (paravus, tardus)					
Baxter *et al.* 1996 [36]	73	AT > 70 ms	16	≥ 70	89/97
Kliewer *et al.* 1993 [37]	57	AT $\geq$ 70 ms	0	≥ 50	82/20
Riehl *et al.* 1997 [38]	214	RI < 0.45 or ΔRI $\geq$ 8%	0	≥ 70	93/96
Schwerk *et al.* 1994 [39]	72	ΔRI $\geq$ 5%	0	≥ 50	82/92
			0	≥ 60	100/94
Speckamp *et al.* 1995 [40]	123	ΔAI $\geq$ 80%	NA	≥ 70	100/94
Stavros *et al.* 1992 [41]	56	Loss of ESP	0	≥ 60	95/97
Strunk *et al.* 1995 [42]	50	AT $\geq$ 70 ms	4	≥ 50	77/46
Combination of direct and indirect stenosis criteria					
Krumme *et al.* 1996 [43]	135	V_{max} > 180 cm/s and/or ΔRI $\geq$ 5%	0	≥ 50	89/92
Radermacher *et al.* 2000 [30]	226	V_{max} >180 cm/s and RRR > 4 and/or AT $\geq$ 70 ms	0	≥ 50	97/98

Abbreviations: AI, acceleration index; AT, acceleration time; RI, resistance index (Pourcelot index); ESP, early systolic peak; RAR, renal aortic ratio; RRR, renal renal ratio.

[a] Only prospective studies with more than 50 patients and used comparison with intra-arterial angiography as the gold standard were considered.

[b] Technical failure: the renal artery or intrarenal arteries could not be visualized by color Doppler ultrasonography.

[c] The lowest degree of stenosis (% diameter stenosis) detected by the respective ultrasound method. NA, data not available.

were small [14]. Future studies should quantify stenoses using either noninvasive Doppler ultrasound, intravascular ultrasound, or a pressure gradient measured by pressure wire (an expensive method) or catheter.

Exclusion of renoparenchymatous disease

Possibly the main reason for a lack of treatment benefit despite successful correction of renal artery stenosis is preexisting renoparenchymatous disease. The two most frequent diseases coexisting with or even causing renal artery stenosis are long-term hypertension and diabetes leading to hypertensive nephrosclerosis and diabetic glomerulosclerosis [48]. Renal biopsy can predict treatment failure but is usually not indicated in these disease entities [49]. Some readily available clinical and angiographic clues as predictors of treatment success have been suggested [50,51] (Table 20.2). However, none of these parameters is sufficiently sensitive or specific, and contradicting data have been published for many of these. Rapidly deteriorating renal function in the presence of renal artery stenosis has been associated with a favorable response after angioplasty [52]; however, follow-up data on renal function are frequently not available. Some screening methods

have been evaluated regarding prediction of treatment success: measurement of renal vein renin, captopril scintigraphy, magnetic resonance tomography, and Doppler ultrasonography. Because a hemodynamically relevant renal artery stenosis should cause increased renin production, renal vein renin measurements have been considered the reference standard for predicting the functional relevance of stenoses. The diagnostic accuracy of this test is, however, disappointing, and the requirement for invasive venous angiography and radiocontrast agents have made this method almost obsolete. Renal scintigraphy without captopril also has only low diagnostic accuracy, but captopril scintigraphy is an established method to predict a treatment effect. Captopril causes a further fall in GFR in the affected kidney. The positive predictive value for blood pressure improvement of a positive captopril scintigraphy is reported to be 92%; however, sensitivity drops to 80% in patients with impaired renal function [29]. This could be due to dependence of renal filtration on vasoconstriction of the efferent arteriole in patients with advanced renoparenchymatous disease, which is impaired after ACEi treatment. A further drawback of captopril scintigraphy is the requirement for meticulous patient preparation in order to obtain reliable results. Patient preparation includes controlled hydration, controlled sodium diet, and removal of diuretics and ACEi 4–14 days before the investigation

Table 20.2 Predictors of a lack of effect of successful correction of renal artery stenosis related to blood pressure and/or renal function.

Patient characteristic	Studies (reference nos.) that found the parameter to be:	
	Predictive	Not predictive
Advanced age, >65 yrs	13, 15, 54, 55	14, 56, 57
Male gender	54	14, 56, 57
Severe atherosclerosis	14, 15, 56	
Proteinuria >1 g/day	15, 58	
Severely impaired renal function (GFR <40 mL/min)	15, 56	14, 55, 57
No sudden appearance of hypertension, or sudden worsening of previously well-controlled hypertension	13	15
Duration of hypertension >10 yrs	14, 54	55
Diastolic blood pressure <80 mmHg	14, 54, 55	57
Systolic blood pressure <160 mmHg	57	55
Diabetes mellitus	14	15, 56
Nonsmoker	14, 15	
Degree of stenosis <70%	14	13, 57
Resistance index >0.80	15	

[29,53]. van Jaarsveld *et al.* did not find a predictive value of captopril scintigraphy for improvement of blood pressure in their study [13].

Gadolinium-assisted magnetic resonance imaging after ACEi treatment has been used to quantify renal filtration and has provided predictive results comparable to captopril scintigraphy [59]. Prospective studies on this fascinating technique as a predictor for renovascular hypertension or azotemia are lacking at present, however.

In two studies with low patient numbers, an increased intrarenal resistance index value measured by Doppler ultrasonography was associated with a rapid loss of renal function [60] and a lack of blood pressure improvement [61], despite correction of renal artery stenosis. A prospective study found that a resistance index

of >0.8 in the interregnal segmental arteries had a sensitivity and specificity of >90% for predicting renal function deterioration and a lack of blood pressure improvement [15] (Figure 20.1).

Correction of renal artery stenosis versus drug treatment

Presently, it is uncertain whether angioplasty or surgery for renal artery stenosis is associated with an improved outcome compared to medical treatment alone. Three randomized controlled trials, with relatively few patients, have been performed and did not show any difference in blood pressure or renal function [13,62,63]. A meta-analysis of these trials found a nonsignificant trend toward blood pressure reduction and lesser requirements for antihypertensive drugs in two of the three trials but no effect on renal function with angioplasty [64]. More studies comparing angioplasty with optimal medical treatment with greater patient numbers are underway (http://www.astral.bham.ac.uk) [65–67]. Until the results of these studies are available, physicians should try to only treat patients for whom there is a high likelihood of a positive response. Drug treatment of renal artery stenosis should include not only antihypertensive drugs but also lipid-lowering drugs, to perhaps prevent progression of renal artery stenosis, and antiplatelet drug treatment to prevent renal artery thrombosis.

Improving short- and long-term results of correction of renal artery stenosis

Ten-year patency rates are still only available for surgically corrected renal artery stenoses, although outcomes may be better after surgery compared to angioplasty [68]. However, angioplasty has become the method of choice because it is less invasive and has a lower mortality rate. Only when an aortic aneurysm or other severe aortic disease requires simultaneous treatment should surgery be the preferred method. Ostial stenoses should always be treated with angioplasty plus stenting; stenoses located >1 cm distally to the aorta or stenoses due to fibromuscular dysplasia can

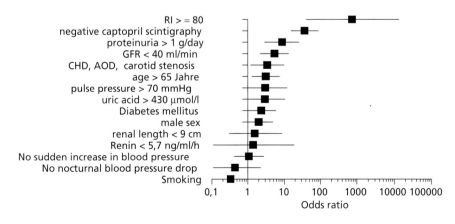

Figure 20.1 Odds ratios for various factors to predict deterioration of renal function. Squares depict odds ratios; lines depict 95% confidence intervals. RI, resistance index; CHD, coronary heart disease; AOD, atheroocclusive disease of the legs.

be treated with angioplasty alone [69]. A randomized controlled study reported better initial patency rates (88% vs. 57%) and lower restenosis rates (14% vs. 48%) 6 months after stent-assisted angioplasty compared to angioplasty alone in ostial stenoses [70]. However, the same study failed to show superiority of stenting regarding blood pressure or renal function improvement. Newer studies report primary patency rates in the range from 94 to 100% [14,57,71,72], but long-term results are less favorable. Restenosis, *de novo* stenosis, or thrombosis rates in the range of 10% per year have been reported both in stent-treated patients and patients who had angioplasty alone [14,15,52,57,71–74]. Revascularization success should therefore be monitored by ultrasonography at 3 months, 6 months, and yearly intervals thereafter. Newer technologies using sirolimus-coated stents are being evaluated [75].

Cholesterol embolism and radiocontrast toxicity

Cholesterol embolism in the renal arterial bed or the aorta is always a dramatic event. It can lead to progressive loss of renal function despite patency of the renal artery. At present there is no reliable method to detect cholesterol embolism. Renal biopsy is invasive and may miss the site of embolism due to sampling error. Blood eosinophilia or the "blue toe" suggest cholesterol embolism but are not sufficiently sensitive or specific to allow the diagnosis of renal cholesterol embolism. Dejani *et al.* found blood eosinophilia of >5% in 7 of 20 patients older than 55 years with impaired renal function (serum creatinine, >2 mg/dL) treated by renal angioplasty [76]. The feasibility of renal protection devices catching cholesterol crystals and other debris has been shown but has not been tested in randomized controlled trials [77].

A further frequent complication associated with renal angiography and renal arterial stenting is radiocontrast toxicity. Treatment of renal artery stenosis may be of greatest benefit in patients with impaired renal function, and these patients are most sensitive to radiocontrast toxicity. Controlled hydration with NaCl at 1 mL/kg/h for 12 h prior to and after angioplasty is considered standard prophylactic therapy. A randomized controlled trial has shown the superiority of this regimen, compared with additional mannitol or furosemide treatment [78]. Prehydration with sodium bicarbonate (154 mmol plus 900 mL 5% glucose solution) instead of saline alone may further lessen the risk. However, these data have not been confirmed in subsequent studies [79]. Acetylcysteine (600–1,200 mg twice a day) has been shown to have an additive protective effect compared with hydration alone for preservation of renal function and prevention of acute kidney failure in several randomized controlled trials [80,81], but a recent meta-analysis including 19 randomized trials failed to show such a protective effect (see chapter 10) [82].

The newer nonionic radiocontrast agents have lessened the risk of toxicity but have not abolished it [83]. Furthermore, the iso-osmolar radiocontrast agent iodixanol has been associated with significantly less contrast nephropathy than the low-osmolar agent iohexol [84]. These results have not been confirmed in other studies. Hemodialysis during or directly after application of radiocontrast agents does not prevent radiocontrast toxicity, but hemofiltration may have a beneficial effect [85]. Here also, confirmatory studies have not been performed, and this method of treatment is invasive and expensive. Calcium channel blockers, ANP [86], dopamine [87], and endothelin receptor antagonist [88] have been proven useless to prevent radiocontrast toxicity. Theophylline may have a protective effect, but its effects are not additive compared to hydration treatment alone [89].

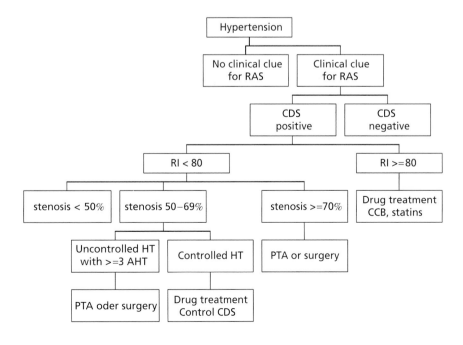

Figure 20.2 Approach to the patient with hypertension and suspected renal artery stenosis.

Conclusions

Patients should only be screened for the presence of renal artery stenosis when the likelihood that they have renal artery stenosis is sufficiently high. Good screening methods are Doppler ultrasonography and captopril scintigraphy, because both of these methods also have some predictive value regarding the likelihood of blood pressure and renal function improvement (RI <80 or positive captopril scintigraphy) following correction of the stenosis. Only patients with a high likelihood for improvement should be treated with angioplasty, because at present the superiority of angioplasty compared to medical treatment alone has not been definitively proven. Future technical improvements regarding prevention of cholesterol embolism and radiocontrast toxicity may increase the proportion of patients who benefit from stenosis correction. Based upon current data, stenoses of >70% should be treated with angioplasty, and stenoses of 50–70% should be treated only if blood pressure cannot be controlled with maximal antihypertensive treatment (opinion). A possible diagnostic and treatment algorithm is shown in Figure 20.2.

References

1 van Ampting JM, Penne EL, Beek FJ, Koomans HA, Boer WH, Beutler JJ. Prevalence of atherosclerotic renal artery stenosis in patients starting dialysis. *Nephrol Dial Transplant* 2003; **18:** 1147–1151.

2 Mailloux LU, Napolitano B, Bellucci AG, Vernace M, Wilkes BM, Mossey RT. Renal vascular disease causing end-stage renal disease, incidence, clinical correlates, and outcomes: a 20-year clinical experience. *Am J Kidney Dis* 1994; **24:** 622–629.

3 Fatica RA, Port FK, Young EW. Incidence trends and mortality in end-stage renal disease attributed to renovascular disease in the United States. *Am J Kidney Dis* 2001; **37:** 1184–1190.

4 Olin JW, Piedmonte MR, Young JR, DeAnna S, Grubb M, Childs MB. The utility of duplex ultrasound scanning of the renal arteries for diagnosing significant renal artery stenosis. *Ann Intern Med* 1995; **122:** 833–838.

5 Zoccali C, Mallamaci F, Finocchiaro P. Atherosclerotic renal artery stenosis: epidemiology, cardiovascular outcomes, and clinical prediction rules. *J Am Soc Nephrol* 2002; **13:** S179–S183.

6 Harding MB, Smith LR, Himmelstein SI, Harrison K, Phillips HR, Schwab SJ et al. Renal artery stenosis: prevalence and associated risk factors in patients undergoing routine cardiac catheterization. *J Am Soc Nephrol* 1992; **2:** 1608–1616.

7 Olin JW, Melia M, Young JR, Graor RA, Risius B. Prevalence of atherosclerotic renal artery stenosis in patients with atherosclerosis elsewhere. *Am J Med* 1990; **88:** 46N–51N.

8 Grim CE, Luft FC, Yune HY, Klatte EC, Weinberger MH. Percutaneous transluminal dilatation in the treatment of renal vascular hypertension. *Ann Intern Med* 1981; **95:** 439–442.

9 Geyskes GG, Puylaert CBAJ, Oei HY, Dorhout Mees EJ. Follow up study of 70 patients with renal artery stenosis treated by percutaneous transluminal dilatation. *BMJ* 1983; **287:** 333–336.

10 Svetkey LP, Kadir S, Dunnick NR, Smith SR, Dunham CB, Lambert M et al. Similar prevalence of renovascular hypertension in selected blacks and whites. *Hypertension* 1991; **17:** 678–683.

11 Fommei E, Ghione S, Hilson AJ, Mezzasalma L, Oei HY, Piepsz A et al. Captopril radionuclide test in renovascular hypertension: a European multicentre study. European Multicentre Study Group. *Eur J Nucl Med* 1993; **20:** 617–623.

12 Mann SJ, Pickering TG, Sos TA, Uzzo RG, Sarkar S, Friend K et al. Captopril renography in the diagnosis of renal artery stenosis: accuracy and limitations. *Am J Med* 1991; **90:** 30–40.

13 van Jaarsveld BC, Krijnen P, Pieterman H, Derkx FH, Deinum J, Postma CT et al. The effect of balloon angioplasty on hypertension in atherosclerotic renal-artery stenosis. Dutch Renal Artery Stenosis Intervention Cooperative Study Group. *N Engl J Med* 2000; **342:** 1007–1014.

14 Giroux MF, Soulez G, Therasse E, Nicolet V, Froment D, Courteau M et al. Percutaneous revascularization of the renal arteries: predictors of outcome. *J Vasc Interv Radiol* 2000; **11:** 713–720.

15 Radermacher J, Chavan A, Bleck J, Vitzthum A, Stoess B, Gebel MJ et al. Use of Doppler ultrasonography to predict the outcome of therapy for renal-artery stenosis. *N Engl J Med* 2001; **344:** 410–417.

16 Johansson M, Jensen G, Aurell M, Friberg P, Herlitz H, Klingenstierna H et al. Evaluation of duplex ultrasound and captopril renography for detection of renovascular hypertension. *Kidney Int* 2000; **58:** 774–782.

17 Meyrier A, Hill GS, Simon P. Ischemic renal diseases: new insights into old entities. *Kidney Int* 1998; **54:** 2–13.

18 van de Ven PJ, Beutler JJ, Kaatee R, Beek FJ, Mali WP, Koomans HA. Angiotensin converting enzyme inhibitor-induced renal dysfunction in atherosclerotic renovascular disease. *Kidney Int* 1998; **53:** 986–993.

19 Buller CE, Nogareda JG, Ramanathan K, Ricci DR, Djurdjev O, Tinckam KJ et al. The profile of cardiac patients with renal artery stenosis. *J Am Coll Cardiol* 2004; **43:** 1606–1613.

20 van Jaarsveld BC, Pieterman H, van Dijk LC, van Seijen AJ, Krijnen P, Derkx FH et al. Inter-observer variability in the angiographic assessment of renal artery stenosis. Dutch Renal Artery Stenosis Intervention Cooperative Study Group. *J Hypertens* 1999; **17:** 1731–1736.

21 Sigmund G, Hettinger M, Block T, Stolben A, Gard R. [Evaluation of renal artery stenosis: comparison of angiography and invasive blood pressure measurement and Doppler ultrasound.] *Rofo Fortschr Geb Rontgenstr Neuen Bildgeb Verfahr* 2000; **172:** 615–622.

22 Selkurt EE. Effective pulse pressure and mean arterial pressure modification on renal hemodynamics and electrolyte and water excretion. *Circulation* 1951; **4:** 541–551.

23 Dawson DL. Noninvasive assessment of renal artery stenosis. *Semin Vasc Surg* 1996; **9:** 172–181.

24 Olbricht CJ, Paul K, Prokop M, Chavan A, Schaefer-Prokop CM, Jandeleit K et al. Minimally invasive diagnosis of renal artery stenosis by spiral computed tomography angiography. *Kidney Int* 1995; **48:** 1332–1337.

25 Elkohen M, Beregi JP, Deklunder G, Artaud D, Mounier-Vehier C, Carre AG. A prospective study of helical computed tomography angiography versus angiography for the detection of renal artery stenoses in hypertensive patients. *J Hypertens* 1996; **14:** 525–528.

26 Vasbinder GB, Nelemans PJ, Kessels AG, Kroon AA, Maki JH, Leiner T et al. Accuracy of computed tomographic angiography and magnetic resonance angiography for diagnosing renal artery stenosis. *Ann Intern Med* 2004; **141:** 674–682.

27 Lenz T, Kia T, Rupprecht G, Schulte KL, Geiger H. Captopril test: time over? *J Hum Hypertens* 1999; **13:** 431–435.

28 Radermacher J, Weinkove R, Haller H. Techniques for predicting a favourable response in patients with renovascular disease. *Curr Opin Nephrol Hypertens* 2001; **10:** 799–805.

29 Taylor A. Functional testing: ACEI renography. *Semin Nephrol* 2000; **20:** 437–444.

30 Radermacher J, Chavan A, Schäffer J, Stoess B, Vitzthum A, Kliem V *et al*. Detection of significant renal artery stenosis with color Doppler sonography: combining extrarenal and intrarenal approaches to minimise technical failure. *Clin Nephrol* 2000; **53:** 333–343.

31 Radermacher J. Ultrasonography in the diagnosis of renovascular hypertension. *Imaging Decisions* 2002; **2:** 15–22.

32 Hansen KJ, Tribble RW, Reavis SW, Canzanello VJ, Craven TE, Plonk GW, Jr., *et al*. Renal duplex sonography: evaluation of clinical utility. *J Vasc Surg* 1990; **12:** 227–236.

33 Karasch T, Strauss AL, Grun B, Worringer M, Neuerburg-Heusler D, Roth FJ *et al*. [Color-coded duplex ultrasonography in the diagnosis of renal artery stenosis.] *Dtsch Med Wochenschr* 1993; **118:** 1429–1436.

34 Postma CT, van Aalen J, de Boo T, Rosenbusch G, Thien T. Doppler ultrasound scanning in the detection of renal artery stenosis in hypertensive patients. *Br J Radiol* 1992; **65:** 857–860.

35 Schäberle W, Strauss A, Neuerburg HD, Roth FJ. Duplex scan in diagnosis of renal artery stenoses and in the assessment of patency following transluminal angioplasty. *Ultraschall Med* 1992; **13:** 271–276.

36 Baxter GM, Aitchison F, Sheppard D, Moss JG, McLeod MJ, Harden PN *et al*. Colour Doppler ultrasound in renal artery stenosis: intrarenal waveform analysis. *Br J Radiol* 1996; **69:** 810–815.

37 Kliewer MA, Tupler RH, Carroll BA, Paine SS, Krieghauser JS, Hertzberg BS *et al*. Renal artery stenosis: analysis of Doppler waveform parameters and tardus-parvus pattern. *Radiology* 1993; **189:** 779–787.

38 Riehl J, Schmitt H, Bongartz D, Bergmann D, Sieberth HG. Renal artery stenosis: evaluation with colour duplex ultrasonography. *Nephrol Dial Transplant* 1997; **12:** 1608–1614.

39 Schwerk WB, Restrepo IK, Stellwaag M, Klose KJ, Schade BC. Renal artery stenosis: grading with image-directed Doppler US evaluation of renal resistive index. *Radiology* 1994; **190:** 785–790.

40 Speckamp F, Vorwerk D, Schurmann K, Risse JH, Kilbinger M, Tacke J *et al*. [Color-coded duplex ultrasonography in the diagnosis of renal artery stenosis.] *Rofo Fortschr Geb Rontgenstr Neuen Bildgeb Verfahr* 1995; **162:** 412–419.

41 Stavros AT, Parker SH, Yakes WF, Chantelois AE, Burke BJ, Meyers PR *et al*. Segmental stenosis of the renal artery: pattern recognition of tardus and parvus abnormalities with duplex sonography. *Radiology* 1992; **184:** 487–492.

42 Strunk H, Jaeger U, Teifke A. [Intrarenal color Doppler ultrasound for exclusion of renal artery stenosis in cases of multiple renal arteries. Analysis of the Doppler spectrum and tardus parvus phenomenon]. *Ultraschall Med* 1995; **16:** 172–179.

43 Krumme B, Blum U, Schwertfeger E, Flugel P, Hollstin F, Schollmeyer P *et al*. Diagnosis of renovascular disease by intra- and extrarenal doppler scanning. *Kidney Int* 1996; **50:** 1288–1292.

44 Radermacher J, Hiss M, Eberhard O, Haller H. High correlation of Doppler sonography with intravascular ultrasound in the assessment of renal artery stenosis. *J Am Soc Nephrol* 2000; **11:** 353A.

45 Kaplan NM. Renal vascular hypertension. In: Bersin J, editor. *Clinical Hypertension*. Lippincott Williams & Wilkins, Philadelphia, 2006; 347–368.

46 Schreiber MJ, Pohl MA, Novick AC. The natural history of atherosclerotic and fibrous renal artery disease. *Urol Clin North Am* 1984; **11:** 383–392.

47 Simon G. What is critical renal artery stenosis? Implications for treatment. *Am J Hypertens* 2000; **13:** 1189–1193.

48 Textor SC, Wilcox CS. Renal artery stenosis: a common, treatable cause of renal failure? *Annu Rev Med* 2001; **52:** 421–442.

49 Wright JR, Duggal A, Thomas R, Reeve R, Roberts IS, Kalra PA. Clinicopathological correlation in biopsy-proven atherosclerotic nephropathy: implications for renal functional outcome in atherosclerotic renovascular disease. *Nephrol Dial Transplant* 2001; **16:** 765–770.

50 Plouin PF, Clement DL, Boccalon H, Dormandy J, Durand-Zaleski I, Fowles G *et al*. A clinical approach to the management of a patient with suspected renovascular disease who presents with leg ischemia. *Int Angiol* 2003; **22:** 333–339.

51 Safian RD. Atherosclerotic renal artery stenosis. *Curr Treat Options Cardiovasc Med* 2003; **5:** 91–101.

52 Muray S, Martin M, Amoedo ML, Garcia C, Jornet AR, Vera M *et al*. Rapid decline in renal function reflects reversibility and predicts the outcome after angioplasty in renal artery stenosis. *Am J Kidney Dis* 2002; **39:** 60–66.

53 Pedersen EB. New tools in diagnosing renal artery stenosis. *Kidney Int* 2000; **57:** 2657–2677.

54 Barri YM, Davidson RA, Senler S, Flynn TC, Seger JM, Harwood TR *et al*. Prediction of cure of hypertension in atherosclerotic renal artery stenosis. *South Med J* 1996; **89:** 679–683.

55 Helin KH, Lepantalo M, Edgren J, Liewendahl K, Tikkanen T, Tikkanen I. Predicting the outcome of invasive treatment of renal artery disease. *J Intern Med* 2000; **247:** 105–110.

56 Paulsen D, Klow NE, Rogstad B, Leivestad T, Lien B, Vatne K *et al*. Preservation of renal function by percutaneous transluminal angioplasty in ischaemic renal disease. *Nephrol Dial Transplant* 1999; **14:** 1454–1461.

57 Burket MW, Cooper CJ, Kennedy DJ, Brewster PS, Angel GM, Moore JA *et al*. Renal artery angioplasty and stent placement: predictors of a favorable outcome. *Am Heart J* 2000; **139:** 64–71.

58 Makanjuola AD, Suresh M, Laboi P, Kalra PA, Scoble JE. Proteinuria in atherosclerotic renovascular disease. *QJM* 1999; **92:** 515–518.

59 Grenier N, Trillaud H, Combe C, Degreze P, Jeandot R, Gosse P *et al*. Diagnosis of renovascular hypertension: feasibility of captopril-sensitized dynamic MR imaging and comparison with captopril scintigraphy. *Am J Roentgenol* 1996; **166:** 835–843.

60 Petersen LJ, Petersen JR, Talleruphuus U, Ladefoged SD, Mehlsen J, Jensen HA. The pulsatility index and the resistive index in renal arteries. Associations with long-term progression in chronic renal failure. *Nephrol Dial Transplant* 1997; **12:** 1376–1380.

61 Frauchiger B, Zierler R, Bergelin RO, Isaacson JA, Strandness DEJ. Prognostic significance of intrarenal resistance indices in patients with renal artery interventions: a preliminary duplex sonographic study. *Cardiovasc Surg* 1996; **4:** 324–330.

62 Plouin PF, Chatellier G, Darne B, Raynaud A. Blood pressure outcome of angioplasty in atherosclerotic renal artery stenosis: a randomized trial. Essai Multicentrique Medicaments vs Angioplastie (EMMA) Study Group. *Hypertension* 1998; **31:** 823–829.

63 Webster J, Marshall F, Abdalla M, Dominiczak A, Edwards R, Isles CG *et al*. Randomised comparison of percutaneous angioplasty vs continued medical therapy for hypertensive patients with atheromatous renal artery stenosis. Scottish and Newcastle Renal Artery Stenosis Collaborative Group. *J Hum Hypertens* 1998; **12:** 329–335.

64 Nordmann AJ, Logan AG. Balloon angioplasty versus medical therapy for hypertensive patients with renal artery obstruction. *Cochrane Database Syst Rev* 2003; **3:** CD002944.

65 Scarpioni R, Michieletti E, Cristinelli L, Ugolotti U, Scolari F, Venturelli C *et al*. Atherosclerotic renovascular disease: medical therapy versus medical therapy plus renal artery stenting in preventing renal failure progression: the rationale and study design of a prospective, multicenter and randomized trial (NITER). *J Nephrol* 2005; **18:** 423–428.

66 Bax L, Mali WP, Buskens E, Koomans HA, Beutler JJ, Braam B *et al.* The benefit of stent placement and blood pressure and lipid-lowering for the prevention of progression of renal dysfunction caused by atherosclerotic ostial stenosis of the renal artery. The STAR study: rationale and study design. *J Nephrol* 2003; **16:** 807–812.

67 Cooper CJ, Murphy TP, Matsumoto A, Steffes M, Cohen DJ, Jaff M *et al.* Stent revascularization for the prevention of cardiovascular and renal events among patients with renal artery stenosis and systolic hypertension: rationale and design of the CORAL trial. *Am Heart J* 2006; **152:** 59–66.

68 Paty PS, Darling RC, III, Lee D, Chang BB, Roddy SP, Kreienberg PB *et al.* Is prosthetic renal artery reconstruction a durable procedure? An analysis of 489 bypass grafts. *J Vasc Surg* 2001; **34:** 127–132.

69 Martin LG, Rundback JH, Sacks D, et al. Quality improvement guidelines for angiography, angioplasty, and stent placement in the diagnosis and treatment of renal artery stenosis in adults. *J Vasc Interv Radiol* 2003; **14:** S297–S310.

70 van de Ven PJ, Kaatee R, Beutler JJ, Beek FJ, Woittiez AJ, Buskens E *et al.* Arterial stenting and balloon angioplasty in ostial atherosclerotic renovascular disease: a randomised trial. *Lancet* 1999; **353:** 282–286.

71 William G, Macaskill P, Chan SF, Karplus TE, Yung W, Hodson E *et al.* Comparative accuracy of renal duplex sonographic parameters in the diagnosis of renal artery stenosis: paired and unpaired analysis. *Am J Roentgenol* 2007; **188:** 798–811.

72 Bush RL, Najibi S, MacDonald MJ, Lin PH, Chaikof EL, Martin LG *et al.* Endovascular revascularization of renal artery stenosis: technical and clinical results. *J Vasc Surg* 2001; **33:** 1041–1049.

73 La Batide-Alanore A, Azizi M, Froissart M, Raynaud A, Plouin PF. Split renal function outcome after renal angioplasty in patients with unilateral renal artery stenosis. *J Am Soc Nephrol* 2001; **12:** 1235–1241.

74 Rodriguez-Lopez JA, Werner A, Ray LI, Verikokos C, Torruella LJ, Martinez E *et al.* Renal artery stenosis treated with stent deployment: indications, technique, and outcome for 108 patients. *J Vasc Surg* 1999; **29:** 617–624.

75 Klugherz BD, Jones PL, Cui X, Chen W, Meneveau NF, DeFelice S *et al.* Gene delivery from a DNA controlled-release stent in porcine coronary arteries. *Nat Biotechnol* 2000; **18:** 1181–1184.

76 Dejani H, Eisen TD, Finkelstein FO. Revascularization of renal artery stenosis in patients with renal insufficiency. *Am J Kidney Dis* 2000; **36:** 752–758.

77 Holden A, Hill A, Jaff MR, Pilmore H. Renal artery stent revascularization with embolic protection in patients with ischemic nephropathy. *Kidney Int* 2006;**70:** 830–832.

78 Solomon R, Werner C, Mann D, D'Elia J, Silva P. Effects of saline, mannitol, and furosemide to prevent acute decreases in renal function induced by radiocontrast agents. *N Engl J Med* 1994; **331:** 1416–1420.

79 Merten GJ, Burgess WP, Gray LV, Holleman JH, Roush TS, Kowalchuk GJ *et al.* Prevention of contrast-induced nephropathy with sodium bicarbonate: a randomized controlled trial. *JAMA* 2004; **291:** 2328–2334.

80 Tepel M, van der Giet M, Schwarzfeld C, Laufer U, Liermann D, Zidek W. Prevention of radiographic-contrast-agent-induced reductions in renal function by acetylcysteine. *N Engl J Med* 2000; **343:** 180–184.

81 Marenzi G, Assanelli E, Marana I, Lauri G, Campodonico J, Grazi M *et al.* N-acetylcysteine and contrast-induced nephropathy in primary angioplasty. *N Engl J Med* 2006; **354:** 2773–2782.

82 Bagshaw SM, McAlister FA, Manns BJ, Ghali WA. Acetylcysteine in the prevention of contrast-induced nephropathy: a case study of the pitfalls in the evolution of evidence. *Arch Intern Med* 2006; **166:** 161–166.

83 Rudnick MR, Goldfarb S, Wexler L, Ludbrook PA, Murphy MJ, Halpern EF *et al.* Nephrotoxicity of ionic and nonionic contrast media in 1196 patients: a randomized trial. The Iohexol Cooperative Study. *Kidney Int* 1995; **47:** 254–261.

84 Aspelin P, Aubry P, Fransson SG, Strasser R, Willenbrock R, Berg KJ. Nephrotoxic effects in high-risk patients undergoing angiography. *N Engl J Med* 2003; **348:** 491–499.

85 Marenzi G, Marana I, Lauri G, Assanelli E, Grazi M, Campodonico J *et al.* The prevention of radiocontrast-agent-induced nephropathy by hemofiltration. *N Engl J Med* 2003; **349:** 1333–1340.

86 Kurnik BR, Allgren RL, Genter FC, Solomon RJ, Bates ER, Weisberg LS. Prospective study of atrial natriuretic peptide for the prevention of radiocontrast-induced nephropathy. *Am J Kidney Dis* 1998; **31:** 674–680.

87 Abizaid AS, Clark CE, Mintz GS, Dosa S, Popma JJ, Pichard AD *et al.* Effects of dopamine and aminophylline on contrast-induced acute renal failure after coronary angioplasty in patients with preexisting renal insufficiency. *Am J Cardiol* 1999; **83:** 260–263, A5.

88 Wang A, Holcslaw T, Bashore TM, Freed MI, Miller D, Rudnick MR *et al.* Exacerbation of radiocontrast nephrotoxicity by endothelin receptor antagonism. *Kidney Int* 2000;**57:** 1675–1680.

89 Erley CM, Duda SH, Rehfuss D, Scholtes B, Bock J, Muller C *et al.* Prevention of radiocontrast-media-induced nephropathy in patients with pre-existing renal insufficiency by hydration in combination with the adenosine antagonist theophylline. *Nephrol Dial Transplant* 1999; **14:** 1146–1149.

21 Diabetes Mellitus

Piero Ruggenenti[1] & Giuseppe Remuzzi[2]

[1]Unit of Nephrology, Azienda Ospedaliera Ospedali Riuniti di Bergamo, 24128 Bergamo, Italy
[2]Clinical Research Center for Rare Diseases "Aldo & Cele Daccò," Mario Negri Institute for Pharmacological Research, 24125 Bergamo, Italy

Introduction

Diabetes mellitus, in particular type 2 diabetes, is a public health concern, and projections for the future are alarming. According to the World Health Organization, diabetes affects over 170 million people worldwide, and this will rise to 300 million people by 2025 [1], about one-third of whom will eventually suffer progressively deteriorating renal function. Ninety to 95% of these patients have type 2 diabetes. The first clinical sign of renal dysfunction in diabetic patients is microalbuminuria (a sign of an endothelial dysfunction not necessarily confined to the kidney), which manifests in 2–5% of patients per year. In 20–40% of cases, microalbuminuria progresses to macroalbuminuria or overt proteinuria, and 10–50% of patients with proteinuria develop chronic kidney disease, which ultimately requires dialysis or transplantation [2]. Of great concern, 40–50% of type 2 diabetic patients with microalbuminuria eventually die of cardiovascular disease. This is threefold more than for diabetic patients without evidence of renal disease [3].

Here we will review the evidence that, in diabetic patients with kidney disease, lowering blood pressure and urinary albumin are effective in reducing the risk of end-stage renal disease (ESRD) as well as of myocardial infarction, heart failure, and stroke and that among antihypertensive medications, angiotensin converting enzyme (ACE) inhibitors or angiotensin II antagonists are the most effective. Although less consistent, data are available that also nondihydropyridine calcium channel blockers (ndCCBs) may lower urinary albumin and slow renal disease progression, and ndCCBs, added to ACE inhibitor therapy, may be more effective. Finally, we will discuss recent evidence that ACE inhibitors can also prevent the onset of microalbuminuria, an early marker of kidney disease, if given to patients with type 2 diabetes and hypertension but normal urinary albumin excretion.

The epidemics of type 2 diabetes and related renal and cardiovascular disease

Diabetes mellitus is the most frequent cause of chronic kidney disease worldwide. Over the past 2 decades, there has been a continuous increase in the incidence of ESRD due to diabetes, predominantly in those with type 2 diabetes [1,2]. In the USA, the proportion of patients with both ESRD and diabetes rose from 27 to 50% between 1982 and 2000, a trend echoed in many developed countries and in non-Caucasian populations (i.e. Afro–Caribbean, Asian, Native American, Australian Aboriginal people, etc.). Until recently, the risk of renal complications was thought to be considerably lower among patients with type 2 diabetes than in those with type 1 diabetes; however, it has now been shown that the risk of nephropathy with progression to ESRD is similar for the two groups [4]. This knowledge has helped to change the perception of type 2 diabetes, and it is now apparent that this disease should be treated with the same seriousness as type 1 diabetes.

The prevalence of type 2 diabetes, and of related kidney disease, is rapidly increasing due to the progressive ageing of the population and the worldwide epidemic of obesity, especially in developing countries. In parallel, the incidence of ESRD within the type 2 diabetes population has increased dramatically. This may be due partly to improved treatments for hypertension and coronary heart disease, allowing more patients with type 2 diabetes to live long enough for nephropathy and ESRD to develop [5], or it may be because the spectrum of diabetes has become more severe. This phenomenon may also be because patients may be treated less optimally than previously as health care systems struggle with the increased load of diabetic patients. For example, a blood pressure target (i.e. $\leq 130/80$ mmHg) is not being achieved as frequently as is ideal, resulting in increased risk of kidney failure. Also, proteinuria may not be treated as a risk factor. Numerous studies have demonstrated that reducing proteinuria is renoprotective [2]. Targeting treatment to both blood pressure and urinary protein is therefore important to limit or prevent kidney disease in people with diabetes.

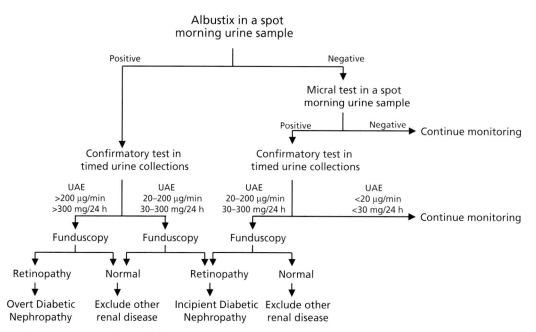

Figure 21.1 A possible algorithm to guide diagnosis of diabetic nephropathy.

Albuminuria is associated with cardiovascular disease mortality independent of other cardiovascular risk factors in both type 1 and type 2 diabetes [5,6]. Diabetic subjects with no evidence of kidney disease have cardiovascular morbidity and mortality comparable to those of age-matched controls without diabetes. In those with albuminuria, the risk increases in parallel with the increase in urinary albumin excretion (UAE). Observational analyses of the UKPDS study found that in patients with type 2 diabetes the incidence of cardiovascular events increases by 2- to 4-fold with the appearance of microalbuminuria (UAE, 20–200 μg/min or 30–300 mg/24 h), by 9- to 10-fold with the progression to macroalbuminuria (UAE, >200 μg/min, or 300 mg/24 h), and by more than 20-fold with the development of renal insufficiency and progression to ESRD [3]. Other studies have found that the incidence of coronary heart disease events increases from 16.4% in type 2 diabetic patients with a urinary protein concentration of <150 mg/L to 34.8% in those with a urinary protein concentration of >300 mg/L, and the incidence of stroke increases from 7.2% to 23% [6]. The excessive

cardiovascular risk means that patient survival is dramatically reduced prior to the development of ESRD, and survival levels fall even further on chronic renal replacement therapy [1–5]. The 5-year survival rates after progression to ESRD are currently 5% in Germany and 27% in Australia.

Diabetic renal disease

Definitions and diagnosis

Clinical diagnosis of diabetic nephropathy is established on the basis of persistent albuminuria in diabetic patients with retinopathy and no evidence of nondiabetic renal disease [8]. In those without retinopathy and with another urinary abnormality, a definite diagnosis can be established only on the basis of a histological evaluation of the kidney (Figure 21.1). Historically, five stages are recognized (Table 21.1) [9]. At the onset of diabetes the

Table 21.1 Stages of diabetic nephropathy.

Stage	Years since diabetes onset	GFR/RPF	UAE (μg/min)	Findings	Histology changes[a]
I Hyperperfusion	0	Elevated	>20[b]	Enlarged kidneys	Glomerular hypertrophy
II Clinical Latency	10–15	Normal-elevated	<20	High-normal BP	Thickening of basement membrane
III Incipient Nephropathy	15–20	Normal-elevated	20–200	Hypertension[c]	Widening of mesangium
IV Overt Nephropathy	20–30	Reduced/decreasing	>200	Worsening hypertension[c]	Diffuse/nodular glomerulosclerosis
V Kidney Failure	>30	Severely reduced	>200	Severe hypertension[c]	Scarring

[a] Less specific changes in type 2 diabetes.

[b] Transient increases.

[c] More frequent and more severe and often preceding the diagnosis of nephropathy in type 2 diabetes.

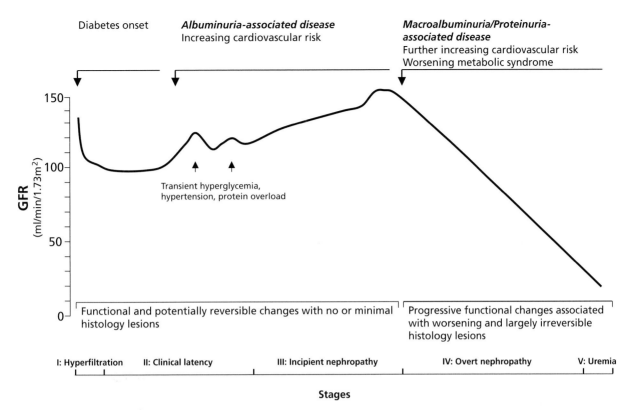

Figure 21.2 Course of diabetic nephropathy according to time-dependent changes in GFR and albuminuria.

glomerular filtration rate (GFR) may be elevated, and there are no evident clinical abnormalities (stage I diabetic nephropathy). Then, with good metabolic control the GFR normalizes (stage II), and over about 10 years microalbuminuria may develop (stage III or incipient nephropathy). Then, albuminuria may increase to the macroalbuminuric range and the GFR starts to decline (stage IV, or overt nephropathy) until kidney failure develops (stage V). More recent evidence, however, suggests that diabetic kidney disease is a continuum. It starts with the appearance of measurable amounts of albumin in the urine and evolves, with a progressive increase in albumin excretion, to a progressive decline in GFR. Not only is this associated with an increased urinary excretion, but also of other plasma components and, without specific treatment, may eventually result in terminal kidney failure (Figure 21.2) [10]. Even with this background, however, here we will use the traditional terminology whenever appropriate to avoid confusion with the earlier literature, in particular, when discussing trials that included patients and evaluated outcomes on the basis of the stages described above.

Thickening of the glomerular basement membrane and diffuse or nodular glomerulosclerosis (diabetic glomerulosclerosis) are the typical features of stage IV diabetic nephropathy, in particular in patients with type 1 diabetes. In those with type 2 diabetes, however, the histology findings may be more heterogeneous, and non-specific changes related to ageing or nephroangiosclerosis, with or without concomitant nodular glomerulosclerosis, may be observed in 30–60% of cases, according to different published case series [11]. Primary glomerular disease, in particular idiopathic membranous nephropathy, is also relatively frequent in older subjects with type 2 diabetes and should always be suspected in those with overt proteinuria but without severe hypertension, renal insufficiency, or retinopathy [11].

Outcome

In early stages of nephropathy, when structural changes are negligible, UAE may increase secondarily to glomerular hyperfiltration, loss of glomerular barrier negative charges and, possibly, reduced albumin reabsorption at the tubular level [10]. In later stages, however, when the structural changes become prominent, albuminuria is largely sustained by an increased permeability of the glomerular barrier, which allows unrestricted ultrafiltration of plasma macromolecules [12]. These macromolecules, most of which are nephrotoxic, may initiate a self-perpetuating process of progressive glomerulosclerosis, tubulo-interstitial inflammation, and scarring, with progressive renal function loss [13]. Ultrafiltered transferrin-iron complexes pH of proximal release iron, which in turn promotes lipid peroxidative damage, causes insulin-like growth factor 1 to dissociate from binding proteins, and stimulates mitogenesis and synthesis of collagen I and IV in proximal tubular cells, lipoproteins, chemotactic lipid factors. Different complement components may promote tubular injury and interstitial inflammation by generating oxygen free radicals and chemotactic gradients (see reference 13 for more details).

The functional and metabolic changes sustained by renal insufficiency and heavy proteinuria, including worsening hypertension, dyslipidemia, endothelial dysfunction, and insulin resistance, eventually accelerate atherosclerosis and cardiovascular disease, which contributes to the dramatic excess cardiovascular morbidity and mortality associated with overt nephropathy [3]. All together, these data support the hypothesis that the appearance in the urine of plasma proteins different from albumin (which usually occurs in parallel with the increase of UAE from micro- to macroalbuminuria) indicates the transition of the disease from a relatively benign stage of functional and potentially reversible abnormalities to a more severe stage of persistent functional and structural changes that, without treatment, sustain a relentless progression to ESRD (see reference 10 for more details). This highlights the importance of early intervention, when the kidney changes are still potentially reversible and renoprotective therapies might have their greatest beneficial effects.

Predisposing conditions

Studies have identified a number of factors that play a part in the development of diabetic nephropathy [14,15]. These include elevated blood pressure and glycosylated hemoglobin and cholesterol concentrations, smoking, advanced age, high level of insulin resistance, male gender (the risk is lower among women, particularly premenopausal women), and Afro–Caribbean, Asian, or Native American races. A family history of cardiovascular events is also an indicator of renal risk. Actually, genetic factors, including some polymorphisms of the ACE gene, appear to play a part in the development of diabetic nephropathy, as familial clustering of diabetes is found among both type 1 and type 2 diabetic patients. In addition to this, the finding of a family history of cardiovascular events is a powerful indicator of renal risk, with clusters of cardiovascular incidents being seen in first-degree nondiabetic relatives of type 1 and type 2 diabetic patients. There is also an interaction between genetic factors and blood glucose levels for the risk of microalbuminuria in newly diagnosed type 2 diabetic patients. The combination of a positive family history and poor glycemic control greatly increases the risk for development of diabetic nephropathy. Hypertension and family history of hypertension are also independent risk factors for subsequent development of microalbuminuria and nephropathy. A study of Pima Indians showed that the risk of developing nephropathy 5 years after the onset of diabetes was nearly threefold higher for those whose blood pressure was in the upper third (i.e. high-normal category) of blood pressure distribution 1 year prior to the development of diabetes [16].

Hypertension, hyperglycemia, and increased cardiovascular morbidity and mortality are typical components of metabolic syndrome, a syndrome of reduced tissue sensitivity to insulin that is often associated with microalbuminuria. Evidence suggests that insulin resistance precedes and probably contributes to the development of microalbuminuria in type 1 diabetic patients [17], as well as in nondiabetic subjects [18]. Until recently, data for type 2 diabetic patients were less clear, since an association between insulin resistance and microalbuminuria was suggested by some

studies but was not confirmed by others. However, the hypothesis of an association between insulin resistance and microalbuminuria was recently revived by a cross-sectional study showing that in a large cohort of type 2 diabetic patients the homeostasis model assessment index, a surrogate of insulin sensitivity, was significantly associated with the albumin/creatinine ratio measured in spot urine samples [19]. To formally test this possibility, Parvanova *et al.* compared the total body glucose disposal rate, quantified by means of a euglycemic hyperinsulinemic clamp technique, in 50 matched pairs of type 2 diabetic patients with micro- or normoalbuminuria [20]. Data showed that subjects with microalbuminuria were more insulin resistant than those with a normal UAE and that the magnitude of insulin resistance was independently associated with microalbuminuria. Of interest, there was also a clear association between more severe insulin resistance and microalbuminuria in the subgroup of patients with normal blood pressure considered separately from those with arterial hypertension. Altogether, these findings lend support to the possibility that insulin resistance is directly associated with microalbuminuria, regardless of its association with arterial hypertension. Another study showed that insulin sensitivity was similar in patients with macro- or microalbuminuria and was not correlated with the degree of UAE, confirming that increased albuminuria is not per se a primary determinant of insulin resistance.

Thus, increased albuminuria could be taken as an indicator of insulin resistance and of the increased renal and cardiovascular risk (the cardio-renal syndrome) associated with the metabolic syndrome.

The cardio-renal syndrome

Several studies have demonstrated a strong association between albuminuria, kidney disease, and increased cardiovascular risk (the so-called cardio-renal syndrome). The investigators of the Reduction of Endpoints in NIDDM with the Angiotensin II Antagonist Losartan (RENAAL) study [21] examined the data focusing on the relationship between albuminuria and cardiovascular end points or hospitalization for heart failure in 1513 patients with type 2 diabetes and overt nephropathy. Patients with high baseline albuminuria (≥ 3 g/g of creatinine) had a 1.92-fold higher risk for the cardiovascular end point and a 2.70-fold higher risk for heart failure compared with patients with low albuminuria (<1.5 g/g). Among all available baseline risk markers, albuminuria was the strongest predictor of cardiovascular outcome. The association between albuminuria and cardiovascular outcome was driven by those patients who also had a renal event (doubling of serum creatinine levels or progression to ESRD). It was also shown that albuminuria reduction was the strongest predictor for cardiovascular outcome: there was an 18% reduction in cardiovascular risk for every 50% reduction in albuminuria and a 27% reduction in heart failure risk for every 50% reduction in albuminuria. Thus, albuminuria is an important factor predicting cardiovascular risk in patients with type 2 diabetes and kidney disease. Reducing albuminuria appears to afford cardiovascular protection in these patients.

With the Irbesartan in Diabetic Nephropathy Trial (IDNT) cohort [22], the investigators examined the baseline characteristics predictive for cardiac events in 1715 individuals with type 2 diabetes, serum creatinine of 1.0–3.0 mg/dL, and UAE rates of $\geq$900 mg/day. A cardiovascular composite end point was used that consisted of cardiovascular death, nonfatal myocardial infarction, hospitalization for heart failure, stroke, amputation, and coronary and peripheral revascularization. Thirty percent of patients had at least one of the cardiovascular composite end points. Older age, male gender, longer duration of diabetes, history of cardiovascular disease, history of congestive heart failure, high urinary albumin/creatinine ratio, and low serum albumin were highly predictive for cardiovascular events; of these, prior history of cardiovascular disease (relative risk [RR], 2.00; 95% confidence interval [CI], 1.63–2.45; $P < 0.0001$) and high urinary albumin/creatinine ratio (RR, 1.29 per natural log unit; 95% CI, 1.13–1.48; $P = 0.0002$) at baseline were the strongest predictors.

Thus, among individuals with diabetes and kidney disease, albuminuria provides prognostic information concerning cardiovascular risk, in addition to that of traditional coronary risk factors. Recent studies, however, have shown that albuminuria has an independent predictive value for cardiovascular events even among subjects without evidence of overt kidney disease and a UAE in normo- or microalbuminuric ranges. Actually, similar to the relationship between blood pressure and risk of cardiovascular events, mounting evidence indicates a continuous relationship between UAE and risk. And like blood pressure, the concept of a threshold level to define normality no longer appears consistent with epidemiological data [23]. Indeed, post hoc analyses of randomized trials in high-risk individuals as well as community-based cohort studies all indicate that incremental increases in albuminuria within the "normal" range carry higher risks of nephropathy or cardiovascular events [24–26]. The Heart Outcome Prevention Evaluation (HOPE) study [24] also showed that the relationship between albuminuria and experiencing a cardiovascular event is not restricted to the microalbuminuric range and extends to as low as 0.5 mg/mmol (albumin/creatinine ratio [A/C]). These observations were confirmed in the Losartan Intervention for End Point Reduction in Hypertension (LIFE) study [25] and several population-based studies [26,27]. In particular, the Framingham Heart Study found that the 6-year risk of cardiovascular disease was threefold higher in nonhypertensive, nondiabetic subjects with urinary A/C ratios above the gender-specific median (3.9 μg/min for men and 7.5 μg/min for women) than in those with urinary A/C ratios below the median [27]. On the basis of the above findings, only negligible amounts of albuminuria below approximately 2 mg/g of urinary creatinine (or an estimated excretion rate of 2 mg/day) should be considered "normal," or as being below a threshold that does not confer excess risk. This corresponds approximately to a urinary concentration of 1–2 μg/ml, that is, below or close to the detection limit of the methods commonly used for the measurement of urinary albumin, such as nephelometry and immunoturbidimetry. Indeed, values above this threshold are significantly associated with risk for overt nephropathy, myocardial infarction, and cardiovascular death. This may have major practical implications, because albuminuria can be ameliorated by decreased insulin sensitivity, weight loss, blood pressure and blood glucose reductions, and renin–angiotensin system (RAS) inhibitor therapy (see reference 10 for more details). In the long-term, these interventions are expected to prevent or delay end-organ damage.

Protecting target organs in people with diabetes and kidney disease

Early studies in type 1 diabetes showed a clear relationship between arterial blood pressure and renal disease progression. This probably reflected the fact that kidneys of subjects with diabetes are more sensitive to the effects of high blood pressure than those of subjects without diabetes, because hyperglycemia may induce a loss of the physiological autoregulation that normally protects the glomerular microcirculation from the variations in systemic blood pressure. In experimental diabetes afferent (preglomerular) vasodilation facilitates the transmission of the aortic pressure to the glomerular vascular bed, thereby increasing glomerular pressure [28]. Thus, intracapillary pressure may be higher than normal, even when the systemic blood pressure is normal, and may further increase when the systemic blood pressure is above "normal." This explains why even small increases in blood pressure (still within the normal range according to the WHO/ISH definition of $\leq$ 130/80 mmHg) can have such a deleterious effect on renal function and why hypertension plays such an important role in the development and progression of diabetic kidney disease.

The first evidence of a beneficial effect of blood pressure reduction was provided by Parving and Mogensen in patients with type 1 diabetes and overt nephropathy [29,30]. They showed that by reducing blood pressure, filtrate loss in diabetic nephropathy could be delayed. Currently, however, it is believed that lowering blood pressure is not enough and that reducing proteinuria is also important [21,22]. Other interventions in addition to lowering blood pressure and proteinuria are important to protect end organs in people with diabetes. Intensified metabolic control reduces the incidence of microalbuminuria and of macrovascular complications in those with no evidence of kidney disease, but there does not seem to be any effect on kidney disease progression in those with established nephropathy. Preliminary evidence suggests that statins, in addition to decreasing cardiovascular events, may reduce proteinuria in diabetic patients with kidney disease. Lifestyle modifications, including weight loss, increased physical activity and, most importantly, smoking cessation, may reduce both micro- and macrovascular complications. Inhibition of the renin–angiotensin–aldosterone system (RAAS) by ACE inhibitors or angiotensin receptor blockers (ARBs) remains, however, the key component of reno- and cardio-protective therapy in people with diabetes [2]. Whether further benefits can be achieved by treatment with nondihydropyridine calcium antagonists or by

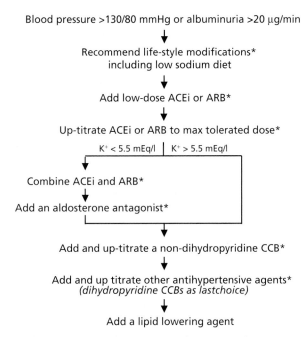

Figure 21.3 A possible algorithm to guide antihypertensive and antiproteinuric therapy in people with diabetes. Treatment should be aimed at achieving systolic and diastolic blood pressure < 130/80 mmHg and the maximal reduction in albuminuria, ideally to <20 μg/min. Consider that a diuretic is almost invariably needed to increase the efficacy of RAAS inhibitor therapy and limit hyperkalemia. Abbreviations: ACEi: ACE inhibitor, ARB: angiotensin receptor blocker, CCB calcium channel blocker, RAAS: Renin Angiotensin Aldosterone System.

intensified blood pressure control has not been clearly established (Figure 21.3 and Table 21.2).

Inhibition of the RAAS

ACE inhibitors

Interest in the role of ACE inhibitors in delaying the progression of diabetic nephropathy began in 1986, when an experimental model of kidney damage, comparing the effects of enalapril with a triple combination of the antihypertensives hydralazine, reserpine, and hydrochlorothiazide, demonstrated that enalapril produced an equally good reduction in mean arterial pressure to the triple therapy [31]. In addition to this, enalapril produced a reduction in proteinuria and less-pronounced glomerulosclerosis.

Table 21.2 Targets of multimodal therapy.

Characteristic	Target
Blood pressure	< 130/80 mmHg
Albuminuria	<20 μg/min
LDL	<100 mg/dL
LDL + VLDL	<130 mg/dL
HbA1c	<7.5%

The antiproteinuric and kidney-protecting effects of the ACE inhibitors were originally thought to be attributable to purely hemodynamic effects, relieving the glomerulus by opening the efferent arterioles (postglomerular), thereby reducing glomerular capillary pressure [31]. However, more recently it has become apparent that ACE inhibitors also affect glomerular function by their effects on glomerular size, glomerular permeability, and the increased negative electrical charge of the glomerular membrane [32,33].

In a study by Mathiesen, normotensive and hypertensive diabetic patients with incipient nephropathy, treated with ACE inhibitors, experienced a reduction in UAE [34]. In addition, a study with metoprolol and enalapril demonstrated greater protection of long-term renal function with the ACE inhibitor [35]. A meta-analysis of 12 trials in 698 type 1 diabetic patients with microalbuminuria who were followed for at least 1 year revealed that ACE inhibitors reduced the risk of progression to macroalbuminuria by 62% compared to that of the placebo group. At 2 years, the UAE rate was 50% lower in the patients taking ACE inhibitors than in those receiving placebo [36]. Parving et al. showed that the beneficial effect of ACE inhibitors on preventing progression from microalbuminuria to overt nephropathy is long lasting (8 years) and is associated with preservation of normal GFR [37].

Data on ACE inhibitors in type 2 diabetes are relatively sparse. Martinez et al. have recently demonstrated that the ACE inhibitor trandolapril can enhance insulin sensitivity (by 17%) and decrease microalbuminuria (by 54%) in hypertensive type 2 diabetic patients [38]. Ravid et al. originally described the beneficial effect of ACE inhibition in normotensive, nonobese microalbuminuric patients with type 2 diabetes by demonstrating that only 12% of the patients in the ACE inhibitor group progressed to macroalbuminuria, compared to 42% in the placebo arm [39]. The blood pressure, however, tended to be lower in the ACE inhibitor group, and the study was not powered to assess whether the improved outcome was due to ACE inhibition therapy or rather to more consistent blood pressure reduction.

However, on the basis of the above findings, there is a general consensus that diabetic patients with micro- or macroalbuminuria, even while they are normotensive, should be treated with ACE inhibitors or combinations thereof [40], as per the National Kidney Foundation algorithm [41].

ARBs

A multinational, randomized, double-blind, placebo-controlled study conducted by Parving et al. [42] examined the effect of RAAS blockade with the ARB irbesartan at a dose of either 150 mg daily or 300 mg daily, compared to placebo, in 590 hypertensive patients with type 2 diabetes and microalbuminuria followed for 2 years. The primary outcome was the time to onset of macroalbuminuria, taken as a marker of overt diabetic nephropathy. Ten of the 194 patients in the 300-mg group (5.2%) and 19 of the 195 patients in the 150-mg group (9.7%) reached the primary end point, compared with 30 of the 201 patients in the placebo group (14.9%) (hazard ratios, 0.30 [95% CI, 0.14–0.61; $P < 0.001$] and 0.61 [95% CI, 0.34–1.08; $P = 0.08$] for the two irbesartan groups, respectively).

Two studies examined the role of angiotensin receptor block-ade on the progression of kidney disease in patients with type 2 diabetes and macroalbuminuria. The RENAAL study [43] showed that, compared with conventional treatment alone (i.e. treatment without ACE inhibitors or ARBs), losartan combined with conventional treatment decreased the level of urinary protein excretion by 35% and reduced the risk of the composite end point (doubled serum creatinine, ESRD, or death) by 22%. This beneficial effect was achieved with comparable blood pressure control in the two treatment arms. In the IDNT study [44] the risk of the combined end point of a doubling of the baseline serum creatinine level, the onset of ESRD, or death from any cause was 20% lower in patients treated with irbesartan than in those treated with conventional therapy and 23% lower than in those treated with amlodipine. These studies also showed a reduction in the rate of heart failure with ARBs but no differences in the overall rate of death or the rate of death from cardiovascular causes.

Angiotensin II blockade was beneficial and well-tolerated regardless of renal function at study entry, a finding that challenges the common belief that RAAS inhibitor therapy should not be offered to individuals who have severe renal insufficiency (i.e. serum creatinine of >3 mg/dL) because of an increased risk of hyperkalemia or acute renal function deterioration, although patients at high risk of adverse effects were ineligible for both trials. In a post hoc, secondary analysis of the RENAAL trial [45], the incidences of ESRD, hospitalizations for heart failure, withdrawals for adverse events, and proteinuria during losartan or conventional treatment were compared within three tertiles of baseline serum creatinine concentrations (highest, 2.1–3.6 mg/dL; middle, 1.6–2.0 mg/dL; lowest, 0.9–1.6 mg/dL). Losartan decreased the risk of ESRD by 24.6, 26.3, and 35.3% in the highest, middle, and lowest tertiles, respectively. For every 100 patients with serum creatinine of >2.0, 1.6–2.0, or <1.6 mg/dL, 4 years of losartan therapy was estimated to save 18.9, 8.4, and 2.9 ESRD events, respectively. Losartan also decreased hospitalizations for heart failure by 50.2 and 45.1 in the highest and middle tertile, respectively. Withdrawals for adverse events other than heart failure were comparable between tertiles and treatment groups. Proteinuria decreased more on losartan than on placebo in all tertiles (highest, 24 vs. −8%; middle, 16 vs. −8%; lowest, 15 vs. −10%).

ACE inhibitors and ARBs: comparative analyses

A meta-analysis of 6167 patients with diabetic kidney disease included in 24 randomized clinical trials of ACE inhibitor or ARB blocker therapy versus placebo or conventional therapy found a similar benefit of both agents on renal outcomes [46]. Indeed, both ACE inhibitors and ARBs slowed progression of kidney disease and promoted regression from micro- to normoalbuminuria. The data, however, showed a reduced all-cause mortality versus conventional therapy or placebo with ACE inhibitors (RR, 0.79, 95% CI, 0.63–0.99), but not with ARBs (RR, 0.99; 95% CI, 0.85–1.17). The relative survival advantage of one class of antihypertensives over the other in this population is, however, still unknown, because only indirect comparisons based on small studies are avail-

able. Indeed, only three trials directly comparing ACE inhibitors with ARBs were included in the meta-analysis. These studies, however, did not report on all-cause mortality, ESRD, or doubling of serum creatinine, which rendered comparative survival analyses impossible. In a more recent study, 250 subjects with type 2 diabetes and early nephropathy were randomly assigned to receive either the ARB telmisartan (80 mg daily, in 120 subjects) or the ACE inhibitor enalapril (20 mg daily, in 130 subjects) [47]. The primary end point was the change in the GFR between the baseline value and the last available value during the 5-year treatment period. After 5 years, the GFR decreased by 17.9 mL/min/1.73 m^2 of body surface area with telmisartan and by 14.9 mL/min/1.73 m^2 with enalapril, with a treatment difference of 3.0 mL/min/1.73 m^2. On the basis of predefined criteria, this difference was not enough to conclude that telmisartan is inferior to enalapril in providing long-term renoprotection in persons with type 2 diabetes. A closer analysis of the data, however, showed that at study end the loss of GFR was 20% more consistent on telmisartan, and that was associated also with a slight excess (22% vs. 16%) of fatal and nonfatal cardiovascular events over enalapril. Thus, altogether, available data suggest a survival benefit and possibly a trend to more-effective renoprotection with ACE inhibitor than with angiotensin II receptor blocker therapy in people with diabetes and kidney disease. Thus, on the basis of available evidence, and also in view of the lower costs, ACE inhibitors should be considered first-line therapy in this population, and ARBs should be considered as second-line or add-on therapy when ACE inhibitors are not tolerated or fail to achieve the target blood pressure.

Combined ACE inhibitor and ARB therapy: preliminary evidence of efficacy

In patients with nondiabetic chronic nephropathies, dual RAS blockade with combined ARB and ACE inhibitor therapy offers greater renoprotective benefits than single-drug RAS blockade with either agent alone. Preliminary evidence indicates that this may apply also to subjects with diabetic kidney disease. The rationale for this approach is based on the consideration that ACE inhibitors and ARBs block the RAS at different levels. Thus, dual RAS blockade may result in a more profound inhibition of the system. Indeed, the Candesartan and Lisinopril Microalbuminuria (CALM) study [48] found that the ACE inhibitor lisinopril and the ARB candesartan achieved similar reductions in blood pressure and albuminuria in 197 patients with type 2 diabetes and incipient nephropathy. A more effective reduction in blood pressure and albuminuria was achieved when the two drugs were used in combination. Several studies have also shown a synergistic antiproteinuric effect in diabetics with overt nephropathy. Whether this translates to more effective renoprotection in the long term is not yet established.

Risks and benefits of antialdosterone therapy

Despite ACE inhibitor or ARB therapy, a substantial proportion of patients with diabetes, in particular type 2, and kidney disease continue to progress or to die prematurely of cardiovascular events. A possible explanation is that enhanced amounts of aldosterone are produced in these patients despite RAS blockade (aldosterone escape). Sato *et al.* [49] observed aldosterone escape in 40% of patients with type 2 diabetes and early nephropathy despite the use of ACE inhibitors. In these patients, the aldosterone antagonist spironolactone decreased UAE and left ventricular mass index without inducing further reduction in arterial blood pressure. Similar benefits, however, were seen also when aldosterone antagonists were used as first-line therapy. In hypertensive patients with type 2 diabetes and microalbuminuria, eplerenone reduced albuminuria even more effectively than enalapril (62% vs. 45% at 6 months vs. baseline), and albuminuria reduction (74%) was even more consistent when the two drugs were used in combination [50]. Altogether, these data provide preliminary evidence that aldosterone has a pathogenic role in diabetic kidney disease and that aldosterone antagonism may be renoprotective. A major drawback, however, of aldosterone antagonism is the increased risk of hyperkalemia. Thus, caution is recommended when aldosterone antagonists are given in combination with ACE inhibitors or ARBs, and this combined therapy should probably be avoided in poorly compliant patients or in those at highest risk because of poorly controlled hyperglycemia and renal insufficiency.

Role of calcium channel blockade: class effects of dihydropyridine and nondihydropyridine calcium antagonists

The results of studies with CCBs in diabetic patients with kidney disease have been mixed, with an increase in albuminuria actually being observed in some studies in which dCCBs such as nifedipine were used [51]. Clearly, differences exist between different classes of calcium antagonists and their effects on reducing proteinuria, thereby providing nephroprotection.

ndCCBs

The ndCCBs have been shown to reduce proteinuria and retard the progression of diabetic nephropathy [52]. These long-term studies show that ndCCBs, such as verapamil and diltiazem, slow progression of nephropathy significantly better than beta-blockers and that their effect in preserving the kidneys is comparable to that of lisinopril, an ACE inhibitor [52]. A meta-analysis of randomized trials of ndCCBs and dCCBs in hypertensive patients with proteinuric kidney disease found that with comparable blood pressure control, ndCCBs reduced proteinuria by about 30% compared to baseline, whereas dCCBs had no appreciable effects on urinary proteins. These findings were taken to suggest ndCCBs as a possible alternative to diuretics as the preferred agents to lower blood pressure in combination with a RAS inhibitor in patients with chronic proteinuric nephropathies [53].

dCCBs

Dihydropyridine calcium antagonists have been found to be less effective than heart rate-lowering calcium antagonists at reducing proteinuria [52]. A long-term study of the effects of ramipril and felodipine therapy alone or in combination for nondiabetic kidney disease found that, with 2-year comparable blood pressure control, proteinuria was reduced to a similar extent by ramipril alone or in combination with felodipine, whereas it was significantly increased with felodipine alone [54]. More recently, the Ramipril Efficacy in Nephropathy 2 (REIN-2) study found that intensified blood pressure control by add-on felodipine treatment in 338 patients with nondiabetic chronic nephropathies on background ACE inhibitor therapy failed to reduce proteinuria or limit progression to ESRD [55].

A direct comparison between an ARB and a dCCB was attempted in the MicroAlbuminuria Reduction with Valsartan (MARVAL) study in type 2 diabetic patients with microalbuminuria [56]. Three hundred thirty-two patients with type 2 diabetes and microalbuminuria, with or without hypertension, were randomly assigned to 80 mg/day valsartan or 5 mg/day amlodipine for 24 weeks. A target blood pressure of 135/85 mmHg was aimed for by dose-doubling followed by addition of bendrofluazide and doxazosin whenever needed. The primary end point was the percent change in albuminuria from baseline to 24 weeks. The albuminuria at 24 weeks was 56% of baseline (95% CI, 49.6–63.0) with valsartan and 92% of baseline (95% CI, 81.7–103.7) with amlodipine, a highly significant between-group effect ($P < 0.001$). Valsartan lowered albuminuria similarly in both the hypertensive and normotensive subgroups. More patients reversed to normoalbuminuria with valsartan (29.9% vs. 14.5%; $P = 0.001$). In summary, for the same level of attained blood pressure and the same degree of blood pressure reduction, valsartan lowered albuminuria in patients with type 2 diabetes and microalbuminuria, including the subgroup with baseline normotension, whereas amlodipine had no effect.

A possible explanation for the above findings is that dCCBs induce a preglomerular vasodilation that facilitates the transmission of systemic blood pressure to the capillary network, which may increase intracapillary pressure, an effect that may offset or even overwhelm the benefits of blood pressure reduction, in particular when the blood pressure is reduced a few millimeters of mercury. Thus, dCCBs should be used as second-line therapy, when the blood pressure is above target despite the use of drugs that inhibit the RAAS or that have neutral effects on albuminuria. A possible exception may be more-recent dihydropyridine calcium antagonists, such as manidipine, that, similarly to ACE inhibitors, may reduce postglomerular resistances and therefore may effectively reduce albuminuria also in people with diabetes.

Role of intensified blood pressure control

In type 2 diabetic patients with overt nephropathy enrolled in the RENAAL [57] or IDNT [58] studies, there was a significant relationship between the blood pressure levels achieved during the follow-up period and the incidence of ESRD or cardiovascular events. Although at any level of achieved blood pressure the overall incidence of events was consistently lower in patients on an ARB than in those on placebo treatment, it was also apparent that the impact of achieved blood pressure on clinical outcomes was independent of patient allocation to ARB or placebo treatment and was consistent within each treatment group [59]. Thus, in type 2 diabetic patients with established nephropathy, both RAS inhibition and blood pressure control have specific and probably additive reno- and cardioprotective effects that may contribute to limit the excess renal and cardiovascular risk via different pathways. Evidence that blood pressure reduction and ACE inhibitor therapy may have an independent and additive protective effect against microalbuminuria is in harmony with current theories on the pathophysiology of diabetic kidney disease [28]. The impact of blood pressure control on the risk of developing microalbuminuria reflects the specific vulnerability of the diabetic kidney to the barotrauma caused by arterial hypertension. Autoregulation of afferent arteriolar tone in response to changes in renal perfusion pressure is defective in diabetes [60], and decreased afferent arteriolar resistance facilitates the transmission of the systemic blood pressure to the glomerular capillary, which increases intracapillary pressure [28,61]. In the long term, these hemodynamic changes may cause endothelial dysfunction, impaired sieving function of the glomerular barrier, increased albumin ultrafiltration, and albuminuria [10]. Thus, reducing systemic blood pressure to normal ranges is crucial to ameliorate glomerular hypertension and prevent glomerular damage. Glomerular hypertension is also ameliorated by drugs, such as ACE inhibitors or ARBs, that dilate the efferent arteriole [61,62]. The incremental benefit of this specific hemodynamic effect would be particularly relevant when arterial hypertension is not effectively controlled [63]. A still-debated issue, however, is whether blood pressure has an independent predictive value also among subjects with blood pressure maintained at usual targets of diastolic pressure of <90 mmHg or mean pressure <107 mmHg and whether further reduction to lower-than-usual targets, according to JCN-7 guidelines [64] of systolic/diastolic pressures of < 130/80 mmHg, may confer additional renoprotection. Whether treatment should target systolic, diastolic, pulse, or mean blood pressure is also far from being established based on controlled studies.

The first evidence that reducing blood pressure to lower-than-usual targets (mean <92 mmHg) may slow the rate of GFR decline in chronic kidney disease was generated by the Modification of Diet in Renal Disease (MDRD) study [65]. As acknowledged by those study authors, however, the proportion of study patients on ACE inhibitor therapy was higher in the low blood pressure group than in the usual blood pressure group. Similarly, the trial by Breyer-Lewis in type 1 diabetic nephropathy patients [66] showed that patients with a lower blood pressure target (mean, <92 mmHg) had an effective reduction in urinary proteins that, by contrast, progressively increased in those with usual target pressure (mean, 100–107 mmHg). Again, however, data were biased by the concomitant treatment with ACE inhibitors that were used at higher doses in patients randomized to the lower-than-usual target group than in those randomized to the usual blood pressure target.

Three other trials comparing the effect of treatment targeted at two different blood pressure levels on similar background RAS inhibitor therapy failed to detect any specific benefit of intensified blood pressure control. The African American Study of Kidney Disease and Hypertension (AASK) found the same rate of GFR decline and the same course of proteinuria in nondiabetic patients in the low (mean, <92 mmHg) or usual (mean, 100–107 mm Hg) blood pressure group [67]. The Appropriate Blood Pressure Control in Diabetes (ABCD) trial showed a similar time-dependent course of creatinine clearance in three large cohorts of type 2 diabetic patients with normo-, micro-, or macroalbuminuria randomized to groups with diastolic blood pressure of <75 mmHg or 80–89 mmHg, respectively [68]. Finally, the REIN-2 study found the same rate of GFR decline, incidence of ESRD, and time-dependent course of proteinuria in two groups of nondiabetic patients with the same ACE inhibitor therapy but who were randomly allocated to low (systolic/diastolic pressures of < 130/80 mmHg) or usual (diastolic pressure <90 mmHg) blood pressure targets [69].

Notably, the above studies targeted therapy to different parameters (mean, diastolic, or systolic blood pressure), and none of them evaluated the impact of blood pressure and its reduction on the risk of developing microalbuminuria. The UK Prospective Diabetes Study (UKPDS) found a lower incidence of macrovascular complications and retinopathy in type 2 diabetic patients randomized to intensified blood pressure control but failed to detect a significant protective effect of lower blood pressure against the risk to develop microalbuminuria [70]. Similarly, the ABCD trial found a trend to a lower incidence of microalbuminuria in type 2 diabetic patients with normal UAE allocated to the low blood pressure group, but the risk reduction versus those in the usual blood pressure group was not significant. Thus, whether and to what extent intensified blood pressure control may have a specific renoprotective effect in people with diabetes remains to be addressed, ideally in a prospective clinical trial in patients on the same background RAS inhibitor therapy and randomly allocated to two different blood pressure targets.

Preventing kidney disease in people with diabetes

Preventing (or delaying) the development of microalbuminuria is a key treatment goal for renal protection and, possibly, cardioprotection. Recent clinical trials suggested that RAS inhibition may actually prevent nephropathy. Post hoc analyses of the Heart Outcomes Prevention Evaluation (HOPE) study [71] and of the Losartan Intervention for Endpoint Reduction in Hypertension (LIFE) study [72] found a lower incidence of overt nephropathy in the subgroup of patients with type 2 diabetes given RAS inhibitor therapy compared to controls. However, these analyses included both patients with normo- or microalbuminuria, and they were not powered to compare the incidence of microalbuminuria between the two treatment groups among patients with normal albumin excretion rate at study entry. A randomized prospective trial of enalapril versus placebo in normotensive patients with type 2 diabetes found a lower incidence of microalbuminuria in those on ACE inhibitor therapy who, however, also had greater blood pressure reduction compared to controls. The design of the trial did not allow the authors to differentiate the beneficial effect of RAS inhibition therapy from that of blood pressure reduction [73].

The Bergamo Nephrologic Diabetes Complication Trial (BENEDICT) was a prospective, randomized, double-blind, parallel group study aimed to compare the protective effect against the development of persistent microalbuminuria (taken as an early marker of diabetic kidney disease) of the ACE inhibitor trandolapril, the ndCCB verapamil, and of the trandolapril plus verapamil combination (VeraTran), compared to placebo in 1204 patients with type 2 diabetes and arterial hypertension but a normal UAE rate [74,75]. Baseline characteristics and simultaneous treatments of patients randomized in the four treatment groups were comparable. Over a median follow-up of 3.6 years, significantly fewer patients in the VeraTran group received additional antihypertensive treatment (in particular, with dCCBs and sympatholytic agents) than in the placebo group ($P < 0.01$). Fewer patients on verapamil than on placebo required concomitant treatment with dCCBs. HbA$_{1C}$ levels were comparable in all four groups and remained below 7% throughout the study, showing that optimal metabolic control was attained in these patients. The blood pressure was relatively well-controlled, with small but statistically significant differences between groups. Microalbuminuria developed in 17 of 300 patients in the group receiving verapamil SR plus trandolapril (5.7%) and in 30 of 300 patients in the placebo group (10%). The Kaplan-Meier curves separated starting at 3 months and continued to diverge. The onset of microalbuminuria was significantly delayed by a factor of 2.6 ($P = 0.02$). The relative reduction of risk of progression from normo- to microalbuminuria with verapamil SR plus trandolapril was 61% (95% CI, 0.19–0.80; $P = 0.01$). The difference between the groups remained significant also after adjustment for follow-up systolic and diastolic blood pressures. Hence, the results exceeded expectations based on blood pressure changes alone. The effect of the two experimental drugs used alone was also analyzed. Microalbuminuria developed in 18 of 301 patients on trandolapril alone (6.0%) and in 36 of 303 patients on verapamil (11.9%). Hence, compared to placebo, trandolapril delayed the onset of microalbuminuria by a factor of 2.1 ($P = 0.01$) and decreased the risk of microalbuminuria by 53% ($P = 0.01$), whereas verapamil had no significant effects.

Three patients in the placebo group one in the trandolapril group, and one in the verapamil group had a fatal cardiovascular event. No fatal cardiovascular events were reported in patients who received VeraTran. These data confirm that, provided that intensified metabolic and blood pressure control is pursued, diabetic patients with normal UAE do not have a substantial excess cardiovascular risk compared to subjects without diabetes. One patient receiving verapamil had a second degree atrioventricular block and one on VeraTran had a sinoatrial block with junctional rhythm. Hospitalization was required in both cases, and the patients recovered fully with treatment withdrawal.

Thus, the BENEDICT study showed that persistent microalbuminuria can be prevented by early intervention. The renoprotective effect of ACE inhibition did not appear to be enhanced by combined ndCCB therapy. These findings suggest that in hypertensive patients with type 2 diabetes and normal renal function, an ACE inhibitor may be the medication of choice for controlling blood pressure. The apparent advantage of ACE inhibitors over other agents includes a protective effect on the kidney against the development of microalbuminuria, which is a major risk factor for cardiovascular events and death in this population.

The findings of the BENEDICT study have been recently extended by a meta-analysis of 7603 patients included in 16 trials of ACE inhibitors or ARBs versus placebo or other antihypertensive agents, showing that only ACE inhibitors effectively prevent microalbuminuria in patients with diabetes and no evidence of kidney disease [76]. Overall, ACE inhibitors reduced the risk of microalbuminuria by 42%. On the basis of these data, it has been calculated that approximately 25 people with diabetes and hypertension should be treated to prevent 1 new case of microalbuminuria over 3–4 years.

Conclusions

Most guidelines recommend any antihypertensive agent in patients with diabetes and hypertension and without nephropathy and only ACE inhibitors or ARBs once nephropathy occurs. The use of any class of antihypertensive agents in patients with diabetes is justified by the significant reduction in mortality and cardiovascular outcomes from the primarily nondiabetic trials of hypertension, but only ACE inhibitors have been proved to reduce the onset of microalbuminuria in this population, and the results of ACE inhibitors look more favorable than those of the other classes of drugs evaluated. Thus, ACE inhibitors have an incremental effect on renal outcomes in patients with diabetes, compared with other agents, and so should be the treatment of choice unless other antihypertensive agents are evaluated against ACE inhibition in the setting of a randomized, controlled trial. Future trials of antihypertensive agents in patients with diabetes and no kidney disease should consider microalbuminuria and other renal outcomes as well as the usually considered outcomes, such as all-cause mortality and cardiovascular end points.

ACE inhibitors should be the key component of a multimodal regimen that includes life-style modifications and optimized control of arterial hypertension, hyperglycemia, and dyslipidemia.

References

1 World Health Organization. The Diabetes Program 2004. http//www. who.int/diabetes/en/ http//www.usrds.org/.

2 Remuzzi G, Schieppati A, Ruggenenti P. Nephropathy in patients with type 2 diabetes. *N Engl J Med* 2002; **346**: 1145–1151.

3 Adler AI, Stevens RJ, Manley SE, Bilous RW, Cull CA, Holman RR *et al*. Development and progression of nephropathy in type 2 diabetes: the United Kingdom Prospective Diabetes Study (UKPDS 64). *Kidney Int* 2003; **63**: 225–232.

4 Hasslacher C, Ritz E, Wahl P, Michael C. Similar risks of nephropathy in patients with type I or type II diabetes mellitus. *Nephrol Dial Transplant* 1989; **4**: 859–863.

5 Keane WF, Eknoyan G. Proteinuria, albuminuria, risk assessment, detection, elimination (PARADE): a position paper of the National Kidney Foundation. *Am J Kidney Dis* 1999; **33**: 1004–1010.

6 Miettinen H, Haffner SM, Lehto S, Ronnemaa T, Pyorala K, Laakso M. Proteinuria predicts stroke and other atherosclerotic vascular disease events in nondiabetic and non-insulin-dependent diabetic subjects. *Stroke* 1996; **27**: 2033–2039.

7 Ritz E, Rychlik I, Locatelli F, Halimi S. End-stage renal failure in type 2 diabetes: a medical catastrophe of worldwide dimensions. *Am J Kidney Dis* 1999; **34**: 795–808.

8 Ruggenenti P, Remuzzi G. The diagnosis of renal involvement in non-insulin-dependent diabetes mellitus. *Curr Opin Nephrol Hypertens* 1997; **6**: 141–145.

9 Mogensen CE, Christensen CK, Vittinghus E. The stages in diabetic renal disease with emphasis on the stage of incipient diabetic nephropathy. *Diabetes* 1983; **32(Suppl 2)**: 64–78.

10 Ruggenenti P, Remuzzi G. Time to abandon microalbuminuria? *Kidney Int* 2006; **70**: 1214–1222.

11 Ruggenenti P, Gambara V, Perna A, Bertani T, Remuzzi G. The nephropathy of non-insulin-dependent diabetes: predictors of outcomes relative to patterns of renal injury. *J Am Soc Nephrol* 1998; **12**: 2336–2343.

12 Lemley KV, Blouch K, Abdullah I, Boothroyd DB, Bennett PH, Myers BD *et al*. Glomerular permselectivity at the onset of nephropathy in type 2 diabetes mellitus. *J Am Soc Nephrol* 2000; **11**: 2095–2105.

13 Abbate M, Benigni A, Bertani T, Remuzzi G. Nephrotoxicity of increased glomerular protein traffic. *Nephrol Dial Transplant* 1999; **14**: 304–312.

14 Gall MA, Rossing P, Skott P, Damsbo P, Vaag A, Bech K *et al*. Prevalence of micro- and macroalbuminuria, arterial hypertension, retinopathy and large vessel disease in European type 2 (noninsulin- dependent) diabetic patients. *Diabetologia* 1991; **34**: 655–661.

15 Ravid M, Brosh D, Ravid-Safran D, Levy Z, Rachmani R. Main risk factors for nephropathy in type 2 diabetes mellitus are plasma cholesterol levels, mean blood pressure, and hyperglycemia. *Arch Intern Med* 1998; **158**: 998–1004.

16 Nelson RG, Pettitt DJ, Baird HR, Charles MA, Liu QZ, Bennett PH *et al*. Pre-diabetic blood pressure predicts urinary albumin excretion after the onset of type 2 (non-insulin-dependent) diabetes mellitus in Pima Indians. *Diabetologia* 1993; **36**: 998–1001.

17 Orchard TJ, Chang YF, Ferrell RE, Petro N, Ellis DE. Nephropathy in type 1 diabetes: a manifestation of insulin resistance and multiple genetic susceptibilities? Further evidence from the Pittsburgh Epidemiology of Diabetes Complication Study. *Kidney Int* 2002; **62**: 963–970.

18 Mykkanen L, Zaccaro DJ, Wagenknecht LE, Robbins DC, Gabriel M, Haffner SM. Microalbuminuria is associated with insulin resistance in nondiabetic subjects: the insulin resistance atherosclerosis study. *Diabetes* 1998; **47**: 793–800.

19 De Cosmo S, Minenna A, Ludovico O, Mastroianno S, Di Giorgio A, Pirro L *et al*. Increased urinary albumin excretion, insulin resistance, and related cardiovascular risk factors in patients with type 2 diabetes: evidence of a sex-specific association. *Diabetes Care* 2005; **28**: 910–915.

20 Parvanova AI, Trevisan R, Iliev IP, Dimitrov BD, Vedovato M, Tiengo A *et al*. Insulin resistance and microalbuminuria: a cross-sectional, case-control study of 158 patients with type 2 diabetes and different degrees of urinary albumin excretion. *Diabetes* 2006; **55**: 1456–1462.

21 de Zeeuw D, Remuzzi G, Parving HH, Keane WF, Zhang Z, Shahinfar S *et al*. Albuminuria, a therapeutic target for cardiovascular protection in type 2 diabetic patients with nephropathy. *Circulation* 2004; **110**: 921–927.

22 Berl T, Hunsicker LG, Lewis JB, Pfeffer MA, Porush JG, Rouleau JL *et al*. Cardiovascular outcomes in the Irbesartan Diabetic Nephropathy Trial of patients with type 2 diabetes and overt nephropathy. *Ann Intern Med* 2003; **138(7)**: 542–549.

23 Forman JP, Brenner BM. "Hypertension" and "microalbuminuria": the bell tolls for thee. *Kidney Int* 2006; **69**: 22–28.

24 Gerstein HC, Mann JF, Yi Q, Zinman B, Dinneen SF, Hoogwerf B *et al*. Albuminuria and risk of cardiovascular events, death, and heart failure in diabetic and nondiabetic individuals. *JAMA* 2001; **286**: 421–426.

25 Wachtell K, Ibsen H, Olsen MH, Borch-Johnsen K, Lindholm LH, Mogensen CE *et al*. Albuminuria and cardiovascular risk in hypertensive patients with left ventricular hypertrophy: the LIFE study. *Ann Intern Med* 2003; **139**: 901–906.

26 Klausen K, Borch-Johnsen K, Feldt-Rasmussen B, Jensen G, Clausen P, Scharling H *et al*. Very low levels of microalbuminuria are associated with increased risk of coronary heart disease and death independently of renal function, hypertension, and diabetes. *Circulation* 2004; **110**: 32–35.

27 Arnlov J, Evans JC, Meigs JB, Wang TJ, Fox CS, Levy D *et al*. Low-grade albuminuria and incidence of cardiovascular disease events in nonhypertensive and nondiabetic individuals: the Framingham Heart Study. *Circulation* 2005; **112**: 969–975.

28 Hostetter TH, Troy JC, Brenner BM. Glomerular haemodynamics in experimental diabetes mellitus. *Kidney Int* 1981; **19**: 410–415.

29 Parving HH, Andersen AR, Smidt UM, Svendsen PA. Early aggressive antihypertensive treatment reduces rate of decline in kidney function in diabetic nephropathy. *Lancet* 1983; **i**: 1175–1179.

30 Mogensen CE. Long-term antihypertensive treatment inhibiting progression of diabetic nephropathy. *Br Med J* 1982; **285**: 685–688.

31 Anderson S, Rennke HG, Brenner BM. Therapeutic advantage of converting enzyme inhibitors in arresting progressive renal disease associated with systemic hypertension in the rat. *J Clin Invest* 1986; **77**: 1993–2000.

32 Amann K, Irzyniec T, Mall G, Ritz E. The effect of enalapril on glomerular growth and glomerular lesions after subtotal nephrectomy in the rat: a stereological analysis. *J Hypertens* 1993; **11**: 969–975.

33 Remuzzi A, Puntorieri S, Battaglia C, Bertani T, Remuzzi G. Angiotensin converting enzyme inhibition ameliorates glomerular filtration of macromolecules and water and lessens glomerular injury in the rat. *J Clin Invest* 1990; **85**: 541–549.

34 Mathiesen ER, Hommel E, Giese J, Parving HH. Efficacy of captopril in postponing nephropathy in normotensive insulin-dependent diabetic patients with microalbuminuria. *Br Med J* 1991; **303**: 81–67.

35 Biorck S, Mulec H, Johnsen SA, Norden G, Aurell M. Renal protective effect of enalapril in diabetic nephropathy. *Br Med J* 1992; **304**: 339–343.

36 ACE Inhibitors in Diabetic Nephropathy Trials Group. Should all patients with type 1 diabetes mellitus and microalbuminuria receive angiotensin converting enzyme inhibitors? *Ann Int Med* 2001; **134**: 370–379.

37 Parving HH, Hovind P. Microalbuminuria in type 1 and type 2 diabetes mellitus: evidence with angiotensin converting enzyme inhibitors and

angiotensin II receptor blockers for treating early and preventing clinical nephropathy. *Curr Hypertens Rep* 2002; **4**: 387–393.

38 Martinez FJ, Diaz AB, Aguilar JA *et al.* Trandolapril enhances insulin sensitivity and decreases microalbuminuria in hypertensive NIDDM patients, abstr. 873. *Diabetologia* 1995; **38(Suppl 1)**: 226.

39 Ravid M, Lang R, Rachmani R, Lishner M. Long-term renoprotective effect of angiotensin-converting enzyme inhibition in non-insulin-dependent diabetes mellitus. *Arch Intern Med* 1996; **156**: 286–289.

40 Bakris GL, Williams M, Dworkin L, Elliott WJ, Epstein M, Toto R *et al.* Preserving renal function in adults with hypertension and diabetes: a consensus approach. *Am J Kidney Dis* 2000; **36**: 646–661.

41 Mogensen CE, Keane WF, Bennett PH, Jerums G, Parving HH, Passa P *et al.* Prevention of diabetic renal disease with special reference to microalbuminuria. *Lancet* 1995; **346**: 1080–1084.

42 Parving H-H, Lehnert H, Bröchner-Mortensen J, Gomis R, Andersen S, Arner P. The effect of irbesartan on the development of diabetic nephropathy in patients with type 2 diabetes. *N Engl J Med* 2001; **345**: 870–878.

43 Brenner BM, Cooper ME, de Zeeuw D, Keane WF, Mitch WE, Parving HH *et al.* Effects of losartan on renal and cardiovascular outcomes in patients with type 2 diabetes and nephropathy. *N Engl J Med* 2001; **345**: 861–869.

44 Lewis EJ, Hunsicker LG, Clarke WR, Berl T, Pohl MA, Lewis JB *et al.* Renoprotective effect of the angiotensin-receptor antagonist irbesartan in patients with nephropathy due to type 2 diabetes. *N Engl J Med* 2001; **345**: 851–860.

45 Remuzzi G, Ruggenenti P, Perna A, Dimitrov BD, de Zeeuw D, Hille DA *et al.* Continuum of renoprotection with losartan at all stages of type 2 diabetic nephropathy: a post hoc analysis of the RENAAL trial results. *J Am Soc Nephrol.* 2004 Dec; **15**: 3117–3125.

46 Strippoli GF, Craig M, Deeks JJ, Schena FP, Craig JC. Effects of angiotensin converting enzyme inhibitors and angiotensin II receptor antagonists on mortality and renal outcomes in diabetic nephropathy: systematic review. *BMJ* 2004; **329**: 828–831.

47 Barnett AH, Bain SC, Bouter P, Karlberg B, Madsbad S, Jervell J *et al.* Angiotensin-receptor blockade versus converting-enzyme inhibition in type 2 diabetes and nephropathy. *N Engl J Med* 2004; **351(19)**: 1952–1961.

48 Mogensen CE, Neldam S, Tikkanen I, Oren S, Viskoper R, Watts RW *et al.* Randomized controlled trial of dual blockade of renin-angiotensin system in patients with hypertension, microalbuminuria, and non-insulin dependent diabetes: the candesartan and lisinopril microalbuminuria (CALM) study. *BMJ* 2000; **321**: 1440–1444.

49 Sato A, Hayashi K, Naruse M, Saruta T. Effectiveness of aldosterone blockade in patients with diabetic nephropathy. *Hypertension* 2003; **41**: 64–68.

50 Epstein M, Buckalew V, Martinez F, *et al.* Antiproteinuric efficacy of eplerenone, enalapril and eplerenone/enalapril combination in diabetic hypertensives with microalbuminuria. *Am J Hypertens* 2002; **15**: 24A.

51 Weidmann P, Boehlen LM, de Courten M. Effects of different antihypertensive drugs on human diabetic proteinuria. *Nephrol Dial Transplant* 1993; **8**: 582–584.

52 Bakris GL, Copley B, Vicknair N, Sadler R, Leurgans S. Calcium channel blockers versus other antihypertensive therapies on progression of NIDDM associated nephropathy. *Kidney Int* 1996; **50**: 1641–1650.

53 Bakris GL, Weir MR, Secic M, Campbell B, Weis-McNulty A. Differential effects of calcium antagonist subclasses on markers of nephropathy progression. *Kidney Int* 2004; **65**: 1991–2002.

54 Herlitz H, Harris K, Risler T, Boner G, Berhheim J, Chanard J *et al.* The effects of an ACE inhibitor and a calcium antagonist on the progression of renal disease: the Nephros study. *Nephrol Dial Transplant* 2001; **16**: 2158–2165.

55 Ruggenenti P, Perna A, Loriga G, Ganeva M, Ene-Iordache B, Turturro M *et al.* Blood-pressure control for renoprotection in patients with non-diabetic chronic renal disease (REIN-2): multicenter, randomised controlled trial. *Lancet* 2005; **365**: 939–946.

56 Viberti G, Wheeldon NM, MicroAlbuminuria Reduction with Valsartan (MARVAL) Study Investigators. Microalbuminuria reduction with valsartan in patients with type 2 diabetes mellitus: a blood pressure-independent effect. *Circulation* 2002 Aug 6; **106(6)**: 672–678.

57 Bakris GL, Weir MR, Shanifar S, Zhang Z, Douglas J, van Dijk DJ *et al.* Effects of blood pressure level on progression of diabetic nephropathy. *Arch Intern Med* 2003; **163**: 1555–1565.

58 Berl T, Hunsicker LG, Lewis JB, Pfeffer MA, Porush JG, Rouleau JL *et al.* Impact of achieved blood pressure on cardiovascular outcomes in the irbesartan diabetic nephropathy trial. *J Am Soc Nephrol* 2005; **16**: 2170–2179.

59 Pohl MA, Blumenthal S, Cordonnier DJ, De Alvaro F, Deferrari G, Eisner G *et al.* Independent and additive impact of blood pressure control and angiotensin II receptor blockade on renal outcomes in the irbesartan diabetic nephropathy trial: clinical implications and limitations. *J Am Soc Nephrol* 2005; **16**: 3027–3037.

60 Hayashi K, Epstein M, Loutzenhiser R, Forster H. Impaired myogenic responsiveness of the afferent arteriole in streptozotocin-induced diabetic rats: role of eicosanoid derangements. *J Am Soc Nephrol* 1992; **2**: 1578–1586.

61 Zatz R, Dunn BR, Meyer TW, Anderson S, Rennke HG, Brenner BM. Prevention of diabetic glomerulopathy by pharmacological amelioration of glomerular capillary hypertension. *J Clin Invest* 1986; **77**: 1925–1930.

62 Anderson S, Rennke HG, Brenner BM. Nifedipine versus fosinopril in uninephrectomized diabetic rats. *Kidney Int* 1992; **41**: 891–897.

63 Weidmann P, Boehlen LM, De Courten M, Ferrari P. Antihypertensive therapy in diabetic patients. *J Hum Hypertens* 1992; **6(Suppl 2)**: S23–S36.

64 Chobanian AV, Bakris GL, Black HR, Cushman WC, Green LA, Izzo JL, Jr., *et al.* The Seventh Report of the Joint National Committee on Prevention, Detection, Evaluation, and Treatment of High Blood Pressure: the JNC 7 report. *JAMA* 2003; **289**: 2560–2572.

65 Peterson JC, Adler S, Burkart JM, Green T, Hebert LA, Hunsicker LG *et al.* Blood pressure control, proteinuria, and the progression of renal disease. The Modification of Diet in Renal Disease Study. *Ann Intern Med* 1995; **123**: 754–762.

66 Breyer-Lewis J, Berl T, Bain RP, Rohde RD, Lewis EJ, and the Collaborative Study Group. Effect of intensive blood pressure control on the course of type 1 diabetic nephropathy. *Am J Kidney Dis* 1999; **34**: 801–817.

67 Wright JT, Bakris G, Grene T, Agodoa LY, Appel LJ, Charleston J *et al.* Effect of blood pressure lowering and antihypertensive drug class on progression of hypertensive kidney disease: results from the AASK trial. *JAMA* 2002; **288**: 2421–2431.

68 Estacio RO, Jeffers BW, Gifford N, Schrier RW. Effect of blood pressure control on diabetic microvascular complications in patients with hypertension and type 2 diabetes. *Diabetes Care* 2000; **23(Suppl 2)**: B54–B64.

69 Ruggenenti P, Perna A, Loriga G, Ganeva M, Ene-Iordache B, Turturro M *et al.* Blood-pressure control for renoprotection in patients with

non-diabetic chronic renal disease (REIN-2): multicentre, ransomised controlled trial. *Lancet* 2005; **365:** 939–946.

70 UK Prospective Diabetes Study Group. Tight blood pressure control and risk of macrovascular and microvascular complications in type 2 diabetes: UKPDS 38. *BMJ* 1998; **317:** 703–713.

71 Heart Outcomes Prevention Evaluation (HOPE) Study Investigators. Effects of ramipril on cardiovascular and microvascular outcomes in people with diabetes melllitus: results of the HOPE study and MICRO-HOPE substudy. *Lancet* 2000; **355:** 253–259.

72 Lindholm LH, Ibsen H, Dahlof B, Devereux RB, Beevers G, de Faire U *et al.* Cardiovascular morbidity and mortality in patients with diabetes in the Losartan Intervention for Endpoint Reduction in Hypertension Study (LIFE): a randomized trial against atenolol. *Lancet* 2002; **359:** 1004–1010.

73 Ravid M, Brosh D, Levi Z, Bar-Dayan Y, Ravid D, Rachmani R. Use of enalapril to attenuate decline in renal function in normotensive, nor-molabuminuric patients with type 2 diabetes mellitus. A randomized controlled trial. *Ann Intern Med* 1998; **128:** 982–988.

74 The BENEDICT group. The Bergamo Nephrologic Diabetes Complications Trial (BENEDICT): design and baselines group. *Control Clin Trials* 2003; **24:** 442–461.

75 Ruggenenti P, Fassi A, Ilieva AP, Bruno S, Iliev IP, Brusegan V*et al.*. Preventing microalbuminuria in type 2 diabetes. *N Engl J Med* 2004; **351:** 1941–1951

76 Strippoli GF, Craig M, Schena FP, Craig JC. Antihypertensive agents for primary prevention of diabetic nephropathy.*J Am Soc Nephrol* 2005; **16:** 3081–3091.

22 Lupus Nephritis

Arrigo Schieppati,[1,2] **Erica Daina,**[2] **& Giuseppe Remuzzi**[1,2]

[1]Division of Nephrology and Dialysis, Ospedali Riuniti di Bergamo, Bergamo, Italy.
[2]Mario Negri Institute for Pharmacological Research, Negri Bergamo Laboratories, Bergamo, Italy.

Definition and epidemiology of lupus nephritis

Systemic lupus erythematosus (SLE) is a disease characterized by autoantibodies directed against self-antigens, immune complex formation, and immune dysregulation and can result in damage to any organ, including the kidney, skin, blood cells, and the nervous system. SLE carries significant mortality and morbidity in the younger, female population. Renal involvement, defined as lupus nephritis, is one of the most serious manifestations of SLE [1]. It usually arises within 5 years of diagnosis, and its prevalence varies, according to published studies, from 30 to 90%. Urinary abnormalities (with or without renal function impairment) are present in approximately 50% of patients at the time of diagnosis and are found in around 75% of patients in the long term [2,3]. Renal impairment eventually develops in 30% of patients with SLE. According to the data of the US Renal Data System [4], lupus nephritis is the cause of about 2% of all end-stage renal disease. Interestingly, the mortality rate at 1 year for this group of patients is 7.7%, or half the mortality rate for the end-stage renal disease population as a whole [5].

Lupus nephritis occurs about nine times more frequently in women than men, but men who develop SLE are more likely to develop renal disease and have a worse prognosis [6]. Most patients develop lupus nephritis early in their disease course. The peak age for the development of SLE is during the third decade of life. SLE is more common in African Americans, Asians, and Hispanic people than in White people, and the spectrum of lupus nephritis also is worse in these groups [7].

Diagnosis and monitoring lupus nephritis

Included among the criteria of the American College of Rheumatology for SLE are minimal criteria for the diagnosis of renal involvement. They are 1) persistent proteinuria greater than 0.5 g/day or greater than 3+ urine dipstick reaction for albumin and 2) cellular casts (may be erythrocytes, granular, tubular, or mixed) [8,9]. Patients with known SLE should be regularly checked for urinary abnormalities by including urinalysis in the panel of laboratory tests, and the test should be repeated during follow-up, because a proportion of patients develop lupus nephritis years after the onset of the disease and because lupus nephritis is often asymptomatic [10].

For a number of patients with SLE, nephritis is the presenting feature of the disease. Proteinuria is the main feature of renal damage in SLE, and the reference standard is the measurement of protein excretion over 24 h. Recently, determination of the protein/creatinine ratio on a random spot sample of urine has emerged as a valid and more feasible test than a timed urine collection [11]. Not only is it a valid method of screening but also it is a reliable index of the effect of treatment in glomerular diseases [12].

Serum creatinine is the screening test for detecting renal function changes, although the normal range is wide. Serum creatinine concentration is affected by factors other than glomerular filtration rate (GFR), such as tubular secretion and generation and extrarenal excretion of creatinine. Due to variation in these processes amongst individuals and over time within individuals, especially for creatinine generation, there is a wide range of serum creatinine levels in people without kidney disease. As a result, there are several significant limitations to estimating kidney function solely from serum creatinine. Creatinine clearance is not accurate in determining the GFR, especially when GFR is only mild to moderately impaired, but more reliable tests, such as clearance of inulin or of a radiolabeled compound, are not routinely available and not practical in the clinical setting. Equations for calculation of GFR are now widely used, such as the Cockcroft-Gault formula, or the Modification of Diet in Renal Disease (MDRD) study formula [13]. However, it is important to note that in most clinical conditions, what matters is not the absolute value of GFR but rather the change in GFR over time in the same individual. For monitoring the kidney function of renal lupus patients therefore it is usually sufficient to monitor serial serum creatinine levels.

Evidence-based Nephrology. Edited by Donald Molony and Jonathan Craig
© 2009 Blackwell Publishing, ISBN: 978-1-4051-3975-5.

The course of the disease may also be monitored with serologic tests. Anti-double-stranded DNA (anti-dsDNA) autoantibody titers correlate roughly, at best, with lupus nephritis activity [14]. Similar to GFR, changes in anti-dsDNA autoantibody titers, rather than absolute values, are more useful clinically. An increase in anti-dsDNA autoantibody titers are a warning sign of possible disease flare but are not accurate enough to justify automatic escalation of the therapy. Rather, an increasing titer suggests the need for strict monitoring for clinical signs of exacerbation. Because methods for measuring anti-dsDNA autoantibodies have not been standardized, it may be difficult to compare data from different laboratories, even for the same patient [15]. Anti-C1q autoantibodies also correlate with disease activity and are a useful test to monitor disease activity and to predict flares [16]. Development of new surrogate markers of disease activity for monitoring long-term outcome of the disease is an interesting field of investigation.

Renal pathology

Lupus nephritis is a term that comprises complex and diverse histopathological manifestations that have different prognoses and require different therapeutic approaches. The different patterns of kidney damage were classified for the first time in a coherent fashion in 1982 (modified in 1995) by the World Health Organization (WHO) [17,18]. Recently under the aegis of the International Society of Nephrology and the Renal Pathology Society (ISN/RPS), a group of renal pathologists, nephrologists, and rheumatologists developed a new classification system, although it is still based on the 1982 WHO classification [19].

Before describing the patterns of kidney damage in lupus nephritis, a few words should be said on the indication for renal biopsy. Renal biopsy is definitely indicated in patients with acute kidney failure, active urinary sediment, or flare-ups of lupus serology with *de novo* renal abnormalities. Although these features are most often associated with diffuse proliferative glomerular disease, a renal biopsy can also reveal other types of lesions that may modify the therapeutic approach. Moreover, an index biopsy allows a clinician to establish activity and chronicity indexes of renal damage and reveal vascular lesions that have unfavorable prognostic value. More often than in other glomerular diseases, a repeat renal biopsy is indicated in lupus nephritis, especially when there is a lack of improvement to appropriate therapy, a relapse, or a late deterioration of renal function. In this case, repeat renal biopsy may help distinguish between active lupus nephritis and chronic sclerotic lesions that are not amenable to aggressive immunosuppression.

The classification of lupus nephritis according to the classic 1982 WHO definitions comprises six classes, defined as follows:

Class I: Normal glomeruli on light microscopy; immune deposits are found on immunofluorescence and electron microscopy

Class II: Pure mesangial alteration; mesangial widening and/or proliferation

Class III: Focal proliferative glomerulonephritis; less than 50% of the glomeruli present segmental or global proliferation with mesangial involvement

Class IV: Diffuse proliferative glomerulonephritis; more than 50% of glomeruli are the site of severe mesangial involvement, endocapillary proliferation, and subendothelial deposits; in both class III and IV, there are subclasses based on the presence of necrotizing lesions and active or chronic lesions

Class V: Membranous glomerulonephritis; may be characterized by pure membranous lesions or may be associated with typical lesions of classes II, III, and IV

Class VI: Advanced sclerosing glomerulonephritis; more than 90% of glomeruli are sclerosed

The recently proposed new classification of the ISN/RPS (Table 22.1) proposes that classes I and II be used for purely mesangial involvement (I, mesangial immune deposits without mesangial hypercellularity; II, mesangial immune deposits with mesangial hypercellularity); class III be used for focal glomerulonephritis (involving <50% of total number of glomeruli) with subdivisions for active and sclerotic lesions; class IV be used for diffuse glomerulonephritis (involving ≥50% of the total number of glomeruli) either with segmental (class IV-S) or global (class IV-G) involvement and also with subdivisions for active and sclerotic lesions; class V be used for membranous lupus nephritis; and class VI be for advanced sclerosing lesions. The aim of this new classification is to provide an unequivocal description of the various lesions and classes of lupus nephritis, allowing a better standardization and lending a basis for further clinicopathologic studies.

We conducted a retrospective analysis of a large cohort of 659 patients with a diagnosis of lupus nephritis followed in 32 nephrology centers in Italy [20]. A renal biopsy had been performed in 82% of patients. Distribution of renal histology classes was as follows. The largest group of patients was in class IV (53.8% of all renal biopsies), followed by class V (16.6%), class III (14.4%), and class II (8.2%). A 6.7% proportion of patients had mixed forms of kidney damage. There was a close relationship between serum creatinine and urinary protein excretion rate at the time of diagnosis and histology class. This distribution may not actually reflect the true incidence of each WHO class, because renal biopsy may not have been performed for milder clinical manifestations of lupus nephritis.

Outcome

Survival of patients with lupus nephritis has improved significantly over the last 40 years, thanks to changes in the specific treatment of lupus nephritis and general medical care. Whereas in the 1950s the 5-year survival rate for patients with lupus nephritis was near 0%, in 1990 patient survival was 83–92% at 5 years and 74–84% at 10 years [1]. Renal survival (living without dialysis) is also reasonably good. Our retrospective analysis of 659 patients with

Table 22.1 WHO and ISN/RPS lupus nephritis classifications.

WHO		ISN/RPS	
CLASS I	Normal glomeruli	CLASS I	Minimal mesangial lupus nephritis
CLASS II	Pure mesangial alterations (mesangiopathy)	CLASS II	Mesangial proliferative lupus nephritis
CLASS III	Focal segmental glomerulonephritis a) Active necrotizing lesions b) Active and sclerosing lesions c) Sclerosing lesions	CLASS III	Focal lupus nephritis A, active lesions A/C, active and chronic lesions C, chronic inactive lesions with glomerular scars
CLASS IV	Diffuse glomerulonephritis a) Without segmental lesions b) Active necrotizing lesions c) Active and sclerosing lesions d) Sclerosing lesions	CLASS IV	Diffuse lupus nephritis A. active lesions A/C, active and chronic lesions C. chronic inactive lesions with glomerular scars
			Each subclass should be further subdivided: S, segmental G, global
CLASS V	Diffuse membranous glomerulonephritis	CLASS V	Membranous lupus nephritis
CLASS VI	Advanced sclerosing glomerulonephritis	CLASS VI	Advanced sclerotic lupus nephritis

lupus nephritis found that the overall probability of renal survival was 80% at 10 years after diagnosis. The probability of maintaining life-supporting kidney function was evaluated according to several variables (clinical characteristics at presentation and WHO histological classification). The presence at the time of diagnosis of hypertension and diffuse proliferative nephritis (WHO class IV) was associated with a worse prognosis [20].

Treatment of lupus nephritis

General principles

The treatment of lupus nephritis is aimed to induce remission of the inflammation, thereby achieving control over renal and extrarenal signs of the disease. Even though there is no universal consent on definitions of remission, the current understanding is that remission of lupus nephritis is characterized by resolution of urinary abnormalities, reduction of proteinuria, and amelioration or stabilization of renal function. Ideally, all these objectives should be achieved with the least possible toxicity [21].

In many patients, irreversible injury may occur that prevents recovery of renal function. Also, healing of the inflammatory process may lead to glomerular sclerosis, for which the hallmark is persistent proteinuria [22]. Therefore, the treatment of lupus nephritis should include supportive, nonimmunological measures in association with immunosuppression.

Supportive therapy

Nonimmunological therapy for lupus nephritis is aimed to reduce proteinuria and to control hypertension. The role of proteinuria as a risk factor for progression of chronic nephropathies has been recognized over the last decade [23]. A number of randomized clinical trials, and substantial noncontrolled evidence, have established angiotensin converting enzyme inhibitors (ACEi) as effective in reducing proteinuria and preventing renal disease progression [24]. They may be used alone or in combination with angiotensin II receptor blockers (ARBs), which have also been demonstrated to exert kidney-protective effects. In general clinical trials assessing the protective role of ACEi or ARBs, patients with lupus nephritis are always excluded, because the concomitant immunosuppressive therapy may complicate the interpretation of results. However, there is no reason to suggest that the trials in non-lupus patients cannot be extrapolated to lupus patients. Moreover, there have been a few uncontrolled studies on small numbers of patients who were treated with aggressive renoprotective therapy that showed that this approach is feasible and probably effective [25,26].

High blood pressure is the other major risk factor for both chronic kidney disease progression and cardiovascular complications. Indeed, in our series of 659 patients, hypertension was associated with a worse prognosis, and cardiovascular events were the primary cause of death in our cohort (24.7% of patients). Again, ACEi and ARBs are the drugs of choice for chronic kidney disease patients, according to many guidelines. The target blood pressure should be <130/80 mmHg, and probably even lower (<120/70 mmHg) if proteinuria exceeds 1 g/day. In non-lupus patients, these goals are usually achieved with a combination of drugs.

Other supportive measures, such as a low-protein diet, blood lipid control, and smoking cessation, even though they have not reached the same degree of evidence compared to the above-mentioned measures, are recommended [28,29].

Immunosuppressive therapy for proliferative lupus nephritis

Although immunosuppressive therapy is not indicated for the treatment of class I and II lupus nephritis, which have an excellent prognosis, it is recommended for proliferative forms of lupus nephritis with the aims of reducing glomerular inflammation and restoring or preserving kidney function.

Treatment regimens have been based on an induction phase aimed to induce remission of the disease in the shortest possible time and a maintenance phase aimed to preserve remission in the long term. The optimal therapy for both phases remains somewhat elusive, for several reasons. There is no consensus on the definition of remission, and as a consequence it is not known how long treatment should be prolonged. Also, the optimal regimen to be instituted in the induction phase is not universally established.

A study conducted at the National Institutes of Health (NIH) 20 years ago showed that kidney function was better-preserved in patients who received various cytotoxic drug therapies, but the difference was statistically significant only for intravenous cyclophosphamide pulses associated with low-dose prednisone compared with high-dose prednisone alone [30]. Treatment of lupus glomerulonephritis with intravenous cyclophosphamide rapidly became standard therapy.

Subsequent studies have focused on the optimal duration of the treatment. This was addressed by studies that compared the effects of short-term versus long-term treatments. Another study of the NIH showed that a regimen of prolonged intravenous cyclophosphamide administration (six monthly pulses followed by pulses every 3 months for 2 years) gave better results in term of preservation of renal function and reduction of the risk of relapses than six monthly pulses of methylprednisolone [31]. Also, this regimen gave better long-term results than a 6-month cycle of intravenous cyclophosphamide. A final study of the same group [32] showed that the combination of intravenous cyclophosphamide pulses with methylprednisolone for 1 year gave better results than either of the drugs given as sole therapy.

Protracted cyclophosphamide regimens, however, carry a significant burden of side effects, most notably a high rate of gonadal toxicity, severe infections, and osteoporosis. In at least one trial the mortality rate was higher in the cyclophosphamide group [33]. The concern over toxicity of these regimens has driven clinicians to investigate whether short-term treatment may be equally effective in controlling renal disease. One important study in this direction was the Euro-Lupus Nephritis Trial, published in 2002 [34]. In this study 90 patients with proliferative lupus nephritis were assigned to a high-dose intravenous cyclophosphamide regimen

Table 22.2 Treatment of patients with class III and IV lupus nephritis based on the available evidence.

Induction phase
Recommended
- Monthly intravenous pulse cyclophosphamide (0.75–1 g/m^2) for 6 mos

associated with
- High-dose prednisone, 1 mg/kg orally, tapered in 4–6 wks

or
- Intravenous pulses of methyprednisolone

Alternative
- MMF, 2–3 g/day in two divided doses for 6 months

associated with
- High-dose prednisone, 1 mg/kg orally, tapered in 4–6 wks

or
- Intravenous pulses of methyprednisolone

Maintenance phase
Optimal therapy for maintenance phase cannot be established by currently available
evidence. Possible choices are:
- MMF, tapered to 1–2 g/day in two divided doses
- Azathioprine, 1–3 mg/kg/day
- Intravenous pulse cyclophosphamide every 3 mos until in complete remission for 1 yr

---

All regimens are associated with low-dose oral prednisone.

(six monthly pulses and two quarterly pulses; initial dose, 0.5 g/m^2, then changed according to white blood cell counts) or a low-dose intravenous cyclophosphamide regimen (a pulse every 2 weeks, for a total of six pulses, at a fixed dose of 500 mg), each of which was followed by azathioprine (2 mg/kg/day). The follow-up period was 41 months. Renal remission was achieved in 71% of the low-dose group and 54% of the high-dose group (not statistically significant). Renal flares were noted in 27% of the low-dose group and 29% of the high-dose group. Although episodes of severe infection were more than twice as frequent in the high-dose group, the difference was not statistically significant. These data, in the authors' opinion, put into question the practice, based on the NIH trials, of treating all lupus nephritis patients with an extended course of intravenous cyclophosphamide. There were, however, evident differences between the populations studied. The European patients had a less severe kidney disease than patients recruited in the NIH trials. According to the authors, this was not due to selection bias of milder cases but represented the spectrum of patients in most European lupus clinics who were referred to the trial. Also, the ethnic composition of the European study, where 84% of patients were Caucasians, compared to a prevalence of 43% black patients in the NIH trials, is an important difference. Nonwhite ethnicity has been recognized as an unfavorable prognostic factor. In conclusion, the results of the European study indicate a promising and probably safer alternative to the traditional NIH regimen, but more data are needed before it becomes the new standard of care for lupus nephritis (Table 22.2).

The most recent systematic review on the treatment of lupus nephritis was published in 2003 by Flanc *et al.* [35]. A total of 920 articles were identified and 25 randomized controlled trials were considered suitable for inclusion, with an overall population of 915 patients. The majority of the studies were comparisons between cyclophosphamide or azathioprine plus steroids versus steroids alone (when the meta-analysis was performed, studies with mycophenolate mofetil (MMF) were under way and so they were not included in the review). Cyclophosphamide plus steroids reduced the risk of doubling of serum creatinine compared to steroids alone but had no impact on end-stage renal failure or mortality. Azathioprine plus steroids reduced the risk of all-cause mortality compared to steroids alone but did not alter renal outcomes. No benefit was found with the addition of plasma exchange to cyclophosphamide or azathioprine plus steroids in terms of risk of mortality, deterioration of kidney function, or uremia. Cyclophosphamide increased the risk of ovarian failure by about twofold (95% confidence interval, 1.10–4.34), while none of the immunosuppressive therapies increased the risk of major infection. The authors of this systematic review concluded that, whereas waiting for new therapeutic agents to be examined in clinical trials, cyclophosphamide combined with steroids remains the best option to preserve kidney function in lupus nephritis and that the smallest effective dose and shortest duration of treatment should be used to minimize gonadal toxicity, without compromising efficacy. The finding that azathioprine reduced all-cause mortality to a greater extent than cyclophosphamide is interesting but should be interpreted with caution. Indeed, this was an indirect comparison, because no study directly compared the two drugs except for one of the NIH studies, which was actually underpowered for this purpose [30]. Moreover, the studies that showed an advantage of azathioprine in terms of mortality (only three studies, for a total of 78 patients) were done in the early 1970s, when mortality for lupus nephritis was very high. Overall, the authors of this meta-analysis found that the quality of the studies was greatly variable. Many of them were done many years ago and presented serious methodological problems. Numbers of subjects enrolled were small in many studies. Moreover, the distribution of ethnic groups and severity of renal involvement varied among studies, making comparisons difficult.

Mycophenolate mofetil

MMF has been proposed as an alternative to cyclophosphamide for the induction of remission of lupus nephritis. As early as 1997 we investigated the effect of MMF in New Zealand Black × New Zealand White (NZBxW) F_1 hybrid mice, a model of genetically determined immune complex disease that mimics SLE in humans [36]. Results showed that the percentage of proteinuric mice was significantly reduced by MMF treatment, and serum blood urea nitrogen levels were also lower than in the vehicle-treated group. MMF had a suppressive effect on autoantibody production and protected animals from leukopenia and anemia. Life survival of MMF-treated lupus mice was significantly improved compared to untreated animals. Thus, MMF delayed kidney function deterioration and prolonged life survival in murine lupus nephritis.

Several clinical studies (not examined in the above-mentioned meta-analysis) have been published since then. The first randomized clinical trial was done in China [37]. In 42 patients with diffuse proliferative lupus nephritis, the efficacy and side effects of a regimen of prednisolone and MMF given for 12 months were compared with those of a regimen of prednisolone and cyclophosphamide given for 6 months followed by prednisolone and azathioprine for 6 months. Eighty-one percent of the 21 patients treated with MMF and prednisolone had a complete remission, and 14% had a partial remission, compared with 76% and 14%, respectively, of the 21 patients treated with cyclophosphamide and prednisolone followed by azathioprine and prednisolone. The improvements in the degree of proteinuria and the serum albumin and creatinine concentrations were similar in the two groups. The rates of relapse were 15% and 11%, respectively, whereas the prevalence of side effects of treatment was greater in the cyclophosphamide group. The follow-up was short, however, and the number of patients was low.

Results from an extended long-term study, with a median follow-up of 63 months, were reported by the same investigators in 2005 [38]. Serum creatinine in both groups remained stable and comparable over time. Creatinine clearance increased significantly in the MMF group, but the between-group difference was not significant. A total of 6.3% in the MMF group and 10.0% of cyclophosphamide-treated patients showed doubling of baseline creatinine during follow-up. The relapse rate was similar in the two groups, while MMF treatment was associated with fewer infections or infections that required hospitalization.

The most recently published trial was done in USA, sponsored by the US Food and Drug Administration [39]. It was a 24-week randomized, open-label, noninferiority trial comparing oral MMF (initial dose, 1000 mg/day, increased to 3000 mg/day) with monthly intravenous cyclophosphamide (0.5 g/m² body surface area, increased to 1.0 g/m²) as induction therapy for active lupus nephritis. A total of 140 patients were recruited; 71 were randomly assigned to receive MMF, and 69 received cyclophosphamide. In the intention-to-treat analysis, 16 of the 71 patients (22.5%) receiving MMF and 4 of the 69 patients (5.8%) receiving cyclophosphamide had complete remission, for an absolute difference of 16.7% ($P = 0.005$), meeting the criterion for noninferiority and demonstrating actually the superiority of MMF to cyclophosphamide.

Partial remission occurred in 21 of the 71 patients (29.6%) and 17 of the 69 patients (24.6%), respectively ($P = 0.51$). Three patients assigned to the cyclophosphamide group died, two during protocol therapy. Fewer severe infections and hospitalizations but more diarrhea occurred among those receiving MMF. This study, however, generated some criticism [40], because patients with relatively mild disease were enrolled, including 20% of patients with membranous nephropathy, a form of lupus nephritis for which optimal treatment has not been established [41].

The efficacy of MMF as a maintenance therapy was assessed in a small trial by Contreras *et al.* [42]. Fifty-nine patients with lupus nephritis received induction therapy consisting of a maximum of seven monthly boluses of intravenous cyclophosphamide plus corticosteroids. Subsequently, the patients were assigned to one of three maintenance therapies: quarterly intravenous injections of cyclophosphamide, oral azathioprine, or oral MMF for 1–3 years. During maintenance therapy, five patients died (four in the cyclophosphamide group and one in the MMF group), and chronic kidney failure developed in five (three in the cyclophosphamide group and one each in the azathioprine and MMF groups). The 72-month event-free survival rate for the composite end point of death or chronic kidney failure was higher in the MMF and azathioprine groups than in the cyclophosphamide group. The rate of relapse-free survival was higher in the MMF group than in the cyclophosphamide group. The incidences of hospitalization, amenorrhea, infections, nausea, and vomiting were significantly lower in the MMF and azathioprine groups than in the cyclophosphamide group.

MMF is clearly less toxic than cyclophosphamide, making it an attractive alternative. However, before it can be adopted as the new standard induction therapy for lupus nephritis, more data are needed. Available studies have had relatively short follow-up periods, and we do not know yet the optimal duration of MMF treatment. Studies are under way to establish the efficacy and safety of a long-term treatment protocol.

Treatment for patients resistant to induction therapy

Some patients do not respond to induction therapy, although it is difficult to define how frequently this occurs, as clinical trials have used different criteria. The optimal therapy for resistant cases is uncertain and cannot established by evidence-based criteria because of the sparse data. In patients resistant to cyclophosphamide after 6 months, a more prolonged course is advisable if side effects are not an obstacle; alternatively, the patient could be switched to MMF [43]. Vice versa, in resistant patients initially treated with MMF, cyclophosphamide should be used. Limited data are available for a number of other treatment modalities, such has intravenous immunoglobulin [44] or high-dose cyclophosphamide with stem cell transplantation [45]. In the previously mentioned systematic review by Flanc *et al.* [35], plasmapheresis did not offer any advantage.

New treatments

Based on new pathogenetic studies, several new therapeutic agents are being tested in preliminary studies or have been simply proposed as potentially effective agents (Table 22.3). Rituximab, a monoclonal antibody directed against the CD20 molecule found on pre-B cells and mature B cells, was introduced in the late 1990s for the treatment of non-Hodgkin's lymphoma [46]. Recently, this antibody has been used to treat glomerular diseases, including lupus [47]. A small study of 10 patients with proliferative nephritis treated with a standard protocol of rituximab and oral steroids was reported by Sfikakis and colleagues [48]. Seven of the 10 patients had already experienced episodes of nephritis requiring steroids plus cyclophosphamide or MMF. Four patients achieved complete remission (normalization of serum creatinine and serum albumin, inactive urinary sediment, and proteinuria of <0.5 g/day) at 1 year. One attained temporary complete remission, and three had partial remission (>50% improvement in all renal parameters). Other series of patients with SLE treated with rituximab have been reported, but these have contained only a proportion of patients with lupus-related kidney disease. Overall, the majority of patients with SLE in whom B-cell depletion is achieved derive some clinical and biochemical benefits [49].

The interaction of B7-related molecules on antigen-presenting cells with CD28 or CTLA-4 antigens on T cells provides a second signal for T-cell activation. Selection inhibition of the B7-CD28 or B7–CTLA-4 interactions produces antigen-specific T-cell unresponsiveness in vitro and suppresses immune function in vivo [50]. A B7-binding protein was generated by genetic fusion of the extracellular domain of murine CTLA-4 to the Fc portion of a mouse immunoglobulin G2a monoclonal antibody (muCTLA4Ig). In lupus-prone NZB/NZW mice, treatment with muCTLA4Ig blocked autoantibody production and prolonged life, even when treatment was delayed until the most advanced stage of clinical illness [51].

Another receptor–ligand pair, CD40 on B cells and CD40 ligand on T cells, is an important costimulatory signal to T- and B-cell activation. Selective blockade of this interaction with an anti-CD40L monoclonal antibody (ruplizumab) ameliorated nephritis in a murine model of lupus [52]. The compound was also tested

Table 22.3 New treatments for lupus nephritis.

Treatment	Type of agent(s)	Mechanism of action	Clinical data
Rituximab	Chimeric antibody directed against CD20 on B lymphocytes	Antibody-dependent cell-mediated cytotoxicity and induction of apoptosis	Clinical benefit reported in patients refractory to conventional therapy in open studies; good tolerability reported.
Abetimus sodium (LJP 394)	Construct of four dsDNA epitopes attached to a polyethylene glycol platform	Induces B-cell tolerance by binding anti-dsDNA antibodies, resulting in B-cell apoptosis or anergy	Reduces number of renal flares and prolongs interval between flares in patients with high-affinity antibodies to its DNA epitope.
Ruplizumab	Anti-CD40 ligand antibody	Blocks costimulatory signal on B cells that induces activation, proliferation, and class switching	A phase II RCT showed improvement in serology and hematuria but was terminated because of thrombotic complications
IDEC-131	Humanized monoclonal antibody against CD154	Blocks costimulatory pathways	In clinical studies, no significant benefit over placebo

in a clinical study of 28 patients with active proliferative lupus nephritis. A reduction of anti-dsDNA antibodies, increase in C3 concentrations, and decrease in hematuria were observed, but the study was terminated prematurely because of thromboembolic events in patients [53].

A humanized monoclonal antibody against CD154 (IDEC-131) was tested in 85 patients with active SLE in a phase II, double-blind, placebo-controlled, multiple-center, multiple-dose study [54]. Efficacy was assessed at week 20, primarily by the Systemic Lupus Erythematosus Disease Activity Index (SLEDAI) and, secondarily, by multiple measures of disease activity. Safety was assessed through week 28 by clinical and laboratory evaluations. SLEDAI scores improved from the baseline levels of disease activity in all groups, including the placebo group. The type and frequency of adverse events were similar between the IDEC-131 and placebo groups.

LJP 394 (Abetimus sodium) is a synthetic toleragen molecule consisting of four double-stranded oligodeoxyribonucleotides attached to nonimmunogenic polyethylene glycol [55]. Abetimus is an immunomodulating agent that induces tolerance in B cells directed against dsDNA. It does this by cross-linking surface antibodies. In a multicenter, partially randomized, placebo-controlled, double-blind, dose-ranging trial, 58 patients were randomly assigned to receive 1, 10, or 50 mg of LJP 394 or placebo [56]. The greatest reductions in mean dsDNA antibody titers were observed in the group of patients who received 50 mg of LJP 394 weekly (38.1% and 37.1% at weeks 16 and 24, respectively). A reduction (29.3%) in dsDNA antibody titers was also observed at week 24 in the group of patients who received 10 mg of LJP 394 weekly. The frequencies of adverse events were comparable in the placebo and active treatment groups. This clinical trial demonstrated the capacity of LJP 394 to reduce dsDNA antibodies.

Another study was designed to determine whether LJP 394 delays or prevents renal flare in patients with lupus renal disease [57]. A total of 230 patients were randomized to receive 16 weekly doses of 100 mg of LJP 394 or placebo, followed by alternating 8-week drug holidays and 12 weekly doses of 50 mg of LJP 394 or placebo. Anti-dsDNA antibodies decreased and C3 levels tended to increase during treatment with LJP 394. In the intent-to-treat population, the time to renal flare was not significantly different between treatment groups, but patients taking LJP 394 had a longer time to institution of high-dose corticosteroids and/or cyclophosphamide and required 41% fewer treatments. In the high-affinity antibody population, the LJP 394 group experienced a longer time to renal flare, 67% fewer renal flares, longer time to institution of high-dose corticosteroids and/or cyclophosphamide, and 62% fewer treatments than the placebo group. Serious adverse events were observed in 25 of the 114 LJP 394-treated patients (21.9%) and 34 of the 116 placebo-treated patients (29.3%). In conclusion, treatment with LJP 394 in patients with high-affinity antibodies to the DNA epitope prolonged the time to renal flare, decreased the number of renal flares, and required fewer high-dose corticosteroids and/or cyclophosphamide treatments compared with placebo.

Membranous nephropathy

Data on treatment of class V (membranous) lupus nephritis are scarce, and optimal therapy for this form of disease is not established. A small study of 41 patients at the NIH showed that patients treated with a combination of cyclophosphamide and steroids or cyclosporine had a higher rate of remission at 1 year than did patients treated with steroids alone [58]. Patients with lupus membranous nephropathy also have been treated by following a regimen of alternate cycles of steroids and chlorambucil, which is used for idiopathic membranous nephropathy [59]. The combination regimen offered a higher rate of remission and lower rate of renal flares, but this study was retrospective.

Recently we have shown that remission can be obtained in idiopathic membranous nephropathy with rituximab [60]. In a prospective, observational study we evaluated the 1-year outcome of eight patients with idiopathic membranous nephropathy and persistent (>6 months) urinary protein excretion greater than 3.5 g/day. They were given four weekly infusions of rituximab (375 mg/m^2). At 3 and 12 months, proteinuria significantly decreased by 51 and 66% from baseline, respectively. At 12 months, two of eight patients were in complete remission (proteinuria of ≤0.5 g/day) and three more had partial remission (proteinuria of ≤3.5 g/day).

Recently, Jacobson and colleagues described a patient with membranous lupus nephritis with persistent nephrotic syndrome despite intensive immunosuppression who had a remission of nephrotic syndrome and recovery of renal function after a course of intravenous rituximab [61].

In the absence of randomized trial data, it is difficult to give a recommendation concerning rituximab. A prudent approach would be to advise to treat conservatively those patients with asymptomatic, nonnephrotic proteinuria. Patients with more aggressive disease (unremitting nephrotic-range proteinuria, declining kidney function) are usually treated as diffuse proliferative forms. However, when a patient known to have membranous lupus nephritis develops such features of worsening disease, a new renal biopsy to ascertain a change of histology class may be warranted. Rituximab is potentially a new effective treatment for resistant cases.

Conclusions

Optimal treatment of lupus nephritis is still a challenge to the clinician, even though there are now more treatment options than in the past. Several questions must be addressed in future studies. First, better definitions of clinical status, remission, and relapse are needed to establish appropriate therapeutic goals. Also, new markers of disease activity for monitoring patients during follow-up are required. Improvement of quality of clinical studies, using more homogeneous clinical and pathological criteria for selection and stratification of patients, is also required.

With regard to newer treatments, the long-term efficacy and safety of MMF as induction therapy have to be established by appropriately designed clinical studies. An important issue that studies have neglected is the optimal dose and duration of steroid therapy. Glucocorticoids lead to substantial long-term toxicity, and studies aimed to identify steroid-sparing strategies are required, although commercially less appealing. The role of the new biological agents, in particular for resistant and rapidly relapsing patients, remains to be explored.

It is interesting that, despite the great deal of knowledge concerning the pathogenesis of lupus nephritis that has been produced in the last decade [61] and the host of new molecules specifically targeted to interfere with the pathogenetic mechanisms, the accepted standard of treatment is based on combinations of old drugs. More independent clinical research is still needed.

References

1 Cameron JS. Lupus nephritis. *J Am Soc Nephrol* 1999; **10**: 413–424.

2 Nossent HC, Henzen-Logmans SC, Vroom TM, Berden JH, Swaak TJ. Contribution of renal biopsy data in predicting outcome in lupus nephritis. Analysis of 116 patients. *Arthritis Rheum* 1990; **33**: 970–977.

3 Korbet SM, Lewis EJ, Schwartz MM, Reichlin M, Evans J, Rohde RD. Factors predictive of outcome in severe lupus nephritis. Lupus Nephritis Collaborative Study Group. *Am J Kidney Dis* 2000; **35**: 904–914.

4 U.S. Renal Data System. *USRDS 2005 Annual Data Report: Atlas of End-Stage Renal Disease in the United States.* National Institute of Diabetes and Digestive and Kidney Diseases, National Institutes of Health, Bethesda, 2005.

5 Huong DL, Papo T, Beaufils H, Wechsler B. Renal involvement in systemic lupus erythematosus. A study of 180 patients from a single center. *Medicine* (Baltimore) 1999; **78**: 148–166.

6 Seligman VA, Lum RF, Olson JL, Li H, Criswell LA. Demographic differences in the development of lupus nephritis: a retrospective analysis. *Am J Med* 2002; **112**: 726–729.

7 Barr RG, Seliger S, Appel GB, Zuniga R, D'Agati V, Salmon J *et al.* Prognosis in proliferative lupus nephritis: the role of socio-economic status and race/ethnicity. *Nephrol Dial Transplant* 2003; **18**: 2039–2046.

8 Tan EM, Cohen AS, Fries JF, Masi AT, McShane DJ, Rothfield NF *et al.* The 1982 revised criteria for the classification of systemic lupus erythematosus. *Arthritis Rheum* 1982; **25**: 1271–1277.

9 Hochberg MC. Updating the American College of Rheumatology revised criteria for the classification of systemic lupus erythematosus. *Arthritis Rheum.* 1997; **40**: 1725.

10 Cameron JS, Turner DR, Ogg CS, Williams DG, Lessof MH, Chantler C *et al.* Systemic lupus with nephritis: a long-term study. *QJM* 1979; **48**: 1–24.

11 Christopher-Stine L, Petri M, Astor BC, Fine D. Urine protein-to-creatinine ratio is a reliable measure of proteinuria in lupus nephritis. *J Rheumatol* 2004; **31**: 1557–1559.

12 Ruggenenti P, Gaspari F, Perna A, Remuzzi G. Cross sectional longitudinal study of spot morning urine protein:creatinine ratio, 24 hour urine protein excretion rate, glomerular filtration rate, and end stage renal failure in chronic renal disease in patients without diabetes. *BMJ* 1998; **316**: 504–509.

13 de Jong PE, Gansevoort RT. Screening techniques for detecting chronic kidney disease. *Curr Opin Nephrol Hypertens* 2005; **14**: 567–572.

14 Hahn BH. Antibodies to DNA. *N Engl J Med* 1998; **338**: 1359–1368.

15 Riboldi P, Gerosa M, Moroni G, Radice A, Allegri F, Sinico A *et al.* Anti-DNA antibodies: a diagnostic and prognostic tool for systemic lupus erythematosus? *Autoimmunity* 2005; **38**: 39–45.

16 Sinico RA, Radice A, Ikehata M, Giammarresi G, Corace C, Arrigo G *et al.* Anti-C1q autoantibodies in lupus nephritis: prevalence and clinical significance. *Ann N Y Acad Sci* 2005 Jun; **1050**: 193–200.

17 Churg J, Sobin LH. *Renal Disease: Classification and Atlas of Glomerular Disease.* Igaku-Shoin, Tokyo, 1982.

18 Churg J, Bernstein J, Glassock RJ. *Renal Disease: Classification and Atlas of Glomerular Diseases,* 2nd edn. Igaky-Shoin, New York, 1995.

19 Weening JJ, D'Agati VD, Schwartz MM, Seshan SV, Alpers CE, Appel GB *et al.* On behalf of International Society of Nephrology Working Group on the Classification of Lupus Nephritis; Renal Pathology Society Working Group on the Classification of Lupus Nephritis. The classification of glomerulonephritis in systemic lupus erythematosus revisited. *Kidney Int* 2004; **65**: 521–530.

20 Lupus nephritis: prognostic factors and probability of maintaining life-supporting renal function 10 years after the diagnosis. Gruppo Italiano per lo Studio della Nefrite Lupica (GISNEL). *Am J Kidney Dis* 1992; **19**: 473–479.

21 Balow JE. Clinical presentation and monitoring of lupus nephritis. *Lupus* 2005; **14**: 25–30.

22 Howie AJ, Turhan N, Adu D. Powerful morphometric indicator of prognosis in lupus nephritis. *QJM* 2003; **96**: 411–420.

23 Remuzzi G, Benigni A, Remuzzi A. Mechanisms of progression and regression of renal lesions of chronic nephropathies and diabetes. *J Clin Invest* 2006; **116**: 288–296.

24 Jafar TH, Stark PC, Schmid CH, Landa M, Maschio G, de Jong PE *et al.* AIPRD Study Group. Progression of chronic kidney disease: the role of blood pressure control, proteinuria, and angiotensin-converting enzyme inhibition: a patient-level meta-analysis. *Ann Intern Med* 2003; **139**: 244–252.

25 Gonzalez-Gay MA, Garcia-Porrua C, Lopez Lazaro L, Olive A. Successful response to captopril in severe nephrotic syndrome secondary to lupus nephritis. *Nephron* 1998; **80**: 353–354.

26 Tse KC, Li FK, Tang S, Tang CS, Lai KN, Chan TM. Angiotensin inhibition or blockade for the treatment of patients with quiescent lupus nephritis and persistent proteinuria. *Lupus* 2005; **14**: 947–952.

27 Ruggenenti P, Brenner BM, Remuzzi G. Remission achieved in chronic nephropathy by a multidrug approach targeted at urinary protein excretion. *Nephron* 2001; **88**: 254–259.

28 Ruggenenti P, Schieppati A, Remuzzi G. Progression, remission, regression of chronic renal diseases. *Lancet* 2001; **357**: 1601–1608.

29 Jadoul M. Optimal care of lupus nephritis patients. *Lupus* 2005; **14**: 72–76.

30 Austin HA, III, Klippel JH, Balow JE, le Riche NG, Steinberg AD, Plotz PH *et al.* Therapy of lupus nephritis. Controlled trial of prednisone and cytotoxic drugs. *N Engl J Med.* 1986; **314**: 614–619.

31 Boumpas DT, Austin HA, III, Vaughn EM, Klippel JH, Steinberg AD, Yarboro CH *et al.* Controlled trial of pulse methylprednisolone versus two regimens of pulse cyclophosphamide in severe lupus nephritis. *Lancet* 1992; **340**: 741–745.

32 Gourley MF, Austin HA, III, Scott D, Yarboro CH, Vaughan EM, Muir J *et al.* Methylprednisolone and cyclophosphamide, alone or in

combination, in patients with lupus nephritis. A randomized, controlled trial. *Ann Intern Med* 1996; **125**: 549–557.

33 Illei GG, Austin HA, Crane M, Collins L, Gourley MF, Yarboro CH *et al.* Combination therapy with pulse cyclophosphamide plus pulse methylprednisolone improves long-term renal outcome without adding toxicity in patients with lupus nephritis. *Ann Intern Med* 2001; **135**: 248–257.

34 Houssiau FA, Vasconcelos C, D'Cruz D, Sebastiani GD, Garrido Ed Fde R, Danieli MG *et al.* Immunosuppressive therapy in lupus nephritis: the Euro-Lupus Nephritis Trial, a randomized trial of low-dose versus high-dose intravenous cyclophosphamide. *Arthritis Rheum* 2002; **46**: 2121–2131.

35 Flanc RS, Roberts MA, Strippoli GF, Chadban SJ, Kerr PG, Atkins RC. Treatment for lupus nephritis. *Cochrane Database Syst Rev* 2004; **1**: CD002922.

36 Corna D, Morigi M, Facchinetti D, Bertani T, Zoja C, Remuzzi G. Mycophenolate mofetil limits renal damage and prolongs life in murine lupus autoimmune disease. *Kidney Int* 1997; **51**: 1583–1589.

37 Chan TM, Li FK, Tang CS, Wong RW, Fang GX, Ji YL *et al.* Efficacy of mycophenolate mofetil in patients with diffuse proliferative lupus nephritis. Hong Kong-Guangzhou Nephrology Study Group. *N Engl J Med* 2000; **343**: 1156–1162.

38 Chan TM, Tse KC, Tang CS, Mok MY, Li FK, Hong Kong Nephrology Study Group. Long-term study of mycophenolate mofetil as continuous induction and maintenance treatment for diffuse proliferative lupus nephritis. *J Am Soc Nephrol* 2005; **16**: 1076–1084.

39 Ginzler EM, Dooley MA, Aranow C, Kim MY, Buyon J, Merrill JT *et al.* Mycophenolate mofetil or intravenous cyclophosphamide for lupus nephritis. *N Engl J Med* 2005; **353**: 2219–2228.

40 McCune WJ. Mycophenolate mofetil for lupus nephritis. *N Engl J Med* 2005; **353**: 2282–2284.

41 Karassa FB. Mycophenolate mofetil or intravenous cyclophosphamide in lupus nephritis. *N Engl J Med* 2006; **354**: 764–765.

42 Contreras G, Tozman E, Nahar N, Metz D. Maintenance therapies for proliferative lupus nephritis: mycophenolate mofetil, azathioprine and intravenous cyclophosphamide. *Lupus* 2005; **14(Suppl 1)**: s33–s38.

43 Glicklich D, Acharya A. Mycophenolate mofetil therapy for lupus nephritis refractory to intravenous cyclophosphamide. *Am J Kidney Dis* 1998; **32**: 318–322.

44 Levy Y, Sherer Y, George J, Rovensky J, Lukac J, Rauova L *et al.* Intravenous immunoglobulin treatment of lupus nephritis. *Semin Arthritis Rheum* 2000; **29**: 321–327.

45 Burt RK, Traynor A, Statkute L, Barr WG, Rosa R, Schroeder J *et al.* Nonmyeloablative hematopoietic stem cell transplantation for systemic lupus erythematosus. *JAMA* 2006; **295**: 527–535.

46 Hainsworth JD, Burris HA, III, Morrissey LH, Litchy S, Scullin DC Jr, Bearden JD, III, *et al.* Rituximab monoclonal antibody as initial systemic therapy for patients with low-grade non-Hodgkin lymphoma. *Blood* 2000; **95**: 3052–3056.

47 Salama AD, Pusey C. Drug insight: rituximab in renal disease and transplantation. *Nat Clin Pract Nephrol* 2006; **2**: 221–230.

48 Sfikakis PP, Boletis JN, Lionaki S, Vigklis V, Fragiadaki KG, Iniotaki A *et al.* Remission of proliferative lupus nephritis following B cell depletion therapy is preceded by down-regulation of the T cell costimulatory molecule CD40 ligand: an open-label trial. *Arthritis Rheum* 2005; **52**: 501–513.

49 Sfikakis PP, Boletis JN, Tsokos GC. Rituximab anti-B-cell therapy in systemic lupus erythematosus: pointing to the future. *Curr Opin Rheumatol* 2005; **17**: 550–557.

50 Judge TA, Tang A, Turka LA. Immunosuppression through blockade of CD28:B7-mediated costimulatory signals. *Immunol Res* 1996; **15**: 38–49.

51 Finck BK, Linsley PS, Wofsy D. Treatment of murine lupus with CTLA4Ig. *Science* 1994; **265**: 1225–1227.

52 Daikh DI, Finck BK, Linsley PS, Hollenbaugh D, Wofsy D. Long-term inhibition of murine lupus by brief simultaneous blockade of the B7/CD28 and CD40/gp39 costimulation pathways. *J Immunol* 1997; **159**: 3104–3108.

53 Boumpas DT, Furie R, Manzi S, Illei GG, Wallace DJ, Balow JE *et al.* BG9588 Lupus Nephritis Trial Group. A short course of BG9588 (anti-CD40 ligand antibody) improves serologic activity and decreases hematuria in patients with proliferative lupus glomerulonephritis. *Arthritis Rheum* 2003; **48**: 719–727.

54 Kalunian KC, Davis JC, Jr., Merrill JT, Totoritis MC, Wofsy D. IDEC-131 Lupus Study Group. Treatment of systemic lupus erythematosus by inhibition of T cell costimulation with anti-CD154: a randomized, double-blind, placebo-controlled trial. *Arthritis Rheum* 2002; **46**: 3251–3258.

55 Abetimus: abetimus sodium, LJP 394. *BioDrugs* 2003; **17**: 212–215.

56 Furie RA, Cash JM, Cronin ME, Katz RS, Weisman MH, Aranow C *et al.* Treatment of systemic lupus erythematosus with LJP 394. *J Rheumatol* 2001; **28**: 257–265.

57 Alarcon-Segovia D, Tumlin JA, Furie RA, McKay JD, Cardiel MH, Strand V *et al.* LJP 394 Investigator Consortium. LJP 394 for the prevention of renal flare in patients with systemic lupus erythematosus: results from a randomized, double-blind, placebo-controlled study. *Arthritis Rheum* 2003; **48**: 442–454.

58 Balow JE, Austin HA, III. Therapy of membranous nephropathy in systemic lupus erythematosus. *Semin Nephrol* 2003; **23**: 386–391.

59 Moroni G, Maccario M, Banfi G, Quaglini S, Ponticelli C. Treatment of membranous lupus nephritis. *Am J Kidney Dis* 1998; **31**: 681–686.

60 Remuzzi G, Chiurchiu C, Abbate M, Brusegan V, Bontempelli M, Ruggenenti P. Rituximab for idiopathic membranous nephropathy. *Lancet* 2002; **360**: 923–924.

61 Jacobson SH, van Vollenhoven R, Gunnarsson I. Rituximab-induced long-term remission of membranous lupus nephritis. *Nephrol Dial Transplant* 2006; **21**: 1742–1743.

62 Houssiau FA. Management of lupus nephritis: an update. *J Am Soc Nephrol* 2004; **15**: 2694–2704.

23 Infection-Related Nephropathies

Monique E. Cho & Jeffrey B. Kopp

Kidney Disease Section, National Institute of Diabetes and Digestive and Kidney Diseases, National Institutes of Health, US Department of Health and Human Services, Bethesda, USA.

Introduction

Kidney disease is an increasingly important complication of human immunodeficiency virus type 1 (HIV-1) infection. The association between HIV-1 infection and kidney disease was first recognized in 1984 by investigators in New York City and Miami; they described a renal syndrome marked by proteinuria and a rapid progression to renal failure [1–3]. Most of these patients had focal segmental glomerulosclerosis with collapsing features, now referred to as HIV-associated collapsing glomerulopathy, or more commonly as HIV-associated nephropathy (HIVAN). In subsequent years, the existence of a specific HIV-associated renal disease remained controversial, partly because of the similarity of HIVAN to heroin nephropathy and the frequent intravenous drug use in this population. Reports demonstrating HIVAN in patients without intravenous drug use, including children, helped to establish HIVAN as a distinct clinical entity and directly linked HIV-1 infection with the development of renal complications [4,5].

Until the advent of highly active antiretroviral therapy (HAART), the annual incidence of end-stage renal disease (ESRD) attributed to HIV-1 infection increased by over 75% between 1990 and 1995 in the USA (Figure 23.1) [6]. Coincident with the widespread use of HAART, however, the incidence of ESRD attributed to HIV reached a plateau in 1996 and even showed a moderate decrease during the years 1995–1999 [7]. Nonetheless, prevalent ESRD cases increased more than twofold during the same period, and this increase in prevalent ESRD cases reflects a longer survival of HIV-infected patients after development of kidney failure [8]. In the era of HAART, therefore, HIV-1 infection has evolved into a chronic disease in patients with access to care, with kidney disease becoming a progressively more significant source of morbidity and mortality.

The prevalence of chronic kidney disease in different stages of HIV-1 infection is unknown. Proteinuria and increased serum creatinine levels have been reported in 7.2–32% of HIV-1-infected patients [9,10]. Although 60% of renal biopsies in HIV-1-infected patients with chronic kidney disease in the USA show HIVAN [11], HIV-1 infection is also associated with other various forms of renal disease. These include HIV-associated glomerulonephritis, thrombotic microangiopathy, and drug-induced nephropathy, with increasing recognition of renal complications of HAART. In addition, renal complications can occur in HIV-infected patients co-infected with hepatitis B or C virus, a topic that has been reviewed elsewhere [12]. This chapter will review renal diseases associated with HIV-1 infection with a central focus on HIV-associated collapsing glomerulopathy and will discuss treatment based on available clinical evidence.

HIVAN and collapsing glomerulopathy

Clinical manifestations and background

Patients of African descent have a striking susceptibility to developing HIV-associated collapsing glomerulopathy, with nearly 90% of cases occurring in African Americans. Estimates of the prevalence of HIV-associated collapsing glomerulopathy in African Americans have ranged from 3.5% to 12% [13,14]. HIV-associated collapsing glomerulopathy is the third leading cause of ESRD in black people ages 20–64 years, after diabetes mellitus and hypertension [7]. Analysis of data from the US Renal Data System (USRDS) indicates that the relative risk for ESRD from HIV-associated nephropathy is approximately 18-fold increased among African American compared to Caucasian patients [15].

Although HIV-associated collapsing glomerulopathy can occur at any stage of the disease, including the time of seroconversion, it is most commonly seen in patients with advanced HIV disease [16]. In patients who are not receiving antiviral therapy, the nephropathy may lead to rapid deterioration to ESRD within weeks to months. Patients with HIV-associated collapsing glomerulopathy present with massive proteinuria and are less likely to have

Evidence-based Nephrology. Edited by Donald Molony and Jonathan Craig
© 2009 Blackwell Publishing, ISBN: 978-1-4051-3975-5.

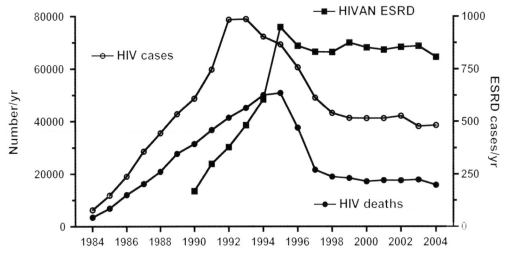

Figure 23.1 Annual incidence of HIV cases, HIV deaths, and ESRD due to HIVAN. The rate of new HIV infections peaked in the early 1990s, probably due to public health campaigns related to blood transfusion, safe sex, and avoiding needle reuse. Since the induction of HAART in 1996, the incidence of HIV deaths (left axis) and ESRD due to HIVAN (right axis) have also declined. All three rates reached a plateau in the past few years, although the prevalence rates for HIV continue to rise (not shown). Data are from the CDC and USRDS.

peripheral edema or hematuria than patients with idiopathic focal segmental glomerulosclerosis. These patients also tend to be normotensive. Urinalysis is remarkable mostly for proteinuria with hyaline casts. Renal ultrasound classically shows enlarged, echogenic kidneys. Renal biopsy is the only method to reliably diagnose HIV-associated collapsing glomerulopathy, as HIV infection may be associated with other renal diseases characterized by proteinuria.

Pathology

Collapsing glomerulopathy, including both HIV-associated and idiopathic varieties, has distinctive histologic features. By light microscopy, the diagnostic features include glomerular capillary collapse combined with podocyte hypertrophy and hyperplasia (Figure 23.2A); one glomerulus with both features is considered sufficient to make the diagnosis of collapsing glomerulopathy [17]. Importantly, these features may be segmental or global, focal or diffuse, and glomerulosclerosis may be absent early in the disease process. Therefore, including HIV-associated collapsing glomerulopathy in the broad category of focal segmental glomerulosclerosis does not seem appropriate [18]. Podocyte proliferation overlying a single capillary loop may appear as "crowning"; more extensive proliferation and detachment from the glomerular basement membrane may appear as a pseudocrescent.

A unique feature of collapsing glomerulopathy is that podocytes undergo dedifferentiation (losing maturity markers, such as synaptopodin and podocin) and transdifferentiation (losing expression of WT-1). Although most investigators have argued that the proliferating cells within Bowman's space are derived from podocytes, it has also been proposed that these cells are parietal epithelial cells [19]. Collapsing glomerulopathy also manifests as extraglomerular disease that often is surprisingly severe

for the extent of glomerular disease, suggesting that this syndrome is a pan-nephropathy. These manifestations include acute and chronic tubular changes, often with microcystic tubular dilatation and an interstitial infiltrate composed of lymphocytes and macrophages (Figure 23.2B). Immunofluorescence analysis of collapsing glomerulopathy typically shows immunoglobulin M (IgM) and C3 in the collapsed and sclerotic segments and also in the mesangium of uninvolved glomeruli. Electron microscopy shows glomerular capillary wrinkling and collapse and podocyte abnormalities, including diffuse foot process effacement and microvillous transformation. Glomerular capillary cells may show tubuloreticular inclusions, which are more common in HIV-associated collapsing glomerulopathy than in idiopathic collapsing glomerulopathy and are never seen in focal segmental glomerulosclerosis.

Pathogenesis of HIV-associated collapsing glomerulopathy

HIV-1 infection of renal epithelium

Possible pathogenic factors in HIVAN are outlined in Table 23.1. Increasing evidence suggests that direct viral infection of renal cells by HIV-1 is at the core of pathogenesis of HIV-associated collapsing glomerulopathy. Until recently, direct infection of renal parenchymal cells by HIV-1 remained controversial because of conflicting data regarding the presence of HIV-1 in renal tissue of patients with HIVAN. Studies using transgenic mouse models of HIV-associated collapsing glomerulopathy have strongly implicated the expression of HIV proteins in the pathogenesis of the renal disease [20–22]. These studies demonstrated that HIV-1 accessory proteins can induce features characteristic of HIV-associated collapsing glomerulopathy, including podocyte hyperplasia and

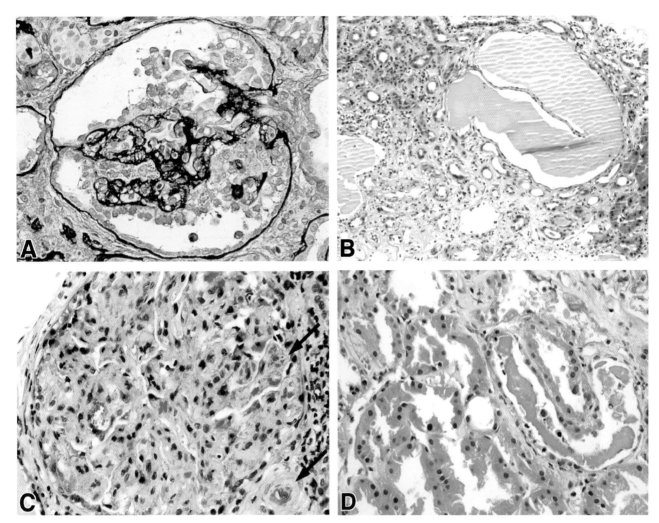

Figure 23.2 Renal pathologic features of HIV-related kidney diseases. (A) Collapsing glomerulopathy (methenamine trichrome stain). The glomerulus shows a collapsed tuft and markedly hyperplastic podocytes partially filling Bowman's space. (B) Collapsing glomerulopathy (methenamine trichrome stain). Microcystic tubular dilatation is present, together with interstitial inflammation and fibrosis. (C) Diffuse proliferative glomerulonephritis with a pattern resembling membranoproliferative glomerulonephritis, type I (Masson trichrome stain). The glomerulus is enlarged with global mesangial and endocapillary hypercellularity and appears mildly hyperlobular. There is partial occlusion of a preglomerular arteriole by thrombus and rare red blood cell fragments within the glomerular tuft (arrows), indicative of thrombotic microangiopathy. (D) Tenofovir-associated tubular injury (hematoxylin and eosin stain). The tubules show degenerative and regenerative changes. Tubular cells have irregular shapes and lack a brush border. Occasional intratubular eosinophilic casts are also noted. Images provided courtesy of Dr. James Balow (panel A), Dr. Laura Barisoni (panels B and D), and Dr. Mark Haas (panel C). Panel C is reprinted with permission from *Kidney International* (Haas *et al.* 2005 [80]).

hypertrophy, microcystic tubular dilatation, mononuclear cell interstitial infiltrate, proteinuria, and renal failure. Bruggeman *et al.* demonstrated that the HIV-1 transgene is expressed in renal glomerular and tubular epithelial cells and that this expression in renal epithelium is required for the development of the HIVAN phenotype [20].

In a further attempt to definitively determine whether HIV-1 infects renal epithelium in HIVAN, Bruggeman *et al.* reported on a renal biopsy series in HIV-1-infected patients with HIVAN [23]. In 11 of 15 patients, HIV-1 was detected in renal epithelial cells by RNA *in situ* hybridization. In many samples, the result was confirmed using riboprobes specific for both the *nef* and *gag* genes and by DNA *in situ* hybridization. HIV-1 RNA was detected in renal tubular epithelial cells, glomerular visceral and parietal epithelial cells, and interstitial leukocytes. Ross *et al.* also discovered that the distribution of HIV-1 infection of renal tubules is similar to the pattern of microcystic tubular disease [24]. These data further support the direct infection of the renal parenchyma by the HIV-1 virus.

The mechanism by which HIV-1 enters renal epithelial cells is unknown. New insights into the pathogenesis of HIV-related disease stem from the recognition that chemokine receptors CCR5 and CXCR4 serve as major coreceptors together with CD4 in

Pathogenic factors	Reference(s)	Evidence
Direct renal infection: • Podocytes • Tubular epithelial cells	[22–26]	Detection of HIV-1 by RNA *in situ* hybridization
Cytotoxicity from HIV proteins • Vpr • Nef	[32–37]	HIV-1 accessory proteins induce HIVAN in transgenic mice
Host factors: genetic susceptibility	[38]	Familiar clustering

Table 23.1 Possible pathogenic factors of HIV-associated collapsing glomerulopathy.

mammalian cells [25,26]. Expression of these receptors appears to be a key to understanding which tissues are permissive for direct HIV infection. No studies, however, have definitively established their constitutive expression in normal renal parenchymal cells or their upregulation in kidney biopsy tissue obtained from HIV-1-infected patients with HIVAN [27,28].

Infection of renal epithelial cells by HIV-1 has an important implication: the kidney may serve as a reservoir for HIV-1. Marras *et al.* detected variations in the HIV-1 envelope sequences in the renal tubular epithelium of HIV-infected patients, indicating that the renal tubular epithelium can support viral replication [29]. Furthermore, the envelope sequences of HIV-1 found in the renal tubular epithelium were distinct from the sequences derived from the same patient's peripheral blood samples, suggesting that the renal epithelium is a distinct reservoir for viral replication from the blood.

Viral genes responsible for HIVAN pathogenesis

Once HIV-1 infects renal tissue, one of the pathways through which the virus inflicts renal injury may be its peptides. The HIV-1 genome contains nine genes (*gag, pol, vif, vpr, vpu, rev, tat, env,* and *nef*) that encode 15 proteins. These viral accessory proteins have pleiotropic effects on cell function and are implicated in renal disease. Vpr, for example, induces G_2 cell cycle arrest, perturbs mitochondrial function, induces (and in some cells prevents) apoptosis, and alters gene transcription by acting as a coactivator or corepressor. Increased levels of apoptosis in renal tissue have been shown in patients with HIVAN compared to non-HIV-infected patients [30], in transgenic models [20], and in proximal tubular epithelial cells infected with HIV-1 [31]. It is unclear if the enhanced apoptosis in HIV-1-infected renal cells predominantly reflects direct toxicity of HIV proteins or indirect effects, such as induction of profibrotic cytokines.

Roles of other accessory proteins inducing renal injury have been investigated. Tat and Nef each induce proliferation of cultured podocytes, a distinctive feature of HIV-associated collapsing glomerulopathy [32,33]. A series of studies using transgenic mice bearing various portions of this genome have suggested which genes may be responsible for renal injury. HIV-1 transgenic mice carrying a replication-defective HIV-1 provirus that lacks *gag* and *pol* develop renal injury characterized by podocyte dysplasia and proliferation, glomerular capillary tuft collapse, and tubular

injury. This characteristic renal injury occurs even in the absence of immunosuppression and viral replication [21,22]. Deletion of *nef* from the transgenic line reduced the severity of interstitial nephritis, but it did not prevent the development of glomerular disease in one transgenic line [34]. More recently, mice bearing *tat* and *vpr* or *vpr* alone developed focal segmental glomerulosclerosis [35]. These data indicate that *vpr* induces focal segmental glomerulosclerosis and that *nef* contributes to interstitial nephritis in transgenic mice [35–37].

Host factors

Although renal parenchymal cell infection and expression of HIV-1 gene products play a crucial role in disease initiation, a variety of host factors likely contribute to the phenotype and the outcome of the disease. The renal epithelial cell proliferation and apoptosis induced by viral products in turn trigger profibrotic pathways. Epidemiologic studies have demonstrated that HIV-1-infected patients do not have equal risk of developing HIVAN. Twenty-five percent of patients with HIV-associated collapsing glomerulopathy have first-degree or second-degree family members with ESRD, suggesting a genetic predisposition to glomerular injury [38]. These data suggest a familial susceptibility to renal injury following diverse stimuli, including HIV-1 infection. The striking predominance of the disease in patients of African descent, particularly in men, is another important observation suggesting inherent risk factors. How the genetic variability or traits may be associated with higher risk of developing HIVAN is unknown. Possible explanations may involve differences in host-specific antibody or cellular responses to viral infection, differences in sclerosing mechanisms, differences in activation of coreceptors for HIV attachment to renal cells and subsequent infectivity, and diminished host ability to repair.

Treatment

Although HIV-associated collapsing glomerulopathy is an important cause of renal failure in the USA, no randomized controlled trials have been carried out to assess various therapies. Thus, recommendations must be based on retrospective or uncontrolled studies or on expert opinion.

Table 23.2 Summary of reports suggesting efficacy of HAART in patients with HIVAN.

Study authors [reference]	Year	Design	Results
Wali *et al.* [42]	1998	Case report	• A patient with HIVAN with dialysis-dependent kidney failure became dialysis-free after 15 wks of triple-agent antiretroviral therapy
Winston *et al.* [16]	2001	Case report	• A patient with HIVAN with dialysis-dependent kidney failure recovered renal function (serum creatinine from 6.3 to 1.4 mg/dL and proteinuria from 17 to 1.5 g/day) after 6 wks of HAART
Betjes *et al.* [39]	2002	Case report	• 3 patients with HIVAN had stable improvement of kidney function after initiating HAART
Szczech *et al.* [41]	2002	Retrospective cohort study of 19 patients	• Use of protease inhibitors as part of HAART regimen significantly slowed decline in GFR compared to group not receiving protease inhibitors
Lucas *et al.* [40]	2004	Retrospective analysis of 12-yr cohort study of 3976 patients with HIV-1 infection in Baltimore, MD	• HIVAN risk was 60% lower in patients treated with HAART • No patient developed HIVAN when HAART was started prior to development of AIDS
Schwartz *et al.* [43]	2005	Analysis of data from CDC and USRDS	• HAART reduced rate of progression to ESRD by 38% in patients with HIVAN

HAART

The abrupt leveling-off in the incident ESRD case rate coincident with the widespread use of HAART suggests that effective antiviral therapy probably prevents the onset or slows progression of HIV-associated collapsing glomerulopathy. Several observational studies have consistently suggested the benefit of HAART in treatment of HIVAN [16,39–42] (Table 23.2). In particular, two case reports have described resolution of HIVAN on antiretroviral therapy, a condition deemed irreversible in the pre-HAART era [16,42]. The authors reported that two patients with dialysis-dependent renal failure associated with HIVAN became dialysis-free following several weeks of HAART. Remarkably, the on-treatment biopsy indicated almost complete resolution of the hypertrophy of podocytes and glomerular collapse and normalization of tubular architecture.

Schwartz *et al.*, using a statistical model to analyze the data from the USRDS and Centers for Disease Control and Prevention (CDC), estimated that HAART had reduced the rate of progression of HIVAN to ESRD by 38% [43]. In addition, HAART may also prevent the development of HIVAN: a retrospective analysis of a 12-year cohort study of 3976 patients with HIV-1 infection suggested that the risk of nephropathy was 60% lower among patients treated with HAART and that no patient developed HIVAN when HAART was started prior to development of AIDS [40].

Angiotensin converting enzyme inhibitors

Available data suggest that angiotensin converting enzyme (ACE) inhibitors may slow the loss of renal function in patients with HIVAN (Table 23.3). In one nonrandomized study of 18 patients with biopsy-proven HIVAN, those treated with captopril had significantly improved renal survival compared to subjects who were not treated with captopril [44]. In another nonrandomized study that evaluated 20 patients with HIVAN, patients treated with fosinopril had a reduction in proteinuria with a small increase in serum creatinine [45]. In contrast, the untreated patients developed marked increases in protein excretion and serum creatinine within 12–24 weeks, suggesting that ACE inhibitors may prolong renal survival. A more recent study of 44 patients with HIVAN also

Table 23.3 Summary of reports suggesting efficacy of ACE inhibitors in patients with HIVAN.

Authors [reference]	Date	Design	Results
Kimmel *et al.* [44]	1996	Case control study of 18 patients	• Improved renal survival in captopril group (mean renal survival, 156 ± 71 vs. 37 ± 5 days)
Burns *et al.* [45]	1997	Prospective cohort study of 20 patients (12 on fosinopril and 8 controls)	• Nonnephrotic patients treated with fosinopril had mild fall in proteinuria (1.7 to 1.3 g/day) and increased serum creatinine (1.3 to 1.5 mg/dL) at 24 wks • Patients without fosinopril deteriorated rapidly with increase in proteinuria (0.8 to 8.5 g/day) and serum creatinine (1.0 to 4.9 mg/dL) • Similar results seen in nephrotic patients within 12 wks
Wei *et al.* [46]	2003	Prospective cohort of 44 patients (28 on fosinopril and 16 controls)	• Risk of kidney failure significantly reduced with ACE inhibitor therapy (risk ratio, 0.003) • Significant mortality benefit also noted with ACE inhibitor therapy (88% of untreated patients died, vs. 33% of treated patients)

found that patients treated with an ACE inhibitor had a 3.3-fold increase in median renal survival time [46].

Immunosuppressive therapy

The role of immunosuppressive therapy is less clear. Studies using prednisone in patients with renal dysfunction and HIV-1 infection show some efficacy in preserving renal function and reducing proteinuria [47,48]. These studies, as with the trials evaluating the efficacy of ACE inhibitors, were not well-controlled, and not all patients underwent renal biopsy. Another retrospective study suggested efficacy of combination therapy with HAART and glucocorticoids [49]. The mean renal survival to ESRD was 26 months for those treated with the combination therapy, 6 months for those given HAART alone, and 3 months for those given neither HAART nor glucocorticoids. Although no studies have suggested efficacy of glucocorticoids in children with HIV-associated collapsing glomerulopathy, a very small study reported remission of proteinuria with cyclosporine therapy in three children who had steroid-resistant renal disease [50]. Again, the study was not a controlled trial and was done before the era of HAART, making it difficult to draw any firm conclusions.

HIV-associated glomerulonephritis

HIV-associated glomerulonephritis is most prevalent among Caucasian, Hispanic, and Asian patients. In the absence of a national registry of renal biopsy findings, the true prevalence of HIV-associated glomerulonephritis is unknown. Several different histologic descriptions have been reported for HIV-associated glomerulonephritis, including IgA nephropathy, a lupus-like pattern, postinfectious glomerulonephritis, membranoproliferative glomerulonephritis, membranous nephropathy, and fibrillary and immunotactoid glomerulonephritis. An example of diffuse proliferative glomerulonephritis is shown in Figure 23.2C. It is not always possible to discern if the renal disease is a consequence of the HIV-1 infection or if it is a coincidental occurrence. For example, patients with HIV disease are often co-infected with hepatitis B virus or hepatitis C virus, each of which have been associated with glomerular diseases such as membranous glomerulopathy and membranoproliferative glomerulonephritis.

The pathogenesis of these forms of HIV-associated glomerulonephritis is not clear. In IgA nephropathy, immune complexes containing HIV proteins have been found in the mesangium, possibly delivered preformed from plasma or forming *in situ*, leading to renal parenchymal inflammation [51]. Guidelines for treatment are limited by the lack of randomized controlled trials, but therapies have included antiretroviral therapy, ACE inhibitors, and prednisone [52,53].

Thrombotic microangiopathy

Since the first report of HIV-associated thrombotic microangiopathy (TMA) in 1984, it has been increasingly recognized in this infection, although clinically evident TMA is infrequent [54]. A retrospective study demonstrated that 15 of 224 AIDS patients (7%) had evidence of TMA at the time of death [55]. The pathologic findings include occlusive thrombi in small arteries and arterioles and detachment of glomerular endothelial cells from the basement membrane. Affected patients typically present with hemolytic uremic syndrome characterized by renal insufficiency, microangiopathic hemolytic anemia, and thrombocytopenia. The mechanisms that account for microvascular damage in HIV-1 infection are poorly understood. There are no data to suggest that HIV-associated TMA should be treated differently from idiopathic or autoimmune forms of TMA. Therapies have included plasmapheresis and/or prednisone, with limited success in HIV-associated TMA.

Drug-induced nephrotoxicity in HIV-1 infection

With the widespread introduction of HAART in 1996, the course of HIV disease has been irrevocably changed. Patients with access to care have benefited from the greatly improved survival associated with HAART, but at a significant cost of increased morbidity from its complications. Acute kidney failure remains common among ambulatory and hospitalized patients with HIV-1 infection, and those with acute kidney failure are more likely to have received HAART [56]. Several antiretroviral agents and medications used to treat complications of HIV-1 infection are known to have nephrotoxicity. Many of these nephrotoxicities stem directly from the processes of drug metabolism, elimination, or drug–drug interactions. In addition, antiretroviral agents may lead to indirect nephrotoxicity by promoting metabolic aberrations, such as insulin resistance, diabetes, dyslipidemia, and hypertension. Renal abnormalities associated with antiretroviral therapy are summarized in Table 23.4. There have been excellent reviews of renal complications of antiretroviral therapy published recently [57–59].

Mechanisms of direct drug nephrotoxicity
Crystallization
Among protease inhibitors, indinavir is most commonly associated with renal or urologic complications, with a 10-fold increase in the incidence of such complications compared to other protease inhibitors in one observational cohort study [60]. Crystallization of indinavir can cause renal colic and acute urinary obstruction due to frank nephrolithiasis or to crystal-laden sludge. Indinavir crystals can also cause dysuria, acute and chronic interstitial nephritis, renal atrophy, and hypertension [61–64]. Indinavir crystalluria is common; in a longitudinal study of 54 patients, 67% developed indinavir crystals on at least one occasion [65]. Therefore, the finding of indinavir crystalluria in an asymptomatic patient is not clinically useful. In addition to indinavir, both saquinavir and nelfinavir have been associated with reports of nephrolithiasis.

Table 23.4 Summary of common renal injuries induced by antiretroviral drugs.

Antiretroviral agent	Metabolism/excretion	Nephrotoxicity	Special consideration
Protease inhibitors			
Indinavir	Liver/kidney	Crystal nephropathy, interstitial nephritis	Maintain urine output >2–3 L/day
Ritonavir	Liver	Acute kidney failure	May potentiate nephrotoxicity of other agents (indinavir, tenofovir)
Nucleoside reverse transcriptase inhibitors			
Abacavir	Liver	Acute kidney failure, interstitial nephritis	Nucleosides are associated with lactic acidosis
Didanosine	Liver/kidney	Acute kidney failure (proximal and distal tubulopathy)	
NRTI			
• Tenofovir	Kidney (elimination via tubular secretion)	Acute kidney failure with prominent proximal tubulopathy	Monitor for Fanconi syndrome
Nonnucleoside reverse transcriptase inhibitors	Liver	None reported	

Drug interactions

Ritonavir has also been associated with acute kidney failure and impaired kidney function, particularly when it is combined with tenofovir and indinavir. The interactions of ritonavir with other drugs metabolized by the cytochrome P450 system have been well-established. Another explanation may involve its inhibition of drug efflux mechanisms in tubular epithelial cells. Ritonavir is a potent inhibitor of P-glycoprotein, a luminal membrane transporter of organic cations, and thus may lead to accumulation of other drugs and potentiate toxicity.

Tubular cytotoxicity

Nucleotide reverse transcriptase inhibitors (NRTIs), such as cidofovir, adefovir, and tenofovir, are eliminated as unchanged drugs in urine by active secretion into the proximal tubule via organic anion transporters. Intracellular accumulation of these nucleotide analogs likely results in cytotoxicity to proximal tubular epithelial cells, resulting in a proximal tubular dysfunction and acute kidney failure. NRTIs may exert cytotoxicity via mitochondrial toxicity. Phosphorylated forms of some NRTIs are potent inhibitors of mitochondrial DNA polymerase [66]. The resulting deficiencies in the mitochondrial oxidative phosphorylation system may lead to disruption in pyruvate oxidation and increased lactic acid production. Thus, organs rich in mitochondria, such as muscle, liver, and kidney (particularly proximal tubules), are at increased risk for clinical toxicities, which can manifest as myopathy, liver steatosis, lactic acidosis, and Fanconi syndrome.

Although tenofovir, a newer NRTI, did not initially demonstrate any significant nephrotoxicity, increasing numbers of reports have described adverse renal outcomes (Figure 23.2D) [67–73]. In these studies, patients had been taking tenofovir at daily doses of 300 mg for varying periods ranging from 2 weeks to 16 months when they developed renal failure. The renal toxicity was predominantly characterized by proximal tubular dysfunction, demonstrated by normoglycemic glucosuria, proteinuria, hematuria, and hypophosphatemia. Some patients also developed signs of distal tubular toxicity, presenting with diabetes insipidus [67,70]. The proteinuria associated with tenofovir is usually mild, but nephrotic-range proteinuria has also been described [73]. Continued administration of tenofovir may lead to chronic kidney disease in some patients. Renal function improves in most patients upon discontinuation of the drug, but patients have experienced persistent glucosuria and proteinuria with elevated creatinine, suggesting irreversible damage. Renal biopsy in these patients has shown acute tubular necrosis, involving particularly the proximal tubules.

Patients taking tenofovir should be monitored regularly, especially those also on ritonavir, which can increase the serum concentration of tenofovir.

Indirect effects of antiretroviral therapy promoting chronic kidney disease

Antiretroviral agents such as protease inhibitors and NRTIs have been associated with insulin resistance, diabetes, dyslipidemia, and hypertension [74–76]. In particular, lipodystrophy, which is most prevalent with protease inhibitor therapy, has been associated with a cluster of metabolic disturbances and hypertension [77,78]. The underlying mechanisms linking HAART with the increased risk for atherosclerotic vascular disease are incompletely understood but may include decreased peroxisome proliferator-activated receptor γ function and altered hormonal status. Given the importance of mitochondrial oxidative stress as the unifying mechanism underlying diabetic complications, the mitochondrial toxicities of NRTIs may also contribute to the pathogenesis or progression of chronic kidney disease. HIV-1-infected individuals thus represent a uniquely challenging population requiring coordination of multiple disciplines for proper care and risk modification.

Conclusions and recommendations

In the era of HAART, HIV-1 infection, once considered a rapidly fatal disease, has now become a chronic illness with increasing morbidity from multiorgan dysfunction due to both the chronic infection of the virus and the complications of antiretroviral therapy. Chronic kidney disease has emerged as a common complication of HIV-1 infection. Despite great success with HAART, renal dysfunction remains a serious clinical challenge, with some therapeutics potentially leading to chronic metabolic derangement or other toxicities.

The HIV Medicine Association of the Infectious Diseases Society of America has recently published guidelines for the management of chronic kidney disease in HIV-1-infected patients [79]. The following are based on those recommendations. It should be noted that, as outlined above, the evidence base for these recommendations is weak and is based largely upon case series and expert opinion.

Screening
• All patients should be examined for renal dysfunction with glomerular filtration rate (GFR) estimation and urinalysis for proteinuria and abnormal urine sediment at the time of diagnosis of HIV-1 infection. This recommendation is based on expert opinion.
• Among those without any evidence of renal dysfunction, individuals at high risk (African Americans, those with CD4 cell counts of <200/µL or HIV RNA levels of >4000 copies/mL, coinfection with hepatitis B or C virus, family history of HIVAN, and other traditional risk factors, such as hypertension and diabetes) should be monitored once yearly at a minimum. These recommendations are based on evidence from observational clinical trials.
• For those with proteinuria (≥2+ by urinalysis) or GFR of <60 mL/min/1.73 m^2, additional evaluations and referral to a nephrologists are recommended. This recommendation is based on clinical observation that early intervention in chronic kidney disease is beneficial.

Management
• In HIV patients with evidence of nephropathy, the target blood pressure should be ≤130/80 mmHg, with initial preferential use of ACE inhibitors or angiotensin receptor blockers, particularly in patients with proteinuria. This recommendation is based on expert opinion from clinical observation.
• Patients with HIVAN and other HIV-associated glomerulonephritis should be treated with HAART at diagnosis, regardless of the severity of renal dysfunction. This recommendation is based on observational studies.
• No specific recommendations regarding use of immunosuppressive medications such as prednisone can be made at this time.
• ACE inhibitors or angiotensin receptor blockers should be added to HAART in patients with proteinuria, especially if the antiretroviral therapy does not lead to improvement in kidney function. This recommendation is based on observational studies.

• Patients receiving tenofovir should be monitored at least semiannually with measurement of renal function, serum phosphorus, and urinalysis for glycosuria and proteinuria. This is particularly important if patients are being treated concurrently with other medications that are eliminated via renal secretion (adefovir, acyclovir, ganciclovir, or cidofovir) or medications that may cause an increased drug level (ritonavir). This recommendation is based on observational studies.
• All patients receiving indinavir should increase fluid intake to achieve a urine output of 2–3 L, with particular attention to this regimen in hot weather or with vigorous exercise. Periodic urinalysis and determination of serum creatinine are indicated in all indinavir-treated patients, perhaps quarterly, in order to identify patients with chronic interstitial nephritis; in such patients indinavir therapy should be promptly discontinued. Certain patients are at increased risk for indinavir stones; these patients include those with prior indinavir stones and those with hepatic dysfunction, which impairs nonrenal clearance.

Acknowledgments. The authors would like to thank Dr. Meryl Waldman (NIDDK, NIH; Bethesda, Maryland) for her thoughtful review of the manuscript and Dr. James Balow (NIDDK, NIH; Bethesda, Maryland), Dr. Laura Barisoni (New York University; New York, New York), and Dr. Mark Haas (Johns Hopkins University; Baltimore, Maryland) for providing the images in Figure 2.

References

1 Gardenswartz MH, Lerner CW, Seligson GR, Zabetakis PM, Rotterdam H, tapper ML *et al.* Renal disease in patients with AIDS: a clinicopathologic study. *Clin Nephrol* 1984; **21**: 197–204.

2 Pardo V, Aldana M, Colton RM, Fischl MA, Jaffe D, Moskowitz L *et al.* Glomerular lesions in the acquired immunodeficiency syndrome. *Ann Intern Med* 1984; **101**: 429–434.

3 Rao TK, Filippone EJ, Nicastri AD, Landesman SH, Frank E, Chen CK *et al.* Associated focal and segmental glomerulosclerosis in the acquired immunodeficiency syndrome. *N Engl J Med* 1984; **310**: 669–673.

4 Pardo V, Meneses R, Ossa L, Jaffe DJ, Strauss J, Roth D *et al.* AIDS-related glomerulopathy: occurrence in specific risk groups. *Kidney Int* 1987; **31**: 1167–1173.

5 Strauss J, Abitbol C, Zilleruelo G, Scott G, Paredes A, Malaga S *et al.* Renal disease in children with the acquired immunodeficiency syndrome. *N Engl J Med* 1989; **321**: 625–630.

6 US Renal Data System. Annual Data Report. National Institute of Diabetes and Digestive and Kidney Diseases, National Institutes of Health, Bethesda, 2001.

7 Ross MJ, Klotman PE. Recent progress in HIV-associated nephropathy. *J Am Soc Nephrol* 2002; **13**: 2997–3004.

8 Eggers PW, Kimmel PL. Is there an epidemic of HIV Infection in the US ESRD program? *J Am Soc Nephrol* 2004; **15**: 2477–2485.

9 Gardner LI, Holmberg SD, Williamson JM, Szczech LA, Carpenter CC, Rompalo AM *et al.* Development of proteinuria or elevated serum creatinine and mortality in HIV-infected women. *J Acquir Immune Defic Syndr* 2003; **32**: 203–209.

10 Szczech LA, Gange SJ, van der Horst C, Bartlett JA, Young M, Cohen MH *et al.* Predictors of proteinuria and renal failure among women with HIV infection. *Kidney Int* 2002; **61**: 195–202.

11 D'Agati V, Appel GB. HIV infection and the kidney. *J Am Soc Nephrol* 1997; **8**: 138–152.

12 Cho ME, Kopp JB. Kidney in viral infections. In: Kher KK, Schnaper HW, Makker SP, eds. *Clinical Pediatric Nephrology*. Informa Healthcare, London, 2006; 275–287.

13 Ahuja TS, Borucki M, Funtanilla M, Shahinian V, Hollander M, Rajaraman S. Is the prevalence of HIV-associated nephropathy decreasing? *Am J Nephrol* 1999; **19**: 655–659.

14 Shahinian V, Rajaraman S, Borucki M, Grady J, Hollander WM, Ahuja TS. Prevalence of HIV-associated nephropathy in autopsies of HIV-infected patients. *Am J Kidney Dis* 2000; **35**: 884–888.

15 Kopp JB, Winkler C. HIV-associated nephropathy in African Americans. *Kidney Int Suppl* 2003; **2003**: S43–S49.

16 Winston JA, Bruggeman LA, Ross MD, Jacobson J, Ross L, D'Agati VD *et al.* Nephropathy and establishment of a renal reservoir of HIV type 1 during primary infection. *N Engl J Med* 2001; **344**: 1979–1984.

17 D'Agati V. Pathologic classification of focal segmental glomerulosclerosis. *Semin Nephrol* 2003; **23**: 117–134.

18 Schnaper HW, Robson AM, Kopp JB. Nephrotic syndrome: minimal change nephropathy, focal segmental glomerulosclerosis, and collapsing glomerulopathy. In: Schrier RW, ed. *Diseases of the Kidney and Urinary Tract: Clinicopathologic Foundations of Medicine*. Lippincott Williams & Wilkins, Philadelphia, 2006; 1585–1672.

19 Nagata M, Hattori M, Hamano Y, Ito K, Saitoh K, Watanabe T. Origin and phenotypic features of hyperplastic epithelial cells in collapsing glomerulopathy. *Am J Kidney Dis* 1998; **32**: 962–969.

20 Bruggeman LA, Dikman S, Meng C, Quaggin SE, Coffman TM, Klotman PE. Nephropathy in human immunodeficiency virus-1 transgenic mice is due to renal transgene expression. *J Clin Invest* 1997; **100**: 84–92.

21 Dickie P, Felser J, Eckhaus M, Bryant J, Silver J, Marinos N *et al.* HIV-associated nephropathy in transgenic mice expressing HIV-1 genes. *Virology* 1991; **185**: 109–119.

22 Kopp JB, Klotman ME, Adler SH, Bruggeman LA, Dickie P, Marinos NJ *et al.* Progressive glomerulosclerosis and enhanced renal accumulation of basement membrane components in mice transgenic for human immunodeficiency virus type 1 genes. *Proc Natl Acad Sci USA* 1992; **89**: 1577–1581.

23 Bruggeman LA, Ross MD, Tanji N, Cara A, Dikman S, Gordon RE *et al.* Renal epithelium is a previously unrecognized site of HIV-1 infection. *J Am Soc Nephrol* 2000; **11**: 2079–2087.

24 Ross MJ, Bruggeman LA, Wilson PD, Klotman PE. Microcyst formation and HIV-1 gene expression occur in multiple nephron segments in HIV-associated nephropathy. *J Am Soc Nephrol* 2001; **12**: 2645–2651.

25 Deng H, Liu R, Ellmeier W, Choe S, Unutmaz D, Burkhart M *et al.* Identification of a major co-receptor for primary isolates of HIV-1. *Nature* 1996; **381**: 661–666.

26 Dragic T, Litwin V, Allaway GP, Martin SR, Huang Y, Nagashima KA *et al.* HIV-1 entry into CD4+ cells is mediated by the chemokine receptor CC-CKR-5. *Nature* 1996; **381**: 667–673.

27 Eitner F, Cui Y, Hudkins KL, Anderson DM, Schmidt A, Morton WR *et al.* Chemokine receptor (CCR5) expression in human kidneys and in the HIV infected macaque. *Kidney Int* 1998; **54**: 1945–1954.

28 Eitner F, Cui Y, Hudkins KL, Stokes MB, Segerer S, Mack M *et al.* Chemokine receptor CCR5 and CXCR4 expression in HIV-associated kidney disease. *J Am Soc Nephrol* 2000; **11**: 856–867.

29 Marras D, Bruggeman LA, Gao F, Tanji N, Mansukhani MM, Cara A *et al.* Replication and compartmentalization of HIV-1 in kidney epithelium of patients with HIV-associated nephropathy. *Nat Med* 2002; **8**: 522–526.

30 Bodi I, Abraham AA, Kimmel PL. Apoptosis in human immunodeficiency virus-associated nephropathy. *Am J Kidney Dis* 1995; **26**: 286–291.

31 Conaldi PG, Biancone L, Bottelli A, Wade-Evans A, Racusen LC, Boccellino M *et al.* HIV-1 kills renal tubular epithelial cells in vitro by triggering an apoptotic pathway involving caspase activation and Fas upregulation. *J Clin Invest* 1998; **102**: 2041–2049.

32 Conaldi PG, Bottelli A, Baj A, Serra C, Fiore L, Federico G *et al.* Human immunodeficiency virus-1 tat induces hyperproliferation and dysregulation of renal glomerular epithelial cells. *Am J Pathol* 2002; **161**: 53–61.

33 Husain M, Gusella GL, Klotman ME, Gelman IH, Ross MD, Schwartz EJ *et al.* HIV-1 Nef induces proliferation and anchorage-independent growth in podocytes. *J Am Soc Nephrol* 2002; **13**: 1806–1815.

34 Kajiyama W, Kopp JB, Marinos NJ, Klotman PE, Dickie P. HIV-transgenic mice lacking gag-pol-nef develop glomerulosclerosis and express viral RNA and protein in glomerular epithelial and tubular cells. *Kidney Int* 2000; **58**: 1148–1159.

35 Dickie P, Roberts A, Uwiera R, Witmer J, Sharma K, Kopp JB. Focal glomerulosclerosis in proviral and c-fms transgenic mice links Vpr expression to HIV-associated nephropathy. *Virology* 2004; **322**: 69–81.

36 Kajiyama W, Kopp JB, Marinos NJ, Klotman PE, Dickie P. Glomerulosclerosis and viral gene expression in HIV-transgenic mice: role of nef. *Kidney Int* 2000; **58**: 1148–1159.

37 Hanna Z, Kay DG, Cool M, Jothy S, Rebai N, Jolicoeur P. Transgenic mice expressing human immunodeficiency virus type 1 in immune cells develop a severe AIDS-like disease. *J Virol* 1998; **72**: 121–132.

38 Freedman BI, Soucie JM, Stone SM, Pegram S. Familial clustering of end-stage renal disease in blacks with HIV-associated nephropathy. *Am J Kidney Dis* 1999; **34**: 254–258.

39 Betjes MG, Verhagen DW. Stable improvement of renal function after initiation of highly active anti-retroviral therapy in patients with HIV-1-associated nephropathy. *Nephrol Dial Transplant* 2002; **17**: 1836–1839.

40 Lucas GM, Eustace JA, Sozio S, Mentari EK, Appiah KA, Moore RD. Highly active antiretroviral therapy and the incidence of HIV-1-associated nephropathy: a 12-year cohort study. *AIDS* 2004; **18**: 541–546.

41 Szczech LA, Edwards LJ, Sanders LL, van der Horst C, Bartlett JA, Heald AE *et al.* Protease inhibitors are associated with a slowed progression of HIV-related renal diseases. *Clin Nephrol* 2002; **57**: 336–341.

42 Wali RK, Drachenberg CI, Papadimitriou JC, Keay S, Ramos E. HIV-1-associated nephropathy and response to highly-active antiretroviral therapy. *Lancet* 1998; **352**: 783–784.

43 Schwartz EJ, Szczech LA, Ross MJ, Klotman ME, Winston JA, Klotman PE. Highly active antiretroviral therapy and the epidemic of HIV+ end-stage renal disease. *J Am Soc Nephrol* 2005; **16**: 2412–2420.

44 Kimmel PL, Mishkin GJ, Umana WO. Captopril and renal survival in patients with human immunodeficiency virus nephropathy. *Am J Kidney Dis* 1996; **28**: 202–208.

45 Burns GC, Paul SK, Toth IR, Sivak SL. Effect of angiotensin-converting enzyme inhibition in HIV-associated nephropathy. *J Am Soc Nephrol* 1997; **8**: 1140–1146.

46 Wei A, Burns GC, Williams BA, Mohammed NB, Wisintainer P, Sivak SL. Long-term renal survival in HIV-associated nephropathy with angiotensin-converting enzyme inhibition. *Kidney Int* 2003; **64**: 1462.

47 Smith MC, Austen JL, Carey JT, Emancipator SN, Herbener T, Gripshover B *et al.* Prednisone improves renal function and proteinuria in human

immunodeficiency virus-associated nephropathy. *Am J Med* 1996; **101**: 41–48.

48 Eustace JA, Nuermberger E, Choi M, Scheel PJ, Jr., Moore R, Briggs WA. Cohort study of the treatment of severe HIV-associated nephropathy with corticosteroids. *Kidney Int* 2000; **58**: 1253–1260.

49 Navarrete JE, Pastan SO. Effect of highly active antiretroviral treatment and prednisone in biopsy-proven HIV-associated nephropathy. *J Am Soc Nephrol* 2000; **11**: 93A.

50 Ingulli E, Tejani A, Fikrig S, Nicastri A, Chen CK, Pomrantz A. Nephrotic syndrome associated with acquired immunodeficiency syndrome in children. *J Pediatr* 1991; **119**: 710–716.

51 Kimmel PL, Phillips TM, Ferreira-Centeno A, Farkas-Szallasi T, Abraham AA, Garrett CT. Brief report: idiotypic IgA nephropathy in patients with human immunodeficiency virus infection. *N Engl J Med* 1992; **327**: 702–706.

52 Mattana J, Siegal FP, Schwarzwald E, Molho L, Sankaran RT, Gooneratne R *et al.* AIDS-associated membranous nephropathy with advanced renal failure: response to prednisone. *Am J Kidney Dis* 1997; **30**: 116–119.

53 Alarcon-Zurita A, Salas A, Anton E, Morey A, Munar MA, Losada P *et al.* Membranous glomerulonephritis with nephrotic syndrome in a HIV positive patient: remarkable remission with triple therapy. *Nephrol Dial Transplant* 2000; **15**: 1097–1098.

54 Alpers CE. Light at the end of the TUNEL: HIV-associated thrombotic microangiopathy. *Kidney Int* 2003; **63**: 385–396.

55 Gadallah MF, el-Shahawy MA, Campese VM, Todd JR, King JW. Disparate prognosis of thrombotic microangiopathy in HIV-infected patients with and without AIDS. *Am J Nephrol* 1996; **16**: 446–450.

56 Franceschini N, Napravnik S, Eron JJ, Jr., Szczech LA, Finn WF. Incidence and etiology of acute renal failure among ambulatory HIV-infected patients. *Kidney Int* 2005; **67**: 1526–1531.

57 Daugas E, Rougier JP, Hill G. HAART-related nephropathies in HIV-infected patients. *Kidney Int* 2005; **67**: 393–403.

58 Izzedine H, Launay-Vacher V, Deray G. Antiviral drug-induced nephrotoxicity. *Am J Kidney Dis* 2005; **45**: 804–817.

59 Wyatt CM, Klotman PE. Antiretroviral therapy and the kidney: balancing benefit and risk in patients with HIV infection. *Expert Opin Drug Saf* 2006; **5**: 275–287.

60 Dieleman JP, Sturkenboom MC, Jambroes M, Gyssens IC, Weverling GJ, ten Venn JH *et al.* Risk factors for urological symptoms in a cohort of users of the HIV protease inhibitor indinavir sulfate: the ATHENA cohort. *Arch Intern Med* 2002; **162**: 1493–1501.

61 Cattelan AM, Trevenzoli M, Naso A, Meneghetti F, Cadrobbi P. Severe hypertension and renal atrophy associated with indinavir. *Clin Infect Dis* 2000; **30**: 619–621.

62 Hanabusa H, Tagami H, Hataya H. Renal atrophy associated with long-term treatment with indinavir. *N Engl J Med* 1999; **340**: 392–393.

63 Kopp JB, Falloon J, Filie A, Abati A, King C, Hortin GL *et al.* Indinavir-associated interstitial nephritis and urothelial inflammation: clinical and cytologic findings. *Clin Infect Dis* 2002; **34**: 1122–1128.

64 Kopp JB, Miller KD, Mican JA, Feurerstein IM, Vaughan E, Baker C *et al.* Crystalluria and urinary tract abnormalities associated with indinavir. *Ann Intern Med* 1997; **127**: 119–125.

65 Gagnon RF, Tecimer SN, Watters AK, Tsoukas CM. Prospective study of urinalysis abnormalities in HIV-positive individuals treated with indinavir. *Am J Kidney Dis* 2000; **36**: 507–515.

66 Martin JL, Brown CE, Matthews-Davis N, Reardon JE. Effects of antiviral nucleoside analogs on human DNA polymerases and mitochondrial DNA synthesis. *Antimicrob Agents Chemother* 1994; **38**: 2743–2749.

67 Verhelst D, Monge M, Meynard JL, Fouqueray B, Mougenot B, Girard PM *et al.* Fanconi syndrome and renal failure induced by tenofovir: a first case report. *Am J Kidney Dis* 2002; **40**: 1331–1333.

68 Coca S, Perazella MA. Rapid communication: acute renal failure associated with tenofovir: evidence of drug-induced nephrotoxicity. *Am J Med Sci* 2002; **324**: 342–344.

69 Creput C, Gonzalez-Canali G, Hill G, Piketty C, Kazatchkine M, Nochy D. Renal lesions in HIV-1-positive patient treated with tenofovir. *AIDS* 2003; **17**: 935–937.

70 Karras A, Lafaurie M, Furco A, Bourgarit A, Droz D, Sereni D *et al.* Tenofovir-related nephrotoxicity in human immunodeficiency virus-infected patients: three cases of renal failure, Fanconi syndrome, and nephrogenic diabetes insipidus. *Clin Infect Dis* 2003; **36**: 1070–1073.

71 Murphy MD, O'Hearn M, Chou S. Fatal lactic acidosis and acute renal failure after addition of tenofovir to an antiretroviral regimen containing didanosine. *Clin Infect Dis* 2003; **36**: 1082–1085.

72 Schaaf B, Aries SP, Kramme E, Steinhoff J, Dalhoff K. Acute renal failure associated with tenofovir treatment in a patient with acquired immunodeficiency syndrome. *Clin Infect Dis* 2003; **37**: e41–e43.

73 Peyriere H, Reynes J, Rouanet I, Daniel N, de Boever CM, Mauboussin JM *et al.* Renal dysfunction associated with tenofovir therapy: report of 7 cases. *J Acquir Immune Defic Syndr* 2004; **35**: 269–273.

74 Brown TT, Cole SR, Li X, Kingsley LA, Palella FJ, Riddler SA *et al.* Antiretroviral therapy and the prevalence and incidence of diabetes mellitus in the multicenter AIDS cohort study. *Arch Intern Med* 2005; **165**: 1179–1184.

75 Friis-Moller N, Weber R, Reiss P, Theibaut R, Kirk O, d'Aminio Monforte A *et al.* Cardiovascular disease risk factors in HIV patients: association with antiretroviral therapy. Results from the DAD study. *AIDS* 2003; **17**: 1179–1193.

76 Walli R, Herfort O, Michl GM, Demant T, Jager H, Dieterle C *et al.* Treatment with protease inhibitors associated with peripheral insulin resistance and impaired oral glucose tolerance in HIV-1-infected patients. *AIDS* 1998; **12**: F167–F173.

77 Jerico C, Knobel H, Montero M, Sorli ML, Guelar A, Gimeno JL *et al.* Hypertension in HIV-infected patients: prevalence and related factors. *Am J Hypertens* 2005; **18**: 1396–1401.

78 Sudano I, Spieker LE, Noll G, Corti R, Weber R, Luscher TF. Cardiovascular disease in HIV infection. *Am Heart J* 2006; **151**: 1147–1155.

79 Gupta SK, Eustace JA, Winston JA, Boydstun II, Ajuga TS, Rodriguez RA *et al.* Guidelines for the management of chronic kidney disease in HIV-infected patients: recommendations of the HIV Medicine Association of the Infectious Diseases Society of America. *Clin Infect Dis* 2005; **40**: 1559–1585.

80 Haas M, Kaul S, Eustace JA. HIV-associated immune complex glomerulonephritis with "lupus-like" features: a clinicopathologic study of 14 cases. *Kidney Int* 2005; **67(4)**: 1381–1390.

24 Hepatitis B Virus

M. Aamir Ali, Scott D. Cohen, & Paul L. Kimmel

Divisions of Nutritional and Gastrointestinal Disease and Renal Diseases and Hypertension, Department of Medicine, George Washington University Medical Center, Washington D.C., USA.

Hepatitis B virus

Hepatitis B virus (HBV) is among the most common chronic infectious diseases, affecting 5% of the world's population [1,2]. In high-prevalence areas, the mode of transmission is primarily vertical, from mother to neonate, as a result of perinatal exposure [3]. Lifetime risk of HBV infection in these regions exceeds 60%, while risk of infection in the USA and Western Europe is less than 20%. However, HBV infection is a significant cause of morbidity and mortality, even in low-prevalence areas. In the USA, there are approximately 1.25 million HBV carriers [4]. Globally, chronic HBV infection is the primary cause of cirrhosis and hepatocellular carcinoma, resulting in up to 1 million deaths each year.

HBV is a small 3.2-kb hepadnavirus whose DNA contains four open reading frames, encoding HBV surface antigen (HbsAg), the HBV e antigen (HBeAg), and the HBV core antigen (HbcAg) [5,6]. HBsAg is detectable in the serum 2–10 weeks after viral exposure. In patients who recover, the antigen becomes undetectable approximately 6 months after it appears. Persistence of HbsAg in the circulation beyond 6 months defines chronic infection. In patients who spontaneously clear infection, anti-HBs antibody is elaborated, usually persisting for life and conferring immunity [3]. HBeAg is a soluble protein whose presence indicates active viral replication. Loss of circulating HbeAg coincides with decreased HBV DNA levels and is a treatment end point. Loss of HBeAg is sometimes due to a precore mutation that suppresses the synthesis of HBeAg, so the antigen is undetectable even while active viral replication occurs [7]. Anti-HBc is present in the circulation in both acute and chronic HBV infection.

Acute HBV infection is subclinical in most patients. Approximately 30% of patients develop symptomatic hepatitis. Patients may experience fever, arthritis, and skin rash during a prodromal period when HBs complexed with anti-HBs activates complement and precipitates in various tissues. This prodrome is followed by elevations in aminotransferase levels and the development of nonspecific symptoms, including fatigue, myalgias, nausea, and vomiting [8]. Ten percent of patients with perinatal infection and nearly all those infected in adulthood recover spontaneously from acute HBV infection [1,8,9], demonstrating that progression to chronicity is markedly decreased in the setting of normal host immunity.

HBV infection and renal disease

HBV infection is associated with a number of renal manifestations (Table 24.1). The association between HBV infection and renal disease was first reported by Combes et al. in 1971 [10]. Subsequently, the field of HBV-associated nephropathy expanded to include other forms of renal disease, including membranoproliferative glomerulonephritis (MPGN), renal disease associated with polyarteritis nodosa (PAN), immunoglobulin A nephropathy (IgAN), and focal segmental glomerulosclerosis (FSGS) [6,11–15]. The incidence of HBV-associated renal disease is far less than that of HBV infection, suggesting viral pathogenic mechanisms, as well as genetic background and host responses, are critical to the development of particular types of nephropathy in susceptible patients. The occurrence of kidney disease associated with HBV infection is often associated with chronic infection [6,16].

Four possible mechanisms for HBV nephropathy have been invoked: 1) direct cytotoxic effects of the virus; 2) deposition of immune complexes consisting of viral antigen and antibody in renal tissue; 3) the action of T lymphocytes and antibodies induced by viral infection; and 4) the effects of cytokines or other virus-induced immune mediators on renal cells [6,11]. The onset and progression of kidney disease in HBV-infected patients is influenced by multiple factors, including age, gender, genetic constitution, immunological profile, and socio-economic status [3,6].

Evidence-based Nephrology. Edited by Donald Molony and Jonathan Craig
© 2009 Blackwell Publishing, ISBN: 978-1-4051-3975-5.

Table 24.1 Reported renal manifestations of HBV infection.

Manifestation
Membranous nephropathy
Membranoproliferative glomerulonephritis
Polyarteritis nodosa
Essential mixed cryoglobulinemia
IgA nephropathy
Focal segmental glomerulosclerosis

Epidemiology

Globally, the prevalence of HBV-associated kidney disease mirrors the prevalence of HBV infection. Well-designed population-based epidemiologic studies, however, are lacking. The age of presentation in children is in infancy among children infected vertically and between 5 and 7 years in those infected horizontally [11]. There is a distinct male predominance in pediatric patients with HBV-associated renal diseases. This predominance is less pronounced in adults, but the underlying reasons are unknown. In the USA, HBV is particularly prevalent in intravenous drug users and in patients with end-stage renal disease (ESRD) treated with hemodialysis [11].

In children with HBV-associated nephropathy, renal disease is most often asymptomatic and is detected by routine laboratory analyses. HBV-associated renal disease in children commonly presents as nephrotic syndrome [11]. A history of acute hepatitis is rarely obtained, as acute HBV infection tends to be subclinical in this population. Spontaneous remission of HBV-associated nephropathy occurred after clearance of HBeAg in 33 of 37 children over a course of 90 months [12]. Renal function was preserved in over 95% of children with HBV-associated renal disease [11]. Adults with HBV-associated renal disease commonly present with nephrotic syndrome and proteinuria and are more likely to recall a history of acute hepatitis. As in children, spontaneous remission is associated with clearance of HBeAg. Progression to kidney failure occurs in one-fourth of adult patients and is associated with failure to clear HBV infection [11].

HBV-associated membranous nephropathy

Pathophysiology

Membranous nephropathy (MN) was the first described, and is the most extensively studied, form of nephropathy in patients with chronic HBV infection [6,17–19]. Combes *et al.* described a patient [10] with nephrotic syndrome and with a history of jaundice after blood transfusion. Circulating Australia antigen was detected by serologic techniques. Examination revealed thickened glomerular capillary basement membranes and mesangial hypercellularity, as well as other features of MN. The Australia antigen was detected in renal tissue by using indirect immunofluorescence. The authors suggested nephropathy was causally linked to the renal deposition of Australia antigen-containing immune complexes. Elution of HBV-associated immune complexes from renal tissue was not performed. Subsequent reports demonstrated detection of HBsAg in renal tissue of patients with MN and HBV infection [15,20].

There are several potential mechanisms for HBV-associated glomerular injury. Deposition of circulating immune complexes in renal tissue is the most widely accepted pathogenic mechanism of injury. Early series defined HBV-associated nephropathy cases in which circulating immune complexes containing HBV antigens were found concurrently with MN, without necessarily demonstrating antigen–antibody complexes in renal tissue [6,17,21]. With technical refinements, it was demonstrated that prior studies in which HBsAg was identified by indirect immunofluorescence were prone to false-positive results [6,17,22]. Glomerular immune deposits in patients with HBV-associated MN contained HBeAg, and not HBsAg, as had been previously accepted [17,23]. In addition to immune complexes, HBV DNA was detectable by *in situ* hybridization in renal tissue of children with HBV-associated glomerulonephritis. Those with HBV DNA detected in renal tubules had a longer duration of proteinuria [24]. HBcAg RNA was found in the nuclei and cytoplasm of both glomerular and tubular cells in more than half of renal biopsies of patients with MN [25]. Persistence of HBV DNA in renal tissue can lead to *de novo* synthesis of viral proteins in the kidney, which can elicit a local immune response with potential immune-mediated cytotoxicity [6,26].

Clinical course

Studies have outlined the clinical characteristics of MN associated with HBV infection [6,17,21,27,28]. Some of these studies predate molecular diagnostic techniques presently available to establish causal relationships between viral infection and renal disease. The diagnosis of HBV-associated MN in many studies was based on one or more of the following criteria: the presence of persistent HBV-associated antigenemia, absence of evidence of other causes of nephropathy, and in some studies the detection of at least one HBV antigen in renal tissue [6]. In the majority of cases, at least one circulating HBV-associated antigen, usually HbsAg, was detected. Inclusion and exclusion criteria for specific renal diseases were variable. Few studies have included renal tissue elution of specific HBV-associated immunoreactants. Therefore, many studies of "HBV-associated renal diseases" have only documented the types of renal diseases present in HBV-infected patients, without establishing causal relationships [6]. Classically, remission of the nephrotic syndrome had been noted in a variable proportion of patients, and the course in patients with persistently elevated urinary protein excretion was often indolent [6]. Clearance of HBV antigenemia has been associated with improvement of signs of renal disease [29–33].

Lai *et al.* [34] reported the clinical features of 21 adults with HBV-associated MN and persistent HBsAg antigenemia and proteinuria. Nephrotic syndrome was present in 57%. Mean urinary protein excretion was 4.1 g/day, one-third had asymptomatic proteinuria, and two patients had chronic kidney failure.

One-fourth of patients had renal insufficiency, and one-third had hypertension.

Lai *et al.* [35] studied 100 consecutive patients with glomerulonephritis and with HBV infection documented by the presence of circulating HBsAg, using appropriate diagnostic criteria for HBV-associated renal disease. Thirty-nine patients had an HBV antigen detected in kidney tissue by monoclonal antibody techniques. HBeAg was the most commonly detected antigen, and 69.2% of patients were found to have an HBV-associated protein present in renal tissue. HBsAg was detected in 53.8% of patients with an HBV protein in renal tissue. MPGN or IgAN was the most common lesion identified in patients with renal HBsAg deposition, but MN was identified in fewer such cases. In contrast, of the patients with renal HBeAg, 55.6% had MN.

Clinical inferences regarding the natural history of HBV-associated MN are hampered because there are few data regarding long-term outcomes in adult patients in whom the diagnosis of HBV-associated MN has been rigorously established. HBV-associated MN has a variable outcome, although the lack of well-controlled longitudinal studies precludes definitive characterizations of outcomes. Progression to advanced chronic kidney disease (CKD) appears to be relatively uncommon [6], and the course may be more favorable in children. Spontaneous remission of nephrotic syndrome has been reported in 30–60% of MN linked to HBV [11]. Development of antibodies to HBeAg has been associated with decreased proteinuria [17]. Clearance of antigenemia appears to be associated with improved renal outcomes, but there are few data available with which to make definitive prognoses.

HBV-associated MPGN

Shortly after the report of MN associated with HBV infection, a study linked a heterogenous set of renal outcomes, including MPGN and FSGS, with HBV [15]. MPGN is also thought to result from deposition of HBV antigen–antibody complexes in mesangial and subendothelial tissues. Lai and colleagues showed MPGN is the most common lesion in patients with HBsAg detected in renal tissue [36]. Lee *et al.* [21] studied 87 patients with chronic HBsAg antigenemia with glomerular disease. One-third had MPGN, but only 21% had MN. MPGN types I and III have been described in association with HBV infection [11]. Caution is necessary in evaluating studies of HBV-associated MPGN preceding the cloning of HCV [6], since coinfection with HCV, which has been well-associated with MPGN, may have been the cause of the renal disease in such cases [6].

The clinical manifestations of HBV-associated MPGN are similar to those of idiopathic MPGN. The most common presentation is nephrotic syndrome with microscopic hematuria. Nearly half the patients have hypertension, and one-fifth have impaired renal function [36]. The prognosis is unfavorable, with a 50% risk of developing ESRD or mortality in 10 years [37].

Treatment

The literature on the treatment of HBV-related MN or MPGN is sparse, consisting primarily of case reports, case series, and treatment studies with historical untreated controls. The large randomized clinical trials that established benefits of various antiviral therapies in chronic HBV infection did not evaluate renal end points. Indeed, patients with renal disease were excluded in several of these trials, as was the case for HCV infection [38]. Despite the lack of a robust evidence-based literature to recommend it, antiviral treatment of HBV-associated nephropathy is warranted in patients with persistent proteinuria, particularly adults, to forestall the initiation of renal disease and progression to ESRD as a complication of the viral illness [11]. Patients at risk for progressing to kidney failure are those with persistent HBe Ag positivity. Eradication of HBV in this population serves the threefold purpose of preventing progression to kidney and liver failure and preventing hepatocellular carcinoma.

Corticosteroids

Success in treatment of idiopathic MN with corticosteroids led to its use in HBV-associated nephropathy. However, although corticosteroids have been used to treat idiopathic MN [39–42], there is currently no clear standard for the treatment of HBV-associated MN. A prospective trial of corticosteroids that compared eight patients treated with a 6-month course of steroids to seven historical controls treated supportively had disappointing results, revealing no improvement in any renal parameter [43]. In addition, corticosteroids were potentially harmful, as increased HBV viral load and persistence of HBeAg were noted in corticosteroid-treated patients [43]. Rapid steroid withdrawal can result in potentially fatal hepatotoxicity in HBV-infected patients maintained on long-term steroids, as the increased viral loads resulting from unchecked viral replication during immunosuppression encounter abruptly reconstituted immune responses. Because of the lack of demonstrable benefits and the potential for adverse events, corticosteroid treatment should not be considered a primary therapy for HBV-associated nephropathy.

Alpha interferon

Alpha interferon (IFN-α) is a cytokine elaborated by B lymphocytes and macrophages and has antiviral and immunomodulatory effects [11]. A randomized, controlled trial of IFN-α was conducted in 40 Taiwanese children with HBV-associated nephropathy [45]. Twenty patients each were randomized to IFN-α treatment or supportive therapy. After 3 months, all patients receiving IFN-α had resolution of proteinuria, whereas all patients receiving supportive treatment had varying degrees of proteinuria. Another study compared 19 children with HBV nephropathy treated with IFN-α for 16 weeks to 20 children with HBV nephropathy treated supportively [45]. Of the IFN-α-treated patients, 53% demonstrated HBeAg clearance and resolution of proteinuria. None of the patients with persistent HBe antigenemia had resolution of proteinuria. While these findings are encouraging, IFN-α treatment involves daily injections and may be poorly tolerated due to flu-like symptoms and leukopenia. As such, this treatment should be weighed against nucleoside analog therapies.

The renal toxicity of IFN therapy has been well-documented [46–55]. Fifteen to 20% of cancer patients treated with IFN had proteinuria that was predominantly mild, clinically insignificant, and reversible on cessation of therapy [56,57]. While the majority of reported nephrotoxicity related to IFN therapy has been in patients with underlying malignancy, there are case reports of its occurrence in patients receiving IFN for chronic viral hepatitis [53,57,58]. Less common presentations of IFN-induced nephrotoxicity in patients with HBV infection are nephrotic syndrome and acute kidney failure [46–54,59]. The histological correlates of acute kidney failure with IFN therapy are variable, including minimal change disease, acute interstitial nephritis, acute tubular necrosis, FSGS, MN, and MPGN [46–54,58]. There is an increased likelihood of nephrotoxicity with IFN therapy in patients with underlying renal disease. Twenty-two of 23 patients with underlying glomerulopathy developed proteinuria while receiving IFN therapy for chronic HCV infection [60]. Proteinuria resolved in the majority after withdrawal of IFN. Although clinically severe renal impairment is rare, these findings underscore the need to monitor renal function closely during IFN therapy.

Pegylated interferon (PEG IFN) is composed of a polyethylene glycol moiety bound to IFN-α [61,62]. The polyethylene glycol increases the IFN half-life and may decrease immunogenicity [61,62]. Because of its prolonged half-life, PEG IFN only needs to be administered weekly. The safety and efficacy of PEG IFN in the treatment of chronic HBV has been demonstrated in several clinical trials, but none of them evaluated renal end points [63–65]. There are currently no reports of the effects of therapy with PEG IFN in HBV-associated renal disease.

Lamivudine

Lamivudine is an orally administered nucleoside analog with efficacy in chronic HBV infection [66]. Since the start of widespread use of lamivudine in the treatment of chronic HBV infection, improvement of HBV-associated renal disease with lamivudine has been the subject of multiple case reports [67–70]. A study comparing 10 patients with HBV-associated MN treated with lamivudine with supportively treated historical controls demonstrated reduction in proteinuria and increased serum albumin concentration in treated patients [66]. Lamivudine at 100 mg daily was administered to the intervention group [66]. At 3 years, 100% of treated patients and 58% of untreated patients had not developed ESRD ($P = 0.024$). In addition, there was a reduction in proteinuria after 6 months in the lamivudine group compared to controls [66]. Unfortunately, relapse of HBV infection after cessation of lamivudine occurs, and there is currently no standard duration of treatment. Therefore, open-ended treatment for a prolonged duration is usual for treatment of chronic HBV infection and may also be required in the setting of HBV-associated renal disease.

With prolonged treatment, however, there is a significant risk of developing viral resistance. After 1 and 5 years of treatment, the risk of resistance was 23 and 65%, respectively [71].

Adefovir dipivoxil

Adefovir dipivoxil is an adenosine triphosphate analog with benefit in chronic HBV infection [72,73]. Nephrotoxicity has been reported at the higher doses of this medication that are used to treat human immunodeficiency virus infection [74]. The dose of adefovir dipivoxil used to treat chronic HBV infection (10 mg daily) is lower and is associated with a risk of nephrotoxicity no greater than placebo [72–74]. The safety of adefovir dipivoxil was demonstrated in 12 patients with lamivudine-resistant HBV infection and varying degrees of renal dysfunction [75]. However, because of the availability of other less nephrotoxic therapeutic options, using adefovir dipivoxil to treat HBV nephropathy should generally be avoided in patients with renal dysfunction.

Adefovir at a 30-mg dose had a 35% incidence of renal toxicity, defined by increased serum creatinine or hypophosphatemia [74]. Adefovir nephrotoxicity is related to proximal tubular accumulation of the drug via an organic anion transporter found on the basolateral membrane of cells [74]. The drug is transported out of the proximal tubule via multidrug resistance-associated protein 2 (MRP2) [74]. Higher doses of the drug may overwhelm the ability of the luminal MRP to transport it out of the proximal tubule cell, resulting in intracellular accumulation and subsequent nephrotoxicity. Larger studies are needed to evaluate the safety and efficacy of adefovir in patients with CKD.

Other agents

Entecavir has been shown in large randomized controlled trials to be superior to lamivudine in the treatment of chronic HBV infection [76,77]. Although there are no reports regarding its use in the treatment of HBV-associated renal disease, it holds promise in view of its high potency and favorable side effects profile. Tenofovir is another nucleoside currently being evaluated for efficacy in treatment of chronic HBV infection. However, tenofovir treatment is associated with renal toxicity via a mechanism similar to adefovir [78,79]. Anelli *et al.* described an HBV-infected patient treated with infliximab, who had rheumatoid arthritis and secondary amyloid-associated amyloidosis [80]. The patient had complete cessation of HBV replication and improvement in creatinine clearance after 1 year of treatment [80]. However, larger clinical trials are needed before conclusions regarding the safety of tumor necrosis factor alpha blockers in HBV infection can be made.

Vaccination

Vaccination against HBV infection has decreased the incidence of HBV-associated renal disease. Prior to widespread vaccination, the incidence of HBV-associated renal disease was 0.3 cases/100,000 children age 0–14 years in 1990–1991 in South Africa. After introduction of widespread vaccination against HBV in 1994–1995, the incidence of HBV-associated renal disease decreased 10-fold in 2000–2001 [1].

HBV and PAN

Epidemiology

PAN is a necrotizing vasculitis involving the medium-sized and small arteries. It is an uncommon complication of HBV infection, affecting 1–5% of those chronically infected [81]. However, older studies suggested as many as 70% of patients with PAN are HBsAg positive [82]. This association has been documented extensively in North America and Europe. In Asia, where HBV is regionally endemic, no association of the viral infection with PAN has been reported [81].

Pathophysiology

The pathophysiology of HBV-associated PAN may be mediated by circulating immune complexes, consisting of HBV-associated antigen, antibody, and complement [83]. Levels of circulating immune complexes have been reported to be proportional to PAN disease activity [84], and complex deposition has been demonstrated histologically in affected arteries [85,86]. HBeAg may be the predominant antigen in immune complexes associated with PAN [87]. The mechanism underlying immune complex tropism to the target vessels is unknown. Antineutrophil cytoplasmic antibodies are rarely found in patients with HBV-associated PAN [88].

PAN-associated vasculitis is notable for necrosis and perivascular inflammation of small and medium-sized blood vessels. The acute polymorphonuclear leukocyte infiltrate promotes a predominantly chronic mononuclear infiltrate that may lead to vascular occlusion and necrosis. Angiography demonstrates microaneurysms, stenosis, and occlusion. Renal angiography typically demonstrates microaneurysms [81].

Clinical course

PAN is a multisystem disease with protean manifestations extending beyond the gastrointestinal tract and the kidneys [81]. Nervous system, rheumatologic, cardiac, and dermatologic involvement have all been described [81]. The initial presentation is often with fever, hypertension, rash, and abdominal and joint pain. Laboratory studies show elevated erythrocyte sedimentation rate, anemia, leukocytosis, and abnormal liver-associated enzymes. Eosinophilia is seen in 10–40% of patients. With progression of disease, as vascular compromise occurs, visceral infarction involving the gastrointestinal tract, kidney, spleen, brain, heart, testicles, and prostate may occur. Gastrointestinal bleeding and perforation have been seen in 16% of patients. Pancreatitis and cholecystitis have also been reported [81].

Although the kidneys are involved in most cases of PAN, there is no classic pathognomonic pattern of renal injury. Hypertension related to renal vessel vasculitis is a common presenting symptom. In classic PAN with large and medium vessel involvement,

renal ischemia and infarction are typical. Fibrinoid necrosis is a frequent pathologic finding. Untreated PAN has a dismal prognosis, with 5-year survival rates of less than 15%. Early mortality results from acute gastrointestinal hemorrhage or ischemia, acute myocardial infarction, or kidney failure. Late mortality is often from complications of ESRD or congestive heart failure [88].

Treatment

Whereas plasma exchange and immunosuppression with corticosteroids and cyclophosphamide are cornerstones of treatment of idiopathic PAN, patients with HBV-associated PAN are at risk of increased viral proliferation and progressive liver disease with prolonged immunosuppression. In addition, rapid withdrawal of immunosuppression in HBV-infected patients may result in the development of fulminant hepatic failure. For these reasons, treatment of the underlying chronic viral infection is important in HBV-associated PAN. Antiviral treatment alone, without addressing the acute vasculitis and its life-threatening consequences, may also be inadequate [89].

There is a dearth of large, well-designed clinical trials evaluating the effectiveness of antiviral therapies in patients with HBV-associated PAN. One approach is to control the acute manifestations of PAN with plasma exchange while treating the underlying viral disease. A study of IFN and plasma exchange therapy in HBV-associated PAN demonstrated HBeAg seroconversion in four patients [90]. In a nonrandomized prospective trial that combined antiviral treatment (vidarabine or IFN) with plasma exchange in 41 patients with HBV-associated PAN, viral replication ceased in over half the patients, and long-term symptom-free survival was achieved in 80% [91]. Because renal disease was present in one-third of these patients and information regarding improvement in renal parameters is unavailable, specific conclusions regarding treatment of nephropathy with this protocol cannot be reached. Another approach is to treat the acute vasculitis with a short course of immunosuppression, followed by plasma exchange and antiviral therapy. Prevention of HBV infection by widespread vaccination has accounted for a remarkable decrease in the proportion of PAN cases associated with HBV infection. In 1972–1976, 38.5% of PAN cases were associated with HBV. In 1997–2002, this proportion decreased to 17.4% [92].

HBV and essential mixed cryoglobulinemia

The association between HBV infection and cryoglobulinemia is controversial. Serologic markers of HBV infection were demonstrated in the cryoproteins of 74% of patients with essential mixed cryoglobulinemia (EMC) [93]. Subsequent larger studies in the post-HCV era have challenged this finding on the basis of study population, accuracy of serologic tests used, and the possibility that HBV was transmitted by transfusion in patients with anemia. A notable challenge came from Ferri and colleagues, who found HBV infection to be causative in only 4 of 231 patients with EMC [94]. In contrast, HCV RNA was detected in 90% of patients with EMC [94]. Furthermore, renal disease in the setting of HBV-associated cryoglobulinemia has never been reliably demonstrated to be caused by HBV antigens. There are no therapeutic trials of antiviral agents in the setting of HBV-associated cryoglobulinemia.

HBV and IgAN

There are increasing cases linking HBs antigenemia with IgAN. However, data are limited to studies of populations where HBV is endemic, which are therefore potentially subject to bias. Wang *et al.* evaluated 50 Chinese patients with IgAN, positive HBV serology, and/or HBV antigens found by renal immunohistochemistry [95]. They concluded HBV infection may have a role in the development of IgAN [95]. However, a Japanese study concluded that there was no association between IgAN and HBV [96]. A total of 130 patients with IgAN were identified. HbsAg was positive in only 4 of 130, or 3.1% [96], which was not different from the general population rate of 2.0% [96]. Lai *et al.* examined the possible role of HBV in the development of IgAN [97]. A total of 125 patients were diagnosed with IgAN [97]. Ten of the 125 patients with IgAN were HBsAg positive. Renal biopsies of these 10 patients were stained with immunoperoxidase for HBsAg, HBcAg, and IgA [97]. There was a control group with renal biopsies from 20 patients with IgAN without HBV antigenemia. Immunoperoxidase staining showed HBcAg in glomerular mesangial cell nuclei in 6 of 10 patients. HbsAg was found in the cytoplasm of one mesangial cell. They concluded that HBsAg and HBcAg in the cytoplasm and nuclei of glomerular cells were potential evidence for a pathogenic role of HBV in IgAN [97].

There are few studies examining the renal outcomes of HBV-infected patients with IgAN. Lai reported a decline in GFR in 19% of patients with IgAN linked to HBV over 40 months [98]. Of these patients, 25% eventually required renal replacement therapy [98]. Further studies are needed to clarify the potential association between HBV and IgAN.

HBV and FSGS

There may be a link between HBV and FSGS; however, research is limited. There is some speculation that FSGS, seen on biopsies of patients with HBV, could be a reflection of the advanced stages of other types of HBV-associated renal diseases [99]. Larger studies are needed to further evaluate this possible association.

HBV and ESRD

There has been a decrease in the incidence of HBV infection among US ESRD patients treated with hemodialysis, largely due to preventive measures implemented since the 1970s [100]. An analysis of data from the Dialysis Outcomes and Practice Patterns Study

(DOPPS) evaluated 308 dialysis units across the world and found a mean HBV prevalence of 3.0% across all centers [101], with 79% of centers having an HBV prevalence of 0–5% [101]. There was a higher prevalence of HBV infection in dialysis patients in France, Germany, and Italy compared to Japan, the UK, and the USA [101]. Universal precautions, including use of gowns and gloves when handling biohazardous materials, monthly testing for HbsAg, and separation of HbsAg-positive patients from negative patients, have all been associated with reduced incidence of HBV in hemodialysis units [100]. Acute infection with HBV tends to show milder clinical manifestations, with decreased levels of aminotransferases compared to patients acutely infected with HBV without ESRD [100]. The development of complications associated with HBV, including cirrhosis and hepatocellular carcinoma, is typically slow and often is longer than the average lifespan of patients maintained on hemodialysis [100]. Nevertheless, it is still essential to prevent transmission of this blood-borne pathogen in hemodialysis units.

Vaccination schedules are important for all patients with CKD, ideally in the predialysis phase, when immune responses to a vaccine may be optimal. In ESRD patients, additional doses beyond the standard three-dose schedule should be considered. Antibody testing for HbsAb to determine the optimal responses may be needed [100].

There have been limited studies on IFN use in hemodialysis patients with HBV. Rodrigues *et al.* studied 13 patients on hemodialysis with HBV and/or HCV infection who were treated with IFN-α 2B [102]. Eight of 13 patients responded to therapy [102]. Nevertheless, the frequency of adverse events with IFN therapy is higher in the ESRD patient population, limiting its use and effectiveness [100].

Several trials have investigated the use of lamivudine in ESRD patients, and these studies noted positive responses with clearance of HbeAg, although the studies were small [100]. Lamivudine therapy may play a role in improving overall patient and graft survival in HBsAg-positive kidney transplant recipients. Lamivudine at 100 mg daily was administered to 11 patients who underwent kidney transplantation between 1996 and 2000 and to 15 patients who had a kidney transplant between 1983 and 1995 [103]. These patients met inclusion criteria, which included rising HBV DNA levels or liver biopsy indicating active inflammation [103]. Patients in the group transplanted between 1996 and 2000 were treated with lamivudine for 32.6 ± 13.3 months, whereas those in the 1983–1995 group were treated for 36.3 ± 11.4 months [103]. Survival of those transplanted between 1996 and 2000 and subsequently treated with lamivudine was similar to HBsAg-negative patients [103]. However, the group transplanted between 1983 and 1995 had a lower survival rate compared to the HBsAg-negative control group [103]. The authors concluded that prompt administration of lamivudine once HBV DNA levels increase may improve survival of HBV-infected kidney transplant recipients [103].

There is concern that immunosuppressive medications used in kidney transplant patients may cause activation of HBV. Calcineurin inhibitors, azathioprine, and steroids may enhance viral replication [100]. Fornairon and colleagues evaluated the effect of kidney transplantation in chronic HBV infection in 151 patients [104]. Over a period of 66 months in which liver biopsies were done, cirrhosis was found in 28% of patients [104]. HBV infection was not associated with differences in survival in this study [104]. However, data are conflicting and further information is needed before conclusions can be reached. Aroldi *et al.* found that death related to hepatic causes was more frequent in HBV-infected transplant patients than in HCV-infected transplant recipients [105].

The incidence of *de novo* glomerulonephritis in HBV-infected kidney transplant recipients was evaluated by Schwarz *et al.* Twenty-one patients of 848 who received a kidney transplant developed *de novo* MN [106]. Eight of these 21 patients also were found to have active infection with either HBV, HCV, or human immunodeficiency virus [106].

Conclusions

Although the incidence of HBV-related renal disease is decreasing with the widespread use of vaccination, it nevertheless remains an important cause of nephropathy, especially in the developing world. HBV infection has been linked to MN, MPGN, PAN, and possibly to IgAN as well as FSGS. MPGN may be an important renal complication of HBV infection. The chronicity of the viral infection and the host responses are likely factors in the pathogenesis of the associated nephropathies. Further studies are needed to determine the exact pathogenic role HBV infection may play in these nephropathies. A number of novel therapeutic approaches exist to treat HBV-related kidney diseases, including IFN-α, lamivudine, and adefovir. However, several of these treatments are associated with the development of nephrotoxicity.

References

1 Lai CL, Ratziu V, Yuen MF, Poynard T. Viral hepatitis B. *Lancet* 2003; **362**: 2089–2094.

2 Levy M, Chen N. Worldwide perspective of hepatitis B-associated glomerulonephritis in the 80s. *Kidney Int* 1991; **40**(**Suppl 35**): S24.

3 Nair S, Perillo RP. Hepatitis B and D. In: Zakim D, Boyer TD, editors. *Hepatology: a Textbook of Liver Disease*, 4th edn. WB Saunders, Philadelphia, 2003; 959–961.

4 Lee WM. Hepatitis B virus infection. *N Engl J Med* 1997; **337**: 1733–1745.

5 Tiollais P, Pourcel C, Dejean A. The hepatitis B virus. *Nature* 1985; **317**: 489.

6 Kimmel PL, Moore J, Jr. Viral glomerular diseases. In: Schrier R, editor. *Diseases of the Kidney and Urinary Tract: Clinicopathologic Foundations of Medicine*, 8th edn. Lippincott, Williams & Wilkins, Baltimore, 2006; 1478–1510.

7 Li J, Buckwold VE, Hon MW, Ou JH. Mechanisms of suppression of hepatitis B virus precore RNA transcription by a frequent double mutation. *J Virol* 1999; **73**: 1239–1244.

8 Mahoney FJ. Update on diagnosis, management, and prevention of hepatitis B virus infection. *Clin Microbiol Rev* 1999; **12**: 351–366.

9 Hyams KC. Risks of chronicity following acute hepatitis B virus infections: a review. *Clin Infect Dis* 1995; **20**: 992–1000.

10 Combes B, Shorey J, Barrera A, Stastny P, Eigenbrodt EH, Hull AR, *et al.* Glomerulonephritis with deposition of Australia antigen-antibody complexes in the glomerular basement membrane. *Lancet* 1971; **ii**: 234–237.

11 Bhimma R, Coovadia HM. Hepatitis B virus-associated nephropathy. *Am J Nephrol* 2004; **24**: 198–211.

12 Gilbert RD, Wiggelinkhuizen J. The clinical course of hepatitis B-associated nephropathy. *Pediatr Nephrol* 1994; **8**: 11–14.

13 Ching-Yuang L. Clinical features and natural course of HBV-related glomerulopathy in children. *Kidney Int* 1991; **40**(**Suppl 35**): 46–53.

14 Johnson RJ, Couser WG. Hepatitis B infection and renal disease: clinical, immunopathogenetic and therapeutic considerations. *Kidney Int* 1990; **37**: 663–676.

15 Kneiser MR, Jenis EH, Lowenthal DT, Bancroft WH, Burns W, Shalhoub R. Pathogenesis of renal disease associated with viral hepatitis. *Arch Pathol* 1974; **97**: 193.

16 Ronco P, Verroust P, Morel-Maroger L. Viruses and glomerulonephritis. *Nephron* 1982; **31**: 97.

17 Lai KN, Lai FM, Chan KW, Chow CB, Tong KL, Vallance-Owen J. The clinico-pathologic features of hepatitis B-associated glomerulonephritis. *QJM* 1987; **63**: 323–333.

18 Coovadia HM, Adhikari M, Morel-Maroger L. Clinico-pathological features of the nephrotic syndrome in South Africa. *QJM* 1979; **48**: 77–91.

19 Slusarczyk J, Michalak T, Nazarewicz-de Mezer T, Krawczynski K, Nowoslawski A. Membranous glomerulonephritis associated hepatitis B core antigen immune complexes. *Am J Pathol* 1980; **98**: 29–39.

20 Kohler PF, Cronin RE, Hammond WS, Olin D, Carr RI. Chronic membranous glomerulonephritis caused by hepatitis B antigen-antibody immune complexes. *Ann Intern Med* 1974; **81**: 448–451.

21 Lee HS, Choi Y, Yu SH, Koh HI, Kim MJ, Ko KW. A renal biopsy study of hepatitis B virus-associated nephropathy in Korea. *Kidney Int* 1988; **34**: 537–543.

22 Maggiore Q, Bartolomeo F, L'Abbate A, Misefari V. HBsAg glomerular deposits in glomerulonephritis: fact or artifact? *Kidney Int* 1981; **19**: 579–586.

23 Hiroshi H, Udo K, Kojima M, Takahashi Y, Miyakawa Y, Miyamoto K *et al.* Deposition of HB e antigen in membranous glomerulonephritis: identification by F(ab')$_2$ fragments of monoclonal antibody. *Kidney Int* 1984; **26**: 338.

24 He XY, Fang LJ, Zhang YE, Sheng FY, Zhang XR, Guo MY. In situ hybridization of hepatitis B DNA in hepatitis B-associated glomerulonephritis. *Pediatr Nephrol* 1998; **12**: 117–120.

25 Lai KN, Ho RT, Tam JS, Lai FM. Detection of hepatitis B virus DNA and RNA in kidneys of HBV-related glomerulonephritis. *Kidney Int* 1996; **50**: 1965–1977.

26 Zhou SD *et al.* The study of the significance of the appearance of HBcAg in glomerulonephritis. *Chin J Nephrol* 1995; **11**: 104–106.

27 Venkataseshan VS, Lieberman K, Kim DU, Thung SN, Dikman S, D'Agati V *et al.* Hepatitis-B-associated glomerulonephritis: pathology, pathogenesis, and clinical course. *Medicine* 1990; **69**: 200.

28 Nagy J, Bajtai G, Brasch H, Sule T, Ambrus M, Deak G *et al.* The role of hepatitis B surface antigen in the pathogenesis of glomerulopathies. *Clin Nephrol* 1979; **12**: 109.

29 Mizushima N, Kanai K, Matsuda H, Matsumoto M, Tamakoshi K, Ishii H *et al.* Improvement of proteinuria in a case of hepatitis B-associated glomerulonephritis after treatment with interferon. *Gastroenterology* 1987; **92**: 524–526.

30 Esteban R, Buti M, Valles M, Allende H, Guardia J. Hepatitis B-associated membranous glomerulonephritis treated with adenine arabinoside monophosphate. *Hepatology* 1986; **6**: 762–763.

31 Takekoshi Y, Tanaka M, Miyakawa Y, Yoshizawa H, Takahashi K, Mayumi M. Free "small" and IgG associated "large" hepatitis B e antigen in the serum and glomerular capillary walls of two patients with membranous glomerulonephritis. *N Engl J Med* 1979; **300**: 814–819.

32 de Man RA, Schalm SW, van der Heijden AJ, ten Kate FW, Wolff ED, Hetjtink RA. Improvement of hepatitis B associated glomerulonephritis after antiviral combination therapy. *J Hepatol* 1989; **8**: 367–372.

33 Schectman JM, Kimmel PL. Remission of hepatitis B-associated membranous glomerulonephritis in human immunodeficiency virus infection. *Am J Kidney Dis* 1991; **17**: 716–718.

34 Lai KN, Li PK, Au TC, Tam JS, Tong KL, Lai FM. Membranous nephropathy related to hepatitis B virus in adults. *N Engl J Med* 1991; **324**: 1457–1463.

35 Lai FM, Lai KN, Tam JS, Lui SF, To KF, Li PK. Primary glomerulonephritis with detectable glomerular hepatitis B virus antigens. *Am J Surg Pathol* 1994; **18**: 175–186.

36 Abbas NA, Pitt MA, Green AT, Solomon LR. Successful treatment of HBV-associated MPGN with alpha interferon. *Nephrol Dial Transplant* 1999; **14**: 1272–1275.

37 Schmitt H, Bohle A, Reineke T, Mayer-Eichberger D, Vogl W. Long-term prognosis of membranoproliferative glomerulonephritis type-I. *Nephron* 1990; **55**: 242–250.

38 Meyers CM, Seeff LB, Stehman-Breen CO, Hoofnagle JH. Hepatitis C and renal disease: an update. *Am J Kidney Dis* 2003; **42**: 631–637.

39 Ponticelli C, Zucchelli P, Passerini P, Cagnoli L, Cesana B, Pozzi C et al. A randomized trial of methylprednisolone and chlorambucil in idiopathic membranous nephropathy. *N Engl J Med* 1989; **320**: 8–13.

40 Tang S, Chan TM, Cheng IK, Lai KN. Clinical features and treatment outcome of idiopathic membranous nephropathy in Chinese patients. *QJM* 1999; **92**: 401–406.

41 Cattran D. Management of membranous nephropathy: when and what for treatment. *J Am Soc Nephrol* 2005; **16**: 1188–1194.

42 Ponticelli C, Altieri P, Scolari F, Passerini P, Roccatello D, Cesana B et al. A randomized study comparing methylprednisolone plus chlorambucil versus methylprednisolone plus cyclophosphamide in idiopathic membranous nephropathy. *J Am Soc Nephrol* 1998; **9**: 444–450.

43 Lai KN, Tam JS, Lin HJ, Lai FM. The therapeutic dilemma of usage of corticosteroids in patients with membranous nephropathy and persistent hepatitis B surface antigenemia. *Nephron* 1990; **54**: 12–17.

44 Lin CY. Treatment of hepatitis B virus-associated membranous nephropathy with recombinant alpha interferon. *Kidney Int* 1991; **47**: 225–230.

45 Bhimma R, Coovadia HM, Kramvis A, Adhikari M, Kew MC. Treatment of hepatitis B virus-associated nephropathy in black children. *Pediatr Nephrol* 2002; **17**: 393–399.

46 Stein DF, Ahmed A, Sunkhara V, Khalbuss W. Collapsing focal segmental glomerulosclerosis with recovery of renal function: an uncommon complication of interferon therapy for hepatitis C. *Dig Dis Sci* 2001; **46**: 530–535.

47 Dressler D, Wright JR, Houghton JB, Kalra PA. Another case of focal segmental glomerulosclerosis in an acutely uremic patient following interferon therapy. *Nephrol Dial Transplant* 1999; **14**: 2049–2050.

48 Haas M, Jager U, Mayer G. Interferon alpha-2c and proteinuria in a patient with focal and segmental glomerulosclerosis. *Lancet* 1997; **349**: 1147–1148.

49 Coreneos E, Petrusevska G, Varghese F, Truong LD. Focal segmental glomerulosclerosis with acute renal failure associated with alpha-interferon therapy. *Am J Kidney Dis* 1996; **28**: 888–892.

50 Auty A. Nephrotic syndrome in a multiple sclerosis patient treated with interferon beta 1a. *Can J Neurological Sci* 2005; **32**: 366–368.

51 Zuber J. Alpha-interferon associated thrombotic microangiopathy. *Medicine* 2002; **81**: 321–331.

52 Herrman J. Membranoproliferative glomerulonephritis in a patient with hairy-cell leukemia treated with alpha-II interferon. *N Engl J Med* 1987; **316**: 112–113.

53 Miranda-Guardiola F. Acute renal failure associated with alpha-interferon therapy for chronic hepatitis B. *Nephrol Dial Transplant* 1995; **10**: 1441–1443.

54 Kimmel PL, Abraham AA, Phillips TM. Membranoproliferative glomerulonephritis in a patient treated with interferon-alpha for HIV infection. *Am J Kidney Dis* 1994; **24**: 858–863.

55 Jones GJ, Itri LM. Safety and tolerance of recombinant interferon alfa-2a (Roferon-A) in cancer patients. *Cancer* 1986; **57**: 1709–1715.

56 Quesada JR, Talpaz M, Rios A, Kurzrock R, Gutterman JU. Clinical toxicity of interferons in cancer patients: a review. *J Clin Oncol* 1986; **4**: 234–243.

57 Ayub A et al. Acute renal failure with alpha interferon therapy: a case report. *Med Sci Res* 1993; **21**: 123–124.

58 Wilson RA. Nephrotoxicity of interferon alfa-ribavirin therapy for chronic hepatitis C. *J Clin Gastroenterol* 2002; **35**: 89–92.

59 Dimitrov Y, Heibel F, Marcellin L, Chantrel F, Moulin B, Hannedouche T. Acute renal failure and nephrotic syndrome with alpha interferon therapy. *Nephrol Dial Transplant* 1997; **12**: 200–203.

60 Ohta S, Yokoyama H, Wada T, Sakai N, Shimizu M, Kato T et al. Exacerbation of glomerulonephritis in subjects with chronic hepatitis C infection after interferon therapy. *Am J Kidney Dis* 1999; **33**: 1040–1048.

61 Cooksley WG. Treatment of hepatitis B with interferon and combination therapy. *Clin Liver Dis* 2004; **8**: 353–370.

62 Cooksley WG. Treatment with interferons (including pegylated interferons) in patients with hepatitis B. *Semin Liver Dis* 2004; **1**: 45–53.

63 Marcellin P, Lau GK, Bonino F, Farci P, Hadziyannis S, Jin R et al. Peginterferon alfa-2a alone, lamivudine alone, and the two in combination in patients with Hbe Ag negative chronic hepatitis B. *N Engl J Med* 2004; **351**: 1206–1217.

64 Lau GK, Piratvisuth T, Luo KX, Marcellin P, Thonsawat S, Cooksley G et al. Peginterferon alfa, lamivudine, and the combination for Hbe Ag positive chronic hepatitis B. *N Engl J Med* 2005; **352**: 2682–2695.

65 Janssen HL, van Zonneveld M, Senturk H, Zeuzem S, Akarca US, Cakaloglu Y et al. Pegylated interferon alfa-2b alone or in combination with lamivudine for HBe Ag positive chronic hepatitis B: a randomised trial. *Lancet* 2005; **365**: 123–129.

66 Tang S, Lai FM, Lui YH, Tank CS, Kung NN, Ho YW et al. Lamivudine in hepatitis B-associated membranous nephropathy. *Kidney Int* 2005; **68**: 1750–1758.

67 Gan SI, Devlin SM, Scott-Douglas NW, Burak KW. Lamivudine for the treatment of membranous glomerulopathy secondary to chronic hepatitis B infection. *Can J Gastroenterol* 2005; **19**: 625–629.

68 Okuse C, Yotsuyanagi H, Yamada N, Ikeda H, Takahashi H, Suzuki M et al. Successful treatment of hepatitis B virus-associated membranous nephropathy with lamivudine. *Clin Nephrol* 2006; **65**: 53–56.

69 Filler G, et al: Another case of HBV associated membranous glomerulonephritis resolving on lamivudine. *Arch Dis Child* 2003; **88**: 460.

70 Connor FL, Rosenberg AR, Kennedy SE, Bohane TD. HBV-associated nephrotic syndrome: resolution with oral lamivudine. *Arch Dis Child* 2003; **88**: 446–449.

71 Lok AS, Lai CL, Leung N, Yao GB, Cui ZY, Schiff ER *et al*. Long term safety of lamivudine treatment in patients with chronic hepatitis B. *Gastroenterology* 2003; **125**: 1714–1722.

72 Marcellin P, Chang TT, Lim SG, Tong MJ, Sievert W, Shiffman ML *et al*. Adefovir dipivoxil for the treatment of HBe Ag positive chronic hepatitis B. *N Engl J Med* 2003; **348**: 808–816.

73 Hadziyannis SJ, et al: Adefovir dipivoxil for the treatment of HBe Ag negative hepatitis B. *N Engl J Med* 2003; **348**: 800–807.

74 Izzedine H, Hulot JS, Launay-Vacher V, Marcellini P, Hadziyannis SJ, Currie G *et al*. Renal safety of adefovir dipivoxil in patients with chronic hepatitis B: two double-blind randomized, placebo-controlled studies. *Kidney Int* 2004; **66**: 1153–1158.

75 Fontaine H, Vallet-Pichard A, Chaix ML, Currie G, Serpaggi J, Verkarre V *et al*. Efficacy and safety of adefovir dipivoxil in kidney recipients, hemodialysis patients, and patients with renal insufficiency. *Transplantation* 2005; **80**: 1086–1092.

76 Chang TT, Gish RG, de Man R, Gadano A, Sollano J, Chao YC *et al*. A comparison of entecavir and lamivudine for HBe Ag positive chronic hepatitis B. *N Engl J Med* 2006; **354**: 1001–1010.

77 Lai CL, Shouval D, Lok AS, Chang TT, Cheinquer H, Goodman Z *et al*. Entecavir versus lamivudine for patients with HBe Ag negative chronic hepatitis B. *N Engl J Med* 2006; **354**: 1011–1020.

78 Izzedine H, Isnard-Bagnis C, Hulot JS, Vittecoq D, Cheng A, Jais CK *et al*. Renal safety of tenofovir in HIV treatment experienced patients. *AIDS* 2004; **18**: 1074–1075.

79 Izzedine H, Launay-Vacher V, Deray G. Antiviral drug-induced nephrotoxicity. *Am J Kidney Dis* 2005; **45**: 804–817.

80 Anneli MG, Torres DD, Manno C, Scioscia C, Iannone F, Covelli M *et al*. Improvement of renal function and disappearance of hepatitis B virus DNA in a patient with rheumatoid arthritis and renal amyloidosis following treatment with infliximab. *Arthritis Rheum* 2005; **52**: 2519–2520.

81 Han SB. Extrahepatic manifestations of chronic hepatitis B. *Clin Liver Dis* 2004; **8**: 403–418.

82 Dienstag JL. Immunopathogenesis of the extrahepatic manifestations of hepatitis B virus infection. *Springer Semin Immunopathol* 1981; **3**: 461–472.

83 Schusterman N, London WT. Hepatitis B and immune complex disease. *N Engl J Med* 1984; **310**: 43–46.

84 Frye KH, Becker MJ, Theofilopoulos AN, Moutsopoulos H, Feldman JL, Talal N. Immune complexes in hepatitis B antigen-associated periarteritis nodosa: detection by antibody dependent cell-mediated cytotoxicity and the Raji cell assay. *Am J Med* 1977; **62**: 783–791.

85 Gocke DJ, Jsu K, Morgan C, Bombardieri S, Lockshin M, Christian CL. Association between polyarteritis and Australia antigen. *Lancet* 1970; **ii**: 1149–1153.

86 Michalak T. Immune complexes of hepatitis B surface antigen in the pathogenesis of periarteritis nodosa: a study of seven necropsy cases. *Am J Pathol* 1978; **90**: 619–632.

87 Trepo C, Guillevin L. Polyarteritis nodosa and extrahepatic manifestations of HBV infection: the case against autoimmune intervention in pathogenesis. *J Autoimmun* 2001; **16**: 269–274.

88 Colmegna I, Maldonado-Coco JA. Polyarteritis nodosa revisited. *Curr Rheumatol Rep* 2005; **7**: 288–296.

89 Deleaval P, Stadler P, Descombes E, Hecker E, Schrago G, Chizzolini C *et al*. Life threatening complications of HBV-related polyarteritis nodosa developing despite interferon alpha-2b therapy: successful treatment with a combination of interferon, lamivudine, plasma exchange and steroids. *Clin Rheumatol* 2001; **20**: 290–292.

90 Guillevin L, Lhote F, Sauvaget F, Deblois P, Rossi F, Levallois D *et al*. Treatment of polyarteritis nodosa related to hepatitis B virus with interferon alpha and plasma exchanges. *Ann Rheum Dis* 1994; **53**: 334–337.

91 Guillevin L, Lhote F, Cohen P, Sauvaget F, Jarrousse B, Lortholary O *et al*. Polyarteritis nodosa related to hepatitis B virus: a prospective study with long term observation of 41 patients. *Medicine* 1995; **74**: 238.

92 Guillevin L, Mahr A, Callard P, Godmer P, Pagnoux C, Leray E *et al*. Hepatitis B virus associated polyarteritis nodosa: clinical characteristics, outcome, and clinical impact of treatment in 115 patients. *Medicine* 2005; **84**: 313–322.

93 Levo Y, Gorevic PD, Kassab HJ, Zucker-Franklin D, Franklin EC. Association between hepatitis B virus and essential mixed cryoglobulinemia. *N Engl J Med* 1977; **296**: 1501–1504.

94 Ferri C, *et al*: Mixed cryoglobulinemia: demographic, clinical, and serologic features and survival in 231 patients. *Semin Arthritis Rheum* 2004; **33**: 355–374.

95 Wang NS, Wu ZL, Zhang YE, Liao LT. Existence and significance of hepatitis B virus DNA in kidneys of IgA nephropathy. *World J Gastroenterol* 2005; **11**: 712–716.

96 Ida H, Izumino K, Asaka M, Fujita M, Takata M, Sasayama S. IgA nephropathy and hepatitis B virus. IgA nephropathy unrelated to hepatitis B surface antigenemia. *Nephron* 1990; **54**: 18–20.

97 Lai KN, Lai FM, Lo S, Ho CP, Chan KW. IgA nephropathy associated with hepatitis B virus antigenemia. *Nephron* 1987; **47**: 141–143.

98 Lai KN, Lai FM. Clinical features and the natural course of hepatitis B virus related glomerulopathy in adults. *Kidney Int* 1991; **40**: S40–S45.

99 Takeda S, Kida H, Katagiri M, Yokoyama H, Abe T, Hattori N. Characteristics of glomerular lesions in hepatitis B virus infection. *Am J Kidney Dis* 1988; **11**: 57–62.

100 Fabrizi F, Bunnapradist S, Martin P. HBV infection in patients with end-stage renal disease. *Semin Liver Dis* 2004; **24**: 63–70.

101 Burdick RA, Bragg-Gresham JL, Woods JD, Hedderwick SA, Kurokawa K, Combe C *et al*. Patterns of hepatitis B prevalence and seroconversion in hemodialysis units from three continents. The DOPPS. *Kidney Int* 2003; **63**: 2222–2229.

102 Rodrigues A, Morgado T, Areias J, Silvestre F, Pinho L, Alves H *et al*. Limited benefits of IFN-alpha therapy in renal graft candidates with chronic viral hepatitis B or C. *Transplant Proc* 1997; **29**: 777–780.

103 Chan TM, Fang GX, Tang CS, Cheng I, Lai KN, Ho SK. Preemptive lamivudine therapy based on HBV DNA level in HBsAg-positive kidney allograft recipients. *Hepatology* 2002; **36**: 1246–1252.

104 Fornairon S, Pol S, Legendre C, Carnot F, Mamzer-Bruneel MF, Brechot C *et al*. The long-term virologic and pathologic impact of renal transplantation on chronic hepatitis B infection. *Transplantation* 1996; **62**: 297–299.

105 Aroldi A, Lampertico P, Montagnino G, Passerini P, Villa M, Campise MR *et al*. Natural history of hepatitis B and C in renal allograft recipients. *Transplantation* 2005; **79**: 1132–1136.

106 106. Schwarz A, Krause PH, Offermann G, Keller F. Impact of de novo membranous glomerulonephritis on the clinical course after kidney transplantation. *Transplantation* 1994; **58**: 650–654.

25 Infection-Related Nephropathies: Hepatitis C Virus

Dirk R. J. Kuypers

Department of Nephrology and Renal Transplantation, University Hospitals Leuven, University of Leuven, Belgium.

Introduction

Hepatitis C virus (HCV) infection not only causes chronic hepatitis and hepatocellular carcinoma but can also lead to extrahepatic disease, like mixed essential cryoglobulinemia (MEC), glomerulonephritides, and lymphoproliferative disorders. Autoimmune disorders and cutaneous and neurological diseases associated with HCV infection are less frequently reported [1]. The prevalence of blood donors carrying anti-HCV antibodies ranges geographically from 0.1 to 2.0% with generally increasing rates as one goes geographically from the north to the south of the globe with the exception of the African continent, in which HCV is more prevalent. HCV infection is also more prevalent in populations at risk of contamination, such as intravenous drug abusers, hemophiliacs, and dialysis patients. The prevalence of anti-HCV-positive patients undergoing maintenance dialysis in developed countries ranges from 3.4% (the Netherlands) to as high as 22.3% (Italy). Several genotypes of HCV (genotypes 1 to 5) have been identified and determine, to some extent, the outcome of liver disease and the response to antiviral therapy. Some genotypes (e.g. genotype 1b) are thought to be more virulent, whereas others are associated with low viremia (e.g. genotype 2). The geographical predominance of the different genotypes is well-documented [2–4].

Glomerular disease associated with HCV infection

The association between HCV infection and glomerulopathy or albuminuria has been extensively demonstrated by surveys of large at-risk populations as well as in autopsy studies, while the presence of cryoglobulinemia is a strong indicator of renal insufficiency in patients with HCV-associated glomerulonephritis [2,5–7]. Not all

types of glomerular disease that have been described in association with HCV infection are actually causally related. HCV infection is prevalent in 15% of patients diagnosed with membranoproliferative glomerulonephritis (MPGN), which is much higher than the expected HCV prevalence, and this number increases to as high as 96% when MPGN is associated with cryoglobulinemia. A much lower prevalence of HCV infection is documented in other types of glomerulonephritis, such as membranous glomerulonephritis (5.5%), minimal change glomerulopathy (4.4%), immunoglobulin A (IgA) nephropathy (2.1%), and focal glomerulosclerosis (4.4%), except when the latter occurs in intravenous drug abusers and HIV/AIDS patients, who are at increased risk for HCV infection. Fibrillar and immunotactoid glomerulopathy and thrombotic microangiopathy have been occasionally described in HCV-positive patients but without any evidence for a causal relationship.

Role of HCV infection in MPGN with type II mixed cryoglobulinemia

HCV-associated MPGN is triggered by the glomerular (subendothelial and mesangial) deposition of circulating immune complexes containing HCV RNA and anti-HCV IgG antibodies, possibly enhanced by impaired clearance of these complexes through the reticuloendothelial system of the HCV-infected liver [8,9]. Several studies have indicated the presence of viral RNA or proteins in renal tissue by using electron microscopy, antibodies against viral proteins, and reverse transcription-PCR (RT-PCR) techniques. Recently, with laser capture microdissection, it has been demonstrated that viral RNA is present in glomeruli of patients affected by different types of HCV-associated glomerulopathies while the viral core protein is predominantly present in the renal tubules [10–12]. It is hypothesized that this viral RNA and protein subsequently activate mesangial cell expression of Toll-like receptors (e.g. TLR3), triggering chemokine/cytokine release (e.g. RANTES, MCP, CCL) and *in situ* complement activation via the lectin (mannose-binding lectin) pathway with engagement of specific Fc receptors on leukocytes, leading to mesangial proliferation, inflammation, and

Evidence-based Nephrology. Edited by Donald Molony and Jonathan Craig
© 2009 Blackwell Publishing, ISBN: 978-1-4051-3975-5.

apoptosis [13–15]. The strong coincidence of MPGN with type II MEC and HCV infection (prevalence of 95% vs. 3% in patients with MPGN without MEC) seems to be the result of the high incidence of cryoglobulins (54%) in the latter group [7]. Some reports suggest that the appearance of cryoglobulins in HCV-infected patients with MPGN is determined by the viral genotype, viral load in peripheral blood leukocytes, anti-HCV IgG titer, and the presence of anti-endothelial cell autoantibodies, but none of these findings has been confirmed in larger controlled studies. Anti-HCV antibodies also bind to the vessel wall in skin biopsies of patients with cryoglobulins and cutaneous vasculitis, further illustrating a causal relationship between these two entities.

Clinical manifestations

Patients with HCV-associated MPGN present with moderate to severe proteinuria, microscopic hematuria, and signs of mild to moderate renal insufficiency in the majority of cases. An acute nephritic syndrome (macroscopic hematuria, severe proteinuria, hypertension, and renal insufficiency) at onset occurs in approximately 25% of cases, while more than 20% of patients are diagnosed with nephrotic syndrome [7,8]. Symptoms of cryoglobulinemia, such as palpable purpura and petechiae (leukocytoclastic vasculitis), arthritis/arthralgia, or peripheral neuropathy (mononeuritis multiplex), Raynaud's phenomenon, weakness, fever, and leg ulcers are present in only half of HCV-associated MPGN cases. Rare cases of pulmonary or myocardial involvement with myocarditis and cardiomyopathy have been reported. Signs of MEC can become manifest years before the renal diagnosis is made or appear concurrently in 10–15% of cases. Extrarenal symptoms fluctuate strongly and can be associated with exacerbations of the renal disease, but they are not always present. Physical signs of liver disease are rare, whereas 60–70% of patients have mildly elevated transaminases. Arterial hypertension requiring therapy occurs in 80% of patients [1,7,8].

The clinical course of HCV-associated MPGN varies, with nearly one-third of patients experiencing a spontaneous remission of renal symptoms. In another one-third of patients urinary abnormalities persist, and renal disease is characterized by an indolent course without progression to kidney failure. About 20% of patients suffer from reversible clinical relapses, sometimes accompanied by signs of systemic involvement. Prognostic factors for MPGN with MEC II are age (>50 years), purpura, high cryocrit (>10%), low serum C3 levels, proteinuria, and high serum creatinine (>1.5 mg/dL). Although some degree of renal function impairment will eventually develop in the course of disease (or is already present at the time of diagnosis), end-stage renal failure occurs in only 10–15% of patients [1,8,16]. A recent large US survey confirmed an age-dependent association between HCV seropositivity and albuminuria, but no association with a low glomerular filtration rate (GFR) [17]. Patients with cryoglobulinemic GN have a 10-year survival of 50–60%; mortality is the result of cardiovascular complications, infections, liver failure, and malignancies.

Cryoglobulins can be detected in about 50–66% of affected patients, and HCV RNA is concentrated over 100-fold relative to serum in the cryoprecipitate. Cryoglobulins are typically composed of polyclonal IgG anti-HCV antibodies and a monoclonal IgMκ rheumatoid factor (type II MEC); occasionally, a type III mixed cryoglobulins is found. Hepatitis C virus RNA and antibodies are detected in more than 90% of affected patients. Hypocomplementemia (low CH50, C4, C1q, and to a lesser extent C3) is present, as is a positive monoclonal IgMκ rheumatoid factor. None of the latter laboratory parameters seems to correlate with clinical disease activity. Other symptoms related to extrahepatic manifestations of HCV infection include monoclonal gammopathy, lymphoma (B-cell non-Hodgkin's lymphoma, immunocytoma, extranodal marginal zone B-cell lymphoma of MALT type), autoimmune hemolytic anemia or thrombocytopenia, porphyria cutanea tarda, lichen planus, necrolytic acral erythema, chronic corneal ulcerations (Mooren's ulcer), polyarteritis nodosa, autoimmune thyroiditis, and other autoimmune disorders like sialadenitis, leading to sicca syndrome and autoimmune hepatitis (with anti-LKM-1 antibodies). Low titers of autoantibodies (ANF, anti-LKM-1, anti-GOR, anti-smooth muscle, and anti-cardiolipin antibodies) are detected in 40–65% of HCV-positive patients but rarely cause clinical disease [1].

Renal pathology

MPGN is the most common type of glomerulonephritis associated with HCV infection, accounting for approximately 54% of patients. The light microscopic histological pattern of HCV-associated type I MPGN, sometimes called "cryoglobulinaemic glomerulonephritis," is that of an exudative type of MPGN with thickening of the glomerular basement membrane with a "double-contour" appearance caused by interposition of monocytes rather than mesangial cells [2]. A picture of lobular glomerulonephritis is sometimes evident in cases of massive mesangial proliferation and infiltration by monocytes together with mesangial matrix expansion. Endocapillary proliferation is usually extensive (monocytes), and a striking feature of MPGN with MEC II is the presence of amorphous eosinophilic periodic acid-Schiff-positive intraluminal deposits that fill or completely obliterate the capillary lumen (intraluminal thrombi) (Figure 25.1A). These deposits are precipitated cryoglobulins of variable sizes and diffusion rates and consist of IgG and IgM, the latter having the identical idiotype of the circulating monoclonal IgM rheumatoid factor. Immunofluorescence shows not only diffuse granular staining of IgG, IgM, and C3 in peripheral glomerular loops, similar to idiopathic MPGN, but also strong intraluminal staining of the intraluminal thrombi (Figure 25.1C and D). Interstitial infiltration by a mixed monocyte–lymphocyte cell population is usually found in the acute stages of disease and can progress to interstitial fibrosis, while about one-third of biopsies show small and medium-size vessels with signs of fibrinoid necrosis and vascular wall infiltration by monocytes (vasculitis), especially in strong exudative forms of MPGN. Electron

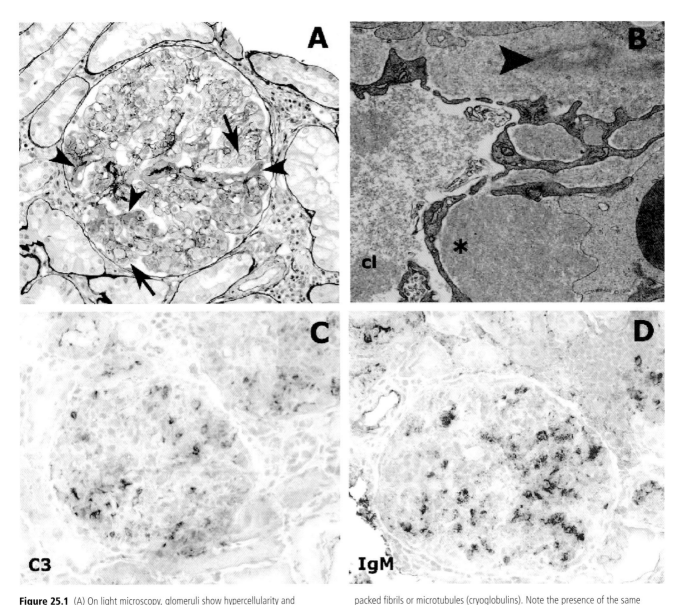

Figure 25.1 (A) On light microscopy, glomeruli show hypercellularity and mesangial expansion. The glomerular capillary walls are thickened with interposition of predominantly monocytes (arrows). Note the intraluminal presence of thrombi consisting of cryoglobulins. (Original magnification, 200×.) (B) On electron microscopy, electron-dense deposits are present in the subendothelial space (asterisk) and the mesangium (arrowhead). These deposits consist of densely packed fibrils or microtubules (cryoglobulins). Note the presence of the same material in the lumen of the glomerular capillary (cl). (Original magnification, 10,000×.) (C) C3 positivity along the capillary walls and in the thrombi. (Original magnification, 200×.) (D) IgM positivity along the capillary walls and in the thrombi. (Original magnification, 200×.) Courtesy of Evelyne Lerut, Department of Pathology, University of Leuven, Belgium.

microscopy can identify the fibrillar structure of the subendothelial cryoglobulin deposits with cylindrical bodies of 0.1–1 μm in length and an annular shape on cross-section consisting of a dense ring with a clear center (Figure 25.1B). A picture of mild mesangial proliferation without significant capillary wall thickening or intraluminal thrombi is encountered in about 10% of patients and is more difficult to distinguish from idiopathic MPGN. Other types of glomerulonephritis associated with HCV infection, like membranous glomerulonephritis, focal glomerulosclerosis, and IgA nephropathy, have been frequently described and their histological appearance does not differ dramatically from the primary glomerulopathies. These types of glomerulonephritis are discussed elsewhere in this textbook.

Treatment

Although specific studies demonstrating an effect of nonimmunosuppressive therapy on HCV-related nephropathy are lacking, symptomatic treatment, similar to that advocated for any proteinuric nephropathy, is advised in all patients with HCV-related glomerulonephritis. It consists of rigorous blood pressure control using salt restriction and angiotensin converting enzyme inhibitors alone or in combination with angiotensin receptor antagonists and loop diuretics. If additional antihypertensive therapy is required, calcium channel blockers might have a theoretical advantage over beta-blockers, as the latter could potentially aggravate extrarenal disease symptoms like Raynaud's phenomenon, necrolytic acral erythema, and leg ulcers. In case of nephrotic syndrome, statins are recommended for the treatment of hyperlipidemia, whereas guidelines concerning routine anticoagulation are lacking. Often, prophylactic dosing of low-molecular-weight heparin is necessary because of the presence of additional prothrombotic risk factors [18].

Antiviral therapy has been extensively tried in HCV-positive patients presenting with glomerulonephritis in an attempt to clear the virus from the serum and thereby improve renal outcome [19,20]. In the 1990s, subcutaneous alpha interferon (IFN-α) was tested in various small uncontrolled studies and described in numerous case reports. The overall results of these trials were disappointing; even with initial clearance of HCV and stabilization or improvement in renal function and/or proteinuria, relapses occurred in the majority of patients as soon as IFN-α therapy, even prolonged therapy lasting 6–12 months, was stopped. The concomitant use of corticosteroids did not significantly alter outcome. The combination of IFN-α or pegylated IFN-α with ribavirin, a guanosine analog with immune-modulating properties, has now become standard treatment for HCV-infected patients without kidney disease, because of a higher efficacy, compared with prolonged IFN-α monotherapy, which resulted in a sustained virological response in only 30% of treated patients [21]. Subsequently, this combination strategy was tested in HCV-related glomerulonephritis. Sabry *et al.* combined IFN-α therapy, 3 million units (MU) three times weekly, with ribavirin at a daily dose of 15 mg/kg body weight for 12 months, in cases where 3 months of IFN-α therapy alone did not clear the virus from serum. Five of 20 patients completely cleared the HCV, while C3 and C4 levels normalized in all patients. Furthermore, proteinuria decreased from 4 to 1.1 g/24 h, and renal function stabilized in the majority of patients (75%). Gastrointestinal and flu-like symptoms attributed to IFN-α were less pronounced in patients receiving combined therapy [22]. Alric *et al.* combined IFN-α (3 MU, three times per week) or pegylated IFN-α (1.5 μg/kg weekly) with ribavirin at 600–1000 mg/day for a mean period of 18 months in 18 patients with HCV-related cryoglobulinemic MPGN after completion of first-line treatment with prednisone or plasmapheresis. During a mean follow-up period of 17 months, a sustained virological response was obtained with this regimen in 67% of patients, whereas renal function stabilized and proteinuria and cryocrit decreased significantly [23]. These and other [24] studies illustrate that it is important to prolong combined IFN-α and ribavirin therapy for a sufficient length of time in order to reduce the number of flare-ups. Until data from controlled studies are available, it is advised that this combination be administered for at least 48 weeks (Table 25.1). Strong dose reductions of ribavirin are frequently necessary because of side effects, like hemolytic anemia, and in the event of impaired renal function. Anemia can occur at therapeutic drug concentrations

Table 25.1 Treatment of HCV-related glomerulonephritis.

Treatment steps

Step I: Symptomatic therapy
- Loop diuretics, angiotensin converting enzyme inhibitors, angiotensin receptor antagonists
- Statins, anticoagulation in case of associated nephrotic syndrome

Step II: Antiviral therapy for 48 wks
- Standard IFN-α therapy, 3×10^6 U, 3 times/wk, or pegylated IFN-α, 1.5 μg/kg/wk in combination with ribavirin, 15 mg/kg/day adapted to creatinine clearance
- Supportive therapy with erythropoietin and low-dose iron when required

Step III: Immunosuppressive induction therapy in cases of severe acute disease
- Methylprednisolone pulse therapy, 0.5–1 g/day for 3 days, followed by oral maintenance therapy and/or cyclophosphamide, 1–2 mg/kg/day
- Plasma exchange, 3 L plasma, 3 times/wk for 2–6 wks
- Rituximab, 375 mg/m^2/wk for 4 wks[a] followed by antiviral therapy for 48 wks (Step II)

[a] See text for details.

(trough plasma concentrations between 10 and 15 μmol/L) and often requires supportive therapy with erythropoietin and low-dose iron.

Acute flares of HCV-related cryoglobulinemic MPGN with rapidly progressive renal function deterioration and/or severe cryoglobulinemic disease will often not respond to antiviral therapy alone and require additional immunosuppressive therapy in order to control inflammatory reactions and vascular manifestations due to cryoglobulin deposition. Short courses of corticosteroids (preferably pulses) with cytotoxic drugs, with or without plasmapheresis, may be needed to decrease cryoglobulin production and deposition [18,19] (Table 25.1). This aggressive induction therapy, although effective, is usually poorly tolerated and is associated with serious infectious complications. Therefore, the judicious use of corticosteroids and cyclophosphamide with or without plasmapheresis should be based on the severity of symptoms and should be reserved for patients with rapid renal function deterioration, nephrotic syndrome, and/or vascular manifestations [8,19]. The clinical indications for plasmapheresis in addition to corticosteroids and cytotoxic agents have not yet been clearly defined. Plasmapheresis is often initiated in order to achieve rapid removal of circulating cryoglobulins, thereby preventing further deposition. The latter is especially important in cases of massive glomerular precipitation, signs of renal vasculitis, and severe extrarenal systemic vasculitis [8]. Prolonged plasmapheresis treatment for 2–6 weeks in combination with immunosuppressive therapy is advised in order to avoid early rebound. After the acute phase is controlled, causative antiviral treatment should be rapidly commenced, especially because prior induction immunosuppressive therapy will have increased HCV viral load with potentially detrimental effects on the underlying liver disease.

Recently, rituximab, a monoclonal anti-CD20 antibody selectively targeting B lymphocytes, has been used successfully in patients with HCV-related cryoglobulinemic MPGN, both as first-line treatment and after failure of conventional therapy [25,26].

Rapid and sustained renal responses were observed in 50–100% of cases, taking into account that only small heterogeneous patient groups were studied until now. Disease relapses seem to respond to rechallenge with the drug, while side effects have been overall limited except in one small study where serious infectious complications (*Cryptococcus neoformans* meningoencephalitis and herpes simplex type 2 pneumonitis) were encountered. Close vigilance for opportunistic infections is therefore warranted. Initial dosing of rituximab is four consecutive weekly intravenous courses of 375 mg/m^2 of body surface. HCV viral load remains remarkably stable or even decreases mildly during rituximab therapy, in contrast to other immunosuppressive therapies. Interestingly, a patient homozygous for the high-affinity (VV) allele of FcγRIIIa (CD16) had a long sustained remission after one course of rituximab, suggesting that, as described for systemic lupus erythematosus, FcγRIIIa genotyping could play a future role in predicting responses to anti-CD20 therapy in HCV-related MPGN. Randomized controlled studies with sufficient prolonged follow-up are of course necessary in order to establish the efficacy of rituximab in HCV-related cryoglobulinemic MPGN in comparison to combined IFN-α–ribavirin therapy. Until efficacy and safety data from these studies are available, rituximab should only be considered in cases of failure of antiviral therapy for moderate HCV-related MPGN or if the combination of corticosteroids and cyclophosphamide (with or without plasmapheresis) cannot control progression of severe disease (kidney failure, nephrotic syndrome, or vascular manifestations) or is poorly tolerated.

References

1 Medina J, Garcia-Buey L, Moreno-Otero R. Review article: hepatitis C virus-related extra-hepatic disease. Aetiopathogenesis and management. *Aliment Pharmacol Ther* 2004; **20:** 129–141.

2 Pouteil-Noble C, Maiza H, Dijoud F, MacGregor B. Glomerular disease associated with hepatitis C virus infection in native kidneys. *Nephrol Dial Transplant* 2000; **15(Suppl 8):** 28–33.

3 Fabrizi F, Pozzi C, Farina M, Dattolo P, Lunghi G, Badalamenti S et al. Hepatitis C virus infection and acute or chronic glomerulonephritis: an epidemiological and clinical appraisal. *Nephrol Dial Transplant* 1998; **13:** 1991–1997.

4 Giannico G, Manno C, Schena FP. Treatment of glomerulonephritides associated with hepatitis C virus infection. *Nephrol Dial Transplant* 2000; **15(Suppl 8):** 34–38.

5 Sabry A, El-Agroudy A, Sheashaa H, El-husseini A, Taha NM, Elbaz M et al. Histological characterization of HCV-associated glomerulopathy in Egyptian patients. *Int Urol Nephrol* 2005; **37:** 355–361.

6 Gopalani A, Ahuja TS. Prevalence of glomerulopathies in autopsies of patients infected with the hepatitis C virus. *Am J Med Sci* 2001; **322(2):** 57–60.

7 Fabrizi F, Colucci P, Ponticelli C, Locatelli F. Kidney and liver involvement in cryoglobulinemia. *Semin Nephrol* 2002; **22(4):** 309–318.

8 D'Amico G. Renal involvement in hepatitis C infection: cryoglobulinemic glomerulonephritis. *Kidney Int* 1998; **54:** 650–671.

9 Roccatello D, Morsica G, Picciotto G, Cesano G, Ropolo R, Bernardi MT et al. Impaired hepatosplenic elimination of circulating cryoglobulins in patients with essential mixed cryoglobulinaemia and hepatitis C virus (HCV) infection. *Clin Exp Immunol* 1997; **110:** 9–14.

10 Hoch B, Juknevicius I, Liapis H. Glomerular injury associated with hepatitis C infection: a correlation with blood and tissue HCV-PCR. *Semin Diagn Pathol* 2002; **19(3):** 175–187.

11 Rodriguez-Inigo E, Casqueiro M, Bartolomé J, Barat A, Caramelo C, Ortiz A et al. Hepatitis C virus RNA in kidney biopsies from infected patients with renal diseases. *J Viral Hepat* 2000; **7:** 23–29.

12 Sansonno D, Lauletta G, Montrone M, Grandaliano G, Schena FP, Dammacco F. Hepatitis C virus RNA and core protein in kidney glomerular and tubular structures isolated with laser capture microdissection. *Clin Exp Immunol* 2005; **140:** 498–506.

13 Smith KD, Alpers CE. Pathogenic mechanisms in membranoproliferative glomerulonephritis. *Curr Opin Nephol Hypertens* 2005; **14:** 396–403.

14 Wörnle M, Schmid H, Banas B, Merkle M, Henger A, Roeder M et al. Novel role of toll-like receptor 3 in hepatitis C-associated glomerulonephritis. *Am J Pathol* 2006; **168(2):** 370–385.

15 Endo M, Ohsawa I, Ohi H, Fujita T, Matsushita M, Fujita T. Mannose-binding lectin contributes to glomerulonephritis induced by hepatitis C virus infection. *Nephron* 2001; **87:** 374–375.

16 Roccattello D, Fornasieri A, Giachino O, Rossi D, Beltrame A, Banfi G et al. Multicenter study on hepatitis C virus-related cryoglobulinemic glomerulonephritis. *Am J Kidney Dis* 2006; **49:** 69–82.

17 Tsui JI, Vittinghoff E, Shlipak MG, O'Hare AM. Relationship between hepatitis C and chronic kidney disease: results from the Third National Health and Nutrition Examination Survey. *J Am Soc Nephrol* 2006; **17(4):** 1168–1174.

18 Kamar N, Rostaing L, Alric L. Treatment of hepatitis C-virus-related glomerulonephritis. *Kidney Int* 2006; **69:** 436–439.

19 Garini G, Allegri L, Vaglio A, Buzio C. Hepatitis C virus-related cryoglobulinemia and glomerulonephritis: pathogenesis and therapeutic strategies. *Ann Ital Med Int* 2005; **20(2):** 71–80.

20 Mazzaro C, Panarello G, Carniello S, Faelli A, Mazzi G, Crovatto M et al. Interferon versus steroids in patients with hepatitis C virus-associated cryoglobulinaemic glomerulonephritis. *Dig Liver Dis* 2000; **32:** 708–715.

21 Manns M, McHuchinson JG, Gordon SC. Peginterferon alfa 2b plus ribavirin compared with interferon alfa 2b plus ribavirin for initial treatment of chronic hepatitis C: a randomized trial. *Lancet* 2001; **358:** 958–965.

22 Sabry AA, Sobh MA, Sheaashaa HA, Kudesia G, Wild G, Fox S et al. Effect of combination therapy (ribavirin and interferon) in HCV-related glomerulopathy. *Nephrol Dial Transplant* 2002; **17:** 1924–1930.

23 Alric L, Plaisier E, Thébault S, Péron J, Rostiang L, Purrat J et al. Influence of antiviral therapy in hepatitis C virus-associated cryoglobulinemic MPGN. *Am J Kidney Dis* 2004; **43(4):** 617–623.

24 Bruchfeld A, Lindahl K, Stahle L, Söderberg M, Schvarcz R. Interferon and ribavirin treatment in patients with hepatitis C-associated renal disease and renal insufficiency. *Nephrol Dial Transplant* 2003; **18:** 1573–1580.

25 Quartuccio L, Soardo G, Romano G, Zaja F, Scott CA, De Marchi G et al. Rituximab treatment for glomerulonephritis in HCV-associated mixed cryoglobulinaemia: efficacy and safety in the absence of steroids. *Rheumatology* 2006; **45:** 842–846.

26 Basse G, Ribes D, Kamar N, Mehrenberger M, Esposito L, Guitard J et al. Rituximab therapy for de novo mixed cryoglobulinemia in renal transplant patients. *Transplantation* 2005; **80(11):** 1560–1564.

26 Polyomavirus-Associated Nephropathy

Fabrizio Ginevri[1] & Hans H. Hirsch[2,3]

[1] Pediatric Nephrology Unit, Istituto G. Gaslini, Genova, Italy
[2] Transplantation Virology & Molecular Diagnostics, Institute for Medical Microbiology, University of Basel, Basel, Switzerland
[3] Infectious Diseases & Hospital Epidemiology, University Hospital Basel, Basel, Switzerland

Introduction

Polyomavirus-associated nephropathy (PVAN) currently represents the most challenging infectious cause of renal dysfunction in kidney transplant recipients. Centers from around the world report PVAN rates of 1–10% during the first 2 years post-transplant [1,2]. Over the following 6–62 months from diagnosis of PVAN, irreversible graft dysfunction and return to dialysis is seen in more than half of the cases [1–4]. Molecular genetic techniques have identified polyomavirus hominis type 1, also called BK virus (BKV), as the principle etiologic agent [5,6]. Less than 10% of PVAN cases with a seemingly milder clinical course have been attributed to the closely related human polyomavirus type 2, also called JC virus [7,8], which is known as the primary cause of a rare demyelinating central nervous system disease in HIV/AIDS, but also occasionally in kidney transplant patients called progressive multifocal leukoencephalopathy [9]. No specific antiviral agent is licensed for treating polyomavirus diseases, and current interventions rely on improving antiviral immunity.

Although single cases of PVAN were reported in the 1970s [10], the recent surge of PVAN after almost 50 years of kidney transplantation is remarkable and, given the unchanged epidemiology of BKV, points to significant changes in current transplant protocols as the cause. BKV infects more than 80% of the world's population during childhood and without specific clinical symptoms. Subsequently, the viral DNA genome persists latently in the reno-urinary tract. In approximately 5% of BKV-infected seropositive adults, asymptomatic BKV shedding is intermittently detectable, typically at low viral loads of $<10^6$ per mL [11,12]. Among patients with impaired immune function, for example, following cancer chemotherapy, advanced HIV infection, or immunosuppression associated with transplant procedures, the prevalence of urinary BKV replication increases to 20–60% and with higher BKV loads of $>10^7$ per mL. Outright BKV disease is rare and almost always associated with significant immune dysfunction in conjunction with specific procedures, such as kidney transplantation for PVAN or bone marrow transplantation for late-onset hemorrhagic cystitis [11]. Here, we review the current evidence and recommendations regarding diagnosis and clinical management of PVAN in kidney transplantation.

Definitions

Grading of the evidence and strength of recommendations is based on a multidisciplinary position paper published in 2005 [1] and standards proposed by the Infectious Diseases Society of America (summarized in Table 26.1) [13]. Note that the grading system in this chapter is different from that presented in the rest of this book, but it has been retained to ensure consistency with how the recommendations were developed. The grading system used for quality is largely study design-based and does not explicitly consider other dimensions of quality of evidence, such as consistency, precision, design, and reporting quality, and relevance of outcomes measured and reported. The strength of recommendations is also largely determined by study design and other components; for example, benefit–harm trade-offs are not explicitly considered. Generally, however, it is likely that a level A recommendation would correspond to a level I recommendation using the GRADE system adopted for this book.

To better compare the results of the various studies, BKV infection, replication, and disease are defined as evidence for past virus exposure, active multiplication, and organ-invasive disease, respectively [14]. Possible PVAN is defined as detectable BKV replication in urine after kidney transplantation. Presumptive PVAN is defined as plasma BKV loads for ≥ 4 weeks of $>10,000$ copies/mL or an equivalent threshold [15], whereas definitive PVAN is defined as histological evidence of BKV replication and cytopathology in tissue samples (Table 26.2) [1].

Evidence-based Nephrology. Edited by Donald Molony and Jonathan Craig
© 2009 Blackwell Publishing, ISBN: 978-1-4051-3975-5.

Table 26.1 Evidence levels and clinical recommendations according to IDSA standards.

Category and grade	Definition
Strength of recommendation	
A	Good evidence to support a recommendation for use
B	Moderate evidence to support a recommendation for use
C	Poor evidence to support a recommendation
D	Moderate evidence to support a recommendation against use
E	Good evidence to support a recommendation against use
Quality of evidence	
I	Evidence from ≥1 properly randomized, controlled trial
II	Evidence from ≥1 well-designed clinical trial, without randomization; from cohort or case-controlled analytic studies (preferably from >1 center); from multiple time series; or dramatic results from uncontrolled experiments
III	Evidence from opinions of respected authorities, based on clinical experience, descriptive studies, or reports of expert committees

Source: Kish 2001 [13].

Abbreviations: IDSA, Infectious Diseases Society of America.

Pathogenesis of PVAN

The pathogenesis of PVAN is not well-understood in detail, but it is undisputed that persistent BKV replication in renal tubular epithelial cells is the central process. Mathematical modeling of BKV dynamics in kidney transplant patients has provided first estimates of fast kinetics with a short BKV half-life of <2 h giving rise to high daily BKV plasma turnover rates of 99% and direct replication-attributable loss of $>10^6$ tubular epithelial cells per day [evidence level II] [16]. Failure to mount and maintain sufficient BKV-specific immune control is viewed as the key permissive factor [level II] [17–20]. In addition, factors (re-)activating BKV replication may come from epithelial injury and regeneration following ischemia, allo-immune responses, drug toxicities,

and drug effects in accordance with murine models [level III] [10,21–23]. Thus, long-lasting disruption of the balance between BKV-activating and -restricting host factors gives rise to progressive organ pathology [24,25] and eventually to outgrowth of more pathogenic BKV variants [26]. In clinics, onset of BKV viruria has been the first indicator of BKV replication which precedes BKV viremia and histologically confirmed "definitive" PVAN by 1–3 months [II] [6,27–29]. Conversely, declining BKV loads in blood and urine are the first marker of resolving PVAN after reducing immunosuppression [evidence level II] [6,27,28]. Thus, quantification of BKV replication has become the pivotal surrogate marker of the risk of PVAN [1].

Risk factors

Various risk factors in the triad of recipient, graft, and virus have been associated with PVAN in kidney transplantation [14]. However, the results of individual studies were often not independently confirmed, making it difficult to interpret the evidence level. In larger retrospective series of more than 60 adult cases, older age (53 vs. 46 years; $P = 0.001$), male recipients, and white ethnicity were found to be associated with PVAN, whereas prior rejection episodes or type of calcineurin inhibitor use were not [2,30]. In a recent adult case–control study matched 1:3 for PVAN in 4-month control biopsies enrolling 19 cases, PVAN was not associated with age, male gender, or white race, but with female donor gender [31]. However, an analysis of a large US database comprising 267 cases of PVAN identified younger age of <20 years, black ethnicity, deceased donor kidney, and prior rejection episodes in addition to male gender as risk factors of PVAN [32]. Despite the large number of patients in this study, uncertainties may have resulted from inclusion of pediatric patients, who are known to develop PVAN at a younger age [33,34]. Preliminary results from a large prospective multicenter study enrolling more than 500 adult *de novo* kidney transplant patients identified no association of BKV viruria, viremia, or viral loads with age, gender, or race but with tacrolimus-compared to cyclosporine-based immunosuppression, and steroid

Table 26.2 PVAN screening, diagnosis, and management in kidney transplant recipients.

Management approach	Testing result	PVAN	Intervention indicated?
Step 1) screening	Positive, with decoy cells in urine cytology, BKV DNA in urine or plasma, BKV RNA in urine	Possible	No [D-III]
Step 2) confirmation	Plasma BKV DNA load >4 $\log_{10}$/mL for >4 weeks Urine BKV VP1 mRNA load >6 $\log_{10}$/mL	Presumptive	Yes [B-II]
Step 3) biopsy	Positive PVAN A: viral cytopathology, mild inflammatory infiltrates, tubular atrophy and fibrosis PVAN B: significant inflammatory infiltrates, mild or moderate tubular atrophy or fibrosis PVAN C: significant fibrosis, variable scores for tubular atrophy, inflammatory infiltrates, or viral cytopathology	Definitive	Yes [A-II]
Step 4) monitoring	Negative Plasma BKV DNA load <2 $\log_{10}$/mL	Resolved	No [D-II]

exposure [35]. Clearly, future validation of risk factors for adult and pediatric kidney transplant recipients will depend on well-designed prospective randomized studies or cohort studies of sufficient sample size.

Intensified immunosuppression with newer, more potent agents has reduced acute rejection episodes in the past decade but also coincided with the emergence of PVAN [1]. With few exceptions, PVAN has been diagnosed in patients receiving triple combinations of immunosuppressive drugs from all classes. However, combinations of tacrolimus and mycophenolate mofetil are more frequently encountered compared to cyclosporine and mycophenolate mofetil [evidence level II] according to retrospective series and case–control studies [5,36,37], cohort studies [38], and large prospectively randomized studies enrolling 200 [28] and >500 patients [35]. The use of steroids [evidence level II] [3,5,27,35,37,39] or antilymphocyte preparations [III] [27,39,40] for the treatment of rejection was associated with BKV replication if maintenance immunosuppression was continued or intensified. This is in contrasted to more favorable courses of PVAN with concurrent acute rejection when steroid treatment for acute rejection is coupled to decreasing maintenance immunosuppression [III] [27,39,41].

Clinical management

Screening for polyomavirus BKV replication

Polyomavirus replication emerged as the single common feature of all kidney transplant patients at risk of PVAN [I] [6,12,25,27,33,42]. The results from prospective studies indicate that BKV replication in the urine examined by either urine cytology or DNA PCR precedes BKV viremia by a median of 4 weeks and histologically documented PVAN by a median of 12 weeks [II] [27,28,35]. Screening for BKV replication may allow for earlier diagnosis and intervention with improved allograft outcome [II] [27–29,43,44]. Conversely, the negative predictive value of polyomavirus replication of >90% is helpful to rule out PVAN [II] [6,8,33]. In a medical decision analysis from North America, screening for BKV viremia was estimated to be cost-saving and to increase the quality of life if PVAN rates exceeded 2.1% [45]. Since transient, self-limiting BKV replication has been observed in renal allograft recipients [II] [6,27,28,43], repeat testing and quantification of BKV DNA load in plasma [27,46] or VP1 mRNA load in urine has been proposed [42]. For viral loads increasing above thresholds, that is, BKV load of >10,000 copies/mL of plasma or VP1 mRNA load of 1,000,000 copies/ng of total urine RNA, a specificity and sensitivity of ≥93% for biopsy-positive PVAN has been reported [II] [1,42,47]. Persisting BKV loads above the threshold equivalents for >3 weeks are highly suggestive of PVAN ("presumptive PVAN") (Table 26.2) [II] [1,46,48], but assay standardization is needed to validate center-specific thresholds [15].

To balance cost and screening efficiency, patients may be screened at least every 3 months during the first 2 years posttransplantation [A-II] and annually thereafter until the fifth year posttransplantation [B-III]. In addition, screening assays ought to be part of the work-up for the subpopulation of kidney transplant patients with allograft dysfunction [A-II] or undergoing allograft biopsy for surveillance [B-II]. Positive screening results ("possible PVAN") (Table 26.2) should be confirmed within 4 weeks [A-II]. For BKV replication above thresholds levels (presumptive PVAN) (Table 26.2), confirmation by allograft biopsy should be sought [A-II] and reduction of maintenance immunosuppression should be considered [B-II]. To monitor the course of BKV replication, quantitative polyomavirus testing in plasma and urine should be performed every 2–4 weeks [B-II], until a decrease below detection is observed [B-III].

Diagnosis of PVAN

PVAN is characterized by intranuclear polyomavirus inclusion bodies in tubular epithelial and/or glomerular parietal cells [I] [3,49,50]. The alterations seen by light microscopy are characteristic, but not pathognomonic, for PVAN and need to be distinguished from other etiologies, for example, cytomegalovirus or adenovirus inclusion, by confirmatory studies, such as immunohistochemistry or *in situ* hybridization to identify polyomavirus proteins like large T-antigen or VP-1, or viral nucleic acids, respectively [I]. Although immunohistochemistry may increase the sensitivity of PVAN diagnosis, discordance of PVAN detection in simultaneously obtained needle biopsy cores may be as high as 30%, pointing to a significant risk of false-negative diagnosis [II] [25]. BKV replication tends to affect nephrons focally with initially predominantly cytopathic changes (PVAN A) followed by more extensive spread with increasing inflammatory infiltrates (PVAN B) and eventually significant tubular atrophy and fibrosis (PVAN C) [II] [25,50]. Clinically, progression from PVAN A to PVAN B and C is associated with increasing rates of kidney transplant loss from 10 to 50% and >90%, respectively [25,46,51]. However, PVAN B and C are morphologically and molecularly difficult to distinguish from acute rejection and chronic allograft nephropathy, respectively [II] [10,54,55].

Thus, the definitive diagnosis of PVAN requires evaluation of a renal biopsy, with demonstration of polyomavirus cytopathic changes and confirmation with an ancillary technique such as immunohistochemistry ("definitive PVAN") (Table 26.2) [A-II]. PVAN histology should be semiquantitatively assessed as PVAN A, B, or C by taking into account the extent of viral cytopathic changes and the extent of inflammatory infiltrates, tubular atrophy, and fibrosis according to the Banff classification [B-II]. Negative biopsy results and signs of acute rejection are best interpreted in the light of BKV load testing in blood and urine [A-II]. In cases with significant BKV replication above threshold levels (presumptive PVA) (Table 26.2) and a negative initial biopsy, adjunct studies (e.g. immunohistochemistry) should be used and, if negative, a rebiopsy should be considered [B-III].

Treatment of PVAN

Antiviral drugs with proven clinical benefit are currently not available for treatment of polyomavirus infection. Nevertheless, control of viral replication has been reported in case series [56] which used sole reduction of immunosuppression [2,4,27,41,51,57], combined treatment of reducing immunosuppression with the antiviral drug cidofovir [51,58–61], with intravenous immunoglobulin preparations (IVIG) [51,62], or with the immunosuppressive drug leflunomide [63,64]. Given the lack of controlled trials and the heterogeneity of intervention protocols, there is as yet no consensus on a "standard" approach to the treatment of PVAN (Table 26.3).

Reduction of immunosuppression

Immunological studies have suggested that reducing immunosuppression allows for recovery of BKV-specific immunity [17,20]. Reduction of calcineurin inhibitor levels or reduction or discontinuation of mycophenolate mofetil dosage prevented progression of persistent BKV viremia ("presumptive PVAN") to histologically proven "definitive PVAN" [II] [28,44]. Rescue of functional allografts could be obtained in more than 90% of prospectively diagnosed cases with definitive PVAN [II] [27,29,44,65], but glomerular filtration rates often remained permanently impaired [II] [4,14,29,51,52,53]. Analysis of plasma BKV load kinetics after reducing immunosuppression indicated a mean efficacy of 20% and suggested biweekly monitoring after a lag of 4–8 weeks until clearance from plasma could be expected over the next 7–13 weeks [II] [16]. Following the reduction of immunosuppression, biopsy-proven acute rejection was rarely observed, but some reported rates of 25% that remain steroid-responsive without recurrence of PVAN [III] [3,39].

The most frequently reported strategies for reducing the immunosuppressive load are as follows:

- Reduce calcineurin inhibitor trough levels. Tacrolimus C_0 trough level are targeted to <6 ng/mL. Cyclosporine C_0 levels are targeted to <125 μg/mL [B-II].
- Reduce antiproliferative agent by 50% of standard dose. Mycophenolate mofetil is then reduced to ≤1 g/day in adult patients or ≤600 mg/m^2/day in pediatric patients. Azathioprine is reduced to <75 mg/day in adult patients or <40 mg/m^2/day in pediatric patients [B-II].
- Switching from mycophenolate mofetil to leflunomide (levels >40 μg/mL) has been advocated because inhibitory activity of leflunomide on BKV replication has been reported in vitro, although with a low selectivity index [66], but a direct comparison with sole immunosuppression reduction has not been reported [B-III].
- Discontinuing components of triple-drug therapies (mostly mycophenolate mofetil) [B-II] [28,44].
- Discontinuing the antiproliferative immunosuppressant and switching from tacrolimus or cyclosporine to sirolimus [B-III] [67].

If allograft dysfunction is present and persists and/or plasma BKV loads fail to show a decrease of >2 $\log_{10}$ over 8–12 weeks, reassessment should be considered, including by allograft biopsy [B-III]. If PVAN persists and acute rejection is ruled out, discontinuing individual components of the maintenance immunosuppression regimen should be considered as a next step [B-III].

Antiviral approaches

Formally, the use of cidofovir is contraindicated in patients with impaired kidney function. However, because cidofovir is selectively concentrated in tubular epithelial cells and urine, off-label use has been proposed at 10- to 20-fold-lower doses than employed to treat cytomegalovirus replication, namely, at (0.25–1 mg/kg every 2 weeks, without concomitant probenecid administration). The success of cidofovir therapy is variable and, as in the case of leflunomide, no data are available to distinguish any antiviral effect from concomitant reduction of immunosuppression. Table 26.3 summarizes reports with ≥4 patients. Thus, off-label use has been proposed for PVAN cases refractory to reduction of immunosuppression [B-III].

Commercially available preparations of IVIG have also been used in PVAN treatment protocols (Table 26.3) [51,62]. However, because the presence of neutralizing antibodies at best reduced, but did not prevent, BKV viremia and PVAN [II] [20,27,68], it is unlikely that IVIG preparations alone provide efficient anti-BKV activity. In the absence of controlled studies, it is at present difficult to dissect the respective role of the different interventions on the outcome of PVAN.

BKV screening and early intervention

Advances in the development of diagnostic tools and a better understanding of PVAN have led to treatment at early stages, before significant renal function deterioration, and this has resulted in improved outcomes (Table 26.4) [25,27,29]. Thus, identification of patients at a "preclinical" stage is paramount for the successful treatment of the disease. Recent data have shown that progression to PVAN can be safely prevented if BKV viremia is used to guide therapeutic intervention [28,44]. In two prospective studies, patients with "presumptive PVAN" cleared BKV viremia upon stopping mycophenolate mofetil or azathioprine, or reducing calcineurin inhibitor levels, without adversely affecting allograft function [28,44]. Hence, in patients with persisting polyomavirus replication (BKV viremia) above thresholds ("presumptive" PVAN) and negative allograft biopsy results, preemptive reduction of immunosuppression should be considered [B-II].

Retransplantation after renal allograft loss due to PVAN

Retransplantation after allograft loss to PVAN has been reported in 17 cases [69,70], with recurrence of BKV viremia in 3 patients (17%). "Definitive" PVAN was diagnosed in two cases (12%), one of which cleared BKV replication but with impaired graft function (6%), whereas recurrent graft loss was observed in the other case (6%). However, the incidence of PVAN after retransplantation cannot be derived from these limited data and may be higher than that seen in primary transplants. In 13 cases (76%), the first allograft had been removed, including in the three cases with PVAN recurrence. Prior to retransplantation, recovery of BKV-specific immunity is viewed as the most critical factor [69,71] and may require a period of 3–12 months of reduced or no immunosuppression.

Table 26.3 Treatment of PVAN with antiviral agents.

Agent and [reference(s)]	No. of cases	Protocol	Notes	Outcome
Cidofovir [2]	41	1.5 mg/kg/wk for 1.5–3 mos 0.25–0.33 mg/kg biweekly	• Lower dosage in a pediatric patient • Associated treatment: ↓ CI and MMF • All patients had advanced PVAN	• 2 graft losses • 2 major functional declines • The pediatric patient stabilized renal function and ↓ viral load
[58]	4	0.25–1 mg/kg bi- or triweekly for 1–4 doses	• Associated treatment: ↓ Tac in 3 pts and IVIG in 1 • All patients had advanced PVAN	• All patients have stable graft function at 6–26 mos posttherapy • Clearance of BK viruria in all but recurrence in 2
[59]	8	0.5–1 mg/kg/wk for 4–10 doses	• Associated treatment: ↓ Tac or switch Tac→CyA; discontinuation or ↓ MMF • Control group treated with ↓ IS alone	• No graft losses vs. 70% graft loss in control group at a median of 24-mo follow-up • No significant effect on BK viruria or viremia
[72]	4	0.25 mg/kg/week for 1 dose	• Associated treatment: ↓ CyA or switch Tac→CyA; discontinuation or ↓ MMF • Control group treated with ↓ IS alone	• No improvement of renal function at a median 35-mo follow-up • Clearance of BK viruria and viremia
[73]	21	0.25–1 mg/kg for ≥3 doses	• Associated treatment: ↓ IS + leflunomide	• 2 graft losses • 9 functional decline • 10 stable graft function
[51]	30	0.25 mg/kg biweekly for 4 doses; if no response, 0.5 mg/kg biweekly for 4–5 doses	• Associated treatment: ↓ Tac or switch Tac→CyA + ↓ MMF in 20 patients; ↓ IS + IVIG in 10 patients • Case–control study	• 50% any renal function decline at a median of 20-mo follow-up • No single intervention (cidofovir, IVIg, and CyA conversion) associated with improved outcome
IVIG [51]	12	1.25 g/kg for 2 doses	• Associated treatment: ↓ Tac or switch Tac→CyA + ↓ MMF; + cidofovir in 10 patients • Case–control study	• 35% any renal function decline at median of 20-mo follow-up • No significant association with improved outcome
[62]	8	Total dose of 2 g/kg in 2–5 divided doses	• Associated treatment: ↓ IS	• 1 graft loss • 7 stabilization of graft function
Leflunomide [63, 64]	26	Starting dose of 100 mg for 5 days; maintenance with 40 mg adjusted to blood levels of 50–100 μg/mL	• Associated treatment: discontinuation of MMF and ↓Tac; + cidofovir in 9 patients	• 4 graft losses • 22 stabilization or improvement of graft functions • 11 patients cleared BK viremia and 8/11 also cleared viruria
[73]	21	Starting dose of 100 mg for 3 days; maintenance with 20 mg; if no response, 40 mg	• Associated treatment: ↓ IS + cidofovir	• 2 graft losses • 9 functional declines • 10 stable graft functions

Abbreviations: CI, calcineurin inhibitors; MMF, mycophenolate mofetil; Tac: tacrolimus; CyA, cyclosporine A; IS, immunosuppression.

Table 26.4 Screening for BKV allows early diagnosis and improves outcome.

Study [reference]	Screening modality	No. of patients with PVAN	S-Crea conc (mg/dL) at diagnosis[a] [controls]	PVAN intervention	Clearance of viremia	S-Crea conc (mg/dL) at follow-up [controls]
Hirsch et al. 2002 [27]	• Screening: decoy cells • Confirm: plasma BKV load • Biopsy, if S-crea >20% or BKV load >10^4 copies/ml	5	2.34 ± 0.96 (1.6–4.0) [NA]	Tailored ↓ IS • ↓Tac or CyA • Switch to Sir • Switch MMF to AZA	5/5	1.72 ± 0.41 (1.4–2.4) [all patients 1.6, 0.8–4.2] No graft loss
Buehrig et al. 2003 [65]	• Routine surveillance biopsy	8	1.7 (1.3–2.5) [3.1; 1.5–5.3]	• ↓Tac or switch to CyA • ↓or taper MMF	NA	1.5 (1.1–2.3) [4.2; 1.7–7.0] No graft loss
Drachenberg et al. 2004 [43]	• Screening: decoy cells • Confirm: plasma BKV load • Biopsy, if S-crea >20% or BKV load >10^4 copies/mL	14	1.5 (1.0–2.2) [2.8; 1.2–5.1]	• ↓Tac or CyA • Stop or ↓ 50% MMF	11/14	2.0 (1.0–4.6) [5.1; 1.5–12.1] No graft loss
Brennan et al. 2005 [28]	• Screening: decoy cells • Confirm: plasma BKV load • Preemptive treatment if plasma BKV load >3 weeks	*23	NA (S-crea at baseline)	• Stop MMF or AZA • ↓Tac or CyA	22/23	1.5 ± 0.42 [1.4 ±0.5]; $P = 0.21$ No PVAN No graft loss
Ginevri et al. 2005 [44]	• Screening with urine BKV DNA • Adjunctive test: Q-DNA blood • Preemptive treatment if plasma BKV load >3 weeks	*5	1.1 (0.7–1.6) [NA]	Protocol defined ↓ IS: • ↓ Tac or CyA • ↓ or stop MMF or AZA	5/5	1.0 (0.8–1.3) No PVAN No graft loss

Abbreviations: S-crea, serum creatinine; NA, not available; IS, immunosuppression; Tac, tacrolimus; CyA, cyclosporine A; Sir, sirolimus; MMF: mycophenolate mofetil; AZA, azathioprine.

[a] Mean serum creatinine concentration (range in parentheses); control values are shown in brackets. Controls were represented by PVAN cohorts identified by biopsy performed after deterioration of renal function rather than surveillance biopsy.

As BKV-specific immunity is not yet available in the clinical routine, a >2-$\log_{10}$ reduction of plasma BKV loads may serve as a surrogate marker [III] [18]. In eight patients (47%), the same immunosuppressive drugs and combinations were used as for the primary graft. In nine patients, tacrolimus, mycophenolate mofetil, and prednisone were used; this group included both cases with "definitive" PVAN.

The success of >80% in this case series indicates that retransplantation remains an option for patients with allograft loss due to PVAN [B-II]. Surgical removal is not a prerequisite for successful retransplantation [D-II]. However, nephrectomy may be appropriate in patients with persisting BKV viremia at the time of retransplantation in order to reduce the risk of superinfection and to better attribute changes in renal function and BKV loads posttransplant to the new allograft [B-III] [69,70]. The same immunosuppressive drugs and combinations may be used [B-III], but intense immunosuppression and allograft injury resulting from toxicity or acute rejection should be avoided [B-III]. No recommendation on the use of induction treatment can be made, but nondepleting anti-interleukin-2 receptor agents may be appropriate [C-III]. Following retransplantation, screening for polyomavirus replication and intervention should be performed, as recommended for patients with a first renal allograft [B-III] [1,69].

Perspective

PVAN still represents a formidable challenge, but as can be gathered from the numerous abstracts presented at the most recent international conferences, high-quality studies are underway and exciting new insights can be expected in the next 12 months in this rapidly moving field.

References

1 Hirsch HH, Brennan DC, Drachenberg CB, Ginevri F, Gordon J, Limaye AP. Polyomavirus-associated nephropathy in renal transplantation: interdisciplinary analyses and recommendations. *Transplantation* 2005; **79:** 1277–1286.

2 Ramos E, Drachenberg CB, Portocarrero M, Wali R, Klassen DK, Fink JC et al. BK virus nephropathy diagnosis and treatment: experience at the University of Maryland Renal Transplant Program. *Clin Transplant* 2002; **2002:** 143–153.

3 Randhawa PS, Finkelstein S, Scantlebury V, Shapiro R, Vivas V, Jordan M et al. Human polyoma virus-associated interstitial nephritis in the allograft kidney. *Transplantation* 1999; **67:**103–109.

4 Vasudev B, Hariharan S, Hussain SA, Zhu YR, Bresnahan BA, Cohen EP. BK virus nephritis: risk factors, timing, and outcome in renal transplant recipients. *Kidney Int* 2005; **68:** 1834–1839.

5 Binet I, Nickeleit V, Hirsch HH, Prince O, Dalquen P, Gudat F et al. Polyomavirus disease under new immunosuppressive drugs: a cause of renal graft dysfunction and graft loss. *Transplantation* 1999; **67**: 918–922.

6 Nickeleit V, Klimkait T, Binet IF, Dalquen P, Del Zenero V, Thiel G et al. Testing for polyomavirus type BK DNA in plasma to identify renal-allograft recipients with viral nephropathy. *N Engl J Med* 2000; **342**: 1309–1315.

7 Kazory A, Ducloux D, Chalopin JM, Angonin R, Fontaniere B, Moret H. The first case of JC virus allograft nephropathy. *Transplantation* 2003; **76**: 1653–1655.

8 Drachenberg CB, Hirsch HH, Papadimitriou JC, Gosert R, Wali RK, Munivenkatappa R, Nogueira J, Cangro CB, Haririan A, Mendley S, Ramos E. Polyomavirus BK versus JC replication and nephropathy in renal transplant recipients: A prospective evaluation. *Transplantation* 2007; **84**: 323–330.

9 Crowder CD, Gyure KA, Drachenberg CB, Werner J, Morales RE, Hirsch HH et al. Successful outcome of progressive multifocal leukoencephalopathy in a renal transplant patient. *Am J Transplant* 2005; **5**: 1151–1158.

10 Hirsch HH. Polyomavirus BK nephropathy: a (re-)emerging complication in renal transplantation. *Am J Transplant* 2002; **2**: 25–30.

11 Hirsch HH. BK virus: opportunity makes a pathogen. *Clin Infect Dis* 2005; **41**: 354–360.

12 Egli A, Infanti L, Stebler C, Gosert R, Hirsch HH. Polyomavirus BK (BKV) and JC (JCV) Replication in Plasma and Urine in Healthy Blood Donors (Abstract# 1058). *Am J Transplant* 2008; **8**: 460.

13 Kish MA. Guide to development of practice guidelines. *Clin Infect Dis* 2001; **32**: 851–854.

14 Hirsch HH, Steiger J. Polyomavirus BK. *Lancet Infect Dis* 2003; **3**: 611–623.

15 Gordon J, Brennan D, Limaye A, Randhawa P, Storch G, Trofe J et al. Multicenter validation of polyomavirus BK quantification for screening and monitoring of renal transplant recipients. *Am J Transplant* 2005; **5**: 381–382.

16 Funk GA, Steiger J, Hirsch HH. Rapid dynamics of polyomavirus type BK in renal transplant recipients. *J Infect Dis* 2006; **193**: 80–87.

17 Comoli P, Azzi A, Maccario R, Basso S, Botti G, Basile G et al. Polyomavirus BK-specific immunity after kidney transplantation. *Transplantation* 2004; **78**: 1229–1232.

18 Binggeli S, Egli A, Schaub S, Binet I, Mayr M, Steiger J, Hirsch HH. Polyomavirus BKV-specific cellular immune response to vp1 and large t-antigen in kidney transplant recipients. *Am J Transplant* 2007; **7**: 1131–1139.

19 Chen Y, Trofe J, Gordon J, Du Pasquier RA, Roy-Chaudhury P, Kuroda MJ et al. Interplay of cellular and humoral immune responses against BK virus in kidney transplant recipients with polyomavirus nephropathy. *J Virol* 2006; **80**: 3495–3505.

20 Comoli P, Binggeli S, Ginevri F, Hirsch HH. Polyomavirus-associated nephropathy: update on BK virus-specific immunity. *Transplant Infect Dis* 2006; **8**: 86–94.

21 Fishman JA. BK virus nephropathy-polyomavirus adding insult to injury. *N Engl J Med* 2002; **347**: 527–530.

22 Atencio IA, Shadan FF, Zhou XJ, Vaziri ND, Villarreal LP. Adult mouse kidneys become permissive to acute polyomavirus infection and reactivate persistent infections in response to cellular damage and regeneration. *J Virol* 1993; **67**: 1424–1432.

23 Han Lee ED, Kemball CC, Wang J, Dong Y, Stapler DC, Jr., Hamby KM et al. A mouse model for polyomavirus-associated nephropathy of kidney transplants. *Am J Transplant* 2006; **6**: 913–922.

24 Nickeleit V, Hirsch HH, Binet IF, Gudat F, Prince O, Dalquen P et al. Polyomavirus infection of renal allograft recipients: from latent infection to manifest disease. *J Am Soc Nephrol* 1999; **10**: 1080–1089.

25 Drachenberg CB, Papadimitriou JC, Hirsch HH, Wali R, Crowder C, Nogueira J et al. Histological patterns of polyomavirus nephropathy: correlation with graft outcome and viral load. *Am J Transplant* 2004; **4**: 2082–2092.

26 Gosert R, Rinaldo CH, Funk GA, Egli A, Ramos E, Drachenberg CB, Hirsch HH. Polyomavirus BK with rearranged noncoding control region emerge in vivo in renal transplant patients and increase viral replication and cytopathology. *J Exp Med* 2008; **205**: 841–852.

27 Hirsch HH, Knowles W, Dickenmann M, Passweg J, Klimkait T, Mihatsch MJ et al. Prospective study of polyomavirus type BK replication and nephropathy in renal-transplant recipients. *N Engl J Med* 2002; **347**: 488–496.

28 Brennan DC, Agha I, Bohl DL, Schnitzler MA, Hardinger KL, Lockwood M et al. Incidence of BK with tacrolimus versus cyclosporine and impact of preemptive immunosuppression reduction. *Am J Transplant* 2005; **5**: 582–594.

29 Ramos E, Drachenberg C, Hirsch HH, Muinvenkatappa R, Papadimitriou J, Nogueira J et al. BK polyomavirus allograft nephropathy (BKPVN): eight-fold decrease in graft loss with prospective screening and protocol biopsy. *Am J Transplant* 2006; **6(S2)**: 121–122.

30 Ramos E, Drachenberg CB, Papadimitriou JC, Hamze O, Fink JC, Klassen DK et al. Clinical course of polyoma virus nephropathy in 67 renal transplant patients. *J Am Soc Nephrol* 2002; **13**: 2145–2151.

31 Amer H, Larson TS, Stengall MD, Cosio FG, Griffin MD. The functional impact of subclinical polyoma virus associated nephrophathy (PVAN) diagnosed on four month kidney transplant protocol biopsy. *Am J Transplant* 2006; **6(S2)**: 91–92.

32 Hayashi RY, Cho YW, Shah T, Peng A, Huand E, Bunnapradist S. Risk factors for polyomavirus nephropathy in renal transplant recipients: an analysis of the OPTN/UNOS database. *Am J Transplant* 2006; **6(S2)**: 92.

33 Ginevri F, De Santis R, Comoli P, Pastorino N, Rossi C, Botti G et al. Polyomavirus BK infection in pediatric kidney-allograft recipients: a single-center analysis of incidence, risk factors, and novel therapeutic approaches. *Transplantation* 2003; **75**: 1266–1270.

34 Smith JM, McDonald RA, Finn LS, Healey PJ, Davis CL, Limaye AP. Polyomavirus nephropathy in pediatric kidney transplant recipients. *Am J Transplant* 2004; **4**: 2109–2117.

35 Hirsch HH, Friman S, Wiecek A, Rostaing L, Pescovitz M. Prospective study of polyomavirus BK viruria and viremia in de novo renal transplantation (abstract #77). *Am J Transplant* 2007; **7**: 150.

36 Mengel M, Marwedel M, Radermacher J, Eden G, Schwarz A, Haller H, Kriepe H. Incidence of polyomavirus-nephropathy in renal allografts: influence of modern immunosuppressive drugs. *Nephrol Dial Transplant* 2003; **18**: 1190–1196.

37 Walker J, Trofe J, Alooway R, Weimert N, Succop P, Buell J et al. Polyomavirus nephropathy: multivariante analysis of risk factors with early corticosteroid cessation. *Am J Transplant* 2006; **6(S2)**: 92.

38 Naesens M, Lerut E, Van Damme B, Snoeck R, Vanrenterghem Y, Kuypers DRJ. Prospective study of BKV viral load, subclinical histology and exposure to tacrolimus and mycophenolic acid in renal allograft recipients. *Am J Transplant* 2006; **6(S2)**: 682–683.

39 Celik B, Shapiro R, Vats A, Randhawa PS. Polyomavirus allograft nephropathy: sequential assessment of histologic viral load, tubulitis, and graft function following changes in immunosuppression. *Am J Transplant* 2003; **3**: 1378–1382.

40 Awadalla Y, Randhawa P, Ruppert K, Zeevi A, Duquesnoy RJ. HLA mismatching increases the risk of BK virus nephropathy in renal transplant recipients. *Am J Transplant* 2004; **4**: 1691–1696.

41 Barri YM, Ahmad I, Ketel BL, Barone GW, Walker PD, Bonsib SM *et al.* Polyoma viral infection in renal transplantation: the role of immunosuppressive therapy. *Clin Transplant* 2001; **15**: 240–246.

42 Ding R, Medeiros M, Dadhania D, Muthukumar T, Kracker D, Kong JM *et al.* Noninvasive diagnosis of BK virus nephritis by measurement of messenger RNA for BK virus VP1 in urine. *Transplantation* 2002; **74**: 987–994.

43 Drachenberg CB, Papadimitriou JC, Wali R, Nogueira J, Mendley S, Hirsch HH *et al.* Improved outcome of polyoma virus allograft nephropathy with early biopsy. *Transplant Proc* 2004; **36**: 758–759.

44 Ginevri F, Azzi A, Hirsch HH, Basso S, Fontana I, Cioni M, Bodaghi S, Salotti V, Rinieri A, Botti G, Perfumo F, Locatelli F, Comoli P. Prospective monitoring of polyomavirus BK replication and impact of pre-emptive intervention in pediatric kidney recipients. *Am J Transplant* 2007; **7**: 2727–2735.

45 Kiberd BA. Screening to prevent polyoma virus nephropathy: a medical decision analysis. *Am J Transplant* 2005; **5**: 2410–2416.

46 Hirsch HH, Drachenberg C, Ramos J, Papadimitriou J, Munivenkatappa R, Nogueira J *et al.* BK viremia level strongly correlates with the extent/pattern of viral nephropathy (BKPVN) implications for a diagnostic cut-off value. *Am J Transplant* 2006; **6(S2)**: 460.

47 Hirsch HH, Drachenberg CB, Steiger J, Ramos E. Polyomavirus-associated nephropathy in renal transplantation: critical issues of screening and management. *Adv Exp Med Biol* 2006; **577**: 160–173.

48 Eid AJ, Viscount HB, Espy MJ, Griffin MD, Smith TF, Razonable RR. The threshold of plasma BK viremia that predicts polyomavirus-associated nephropathy (PVAN). *Am J Transplant* 2006; **6(S2)**: 686.

49 Nickeleit V, Singh HK, Mihatsch MJ. Latent and productive polyomavirus infections of renal allografts: morphological, clinical, and pathophysiological aspects. *Adv Exp Med Biol* 2006; **577**: 190–200.

50 Drachenberg CB, Papadimitriou JC. Polyomavirus-associated nephropathy: update in diagnosis. *Transplant Infect Dis* 2006; **8**: 68–75.

51 Wadei HM, Rule AD, Lewin M, Mahale AS, Khamash HA, Schwab TR *et al.* Kidney transplant function and histological clearance of virus following diagnosis of polyomavirus-associated nephropathy (PVAN). *Am J Transplant* 2006; **6**: 1025–1032.

52 Vasudev B, Hariharan S, Hussain SA, Zhu YR, Bresnahan BA, Cohen EP. BK virus nephritis: Risk factors, timing, and outcome in renal transplant recipients. *Kidney Int* 2005; **68**: 1834–1839.

53 Saad ER, Bresnahan BA, Cohen EP, Lu N, Orentas RJ, Vasudev B, Hariharan S. Successful treatment of BK viremia using reduction in immunosuppression without antiviral therapy. *Transplantation* 2008; **85**: 850–854.

54 Mannon RB, Hoffmann SC, Kampen RL, Cheng OC, Kleiner DE, Ryschkewitsch C *et al.* Molecular evaluation of BK polyomavirus nephropathy. *Am J Transplant* 2005; **5**: 2883–2893.

55 Nickeleit V, Hirsch HH, Zeiler M, Gudat F, Prince O, Thiel G *et al.* BK-virus nephropathy in renal transplants-tubular necrosis, MHC-class II expression and rejection in a puzzling game. *Nephrol Dial Transplant* 2000; **15**: 324–332.

56 Trofe J, Hirsch HH, Ramos E. Polyomavirus-associated nephropathy: update of clinical management in kidney transplant patients. *Transplant Infect Dis* 2006; **8**: 76–85.

57 Trofe J, Cavallo T, First MR, Weiskittel P, Peddi VR, Roy-Chaudhury P *et al.* Polyomavirus in kidney and kidney-pancreas transplantation: a defined protocol for immunosuppression reduction and histologic monitoring. *Transplant Proc* 2002; **34**: 1788–1789.

58 Vats A, Shapiro R, Singh Randhawa P, Scantlebury V, Tuzuner A, Saxena M *et al.* Quantitative viral load monitoring and cidofovir therapy for the management of BK virus-associated nephropathy in children and adults. *Transplantation* 2003; **75**: 105–112.

59 Kuypers DR, Vandooren AK, Lerut E, Evenepoel P, Claes K, Snoeck R *et al.* Adjuvant low-dose cidofovir therapy for BK polyomavirus interstitial nephritis in renal transplant recipients. *Am J Transplant* 2005; **5**: 1997–2004.

60 Araya CE, Lew JF, Fennell RS, III, Neiberger RE, Dharnidharka VR. Intermediate-dose cidofovir without probenecid in the treatment of BK virus allograft nephropathy. *Pediatr Transplant* 2006; **10**: 32–37.

61 Trofe J, Gaber LW, Stratta RJ, Shokouh-Amiri MH, Vera SR, Alloway RR *et al.* Polyomavirus in kidney and kidney-pancreas transplant recipients. *Transplant Infect Dis* 2003; **5**: 21–28.

62 Sener A, House AA, Jevnikar AM, Boudville N, McAlister VC, Muirhead N *et al.* Intravenous immunoglobulin as a treatment for BK virus associated nephropathy: one-year follow-up of renal allograft recipients. *Transplantation* 2006; **81**: 117–120.

63 Rinaldo CH, Hirsch HH. Antivirals for the treatment of polyomavirus BK replication. *Expert Rev Anti Infect Ther* 2007; **5**: 105–115.

64 Josephson MA, Gillen D, Javaid B, Kadambi P, Meehan S, Foster P *et al.* Treatment of renal allograft polyoma BK virus infection with leflunomide. *Transplantation* 2006; **81**: 704–710.

65 Buehrig CK, Lager DJ, Stegall MD, Kreps MA, Kremers WK, Gloor JM *et al.* Influence of surveillance renal allograft biopsy on diagnosis and prognosis of polyomavirus-associated nephropathy. *Kidney Int* 2003; **64**: 665–673.

66 Farasati NA, Shapiro R, Vats A, Randhawa P. Effect of leflunomide and cidofovir on replication of BK virus in an in vitro culture system. *Transplantation* 2005; **79**: 116–118.

67 Wali RK, Drachenberg C, Hirsch HH, Papadimitriou J, Nahar A, Mohanlal V *et al.* BK virus-associated nephropathy in renal allograft recipients: rescue therapy by sirolimus-based immunosuppression. *Transplantation* 2004; **78**: 1069–1073.

68 Bohl DL, Storch GA, Ryschkewitsch C, Gaudreault-Keener M, Schnitzler MA, Major EO *et al.* Donor origin of BK virus in renal transplantation and role of HLA C7 in susceptibility to sustained BK viremia. *Am J Transplant* 2005; **5**: 2213–2221.

69 Hirsch HH, Ramos E. Retransplantation after polyomavirus-associated nephropathy: just do it? *Am J Transplant* 2006; **6**: 7–9.

70 Womer KL, Meier-Kriesche HU, Patton PR, Dibadj K, Bucci CM, Foley D *et al.* Preemptive retransplantation for BK virus nephropathy: successful outcome despite active viremia. *Am J Transplant* 2006; **6**: 209–213.

71 Ginevri F, Pastorino N, de Santis R, Fontana I, Sementa A, Losurdo G *et al.* Retransplantation after kidney graft loss due to polyoma BK virus nephropathy: successful outcome without original allograft nephrectomy. *Am J Kidney Dis* 2003; **42**: 821–825.

72 Lipshutz GS, Mahanty H, Feng S, Hirose R, Stock PG, Kang SM *et al.* BKV in simultaneous pancreas-kidney transplant recipients: a leading cause of renal graft loss in first 2 years post-transplant. *Am J Transplant* 2005; **5**: 366–373.

73 Barri YM, Rice PS, Melton L, Fischbach B, Corpier C, Nesser D. Improved renal transplant outcome in polyoma viral infection with the combination of low-dose cidofovir and leflunomide. *J Am Soc Nephrol* 2005; **16**: 699A.

Toxic Nephropathies

27 Toxic Nephropathies: Nonsteroidal Anti-Inflammatory Drugs

Wai Y. Tse[1] & Dwomoa Adu[2]

[1]Department of Nephrology, Derriford Hospital, Plymouth PL6 8DH, UK.
[2]Department of Nephrology, Queen Elizabeth Hospital, Birmingham B15 2TH, UK.

Introduction

Nonsteroidal anti-inflammatory drugs (NSAIDs) are one of the most commonly prescribed groups of drugs for the treatment of pain and inflammation. It is estimated that, worldwide, more than 30 million people take NSAIDs daily [1]. The widespread use of NSAIDs means that renal complications are likely to be seen frequently. These include salt and water retention, acute tubular necrosis, acute interstitial nephritis, hyperkalemia, and acute and chronic kidney failure [2–6].

In addition to renal side effects, NSAID use risks also include significant gastrointestinal complications and cardiac events, such as myocardial infarction and acute coronary syndromes. Nonselective NSAIDs inhibit both constitutive cyclooxygenase 1 (COX-1) and inducible COX-2, the rate-limiting enzymes that are involved in production of prostaglandins and thromboxane A_2. It was hoped that COX-2-selective NSAIDs would have anti-inflammatory activity but lack the deleterious effects on homeostatic functions mediated by COX-1 activation. Three highly selective COX-2 NSAIDs were originally approved by the US Food and Drug Administration, namely, celecoxib, rofecoxib, and valdecoxib. However, increased myocardial infarction and ischemic strokes seen with rofecoxib [7] and increased cardiovascular events in patients who underwent coronary artery bypass surgery and received valdecoxib [8] led to the withdrawal of these two COX-2 inhibitors in 2004 and 2005, respectively. Low-dose aspirin irreversibly inhibits platelet COX-1, thereby blocking the synthesis of thromboxane A_2, a prothrombotic factor, and has little effect on endothelial COX-2-derived prostacyclin. Prostacyclin inhibits platelet aggregation and leads to vasodilatation. Due to its selectivity, low-dose aspirin is the drug of choice for the prevention of thrombotic events, even for those patients with underlying kidney disease, without the risk of jeopardizing prostaglandin-dependent kidney function. By con-

trast, higher doses of aspirin can inhibit COX-2-derived prostacyclin production. Prostacyclin is mainly COX-2 derived and is inhibited by both nonselective NSAIDs as well as COX-2-selective NSAIDs. Therefore, a potential cardiovascular risk is seen with nonselective NSAIDs as well as COX-2-selective drugs [9–11].

Cyclooxygenases in the kidney

The enzyme phospholipase A_2 converts phospholipids into arachidonic acid, which is the substrate for three different enzymes: COX, which is inhibited by NSAIDs, cytochrome P450 monooxygenase, and lipoxygenase (Figure 27.1). Phospholipase A_2 is activated by kinins, vasopressin, angiotensin II, and extracellular hyperosmolarity and increases prostaglandin synthesis through the three pathways [12]. Each pathway influences some aspects of renal hemodynamics or tubular function. Two isoforms of COX (COX-1 and COX-2) have been identified in mammalian cells [13,14]. COX-1, which is constitutively expressed, mediates gastric cytoprotection and vascular homeostasis [15]. COX-2 expression is regulated by salt and water intake, medullary tonicity, growth factors, cytokines, and adrenal steroids [16] and produces prostaglandins in inflamed tissues [15]. COX-2-dependent prostaglandin formation is also necessary for normal kidney development [17]. In mice, the complete absence of COX-2 resulted in severe renal dysplasia characterized by a postnatal arrest of maturation in the subcapsular nephrogenic zone and progressive deterioration with increasing age [18]. Antenatal exposure of both mice and rats to an inhibitor of COX-2, but not of COX-1, had similar effects [19].

Constitutive COX-2 mRNA as well as inducible COX-2 mRNA are present in the kidney [20]. In the human kidney, COX-2 is present in podocytes, endothelium, proximal convoluted tubule and collecting duct, renal vasculature, the macula densa, and the medullary interstitial cells [21], whereas COX-1 is found in the vasculature, the collecting ducts, glomeruli, and medullary interstitial cells [22].

Evidence-based Nephrology. Edited by Donald Molony and Jonathan Craig
© 2009 Blackwell Publishing, ISBN: 978-1-4051-3975-5.

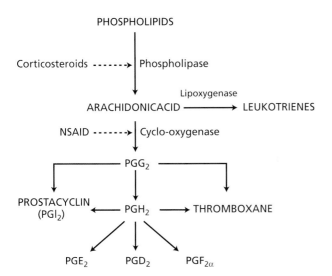

Figure 27.1 Pathway of arachidonic acid metabolism. The lipoxygenase pathway results in the production of leukotrienes; the role of these compounds in the kidney is unclear. The cyclo-oxygenase pathways leads to the production of the unstable cyclic endoperoxidase PGG2. Subsequent enzymatic conversion results in the production of the classical 2-series prostaglandins PGI$_2$, PGE$_2$, PGD$_2$, PGF$_{2\alpha}$, and thromboxane A$_2$.

Actions of renal prostaglandins

The kidney produces the vasodilator prostaglandins PGE$_2$, PGF$_{2\alpha}$, and PGI$_2$ and the vasoconstrictor thromboxane A$_2$. These autocoids, synthesized and metabolized by the kidney, autoregulate renal blood flow, renin release, tubular ion transport, and water metabolism [23–26]. PGI$_2$, which is mainly present in the afferent arteriole and glomerulus, plays a major role in controlling glomerular hemodynamics [27]. In contrast, PGE$_2$, which is predominantly produced in the collecting tubule and within the interstitium, regulates medullary hemodynamics [26].

Effects on COX-2 NSAIDs on renal prostaglandins

The urinary excretion of PGE$_2$ and 6-keto-PGF1$_a$, the stable metabolite of PGI$_2$, reflects renal synthesis of PGE$_2$ and PGI$_2$, respectively. In healthy older adults, rofecoxib reduces baseline urinary 6-keto-PGF$_{1\alpha}$ by 47%, and this was comparable to the 53% reduction induced by indomethacin [28]. In another study, rofecoxib reduced urinary PGE$_2$ and 6-keto-PGF1$_\alpha$ excretion in healthy volunteers by approximately 40–50%, similar to that induced by meloxicam or diclofenac [29]. Furthermore, excretion of urinary 6-keto-PGF$_{1\alpha}$ was comparable in response to celecoxib and traditional NSAIDs [30]. In a trial of healthy elderly volunteers on a normal sodium intake, multiple doses of twice-daily celecoxib reduced PGE$_2$ and 6-keto-PGF$_{1\alpha}$ excretion to the same degree as naproxen, by approximately 65 and 80%, respectively [31]. These data suggest that the COX-2 isoform plays an important role in renal prostaglandin biosynthesis. It is thus likely that COX-2 inhibitors will impact renal function just as nonselective NSAIDs do.

Maintenance of renal blood flow and glomerular filtration rate

Prostaglandins maintain renal blood flow and the glomerular filtration rate despite vasoconstrictor stimuli, such as leukotrienes, thromboxane A$_2$, angiotensin II, vasopressin, endothelin, and catecholamines. Catecholamines also stimulate the local production of prostaglandins, resulting in a feedback loop between vasoconstrictors and vasodilatory prostaglandins [32–34]. PGF$_{2\alpha}$-like peroxidation products also have major vasoconstrictive effects [35]. Thus, in patients with underlying ischemic or inflammatory renal injury, the addition of a nonselective or COX-2-selective NSAID not only decreases the production of vasodilatory prostaglandins but also results in the nonenzymatic formation of vasoconstrictor metabolites of arachidonic acid, which further jeopardizes renal blood flow and glomerular filtration. Under normal, euvolemic conditions, NSAIDs produce negligible effects on renal hemodynamics [36,37]. However, in the presence of salt depletion, an ineffective circulating plasma volume, or under conditions characterized by high circulating levels of vasoconstrictor hormones, NSAIDs may be nephrotoxic. Such conditions include cirrhosis, hypovolemia, cardiac disease, renal disease, septic shock, advanced age, diuretic use, diabetes mellitus, and following surgery [38].

In elderly, salt-replete subjects, both indomethacin and rofecoxib decreased sodium excretion, but only indomethacin reduced the glomerular filtration rate [28]. Celecoxib, like rofecoxib, affects renal function in selected groups of subjects. Whelton *et al.* in 2000 compared celecoxib with naproxen in 29 healthy elderly subjects in a single blind, randomized, crossover study [39]. Subjects were given either celecoxib at 200 mg twice daily for 5 days followed by celecoxib at 400 mg twice daily for the next 5 days or they received naproxen at 500 mg twice daily for 10 days. After a 7-day washout, subjects were crossed over to the other regimen. Glomerular filtration rate fell more with naproxen than with celecoxib, although urinary excretion of prostaglandin E$_2$, 6-keto-PGF1$_\alpha$, and sodium was comparable. In another study involving salt-depleted elderly subjects rofecoxib and indomethacin induced a comparable reduction of glomerular filtration rate [40]. These studies illustrate that COX-2 inhibitors and nonselective NSAIDs have similar effects on renal hemodynamics.

Postoperative use of NSAIDs

A meta-analysis of 19 trials showed that the postoperative use of NSAIDs in adults with normal preoperative renal function resulted in a 16-mL/min fall in creatinine clearance (95% confidence interval [CI], 5–28) and potassium excretion by 38 mmol/day (95% CI, 19–56) on the first day after surgery compared with placebo [41]. No cases of postoperative acute kidney failure requiring dialysis were seen. The conclusions were that NSAIDs caused a clinically unimportant reduction in kidney function in the early postoperative period in patients with normal kidney function and that these drugs should not be withheld in such patients. Others have reported, however, an overall incidence of postoperative renal insufficiency of 18% after major surgery, with a subsequent hospital mortality rate of 13% [42].

Renal dysfunction in COX-2 trials

In one study, renal adverse events were reported in 24.3% of 144 patients receiving celecoxib and in 30.8% of 143 patients receiving diclofenac and omeprazole. Kidney failure (defined as a rise in serum creatinine to above 200 μmol/L) was seen in 5.6 and 6.3% of patients, respectively [43]. Overall, renal adverse events were more common in patients with renal impairment (celecoxib, 51.4%; diclofenac plus omeprazole, 40.7%). In another study, adverse effects related to kidney function occurred in about 1% of naproxen- and rofecoxib-treated patients [44]. In a review of randomized clinical trials lasting 2 weeks or more involving celecoxib, a rise in serum creatinine was seen in 0.7% of patients treated with celecoxib and in 1.2% of patients treated with diclofenac ($P < 0.05$) [45]. In a meta-analysis of data from company clinical trial reports, there was no difference in the incidence of renal adverse events (defined as an increase in serum creatinine >1.3 times the upper limit of normal) in 15,319 patients treated with celecoxib (0.3%) or other NSAIDs (0.5%) (relative risk [RR], 0.78; 95% CI, 0.48–1.3) [46].

In summary, from these trials there are no differences in renal side effects between COX-2-selective inhibitors and nonselective inhibitors.

Renin release and potassium homeostasis

PGE_2, PGI_2, and arachidonic acid are potent stimuli of renin release [23]. Both nonselective and COX-2-selective NSAIDs can inhibit renin secretion and under some circumstances lead to hyporeninemia and hypoaldosteronism with attendant hyperkalemia. This is particularly common in patients with preexisting renal impairment [47–49]. Inhibition of prostaglandin synthesis can also lead to hyperkalemia by decreasing distal tubular flow rate and sodium delivery, both of which limit potassium secretion [50,51].

Natriuresis and diuresis

Renal prostaglandins are natriuretic and diuretic. They inhibit sodium and chloride reabsorption in the proximal and distal nephrons and in the loop of Henle [52,53], reduce the renal cortico-medullary solute gradient, and antagonize the action of vasopressin *in vivo* [54]. Although prostaglandins acutely influence salt and water excretion, they do not regulate it under normal conditions.

Clinical syndromes associated with nonselective and COX-2-selective NSAIDs

Acute renal impairment and acute tubular necrosis

Under circumstances where there is poor renal perfusion with high renin levels, nonselective and COX-2-selective NSAIDs can reduce glomerular filtration rate, resulting in acute kidney failure. This complication has been reported with most NSAIDs but only rarely with aspirin. Kidney failure has also been described after administration of topical and intramuscular NSAIDs [55–57].

A multicenter study in France examined the incidence and subsequent outcome of patients with drug-induced acute kidney failure [58]. Of the 398 patients with acute kidney failure, 147 (36.9%) had taken NSAIDs. One-third of them required dialysis, and 71.4% recovered or regained previous renal function. A renal biopsy obtained in 25 patients with NSAID-associated kidney failure disclosed acute tubular necrosis and acute interstitial nephritis in 21 patients and either minimal change nephropathy or chronic renal damage in 4. A nested case–control study using the United Kingdom General Practice Research Database reported that current users had an RR of developing acute kidney failure of 3.2 (95% CI, 1.8–5.8) compared with non-NSAID users [59]. This increased risk was higher in patients with heart failure, hypertension, or diabetes. Thus, although renal side effects from NSAID use are relatively rare, renal damage can be irreversible and the outcome can be fatal. Renal function usually improves upon drug withdrawal, although in some cases permanent renal damage may occur [60].

Acute kidney failure and hyperkalemia have been observed after the administration of COX-2-selective inhibitors to patients with risk factors for NSAID-induced acute renal insufficiency, including underlying chronic renal impairment and volume depletion [61]. Acute kidney failure was also reported in a patient with a kidney transplant 4 weeks after starting rofecoxib [62].

Acute tubulo-interstitial nephritis

NSAIDs of different classes have been associated with acute tubulo-interstitial nephritis and kidney failure [2,60,63,64]. Acute allergic tubulo-interstitial nephritis due to NSAIDs is much less common than hemodynamic kidney failure. The patients are often elderly, and the drug may have been taken for months or years before the development of acute interstitial nephritis. Clinical evidence of an allergic reaction, such as fever, rash, arthralgia, eosinophilia, or eosinophiluria, is uncommon. Of note, proteinuria, often in the nephrotic range, may occasionally appear, especially in fenoprofen-induced tubulo-interstitial nephritis [63,65,66]. Cases of interstitial nephritis have been reported with both celecoxib and rofecoxib [67–73]. In two cases, interstitial nephritis was associated with glomerulopathies, one case with minimal change disease [71] and the other one with membranous nephropathy [67]. Thus, there is little evidence that suggests a major difference between NSAIDs and COX-2 inhibitors in the incidence of acute interstitial nephritis.

NSAID-induced acute tubulo-interstitial nephritis is formally diagnosed by renal biopsy. A patchy acute tubular damage coexists with tubulo-interstitial infiltrate predominantly of T lymphocytes and, to a lesser extent, monocytes/macrophages, B lymphocytes, plasma cells, and eosinophils [66,74]. Rarely, a granulomatous interstitial nephritis is seen [75]. Immunofluorescence microscopy is usually negative or nonspecific. The predominance of T lymphocytes in the interstitial infiltrate has been taken to indicate that T-lymphocyte activation mediates this syndrome, rather than a humoral mechanism, as in other forms of drug-induced acute interstitial nephritis [65,66]. Inhibition of renal COX has also been incriminated in the genesis of NSAID-induced acute tubulo-interstitial nephritis. The resulting stimulation of the lipoxygenase pathway of arachidonic acid metabolism produces leukotrienes, which are potent chemotactic factors for lymphocytes. Recovery of renal function may be only partial [74], and chronic interstitial fibrosis may progress to chronic renal failure [76]. Prednisolone has been successfully used in anecdotal reports, but there is no conclusive evidence that corticosteroids hasten the resolution of the renal lesion [2].

Glomerulonephritis

Membranous nephropathy with nephrotic syndrome may occur as an idiosyncratic reaction to various classes of NSAIDs [77–79]. The temporal association with the intake of NSAIDs, the prompt and complete recovery after drug discontinuation, and the absence of recurrent disease may help distinguish NSAID-associated membranous nephropathy from the idiopathic form [80]. As with NSAIDs, glomerulopathies with the nephrotic syndrome can occur with COX-2 inhibitors [72]. Membranous nephropathy with acute interstitial nephritis secondary to celecoxib has been described [67].

Renal papillary necrosis

Renal papillary necrosis has been infrequently reported in patients treated with ibuprofen, indomethacin, phenylbutazone, fenoprofen, or mefenamic acid [60,76,81–83] or with paracetamol [84,85]. One case of celecoxib-related renal papillary necrosis has been reported [86].

Chronic kidney failure

Sandler *et al.* in 1991 evaluated the risk for chronic kidney disease associated with regular use of non-aspirin NSAIDs in 554 patients with newly diagnosed chronic renal dysfunction [5]. They found a twofold-increased risk for chronic kidney disease in patients with a history of previous daily use of NSAIDs (adjusted odds ratio, 2.1; 95% CI, 1.1–4.1). The increased risk was predominantly limited to men older than 65 years, for whom the odds ratio was 10.0 (95% CI, 1.2–82.7) after adjusting for use of other analgesics. The NSAID-associated risk was also greater among those with a history of conditions that might indicate an enhanced susceptibility to the effects of NSAIDs, including previous myocardial infarction, congestive heart failure, heavy alcohol consumption (as a surrogate for cirrhosis), or diuretic use. These observations were confirmed in a recent case–control study of 716 patients with end-stage renal failure and 361 controls [6]. In this study a high cumulative intake of NSAIDs (>5000 tablets) was associated with a 4.5-fold excess risk of end-stage renal failure, although the CI was wide (1.0–19.5) and, curiously, this excess risk was not seen when an average annual intake of NSAIDs was examined. Other studies of NSAID usage in hospitalized patients [87,88] and also cohort studies, however, did not show this association [89,90]. The reasons for these discrepant findings are unclear. On balance, it seems likely that chronic usage of NSAIDs may be associated with a slightly increased risk for the development of chronic kidney failure.

Some patients with chronic kidney failure rely on prostaglandin-mediated vasodilatation to maintain renal blood flow [91–93]. Addition of NSAIDs may cause further deterioration of renal function [48,91,93,94].

Salt and water retention

NSAID therapy may aggravate the sodium retention induced by renal hypoperfusion in heart failure, cirrhosis, or nephrotic syndrome [3]. Hyponatremia may occur if water retention is disproportionate to sodium retention [95], especially when thiazide diuretics are given simultaneously [2].

Hypertension

Two large meta-analyses encompassing more than 90 studies have demonstrated that NSAIDs may increase blood pressure, especially in previously hypertensive patients [96,97]. NSAIDs elevate supine mean blood pressure by 5 mmHg [97], a rise known to increase hypertension-related morbidity and mortality [98]. This complication is of importance in the elderly, who are frequently prescribed NSAIDs for musculoskeletal disorders and also have a high prevalence of other chronic disorders, including hypertension.

Whelton *et al.* performed a post hoc analysis on the renal safety of celecoxib, incorporating more than 50 clinical studies with more than 13,000 subjects [31]. The most common events, peripheral edema (2.1%), hypertension (0.8%), and exacerbation of preexisting hypertension (0.6%), were not dose or time related. Their incidence and profile were similar to those of nonselective NSAIDs. A similar post hoc analysis of rofecoxib revealed peripheral edema in 3.8% of the patients [99].

Whelton *et al.* also compared the effects of celecoxib at 200 mg and rofecoxib at 25 mg over a 6-week period in 810 hypertensive patients with osteoarthritis, aged over 65 years [100]. Edema developed in nearly twice as many rofecoxib-treated than celecoxib-treated patients (9.5% vs. 4.9%; $P = 0.014$). Systolic blood pressure increased significantly in 17% of rofecoxib-treated patients, compared with 11% of celecoxib-treated patients ($P = 0.032$). In conclusion, celecoxib induces edema less frequently and results in smaller rises in blood pressure than rofecoxib. A meta-analysis of COX-2 inhibitors and their effects on blood pressure showed that they were associated with a nonsignificant higher risk of causing hypertension compared with placebo (RR, 1.61; 95% CI, 0.91–2.84) or nonselective NSAIDs (RR, 1.25; 95% CI, 0.87–1.78) [101]. Thus, both NSAIDs and COX-2 inhibitors can raise blood pressure, especially in hypertensive, elderly patients, and there is no substantial evidence to suggest that COX-2 inhibitors are safer in this respect.

Hyperkalemia and hyporeninemic hypoaldosteronism

NSAIDs may cause hyperkalemia, and this is seen more commonly in patients with chronic kidney failure, diabetes mellitus, and type IV tubular acidosis through previously outlined mechanisms [48,102,103]. Increases in potassium levels are also expected to occur with COX-2 inhibitors. Indeed, rofecoxib raises serum potassium levels by more than 0.8 mM, with a similar incidence as NSAIDs [104]. NSAIDs must be used with caution in patients taking other drugs known to decrease renal potassium excretion, such as potassium-sparing diuretics, angiotensin converting enzyme inhibitors, and β-blockers.

Therapeutic use of NSAIDs in nephrotic syndrome

NSAIDs reduce proteinuria in patients with nephrotic syndrome [105,106], probably by reducing renal blood flow and glomerular filtration rate [107]. The occurrence of irreversible kidney failure in patients with a nephrotic syndrome treated with NSAIDs [58] suggests great caution for the use of these drugs in this clinical setting.

Conclusions

The increasing use of NSAIDs both by prescription and from over-the-counter sales has increased the prevalence of nephrotoxicity. A history of NSAID use should be sought in all patients with unexplained impairment of renal function and/or proteinuria. In patients with volume depletion or decreased organ perfusion, the use of NSAIDs should be avoided. NSAIDs should not be prescribed in patients with chronic renal impairment or with a functioning kidney transplant. Patients with an NSAID-induced, interstitial nephritis or papillary necrosis should not be given NSAIDs again. In some individuals who have developed NSAID-induced acute kidney failure and who have recovered kidney function, NSAIDs may be reintroduced if clinically necessary, provided that the risk factors for enhanced susceptibility have been corrected and that renal function is closely monitored. COX-2-selective inhibitor use requires the same cautions as with traditional NSAIDs.

References

1 Singh G, Triadafilopoulos G. Epidemiology of NSAID induced gastrointestinal complications. *J Rheumatol Suppl* 1999; **56**: 18–24.

2 Clive DM, Stoff JS. Renal syndromes associated with anti-inflammatory drugs. *N Engl J Med* 1984; **310**: 563–572.

3 Blackshear JL, Napier JS, Davidman M, Stillman MT. Renal complications of non-steroidal anti-inflammatory drugs: identification and monitoring of those at risk. *Semin Arthritis Rheum* 1985; **14**: 163–175.

4 Henrich WL. Southwestern Internal Medicine Conference: Analgesic nephropathy. *Am J Med Sci* 1988; **295**: 561–568.

5 Sandler DP, Burr FR, Weinberg CR. Nonsteroidal anti-inflammatory drugs and the risk for chronic renal disease. *Ann Intern Med* 1991; **115**: 165–172.

6 Perneger TV, Whelton PK, Klag MJ. Risk of kidney failure associated with the use of acetaminophen, aspirin, and nonsteroidal anti-inflammatory drugs. *N Engl J Med* 1994; **331**: 1675–1679.

7 Bresalier RS, Sandler RS, Quan H, Bolognese JA, Oxenius B, Horgan K *et al.* Cardiovascular events associated with rofecoxib in a colorectal adenoma chemoprevention trial. *N Engl J Med* 2005; **352**: 1092–1102.

8 Nussmeier NA, Whelton AA, Brown MT, Langford RM, Hoeft A, Parlow JL *et al.* Complications of the COX-2 inhibitors parecoxib and valdecoxib after cardiac surgery. *N Engl J Med* 2005; **352**: 1081–1091.

9 Johnsen SP, Larsson H, Tarone RE, McLaughlin JK, Norgard B, Friis S *et al.* Risk of hospitalisation for myocardial infarction among users of rofecoxib, celecoxib, and other NSAIDs: a population based case control study. *Arch Intern Med* 2005; **165**: 978–984.

10 Hippisley-Cox J, Coupland C. Risk of nyocardial infarction in patients taking cyclo-oxygenase-2 inhibitors or conventional non-steroidal anti-inflammatory drugs: Population based nested case-control analysis. *BMJ* 2005; **330**: 1366.

11 Kearney PM, Baigent C, Godwin J, Halls H, Emberson JR, Patron C. Do selective cyclo-oxygenase-2 inhibitors and traditional non-steroidal anti-inflammatory drugs increase the risk of atherothrombosis? Meta-analysis of randomised trials. *BMJ* 2006; **332(7533)**: 1302–1308.

12 Aiken JW, Vane JR. Intrarenal prostaglandin release attenuates the renal vasoconstrictor activity of angiotensin. *J Pharmacol Exp Ther* 1973; **184**: 678–687.

13 Kujubu D, Fletcher B, Varnum, BC, Lim R, Herschman H. TIS 10, a phorbol ester tumor promoter-inducible mRNA from Swiss 3T3 cells, encodes a novel prostaglandin synthase/cyclooxygenase homologue. *J Biol Chem* 1991; **266**: 12866–12872.

14 O'Banion M, Sadowski K, Winn V, Young D. A serum- and glucocorticoid-regulated 4-kilobase mRNA encodes a cyclooxygenase-related protein. *J Biol Chem* 1991; **266**: 23261–23267.

15 Jones DA, Carlton DP, McIntyre TM, Zimmerman GA, Prescott SM. Molecular cloning of human prostaglandin endoperoxide synthase type II and demonstration of expression in response to cytokines. *J Biol Chem* 1993; **268**: 9049–9054.

16 Harris RC, McKanna JA, Alcai Y, Jacobson HR, Dubois RN, Breyer MD. Cyclo-oxygenase-2 is associated with the macula densa of rat kidney and increases with salt restriction. *J Clin Invest* 1994; **94**: 2504–2510.

17 Zhang MZ, Wang JL, Cheng HF, Harris RC, McKanna JA. Cyclooxygenase-2 in rat nephron development. *Am J Physiol* 1997; **273**: F994–F1002.

18 Dinchuk JE, Car BD, Focht RJ, Johnston JJ, Jaffee BD, Covington MB *et al.* Renal abnormalities and an altered inflammatory response in mice lacking cyclooxygenase II. *Nature* 1995; **378**: 406–409.

19 Komhoff M, Wang JL, Cheng HF, Langenbach R, McKanna JA, Harris RC *et al.* Cyclooxygenase-2-selective inhibitors impair glomerulogenesis and renal cortical development. *Kidney Int* 2000; **57**: 414–422.

20 O'Neill GP, Ford-Hutchinson AW. Expression of mRNA for cyclooxygenase-1 and cyclooxygenase-2 in human tissues. *FEBS Lett* 1993; **330**: 156–160.

21 Komhoff M, Grone HJ, Klein T, Seeyberth H, Nusing R. Localization of cyclooxygenase-1 and -2 in adult and fetal human kidney: implication for renal function. *Am J Physiol* 1997; **272**: F460–F468.

22 Nantel F, Meadows E, Denis D, Connolly B, Metters KM, Giaid A. Immunolocalization of cyclooxygenase 2 in the macula densa of human elderly. *FEBS Lett* 1999; **457**: 475–477.

23 Henrich WL. Role of the prostaglandins in renin secretion. *Kidney Int* 1981; **19**: 822–830.

24 Lifschitz MD. Prostaglandins and renal blood flow: in vivo studies. *Kidney Int* 1981; **19**: 781–785.

25 Schnermann J, Briggs JP. Participation of renal cortical prostaglandins in the regulation of glomerular filtration rate. *Kidney Int* 1981; **19**: 802–815.

26 Dunn MJ. Nonsteroidal anti-inflammatory drugs and renal function. *Annu Rev Med* 1984; **35**: 411–428.

27 Patrono C, Ciabattoni G, Remuzzi G, Gotti E, Bombardieri S, Di Munno O *et al.* Functional significance of renal prostacyclin and thromboxane A2 production in patients with systemic lupus erythematosus. *J Clin Invest* 1985; **76**: 1011–1018.

28 Catella-Lawson F, McAdam B, Morrison BW, Kapoor S, Kujubu D, Antes L *et al.* Effects of specific inhibition of cyclooxygenase-2 on sodium balance, hemodynamics and vasoactive eicosanoids. *J Pharmacol Exp Ther* 1999; **289**: 735–741.

29 Van Hecken A, Schwartz JI, Depré M, De Lepeleire I, Dallob A, Tanaka W *et al.* Comparative inhibitory activity of rofecoxib, meloxicam, diclofenac, ibuprofen and naproxen on COX-2 versus COX-1 in healthy volunteers. *J Clin Pharmacol* 2000; **40**: 1109–1120.

30 McAdam BF, Catella-Lawson F, Mardini IA, Kapoor S, Lawson JA, FitzGerald GA. Systemic biosynthesis of prostacyclin by cyclooxygenase (COX)-2: the human pharmacology of a selective inhibitor of COX-2. *Proc Natl Acad Sci USA* 1999; **96**: 272–277.

31 Whelton A, Maurath CJ, Verburg KM, Geis GS. Renal safety and tolerability of celecoxib, a novel cyclooxygenase-2 inhibitor. *Am J Ther* 2000; **7**(**3**): 159–175.

32 Dibona GF. Prostaglandins and non-steroidal anti-inflammatory drugs: effects on renal haemodynamics. *Am J Med* 1986; **80**(**Suppl 1A**): 12–21.

33 Scharschmidt LA, Simonson MS, Dunn MJ. Glomerular prostaglandins, angiotensin II, and nonsteroidal antiinflammatory drugs. *Am J Med* 1986; **81**(**2B**): 30–42.

34 Pelayo JC. Renal adrenergic effector mechanisms: glomerular sites for prostaglandin interaction. *Am J Physiol* 1988; **254**(**23**): F184–1F90.

35 Takahashi K, Nammour TM, Fukunaga M, Ebert J, Morrow JD, Roberts LJ, II, *et al.* Glomerular action of a free radical-generated novel prostaglandin, 8-epi-prostaglandin F2 alpha in the rat. *J Clin Invest* 1992; **90**: 136–141.

36 Donker AJM, Arisz L, Brentjens JRH, van der Hem GK, Hollemans HJG. The effect of indomethacin on kidney function and plasma renin activity in man. *Nephron* 1976; **17**: 288–296.

37 Muther RS, Bennett WM. Effect of aspirin on glomerular filtration rate in normal humans. *Ann Intern Med* 1980; **92**: 386–387.

38 Garella S, Matarese RA. Renal effects of prostaglandins and clinical adverse effects of non-steroidal anti-inflammatory drugs. *Medicine* 1984; **63**: 165–181.

39 Whelton A, Schulman G, Wallemark C, Drower EJ, Isakson PC, Verburg KM *et al.* Effects of celecoxib and naproxen on renal function in the elderly. *Arch Intern Med* 2000; **160**(**10**): 1465–1470.

40 Swan SK, Rudy DW, Lasseter KC, Ryan CF, Buechel KL, Lambrecht LJ *et al.* Effect of cyclooxygenase-2 inhibition on renal function in elderly persons receiving a low salt diet. A randomised, controlled trial. *Ann Intern Med* 2000; **133**(**1**): 1–9.

41 Lee A, Cooper MC, Craig JC, Knight JF, Keneally JP. Effects of non-steroidal anti-inflammatory drugs on postoperative renal function in adults with normal renal function. *Cochrane Database Syst Rev* 2004; **2**: CD002765.

42 Hou S, Bushinsky D, Wish J, Cohen J, Harrington J. Hospital-acquired renal insufficiency: a prospective study. *Am J Med* 1983; **1983**(**74**): 243–248.

43 Chan FK, Hung LC, Suen BY, Wu JC, Lee KC, Leung VK *et al.* Celecoxib versus diclofenac and omeprazole in reducing the risk of recurrent ulcer bleeding in patients with arthritis. *N Engl J Med* 2002; **347**(**26**): 2104–2110.

44 Bombardier C, Laine L, Reicin A, Shapiro D, Burgos-Vargas R, Davis B *et al.* Comparison of upper gastrointestinal toxicity of rofecoxib and naproxen in patients with rheumatoid arthritis. VIGOR Study Group. *N Engl J Med* 2000; **343**(**21**): 1520–1528.

45 Silverstein FE, Faich G, Goldstein JL, Simon LS, Pincus T, Whelton A *et al.* Gastrointestinal toxicity with celecoxib vs nonsteroidal anti-inflammatory drugs for osteoarthritis and rheumatoid arthritis. The CLASS study: a randomized controlled trial. Celecoxib Long-term Arthritis Safety Study. *JAMA* 2000; **284**(**10**): 1247–1255.

46 Moore RA, Derry S, Makinson GT, McQuay HJ. Tolerability and adverse events in clinical trials of celecoxib in osteoarthritis and rheumatoid arthritis: systematic review and meta-analysis of information from company clinical trial reports. *Arthritis Res Ther* 2005; **7**(**3**): R644–R665.

47 Goldzer RC, Coodley EL, Rosner MJ, Simons WM, Schwartz AM. Hyperkalaemia associated with indomethacin. *Arch Intern Med* 1980; **141**: 802–804.

48 Galler M, Folkert VW, Schlondorff D. Reversible acute renal insufficiency and hyperkalemia following indomethacin therapy. *JAMA* 1981; **246**: 154–155.

49 Brater D, Harris C, Redfern J, Gertz B. Renal effects of COX-2 selective inhibitors. *Am J Nephrol* 2001; **2001**(**21**): 1–15.

50 Tannen RL. Potassium in cardiovascular and renal medicine, arrhythmias, myocardial infarction and hypertension. In: Whelton PK, Whelton A, Walker WG, editors. *Drug Interactions Causing Hyperkalaemia.* Marcel Dekker, New York, 1986.

51 Field MJ, Giebisch G. Mechanisms of segmental potassium reabsorption and secretion. In: Seldin DW, Giebisch G, editors. *The Regulation of Potassium Balance.* Raven, New York, 1989.

52 Stokes JB. Effect of prostaglandin E2 on chloride transport across the rabbit thick ascending limb of Henle. Selective inhibition of the medullary portion. *J Clin Invest* 1979; **64**: 495–502.

53 Kinoshita Y, Romero JC, Knox F. Effect of renal interstitial infusion of arachidonic acid on proximal sodium reabsorption. *Am J Physiol* 1989; **26**: F237–F242.

54 Lum GM, Aisenberg GA, Dunn MJ, Berl T, Schrier RW, McDonald KM. In vivo effect of indomethacin to potentiate the renal medullary cyclic AMP response to vasopressin. *J Clin Invest* 1977; **59**: 8–13.

55 Pearce CJ, Gonzalez FM, Wallin JD. Renal failure and hyperkalemia associated with ketorolac tromethamine. *Arch Intern Med* 1993; **153**: 1000–1002.

56 Smith K, Halliwell RMT, Lawrence S, Klineberg PL, O'Connell P. Acute renal failure associated with intramuscular ketorolac. *Anaesthesia Intensive Care* 1993; **21**: 700–703.

57 O'Callaghan CA, Andrews PA, Ogg CS. Renal disease and use of topical non-steroidal anti-inflammatory drugs. *Br Med J* 1994; **308**: 110–111.

58 Kleinknecht D, Landais P, Goldfarb B. Analgesic and non-steroidal anti-inflammatory drug-associated acute renal failure: a prospective collaborative study. *Clin Nephrol* 1986; **25**: 275–281.

59 Huerta C, Castellsague J, Varas-Lorenzo C, Garcia Rodriguez LA. Nonsteroidal anti-inflammatory drugs and risk of ARF in the general population. *Am J Kidney Dis* 2005; **45**(**3**): 531–539.

60 Carmichael T, Shankel SW. Effects of non-steroidal anti-inflammatory drugs on prostaglandins and renal function. *Am J Med* 1985; **78**: 992–1000.

61 Parazella M, Eras J. Are selective COX-2 inhibitors nephrotoxic. *Am J Kidney Dis* 2000; **35(5)**: 937–940.

62 Wolf G, Porth J, Stahl RA. Acute renal failure associated with rofecoxib. *Ann Intern Med* 2000; **133(5)**: 394.

63 Brezin JH, Katz SM, Schwartz AB, Chinitz JL. Reversible renal failure and nephrotic syndrome assiciated with nonsteroidal anti-inflammatory drugs. *N Engl J Med* 1979; **310**: 1271–1273.

64 Abraham PA, Keane WF. Glomerular and interstiti disease induced by nonsteroidal anti-inflammatory drugs. *Am J Nephrol* 1984; **4**: 1–6.

65 Finkelstein A, Fraley DS, Stachura I, Feldman HA, Grandy DR, Bourke E. Fenoprofen nephropathy: lipoid nephrosis and interstitial nephritis: a possible T lymphocyte disorder. *Am J Med* 1982; **72**: 81–87.

66 Bender WL, Whelton A, Beschorner WE, Darwish MO, Hall-Craggs M, Solez K. Interstitial nephritis, proteinuria and renal failure caused by non-steroidal anti-inflammatory drugs. Immunological characterisation of the infiltrate. *Am J Med* 1984; **1984**: 1006–1012.

67 Alper ABJ, Meleg-Smith S, Krane NK. Nephrotic syndrome and interstitial nephritis associated with celecoxib. *Am J Kidney Dis* 2002; **40**: 1886–1890.

68 Alim N, Peterson L, Zimmerman S, Updike S. Rofecoxib-induced acute interstitial nephritis. *Am J Kidney Dis* 2003; **41**: 720–721.

69 Brewster UC, Perazella MA. Acute tubulointerstitial nephritis associated with celecoxib. *Nephrol Dial Transplant* 2004; **18**: 1017–1018.

70 Chow KM, Szeto CC, Li P, Lai FM. Acute interstitial nephritis and COX-2 inhibition. *Hospital Med* 2003; **64**: 429.

71 Demke D, Zhao S, Arellano FM. Interstitial nephritis associated with celecoxib. *Lancet* 2001; **358**: 1726–1727.

72 Markowitz GS, Falkowitz DC, Isom R, Zaki M, Imaizumi S, Appel GB *et al.* Membranous glomerulopathy and acute interstitial nephritis following treatment with celecoxib. *Clin Nephrol* 2003; **59**: 137–142.

73 Rocha JL, Fernando-Alonso J. Acute tubulointerstitial nephritis associated with the selective COX-2 enzyme inhibitor, rofecoxib. *Lancet* 2001; **357**: 1946–1947.

74 Cameron JS. Allergic interstitial nephritis: clinical features and pathogenesis. *QJM* 1988; **66(250)**: 97–115.

75 Schwartz A, Krause PH, Keller T, Offerman G, Mihatsch MJ. Granulomatous interstitial nephritis after non-steroidal anti-inflammatory drugs. *Am J Nephrol* 1988; **8**: 410–416.

76 Adams DH, Howie AJ, Micheal J, McConkey B, Bacon PA, Adu D. Non-steroidal anti-inflammatory drugs and renal failure. *Lancet* 1986; **i**: 57–60.

77 Campistol JM, Galofre J, Botey A, Torras A, Revert LI. Reversible membranous nephropathy associated with diclofenac. *Nephrol Dial Transplant* 1989; **4**: 393–395.

78 Tattersall J, Greenwood R, Farrington K. Membranous nephropathy associated with diclofenac (letter). *Postgrad Med J* 1992; **68(799)**: 392–393.

79 Grcevska L, Polenakovi M, Ferluga D, Vizjak A, Stavric G. Membranous nephropathy with severe tubulointerstitial and vascular changes in a patient with psoriatic arthritis treated with non-steroidal anti-inflammatory drugs. *Clin Nephrol* 1993; **39**: 250–253.

80 Radford MG, Holley KE, Grande JP, Larson TS, Wagoner RD, Donadio JV *et al.* Reversible membranous nephropathy associated with the use of nonsteroidal antiinflammatory drugs. *JAMA* 1996; **276**: 466–469.

81 Munn E, Lynn KL, R BR. Renal papillary necrosis following regular consumption of NSAIDs. *N Z J Med* 1976; **95**: 213–214.

82 Shah GM, Muhalwas KK, Winer RL. Renal papillary necrosis due to ibuprofen. *Arthritis Rheum* 1981; **24**: 1208–1210.

83 Segasothy M, Thyaparan A, Kamal A, Sivalingam S. Mefamanic acid nephropathy. *Nephron* 1987; **45**: 156–157.

84 Krikler DM. Paracetamol and the kidney. *Br J Med* 1967; **2**: 615.

85 Master DR, Krikler DM. Analgesic nephropathy associated with paracetamol. *Proc R Soc Med* 1973; **66**: 904.

86 Akhund L, Quinet RJ, Ishaq S. Celecoxib-related renal papillary necrosis. *Arch Intern Med* 2003; **163**: 114–115.

87 Fox DA, Jick H. Non-steroidal anti-inflammatory drugs and renal disease. *JAMA* 1984; **151**: 1299–1300.

88 Beard K, Perera DR, Jick H. Drug-induced parenchymal renal disease in outpatients. *J Clin Pharmacol* 1988; **28(5)**: 431–435.

89 Rexrode KM, Buring JE, Glynn RJ, Stampfer MJ, Youngman LD, Gaziano JM. Analgesic use and renal function in men. *JAMA* 2001; **286(3)**: 315–321.

90 Curhan GC, Knight EL, Rosner B, Hankinson SE, Stampfer MJ. Lifetime nonnarcotic analgesic use and decline in renal function in women. *Arch Intern Med* 2004; **164(14)**: 1519–1524.

91 Ciabattoni G, Cinotti GA, Pierucci A. Effects of sulindac and ibuprofen in patients with chronic glomerular disease: evidence for the dependence of renal function on prostacyclin. *N Engl J Med* 1984; **310**: 279–288.

92 Patrono C, Pierucci A. Renal effects of nonsteroidal antiinflammatory drugs in chronic glomerular disease. *Am J Med* 1986; **82(Suppl 2B)**: 71–83.

93 Brandstetter RD, Mar DD. Reversible oliguric renal failure associated with ibuprofen treatment. *Br Med J* 1978; **2**: 1194–1195.

94 Tan SY, Shapiro R, Kish MA. Reversible acute renal failure induced by indomethacin. *JAMA* 1979; **241**: 2732–2733.

95 Blum M, Aviram A. Ibuprofen-induced hyponatraemia. *Rheumatol Rehab* 1980; **19**: 258–259.

96 Pope JE, Anderson JJ, Felson DT. A meta-analysis of the effects of nonsteroidal anti-inflammatory drugs on blood pressure. *Arch Intern Med* 1994; **21**: 289–300.

97 Johnson AG, Nguyen TV, Day RO. Do nonsteroidal anti-inflammatory drugs affect blood pressure? *Ann Intern Med* 1994; **121**: 289–300.

98 Collins R, Peto R, Godwin J, MacMahon S. Blood pressure, stroke, and coronary heart disease. Part 2. Short-term reductions in blood pressure: overview of randomised drug trials in their epidemiological context. *Lancet* 1990; **335**: 827–838.

99 Whelton A. Renal aspects of treatment with conventional nonsteroidal anti-inflammatory drugs versus cyclooxygenase-2 inhibitor. *Am J Med* 2001; **110(Suppl 1)**: 33–42.

100 Whelton A, Fort JG, Puma JA, Normandin D, Bello AE, Verburg KM *et al.* Cyclooxygenase-2 specific inhibitors and cardiorenal function: a randomized, controlled trial of celecoxib and refecoxib in older hypertensive osteoarthritis patients. *Am J Ther* 2001; **8(2)**: 85–95.

101 Aw TJ, Haas SJ, Liew D, Krum H. Meta-analysis of cyclooxygenase-2 inhibitors and their effects on blood pressure. *Arch Intern Med* 2005; **165(5)**: 490–496.

102 Kutyrina IM, Androsova SO, Tareyeva IE. Indomethacin-induced hyporeninaemic hypoaldosterism. *Lancet* 1979; **i**: 785.

103 Findling JW, Beckstrom D, Rawsthorne L, Kozin F, Itskovitz H. Indomethacin-induced hyperkalaemia in three patients with gouty arthritis. *JAMA* 1980; **244**: 1127–1128.

104 Brater DC, Harris C, Redfern JS, Gertz BJ. Renal effects of COX-2 selective inhibitors. *Am J Nephrol* 2001; **21**: 1–15.

105 Donker AJM, Brentjens JRH, van der Hem GK, Arisz L. Treatment of the nephrotic syndrome with indomethacin. *Nephron* 1978; **22**: 374–381.

106 Gansevoort RT, Heeg JE, Vriesendorp R, de Zeeuw D, de jong PE. Antiproteinuric drugs in patients with idiopathic membranous glomerulopathy. *Nephrol Dial Transplant* 1992; **7**(**Suppl 1**): 91–96.

107 Tiggeler RGWL, Hulme B, Wijdeveld PGAB. Effect of indomethacin on glomerular permeability in the nephrotic syndrome. *Kidney Int* 1979; **16**: 312–321.

Toxic Nephropathies: Environmental Agents and Metals

Richard P. Wedeen

Department of Veterans Affairs New Jersey Health Care System, 385 Tremont Avenue, East Orange, New Jersey, USA; University of Medicine and Dentistry of New Jersey, The New Jersey Medical School, 185 South Orange Avenue, Newark, New Jersey, USA

Introduction

Environmental nephrotoxins include materials found in the workplace and pharmaceutical agents used for the diagnosis and treatment of disease (Table 28.1). In this chapter, I will not review the long list of drugs for which renal damage is a side effect. Nonpharmaceutical toxins recognized as producing kidney disease are those substances that cause occupational kidney diseases. Kidney diseases resulting from high-dose occupational exposure in a few workers serve as models for understanding kidney disease among whole populations exposed to low doses of toxins. The clinically important industrial nephrotoxins include lead, mercury, cadmium, silica, and a variety of (sometimes poorly defined) organic hydrocarbons (aliphatic, aromatic, and halogenated). Uranium, chromium, and arsenic rarely produce kidney disease and will not be discussed further.

It should be recognized that there are no randomized controlled trials for the treatment of kidney diseases caused by these environmental agents. The cornerstone of treatment is prevention and the termination of exposure.

Heavy metals

Lead

Severe acute lead poisoning occurring over days or weeks was common among poor urban children in the USA in the early part of the 20th century. Blood lead levels exceeded 70 μg/dL (current mean blood lead in the USA is <2 μg/dL). Acute childhood lead poisoning usually occurred because of the ingestion of lead-based paint in deteriorated housing (pica). Renal symptoms of acute lead poisoning, called the Fanconi syndrome, consist of transient proximal tubular reabsorptive defects manifested by aminoaciduria, phosphaturia, and glycosuria. The Fanconi

syndrome is regularly reproducible in experimental animals exposed to sufficiently high doses of lead and is reversed by chelation therapy or removal from exposure [1].

Acute symptomatic lead poisoning with encephalopathy, abdominal colic, peripheral motor neuropathy, and anemia is distinctly uncommon today. Far more common is chronic lead poisoning, which is either asymptomatic or accompanied by nonspecific complaints. Long-term, low-dose exposure in adults is also associated with hypertension, gout, and tubulo-interstitial nephritis that is histologically indistinguishable from hypertensive nephrosclerosis. In the past, lead nephropathy was identified in lead workers after many years of exposure to lead dust in the industry. Blood lead in these workers was often above 40 μg/dL on the job, which is the exposure limit promulgated in the federal occupational lead standard. It was widely assumed that blood lead levels of 60 μg/dL or higher, sustained for many years, were required to induce lead nephropathy. However, recent epidemiologic evidence using blood and bone lead measurements (by noninvasive in vivo K X-ray fluorescence) indicate that the adverse effects of lead on blood pressure and kidney function occur at much lower levels than previously recognized. Ninety-five percent of the body stores of lead are retained in bone, with a biological half-life approximating 2 decades, whereas blood lead has a biological half-life of about 30 days. Bone lead therefore reflects cumulative lead absorption, whereas blood lead primarily reflects recent exposure.

Blood lead and bone lead predict blood pressure even when both are within the range traditionally considered "normal." Epidemiologic evidence that low-level lead absorption (blood lead of <10 μg/dL) has deleterious effects on blood pressure and renal function was obtained from National Health and Nutrition Evaluation Survey III, 1988–1994. Analysis of data on over 15,000 Americans showed that hypertensive people had significantly higher blood lead levels (4.21 vs. 3.30 μg/dL) than people without hypertension [2]. Two large, cross-sectional studies also reported a significant association between low-level lead exposure and serum creatinine [3,4]. The adverse effects of low-level lead exposure on renal function are further supported by longitudinal observations [5]. Because lead does not accumulate in patients with kidney

Evidence-based Nephrology. Edited by Donald Molony and Jonathan Craig
© 2009 Blackwell Publishing, ISBN: 978-1-4051-3975-5.

Table 28.1 Environmental nephrotoxins.

Substance	Pathology			Comments
	ATN	TIN	G	
Metals				
Pb	+	+	−	Fanconi syndrome, tubular proteinuria, hypertension, gout
Cd	−	+	−	Fanconi syndrome, Ca^{++} wasting, tubular proteinuria
Hg[1]	+	+	+	G →immune, genetic control, nephrotic syndrome; $HgCl_2 \rightarrow$ ATN
As	+	+	−	AsH_3, hemolysis
Cr[1]	+	+	−	$Cr^{+++} \rightarrow$ tubular proteinuria, nasal perforation, cancer; $Cr^{+++++} \rightarrow$ ATN
U	+	+	−	tubular proteinuria
Si	−	−	+	immune adjuvant, immune complexes, ANCA, Wegener's granulomatosis
Organics				
CCl^4	+	+	−	liver damage, alcohol enhanced, dry cleaner
Toluene	−	−	−	tubular proteinuria, glue sniffing
Solvents	−	−	+	immune G, tubular proteinuria
Selected Drugs[2]				
Aminoglycosides	+	+	−	ARF after 8 days, lysosomal accumulation S_1 and S_2
Amphotericin B	−	+	−	distal RTA, $K^+\downarrow$, $Mg^{++}\downarrow$, Uosm ↓, tubular calcification
Penicillins	−	+	−	allergic component, acute, after 15 days, interstitial edema, lymphocytic infiltration
Vancomycin	+	+	−	ARF
Sulfonamides	−	+	−	intra-luminal crystals, kidney stones, ARF, microhematuria, soluble in alkaline urine
Acyclovir	−	+	−	intraluminal crystal deposition, flank pain, microhematuria
Cyclosporin A Tacrolimus	+	+	−	ARF, vasomotor, proximal tubule vacuolization, striped fibrosis, arteriolar hyalinosis
Gold salts	−	+	+	membranous glomerulopthy, gold in tubular epithelium, separate tubular disease
D-penicillamine	−	−	−	membranous glomerulopthy, vasculitis
Cis-platinum	+	+	−	ARF, usually reversible
Mitomycin	−	+	−	thrombosis, hemolytic uremic syndrome

1. Depends on valance and organic form.
2. Often in clinically complex settings with multicausal renal damage.
Abbreviations: ATN, acute tubular necrosis; TIN, tubular interstitial nephritis; G, glomerulopathy; ARF, acute renal failure; RTA, renal tubular acidosis.

failure of nonlead etiology, these observations point to low-level lead exposure as a contributor to hypertension and kidney disease.

Bone lead levels were found to be significant predictors of hypertension in community-exposed men [6]. The mean blood lead level in these men was 6 μg/dL. Similarly, bone lead levels were found to be a significant predictor of hypertension in nurses [7]. A study in pregnant women with a geometric mean blood lead level of 1.9 μg/dL found increases in bone lead were associated with an increased risk of pregnancy hypertension [8]. Increases in both diastolic and systolic blood pressures in pregnant women were significantly associated with blood lead, and the major portion of the effect was found with blood lead levels under 5 μg/dL. These observations on the adverse effects at blood lead levels below

10 μg/dL in diverse groups indicate that, even at levels traditionally considered acceptable, important adverse health effects occur.

Treatment of lead-induced hypertension and kidney failure with calcium ethylenediaminetetraacetic acid ($CaNa_2$–EDTA; also called calcium disodium versenate or edetate calcium disodium) may improve the glomerular filtration rate (GFR) or reduce the rate of progression of kidney failure. The reversible component of lead nephropathy reported following $CaNa_2$–EDTA therapy in lead workers (mean blood lead, 18 μg/dL) may have resulted from the correction of acute lead absorption superimposed on chronic lead nephropathy [9]. Similar therapeutic effects have been noted in kidney failure at much lower levels of lead exposure. Lin *et al.* [10] treated kidney patients (mean creatinine, 2.1 mg/dL; mean blood lead, 5.3 μg/dL) with CaNa$_2$–EDTA , 4–13 g intravenously, over 2 years. The treated group had an increase in GFR averaging 3.4 mL/min, whereas untreated controls had a decrease in GFR of 1.0 mL/min during this period. The same laboratory demonstrated that low levels of lead absorption correlate significantly with the rate of progression of kidney failure in type 2 diabetics and that CaNa$_2$–EDTA therapy, averaging 7 g over 3 months, significantly reduced the rate of progression of kidney failure compared to untreated diabetic controls [11]. These results suggest that reducing even very low levels of lead may improve GFR in a variety of non-lead-related kidney diseases. Moreover, if the beneficial effect of CaNa$_2$–EDTA is, in fact, due to the removal of lead from the body, these observations indicate that there is no threshold for the deleterious effects of lead on kidneys.

However, the mechanism of the beneficial effect of CaNa$_2$–EDTA on the kidneys is by no means clear. There were no controls with normal renal function or with minimal body lead stores in Lin's studies. The effect of chelating lead on subjects with low-level lead absorption by succimer has not been evaluated. It therefore remains possible that the beneficial effect of CaNa$_2$–EDTA on GFR is due to actions other than the removal of lead. Modification of potential mediators of hypertension and reduced GFR, such as other cations, reactive oxygen species [12], or uric acid [13], may have accounted for the improvement in GFR found by Lin *et al.*

Prevention remains the most effective method of treatment of lead poisoning. Chelation transiently increases the rate of removal of lead, causing the urinary excretion of up to several milligrams of lead in heavily exposed individuals within a few days. If, on the other hand, excessive exposure is terminated, the expected urinary excretion of 100–200 μg of lead/day will achieve a negative balance of 35–70 mg/year. Because a lifetime of occupational exposure can result in bone lead stores of 500 mg or more, a course of chelation therapy (e.g. 1–2 g CaNa$_2$–EDTA) eliminates only about 0.2–0.4 % of the body burden, whereas terminating exposure reduces bone stores by about 10% per year. Although it is not feasible to eliminate all lead intake, similar calculations for individuals with low-level exposure indicate that, in the long term, prevention is more effective than chelation in lowering the body lead stores. In summary, chelation therapy is justified in cases of symptomatic lead poisoning or when the blood lead exceeds about 70 μg/dL, but when no symptom end point is clearly defined, chelation for blood lead of <70 μg/dL is not usually justified.

Mercury

The toxicity of mercury depends on both its chemical form and the route of absorption. Although preferentially accumulated in the kidney, neurologic disease, but not kidney disease, regularly follows exposure to elemental mercury. Once in the environment, elemental mercury undergoes biotransformation to both organic and inorganic salts, which are absorbed by living organisms and thus enter the food chain. Methyl, ethyl, and phenoxyethyl mercury are important organomercurial contaminants arising from industrial and agricultural processes. Whereas certain organomercurials (e.g. chlormerodrin) are potent diuretics, others that are also con-

centrated in the proximal tubule (e.g. *p*-chloromercuribenzoate) have no diuretic effect. In contrast, the mercuric salt, corrosive sublimate (mercury bichloride [HgCl$_2$]), is highly nephrotoxic and, at 1 mg/kg, uniformly produces acute tubular necrosis [14]. Similar nephrotoxicity is induced by phenyl and methoxy methyl mercuric salts. Another mercurous salt (calomel [Hg$_2$Cl$_2$]) was widely used for therapy until the 20th century and is relatively nontoxic.

In addition to diuresis and acute tubular necrosis, mercury has been sporadically reported to cause nephrotic syndrome in what has usually been considered an idiosyncratic response. Observations in rats may provide a framework for understanding mercury-induced glomerular disease in humans. In 1971, Bariety *et al.* [15] reported that multiple subcutaneous injections of HgCl$_2$ in specific rat strains, in doses too small to produce tubular necrosis, induced membranous nephropathy. Kidney disease characterized by glomerular deposition of immune complexes and heavy proteinuria developed in about 2 months. Subsequent studies showed that the immune response is actually biphasic; immune complex deposition is preceded by anti-glomerular basement membrane antibody and complement deposition. The response to mercury in the rat is under precise genetic control. As little as 0.05 mg/kg of body weight will elicit immunologically mediated glomerular disease in selected strains. As in humans, mercury-induced glomerular disease in rats is self-limited.

There are no randomized clinical trials for the treatment of acute tubular necrosis or nephrotic syndrome due to mercury. Chelation therapy has been employed for excessive mercury exposure, often defined as more than 5 μg Hg/dL in blood or 50 μg Hg/L in urine, but evidence for the effectiveness of chelation therapy is lacking. Traditional use of BAL (British antilewisite, dimercaprol) for chelating mercury is currently being replaced by its soluble congeners, dimercaptopropane sulfonic acid (unithiol, or Dimaval) and succimer (dimercaptosuccinic acid; Chemet). Dimercaptopropane sulfonic acid is the chelator of choice for inorganic mercury intoxication, whereas succimer is the agent of choice for organic mercury [16]. Case reports suggest that in the presence of severe kidney failure the mercury-chelate complex can be removed by hemodialysis or hemofiltration.

Cadmium

Acute absorption of as little as 10 mg of cadmium as dust or fumes induces severe gastrointestinal symptoms and, after a delay of 8–24 h, fatal pulmonary edema. Chronic low-dose exposure causes slowly progressive emphysema, anosmia, and proximal tubular reabsorptive defects characterized by hypercalciuria, low-molecular-weight proteinuria, enzymuria, aminoaciduria, and renal glycosuria [17]. Hypercalciuria (with normocalcemia), phosphaturia, and distal renal tubular acidosis result in clinically important osteomalacia, pseudofractures, and urinary tract stones [18]. Proximal tubular dysfunction is followed by interstitial nephritis, which can progress to chronic kidney failure. The biologic half-life of cadmium in humans exceeds 15 years, and one-third of the total body stores (10–20 mg) is retained in the kidneys. Absorbed cadmium is initially sequestered in the liver and kidney, where it is bound to a cysteine-rich apoprotein, metallothionein. Although uptake in the liver initially exceeds that in the kidney, most of the cadmium is eventually bound to protein in the proximal tubules, where it is accumulated until a "critical concentration," approximately $200 \, \mu g/g$ of renal cortex, is achieved. At this tissue level, adverse renal effects become evident, including tubular proteinuria and increased cadmium excretion. Significant abnormalities of proximal tubular function are associated with urinary cadmium excretion in excess of $30 \, \mu g/day$.

Clinical symptoms associated with cadmium nephropathy derive primarily from the increased calcium excretion that accompanies the renal tubular dysfunction. Hypouricemia, hypophosphatemia, intermittent renal glycosuria, or elevated serum alkaline phosphatase (in the absence of kidney failure or hyperparathyroidism) may bring the acquired Fanconi syndrome to a clinician's attention, but ureteral colic is more likely to be a cadmium worker's chief complaint. Although both osteomalacia and kidney failure are distinctly uncommon in cadmium workers, urinary calculi have been reported in up to 40% of those subjected to industrial exposure [19].

Itai-itai disease

In Japan, a painful bone disease associated with pseudofractures due to cadmium-induced renal calcium wasting was recognized in the 1950s. Attributed to local contamination of food staples by river water polluted with industrial effluents, the syndrome known as itai-itai, or "ouch-ouch" disease, primarily afflicted postmenopausal, multiparous women. Sustained deficiencies in iron, zinc, calcium, and vitamin D rendered these women particularly vulnerable to cadmium toxicity. The women with itai-itai disease tended to have reduced GFR, anemia, lymphopenia, and hypotension as well as osteomalacia. They exhibited a waddling gait, short stature, anemia, glycosuria, and elevated serum alkaline phosphatase levels. Hypertension was absent. β_2-Microglobulin excretion exceeded the normal maximum (1 mg/g of creatinine) by 100-fold, and GFR was substantially reduced in the most severely affected individuals. Long-term follow-up studies showed that excessive urinary excretion of the low-molecular-weight protein β_2-microglobulin predicts the later development of kidney failure in patients with itai-itai disease and that kidney damage progresses even after exposure has ceased. Succimer is effective for chelation in acute cadmium poisoning [16]. No agent has been found effective for mobilizing hepatic or renal stores of cadmium.

Silicon

Silicon is a semi-metal found as the dioxide (SiO_2, silicon dioxide) in 28% of the earth's crust. It has been reported to induce interstitial nephritis by direct deposition of crystalline material in the renal parenchyma [20] and by immunologic mechanisms, acting as an adjuvant to stimulate the immune response [21]. Tubular proteinuria is found in workers exposed to silica dust. The odds of a sandblaster developing end-stage renal disease is 3.8 compared to matched controls. In the accelerated form of silicosis known as silicoproteinosis, silicon dust appears to be indirectly responsible for

rapidly progressive, immune complex-mediated focal glomerulosclerosis [22]. In addition to severe pulmonary disease, these patients develop an overwhelming autoimmune response that frequently includes lupus erythematosus [23] or rheumatoid arthritis (Caplan's syndrome). Glomerular disease, sometimes in association with silica-induced systemic sclerosis, systemic lupus erythematosus, and small vessel vasculitis, has also been described as a result of exposure to silica dust independent of silicosis [24]. Antineutrophil cytoplasmic antibody (c-ANCA)-positive Wegener's granulomatosis has been associated with exposure to silica dust as well as to silica-containing compounds, such as grain dust. No specific therapies have been reported for silica-induced glomerular disease other than those in current use for immunologically medicated glomerular disease.

Solvent nephropathy

Halogenated hydrocarbons have often been implicated in the induction of acute tubular necrosis or Fanconi syndrome in both humans and experimental animals. Low-level occupational absorption by inhalation of volatile hydrocarbons or absorption through the skin may also induce tubular proteinuria, which does not necessarily signify the presence of clinical kidney failure.

At least 40 case–control studies have examined the relationship between glomerulonephritis and exposure to organic solvents. A number of these studies concluded that patients with chronic glomerulonephritis had been exposed to organic solvents (aliphatic and aromatic) more frequently than patients with other diseases. Initially, solvent nephropathy was associated with antiglomerular basement membrane antibody-mediated glomerulonephritis and pulmonary hemorrhage, i.e. Goodpasture's syndrome, but later reports of solvent nephropathy have included many different types of glomerulonephritis [25].

The etiologic role of solvents remains controversial because the dose and exact chemical composition of industrial solvents are usually unknown. Moreover, of the thousands of workers exposed, very few develop immunologically mediated glomerular disease. The genetic and environmental factors that make specific individuals susceptible to solvent nephropathy have not been delineated. The experimental mercury-induced immunologically mediated glomerular disease in rodents described above may provide a model for understanding solvent nephropathy in humans. No specific therapies have been recommended for solvent nephropathy. Avoidance of exposure to volatile hydrocarbons and their derivatives remains an essential preventive approach.

References

1 Chisolm JJ. The use of chelating agents in the treatment of acute and chronic lead intoxication in childhood. *Pediatrics* 1968; **73**(1): 1–38.

2 Munter P, He J, Vupputuri S, Coresh J, Batuman V. Blood lead and chronic kidney disease in the general United States population: results from NHANES III. *Kidney Int* 2003; **63**: 1044–1050.

3 Payton M, Hu H, Sparrow D, Young JB, Landsberg L, Weiss S. Relation between blood lead and urinary biogenic amines in community-exposed men. *Am J Epidemiol* 1993; **138(10):** 815–825.

4 Staessen J, Lauwerys RR, Buchet J-P, Bulpitt CJ, Rondia D, Vanenterghem Y *et al.* Impairment of renal function with increasing blood lead concentration in the general population. The Cadmibel Study Group. *N Engl J Med* 1994; **327:** 151–156.

5 Kim R, Rotnitski A, Parrow D, Weiss ST, Wager C, Hu H. A longitudinal study of low-level lead exposure and impairment of renal function. The normative aging study. *JAMA* 1996; **275:** 1177.

6 Cheng Y, Schwartz J, Sparrow D, Aro A, Weiss, ST, Hu H. Bone lead and bone lead levels in relation to baseline blood pressure and the prospective development of hypertension: The Normative Aging Study. *Am J Epidemiol* 2001; **153(2):** 164–171.

7 Korrick SA, Hunter DJ, Rotnitzky A, Hu H, Speizer FE. Lead and hypertension in a sample of middle-aged women. *Am J Public Health* 1999; **89(3):** 330–335.

8 Rothenberg S, Khondrashov V, Manalo M, Jiang J, Cuellar R, Garcia M *et al.* Increases in hypertension and blood pressure during pregnancy with increased bone lead levels. *Am J Epidemiol* 2002; **156(12):** 1079–1087.

9 Wedeen RP, Mallik DK, Batuman V. Detection and treatment of occupational lead nephropathy. *Arch Intern Med* 1979; **139:** 53–57.

10 Lin J-L, Lin-Tan D-T, Hsu K-H, Yu C-C. Environmental lead exposure and progression of chronic renal diseases in patients without diabetes. *N Eng J Med* 2003; **348(4):** 277–286.

11 Lin J-L, Lin-Tan D-T, Yu C-C, Li Y-J, Huang Y-Y, Li K-L. Environmental exposure to lead and progressive diabetic nephropathy in patients with type II diabetes. *Kidney Int* 2006; **69:** 2049–2056.

12 Ding Y, Vazari ND, Gonick HC. Lead-induced hypertension. II. Response to sequential infusions of L-arginine, superoxide dismutase and nitroprusside. *Environ. Res.* 1998; **76:** 107–113.

13 Kang D-H, Nakagawa T, Feng L, Watanabe S, Lin H, Mazzali M *et al.* Role for uric acid in the progression of renal disease. *J Am Soc Nephrol* 2002; **13:** 2888–2897.

14 Biber TUL, Mylie M, Baines AD, Gottschalk CW, Oliver JR, MacDowel MC. A study by micropuncture and microdissection of acute renal damage in rats. *Am J Med* 1968; **44:** 664–705.

15 Bariety J, Druet P, Laliberte F, Sapin C. Glomerulonephritis with α and β_1 C-globulin deposits induced in rats by mercuric chloride. *Am J Pathol* 1971; **65:** 293–300.

16 Andersen O. Chemical and biologic considerations in the treatment of metal intoxication by chelating agents. *Med Chem* 2004; **4:** 11–23.

17 Nordberg GF, Kjellstrom T, Nordberg M. Kinetics and metabolism: other toxic effects. In: Friberg L, Elinder C-G, Kjellström, Nordberg GF, editors. *Cadmium and Health: a Toxicological and Epidemiological Appraisal.* CRC Press, Boca Raton, 1986.

18 Jarup L, Elinder CG. Incidence of renal stones among cadmium exposed battery workers. *Br J Ind Med* 1993; **50:** 598–602.

19 Thun MJ, Osorio AM, Schober S, Hannon WH, Lewis B, Halperin W. Nephropathy in cadmium workers: assessment of risk from airborne occupational cadmium exposure. *Br J Ind Med* 1989; **46:** 689–697.

20 Dobbie JW, Smith MJB. Silicate nephrotoxicity in the experimental animal: the missing factor in analgesic nephropathy. *Scottish Med J* 1982; **27:** 10–16.

21 Parks CG, Conrad K, Cooper RS. Occupational exposure to crystalline silica and autoimmune disease. *Environ Health Perspect* 1999; **107(Suppl 5):** 793–798.

22 Osorio AM, Thun MJ, Novak RF, Cura JV, Avner ED. Silica and glomerulonephritis: a case report and review of the literature. *Am J Kidney Dis* 1987; **9:** 224–230.

23 Calvert GM, Steenland K, Palu S. End stage renal disease among silica-exposed gold miners. A new method for assessing incidence among epidemiologic controls. *JAMA* 1995; **277:** 1219–1224.

24 Nuyts GD, Van Vlem E, De Vos A, Daelemans RA, Rorive G, Elseviers MM *et al.* Wegener granulomatosis is associated to exposure to silicon compounds: a case-control study. *Nephrol Dial Transplant* 1995; **10:** 162–167.

25 Wedeen RP. Occupational renal diseases. *Am J Kidney Dis* 1984; **3:** 241–357.

29 The Kidney in Pregnancy

Phyllis August[1] & Tiina Podymow[2]
[1]Weill Medical College of Cornell University, New York, New York
[2]Division of Nephrology, McGill University, Montreal, Quebec, Canada

Pregnancy, in the setting of significant maternal kidney disease, is hazardous and frequently unsuccessful, due in part to the failure to adapt to pregnancy-associated hemodynamic alterations. Pregnancy imposes a hemodynamic strain on maternal renal function, so that in some women with preexisting kidney disease, renal function deteriorates during or after pregnancy. Alterations in immune function and increased inflammation associated with pregnancy may also contribute to worsening of kidney disease during gestation. In general, the closer to normal the glomerular filtration rate (GFR) and blood pressure are, the greater the chance of a successful pregnancy. Management of gravidas with kidney disease may be complicated and requires an understanding of the physiologic changes associated with pregnancy, as well as close cooperation between obstetrician and nephrologist. This chapter will focus mainly on clinical issues related to kidney disease in pregnant women. Although some areas in obstetric medicine have been extensively studied with randomized controlled trials (e.g. prevention of preeclampsia), kidney disease in pregnancy is less common, and the quality of the evidence guiding clinical practice in this field of medicine is not of the highest level. There are, however, many clinical questions which have been studied well with randomized controlled trials. Summaries of these trials can be found in the pregnancy and childbirth module of the Cochrane Library, the largest single section of the Cochrane Library. Most evidence consists of case series with modest numbers of subjects. Recent epidemiologic surveys have highlighted the problem of unrecognized chronic kidney disease in the US population [1] and, based on extrapolation of these data, the prevalence of chronic kidney disease in women of childbearing age may be only approximately 0.2% .

Renal anatomy and physiology in pregnancy

A brief review of some of the important physiological alterations in pregnancy is useful for guiding therapeutic principles. Much of the data on renal function and physiology during pregnancy were collected more than 25 years ago. More recent studies in animal models of pregnancy have begun to examine some of the mediators of the renal alterations, including steroid hormones, nitric oxide, and relaxin. The difficulties in studying pregnant women have clearly been an impediment in this field.

Anatomic and functional changes in the urinary tract

Kidney length increases approximately 1 cm during normal gestation, and overall kidney volume increases by up to 30% [2]. The major anatomic alterations of the urinary tract during pregnancy, however, are seen in the collecting system, where calyces, renal pelves, and ureters dilate, often giving the erroneous impression of obstructive uropathy. The cause of the ureteral dilation is disputed and has been attributed to hormonal mechanisms [3] as well as mechanical obstruction by the enlarging uterus. These morphologic changes result in stasis in the urinary tract and a propensity of pregnant women with asymptomatic bacteriuria to develop frank pyelonephritis, particularly in women with a history of prior urinary tract infection [4].

Renal hemodynamics

Pregnancy is characterized by marked vasodilatation, which is detectable early in the first trimester, by 6 weeks of gestation. In fact, recent studies of the menstrual cycle demonstrated that vasodilation is also present in the late luteal phase, prior to conception [5]. This early vasodilation is accompanied by a decrease in blood pressure, increase in cardiac output, and increases in renal plasma flow and glomerular filtration, all of which persist until late gestation. Since renal plasma flow increases slightly more than GFR, the filtration fraction remains constant or slightly lower in pregnancy [6]. Increases in renal hemodynamics reach a maximum during the first trimester and are approximately 50% greater than nonpregnancy levels [7]. Micropuncture studies performed in the gravid rat suggest that renal vasodilatation and increased glomerular plasma flow are the primary determinants of the increased renal hemodynamics in pregnancy. In humans, using clearance techniques (inulin, PAH, and neutral dextrans), the increment in GFR has

Evidence-based Nephrology. Edited by Donald Molony and Jonathan Craig
© 2009 Blackwell Publishing, ISBN: 978-1-4051-3975-5.

been largely attributed to increased renal plasma flow, decreased oncotic pressure, and an increased glomerular ultrafiltration coefficient, but not with increments in transglomerular hydrostatic pressure difference. The implications of these observations are that although GFR is significantly increased throughout the duration of normal pregnancy, there is little evidence for increased intraglomerular pressure and, therefore, little risk that the hyperfiltration associated with gestation is associated with additional strain on diseased kidneys, a conclusion that has not been tested in clinical trials. Increased progesterone, estrogen, nitric oxide, and relaxin have all been implicated as mediators of the systemic and renal vasodilation of pregnancy [8–10].

Creatinine production is unchanged during pregnancy; thus, increments in clearance result in decreased serum levels. There is also increased excretion of glucose, amino acids, calcium, and urinary protein, resulting in an increase in the upper limit of normal for urinary protein excretion (from 150 to 300 mg/day).

Acid–base regulation in pregnancy

In the resting state there are increases in respiratory rate, tidal volume, and alveolar ventilation, all of which result in a reduced arterial PCO_2 [11]. Augmented respiratory sensitivity in pregnancy has been attributed to the increased circulating level of progesterone, which directly stimulates the medullary respiratory center. There is a partly compensated respiratory alkalosis, with reductions in hydrogen ion concentration, PCO_2, and serum bicarbonate, changes that are apparent in the first trimester [12]. It has recently been demonstrated that exercise-induced increases in acid concentration are similar in pregnancy and nonpregnancy [11]. Finally, it should be appreciated that a PCO_2 of 40 mmHg signifies considerable carbon dioxide retention in pregnancy.

Water metabolism

Pregnancy is associated with a decrease in plasma osmolality of 5–10 mOsm/kg below that of nongravid women. This decrease in plasma osmolality is associated with appropriate responses to water loading and dehydration and suggests a resetting of the osmoreceptor system and thirst occurring at lower serum osmolality. Clinical studies demonstrating decreased osmotic thresholds for thirst and arginine vasopressin (AVP) release in pregnant women support this hypothesis [13,14]. In addition, pregnant women metabolize AVP more rapidly as a consequence of increased production of placental vasopressinases [14]. Pregnant women may develop syndromes of transient diabetes insipidus due to the increased metabolism of AVP. These syndromes may be treated with dDAVP, which is effective owing to a different N terminus that is resistant to the circulating vasopressinases.

Along with decreased serum osmolality, serum sodium is also lower in pregnancy. This may be due in part to relaxin, a peptide hormone in the insulin family, secreted by the corpus luteum and placenta during human gestation [15,16]. Relaxin is associated with early pregnancy osmoregulatory changes, as well as increases in GFR and vasodilatation [15]. β-Human chorionic gonadotropin appears to cause release of relaxin, which then stim-

ulates the hypothalamus, resulting in thirst and AVP secretion [17]. Chronic administration of relaxin to rats mimics several of the hemodynamic and osmotic changes of pregnancy, whereas antirelaxin antibodies reverse these changes.

Volume regulation

Total body water increases by 6–8 L during pregnancy, 4–6 L of which is extracellular. Plasma volume increases 50% during gestation, the largest rate of increase occurring in mid-pregnancy [5]. There is a gradual cumulative retention of about 900 mEq of sodium during pregnancy, which is distributed between the products of conception and the maternal extracellular space. Despite the increase in plasma volume during pregnancy, there is no evidence for a hypervolemic (i.e. overfilled circulation) state during pregnancy. Indeed, the marked vasodilation that is observed as early as the first trimester may be the stimulus for increased sodium retention and increased plasma volume. The observations that blood pressure is significantly lower and that the renin–angiotensin system is stimulated during normal pregnancy are consistent with primary vasodilation preceding and causing the increase in plasma volume.

Blood pressure regulation

Normal pregnancy is characterized by generalized vasodilation so marked that despite increases in cardiac output and plasma volume in the range of 40%, mean arterial pressures decrease approximately 10 mm [18]. The decrement in blood pressure is apparent in the first trimester, reaching a nadir by mid-pregnancy and then increasing gradually to approach prepregnancy values at term. Potential mediators of the vasodilation of pregnancy include placental hormones, nitric oxide, relaxin, prostacylin, and vascular endothelial growth factor. In response to the vasodilation and lower blood pressure, the renin–angiotensin system is markedly stimulated in pregnancy. Increases in plasma renin activity are apparent early in pregnancy, and levels increase to reach a maximum of about four times nonpregnant values by mid-pregnancy [18]. The increase in plasma renin activity is accompanied by increases in aldosterone secretion. Angiotensin II levels have not been studied extensively in pregnancy but are likely to be increased as well. Despite the increased renin and aldosterone levels, blood pressure and electrolytes are normal during pregnancy. Indeed, normotensive gravidas demonstrates exaggerated responses to *acute* converting enzyme inhibition, suggesting that the stimulated renin–angiotensin system is an important defense against hypotension during pregnancy [19].

Assessment of renal function in pregnancy

The GFR increases by 40–65% in pregnancy, but creatinine production is unchanged, resulting in decreased serum creatinine levels. One study reported average values of 0.83 mg/dL (73 μmol/L) in nonpregnant women and 0.74, 0.58, and 0.53 mg/dL (65, 51, and 46 μmol/L) in the first, second, and third trimesters of pregnancy, respectively, with values for the upper limit of normal of 0.96, 0.9, and 1.02 mg/dL (85, 80, and 90 μmol/L) [20]. Calculation of GFR by creatinine-based formulae is challenged by increasing maternal weight that is not muscle weight, and neither the MDRD formula nor Cockroft-Gault GFR estimates have been validated in pregnancy [21]. Measurement of serum cystatin C had been proposed as a more sensitive marker for GFR, as it was thought to be independent of age, weight, height, or muscle mass; however, this has not been found when studied in pregnancy [22]. At this time, creatinine clearance measured by 24-h urine collection remains the most-well-validated method for measuring renal function.

Proteinuria is measured using 24-h urine collection, urine dipstick, and the protein/creatinine ratio, but the gold standard remains the 24-h urine protein measurement. A 24-h protein level greater than 300 mg is abnormal in pregnancy and correlates with a urine dipstick protein measurement of 1+. Although commonly used to detect significant proteinuria, urine dipstick testing is susceptible to error due to variations in urine concentration and may miss up to 10% of hypertensive pregnant women with true proteinuria [23]; thus, if the level of suspicion is high, 24-h urine testing should be performed. The total protein/creatinine ratio has been shown to estimate 24-h urine protein in nonpregnant patients; however, in pregnancy it does not appear to exclude the equivalent of 0.3 g/24 h proteinuria and underestimates severe proteinuria, so it cannot be recommended as an alternative to 24-h measurement [24].

Kidney disease in pregnancy

Kidney disease during pregnancy may be due to 1) preexisting kidney disease that was diagnosed prior to conception, 2) chronic kidney disease that was unappreciated prior to pregnancy and diagnosed for the first time during pregnancy, or 3) kidney disease that develops for the first time during pregnancy. Overlapping categories occur with some diseases. For example, lupus nephritis may be a chronic condition or it may develop for the first time during pregnancy.

Chronic kidney disease: general principles

Fertility and ability to sustain an uncomplicated pregnancy are related to the degree of renal functional impairment, rather than to the specific underlying disorder. The greater the functional impairment, and/or the higher the blood pressure, the less likely the pregnancy will be successful. Patients with preserved renal function and normal or well-controlled blood pressure have favorable maternal and fetal outcomes. Those with moderate renal insufficiency (serum creatinine of 1.2–2.5 mg/dL [110–220 μmol/L]) are at increased risk for preeclampsia (20–30%) and preterm delivery. Women with moderate or severe renal dysfunction should be discouraged from conceiving, because up to 40% of these pregnancies are complicated by hypertension or deterioration in renal function that may be irreversible [25]. The level of blood pressure at the time of conception is an important variable in pregnancy outcome. In the absence of hypertension there is significantly less chance of irreversible deterioration in renal function during pregnancy. When hypertension is present, and especially when it is severe, pregnancy outcome is rarely uncomplicated. Premature delivery and deterioration in renal function are expected. Urine protein excretion may increase markedly in pregnant women with underlying kidney disease. Although the increments in protein excretion during pregnancy may not necessarily reflect worsening of underlying kidney disease, increased proteinuria is associated with worse fetal prognosis.

Kidney diseases associated with systemic illness

Diabetes is one of the most common medical disorders encountered during pregnancy, and the majority of cases are due to gestational diabetes. Preexisting diabetes poses significant risks to pregnancy. Many younger women with pregestational diabetes have type 1 diabetes, and if their disease has been present for 10–15 years, they may show early signs of diabetic nephropathy. Women with microalbuminuria (compared to macroalbuminuria), well-preserved renal function, and normal blood pressure have a good prognosis for pregnancy, although they are at increased risk for preeclampsia and urinary tract infection [26,27]. In one prospective cohort study from Denmark, 240 pregnant women with type 1 diabetes were followed during pregnancy, of whom 26 (11%) had microalbuminuria and 11 (5%) had diabetic nephropathy. A 62% proportion of women with microalbuminuria and 91% of women with diabetic nephropathy had preterm deliveries (compared with 35% of women with normal albumin excretion). Preeclampsia developed in 6% of women with normal albumin excretion compared with 42% and 64% of women with microalbuminuria and diabetic nephropathy, respectively [27]. In another study of 72 pregnancies in 58 women with diabetic nephropathy, high serum creatinine at enrollment, independent of urinary protein excretion, was associated with preterm delivery, very low birth weight, and neonatal hypoglycemia. With respect to progression of maternal kidney disease as a consequence of pregnancy, one study from Denmark reported that 26 women with type 1 diabetes who became pregnant had similar rates of deterioration in renal function over a 16-year follow-up, compared to 67 control subjects with comparable disease who had never been pregnant [28]. Thus, when baseline renal function and blood pressure are still normal, pregnancy is not likely to accelerate the progression of early diabetic nephropathy [28], although it is not unusual for urinary protein excretion to increase significantly during pregnancy, and there are only limited data that have specifically addressed this problem. Women with non-nephrotic-range proteinuria preconception may develop nephrotic-range proteinuria during pregnancy, but it is usually reversible. Women with overt nephropathy preconception, particularly those with impaired renal function and hypertension, have a high incidence of premature delivery and deterioration in maternal renal function [26]. Women with type 1 diabetes with microalbuminuria and normal renal function and normotension should be encouraged *not* to postpone pregnancy because of the worse prognosis once overt nephropathy develops.

There are no published studies of pregnancy and nephropathy associated with type 2 diabetes; however, given the increasing prevalence of this condition, it is an important area for future study.

Tight glucose control is critical because of the established association between glucose control and fetal outcome [29]. Thus, all women with diabetes should be managed by physicians experienced with diabetes in pregnancy. Blood pressure control is also important; however, because angiotensin converting enzyme inhibitors and angiotensin receptor blockers are contraindicated during pregnancy, women should be switched to other agents prior to conception.

Women with lupus nephritis during pregnancy present unique problems. Although similar considerations apply regarding the relationship between level of renal function and blood pressure to pregnancy outcome, in general, lupus is a much more unpredictable illness because of the tendency of the disease to flare. Recent data suggest that pregnancy duration, total disease duration, and disease activity and damage prior to pregnancy are associated with increased organ damage following pregnancy in women with lupus [30]. Whether or not pregnancy per se is a risk factor for lupus flares has been disputed [31]. Although some studies report no increase in flares attributable to pregnancy in patients in remission [32], prospective data from other studies suggest that pregnancy is associated with a greater chance of disease exacerbation [33,34]. Women with lupus are advised not to conceive unless their disease has been "inactive" for the preceding 6 months, as there is a higher incidence of fetal demise with active disease [35]. Additional complications associated with lupus and pregnancy include placental transfer of maternal autoantibodies, which can cause a neonatal lupus syndrome characterized by heart block, transient cutaneous lesions, or both. Women with lupus are also more likely to have clinically significant titers of antiphospholipid antibodies and the lupus anticoagulant, which are associated with spontaneous fetal loss, hypertensive syndromes indistinguishable from preeclampsia, and thrombotic events including deep vein thrombosis, pulmonary embolus, myocardial infarction, and strokes [36]. Thus, all women with systemic lupus erythematosus should be screened for antiphospholipid antibodies early in gestation. When titers are elevated (more than 40 GPL), daily aspirin (80–325 mg) is recommended. If there is a history of thrombotic events, then heparin in combination with aspirin is recommended [37].

One of the difficulties in managing lupus nephritis during pregnancy is that increased activity of lupus may be difficult to distinguish from preeclampsia. Both are characterized by an increase in proteinuria, a decrease in GFR, and hypertension. Thrombocytopenia may also be observed in both conditions. Hypocomplementemia is not a feature of preeclampsia, whereas increases in liver function tests may be observed in preeclampsia but are not characteristic of lupus activity. If disease activity is present before 20 weeks of gestation, then the diagnosis is more likely to be a lupus flare. In the latter half of pregnancy, it may be impossible to distinguish between a renal lupus flare and preeclampsia. In fact, frequently both are present simultaneously, and what starts as increased lupus activity appears to trigger preeclampsia. Spun urine microscopy for red blood cell casts can also signal lupus nephritis activity. Unfortunately, delivery may be necessary if immunosuppressive therapy and supportive care fail to stabilize the condition. The approach to treatment of lupus nephritis during pregnancy is based largely on anecdotal experience and knowledge regarding treatment of lupus in nonpregnant patients, as well as information on fetal toxicity of immunosuppressants that has been gained from treatment of other conditions, such as organ transplantation. Steroids and azathioprine are the mainstays of treatment. A recent prospective, observational study of women with lupus exposed to hydroxychloroquine during pregnancy suggested that this agent was associated with improved outcomes and absence of fetal toxicity [38]. Cyclophosphamide is generally not recommended during pregnancy, because of potential fetal toxicity [39], and should only be used when the mother's life is in jeopardy. We are unaware of published data regarding use of mycophenolate mofetil during pregnancy for treatment of lupus nephritis. It is embryotoxic in animal studies and has been associated with fetal malformations in humans [40].

Chronic glomerulonephritis

Child-bearing women may be afflicted with any of the forms of chronic glomerulonephritis common in this age group. These include immunoglobulin A nephropathy, focal and segmental glomerulosclerosis, membranoproliferative glomerulonephritis, minimal change nephritis, and membranous nephropathy. We are unaware of data that would support the notion that histologic subtype confers a specific prognosis for pregnancy. Rather, the previously mentioned principles are applicable to women with chronic glomerulonephritis; when renal function is normal and hypertension is absent, the prognosis is good.

Polycystic kidney disease

Young women with autosomal dominant polycystic kidney disease are frequently asymptomatic, with normal renal function and normal blood pressure, and indeed they may be unaware of their diagnosis. Little has been written about polycystic kidney disease and pregnancy, because many patients with this condition have well-preserved kidney function until after childbearing. A series consisting of 235 women with autosomal dominant polycystic kidney disease and 108 unaffected family members evaluated pregnancy outcomes and reported an increased incidence of maternal complications in affected compared to unaffected women [41]. Preexisting hypertension was the most common risk factor for maternal complications during pregnancy [41]. Pregnant women with polycystic kidney disease should be considered at increased risk of urinary tract infection. Estrogen is reported to cause liver cysts to enlarge, and repeated pregnancies may result in symptomatic enlargement of liver cysts. Given the association between cerebral aneurysms and autosomal dominant polycystic kidney disease in some families, screening for such aneurysms should be considered prior to natural labor. All patients should undergo genetic counseling before pregnancy to ensure they are aware that their offspring have a 50% chance of being affected.

Chronic pyelonephritis

Dilation and stasis in the urinary tract make chronic pyelonephritis (nephropathies associated with recurrent urinary tract infection, often in association with urinary tract abnormalities, e.g. vesicoureteral reflux) in gravidas more prone to exacerbation. These women should have a high fluid intake and should be screened frequently for bacteriuria. Women with reflux nephropathy have been reported to have an adverse prognosis during pregnancy. A prospective study of 54 pregnancies in 46 women with reflux nephropathy found that preeclampsia was present in 24% and more common in women with preexisting hypertension [42]. Nine (18%) experienced deterioration in renal function during pregnancy, and those with preexisting reduced renal function were at greater risk. One-third of the infants were delivered preterm, and 43% had vesicoureteral reflux. These high-risk women should be screened with urine cultures and should be treated promptly when infections are present, with consideration to suppressive antibiotic therapy for the duration of pregnancy in some cases.

Chronic kidney diseases that may be first diagnosed during pregnancy

The presence of chronic kidney disease may be diagnosed for the first time during pregnancy, in part because pregnant women are scrutinized more closely and also because the renal hemodynamic alterations during pregnancy may cause proteinuria to increase and be clinically detectable for the first time. Frequent measurement of blood pressure may also lead to diagnosis of kidney diseases accompanied by hypertension. Furthermore, the presence of even mild preexisting kidney disease is associated with an increased risk of preeclampsia; thus, underlying kidney disease may first become apparent after preeclampsia has developed in later pregnancy. Kidney diseases that may have been relatively silent preconception but that may "present" during pregnancy include immunoglobulin A nephropathy, focal and segmental glomerulosclerosis, polycystic kidney disease, and reflux nephropathy. Renal diagnostic testing during pregnancy can include blood and urine testing and ultrasonography. Renal biopsy is usually deferred until after delivery, unless there is acute deterioration in renal function or morbid nephrotic syndrome. Although experienced operators have reported few complications of renal biopsy during pregnancy, increased renal blood flow, hypertension, and difficulty positioning the patient are concerns [43–45]. The timing of renal biopsy after delivery depends on the clinical circumstances. If renal function is normal, and only proteinuria is present, it is reasonable to delay biopsy by at least 1–2 months, because proteinuria may improve once the hemodynamic alterations associated with pregnancy have resolved. If renal function is impaired, then biopsy should be considered within a few weeks of delivery.

Kidney diseases that develop for the first time during pregnancy

Pregnant women are at risk for any of the kidney diseases that occur in childbearing-age women, including pyelonephritis, glomerulonephritis, interstitial nephritis, and acute kidney failure.

Pyelonephritis in pregnant women is more likely to be associated with significant azotemia compared with nonpregnant women and should be treated aggressively. Glomerulonephritis and interstitial nephritis are not more likely to develop during pregnancy, although they do occur. Acute kidney failure in association with pregnancy, a rare complication in developed countries, is also decreasing in incidence in the developing world, with only 190 cases observed in a 20-year period in eastern India [46]. Recent estimates suggest that the incidence of acute kidney failure from obstetric causes is less than 1/20,000 pregnancies [47].

When acute kidney failure occurs early in pregnancy (12–18 weeks), it is usually in association with septic abortion or prerenal azotemia due to hyperemesis gravidarium. Most cases of acute kidney failure in pregnancy occur between gestational week 35 and the puerperium and are primarily due to preeclampsia and bleeding complications. Preeclampsia, particularly the HELLP variant (*h*emolysis, *e*levated *l*iver enzymes, *l*ow *p*latelet count) is an important cause of acute kidney failure in pregnancy [26]. Although most cases of preeclampsia are not usually associated with kidney failure, the HELLP syndrome may be associated with significant renal dysfunction, especially if not treated promptly. Most women without preexisting kidney or hypertensive disease do not require long-term renal replacement therapy. Additional important clinical entities causing kidney failure during pregnancy are discussed next.

Thrombotic microangiopathy

Although rare, thrombotic microangiopathies (thrombotic thrombocytopenic purpura [TTP] and hemolytic uremic syndrome [HUS]) are an important cause of pregnancy-associated acute kidney failure because they are associated with considerable morbidity. They also share several clinical and laboratory features with pregnancy-specific disorders, such as the HELLP variant of preeclampsia and acute fatty liver of pregnancy; thus, distinction of these syndromes is important for therapeutic and prognostic reasons. Features that may be helpful in making the correct diagnosis include timing of onset and the pattern of laboratory abnormalities. Preeclampsia typically develops in the third trimester, with only a few cases developing in the postpartum period, usually within a few days of delivery. TTP usually occurs antepartum, with many cases developing in the second trimester, as well as the third. HUS is usually a postpartum disease. Symptoms may begin antepartum, but most cases are diagnosed postpartum.

Preeclampsia is much more common than TTP or HUS, and it is usually preceded by hypertension and proteinuria. Kidney failure is unusual, even with severe cases, unless significant bleeding or hemodynamic instability or marked disseminated intravascular coagulation (DIC) occurs. In some cases, preeclampsia develops in the immediate postpartum period, and when thrombocytopenia is severe, it may be indistinguishable from HUS. However, preeclampsia spontaneously recovers, whereas TTP or HUS is often associated with persistent renal insufficiency and hypertension, with many patients requiring long-term dialysis or transplantation [48].

In contrast to TTP and HUS, preeclampsia may be associated with mild DIC and prolongation of prothrombin and partial thromboplastin times. Another laboratory feature of preeclampsia and HELLP syndrome that is not usually associated with TTP or HUS is marked elevation in liver enzymes. The presence of fever is more consistent with a diagnosis of TTP than preeclampsia or HUS. The main distinctive features of HUS are its tendency to occur in the postpartum period and the severity of the associated kidney failure. Treatment of preeclampsia and HELLP syndrome is delivery and supportive care. More aggressive treatment is rarely indicated. Some centers have reported the use of steroids in cases of severe HELLP syndrome, although this therapy has not been rigorously evaluated in placebo-controlled clinical trials [49]. Treatment of TTP and HUS includes plasma infusion or exchange and other modalities used in nonpregnant patients with these disorders.

Acute tubular necrosis

Acute tubular necrosis, either induced by volume depletion or exposure to nephrotoxins, may occur during pregnancy, although the incidence is low. In the first trimester, acute tubular necrosis is usually associated with hyperemesis gravidarium, whereas later in pregnancy and in the peripartum period, it is usually associated with abruptio placenta or other causes of obstetric hemorrhage. Occasionally, nonsteroidal anti-inflammatory agents, used for postpartum analgesia, may precipitate acute kidney failure in patients who are volume depleted from either hemorrhage, decreased fluid intake, or both. In severe cases of obstetric hemorrhage, acute cortical necrosis with associated DIC may be present, and ultrasonography or computed tomography may demonstrate hyperechoic or hypodense areas in the renal cortex. Most patients ultimately require dialysis, but 20–40% with cortical necrosis have partial recovery of renal function.

Acute fatty liver of pregnancy

Acute fatty liver is a rare complication of late pregnancy that is characterized by rapidly progressive liver failure. Women usually present with nausea, vomiting, and anorexia, and many patients have coincident diagnoses of preeclampsia or HELLP syndrome [50]. Other laboratory abnormalities (in addition to marked elevations in aspartate aminotransferase and alanine aminotransferase) frequently observed include elevated bilrubin, hypofibrinigemia, prolonged partial thromboplastin time, hypoglycemia, anemia, and low platelet count [51]. Many cases are associated with significant azotemia, and one series compared AFLP to HELLP syndrome and observed that acute kidney failure was significantly more common with AFLP [52]. Those authors hypothesized that because AFLP is believed to be a disease of mitochondrial dysfunction [53], it is possible that the kidney dysfunction associated with AFLP reflects inhibition of β-oxidation of fats in the kidney. Autopsy data have demonstrated microvesicular fat in the kidneys of women with AFLP. Delivery is indicated, and most patients improve shortly afterwards. This disorder was formerly associated with a more ominous outcome, which may have been a conse-

quence of late diagnosis, although in a recent case series maternal mortality was reported in two of six cases [51]. When diagnosed early, long-term morbidity is reduced.

Urinary tract obstruction

Pregnancy is associated with dilation of the collecting system, which is not usually accompanied by renal dysfunction. Rarely, complications such as large uterine fibroids that enlarge in the setting of pregnancy can lead to obstructive uropathy. Occasionally, acute urinary tract obstruction in pregnancy is caused by a kidney stone. Diagnosis can usually be made by ultrasonography. Often the stone will pass spontaneously, but occasionally cystoscopy is necessary for insertion of a stent to remove a fragment of stone and relieve obstruction, particularly if there is sepsis or a solitary kidney. ESW lithotripsy is contraindicated during pregnancy because of the possibility of adverse effects on the fetus.

Acute renal failure during pregnancy

Management of acute kidney failure occurring in pregnancy or immediately postpartum is similar to that in nongravid subjects, although there are several important considerations unique to pregnancy. Uterine hemorrhage near term may be concealed and blood loss underestimated; thus, any overt blood loss should be replaced early. Both peritoneal dialysis and hemodialysis have been used successfully in patients with obstetric acute kidney failure. Neither pelvic peritonitis nor the enlarged uterus is a contraindication to the former method. In fact, this form of treatment is more gradual than hemodialysis and thus less likely to precipitate labor. Because urea, creatinine, and other metabolites that accumulate in uremia traverse the placenta, dialysis should be undertaken early, with the aim of maintaining the blood urea nitrogen at approximately 50 mg/dL (8 μmol/L). In essence, the advantages of early dialysis in nongravid patients are even more important for the pregnant patient. Excessive fluid removal should be avoided, because it may contribute to hemodynamic compromise, reduction of uteroplacental perfusion, and premature labor. On the other hand, polyhydramnios is also thought to contribute to premature labor. In some cases it may be advisable to perform continuous fetal monitoring during dialysis, particularly after mid-pregnancy.

Therapy of end-stage renal disease during pregnancy

Dialysis

Fertility is reduced in dialysis patients, due to abnormalities of pituitary leutinizing hormone release leading to anovulation. Pregnancy that does occur in patients undergoing maintenance dialysis is extremely high risk, and conception should not be encouraged due to very high fetal mortality; in large surveys, only 42–60% of such pregnancies resulted in a live-born infant. Prematurity, very low birth weight, and intrauterine growth restriction are common, and approximately 85% of infants born to women who conceive after starting dialysis are born before 36 weeks of gestation.

Management of patients on dialysis who are pregnant includes several considerations, but the single most important factor influencing fetal outcome is the maternal plasma urea level [54]. In patients undergoing hemodialysis, both the number of dialysis sessions per week as well as the time per session must be increased to a minimum of 20 h/week, aiming for a predialysis urea of 30–50 mg/dL (5–8 mmol/L) [54,55]. Heparinization should be minimal, to prevent obstetric bleeding. Dialysate bicarbonate should be decreased to 25 mEq/L, in keeping with the expected physiologic metabolic acidosis of pregnancy. If peritoneal dialysis is being used, decreased exchange volumes by increasing exchange frequency or cycler use are recommended [56]. Adequate calorie and protein intakes are required; 1 g/kg/day protein intake plus an additional 20 g/day has been suggested [57]. After the first trimester, maternal "dry" weight should be increased by ~1 lb. (400 g)/week to adjust for the expected progressive weight increase in pregnancy. Antihypertensive therapy should be adjusted for pregnancy by discontinuing angiotensin converting enzyme inhibitors and angiotensin receptor blockers and aiming for maintenance of maternal diastolic pressure of 80–90 mmHg by using methyl-DOPA, labetalol, and sustained-release nifedipine in standard doses to achieve the target. Anemia should be treated with supplemental iron, folic acid, and erythropoietin. Erythropoietin is safe in pregnancy, and pregnancy-related erythropoietin resistance requires a dose increase of approximately 50% to maintain hemoglobin target levels of 10–11 g/dL. Frequent monitoring of iron stores and treatment with intravenous iron should be prescribed as necessary [57]. Due to placental 25(OH)-vitamin D_3 conversion, decreased supplemental vitamin D may be required and should be guided by levels of vitamin D, parathyroid hormone, calcium, and phosphorus. Magnesium supplementation may be needed to maintain serum magnesium levels at 5–7 mg/dL (2–3 mmol/L). Low-dose aspirin to prevent preeclampsia has been suggested. Babies born to mothers on dialysis may require monitoring for osmotic diuresis in the immediate postpartum period if maternal urea was high at the time of delivery.

Kidney transplantation

Menstruation and fertility resumes in most women from 1–12 months post-kidney transplantation. Several thousand women have undergone pregnancy following kidney transplantation, and pregnancy in this population appears to involve much lower risk to mother and baby than pregnancy in patients on dialysis. Although pregnancy has become more common after transplantation, there have been little more than case reports and cases series to guide practice decisions; a Consensus Conference generated a report in 2005 summarizing the literature and provided practice guidelines as well as identified gaps in knowledge [58]. Most pregnancies (greater than 90%) that proceed beyond the first trimester succeed; however, there are maternal and fetal complications due to immunosuppressant effects, preexisting hypertension, and renal dysfunction. These include maternal complications of steroid therapy, such as impaired glucose tolerance, hypertension (47–73%), preeclampsia (30%), and increased infection. Fetal complications include a higher incidence of premature delivery and intrauterine growth restriction with lower birth weight. Best practice guidelines have outlined criteria for considering pregnancy in kidney transplant recipients [58–60], and it is suggested that those contemplating pregnancy should meet the following criteria:

1) Good health and stable renal function for 1–2 years after transplantation with no recent acute or ongoing rejection or infections
2) Absent or minimal proteinuria (<0.5 g/day)
3) Normal blood pressure or easily managed hypertension
4) No evidence of pelvicalyceal distention on ultrasonography prior to conception
5) Serum creatinine less than 1.5 mg/dL (133 μmol/L)
6) Drug therapy of prednisone at 15 mg/day or less, azathioprine at 2 mg/kg or less, cyclosporine at >5 mg/kg/day.

Management of all pregnant transplant patients should be by a high-risk obstetrician, due to risk of intrauterine growth restriction and preeclampsia. Future studies are required to address optimal immunosuppression in pregnancy. Although cyclosporine levels tend to decrease during pregnancy, there is no information regarding whether the drug dosage should be increased. Experience with tacrolimus is increasing, but it has not been used as widely in pregnancy as cyclosporine, although growing experience suggests that is safe, with a similar side effect profile to cyclosporine. Considerations regarding hypertension and growth restriction are important; there is no established blood pressure target, although 140/90 mmHg is suggested by the authors, and antihypertensives should be switched to those safe in pregnancy. Pregnancy safety has not been established for either mycophenolate mofetil or sirolimus [61]. Mycophenolate mofetil has been reported to be embryotoxic in animals and is associated with ear and other deformities in humans. This drug should be discontinued during pregnancy, and women should be switched to azathioprine if indicated. Sirolimus has caused delayed ossification in animal studies and although successful live-born human outcomes have been reported, its use is contraindicated in humans until more data are available. Finally, data from the National Transplantation Pregnancy Registry and the European Dialysis and Transplant Association suggest that pregnancy rarely negatively affects the graft, though there may be minor increases in serum creatinine postpartum compared with prepregnancy creatinine [59,61]. Rejection is difficult to diagnose in pregnancy, and renal biopsy may be required; the consensus opinion was that steroids are a safe treatment, as is intravenous immunoglobulin, but the safety of antilymphocyte globulins or rituximab in pregnancy is unknown [58].

Hypertensive disorders of pregnancy

A comprehensive discussion of hypertensive disorders of pregnancy is beyond the scope of this chapter, but preeclampsia will be briefly discussed because renal manifestations are an important feature. Although maternal death is a rare event in most Western nations where access to prenatal care is adequate, hypertensive disorders are one of the leading causes of maternal death worldwide, accounting for 15–20% of all maternal deaths in the developing as well as the developed world [62]. In the USA, approximately 8–10% of all pregnancies are complicated by hypertension, with half of these cases attributable to the pregnancy-specific disorder preeclampsia. Hypertensive disorders in pregnancy are significantly more common than kidney disease in pregnancy, and because of the burden on both maternal as well as neonatal health, there are many examples of well-controlled multicenter randomized controlled trials and meta-analyses that have addressed such issues as prevention of preeclampsia, treatment and prevention of eclamptic seizures, and to a lesser degree, use of antihypertensive agents in pregnancy.

The classification scheme of hypertensive disorders in pregnancy is one that has been in use for many years in the USA and has been endorsed by The National High Blood Pressure Education Program and the American College of Obstetricians and Gynecologists. It includes four designations: chronic or preexisting hypertension, preeclampsia/eclampsia, preeclampsia superimposed on chronic hypertension, and gestational hypertension.

Screening tests for preeclampsia

Because most of the morbidity attributable to hypertension in pregnancy is due to preeclampsia or superimposed preeclampsia, considerable efforts have been made to evaluate various clinical, hormonal, and biochemical tests to identify early in pregnancy those at risk for the condition later in pregnancy or for those who manifest early, "preclinical" signs of the disorder. Although there are currently no effective preventive strategies for most women, the argument has been made that early identification would lead to closer surveillance and institution of certain lifestyle adjustments (e.g. stopping work, increased rest). To date, no single test has been shown to meet standard criteria for a useful screening test, and a recent comprehensive review of the subject emphasized this point [63].

Prevention of preeclampsia

Many strategies have been investigated in well-conducted clinical trials (including thousands of women) on the use of antiplatelet therapy, nutritional supplementation, and antioxidant vitamins for the prevention of preeclampsia. These trials, and subsequent meta-analyses, demonstrated a small benefit (10–15% reduction in relative risk) for low-dose aspirin in the prevention of preeclampsia and its clinically important adverse maternal and fetal outcomes [64]. With respect to nutritional strategies, calcium supplementation appears to have some benefit in women ingesting a baseline low-calcium diet [65], whereas to date, antioxidant supplementation with vitamins C and E has not shown benefit in two large randomized controlled trials [66,67].

Antihypertensive therapy during pregnancy

There remain many unanswered questions regarding the appropriate use of antihypertensive treatments in pregnant women. Neither the indications for antihypertensive therapy, the target blood pressures after treatment is initiated, the optimal antihypertensive agent, nor the role of lowered blood pressure in preventing complications has been adequately assessed. The reader is referred to recently published reviews of this subject [68].

Anticonvulsant therapy in women with eclampsia

There is strong evidence from randomized trials to support the use of magnesium sulfate for prevention and treatment of eclampsia [69]. This agent reduces the incidence of eclampsia in women with preeclampsia and lowers the risk of maternal death in women with eclampsia. It is superior to other agents, such as phenytoin and diazepam.

Conclusions

Kidney disease in pregnancy poses considerable risk to maternal as well as fetal health. Based on case series published over the last several decades, pregnancy outcome appears directly related to the level of baseline renal function and degree of hypertension. Because the kidney disorders discussed in this chapter are relatively uncommon, multicenter efforts are needed to better identify risks and determine optimal therapeutic strategies.

References

1 Coresh J, Byrd-Holt D, Astor BC, Briggs JP, Eggers PW, Lacher DA et al. Chronic kidney disease awareness, prevalence, and trends among U.S. adults, 1999 to 2000. *J Am Soc Nephrol* 2005; **16(1)**: 180–188.

2 Christensen T, Klebe JG, Bertelsen V, Hansen HE. Changes in renal volume during normal pregnancy. *Acta Obstet Gynecol Scand* 1989; **68(6)**: 541–543.

3 Guyer PB, Delany D. Urinary tract dilatation and oral contraceptives. *Br Med J* 1970; **4(5735)**: 588–590.

4 Weissenbacher ER, Reisenberger K. Uncomplicated urinary tract infections in pregnant and non-pregnant women. *Curr Opin Obstet Gynecol* 1993; **5(4)**: 513–516.

5 Chapman AB, Zamudio S, Woodmansee W, Merouani A, Osorio F, Johnson A et al. Systemic and renal hemodynamic changes in the luteal phase of the menstrual cycle mimic early pregnancy. *Am J Physiol* 1997; **273(5 Pt 2)**: F777–F782.

6 Sturgiss SN, Wilkinson R, Davison JM. Renal reserve during human pregnancy. *Am J Physiol* 1996; **271(1 Pt 2)**: F16–F20.

7 Sturgiss SN, Dunlop W, Davison JM. Renal haemodynamics and tubular function in human pregnancy. *Baillieres Clin Obstet Gynaecol* 1994; **8(2)**: 209–234.

8 Hart MV, Hosenpud JD, Hohimer AR, Morton MJ. Hemodynamics during pregnancy and sex steroid administration in guinea pigs. *Am J Physiol* 1985; **249(2 Pt 2)**: R179–R185.

9 Debrah DO, Novak J, Matthews JE, Ramirez RJ, Shroff SG, Conrad KP. Relaxin is essential for systemic vasodilation and increased global arterial compliance during early pregnancy in conscious rats. *Endocrinology* 2006; **147(11)**: 5126–5131.

10 Cadnapaphornchai MA, Ohara M, Morris KG, Jr., Knotek M, Rogachev B, Ladtkow T et al. Chronic NOS inhibition reverses systemic vasodilation

and glomerular hyperfiltration in pregnancy. *Am J Physiol Renal Physiol* 2001; **280(4)**: F592–F598.

11 Heenan AP, Wolfe LA. Plasma acid-base regulation above and below ventilatory threshold in late gestation. *J Appl Physiol* 2000; **88(1)**: 149–157.

12 Wolfe LA, Kemp JG, Heenan AP, Preston RJ, Ohtake PJ. Acid-base regulation and control of ventilation in human pregnancy. *Can J Physiol Pharmacol* 1998; **76(9)**: 815–827.

13 Lindheimer MD, Davison JM. Osmoregulation, the secretion of arginine vasopressin and its metabolism during pregnancy. *Eur J Endocrinol* 1995; **132(2)**: 133–143.

14 Davison JM, Sheills EA, Philips PR, Barron WM, Lindheimer MD. Metabolic clearance of vasopressin and an analogue resistant to vasopressinase in human pregnancy. *Am J Physiol* 1993; **264(2 Pt 2)**: F348–F353.

15 Danielson LA, Conrad KP. Time course and dose response of relaxin-mediated renal vasodilation, hyperfiltration, and changes in plasma osmolality in conscious rats. *J Appl Physiol* 2003; **95(4)**: 1509–1514.

16 Conrad KP, Debrah DO, Novak J, Danielson LA, Shroff SG. Relaxin modifies systemic arterial resistance and compliance in conscious, nonpregnant rats. *Endocrinology* 2004; **145(7)**: 3289–3296.

17 Davison JM, Shiells EA, Philips PR, Lindheimer MD. Serial evaluation of vasopressin release and thirst in human pregnancy. Role of human chorionic gonadotrophin in the osmoregulatory changes of gestation. *J Clin Invest* 1988; **81(3)**: 798–806.

18 Wilson M, Morganti AA, Zervoudakis I, Letcher RL, Romney BM, Von Oeyon P *et al.* Blood pressure, the renin-aldosterone system and sex steroids throughout normal pregnancy. *Am J Med.* 1980; **68(1)**: 97–104.

19 August P, Mueller FB, Sealey JE, Edersheim TG. Role of renin-angiotensin system in blood pressure regulation in pregnancy. *Lancet* 1995; **345(8954)**: 896–897.

20 Girling JC. Re-evaluation of plasma creatinine concentration in normal pregnancy. *J Obstet Gynaecol* 2000; **20(2)**: 128–131.

21 Quadri KH, Bernardini J, Greenberg A, Laifer S, Syed A, Holley JL. Assessment of renal function during pregnancy using a random urine protein to creatinine ratio and Cockcroft-Gault formula. *Am J Kidney Dis* 1994; **24(3)**: 416–420.

22 Akbari A, Lepage N, Keely E, Clark HD, Jaffey J, MacKinnon M *et al.* Cystatin-C and beta trace protein as markers of renal function in pregnancy. *BJOG* 2005; **112(5)**: 575–578.

23 Phelan LK, Brown MA, Davis GK, Mangos G. A prospective study of the impact of automated dipstick urinalysis on the diagnosis of preeclampsia. *Hypertens Pregnancy* 2004; **23(2)**: 135–142.

24 Durnwald C, Mercer B. A prospective comparison of total protein/creatinine ratio versus 24-hour urine protein in women with suspected preeclampsia. *Am J Obstet Gynecol* 2003; **189(3)**: 848–852.

25 Jones DC, Hayslett JP. Outcome of pregnancy in women with moderate or severe renal insufficiency. *N Engl J Med* 1996; **335(4)**: 226–232.

26 Khoury JC, Miodovnik M, LeMasters G, Sibai B. Pregnancy outcome and progression of diabetic nephropathy. What's next? *J Matern Fetal Neonatal Med* 2002; **11(4)**: 238–244.

27 Ekbom P, Damm P, Feldt-Rasmussen B, Feldt-Rasmussen U, Molvig J, Mathiesen ER. Pregnancy outcome in type 1 diabetic women with microalbuminuria. *Diabetes Care* 2001; **24(10)**: 1739–1744.

28 Rossing K, Jacobsen P, Hommel E, Mathiesen E, Svenningsen A, Rossing P *et al.* Pregnancy and progression of diabetic nephropathy. *Diabetologia* 2002; **45(1)**: 36–41.

29 Jensen DM, Damm P, Moelsted-Pedersen L, Ovesen P, Westergaard JG, Moeller M *et al.* Outcomes in type 1 diabetic pregnancies: a nationwide, population-based study. *Diabetes Care* 2004; **27(12)**: 2819–2823.

30 Andrade RM, McGwin G, Jr., Alarcon GS, Sanchez ML, Bertoli AM, Fernandez M *et al.* Predictors of post-partum damage accrual in systemic lupus erythematosus: data from LUMINA, a multiethnic US cohort (XXXVIII). *Rheumatology* (Oxford) 2006; **45(11)**: 1380–1384.

31 Lockshin MD. Pregnancy associated with systemic lupus erythematosus. *Semin Perinatol* 1990; **14(2)**: 130–138.

32 Derksen RH, Bruinse HW, de Groot PG, Kater L. Pregnancy in systemic lupus erythematosus: a prospective study. *Lupus* 1994; **3(3)**: 149–155.

33 Petri M, Howard D, Repke J. Frequency of lupus flare in pregnancy. The Hopkins Lupus Pregnancy Center experience. *Arthritis Rheum* 1991; **34(12)**: 1538–1545.

34 Ruiz-Irastorza G, Lima F, Alves J, Khamashta MA, Simpson J, Hughes GR *et al.* Increased rate of lupus flare during pregnancy and the puerperium: a prospective study of 78 pregnancies. *Br J Rheumatol* 1996; **35(2)**: 133–138.

35 Julkunen H. Pregnancy and lupus nephritis. *Scand J Urol Nephrol* 2001; **35(4)**: 319–327.

36 Erkan D. The relation between antiphospholipid syndrome-related pregnancy morbidity and non-gravid vascular thrombosis: a review of the literature and management strategies. *Curr Rheumatol Rep* 2002; **4(5)**: 379–386.

37 Empson M, Lassere M, Craig JC, Scott JR. Recurrent pregnancy loss with antiphospholipid antibody: a systematic review of therapeutic trials. *Obstet Gynecol* 2002; **99**: 135–144

38 Clowse ME, Magder L, Witter F, Petri M. Hydroxychloroquine in lupus pregnancy. *Arthritis Rheum* 2006; **54(11)**: 3640–3647.

39 Clowse ME, Magder L, Petri M. Cyclophosphamide for lupus during pregnancy. *Lupus* 2005; **14(8)**: 593–597.

40 Le Ray C, Coulomb A, Elefant E, Frydman R, Audibert F. Mycophenolate mofetil in pregnancy after renal transplantation: a case of major fetal malformations. *Obstet Gynecol* 2004; **103(5 Pt 2)**: 1091–1094.

41 Chapman AB, Johnson AM, Gabow PA. Pregnancy outcome and its relationship to progression of renal failure in autosomal dominant polycystic kidney disease. *J Am Soc Nephrol* 1994; **5(5)**: 1178–1185.

42 North RA, Taylor RS, Gunn TR. Pregnancy outcome in women with reflux nephropathy and the inheritance of vesico-ureteric reflux. *Aust N Z J Obstet Gynaecol* 2000; **40(3)**: 280–285.

43 Packham D, Fairley KF. Renal biopsy: indications and complications in pregnancy. *Br J Obstet Gynaecol* 1987; **94(10)**: 935–939.

44 Chen HH, Lin HC, Yeh JC, Chen CP. Renal biopsy in pregnancies complicated by undetermined renal disease. *Acta Obstet Gynecol Scand* 2001; **80(10)**: 888–893.

45 Kuller JA, D'Andrea NM, McMahon MJ. Renal biopsy and pregnancy. *Am J Obstet Gynecol* 2001; **184(6)**: 1093–1096.

46 Prakash J, Kumar H, Sinha DK, Kedalaya PG, Pandey LK, Srivastava PK *et al.* Acute renal failure in pregnancy in a developing country: twenty years of experience. *Ren Fail* 2006; **28(4)**: 309–313.

47 Gammill HS, Jeyabalan A. Acute renal failure in pregnancy. *Crit Care Med* 2005; **33(10 Suppl)**: S372–S384.

48 Dashe JS, Ramin SM, Cunningham FG. The long-term consequences of thrombotic microangiopathy (thrombotic thrombocytopenic purpura and hemolytic uremic syndrome) in pregnancy. *Obstet Gynecol* 1998; **91(5 Pt 1)**: 662–668.

49 van Runnard Heimel PJ, Franx A, Schobben AF, Huisjes AJ, Derks JB, Bruinse HW. Corticosteroids, pregnancy, and HELLP syndrome: a review. *Obstet Gynecol Surv* 2005; **60**(1): 57–70.

50 Castro MA, Fassett MJ, Reynolds TB, Shaw KJ, Goodwin TM. Reversible peripartum liver failure: a new perspective on the diagnosis, treatment, and cause of acute fatty liver of pregnancy, based on 28 consecutive cases. *Am J Obstet Gynecol* 1999; **181**(2): 389–395.

51 Fesenmeier MF, Coppage KH, Lambers DS, Barton JR, Sibai BM. Acute fatty liver of pregnancy in 3 tertiary care centers. *Am J Obstet Gynecol* 2005; **192**(5): 1416–1419.

52 Vigil-De Gracia P. Acute fatty liver and HELLP syndrome: two distinct pregnancy disorders. *Int J Gynaecol Obstet* 2001; **73**(3): 215–220.

53 Ibdah JA, Bennett MJ, Rinaldo P, Zhao Y, Gibson B, Sims HF *et al.* A fetal fatty-acid oxidation disorder as a cause of liver disease in pregnant women. *N Engl J Med* 1999; **340**(22): 1723–1731.

54 Haase M, Morgera S, Budde K. A systematic approach to managing pregnant dialysis patients: the importance of an intensified haemodiafiltration protocol. *Nephrol Dial Transplant* 2006. (Epub ahead of print; 27 Feb 2006 posting date.)

55 Shemin D. Dialysis in pregnant women with chronic kidney disease. *Semin Dial* 2003; **16**(5): 379–383.

56 Smith WT, Darbari S, Kwan M, O'Reilly-Green C, Devita MV. Pregnancy in peritoneal dialysis: a case report and review of adequacy and outcomes. *Int Urol Nephrol* 2005; **37**(1): 145–151.

57 Holley JL, Reddy SS. Pregnancy in dialysis patients: a review of outcomes, complications, and management. *Semin Dial* 2003; **16**(5): 384–388.

58 McKay DB, Josephson MA, Armenti VT, August P, Coscia LA, Davis CL *et al.* Reproduction and transplantation: report on the AST Consensus Conference on Reproductive Issues and Transplantation. *Am J Transplant* 2005; **5**(7): 1592–1599.

59 European Best Practice Guidelines for Renal Transplantation. Section IV: Long-term management of the transplant recipient. IV.10. Pregnancy in renal transplant recipients. *Nephrol Dial Transplant* 2002; **17**(**Suppl 4**): 50–55.

60 McKay DB, Josephson MA. Pregnancy in recipients of solid organs: effects on mother and child. *N Engl J Med* 2006; **354**(12): 1281–1293.

61 Armenti VT, Radomski JS, Moritz MJ, Gaughan WJ, McGrory CH, Coscia LA. Report from the National Transplantation Pregnancy Registry (NTPR): outcomes of pregnancy after transplantation. *Clin Transplant* 2004; **2004**: 103–114.

62 Khan KS, Wojdyla D, Say L, Gulmezoglu AM, Van Look PF. WHO analysis of causes of maternal death: a systematic review. *Lancet* 2006; **367**(9516): 1066–1074.

63 Conde-Agudelo A, Villar J, Lindheimer M. World Health Organization systematic review of screening tests for preeclampsia. *Obstet Gynecol* 2004; **104**(6): 1367–1391.

64 Duley L, Henderson-Smart DJ, Knight M, King JF. Antiplatelet agents for preventing pre-eclampsia and its complications. *Cochrane Database Syst Rev* 2004; **1**: CD004659.

65 Hofmeyr GJ, Atallah AN, Duley L. Calcium supplementation during pregnancy for preventing hypertensive disorders and related problems. *Cochrane Database Syst Rev* 2006; **3**: CD001059.

66 Rumbold AR, Crowther CA, Haslam RR, Dekker GA, Robinson JS. Vitamins C and E and the risks of preeclampsia and perinatal complications. *N Engl J Med* 2006; **354**(17): 1796–1806.

67 Poston L, Briley AL, Seed PT, Kelly FJ, Shennan AH. Vitamin C and vitamin E in pregnant women at risk for pre-eclampsia (VIP trial): randomised placebo-controlled trial. *Lancet* 2006; **367**(9517): 1145–1154.

68 Podymow T, August P, Umans JG. Antihypertensive therapy in pregnancy. *Semin Nephrol* 2004; **24**(6): 616–625.

69 Duley L. Evidence and practice: the magnesium sulphate story. *Best Pract Res Clin Obstet Gynaecol* 2005; **19**(1): 57–74.

5 Chronic Kidney Disease, Chronic Renal Failure

30 Progression of Kidney Disease: Diagnosis and Management

Anil K. Agarwal, Nabil Haddad, & Lee A. Hebert

Department of Internal Medicine, The Ohio State University Medical Center, Columbus, USA

Introduction

Progression of kidney disease refers to irreversible loss of glomerular filtration rate (GFR) due to structural damage to the kidney. Progression to end-stage renal disease (ESRD) usually involves two mechanisms: those of the primary kidney disease, and those of "natural progression." The latter refers to a vicious cycle in which GFR loss begets more GFR loss. The vicious cycle is induced by the systemic hypertension, glomerular hyperperfusion, proteinuria, and systemic metabolic dysfunctions set in motion by nephron loss [1]. Details of the mechanisms of natural progression are discussed in chapter 3. This chapter focuses on therapies to slow natural progression [1–3], which should be used along with the therapies to treat the primary kidney disease. The goal is to preserve enough nephron function to avoid the vicious cycle of natural progression.

GFR loss and risk of natural progression

The threshold for natural progression attributable to GFR loss appears to be crossed when loss of nephron function exceeds 50%. For example, unilateral nephrectomy, as with living kidney donors, does not usually lead to natural progression [4]. However, partial nephrectomy of a solitary kidney does lead to natural progression [5]. A normal solitary kidney can be vulnerable to natural progression if it is congenital or acquired early in life [6] or if it is accompanied by hypertension, obesity, hyperlipidemia, or hyperglycemia [2–4,7]. A patient with a 50% loss of nephron function may also be vulnerable to natural progression if the nephron loss is the result of hypertension, as observed in black people [8] or as the result of glomerulonephritis (GN) [9]. The latter is suggested by scenarios in which the clinical manifestations of biopsy-proven severe acute

GN resolve, based on return of serum creatinine and proteinuria to near normal levels. Over the ensuing years, however, proteinuria increases, hypertension develops, and serum creatinine begins to rise. A repeat kidney biopsy shows complete resolution of the inflammatory GN, but it is replaced by a segmental sclerosing glomerulopathy [9]. This is now recognized as secondary focal and segmental glomerulosclerosis attributed to natural progression [10] (see chapter 13). These observations suggest that a 50% GFR loss in which the surviving glomeruli show diffuse segmental damage (e.g. resolved GN) carries a higher risk of natural progression than a 50% GFR loss in which the surviving nephrons are normal (e.g. unilateral nephrectomy in a live donor).

Proteinuria magnitude and risk of natural progression

In most chronic kidney diseases (CKDs), proteinuria magnitude is the single strongest risk factor for progression [2,3,11]. The threshold for natural progression attributable to proteinuria appears to be crossed when proteinuria exceeds 500 mg/day [12]. Nonselective proteinuria (large amounts of protein with molecular weights exceeding that of albumin) is mainly responsible for the natural progression attributed to proteinuria [2]. Indeed, highly selective proteinuria (when urine protein is almost entirely albumin) can persist in the nephrotic range for more than 10 years without causing structural damage to the kidney [13].

Monitoring kidney disease progression

Progression represents irreversible kidney damage. Generally it is not feasible to monitor the damage itself [14]. Instead, surrogate measures, especially changes in proteinuria and GFR, are used. In most CKD patients the first evidence of natural progression is a progressive increase in proteinuria. Only later does evidence of declining GFR appear [9]. Important exceptions are the nephropathy

Evidence-based Nephrology. Edited by Donald Molony and Jonathan Craig
© 2009 Blackwell Publishing, ISBN: 978-1-4051-3975-5.

of type 2 diabetes mellitus [15] and hypertensive nephrosclerosis in African Americans [16]. Under these conditions serum creatinine can increase to 2.0 mg/dL with only minimal proteinuria.

Monitoring proteinuria trends

Accurate monitoring of a patient's proteinuria trends is critically important to CKD management, because proteinuria magnitude predicts progression and therapy that reduces proteinuria slows progression [2,3,11]. The reason for these associations is that proteinuria is likely nephrotoxic, probably through multiple mechanisms [2]. The MDRD study and the REIN trial showed that for each 1.0-g/day reduction in proteinuria achieved by 4–6 months of therapy, subsequent GFR decline was slowed by 1–2 mL/min/year [2]. GFR loss in CKD usually occurs at about 4–10 mL/min/year [2,3]. Thus, each therapy-induced 1.0-g/day proteinuria reduction should substantially prolong time to onset of ESRD (Figure 30.1).

The recommended method for assessing proteinuria trends is from the urine protein/creatinine (P/C) ratio of intended 24-h urine collections [2,17]. The National Kidney Foundation's Kidney Disease Outcomes Quality Initiative (K/DOQI) guidelines recommend the spot urine P/C ratio to monitor proteinuria trends [18]; however, the spot urine P/C ratio is reliable only for detecting large changes in 24-h proteinuria. For moderate proteinuria changes (e.g. 0.5–3.0 g/day) a more reliable measure is the P/C ratio of intended 24-h urine collections that are 50% or more complete based on creatinine content [19].

Once it is established that the proteinuria is glomerular in origin (i.e. most of the protein is albumin), it is acceptable to monitor proteinuria trends by measuring urine total protein rather than urine albumin. The two measures are highly correlated, and measuring urine total protein is less expensive than measuring urine albumin [20].

Monitoring GFR trends

In individual patients, it is usually sufficient to monitor GFR trends by measuring serum creatinine serially. However, if the serum creatinine level changes, one must keep in mind the conditions that can increase serum creatinine by increasing creatinine production (eating cooked meat, creatine ingestion, increased exercise, or increased muscle mass) or can decrease creatinine production (vegetarian diet, muscle wasting, or decreased exercise) [2]. If a chronic change in creatinine production is occurring (e.g. muscle wasting), GFR trends can be monitored by measuring serial 24-h urine creatinine clearance, which is not affected by changes in creatinine production. If creatinine clearance is used, an accurate 24-h collection is essential [2].

The MDRD-4 equation is now widely used to monitor GFR trends in individual patients. Its strengths are its simplicity (the required variables are age, sex, race, and serum creatinine), accuracy in many CKD patients, and the ability to take into account the influence of age. The latter is important in assessing a patient's GFR trend over 10 years or more [21]. MDRD-4 shortcomings include inaccuracy in K/DOQI CKD stages 1 and 2, which includes the majority of CKD patients [18]. As discussed above, in these patients, trends in GFR can be inferred from serial measurement of serum creatinine, ideally expressed to the second decimal point (in milligrams per deciliter) or the nearest whole number (in micromoles per liter). MDRD-4 is also inaccurate in those with high-normal creatinine production (GFR is underestimated) or low-normal creatinine production (GFR is overestimated) [22]. The Cockroft-Gault equation takes into account body weight and its effect on creatinine clearance. However, in general, the Cockroft-Gault and MDRD-4 equations provide similar estimates of GFR, especially in the mid-range of estimated GFR values [21]. Nevertheless, MDRD-4 is easier for clinical laboratories to implement

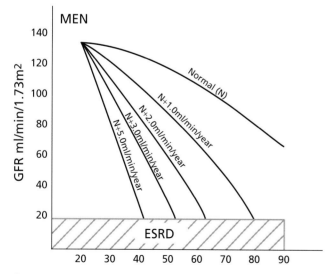
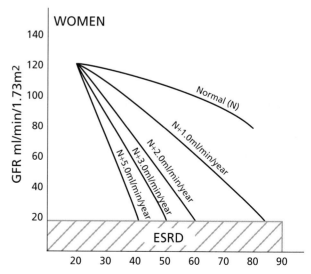

Figure 30.1 Average rate of GFR decline due to aging (top curve) in comparison to hypothetical patients each with onset of a progressive kidney disease at age 25 years but with different rates of GFR decline superimposed on the GFR decline of aging (left panel, men; right panel, women). Note that small differences in the GFR decline rate can result in large differences in time to onset of ESRD. The top curves are adapted from Stevens [21] with permission.

because its calculation does not require body weight. The role of cystatin C in monitoring GFR trends remains to be established [23,24].

Therapy of natural progression

Because of the gravity of ESRD and the benefit of even small decreases in CKD progression rate (Figure 30.1), a strong argument can be made for the general use of an aggressive, multiple risk factor intervention involving both the therapies that are of proven benefit and those that are of plausible benefit but considered prudent to use [1–3]. However, we do not recommend an aggressive approach in those with kidney conditions with low ESRD risk. These patients include those with steroid-responsive minimal change disease, a solitary kidney that is normal, was acquired in adulthood, and not accompanied by other CKD risk factors, hereditary nephritis, or thin glomerular basement membrane disease in a normotensive adult whose only renal manifestation is microscopic hematuria or in an elderly patient with idiopathic and moderately elevated serum creatinine (1.30–2.00 mg/dL) and minor proteinuria (24-h urine P/C ratio of <1.0) and whose renal parameters have been stable for at least 1 year. The latter group is much more likely to die of cardiovascular disease (CVD) than progress to ESRD [25,26].

Described next are the recommended therapies, listed according to level of recommendation. A level 1 (highest) recommendation is based on one or more large randomized clinical trials (RCTs) that have documented effects on GFR decline. Level 2 recommendations are based on secondary analyses of the level 1 RCTs, or on RCTs that have documented effects on proteinuria but not GFR decline, or that appear to be of high quality but may not be definitive because therapy involved a relatively small number of patients.

The goals of progression therapy are 1) to reduce proteinuria as much as possible, ideally to <500 mg/day, which appears to approach the maximum benefit of proteinuria reduction [12], and 2) to slow GFR decline as much as possible, ideally to about 1 ml/min/year, which is the rate of GFR decline attributable to aging [21] (Figure 30.1).

Level 1 recommendations to slow natural progression
Recommendation 1: Control blood pressure
The "low BP goal" is recommended [2,3,18,27–29]. Based on the relevant RCTs, we suggest a sitting systolic blood pressure (BP) in the 120s or less, if tolerated [2,3]. The qualification "or less, if tolerated" is based on the evidence that "optimal" BP (systolic BP of <120 mmHg) is associated with significantly lower CVD risk than "normal" BP (systolic BP of 120–129 mmHg) [30], and there is no convincing evidence that systolic BP of <120 mmHg is harmful to CKD function [12,29]. Sitting is the recommended position for measuring BP, because it is the position that was used in the relevant RCTs. Systolic BP is the recommended goal because in the relevant RCTs, achieved systolic BP strongly correlated with GFR decline but achieved diastolic BP did not [2,31]. Specifying a goal with both a systolic and diastolic BP component

is not recommended. It can be confusing to the physician and the patient and can lead to overtreatment [32]. For example, under current guidelines [18], a CKD patient with BP of 108/86 mmHg would require more antihypertensive therapy. However, the "optimal" systolic BP likely places the patient at low CV and renal risk, and the modestly increased diastolic BP (isolated diastolic hypertension) likely represents an artifact, particularly in white hypertensive patients [32].

The greater the proteinuria the greater the benefit of the low BP goal in slowing GFR decline [2,3]. In addition, in CKD patients with low-level proteinuria, the low BP goal slows the progression of proteinuria from low levels to high levels more than the usual BP goal (135/85 mmHg) and likely reduces CVD risk more than the usual BP goal [2,3]. Thus, the low BP goal can also be recommended in those with low-level proteinuria, even though the current guidelines do not recommend that [18,27].

Home BP monitoring is recommended to assess whether the patient is achieving the BP goal [33]. Treating nocturnal hypertension, assessed by ambulatory BP monitoring, may also provide benefit [34]. An evidence-based and experienced-based algorithm for BP control is shown in Figure 30.2. The low BP goal should be achieved early in the course of CKD. Delay in achieving the low BP goal increases the risk for progression to ESRD [28]. If the systolic BP is 20 mmHg or more above goal, generally two or more antihypertensive agents will be needed to bring the blood pressure to goal [18].

Recommendation 2: ACE inhibitor
The drug class of angiotensin converting enzyme inhibitors (ACEi) is recommended as first-line therapy in all CKD patients [1,2]. It has been suggested, however, that a diuretic should be first-line therapy for CKD in those with low-level proteinuria [18,35]. This recommendation is based on the ALLHAT study [35]. However, ALLHAT's protocol did not use ACEi optimally (with diuretic, if needed). As a consequence ALLHAT's design may have biased the outcome in favor of diuretics, particularly at the expense of ACEi [36]. Also, a diuretic as monotherapy may induce metabolic dysfunctions that include hypokalemia, hyperglycemia, hyperuricemia, and stimulation of the renin–angiotensin–aldosterone system [2,3,36]. However, if the diuretic is used along with an ACEi (or angiotensin II receptor blocker [ARB]), most of the metabolic dysfunctions that have been associated with diuretic use in observational studies and which are felt to increase CVD risk appear to be largely mitigated [36,37].

Although both ACEi and ARB are kidney protective [2], ACEi is the first choice because it is not clear if ARB are cardioprotective to the level of ACEi [2,38–41]. ACEi should be used even if the patient is not clinically hypertensive [2,12]. Measures that may increase ACEi kidney protection include a low-salt and reduced-protein diet [2], diuretic therapy [2,42], the low BP goal [2,3], and statin therapy [2]. ACEi are antiproteinuric even in inflammatory glomerulonephritis [2]. ACEi should be continued even though GFR declines to stage 4 CKD (15–29 mL/min/1.73 m^2) [43]. To prevent hyperkalemia, dietary potassium restriction and

Algorithm 1. Initial antihypertensive therapy[a]

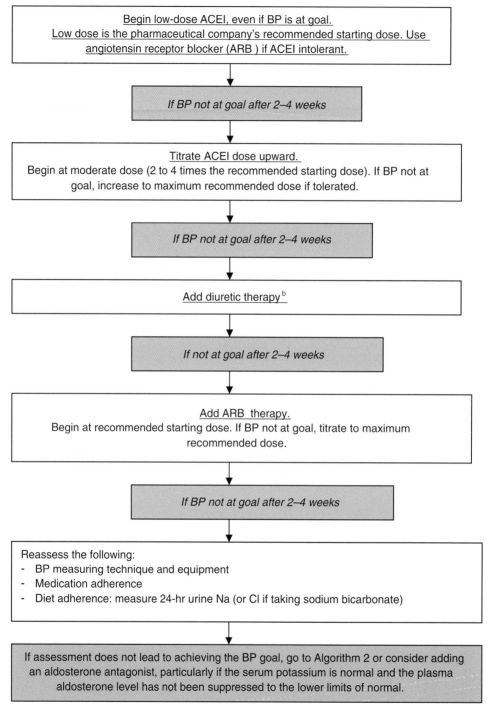

Figure 30.2 Antihypertensive regimens in CKD

[a] Assumes nonpharmacologic therapy to control BP is in place (see text) and that the patient does not have renovascular hypertension, congestive heart failure, ischemic heart disease, or hypertensive urgency. The above approach focuses on BP control in proteinuric nephropathies, but is also appropriate for nephrosclerosis, polycystic kidney disease, and interstitial nephropathies.

[b] The suggestion to add diuretic before ARB is arbitrary but can be justified by the evidence that diuretic increases the antihypertensive effect of angiotensin-converting-enzyme inhibitor (ACE inhibitor), is often needed in chronic kidney disease (CKD) to control fluid retention, is inexpensive, and may increase the renoprotective effects of ACE inhibitor, angiotensin receptor blocker (ARB), or the combination [57]. Emphasize salt restriction in autosomal dominant polycystic kidney disease (ADPKD) rather than diuretic therapy, which may promote cyst growth [3]. Details of diuretic therapy are discussed previously [3].

Algorithm 2. Recommended therapy if Algorithm 1 fails to control BP.

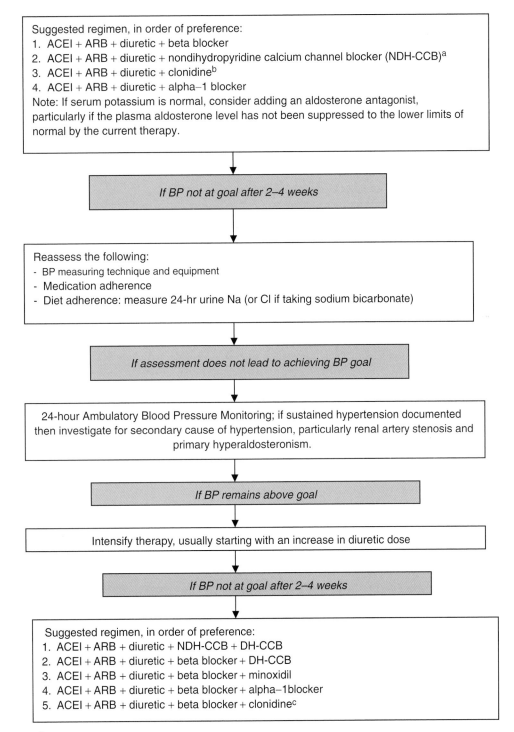

Suggested regimen, in order of preference:
1. ACEI + ARB + diuretic + beta blocker
2. ACEI + ARB + diuretic + nondihydropyridine calcium channel blocker (NDH-CCB)[a]
3. ACEI + ARB + diuretic + clonidine[b]
4. ACEI + ARB + diuretic + alpha–1 blocker

Note: If serum potassium is normal, consider adding an aldosterone antagonist, particularly if the plasma aldosterone level has not been suppressed to the lower limits of normal by the current therapy.

If BP not at goal after 2–4 weeks

Reassess the following:
- BP measuring technique and equipment
- Medication adherence
- Diet adherence: measure 24-hr urine Na (or Cl if taking sodium bicarbonate)

If assessment does not lead to achieving BP goal

24-hour Ambulatory Blood Pressure Monitoring; if sustained hypertension documented then investigate for secondary cause of hypertension, particularly renal artery stenosis and primary hyperaldosteronism.

If BP remains above goal

Intensify therapy, usually starting with an increase in diuretic dose

If BP not at goal after 2–4 weeks

Suggested regimen, in order of preference:
1. ACEI + ARB + diuretic + NDH-CCB + DH-CCB
2. ACEI + ARB + diuretic + beta blocker + DH-CCB
3. ACEI + ARB + diuretic + beta blocker + minoxidil
4. ACEI + ARB + diuretic + beta blocker + alpha–1blocker
5. ACEI + ARB + diuretic + beta blocker + clonidine[c]

[a]Diltiazem and verapamil sustained release preparations are recommended.

[b]Clonidine recommended for individuals receiving insulin, because it does not importantly affect glucoregulation, and for those who have difficulty with beta blocker (eg., bronchospasm, cardiac conduction).

[c]Beta blocker/clonidine combination is usually well tolerated, but may cause bradycardia.

Figure 30.2 (*Continued,*)

the concomitant use of furosemide and sodium bicarbonate may be indicated [44].

The benefits of ACEi appear to be shared by all ACEi [2,45]. The longer-acting ACEi are preferred over captopril [38,44]. Advancing the ACEi dose to tolerance increases its antiproteinuric effect [2] and decreases the likelihood of aldosterone escape (increasing plasma aldosterone levels during stable ACEi therapy), which could in turn diminish the ACEi renoprotection [46].

A recent meta-analysis suggested that ACEi may not have kidney-protective effects apart from BP control [47]. However, that analysis included the ALLHAT study, which did not use ACEi optimally, and 126 other RCTs of varying sizes, many of which may not have had the same methodologic rigor of the large RCTs discussed above. Also, a recent retrospective analysis of ACEi use in diabetic patients suggested more rapid progression in those receiving ACEi than those not receiving ACEi [48]. However, that study lacked BP measures and contradicted the long-term results of trials of diabetic nephropathy [49,50].

Recommendation 3: ARB therapy

ARB are kidney protective in the nephropathy of type 2 diabetes and likely in other nephropathies as well [2]. ARB are recommended as first-line therapy in those who are ACEi intolerant (with cough, angioedema, or allergy). In CKD, ARB may raise serum potassium less than ACEi [2], perhaps because in usual doses ARB do not suppress aldosterone as much as ACEi [51]. The highest tolerated ARB dose is recommended because it is the most antiproteinuric [52,53] and more likely to result in regression of left ventricular hypertrophy [54] than usual ARB doses. ARB may be especially effective in those who are homozygous for deletion of the ACE gene (DD genotype) [55].

Recommendation 4: Combination ACEi and ARB

The combination of the ACEi and ARB classes of medications is more antiproteinuric [56] and slows progression better than either drug alone [57]. Combination therapy generally improves BP control [58,59], although the effect may not be large [58]. Combination ACEi and ARB is recommended as the next step if the CKD patient fails to achieve the BP and proteinuria goals after 2 months of ACEi-plus-diuretic therapy (Figure 30.2). Diuretic therapy may increase the renoprotective effects of combination ACEi and ARB therapy [57].

An alternative to adding an ARB to ACEi-plus-diuretic therapy is the addition of a nondihydropyridine calcium channel blocker (NDHCCB; verapamil or cardiazem) [60–62].

Recommendation 5: Avoid dihydropyridine calcium blockers unless needed for BP control

Generally, the dihydropyridine CCB (DHCCB) amlodipine lowers BP better than an ACEi or a beta blocker; however, in those with hypertensive nephrosclerosis, it can lead to accelerated GFR decline and an increased risk of the composite end point of doubling of serum creatinine, ESRD, or death [2]. There are other lines of evidence that DHCCB are not kidney protective [2]. However,

the clearest evidence has come from the recent REIN-2 trial [31], in which nondiabetic proteinuric renal disease patients receiving ramipril were randomized to the usual or the low BP goal. DHCCB (felodipine) was used to achieve the low BP goal. Despite achieving the low BP goal, the DHCCB group did not experience slower GFR decline or proteinuria reduction compared to those maintained at the usual BP goal. This suggests that the DHCCB group had sustained glomerular hypertension, despite concomitant ramipril therapy and despite achieving the low BP goal [44,60,61]. It is likely the DHCCB provided cardiovascular protection because it lowered systemic BP. Its addition to ramipril did not, however, provide additional kidney protection (proteinuria reduction or slowed GFR decline) beyond that achieved with the baseline dose of ramipril in this study. For alternatives to DHCCB that should provide systemic BP control and kidney protection, see recommended therapies 2–4, 7–12, and 15 in the context of the algorithm shown in Figure 30.2. Further insight into the kidney-protective effects of the combination ACEi plus DHCCB should be forthcoming from the Avoiding Cardiovascular Events through Combination Therapy in Patients Living with Systolic Hypertension (ACCOMPLISH) trial [63].

Recommendation 6: Control protein intake

Reducing dietary protein intake from the usual level (about 1–1.5 g/kg of ideal body weight/day) to about 0.7 g/kg ideal body weight/day (low-protein diet) slows GFR decline in those with proteinuria of >1 g/day [2]. A further benefit of the lower protein intake is that it slows proteinuria progression in CKD, even in those who at baseline have low-level proteinuria (e.g. <250 mg/day) [2]. Soy proteins may be less proteinuric than animal proteins [2,64]. Dietary protein intake should be monitored periodically, for example, every 4–6 months, by urine urea excretion in 24-h urine collections [2,17]. Monitoring urine protein intake is particularly important in those who are not achieving their proteinuria goal. CKD patients who are men or who have glomerular disease may particularly benefit from the low-protein diet [65].

Level 2 recommendations to slow natural progression
Recommendation 7: Restrict NaCl intake, diuretic therapy

A high salt intake (e.g. 200 mmol NaCl/day; 4.6 g sodium) can completely override the antiproteinuria effects of ACEi, ARB, or NDHCCB therapy [2,66]. The recommended NaCl intake in CKD (assuming that renal salt wasting is not present) is about 80–120 mmol/day (2 to 3 g Na). The NaCl intake of the average North American adult is about 170 mmol/day (3.9 g Na). Salt intake should be monitored periodically (e.g. every 4–6 months) by 24-h urine collection [2,17]. The monitoring of 24-h urine sodium content is particularly important in those not achieving the BP or proteinuria goal. In patients receiving $NaHCO_3$ therapy, urine chloride rather than sodium should be monitored. Concomitant KCl therapy needs to be taken into account in assessing NaCl intake in such patients [2]. Diuretic therapy improves BP control and proteinuria reduction in those receiving ACEi or ARB [2,42,57]. Nevertheless, the ideal treatment may be to avoid use of a diuretic, if possible, because of multiple metabolic dysfunctions [41]. These metabolic dysfunctions, however, may be mitigated by concomitant ACEi–ARB therapy. Note that 40% of the AASK and 60% of the MDRD patients did not receive a diuretic, and they generally achieved their BP goals [2].

Recommendation 8: Control fluid intake

A retrospective analysis of MDRD Study A showed that urine volumes exceeding 2 L/day were associated with faster GFR decline, especially in polycystic kidney disease patients [67]. The patients with the higher urine volumes showed higher BP, lower serum sodium, and frankly hypotonic urine, suggesting that they were "pushing fluids." It is not uncommon that CKD patients are advised to increase fluid intake [68]. However, in patients with CKD there is no evidence of benefit, and it may cause harm based on data from both the MDRD [67] and AASK [69] studies.

Recommendation 9: NDHCCB therapy

The class of NDHCCB drugs, which includes diltiazem and verapamil, is antiproteinuric and may be renoprotective [2,60–63]. NDHCCB used together with a DHCCB is a potent antihypertensive combination when used along with other antihypertensive therapies. It can be recommended in CKD patients with poorly controlled hypertension that is resistant to the usual measures [2].

Recommendation 10: Control each component of metabolic syndrome

The metabolic syndrome is defined as any three of the following conditions [70,71]:

1 BP of $\geq$135/85 mmHg or BP requiring therapy for hypertension
2 Fasting blood glucose of >110 mg/dL, or treatment for hyperglycemia
3 Serum high-density lipoprotein cholesterol of <40 mg/dL for men or <50 mg/dL for women
4 Serum triglycerides of $\geq$150 mg/dL or drug therapy needed to control hypertriglyceridemia
5 Waist circumference of >40 in. (102 cm) in men or above 35 in. (88 cm) in women.

Each component of the metabolic syndrome has been found to be a risk factor for CKD progression. Also, the prevalence of microalbuminuria and CKD increases proportionately with the number of components of the metabolic syndrome that are present in a given patient [71].

Obesity increases the risk of CKD and is associated with glomerulomegaly, focal and segmental glomerulosclerosis, and proteinuria, which can be progressive [2]. Reducing even moderate obesity can reduce proteinuria [2]. In a randomized trial in moderately obese CKD patients (mean body mass index, 32; mean proteinuria, 2.8 g/day) a 4% decrease in body weight over 5 months reduced proteinuria by 31% [2].

With regard to statins, there have been numerous trials showing that statins have antiproteinuric effects and appear to be kidney protective. However, it is widely believed that the definitive trial has not been done [72]. This is discussed in greater detail in chapter 32. However, in progress is the SHARP trial, in which CKD patients are being randomized to placebo or combined simvastatin–ezetimibe therapy [72].

With respect to kidney protection by fibrates, gemfibrozil does not appear to slow progression of CKD [73]. However, fenofibrate has an antiproteinuric effect in diabetic humans and animal models [74]. This drug, however, causes an increase in serum creatinine in CKD patients. The mechanism is unclear. It has been suggested that fenofibrate is nephrotoxic or that it increases creatinine production. However, our recent analysis of 13 fenofibrate-treated patients followed for up to 5 years did not find evidence for either of those mechanisms. Indeed, although serum creatinine increased acutely during follow-up, when the fenofibrate was discontinued, the serum creatinine returned to or below baseline, which is remarkable because each patient previously showed evidence of progression [75].

Some authors advise against the routine use of lipid-lowering therapy in CKD because of lack of proof of a kidney-protective effect [72]. We suggest, however, that given the clear evidence that CKD itself is a CVD risk factor and that there is substantial evidence that statins are antiproteinuric and kidney protective by means of their lipid-lowering effect or anti-inflammatory, antithrombotic, "pleiotropic" effects [76–78], a strong argument can be made for the routine use of lipid-lowering therapy in CKD with a goal of reducing low-density lipoprotein cholesterol to <100 mg/dL and raising high-density lipoprotein cholesterol as much as feasible [2,3]. With regard to statin dose, in general, high-dose statin therapy shows better cardiovascular protection than low-dose therapy (typical starting dose of statins) [79] and generally is as well-tolerated as the low doses [80]. A complete discussion of this topic is found in chapter 32.

Recommendation 11: Aldosterone antagonists

Spironolactone and the more selective aldosterone antagonist eplerenone have substantial antihypertensive [81], cardioprotective [2], and antiproteinuric effects even when administered in low doses and in the presence of ACEi therapy [46,82]. The mechanism is not clear. However, it could involve effects of aldosterone blockade on the endothelium and the profibrotic effects of aldosterone [46]. If these drugs are used in combination with an ACEi or ARB, careful monitoring to avoid hyperkalemia is in order. Spironolactone may increase the risk of upper gastrointestinal bleeding [83].

Recommendation 12: Beta blocker therapy

The AASK study showed that beta blocker therapy is more antiproteinuric and slows GFR decline better than amlodipine [2]. However, beta blockers increase the likelihood of diabetes and, as monotherapy or combined with a diuretic, increase the mortality rate of hypertension management compared to ACEi plus a diuretic [84]. Thus, beta blockers should be avoided in CKD unless required to manage heart disease [85]. Carvedilol, however, may be better tolerated [86].

Recommendation 13: Smoking cessation

There is strong epidemiologic evidence that cigarette smoking promotes progression of all forms of kidney disease and that this effect may be of greater magnitude in African Americans [2]. Also, cigarette smoking combined with obesity increases CVD mortality by 6- to 11-fold [87].

Recommendation 14: Correct severe anemia

Correction of anemia by erythropoietin-stimulating agents (ESAs) has the potential to slow progression of CKD by multiple mechanisms, including mitigation of renal hypoxia and increasing the antioxidant activity of blood [88]. Erythropoietin can prevent apoptosis of cells by altering cell signaling pathways [89]. Additionally, erythropoietin inhibits proinflammatory cytokines and has a protective effect on endothelial cells [90,91].

Low hematocrit has been shown to be an independent predictor of progression of nephropathy in type 1 diabetes mellitus [92], type 2 diabetes mellitus [93], and nondiabetic renal disease [94–96]. Lower hematocrit is linked, in a linear fashion, to development of ESRD [97–99]. ESA treatment of CKD anemia in observational studies is associated with slowing of GFR decline, especially in nondiabetic CKD patients [100–104]. In a small RCT involving ESA treatment of anemic nondiabetic CKD patients, the ESA showed a 60% reduction in death or the need for renal replacement in patients in the early treatment arm [105].

Recently, the Correction of Hemoglobin and Outcomes in Renal Insufficiency (CHOIR) study, which used erythropoietin alpha therapy in 1432 CKD patients randomized to either a high hemoglobin goal (13.5 g/dL) or a low hemoglobin goal (11.3 g/dL) was stopped prematurely because of increased CV events in the patients assigned to the high hemoglobin goal group. The Cardiovascular Reduction Early Anemia Treatment with Epoetin Beta (CREATE) study randomized 603 anemic CKD patients in an open-label fashion to receive epoetin beta to achieve target hemoglobin levels of 13–15 or 10.5–11.5 g/dL. During the 3-year follow-up, the primary end point of a composite of eight CV events was not significantly different between the two groups. The estimated GFR decline was similar, although dialysis was required in more patients in the high hemoglobin target group. Still ongoing in Europe and North America is the Trial to Reduce Cardiovascular Events with Aranesp Therapy (TREAT) study. This double-blind, randomized, placebo-controlled study has enrolled 4000 diabetic patients with nephropathy to assess the effect of anemia correction on CV and renal outcomes.

Until the results of the TREAT study become fully available, treatment of anemia in CKD can be recommended if the hemoglobin level is <9.0 g/dL, because of the documented improvement in quality of life. The recent update of the K/DOQI anemia recommendations suggests a target hemoglobin of 11–12 g/dL that should not exceed 13 g/dL [106]. A more complete discussion of this topic is found in chapter 31.

Recommendation 15: Control elevated uric acid levels

In a placebo-controlled, randomized trial, allopurinol therapy resulted in a 40% lesser increase in serum creatinine over 1 year of follow-up and improved BP control (~13-mmHg-lower systolic BP) [107]. The mechanisms may involve inhibition of uric acid effects that induce arteriopathy, which may induce CV and kidney disease [108].

Recommendation 16: Renin inhibition

Aleskiren, a direct renin inhibitor, is antiproteinuric, appears to be kidney protective alone or in combination with ARB, and is well-tolerated [109,110]. Its role in kidney protection remains to be established.

Other measures to consider to slow CKD progression

It should be noted that the strength of the evidence for the application of the following for slowing progression of CKD is not as strong as data for BP control, proteinuria control, and renin–angiotensin–aldosterone system blockade.

- Avoid multiple daily doses of acetaminophen, particularly in women, because of the evidence that it is significantly associated with rising serum creatinine during prolonged follow-up [111]
- Avoid nonsteroidal anti-inflammatory drugs altogether, or at most take them no more than once or twice weekly, because of their known nephrotoxicity [2]; daily low-dose (baby) aspirin, however, appears to provide net benefit in CKD [112]
- Avoid herbal therapy unless the safety of the herb has been proved; many herbal products appear to be nephrotoxic [113]
- Avoid prolonged severe hypokalemia because it can cause progressive renal interstitial fibrosis [2]
- $NaHCO_3$ to correct metabolic acidosis should be considered because of its anticatabolic effects [2]. Also, the nephrotoxicity of nonselective proteinuria appears to be strongly related to activation of the alternative complement pathway in the renal tubular compartment [2,114]. $NaHCO_3$ inhibits this process by raising tubular fluid pH [2]
- Control hyperphosphatemia and hyperparathyroidism; in animal models and in human studies, controlling hyperphosphatemia slows CKD progression. Also, active 1,25-(OH)-vitamin D therapy, which has effects on calcium, phosphorus, and parathyroid hormone, was found to be potentially antiproteinuric (dipstick protein) in CKD in one post hoc analysis of an RCT, and by this mechanism it might be kidney protective [115].

References

1 Haddad N, Brown C, Hebert LA. Retarding progression of kidney disease. In: Feehally J, Floege J, Johnson RJ, editors, *Comprehensive Clinical Nephrology*, 3rd edn. Mosby/Elsevier, Philadelphia, 2007, p 823–830.
2 Wilmer WA, Rovin BH, Hebert CJ, Rao SV, Hebert LA. Management of glomerular proteinuria: a commentary. *J Am Soc Nephrol* 2003; **14:** 3217–3232.

3 Hebert LA, Wilmer WA, Falkenhain ME, Ladson-Wofford SE, Nahman NS, Jr., Rovin BH. Renoprotection: one or many therapies? *Kidney Int* 2001; **59:** 1211–1226.

4 Davis CL. Evaluation of the living kidney donor: current perspectives. *Am J Kidney Dis* 2004; **43:** 508–530.

5 Novick AC, Gephardt G, Guz B, Steinmuller D, Tubbs RR. Long-term follow-up after partial removal of a solitary kidney. *N Engl J Med* 1991; **325:** 1058–1062.

6 Bay WH, Hebert LA. The living donor in kidney transplantation. *Ann Intern Med* 1987; **106:** 719–727.

7 Praga M, Hernandez E, Herrero JC, Morales E, Revilla Y, Diaz-Gonzalez R *et al.* Influence of obesity on the appearance of proteinuria and renal insufficiency after unilateral nephrectomy. *Kidney Int* 2000; **58:** 2111–2118.

8 Hebert LA, Kusek JW, Greene T, Adodoa LY, Jones CA, Levey AS *et al.* Effects of blood pressure control on progressive renal disease in blacks and whites. Modification of Diet in Renal Disease Study Group. *Hypertension* 1997; **30:** 428–435.

9 Baldwin DS. Chronic glomerulonephritis: nonimmunologic mechanisms of progressive glomerular damage. *Kidney Int* 1982; **21:** 109–120.

10 D'Agati VD, Fogo AB, Bruijn JA, Jennette JC. Pathologic classification of focal segmental glomerulosclerosis: a working proposal. *Am J Kidney Dis* 2004; **43:** 368–382.

11 Lea J, Greene T, Hebert L, Lipkowitz M, Massry S, Middleton J *et al.* The relationship between magnitude of proteinuria reduction and risk of end-stage renal disease: results of the African American Study of Kidney Disease and Hypertension. *Arch Intern Med* 2005; **165:** 947–953.

12 Jafar TH, Stark PC, Schmid CH, Landa M, Maschio G, de Jong PE *et al.* Progression of chronic kidney disease: the role of blood pressure control, proteinuria, and angiotensin-converting enzyme inhibition: a patient-level meta-analysis. *Ann Intern Med* 2003; **139:** 244–252.

13 Branten AJ, van den Born J, Jansen JL, Assmann KJ, Wetzels JF. Familial nephropathy differing from minimal change nephropathy and focal glomerulosclerosis. *Kidney Int* 2001; **59:** 693–701.

14 Moghazi S, Jones E, Schroepple J, Arya K, McClellan W, Hennigar RA *et al.* Correlation of renal histopathology with sonographic findings. *Kidney Int* 2005; **67:** 1515–1520.

15 Rigalleau V, Lasseur C, Raffaitin C, Beauvieux MC, Barthe N, Chauveau P *et al.* Normoalbuminuric renal-insufficient diabetic patients: a lower-risk group. *Diabetes Care* 2007; **30:** 2034–2039.

16 Appel LJ, Wright JT, Greene T, Kusek JW, Lewis JB, Wang X *et al.* Long-term effects of renin-angiotensin system-blocking therapy and a low blood pressure goal on progression of hypertensive chronic kidney disease in African Americans. *Arch Intern Med* 2008; **168:** 832–839.

17 Shidham G, Hebert LA. Controversies in nephrology. Timed urine collections are not needed to measure urine protein excretion in clinical practice. *Am J Kidney Dis* 2006; **47:** 8–14.

18 National Kidney Foundation. K/DOQI clinical practice guidelines on hypertension and antihypertensive agents in chronic kidney disease. *Am J Kidney Dis* 2004; **43(Suppl 291):** S1–S290.

19 Birmingham DJ, Rovin BH, Shidham G, Nagaraja HN, Zou X, Bissell M *et al.* Spot urine protein/creatinine ratios are unreliable estimates of 24 h proteinuria in most systemic lupus erythematosus nephritis flares. *Kidney Int* 2007; **72:** 865–870.

20 Birmingham DJ, Rovin BH, Shidham G, Bissell M, Nagaraja HN, Hebert LA *et al.* Relationship between albuminuria and total proteinuria in SLE nephritis: diagnostic and therapeutic implications. *Clin J Am Soc Nephrol* 2008. [Epub ahead of print.]

21 Stevens LA, Coresh J, Greene T, Levey AS. Assessing kidney function: measured and estimated glomerular filtration rate. *N Engl J Med* 2006; **354:** 2473–2483.

22 Hebert LA, Nori U, Hebert PL. Measured and estimated glomerular filtration rate. *N Engl J Med* 2006; **355:** 1068. [Author reply, **355:** 1069–1070.]

23 Macdonald J, Marcora S, Jibani M, Roberts G, Kumwenda M, Glover R *et al.* GFR estimation using cystatin C is not independent of body composition. *Am J Kidney Dis* 2006; **48:** 712–719.

24 Ix JH, Shlipak MG, Chertow GM, Whooley MA. Association of cystatin C with mortality, cardiovascular events, and incident heart failure among persons with coronary heart disease: data from the Heart and Soul Study. *Circulation* 2007; **115:** 173–179.

25 Brosius FC, III, Hostetter TH, Kelepouris E, Mitsnefes MM, Moe SM, Moore MA *et al.* Detection of chronic kidney disease in patients with or at increased risk of cardiovascular disease: a science advisory from the American Heart Association Kidney and Cardiovascular Disease Council; the Councils on High Blood Pressure Research, Cardiovascular Disease in the Young, and Epidemiology and Prevention; and the Quality of Care and Outcomes Research Interdisciplinary Working Group: developed in collaboration with the National Kidney Foundation. *Circulation* 2006; **114:** 1083–1087.

26 Collins AJ, Li S, Gilbertson DT, Liu J, Chen SC, Herzog CA. Chronic kidney disease and cardiovascular disease in the Medicare population. *Kidney Int Suppl* 2003; **87:** S24–S31.

27 Levey AS, Mulrow CD. An editorial update: what level of blood pressure control in chronic kidney disease? *Ann Intern Med* 2005; **143:** 79–81.

28 Sarnak MJ, Greene T, Wang X, Beck G, Kusek JW, Collins AJ *et al.* The effect of a lower target blood pressure on the progression of kidney disease: long-term follow-up of the modification of diet in renal disease study. *Ann Intern Med* 2005; **142:** 342–351.

29 Pohl MA, Blumenthal S, Cordonnier DJ, De Alvaro F, Deferrari G, Eisner G *et al.* Independent and additive impact of blood pressure control and angiotensin II receptor blockade on renal outcomes in the irbesartan diabetic nephropathy trial: clinical implications and limitations. *J Am Soc Nephrol* 2005; **16:** 3027–3037.

30 Vasan RS, Larson MG, Leip EP, Evans JC, O'Donnell CJ, Kannel WB *et al.* Impact of high-normal blood pressure on the risk of cardiovascular disease. *N Engl J Med* 2001; **345:** 1291–1297.

31 Ruggenenti P, Perna A, Loriga G, Ganeva M, Ene-Iordache B, Turturro M *et al.* Blood-pressure control for renoprotection in patients with non-diabetic chronic renal disease (REIN-2): multicentre, randomised controlled trial. *Lancet* 2005; **365:** 939–946.

32 Hebert CJ, Shidham G, Hebert LA. Should the target for blood pressure control specify both a systolic and a diastolic component? *Curr Hypertens Rep* 2005; **7:** 360–362.

33 Verberk WJ, Kroon AA, Kessels AG, deLeeuw PW. Home blood pressure measurement: a systematic review. *J Am Coll Cardiol* 2005; **46:** 743–751.

34 Fagard RH, Celis H, Thijs L, Staessen JA, Clement DL, De Buyzere ML *et al.* Daytime and nighttime blood pressure as predictors of death and cause-specific cardiovascular events in hypertension. *Hypertension* 2008; **51:** 55–61.

35 Levey AS, Uhlig K. Which antihypertensive agents in chronic kidney disease? *Ann Intern Med* 2006; **144:** 213–215.

36 Hebert LA, Rovin BH, Hebert CJ. The design of ALLHAT may have biased the study's outcome in favor of the diuretic cohort. *Nat Clin Pract Nephrol* 2007; **3**: 60–61.

37 Kjeldsen SE, Julius S, Mancia G, McInnes GT, Hua T, Weber MA *et al.* Effects of valsartan compared to amlodipine on preventing type 2 diabetes in high-risk hypertensive patients: the VALUE trial. *J Hypertens* 2006; **24**: 1405–1412.

38 Hebert LA, Rovin BH, Hebert CJ. Response to Dr. Brenner's comments. *J Am Soc Nephrol* 2004; **15**: 1356–1357.

39 Strauss MH, Hall AS. Angiotensin receptor blockers may increase risk of myocardial infarction: unraveling the ARB-MI paradox. *Circulation* 2006; **114**: 838–854.

40 Wang JG, Li Y, Franklin SS, Safar M. Prevention of stroke and myocardial infarction by amlodipine and angiotensin receptor blockers: a quantitative overview. *Hypertension* 2007; **50**: 181–188.

41 Rovin BH, Hebert LA. Thiazide diuretic monotherapy for hypertension: diuretic's dark side just got darker. *Kidney Int* 2007; **72**: 1423–1426.

42 Esnault VL, Ekhlas A, Delcroix C, Moutel MG, Nguyen JM. Diuretic and enhanced sodium restriction results in improved antiproteinuric response to RAS blocking agents. *J Am Soc Nephrol* 2005; **16**: 474–481.

43 Hou FF, Zhang X, Zhang GH, Xie D, Chen PY, Zhang WR *et al.* Efficacy and safety of benazepril in advanced chronic renal insufficiency. *N Engl J Med* 2006; **354**: 131–140.

44 Hebert LA. Optimizing ACE inhibitor therapy for CKD. *N Engl J Med* 2006; **354**: 189–191.

45 Tu K, Gunraj N, Mamdani M. Is ramipril really better than other angiotensin-converting enzyme inhibitors after acute myocardial infarction? *Am J Cardiol* 2006; **98**: 6–9.

46 Schjoedt KJ, Rossing K, Juhl TR, Boomsma F, Rossing P, Tarnow L *et al.* Beneficial impact of spironolactone in diabetic nephropathy. *Kidney Int* 2005; **68**: 2829–2836.

47 Casas JP, Chua W, Loukogeorgakis S, Vallance P, Smeeth L, Hingorani AD *et al.* Effect of inhibitors of the renin-angiotensin system and other antihypertensive drugs on renal outcomes: systematic review and meta-analysis. *Lancet* 2005; **366**: 2026–2033.

48 Suissa S, Hutchinson T, Brophy JM, Kezouh A. ACE-inhibitor use and the long-term risk of renal failure in diabetes. *Kidney Int* 2006; **69**: 913–919.

49 Wilmer WA, Hebert LA, Lewis EJ, Rohde RD, Whittier F, Cattran D *et al.* Remission of nephrotic syndrome in type 1 diabetes: long-term follow-up of patients in the Captopril Study. *Am J Kidney Dis* 1999; **34**: 308–314.

50 So WY, Ma RC, Ozaki R, Tong PC, Ng MC, Ho CS *et al.* Angiotensin-converting enzyme (ACE) inhibition in type 2, diabetic patients: interaction with ACE insertion/deletion polymorphism. *Kidney Int* 2006; **69**: 1438–1443.

51 Haddad N, Rajan J, Agarwal A, *et al.* In chronic kidney disease ACE inhibition therapy suppresses plasma aldosterone levels better than angiotensin receptor blocker. *J Am Soc Nephrol* 2005; **10**: 616A.

52 Rossing K, Schjoedt KJ, Jensen BR, Boomsma F, Parving HH. Enhanced renoprotective effects of ultrahigh doses of irbesartan in patients with type 2 diabetes and microalbuminuria. *Kidney Int* 2005; **68**: 1190–1198.

53 Schmieder RE, Klingbeil AU, Fleischmann EH, Veelken R, Delles C. Additional antiproteinuric effect of ultrahigh dose candesartan: a double-blind, randomized, prospective study. *J Am Soc Nephrol* 2005; **16**: 3038–3045.

54 Malmqvist K, Kahan T, Edner M, Held C, Hagg A, Lind L *et al.* Regression of left ventricular hypertrophy in human hypertension with irbesartan. *J Hypertens* 2001; **19**: 1167–1176.

55 Parving HH, de Zeeuw D, Cooper ME, Remuzzi G, Liu N, Lunceford J *et al.* ACE gene polymorphism and losartan treatment in type 2 diabetic patients with nephropathy. *J Am Soc Nephrol* 2008; **19**: 771–779.

56 Wolf G, Ritz E. Combination therapy with ACE inhibitors and angiotensin II receptor blockers to halt progression of chronic renal disease: pathophysiology and indications. *Kidney Int* 2005; **67**: 799–812.

57 Nakao N, Yoshimura A, Morita H, Takeda M, Kayano T, Ideura T. Combination treatment of angiotensin-II receptor blocker and angiotensin-converting-enzyme inhibitor in non-diabetic renal disease (COOPERATE): a randomised controlled trial. *Lancet* 2003; **361**: 117–124.

58 Yusuf S, Teo KK, Pogue J, Dyal L, Copland I, Schumacher H *et al.* Telmisartan, ramipril, or both in patients at high risk for vascular events. *N Engl J Med* 2008; **358**: 1547–1559.

59 Doulton TW, He FJ, MacGregor GA. Systematic review of combined angiotensin-converting enzyme inhibition and angiotensin receptor blockade in hypertension. *Hypertension* 2005; **45**: 880–886.

60 Khosla N, Bakris GL. Lessons learned from recent hypertension trials about kidney disease. *Clin J Am Soc Nephrol* 2006; **1**: 229–235.

61 Remuzzi G, Macia M, Ruggenenti P. Prevention and treatment of diabetic renal disease in type 2 diabetes: the BENEDICT study. *J Am Soc Nephrol* 2006; **17**: S90–S97.

62 PROCOPA. Dissociation between blood pressure reduction and fall in proteinuria in primary renal disease: a randomized double-blind trial. *J Hypertens* 2002; **20**: 729–737.

63 Jamerson KA, Bakris GL, Wun CC, Dahlof B, Lefkowitz M, Manfreda S *et al.* Rationale and design of the avoiding cardiovascular events through combination therapy in patients living with systolic hypertension (ACCOMPLISH) trial: the first randomized controlled trial to compare the clinical outcome effects of first-line combination therapies in hypertension. *Am J Hypertens* 2004; **17**: 793–801.

64 Teixeira SR, Tappenden KA, Carson L, Jones R, Prabhudesai M, Marhsall WP *et al.* Isolated soy protein consumption reduces urinary albumin excretion and improves the serum lipid profile in men with type 2 diabetes mellitus and nephropathy. *J Nutr* 2004; **134**: 1874–1880.

65 Levey AS, Greene T, Sarnak MJ, Wang X, Beck GJ, Kusek JW *et al.* Effect of dietary protein restriction on the progression of kidney disease: long-term follow-up of the Modification of Diet in Renal Disease (MDRD) Study. *Am J Kidney Dis* 2006; **48**: 879–888.

66 Jones-Burton C, Mishra SI, Fink JC, Brown J, Gossa W, Bakris GL *et al.* An in-depth review of the evidence linking dietary salt intake and progression of chronic kidney disease. *Am J Nephrol* 2006; **26**: 268–275.

67 Hebert LA, Greene T, Levey AS, Falkenhain ME, Klahr S. High urine volume and low urine osmolality are risk factors for faster progression of renal disease. *Am J Kidney Dis* 2003; **41**: 962–971.

68 Wenzel UO, Hebert LA, Stahl RAK, Krenz I. My doctor said I should drink a lot! Recommendations for fluid intake in patients with chronic renal disease. *Clin J Am Soc Nephrol* 2006; **1**: 344–346.

69 Wang X, Lewis J, Appel L, Cheek D, Contreras G, Faulkner M *et al.* Validation of creatinine-based estimates of GFR when evaluating risk factors in longitudinal studies of kidney disease. *J Am Soc Nephrol* 2006; **17**: 2900–2909.

70 Ford ES, Giles WH, Dietz WH. Prevalence of the metabolic syndrome among US adults: findings from the third National Health and Nutrition Examination Survey. *JAMA* 2002; **287**: 356–359.

71 Kurella M, Lo JC, Chertow GM. Metabolic syndrome and the risk for chronic kidney disease among nondiabetic adults. *J Am Soc Nephrol* 2005; **16:** 2134–2140.

72 Tonelli M. Do statins protect the kidney by reducing proteinuria? *Ann Intern Med* 2006; **145:** 147–149.

73 Tonelli M, Collins D, Robins S, Bloomfield H, Curhan GC. Effect of gemfibrozil on change in renal function in men with moderate chronic renal insufficiency and coronary disease. *Am J Kidney Dis* 2004; **44:** 832–839.

74 Ansquer JC, Foucher C, Rattier S, Taskinen MR, Steiner G *et al.* Fenofibrate reduces progression to microalbuminuria over 3 years in a placebo-controlled study in type 2 diabetes: results from the Diabetes Atherosclerosis Intervention Study (DAIS). *Am J Kidney Dis* 2005; **45:** 485–493.

75 Khanna B, Valentine C, Nagaraja H, *et al.* Fenofibrate (FF)-induced increase in serum creatinine (SCr) in chronic kidney disease (CKD) does not appear to be the result of nephrotoxicity or increased creatinine production. National Meeting, American Society of Nephrology, San Diego, 2006.

76 Epstein M, Campese VM. Pleiotropic effects of 3-hydroxy-3-methylglutaryl coenzyme a reductase inhibitors on renal function. *Am J Kidney Dis* 2005; **45:** 2–14.

77 Chang JW, Yang WS, Min WK, Lee SK, Park JS, Kim SB. Effects of simvastatin on high-sensitivity C-reactive protein and serum albumin in hemodialysis patients. *Am J Kidney Dis* 2002; **39:** 1213–1217.

78 D'Amico G. Statins and renal diseases: from primary prevention to renal replacement therapy. *J Am Soc Nephrol* 2006; **17:** S148–S152.

79 Nissen SE, Nicholls SJ, Sipahi I, Libby P, Raichlen JS, Ballantyne CM *et al.* Effect of very high-intensity statin therapy on regression of coronary atherosclerosis: the ASTEROID trial. *JAMA* 2006; **295:** 1556–1565.

80 Newman C, Tsai J, Szarek M, Luo D, Gibson E. Comparative safety of atorvastatin 80 mg versus 10 mg derived from analysis of 49 completed trials in 14,236 patients. *Am J Cardiol* 2006; **97:** 61–67.

81 Calhoun DA. Use of aldosterone antagonists in resistant hypertension. *Prog Cardiovasc Dis* 2006; **48:** 387–396.

82 Schjoedt KJ, Rossing K, Juhl TR, Boomsma F, Tarnow L, Rossing P *et al.* Beneficial impact of spironolactone on nephrotic range albuminuria in diabetic nephropathy. *Kidney Int* 2006; **70:** 536–542.

83 Verhamme K, Mosis G, Dieleman J, Stricker B, Sturkenboom M. Spironolactone and risk of upper gastrointestinal events: population based case-control study. *BMJ* 2006; **333:** 330.

84 Beevers DG. The end of beta blockers for uncomplicated hypertension? *Lancet* 2005; **366:** 1510–1512.

85 Messerli FH, Bangalore S. Beta-blocker therapy in hypertension: a need to pause and reflect. *J Am Coll Cardiol* 2008; **51:** 517–518 (reply).

86 Giles TD, Bakris GL, Weber MA. Beta-blocker therapy in hypertension: a need to pause and reflect. *J Am Coll Cardiol* 2008; **51:** 516–517. (author reply, **51:** 517–518.)

87 Freedman DM, Sigurdson AJ, Rajaraman P, Doody MM, Linet MS, Ron E. The mortality risk of smoking and obesity combined. *Am J Prev Med* 2006; **31:** 355–362.

88 Grune T, Sommerburg O, Siems WG. Oxidative stress in anemia. *Clin Nephrol* 2000; **53:** S18–S22.

89 Maiese K, Li F, Chong ZZ. New avenues of exploration for erythropoietin. *JAMA* 2005; **293:** 90–95.

90 Chong ZZ, Kang JQ, Maiese K. Angiogenesis and plasticity: role of erythropoietin in vascular systems. *J Hematother Stem Cell Res* 2002; **11:** 863–871.

91 Kuriyama S, Hopp L, Yoshida H, Hikita M, Tomonari H, Hashimoto T *et al.* Evidence for amelioration of endothelial cell dysfunction by erythropoietin therapy in predialysis patients. *Am J Hypertens* 1996; **9:** 426–431.

92 Breyer JA, Bain RP, Evans JK, Nahman NS, Jr., Lewis EJ, Cooper M *et al.* Predictors of the progression of renal insufficiency in patients with insulin-dependent diabetes and overt diabetic nephropathy. The Collaborative Study Group. *Kidney Int* 1996; **50:** 1651–1658.

93 Yokoyama H, Tomonaga O, Hirayama M, Ishii A, Takeda M, Babazono T *et al.* Predictors of the progression of diabetic nephropathy and the beneficial effect of angiotensin-converting enzyme inhibitors in NIDDM patients. *Diabetologia* 1997; **40:** 405–411.

94 Muirhead N. The rationale for early management of chronic renal insufficiency. *Nephrol Dial Transplant* 2001; **16(Suppl 7):** 51–56.

95 Klahr S. Prevention of progression of nephropathy. *Nephrol Dial Transplant* 1997; **12(Suppl 2):** 63–66.

96 Peterson JC, Adler S, Burkart JM, Greene T, Hebert LA, Hunsicker LG *et al.* Blood pressure control, proteinuria, and the progression of renal disease. The Modification of Diet in Renal Disease Study. *Ann Intern Med* 1995; **123:** 754–762.

97 Iseki K, Ikemiya Y, Iseki C, Takishita S. Haematocrit and the risk of developing end-stage renal disease. *Nephrol Dial Transplant* 2003; **18:** 899–905.

98 Keane WF, Brenner BM, de Zeeuw D, Grunfeld JP, McGill J, Mitch WE *et al.* The risk of developing end-stage renal disease in patients with type 2 diabetes and nephropathy: the RENAAL study. *Kidney Int* 2003; **63:** 1499–1507.

99 Cusick M, Chew EY, Hoogwerf B, Agron E, Wu L, Lindley A *et al.* Risk factors for renal replacement therapy in the Early Treatment Diabetic Retinopathy Study (ETDRS), report no. 26. *Kidney Int* 2004; **66:** 1173–1179.

100 Jungers P, Choukroun G, Oualim Z, Robino C, Nguyen AT, Man NK. Beneficial influence of recombinant human erythropoietin therapy on the rate of progression of chronic renal failure in predialysis patients. *Nephrol Dial Transplant* 2001; **16:** 307–312.

101 Dean BB, Dylan M, Gano A, Jr., Knight K, Ofman JJ, Levine BS. Erythropoiesis-stimulating protein therapy and the decline of renal function: a retrospective analysis of patients with chronic kidney disease. *Curr Med Res Opin* 2005; **21:** 981–987.

102 Tapolyai M, Kadomatsu S, Perera-Chong M. rHu-erythropoietin (EPO) treatment of pre-ESRD patients slows the rate of progression of renal decline. *BMC Nephrol* 2003; **4:** 3.

103 Roth D, Smith RD, Schulman G, Steinman TI, Hatch FE, Rudnick MR *et al.* Effects of recombinant human erythropoietin on renal function in chronic renal failure predialysis patients. *Am J Kidney Dis* 1994; **24:** 777–784.

104 Kuriyama S, Tomonari H, Yoshida H, Hashimoto T, Kawaguchi Y, Sakai O. Reversal of anemia by erythropoietin therapy retards the progression of chronic renal failure, especially in nondiabetic patients. *Nephron* 1997; **77:** 176–185.

105 Gouva C, Nikolopoulos P, Ioannidis JP, Siamopoulos KC. Treating anemia early in renal failure patients slows the decline of renal function: a randomized controlled trial. *Kidney Int* 2004; **66:** 753–760.

106 KDOQI clinical practice guideline and clinical practice recommendations for anemia in chronic kidney disease: 2007 update of hemoglobin target. *Am J Kidney Dis* 2007; **50:** 471–530.

107 Mohanram A, Zhang Z, Shahinfar S, Keane WF, Brenner RM, Toto RD. Anemia and end-stage renal disease in patients with type 2 diabetes and nephropathy. *Kidney Int* 2004; **66:** 1131–1138.

108 Fang J, Alderman MH. Serum uric acid and cardiovascular mortality the NHANES I epidemiologic follow-up study, 1971–1992. National Health and Nutrition Examination Survey. *JAMA* 2000; **283:** 2404–2410.

109 Persson F, Rossing P, Schjoedt KJ, Juhl T, Tarnow L, Stehouwer CD *et al.* Time course of the antiproteinuric and antihypertensive effects of direct renin inhibition in type 2 diabetes. *Kidney Int* 2008; **73:** 1419–1425.

110 Parving HH, Lewis JB, Lewis EJ, *et al.* Aliskiren in the evaluation of proteinuria in diabetes (AVOID). *J Am Soc Nephrol* 2007; **18:** SA-PO1051 (abstract).

111 Curhan GC, Knight EL, Rosner B, Hankinson SE, Stampfer MJ. Lifetime nonnarcotic analgesic use and decline in renal function in women. *Arch Intern Med* 2004; **164:** 1519–1524.

112 Fored CM, Nyren O. Acetaminophen, aspirin, and renal failure (letter). *N Engl J Med* 2002; **346:** 1588–1589.

113 Isnard Bagnis C, Deray G, Baumelou A, Le Quintrec M, Vanherweghem JL. Herbs and the kidney. *Am J Kidney Dis* 2004; **44:** 1–11.

114 Rangan GK, Pippin JW, Coombes JD, Couser WG. C5b-9 does not mediate chronic tubulointerstitial disease in the absence of proteinuria. *Kidney Int* 2005; **67:** 492–503.

115 Agarwal R, Acharya M, Tian J, Hippensteel RL, Melnick JZ, Qiu P *et al.* Antiproteinuric effect of oral paricalcitol in chronic kidney disease. *Kidney Int* 2005; **68:** 2823–2828.

31 Treatment of Anemia in Chronic Kidney Disease, Stages 3–5

Robert N. Foley

Chronic Disease Research Group, Minneapolis, USA

Introduction

Anemia is common in chronic kidney disease (CKD), and a dose-dependent relationship exists between the severities of both conditions. Recombinant technology has revolutionized the therapy of anemia in CKD, and many controlled trials, primarily examining hemoglobin targets and how to achieve these targets, have been performed. For many other components of anemia management, clinical precedent, opinion, and observational studies have been the foundation for treatment.

Evaluation of anemia in CKD

Anemia is virtually the rule in late-stage CKD, irrespective of the underlying primary disease process [1]. Although anemia is often multifactorial, erythropoietin deficiency and resistance are thought to be major contributing factors, and most guidelines are primarily based upon these beliefs. This being said, it is vital that other potential causes be considered when treating anemia in CKD. As the differential diagnosis of anemia can be extremely wide, most guidelines take a pragmatic approach and clearly cannot replace expert hematological opinion with regard to identifying other contributing or exacerbating factors. Hints that anemia is caused by conditions other than CKD include anemia severity that is not commensurate with the level of kidney function, iron deficiency, and the presence of leukopenia or thrombocytopenia.

Few clinical trials have been performed to test the effectiveness of different anemia evaluation strategies in CKD populations. Several national guidelines suggest that glomerular filtration rates (GFRs) of less than 60 mL/min/1.73 m^2 should stimulate a search for anemia. It is likely that this opinion is based on experience from referral populations, and the utility of this approach in other

settings is unknown. Typical guidelines for initial assessment of anemia are as follows [2]:
- Complete blood counts, including hemoglobin concentration, mean corpuscular hemoglobin, mean corpuscular volume, mean corpuscular hemoglobin concentration, white blood cell count (and differential), and platelet count
- Absolute reticulocyte count
- Serum ferritin to assess iron stores
- Serum transferrin saturation (or reticulocyte hemoglobin content or percent hypochromic red cells, where available) to gauge the adequacy of iron available for erythropoiesis

Fluid retention and expansion of extracellular fluid volume are typical features of advancing kidney disease, and hemodilution can affect hemoglobin concentrations. Hence, in patients receiving hemodialysis, interdialytic fluid shifts need to be considered when evaluating hemoglobin levels. Several guidelines recommend that hemoglobin levels be measured before dialysis, midweek, partly reflecting the fact that virtually all the observational and trial data are based on this parameter [2].

Serum ferritin is the main marker of storage iron in common use. Several tests for assessing the adequacy of iron availability for erythropoiesis are available, such as transferrin saturation, percent hypochromic red blood cells, and reticulocyte hemoglobin content. In practice, only the first of these tests, iron availability, is in routine clinical use.

Several definitions of anemia have been used in national guidelines for CKD anemia management. For example, the US National Kidney Foundation Disease Outcomes Quality Initiative (K/DOQI) guidelines recommend a minimum frequency of hemoglobin testing of once per year in all patients known to have CKD, irrespective of disease severity [2]. Unfortunately, no controlled studies are available to guide the optimum frequency for anemia testing.

In the K/DOQI guidelines, anemia was defined as hemoglobin values of <13.5 g/dL in adult men and 12.5 g/dL in women [2]. The relationship between hemoglobin and estimated GFR (eGFR) was investigated in the National Health and Nutrition and Examination Survey III (NHANES III), a cross-sectional survey of

Evidence-based Nephrology. Edited by Donald Molony and Jonathan Craig
© 2009 Blackwell Publishing, ISBN: 978-1-4051-3975-5.

nutritional and health status in 15,419 individuals approximately randomly selected from the general US population [3,4]. This survey showed that hemoglobin levels declined when GFR fell below 75 mL/min/1.73 m^2 in men and 45 mL/min/1.73 m^2 in women. As expected, the prevalence of anemia depended heavily on the hemoglobin levels used to define it. For example, when hemoglobin levels of less than 13 g/dL were used to define anemia, a relationship with eGFR became apparent below 60 mL/min/1.73 m^2 in men and 45 mL/min/1.73 m^2 in women. For hemoglobin levels less than 11, a relationship with GFR was not apparent until eGFR values fall below 30 mL/min/1.73 m^2, with no apparent gender differences. It is likely that the prevalence of anemia is much higher in populations referred for specialist nephrology care [5,6]. In addition, studies from referral populations suggest that patients with diabetes mellitus develop anemia at higher eGFR levels and sooner than otherwise expected [7–12].

The relationship between serum ferritin and hemoglobin levels has also been studied in general population settings. In subjects with CKD, abnormally low hemoglobin levels are not apparent until ferritin levels fall below 25 ng/mL in men or 11 ng/mL in women, closely paralleling findings in the general population without overt kidney disease [13]. In patients on maintenance hemodialysis, the association profile between ferritin and hemoglobin is less straightforward, in part because inflammation is so common (with high ferritin levels acting as an acute phase reactant). In the latter group, while low ferritin levels imply deficient iron stores, high levels do not exclude this possibility. The association between transferrin saturation and hemoglobin appears to be continuous and approximately linear in nature [13]. In other words, no single threshold value for transferrin saturation appears to discriminate anemic from nonanemic hemoglobin values.

Hemoglobin targets in CKD

Hemoglobin target trials suffer from all the limitations of randomized trial designs, including cost, use of selected populations, and problems with generalizability of trial results to latter-day patients, because time must elapse before sufficient outcomes can be accumulated to identify between-group differences. Hemoglobin target trials also have limitations that are not present with typical placebo-controlled trials in which the experimental intervention is not defined by physiological variables, like hemoglobin. Most hemoglobin target trials suffer from this unattractive design feature, in that they randomly assign subjects to hemoglobin targets and not to treatments; in contrast, the anemia treatment is typically not part of the experimental design. In these trials, therefore, one is left in a situation where the main treatment is a co-intervention. This leads to the unfortunate possibility that hemoglobin target trials may not be completely comparable, because anemia treatment becomes a variable that is outside the control of the experimental design. Although this may be unavoidable, it is unfortunate because it becomes difficult to decide whether differences in out-

comes in different trials reflect differences in hemoglobin targets or in the methods used to achieve these targets.

Another typical trial strategy involves studying patients with declining hemoglobin levels; one group is randomly assigned to receive anemia treatment to maintain current hemoglobin levels ("now"), while hemoglobin levels are allowed to continue to decline in the other group until they reach a predefined low value which triggers salvage treatment ("later"). The later arm differs in several ways from the early intervention arm, including hemoglobin level at which treatment is instituted, severity of kidney disease at which treatment is instituted, and era of time. Critically, none of these variables is completely controlled by the experimental process, so that the nature of the intervention, by design, is allowed to vary from patient to patient.

In summary, although experimental designs appear to be the best way forward, target hemoglobin trials may have unique limitations not shared by other trials.

Many trials of hemoglobin targets, or erythropoiesis-stimulating agent (ESA) dose, have included death, cardiovascular events, left ventricular size, quality of life, and rates of loss of kidney function as outcomes [14–38]. Table 31.1 summarizes major findings from those studies with 100 or more subjects and at least 6 months of follow-up. When one examines these trials, a noteworthy overall finding is the heterogeneous nature of hemoglobin target effects, with the possible exception of quality of life, and even that outcome is not entirely homogenous in direction. Another notable feature of Table 31.1 is that most of the larger recent trials have compared intermediate to high targets, without an untreated (or placebo or low hemoglobin) arm. Lack of no-treatment arms naturally generates a degree of caution. For example, showing that intermediate and high target hemoglobin levels have similar treatment effects cannot refute the hypothesis that the effects of low targets are intrinsically different from those of intermediate and high targets. This situation is somewhat clearer for quality of life assessments, because initial trials included untreated arms and an earlier generation of trials showed superiority of treatment with respect to quality of life [23].

Mortality and major cardiovascular events

Many of the studies reported to date have been underpowered to detect differences in major outcomes like death and cardiovascular events. The US Normal Hematocrit Study and the Correction of Hemoglobin and Outcomes in Renal Insufficiency trial are the most obvious exceptions [14,31]. The first of these studies examined hemodialysis patients with symptomatic cardiac disease. The finding that patients assigned to the higher hemoglobin target of 14 g/dL had increased rates of the primary outcome (death or nonfatal myocardial infarction) did not reach statistical significance when the multiple interim analyses used in the trial were considered. In the second of these trials, involving patients with CKD not on dialysis, neither futility nor efficacy boundaries were crossed at the time the study was terminated early. When all events were subsequently examined, increased rates of the primary outcome variable were observed with the higher hemoglobin target.

Table 31.1 Major findings from randomized trials with at least 100 subjects and 6 months of follow-up, reporting on death, cardiovascular events, left ventricular size, quality of life, or rates of change of renal function.

Study [reference], CKD type, sample size	Target Hgb (g/dL) or EPO or ESA dose and treatment group allocation	Major entry criterion	Base Hgb	Completed as planned?	Achieved Hgb (g/dL)[a]	Death	CV event	LVH/LVD	URR Kt/V	Transfusion	QoL overall	QoL fatigue	BP	BP meds	Access loss	Δ GFR
Singh 2006 [36], ND, n = 1432	Hgb 13.5 vs. 11.3, open label		10.1	No	12.6 vs. 11.3	↑↔ ?[b,c]	↑↔?[c]				↔	↔	↑			↔
Besarab 1998 [14], HD, n = 1233	Hgb 14.0 vs. 10.0, allocation concealed	CVD	10.2	No	13.0 vs. 10.0	↔↑[d]	↔↑[d]		→	→			↔		↑	
Drueke 2006 [36], ND, n = 603	Hgb 13.5–15.0 vs. 10.5–11.5, open label	CVD <3 mos	11.6	No	13.3 vs. 11.6	↔↑[e]	↔↑[e]	↔			↑	↑	↔	↔		↔↑[f]
Parfrey 2005 [17], HD, n = 596	Hgb 13.5–14.5 vs. 9.5–11.5, allocation concealed	No CVD No LVD	11.0	Yes	13.0 vs. 10.9	↔	CVA ↑	↔	→		↔	↑	↔	↑	↔	
Furuland 2003 [15],9 HD, n = 416	Hgb 13.5–16.0 vs. 9.0–12.0, open label	No CVD[h]	10.9	Yes	14.3 vs. 10.9	↔	↔		→		↑		↔	↔	↔	
Rossert 2006 [37], ND, n = 390	Hgb 13.0–15.0 vs. 11–12, open label	Anemia and GFR decline <0.6 mL/min/mo.	11.5	No	11.7 vs. 13.9	↔					↔					↔
Macdougall 2006 [38] ND, n = 197	Start EPO alfa when Hgb declines to 11 vs. when Hgb declines to 9; open label		10.8	No	11.0 vs. 10.5	↔		↔								↔
Roger 2004 [20], ND, n = 155	Early EPO, Hgb 12.0–13.0 vs. late EPO, Hgb 9.0–10.0; allocation concealed	Hgb decline ≥1.0 g/dL, 1 yr	11.2	Yes	12.1 vs. 10.8			↔			↔	↔	↔			↔

(continued)

Table 31.1 (*Cont.*)

Study [reference], CKD type, sample size	Target Hgb (g/dL) or EPO or ESA dose and treatment group allocation	Major entry criterion	Base Hgb	Completed as planned?	Achieved Hgb (g/dL)[a]	Death	CV event	LVH/LVD	URR Kt/V	Transfusion	QoL overall	fatigue	BP	BP meds	Access loss	Δ GFR
Levin 2005 [18], ND, n = 152	Early EPO, Hgb 12.0–14.0 vs. late EPO Hgb 9.0–10.5; allocation concealed	Hgb decline ≥1.0 g/dL, 1 yr	11.8	No	12.8 vs. 11.5	↔	↔	↕				↑	↑			↕
Nissenson 1995 [21], PD, n = 152	ESA vs. placebo, allocation concealed		8.0	Yes	11.2 vs. 7.0	↔				→		↑	↑			
Foley 2000 [16], HD, n = 146	Hgb 13.0–14.0 vs. 9.5–10.5, open label	No CVD, LVH, or LVD	10.4	Yes	13.0 vs. 10.5	↔	↔	↕	→		↕	↑		↑	↕	
Bahlmann 1991 [22], HD, n = 129	EPO vs. placebo, allocation concealed		7.7	Yes	10.7 vs. 7.8	↔				→						
CESG 1990 [23], HD, n = 118	High EPO vs. low EPO vs. placebo, allocation concealed	No major comorbidity	7.0	Yes	11.7 vs. 10.2 vs. 7.4	↔				→	↑	↑	↑		↑	

Abbreviations: ND, nondialysis; HD, hemodialysis; PD, peritoneal dialysis; EPO, epoetin; Hgb, hemoglobin; CESG, Canadian Erythropoietin Study Group; CVA, cerebrovascular accident; LVH, left ventricular hypertrophy; LVD, left ventricular dilation; URR, urea reduction ratio; QoL, quality of life.

a Among the studies, Hgb levels were reported in many ways; values reported here (in grams per deciliter) are indicative.

b An asterisk denotes the primary outcome. ↑, better or higher; ↔, equivalent; ↓ worse or lower.

c The primary end point was a composite of death, myocardial infarction, hospitalization for congestive heart failure (without renal replacement therapy), and stroke. The study was terminated early, even though futility and efficacy boundaries had not been reached. When further events were considered, primary outcome rates were higher in the high target group.

d The primary outcome was a composite of death or nonfatal myocardial infarction.

e The primary efficacy end point was a composite for first cardiovascular event, including sudden death, myocardial infarction, acute heart failure, stroke, transient ischemic attack, angina pectoris, peripheral vascular disease with amputation or necrosis, or cardiac arrhythmia.

f Even though rates of loss of GFR were identical, patients in the high target group had higher rates of need for dialysis.

g The sample included hemodialysis, peritoneal dialysis, and nondialysis CKD patients. A total of 70% were on hemodialysis.

h Criterion added during the progress of the trial, in response to the findings of the US Normal Hematocrit Study [13].

The latter trial had some issues that could potentially threaten validity and generalizability, not the least of which were the use of an initial dose of ESA far larger than typical for a population with non-dialysis CKD and a large rate of unexpected dropouts. In another trial of hemodialysis patients without symptomatic heart disease or dilated left ventricles, the 13.5–14.5 g/dL group had unexpectedly higher rates of cerebrovascular events compared to the control arm (9.5–11.5 g/dL). This latter trial showed no differences in the rates of other cardiovascular events or death [17].

Left ventricle size

There is little evidence for the widely held belief that partial treatment of anemia improves left ventricular hypertrophy in CKD patients. In fact, the controlled evidence for this belief appears to have come from three trials that involved approximately 50 patients [27,34]. As shown in Table 31.1, most of the evidence has been generated from trials of intermediate or high targets and, so far, the available evidence suggests neutral effects.

Quality of life

Most, but not all, studies have shown that higher hemoglobin targets improve quality of life in patients with CKD. These effects have been most obvious in the domains of vitality and fatigue and have been seen with hemoglobin targets up to 15 g/dL and achieved hemoglobin values up to approximately 13 g/dL (Table 31.1).

Hemodialysis access

Some studies have shown that higher hemoglobin targets lead to higher rates of vascular access problems in hemodialysis patients. These effects have been less obvious in recent trials that have excluded hemodialysis patients with ongoing vascular access problems. For example, in the US Normal Hematocrit Study, vascular access thrombosis rates were approximately one-third higher in the higher hemoglobin group [14].

Blood pressure

Several of the trials reported to date have shown that higher hemoglobin targets lead to higher blood pressure levels or greater antihypertensive requirements for antihypertensive therapy (Table 31.1). Whereas this effect was more apparent in earlier trials, two recent trials in CKD patients not on dialysis showed discordant effects with respect to raising blood pressure levels [35,36].

Dialysis adequacy and change in GFR

Compared to intermediate hemoglobin targets, higher hemoglobin targets have been associated with lower measures of intradialytic urea clearance in several studies of hemodialysis patients (Table 31.1). In general, the between-target differences were small, and the clinical significance of these differences is unclear [39].

The effect of hemoglobin targets on rates of progression of CKD is unclear. Whereas the larger, more recently published studies (Table 31.1) have not shown an effect in either a harmful or beneficial direction, it is likely that the currently available evidence does not allow definitive conclusions. It should be noted that one recent large trial showed that patients in the high hemoglobin arm were more likely to require hemodialysis earlier than controls, even though rates of loss of kidney function were identical in the two arms [35]. Good clinical practice would mandate that higher hemoglobin targets not be attempted without frequent clinical monitoring and should probably be avoided in comparatively noncompliant patients.

Transfusions

Avoidance of blood transfusions is highly desirable for many reasons, and it is clear from the studies performed to date that higher hemoglobin targets are associated with lower transfusion rates (Table 31.1).

Target recommendations

The available evidence suggests that an initial hemoglobin target of ≥ 11.0 g/dL has a reasonable evidence base [2,40]. Beyond this, a clear-cut upper bound for hemoglobin target is difficult to define from the current evidence base, especially given the divergence between benefits in quality of life and potentially harmful effects. It is also apparent that hemoglobin levels vary considerably and that keeping levels within narrow ranges is extremely difficult among individuals. Safety issues, considered in isolation, clearly suggest that hemoglobin levels above 12 g/dL should not be a routine recommendation. However, many patients might accept the potential incremental risk associated with higher hemoglobin levels in return for quality-of-life benefits. With this approach, lengthy risk–benefit discussions with patients, families, and caregivers are needed. One fervently hopes that this unsatisfactory situation, where an upper hemoglobin target remains unclear, even after almost 20 years of target hemoglobin trials, will be clarified by the completion of ongoing intervention trials.

Use of ESAs

ESAs are molecules that increase rates of red blood cell production, acting through the erythropoietin receptor, either directly or indirectly. At present, the ESAs in clinical use include epoetin alfa, epoetin beta, and darbepoetin. Although the first two entities are very similar to endogenous erythropoietin in terms of molecular structure and biological activity, the third of these entities, in contrast, has a longer half-life than the native hormone.

The optimum frequency of hemoglobin measurement under ESA therapy is unknown. In particular, no trial has been performed in which the primary intervention was randomization to different frequencies of hemoglobin monitoring, without alteration of ESA therapy. Clinical judgment should be exercised in less stable situations, such as initiation of ESA therapy, hemoglobin levels above or below target, rapid changes in hemoglobin level, and unstable clinical circumstances. Similarly, no trial has been performed among patients initiating ESA therapy in which the intervention has been

Table 31.2 Major findings from trials with at least 50 subjects comparing subcutaneous or intravenous administration of a single ESA.

Study [reference], CKD type, sample size	Intervention, ESA strategy, treatment group allocation	Target hemoglobin (g/dL)	Single ESA dose?	Iron replete?	Duration	Result
Kaufman 1998 [41], HD, n = 208	i.v. vs. s.c. epoetin alfa 3 times weekly, open label	10–11	No	Ferritin >100 ng/mL	26 wks	Lower epoetin dose with s.c.
Muirhead 1992 [42], HD, n = 128	i.v. vs. s.c. epoetin alfa 3 times weekly, open-label	10.5–12.5	No	TSAT >20%	24 wks	Lower epoetin dose with s.c.
Leikis 2004 [43], HD, n = 81	i.v. vs. s.c. epoetin alfa (and 1 vs. 2 vs. 3 times per wk), crossover, open label	None, withdrawn if <9 or >14	Yes	Ferritin 300–800 ng/mL and TSAT 25–50%	3 mos/treatment	Higher hemoglobin with s.c.
Aarup 2006 [44], HD, n = 71	i.v. vs. s.c. darbepoetin once weekly, crossover, open label	11.0–13.7	No		20 wks/treatment	No difference in darbepoetin dose
Cervelli 2005 [45], HD, n = 53	i.v. vs. s.c. darbepoetin once weekly, crossover, allocation concealed	11.0–13.0	No	Ferritin ≥200 ng/mL and TSAT ≥25 %	6 mos/treatment	No difference in darbepoetin dose

Abbreviations: HD, hemodialysis; i.v., intravenous; s.c., subcutaneous; TSAT, transferrin saturation.

different target rates of change of hemoglobin level. Finally, no trials have compared different frequencies of dose adjustment of ESA. In the absence of such information, most guidelines have recommended a minimum frequency for hemoglobin measurement of at least monthly measurements in stable patients and have suggested rates of increase in hemoglobin levels of 1–2 g/dL/month during the initiation phase.

Table 31.2 summarizes findings from trials that have compared subcutaneous and intravenous routes of administration of ESAs [41–45]. These studies suggest that the subcutaneous route is associated with lower epoetin alfa dose among hemodialysis patients. They also suggest that darbepoetin is equally efficacious with regard to hemoglobin level attainment whether used subcutaneously or intravenously. In practice, concerns that subcutaneous epoetin may cause pure red cell aplasia in hemodialysis patients has led to the recommendation, in many guidelines, that it be given intravenously in this population [46], even though pure red cell aplasia rates appeared to have declined worldwide since 2003 [47].

Table 31.3 summarizes findings from trials comparing different frequencies of administration of subcutaneous epoetin [28,48–50]. These trials suggest equivalent efficacy regarding attained hemoglobin levels, whether epoetin is administered once, twice, or three times per week or once every 2 weeks.

Table 31.4 summarizes findings from major trials that compared different ESAs with hemoglobin level as the outcome variable. These studies suggest that darbepoetin once per week is as efficacious as epoetin two or three times per week, and darbepoetin once every 2 weeks is as efficacious as epoetin once per week in dialysis patients.

In practice, the use of ESAs varies widely according to factors like practice setting and patient preference. In addition, hemoglobin levels alone have been the major efficacy criterion in the trials performed to date. Clearly, structurally different biological molecules

may have different actions at many sites beyond the bone marrow, and the comparative safety profiles of different ESAs and how they are used remain to be determined in adequately powered randomized trials.

Iron therapy

No iron intervention trials have been performed that had sufficient power to adequately examine safety issues, which is unfortunate, given the fact that iron is a potent oxidizing agent, in addition to being an essential component of heme. The optimum frequency for iron testing has never been determined using experimental methods. As a result, guidelines that suggest that the minimum frequency should be at least once per month in stable patients are only opinion-based.

Iron status markers

Although small studies in hemodialysis patients have suggested that intravenous iron-based treatment based on transferrin saturation targets between 30 and 50% lowered the epoetin dose (vs. 20–30%) [51], as did a ferritin target of 400 ng/mL (vs. 200 ng/mL) [52], the evidence base appears to be inadequate for formulation of firm recommendations. Hence, recommendations that lower bounds for ferritin and transferrin saturation levels should be 200 ng/mL and 20% [2], respectively, probably should be viewed as less than definitive, and further trials are clearly needed. An even stronger disclaimer may be required for establishing upper bounds for optimum ferritin and transferrin saturation targets, if these are to be based, ideally, on evidence from randomized controlled trials.

Two randomized trials have used reticulocyte hemoglobin content as an indicator of iron status in hemodialysis patients. In the first of these trials, 157 patients were randomly assigned to iron

Table 31.3 Major findings from trials with at least 50 subjects comparing different frequencies of administration of a single ESA.

Study [reference], CKD type, sample size	Intervention, ESA strategy, treatment group allocation	Target Hgb (g/dL)	Iron replete?	Duration (wks)	Result
Provenzano 2006 [48], ND, n = 519	QW, Q2W, Q3W, or Q4W, open label	>11		16	Similar hemoglobin with QW and Q2W, lower with Q3W and Q4W
Covic 2006 [49], HD, n = 207	Epoetin beta s.c., QW vs. Q2W, open label	10–12	Ferritin 100–800 ng/mL and TSAT 20–50%	24	No difference in Hgb or epoetin beta dose
Locatelli 2002 [50], HD, n = 173	Epoetin beta s.c., QW vs 3 times/wk, open label	9.3	Ferritin 100–800 ng/mL and TSAT 20–50%	24	No difference in Hgb or epoetin beta dose
Weiss 2000 [28], HD, n = 158	Epoetin beta s.c., QW vs. 2 or 3 times/wk, open label	10–13	Ferritin 200–500 ng/mL	24	No difference in Hgb or epoetin beta dose

Abbreviations: ND, nondialysis; HD, hemodialysis; QW, once every week; Q2W, once every 2 weeks; Q3W, once every 3 weeks, Q4W, once every 4 weeks; s.c., subcutaneous; Hgb, hemoglobin; TSAT, transferrin saturation.

management based on serum ferritin level (treatment threshold of <100 ng/mL) and transferrin saturation (threshold of <20%), or on reticulocyte hemoglobin content (threshold, 29 pg), with 6 months follow-up and intravenous iron dextran (100 mg for 10 consecutive treatments) as iron therapy. Although hemoglobin levels and epoetin doses were the same in both groups, weekly doses of iron dextran were lower when reticulocyte hemoglobin content was used to determine therapy [53]. The other trial used a reticulocyte hemoglobin content of <32.5 pg or a transferrin saturation of <20% to diagnose iron deficiency and used 240 mg of iron colloid intravenously over 2 weeks as treatment, with follow-up lasting 16 weeks. In this study, use of transferrin saturation as a trigger for iron therapy led to lower epoetin doses to achieve equivalent hemoglobin levels [54]. Hence, the available literature does not definitively support the use of reticulocyte hemoglobin content as an indicator of iron deficiency, and more randomized trials are needed. Similar comments apply to other markers of this deficiency, including hypochromic red blood cells, zinc protoporphyrin, and soluble transferrin receptors.

Modes of administration of iron

Although several trials [55–62] have studied the effect of iron on hemoglobin levels in patients with CKD, the patient populations and methodologies employed have been quite heterogeneous, especially with regard to proportions with overt iron deficiency, simultaneous use of ESAs, use of untreated control arms, sample sizes, and study durations. Table 31.4 shows findings from the larger trials that compared different modes of iron therapy, or one mode of iron therapy versus no iron therapy (as opposed to different doses of the same therapy without a control arm). Although much evidence remains to be gathered, these trials tend to show that intravenous iron therapy is more efficacious than oral iron therapy for achieving target hemoglobin levels in hemodialysis patients. The situation is less clear in CKD patients not requiring

Table 31.4 Major findings from trials with at least 50 subjects comparing different formulations of iron.

Study [reference], CKD type, sample size	Intervention, treatment group allocation	Iron critria	ESA	Duration	Result
Van Wyck 2005 [56], ND, n = 188	i.v. iron sucrose, 1 g in divided doses (2 or 5) over 14 days vs. ferrous sulfate 325 mg orally t.i.d. for 56 days; open label	Ferritin ≤300 ng/mL and TSAT ≤25%	Epoetin or darbepoetin at constant dose	56 days	Higher hemoglobin with i.v. iron
Charytan 2005 [57], ND, n = 96	i.v. iron sucrose, 5 doses of 200 mg weekly vs. 29 days of oral FeSO4, 325 mg t.i.d.		Epoetin	42 days	Similar hemoglobin with oral and i.v. iron
Agarwal 2006 [55], ND, n = 75	i.v. sodium ferric gluconate complex 250 mg wkly x 4 vs. oral ferrous sulfate 325 mg t.i.d. x 42 days; open label	Ferritin <100 ng/mL or TSAT <20%	None	42 days	Similar hemoglobin with oral and i.v. iron
Fishbane 1995 [60], HD, n = 52	i.v. iron dextran 100 mg twice wkly	Ferritin >100 ng/mL and TSAT >15%	Epoetin	4 mos	Higher hemoglobin and lower epoetin dose with i.v. iron

Search strategy employed: randomized trial, iron, intravenous or oral, dialysis, or kidney or renal.

Abbreviations: ND, nondialysis; HD, hemodialysis; i.v., intravenous, t.i.d., three times/day; TSAT, transferrin saturation.

dialysis, and it seems reasonable to recommend either oral or intravenous iron therapy if achieving target hemoglobin levels with the lowest possible ESA dose is the therapeutic objective.

Limitations of body of evidence

All the studies of iron therapy described above have used early surrogate markers as primary outcomes, including hemoglobin, ferritin levels, transferrin saturation levels, and ESA doses. Given the nature of the therapy, however, there is clearly a requirement for randomized trials evaluating long-term safety parameters, including death, progression of kidney disease, and natural history of adverse events. These trials should include placebo-controlled trials of individual agents and placebo-controlled trials of multiple agents, so that safety and efficacy can truly be determined.

References

1 Eschbach JW, Adamson JW. Anemia of end-stage renal disease (ESRD). *Kidney Int* 1985; **28:** 1–5.

2 NKF. K/DOQI guidelines, anemia. http://www.kidney.org/professionals/KDOQI /guidelines_anemia/cpr12.htm

3 Hsu CY, Bates DW, Kuperman GJ, Curhan GC. Relationship between hematocrit and renal function in men and women. *Kidney Int* 2001; **59:** 725–731.

4 Astor BC, Muntner P, Levin A, Eustace JA, Coresh J. Association of kidney function with anemia: the Third National Health and Nutrition Examination Survey (1988-1994). *Arch Intern Med* 2002; **162:** 1401–1408.

5 McClellan W, Aronoff SL, Bolton WK, Hood S, Lorber DL, Tang KL *et al.* The prevalence of anemia in patients with chronic kidney disease. *Curr Med Res Opin* 2004; **20:** 1501–1510.

6 Levin A, Thompson CR, Ethier J, Carlisle EJ, Tobe S, Mendelssohn D *et al.* Left ventricular mass index increase in early renal disease: Impact of decline in hemoglobin. *Am J Kidney Dis* 1999; **34:** 125–134.

7 Guralnik JM, Eisenstaedt RS, Ferrucci L, Klein HG, Woodman RC. Prevalence of anemia in persons 65 years and older in the United States: Evidence for a high rate of unexplained anemia. *Blood* 2004; **104:** 2263–2268.

8 Ishimura E, Nishizawa Y, Okuno S, *et al.* Diabetes mellitus increases the severity of anemia in non-dialyzed patients with renal failure. *J Nephrol* 1998; **11:** 83–86.

9 Bosman DR, Winkler AS, Marsden JT, Macdougall IC, Watkins PJ. Anemia with erythropoietin deficiency occurs early in diabetic nephropathy. *Diabetes Care* 2001; **24:** 495–499.

10 Thomas MC, MacIsaac RJ, Tsalamandris C, Power D, Jerums G. Unrecognized anemia in patients with diabetes: A cross-sectional survey. *Diabetes Care* 2003; **26:** 1164–1169.

11 Thomas MC, MacIsaac RJ, Tsalamandris C, *et al.* The burden of anaemia in type 2 diabetes and the role of nephropathy: A cross-sectional audit. *Nephrol Dial Transplant* 2004; **19:** 1792–1797.

12 El-Achkar TM, Ohmit SE, McCullough PA, *et al.* Higher prevalence of anemia with diabetes mellitus in moderate kidney insufficiency: The Kidney Early Evaluation Program. *Kidney Int* 2005; **67:** 1483–1488.

13 Hsu CY, McCulloch CE, Curhan GC. Epidemiology of anemia associated with chronic renal insufficiency among adults in the United States: results from the Third National Health and Nutrition Examination Survey. *J Am Soc Nephrol* 2002; **13:** 504–510.

14 Besarab A, Bolton WK, Browne JK, Egrie JC, Nissenson AR, Okamoto DM *et al.* The effects of normal as compared with low hematocrit values in patients with cardiac disease who are receiving hemodialysis and epoetin. *N Engl J Med* 1998; **339:** 584–590.

15 Furuland H, Linde T, Ahlmen J, Christensson A, Strombom U, Danielson BG. A randomized controlled trial of haemoglobin normalization with epoetin alfa in pre-dialysis and dialysis patients. *Nephrol Dial Transplant* 2003; **18:** 353–361.

16 Foley RN, Parfrey PS, Morgan J, Barre PE, Campbell P, Cartier P *et al.* Effect of hemoglobin levels in hemodialysis patients with asymptomatic cardiomyopathy. *Kidney Int* 2000; **58:** 1325–1335.

17 Parfrey PS, Foley RN, Wittreich BH, Sullivan DJ, Zagari MJ, Frei D. Double-blind comparison of full and partial anemia correction in incident hemodialysis patients without symptomatic heart disease. *J Am Soc Nephrol* 2005; **16:** 2180–2189.

18 Levin A, Djurdjev O, Thompson C, Barrett B, Ethier J, Carlisle E *et al.* Canadian randomized trial of hemoglobin maintenance to prevent or delay left ventricular mass growth in patients with CKD. *Am J Kidney Dis* 2005; **46:** 799–811.

19 Suzuki M, Hirasawa Y, Hirashima K, Arakawa M, Odaka M, Ogura Y *et al.* Dose-finding, double-blind, clinical trial of recombinant human erythropoietin (Chugai) in Japanese patients with end-stage renal disease. Research Group for Clinical Assessment of rhEPO. *Contrib Nephrol* 1989; **76:** 179–192.

20 Roger SD, McMahon LP, Clarkson A, Disney A, Harris D, Hawley C *et al.* Effects of early and late intervention with epoetin alpha on left ventricular mass among patients with chronic kidney disease (stage 3 or 4): results of a randomized clinical trial. *J Am Soc Nephrol* 2004; **15:** 148–156.

21 Nissenson AR, Korbet S, Faber M, Burkart J, Gentile D, Hamburger R *et al.* Multicenter trial of erythropoietin in patients on peritoneal dialysis. *J Am Soc Nephrol* 1995; **5:** 1517–1529.

22 Bahlmann J, Schoter KH, Scigalla P, Gurland HJ, Hilfenhaus M, Koch KM *et al.* Morbidity and mortality in hemodialysis patients with and without erythropoietin treatment: a controlled study. *Contrib Nephrol* 1991; **88:** 90–106.

23 Canadian Erythropoietin Study Group. Association between recombinant human erythropoietin and quality of life and exercise capacity of patients receiving haemodialysis. *BMJ* 1990; **300:** 573–578.

24 Roth D, Smith RD, Schulman G, Steinman TI, Hatch FE, Rudnick MR *et al.* Effects of recombinant human erythropoietin on renal function in chronic renal failure predialysis patients. *Am J Kidney Dis* 1994; **24:** 777–784.

25 Revicki DA, Brown RE, Feeny DH, Henry D, Teehan BP, Rudnick MR *et al.* Health-related quality of life associated with recombinant human erythropoietin therapy for predialysis chronic renal disease patients. *Am J Kidney Dis* 1995; **25:** 548–554.

26 Kuriyama S, Tomonari H, Yoshida H, Hashimoto T, Kawaguchi Y, Sakai O. Reversal of anemia by erythropoietin therapy retards the progression of chronic renal failure, especially in nondiabetic patients. *Nephron* 1997; **77:** 176–185.

27 Sikole A, Polenakovic M, Spirovska V, Polenakovic B, Masin G. Analysis of heart morphology and function following erythropoietin treatment of anemic dialysis patients. *Artif Organs* 1993; **17:** 977–984.

28 Weiss LG, Clyne N, Divino Fihlho J, Frisenette-Fich C, Kurkus J, Svensson B. The efficacy of once weekly compared with two or three times

weekly subcutaneous epoetin beta: results from a randomized controlled multicentre trial. Swedish Study Group. *Nephrol Dial Transplant* 2000; **15:** 2014–2019.

29 Lim VS, DeGowin RL, Zavala D, Kirchner PT, Abels R, Perry P *et al.* Recombinant human erythropoietin treatment in pre-dialysis patients. A double-blind placebo-controlled trial. *Ann Intern Med* 1989; **110:** 108–114.

30 Kleinman KS, Schweitzer SU, Perdue ST, Bleifer KH, Abels RI. The use of recombinant human erythropoietin in the correction of anemia in pre-dialysis patients and its effect on renal function: a double-blind, placebo-controlled trial. *Am J Kidney Dis* 1989; **14:** 486–495.

31 McMahon LP, McKenna MJ, Sangkabutra T, Mason K, Sostaric S, Skinner SL *et al.* Physical performance and associated electrolyte changes after haemoglobin normalization: a comparative study in haemodialysis patients. *Nephrol Dial Transplant* 1999; **14:** 1182–1187.

32 McMahon LP, Johns JA, McKenzie A, Austin M, Fowler R, Dawborn JK. Haemodynamic changes and physical performance at comparative levels of haemoglobin after long-term treatment with recombinant erythropoietin. *Nephrol Dial Transplant* 1992; **7:** 1199–1206.

33 Watson AJ, Gimenez LF, Cotton S, Walser M, Spivak JL. Treatment of the anemia of chronic renal failure with subcutaneous recombinant human erythropoietin. *Am J Med* 1990; **89:** 432–435.

34 Morris KP, Skinner JR, Hunter S, Coulthard MG. Short term correction of anaemia with recombinant human erythropoietin and reduction of cardiac output in end stage renal failure. *Arch Dis Child* 1993; **68:** 644–648.

35 Drueke TB, Locatelli F, Clyne N, Eckardt KU, Macdougall IC, Tsakiris D *et al.* Normalization of hemoglobin level in patients with chronic kidney disease and anemia. *N Engl J Med* 2006; **355:** 2071–2084.

36 Singh AK, Szczech L, Tang KL, Barnhart H, Sapp S, Wolfson M *et al.* Correction of anemia with epoetin alfa in chronic kidney disease. *N Engl J Med* 2006; **355:** 2085–2098.

37 Rossert J, Levin A, Roger SD, Horl WH, Fouqueray B, Gassmann-Mayer C *et al.* Effect of early correction of anemia on the progression of CKD. *Am J Kidney Dis* 2006; **47:** 738–750.

38 Macdougall IC, Temple RM, Kwan JT. Is early treatment of anaemia with epoetin-α beneficial to pre-dialysis chronic kidney disease patients? Results of a multicentre, open-label, prospective, randomized, comparative group trial. *Nephrol Dial Transplant* 2006; **22:** 784–793.

39 Eknoyan G, Beck GJ, Cheung AK, Daugirdas JT, Greene T, Kusek JW *et al.* Effect of dialysis dose and membrane flux in maintenance hemodialysis. *N Engl J Med* 2002; **347:** 2010–2019.

40 Locatelli F, Aljama P, Barany P, Canaud B, Carrera F, Eckardt KU *et al.* Revised European best practice guidelines for the management of anaemia in patients with chronic renal failure. *Nephrol Dial Transplant* 2004; **19(Suppl 2):** ii1–ii47.

41 Kaufman JS, Reda DJ, Fye CL, Goldfarb DS, Henderson WG, Kleinman JG *et al.* Subcutaneous compared with intravenous epoetin in patients receiving hemodialysis. Department of Veterans Affairs Cooperative Study Group on Erythropoietin in Hemodialysis Patients. *N Engl J Med* 1998; **339:** 578–583.

42 Muirhead N, Churchill DN, Goldstein M, Nadler SP, Posen G, Wong C *et al.* Comparison of subcutaneous and intravenous recombinant human erythropoietin for anemia in hemodialysis patients with significant comorbid disease. *Am J Nephrol.* 1992; **12:** 303–310.

43 Leikis MJ, Kent AB, Becker GJ, McMahon LP. Haemoglobin response to subcutaneous versus intravenous epoetin alfa administration in iron-replete haemodialysis patients. *Nephrology* (Carlton) 2004; **9:** 153–160.

44 Aarup M, Bryndum J, Dieperink H, Joffe P. Clinical implications of converting stable haemodialysis patients from subcutaneous to intravenous administration of darbepoetin alfa. *Nephrol Dial Transplant* 2006; **21:** 1312–1316.

45 Cervelli MJ, Gray N, McDonald S, Gentgall MG, Disney AP. Randomized cross-over comparison of intravenous and subcutaneous darbepoetin dosing efficiency in haemodialysis patients. *Nephrology* (Carlton) 2005; **10:** 129–135.

46 Casadevall N, Nataf J, Viron B, Kolta A, Kiladjian JJ, Martin-Dupont P *et al.* Pure red-cell aplasia and antierythropoietin antibodies in patients treated with recombinant erythropoietin. *N Engl J Med* 2002; **346:** 469–475.

47 Bennett CL, Luminari S, Nissenson AR, Tallman MS, Klinge SA, McWilliams N *et al.* Pure red-cell aplasia and epoetin therapy. *N Engl J Med* 2004; **351:** 1403–1408.

48 Provenzano R, Bhaduri S, Singh AK, PROMPT Study Group. Extended epoetin alfa dosing as maintenance treatment for the anemia of chronic kidney disease: the PROMPT study. *Clin Nephrol* 2005; **64:** 113–123.

49 Mircescu G, Garneata L, Ciocalteu A, Golea O, Gherman-Caprioara M, Capsa D *et al.* Once-every-2-weeks and once-weekly epoetin beta regimens: equivalency in hemodialyzed patients. *Am J Kidney Dis* 2006; **48:** 445–455.

50 Locatelli F, Baldamus CA, Villa G, Ganea A, Martin de Francisco AL. Once-weekly compared with three-times-weekly subcutaneous epoetin beta: results from a randomized, multicenter, therapeutic-equivalence study. *Am J Kidney Dis* 2002; **40:** 119–125.

51 Besarab A, Amin N, Ahsan M, Vogel SE, Zazuwa G, Frinak S *et al.* Optimization of epoetin therapy with intravenous iron therapy in hemodialysis patients. *J Am Soc Nephrol* 2000; **11:** 530–538.

52 DeVita MV, Frumkin D, Mittal S, Kamran A, Fishbane S, Michelis MF. Targeting higher ferritin concentrations with intravenous iron dextran lowers erythropoietin requirement in hemodialysis patients. *Clin Nephrol* 2003; **60:** 335–340.

53 Fishbane S, Shapiro W, Dutka P, Valenzuela OF, Faubert J. A randomized trial of iron deficiency testing strategies in hemodialysis patients. *Kidney Int* 2001; **60:** 2406–2411.

54 Kaneko Y, Miyazaki S, Hirasawa Y, Gejyo F, Suzuki M. Transferrin saturation versus reticulocyte hemoglobin content for iron deficiency in Japanese hemodialysis patients. *Kidney Int* 2003; **63:** 1086–1093.

55 Agarwal R, Rizkala AR, Bastani B, Kaskas MO, Leehey DJ, Besarab A. A randomized controlled trial of oral versus intravenous iron in chronic kidney disease. *Am J Nephrol* 2006; **26:** 445–454.

56 Van Wyck DB, Roppolo M, Martinez CO, Mazey RM, McMurray S, United States Iron Sucrose (Venofer) Clinical Trials Group. A randomized, controlled trial comparing IV iron sucrose to oral iron in anemic patients with nondialysis-dependent CKD. *Kidney Int* 2005; **68:** 2846–2856.

57 Charytan C, Qunibi W, Bailie GR, Venofer Clinical Studies Group. Comparison of intravenous iron sucrose to oral iron in the treatment of anemic patients with chronic kidney disease not on dialysis. *Nephron Clin Pract* 2005; **100:** c55–c62.

58 Aggarwal HK, Nand N, Singh S, Singh M, Hemant, Kaushik G. Comparison of oral versus intravenous iron therapy in predialysis patients of chronic renal failure receiving recombinant human erythropoietin. *J Assoc Physicians India* 2003; **51:** 170–174.

59 Stoves J, Inglis H, Newstead CG. A randomized study of oral vs intravenous iron supplementation in patients with progressive renal insufficiency treated with erythropoietin. *Nephrol Dial Transplant* 2001; **16:** 967–974.

60 Fishbane S, Frei GL, Maesaka J. Reduction in recombinant human erythropoietin doses by the use of chronic intravenous iron supplementation. *Am J Kidney Dis* 1995; **26:** 41–46.

61 Fudin R, Jaichenko J, Shostak A, Bennett M, Gotloib L. Correction of uremic iron deficiency anemia in hemodialyzed patients: a prospective study. *Nephron* 1998; **79:** 299–305.

62 Markowitz GS, Kahn GA, Feingold RE, Coco M, Lynn RI. An evaluation of the effectiveness of oral iron therapy in hemodialysis patients receiving recombinant human erythropoietin. *Clin Nephrol* 1997; **48(1):** 34–40.

32 Dyslipidemia in Chronic Kidney Disease

Vera Krane & Christoph Wanner

Department of Medicine, Division of Nephrology, University of Würzburg, Würzburg, Germany

Introduction

Today, clinicians use serum total cholesterol, low-density lipoprotein (LDL) cholesterol, high-density lipoprotein (HDL) cholesterol, and triglycerides (lipid profile) for diagnosis and treatment of hyper- or dyslipidemia. These lipids are transported within lipoproteins, which have been isolated and used in patient-oriented research and for in vitro experiments. Lipoproteins not only contain lipids but also proteins, so-called apolipoproteins. Integrating all these components into the discussion, lipidologists use terms such as "composition of lipoprotein particles" that may not be familiar or routinely understood by clinicians. Quite often, statins are mistakenly prescribed for patients with very high triglycerides that arise from triglyceride-rich lipoproteins. This is unfortunate, because statins work via receptors that mediate absorption of cholesterol-rich lipoproteins by the liver. Therefore, it is of advantage for nephrologists to have some basic knowledge about lipids, lipoproteins, and apolipoproteins in order to diagnose and treat lipid disorders adequately in a patient population prone to suffer from complex forms of dyslipidemia as well as significant cardiovascular disease (CVD). For a better understanding, Figure 32.1 and Table 32.1 are provided. This figure and table are complementary, as they combine knowledge about lipoproteins and the lipid components.

Types of dyslipidemia in different stages of chronic kidney disease and renal replacement therapy

General aspects

Qualitative characteristics of dyslipoproteinemia are similar in early renal insufficiency and in advanced kidney failure. Hypertriglyceridemia and delayed catabolism of triglyceride-rich lipoproteins resulting in increased concentrations of very low density lipoproteins (VLDLs) and intermediate density lipoproteins (IDLs) and reduced levels of HDL appear to be the main metabolic abnormality. Plasma cholesterol concentration is usually normal, even reduced, and only occasionally elevated. Dyslipidemia is detected in an early stage of chronic kidney disease (CKD, stage 2) and is best characterized by abnormalities in the composition of apolipoproteins. Increased levels of apoC-III and decreased levels of the apoA-I/apoC-III ratio are considered to be the hallmarks of an altered apolipoprotein profile in kidney disease [1].

CKD and proteinuria: impact on serum lipids and lipoproteins

Dyslipidemia is present in 70–90% of patients with nephrotic syndrome. Combined hyperlipidemia, with an increase in the serum total cholesterol/LDL cholesterol ratio and increased serum triglycerides, is the most common form (50%) [2–4]. One-third of patients have an exclusive elevation of LDL cholesterol, whereas only 4% of patients show pure hypertriglyceridemia. Changes in the composition of lipoprotein particles also have been described, with cholesterol enrichment in IDL but not LDL [5,6]. The levels of HDL cholesterol may vary [7,8]. This could be due to high serum lipoprotein (a) [Lp(a)] contaminating the HDL samples when cholesterol is assayed. The reasons why patients with nephrotic syndrome present different accumulations of triglycerides and cholesterol may include factors such as genetic apolipoprotein phenotypes, concomitant drug therapy, and the catabolic state of the individual. Two separate processes impede the removal of triglyceride-rich lipoproteins in nephrotic syndrome. One is an abnormality in VLDL that decreases the ability to bind to endothelial surfaces in the presence of saturating Lipoprotein Lipase (LPL) [9]. This defect in VLDL function, and presumably structure, results from proteinuria [10]. The second defect is the inability of LPL to bind effectively to vascular endothelium [11]. Whereas VLDL levels are high due to reduced catabolism, LDL levels are increased because of increased synthesis[12]. The presence of uremia in nephrotic patients leads to further changes [13].

Evidence-based Nephrology. Edited by Donald Molony and Jonathan Craig
© 2009 Blackwell Publishing, ISBN: 978-1-4051-3975-5.

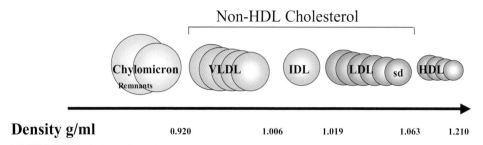

Figure 32.1 Relative density of lipoproteins in human plasma.

Markedly elevated Lp(a) concentrations have been found in the majority of patients with proteinuria [14,15] and nephrotic syndrome and resolve when remission of the nephrotic syndrome is induced [16,17]. There are data that suggest increased synthesis, rather than decreased catabolism, causes elevated plasma Lp(a) concentrations in nephrotic syndrome [18].

Hemodialysis and dyslipidemia

Dyslipidemia in hemodialysis patients is more frequent than in the general population [19,20] and is characterized by hypertriglyceridemia and low levels of HDL [21–29]. However, levels of total cholesterol and LDL usually are normal [30–34]. This translates into the most characteristic feature of the end-stage renal disease (ESRD)-associated dyslipidemia represented by an accumulation of triglyceride-rich lipoproteins (VLDL remnants) and IDL [23,31,35]. Catabolism of IDL and LDL is severely impaired, resulting in a markedly prolonged residence time of both particles [36]. Additionally, qualitative changes of LDL with formation of small dense LDL are found [37–40]. On the level of apolipoproteins, the dyslipidemia can also be classified as an accumulation of apoB-containing triglyceride-rich lipoprotein particles containing apoC-III and Lp(a) or lipoprotein B complex particles [41–43]. Besides a defect in postprandial chylomicron remnant clearance, abnormal HDL apoA-I and apoA-II kinetics have been described, with increased catabolism of apoA-I and decreased production rate of apoA-II resulting in reduced plasma levels of both apolipoproteins [44,45].

Continuous ambulatory peritoneal dialysis and dyslipidemia

Continuous ambulatory peritoneal dialysis (CAPD) patients present with higher plasma cholesterol, triglyceride, LDL, and Lp(a) levels than hemodialysis patients [46–52]. This additional increase is most likely due to two factors [53]: 1) loss of protein (7–14 g/day) into the peritoneal dialysate [54], and 2) absorption of glucose (150–200 g/day) from the dialysis fluid [55–57]. This was in part reflected in the data from Prinsen *et al.*, who reported VLDL-1 apoB100 and VLDL-2 apoB100 pool sizes were increased due to disturbances in both synthesis and catabolism. VLDL-1 apoB100 production is, at least partially, explained by increased free fatty acid availability secondary to peripheral insulin resistance; thus, insulin resistance might be a potential therapeutic target in peritoneal dialysis patients [58]. In general, qualitative lipoprotein abnormalities are similar to those found in hemodialysis patients, and most mechanisms altering lipoprotein metabolism are probably also qualitatively the same [59,60], even though a study in normolipidemic CAPD patients demonstrated less-pronounced abnormalities of cholesterol transport in normolipidemic CAPD patients than in hemodialysis patients [61].

Lipid abnormalities after kidney transplantation

Posttransplant dyslipidemia is qualitatively and quantitatively dependent on age, gender, body weight, and type, and dose of immunosuppressive agents [62]. The prevalence of lipid changes in

Table 32.1 Lipoprotein classes of human plasma.

Lipoprotein	Density g/mL	Particle(s)	Composition (% mass)				
			TG	FC	CE	PL	Pr
Chylomicrons	<0.95	AI, AIV,B-48 C,E	90	1	2	5	2
VLDL	<1.006	B-100,C,E	54	7	13	16	10
IDL	1.006–1019	B-100,C,E	20	9	34	20	17
LDL	1.019–1.063	B-100	4	9	34	20	17
HDL	1.063–1.210	AI, AII,E,C	4	4	14	29	49
Lp(a)	1.080–1.100	B-100,(a)	3	9	36	18	34

Abbreviations: TG, triglyceride; FC, free cholesterol; CE, cholesteryl ester; PL, phospholipids; Pr, protein.

kidney transplant recipients is very high. Particularly common are increases in cholesterol and LDL. HDL is usually normal, and triglycerides are often increased [63–66].

Dyslipidemia and impact on CVD

The risks of cardiovascular morbidity and mortality are profoundly increased in patients with CKD [67]. For instance, the majority of patients with CKD die of cardiovascular events before reaching ESRD [68].

Nephrotic syndrome

There is no reason to doubt that the severe, persistent elevation of cholesterol, LDL, IDL, and Lp(a) represent a highly atherogenic condition. Relatively little and conflicting information has been published on the risk of atherosclerotic vascular disease [69–71]. All of these studies were retrospective, however, and flawed by small sample numbers, selection bias, and lack of control for other atherosclerotic risk factors. Some studies included patients with minimal change disease, and these patients would most likely not remain nephrotic and hence not remain at risk for the long-term complications of hyperlipidemia. According to Ordonez et al., the adjusted relative risks of myocardial infarction and coronary death in nephrotic syndrome are 5.5 and 2.8, respectively. Data were obtained for 142 patients matched with healthy controls and followed prospectively for 5.6 and 1.2 years [72].

Dialysis

CVD is the leading cause of morbidity and mortality in hemodialysis patients; cardiac disease accounts for 44% of overall mortality [73,74]. Approximately 22% of these deaths from cardiac causes are attributed to acute myocardial infarction. In patients who survive a myocardial infarction, the mortality from cardiac causes is 59% at 1 year, 73% at 2 years, and nearly 90% at 3 years [75,76]. After adjusting for age, gender, race, and diagnosis of diabetes, mortality from CVD is far greater in hemodialysis patients than in the general population. It ranges from 500-fold in individuals aged 25–35 years to 5-fold in individuals aged >85 years [77]. This might be due to an increased prevalence of traditional and further kidney disease-related risk factors [78]. In this context, lipid abnormalities have been suggested as a major cause of vascular disease in hemodialysis patients [79–81]. Whereas the log-linear relation between risk of coronary artery disease and blood cholesterol is well-established in the general population, most cross-sectional studies with longitudinal follow-up have failed to demonstrate that plasma total cholesterol, LDL cholesterol, and triglycerides are associated with increased cardiovascular mortality in hemodialysis patients [82,83]. Even inverse associations have been observed among hemodialysis patients between blood cholesterol and all-cause or cardiovascular mortality. The relationship

between serum cholesterol and mortality has been described as U-shaped and, recently, as a J-shaped curve. The risk of death is 4.3 times greater in hemodialysis patients with serum cholesterol of <100 mg/dL (<2.6 mmol/L) than in those with values between 200 and 250 mg/dL (5.2–6.5 mmol/L) [84,85]. This phenomenon is known as reverse risk factor causality and is embedded in the condition of reverse epidemiology [86]. Concomitant chronic illnesses that induce a compensatory decrease in cholesterol synthesis are also associated with an increased risk of death, producing artifactual negative associations (confounding) between cholesterol and mortality [87]. This hypothesis was supported by Liu et al., who demonstrated that hypercholesterolemia was an independent risk factor for all-cause and cardiovascular mortality in a subgroup of ESRD patients without serologic evidence of inflammation or malnutrition but not in patients with inflammation [88]. In another prospective study of 1167 hemodialysis patients, low serum cholesterol levels were associated with all-cause mortality in patients with low serum albumin [89]. These effects may limit the extent to which standard observational studies can identify the true impact of serum cholesterol on the development of vascular disease in this and other populations [90,91]. In the largest and longest study to date, 419 dialysis patients were followed prospectively over a 21-year period. During this time 49% died of CVD and 23% experienced fatal or nonfatal ischemic events. Smoking, hypertension, and hypertriglyceridemia were identified as independent risk factors for CVD [92]. Another "positive" study in a group of 196 diabetic patients receiving hemodialysis demonstrated elevated cholesterol levels with high LDL/HDL ratios that were associated with an increased risk of cardiac death during a 45-month follow-up [93].

Data on the effects of lipids on cardiovascular risk in peritoneal dialysis patients are sparse. Only two studies that examined the relationship between dyslipidemia and CVD were identified. Both had major design limitations [94,95].

Kidney transplantation

Kidney transplant recipients suffer from a high morbidity and mortality due to premature CVD [96]. Several studies have reported a positive association between total cholesterol and CVD, but unfortunately few of them have examined the relationship between LDL and CVD. Lower levels of HDL were associated with CVD in most studies. In about half of the studies higher levels of triglycerides were associated with CVD [97–106]. Recently, the findings of an observational study of 1200 patients up to 15 years after kidney transplantation were in line with these results, showing associations between diabetes, prior transplant, body mass index at the time of transplant, cholesterol level, and LDL level with early acute coronary syndrome [107]. Another recent observational study did not prove these findings [108]. No significant association between triglyceride and total cholesterol levels with patient mortality has been observed. Similarly, no associations were found with allograft loss. This study was done in a much smaller cohort (154 patients) with clearly shorter follow-up (6.1 years).

Cardiovascular end point studies on lipid-lowering therapy in CKD patients

CKD stages 1–4

Until now, no prospective, randomized, controlled trials on lipid-lowering therapy in patients with CKD stages 1–4 have been published. The effect of lipid-lowering therapy on cardiovascular, cerebrovascular, and renal outcomes in patients with CKD stages 2 and 3 was investigated in post hoc subgroup analyses of the Pravastatin Pooling Project. In this trial, a total of 12,333 subjects with estimated glomerular filtration rates (GFRs) determined by the Cockcroft-Gault equation of 60–89.9 mL/min/1.73 m^2 and 4491 subjects with estimated GFRs of 30–59.9 mL/min/1.73 m^2 were analyzed; the results showed that 40 mg/day pravastatin produced a significant 23% relative risk reduction for the combined risk of nonfatal myocardial infarction, coronary mortality, and coronary revascularization in people with moderate CKD. Similar results were obtained in patients with mild CKD. In the subgroup of diabetic patients (i.e. the patients with the highest baseline risk), the highest absolute risk reduction was observed (6.4%) [109,110].

Furthermore, a prespecified subgroup analysis of 6517 patients with kidney dysfunction from the ASCOT study revealed that atorvastatin significantly reduced the risk of the combined primary end point of nonfatal myocardial infarction and cardiac death [111]. Of the 1329 patients with serum creatinine levels of 110–200 μmol/L (1.21–2.26 mg/dL) who entered the Heart Protection Study, 182 of those who received simvastatin and 268 of those in the placebo group experienced a vascular event, indicating a proportional risk reduction with simvastatin treatment of about one-fourth [112]. Finally, a recent pooled analysis of 30 double-blind, randomized trials testing fluvastatin versus placebo in patients with moderate (creatinine clearance of ≥50 mL/min) to severe (creatinine clearance of ≤50 mL/min) renal insufficiency described a 41% and 30% reductions in the relative risk of cardiac death and nonfatal myocardial infarction in patients with severe and moderate renal impairment [113]. The analysis of adverse effects in the above-mentioned trials showed no special safety concerns in patients with CKD. Serum lipids were adequately lowered.

Other lipid-lowering agents to be considered are fibrates. Gemfibrozil has been shown to lower the risk of coronary death or nonfatal myocardial infarction in 1046 patients of the VA-HIT trial with impaired renal function, but the risk of sustained increases in serum creatinine was elevated in gemfibrozil-treated participants compared with placebo [114].

In conclusion, there is indirect evidence that patients with CKD stages 2 and 3 may benefit from statin therapy with respect to cardiovascular events. Patients with stage 4 CKD (GFR of <30 mL/min/1.73 m^2) were either absent or their numbers were too small to be analyzed.

CKD stage V: dialysis

In light of the findings described above, the results of the 4D study came as a surprise. A total of 1255 patients with type 2 diabetes on maintenance hemodialysis were randomized to receive 20 mg atorvastatin or matching placebo. After a median follow-up of 4 years, a nonsignificant 8% relative risk reduction in the primary composite end point (cardiac death, nonfatal myocardial infarction, and stroke) was observed. Atorvastatin reduced the rate of all cardiac events combined (relative risk, 0.82; 95% confidence interval, 0.68–0.99; $P = 0.03$, nominally significant) but did not reduce the rate of all cerebrovascular events combined or total mortality. Of note, there was a higher incidence of fatal stroke in the atorvastatin group compared with placebo (27 versus 13; relative risk, 2.03; $P = 0.04$). The overall incidence of adverse events was comparable between groups [115].

According to these data, we would not recommend initiation of statin treatment in patients with type 2 diabetes mellitus undergoing hemodialysis and with LDL levels of <190 mg/dL. Large-scale randomized controlled trials on lipid-lowering therapy in peritoneal dialysis patients and nondiabetic hemodialysis patients are currently under way: the AURORA study, comparing rosuvastatin with placebo in more than 2750 hemodialysis patients [116], and the SHARP trial [117], which is a randomized study of about 9000 patients with CKD (including kidney transplant recipients) partly on dialysis treatment (hemodialysis and peritoneal dialysis) and receiving either simvastatin in combination with ezetimibe or a placebo. Results from both trials are anticipated in the next few years.

CKD stages 1–4 T, kidney transplant recipients

The final CKD subpopulation considered in this chapter is kidney transplant recipients. The ALERT study [118] was the first large-scale cardiovascular outcome trial to be conducted in kidney transplant recipients and compared fluvastatin with placebo in 2102 patients followed for 5–6 years. Fluvastatin showed no significant reduction in the composite primary end point of cardiac death, nonfatal myocardial infarction, and coronary intervention procedure. The reductions observed in two of three subcomponents of the primary end point, cardiac death or nonfatal myocardial infarction, were interpreted as a great success for this therapy. Notably, the overall incidence of adverse events and study discontinuations with fluvastatin treatment was similar to placebo. The authors suggested that the trial was too small to detect a significant effect on the composite primary end point because the event rate was lower than expected. Therefore, an extension study was performed in which 1652 patients were treated with open-label fluvastatin for 2 years. A 31% relative reduction in major adverse cardiac events and a 29% relative reduction in cardiac death or definite nonfatal myocardial infarction were found. Total mortality and graft loss did not differ significantly between groups [119]. Another subgroup analysis supported an early introduction of fluvastatin therapy in kidney transplant recipients and suggested a greater benefit with respect to cardiac death and myocardial infarction in patients treated earlier [120]. Clearly, studies in patients who have received kidney transplants require a high number-needed-to-treat in their design, in line with primary prevention trials.

In summary, the results of the 4D and ALERT studies do not necessarily cast doubt on the validity of the subgroup analyses done for patients with CKD stages 2 and 3, in whom statins appear to be just as effective as in patients with normal kidney function. The issue remains undecided whether statins are still effective for reducing cardiovascular risk in those with more advanced stages of CKD.

Renal end point studies of lipid-lowering therapy in CKD patients

In addition to the effects of lipid-lowering drugs on cardiovascular and cerebrovascular outcomes, there are data that suggest that lipid lowering may slow the rate of decline in kidney function and lower urinary protein excretion. Recently, a meta-analysis of 27 studies, including 39,704 participants with a baseline mean GFR of 41–99 mL/min, addressed these questions. It showed that statin therapy leads to a small reduction in the rate of kidney function loss in patients with CVD (loss of estimated GFR, 1.22 mL/min/year slower in statin recipients) but not a significant effect based on studies of subjects with diabetic or hypertensive kidney disease or glomerulonephritis [121]. Proteinuria appeared to be modestly reduced. Gemfibrozil did not exert a clinically relevant effect on rates of kidney function loss in a comparable analysis [122].

Treatment guidelines

General remarks

Guidelines for management of dyslipidemia in CKD have been issued, including the European Best Practices guidelines (EBPG) [123] and the US National Kidney Foundation's Kidney Disease Outcomes Quality Initiative (K/DOQI) guidelines [124]. Guidelines on lipid-lowering therapy in CKD patients were difficult to define because of the lack of randomized controlled interventional trials showing that the treatment of dyslipidemia reduces the incidence of vascular events. Furthermore, it is possible that in some subpopulations of CKD treatment of dyslipidemia may not be as safe or as effective in reducing the incidence of vascular disease as it is in the general population. When these guidelines were prepared, the 4D and ALERT trials were still under way. Therefore, both working groups, EBPG and K/DOQI, concluded that additional trials are needed to fill this gap and advised randomization of patients into controlled clinical trials. In the following section, the main aspects of the EBPG guidelines for the treatment of hemodialysis patients and the K/DOQI guidelines are summarized.

Principles of lipid-lowering therapy for CKD patients

As patients with CKD have a very high prevalence of dyslipidemia and CVD [125–128], the EBPG working group concluded that hemodialysis patients should be treated according to existing guidelines of lipid-lowering therapy for the general population, applying a high-risk strategy. The K/DOQI working group recommended that the NCEP/ATP III guidelines [129] were generally applicable to patients with CKD stages 1–4. Some additional specific aspects of the management of dyslipidemias in CKD should be considered. These include the following:

1) CKD should be classified as a CVD risk equivalent.

2) Complications of lipid-lowering therapies resulting from reduced kidney function should be anticipated.

3) Indications for the treatment of dyslipidemia other than preventing CVD should be considered when deciding on specific treatment strategies.

4) Treatment of proteinuria as an alternative treatment of dyslipidemia may prove beneficial.

In conjunction with dyslipidemia, the assessment and management of other modifiable, conventional risk factors (hypertension, smoking, obesity, and diabetes) should be performed.

Assessment and diagnosis of dyslipidemia

A complete fasting lipid profile with total cholesterol, LDL, HDL, and triglycerides is recommended for patients with CKD. For patients with stage 5 CKD, dyslipidemia should be evaluated upon presentation, at 2–3 months after a change in treatment, or with other conditions known to cause dyslipidemia (change in proteinuria, GFR, etc.) and at least annually thereafter. The EBPG advises measurement of cholesterol, HDL, and triglycerides more frequently. LDL should be calculated according to the Friedewald formula if triglycerides are <400 mg/dL; otherwise, direct LDL measurement is recommended. If triglycerides are >800 mg/dL, no LDL measurement needs to be performed. Whenever possible in patients with CKD stage 5, lipid profiles should be measured after an overnight fast, because eating increases especially triglycerides and also total cholesterol. However, it is better to obtain nonfasting lipid profiles than to forgo evaluation altogether. In hemodialysis patients blood should be taken either before dialysis or on nondialysis days, at least 12 h after hemodialysis treatment, because the hemodialysis procedure may acutely alter plasma lipids [130]. Patients with dyslipidemia should be evaluated for secondary causes. Acute medical conditions (e.g. serious infections or myocardial infarction) may alter plasma lipids. It is best to wait until these conditions have resolved. Immunosuppressive medications may cause dyslipidemia. The recommendation is to assess the lipid profile 2–3 months after starting or stopping an agent that is known to influence plasma lipids.

Treatment of dyslipidemia

Three patient groups are to be distinguished:

1 In adults with stage 5 CKD and fasting triglycerides of ≥500 mg/dL (≥5.65 mmol/L) that cannot be ameliorated by correcting an underlying cause, treatment with therapeutic life-style changes (TLC) and a triglyceride-lowering agent should be considered to prevent acute pancreatitis. Only when triglycerides are <500 mg/dL (<5.65 mmol/L) should attention be focused on LDL cholesterol reduction. According to EBPG, in patients with triglycerides of >800 mg/dL (>9 mmol/L) who are resistant to any intervention, the administration of fish oil and/or a switch to low-molecular-weight heparin as anticoagulant during hemodialysis therapy should be considered.

2 For adults with stage 5 CKD and LDL of ≥100 mg/dL (≥2.59 mmol/L), treatment should be considered to reduce LDL to <100 mg/dL (<2.59 mmol/L).

3 For adults with stage 5 CKD and LDL of <100 mg/dL (<2.59 mmol/L), fasting triglycerides of ≥200 mg/dL (≥2.26 mmol/L), and non-HDL cholesterol (total cholesterol minus HDL cholesterol) of ≥130 mg/dL (≥3.36 mmol/L), treatment should be considered to reduce non-HDL cholesterol to <130 mg/dL (<3.36 mmol/L). The EBPG chose a lower threshold for initiation of therapy with triglycerides ≥180 mg/dL (≥2 mmol/L).

Treatment of very high triglycerides

TLC is the therapy of first choice and includes diet, weight reduction, increased physical activity, abstinence from alcohol, and treatment of hyperglycemia, if present. For patients with fasting triglycerides of ≥1000 mg/dL (≥11.29 mmol/L), the NCEP/ATP III diet recommendations include a very low fat diet (<15% total calories), medium-chain triglycerides, and fish oils. Diet should be used judiciously, if at all, in individuals who are malnourished. If TLC is not sufficient to reduce triglycerides to <500 mg/dL (<5.65 mmol/L), treatment with a fibrate or nicotinic acid should be considered. Statins cause less triglyceride lowering, and bile acid sequestrants (BASs) may actually increase triglyceride levels. In any case, the benefits of drug therapy for hypertriglyceridemia should be weighed against the increased risks (particularly for myositis and rhabdomyolysis) in CKD.

Treatment of high LDL
Treatment with TLC
It may be possible to reduce the level of proteinuria and thereby improve a patient's lipid profile [131,132]. For patients with LDL of 100–129 mg/dL (2.59–3.34 mmol/L), it is reasonable to attempt dietary changes for 2–3 months before beginning drug treatment. Diet changes should be used judiciously, if at all, however, when there is evidence of protein–energy malnutrition [133], because there have been no randomized trials that have examined the safety and efficacy of a low-fat, low-cholesterol diet in patients with CKD. There are data that suggest that exercise improves cardiovascular function in hemodialysis patients [134] and decreases triglycerides in CKD patients [135]. The role of weight reduction in CKD patients [133] is unclear. Additional studies are needed to define the role of diet, exercise, and weight reduction in patients with CKD.

Treatment with a statin
In patients who cannot reduce LDL to <100 mg/dL (<2.59 mmol/L) by TLC, a statin should be added because of the strong evidence from studies in the general population that statins reduce CVD and all-cause mortality and the lack of any strong evidence to the contrary in patients with CKD. Whether statins cause hepatotoxicity is controversial. EBPG recommend liver function tests every 6 weeks. Patients should be monitored for signs and symptoms of myopathy. Creatine kinase monitoring is mandatory if muscle symptoms develop. The risk of myopathy from statins is increased by CKD, advanced age, small body frame, and concomitant medications [136]. Patients who develop muscle pain or tenderness should discontinue statin therapy immediately and have a creatine kinase level determined. Doses of lovastatin, fluvastatin, or simvastatin are recommended to be reduced by approximately 50% in patients with CKD stages 4 and 5 according to K/DOQI, whereas the EBPG states that statin doses are usually the same in hemodialysis patients as in the general population.

Medications known to increase statin blood levels should either be avoided or the statin should be reduced or stopped. Cyclosporine has been shown to increase the blood levels of virtually every statin. Even fluvastatin and pravastatin, which are not metabolized by cytochrome P450 3A4, show two- and fivefold increased plasma levels. Accumulating evidence suggests that statins can be used safely with cyclosporine if the dose of the statin is reduced [137–140]. The addition of a third agent that is also metabolized by the cytochrome P450 system increases the risk of myositis and rhabdomyolysis. Such combinations should be avoided. Because of the lack of sufficient data, it should also be assumed that tacrolimus may cause elevations in statin blood levels [141]. Everolimus has minimal effects on blood levels of atorvastatin and pravastatin [142]. The effects of sirolimus on statins are not well known.

Adding a second LDL-lowering agent to a statin
There are very few data on the safety and efficacy of combination therapies in patients with CKD. The K/DOQI guidelines state that in general, it is wise to avoid the use of a fibrate together with a statin. EBPG recommended avoiding combining a fibric acid analog with a statin due to the high risk of rhabdomyolysis. BASs can be considered in combination with a statin in patients with LDL of ≥100 mg/dL (≥2.59 mmol/L) despite TLC and optimal treatment with a statin [143]. They are contraindicated in patients with triglycerides of ≥400 mg/dL (≥4.52 mmol/L) because they may increase triglycerides in some patients. Sevelamer hydrochloride lowers lipid levels by mechanisms similar to those of BASs [144]. Furthermore, nicotinic acid can be considered an alternative second agent in combination with a statin for patients with high triglycerides or for those not tolerating a BAS. There are no data on the use of a combination therapy with a statin and nicotinic acid in patients with CKD.

Treating high LDL in patients who cannot take a statin
Patients with minor adverse effects from a statin may tolerate a reduced dose or a different statin; sometimes a second-line agent needs to be used. BASs, nicotinic acid, and sevelamer [145,146] are possible alternatives.

Use of BASs in kidney transplant recipients

Using BASs in kidney transplant recipients may be difficult because of a possible interference with the absorption of immunosuppressive medications that bind to lipids. Even though two small studies did not find a reduction in cyclosporine levels [147,148], it may be prudent to avoid administering a BAS from 1 h before until 4 h after the administration of cyclosporine and to monitor blood levels of cyclosporine. For many patients, the potential risk of transplant rejection resulting from poor absorption of immunosuppressive medication may outweigh the benefits of a further reduction in LDL.

For kidney transplant recipients who have LDL levels of ≥100 mg/dL (≥2.59 mmol/L) despite maximal medical management, consideration should be given to changing the immunosuppression protocol. In deciding whether to change immunosuppressive agents, the risk of rejection should be weighed against the risk of CVD. Moreover, the effects of immunosuppression on overall CVD risk should be taken into account, not just their effects on dyslipidemia. For example, different immunosuppressive agents have different effects on blood pressure and posttransplant diabetes, both of which can affect the incidence of CVD.

Treating non-HDL cholesterol in patients with high triglycerides

Non-HDL cholesterol is defined as total cholesterol minus HDL. High fasting triglycerides (180–499 mg/dL; 2–5.7 mmol/L) are not used as goals of therapy, but they are markers of increased coronary risk and should be treated in the absence of increased LDL [129]. The finding that elevated triglycerides were an independent cardiovascular risk factor in some studies suggests that some triglyceride-rich lipoproteins are atherogenic [149,150]. The latter are partially degraded VLDL, commonly called remnant lipoproteins. Non-HDL cholesterol was demonstrated to remain one of the strongest predictors for intima media thickness in 897 hemodialysis patients [151]. Non-HDL cholesterol also was a predictor of aortic atherosclerosis in a cohort of 205 hemodialysis patients [152]. Therefore, non-HDL cholesterol is an independent factor affecting arterial wall thickening and stiffness. Recent data suggest that non-HDL cholesterol may actually be a better predictor of coronary mortality than LDL [153]. Non-HDL cholesterol is also a reasonable surrogate marker for apoB, the major apolipoprotein of all atherogenic lipoproteins [154]. In one study, hemodialysis patients showed higher levels of VLDL and IDL, and lower levels of HDL, than age- and sex-matched controls with similar levels of plasma triglycerides [155]. However, so far no evidence has linked low HDL, high fasting triglycerides, and increased non-HDL cholesterol directly to CVD in patients with CKD. Clearly, additional studies are needed to establish whether therapy targeting lower levels of VLDL and IDL is safe and effective in patients with CKD.

TLC for high triglycerides and non-HDL cholesterol

There are virtually no studies on the effects of alcohol consumption in patients with CKD. Even if studies from the general population have produced conflicting results as to whether intensive glycemic control reduces the risk for CVD, CKD patients with low HDL and or high triglycerides should be assessed for diabetes, and diabetic patients with this lipid profile should have as good glycemic control as possible without causing excessive hypoglycemia. Obesity is associated with low HDL and/or high triglycerides. There are a few studies demonstrating successful weight reduction in obese patients with CKD. A limited number of studies suggest that low-fat diets [156] and increased physical activity [135] may be effective in patients with CKD. A few studies have examined the effects of fish oil supplements on lipoproteins in patients with CKD; their results have been inconclusive [157–161].

Drug therapy for high triglycerides and non-HDL cholesterol

Patients who are not already receiving a statin for treatment of LDL cholesterol who have fasting triglycerides of ≥200 mg/dL (≥2.26 mmol/L) (K/DOQI) or ≥180 mg/dL (≥2 mmol/L) (EBPG) and non-HDL cholesterol of ≥130 mg/dL (≥3.36 mmol/L) and who do not have liver disease should be started on a statin along with TLC. The safety and efficacy of statins for preventing CVD have been more conclusively established in randomized trials in the general population. If a statin cannot be used, a fibrate may be considered. The blood levels of bezafibrate, clofibrate, and fenofibrate are increased in patients with decreased kidney function compared to controls with normal kidney function [162–165]. In contrast, blood levels of gemfibrozil do not appear to be altered by decreased kidney function. Bezafibrate, ciprofibrate, fenofibrate, and gemfibrozil have been reported to cause increased serum creatinine and blood urea nitrogen levels [166,167]. Since dose modification for decreased kidney function is not required for gemfibrozil, unlike other fibrates, gemfibrozil should probably be considered the fibrate of choice for most CKD patients. Nicotinic acid can be used in place of fibrates for patients with elevated triglycerides. However, there are almost no data on blood levels of nicotinic acid in patients with CKD. Furthermore, the use of polysulfone or polyamide high-flux dialysis has been shown to ameliorate hypertriglyceridemia in some patients [168–171]. Treatment of renal anemia with erythropoietin in hemodialysis patients has beneficial effects on plasma lipid concentrations [172].

Isolated low HDL cholesterol

Patients with isolated low HDL cholesterol should be treated with TLC. Pharmacological treatment of isolated low HDL cholesterol is not recommended because the risks of pharmacological therapy to raise HDL probably outweigh the benefits.

Other lipid-lowering agents

Ezetimibe was approved after publication of the above-presented guidelines. There are data on ezetimibe treatment in patients, including peritoneal dialysis, hemodialysis, and CKD patients [173,174] as well as kidney transplant recipients [175] that show it to be an effective lipid-lowering agent when added to other lipid-lowering therapies as well as to be safe in patients with reduced renal function and in patients who do not tolerate statin therapy.

At this time, there are no data about its influence on cardiovascular events.

References

1 Samuelsson O, Attmann PO, Knight-Gibson C, Kron B, Larsson R, Mulec H et al. Lipoprotein abnormalities without hyperlipidemia in moderate renal insufficiency. *Nephrol Dial Transplant* 1991; **9:** 1580–1585.

2 Joven J, Villabona C, Vilella E, Masana L, Alberti R, Valles M. Abnormalities of lipoprotein metabolism in patients with the nephrotic syndrome. *N Engl J Med* 1990; **323:** 579–584.

3 Ohta T, Matsuda I. Lipid and apolipoprotein levels in patients with nephrotic syndrome. *Clin Chem Acta* 1981; **117:** 133–143.

4 Gherardi E, Rota E, Calandra S, Genova R, Tamborino A. Relationship among the concentrations of serum lipoproteins and changes in their chemical composition in patients with untreated nephrotic syndrome. *Eur J Clin Invest* 1977; **7:** 563–570.

5 Krämer-Guth A, Nauck M, Pavenstädt H, Königer M, Wieland H, Schollmeyer P et al. Preferential uptake of intermediate-density lipoproteins from nephrotic patients by human mesangial and liver cells. *J Am Soc Nephrol* 1994; **5:** 1081–1090.

6 Krämer A, Nauck M, Pavenstädt H, Schwedler S, Wieland H, Schollmeyer P et al. Receptor-mediated uptake of IDL and LDL from nephrotic patients by glomerular epithelial cells. *Kidney Int* 1993; **44:** 1341–1351.

7 Short CD, Durrington PN, Mallick NP, Hunt LP, Tetlow L, Ishola M. Serum and urinary high-density lipoproteins in glomerular disease with proteinuria. *Kidney Int* 1986; **29:** 1224–1228.

8 Appel GB, Blum CB, Chien S, Kunis CL, Appel AS. The hyperlipidemia of the nephrotic syndrome. *N Engl J Med* 1985; **312:** 1544–1548.

9 Kaysen GA, Pan X-M, Couser WG, Staprans I. Defective lipolysis persists in hearts of rats with Heymann nephritis in the absence of nephrotic plasma. *Am J Kidney Dis* 1993; **22:** 128–134.

10 Davies RW, Staprans I, Hutchison FN, Kaysen GA. Proteinuria, not altered albumin metabolism, affects hyperlipidemia in the nephrotic rat. *J Clin Invest* 1990; **86:** 600–605.

11 Shearer GC, Kaysen GA. Proteinuria and plasma compositional changes contribute to defective lipoprotein catabolism in the nephrotic syndrome by separate mechanisms. *Kidney Int* 2001; **37(Suppl 2):** S119–S122.

12 de Sain-van der Velden MG, Kaysen GA, Barrett HA, Stellaard F, Gadellaa MM, Voorbij HA et al. Increased VLDL in nephrotic patients results from a decreased catabolism while increased LDL results from increased synthesis. *Kidney Int* 1998; **53(4):** 994–1001.

13 Joven J, Villabona C, Viletta E. Pattern of hyperlipoproteinemia in human nephrotic syndrome: influence of renal failure and diabetes mellitus. *Nephron* 1993; **64:** 565–569.

14 Karadi I, Romics L, Palos G, Doman J, Kaszas I, Hesz A et al. Lp(a) lipoprotein concentration in serum of patients with heavy proteinuria of different origin. *Clin Chem* 1989; **35:** 2121–2123.

15 Thomas ME, Freestone A, Varghese Z, Persaud JW, Moorhead JF. Lipoprotein(a) in patients with proteinuria. *Nephrol Dial Transplant* 1992; **7:** 597–601.

16 Stenvinkel P, Berglund L, Heimbürger O, Petterson E, Alvestrand A. Lipoprotein (a) in nephrotic syndrome. *Kidney Int* 1993; **44:** 1116–1123.

17 Wanner C, Rader D, Bartens W, Krämer J, Brewer HB, Schollmeyer P et al. Elevated plasma lipoprotein(a) in patients with the nephrotic syndrome. *Ann Intern Med* 1993; **119:** 263–269.

18 De Sain-Van Der Velden MG, Reijngoud DJ, Kaysen GA, Gadellaa MM, Voorbij H, Stellaard F et al. Evidence for increased synthesis of lipoprotein(a) in the nephrotic syndrome. *J Am Soc Nephrol* 1998; **9(8):** 1474–1481.

19 Kasiske BL. Hyperlipidemia in patients with chronic renal disease. *Am J Kidney Dis* 1998; **32:** S142–S156.

20 Brunzell JD, Albers JJ, Haas LB, Goldberg AP, Agadoa L, Sherrard DJ. Prevalence of serum lipid abnormalities in chronic haemodialysis. *Metabolism* 1977; **26:** 903–910.

21 Pedro BJ, Senti M, Rubies PJ, Pelegri A, Romero R. When to treat dyslipidaemia of patients with chronic renal failure on haemodialysis? A need to define specific guidelines. *Nephrol Dial Transplant* 1996; **11:** 308–313.

22 Lacour B, Roullet JB, Beyne P, Kreis H, Thevenin M, Drueke T. Comparison of several atherogenicity indices by the analysis of serum lipoprotein composition in patients with chronic renal failure with or without haemodialysis, and in renal transplant patients. *J Clin Chem Clin Biochem* 1985; **23:** 805–810.

23 Cheung AK, Wu LL, Kablitz C, Leypoldt JK. Atherogenic lipids and lipoproteins in haemodialysis patients. *Am J Kidney Dis* 1993; **22:** 271–276.

24 Rapoport J, Aviram M, Chaimovitz C, Brook JG. Defective high-density lipoprotein composition in patients on chronic haemodialysis. A possible mechanism for accelerated atherosclerosis. *N Engl J Med* 1978; **299:** 1326–1329.

25 Rubies-Prat J, Espinel E, Joven J, Ras MR, Pira L. High-density lipoprotein cholesterol subfractions in chronic uremia. *Am J Kidney Dis* 1987; **9:** 60–65.

26 Atger V, Duval F, Frommherz K, Drueke T, Lacour B. Anomalies in composition of uremic lipoproteins isolated by gradient ultracentrifugation: relative enrichment of HDL in apolipoprotein C-III at the expense of apolipoprotein A-I. *Atherosclerosis* 1988; **74:** 75–83.

27 Joven J, Rubies-Prat J, Espinel E, Chacon P, Olmos A, Masdeu S. Apoprotein A-I and high density lipoprotein subfractions in patients with chronic renal failure receiving haemodialysis. *Nephron* 1985; **40:** 451–454.

28 Parsy D, Dracon M, Cachera C, Parra HJ, Vanhoutte G, Tacquet A et al. Lipoprotein abnormalities in chronic haemodialysis patients. *Nephrol Dial Transplant* 1988; **3:** 51–56.

29 Senti M, Romero R, Pedro-Botet J, Pelegri A, Nogues X, Rubies-Prat J. Lipoprotein abnormalities in hyperlipidemic and normolipidemic men on haemodialysis with chronic renal failure. *Kidney Int* 1992; **41:** 1394–1399.

30 Attman PO, Alaupovic P. Lipid and apolipoprotein profiles of uremic dyslipoproteinemia: relation to renal function and dialysis. *Nephron* 1991; **57:** 401–410.

31 Oi K, Hirano T, Sakai S, Kawaguchi Y, Hosoya T. Role of hepatic lipase in intermediate-density lipoprotein and small, dense low-density lipoprotein formation in haemodialysis patients. *Kidney Int* 1999; **56(Suppl 71):** S227–S228.

32 Attman PO, Samuelsson O, Alaupovic P. Lipoprotein metabolism and renal failure. *Am J Kidney Dis* 1993; **21:** 573–592.

33 Oda H, Keane WF. Lipid abnormalities in end stage renal disease. *Nephrol Dial Transplant* 1998; **13(Suppl 1):** S45–S49.

34 Deighan CJ, Caslake MJ, McConnell M, Boulton-Jones JM, Packard CJ. Atherogenic lipoprotein phenotype in end-stage renal failure: origin and extent of small dense low-density lipoprotein formation. *Am J Kidney Dis* 2000; **35:** 852–862.

35 Joven J, Vilella E, Ahmad S, Cheung MC, Brunzell JD. Lipoprotein heterogeneity in end-stage renal disease. *Kidney Int* 1993; **43:** 410–418.

36 Ikewaki K, Schaefer JR, Frischmann ME, Okubo K, Hosoya T, Mochizuki S et al. Delayed in vivo catabolism of intermediate-density lipoprotein and low-density lipoprotein in hemodialysis patients as potential cause of premature atherosclerosis. *Arterioscler Thromb Vasc Biol* 2005; **25:** 2615–2622.

37 Quaschning T, Schomig M, Keller M, Thiery J, Nauck M, Schollmeyer P et al. Non-insulin-dependent diabetes mellitus and hypertriglyceridaemia impair lipoprotein metabolism in chronic haemodialysis patients. *J Am Soc Nephrol* 1999; **10:** 332–341.

38 Rajman I, Harper L, McPake D, Kendall MJ, Wheeler DC. Low-density lipoprotein subfraction profiles in chronic renal failure. *Nephrol Dial Transplant* 1998; **13:** 2281–2287.

39 O'Neal D, Lee P, Murphy B, Best J. Low-density lipoprotein particle size distribution in end-stage renal disease treated with haemodialysis or peritoneal dialysis. *Am J Kidney Dis* 1996; **27:** 84–91.

40 Ambrosch A, Domroese U, Westphal S, Dierkes J, Augustin W, Neumann KH et al. Compositional and functional changes of low-density lipoprotein during haemodialysis in patients with ESRD. *Kidney Int* 1998; **54:** 608–617.

41 Attman PO, Samuelsson OG, Moberly J, Johansson AC, Ljungman S, Weiss LG et al. Apolipoprotein B-containing lipoproteins in renal failure: the relation to mode of dialysis. *Kidney Int* 1999; **55:** 1536–1542.

42 Wakabayashi Y, Okubo M, Shimada H, Sato N, Koide A, Marumo F et al. Decreased VLDL apoprotein CII/apoprotein CIII ratio may be seen in both normotriglyceridemic and hypertriglyceridemic patients on chronic haemodialysis treatment. *Metabolism* 1987; **36:** 815–820.

43 Kandoussi AM, Hugue V, Parra HJ, Dracon M, Fruchart JC, Tacquet A et al. Apolipoprotein AI and apolipoprotein B containing particle analysis in normolipidemic hemodialyzed patients: evidence of free apolipoprotein E. *Am J Nephrol* 1996; **16:** 287–292.

44 Weintraub M, Burstein A, Rassin T, Liron M, Ringel Y, Cabili S et al. Severe defect in clearing postprandial chylomicron remnants in dialysis patients. *Kidney Int* 1992; **42:** 1247–1252.

45 Okubo K, Ikewaki K, Sakai S, Tada N, Kawaguchi Y, Mochizuki S. Abnormal HDL apolipoprotein A-I and A-II kinetics in hemodialysis patients: a stable isotope study. *J Am Soc Nephrol* 2004; **15:** 1008–1015.

46 Sniderman A, Cianflone K, Kwiterovich PO, Jr., Hutchinson T, Barre P, Prichard S. Hyperapobetalipoproteinemia: the major dyslipoproteinemia in patients with chronic renal failure treated with chronic ambulatory peritoneal dialysis. *Atherosclerosis* 1987; **65:** 257–264.

47 Ramos JM, Heaton A, McGurk JG, Ward MK, Kerr DN. Sequential changes in serum lipids and their subfractions in patients receiving continuous ambulatory peritoneal dialysis. *Nephron* 1983; **35:** 20–23.

48 Roncari DAK, Breckenridge WC, Khanna R, Oreopoulos DG. Rise in high-density lipoprotein cholesterol in some patients treated with CAPD. *Perit Dial Bull* 1988; **1:** 136–141.

49 Boeschoten EW, Zuyderhoudt FMJ, Krediet RT, Arisz L. Changes in weight and lipid concentrations during CAPD treatment. *Perit Dial Bull* 1988; **19:** 8–13.

50 Shoji T, Nishizawa Y, Nishitani H, Yamakawa M, Morii H. High serum-lipoprotein(a) concentration in uremic patients treated with continuous ambulatory peritoneal dialysis. *Clin Nephrol* 1992; **38:** 271–276.

51 Anwar N, Bhatnager D, Short CD, Mackness MI, Durrington PN, Prais H et al. Serum lipoprotein(a) concentrations in patients undergoing continuous ambulatory peritoneal dialysis. *Nephrol Dial Transplant* 1993; **8:** 71–74.

52 Webb AT, Reaveley DA, O'Donnell M, O'Connor B, Seed M, Brown EA. Lipoprotein(a) in patients on maintenance haemodialysis and continuous ambulatory peritoneal dialysis. *Nephrol Dial Transplant* 1993; **8:** 609–613.

53 Morrison G. Metabolic effects of continuous ambulatory peritoneal dialysis. *Ann Rev Med* 1989; **40:** 163–172.

54 Saku K, Sasaki J, Naito S, Arakawa K. Lipoprotein and apolipoprotein losses during continuous ambulatory peritoneal dialysis. *Nephron* 1989; **51:** 220–224.

55 Lameire N, Matthys D, Matthys E, Beheydt R. Effect of long-term CAPD on carbohydrate and lipid metabolism. *Clin Nephrol* 1988; **30:** S53–S58.

56 Breckenridge WC, Roncari DAK, Khanna R, Oreopoulos DG. The influence of continuous ambulatory peritoneal dialysis on plasma lipoproteins. *Atherosclerosis* 1992; **45:** 249–258.

57 Haas LB, Wahl PW, Sherrard DJ. A longitudinal study of lipid abnormalities in renal failure. *Nephron* 1983; **33:** 145–159.

58 Prinsen BH, Rabelink TJ, Romijn JA, Bisschop PH, de Barse MM, de Boer J et al. A broad-based metabolic approach to study VLDL apoB100 metabolism in patients with ESRD and patients treated with peritoneal dialysis. *Kidney Int* 2004; **65:** 1064–1075.

59 Lindholm B, Norbeck HE. Serum lipids and lipoproteins during continuous ambulatory peritoneal dialysis. *Acta Med Scand* 1986; **220:** 143–151.

60 Thomas ME, Moorhead JF. Lipids in CAPD: a review. *Contrib Nephrol* 1990; **85:** 92–99.

61 Dieplinger H, Schoenfeld PY, Fielding CJ. Plasma cholesterol metabolism in end-stage renal disease. *J Clin Invest* 1986; **77:** 1071–1083.

62 Kasiske BL. Risk factors for accelerated atherosclerosis in renal transplant recipients. *Am J Med* 1988; **84:** 985–992.

63 Aakhus S, Dahl K, Widerøe TE. Hyperlipidaemia in renal transplant patients. *J Intern Med* 1996; **239:** 407–415.

64 Gonyea JE, Anderson CF. Weight change and serum lipoproteins in recipients of renal allografts. *Mayo Clin Proc* 1992; **67:** 653–657.

65 Brown JH, Murphy BG, Douglas AF, Short CD, Bhatnagar D, Mackness MI et al. Influence of immunosuppressive therapy on lipoprotein(a) and other lipoproteins following renal transplantation. *Nephron* 1997; **75:** 277–282.

66 Moore R, Thomas D, Morgan E, Wheeler D, Griffin P, Salaman J et al. Abnormal lipid and lipoprotein profiles following renal transplantation. *Transplant Proc* 1993; **25:** 1060–1061.

67 Go AS, Chertow GM, Fan D, McCulloch CE, Hsu CY. Chronic kidney disease and the risks of death, cardiovascular events, and hospitalization. *N Engl J Med* 2004; **351:** 1296–1305.

68 Keith DS, Nichols GA, Gullion CM, Brown JB, Smith DH. Longitudinal follow-up and outcomes among a population with chronic kidney disease in a large managed care organization. *Arch Intern Med* 2004; **164:** 659–663.

69 Berlyne GM, Mallick NP. Ischemic heart disease as a complication of nephrotic syndrome. *Lancet* 1969; **ii:** 399–400.

70 Curry RC, Roberts WC. Status of the coronary arteries in the nephrotic syndrome. *Am J Med* 1977; **63**: 183–192.

71 Wass V, Cameron JS. Cardiovascular disease and the nephrotic syndrome: the other side of the coin. *Nephron* 1981; **27**: 58–61.

72 Ordonez JD, Hiatt R, Killebrew E, Fireman BH. The increased risk of coronary heart disease associated with nephrotic syndrome. *Kidney Int* 1993; **44**: 638–642.

73 US Renal Data System. Causes of death. *Am J Kidney Dis* 1997; **30**: S107–S117.

74 US Renal Data System. The USRDS Dialysis Morbidity and Mortality Study: Wave 2. *Am J Kidney Dis* 1997; **30**: S67–S85.

75 Herzog CA, Ma JZ, Collins AJ. Poor long-term survival after acute myocardial infarction among patients on long-term dialysis. *N Engl J Med* 1998; **339**: 799–805.

76 Chantrel F, Enache I, Bouiller M, Kolb I, Kunz K, Petitjean P *et al.* Abysmal prognosis of patients with type 2 diabetes entering dialysis. *Nephrol Dial Transplant* 1999; **14**: 129–136.

77 Foley RN, Parfrey PS, Sarnak MJ. Clinical epidemiology of cardiovascular disease in chronic renal disease. *Am J Kidney Dis* 1998; **32**: S112–S119.

78 Parfrey PS, Foley RN. The clinical epidemiology of cardiac disease in chronic renal failure. *J Am Soc Nephrol* 1999; **10**: 1606–1615.

79 Hahn R, Oette K, Mondorf H, Finke K, Sieberth HG. Analysis of cardiovascular risk factors in chronic haemodialysis patients with special attention to the hyperlipoproteinemias. *Atherosclerosis* 1983; **48**: 279–288.

80 Avram MM, Fein PA, Antignani A, Mittman N, Mushnick RA, Lustig AR *et al.* Cholesterol and lipid disturbances in renal disease: the natural history of uremic dyslipidaemia and the impact of haemodialysis and continuous ambulatory peritoneal dialysis. *Am J Med* 1989; **87**: 55N–60N.

81 Attman PO. Hyperlipoproteinaemia in renal failure: pathogenesis and perspectives for intervention. *Nephrol Dial Transplant* 1993; **8**: 294–295.

82 Ma KW, Greene EL, Raij L. Cardiovascular risk factors in chronic renal failure and haemodialysis populations. *Am J Kidney Dis* 1992; **19**: 505–513.

83 Zimmermann J, Herrlinger S, Pruy A, Metzger T, Wanner C. Inflammation enhances cardiovascular risk and mortality in haemodialysis patients. *Kidney Int* 1999; **55**: 648–658.

84 Lowrie EG, Lew NL. Death risk in haemodialysis patients: the predictive value of commonly measured variables and an evaluation of death rate differences between facilities. *Am J Kidney Dis* 1990; **15**: 458–482.

85 Degoulet P, Legrain M, Reach I, Aime F, Devries C, Rojas P *et al.* Mortality risk factors in patients treated by chronic haemodialysis. Report of the Diaphane Collaborative Study. *Nephron* 1982; **31**: 103–110.

86 Kalantar-Zadeh K, Block G, Humphreys MH, Kopple JD. Reverse epidemiology of cardiovascular risk factors in maintenance dialysis patients. *Kidney Int* 2003; **63**: 793–808.

87 Corti MC, Guralnik JM, Salive ME, Harris T, Ferrucci L, Glynn RJ *et al.* Clarifying the direct relation between total cholesterol levels and death from coronary heart disease in older persons. *Ann Intern Med* 1997; **126**: 753–760.

88 Liu Y, Coresh J, Eustace JA, Longenecker JC, Jaar B, Fink NE *et al.* Association between cholesterol level and mortality in dialysis patients: role of inflammation and malnutrition. *JAMA* 2004; **291**: 451–459.

89 Iseki K, Yamazato M, Tozawa M, Takishita S. Hypocholesterolemia is a significant predictor of death in a cohort of chronic haemodialysis patients. *Kidney Int* 2002; **61**: 1887–1893.

90 Baigent C, Burbury K, Wheeler D. Premature cardiovascular disease in chronic renal failure. *Lancet* 2000; **356**: 147–152.

91 Ishani A, Collins AJ, Herzog CA, Foley RN. Septicemia, access and cardiovascular disease in dialysis patients: The USRDS Wave 2 study. *Kidney Int* 2005; **68**: 311–318.

92 Kates DM, Haas L, Brunzell J, Sherrard DJ. Risk factors for cardiovascular disease in end-stage renal failure patients: a 21 year study. *J Am Soc Nephrol* 1995; **6**: 540 A.

93 Tschope W, Koch M, Thomas B, Ritz E. Serum lipids predict cardiac death in diabetic patients on maintenance haemodialysis. Results of a prospective study. The German Study Group Diabetes and Uremia. *Nephron* 1993; **64**: 354–358.

94 Webb AT, Brown EA. Prevalence of symptomatic arterial disease and risk factors for its development in patients on continuous ambulatory peritoneal dialysis. *Perit Dial Int* 1993; **13**: S406–S408.

95 Olivares J, Cruz C, Gas JM, Prados MC, Perdiquero M, Caparros G *et al.* Evolution of lipid profiles in long-term peritoneal dialysis. *Adv Perit Dial* 1992; **8**: 373–375.

96 Raine AE. Hypertension and ischaemic heart disease in renal transplant recipients. *Nephrol Dial Transplant* 1995; **10(Suppl 1)**: 95–100.

97 Quaschning T, Mainka T, Nauck M, Rump LC, Wanner C, Kramer-Guth A. Immunosuppression enhances atherogenicity of lipid profile after transplantation. *Kidney Int Suppl* 1999; **71**: S235–S237.

98 Kasiske BL, Guijarro C, Massy ZA, Wiederkehr MR, Ma JZ. Cardiovascular disease after renal transplantation. *J Am Soc Nephrol* 1996; **7**: 158–165.

99 Aker S, Ivens K, Grabensee B, Heering P. Cardiovascular risk factors and diseases after renal transplantation. *Int Urol Nephrol* 1998; **30**: 777–788.

100 Aakhus S, Dahl K, Wideroe TE. Cardiovascular morbidity and risk factors in renal transplant patients. *Nephrol Dial Transplant* 1999; **14**: 648–654.

101 Kasiske BL, Chakkera H, Roel J. Explained and unexplained ischemic heart disease risk after renal transplantation. *J Am Soc Nephrol* 2000; **11**: 1735–1743.

102 Ong CS, Pollock CA, Caterson RJ, Mahony JF, Waugh DA, Ibels LS. Hyperlipidemia in renal transplant recipients: natural history and response to treatment. *Medicine* 1994; **73**: 215–223.

103 Barbagallo CM, Pinto A, Gallo S, Parrinello G, Caputo F, Sparacino V *et al.* Carotid atherosclerosis in renal transplant recipients: relationships with cardiovascular risk factors and plasma lipoproteins. *Transplantation* 1999; **67**: 366–371.

104 Roodnat JI, Mulder PG, Zietse R, Rischen-Vos J, van Riemsdijk JC, Ijzermans JN *et al.* Cholesterol as an independent predictor of outcome after renal transplantation. *Transplantation* 2000; **69**: 1704–1710.

105 Massy ZA, Mamzer-Bruneel MF, Chevalier A, Millet P, Helenon O, Chadefaux-Vekemans B *et al.* Carotid atherosclerosis in renal transplant recipients. *Nephrol Dial Transplant* 1998; **13**: 1792–1798.

106 Biesenbach G, Margreiter R, Konigsrainer A, Bosmuller C, Janko O, Brucke P *et al.* Comparison of progression of macrovascular diseases after kidney or pancreas and kidney transplantation in diabetic patients with end-stage renal disease. *Diabetologia* 2000; **43**: 231–234.

107 Fazelzadeh A, Mehdizadeh AR, Ostovan MA, Raiss-Jalali GA. Predictors of cardiovascular events and associated mortality of kidney transplant recipients. *Transplant Proc* 2006; **38**: 509–511.

108 Schaeffner ES, Fodinger M, Kramar R, Frei U, Horl WH, Sunder-Plassmann G *et al.* Prognostic associations between lipid markers and outcomes in kidney transplant recipients. *Am J Kidney Dis* 2006; **47**: 509–517.

109 Tonelli M, Isles C, Curhan GC, Tonkin A, Pfeffer MA, Shepherd J *et al.* Effect of pravastatin on cardiovascular events in people with chronic kidney disease. *Circulation* 2004; **110:** 1557–1563.

110 Tonelli M, Keech A, Shepherd J, Sacks F, Tonkin A, Packard C *et al.* Effect of pravastatin in people with diabetes and chronic kidney disease. *J Am Soc Nephrol* 2005; **16:** 3748–3754.

111 Sever PS, Dahlof B, Poulter NR, Wedel H, Beevers G, Caulfield M *et al.* Prevention of coronary and stroke events with atorvastatin in hypertensive patients who have average or lower-than-average cholesterol concentrations, in the Anglo-Scandinavian Cardiac Outcomes Trial Lipid Lowering Arm (ASCOT-LLA): a multicentre randomised controlled trial. *Lancet* 2003; **361:** 1149–1158.

112 Heart Protection Study Collaborative Group. MRC/BHF Heart Protection Study of cholesterol lowering with simvastatin in 20,536 high-risk individuals: a randomised placebo-controlled trial. *Lancet* 2002; **360:** 7–22.

113 Holdaas H, Wanner C, Abletshauser C, Gimpelewicz C, Isaacsohn J. The effect of fluvastatin on cardiac outcomes in patients with moderate to severe renal insufficiency: a pooled analysis of double-blind, randomized trials. *Int J Cardiol* 2007; **117:** 64–74.

114 Tonelli M, Collins D, Robins S, Bloomfield H, Curhan GC *et al.* Veterans' Affairs High-Density Lipoprotein Intervention Trial (VA-HIT) Investigators. Gemfibrozil for secondary prevention of cardiovascular events in mild to moderate chronic renal insufficiency. *Kidney Int* 2004; **66:** 1123–1130.

115 Wanner C, Krane V, Marz W, Olschewski M, Mann JF, Ruf G *et al.* German Diabetes and Dialysis Study Investigators. Atorvastatin in patients with type 2 diabetes mellitus undergoing haemodialysis. *N Engl J Med* 2005; **353:** 238–248.

116 Fellstrom BC, Holdaas H, Jardine AG. Why do we need a statin trial in haemodialysis patients? *Kidney Int Suppl* 2003; **84(Suppl):** S204–S206.

117 Baigent C, Landray M. Study of Heart and Renal Protection (SHARP). *Kidney Int* 2003; **84(Suppl 81):** S207–S210.

118 Holdaas H, Fellstrom B, Jardine AG, Holme I, Nyberg G, Fauchald P *et al.* Assessment of LEscol in Renal Transplantation (ALERT) Study Investigators. Effect of fluvastatin on cardiac outcomes in renal transplant recipients: a multicentre, randomised, placebo-controlled trial. *Lancet* 2003; **361:** 2024–2031.

119 Holdaas H, Fellstrom B, Cole E, Nyberg G, Olsson AG, Pedersen TR *et al.* Assessment of LEscol in Renal Transplantation (ALERT) Study Investigators. Long-term cardiac outcomes in renal transplant recipients receiving fluvastatin: the ALERT extension study. *Am J Transplant* 2005; **5:** 2929–2936.

120 Holdaas H, Fellstrom B, Jardine AG, Nyberg G, Gronhagen-Riska C, Madsen S *et al.* ALERT Study Group. Beneficial effect of early initiation of lipid-lowering therapy following renal transplantation. *Nephrol Dial Transplant* 2005; **20:** 974–980.

121 Sandhu S, Wiebe N, Fried LF, Tonelli M. Statins for improving renal outcomes: a meta-analysis. *J Am Soc Nephrol* 2006; **17:** 2006–2016.

122 Tonelli M, Collins D, Robins S, Bloomfield H, Curhan GC. Effect of gemfibrozil on change in renal function in men with moderate chronic renal insufficiency and coronary disease. *Am J Kidney Dis* 2004; **44:** 832–839.

123 European Best Practice guidelines for haemodialysis (part 1). Section VII. Vascular disease and risk factors. *Nephrol Dial Transplant* 2002; **17(Suppl 7):** 88–109.

124 National Kidney Foundation. K/DOQI clinical practice guidelines for managing dyslipidemias in chronic kidney disease. *Am J Kidney Dis* 2003; **41(Suppl 3):** S1–S92.

125 Jungers P, Massy ZA, Nguyen Khoa T, Fumeron C, Labrunie M, Lacour B *et al.* Incidence and risk factors of atherosclerotic cardiovascular accidents in predialysis chronic renal failure patients: a prospective study. *Nephrol Dial Transplant* 1997; **12:** 2597–2602.

126 Landray MJ, Thambyrajah J, McGlynn FJ, Jones HJ, Baigent C, Kendall MJ *et al.* Epidemiological evaluation of known and suspected cardiovascular risk factors in chronic renal impairment. *Am J Kidney Dis* 2001; **38:** 537–546.

127 Tonelli M, Bohm C, Pandeya S, Gill J, Levin A, Kiberd BA. Cardiac risk factors and the use of cardioprotective medications in patients with chronic renal insufficiency. *Am J Kidney Dis* 2001; **37:** 484–489.

128 Levin A, Djurdjev O, Barrett B, Burgess E, Carlisle E, Ethier J *et al.* Cardiovascular disease in patients with chronic kidney disease: getting to the heart of the matter. *Am J Kidney Dis* 2001; **38:** 1398–1407.

129 Executive Summary of the Third Report of The National Cholesterol Education Program (NCEP) Expert Panel on Detection, Evaluation, and Treatment of High Blood Cholesterol In Adults (Adult Treatment Panel III). *JAMA* 2001; **285:** 2486–2497.

130 Ingram AJ, Parbtani A, Churchill DN. Effects of two low-flux cellulose acetate dialysers on plasma lipids and lipoproteins: a cross-over trial. *Nephrol Dial Transplant* 1998; **13:** 1452–1457.

131 Keilani T, Schlueter WA, Levin ML, Batlle DC. Improvement of lipid abnormalities associated with proteinuria using fosinopril, an angiotensin-converting enzyme inhibitor. *Ann Intern Med* 1993; **118:** 246–254.

132 Ravid M, Neumann L, Lishner M. Plasma lipids and the progression of nephropathy in diabetes mellitus type II: effect of ACE inhibitors. *Kidney Int* 1995; **47:** 907–910.

133 National Kidney Foundation Kidney Disease Outcomes Quality Initiative (K/DOQI). Clinical practice guidelines for nutrition in chronic renal failure. *Am J Kidney Dis* 2000; **35:** S1–S140.

134 Deligiannis A, Kouidi E, Tassoulas E, Gigis P, Tourkantonis A, Coats A. Cardiac effects of exercise rehabilitation in haemodialysis patients. *Int J Cardiol* 1999; **70:** 253–266.

135 Goldberg AP, Geltman EM, Hagberg JM, Gavin JR, III, Delmez JA, Carney RM et al. Therapeutic benefits of exercise training for haemodialysis patients. *Kidney Int Suppl* 1983; **16:** S303–S309.

136 Pasternak RC, Smith SC, Jr., Bairey-Merz CN, Grundy SM, Cleeman JI, Lenfant C. ACC/AHA/NHLBI clinical advisory on the use and safety of statins. *Stroke* 2002; **33:** 2337–2341.

137 Holdaas H, Jardine AG, Wheeler DC, Brekke IB, Conlon PJ, Fellstrom B *et al.* Effect of fluvastatin on acute renal allograft rejection: a randomized multicenter trial. *Kidney Int* 2001; **60:** 1990–1997.

138 Kasiske BL, Heim-Duthoy KL, Singer GG, Watschinger B, Germain MJ, Bastani B. The effects of lipid-lowering agents on acute renal allograft rejection. *Transplantation* 2001; **72:** 223–227.

139 Katznelson S, Wilkinson AH, Kobashigawa JA, Wang XM, Chia D, Ozawa M *et al.* The effect of pravastatin on acute rejection after kidney transplantation: a pilot study. *Transplantation* 1996; **61:** 1469–1474.

140 Renders L, Mayer-Kadner I, Koch C, Scharffe S, Burkhardt K, Veelken R *et al.* Efficacy and drug interactions of the new HMG-CoA reductase inhibitors cerivastatin and atorvastatin in CsA-treated renal transplant recipients. *Nephrol Dial Transplant* 2001; **16:** 141–146.

141 Ichimaru N, Takahara S, Kokado Y, Wang JD, Hatori M, Kameoka H *et al.* Changes in lipid metabolism and effect of simvastatin in renal transplant

recipients induced by cyclosporine or tacrolimus. *Atherosclerosis* 2001; **158:** 417–423.

142 Kovarik JM, Hartmann S, Hubert M, Berthier S, Schneider W, Rosenkranz B et al. Pharmacokinetic and pharmacodynamic assessments of HMG-CoA reductase inhibitors when coadministered with everolimus. *J Clin Pharmacol* 2002; **42:** 222–228.

143 Hunninghake D, Insull W, Jr., Toth P, Davidson D, Donovan JM, Burke SK. Coadministration of colesevelam hydrochloride with atorvastatin lowers LDL cholesterol additively. *Atherosclerosis* 2001; **158:** 407–416.

144 Braunlin W, Zhorov E, Guo A, Apruzzese W, Xu Q, Hook P et al. Bile acid binding to sevelamer HCl. *Kidney Int* 2002; **62:** 611–619.

145 Chertow GM, Burke SK, Lazarus JM, Stenzel KH, Wombolt D, Goldberg D et al. Poly[allylamine hydrochloride] (RenaGel): a noncalcemic phosphate binder for the treatment of hyperphosphatemia in chronic renal failure. *Am J Kidney Dis* 1997; **29:** 66–71.

146 Chertow GM, Burke SK, Raggi P. Sevelamer attenuates the progression of coronary and aortic calcification in haemodialysis patients. *Kidney Int* 2002; **62:** 245–252.

147 Jensen RA, Lal SM, Diaz-Arias A, James-Kracke M, Van Stone JC, Ross G, Jr. Does cholestyramine interfere with cyclosporine absorption? A prospective study in renal transplant patients. *ASAIO J* 1995; **41:** M704–M706.

148 Keogh A, Day R, Critchley L, Duggin G, Baron D. The effect of food and cholestyramine in the absorption of cyclosporine in cardiac transplant recipients. *Transplant Proc* 1988; **20:** 27–30.

149 Hodis HN. Triglyceride-rich lipoprotein remnant particles and risk of atherosclerosis. *Circulation* 1999; **99:** 2852–2854.

150 Byrne CD. Triglyceride-rich lipoproteins: are links with atherosclerosis mediated by a procoagulant and proinflammatory phenotype? *Atherosclerosis* 1999; **145:** 1–15.

151 Shoji T, Kawagishi T, Emoto M, Maekawa K, Taniwaki H, Kanda H et al. Additive impacts of diabetes and renal failure on carotid atherosclerosis. *Atherosclerosis* 2000; **153:** 257–258.

152 Shoji T, Nishizawa Y, Kawagishi T, Taniwaki H, Tabata T, Inoue T et al. Intermediate-density lipoprotein as an independent risk factor for aortic atherosclerosis in hemodialysis patients. *J Am Soc Nephrol* 1998; **9:** 1277–1284.

153 Cui Y, Blumenthal RS, Flaws JA, Whiteman MK, Langenberg P, Bachorik PS et al. Non-high-density lipoprotein cholesterol level as a predictor of cardiovascular disease mortality. *Arch Intern Med* 2001; **161:** 1413–1419.

154 Abate N, Vega GL, Grundy SM. Variability in cholesterol content and physical properties of lipoproteins containing apolipoprotein B-100. *Atherosclerosis* 1993; **104:** 159–171.

155 Shoji T, Nishizawa Y, Kawagishi T, Tanaka M, Kawasaki K, Tabata T et al. Atherogenic lipoprotein changes in the absence of hyperlipidemia in patients with chronic renal failure treated by haemodialysis. *Atherosclerosis* 1997; **131:** 229–236.

156 Soroka N, Silverberg DS, Greemland M, Birk Y, Blum M, Peer G et al. Comparison of a vegetable-based (soya) and an animal-based low-protein diet in predialysis chronic renal failure patients. *Nephron* 1998; **79:** 173–180.

157 Khajehdehi P. Lipid-lowering effect of polyunsaturated fatty acids in hemodialysis patients. *J Ren Nutr* 2000; **10:** 191–195.

158 Seri S, D'Alessandro A, Acitelli S, Giammaria U, Cocchi M, Noble RC. Effect of dietary supplementation by alternative oils on blood lipid levels of hemodialysed patients. *Med Sci Res* 1993; **21:** 315–316.

159 Urakaze M, Hamazaki T, Yano S, Kashiwabara H, Oomori K, Yokoyama T. Effect of fish oil concentrate on risk factors of cardiovascular complications in renal transplantation. *Transplant Proc* 1989; **21:** 2134–2136.

160 Maachi K, Berthoux P, Burgard G, Alamartine E, Berthoux F. Results of a 1-year randomized controlled trial with omega-3 fatty acid fish oil in renal transplantation under triple immunosuppressive therapy. *Transplant Proc* 1995; **27:** 846–849.

161 Castro R, Queiròs J, Fonseca I, Pimentel JP, Henriques AC, Sarmento AM et al. Therapy of post-renal transplantation hyperlipidaemia: comparative study with simvastatin and fish oil. *Nephrol Dial Transplant* 1997; **12:** 2140–2143.

162 Abshagen U, Kösters W, Kaufman B, Lang PD. Pharmacokinetics of bezafibrate after single and multiple doses in the presence of renal failure. *Klin Wochenschr* 2001; **58:** 889–896.

163 Goldberg AP, Sherrard DJ, Haas LB, Brunzell JD. Control of clofibrate toxicity in uremic hypertriglyceridaemia. *Clin Pharmacol Ther* 1977; **21:** 317–325.

164 Desager JP, Costermans J, Verberckmoes R, Harvengt C. Effect of hemodialysis on plasma kinetics of fenofibrate in chronic renal failure. *Nephron* 1982; **31:** 51–54.

165 Knauf H, Kolle EU, Mutschler E. Gemfibrozil absorption and elimination in kidney and liver disease. *Klin Wochenschr* 1990; **68:** 692–698.

166 Broeders N, Knoop C, Antoine M, Tielemans C, Abramowicz D. Fibrate-induced increase in blood urea and creatinine: is gemfibrozil the only inonocuous agent? *Nephrol Dial Transplant* 2000; **15:** 1993–1999.

167 Lipscombe J, Lewis GF, Cattran D, Bargman JM. Deterioration in renal function associated with fibrate therapy. *Clin Nephrol* 2001; **55:** 39–44.

168 Seres DS, Strain GW, Hashim SA, Goldberg IJ, Levin NW. Improvement of plasma lipoprotein profiles during high-flux dialysis. *J Am Soc Nephrol* 1993; **3:** 1409–1415.

169 de Precigout V, Higueret D, Larroumet N, Combe C, Iron A, Blanchetier V et al. Improvement in lipid profiles and triglyceride removal in patients on polyamide membrane hemodialysis. *Blood Purif* 1996; **14:** 170–176.

170 Goldberg IJ, Kaufman AM, Lavarias VA, Vanni-Reyes T, Levin NW. High flux dialysis membranes improve plasma lipoprotein profiles in patients with end-stage renal disease. *Nephrol Dial Transplant* 1996; **11(Suppl 2):** 104–107.

171 Blankestijn PJ, Vos PF, Rabelink TJ, van Rijn HJ, Jansen H, Koomans HA et al. High-flux dialysis membranes improve lipid profile in chronic haemodialysis patients. *J Am Soc Nephrol* 1995; **5:** 1703–1708.

172 Pollock CA, Wyndham R, Collett PV, Elder G, Field MJ, Kalowski S et al. Effects of erythropoietin therapy on the lipid profile in end-stage renal failure. *Kidney Int* 1994; **45:** 897–902.

173 Baigent C, Landray M, Leaper C, Altmann P, Armitage J, Baxter A et al. First United Kingdom Heart and Renal Protection (UK-HARP-I) study: biochemical efficacy and safety of simvastatin and safety of low-dose aspirin in chronic kidney disease. *Am J Kidney Dis* 2005; **45:** 473–484.

174 Landray M, Baigent C, Leaper C, Adu D, Altmann P, Armitage J et al. The second United Kingdom Heart and Renal Protection (UK-HARP-II) Study: a randomized controlled study of the biochemical safety and efficacy of adding ezetimibe to simvastatin as initial therapy among patients with CKD. *Am J Kidney Dis* 2006; **47:** 385–395.

175 Buchanan C, Smith L, Corbett J, Nelson E, Shihab F. A retrospective analysis of ezetimibe treatment in renal transplant recipients. *Am J Transplant* 2006; **6:** 770–774.

176 Quaschning T, Krane V, Metzger T, Wanner C. Abnormalities in uremic lipoprotein metabolism and its impact on cardiovascular disease. *Am J Kidney Dis* 2001; **38(Suppl1):** S14–S19.

33 Chronic Kidney Disease and Hypertension

Sangeetha Satyan[1] & Rajiv Agarwal[1,2]
[1] Division of Nephrology, Department of Medicine, Indiana University School of Medicine, Indianapolis, USA
[2] Richard L. Roudebush, VA Medical Center, Indianapolis, USA

Hypertension (HTN) is very common among patients with chronic kidney disease (CKD). Using ambulatory blood pressure (BP) monitoring in patients with CKD, Andersen *et al.* [1] found that in 232 veterans, 35% had isolated systolic HTN, 3% had isolated diastolic HTN, 27% had combined systolic and diastolic HTN, and 35% had normotension or well-controlled BP. Elevated BP is an important cardiovascular (CV) risk factor in the general population as well as in those with CKD. In addition, high BP is a well-recognized risk factor for the development and progression of kidney disease. The prevalence of end-stage renal disease (ESRD) is rising rapidly. Physicians are confronted with a major challenge of preventing ESRD among patients with CKD, and treatment of HTN is a cornerstone for such intervention. Several prospective trials have been performed to determine the goal BP, outcome, and choice of antihypertensive therapy in patients with HTN and CKD. The optimal level of BP in CKD is still unclear despite the numerous studies. Based on the available data, the National Kidney Foundation (NKF) [2] and the Joint National Committee (JNC) [3] have recommended a goal BP of less than 130/80 mmHg in patients with CKD. In this chapter we discuss the rationale for these recommendations.

CKD burden in the general population

The burden of CKD in the general population is increasingly acknowledged. In a cross-sectional study of 16,589 adults aged 17 years and older (Third National Health and Nutrition Examination Survey, conducted from 1988 to 1994), 3% had elevated serum creatinine, defined as ≥ 1.6 mg/dL for men and ≥ 1.4 mg/dL for women [4]. HTN, defined as BP of $\geq 140/90$ mmHg or use of antihypertensive medications, was noted in 70% of these individuals. What was more astonishing was the fact that among the hypertensive individuals, only 11% had a BP of <130/85 mmHg (the goal

Evidence-based Nephrology. Edited by Donald Molony and Jonathan Craig
© 2009 Blackwell Publishing, ISBN: 978-1-4051-3975-5.

BP for CKD without proteinuria, as recommended by JNC-6). In each category of BP, elevated serum creatinine was more prevalent among treated than untreated individuals with HTN, and the relationship between elevated serum creatinine and BP was linear among untreated individuals and was J-shaped among treated individuals. Despite the inherent limitations of this cross-sectional study and that the data signified an association rather than causation, the study revealed a high burden of CKD in the general population and the suboptimal control of BP in such individuals.

Misclassification of HTN with BP monitoring in clinic

Measurement of BP via a sphygmomanometer and a stethoscope is the most common method for estimation of arterial pressure in a clinical practice. Clinical diagnosis and HTN management are based almost entirely on office measurements. However, these measurements may be prognostically less reliable than BP obtained outside the office setting. When home BP monitoring (self-measured BP) is performed, HTN is less frequently misclassified and better correlation is achieved with putative markers of kidney disease progression [5]. Masked HTN, that is, normotension in the clinic and HTN at home, is associated with higher risk of ESRD in patients with CKD [5]. Conversely, "white coat" HTN, which is HTN in the clinic and normotension at home, is associated with better renal outcomes. Ambulatory BP monitoring is also prognostically superior to clinic BP but does not further refine the prognosis made by home BP monitoring [6]. In patients on hemodialysis, home BP, not the predialysis and postdialysis BP values, shares a combination of high sensitivity and high specificity of greater than 80% to make a diagnosis of HTN with the reference standard of ambulatory BP monitoring [7]. In addition, home BP is a better predictor of left ventricular hypertrophy in patients on hemodialysis compared with peridialysis BP [8]. These data suggest that self-measurement of BP by patients with CKD can serve as a useful addition to assessing the level of HTN control and prognosis.

Role of angiotensin converting enzyme inhibitors and angiotensin II receptor blockers in CKD and HTN

A significant interaction between proteinuria and BP has been delineated among patients with CKD and HTN that seems to be important especially with reference to outcomes. The introduction of agents blocking the renin–angiotensin–aldosterone system was an important milestone in the management of patients with CKD and HTN, particularly in those with diabetes mellitus and proteinuria. Drugs inhibiting the renin–angiotensin system have the added benefit of reducing glomerular HTN and other nonhemodynamic benefits. In addition, angiotensin converting enzyme inhibitors (ACEi) preferentially improve arterial stiffness and lower central aortic pressures more than beta-blockers or calcium channel blockers, which may offer an additional mechanism of improvement in CV outcomes seen with this class of drugs [9].

Diabetic nephropathy is a major cause of ESRD and enhances the mortality rate in the diabetic population. A landmark study by Lewis *et al.* [10] provided initial evidence that use of an ACEi (captopril) in patients with type 1 diabetes mellitus and proteinuria of $\geq$500 mg/day was superior to placebo in preventing the progression of kidney disease and lessened the mortality and ESRD rates. There was no significant difference in BP control in the two groups. Proteinuria reduction was overall greater in the captopril group than in the placebo group. The study led to the widespread use of ACEi in diabetic nephropathy. Whether ACEi would be equally beneficial in those with less or no proteinuria was not answered by this study.

The benefit of ACEi in nondiabetic nephropathies has been shown in several studies. The Italian investigators of the Ramipril Efficacy in Nephropathy (REIN) study reported that among patients with chronic nondiabetic nephropathies, ramipril was superior to conventional antihypertensive therapy in attenuating the loss of renal function over the long term [11,12]. The GFR decline per month was significantly lowered with ramipril among patients with baseline proteinuria of >3 g/day, even during the short follow-up, but not in those with baseline proteinuria of 1–2.9 g/day. However, ramipril was more effective in reducing proteinuria and progression to ESRD, even in patients with non-nephrotic-range proteinuria. The goal BP in this study was <90 mmHg diastolic BP, which at the time of the study was the recommended target for these patients. Thus, pretreatment proteinuria is highly predictive of the benefit of ACEi on long-term kidney function, with a greater benefit in those with higher proteinuria. ACEi gained a pivotal role in preventing progression of CKD in both diabetic and nondiabetic nephropathies, with benefits extending beyond BP reduction and became the mainstream treatment in CKD.

The Irbesartan Diabetic Nephropathy Trial (IDNT) assessed the role of irbesartan, an angiotensin II receptor blocker (ARB), in slowing the progression of nephropathy (median urine protein excretion of 2.9 g/day) in patients with type 2 diabetes [13]. Irbesartan, compared to placebo and amlodipine, significantly lowered the risk of doubling of serum creatinine and development of ESRD. These results could not be explained by differences in the mean arterial pressure (MAP) during follow-up. The MAP was significantly higher by 3.3 mmHg in the placebo group than the irbesartan and amlodipine groups. Proteinuria reduction on average was 33, 6, and 10% in the irbesartan, amlodipine, and placebo groups, respectively. The overall mortality and CV event rates were not significantly different between the groups. Irbesartan was well-tolerated.

In another study of patients with nephropathy and HTN associated with type 2 diabetes (RENAAL), losartan, compared to placebo, resulted in a 16% risk reduction in the composite end point of doubling of serum creatinine, ESRD, or death [14]. Overall mortality and morbidity and mortality from CV causes were similar in the two groups. There was no significant difference in the BP between the two groups at the end of the study, although the losartan group had a significantly lower MAP at the end of 1 year. Albuminuria reduction on average was about 35% in the losartan group, whereas it increased in the placebo group ($P < 0.001$ between the groups). The ARBs in these two studies involving patients with nephropathy from type 2 diabetes led to significant improvement in the renal outcomes that was beyond that attributable to BP reduction and appeared to be in part related to albuminuria reduction. Two post hoc analyses from this trial demonstrated that baseline albuminuria and reduction in albuminuria were predictive of primary outcome, ESRD outcome, CV outcomes, and hospitalization due to heart failure [15,16]. Whether ARB is superior to ACEi in patients with nephropathy from type 2 diabetes is unclear, but certainly remains an obvious alternative to those who do not tolerate ACEi. ACEi could be used when ARBs are cost prohibitive.

BP level and progression of nephropathy

Post hoc analysis of the RENAAL study was also done to evaluate the impact of systolic BP on renal outcomes [17]. A baseline systolic BP of 140–159 mmHg, compared to <130 mmHg, increased the risk of ESRD or death by 38%. In a multivariate model that also included the urinary albumin/creatinine ratio, each 10-mmHg rise in baseline systolic BP increased the risk for ESRD or death by 6.7%; a similar rise in diastolic BP decreased the risk by 10.9%. Thus, the predictive capability for renal outcomes is stronger for baseline systolic BP and widening pulse pressure in patients with nephropathy from type 2 diabetes. Among patients with a baseline pulse pressure of >90 mmHg, the losartan group compared to the placebo group had a 53.5% and 35.5% risk reduction for ESRD alone and ESRD or death, respectively. One explanation for these favorable results may be the known effects of ARBs on improvement in central pressures and arterial stiffness [18].

Goal BP in CKD and HTN

The Modification of Diet in Renal Disease (MDRD) study tested whether dietary protein restriction and BP control delayed the progression of renal disease [19,20] (Table 33.1). Patients with insulin-requiring diabetes were excluded, and ACEi use was encouraged but was not mandatory. Although the mean decline in the GFR was overall not significantly different between the two groups in either study (Table 33.1), a higher follow-up MAP was significantly associated with a faster decline in GFR. In the first study, GFR decline was steeper for MAP of >98 mmHg in those with baseline proteinuria of 0.25–3.0 g/day and for MAP of >92 mmHg in those with proteinuria of ≥3 g/day. In the second study (more advanced CKD), GFR decline demonstrated an inverse relationship with follow-up BP only for patients with baseline proteinuria of ≥1 g/day. In addition, there was a significant reduction in proteinuria in the low-BP groups in both studies. The studies signified the importance of BP control in ameliorating GFR decline, particularly in those with proteinuria, even in patients without insulin-requiring diabetes. This led to the JNC-6 guideline of target BP of <125/75 mmHg in those with proteinuria of ≥1 g/day. However, there was a disproportionate use of ACEi in the usual BP and low target BP groups, 32% and 51%, respectively, which could have contributed to the observed results.

After the completion of the MDRD study, which was conducted from 1989 to 1993, those patients were followed long-term through 2000 in an observational fashion, and no specific target BP was mandated [21]. ESRD developed in 62% in the low BP target (MAP <92 mmHg) and 70% in the usual BP target (MAP 102–107 mmHg) groups. The adjusted hazard ratios in the low BP group for ESRD and the composite outcome of ESRD or all-cause death were 0.68 ($P < 0.001$) and 0.77 ($P = 0.0024$), respectively. These results did not vary considerably after adjustment for ACEi use. However, there were no BP measurements during the long-term follow-up, and therefore the exact mechanism by which assignment to the low BP group resulted in these better outcomes is unclear.

The REIN-2 trial tested whether BP lowering in addition to ACE inhibition is beneficial in CKD [22]. Patients with nondiabetic proteinuric nephropathies who were already being treated with ramipril were randomized to either conventional (diastolic BP <90 mmHg) or intensified (BP < 130/80 mmHg) BP control. Felodipine was used in the intensive treatment group to further lower the BP. Concomitant antihypertensive drugs were used in both groups as needed to attain target BP. Urinary protein excretion was similar in both groups at baseline and throughout follow-up. BP decreased from 137/84 to 130/80 mmHg ($P < 0.0001$) in the intensified BP control group and from 136/84 to 134/82 mmHg in the conventional control group ($P = 0.02$ for systolic and 0.03 for diastolic BP). A separation in MAP by about 3 mmHg was maintained throughout the study. The study was stopped after a short follow-up based on futility. There was no significant difference in the percentage of patients reaching ESRD in the two groups (23% vs. 20%; $P = 0.99$). The median rate of GFR decline was similar in both groups throughout the study period. However, as expected, GFR decline was slower in patients with <3-g/day proteinuria than in those with >3-g/day proteinuria (0.19 mL/min/month vs. 0.49 mL/min/month; $P = 0.001$). These results suggest that the use of felodipine to further lower the BP does not confer renal protection in nondiabetic patients with overt proteinuria. The study provokes the thought that perhaps one should focus on variables other than BP, such as protein excretion, to evaluate the renoprotective effects of drugs.

In the African American Study of Kidney disease and HTN (AASK), patients with hypertensive renal disease were assigned to MAP goals of 102–107 mmHg and ≤92 mmHg [23]. The achieved BP was on average 128/78 mmHg and 141/85 mmHg, respectively, in the low and usual BP groups, with a mean separation in MAP of approximately 10 mmHg throughout the follow-up. There was no significant difference between the two groups in the GFR slope or the composite outcome (GFR decline of ≥50% from baseline, ESRD, or death). Thus, the low BP goal in this study had no added benefit in improving renal outcome. GFR decline was significantly lower in patients with baseline urinary protein/creatinine ratios of ≤0.22 compared to those with a ratio of >0.22. No significant differences in all-cause and cardiovascular mortality were noted between the groups. The results of this study do not support the low BP goal in African Americans with hypertensive renal disease in terms of decreasing the rate of GFR decline and the composite outcome. However, the study did not have sufficient power to identify differences in mortality and ESRD. Although cardiovascular outcomes were not an end point of the study, subsequent analyses of the AASK trial did not show a significant effect of BP level on cardiovascular events [24]. The hazard ratios in the low versus usual BP goal comparison for CV deaths, CV composite outcome (first CV hospitalizations and CV deaths), CV composite outcome or ESRD, and all CV events, respectively, were 0.98 (95% confidence interval [CI], 0.48–2.01; $P = 0.96$), 0.84 (95% CI, 0.61–1.16; $P = 0.29$), 0.91 (95% CI, 0.72–1.15; $P = 0.42$), and 1.06 (95% CI, 0.76–1.49; $P = 0.73$). These findings of no apparent benefit could have been due to the inadequate power of the study.

The NKF guidelines for HTN recommend a goal BP of < 130/80 mmHg for all patients with CKD and HTN [2]. A patient-level meta-analysis supports the need for systolic BP control to 110–129 mmHg in patients with CKD and proteinuria of greater than 1 g/day [25]. These guidelines seem reasonable considering the available data. However, an individualized approach needs to be taken for each patient with CKD in determining the goal BP. For example, a more aggressive reduction in BP and nonpharmacologic measures may be attempted in patients who have persistent proteinuria or increasing proteinuria.

Choice of antihypertensive therapy in CKD and HTN

The benefits of ACEi and ARB in CKD among diabetic and nondiabetic patients with proteinuria and HTN were described above.

Table 33.1 Trials reporting outcomes in patients with HTN and CKD

Study	Primary Aim	Total number of patients randomized n	Study Population	Study Design	Outcomes evaluated	Duration of follow-up	Results	Reference
The effect of Angiotensin-Converting Enzyme Inhibition on Diabetic Nephropathy	To determine whether captopril has kidney-protecting properties independent of its effect on BP in diabetic nephropathy	409	Age: 18–49; IDDM for at least 7 years; serum creatinine $\leq$2.5 mg/dl; Urine protein excretion $\geq$ 500 mg/24 hours	DBRCT in 30 centers; Captopril 25 mg po tid (n = 207), Placebo (n = 202); Goal SBP < 140 mm Hg, DBP < 90 mm Hg	Primary end point -Doubling of baseline serum creatinine to at least 2.0 mg/dl ; Secondary end points - Length of time to the combined end points of death, dialysis, and transplantation and changes in renal function	Median: 3 years	Serum creatinine doubled in 25 patients in the captopril gp, vs 43 patients in the placebo gp (P = 0.007). The risk reduction in the captopril gp was 48% as a whole, and 78% in the subset of patients with a baseline serum creatinine of 2.0 mg/dl. Risk reduction was 50% for the combined end point in the captopril group.	10
The effects of dietary protein restriction and BP control on the progression of CKD (MDRD)	To test whether restricting protein and controlling HTN delay the progression of renal disease	Study 1–585; Study 2–255	Age: 18–70; Serum creatinine: (M) 1.4–7.0; (F) 1.2–7.0 mg/dl; MAP $\leq$ 125 mm Hg; Study 1–GFR–25–55 ml/min, Study 2–GFR–13–24 ml/min. Insulin requiring diabetics and those with proteinuria > 10 g/d were excluded.	RCT in 15 centers. Assigned to a usual (MAP $\leq$ 107 mm hg) or low (MAP $\leq$ 92 mm Hg) BP group; to usual or low-protein diet (study 1) and low and verylow protein diet (study 2) groups. Step-wise approach of pharmacologic therapy for BP was used, and ACEI were encouraged as agents of first choice	Primary outcome: Decline in GFR measured by i-iothalamate clearance, stratified by BP and proteinuria	Mean: 2.2 years	The mean decline in GFR was overall not significantly different in both studies. Among patients with higher baseline proteinuria, the low-BP group had a significantly slower rate of GFR decline in both studies.	20
Effect of Ramipril on decline in GFR and risk of terminal renal failure in proteinuric, non-diabetic nephropathy (REIN)	To test the hypothesis that glomerular protein traffic, and its modification by an ACEI, influences renal disease progression	352	Age : 18–70; Cr Cl 20–70 ml/min with variation < 30% in previous 3 months, Urine protein excretion > 1g/24 hrs for at least 3 months, no ACEI for at least 2 months before study	DBRCT; Urine protein 1–2.9g/24h (stratum 1, n = 186); $\geq$ 3g/24h (stratum 2, n = 166); Randomized to ramipril (1.25 mg) or placebo. Dose increased every 2 weeks for a goal DBP < 90 mm Hg. Other agents used as needed to achieve goal BP	Primary outcome: Rate of GFR decline measured by iohxol clearance. Secondary outcomes: urinary protein excretion, and serum creatinine concentration. Intention to treat analyses.	Mean: 16 months (stratum 2); Median : 31 months (stratum 1)	Stratum 2 : The GFR decline per month was significantly lower in the ramipril than the placebo group (0.53 vs 0.88 ml/min, p = 0.03). Significant reduction in proteinuria in the ramipril group that correlated inversely with GFR decline. Stratum 1: The GFR decline per month not significantly different (ramipril 0.26 vs. placebo 0.29 ml/min, p = 0.06). Significant reduction in proteinuria and progression to ESRD in the ramipril group.	11,12
Renoprotective effect of irbesartan in patients with nephropathy due to type-2 diabetes (IDNT)	To determine whether the use of an ARB or a CCB would provide protection against the progression of nephropathy due to type 2 diabetes beyond that attributable to the lowering of the BP	1715	Age: 30–70; type 2 DM, HTN–BP > 135/85 or use of antihypertensive agents, urinary protein excretion of at least 900 mg/24 hours, serum creatinine–(M) 1.2–3.0 mg/dl, (F) 1–3 mg/dl	DBRCT in 210 clinical centers; Randomized to irbesartan (n = 579, dose titration 75–300 mg/day); Amlodipine (n = 567, dose titration 2.5–10 mg/day); or placebo (n = 569)	Primary end point: Composite of a doubling of the base-line serum creatinine, onset of ESRD, or death. Secondary outcome: combined cardiovascular end point.	Mean: 2.6 years	The risk of the primary composite end point in the irbesartan group was 20% and 23% lower than the placebo (p = 0.02) and amlodipine (P = 0.006) groups respectively. No significant differences in death rates from any cause or the CV composite end point.	13

Study	n	Objective	Population	Design	Endpoints	Duration	Results	Ref
Effects of BP level on progression of diabetic nephropathy (RENAAL)	1513	To assess the role of the angiotensin-II-receptor antagonist losartan in patients with type 2 diabetes and nephropathy	Age–31–70, type 2 diabetes and nephropathy (urine albumin/creatinine ratio of atleast 300 mg/g or proteinuria of at least 0.5 g/day), serum creatinine 1.3–3.0 mg/dl	DBRCT, multinational study, randomized to losartan (50 mg–100 mg daily) or placebo, stratified by baseline protenuria (urine albumin-to-creatinine ratio <2000 mg/g or ≥ 2000 mg/g). Additional open-label agents used as needed for goal BP <140/90 mm Hg.	Primary composite end point: Time to doubling of serum creatinine, ESRD, or death, whichever occurred first. Secondary end points: composite of morbidity and mortality from cardiovascular causes, protenuria, and the rate of progression of renal disease.	Mean: 3.4 years	Osartan had a 16% risk reduction in the primary end point than placebo (p = 0.02). Similar rates of death, and cardiovascular morbidity and mortality in the 2 groups. Losartan had a 35% reduction in proteinuria (p < 0.001, compared to placebo)	14
Effect of BP lowering and antihypertensive drug class on progression of hypertensive kidney disease (AASK)	1094	To compare effects of 2 levels of BP control and 3 antihypertensive drug classes on GFR decline in African Americans with HTN	Age–17–80; African Americans; HTN; GFR 20–65 ml/min; non-diabetics.	3 × 2 factorial design; randomized to usual (102–107 mm Hg) or lower (<92 mm Hg) MAP goal. Treatment with metoprolol, 50–200 mg/d; ramipril, 2.5–10 mg/d; or amlodipine, 5–10 mg/d assigned in 2:2:1 ratio. Additional open-labeled agents added sequentially.	Primary: Rate of change in GFR (GFR slope–acute and chronic). Secondary clinical composite outcome: GFR reduction by 50% or by 25 ml/min from baseline, ESRD, or death.Other secondary outcomes: urine protein excretion, all CVE.	3–6.4 years	There was no significant difference in mean GFR slope from baseline through 4 years in the 2 BP gps and the drug gp comparisons. The secondary clinical composite outcome was similar in the 2 BP groups, but the ramipril gp had a 22% reduction compared to the other drug gps.	23, 26
Effects of BP level on progression of diabetic nephropathy (post hoc analyses of RENAAL)	1513	To evaluate the impact of baseline and treated SBP, DBP, and PP, to assess the specific effect of losartan, and the implications of dihydropyridine calcium channel blockers as concurrent therapy on composite and individual outcomes in patients with type 2 diabetes and nephropathy	Age–31–70, type 2 diabetes and nephropathy (urine albumin/creatinine ratio of atleast 300 mg/g or proteinuria of at least 0.5 g/day), serum creatinine 1.3–3.0 mg/dl	DBRCT, multinational study, randomized to losartan (50 mg–100 mg daily) or placebo, stratified by baseline proteinuria (urine albumin-to-creatinine ratio <2000 mg/g or ≥ 2000 mg/g). Additional open-label agents used as needed for goal BP < 140/90 mm Hg.	Primary composite end point: Time to doubling of serum creatinine, ESRD, or death, whichever occurred first.	Mean: 3.4 years	Baseline SBP of 140-159 mm Hg, compared to SBP <130 mm Hg increased risk for ESRD or death by 38% (p = 0.05). Patients randomized to the losartan group with a baseline PP > 90 mm hg had a 35.5% risk reduction for ESRD or death (p = 0.02) compared to the placebo gp.	17
Blood-pressure control for renoprotection in patients with non-diabetic chronic renal disease (REIN -2)	338	To assess the effect of intensified vs. conventional BP control on progression to ESRD in patients with non-diabetic proteinuric nephropathies	Age 18–70, non-diabetic nephropathy with persistent proteinuria (> 1g/24 hours for at least 3 months). Proteinuria of 1-3 g if cr cl <45 ml/min, and proteinuria ≥ 3 g if cr cl <70 ml/min	Multicenter RCT. All received background ACEI therapy with ramipril. Randomized to conventional (DBP <90 mm Hg) or intensified (BP <130/80 mm Hg) BP control. Add-on therapy with felodipine in the intensified BP group.	Primary outcome: Time to ESRD over 36 months follow-up. Secondary aims: To compare the effects of two different levels of BP control on GFR decline, residual proteinuria, and fatal and non-fatal CVE.	Median: 19 months	No significant difference in the progression to ESRD in the 2 BP gps (p = 0.99). No difference in the secondary outcomes between the two groups.	22

(continued)

Table 33.1 (cont.)

Study	Total number of patients randomized n	Primary Aim	Study Population	Study Design	Outcomes evaluated	Duration of follow-up	Results	Reference
Renal outcomes in high-risk hypertensive patients treated with an ACEI or a CCB vs a diuretic (ALLHAT post hoc analyses)	33357	To determine whether, in high-risk hypertensive patients with a reduced GFR, treatment with a CCB or an ACEI lowers the incidence of renal disease outcomes compared with treatment with a diuretic	Age ≥ 55, Stage 1 or 2 HTN with at least 1 other CAD risk factor, serum creatinine <2 mg/dl	DBRCT, post hoc analyses, randomized to receive chlorthalidone (12.5–25 mg/d), amlodipine (2.5–10 mg/d), or lisinopril (10–40 mg/d) in a 1.7:1:1 ratio. Goal BP < 140/90 in each arm by adding open-label agents as needed. Stratified by baseline e GFR.	Clinical renal outcomes: Development of ESRD or death from kidney disease; composite end point of ESRD or ≥ 50% decline in GFR from baseline; mean GFR during study follow-up.	Mean: 4.9 years	No significant difference in the outcomes in patients taking chlorthalidone compared to those who received lisinopril or amlodipine, irrespective of the baseline GFR.	27
Effect of a lower target BP on the progression of kidney disease: Long-term follow-up of the MDRD study (post hoc analyses)	840	To assess the effects of a low target BP on kidney failure and all-cause mortality	Age: 18–70; Serum creatinine: (M) 1.4–7.0; (F) 1.2–7.0 mg/dl; MAP ≤ 125 mm Hg; Study A–GFR–25–55 ml/min, Study B–GFR–13–24 ml/min	Long term follow-up of patients from 1993 to 2000, after the MDRD study ended (See above for MDRD study design).	Outcomes: Kidney failure and a composite outcome of kidney failure or all-cause mortality, through extended follow-up	Approx. 7 years (1993–2000)	The adjusted hazard ratios in the low target BP group compared with the usual target BP group were 0.68 and 0.77 for development of kidney failure and the composite outcome respectively.	21

In the AASK trial (Table 33.1), patients were randomized to initial treatment with a beta blocker (metoprolol), ACEi (ramipril), or a dihydropyridine calcium channel blocker (amlodipine) [23,26]. Additional open-label agents were used to achieve the BP goals. In an interim analysis following discontinuation of the amlodipine intervention for safety reasons [26], ramipril compared to amlodipine was associated with a 36% slower mean GFR decline over 3 years and a 48% risk reduction of the clinical end points. However, the risk reduction was profoundly influenced by the subgroup of patients with baseline proteinuria. Among patients with no baseline proteinuria or with GFR of ≥ 40 mL/min, there was no difference in the GFR decline between the two groups at the end of the follow-up and GFR remained slightly higher in the amlodipine group than the ramipril group. Follow-up systolic BP was 2 mmHg lower for the amlodipine group than the other groups.

In the ramipril versus metoprolol comparison following the completion of the study [23], the mean GFR decline was slower during the acute phase with ramipril than with metoprolol (ramipril, -0.23 vs. metoprolol, -1.73 mL/min/1.73 m^2; $P = 0.01$). During the 4-year follow-up, GFR decline was marginally better in the ramipril group (-1.81 vs. 2.42 mL/min/1.73 m^2/year; $P = 0.07$). However, the chronic GFR slopes were similar between the two groups (ramipril, -1.87, vs. metoprolol, -2.12; $P = 0.25$). In the amlodipine versus metoprolol comparison, GFR increased in the amlodipine group during the acute phase (4.03 mL/min/1.73 m^2 -1.73 mL/min/1.73 m^2; $P < 0.001$). However, the decline in GFR was faster during the chronic phase in the amlodipine group (-3.22 mL/min/1.73 m^2) compared to the metoprolol group (-2.33 mL/min/1.73 m^2; $P = 0.02$).

GFR decline was significantly slower during the 3-year follow-up in the amlodipine group than the metoprolol group (1.60 vs. 2.68 mL/min/year; $P = 0.004$), which was primarily a reflection of the change during the acute phase, which was likely a hemodynamic response. The beneficial effect on GFR in the amlodipine group during the acute phase and total GFR slopes was significantly related to baseline proteinuria and occurred only if the baseline urine protein/creatinine ratio was 0.22 or less. This interaction of baseline proteinuria was not significant for the chronic slope or the clinical composite outcome. However, among patients with baseline urine protein/creatinine ratios of > 0.22, the metoprolol group compared with the amlodipine group had a risk reduction of 38% ($P = 0.03$) for the main composite outcome. In addition, mean declines in GFR were smaller for patients with higher baseline GFR but larger for those with lower baseline GFR in the amlodipine group compared with metoprolol groups. The risk reduction for the main clinical composite outcome with ramipril was 22% compared to metoprolol. Overall, although there was no difference among the three drug regimens in the primary analysis of the GFR slope, ramipril was more beneficial than the other two drugs in slowing progression of hypertensive kidney disease based on the results of secondary analyses. Metoprolol may be superior to amlodipine in improving renal outcomes, particularly among those with higher proteinuria and lower baseline GFR in African Americans with hypertensive kidney disease. Subsequent

analyses showed no difference in CV outcomes in the three drug groups [24]. The hazard ratios for CV deaths in the ramipril versus metoprolol, amlodipine versus metoprolol, and ramipril versus amlodipine comparisons were 1.06 (95% CI, 0.47–2.39), 1.18 (95% CI, 0.46–3.04), and 0.90 (95% CI, 0.35–2.30), respectively. The hazard ratios for CV composite outcomes (first CV hospitalizations and CV deaths) in the respective comparisons were 0.98 (95% CI, 0.69–1.39), 0.77 (95% CI, 0.48–1.24), and 1.27 (95% CI, 0.78–2.06) (P not significant, all comparisons).

In the REIN-2 trial [121], addition of the dihydropyridine calcium channel blocker felodipine for treatment of patients with nondiabetic proteinuric nephropathies receiving ACEi therapy (ramipril) did not slow the progression to ESRD or GFR decline and did not reduce proteinuria. The patients had a baseline GFR of about 35 mL/min and urine protein excretion of about 2.9 g/day.

Post hoc analysis of the ALLHAT study [27] assessed whether therapy with a calcium channel blocker (amlodipine) or an ACEi (lisinopril) improved the renal outcomes compared to a diuretic (chlorthalidone) among patients with HTN stratified by baseline estimated GFR (GFR, ≥ 90 mL/min, 60–89 mL/min, and < 60 mL/min). All three groups required additional antihypertensive medications to achieve a target BP of $< 140/90$ mmHg. The ALLHAT study had 33,357 participants, of whom about 17% had CKD. Proteinuria was not measured, and patients with baseline creatinine of > 2 mg/dL were excluded. The baseline estimated GFR was 3–6 mL/min higher in the amlodipine group than the other two groups. Compared with the chlorthalidone group, the incidence of ESRD was not significantly different in the lisinopril or amlodipine groups across the three GFR groups for the total group or for participants who had diabetes at baseline. The major limitation of this analysis is the lack of information on baseline proteinuria.

The results, however, do not nullify conclusions from several other studies that ACEi or ARBs, usually in combination with a diuretic, slow the progression of kidney disease better than the other hypertensive agents. Moreover, BP control in CKD usually requires two or more antihypertensive agents.

Conclusions

Renoprotective strategies include both BP and proteinuria reduction in addition to others. Nonpharmacologic therapies, such as sodium restriction, weight loss, and increased physical activity, play a significant role in BP reduction in such patients. Proper use of diuretics is important for regulating the volume status and thus improving BP in these patients. Although ACEi and ARBs have a key role in BP and proteinuria reduction in CKD, they almost always require the addition of diuretics and other agents to achieve adequate BP. We need novel therapies and innovative approaches to prevent ESRD and to decrease mortality in patients with CKD. An individualized approach is recommended in managing patients with CKD and HTN. Studies determining outcomes in CKD using home BP and ambulatory BP measurements would be very informative.

References

1 Andersen MJ, Khawandi W, Agarwal R. Home blood pressure monitoring in CKD. *Am J Kidney Dis* 2005; **45(6):** 994–1001.

2 K/DOQI clinical practice guidelines on hypertension and antihypertensive agents in chronic kidney disease. *Am J Kidney Dis* 2004; **43(5 Suppl 1):** S1–S290.

3 Chobanian AV, Bakris GL, Black HR, Cushman WC, Green LA, Izzo JL, Jr., *et al.* Seventh report of the Joint National Committee on Prevention, Detection, Evaluation, and Treatment of High Blood Pressure. *Hypertension* 2003; **42(6):** 1206–1252.

4 Coresh J, Wei GL, McQuillan G, Brancati FL, Levey AS, Jones C *et al.* Prevalence of high blood pressure and elevated serum creatinine level in the United States: findings from the third National Health and Nutrition Examination Survey (1988–1994). *Arch Intern Med* 2001; **161(9):** 1207–1216.

5 Agarwal R, Andersen MJ, Bishu K, Saha C. Home blood pressure monitoring improves the diagnosis of hypertension in hemodialysis patients. *Kidney Int* 2006; **69(5):** 900–906.

6 Agarwal R, Andersen MJ. Prognostic importance of ambulatory blood pressure recordings in patients with chronic kidney disease. *Kidney Int* 2006; **69(7):** 1175–1180.

7 Agarwal R, Andersen MJ, Bishu K, Saha C. Home blood pressure monitoring improves the diagnosis of hypertension in hemodialysis patients. *Kidney Int* 2006; **69(5):** 900–906.

8 Agarwal R, Brim NJ, Mahenthiran J, Andersen MJ, Saha C. Out-of-hemodialysis-unit blood pressure is a superior determinant of left ventricular hypertrophy. *Hypertension* 2006; **47(1):** 62–68.

9 Guerin AP, Blacher J, Pannier B, Marchais SJ, Safar ME, London GM. Impact of aortic stiffness attenuation on survival of patients in end-stage renal failure. *Circulation* 2001; **103(7):** 987–992.

10 Lewis EJ, Hunsicker LG, Bain RP, Rohde RD. The effect of angiotensin-converting-enzyme inhibition on diabetic nephropathy. The Collaborative Study Group. *N Engl J Med* 1993; **329(20):** 1456–1462.

11 The GISEN Group (Gruppo Italiano di Studi Epidemiologici in Nefrologia). Randomised placebo-controlled trial of effect of ramipril on decline in glomerular filtration rate and risk of terminal renal failure in proteinuric, non-diabetic nephropathy. *Lancet* 1997; **349(9069):** 1857–1863.

12 Ruggenenti P, Perna A, Gherardi G, Garini G, Zoccali C, Salvadori M *et al.* Renoprotective properties of ACE-inhibition in non-diabetic nephropathies with non-nephrotic proteinuria. *Lancet* 1999; **354(9176):** 359–364.

13 Lewis EJ, Hunsicker LG, Clarke WR, Berl T, Pohl MA, Lewis JB *et al.* Renoprotective effect of the angiotensin-receptor antagonist irbesartan in patients with nephropathy due to type 2 diabetes. *N Engl J Med* 2001; **345(12):** 851–860.

14 Brenner BM, Cooper ME, de Zeeuw D, Keane WF, Mitch WE, Parving HH *et al.* Effects of losartan on renal and cardiovascular outcomes in patients with type 2 diabetes and nephropathy. *N Engl J Med* 2001; **345(12):** 861–869.

15 de Zeeuw D., Remuzzi G, Parving HH, Keane WF, Zhang Z, Shahinfar S *et al.* Albuminuria, a therapeutic target for cardiovascular protection in type 2 diabetic patients with nephropathy. *Circulation* 2004; **110(8):** 921–927.

16 de Zeeuw D, Ramjit D, Zhang Z, Ribeiro AB, Kurokawa K, Lash JP *et al.* Renal risk and renoprotection among ethnic groups with type 2 diabetic nephropathy: a post hoc analysis of RENAAL. *Kidney Int* 2006; **69(9):** 1675–1682.

17 Bakris GL, Weir MR, Shanifar S, Zhang Z, Douglas J, van Dijk DJ *et al.* Effects of blood pressure level on progression of diabetic nephropathy: results from the RENAAL study. *Arch Intern Med* 2003; **163(13):** 1555–1565.

18 Ichihara A, Kaneshiro Y, Takemitsu T, Sakoda M, Itoh H. Benefits of candesartan on arterial and renal damage of non-diabetic hypertensive patients treated with calcium channel blockers. *Am J Nephrol* 2006; **26(5):** 462–468.

19 Peterson JC, Adler S, Burkart JM, Greene T, Hebert LA, Hunsicker LG *et al.* Blood pressure control, proteinuria, and the progression of renal disease. The Modification of Diet in Renal Disease Study. *Ann Intern Med* 1995; **123(10):** 754–762.

20 Klahr S, Levey AS, Beck GJ, Caggiula AW, Hunsicker L, Kusek JW *et al.* The effects of dietary protein restriction and blood-pressure control on the progression of chronic renal disease. Modification of Diet in Renal Disease Study Group. *N Engl J Med* 1994; **330(13):** 877–884.

21 Sarnak MJ, Greene T, Wang X, Beck G, Kusek JW, Collins AJ *et al.* The effect of a lower target blood pressure on the progression of kidney disease: long-term follow-up of the modification of diet in renal disease study. *Ann Intern Med* 2005; **142(5):** 342–351.

22 Ruggenenti P, Perna A, Loriga G, Ganeva M, Ene-Iordache B, Turturro M *et al.* Blood-pressure control for renoprotection in patients with non-diabetic chronic renal disease (REIN-2): multicentre, randomised controlled trial. *Lancet* 2005; **365(9463):** 939–946.

23 Wright JT, Jr., Bakris G, Greene T, Agodoa LY, Appel LJ, Charleston J *et al.* Effect of blood pressure lowering and antihypertensive drug class on progression of hypertensive kidney disease: results from the AASK trial. *JAMA* 2002; **288(19):** 2421–2431.

24 Norris K, Bourgoigne J, Gassman J, Hebert L, Middleton J, Phillips RA *et al.* Cardiovascular outcomes in the African American Study of Kidney Disease and Hypertension (AASK) Trial. *Am J Kidney Dis* 2006; **48(5):** 739–751.

25 Jafar TH, Stark PC, Schmid CH, Landa M, Maschio G, de Jong PE *et al.* Progression of chronic kidney disease: the role of blood pressure control, proteinuria, and angiotensin-converting enzyme inhibition: a patient-level meta-analysis. *Ann Intern Med* 2003; **139(4):** 244–252.

26 Agodoa LY, Appel L, Bakris GL, Beck G, Bourgoignie J, Briggs JP *et al.* Effect of ramipril vs amlodipine on renal outcomes in hypertensive nephrosclerosis: a randomized controlled trial. *JAMA* 2001; **285(21):** 2719–2728.

27 Rahman M, Pressel S, Davis BR, Nwachuku C, Wright JT, Jr., Whelton PK *et al.* Renal outcomes in high-risk hypertensive patients treated with an angiotensin-converting enzyme inhibitor or a calcium channel blocker vs a diuretic: a report from the Antihypertensive and Lipid-Lowering Treatment to Prevent Heart Attack Trial (ALLHAT). *Arch Intern Med* 2005; **165(8):** 936–946.

34 Recognition and Management of Mineral and Bone Disorder of Chronic Kidney Disease and End-Stage Renal Disease

Donald A. Molony

Division of Renal Diseases and Hypertension and Center for Clinical Research and Evidence-Based Medicine, University of Texas Houston Medical School, Houston, USA

The recognition and therapeutic management of the metabolic bone disease of chronic kidney failure occupies a central place in the overall treatment of end-stage renal disease (ESRD) patients and is one of the unique activities that differentiates, in practice, chronic kidney disease (CKD) specialized care from the routine care of patients provided by the general internist. Much of the rationale for current treatment of chronic kidney disease mineral and bone disorder (MBD) has been based on biological reasoning: the view that if abnormalities in the hormone systems that regulate bone health and calcium and phosphorus metabolism can be corrected, then the disease states that result from these abnormalities can be treated and survival and quality of health improved. Figure 34.1 illustrates some of the important relationships between these hormone systems [1–11]. The validity for patients with CKD and ESRD of a therapeutic approach based on such pathophysiological reasoning and on evidence from animal models has been supported mostly by results from epidemiologic, observational studies; evidence arising from randomized controlled trials (RCTs) is more limited [1,12,13].

Thus, current therapies rely on a combination of approaches, including hormone replacement where hormone deficiencies are recognized [e.g. 25(OH)-vitamin D and 1,25(OH)$_2$-vitamin D] and suppression where excesses occur (e.g. parathyroid hormone [PTH]) and direct modulation of serum and/or whole-body phosphorus and calcium. This chapter will examine the evidence that supports current practice in adult patients with CKD and with ESRD. The evidence as it relates to pedeatric patients is covered in chapter 60. The biochemical targets for management of MBD recommended by national guideline committees are compared in Table 34.1 [14–23]. The oldest of these guidelines, the Kidney Disease Outcomes Quality Initiative (K/DOQI), was last updated with evidence prior to January 2001, and there have been some calls for revisions to reflect new data [24–26]. It is anticipated that the Kidney Disease: Improving Global Outcomes (KDIGO) guidelines will address some of the expressed concerns [27]. Table 34.1 does not include KDIGO targets, as these guidelines are still under review.

It should be noted that the recommendations regarding treatment of MBD during CKD stages 3 and 4 or in earlier stages of CKD have been determined commonly by expert opinion and by the extrapolation of evidence from ESRD [13]. Furthermore, there are, to date, no published well-designed clinical trials in either ESRD or CKD that have evaluated the impact of concurrent modulation of multiple interrelated therapies (e.g. phosphate binders along with vitamin D and calcimetics) on the long-term outcomes of mortality and non-bone-related morbidity. Trials examining a limited number of these combined strategies are currently in progress [1,28].

Lending credence to an approach of arbitrating clinical decision making on the basis of biological plausibility and a mechanistic view of the disease processes responsible for MBD is the epidemiological and observational evidence that MBD is associated with bone demineralization and more importantly, clinically, with overt symptomatic bone disease and potentially with nonosseous calcification, including calcification of the vasculature. The latter is thought to contribute to the increased premature cardiovascular and all-cause mortality that occurs in CKD [29–50]. The causal link between vitamin D deficiency in CKD, secondary hyperparathyroidism, dysregulation of Ca and PO$_4$, demineralizing bone diseases of low or high turnover, MBD, and vascular disease is based principally on this epidemiologic and observational evidence [29,51–59]. Recently, some RCT evidence in ESRD patients has been obtained that supports a causal link between MBD and mortality and the potential benefits of the therapeutic interruption of this causal pathway [60]. Similarly, the evaluation of outcomes of the currently recommended therapies for management of MBD in CKD and ESRD is based principally on results from observational studies, and therefore the conclusions regarding therapy that can be drawn from these studies are subject to some uncertainty. The individual therapies or, more importantly, combinations of these therapies, should be scrutinized with well-designed RCTs of sufficient size evaluating patient-centered outcomes in patients with both ESRD and CKD [61].

Evidence-based Nephrology. Edited by Donald Molony and Jonathan Craig
© 2009 Blackwell Publishing, ISBN: 978-1-4051-3975-5.

Table 34.1 Comparison of guidelines and recommendations regarding targets for biochemical parameters of MBD of CKD and ESRD.

Biochemical parameter	Disease status	Recommendation from national body (yr of publication)				
		Caring for Australians with Renal Impairment (2005)	Canadian Society of Nephrology Hemodialysis Clinical Practice Guidelines (2006)	European Best Practice Guidelines (2006)	K/DOQI US National Kidney Foundation (2003)	UK Renal Assoc. (2006)
PO_4, mg/dL	CKD stages 3 & 4	Target within normal range			2.7–4.6	2.8–4.7
	ESRD	2.5–5.0		2.5–5.5	3.5–5.5	3.4–5.6
Ca, mg/dL	CKD stages 3 & 4	Target normal range			Target normal range	Target normal range
	ESRD	8.4–9.5	Target normal range		8.4–9.5	8.8–10.4
$Ca \times PO_4$, mg^2/dL^2	CKD stages 3 & 4			<55		<60, ideally <52
	ESRD	<50		<55	<55	<60, ideally <52
iPTH, pg/mL	CKD stage 3				35–70	Within normal range
	CKD stage 4				70–110	<2× normal upper limit of assay
	ESRD	2–3× upper limit of normal	Avoid PTH <100, treat if >500 and symptoms		150–300	<4× nomal upper limit of assay

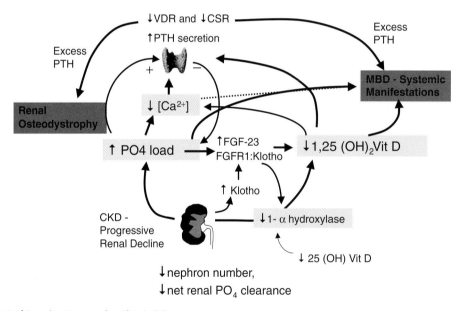

Figure 34.1 Pathogenesis of Secondary Hyperparathyroidism in CKD.

This figure illustrates some of the complex relationships between calcium, phosphorus, vitamin D, and PTH that determine normal mineral metabolism and some of the ways in which these relationships may be altered in CKD leading to the development of secondary hyperparathyroidism and the MBD of CKD. Two processes mediate the early events in the pathogenesis of SHPTH in early CKD; the renal and systemic response to excess phosphorus and the fall in active 1,25 diydroxy-vitamin D levels. The number of functioning nephron units decline as renal function worsens. The maintenance of normal serum phosphorus levels in CKD patients is dependent on an increase in phosphate excretion per nephron. High PTH and low active vitamin D levels inhibit tubular phosphate transport by decreasing sodium-dependent phosphate cotransporter activity. FGF-23 and the FGF-23 FGFR-Klotho complex may be important modulators of renal phosphate. In addition, FGF-23 appears to reduce 1,25(OH)₂ vitamin D in part by reductions in 1-α-hydroxylase activity. The fall in 1-α-hydroxylase activity in CKD is most likely secondary to multiple mechanisms. Active vitamin D is also reduced in many patients because of insufficiency in 25 hydroxyvitamin D. Low levels of active vitamin D reduce calcium absorption from the GI tract and stimulate secretion of PTH. Additionally, low calcium levels stimulate PTH secretion; as a result calcium levels are partially restored by release of calcium from the bone. Excess PTH, hyperphosphatemia, and vitamin D deficiency each appear to contribute to the development of the systemic manifestations of CKD-MBD.

The results of a limited number of such studies have been reported.

Definition of MBD in CKD

The traditional views of bone disease in renal insufficiency (CKD) and renal failure (ESRD) have emphasized dimineralizing bone diseases representing a spectrum of bone pathologies ranging from osteitis fibrosa of secondary hyperparathyroidism to adynamic bone disease [62–65]. These definitions have been based largely on observational cross-sectional studies in CKD patient populations. Distinct bone histological patterns or disease states classified according to the American Society for Bone and Mineral Research criteria have been to varying degrees correlated to PTH, vitamin D, and mineral metabolism status [65]. The bone classification definitions and the utility of bone biopsy in identifying individuals with high-turnover and low-turnover metabolic bone disease and in monitoring treatment effects have been reviewed extensively [62–65].

The KDIGO guidelines have proposed an expansion of the definition of MBD that occurs in CKD (CKD-MBD) [27]. This new definition is necessitated by the emerging view that CKD-MBD is a systemic pathologic process that results both in bone pathology (renal osteodystrophy) and in other nonosseous abnormalities, including vascular and soft tissue calcification. This body recommended the following:

> The term *renal osteodystrophy* [should] be used exclusively to define the bone pathology associated with CKD. The many clinical, biochemical, and imaging abnormalities that have heretofore been identified as correlates of renal osteodystrophy should be defined more broadly as a clinical entity or syndrome to be called *chronic kidney disease-mineral and bone disorder.*

The latter then is a systemic disorder of mineral and bone metabolism due to CKD with one or more of the following: abnormalities in calcium, phosphorus, PTH, or vitamin D metabolism or of bone turnover, mineralization, volume, linear growth or strength, or vascular or other soft tissue calcification [27]. This revised definition of MBD of CKD is based on evidence from observational studies reported over the last 30 years. These studies have underscored the central role of secondary hyperparathyroidism in the pathogenesis of MBD; hence, the definition of the disease in large part is related to the occurrence and consequences of this secondary hyperparathyroidism. As potential biomarkers of early mineral metabolism are identified and validated, such as FGF23, the definition of MBD may need to be reframed [11,66–68].

MBD can also be framed in terms of specific vitamin D deficiency states recognized in CKD. Vitamin D deficiency [both that of 25(OH)- and "active" $1,25(OH)_2$-vitamin D] plays a central role in the development of secondary hyperparathyroidism and may antedate by some time in individuals experiencing progressive loss of renal function measurable elevations in serum intact PTH (iPTH) levels [69–73]. Thus, vitamin D deficiency has been considered a potential target for early therapeutic intervention.

Table 34.2 Vitamin D preparations evaluated with multiple cohort or RCTs in patients with CKD or ESRD.

Vitamin D class	Agent
Vitamin D	Cholecalciferol, D_3
Vitamin D, "vitamin"	Ergocalciferol, D_2
Active vitamin D, "hormone"	$1,25(OH)_2$-vitamin D
Established Active vitamin D	Calcitriol, $1,25(OH)_2$-vitamin D_3
Active vitamin D analogs	Alfacalcidiol Paricalcitol, 19-*nor*-$1,25(OH)_2$-vitamin D_2 Doxecalciferol, 1-α-(OH)-vitamin D_2

The RCT and observational study evidence supporting replacement strategies for CKD and ESRD patients deficient in vitamin D with cholecalciferol (vitamin D_3), ergocalciferol [vitamin D_2], and active forms of vitamin D_3 or D_2 [$1,25(OH)_2$-vitamin D or an equivalent] will be reviewed below. Table 34.2 lists the forms of vitamin D that have been evaluated in clinical trials in patients with either CKD or ESRD [74].

The relative contributions of 25(OH)-vitamin D and $1,25(OH)_2$-vitamin D in the pathogenesis of MBD are unknown, and to date no RCTs comparing treatment outcomes in a head-to-head study of both hydroxylated forms of vitamin D or evaluating their concurrent use have been reported. The evidence in CKD and ESRD is principally related to the effects of active 1,25-hormone on parameters of bone health and on Ca and PO_4 metabolism; fewer studies have evaluated the effects of cholecalciferol or calcidiol replacement on PTH and active vitamin D levels in ESRD [3,75–82]. By current customary practice, there is a general consensus that active vitamin D "hormone" [active $1,25(OH)_2$-vitamin D] deficiency is part of the clinical spectrum of MDB, and there is an emerging view that vitamin D deficiency [25(OH)-vitamin D] is also important in CKD and ESRD.

One of the important limitations of conducting clinical trials is the challenge of determining noninvasively, using a measure that can be employed in routine clinical practice, when MBD begins and the effectiveness of the treatment under investigation in modulating the MBD. Current assays for iPTH and vitamin D may have somewhat more limited reliability and reproducibility, as has been demonstrated when the same sample is tested in multiple different reference laboratories [83,84]. Furthermore, evidence has emerged from some investigations (but not all) that indicates that iPTH measurements may not always allow for accurate classification of a significant number of patients into those with low- versus high-turnover bone disease or to identify patients with a significant osteoporosis component [85–91]. Correct classification of patients is likely to have important implications for response to therapy [23,92]. None of the currently recommended testing regimens has been evaluated in an RCT for its utility in impacting long-term clinical outcomes. The clinical trials evidence reviewed in this chapter that relies on PTH or vitamin D levels as the primary outcome may need to be reconsidered as more sophisticated tests are developed and validated. Ideally, therapy for treatment and/or prevention of MBD and its complications should be evaluated in terms of its effects on bone pathology, clinically relevant bone disease outcomes such as fracture risk, and on vascular health, patient survival, and the preservation of a state of optimal health [13,61]. In current practice, therapeutic success is often monitored by achievement of target PTH, PO_4 and Ca levels and, thus, this chapter will also review the therapies of MBD in terms of their effects on these biochemical disease-centered surrogate outcomes.

In the development of CKD, when does MBD begin?

If MBD is a systemic disease with severe consequences, it makes sense that initiation of specific targeted therapies either before the disease begins (primary prevention) or early in the course of disease (secondary prevention) might be able to reduce morbidity and improve overall survival among CKD patients. The most proximate initiating events in the pathogenesis of MBD of CKD are currently the focus of intense investigation. These investigations are clinically relevant in that they may allow for the development of early biomarkers of disease, allow for earlier treatment at a stage where treatment is presumably more effective, and suggest new loci for therapeutic interventions. Likely candidates include FGF-23, klotho, and phosphatonins, all of which may participate in the early pathogenesis of secondary hyperparathyroidism and MBD of CKD [6,9,10,67,68,93,94]. The utility of these "early" biomarkers of MBD in CKD has not been confirmed with cohort, epidemiologic, or RCT evidence, either as diagnostic tests that efficiently identify patients with MBD or as a way of directing therapeutic interventions and monitoring the effectiveness of these interventions. Despite the potential promise of these early biomarkers, clinical trials evidence is lacking to support the routine use of vitamin D in CKD for the prevention of MBD before overt vitamin D deficiency itself is identified. The clinical trials evidence on early recognition and treatment of MBD in the CKD patient is limited to the recognition of vitamin D deficiency and replacement strategies with vitamin D once deficiency is confirmed.

Epidemiology and definition of vitamin D deficiency

A number of recent studies have reported the frequency of vitamin D deficiency for both calcidiol [25(OH)-vitamin D] and calcitriol [$1,25(OH)_2$-vitamin D_3] and their respective vitamin D_2 counterparts for the normal adult population and for those with CKD or ESRD [72,95–104]. These studies have used definitions of vitamin D adequacy, insufficiency, and deficiency for both 25(OH)-vitamin D and $1,25(OH)_2$-vitamin D metabolites that have been determined principally from an examination of the effects of these deficiencies on PTH levels and on bone health and histology, clin-

ical phenomena that are regulated largely by active $1,25(OH)_2$-vitamin D hormone [105]. These definitions tell us little about the effects of vitamin D deficiency on nonosseous tissues. It is quite possible that higher levels are required to treat optimally the potential non-bone-related effects of vitamin D in patients with CKD [106,107]. Although epidemiologic studies demonstrate a strong association between vitamin D deficiency either assumed because of place of residence (northern climes) or measured using the normal values defined as above and a number of cellular, developmental, and immune dysfunctions, including myopathy, multiple sclerosis, psoriasis, infections, and malignancies, the converse has not been formally demonstrated, with a few exceptions [107–118], specifically, that the replacement of vitamin D either as 25(OH)-vitamin D or as active $1,25(OH)_2$-vitamin D hormone results in a reduction in cancer risk, infection risk, myopathy, anemia, and renal fibrosis in patient populations where vitamin D deficiency is the consequence of CKD.

$1,25(OH)_2$-vitamin D deficiency has long been recognized to occur in an increasing proportion of subjects as renal function levels decline. At an estimated glomerular filtration rate (eGFR) of <60 mL/min/1.73 m^2, most studies report that 50% of patients with CKD will be vitamin D hormone insufficient or deficient [69,70,72]. Recently, Levin and coworkers reconfirmed the topology of the decline in 25(OH)- and $1,25(OH)_2$-vitamin D in CKD and a correlation between the increasing prevalence of vitamin D deficiency and secondary hyperparathyroidism [72]. They reported a direct relationship of declining GFR with declining $1,25(OH)_2$-vitamin D_3 ($R^2 = 0.3827$; $P < 0.0001$), but not with 25(OH)-vitamin D levels. They also reported onset of overt hyperparathyroidism at eGFR levels of <45 mL/min/1.73 m^2, at a level where roughly 50% of the subjects in their survey population were deficient in $1,25(OH)_2$-vitamin D_3. The relationship of vitamin D deficiency and the development of hyperparathyroidism was strongest for $1,25(OH)_2$-vitamin D. They also reconfirmed that abnormal serum values for calcium and phosphorus do not occur until late in the course of CKD and as such are not good markers for either secondary hyperparathyroidism or vitamin D deficiency. Recently, Wolf and coworkers demonstrated that PTH status, late in CKD, provided a poor marker of an individual patient's vitamin D status [118]. LeClair and coworkers demonstrated significant calcidiol [25(OH)-vitamin D] deficiency in CKD, with only 17% of patients with CKD stage 3 and 12% of patients with CKD stage 4 having sufficient levels [101]. In this cohort of CKD patients, vitamin D levels did not increase during the summer months, implying that sunlight exposure was not sufficient for ensuring adequate levels of calcidiol. A cross-sectional study conducted in Hawaii demonstrated a significant number of healthy individuals with calcidiol insufficiency despite more than 30 h of sunlight/week [103]. Thus, sufficient levels of calcidiol cannot be assumed without a direct measurement in CKD patients, even among those with adequate sun exposure.

Although is it clear that patients with CKD are at significant risk for calcidiol and calcitriol deficiency and, consequently, secondary hyperparathyroidism and MBD, the full benefits from the various vitamin D replacement strategies have not been investigated with well-designed RCTs. The hypothesis that pharmacological replacement of either calcidiol or of active $1,25(OH)_2$-vitamin D hormone will result in improvements in survival has not been evaluated with a rigorous RCT in subjects with CKD or ESRD. Vitamin D therapy in CKD and ESRD has been evaluated in terms of the effects on bone histology and fracture risk and on PTH and metabolic parameters.

Data from non-CKD patients have been reviewed in recent meta-analyses analyzing the evidence for prevention of fractures and for improvement in survival [120–128]. These clinical trials focused mainly on elderly individuals with osteoporosis. These studies included elderly individuals with unrecognized CKD. Consideration of these results might have relevance to the CKD population in the absence of similar specific CKD trials. The findings reported from RCTs in "normal" elderly subjects are similar to the findings that arise from the observational studies in CKD patients.

Vitamin D supplementation does appear to reduce the risk of hip or other clinically significant fractures in elderly women and men who have osteoporosis or are at risk for this disease. Bischoff-Ferrari conducted a meta-analysis of RCTs in which cholecalciferol was administered to elderly patients for prevention of hip or nonvertebral fractures [128]. They found five and seven RCTs that met their inclusion criteria where vitamin D therapy was evaluated for the prevention of hip and nonvertebral fractures, respectively. All of the studies identified used cholecalciferol as the active agent. They noted significant heterogeneity that disappeared when the studies employing high doses of vitamin D were analyzed separately from low-dose trials. They found that a higher dose of vitamin D (700–800 IU/day) reduced the relative risk (RR) of hip fracture by 26% (95% confidence interval [CI], 0.61–0.88) and nonvertebral fractures by 23% (95% CI, 0.68–0.87) versus either calcium or placebo. Vitamin D at a low dose (400 IU/day) did not confer benefit in these studies. In a more recent analysis that combined the low-dose and higher-dose studies, Jackson et al. did not demonstrate a similar benefit from vitamin D in preventing falls to that reported by Bishoff-Ferrair [124]. From recent studies it is uncertain whether a benefit is seen with customary doses of vitamin D or only with supraphysiologic doses and whether a benefit is seen in the absence of supplementation of dietary calcium [126,129]. In order to determine the impact of calcium supplementation, Boonen et al. recently updated the meta-analysis of Bischoff-Ferrari and found a favorable effect on hip fracture prevention with vitamin D when administered with calcium supplementation but, in contrast to the earlier meta-analysis, an absence of a significant overall benefit when cholecalciferol, even in the higher doses, was used alone. Others have also evaluated in a systematic review the benefits of achieving high serum levels of 25(OH)-vitamin D in non-renal failure patients and demonstrated limited benefits for subsets of the population, but the studies could not separate the benefits from those related to calcium and were inadequately designed to address the question of harm [123].

Does vitamin D supplementation improve other aspects of health and survival in the non-CKD population?

The observations that measured 25(OH)-vitamin D deficiency or, alternatively, residence in northern latitudes is associated epidemiologically with increased risk of infection, malignancy, myeloproliferative disorders, myopathy, neurodegenerative disorders, etc., have resulted in the recommendation that vitamin D supplementation be administered to the general population and that this might result in reduced mortality [107,110]. Autier and Gandini performed a meta-analysis of RCTs with vitamin D and demonstrated a significant survival advantage for subjects on vitamin D, especially at higher doses [130]. The effect was associated with a fivefold increase in 25(OH)-vitamin D levels in the treatment groups and was most robustly demonstrated in the RCTs that compared cholecalciferol administration to placebo rather than ergocalciferol to placebo. This differential benefit was somewhat attenuated in trials that used vitamin D in combination with calcium supplementation. Overall for all of the vitamin D trials, an RR reduction for death of 7% was determined with a number needed to treat of 169 (95% CI, 91–1178). More recently, Lappe et al. in a three-armed RCT of vitamin D plus calcium versus calcium alone or versus placebo demonstrated a substantially decreased risk for the development of cancer for the women assigned to the vitamin D plus calcium group compared to the other two study arms when the women were followed beyond the first year of therapy [111]. Whether these health benefits are attenuated or magnified in CKD patients on vitamin D supplementation has not been tested with an RCT.

Evidence from observational and epidemiological studies does support the hypothesis of a survival advantage in CKD stage 5 and likely late stage 4 from the use of active vitamin therapies. Some of this evidence as it pertains to cardiovascular risk has been summarized by Levin and Li [131]. More recently, Wolf et al. demonstrated in a prospective cohort of patients new to dialysis that those who were treated with active vitamin D (either continuing on active vitamin D started during predialysis with CKD stage 4 or initiated on vitamin D concurrent with initiation of dialysis) experienced a significant 90-day survival advantage compared to those who were not treated with active $1,25(OH)_2$-vitamin D (or its equivalent) [119]. The survival advantage in this population appeared to be obtained whether patients were deficient in 25(OH)- or $1,25(OH)_2$-vitamin D. Whether a similar survival benefit would have been observed in incident dialysis patients who were deficient in 25(OH)-vitamin D had they been treated with ergocalciferol or other forms of active vitamin D precursors could not be evaluated in this observational study.

The association of active vitamin D therapies with improved survival in ESRD has been observed in multiple cohorts of prevalent ESRD patients on dialysis [132–140]. Tang and coworkers observed that patients on hemodialysis who received active vitamin D had a lower mortality than those who did not, irrespective of their serum PTH, PO_4, or calcium status [132]. Furthermore, they reported that those who received active vitamin D_2 (paricalcitol) appeared to do better than those treated with vitamin D_3 (calcitriol) [133]. Tentori and coworkers reported similar survival patterns with active vitamin D therapy in a different cohort in a later time period [134]. They also observed a survival advantage when active vitamin D_2 forms (paricalcitol and doxecalciferol) were compared to vitamin D_3 (calcitriol). The survival curves for paricalcitol and doxecalciferol were superimposed. In each of these observational studies the apparent survival advantage was relatively small. No head-to-head comparison in an RCT of sufficient duration of one form of vitamin D versus another or versus placebo has been performed to determine the true survival benefit of a specific vitamin D therapy for patients on dialysis. Despite sophisticated and appropriate statistical adjustments, the observational studies cannot be assumed to be entirely free of bias. Given that the magnitude of the observed benefit is small, it cannot be assumed that if this question were to be examined with an RCT that a similar survival benefit for vitamin D would be found [142]. However, in the absence of multiple robust RCTs, it is appropriate to acknowledge that a survival benefit for vitamin D sufficiency and/or its therapeutic restoration is supported by multiple lines of epidemiological reasoning. This body of evidence fulfills the major considerations attributed to Sir Austin Bradford-Hill, by which one can infer likely causal linkage between an exposure (active vitamin D deficiency) and an outcome (increased mortality), including dose response, strength of association, consistency, and biological plausibility, among others [1,143,144].

What is the evidence then that vitamin D replacement in patients with CKD results in meaningful clinical patient-centered outcomes?

Whenever possible, therapy should be informed by patient-centered outcomes that include improved survival, reduced risk of hospitalization, reductions in cardiovascular disease and cardiovascular events, reduced risk of fractures, and improved quality of life. Most of the clinical trials evaluating vitamin D therapy and informing its current clinical use in CKD measure disease-oriented and/or surrogate outcomes, such as changes in serum phosphorus, calcium concentrations, bone histology by biopsy or noninvasive measures, and serum PTH levels. The evidence that vitamin D therapies improve both patient-centered and disease-oriented outcomes is reviewed.

Before examining a recent meta-analysis of the RCT evidence, it may be useful to examine briefly the data that historically resulted in the current recommendations for use of vitamin D in CKD and ESRD. Renal osteodystrophy was recognized as a significant and progressive disease in patients with ESRD soon after effective renal replacement therapy became generally available in North American, Europe, and Asia. The disease state was recognized as demineralizing and debilitating bone disease, hypocalcemia, and

hyperphosphatemia. It was observed to be more prevalent in patients with prolonged kidney failure, especially those with chronic diseases of the renal tubulo-interstitium [145]. Bone biopsy studies demonstrated that the degree of disordered bone architecture was associated directly with the degree of hyperparathyroidism and that the latter correlated in some studies to 25(OH)-vitamin D deficiency or to 1,25(OH)$_2$-vitamin D deficiency [105,146–148].

The first clinical trials with vitamin D replacement in CKD were conducted, prior to the availability of significant quantities of active vitamin D, with either supraphysiologic doses of cholecalciferol or 25(OH)-vitamin D_3 [75,76,78,79]. When these studies were performed in patients with ESRD, they were generally short term (typically 12 weeks) and included small numbers of subjects. Typically, improvements in bone pain, alkaline phosphatase, and PTH levels in patients with severe secondary hyperparathyroidism were evaluated. Typically, these early studies in ESRD cohorts did not include a control group and none evaluated hard patient outcomes, such as fracture rates and mortality. Some of these early cohort studies did include evaluations of bone histomorphology by biopsy.

Some of the earliest investigations of 1,25(OH)$_2$-vitamin D therapy reported two findings that have subsequently proven to be causes for concern. First, Berl *et al.* conducted an RCT on a small number of hemodialysis patients [75], comparing the biochemical effects of oral therapy with calcitriol versus cholecalcerferol. They reported a prompt development of hypercalcemia in nearly all of their subjects receiving calcitriol (maximum dose, 1.5 μg/day), even though these patients were receiving aluminum and not calcium salts as a phosphate binder. Second, Christiansen and coworkers examined the effects of calcitriol in CKD patients [149–151]. They reported that calcitriol produced significant and abrupt increases in serum calcium levels and a doubling of renal calcium excretion. Importantly, in these studies oral calcitriol therapy significantly accelerated the rate of decline of renal function. Others have reported that calcitriol is safe without any adverse effect on renal function when used in very low doses that do not invoke a hypercalcemic response but that are sufficient to manage the early stages of secondary hyperparathyroidism in CKD [152,153]. Calcitriol is currently commonly used in CKD patients. More recently, Coburn and Coyne reported the effects of newer vitamin D analogs on urinary calcium excretion and renal function [154,155]. These investigators did not see elevations in urinary calcium excretion comparable to those reported by Christainsen *et al.* nor changes in the GFR with 6 months of oral therapy with the newer agents.

The widespread adoption of vitamin D therapy in ESRD more than 2 decades ago was based on two lines of evidence: on the effects of vitamin D replacement in ESRD patients on biochemical markers of MBD, such as PTH, PO_4, Ca, and alkaline phosphatase, that were reported from multiple mainly short-term nonrandomized trials, and on the clinical reasoning that emerged from experimental studies in laboratory animals. One of the principal initial goals of this therapy was correction of the hypocalcemia and consequent suppression of PTH based on mechanistic reasoning. This mechanistic rationale for therapy has been summarized elsewhere [76,156].

Most recently, Palmer and colleagues reevaluated the clinical trials evidence regarding vitamin D use in ESRD and CKD using the formal analytical methods specified by the Cochrane collaboration, therefore limiting their analysis to evidence from RCTs [157,158]. They evaluated the effects of vitamin D on the magnitude of suppression of PTH and on the treatment of hyperphosphatemia, as well as the impact of vitamin D therapy on renal function, hypercalcemia, and on mortality. This analysis of the published literature demonstrated a number of findings.

Despite the promise of benefit from the observational studies in CKD patients and from the RCT results in the general population and the biological plausibility for a survival benefit, there have been no clinical RCTs specifically designed to demonstrate this survival benefit in patients treated with vitamin D in either the ESRD or the CKD population. In their meta-analysis, Palmer et al. referred to eight trials that reported on mortality as part of reporting of adverse events. The shortest of these trials was 12 weeks, and the longest in CKD patients, 2 years; the weighted average follow-up for the six trials that compared vitamin D to non-vitamin D therapy was approximately 1.2 years. Many of these trials excluded diabetic patients, and the average age of participants was less than 50 years. In these trials, there were a total of 16 deaths, 10 in those receiving vitamin D and 6 in the placebo group, or approximately 2 deaths for every 100 patient-years of follow-up. Thus, these trials were significantly underpowered to demonstrate any survival difference with vitamin D therapy and generally examined a healthier-than-typical hemodialysis population.

From their meta-analysis, Palmer et al. did conclude that active vitamin D therapy with newer agents reduced end-of-treatment PTH levels but that this potential therapeutic benefit was associated with potentially problematic albeit small increases in serum calcium and to a lesser degree with increases in PO_4 levels, but not with increased episodes of overt hypercalcemia or hyperphosphatemia. These findings of benefit versus the harm of generating hypercalcemia were more robust when a single trial using 22-oxacalcitriol, in which the rate of hypercalcemia was unusually high, was excluded from the analysis. The benefits on PTH control of therapy with an "established" vitamin D (1,25-dihydroxycholecalciferol) were not confirmed in this systematic review. Furthermore, the use of an established agent was associated with an increased risk of hypercalcemia and hyperphosphatemia. The conclusions that arise from this meta-analysis are somewhat tempered by the significant interstudy heterogeneity and by the less-than-robust methodologic quality of some of the available studies.

One of the principle findings from this meta-analysis is that there is a surfeit of robust RCT evidence underlying some of the assumptions regarding therapeutic benefits of vitamin D in CKD and ESRD. There are few direct comparisons of treatment with one form of vitamin D versus another or with a placebo. In a single RCT with 263 ESRD patients comparing head to head calcitriol versus paricalcitol, Sprague et al. demonstrated a more rapid reduction in PTH and less hypercalcemia with the paricalcitol treatment [159].

Much of the evidence to support the use of vitamin D comes from longitudinal studies, in which patients serve as their own control and where suppression of PTH and/or improvements in bone histomorphometry on biopsy have been the primary outcomes evaluated, or from comparisons of one active vitamin D with another [160–192]. Because many of these studies did not include random allocation, many of these would not normally be included in systematic reviews such as that performed by Palmer et al. Nonetheless, these studies provide some rationale for use of active vitamin D preparations to ameliorate the most severe effects of secondary hyperparathyroidism pending additional RCT evidence regarding the optimal dosing, route, and form of vitamin D for prevention of renal MBD and mortality.

The K/DOQI recommends that dialysis patients with iPTH levels of >300 pg/mL should receive active vitamin D to reduce PTH to target, that intermittent intravenous calcitriol is more effective than daily oral dosing, and that paricalcitol or doxercalciferol should be considered for patients who become more hypercalcemic or hyperphophatemic with calcitriol.

25(OH)-Vitamin D

Epidemiologic studies have identified significant 25(OH)-vitamin D deficiency in CKD populations. Clinical trials have provided evidence for the utility of vitamin D replacement therapy with cholecalciferol or ergocalciferol in the general population, where replacement therapy corrects secondary hyperparathyroidism, improves bone mineralization, reduces fracture risk, and improves motor and immune functions and may even delay the development of type 2 diabetes [104,105,109,111–120]. The epidemiologic and RCT data supporting these benefits of vitamin D replacement therapy in the general population have been extensively reviewed by Hollick and others [107,120,123]. The use of ergocalciferol or cholecalciferol in the CKD and ESRD population are less well studied. Prior to the introduction of active forms of vitamin D (calcitriol, etc.), correction of vitamin D deficiency in ESRD populations with significant renal osteodystrophy was attempted with pharmacologic doses of ergocalciferol or cholecalciferol. The results were variable. A number of the early studies failed to demonstrate a significant effect of suprapharmacologic doses of cholecalciferol or ergocalciferol on biochemical markers of MBD. Significant side effects were noted. Improvement in bone mineralization was rarely measured or reported.

Recently, Saab et al. reexamined the use of ergocalciferol in a prevalent dialysis cohort of 119 patients [82]. They noted no significant change in the biochemical parameters (serum calcium, PO_4, and Ca–PO_4 product) after 6 months of therapy with 50,000 IU of ergocalciferol monthly despite significant improvements in 25(OH)-vitamin D levels. They did not probe the long-term impact of this therapy on the patient-centered outcomes of bone health and survival. Zisman et al. demonstrated a modest improvement in PTH control in CKD stage 3 patients treated with ergocalciferol long term but no similar benefit for patients with CKD stage 4 and more severe secondary hyperparathyroidism [193]. The implications of their findings for ESRD patients warrant further exploration. The exact role of ergocalciferol or cholecalciferol supplementation in the treatment of dialysis patients in the current era has, to date, not been evaluated with clinical RCTs.

Hyperphosphatemia

Many of the therapeutic efforts directed towards the management of the systemic disease of MBD of CKD are focused on the management of the excess phosphorus retention that is a consequence of CKD. In this regard, it is prudent to first examine the evidence that phosphorus itself contributes to increased mortality and morbidity in CKD and to examine whether reduction in phosphorus absorption either by dietary restriction or the use of phosphate binders results in improvements in this excess mortality and these morbidities.

The hypothesis that excess phosphorus retention and hyperphosphatemia result in significant human disease arises from two lines of evidence. These include experimental data from animal experiments and *in vitro* cell culture models and epidemiological data from human populations. The latter have included studies both in populations of dialysis patients and in cohorts of subjects with normal renal function or mild to moderate CKD. In studies first performed more than 20 years ago, Slatopolsky and colleagues demonstrated in animal models of renal insufficiency that secondary hyperparathyroidism, renal bone disease, and even renal failure progression could be attenuated after a 5/6 nephrectomy or other causes of acute renal failure if the animals were fed a very low phosphate diet. This body of evidence has been summarized elsewhere [194,195]. More recently the laboratories of Giachelli, Shannahan, Moe, and others have reported findings that provided a potential molecular mechanism for both direct and indirect effects of increased extracellular phosphorus (and often calcium in a synergistic manner) on fibrosis, MBD, and vascular calcification. These studies have been summarized by these three investigators in recent reviews [196–204].

Epidemiologic studies of patients with ESRD have demonstrated that there is a strong association between elevations in serum phosphorus levels, MBD of CKD, and mortality. These studies are summarized in Table 34.3 [44,205–220]. Block and coworkers analyzed a large data set of prevalent hemodialysis patients. They demonstrated that patients with baseline serum PO_4 levels of greater than 5.5 mg/dL experienced a significant dose-dependent increase in mortality over the subsequent 2 years of follow-up [207]. Block *et al.* have more recently replicated these findings [210]. Similar results have emerged from the DOPPS and other large dialysis patient cohorts [211]. Kalantar-Zadeh and coworkers, examining a large database of prevalent dialysis patients in the USA, demonstrated a similar relationship between PO_4 and mortality [44]. Kalantar-Zadeh's analysis differed from those conducted by Block and others in that they examined the time-dependent effect of PO_4 on mortality. In their fully adjusted

model (adjusted for significant comorbidities, age, gender, and nutritional status), serum PO_4 levels greater than 5.5 mg/dL and less than 2.8 were independently associated with increased mortality. On the basis of these findings, the K/DOQI and other consensus evidence-based guidelines have recommended that phosphorus levels in patients be targeted to relatively narrow ranges. A summary of the major recommendations with regards to the biochemical targets for therapy from some of the principal national bodies are shown in Table 34.1.

It should be noted that reduced survival in ESRD patients with MBD cannot be fully described by any single biochemical parameter, such as phosphorus, or by multiple parameters taken together where the target levels for these parameters have been largely determined separately. Stevens, Levin, and coworkers demonstrated in a prospective cohort the complex interplay between each of the MBD biochemical and clinical parameters and mortality [73]. Their analysis supports the hypothesis that patients may require different targets depending on their duration on dialysis. It is not surprising that the optimal calcium, phosphorus, and PTH targets for best cardiovascular and mortality outcomes might evolve as the vascular disease burden changes with duration of ESRD and time on dialysis. It is also likely that the optimal serum calcium and phosphorus targets and response to therapy might be different for individuals with some preservation of renal clearance [49,74].

Evidence is now emerging to implicate high phosphorus burdens with increased mortality risk in individuals with more normal renal function. Using a time-dependent model and the Framingham offspring cohort, Dhingra *et al.* demonstrated a significant association of serum phosphorus levels at the high end of the "normal" range, namely, above 3.5 mg/dL, with increased cardiovascular morbidity and mortality among healthy individuals with GFRs greater than 90 mL/min/1.73 m^2 followed for an average of 16 years [220]. They were also able to demonstrate an association of an increased Ca–PO_4 product with cardiovascular events. Tonelli *et al.* demonstrated a similar impact of a higher serum PO_4, albeit still within the normal range, on cardiovascular events among survivors of a myocardial infarction who participated in a secondary prevention trial [221]. The eGFRs (mean for the entire cohort, 71.95 mL/min/1.73 m^2) were similar across the spectrum of PO_4 levels, and a separate analysis conducted among participants with and without eGFRs of <60 mL/min/1.73 m^2 did not change the overall findings. In this cohort of individuals with pre-existing coronary artery disease and dyslipidemia, a fasting serum PO_4 value of >3.5 mg/dL was associated with an increased risk of mortality, and a value of >4.0 mg/dL was associated with a second myocardial infarction or congestive heart failure.

In a retrospective cohort study conducted in Veterans Affairs' (VA) Medical Centers located in the Pacific Northwest, Kestenbaum *et al.* demonstrated a linear increase in risk of mortality among patients with CKD with baseline serum PO_4 levels of >3.5 mg/dL or higher [218]. In an analysis of a separate VA population, Schwarz and coworkers observed in subjects identified with CKD by eGFRs on two separate occasions that serum PO_4 values of

Table 34.3 Observational studies identifying associations with biochemical parameters of mineral metabolism and mortality and morbidity in prevalent and incident dialysis patients and in patients with CKD.

Study and no. of subjects	Population	Level at which increased risk of mortality observed					Comments
		Calcium (mg/dL)	Phosphorus (mg/dL)	Ca × PO$_4$ (mg^2/dL^2)	iPTH (pg/mL)		
Dialysis population cohorts, incident or prevalent							
Lowrie (1990), $n = 12{,}000$	US prevalent dialysis patients, large dialysis provider (LDO, Fresenius)	<9.0; >12.0	>7.0	Not shown	Not evaluated		Principal goal of study to demonstrate association of low albumin with mortality
Leggat (1998) $n = 6251$	National samples of US prevalent HD patients (CMAS, DMMS)		>7.5				Population dichotomized into those with PO$_4$ above or below 7.5, as measure of nutritional and binder compliance
Block (1998) $n = 6407$	National samples of US prevalent HD patients (CMAS, DMMS)	No relationship observed	>6.5	>52			Prevalent patients with dialysis >1 yr only, values divided by quintiles
Ganesh (2001) $n = 14{,}829$	National sample of US prevalent dialysis patients	Not evaluated	>6.5		<33; >495		
Marco (2003) $n = 143$	Prevalent Spanish HD patients	Not separately evaluated	>6.5	>52	>476		End points: cardiovascular events and all-cause mortality; follow-up 6 yrs; calcium-based phosphate binders standard
Block (2004) $n = 40{,}538$	US prevalent HD patients, large dialysis provider (LDO, Fresenius)	>9.5	>5.0	>50	>600		Case mix and multivariable adjusted results, baseline data
Young (2005) $n = 17{,}236$	Worldwide survey of prevalent dialysis patients (DOPPS)	>11.4, <7.8 (albumin-corrected calcium level)	>6.5, <3.5	>65	Not reported		
Slinin (2005), all-cause mortality $n = 14{,}829$	National sample of US prevalent dialysis patients	>9.7	>6.4	>59.3	>480		
Slinin (2005), CVD, fatal and nonfatal MI, CHF		>10.2	>4.5	>50.2	>480		
Rodriguez-Benot (2005) $n = 385$	Incident Spanish HD patients		>5.0				
Kalantar (2006), fixed model, time-dependent model $n = 58{,}058$	US prevalent HD patients, large dialysis provider (LDO, DaVita)	< 8.5; > 10.5	<3.0; >7.0	>55; >70	<200; >400		Case mix and multivariable adjusted results, time-dependent hazard; strong association between elevations in alkaline phosphatase and mortality

(continued)

Table 34.3 (*continued*)

Study and no. of subjects	Population	Level at which increased risk of mortality observed					Comments
		Calcium (mg/dL)	Phosphorus (mg/dL)	Ca × PO$_4$ (mg^2/dL^2)	iPTH (pg/mL)		
Melamed (2006) $n = 1007$	Incident cohort of US HD and PD patients	> 9.7	>6.0	>56	>308		
Noordzji (2006) $n = 1629$	Incident cohort of Dutch HD and PD patients	No increase in mortality observed for entire group but increased in HD patients with Ca values above target	>5.5	>55	No increased mortality observed		Cardiovascular mortality reported; hospitalizations increased in association with Ca levels outside target range
Noordzji (2008) $n = 1621$	Incident cohort of Dutch HD and PD patients	>9.5 in HD patients only; calcium <8.4 protective	>4.5	>55	No effect observed		Effect of increased calcium on mortality greatest in patients with low PO$_4$
Nakai (2008) $n = 27,404$	Japanese prevalent adult HD patients on dialysis >2 yrs	>10.0	>5.0		>119		
CKD, predialysis populations: mortality or morbidity outcomes							
Kestenbaum (2005) $n = 3490$	US VA Medical System		>3.5				
Schwarz (2006) $n = 1012$	US VA Medical System		>4.3	>40			Outcome of study renal progression and not mortality
Dhingra (2007) $n = 3368$	Framingham offspring cohort	No correlation found in normal range for Ca	>3.5	Correlated with PO$_4$	Not reported		16 yrs follow-up

Abbreviations: HD, hemodialysis; PD, peritoneal dialysis; CVD, cardiovascular disease; MI, myocardial infarction; CHF, congestive heart failure.

>4.3 mg/dL were associated with a more rapid progression of CKD to either a doubling of creatinine or ESRD [219].

Treatment strategies for hyperphosphatemia

Whereas serum PO_4 levels of greater than 4.5 and 5.5 mg/dL in CKD and ESRD populations, respectively, have been associated in observational studies with increased mortality, it cannot be assumed *a priori* that all therapeutic interventions to lower serum phosphorus levels in patients with CKD or ESRD to a specified "normal" range will result in similar levels of improved outcomes. Clinical trials comparing different strategies that lower PO_4, including dietary phosphorus restriction, the use of phosphate binders, and direct measures to control hyperparathyroidism, are required to determine absolutely the optimal strategies at each level of renal function and the optimal serum phosphorus targets to achieve with such treatments. Some but not all of the aspects of this clinical question are addressed by evidence that will be reviewed. Importantly, very few RCTs have examined the impact of multiple simultaneous interventions on patient-oriented "hard" outcomes.

Phosphate-restricted diet

An important component of any approach to hyperphosphatemia and the net positive phosphorus balance that occurs as a result of reduced renal excretion is the prescription of a phosphate-restricted diet. This approach is further supported by the observation from animal studies that phosphate restriction can significantly attenuate the development of secondary hyperparathyroidism [194,195]. In observations of CKD patients, renal phosphorus elimination in CKD stage 3 and early stage 4 is typically maintained as a result of compensatory changes, importantly, increased PTH secretion and consequent increased PO_4 elimination per functioning nephron. The observational data reviewed above, however, suggest that an increased phosphorus burden with normal serum phosphorus levels in the CKD patient nevertheless may result in diminished survival, mainly through premature cardiovascular events. There is no RCT that has examined the effects of phosphorus dietary restriction in CKD patients who have normal serum phosphorus levels. The focus of the evaluation of dietary phosphorus restriction has been on CKD and ESRD patients with overt elevations in serum phosphorus.

The typical North American and European daily diet contains between 800 and 1500 mg of phosphorus (800–1000 mg on a 1.2-g/kg protein-replete diet), of which approximately 50–60% is absorbed for an average weekly phosphorus load of approximately 4200 mg (2800–6300 mg) [222,223]. Judicious dietary restriction can reduce PO_4 to the lower end of this range [224]. In early stages of CKD, random serum PO_4 levels are normal but postprandial PO_4 levels may be elevated [225,226]; the latter may play a role in the pathogenesis of secondary hyperparathyroidism and in the excess mortality observed among CKD patients [227,228].

As CKD progresses, residual functioning nephrons increase net PO_4 excretion. Although PO_4 metabolism is altered early in CKD, it is only during late stage 4 and early stage 5 CKD that the GFR declines sufficiently such that this compensatory process no longer suffices and observed serum PO_4 levels increase. Patients on dialysis have negligible renal excretion of absorbed phosphorus, and a neutral phosphorus balance depends on reductions of ingested PO_4 and on augmented gastrointestinal (GI) and dialysis-related elimination [229]. Conventional thrice-weekly hemodialysis (12 h/week) will typically eliminate roughly 2400 mg of phosphorus. A net positive PO_4 balance can be greater than 1800 mg/week [230,231]. Although PO_4 elimination by dialysis is increased somewhat by newer modalities of dialysis (hemodiafiltration [232], daily dialysis [233], nocturnal dialysis [234–236], etc.), the limited availability and acceptance of the latter modalities that increase duration of dialysis, requires, that most patients rely principally on diet and on reduction of PO_4 absorption with phosphate binders to manage the PO_4 load. The latter works best to control PO_4 when some meaningful dietary PO_4 restriction is achieved [237–239].

Murphy-Gutekunst and others have evaluated sources of phosphorus in commercially available foods and demonstrated multiple sources of hidden PO_4, principally as food additives. They have addressed the impact of these sources on the PO_4 burden and the resultant challenges for PO_4 control in CKD patients [240–244]. Adequate dietary PO_4 restriction may increase the risk of protein malnutrition [245]. The safety of this excess PO_4 in the form of food additives for the general population has been called into question [246–248]. Although the impact of such food additives on the health of the CKD population is unknown, it is argued that the excess PO_4 could contribute importantly to cardiovascular disease [222,249], development of secondary hyperparathyroidism, vitamin D deficiency, and accelerated renal failure progression [195,248,250]. The inability of dialysis to adequately control PO_4 balance speaks to the inevitability of the need for phosphate binders for the majority of patients with ESRD [251,252].

Phosphate binders

Another pillar of treatment of MBD in late-stage CKD and in ESRD has been the prevention and treatment of hyperphosphatemia through reduction in PO_4 absorption from food with dietary manipulation in combination with oral PO_4 binders. The currently available phosphate binders have each been demonstrated to reduce PO_4 absorption from the GI tract and control serum PO_4 concentrations to targeted levels when utilized in recommended doses. This evidence has been reviewed by a number of investigators [253,254]. Agents currently in use for which there is either observational or study trial data demonstrating their efficacy as phosphate binders are shown in Table 34.4. Because each of these agents is effective in lowering phosphorous, the question of their appropriate use rests on whether it results in improved bone and cardiovascular health and reduced overall morbidity and mortality

Class	Agent	Comments
Mineral salts	Calcium carbonate	Extensive clinical experience in CKD and ESRD populations; limited RCT comparison to placebo
	Calcium acetate	Extensive clinical experience in CKD and ESRD populations; RCT evidence compared to other phosphate binders
	Calcium citrate	Limited trials evidence in ESRD
	Magnesium hydroxide	Limited trials evidence in ESRD and CKD
	Magnesium carbonate	Short-term RCT evidence in ESRD
Metal-based compounds	Aluminum hydroxide	Extensive clinical experience in CKD and ESRD populations; no RCT comparison with placebo
	Lanthanum carbonate	Extensive prospective cohort evidence in ESRD populations; RCT evidence compared to other phosphate binders
	Iron salts	Limited clinical trials evidence
Nonabsorbed polymers and resins	Sevelamer-HCl	Extensive prospective cohort evidence in ESRD populations; RCT evidence compared to other phosphate binders; surrogate and patient-centered outcomes.
	Sevelamer carbonate	RCT evidence compared to other phosphate binders; equivalency study compared to sevelamer-HCl

Table 34.4 Agents used as phosphate binders in CKD and ESRD patients.

in individuals with CKD and ESRD. Additionally, for the individual patient, decisions on their use might also be influenced by tolerability and overt side effects.

The question of cost-effectiveness of one phosphate binder versus another, a public policy question of relevance for health authorities, will not be addressed in this chapter, even though this consideration has influenced importantly some of the decisions regarding the development of national guidelines. To better appreciate the potential and the limitations of such analyses, the reader is referred to four recent cost-effectiveness analyses comparing two phosphate binders, in which the analyses arrive at largely opposite conclusions [255–259]. The cost-effectiveness analysis by Manns *et al.* argues that substantial clinical benefit has not been demonstrated for any particular binder strategy, hence, the "cost minimalization" approach reported by this group [255]. Their findings are in contrast to the systematic review and cost-effectiveness analysis of Nadin and the cost-effectiveness analyses of Taylor *et al.* and of Huybrechts and coworkers [257–259].

Given the strong association between the severe elevations in PO₄ that occur in late stages of CKD and nonosseous or metastatic calcification, phosphate binders have been universally adopted into routine care of the ESRD patient without supporting RCT evidence in which outcomes with phosphate binders have been compared to outcomes with treatment strategies not including binders. This

acceptance of phosphate binders without RCT evidence, in general, seems prudent for the severely hyperphosphatemic ESRD patient with severe secondary hyperparathyroidism. The evidence that has emerged from observational studies in ESRD populations does not help with the questions of when, along the spectrum of CKD, phosphate binders should be initiated, what level of serum or total body phosphorus should be targeted to obtain the best health outcomes, and whether all phosphate binders are equivalent in terms of long-term outcomes if they achieve equivalent PO₄ control. This last question drives the attention that has been paid to measuring, in short-term clinical trials, the efficacy of one binder compared to another in terms of biochemical parameters, but it begs entirely the related questions regarding the optimal PO₄ target along the continuum of CKD and whether the use of some PO₄ binders at particular stages of CKD might produce unintended adverse consequences. The uncertainty that arises from the sparseness of RCT data in CKD stages 3 and 4 has led most national guidelines groups to recommend achievement of normal PO₄ levels in these patients by relying principally on diet. These recommended target PO₄ levels, where available, are listed in Table 34.1.

This chapter will attempt to summarize the efficacy trials evidence insofar as these data inform one or more of the potential harms, namely, of hypercalcemia, hypercaluria,

Table 34.5 Comparison of epidemiologic criteria supporting a causal link of adverse outcomes for three elements.

Epidemiologic criterion	Aluminum	Calcium	Lanthanum
Strength of association	Strong	Strong	Unknown
Consistency, unbiasedness of findings	Criteria met	Criteria met	Unknown
Specificity	Criteria meet	Criteria met	Unknown
Temporality	Yes	Yes	Unknown
Epidemiology in human populations	Yes, strong	Yes moderate	Not yet demonstrated
Biological gradient, dose-effect relationship	Yes	Yes	Yes, increased accumulation with increased duration of use
Biological plausibility	Yes	Yes	Yes
Experimental evidence from animal studies	Yes	Yes	Yes
Analogy	Yes	Yes	Yes

hyperphosphatemia, renal failure progression, reduced survival, and oversuppression of PTH and development of adynamic bone disease. The focus of this section will be on a review of the evidence that relates phosphate binder choice to changes in patient-centered outcomes, focusing principally on hard outcomes, such as mortality and hospitalization rates rather than on surrogate outcomes, such as measures of vascular calcification and pulse-wave velocity.

Metal salts as phosphate binders

Aluminum salts

Aluminum hydroxide is an effective phosphate binder according to results from experience in the mid- to late 1970s, when use of aluminum hydroxide came into widespread use [260]. Aluminium hydroxide was adopted in part because of concerns with the potential for the development of hypercalcemia with the use of calcium carbonate and other calcium salts, and these concerns emerging from expert opinion in the absence of cohort or RCT evidence drove much of the change in therapy [260]. Subsequently, aluminum hydroxide fell out of favor because of case series that associated aluminum accumulation with neurotoxicity and other toxicities [261–269]. These concerns received further impetus from epidemiological data, in particular the well-studied disease outbreaks associated with parenteral aluminum from dialysate, from animal models of aluminum toxicity, and finally from the observation that chelation therapy appeared to modify the natural history of this toxicity in cases attributed to oral aluminum exposure. Chelation therapy was administered with significant associated morbidity and resource utilization. The more fulminant forms of overt dialysis dementia and aluminum-associated osteomalatia appeared to disappear in the USA after general abandonment of aluminum salts as a phosphate binder [277–280]. Whether this was due to a true therapeutic benefit from avoidance of exposure to aluminum or an issue with case identification is unknown. Clearly, given the widely held view by many that aluminum is harmful, an RCT to interrogate its benefits and its toxicities is not feasible. The best one can do is to assess its potential for harm using the accepted criteria for determining that an exposure is likely linked causally to an adverse outcome. These criteria, attributed to Sir Bradford-Hill, are listed in Table 34.5. The evidence supporting the view that aluminum salts as a phosphate binder are harmful has been reviewed elsewhere [260,263,264,266]. These data do not allow one to conclude that there is some low level of aluminum exposure that is safe with chronic use [274,275,277]. There is significant absorption of aluminum even in individuals with normal renal function, where this excess is excreted in the urine [281]. In the patient with ESRD, this absorbed aluminum is retained.

The current K/DOQI recommends that the use of aluminum salts as phosphate binders be considered (guideline 5.8) if an individual with ESRD has a serum phosphorus level of >7.0 mg/dL (2.26 mmol/L). Furthermore, the K/DOQI recommendations state that aluminum-based phosphate binders may be used as a short-term therapy (4 weeks), and for one course only, to be replaced thereafter by other phosphate binders and where other modalities such as more frequent dialysis are also considered [22].

Lanthanum-carbonate

Other metal salts that are effective in reducing phosphate absorption from the GI tract and improving circulating phosphorus levels in short-term efficacy trials include iron salts (ferrous sulfate) and the lanthanum salt La-carbonate. These metal-based phosphate binders have been advanced as alternatives to calcium-based phosphate binders. In *in vitro* studies lanthanum carbonate was demonstrated to be a highly efficient binder of PO_4, with well-preserved effectiveness across a wide pH range [282]. Lanthanum carbonate has been widely studied in patients and in animals for its efficacy and safety [283–287].

The available evidence on the safety and effectiveness of lanthanum carbonate, currently approved in many countries including the USA, Canada, and Europe under the brand name Fosrenol, has been reviewed. Most of the information regarding long-term safety of lanthanum has been culled from cohort studies, open-label extensions of shorter-term RCTs in which the control arm is dropped and study subjects were followed over years on La-carbonate phosphate binder therapy. These studies have included hemodialysis patients in Europe, Japan, and the USA, with some followed for more than 3 years while on lanthanum carbonate [284,286–292]. Short-term studies that have probed patient outcomes with use of lanthanum carbonate compared to placebo have shown that lanthanum is associated with substantial improvements in biochemical markers of MBD in ESRD patients, including substantial reductions in PO_4, the Ca–PO_4 product, and improvements in iPTH and bone histomorphometry [288,293,294]. When lanthanum carbonate has been evaluated in RCTs with calcium carbonate as the control phosphate binder, investigators have reported equivalent control of PO_4 with improved Ca–PO_4 product, iPTH levels, and markedly less hypercalcemia [284,286–288,292] compared to calcium carbonate phosphate binders.

In animal models, lanthanum carbonate accumulates prominently in the liver and bone, and less significantly in the kidney and other soft tissues [295–298]. Similar accumulation is noted in patients after long-term exposure despite very minimal GI absorption of lanthanum. Spasovski noted that although lanthanum accumulation in bone is low, release of lanthanum from the bones of these dialysis patients continued even 2 years after discontinuation of the lanthanum [290]. These authors and others have observed that lanthanum does not disrupt normal bone architecture in a manner analogous to aluminum [290,294,295]. Deposition of lanthanum into the liver is not associated with elevations in liver transaminases or in reductions in hepatic synthetic function, but the results of systematic liver biopsies performed in lanthanum study subjects have not been reported, so the possibility of some long-term liver damage cannot be absolutely excluded [286,291]. Lanthanum absorption appears to be principally as La-Cl salts and not as the much less soluble La-carbonate [299]. The absorption of La from the GI tract after oral administration and its accumulation appear to be accentuated by uremia in most animal models.

Some but certainly not all investigators have reported measurable accumulations of La in the brains of uremic animals [296,297]. One group has challenged this evidence, arguing that the measurement of La in animal brain tissue is due to contamination from peripheral blood during the processing and that work completed almost 20 years ago demonstrated that the normal blood-brain barrier was impermeable to lanthanum [300]. In these earlier studies summarized by Evans, La was evaluated as a potential radiographic imaging marker, and the chemical and biological properties of La were evaluated after either a single administration or a limited number of exposures [299]. These studies demonstrated that La typically was excluded by the tight junction of the blood-brain

barrier after a single exposure, but in animal models of osmotic injury or after repeated exposure, limited lanthanum passage could be demonstrated [301,302].

Recently, Feng provided more direct evidence that La may indeed cross the blood-brain barrier in sufficient albeit still minute quantities to affect rat brain function and composition [303,304]. In a series of experimental studies that did not require direct measurement of La in the brain, they demonstrated by magnetic resonance imaging significant changes in the normal brain ion content (Ca, Fe, and Zn) and distribution in rats given lanthanum chloride in their drinking water. If such events are occurring in patients, even to a much lower degree, it would be worrisome especially in light of the stated objective of using phosphate binders in the first place, that is, extending survival and improving quality of life of ESRD patients.

An RCT comparing cognitive function in patients randomized to La-carbonate versus calcium carbonate over 24 months has been reported [305]. The authors reported no difference in cognitive function at 24 months in patients remaining in the two groups. The results, however, may have been biased by the investigators' choice to exclude from the analysis only those patients randomized to lanthanum who were withdrawn from taking La for any reason including adverse side effects but to include in the analysis all patients in the comparison group randomized to receive conventional therapy, whether they were maintained on the originally specified calcium carbonate binder or were switched to an alternative binder because of side effects. In other words, the investigators chose to compare a potentially less-healthy control group of patients to healthy La survivors group. Their observation that the patients in the La group did not perform profoundly better in the final cognitive function studies is somewhat concerning. Thus, the long-term safety of lanthanum in uremic patients has not been unambiguously established.

Non-metal-based phosphate binders

The non-metal-based phosphate binders can be divided into two categories. The first category contains the mineral salts, such as calcium carbonate and calcium acetate or magnesium hydroxide and magnesium carbonate, where some of the mineral is absorbed as part of normal physiologic processes and some remains in the GI tract to form nonabsorbable salts with phosphorus. The second of the categories consists of nonabsorbed polymer resins that bind phosphorus in the GI tract and are excreted in the feces (Sevelamer HCl and Sevelamer carbonate).

Magnesium salts
Magnesium carbonate, Mg-hydroxide, and other magnesium salts will bind phosphorus [306–310]. Magnesium has been used intermittently in ESRD patients for this purpose, but has not been widely studied because of concerns about the potential adverse effects from excessive Mg absorption in individuals with kidney failure [311,312]. Recently Spiegel *et al.* compared the efficacy for

controlling hyperphosphatemia of magnesium carbonate to calcium acetate and found that both were well-tolerated and effective [313]. This was a short-term study, so long-term events could not be evaluated and await additional clinical trials.

Calcium carbonate and calcium acetate

Both calcium carbonate and calcium acetate have been demonstrated as effective in controlling hyperphosphatemia in ESRD patients in large cohort studies and smaller controlled clinical trials. The latter was introduced approximately 20 years ago, as it was observed to result in less calcium absorption from the GI tract in animal experiments and in human balance studies, and it was advocated as superior because of a potential reduced risk of hypercalcemia [314]. Most balance studies have demonstrated a substantially lower albeit significant net positive calcium balance in ESRD patients treated with calcium acetate compared to carbonate [315–317], but many have reported equivalent rates of hypercalcemia [317,318]. In addition, patient adherence with calcium carbonate appeared in general to be better [317,319].

Calcium carbonate was recognized as a potential therapeutic agent in ESRD more than 40 years ago based on its ability to result in a net positive calcium balance and in reduced phosphorus absorption in uremic patients [320]. In comparison to aluminum hydroxide, it was equally effective in controlling the latter [229], although in one study some patients required addition of aluminum to achieve target control of PO_4 [321]. Additionally, $CaCO_3$ has been associated with an increased incidence of hypercalcemia compared either to aluminum or to calcium acetate [254,322], in part due to a relative increased GI absorption when administered with [323] or without [324] food, even though net absorption of calcium in kidney failure in the absence of vitamin D was substantially reduced [325].

It is current practice to administer vitamin D to patients with CKD usually at a point in the progression of their disease that antedates the need to initiate PO_4 binders, and virtually all ESRD patients require both agents. Shortly after Clarkson, Ginsburg *et al.* reported clinically significant hypercalcemia in dialysis patients receiving 2–6 g/day of $CaCO_3$ orally [326]. Furthermore, it was quickly established that individuals dialyzed against a higher calcium dialysate concentration (during either hemodialysis or peritoneal dialysis) experienced increased episodes of hypercalcemia and increased suppression of PTH when they received $CaCO_3$ as their binder [327–330]. These effects could be somewhat mitigated by use of lower bath calcium concentrations [297,322,331] or more $Al(OH)_3$ or $Mg(OH)_2$ as phosphate binders [310]. In the current era of dialysis, Salusky and coworkers have demonstrated that coadministration of vitamin D with $CaCO_3$ as the phosphate binder results in a significant increase in hypercalcemic episodes in pediatric peritoneal dialysis patients compared to patients not receiving calcium orally [332]. Use of $CaCO_3$ in patients with CKD stages 3 and 4 may result in a lower number of hypercalcemic episodes and produce significant suppression of PTH [333], but recent studies support the notion that long-term use of calcium carbonate might contribute to vascular calcification even in predialysis patients [47,334–336].

Calcium acetate was introduced as a phosphate binder with a potential for reduced GI calcium absorption in part because of the exposure to roughly one-half of the elemental calcium for equivalent PO_4 binding capacity [253,254]. It was hoped that this would result in less hypercalcemia. Some of the initial clinical trials demonstrated the expected favorable serum calcium result [315,316,337]. Other investigators, however, either did not demonstrate a difference in the risk of hypercalcemia with the acetate salt compared with the carbonate in either crossover RCTs or longitudinal cohort studies [317,338,339] or found an actual worsening of hypercalcemia with calcium acetate, albeit with improved PO_4 control [313]. In the latter studies, hypercalcemia appeared to be most likely in patients who were receiving vitamin D and less likely when dialysate calcium was reduced [339]. Medication adherence appeared to be better with the carbonate than with the acetate [313,317]. It should also be noted that in healthy volunteers, calcium acetate does not increase aluminum absorption when these are administered together, whereas citrate does [340]. The latter may be an issue for CKD patients who are receiving citrate to correct metabolic acidosis [271].

The long-term consequences of the oral calcium loads at the doses typically used for binding phosphorus in ESRD patients have been debated extensively [341–344]. The evidence that informs this debate arises both from observational studies and from a limited number of RCTs, with the latter comparing the effects of different phosphate binders on long-term patient-centered outcomes. The observational data are reviewed in the next section.

Calcium-based phosphate binders: are they safe?

A general assumption that followed from the widespread use of calcium salts as PO_4 binders was that, short of causing overt hypercalcemia, some net positive calcium absorption would be beneficial as it might improve bone health and reduce cardiovascular risk. Both of these assumptions have been challenged recently by new RCT evidence in the general population. Bollard and colleagues randomly assigned postmenopausal women with sufficient vitamin D levels to receive 1 g of elemental calcium daily as calcium citrate versus placebo and followed these women for 5 years [345]. The women who were assigned to the calcium group experienced a higher rate of myocardial infarction and a trend towards reduced survival compared to women not receiving calcium. The population was principally individuals with mild CKD by virtue of their age and mild baseline elevations in creatinine. The benefits of calcium supplementation on preventing osteoporosis have been challenged by the negative results of the Women's Health Study [346]. A recent meta-analysis of the effects of calcium alone without vitamin D on bone health concluded that neither the pooled analysis of prospective cohort studies nor that of RCTs demonstrated a reduction in fracture risk. Furthermore, there was no observed treatment benefit in RCTs for hip or vertebral fractures from calcium supplementation [347].

In patients with ESRD, it is recognized that oral calcium administration both reduces phosphorus absorption and modestly increases serum calcium in such patients with hypocalcemia. Both of these effects were previously thought to be beneficial, as they both result in suppression of PTH. Calcium salts were widely adopted as phosphate binders in an era when the correction of hypocalcemia in ESRD patients was already a specific goal of multiple simultaneous interventions, including use of high dialysate calcium concentrations [348]. The last decade has seen a significant shift away from this approach, largely due to an appreciation of a significant incidence of postdialysis hypercalcemia and the emergence of adynamic bone disease thought, in part, to be due to oversuppression of PTH by hypercalcemia [349–352]. Furthermore, a number of observational studies have demonstrated an association of decreased survival in ESRD patients with higher predialysis serum calcium concentrations. These observations further accelerated the abandonment of strategies to raise serum calcium levels after 1997. The results of these observational studies are summarized in Table 34.3.

In a seminal study, Block *et al.* reported increases in observed mortality independently associated in ESRD patients with abnormalities in the biochemical parameters of MBD [207]. Mortality was associated with elevations in baseline serum phosphorus levels (reviewed above) and the calcium–phosphorus product. These observations have been replicated by Block *et al.* and by other groups independently examining dialysis patient population data [44,208–217]. In a follow-up analysis of a large dialysis cohort, Block demonstrated that mortality increased significantly with serum calcium levels of >9.5 mg/dL and a calcium–phosphorus product of >50–55 mg^2/dL [210]. In this second analysis, they observed a continuous relationship between increasing serum calcium and mortality, and the highest survival rates were seen in patients with the lowest baseline calcium levels. Klantar-Zadeh, using a somewhat different analytical methodology, demonstrated a similar relationship between high serum calcium levels and mortality [44]. In their maximally adjusted model, patients with the highest serum calcium levels experienced the highest mortality risk, and patients with serum calcium levels of between 8.2 and 9.5 demonstrated the most favorable survival. The observations arising from all of these studies have been relatively consistent; higher levels of serum calcium, serum phosphorus, and Ca–PO$_4$ product are each independently associated with reduced survival, even if the magnitude of impact or the threshold for the effect reported from each study differ somewhat (Table 34.3). Based on these observational studies, current K/DOQI guidelines recommend targeting a serum calcium level of 8.4–9.5 mg/dL.

London and others have provided evidence that it is not simply the serum calcium level but rather the total calcium exposure that may determine the mortality risk. They have demonstrated from longitudinal cohort studies performed in ESRD populations that increased exogenous calcium loads are associated with increased vascular calcification [31,32,41,42] and in independent observa-

tions, with increased mortality [37,39]. Most recently this group has reported that in patients with adynamic bone disease as might occur with oversuppression of PTH by exogenous calcium loading compared to those with high-turnover bone disease, the relationship between exogenous calcium burden and mortality is strongest [51].

Although the classic Bradford-Hill considerations for a possible causal relationship between exposure to calcium and adverse outcomes are largely fulfilled (Table 34.5), there are no RCTs with masked allocation evaluating the long-term patient-oriented outcomes of phosphate binder therapy compared to placebo, therewith addressing this question with the lowest opportunity for bias and confounding. Despite a significant number of observational studies in which the use of calcium-based phosphate binders is associated with vascular calcification and premature cardiovascular disease, some equipoise with respect to the safety of calcium-based phosphate binders compared to non-calcium-based binders exists. This has permitted completion of RCTs comparing outcomes with calcium-based phosphate binders to outcomes with the non-calcium-based phosphate binder sevelamer. These studies have compared calcium-based binders to sevelamer principally in ESRD patients and have not investigated the incremental benefit of either phosphate binder compared to a no-phosphate binder control. In patients with ESRD who manifest the most severe dysregulation of PO$_4$ metabolism and the highest levels of serum PO$_4$, inclusion of a placebo arm to a phosphate binder trial is probably not ethically sustainable. However, the use of any of the currently available phosphate binders in CKD stages 3 and 4 has not been studied rigorously with multiple RCTs evaluating mortality and cardiovascular outcomes, and the benefits from these medicines in this patient population are less certain. Thus, RCTs with appropriate controls are appropriate and required in CKD stages 3 and 4 to address the following questions: 1) when to initiate phosphate binders as an individual progresses through the stages of CKD; 2) what target levels of PO$_4$ and PTH should be recommended at each stage of CKD to achieve optimal benefit on mortality and morbidities, including renal failure progression; 3) how to use the binders optimally in conjunction with vitamin D; and 4) what binders might be most effective in maintaining health and survival.

It is plausible that patients with moderate to moderately severe CKD (CKD stage 3 and early stage 4) might behave either similarly or differently than ESRD patients when exposed to phosphate binders. The epidemiologic and observational data and the limited RCT evidence available in CKD patients support the hypothesis that patients with late CKD stage 4 behave similarly to CKD stage 5 and ESRD patients. Thus, data from ESRD population-based studies have been used in the absence of more direct RCT evidence for CKD stage 4 to inform practice. Observational studies have identified a significant degree of vascular calcification in CKD patients [50,331,335,353], especially in those patients with diabetes or increased markers of inflammation, and that this vascular calcification is associated with a number of factors, including the quantity of calcium ingested [47,50,334,335].

What is the evidence that exposure to calcium salts in the form of phosphate binders may result in less favorable outcomes when compared to non-calcium-based binders? These data are of four types: 1) epidemiological data that demonstrate a strong positive association between calcium exposure and adverse outcomes (Table 34.3); 2) whole-animal studies and experimental models using human cells in culture; 3) short-term human trials reporting serum and urine calcium levels, PO_4, and PTH; and 4) the results of long-term RCTs comparing calcium-based phosphate binders to sevelamer and evaluating hard outcomes. The evidence from each of these sources when evaluated in the context of the totality of evidence is consistent with the remainder of this evidence. The RCT evidence is considered below.

Sevelamer

Sevelamer is a cross-linked poly(allylamine)-hydrochloride or carbonate, a calcium-free, metal-free, nonmineral, nonabsorbed polymer that binds phosphorus in the proximal intestine and bile acid more distally [354–360]. This first characteristic permits sevelamer to perform as an efficacious binder of PO_4 in the more proximal portions of the GI tract, the second as a sequestrant acting more distally to decrease low-density lipoprotein (LDL) cholesterol and triglyceride levels [356–362]. It is available in most countries as the hydrochloride. A newer form of sevelamer polymer as the carbonate is available in a limited but growing number of countries [360]. These phosphate binders have been evaluated in patients with ESRD [354–356,359–361,363,364] and CKD [336,362] with hyperphosphatemia in comparison to calcium-based phosphate binders or in comparisons of one form of sevelamer to the other. There have been three crossover trials that have probed the use of sevelamer to control phosphorus in combination with a calcium-based phosphate binder [365–369]. The principal goal of the efficacy studies has been the control of hyperphosphatemia. In addition, long-term clinical RCTs have been conducted comparing sevelamer to calcium-based phosphate binders on coronary artery and vascular calcification, on pulse wave velocity [370,371], on mortality, and on hospitalization rates. The studies of 52 weeks or longer in duration are shown in Table 34.6 [60,335,364,372–379]. RCT evidence of potentially favorable effects of sevelamer compared to calcium-based phosphate binders on biochemical parameters, including LDL and high-density lipoprotein (HDL) cholesterol levels, C-reactive protein, fetuin, FGF-23, and uric acid (many of which are candidate markers of inflammation) has also been reported [380–382]. These "pleiotropic" effects of sevelamer theoretically may provide additional long-term health benefits from sevelamer use, but the magnitude of these potential benefits has yet to be established [383].

It should be noted that most clinical trials (observational studies, single-arm efficacy trials, and RCTs) with sevelamer-HCl report consistently lower serum bicarbonate levels in patients on sevelamer-HCl for longer than a few weeks compared to the level in the same patients prior to sevelamer-HCl therapy or in comparison to patients on other phosphate binders, including sevelamer-carbonate, aluminum hydroxide, calcium-carbonate, and calcium acetate. In sevelamer-treated patients, observed serum bicarbonate levels range from 18 to 21.5 mEq/L (commonly 18.5–20.5) compared to levels of close to 22 mEq/L reported in most patients treated with other PO_4 binders. The mild acidosis is thought to be due to the absorption of additional Cl^- released from sevelamer-HCl and not an effect of the sevelamer polymer itself, since use of sevelamer as the carbonate results in correction of this acidosis [384]. The long-term clinical implication of the mild metabolic acidosis seen in patients treated with sevelamer-HCl is uncertain; to date there have been no clinical trials that have implicated the mild acidosis per se as causal of significant adverse events.

Both the HCl and the carbonate forms of sevelamer reduce phosphorus absorption and serum phosphorus levels in an identical dose-dependent fashion, as reported in two recent clinical trials. In the first trial, the investigators determined that sevelamer carbonate and sevelamer HCl were equipotent and efficacious as phosphate binders [384]. They also demonstrated that the carbonate form of sevelamer was associated with fewer GI side effects of any type (15 vs. 28%; $P < 0.007$) and with normalization of serum HCO_3 levels (22.4 vs 20.8 mEq/L) [384]. A second trial conducted in patients with CKD or ESRD demonstrated that once-daily dosing of sevelamer carbonate with a meal was not as effective in reducing PO_4 in those patients with the most severe elevations in baseline PO_4 as thrice-daily dosing with meals and/or snacks but did control PO_4 to target in some patients with more moderate degrees of hyperphosphatemia [360,385].

Both forms of sevelamer also bind bile salts and improve LDL and HDL cholesterol and triglyceride levels in these patients. The impact of the observed improvements in lipid profiles with sevelamer on patient-oriented clinical outcomes is unknown. Similar degrees of improvement in lipid profiles did not result in substantial improvements in vascular outcomes in one large RCT [386], but a meta-analysis by Stripolli *et al.* that also included these trial results supported the view that the pharmacologic modulation in lipid profiles in CKD patients is beneficial [387]. The recent CARE II trial of Qunibi and coworkers that included a lipid-lowering intervention (atorvastatin) did not evaluate patient-oriented outcomes and therefore does not add to the evidence informing this specific question [364].

Long-term RCT comparisons of sevelamer with other phosphate binders

The important long-term risks and benefits of sevelamer as a phosphate binder have been probed with RCTs virtually exclusively in comparison to calcium-based phosphate binders. These RCTs have evaluated the effects of a phosphate binder on disease-oriented outcomes, including coronary artery calcification, pulse wave velocity, bone mineral density, and bone histomorphology, and on patient-centered outcomes, including mortality and hospitalization rates. A single case report of reversal of calciphylaxis with high-dose sevelamer is intriguing but has not been corroborated in an RCT [388]. Table 34.6 lists RCTs of at least 12 months in duration

Table 34.6 Long-term clinical trials comparing calcium-based phosphate binders to sevelamer.

Clinical study (yr)	Calcium-based phosphate binder used	Outcome measured	Outcome reported	Duration of follow-up: no. of subjects
Studies using surrogate outcomes				
Chertow (TTG) (2004)	Acetate and carbonate	Change in CAC score	Significantly slower progression of coronary artery, aortic, and mitral valve calcification by EBCT in sevelamer group	1 yr; 200 prevalent HD patients
Braun (2004)	Carbonate	Change in CAC score	Significant progression of coronary artery and aortic valve calcification by EBCT in calcium group, no progression in sevelamer group	2 yrs; 114 prevalent HD patients
Raggi (TTG, 1 yr of follow-up) (2005)	Acetate and carbonate	Bone mineralization	Stability or improvement in trabecular bone mineralization in sevelamer group, progression of demineralization in calcium group	1 yr; 111 prevalent HD patients
Asmus (TTG, 2 yrs of follow-up, Germany and Austria) (2005)	Carbonate	Bone mineralization	Stability or improvement in trabecular bone mineralization in sevelamer group, progression of demineralization in calcium group	2 yrs; 72 prevalent HD patients
Block (RIND-18 primary study) (2005)	Carbonate and acetate	Change in CAC score	More rapid progression of coronary calcification in calcium group among those with calcification at baseline	18 mos; 127 incident HD patients
Russo (2007)	Carbonate	Change in CAC score in CKD	More rapid progression of coronary calcification in calcium group or those treated with diet only compared to sevelamer	2 yrs; 90 predialysis patients
Ferreira (2008)	Carbonate	Bone mineralization	Bone formation rate per surface area increased by sevelamer in HD patients with mostly adynamic bone disease	1 yr; 119 prevalent HD patients
Qunibi (CARE-2) (2008)	Acetate	Change in CAC score	Noninferiority (within 1.8 SD) of calcium-acetate plus atorvastatin compared to sevelamer for slowing the rate of vascular calcification by CT	1 yr; 203 prevalent HD patients
Studies using hard outcomes				
Block (RIND; 5 yrs follow-up) (2007)	Carbonate and acetate	Mortality in incident dialysis	Increased survival over 5 yrs in subjects allocated to sevelamer arm at randomization	5 yrs; 127 incident HD patients
Suki (DCOR) (2007)	Acetate 70%, carbonate 30%	Mortality	Inconclusive result for overall mortality; mortality benefit for strata over age 65 yrs	3.5 yrs; 2103 prevalent HD patients
St. Peter (DCOR) (2008)	Acetate 70%, carbonate 30%	Hospitalization rate	Reduced number of hospitalizations and hospital days in sevelamer arm; no observed difference in overall mortality between the two arms	4 yrs; 2103 prevalent HD patients

Abbreviations: HD, hemodialysis.

that compared outcomes in patients treated with sevelamer or calcium-based phosphate binders [60,335,364,372–379]. The first eight reports are from six trials that evaluated disease-oriented outcomes, and the remaining three are from two trials reporting on patient-centered outcomes. These trials demonstrated a statistically significant increase in vascular calcification (coronary arteries, heart valves, and/or aorta) in predialysis, incident dialysis, and prevalent dialysis patients treated with either diet alone or calcium-based phosphate binders alone compared to sevelamer-treated patients. In the prevalent hemodialysis patients studied in the treat-to-goal trial reported by Chertow and coworkers [372] and by Asmus et al. [375], vascular calcification progressed significantly more in the calcium-treated group compared to the sevelamer group at 1 year and yet further again at 2 years. The benefit from sevelamer treatment was greatest for those with the most intense calcification at study entry.

Most recently, Qunibi [364] compared vascular calcification scores in prevalent hemodialysis patients treated either with sevelamer-HCl or with calcium-acetate plus atorvastatin where the atorvastatin was titrated in both arms of the study to achieve the same lipid profile with both binders. They observed that the between-binder group difference in calcification scores in the patients followed for 12 months was no greater than the predetermined margin of 1.8. The authors argued that calcium acetate is not inferior to sevelamer in modulating coronary artery calcification (CAC) scores when both are used along with a statin. The study was limited by its short duration and substantial and differential dropout rates: 28 and 43% in the calcium-acetate group prior to 6 months and prior to 1 year, respectively, and 13 and 30% for the same periods in sevelamer-treated participants. There were 7 deaths during approximately 75 patient-years of observation in the calcium arm of the trial (actuarial method) compared to 3 deaths during approximately 86 patient-years in the sevelamer arm. The authors did not report whether these death rates were different statistically.

The three remaining studies in Table 34.6 report as their primary or secondary outcomes patient-centered outcomes. Block and coworkers followed the original RIND trial cohort for a total of 60 months from the date of first enrollment [60]. They demonstrated two important findings in this planned extension of the RIND trial. First, they provided the first prospective validation in ESRD patients of the CAC score as a predictor of future mortality. Second, the authors reported a statistically significant, more favorable hazard ratio (lower mortality) over the entire survival curve for study subjects enrolled in the sevelamer arm at initiation of dialysis compared to patients randomized to receive the calcium-based phosphate binders for the first 18 months of hemodialysis treatment. The difference in the annualized hazard ratio if extrapolated over 5 years might result in a substantial absolute risk reduction for mortality. (A crude estimate for the absolute risk reduction over 5 years of roughly 28% can be made with a degree of uncertainty.) Block et al. provided evidence of a potential survival benefit from using sevelamer in place of calcium-based phosphate binders that is consistent with the epidemiologic data.

Suki et al. conducted the largest trial to date comparing outcomes in prevalent dialysis patients treated either with sevelamer or calcium-based phosphate binders (70% calcium acetate, 30% calcium carbonate) [378]. This trial was inconclusive for the primary outcome of all-cause mortality for the entire study population because of a 30% lower than predicted mortality rate and the uncertainty introduced by an approximately 50% dropout rate at 2 years. For the strata of patients older than 65 years, however, a preplanned analysis revealed a significant survival advantage for those elderly patients allocated to the sevelamer arm of the trial. St. Peter and colleagues used the Centers for Medicare and Medicaid Services medical billings to determine the hospitalization rates and length of stay and overall mortality for all DCOR study subjects whether actively enrolled or lost to follow-up [379]. They demonstrated a statistically significant reduction in multiple hospitalizations and hospital days for those individuals originally allocated to sevelamer rather than calcium-based phosphate binders.

The RCT evidence does not eliminate some of the uncertainty regarding the magnitude and the topography of the survival benefit from the use of sevelamer and/or elimination of calcium salts as phosphate binders. Further clinical trials may be required. It should be noted, however, that the hypothesis that excessive calcium ingestion is associated with reduced survival is supported by substantial epidemiologic and observational data in addition to the RCTs reviewed. Furthermore, a recent observational study by Borzecki et al. demonstrated that incident dialysis patients in the VA medical system had a 33% (multivariant-adjusted) to 35% (propensity score-adjusted) improved 18-month survival if they were treated with sevelamer rather than calcium acetate or carbonate [389]. Although the magnitude of the benefit was greater in this observational study than that reported for the elderly subjects in the RCT by Suki, the effect size in the Borzecki study is large enough that it is likely that a benefit would persist were the same question interrogated in this incident dialysis population under RCT conditions [142].

Sevelamer effects on bone histology

In addition to a potential survival benefit, findings from a number of RCTs in prevalent hemodialysis patients support the hypothesis that sevelamer improves bone health in patients with MBD of CKD more than comparable control of PO_4 with calcium-based phosphate binders [332,366,374,375,377]. Each of these studies reported improvement in some measure of bone mineralization and biochemical parameters associated with improved bone health, such as alkaline phosphatase. Raggi and Asmus demonstrated increases in trabecular bone mineralization that were significantly greater in sevelamer-treated subjects [374,375]. Kokuho et al. evaluated patients with low-turnover bone disease and low iPTH and demonstrated improved biochemical bone parameters when sevelamer was used either alone or in combination with calcium carbonate in a strategy designed to reduce overall calcium exposure [366]. In an RCT in prevalent hemodialysis patients, Ferriera et al. evaluated the effects of sevelamer versus calcium carbonate on bone histomorphometry [377]. A majority (59%) of their population (prevalent hemodialysis patients) demonstrated features of adynamic bone disease at study entry. Over the 1 year of the study, the patients randomized to receive sevelamer demonstrated improvements in their bone formation rate per bone surface area that were not seen in the opposite arm of the study. None of these studies evaluated changes in fracture rates.

Sevelamer: when should it be used

K/DOQI guidelines recommend that clinicians consider using sevelamer as a phosphate binder in place of calcium-based binders in those patients who cannot tolerate calcium binders due to the development of hypercalcemia or in those patients who already demonstrate vascular calcification or who are at high future risk of developing vascular calcification. The latter group includes elderly dialysis patients, those with long-standing kidney failure on dialysis for more than 2 years, and those with diabetes mellitus [50,353,382]. For the remainder of the dialysis and CKD populations, reliable simple measures are available that have been shown in clinical trials to identify most individuals with significant vascular calcification. Sophisticated approaches using computed tomography technology have been developed [390–393] and validated for the general and dialysis populations [60,394–403]. Potentially of greater broad clinical applicability are those techniques that have been developed and validated that utilize X-ray or ultrasound to identify the presence of vascular calcification [404–406].

Meta-analyses comparing sevelamer and other binders

Meta-analyses on the effectiveness of sevelamer as a PO_4 binder have been performed. It should be noted that because most of the clinical trials used either PO_4 levels or the $Ca–PO_4$ product to titrate the dose of the binders, substantial differences in end-of-trial PO_4 levels should not be expected. Any differences might reasonably be assumed to be due to potential protocol failure. On the other hand, meta-analyses could reasonably evaluate differences in control of hyperparathyroidism, frequency of hypercalcemic events, changes in coronary artery calcification, mortality, and morbidities such as hospitalization rates. Attempts at compiling such comprehensive summaries have been limited by the availability of robust RCT evidence of long-term hard outcomes in CKD and ESRD patients and the significant important differences in trial design including duration of follow-up, resulting in significant between-study heterogeneity.

Burke *et al.* conducted a systematic review of the literature on sevelamer-HCl reported through October 2002 (68 published reports, 46 abstracts evaluated, and 17 included in the final analysis) to evaluate the question of the effect of ingestion of sevelamer as a phosphate binder on lipid profiles and on the biochemical parameter of MBD in ESRD, specifically, on serum PO_4, Ca, Ca–PO_4 product, and iPTH [407]. They did not evaluate the literature for comparisons of sevelamer with any other phosphate binder. Burke *et al.* demonstrated a significant fall in serum PO_4 (average

reduction of 2.1 mg/dL; 95% CI, 3.1–1.2), in the Ca–PO_4 product (15.9 mg²/dL; 95% CI, 121.4–10.4), in iPTH (36.0 mg/dL; 95% CI, 67.7–4.28) and in triglycerides (22.0 mg/dL) and total and LDL cholesterol (30.6 mg/dL [95% CI, 35.4–25.8] and 31.4 mg/dL [95% CI, 35.5–27.3], respectively), and a concomitant rise in HDL cholesterol (4.1 mg/dL). Serum calcium levels did not change (0.09 mg/dL; 95% CI, −0.10 to 0.14).

Nadin conducted a similar evaluation in 2005 but also included an assessment of morbidity and mortality outcomes and cost-effectiveness in comparison to other binders. She included studies identified through January 21, 2005, evaluated 177 reports, and included 53 in the final analysis [408]. She concluded that the evidence demonstrates that sevelamer is as effective as calcium salts in lowering PO_4 and product, with a lower risk of hypercalcemia. She also noted substantial evidence on vascular calcification and more limited evidence on patient-oriented outcomes related to morbidity and mortality.

Most recently, Tonelli and coworkers evaluated the clinical efficacy and safety of sevelamer versus calcium-based phosphate binders [209]. This review represents an update of a prior report from the same investigators [210]. Tonelli *et al.* reported that hypercalcemia was more likely in patients treated with calcium-based phosphate binders, with an absolute risk reduction of 21% (95% CI, 13–29%) with sevelamer for a number needed to harm with the use of calcium-based phosphate binders of 5. Hypercalcemia was the only significant risk difference that emerged from this meta-analysis. These findings reiterate findings reported in the analysis by Nadin and others [208]. Tonelli *et al.* also reported an effect of binder choice on end-of-study phosphorus levels that favored calcium-based binders. They combined studies that used the calcium–phosphorus product as the end point for titration of binder dose with studies that used a serum PO_4 target as the dosing determinant. The former dosing protocol if successful would require lower serum PO_4 levels in those patients allocated to calcium-based PO_4 binders, given the nearly universal observation of higher calcium levels in these patients, and this difference in protocol dosing targets might account for the large heterogeneity reported by Tonelli and could account for the difference in PO_4 levels achieved rather than any difference in intrinsic efficacy of the binders. Indeed, when the DCOR results were eliminated from the meta-analysis, the observed effect of binder class on end-of-study PO_4 levels achieved was magnified.

Tonelli and coworkers also reported an absence of benefit in patient-oriented outcomes when sevelamer was used in place of calcium-based binders. Their finding of an equivalency of survival benefits with either calcium-based phosphate binders or sevelamer is based on their meta-analysis of five RCTs [60,372,378,411,412]. Only two of these studies had mortality as a primary [378] or secondary [60] outcome of the trial and were sufficiently long in duration to observe potential effects of a "vascular sparing" intervention on mortality. Results from the largest study were only available in abstract form at the time of the analysis. Tonelli *et al.* included results from an 8-week crossover study in which no deaths were reported in 20 subjects [412] and results from a

5-month study in which multiple interventions were performed simultaneously (including changes in dialysate calcium content and vitamin D) [411]. Some of the limitations of this analysis have been reviewed recently by Frazao and others [413].

Hyper- and hypoparathyroidism

Evidence that hyper- and hypothyroidism result in increased mortality and morbidity

The clinical benefits that arise from vitamin D therapies and from the management of the dysregulation of phosphorus and calcium metabolism in CKD may be due, in part, to prevention or correction of hyperparathyroidism. Evidence supporting the view that hyperparathyroidism itself leads to increased mortality and morbidity has arisen from epidemiologic studies in "normal" populations with hyperparathyroidism due to vitamin D deficiency [414–422], in cohorts of CKD patients [74], and in prevalent dialysis cohorts and from observational studies and RCTs comparing the long-term outcomes of surgical treatment versus conservative management of primary hyperparathyroidism 423–434].

Epidemiological studies in populations of chronic dialysis patients and of patients with CKD not yet on dialysis have identified an independent association of both hyperparathyroidism and oversuppression of PTH secretion with an increase in mortality. The largest of such studies are included in Table 34.3. This association is most evident in those studies where sensitive and stable PTH assays were employed [86]. Block and coworkers analyzed a large data set of prevalent hemodialysis patients and demonstrated that patients with an initial iPTH level of >300 pg/mL experienced a significant "dose-dependent" increase in mortality over the subsequent 2 years of follow-up [207,210]. Similar observations have emerged from the DOPPS and other large dialysis cohorts [211–220]. Kalantar-Zadeh and coworkers, examining a large data set of prevalent dialysis patients in the USA, demonstrated a similar relationship between PTH and mortality. In their fully adjusted model, adjusted for significant comorbidities, age, gender, and nutritional status, PTH levels of >600 pg/mL were independently associated with increased mortality [44]. The analyses of Kalantar-Zadeh and others have also identified an increase in mortality with achievement of low PTH in dialysis patients, most commonly with levels of iPTH of <100–150 pg/mL. Both high and low PTH levels are also associated with increased risk of fracture in CKD patients [432,433], and primary hyperparathyroidism is associated with increased mortality risk in the general population [414–422].

Studies that have included bone biopsy have identified that a significant number of patients with low iPTH levels have adynamic bone disease. The potential causes of adynamic bone disease have been reviewed elsewhere [85,87,92,349,434]. It is relevant to the optimal management of MBD of CKD that adynamic bone disease may occur in the setting of oversuppression of PTH potentially from vitamin D therapies and excess calcium loads and theoretically with calcimimetics. Kalantar-Zadeh provided evidence that adynamic bone disease occurs principally in patients who

demonstrate clinical or laboratory measures of malnutrition [60]. The relative contribution of malnutrition versus pharmacologic oversuppression of PTH on the development of adynamic bone disease awaits clarification by further study.

Adynamic bone disease may increase mortality risk or, as shown recently by London and others, may accentuate the mortality and cardiovascular disease risks associated with an increased calcium intake [51,436,437]. Given the importance of properly identifying patients with adynamic bone disease when determining optimal therapy for an individual patient, it should be noted that Malluche and others reported that conventional iPTH assays may lead to the misclassification of bone disease in a significant number of patients, particularly those with low-turnover disease [63,83,352]. The potential for misclassification is further complicated by the finding that PTH assays vary significantly from one reference laboratory to the next [84]. Nonetheless, at the present time the iPTH assay remains a standard for directing therapy of MBD.

In the absence of overt kidney disease, both primary hyperparathyroidism and secondary hyperparathyroidism that is the result of 25(OH)-vitamin D deficiency are associated with increased cardiovascular mortality. Outcomes data from a prospectively followed Swedish cohort demonstrate that individuals newly identified with primary hyperparathyroidism have a significantly increased risk of death over the next 14 years compared to healthy individuals in the population [422]. These findings have been reproduced in other populations that have included subjects with symptomatic hyperparathyroidism as a consequence of hypercalcemia as well as those who are entirely "asymptomatic" [422]. Sambrook et al. observed an increased mortality associated with elevations in serum PTH levels in a cohort of elderly frail Australian men and women that was independent of vitamin D status, bone mass, or renal function [417].

These studies do not permit an unambiguous separation of the causal influence of a high PTH on mortality from other potential confounders, such as renal insufficiency and mineral dysregulation, in CKD patients. However, preliminary evidence from an RCT does support the view that has emerged from observational studies that PTH in excess can lead directly to an increase in mortality, principally from cardiovascular causes [423,424,426]. Patients with "asymptomatic" primary hyperparathyroidism were randomized to undergo minimally invasive parathyroidectomy versus medical management without surgery. Those with parathyroidectomy demonstrated an improvement in cognitive function and quality of life and improved survival [423,424].

Targets for PTH levels

On the basis of the observational data from dialysis populations, K/DOQI guidelines recommend that therapies be initiated to maintain iPTH levels in dialysis-dependent patients of 150–300 pg/mL, in CKD stage 3 patients of 35–70 pg/mL, and in CKD stage 4 patients of 70–110 pg/mL [22]. The recommendations for target PTH levels in CKD stages 3 and 4 are based principally on expert opinion. To date, there is no evidence from RCTs that provides definitive proof for the recommended PTH target levels in patients with CKD stages 3 and 4, nor are there any RCTs that demonstrate that treatment of patients with CKD stage 3 or 4 with hyperparathyroidism to the recommended PTH target for each stage improves survival.

Treatments for secondary hyperparathyroidism of CKD

There are five modalities of treatment (four of which have practical clinical application) that have been demonstrated with either observational studies or clinical RCTs to help prevent or manage secondary hyperparathyroidism. Vitamin D and phosphate reduction therapies, which may have other important therapeutic benefits in patients with CKD beyond their effect on PTH, are reviewed above. Other modalities that will suppress PTH include induction of hypercalcemia, surgical parathyroidectomy, and calcimimetic administration. The latter is sometimes referred to as a medical parathyroidectomy.

It was recognized more than 4 decades ago that elevations in serum calcium levels in dialysis-dependent patients result in reductions in PTH levels. This led to adoption of higher dialysate calcium concentrations as the standard of care and facilitated the widespread adoption of vitamin D therapies and oral calcium supplementation. More recently, attention has been directed towards the risks associated with increased calcium burdens, including the oversuppression of parathyroid function and the development of low-turnover bone disease. This led to a major shift in the choice of dialysate composition; currently, lower bath ionized calcium concentrations are the standard [1]. Thus, although PTH secretion remains somewhat responsive to serum calcium levels in patients with secondary hyperparathyroidism of CKD, strategies to intentionally increase serum ionized calcium concentrations to hypercalcemic levels are no longer considered safe or prudent. Intentional calcium loading as a means of controlling PTH will not be considered further in this chapter as a practical therapy for secondary hyperparathyroidism. The clinical trial evidence for the two remaining therapies for reduction of hyperparathyroidism, namely, surgical parathyroidectomy and cinacalcet administration, are considered.

Surgical parathyroidectomy

Numerous case series and cohort studies have demonstrated that surgical parathyroidectomy does reduce PTH levels in dialysis patients with secondary hyperparathyroidism. Prospective surgical cohorts have also described the rate of complications, the "optimal" surgical technique to increase the probability of maintaining target PTH levels postoperatively, and the effects of parathyroidectomy on the bone component of MBD, on postoperative serum calcium levels, and the need for vitamin D supplementation [425426,431,438–440]. Surgical parathyroidectomy has been advocated principally as a means of controlling severe hyperparathyroidism in dialysis patients who are refractory to medical management. There have been, to date, no long-term RCTs

comparing parathyroidectomy to other modalities of controlling PTH in ESRD patients with respect to mortality and significant morbidities, including pathologic fractures and cardiovascular events [427–434,441–443]. Parathyroidectomy has not been evaluated either with observational studies or with an RCT as a modality of treatment for secondary hyperparathyroidism in patients not yet on dialysis. Surgical parathyroidectomy has not been evaluated in comparison to medical approaches such as the use of calcimimetics. The latter medical approach has displaced surgical parathyroidectomy in many areas of the world.

Calcimimetic therapy

The fourth modality of treatment for MBD in ESRD that is gaining in usage in many countries is the suppression of excess PTH secretion with a calcimimetic [444]. Currently the only calcimimetic that has been approved for use in the USA and elsewhere is cinacalcet. Cinacalcet has been approved by the US Food and Drug Administration for treatment of secondary hyperparathyroidism in ESRD only. Therapy with cinacalcet is not currently included in any of the major national guidelines, most of which were written prior to its clinical introduction. Clinicians have investigated cinacalcet's actions with prospective cohorts [445,446] and RCTs [447–451] and have demonstrated its efficacy in lowering elevated PTH levels in patients with secondary hyperparathyroidism. With the reduction in PTH levels, serum calcium, and to a lesser degree PO_4, levels fall as calcium moves into bone. A number of these clinical trials have demonstrated that patients treated with cinacalcet as part of their MBD therapy are much more likely to achieve K/DOQI targets than patients receiving more conventional therapy [447,448,450]. Attainment of target biochemical parameters may be specifically enhanced by a dose optimization algorithm that adjusts doses of vitamin D and cinacalcet simultaneously [450,452].

The short-term clinical trials address, only partially, patient-centered outcomes such as any mortality benefit from cinacalcet and long-term safety of its use. Ongoing clinical trials are currently addressing the former issue [453]. To address the latter question, Cunningham combined the results from four trials of 6–12 months in duration [454]. The majority of study subjects were observed for 6 months. Cunningham reported that patients assigned to cinacalcet treatment were less likely to be hospitalized for a cardiovascular event (RR, 0.61; 95% CI, 0.43–0.86) or sustain a fracture (RR, 0.46; 95% CI, 0.22–0.95) compared to control study subjects. Furthermore, cinacalcet-treated patients reported improvements in their quality of life as measured by the SF-36 and KDQOL-CF. No difference in mortality was noted.

These studies did not address the potential risk of low-turnover bone disease from excess suppression of PTH with cinacalcet. Lien et al. evaluated the effects of cinacalcet on BMD over 26 weeks in 14 patients randomly assigned to conventional therapy ($n = 6$) or cinacalcet ($n = 8$) [448]. They reported an improvement in BMD of the proximal femur with cinacalcet from a pooled analysis using

Student's *t* test rather than more conservative nonparametric methods. Although their conclusion that cinacalcet reverses bone loss cannot be supported with their small sample size, their observation that the changes in bone mineral density if present with cinacalcet are much smaller than those following surgical parathyroidectomy does suggest that medical parathyroidectomy with cinacalcet might be quite different from its surgical counterpart.

Recently, Strippoli and coworkers completed a meta-analysis of high-quality studies examining calcimimetic use in CKD and ESRD [455,456]. Garside *et al.* have conducted a similar analysis as part of their Health Technology Assessment 2007 [457]. Both groups reported similar findings. Both groups reported that the studies included in their final meta-analyses were conducted principally in patients with ESRD on dialysis. They concluded that cinacalcet when administered with standard therapy was more effective at achieving PTH target levels than placebo (40 vs. 5% in the pooled analysis by Garside; $P < 0.001$) and was more effective than standard therapy for patients with moderate to severe hyperparathyroidism. Among study subjects that achieved the PTH target, 90% of those treated with cinacalcet exhibited a fall in the $Ca-PO_4$ product, versus 1% of those treated with placebo. Pooled incidences of serious adverse effects for cinacalcet versus placebo were not different [455,457]. Significantly more episodes of nausea (31 vs. 19%; $P < 0.001$) and vomiting (27 vs. 15%; $P < 0.001$) were reported for patients treated with cinacalcet and these increases were dose dependent [457]. Strippoli noted in a meta-analysis that no significant effects on patient-oriented outcomes such as mortality were demonstrated [455].

These two meta-analyses did not address the use of calcimimetics in CKD stages 3 and 4 prior to the initiation of renal replacement therapy. To date there has been only one 18-week RCT exclusively in pre-ESRD patients treated with calcimimetics compared to other modalities of secondary hyperparathyroidism management. Charytan *et al.* reported that cinacalcet improved PTH levels without producing significant changes in serum PO_4 and Ca levels [449]. They reported modest GI side effects. Lien *et al.* included four CKD stage 4 patients in their RCT on bone mineral density [448]. Neither of these studies permits firm conclusions about the possible benefits or harms of cinacalcet in predialysis patients. Trials in CKD stages 3 and 4 are in progress. Trials in pre-ESRD patients should address issues related to the impact of calcimimetics on mortality and on morbidity, including whether suppression of PTH with cinacalcet in this patient population increases the subsequent risk of low-turnover bone disease, especially when these patients progress to ESRD. Although there is potential promise with the use of cinacalcet in pre-ESRD patients, pending the results of the ongoing studies, cinacelcet cannot be recommended as either safe or effective in patients with the CKD stage 3 or 4.

Bisphosphonates

Bisphosphonates are used widely for the treatment and/or prevention of osteoporosis and its complications in the general popula-

tion. These agents are eliminated importantly via renal excretion [458,459]. The efficacy of these agents in the treatment of osteoporosis in individuals without renal function has been confirmed with robust RCT evidence from multiple trials [460]. Their use in individuals with CKD is less well studied. In multiple large RCTs, elderly individuals with osteoporosis experienced fewer significant fractures when treated with bisphosphonates than those in control groups treated with customary care (typically, calcium supplementation). These RCTs, however, have not included by design significant numbers of individuals with known CKD, and none of these studies stratified subjects by baseline kidney function. Many elderly patients with CKD are identified as at risk for osteoporosis [461]. This risk appears to be much higher than for age- and gender-matched controls [462,463]. Alem *et al.* described a much-increased risk of hip fractures in Caucasian ESRD patients with an overall odds ratio of fracture of 4.44 (95% CI, 4.16–4.75) [464,465]. In patients with CKD the degree of demineralization is directly correlated to the degree (stage) and/or duration of CKD [461,466]. Additionally, demineralization may be accelerated in certain CKDs, such as those typically treated with steroids (e.g. glomerulonephritis, lupus nephritis, etc.) and those with chronic metabolic acidosis associated with renal tubular acidosis [467].

It is likely that the osteoporosis risk in elderly patients with mild to moderate CKD will be recognized by these patients' primary care physician long before they are identified with CKD and referred to a nephrologist [466]. Thus, it is relevant to review the data regarding the use of bisphosphantes in the CKD and ESRD populations. There are five questions that need to be addressed. Because bisphosphonates are principally metabolized via renal excretion, are they safe for use in patients with CKD and ESRD? Do they contribute to low-turnover bone disease in CKD, as suggested by case series arising from the non-CKD population [468]? If used to treat osteoporosis, are they effective in this population in improving bone health and reducing morbidity and/or mortality? If they are to be used in treating osteoporosis, how can patients with osteoporosis best be identified? And if they are useful for treatment of osteoporosis, do they have any role in preventing the bone mineral loss that occurs in transplant patients receiving corticosteroids?

The risk of adynamic bone disease and the effectiveness of these agents in individuals with both osteoporosis and MBD can be determined best by clinical RCTs. No such trials have been conducted that have been specifically designed to address the risk of adynamic bone disease in CKD and/or dialysis-dependent patients. Recently, Miller and coworkers evaluated the safety of bisphosphonates in patients with CKD stages 3 and 4 [469,470]. They reanalyzed and combined by meta-analysis data from nine large RCTs examining the use of the bisphosphonate risedronate (5 mg daily) to treat or prevent osteoporosis or to treat or prevent steroid-induced bone disease. Some subjects were included in these RCTs who had significant levels of CKD that was initially unrecognized because these subjects had near-normal serum creatinine levels but significant CKD when estimated GFRs (eGFRs) were calculated in retrospect. In this post hoc secondary analysis of patients with CKD treated in these RCTs with risedronate compared to control treatment, Miller and coworkers demonstrated that CKD patients treated with risedronate did not experience an increase in reported adverse events. Furthermore, they did not see an acceleration of decline in renal function or an increase in low-turnover bone disease for patients in any of the three CKD strata evaluated.

These findings are limited because the clinical trials were not specifically designed to evaluate the kidney injury outcomes in CKD patients. Furthermore, patients with CKD were not separately randomized. Nonetheless, this analysis supports the view that in patients with eGFRs of greater than 30 mL/min/1.73 m^2 that risedronate is safe and may be safe for patients with even more severely impaired renal function after dose adjustment. In a similar manner, Jamal et al. evaluated the effects of alendronate in women in the FIT study who had reduced renal function [471]. They too indentified no differences in reported adverse events. Furthermore, from their post hoc analysis of RCT results, these authors provided some data supporting the efficacy of alendronate in women with CKD. In the women with eGFRs of <45 mL/min/1.73 m^2, bone mineral density increased with treatment by 5.6% (95% CI, 4.8–6.5%) compared to an increase in bone mineral density in treated women with normal or near-normal renal function of 4.8% (95% CI, 4.6–5.0). Each group demonstrated a similar reduction in clinically important fractures with alendronate therapy. These results arise from a retrospective analysis.

Three small prospective trials have provided additional preliminary evidence that oral bisphosphonates might result in beneficial clinical outcomes in patients with CKD and ESRD [472–474]. In a case–control study, Hansen et al. reported that the risk of changes in bone mass of the spine, femur, and radius were similar in men in the low versus the normal renal function groups [472]. Nitta followed 35 hemodialysis patients for 15 months, including 6 months on standard therapy and 9 months of etidronate therapy (200 mg/day for 14 days every 3 months for three cycles) and reported that coronary calcification scores were improved and markers of inflammation diminished during etidronate therapy [473]. In a small RCT, Aryoshi et al. compared arterial calcification progression in dialysis patients assigned to receive 400 mg/day of etidronic acid versus customary care over 24 weeks [474]. Patients assigned to the bisphosphonate therapy demonstrated no progression of CAC and a decline in aorta calcification, whereas aorta calcification in the control group increased significantly. There was no difference in other biochemical parameters or CAC scores. These latter two studies raise the possibility, yet to be proven, that bisphosphonates might have therapeutic benefits for patients with ESRD. Current guidelines recommend that these agents not be used in individuals with moderate to severe CKD (GFR of <30 mL/ min/1.73 m^2). Furthermore, certain bisphosphonates classically used in patients with the hypercalcemia of malignancy (zoledronate and pamidronate, but not ibandronate) have been reported to cause either acute kidney failure or a focal and segmental glomerulosclerosis-like lesion when given in higher doses acutely to patients with renal insufficiency [475]. From the case reports of acute kidney injury with zoledronate, the kidney failure occurred after some delay and was not always fully reversible

with cessation of the medication. In the posttransplant period, the use of zolendronate has not been associated with acute renal failure in small clinical trials [476,477].

A number of clinical trials have evaluated the use of bisphosphonates in the post-kidney transplant patient. These patients present a mixed picture; they often have secondary hyperparathyroidism and MBD as a consequence of long-term dialysis treatment antecedent to their transplantation and they are at increased risk in the posttransplant period for steroid-induced osteoporosis. This patient population might shed some light on the potential efficacy and safety of bisphosphonates in a kidney failure population. A number of RCTs have examined the effects of bisphosphonates on renal function and on bone mineral density after transplant for up to 2 years [478–480]. These clinical trial results have been summarized by Mitterbauer et al. and by Palmer et al. [476,477] and will not be addressed further in this chapter. However, it may be significant that even though renal function in transplant patients was substantially restored, adynamic bone disease was identified in the clinical trial that included evaluation of bone histomorphology [480].

Ideally, individuals with CKD without osteoporosis should not be given bisphosphonates, because these agents suppress bone turnover and thereby could potentially complicate in this patient population any adynamic bone disease that has arisen from other causes. Noninvasive methods typically used to identify patients with osteoporosis are problematic. In particular, dual-energy X-ray absorption methodologies do not differentiate well between demineralization due to renal osteodystrophy and osteoporosis. Alternative noninvasive measures, such as peripheral quantitative computed tomography, might better identify individuals with demineralization, but the only reliable method for differentiating osteoporosis from the MBD of CKD is with a bone biopsy [481,482].

At present, bisphosphonates are not approved for use in patients with significant renal impairment. Evidence does suggest that these agents, especially oral agents such as risedronate and alendronate, are safe and may result in improved bone health when used in patients with milder degrees of CKD (eGFR of >30 mL/min/1.73 m^2). The study by Nitta and colleagues raises the possibility that these agents might also benefit patients with ESRD, but these investigators' findings await confirmation in larger RCTs.

References

1 Kovesdy CP, Mehrotra R, Kalantar-Zadeh K. Battleground: chronic kidney disorders mineral and bone disease: calcium obsession, vitamin D, and binder confusion. *Clin J Am Soc Nephrol* 2008; **3(1):** 168–173.

2 Kovesdy CP, Kalantar-Zadeh K. Bone and mineral disorders in predialysis CKD. *Int Urol Nephrol* 2008; **40(2):** 427440.

3 Andress DL. Vitamin D in chronic kidney disease: a systemic role for selective vitamin D receptor activation. *Kidney Int* 2006; **69:** 33–43.

4 Berndt TJ, Schiavi S, Kumar R. "Phosphatonins" and the regulation of phosphorus homeostasis. *Am J Physiol Renal Physiol* 2005; **289(6)**: F1170–F1182.

5 Felsenfeld A, Rodriguez M, Aguilera-Tejero E. Dynamics of parathyroid hormone secretion in health and secondary hyperparathyroidism. *Clin J Am Soc Neph* 2007; **2**: 1283–1305.

6 Goodman WG, Quarles LD. Development and progression of secondary hyperparathyroidism in chronic kidney disease: lessons from molecular genetics. *Kidney Int* 13 June 2007 posting date [Epub ahead of print].

7 Locatelli F, Cannata-Andia JB, Drueke TB, Horl WH, Fouque D, Heimburger O, Ritz E. Management of disturbances of calcium and phosphate metabolism in chronic renal insufficiency, with emphasis on the control of hyperphosphatemia. *Nephrol Dial Transplant* 2002; **17**: 723–731.

8 Prosser DE, Jones G. Enzymes involved in the activation and inactivation of vitamin D. *Trends Biochem Sci* 2004; **29(12)**: 664–673.

9 Liu S, Quarles LD. How fibroblast growth factor 23 works. *J Am Soc Nephrol* 2007; **18(6)**: 1637–1647.

10 Shaikh A, Brendt T, Kumar R. Regulation of phosphate homeostasis by the phosphatonins and other novel mediators. *Pediatr Nephrol* 2008; **23**: 1203–1210.

11 Torres PU, Prie D, Molina-Bletry1 V, Beck L, Silve C, Friedlander G. Klotho: an antiaging protein involved in mineral and vitamin D metabolism. *Kidney Int* 2007; **71**: 730–737.

12 Wolf M, Thadhani R. Vitamin D in patients with renal failure: a summary of observational mortality studies and steps moving forward. *J Steroid Biochem Mol Biol* 2007; **103(3–5)**: 487–490.

13 Andress DL, Coyne DW, Kalantar-Zadeh K, Molitch ME, Zangeneh F, Sprague SM. Management of secondary hyperparathyroidism in stages 3 and 4 chronic kidney disease. *Endocr Pract* 2008; **14(1)**: 18–27.

14 Branley P. Use of phosphate binders in chronic kidney disease. The CARI guidelines. *Nephrology* 2006; **11(Suppl 1)**: S245–S262.

15 Elder G. Parathyroid hormone. The CARI guidelines. *Nephrology* 2006; **11(Suppl 1)**: S209–S216.

16 Elder G. Use of calcimimetic drugs. The CARI guidelines. *Nephrology* 2006; **11(Suppl 1)**: S240–S244.

17 Hawley C, Elder G. Calcium. The CARI guidelines. *Nephrology* 2006; **11(Suppl 1)**: S198–S200.

18 Hawley C. Calcium x phosphate product. The CARI guidelines. *Nephrology* 2006; **11(Suppl 1)**: S206–S208.

19 Hawley C. Serum phosphate. The CARI guidelines. *Nephrology* 2006; **11(Suppl 1)**: S201–S205.

20 Jindal K, Chan CT, Deziel C, Hirsch D, Soroka SD, Tonelli M *et al.* Mineral metabolism. CSN Hemodialysis Clinical Practice Guidelines. *J Am Soc Nephrol* 2006; **17**: S11–S15.

21 European Best Practice Guidelines for Haemodialysis (Part 1). Section VII. Vascular disease and risk factors: hyperphosphataemia and calcium-phosphorus ion product. *Nephrol Dial Transplant* 2002; **17(Suppl 7)**: 95–96.

22 National Kidney Foundation. K/DOQI clinical practice guidelines for bone metabolism and disease in chronic kidney disease. *Am J Kidney Dis* 2003; **42(Suppl 3)**: S1–S201.

23 Martin KJ, Olgaard K, Bone Turnover Work Group. Diagnosis, assessment, and treatment of bone turnover abnormalities in renal osteodystrophy. *Am J Kidney Dis* 2004; **43(3)**: 558–565.

24 Andress DL. Bone and mineral guidelines for patients with chronic kidney disease: a call for revision. *Clin J Am Soc Nephrol* 2008; **3**: 179–183.

25 Monge M, Shahapuni I, Oprisiu R, Esper N, Morinière P, Massy Z *et al.* Reappraisal of 2003 NKF-K/DOQI guidelines for management of hyperparathyroidism in chronic kidney disease patients. *Nat Clin Pract Nephrol* 2006; **2(6)**: 326–336.

26 Ix HI, Quarles LD, Chertow GM. Guidelines for disorders of mineral metabolism and secondary hyperparathyroidism should not yet be modified. *Nat Clin Pract Nephrol* 2006; **2(6)**: 337–339.

27 Moe S, Drüeke T, Cunningham J, Goodman W, Martin K, Olgaard K *et al.* Definition, evaluation, and classification of renal osteodystrophy: a position statement from Kidney Disease: Improving Global Outcomes (KDIGO). *Kidney Int* 2006; **69**: 1945–1953.

28 Palmer SC, Craig JC, Strippoli GF. Sevelamer: a promising but unproven drug. *Nephrol Dial Transplant* 2007; **22(10)**: 2742–2745.

29 London GM, Marty C, Marchais SJ, Guerin AP, Metivier F, de Vernejoul MC. Arterial calcifications and bone histomorphometry in end-stage renal disease. *J Am Soc Nephrol* 2004; **15(7)**: 1943–1951

30 London GM. Cardiovascular calcifications in uremic patients: clinical impact on cardiovascular function. *J Am Soc Nephrol* 2003; **14(Suppl 9)**: S305–S309.

31 London GM, Guerrin AP, Marchais SJ, Metivier F, Pannier B, Adda H. Arterial media calcification in end-stage renal disease: impact on all-cause and cardiovascular mortality. *Nephrol Dial Transplant* 2003; **18**: 1731–1740.

32 London GM, Marchais SJ, Guérin AP, Métivier F. Arteriosclerosis, vascular calcifications and cardiovascular disease in uremia. *Curr Opinion Nephrol Hypertens* 2005; **14(6)**: 525–531.

33 Raggi P, Kleerekoper M. Contribution of bone and mineral abnormalities to cardiovascular disease in patients with chronic kidney disease. *Clin J Am Soc Nephrol* 2008; **3**: 836–843.

34 Raggi P, Boulay A, Chasan-Taber S, Amin N, Dillon M, Burke SK *et al.* Cardiac calcification in adult hemodialysis patients. A link between end-stage renal disease and cardiovascular disease? *J Am Coll Cardiol* 2002; **39**: 695–701.

35 Raggi P, Giachelli C, Bellasi A. Interaction of vascular and bone disease in patients with normal renal function and patients undergoing dialysis. *Nat Clin Pract Cardiovasc Med* 2007; **4(1)**: 26–33.

36 Blacher J, Guerin AP, Pannier B, *et al.* Arterial calcifications, arterial stiffness, and cardiovascular risk in end-stage renal disease. *Hypertension* 2001; **38**: 938–942.

37 Blacher J, Guerin AP, Pannier B, *et al.* Impact of aortic stiffness on survival in end-stage renal disease. *Circulation* 1999; **99**: 2434–2439.

38 Braun J, Oldendorf M, Moshage W, Heidler R, Zeitler E, Luft FC. Electron beam computed tomography in the evaluation of cardiac calcification in chronic dialysis patients. *Am J Kidney Dis* 1996; **27(3)**: 394–401.

39 Matsuoka M, Iseki K, Tamashiro M, Fujimoto N, Higa N, Touma T *et al.* Impact of high coronary artery calcification score (CACS) on survival in patients on chronic hemodialysis. *Clin Exp Nephrol* 2004; **8(1)**: 54–58.

40 Ketteler M, Schlieper G, Floege J. Calcification and cardiovascular health: new insights into an old phenomenon. *Hypertension* 2006; **47(6)**: 1027–1034.

41 Guerin AP, London GM, Marchais SJ, Metivier F. Arterial stiffening and vascular calcifications in end-stage renal disease. *Nephrol Dial Transplant* 2000; **15**: 1014–1021.

42 Guerin AP, Blacher J, Pannier B, Marchais SJ, Safar ME, London GM. Impact of aortic stiffness attenuation on survival of patients in end-stage renal failure. *Circulation* 2001; **103(7)**: 987–992.

43 Haydar AA, Hujairi NM, Covic AA, Pereira D, Rubens M, Goldsmith DJ. Coronary artery calcification is related to coronary atherosclerosis

in chronic renal disease patients: a study comparing EBCT-generated coronary artery calcium scores and coronary angiography. *Nephrol Dial Transplant* 2004; **19(9):** 2307–2312.

44 Kalantar-Zadeh K, Kuwae N, Regidor DL, Kovesdy CP, Kilpatrick RD, Shinaberger CS *et al.* Survival predictability of time-varying indicators of bone disease in maintenance hemodialysis patients. *Kidney Int* 2006; **70(4):** 771–780.

45 Kalpakian M, Mehrotra R. Vascular calcification and disordered mineral metabolism in dialysis patients. *Semin Dial* 2007; **20(2):** 139–143.

46 Rostand SG, Sanders C, Kirk KA, Rutsky EA, Fraser RG. Myocardial calcification and cardiac dysfunction in chronic renal failure. *Am J Med* 1988; **85(5):** 651–657.

47 Sigrist M, Taal M, Bungay P, McIntyre C. Progressive vascular calcification over 2 years is associated with arterial stiffening and increased mortality in patients with stages 4 and 5 chronic kidney disease. *Clin J Am Soc Nephrol* 2007; **2:** 1241–1248.

48 Toussaint ND, Lau KK, Strauss BJ, Polkinghorne KR, Kerr PG. Associations between vascular calcification, arterial stiffness and bone mineral density in chronic kidney disease. *Nephrol Dial Transplant* 2008; **23(2):** 586–593.

49 Mehrota R. Disordered mineral metabolism and vascular calcification in nondialyzed chronic kidney disease patients. *J Ren Nutr* 2006; **26:** 100–118.

50 Mehrotra R, Budoff M, Hokanson JE, Ipp E, Takasu J, Adler S. Progression of coronary artery calcification in diabetics with and without chronic kidney disease. *Kidney Int* 2005; **68(3):** 1258–1266.

51 London GM, Marchais SJ, Guérin AP, Boutouyrie P, Métivier F, de Vernejoul MC. Association of bone activity, calcium load, aortic stiffness, and calcifications in ESRD. *J Am Soc Nephrol* 14 May 2008 [Epub ahead of print].

52 Taal MW, Roe S, Masud T, Green D, Porter C, Cassidy MJ. Total hip bone mass predicts survival in chronic hemodialysis patients. *Kidney Int* 2003; **63(3):** 1116–1120.

53 Taal MW, Masud T, Green D, Cassidy MJ. Risk factors for reduced bone density in haemodialysis patients. *Nephrol Dial Transplant* 1999; **14(8):** 1922–1928.

54 Galassi A, Spiegel DM, Bellasi A, Block GA, Raggi P. Accelerated vascular calcification and relative hypoparathyroidism in incident haemodialysis diabetic patients receiving calcium binders. *Nephrol Dial Transplant* 2006; **21(11):** 3215–3222.

55 Goodman WG, London G, Amann K, Block GA, Giachelli C, Hruska KA *et al.* Vascular calcification in chronic kidney disease. *Am J Kidney Dis* 2004; **43(3):** 572–579.

56 Mathew S, Tustison KS, Sugatani T, Chaudhary LR, Rifas L, Hruska KA. The mechanism of phosphorus as a cardiovascular risk factor in CKD. *J Am Soc Nephrol* 2008; **19(6):** 1092–1105.

57 Meema HE, Oreopoulos DG, de Veber GA. Arterial calcifications in severe chronic renal disease and their relationship to dialysis treatment, renal transplant and parathyroidectomy. *Radiology* 1976; **121:** 315–321.

58 Tomiyama C, Higa A, Dalboni MA, Cendoroglo M, Draibe SA, Cuppari L *et al.* The impact of traditional and non-traditional risk factors on coronary calcification in pre-dialysis patients. *Nephrol Dial Transplant* 2006; **21(9):** 2464–2471.

59 Yamada K, Fujimoto S, Nishiura R, Komatsu H, Tatsumoto M, Sato Y *et al.* Risk factors of the progression of abdominal aortic calcification in patients on chronic haemodialysis. *Nephrol Dial Transplant* 2007; **22(7):** 2032–2037.

60 Block GA, Raggi P, Bellasi A, Kooienga L, Spiegel DM. Mortality effect of coronary calcification and phosphate binder choice in incident hemodialysis patients. *Kidney Int* 2007; **71:** 438–441.

61 Manns B, Owen WF, Winkelmayer WC, Devereaux PJ, Tonelli M. Surrogate markers in clinical studies: Problems solved or created? *Am J Kidney Dis* 2006; **48:** 159–166.

62 Parfitt AM. Renal bone disease: a new conceptual framework for the interpretation of bone histomorphometry. *Curr Opin Nephrol Hypertens* 2003; **12:** 387–403.

63 Trueba D, Sawaya BP, Mawad H, Malluche HH. Bone biopsy: indications, techniques, and complications. *Semin Dial* 2003; **16(4):** 341–345.

64 Lerma EV. Definition and classification of renal osteodystrophy. *Clin Rev Bone Min Metabol* 2007; **5(1):** 3–9.

65 Recker RR, Barger-Lux J, Langman CB, Jan de Beur J. Bone biopsy and histomorphometry in clinical practice. *In:* Favus MJ, editor, *AS-BMR: Primer on the Metabolic Bone Diseases and Disorders of Mineral Metabolism,* 6th edn., 2006; 161–169.

66 Gupta A, Winer K, Econs MJ, Marx SJ, Collins MT. FGF-23 is elevated by chronic hyperphosphatemia. *J Clin Endocrinol Metab* 2004; **89(9):** 4489–4492.

67 Gutierrez O, Isakova T, Rhee E, Shah A, Holmes J, Collerone G *et al.* Fibroblast growth factor-23 mitigates hyperphosphatemia but accentuates calcitriol deficiency in chronic kidney disease. *J Am Soc Nephrol* 2005; **16(7):** 2205–2215.

68 Masuyama R, Stockmans I, Torrekens S, van Looveren R, Maes C, Carmeliet P *et al.* Vitamin D receptor in chondrocytes promotes osteoclastogenesis and regulates FGF 23 production in osteoblasts. *J Clin Invest* 2006; **116:** 3150–3159.

69 Martinez I, Saracho R, Montenegro J, Llach F. A deficit of calcitriol synthesis may not be the initial factor in the pathogenesis of secondary hyperparathyroidism. *Nephrol Dial Transplant* 1996; **11(Suppl 3):** 22–8.

70 Llach F, Yudd M. Pathogenic, clinical, and therapeutic aspects of secondary hyperparathyroidism in chronic renal failure. *Am J Kidney Dis* 1998; **32(2 Suppl 2):** S3–S12.

71 Craver L, Marco MP, Martínez I, Rue M, Borràs M, Martín ML *et al.* Mineral metabolism parameters throughout chronic kidney disease stages 1-5-achievement of K/DOQI target ranges. *Nephrol Dial Transplant* 2007; **22(4):** 1171–1176.

72 Levin A, Bakris GL, Molitch M, Smulders M, Tian J, Williams LA *et al.* Prevalence of abnormal serum vitamin D, PTH, calcium, and phosphorus in patients with chronic kidney disease: Results of the study to evaluate early kidney disease. *Kidney Int* 2007; **71:** 31–38.

73 Stevens LA, Djurdjev O, Cardew S, Cameron EC, Levin A. Calcium, phosphate, and parathyroid hormone levels in combination and as a function of dialysis duration predict mortality: evidence for the complexity of the association between mineral metabolism and outcomes. *J Am Soc Nephrol* 2004; **15:** 770–779.

74 Kestenbaum B, Belozeroff V. Mineral metabolism disturbances in patients with chronic kidney disease. *Eur J Clin Invest* 2007; **37(8):** 607–622.

75 Berl T, Berns AS, Hufer WE, Hammill K, Alfrey AC, Arnaud CD *et al.* 1,25-Dihydroxycholecalciferol effects in chronic dialysis: a double-blind controlled study. *Ann Intern Med* 1978; **88(6):** 774–780.

76 Coburn JW, Hartenbower DL, Brickman AS. Advances in vitamin D metabolism as they pertain to chronic renal disease. *Am J Clin Nutr* 1976; **29:** 1283–1299.

77 Dahl E, Nordal KP, Halse J. Predialysis calcitroil administration: effects on pre- and post-transplant renal osteodystrophy. *J Intern Med* 1996; **239(6):** 537–540.

78 DeLuca HF, Avioli LV. Treatment of renal osteodystrophy with 25-hydroxycholecalciferol. *Arch Int Med* 1970; **126:** 896–899.

79 Slatopolsky E, Weerts C, Thielan J, Horst R, Harter H, Martin KJ. Marked suppression of secondary hyperparathyroidism by intravenous administration of 1,25-dihydroxy-cholecalciferol in uremic patients. *J Clin Invest* 1984; **74:** 2136–2143.

80 Al-Aly Z, Qazi RQ, Gonzalez EA, Zeringue A, Martin KJ. Changes in serum 25-hydroxyvitamin D and plasma intact PTH levels following treatment with ergocalciferol in patient with CKD. *Am J Kidney Dis* 2007; **50:** 59–68.

81 Heaney RP, Davies KM, Chen TC, Holick MF, Barger-Lux MJ. Human serum 25-hydorxycholecalciferol responses to extended oral dosing with cholecalciferol. *Am J Clin Nutri* 2003; **77:** 204–210.

82 Saab G, Young DO, Gincherman Y, Giles K, Norwood K, Coyne DW. Prevalence of vitamin D deficiency and the safety and effectiveness of monthly ergocalciferol in hemodialysis patients. *Nephron Clin Pract* 2007; **105:** c132–c138.

83 Cantor T, Yang Z, Caraiani N, Ilamathi E. Lack of comparability of intact parathyroid hormone measurements among commercial assays for end-stage renal disease patients: implication for treatment decisions. *Clin Chem* 2006; **52(9):** 1771–1776.

84 Souberbielle JC, Boutten A, Carlier MC, Chevenne D, Coumaros G, Lawson-Body E *et al.* Inter-method variability in PTH measurement: implication for the care of CKD patients. *Kidney Int* 2006; **70(2):** 345–350.

85 Barreto FC, Barreto DV, Moyses RMA, Neves KR, Canziani MEF, Draibe SA *et al.* K/DOQI-recommended intact PTH levels do not prevent low-turnover bone disease in hemodialysis patients. *Kidney Int* 2008; **73:** 771–777.

86 Melamed ML, Eustace JA, Plantinga LC, Jaar BG, Fink NE, Parekh RS *et al.* Third-generation parathyroid hormone assays and all-cause mortality in incident dialysis patients: the CHOICE study. *Nephrol Dial Transplant* 2008; **23(5):** 1650–1658.

87 Coen G, Ballanti P, Bonucci E, Calabria S, Costantini S, Ferrannini M *et al.* Renal osteodystrophy in predialysis and hemodialysis patients: comparison of histologic patterns and diagnostic predictivity of intact PTH. *Nephron* 2002; **91(1):** 103–111.

88 Coen G, Ballanti P, Bonucci E, Calabria S, Centorrino M, Fassino V *et al.* Bone markers in the diagnosis of low turnover osteodystrophy in haemodialysis patients. *Nephrol Dial Transplant* 1998; **13(9):** 2294–2302.

89 Coen G, Bonucci E, Ballanti P, Balducci A, Calabria S, Nicolai GA *et al.* PTH 1-84 and PTH "7-84" in the noninvasive diagnosis of renal bone disease. *Am J Kidney Dis* 2002; **40:** 348–354.

90 Lehman G, Stein G, Hüller M, Schemer R, Ramakrishnan K, Goodman WG. Specific measurement of PTH (1-84) in various forms of renal osteodystrophy (ROD) as assessed by bone histomorphometry. *Kidney Int* 2005; **68:** 1206–1214.

91 Quarles LD, Lobaugh B, Murphy G. Intact parathyroid hormone overestimates the presence and severity of parathyroid-mediated osseous abnormalities in uremia. *J Clin Endocrinol Metab* 1992; **75:** 145–150.

92 Brandenburg VM, Floege J. Adynamic bone disease-bone and beyond. *NDT Plus* 2008; **1(3):** 135–147.

93 Barthel TK, Mathern DR, Whitefield K, Haussler CA, Hopper HA, Hsieh J-C *et al.* 1,25-Dihydroxyvitamin D3/VDR-mediated induction of FGF23 as well as transcriptional control of other bone anabolic and catabolic genes that orchestrate the regulation of phosphate and calcium mineral metabolism. *J Steriod Biochem Mol Biol* 2007; **103(3–5):** 381–388.

94 Fliser D, Kollerits B, Neyer U, Ankerst DP, Lhotta K, Lingenhel A *et al.* Fibroblast growth factor 23 (FGF23) predicts progression of chronic kidney disease: The Mild to Moderate Kidney Disease (MMKD) Study. *J Am Soc Nephrol* 2007; **18:** 2601–2608.

95 Chonchol M, Scragg R. 25-Hydroxyvitamin D, insulin resistance, and kidney function in the third National Health and Nutrition Examination Survey. *Kidney Int* 2006; **71:** 134–139.

96 Coen G, Mantella D, Manni M, Balducci A, Nofroni I, Sardella D *et al.* 25-Hydroxyvitamin D levels and bone histomorphometry in hemodialysis renal osteodystrophy. *Kidney Int.* 2005; **68(4):** 1840–1848.

97 Hyppönen E, Boucher BJ, Berry DJ, Power C. 25-Hydroxyvitamin D, IGF-1, and metabolic syndrome at 45 years of age. A cross-sectional study in the 1958 British Birth Cohort. *Diabetes* 2008; **57:** 298–305.

98 London GM, Guerin AP, Verbeke FH, Pannier B, Boutouyrie P, Marchais SJ *et al.* Mineral metabolism and arterial functions in end-stage renal disease: potential role of 25-hydroxyvitamin D deficieincy. *J Am Soc Nephrol* 2007; **18:** 613–620.

99 Looker AC, Dawson-Hughes B, Calvo MS, Gunter EW, Sahyoun NR. Serum 25-hydoxyvitamin D status of adolescents and adults in two seasonal subpopulations from NHANES III. *Bone* 2002; **30(5):** 771–777.

100 Roddam AW, Neale R, Appleby P, Allen NE, Tipper S, Key TJ. Association between plasma 25-hydoxyvitamin D levels and fracture risk. The EPIC-Oxford study. *Am J Epidemiol* 2007; **166:** 1327–1336.

101 LeClair RE, Hellman RN, Karp SL, Kraus M, Ofner S, Li Q *et al.* Prevalence of calcidiol deficiency in CKD: a cross-sectional study across latitudes in the United States. *Am J Kidney Dis* 2005; **45(5):** 1026–1033.

102 Martins D, Wolf M, Pan D, Zadshir A, Tareen N, Thadhani R *et al.* Prevalence of cardiovascular risk factors and the serum levels of 25-hydroxyvitamin D in the United States: data from the Third National Health and Nutrition Examination Survey. *Arch Intern Med* 2007; **167(11):** 1159–1165.

103 Binkley N, Novotny R, Krueger D, Kawahara T, Daida YG, Lensmeyer G *et al.* Low vitamin D status despite abundant sun exposure. *J Clin Endocrinol Metab* 2007; **92(6):** 2130–2135.

104 Allain TJ, Dhesi J. Hypovitaminosis D in older adults. *Gerontology* 2003; **49:** 273–278.

105 Ghazali A, Fardellone P, Prun A, Atik A, Achard J-M, Oprisiu R *et al.* Is low plasma 25-(OH) vitamin D a major risk factor for hyperparathyroidism and Looser's zones independent of calcitriol? *Kidney Int* 1999; **55:** 2169–2177.

106 Vieth R. Vitamin D supplementation, 25-hydroxyvitamin D concentrations, and safety. *Am J Clin Nutr* 1999; **69:** 842–856.

107 Holick MF. Vitamin D deficiency. *N Engl J Med* 2007; **357(3):** 266–281.

108 Gross MD. Vitamin D and calcium in the prevention of prostate and colon cancer: new approaches for the identification of needs. *J Nutr* 2005; **135:** 326–331.

109 Holick MF. Vitamin D: importance in the prevention of cancers, type 1 diabetes, heart disease, and osteoporosis. *Am J Clin Nutr* 2004; **79:** 362–371.

110 Holick MF. Sunlight and vitamin D for bone health and prevention of autoimmune diseases, cancers, and cardiovascular disease. *Am J Clin Nutr* 2004; **80(Suppl):** 167S–188S.

111 Lappe JM, Travers-Gustafson D, Davies KM, Recker RR, Heaney RP. Vitamin D and calcium supplementation reduces cancer risk: results of a randomized trial. *Am J Clin Nutr* 2007; **85:** 1586–1591.

112 Lim W-C, Hanauer SB, Li Y-C. Mechanisms of disease: vitamin D and inflammatory bowel disease. *Nat Clin Pract Gastroenterol Hepatol* 2005; **2(7):** 308–315.

113 Lips P, Wiersinga A, van Ginkel FC, Jongen MJ, Netelenbos JC, Hackeng WH *et al.* The effect of vitamin D supplementation on vitamin D status and parathyroid function in elderly subjects. *J Clin Endocrinol Metab* 1988; **67:** 644–650.

114 Lips P. Vitamin D deficiency and secondary hyperparathyroidism in the elderly: consequences for bone loss and fractures and therapeutic implications. *Endocr Rev* 2001; **22(4):** 477–501.

115 Mark BL, Carson AS. Vitamin D and autoimmune disease: implications for practice from the multiple sclerosis literature. *J Am Diet Assoc* 2006; **106:** 418–424.

116 Newmark HL, Newmark J. Vitamin D and Parkinson's disease: a hypothesis. *Movement Disorders* 2007; **22:** 461–468.

117 Pittas AG, Lau J, Hu FB, Dawson-Hughes B. The role of vitamin D and calcium in type 2 diabetes. A systematic review and meta-analysis. *J Clin Endocrinol Metab* 2007; **92:** 2017–2029.

118 Watson KE, Abrolat, ML, Malone, LL, *et al.* Active serum vitamin D levels are inversely correlated with coronary calcification. *Circulation* 1997; **96:** 1755–1760.

119 Wolf M, Shah A, Gutierrez O, Ankers E, Monroy M, Tamez H *et al.* Vitamin D levels and early mortality among incident hemodialysis patients. *Kidney Int* 2007; **72(8):** 1004–1013.

120 Bischoff-Ferrari H A, Giovannucci E, Willett WC, Dietrich T, Dawson-Hughes B. Estimation of optimal serum concentrations of 25-hydroxyvitamin D for multiple health outcomes. *Am J Clin Nutr* 2006;**84:** 18–28.

121 Björkman M, Sorva A, Tilvis R. Responses of parathyroid hormone to vitamin D supplementation: a systematic review of clinical trials. *Arch Gerontol Geriatr* 1 Feb 2008 [Epub ahead of print].

122 Boonen S, Vanderschueren D, Haentjens P, Lips P. Calcium and vitamin D in the prevention and treatment of osteoporosis. *J Intern Med* 2006;**259:** 539–552.

123 Cranney A, Horsley T, O'Donnell S, Weiler H, Pui L, Ooi D *et al.* Effectiveness and safety of vitamin D in relation to bone health. *Evid Rep Technol Assess* 2007; **158:** 1–235.

124 Jackson C, Gaugris S, Sen SS, Hosking D. The effect of cholecalciferol (vitamin D3) on the risk of fall and fracture: a meta-analysis. *Q J Med* 2007; **100:** 185–192.

125 Richy F, Schacht E, Bruyere O, Ethgen O, Gourlay M, Reginster J-Y. Vitamin D analogs versus native vitamin D in preventing bone loss and osteoporosis-related fractures: a comparative meta-analysis. *Calcif Tissue Int* 2005; **76:** 176–186.

126 Tang BMP, Eslick GD, Nowson C, Smith C, Bensoussan A. Use of calcium or calcium in combination with vitamin D supplementation to prevent fractures and bone loss in people aged 50 years and older: a meta-analysis. *Lancet* 2007; **370:** 657–666.

127 Bischoff-Ferrari HA, Dawson-Hughes B, Willett WC, Staehelin HB, Bazemore MG, Zee RY *et al.* Effect of vitamin D on falls: a meta-analysis. *JAMA* 2004; **291(16):** 1999–2006.

128 Bischoff-Ferrari HA, Willett WC, Wong JB, Giovannucci E, Dietrich T, Dawson-Hughes B. Fracture prevention with vitamin D supplementation: a meta-analysis of randomized controlled trials. *JAMA* 2005; **293(18):** 2257–2264.

129 Boonen S, Lips P, Bouillon R, Bischoff-Ferrari HA, Vandershueren D, Haentjens P. Need for additional calcium to reduce the risk of hip fracture with vitamin D supplementation: evidence from a comparative

130 Autier P, Gandini S. Vitamin D supplement and total mortality: a meta-analysis of randomized controlled trials. *Arch Intern Med* 2007; **167(16):** 1730–1737.

131 Levin A, Li YC. Vitamin D and its analogues: do they protect against cardiovascular disease in patients with kidney disease? *Kidney Int* 2005; **68(5):** 1973–1981.

132 Teng M, Wolf M, Lowrie E, Ofsthun N, Lazarus JM, Thadhani R. Survival of patients undergoing hemodialysis with paricalcitol or calcitriol therapy. *N Engl J Med* 2003; **349(5):** 446–456.

133 Teng M, Wolf M, Ofsthun MN, Lazarus JM, Hernán MA, Camargo CA, Jr., *et al.* Activated injectable vitamin D and hemodialysis survival: a historical cohort study. *J Am Soc Nephrol* 2005; **16(4):** 1115–1125.

134 Tentori F, Hunt WC, Stidley CA, Rohrscheib MR, Bedrick EJ, Meyer KB. Mortality risk among hemodialysis patients receiving different vitamin D analogs. *Kidney Int* 2006; **70(10):** 1858–1865

135 Tentori F, Blayney MJ, Albert JM, Gillespie BW, Kerr PG, Bommer J *et al.* Mortality risk for dialysis patients with different levels of serum calcium, phosphorus, and PTH: the Dialysis Outcomes and Practice Patterns Study (DOPPS). *Am J Kidney Dis* 30 May 2008 [Epub ahead of print].

136 Thadhani R, Wolf M. Vitamin D in patients with kidney disease: cautiously optimistic. *Adv Chronic Kidney Dis* 2007; **14(1):** 22–26.

137 Wolf M, Thadhani R. Beyond minerals and parathyroid hormone: role of active vitamin D in end-stage renal disease. *Semin Dial* 2005; **18:** 302–306.

138 Shoji T, Shinohara K, Kimoto E, *et al.* Lower risk for cardiovascular mortality in oral 1α-hydroxy vitamin D3 users in a haemodialysis population. *Nephrol Dial Transplant* 2004; **19:** 179–184.

139 Kovesdy CP, Kalantar-Zadeh K. Vitamin D receptor activation and survival in chronic kidney disease. *Kidney Int* 2008; **73(12):** 1355–1363.

140 Kovesdy CP, Ahmadzadeh S, Anderson JE, Kalantar-Zadeh K. Association of activated vitamin D treatment and mortality in chronic kidney disease. *Arch Intern Med* 2008; **168(4):** 397–403.

141 Holick MF. Vitamin D for health and in chronic kidney disease. *Semin Dial* 2005; **18:** 266–275.

142 Kunz R, Vist GE, Oxman AD. Randomisation to protect against selection bias in healthcare trials. *Cochrane Database Syst Rev* 2007; **2:** MR000012.

143 Bradford-Hill A. The environment and disease: association or causation? *Proc R Soc Med London* 1965, **58:** 295–300.

144 Phillips CV, Goodman KJ. The missed lessons of Sir Austin Bradford Hill. *Epidemiol PerspectInnov* 2004; **1:**3.

145 Cundy T, Hand DJ, Oliver DO, Woods CG, Wright FW, Kanis JA. Who gets renal bone disease before beginning dialysis? *Br Med J* 1985; **290:** 271–275.

146 Clair F, Leenhardt L, Bourdeau A, Zingraff J, Robert D, Dubost C *et al.* Effect of calcitriol in the control of plasma calcium after parathyroidectomy. A placebo-controlled, double-blind study in chronic hemodialysis patients. *Nephron* 1987; **46(1):** 18–22.

147 Andress DL, Norris KC, Coburn JW, Slatopolsky EA, Sherrard DJ. Intravenous calcitriol in the treatment of refractory osteitis fibrosa of chronic renal failure. *N Engl J Med* 1989; **321:** 274–279.

148 Hamdy NA, Kanis JA, Beneton MN, Brown CB, Juttmann JR, Jordans JG *et al.* Effect of alfacalcidol on natural course of renal bone disease in mild to moderate renal failure. *Br Med J* 1995; **310(6976):** 358–363.

149 Christiansen C, Rodbro P, Christensen MS, Hartnack B, Transbol I. Deterioration of renal function during treatment of chronic renal failure with 1,25-dihydroxycholecalciferol. *Lancet* 1978; **ii(8092):** 700–703.

150 Christiansen C, Rodbro P, Christensen MS, Hartnack B. Is 1,25-dihydroxy-cholecalciferol harmful to renal function in patients with chronic renal failure? *Clin Endocrinol* 1981; **15:** 229–236.

151 Christiansen C, Røodbro P, Christensen MS, Naestoft J, Hartnack B, Transbøol I. Decreased renal function in association with administration of 1,25-dihydroxyvitamin D3 to patients with stable, advanced renal failure. *Contrib Nephrol* 1980; **18:** 139–146.

152 Ritz E, Küster S, Schmidt-Gayk H, Stein G, Scholz C, Kraatz G *et al.* Low-dose calcitriol prevents the rise in 1,84-iPTH without affecting serum calcium and phosphate in patients with moderate renal failure (prospective placebo-controlled multicentre trial). *Nephrol Dial Transplant* 1995; **10(12):** 2228–2234.

153 Sprague SM, Moe SM. Safety and efficacy of long-term treatment of secondary hyperparathyroidism by low-dose intravenous calcitriol. *Am J Kidney Dis* 1992; **19(6):** 532–539.

154 Coburn JW, Maung HM, Elangovan L, Germain MJ, Lindberg JS, Sprague SM *et al.* Doxercalciferol safely suppresses PTH levels in patients with secondary hyperparathyroidism associated with chronic kidney disease stages 3 and 4. *Am J Kidney Dis* 2004; **43(5):** 877–890.

155 Coyne D, Acharya M, Qui P, Abboud H, Batlle D, Rosansky S *et al.* Paricalcitol capsule for the treatment of secondary hyperparathyroidism in stages 3 and 4 CKD. *Am J Kidney Dis* 2006; **47:** 263–276.

156 Kim G, Sprague SM. Use of vitamin D analogs in chronic renal failure. *Adv Ren Replace Ther* 2002; **9:** 175–183.

157 Palmer SC, McGregor DO, Craig JC, Elder G, Strippoli GF. Vitamin D analogues for treatment and prevention of bone disease in chronic kidney disease (protocol). *Cochrane Database Syst Rev* 2006; **1:** CD005633.

158 Palmer SC, McGregor DO, Macaskill P, Craig JC, Elder GJ, Strippoli GF. Meta-analysis: vitamin D compounds in chronic kidney disease. *Ann Intern Med* 2007; **147(12):** 840–853.

159 Sprague SM, Llach F, Amdahl M, Taccetta C, Batlle D. Paricalcitol versus calcitriol in the treatment of secondary hyperparathyroidism. *Kidney Int* 2003; **63:** 1483–1490.

160 Coyne DW, Grieff M, Ahya SN, Giles K, Norwood K, Slatopolsky E. Differential effects of acute administration of 19-nor-1,25-dihydroxy-vitamin D2 and 1,25-dihydroxy-vitamin D3 on serum calcium and phosphorus in hemodialysis patients. *Am J Kidney Dis* 2002; **40(6):** 1283–1288.

161 Dobrez DG, Mathes A, Amdahl M, Marx SE, Melnick JZ, Sprague SM. Paricalcitol-treated patients experience improved hospitalization outcomes compared with calcitriol-treated patients in real-world clinical settings. *Nephrol Dial Transplant* 2004; **19:** 1174–1181.

162 Greenbaum LA, Benador N, Goldstein SL, Paredes A, Melnick JZ, Mattingly S *et al.* Intravenous paricalcitol for treatment of secondary hyperparathyroidism in children on hemodialysis. *Am J Kidney Dis* 2007; **49(6):** 814–823.

163 Gordon PL, Sakkas GK, Doyle JW, Shubert T, Johansen KL. Relationship between vitamin D and muscle size and strength in patients on hemodialysis. *J Renal Nutr* 2007; **6:** 397–407.

164 Lindberg J, Martin KJ, González EA, Acchiardo SR, Valdin JR, Soltanek C. A long-term, multicenter study of the efficacy and safety of paricalcitol in end-stage renal disease. *Clin Nephrol* 2001; **56(4):** 315–323.

165 Llach F, Yudd M. Paricalcitol in dialysis patients with calcitriol-resistant secondary hyperparathyroidism. *Am J Kidney Dis* 2001; **38(Suppl 5):** S45–S50.

166 Llach F, Keshav G, Goldblat MV, Lindberg JS, Sadler R, Delmez J *et al.* Suppression of parathyroid hormone secretion in hemodialysis patients by a novel vitamin D analogue: 19-nor-1,25-dihydroxyvitamin D2. *Am J Kidney Dis* 1998; **32(2 Suppl):** S48–S54.

167 Martin KJ, Gonzalez EA, Gellens M, Hamm LL, Abboud H, Lindberg J. 19-Nor-1-alpha-25-dihydroxyvitamin D2 (paricalcitol) safely and effectively reduces the levels of intact parathyroid hormone in patients on hemodialysis. *J Am Soc Nephrol* 1998; **9:** 1427–1432.

168 Martin KJ, González EA, Gellens ME, Hamm LL, Abboud H, Lindberg J. Therapy of secondary hyperparathyroidism with 19-nor-1α,25-dihydroxyvitamin D2. *Am J Kidney Dis* 1998; **32(2 Suppl 2):** S61–S66.

169 Ross EA, Tian J, Abboud H, Hippensteel R, Melnick JZ, Pradhan RS *et al.* Oral paricalcitol for the treatment of secondary hyperparathyroidism in patients on hemodialysis or peritoneal dialysis. *Am J Nephrol* 2008; **28(1):** 97–106.

170 Bacchini G, Fabrizi F, Pontoriero G, Marcelli D, Di Filippo S, Locatelli F. 'Pulse oral' versus intravenous calcitriol therapy in chronic hemodialysis patients. A prospective and randomized study. *Nephron* 1997; **77(3):** 267–272.

171 Chandra P, Binongo JN, Ziegler TR, Schlanger LE, Wang W, Someren JT *et al.* Cholecalciferol (vitamin D3) therapy and vitamin D insufficiency in patients with chronic kidney disease: a randomized controlled pilot study. *Endocr Pract* 2008; **14(1):** 10–17.

172 Dunlay R, Rodriguez M, Felsenfeld AJ, Llach F. Direct inhibitory effect of calcitriol on parathyroid function (sigmoidal curve) in dialysis. *Kidney Int* 1989; **36(6):** 1093–1098.

173 Fischer ER, Harris DC. Comparison of intermittent oral and intravenous calcitriol in hemodialysis patients with secondary hyperparathyroidism. *Clin Nephrol* 1993; **40:** 216–220.

174 Gallieni M, Brancaccio D, Padovese P, Rolla D, Bedani P, Colantonio G *et al.* Low-dose intravenous calcitriol treatment of secondary hyperparathyroidism in hemodialysis patients. Italian Group for the Study of Intravenous Calcitriol. *Kidney Int* 1992; **42(5):** 1191–1198.

175 Goodman WG, Ramirez JA, Belin TR, Chon Y, Gales B, Segre GV *et al.* Development of adynamic bone in patients with secondary hyperparathyroidism after intermittent calcitriol therapy. *Kidney Int* 1994; **46:** 1160–1166.

176 Gordon PL, Sakkas GK, Doyle JW, Shubert T, Johansen KL. Relationship between vitamin D and muscle size and strength in patients on hemodialysis. *J Renal Nutr* 2007; **6:** 397–407.

177 Hayashi M, Tsuchiya Y, Itaya Y, Takenaka T, Kobayashi K, Yoshizawa M *et al.* Comparison of the effects of calcitriol and maxacalcitol on secondary hyperparathyroidism in patients on chronic haemodialysis: a randomized prospective multicentre trial. *Nephrol Dial Transplant* 2004; **19:** 2067–2073.

178 Indridason OS, Quarles LD. Comparison of treatments for mild secondary hyperparathyroidism in hemodialysis patients. Durham Renal Osteodystrophy Study Group. *Kidney Int* 2000; **57:** 282–292.

179 Koshikawa S, Akizawa T, Kurokawa K, Marumo F, Sakai O, Arakawa M *et al.* Clinical effect of intravenous calcitriol administration on secondary hyperparathyroidism. A double-blind study among 4 doses. *Nephron* 2002; **90(4):** 413–423.

180 Memmos DE, Eastwood JB, Talner LB, Gower PE, Curtis JR, Phillips ME *et al.* Double-blind trial of oral 1,25-dihydroxy vitamin D3 versus placebo in asymptomatic hyperparathyroidism in patients receiving maintenance hemodialysis. *Br Med J* 1981; **282:** 1919–1924.

181 Malberti F, Surian M, Cosci P. Improvement of secondary hyperparathyroidism and reduction of the set point of calcium after intravenous calcitriol. *Kidney Int Suppl* 1993; **41:** S125–S130.

182 Moe S, Wazny LD, Martin JE. Oral calcitriol versus oral alfacalcidol for the treatment of secondary hyperparathyroidism in patients receiving hemodialysis: a randomized, crossover trial. *Can J Clin Pharmacol* 2008; **15(1):** e36–e43.

183 Quarles LD, Yohay DA, Carroll BA, Spritzer CE, Minda SA, Bartholomay D *et al.* Prospective trial of pulse oral versus intravenous calcitriol treatment of hyperparathyroidism in ESRD. *Kidney Int* 1994; **45:** 1710–1721.

184 Rodriguez M, Caravaca F, Fernandez E, Borrego MJ, Lorenzo V, Cubero J *et al.* Parathyroid function as a determinant of the response to calcitriol treatment in the hemodialysis patient. *Kidney Int* 1999; **56(1):** 306–317.

185 Akiba T, Marumo F, Owada A, Kurihara S, Inoue A, Chida Y *et al.* Controlled trial of falecalcitriol versus alfacalcidol in suppression of parathyroid hormone in hemodialysis patients with secondary hyperparathyroidism. *Am J Kidney Dis* 1998; **32:** 238–246.

186 Ala-Houhala M, Holmberg C, Rönnenholm K, Paganus A, Laine J, Koskimies O. Alphacalcidol oral pulses normalize uremic hyperparathyroidism prior to dialysis. *Pediatr Nephrol* 1995;**9:** 737–741.

187 Mochizuki T, Naganuma S, Tanaka Y, Iwamoto Y, Ishiguro C, Kawashima Y *et al.* Prospective comparison of the effects of maxacalcitol and calcitriol in chronic hemodialysis patients with secondary hyperparathyroidism: a multicenter, randomized crossover study. *Clin Nephrol* 2007; **67(1):** 12–19.

188 Tarrass F, Yazidi A, Sif H, Zamd M, Benghanem MG, Ramdani B. A randomized trial of intermittent versus continuous oral alfacalcidol treatment of hyperparathyroidism in end-stage renal disease. *Clin Nephrol* 2006;**65(6):** 415–418.

189 Hayashi M, Tsuchiya Y, Itaya Y, Takenaka T, Kobayashi K, Yoshizawa M *et al.* Comparison of the effects of calcitriol and maxacalcitol on secondary hyperparathyroidism in patients on chronic haemodialysis: a randomized prospective multicentre trial. *Nephrol Dial Transplant* 2004; **19(8):** 2067–2073.

190 Maung HM, Elangovan L, Frazao JM, Bower JD, Kelley BJ, Acchiardo SR *et al.* Efficacy and side effects of intermittent intravenous and oral doxercalciferol (1α-hydroxyvitamin D_2) in dialysis patients with secondary hyperparathyroidism: a sequential comparison. *Am J Kidney Dis* 2000; **37:** 532–543.

191 Frazao JM, Elangovan L, Maung HM, Chesney RW, Acchiardo SR, Bower JD *et al.* Intermittent doxercalciferol (1α-hydroxyvitamin D_2) therapy for secondary hyperparathyroidism. *Am J Kidney Dis* 2000; **36:** 550–561.

192 Tan AU, Levine BS, Mazess RB, Kyllo DM, Bishop CW, Knutson JC *et al.* Effective suppression of parathyroid hormone by 1α-hydroxyvitamin D_2 in hemodialysis patients with moderate to severe secondary hyperparathyroidism. *Kidney Int* 1997; **51:** 317–323.

193 Zisman AL, Hristova M, Ho LT, Sprague SM. Impact of ergocalciferol treatment of vitamin D deficiency on serum parathyroid hormone concentrations in chronic kidney disease. *Am J Nephrol* 2007; **27(1):** 36–43.

194 Lopez-Hilker S, Dusso AS, Rapp NS, Martin KJ, Slatopolsky E. Phosphorus restriction reverses hyperparathyroidism in uremia independent of changes in calcium and calcitriol. *Am J Physiol* 1990; **259(3):** F432–F437.

195 Slatopolsky E, Finch J, Denda M, Ritter C, Zhong M, Dusso A *et al.* Phosphorus restriction prevents parathyroid gland growth. *J Clin Invest* 1996; **97:** 2534–2540.

196 Giachelli CM. Vascular calcification: in vitro evidence for the role of inorganic phosphate. *J Am Soc Nephrol* 2003; **14(Suppl 9):** S300–S304.

197 Giachelli CM, Speer MY, Li X, Rajachar RM, Yang H. Regulation of vascular calcification: roles of phosphate and osteopontin. *Circ Res* 2005; **96(7):** 717–722

198 Li X, Yang HY, Giachelli CM. Role of the sodium-dependent phosphate cotransporter, Pit-1, in vascular smooth muscle cell calcification. *Circ Res* 2006; **98(7):** 905–912.

199 El-Abbadi M, Giachelli CM. Mechanisms of vascular calcification. *Adv Chronic Kidney Dis* 2007; **14(1):** 54–66.

200 Li X, Giachelli CM. Sodium-dependent phosphate cotransporters and vascular calcification. *Curr Opin Nephrol Hypertens* 2007; **16(4):** 325–328.

201 Moe SM, Chen NX. Pathophysiology of vascular calcification in chronic kidney disease. *Circ Res* 2004; **95:** 560–567.

202 Proudfoot D, Skepper JN, Hegyi L, Bennett MR, Shanahan CM, Weissberg PL. Apoptosis regulates human vascular calcification *in vitro*: Evidence for initiation of vascular calcification by apoptotic bodies. *Circ Res* 2000; **87:** 1055–1062.

203 Shroff RC, Shanahan CM. The vascular biology of calcification. *Semin Dial* 2007; **20(2):** 103–109.

204 Ketteler M, Giachelli C. Novel insights into vascular calcification. *Kidney Int* 2006; **105:** S5–S9.

205 Lowrie EG, Lew NL. Death risk in hemodialysis patients: the predictive value of commonly measured variables and an evaluation of death rate differences between facilities. *Am J Kidney Dis* 1990; **15(5):** 458–482.

206 Leggat JE, Orzol SM, Hulbert-Shearson TE, Golper TA, Jones CA, Held PJ *et al.* Noncompliance in hemodialysis: predictors and survival analysis. *Am J Kidney Dis* 1998; **32:** 139–145.

207 Block GA, Hulbert-Shearon TE, Levin NW, Port FK. Association of serum phosphorus and calcium x phosphate product with mortality risk in chronic hemodialysis patients: a national study. *Am J Kidney Dis* 1998; **31(4):** 607–617.

208 Ganesh S, Stack A, Levin N, Hulbert-Sheron T, Port F. Assocation of elevated serum PO_4, Ca x PO_4 product, and parathyroid hormone with cardiac mortality risk in chronic hemodialysis patients. *J Am Soc Nephrol* 2001; **12:** 2131–2138.

209 Marco MP, Craver L, Betriu A, Belart M, Fibla J, Fernández E. Higher impact of mineral metabolism on cardiovascular mortality in a European hemodialysis population. *Kidney Int* 2003; **85:** S111–S114.

210 Block GA, Klassen PS, Lazarus JM, Ofsthun N, Lowrie EG, Chertow GM. Mineral metabolism, mortality, and morbidity in maintenance hemodialysis. *J Am Soc Nephrol* 2004; **15(8):** 2208–2218.

211 Young EW, Albert JM, Satayathum S, Goodkin DA, Pisoni RL, Akiba T *et al.* Predictors and consequences of altered mineral metabolism: the Dialysis Outcomes and Practice Patterns Study. *Kidney Int* 2005; **67(3):** 1179–1187.

212 Slinin Y, Foley RN, Collins AJ. Calcium, phosphorus, parathyroid hormone, and cardiovascular disease in hemodialysis patients: the USRDS Waves 1, 3, and 4 study. *J Am Soc Nephrol* 2005; **16:** 1788–1793.

213 Rodriguez-Benot A, Martin-Malo A, Alvarez-Lara MA, Rodriguez M, Aljama P. Mild hyperphosphatemia and mortality in hemodialysis patients. *Am J Kidney Dis* 2005; **46(1):** 68–77.

214 Melamed ML, Eustace JA, Plantinga L, Jaar BG, Fink NE, Coresh J *et al.* Changes in serum calcium, phosphate, and PTH and the risk of death in incident dialysis patients: a longitudinal study. *Kidney Int* 2006; **70:** 351–357.

215 Nakai S, Akiba T, Kazama J, Yokoyama K, Fukagawa M, Tominaga Y et al. Effects of serum calcium, phosphorus, and intact parathyroid hormone levels on survival in chronic hemodialysis patients in Japan. *Ther Apher Dial* 2008; **12**(1): 49–54.

216 Noordzij M, Korevaar JC, Bos WJ, Boeschoten EW, Dekker FW, Bossuyt PM et al. Mineral metabolism and cardiovascular morbidity and mortality risk: peritoneal dialysis patients compared with haemodialysis patients. *Nephrol Dial Transplant* 2006; **21**(9): 2513–2520.

217 Noordzij M, Korevaar JC, Dekker FW, Boeschoten EW, Bos WJ, Krediet RT et al. Mineral metabolism and mortality in dialysis patients: a reassessment of the K/DOQI guideline. *Blood Purif* 2008; **26**(3): 231–237.

218 Kestenbaum B, Sampson JN, Rudser KD, Patterson DJ, Seliger SL, Young B et al. Serum phosphate levels and mortality risk among people with chronic kidney disease. *J Am Soc Nephrol* 2005; **16**(2): 520–528.

219 Schwarz S, Trivedi BK, Kalantar-Zadeh K, Kovesdy CP. Association of disorders in mineral metabolism with progression of chronic kidney disease. *Clin J Am Soc Nephrol* 2006; **1**: 825–831.

220 Dhingra R, Sullivan LM, Fox CS, Wang TJ, D'Agostino RB, Sr., Gaziano JM et al. Relations of serum phosphorus and calcium levels to the incidence of cardiovascular disease in the community. *Arch Intern Med* 2007; **167**(9): 879–885.

221 Tonelli M, Sacks F, Pfeffer M, Gao Z, Curhan G, Cholesterol and Recurrent Events Trial Investigators. Relation between serum phosphate level and cardiovascular event rate in people with coronary disease. *Circulation* 2005; **112**(17): 2627–2633.

222 Coladonato JA. Control of hyperphosphatemia among patients with ESRD. *J Am Soc Nephrol* 2005; **16**: S107–S114.

223 Willett WC, Buzzard M. *Nature of Variation in Diet in Nutritional Epidemiology*, 2nd edn. Oxford University Press, New York, 1998; 33–49.

224 Cupisti A, Morelli E, Meola M, Barsotti M, Barsotti G. Vegetarian diet alternated with conventional low-protein diet for patients with chronic renal failure. *J Ren Nutr* 2002; **12**: 32–37.

225 Craver L, Marco MP, Martínez I, Rue M, Borras M, Martín ML et al. Mineral metabolism parameters throughout chronic kidney disease stages 1–5: achievement of K/DOQI target ranges. *Nephrol Dial Transplant* 2002; **22**: 1171–1176.

226 Isakova T, Gutierrez O, Shah A, Castaldo L, Holmes J, Lee H et al. Postprandial mineral metabolism and secondary hyperparathyroidism in early CKD. *J Am Soc Nephrol* 2008; **19**: 615–623.

227 Martinez I, Saracho R, Montenegro J, Llach F. The importance of dietary calcium and phosphorus in the secondary hyperparathyroidism of patients with early renal failure. *Am J Kidney Dis* 1997; **29**: 496–502.

228 Onufrak SJ, Bellasi A, Shaw LJ, Herzog CA, Cardarelli F, Wilson PW et al. Phosphorus levels are associated with subclinical atherosclerosis in the general population. *Atherosclerosis* 17 Dec 2007 [Epub ahead of print].

229 Ramirez JA, Emmett M, White MG, Fathi N, Santa Ana CA, Morawski SG et al. The absorption of dietary phosphorus and calcium in hemodialysis patients. *Kidney Int* 1986; **30**: 753–759.

230 Gotch FA, Panlilio F, Sergeyeva O, Rosales L, Folden T, Kaysen G et al. A kinetic model of inorganic phosphorus mass balance in hemodialysis therapy. *Blood Purif* 2003; **21**: 51–57.

231 Kuhlmann MK. Management of hyperphosphatemia. *Hemodial Int* 2006; **10**: 338–345.

232 Minutolo R, Bellizzi V, Cioffi M, Iodice C, Giannattasio P, Andreucci M et al. Postdialytic rebound of serum phosphorus: pathogenetic and clinical insights. *J Am Soc Nephrol* 2002; **13**: 1046–1054.

233 Achinger SG, Ayus JC. The role of daily dialysis in the control of hyperphosphatemia. *Kidney Int* 2005; **67**(Suppl 95): S28–S32.

234 Mucsi I, Hercz G, Uldall R, Ouwendyk M, Francoeur R, Pierratos A. Control of serum phosphate without any phosphate binders in patients treated with nocturnal hemodialysis. *Kidney Int* 1998; **53**: 1399–1404.

235 Walsh M, Culleton B, Tonelli M, Manns B. A systematic review of the effect of nocturnal hemodialysis on blood pressure, left ventricular hypertrophy, anemia, mineral metabolism, and health-related quality of life. *Kidney Int* 2005; **67**(4): 1500–1508.

236 Culleton BF, Walsh M, Klarenbach SW, Mortis G, Scott-Douglas N, Quinn RR et al. Effect of frequent nocturnal hemodialysis vs conventional hemodialysis on left ventricular mass and quality of life: a randomized controlled trial. *JAMA* 2007; **298**(11): 1291–1299.

237 Barsotti G, Cupisti A. The role of dietary phosphorus restriction in the conservative management of chronic renal disease. *J Ren Nutr* 2005; **15**: 189–192.

238 Barsotti G, Cupisti A, Morelli E, Meola M, Cozza V, Barsotti M et al. Secondary hyperparathyroidism in severe chronic renal failure is corrected by very-low dietary phosphate intake and calcium carbonate supplementation. *Nephron* 1998; **79**(2): 137–141.

239 Uribarri J. Phosphorus homeostasis in normal health and in chronic kidney disease patients with special emphasis on dietary phosphorus intake. *Semin Dial* 2007; **20**(4): 295–301.

240 Murphy-Gutekunst L, Barnes K. Hidden phosphorus at breakfast: part 2. *J Ren Nutr* 2005; **15**: E1–E6.

241 Murphy-Gutekunst L, Uribarri J. Hidden phosphorus enhanced meats: part 3. *J Ren Nutr* 2005; **15**: E1–E4.

242 Murphy-Gutekunst L. Hidden phosphorus in popular beverages: part 1. *J Ren Nutr* 2005; **15**: E1–E6.

243 Murphy-Gutekunst L. Hidden phosphorus: where do we go from here? *J Ren Nutr* 2007; **17**: E31–E36.

244 Uribarri J, Calvo MS. Hidden sources of phosphorus in the typical American diet: does it matter in nephrology? *Semin Dial* 2003; **16**: 186–188.

245 Kopple JD, Coburn JW. Metabolic studies of low protein diets in uremia. II. Calcium, phosphorus, and magnesium. *Medicine* 1973; **52**: 597–607.

246 Calvo MS, Kumar R, Heath H. Persistently elevated parathyroid hormone secretion and action in young women after four weeks of ingesting high phosphorus, low calcium diets. *J Clin Endocrinol Metab* 1990; **70**: 1334–1340.

247 Calvo MS, Kumar R. Elevated secretion and action of serum parathyroid hormone in young adults consuming high phosphorus, low calcium diets assembled from common foods. *J Clin Endocrinol Metab* 1988; **66**: 823–829.

248 Sax L. Commentary. The Institute of Medicine's "dietary reference intake" for phosphorus: a critical perspective. *J Am Coll Nutr* 2001; **20**: 271–278.

249 Ritz E, Gross ML. Hyperphosphatemia in renal failure. *Blood Purif* 2005; **23**: 6–9.

250 Lumlertgul D, Burke TJ, Gillum DM, Afrey AC, Harris DC, Hammond WS et al. Phosphate depletion arrests progression of chronic renal failure independent of protein intake. *Kidney Int* 1986; **29**: 658–666.

251 Hsu CH. Are we mismanaging calcium and phosphate metabolism in renal failure? *Am J Kidney Dis* 1997; **29**: 641–649.

252 Rufino M, De Bonis E, Martin M, et al. Is it possible to control hyperphosphatemia with diet, without introducing protein malnutrition? *Nephrol Dial Transplant* 1998; **13**: 65–67.

253 Emmett M. A comparison of clinically useful phosphorus binders for patients with chronic kidney failure. *Kidney Int* 2004; **66(Suppl 90):** S25–S32.

254 Sheikh MS, Maguire JA, Emmett M, Santa Ana CA, Nicar MJ, Schiller LR *et al.* Reduction of dietary phosphorous absorption by phosphorous binders. A theoretical, in vitro, and in vivo study. *J Clin Invest* 1989; **83(1):** 66–73.

255 Manns B, Klarenbach S, Lee H, Culleton B, Shrive F, Tonelli M. Economic evaluation of sevelamer in patients with end-stage renal disease. *Nephrol Dial Transplant* 2007; **22:** 2867–2878.

256 Huybrechts KF, Caro JJ, London GM. Modeling the implications of changes in vascular calcification in patients on hemodialysis. *Kidney Int* 2005; **67:** 1532–1538.

257 Huybrechts KF, Caro JJ, Wilson DA, O'Brien JA. Health and economic consequences of sevelamer use for hyperphosphatemia in patients on hemodialysis. *Value Health* 2005; **8(5):** 549–561.

258 Nadin C. Sevelamer as a phosphate binder in adult hemodialysis patients: an evidence-based review of its therapeutic value. *Core Evidence* 2005; **1:** 43–63.

259 Taylor M J, Elgazzar HA, Chaplin S, Goldsmith D, Molony DA. An economic evaluation of sevelamer in patients new to dialysis. *Curr Med Res Opin* 2008; **24:** 601–608.

260 Molony DA, Murthy BVR. Accumulation of metals and minerals from phosphate binders. *Blood Purif* 2005; **23(Suppl 1):** 2–9.

261 Alfrey AC. Aluminum toxicity in patients with chronic renal failure. *Ther Drug Monit* 1993; **15:** 593–597.

262 de Wolff FA. Toxicological aspects of aluminum poisoning in clinical nephrology. *Clin Nephrol* 1985; **24(Suppl 1):** S9–S14.

263 Cannata-Andía JB, Fernández-Martín JL. The clinical impact of aluminium overload in renal failure. *Nephrol Dial Transplant* 2002; **17(Suppl 2):** 9–12.

264 Campbell A. The potential role of aluminium in Alzheimer's disease. *Nephrol Dial Transplant* **17(Suppl 2):** 17–20.

265 Alfrey AC, LeGendre GR, Kaehny WD. The dialysis encephalopathy syndrome. Possible aluminum intoxication. *N Engl J Med* 1976; **294:** 184–188.

266 Malluche HH. Aluminium and bone disease in chronic renal failure. *Nephrol Dial Transplant* **17(Suppl 2):** 21–24.

267 Parkinson IS, Ward MK, Feest TG, Fawcett RW, Kerr DN. Fracturing dialysis osteodystrophy and dialysis encephalopathy. An epidemiological survey. *Lancet* 1979; **i(8113):** 406–409.

268 Jeffery EH, Abreo K, Burgess E, *et al.* Systemic aluminum toxicity: effects on bone, hematopoietic tissue, and kidney. *J Toxicol Environ Health* 1996; **48:** 649–665.

269 Andreoli SP, Bergstein JM, Sherrard DL. Aluminum intoxication from aluminum-containing phosphate binders in children with azotemia not undergoing dialysis. *N Engl J Med* 1984; **310:** 1079–1084.

270 Drüeke TB. Intestinal absorption of aluminium in renal failure. *Nephrol Dial Transplant* 2002; **17(Suppl 2):** 13–16

271 Coburn JW, Mischel MG, Goodman WG, Salusky IB. Calcium citrate markedly enhances aluminum absorption from aluminum hydroxide. *Am J Kidney Dis* 1991; **17(6):** 708–711.

272 Beynon H, Cassidy MJ. Gastrointestinal absorption of aluminium. *Nephron* 1990; **55:** 235–236.

273 Lote CJ, Saunders H. Aluminium: gastrointestinal absorption and renal excretion. *Clin Sci* 1991; **81:** 289–295.

274 Ittel TH, Kluge R, Sieberth HG. Enhanced gastrointestinal absorption of aluminium in uraemia: time course and effect of vitamin D. *Nephrol Dial Transplant* 1988; **3:** 617–623.

275 Wilhelm M, Jager DE, Ohnesorge FK. Aluminium toxicokinetics. *Pharmacol Toxicol* 1990; **66:** 4–9.

276 de Wolff FA. Toxicological aspects of aluminum poisoning in clinical nephrology. *Clin Nephrol* 1985; **24(Suppl 1):** S9–S14.

277 Cannata-Andia JB. Reconsidering the importance of long-term low-level aluminum exposure in renal failure patients. *Semin Dial* 2001; **14:** 5–7.

278 Berlyne GM, Ben-Ari J, Pest D, Weinberger J, Stern M, Levine R *et al.* Hyperaluminaemia from aluminum resins in renal failure. *Lancet* 1970; **ii(7671):** 494–496

279 Salusky IB, Coburn JW, Paunier L, Sherrard DJ, Fine RN. Role of aluminum hydroxide in raising serum aluminum levels in children undergoing continuous ambulatory peritoneal dialysis. *J Pediatr* 1984; **105(5):** 717–720.

280 Salusky IB, Foley J, Nelson P, *et al.* Aluminum accumulation during treatment with aluminum hydroxide and dialysis in children and young adults with chronic renal disease. *N Engl J Med* 1991; **324:** 527–531.

281 Weberg R, Berstad A. Gastrointestinal absorption of aluminium from single doses of aluminium containing antacids in man. *Eur J Clin Invest* 1986; **16(5):** 428–432.

282 Autissier V, Damment SJ, Henderson RA. Relative in vitro efficacy of the phosphate binders lanthanum carbonate and sevelamer hydrochloride. *J Pharm Sci* 2007; **96(10):** 2818–2827.

283 Nelson R. Novel phosphate binder is effective in patients on haemodialysis. *Lancet* 2002; **360:** 1483.

284 Hutchison AJ, Maes B, Vanwalleghem J, Asmus G, Mohamed E, Schmieder R. Efficacy, tolerability, and safety of lanthanum carbonate in hyperphosphatemia: a 6-month, randomized, comparative trial versus calcium carbonate. *Nephron Clin Pract* 2005; **100(1):** C8–C19.

285 Hutchison AJ, Speake M, Al-Baaj F. Reducing high phosphate levels in patients with chronic renal failure undergoing dialysis: a 4-week, dose-finding, open-label study with lanthanum carbonate. *Nephrol Dial Transplant* 2004; **19:** 1902–1906.

286 Hutchison AJ, Maes B, Vanwalleghem J, Asmus G, Mohamed E, Schmieder R *et al.* Long-term efficacy and tolerability of lanthanum carbonate: results from a 3-year study. *Nephron Clin Pract* 2006; **102(2):** C61–C71.

287 D'Haese PC, Spasovski GB, Sikole A, Hutchison A, Freemont TJ, Sulkova S *et al.* A multicenter study on the effects of lanthanum carbonate (Fosrenol) and calcium carbonate on renal bone disease in dialysis patients. *Kidney Int* 2003; **63:** S73–S78.

288 Joy MS, Finn WF. Randomized, double blind, placebo-controlled, dose-titration, phase III study assessing the efficacy and tolerability of lanthanum carbonate: a new phospate binder for the treatment of byperphosphatemia. *Am J Kid Dis* 2003; **42:** 96–107.

289 Finn WF, Joy MS. A long-term, open-label extension study on the safety of treatment with lanthanum carbonate, a new phosphate binder, in patients receiving hemodialysis. *Curr Med Res Opin* 2005; **21(5):** 657–664.

290 Spasovski GB, Sikole A, Gelev S, Masin-Spasovska J, Freemont T, Webster I *et al.* Evolution of bone and plasma concentration of lanthanum in dialysis patients before, during 1 year of treatment with lanthanum carbonate and after 2 years of follow-up. *Nephrol Dial Transplant* 2006; **21(8):** 2217–2224.

291 Cozzolino M, Brancaccio D. Lanthanum carbonate-new data on parathyroid hormone control without liver damage. *Nephrol Dial Transplant* 2007; **22(2):** 316–318.

292 Shigematsu T, Lanthanum Carbonate Research Group. Lanthanum carbonate effectively controls serum phosphate without affecting serum calcium levels in patients undergoing hemodialysis. *Ther Apher Dial* 2008; **12(1):** 55–61.

293 Freemont T, Malluche HH. Utilization of bone histomorphometry in renal osteodystrophy: demonstration of a new approach using data from a prospective study of lanthanum carbonate. *Clin Nephrol* 2005; **63(2):** 138–145.

294 Freemont AJ, Hoyland JA, Denton J. The effects of lanthanum carbonate and calcium carbonate on bone abnormalities in patients with end-stage renal disease. *Clin Nephrol* 2005; **64(6):** 428–437.

295 Behets GJ, Dams G, Vercauteren SR, Damment SJ, Bouillon R, De Broe ME et al. Does the phosphate binder lanthanum carbonate affect bone in rats with chronic renal failure? *J Am Soc Nephrol* 2004; **15(8):** 2219–2228

296 Lacour B, Lucas A, Auchère D, Ruellan N, de Serre Patey NM, Drüeke TB. Chronic renal failure is associated with increased tissue deposition of lanthanum after 28-day oral administration. *Kidney Int* 2005;**67(3):** 1062–1069.

297 Slatopolsky E, Liapis H, Finch J. Progressive accumulation of lanthanum in the liver of normal and uremic rats. *Kidney Int* 2005; **68(6):** 2809–2813.

298 Huang J, Zhang T-L, Xu S-J, Li R-C, Wang K, Zhang J et al. Effects of lanthanum on composition, crystal size, and lattice structure of femur bone mineral of Wistar rats. *Calcif Tissue Int* 2006; **78:** 241–247.

299 Evans CH. *Biochemistry of the Lanthanides*. Plenum Press, New York, 1990.

300 Damment SJ, De Broe ME, D'Haese PC, Bramall N, Cox AG, McLeod CW. Incredulous effects of lanthanum? *Toxicol Lett* 2007; **168(2):** 186–189.

301 Bouldin TW, Krigman MR. Differential permeability of cerebral capillary and choroid plexus to lanthanum ion. *Brain Res* 1975; **99(2):** 444–448.

302 Dorovini-Zis K, Sato M, Goping G, Rapoport S, Brightman M. Ionic lanthanum passage across cerebral endothelium exposed to hyperosmotic arabinose. *Acta Neuropathol* 1983; **60(1–2):** 49–60.

303 Feng L, Xiao H, He X, Li Z, Li F, Liu N et al. Long-term effects of lanthanum intake on the neurobehavioral development of the rat. *Neurotoxicol Teratol* 2006; **28(1):** 119–124.

304 Feng L, Xiao H, He X, Li Z, Li F, Liu N et al. Neurotoxicological consequence of long-term exposure to lanthanum. *Toxicol Lett* 2006; **165(2):** 112–120.

305 Altamnn P, Barnett ME, Winn WF, SDP405-307 Lanthanum Carbonate Study. Cognitive function in stage 5 chronic kidney disease patients on hemodialysis: No adverse effectrs of lanthanum carbonate compared with standard phosphate-binder therapy. *Kidney Int* 2006; **71(3):** 252–259.

306 Brunner FP, Thiel G. Re: the use of magnesium-containing phosphate binders in patients with end-stage renal disease on maintenance haemodialysis. *Nephron* 1982; **32:** 266.

307 Guillot AP, Hood VL, Runge CF, Gennari FJ. The use of magnesium-containing phosphate binders in patients with end-stage renal disease on maintenance hemodialysis. *Nephron* 1982; **30:** 114–117.

308 Delmez JA, Kelber J, Norword KY, Giles KS, Slatopolsky E. Magnesium carbonate as a phosphorus binder: a prospective, controlled, crossover study. *Kidney Int* 1996; **49:** 163–167.

309 Oe PL, Lips P, van der Meulen J, et al. Long-term use of magnesium hydroxide as a phosphate binder in patients on hemodialysis. *Clin Nephrol* 1987; **28:** 180–185.

310 Moriniere P, Vinatier I, Westeel PF, Cohemsolal M, Belbrik S, Abdulmassih Z et al. Magnesium hydroxide as a complementary aluminium-free phosphate binder to moderate doses of oral calcium in uraemic patients on chronic haemodialysis: lack of deleterious effect on bone mineralisation. *Nephrol Dial Transplant* 1988; **3:** 651–656.

311 Loghman-Adham M. Safety of new phosphate binders for chronic renal failure. *Drug Saf* 2003; **26(15):** 1093–1115.

312 Navarro JF, Mora C, Jiménez A, Torres A, Macía M, García J. Relationship between serum magnesium and parathyroid hormone levels in hemodialysis patients. *Am J Kidney Dis* 1999; **34(1):** 43–48.

313 Spiegel DM, Farmer B, Smits G, Chonchol M. Magnesium carbonate is an effective phosphate binder for chronic hemodialysis patients: a pilot study. *J Ren Nutr* 2007; **17(6):** 416–422.

314 Mai ML, Emmett M, Sheikh MS, Santa Ana CA, Schiller L, Fordtran JS. Calcium acetate, an effective phosphorous binder in patients with renal failure. *Kidney Int* 1989; **36:** 690–695.

315 Emmett M, Sirmon MD, Kirkpatrick WG, Nolan CR, Schmitt GW, Cleveland MB. Calcium acetate control of serum phosphorus in hemodialysis patients. *Am J Kidney Dis* 1991; **17(5):** 544–550.

316 Schaefer K, Scheer J, Asmus G, Umlauf E, Hagemann J, von Herrath D. The treatment of uraemic hyperphosphataemia with calcium acetate and calcium carbonate: a comparative study. *Nephrol Dial Transplant* 1991; **6(3):** 170–175.

317 Delmez JA, Tindira CA, Windus DW, Norwood KY, Giles KS, Nighswander TL et al. Calcium acetate as a phosphorus binder in hemodialysis patients. *J Am Soc Nephrol* 1992; **3(1):** 96–102.

318 Ring T, Nielsen C, Andersen SP, Behrens JK, Sodemann B, Kornerup HJ. Calcium acetate versus calcium carbonate as phosphorus binders in patients on chronic haemodialysis: a controlled study. *Nephrol Dial Transplant* 1993; **8:** 341–346.

319 Pflanz S, Henderson IS, McElduff N, Jones MC. Calcium acetate versus calcium carbonate as phosphate-binding agents in chronic haemodialysis. *Nephrol Dial Transplant* 1994; **9(8):** 1121–1124.

320 Clarkson EM, McDonald SJ, De Wardener WE. The effect of a high intake of calcium carbonate in normal subjects and patients with chronic renal failure. *Clin Sci* 1966; **30:** 425–438.

321 Slatopolsky E, Weerts C, Lopez-Hilker S, Norwood K, Zink M, Windus D. Calcium carbonate as a phosphate binder in patients with chronic renal failure undergoing dialysis. *N Engl J Med* 1986; **315:** 157–161.

322 Hercz G, Kraut JA, Andress DA, Howard N, Roberts C, Shinaberger JH et al. Use of calcium carbonate as a phosphate binder in dialysis patients. *Miner Electrolyte Metab* 1986; **12:** 314–319.

323 Heaney RP, Smith KT, Recker RR, Hinders SM. Meal effects on calcium absorption. *Am J Clin Nutr* 1989; **49(2):** 372–376.

324 Schiller LR, Santa Ana CA, Sheikh MS, Emmett M, Fordtran JS. Effect of the time of administration of calcium acetate on phosphorus binding. *N Engl J Med* 1989; **320(17):** 1110–1113.

325 Coburn JW, Koppel MH, Brickman AS, Massry SG. Study of intestinal absorption of calcium in patients with renal failure. *Kidney Int* 1973; **3(4):** 264–272.

326 Ginsburg DS, Kaplan EL, Katz AI. Hypercalcaemia after oral calcium-carbonate therapy in patients on chronic haemodialysis. *Lancet* 1973; **i(7815):** 1271–1274.

327 Moriniere P, el Esper N, Viron B, Judith D, Bourgeon B, Farquet C *et al.* Improvement in severe secondary hyperparathyroidism in dialysis patients by intravenous 1 alpha (OH) vitamin D3, oral CaCO3 and low dialysate calcium. *Kidney Int Suppl* 1993; **41:** S121–S124.

328 Weinreich T, Ritz E, Passlick-Deetjen J. Long-term dialysis with low-calcium solution (1.0 mmol/L) in CAPD: effects on bone mineral metabolism. Collaborators in the Multicenter Study Group. *Perit Dial Int* 1996; **16(3):** 260–268.

329 Weinreich T, Passlick-Deetjen J, Ritz E. Low dialysate calcium in continuous ambulatory peritoneal dialysis: a randomized controlled multicenter trial. The Peritoneal Dialysis Multicenter Study Group. *Am J Kidney Dis* 1995; **25(3):** 452–460.

330 Drüeke T, Bordier PJ, Man NK, Jungers P, Marie P. Effects of high dialysate calcium concentration on bone remodelling, serum biochemistry, and parathyroid hormone in patients with renal osteodystrophy. *Kidney Int* 1977; **11(4):** 267–274.

331 Spasovski G, Gelev S, Masin-Spasovska J, Selim G, Sikole A, Vanholder R. Improvement of bone and mineral parameters related to adynamic bone disease by diminishing dialysate calcium. *Bone* 2007; **41(4):** 698–703.

332 Salusky IB, Goodman WG, Sahney S, Gales B, Perilloux A, Wang HJ *et al.* Sevelamer controls parathyroid hormone-induced bone disease as efficiently as calcium carbonate without increasing serum calcium levels during therapy with active vitamin D sterols. *J Am Soc Nephrol* 2005; **16(8):** 2501–2508.

333 Tsukamoto Y, Moriya R, Nagaba Y, Morishita T, Izumida I, Okubo M. Effect of administering calcium carbonate to treat secondary hyperparathyroidism in nondialyzed patients with chronic renal failure. *Am J Kidney Dis* 1995; **25(6):** 879–886.

334 Russo D, Palmiero G, De Blasio AP, Balletta MM, Andreucci VE. Coronary artery calcification in patients with CRF not undergoing dialysis. *Am J Kidney Dis* 2004; **44(6):** 1024–1030.

335 Russo D, Corrao S, Miranda I, Ruocco C, Manzi S, Elefante R *et al.* Progression of coronary artery calcification in predialysis patients. *Am J Nephrol* 2007; **27(2):** 152–158.

336 Russo D, Miranda I, Ruocco C, Battaglia Y, Buonanno E, Manzi S *et al.* The progression of coronary artery calcification in predialysis patients on calcium carbonate or sevelamer. *Kidney Int* 2007; **72(10):** 1255–1261.

337 Janssen MJ, van der KA, ter Wee PM, van Boven WP. Aluminum hydroxide, calcium carbonate and calcium acetate in chronic intermittent hemodialysis patients. *Clin Nephrol* 1996; **45(2):** 111–119.

338 Fournier A, Moriniere P, Ben Hamida F, el Esjer N, Shenovda M, Ghazali A *et al.* Use of alkaline calcium salts as phosphate binders in uremic patients. *Kidney Int Suppl* 1992; **38:** S50–S61.

339 Oettinger CW, Oliver JC, Macon EJ. The effects of calcium carbonate as the sole phosphate binder in combination with low calcium dialysate and calcitriol therapy in chronic hemodialysis patients. *J Am Soc Nephrol* 1992; **3:** 995–1001.

340 Nolan CR, Califano JR, Butzin CA. Influence of calcium acetate or calcium citrate on intestinal aluminum absorption. *Kidney Int* 1990; **38:** 937–941.

341 Qunibi WY, Nolan CA, Ayus JC. Cardiovascular calcification in patients with end-stage renal disease: a century-old phenomenon. *Kidney Int Suppl* 2002; **82:** S73–S80.

342 Moe SM, Chertow GM. The case against calcium-based phosphate binders. *Clin J Am Soc Nephrol* 2006;**1(4):** 697–703.

343 Friedman E. Calcium-based phosphate binders are appropriate in chronic renal failure. *Clin J Am Soc Nephrol* 2006; **1:** 704–709.

344 Spiegel DM, Block GA. Should we be using calcium-containing phosphate binders in patients on dialysis? *Nat Clin Pract Nephrol* 2008; **4(3):** 118–119.

345 Bolland MJ, Barber PA, Doughty RN, Mason B, Horne A, Ames R *et al.* Vascular events in healthy older women receiving calcium supplementation: randomised controlled trial. *BMJ* 2008; **336(7638):** 262–266.

346 Jackson RD, LaCroix AZ, Gass M, Wallace RB, Robbins J, Lewis CE *et al.* Calcium plus vitamin D supplementation and the risk of fractures. *N Engl J Med* 2006; **354(7):** 669–683.

347 Bischoff-Ferrari HA, Dawson-Hughes B, Baron JA, Burckhardt P, Li R, Spiegelman D *et al.* Calcium intake and hip fracture risk in men and women: a meta-analysis of prospective cohort studies and randomized controlled trials. *Am J Clin Nutr* 2007; **86(6):** 1780–1790.

348 Perez-Mijares R, Gomez-Fernandez P, Almaraz-Jimenez M, Ramos-Diaz M, Rivero-Bohorquez J. Treatment of severe secondary hyperparathyroidism with administration of calcium carbonate, intermittent high oral doses of 1,25-dihydroxyvitamin D3 and dialysate with 3 mEq/1 calcium concentration. *Am J Nephrol* 1993; **13(2):** 149–154.

349 Coen G. Adynamic bone disease: an update and overview. *J Nephrol* 2005; **18(2):** 117–122.

350 Goodman WG, Ramirez JA, Belin TR, Chon Y, Gales B, Segre GV *et al.* Development of adynamic bone in patients with secondary hyperparathyroidism after intermittent calcitriol therapy. *Kidney Int* 1994; **46:** 1160–1166.

351 Hercz G, Pei Y, Greenwood C, Manuel A, Saiphoo C, Goodman WG *et al.* Aplastic osteodystrophy without aluminum: the role of "suppressed" parathyroid function. *Kidney Int* 1993; **44:** 860–866.

352 Kurz P, Monier-Faugere MC, Bognar B, Werner E, Roth P, Vlachojannis J *et al.* Evidence for abnormal calcium homeostasis in patients with adynamic bone disease. *Kidney Int* 1994; **46:** 855–861.

353 Kramer H, Toto R, Peshock R, Cooper R, Victor R. Association between chronic kidney disease and coronary artery calcification: the Dallas Heart Study. *J Am Soc Nephrol* 2005; **16(2):** 507–513

354 Burke SK, Slatopolsky EA, Goldberg DI. RenaGel, a novel calcium- and aluminium-free phosphate binder, inhibits phosphate absorption in normal volunteers. *Nephrol Dial Trans* 1997; **12(8):** 1640–1644.

355 Goldberg DI, Dillon MA, Slatopolsky EA, Garrett B, Gray JR, Marbury T *et al.* Effect of RenaGel, a non-absorbed, calcium- and aluminium-free phosphate binder, on serum phosphorus, calcium, and intact parathyroid hormone in end-stage renal disease patients. *Nephrol Dial Transplant* 1998; **13:** 2303–2310.

356 Slatopolsky EA, Burke SK, Dillon MA. RenaGel, a nonabsorbed calcium- and aluminum-free phosphate binder, lowers serum phosphorus and parathyroid hormone. The RenaGel Study Group. *Kidney Int* 1999; **55:** 299–307.

357 Swearingen RA, Chen X, Petersen JS, Riley KS, Wang D, Zhorov E. Determination of the binding parameter constants of Renagel capsules and tablets utilizing the Langmuir approximation at various pH by ion chromatography. *J Pharm Biomed Anal* 2002; **29(1–2):** 195–201.

358 Braunlin W, Zhorov E, Guo A, Apruzzese W, Xu Q, Hook P *et al.* Bile acid binding to sevelamer HCl. *Kidney Int* 2002; **62(2):** 611–619.

359 Bleyer AJ, Burke SK, Dillon M, Garrett B, Kant KS, Lynch D *et al.* A comparison of the calcium-free phosphate binder sevelamer hydrochloride

with calcium acetate in the treatment of hyperphosphatemia in hemodialysis patients. *Am J Kidney Dis* 1999; **33**: 694–701.

360 Duggal A, Hanus M, Zhorov E, Dagher R, Plone MA, Goldberg J *et al.* Novel dosage forms and regimens for sevelamer-based phosphate binders. *J Ren Nutr* 2006; **16(3)**: 248–252.

361 Castro R, Herman A, Ferreira C, Travassos F, Nunes-Azevedo J, Oliveira M. RenaGel efficacy in severe secondary hyperparathyroidism. *Nefrologia* 2002; **22(5)**: 448–455.

362 Pieper AK, Haffner D, Hoppe B, Dittrich K, Offner G, Bonzel KE *et al.* A randomized crossover trial comparing sevelamer with calcium acetate in children with CKD. *Am J Kidney Dis* 2006; **47(4)**: 625–663.

363 Qunibi WY, Hootkins RE, McDowell LL, Meyer MS, Simon M, Garza RO *et al.* Treatment of hyperphosphatemia in hemodialysis patients: the Calcium Acetate Renagel Evaluation (CARE Study). *Kidney Int* 2004; **65**: 1914–1926.

364 Qunibi W, Moustafa M, Muenz LR, He DY, Kessler PD, Diaz-Buxo JA *et al.* A 1-year randomized trial of calcium acetate versus sevelamer on progression of coronary artery calcification in hemodialysis patients with comparable lipid control: the Calcium Acetate Renagel Evaluation-2 (CARE-2) study. *Am J Kidney Dis* 2008; **51(6)**: 952–965.

365 Sturtevant JM, Hawley CM, Reiger K, Johnson DW, Campbell SB, Burke JR *et al.* Efficacy and side-effect profile of sevelamer hydrochloride used in combination with conventional phosphate binders. *Nephrology* (Carlton) 2004; **9**: 406–413.

366 Kokuho T, Toya Y, Kawaguchi Y, Tamura K, Iwatsubo K, Dobashi Y *et al.* Sevelamer hydrochloride improves hyperphosphatemia in hemodialysis patients with low bone turnover rate and low intact parathyroid hormone levels. *Ther Apher Dial* 2007; **11(6)**: 442–448.

367 Koiwa F, Onoda N, Kato H, Tokumoto A, Okada T, Fukagawa M *et al.* Prospective randomized multicenter trial of sevelamer hydrochloride and calcium carbonate for the treatment of hyperphosphatemia in hemodialysis patients in Japan. *Ther Apher Dial* 2005; **9(4)**: 340–346.

368 Koiwa F, Kazama JJ, Tokumoto A, Onoda N, Kato H, Okada T *et al.* Sevelamer hydrochloride and calcium bicarbonate reduce serum fibroblast growth factor 23 levels in dialysis patients. *Ther Apher Dial* 2005; **9(4)**: 336–339.

369 Ogata H, Koiwa F, Shishido K, Kinugasa E. Combination therapy with sevelamer hydrochloride and calcium carbonate in Japanese patients with long-term hemodialysis: alternative approach for optimal mineral management. *Ther Apher Dial* 2005; **9(1)**: 11–15.

370 Takenaka T, Suzuki H. New strategy to attenuate pulse wave velocity in haemodialysis patients. *Nephrol Dial Transplant* 2005; **20(4)**: 811–816.

371 Othmane Tel H, Bakonyi G, Egresits J, Fekete BC, Fodor E, Jarai Z *et al.* Effect of sevelamer on aortic pulse wave velocity in patients on hemodialysis: a prospective observational study. *Hemodial Int* 2007; **11(Suppl 3)**: S13–S21.

372 Chertow GM, Burke SK, Raggi P, Treat to Goal Working Group. Sevelamer attenuates the progression of coronary and aortic calcification in hemodialysis patients. *Kidney Int* 2002; **62(1)**: 245–252.

373 Braun J, Asmus HG, Holzer H, Brunkhorst R, Krause R, Schulz W *et al.* Long-term comparison of a calcium-free phosphate binder and calcium carbonate - phosphorus metabolism and cardiovascular calcification. *Clin Nephrol* 2004; **62(2)**: 104–115.

374 Raggi P, James G, Burke SK, Bommer J, Chasan-Taber S, Holzer H *et al.* Decrease in thoracic vertebral bone attenuation with calcium-based phosphate binders in hemodialysis. *J Bone Miner Res* 2005; **20(5)**: 764–772.

375 Asmus HG, Braun J, Krause R, Brunkhorst R, Holzer H, Schulz W *et al.* Two year comparison of sevelamer and calcium carbonate effects on cardiovascular calcification and bone density. *Nephrol Dial Transplant* 2005; **20(8)**: 1653–1661.

376 Block GA, Spiegel DM, Ehrlich J, *et al.* Effects of sevelamer and calcium on coronary artery calcification in patients new to hemodialysis. *Kidney Int* 2005; **68(4)**: 1815–1824.

377 Ferreira A, Frazao JM, Monier-Fauger M-C, Gil C, Galvao J, Oliveira C *et al.* Effects of sevelamer hydrochloride and calcium carbonate on renal osteodystrophy in hemodialysis patients. *J Am Soc Nephrol* 2008; **19**: 405–412.

378 Suki WN, Zabaneh R, Cangiano JL, Reed J, Fischer D, Garrett L *et al.* Effects of sevelamer and calcium-based phosphate binders on mortality in hemodialysis patients. *Kidney Int* 2007; **72(9)**: 1130–1137.

379 St Peter WL, Liu J, Weinhandl E, Fan Q. A comparison of sevelamer and calcium-based phosphate binders on mortality, hospitalization, and morbidity in hemodialysis: a secondary analysis of the Dialysis Clinical Outcomes Revisited (DCOR) randomized trial using claims data. *Am J Kidney Dis.* 2008; **51(3)**: 445–454.

380 Cagler K, Yilmaz MI, Saglam M, Cakir E, Acikel C, Eyileten T *et al.* Short-term treatment with sevelamer increases serum Fetuin-A concentration and improves endothelial dysfunction in chronic kidney disease stage 4 patients. *Clin J Am Soc Nephrol* 2008; **3**: 61–68.

381 Garg JP, Chasan-Taber S, Blair A, Plone M, Bommer J, Raggi P *et al.* Effects of sevelamer and calcium-based phosphate binders on uric acid concentrations in patients undergoing hemodialysis: a randomized clinical trial. *Arthritis Rheum* 2005; **52**: 290–295.

382 Shantouf R, Budoff MJ, Ahmadi N, Tiano J, Flores F, Kalantar-Zadeh K. Effects of sevelamer and calcium-based phosphate binders on lipid and inflammatory markers in hemodialysis patients. *Am J Nephrol* 2008; **28**: 275–279.

383 Nikolov IG, Joki N, Maizel J, Lacour B, Drueke TB, Massy ZA. Pleiotropic effects of the non-calcium phosphate binder sevelamer. *Kidney Int* 2006; **70**: S16–S23.

384 Delmez J, Block G, Robertson J, Chasan-Taber S, Blair A, Dillon M *et al.* A randomized, double-blind, crossover design study of sevelamer hydrochloride and sevelamer carbonate in patients on hemodialysis. *Clin Nephrol* 2007; **68**: 386–391.

385 Fischer D, Cline K, Plone MA, Dillon M, Burke SK, Blair AT. Results of a randomized crossover study comparing once-daily and thrice-daily sevelamer dosing. *Am J Kidney Dis* 2006; **48(3)**: 437–444.

386 Wanner C, Krane V, März W, Olschewski M, Mann JF, Ruf G *et al.* Atorvastatin in patients with type 2 diabetes mellitus undergoing hemodialysis. *N Engl J Med* 2005; **353(3)**: 238–248.

387 Strippoli GF, Navaneethan SD, Johnson DW, Perkovic V, Pellegrini F, Nicolucci A *et al.* Effects of statins in patients with chronic kidney disease: meta-analysis and meta-regression of randomised controlled trials. *BMJ* 2008; **336(7645)**: 645–651.

388 Al-Hwiesh A. Calciphylaxis of both proximal and distal distribution. *Saudi J Kidney Dis Transpl* 2008; **19(1)**: 82–86.

389 Borzecki AM, Lee A, Wang SW, Brenner L, Kazis LE. Survival in end stage renal disease: calcium carbonate vs. sevelamer. *J Clin Pharm Ther* 2007; **32(6)**: 617–624.

390 Rumberger JA, Brundage BH, Rader DJ *et al.* Electron beam computed tomographic coronary calcium scanning: a review and guidelines for use in asymptomatic persons. *Mayo Clin Proc* 1999; **74**: 243–252.

391 Greenland P, Bonow RO, Brundage BH, Budoff MJ, Eisenberg MJ, Grundy SM *et al.* ACCF/AHA 2007 clinical expert consensus document on coronary artery calcium scoring by computed tomography in global cardiovascular risk assessment and in evaluation of patients with chest pain: a report of the American College of Cardiology Foundation Clinical Expert Consensus Task Force (ACCF/AHA Writing Committee to Update the 2000 Expert Consensus Document on Electron Beam Computed Tomography) developed in collaboration with the Society of Atherosclerosis Imaging and Prevention and the Society of Cardiovascular Computed Tomography. *J Am Coll Cardiol* 2007; **49(3):** 378–402.

392 Bellasi A, Raggi P. Techniques and technologies to assess vascular calcification. *Semin Dial* 2007; **20(2):** 129–133.

393 Moe SM, O'Neill KD, Fineberg N, Persohn S, Ahmed S, Garrett P *et al.* Assessment of vascular calcification in ESRD patients using spiral CT. *Nephrol Dial Transplant* 2003; **18:** 1152–1158.

394 Raggi P, Shaw LJ. Epidemiologic guidance with coronary artery calcium scoring. *Curr Cardiol Rep* 2008; **10(1):** 60–66.

395 Bellasi A, Lacey C, Taylor AJ, Raggi P, Wilson PW, Budoff MJ *et al.* Comparison of prognostic usefulness of coronary artery calcium in men versus women (results from a meta- and pooled analysis estimating all-cause mortality and coronary heart disease death or myocardial infarction). *Am J Cardiol* 2007; **100(3):** 409–414.

396 Blacher J, Guerin AP, Pannier B *et al.* Arterial calcifications, arterial stiffness, and cardiovascular risk in end-stage renal disease. *Hypertension* 2001; **38:** 938–942.

397 Blacher J, Guerin AP, Pannier B *et al.* Impact of aortic stiffness on survival in end-stage renal disease. *Circulation* 1999; **99:** 2434–2439.

398 Budoff MJ, Shaw LJ, Liu ST, Weinstein SR, Mosler TP, Tseng PH *et al.* Long-term prognosis associated with coronary calcification: observations from a registry of 25,253 patients. *J Am Coll Cardiol* 2007; **49(18):** 1860–1870.

399 Goodman W, London G, Amman K *et al.* Vascular calcification in chronic kidney disease. *Am J Kidney Dis* 2004; **43(3):** 572–579.

400 Raggi P, Bellasi A, Ferramosca E, Islam T, Muntner P, Block GA. Association of pulse wave velocity with vascular and valvular calcification in hemodialysis patients. *Kidney Int* 2007; **71(8):** 802–807.

401 Raggi P, Giachelli C, Bellasi A. Interaction of vascular and bone disease in patients with normal renal function and patients undergoing dialysis. *Nat Clin Pract Cardiovasc Med* 2007; **4(1):** 26–33.

402 Shaw LJ, Raggi P, Schisterman E, Berman DS, Callister TQ. Prognostic value of cardiac risk factors and coronary artery calcium screening for all-cause mortality. *Radiology* 2003; **228(3):** 826–833.

403 Wang AY, Wang M, Woo J *et al.* Cardiac valve calcification as an important predictor for all-cause mortality and cardiovascular mortality in long-term peritoneal dialysis patients: a prospective study. *J Am Soc Nephrol* 2003; **14:** 159–168.

404 Adragao T, Pires A, Lucas C, Birne R, Magalhaes L, Gonçalves M *et al.* A simple vascular calcification score predicts cardiovascular risk in haemodialysis patients. *Nephrol Dial Transplant* 2004; **19(6):** 1480–1488.

405 Bellasi A, Ferramosca E, Muntner P, Ratti C, Wildman RP, Block GA *et al.* Correlation of simple imaging tests and coronary artery calcium measured by computed tomography in hemodialysis patients. *Kidney Int* 2006; **70(9):** 1623–1628.

406 Muntner P, Ferramosca E, Bellasi A, Block GA, Raggi P. Development of a cardiovascular calcification index using simple imaging tools in haemodialysis patients. *Nephrol Dial Transplant* 2007; **22(2):** 508–514.

407 Burke SK, Dillon MA, Hemken DE, Rezabek MS, Balwit JM. Meta-analysis of the effect of sevelamer on phosphorus, calcium, PTH, and serum lipids in dialysis patients. *Adv Ren Replace Ther* 2003; **10(2):** 133–145.

408 Nadin C. Sevelamer as a phosphate binder in adult hemodialysis patients: an evidence-based review of its therapeutic value. *Core Evidence* 2005; **1(1):** 43–63.

409 Tonelli M, Wiebe N, Culleton B, Lee H, Klarenbach S, Shrive F *et al.* Systematic review of the clinical efficacy and safety of sevelamer in dialysis patients. *Nephrol Dial Transplant* 2007; **22:** 2856–2866.

410 Manns B, Stevens L, Miskulin D, Owen WF, Jr., Winkelmayer WC, Tonelli M. A systematic review of sevelamer in ESRD and an analysis of its potential economic impact in Canada and the United States. *Kidney Int* 2004; **66(3):** 1239–1247.

411 Sadek T, Mazouz H, Bahloul H, Oprisiu R, El Esper N, El Esper I *et al.* Sevelamer hydrochloride with or without alphacalcidol or higher dialysate calcium vs calcium carbonate in dialysis patients: An open-label, randomized study. *Nephrol Dial Transplant* 2002; **8:** 582–588.

412 Shaheen FA, Akeel NM, Badawi LS, Souqiyyeh MZ. Efficacy and safety of sevelamer: comparison with calcium carbonate in the treatment of hyperposphatemia in hemodialysis patients. *Saudi Med J* 2004; **25(6):** 785–791.

413 Frazao JM. Treatment of hyperphosphataemia with sevelamer hydrochloride in dialysis patients: is there a survival advantage? A close look into a meta-analysis. *Port J Nephrol Hypertens* 2008; **22:** 165–167.

414 Björkman MP, Sorva AJ, Tilvis RS. Elevated serum parathyroid hormone predicts impaired survival prognosis in a general aged population. *Eur J Endocrinol* 2008; **158(5):** 749–753.

415 Kamycheva E, Sundsfjord J, Jorde R. Serum parathyroid hormone levels predict coronary heart disease: the Tromsø Study. *Eur J Cardiovasc Prev Rehabil.* 2004;**11(1):** 69–74.

416 Saleh F, Jorde R, Svartberg J, Sundsfjord J. The relationship between blood pressure and serum parathyroid hormone with special reference to urinary calcium excretion: the Tromsø Study. *J Endocrinol Invest* 2006; **29:** 214–220.

417 Sambrook PN, Chen JS, March LM, Cameron ID, Gummin RG, Lord SR *et al.* Serum parathyroid hormone is associated with increased mortality independent of 25-hydroxy vitamin D status, bone mass, and renal function in the frail and very old: a cohort study. *J Clin Endocrinol Metab* 2004; **89:** 5477–5481.

418 Øgard CG, Engholm G, Almdal TP, Vestergaard H. Increased mortality in patients hospitalized with primary hyperparathyroidism during the period 1977-1993 in Denmark. *World J Surg* 2004; **28(1):** 108–111.

419 Hedbäck G, Odén A. Increased risk of death from primary hyperparathyroidism: an update. *Eur J Clin Invest* 1998; **28(4):** 271–276.

420 Kiernan TJ, O'Flynn AM, McDermott JH, Kearney P. Primary hyperparathyroidism and the cardiovascular system. *Int J Cardiol* 2006; **113:** e89–e92.

421 Perrier ND. Impact of 25 hydroxyvitamin D deficiency in perioperative parathyroid hormone kinetics and results in patients with primary hyperparathyroidism. *Surgery* 2007; **142(6):** 1027–1029.

422 Nilsson IL, Wadsten C, Brandt L, Rastad J, Ekbom A. Mortality in sporadic primary hyperparathyroidism: nationwide cohort study of multiple parathyroid gland disease. *Surgery* 2004; **136(5):** 981–987.

423 Nilsson IL, Aberg J, Rastad J, Lind L. Maintained normalization of cardiovascular dysfunction 5 years after parathyroidectomy in primary hyperparathyroidism. *Surgery* 2005; **137(6):** 632–638.

424 Sheldon DG, Lee FT, Neil NJ, Ryan JA, Jr. Surgical treatment of hyperparathyroidism improves health-related quality of life. *Arch Surg* 2002; **137(9)**: 1022–1026.

425 Palazzo FF, Sadler GP. Minimally invasive parathyroidectomy. *Br Med J* 2004; **328(7444)**: 849–850.

426 Sejean K, Calmus S, Durand-Zaleski I, Bonnichon P, Thomopoulos P, Cormier C *et al.* Surgery versus medical follow-up in patients with asymptomatic primary hyperparathyroidism: a decision analysis. *Eur J Endocrinol* 2005; **153(6)**: 915–927.

427 Foley RN, Li S, Liu J, Gilbertson DT, Chen SC, Collins AJ. The fall and rise of parathyroidectomy in U.S. hemodialysis patients, 1992 to 2002. *J Am Soc Nephrol* 2005; **16(1)**: 210–218.

428 Trombetti A, Stoermann C, Robert JH, Herrmann FR, Pennisi P, Martin PY *et al.* Survival after parathyroidectomy in patients with end-stage renal disease and severe hyperparathyroidism. *World J Surg* 2007; **31(5)**: 1014–1021.

429 Slinin Y, Foley RN, Collins AJ. Clinical epidemiology of parathyroidectomy in hemodialysis patients: the USRDS Waves 1, 3, and 4 study. *Hemodialysis Int* 2007; **11**: 62–71.

430 Kestenbaum B, Andress DL, Schwartz SM, Gillen DL, Seliger SL, Jadav PR *et al.* Survival following parathyroidectomy among United States dialysis patients. *Kidney Int* 2004; **66**: 2010–2016.

431 Coen G, Calabria S, Bellinghieri G, Pecchini F, Conte F, Chiappini MG *et al.* Parathyroidectomy in chronic renal failure: short- and long-term results on parathyroid function, blood pressure and anemia. *Nephron* 2001; **88(2)**: 149–155.

432 Rudser KD, de Boer IH, Dooley A, Young B, Kestenbaum B. Fracture risk after parathyroidectomy among chronic hemodialysis patients. *J Am Soc Nephrol* 2007; **18(8)**: 2401–2407.

433 Danese MD, Kim J, Doan QV, Dylan M, Griffiths R, Chertow GM. PTH and the risks for hip, vertebral, and pelvic fractures among patients on dialysis. *Am J Kidney Dis* 2006; **47(1)**: 149–156.

434 Evenepoel P, Claes K, Kuypers D, Maes B, Vanrenterghem Y. Impact of parathyroidectomy on renal graft function, blood pressure and serum lipids in kidney transplant recipients: a single centre study. *Nephrol Dial Transplant* 2005; **20(8)**: 1714–1720.

435 Andress DL. Adynamic bone in patients with chronic kidney disease. *Kidney Int* 2008; **73(12)**: 1345–1354.

436 Avram MM, Mittman N, Myint MM, Fein P. Importance of low serum intact parathyroid hormone as a predictor of mortality in hemodialysis and peritoneal dialysis patients: 14 years of prospective observation. *Am J Kidney Dis* 2001; **38**: 1351–1357.

437 Matsubara K, Suliman ME, Qureshi AR, Axelsson J, Martola L, Heimbürger O *et al.* Bone mineral density in end-stage renal disease patients: association with wasting, cardiovascular disease and mortality. *Blood Purif* 2008; **26(3)**: 284–290.

438 Gagné ER, Ureña P, Leite-Silva S, Zingraff J, Chevalier A, Sarfati E *et al.* Short- and long-term efficacy of total parathyroidectomy with immediate autografting compared with subtotal parathyroidectomy in hemodialysis patients. *J Am Soc Nephrol* 1992; **3(4)**: 1008–1017.

439 Lorenz K, Ukkat J, Sekulla C, Gimm O, Brauckhoff M, Dralle H. Total parathyroidectomy without autotransplantation for renal hyperparathyroidism: experience with a qPTH-controlled protocol. *World J Surg* 2006; **30(5)**: 743–751.

440 Rothmund M, Wagner PK, Schark C. Subtotal parathyroidectomy versus total parathyroidectomy and autotransplantation in secondary hyperparathyroidism: a randomized trial. *World J Surg* 1991; **15(6)**: 745–750.

441 Mazzaferro S, Chicca S, Pasquali M, Zaraca F, Ballanti P, Taggi F *et al.* Changes in bone turnover after parathyroidectomy in dialysis patients: role of calcitriol administration. *Nephrol Dial Transplant* 2000; **15(6)**: 877–882.

442 Nichols P, Owen JP, Ellis HA, Farndon JR, Kelly PJ, Ward MK. Parathyroidectomy in chronic renal failure: a nine-year follow-up study. *Q J Med* 1990; **77**: 1175–1193.

443 Almqvist EG, Becker C, Bondeson AG, Bondeson L, Svensson J. Early parathyroidectomy increases bone mineral density in patients with mild primary hyperparathyroidism: a prospective and randomized study. *Surgery* 2004; **136(6)**: 1281–1288.

444 Reichel H. Current treatment options in secondary renal hyperparathyroidism: a critical review. *Nephrol Dial Transplant* 2006; **21**: 23–28.

445 Chertow GM, Blumenthal S, Turner S, Roppolo M, Stern L, Chi EM *et al.* Cinacalcet hydrochloride (Sensipar) in hemodialysis patients on active vitamin D derivatives with controlled PTH and elevated calcium X phosphate. *Clin J Am Soc Nephrol* 2006; **1**: 305–312.

446 Moe SM, Chertow GM, Coburn JW, Quarles LD, Goodman WG, Block GA *et al.* Achieving NKF-K/DOQI bone metabolism and disease treatment goals with cinacalcet HCl. *Kidney Int* 2005; **76**: 760–771.

447 Lindberg JS, Culleton B, Wong G, Borah MF, Clark RV, Shapiro WB *et al.* Cinacalcet HCl, an oral calcimimetic agent for the treatment of secondary hyperparathyroidism in hemodialysis and peritoneal dialysis: a randomized, double-blind, multicenter study. *J Am Soc Nephrol* 2005; **16(3)**: 800–807.

448 Lien YH, Silva AL, Whittman D. Effects of cinacalcet on bone mineral density in patients with secondary hyperparathyroidism. *Nephrol Dial Transplant* 2005; **20(6)**: 1232–1237.

449 Charytan C, Coburn J, Chonchol M, Herman J, Lien YH, Liu W *et al.* Cinacalcet hydrochloride is an effective treatment for secondary hyperparathyroidism in patients with CKD not receiving dialysis. *Am J Kidney Dis* 2005; **46(1)**: 58–67.

450 Messa P, Macário F, Yaqoob M, Bouman K, Braun J, von Albertini B *et al.* The OPTIMA study: assessing a new cinacalcet (Sensipar/Mimpara) treatment algorithm for secondary hyperparathyroidism. *Clin J Am Soc Nephrol* 2008; **3(1)**: 36–45.

451 Sterrett JR, Strom J, Stummvoll HK, Bahner U, Disney A, Soroka SD *et al.* Cinacalcet HCI (Sensipar/Mimpara) is an effective chronic therapy for hemodialysis patients with secondary hyperparathyroidism. *Clin Nephrol* 2007; **68(1)**: 10–17.

452 Block GA, Zeig S, Sugihara J, Chertow GM, Chi EM, Turner SA *et al.* Combined therapy with cinacalcet and low doses of vitamin D sterols in patients with moderate to severe secondary hyperparathyroidism. *Nephrol Dial Transplant* 2008; **23**: 1–8.

453 Chertow GM, Pupim LB, Block GA, Correa-Rotter R, Drueke TB, Floege J *et al.* Evaluation of Cinacalcet Therapy to Lower Cardiovascular Events (EVOLVE): rationale and design overview. *Clin J Am Soc Nephrol* 2007; **2(5)**: 898–905.

454 Cunningham J, Danese M, Olson K, Klassen P, Chertow GM. Effects of the calcimimetic cinacalcet HCl on cardiovascular disease, fracture, and health-related quality of life in secondary hyperparathyroidism. *Kidney Int* 2005; **68**: 1793–1800.

455 Strippoli GF, Palmer S, Tong A, Elder G, Messa P, Craig JC. Meta-analysis of biochemical and patient-level effects of calcimimetic therapy. *Am J Kidney Dis* 2006; **47(5)**: 715–726.

456 Strippoli GF, Tong A, Palmer SC, Elder G, Craig JC. Calcimimetics for secondary hyperparathyroidism in chronic kidney disease patients. *Cochrane Database Syst Rev* 2006; **4**: CD006254.

457 Garside R, Pitt M, Anderson R, Mealing S, Roome C, Snaith A *et al.* The effectiveness and cost-effectiveness of cinacalcet for secondary hyperparathyroidism in end-stage renal disease patients on dialysis: a systematic review and economic evaluation. *Health Technol Assess* 2007; **11(18):** iii, xi–xiii, 1–167.

458 Rodan GA, Fleisch HA. Bisphosphonates: mechanism of action. *J Clin Invest* 1996; **97(12):** 2692–2696.

459 Saha H, Castren-Kortekangas P, Ojanen S, Juhakoski A, Tuominen J, Tokola O, Pasternack A. Pharmacokinetics of clodronate in renal failure. *J Bone Miner Res* 1994; **9(12):** 1953–1958.

460 Barone A, Giusti A, Pioli G, Girasole G, Razzano M, Pizzonia M *et al.* Secondary hyperparathyroidism due to hypovitaminosis D affects bone mineral density response to alendronate in elderly women with osteoporosis: a randomized controlled trial. *J Am Geriatr Soc* 2007; **55(5):** 752–757.

461 Klawansky S, Komaroff E, Cavanaugh PF, Jr., Mitchell DY, Gordon MJ, Connelly JE *et al.* Relationship between age, renal function and bone mineral density in the US population. *Osteoporos Int* 2003; **14:** 570–576.

462 Weisinger JR, Bellorin-Font E. Postmenopausal osteoporosis in the dialysis patient. *Curr Opin Nephrol Hypertens* 2003; **12(4):** 381–386.

463 Ensrud KE, Lui LY, Taylor BC, Ishani A, Shlipak MG, Stone KL *et al.* Renal function and risk of hip and vertebral fractures in older women. *Arch Intern Med* 2007; **167:** 133–139.

464 Alem AM, Sherrard DJ, Gillen DL, Weiss NS, Beresford SA, Heckbert SR *et al.* Increased risk of hip fracture among patients with end-stage renal disease. *Kidney Int* 2000; **58(1):** 396–399.

465 Stehman-Breen C. Risk of hip fracture among dialysis and renal transplant recipients. *JAMA* 2002; **288(23):** 3014–3018.

466 Cunningham J, Sprague SM, Cannata-Andia J, Coco M, Cohen-Solal M, Fitzpatrick L *et al.* Osteoporosis in chronic kidney disease. *Am J Kidney Dis* 2004; **43(3):** 566–571.

467 Domrongkitchaiporn S, Pongsakul C, Stitchantrakul W, Sirikulchayanonta V, Ongphiphadhanakul B, Radinahamed P *et al.* Bone mineral density and histology in distal renal tubular acidosis. *Kidney Int* 2001; **59:** 1086–1093.

468 Odvina CV, Zerwekh JE, Rao DS, Maalouf N, Gottschalk FA, Pak CY. Severely suppressed bone turnover: a potential complication of alendronate therapy. *J Clin Endocrinol Metab* 2005; **90(3):** 1294–1301.

469 Miller PD, Roux C, Boonen S, Barton IP, Dunlap LE, Burgio DE. Safety and efficacy of Risedronate in patients with age-related reduced renal function as estimated by the Cockcroft and Gault method: a pooled analysis of nine clinical trials. *J Bone Miner Res* 2005; **20:** 2105–2115.

470 Miller P, Schwartz E, Chen P, Misurski A, Krege J. Teriparatide in postmenopausal women with osteoporosis and mild or moderate renal impairment. *Ostoeporosis Int* 2007; **18:** 59–68.

471 Jamal SA, Bauer DC, Ensrud KE, Cauley JA, Hochberg M, Ishani A *et al.* Alendronate treatment in women with normal to severely impaired renal function: an analysis of the fracture intervention trial. *J Bone Miner Res* 2007; **22(4):** 503–508.

472 Hansen KE, Hofmann RM, Drake RK, Argall TR, Bier HA, Grigg KT *et al.* An exploratory analysis of alendronate in older men with low glomerular filtration rate. *J Aging Pharmacother* 2006; **13:** 21–44.

473 Nitta K, Akiba T, Suzuki K, Uchida K, Watanabe RI, Majima K *et al.* Effects of cyclic intermittent etidronate therapy on coronary artery calcification in patients receiving long-term hemodialysis. *Am J Kidney Dis* 2004; **44:** 680–688.

474 Aryoshi T, Eishi K, Sakamoto I, Matsukuma S, Odate T. Effect of etidronic acid on arterial calcification in dialysis patients. *Clin Drug Invest* 2006; **26:** 215–222.

475 Markowitz GS, Appel GB, Fine PL, Fenves AZ, Loon NR, Jagannath S *et al.* Collapsing focal segmental glomerulosclerosis following treatment with high-dose pamidronate. *J Am Soc Nephrol* 2001; **12(6):** 1164–1172.

476 Mitterbauer C. Schwartz C, Haas M, Oberbauer R. Effects of bisphosphonates on bone loss in the first year after renal transplantation-a meta-analysis of randomized controlled trials. *Nephrol Dial Transplant* 2006; **21(8):** 2275–2281.

477 Palmer SC, McGregor DO, Strippoli GF. Interventions for preventing bone disease in kidney transplant recipients. *Cochrane Database Syst Rev* 2007; **3:** CD005015.

478 Schwarz C, Mitterbauer C, Heinze G, Woloszczuk W, Haas M, Oberbauer R. Nonsustained effect of short-term bisphosphonate therapy on bone turnover three years after renal transplantation. *Kidney Int* 2004; **65(1):** 304–309.

479 Coco M, Glicklich D, Faugere MC, Burris L, Bognar I, Durkin P *et al.* Prevention of bone loss in renal transplant recipients: a prospective, randomized trial of intravenous pamidronate. *J Am Soc Nephrol* 2003; **14(10):** 2669–2676.

480 Grotz W, Nagel C, Poeschel D, Cybulla M, Petersen KG, Uhl M *et al.* Effect of ibandronate on bone loss and renal function after kidney transplantation. *J Am Soc Nephrol* 2001; **12(7):** 1530–1537.

481 Jamal SA, Gilbert J, Gordon C, Bauer DC. Trabecular density vs cortical density in fracture prediction in HD patients. *J Bone Miner Res* 2006; **21:** 543–548.

482 Grabe DW, Chan M, Eisele G. Open-label pilot study compariing quantitative ultrasound and dual-energy X-ray absorptiometry to assess corticosteroid-induced osteoporosis in patients with chronic kidney disease. *Clin Ther* 2006; **28:** 255–263.

35 Preparation for Dialysis

Mark G. Parker[1] & Jonathan Himmelfarb[2]

[1] Maine Medical Center, Portland, ME, USA
[2] University of Washington, Seatle, WA, USA

Proper preparation of chronic kidney disease (CKD) patients for renal replacement therapy is a multidisciplinary process orchestrated by the nephrologist. The National Kidney Foundation Kidney Disease Outcomes Quality Initiative (K/DOQI) guidelines state "preparation for kidney replacement therapy" as the principle clinical action of stage 4 (glomerular filtration rate, 15–29 mL/min/1.73 m^2) of CKD [1]. Current prevalence estimates suggest that this group comprises 400,000 individuals in the adult population in the USA [2]. Over 8 million people are thought to have stage III CKD or worse. Indeed, many nephrologists introduce discussions of replacement therapy preparation in the latter portions of stage III CKD in concert with ongoing care directed at ameliorating the metabolic derangements of declining renal function. Strategies for slowing renal disease progression and treating complications of CKD, such as hypervolemia, hyperkalemia, metabolic acidosis, renal osteodystrophy, hypertension, and anemia, are explored in detail in chapters 30 to 34. The subsequent discussion focuses on the approach to dialysis modality selection and preparation for specific modalities.

Timeliness of nephrology referral and outcomes

A significant body of literature has emerged over the past decade pertaining to the timing of referral of the CKD patient to a nephrologist and its impact on outcomes. The importance of timely referral may be related to intensified progression delay strategies and expert treatment of CKD complications but has been studied more specifically in relation to adequate preparation for renal replacement therapy.

The earliest study of the impact of timing of referral on outcome was performed on a small patient cohort over 20 years ago [3] in Oxford, England. Fifty-five patients who started maintenance dialysis in 1981 were divided into two groups: those meeting the nephrologist less than 1 month before initiation of renal replacement therapy (late referral), and all others (early referral). All dialysis was initiated in acute hospital care. The primary outcome was severe complications protracting hospital stay. Sixteen of 23 patients (70%) in the late referral group fulfilled the outcome definition, as opposed to only 3 members (9%) of the early referral group.

Little was published on this topic again until a series of articles appeared beginning in the late 1990s. The majority of these studies followed patients prospectively from the time of entry into dialysis but relied on retrospective record review and patient recall to characterize the nature of each individual's pre-end-state renal disease (ESRD) care. The principle outcomes reported were mortality or, in the case of incident hemodialysis patients, type and timing of permanent vascular access use. A single-center study from the UK [4] of 198 patients reported shorter hospital stays upon initiation of dialysis (median hospital days, 9.7 vs. 25 for patients referred >3 months prior to the start of dialysis compared to those referred later) but did not demonstrate a survival benefit. This study may not have been adequately powered with regard to mortality. Cohorts studied from much larger databases have repeatedly demonstrated a survival disadvantage for late referral, however [5–8].

The Choices for Healthy Outcomes in Caring for End-Stage Renal Disease (CHOICE) investigators studied a cohort of over 800 patients at 81 centers from 1995 to 1998 [6], 25% initiating with peritoneal dialysis and 75% starting with hemodialysis. Patients were characterized by time of nephrology referral as >12 months (early), 4–12 months (intermediate), and <4 months (late). Thirty percent of patients were referred late. First-year mortality in the three groups was 4.3, 9.5, and 13.3%, and separation in mortality in the three groups persisted through 3 years of follow-up (Figure 35.1). A graded increase in hazard ratio persisted after adjustment for comorbidities and demographics. In this US study, late referral patients were more likely to be black, uninsured, and have a greater burden of comorbidity. A similar gradation of worsening mortality from early through intermediate to late referral was reported in EPIREL, a multicenter study in Lorraine, a metropolitan administrative region of France [5]. With early referral patients as the reference group, the odds ratio for death within 90 days

Evidence-based Nephrology. Edited by Donald Molony and Jonathan Craig
© 2009 Blackwell Publishing, ISBN: 978-1-4051-3975-5.

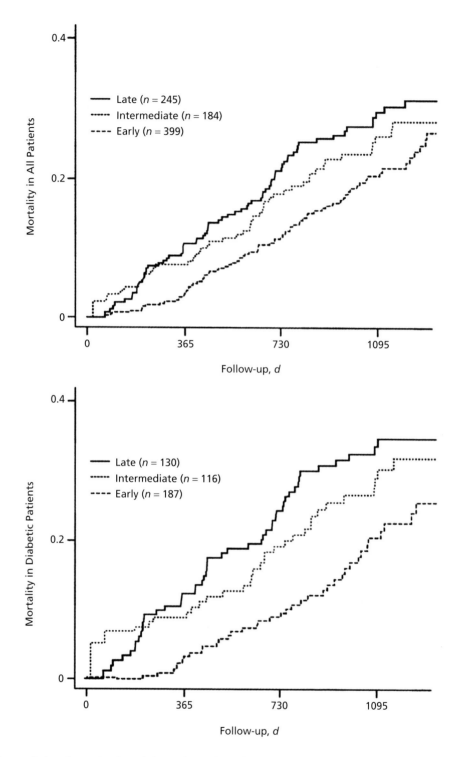

Figure 35.1 Cumulative mortality in patients undergoing early, intermediate, or late evaluation by a nephrologist. (Reprinted with permission from reference 6.)

of initiation of dialysis was 2.7 in the intermediate group and 4.9 in the late referral group. The EPIREL investigators also reported "emergency" first dialysis and temporary vascular access catheter use for first dialysis in over 80% of late referrals, compared with approximately 30% of the early referral patients. Stack [7] reported on the Dialysis Morbidity and Mortality Study (DMMS) Wave 2 patient cohort, demonstrating an adjusted relative risk of death for late referral (<4 months before dialysis initiation) versus early referral of 1.68 at 1 year into ESRD and 1.23 at 2 years. He also found that late referral patients were more likely to be black or Hispanic, less frequently had permanent vascular access, and had poorer metabolic and nutritional characteristics at entry into dialysis. The largest cohort study of this type utilized claims data from the Centers for Medicare & Medicaid Services (CMS) database and was a retrospective assessment of 109,321 Medicare-eligible patients (>66 years old) entering dialysis in the USA from 1995 to 1998 [8]. Pre-ESRD care was characterized by duration and frequency of nephrology contact. Of these patients, 50% had no nephrology specialist care prior to dialysis initiation and 37% had their first nephrology visit within 6 months prior to ESRD. Overall first-year mortality was 36%, and the adjusted hazards ratio was greatest, 1.51, for the group with no significant pre-ESRD nephrology contact.

Several investigators have focused on the timing and type of vascular access for hemodialysis as the principle outcome measure of referral timing studies. Clearly, catheter use is associated with increased morbidity and mortality [9,10]. Late referral patients are more likely to initiate dialysis with a vascular access catheter. The CHOICE investigators demonstrated this finding in the subgroup of their study patients who initiated hemodialysis therapy [11]. Only 10% of patients referred <1 month prior to ESRD initiated with an arteriovenous access, as opposed to 30% of patients referred between 1 and 12 months and 46% referred at >12 months. The median duration of catheter use was 202 days in the late referral group compared to 57 days for those requiring catheters in the earliest referral group. Early referral patients were far more likely to have an arteriovenous access in use within the first 6 months of dialysis than the latest referrals (82% vs. 56%). Similar findings were reported previously in a smaller cohort from the New England Medical Center [12]. These investigators also noted that patients from health maintenance organizations had a 4.5 times greater odds of being referred late compared to Medicare patients. This observation may have been unique to the regional practice patterns of the era (1992–1997), however.

A lingering uncertainty of the foregoing studies is the possibility that late referral is not an independent variable that influences outcome; rather, late referral is merely a surrogate for poor access to health care in general. Winkelmayer et al. [13] have attempted to address this through propensity analysis, a scoring system that attempts to discern the expected probability of receiving a treatment based on a patient's baseline characteristics. Studying a group of over 3000 New Jersey Medicare and Medicaid patients incident to dialysis from 1991 to 1996, these investigators concluded that

overall mortality was indeed markedly higher in the late referral group, but the effect appeared to be limited to the first 3 months after initiation of dialysis.

The economic implications of late referral were assessed by McLaughlin et al. using decision analytic modeling with a simulated cohort of 1000 typical incident dialysis patients [14]. Allowing fixed assumptions about rates of CKD progression, hospitalization, initiation of dialysis, modality switching, and death, the model predicted a 20.3% cost savings over a 5-year period for early referral compared to late referral.

Modality selection

Counseling CKD patients about renal replacement therapy options for ESRD is a distinct educational process. Patients in late stage 3 and stage 4 CKD should be instructed about a range of potential options, including home and in-center dialysis modalities, transplantation, and in appropriate cases, withholding of renal replacement therapy. It is particularly important to note that there is an allograft survival advantage when kidney transplantation is performed preemptively, that is, without previous initiation of dialysis [15]. Moreover, early consideration of transplantation is of prime importance for diabetic patients, who stand to gain a substantial survival benefit compared to long-term dialysis therapy [16,17]. Preparation for transplantation is addressed elsewhere in this textbook. Unless there is absolute certainty about a patient's prospect for preemptive live donor kidney transplantation, it is preferable to provide dialysis preparation in parallel with or as an alternative to transplantation evaluation.

A small body of literature has evolved on the value of pre-ESRD patient education and subsequent outcomes. Some of this work has focused on specific predialysis interventional programs, while other studies have encompassed dialysis-specific education in a broader paradigm of CKD indoctrination. Two multicenter studies in Spain addressed the value of predialysis education. Gomez et al. [18] provided over 200 patients with a standard informational package that included a flip chart presentation, books, and video. Using pre- and postinformational questionnaires, these investigators demonstrated a substantial improvement in knowledge about treatment options. In particular, subjects gained knowledge about peritoneal dialysis, the modality least familiar to patients prior to the formal instruction program. Marron et al. [19] studied 621 patients from 24 centers for the effect of pre-ESRD care and patient education on the nature of dialysis initiation. They characterized initiation as either "planned" (outpatient start with the use of a permanent vascular or peritoneal access) or "unplanned" (defined as uremia requiring emergency dialysis). Although three-fourths of the patient population had received nephrology care for at least 3 months pre-ESRD, only half had received a specific educational program on dialysis modalities. Nonplanned starts occurred 49% of the time. Even patients with early nephrology referral had nonplanned entry into dialysis in 33% of cases, a somewhat startling

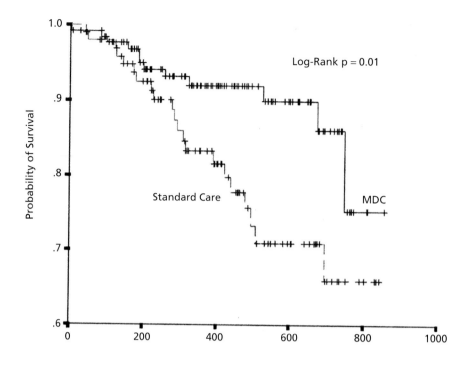

Figure 35.2 Kaplan-Meier survival curves for patients after starting chronic dialysis therapy: comparison of patients seen prior to dialysis initiation in the multidisiciplinary clinic versus standard nephrology care. (Reprinted with permission from reference 22.)

commentary on the fractured care that continues to exist in the nephrology community despite increased efforts to provide coordinated care. Among patients receiving dialysis-specific pre-ESRD education, however, a planned start happened in 73.4%. Dialysis-specific programs were also associated with a higher number of pre-ESRD visits and increased probability of choosing peritoneal dialysis as treatment modality: 31% versus 8% in the "uneducated" group.

Broader multidisciplinary educational and care team approaches, termed by some as "psychoeducational intervention" [20,21], for CKD and pre-ESRD care have been evaluated and the results have been published [20–23]. Most of these studies have originated in Canada. Such teams typically include a nephrologist, nurse educator, social worker, dietician, pharmacist, and peer support. The information that is provided is specific to ongoing CKD care and renal replacement therapy counseling when appropriate. Positive outcomes have generally been described with regard to biochemical indices, dialysis access preparation, and survival, although none of these studies was performed in a prospective, randomized, controlled fashion. A Canadian–Italian cooperative case–control study of this type, the Can-It Impact study [22], demonstrated a significant survival advantage (Figure 35.2) for incident dialysis patients who had received multidisciplinary clinic care as opposed to "standard" nephrology care.

Evidence indicates that it is prudent to educate patients and selected family or friends in a systematic manner using some combination of multidisciplinary renal team personnel. Potential dialysis

patients need information not only about the mechanics of specific dialysis modalities but also the associated features of such therapy to help make informed choices. Factors such as modality-specific dietary restrictions, travel and time commitments for in-center therapy, nature of the home environment and self-care capability for home therapy, and adaptability of a modality to particular career or recreational life-styles all play a role in the choice of therapy. Furthermore, utilizing the expertise of the extended care team to assess the suitability of an individual patient for a specific modality may help guide the nephrologist in counseling the patient.

Patients often wish to know if a specific dialysis modality conveys a beneficial health outcome advantage. A number of observational studies, both small and large in scope, have attempted to answer this question and have been inconclusive. Several studies have suggested a slight survival advantage in the first 2 years after ESRD for patients on peritoneal dialysis compared to hemodialysis [24–26]. Speculation on the reason for this result has centered on the importance of preserved residual renal function for peritoneal dialysis patients early after ESRD onset. Other investigators demonstrated no difference in mortality between the two modalities [27–29] or a lack of early outcome difference (1–2 years) followed by a relative mortality risk in favor of hemodialysis [30,31]. Still other investigators have concluded that the results vary by analytical method [32] or by stratification of patients according to risk factors [33]. In the latter example, an analysis of 398,940 US Medicare incident dialysis patients from 1995 to 2000 suggested that mortality risk favored peritoneal dialysis for nondiabetic patients in aggregate and young diabetic patients without significant comorbidity but favored hemodialysis in older diabetic patients. Outcomes were neutral among nondiabetic and diabetic patients with significant comorbidities, as well as the nondiabetic elderly.

Importance of comorbidities

The importance of comorbidity at entry into dialysis cannot be overlooked. In a Canadian multicenter observational study, Murphy *et al.* [34] concluded that apparent survival rates favoring peritoneal dialysis disappeared when adjusted for the overall lower comorbidity burden of the peritoneal dialysis cohort. Similarly, the CHOICE investigators concluded that the number and severity of comorbid conditions tended to be lower in patients choosing peritoneal dialysis in their cohort [35], again, possibly explaining mortality differences. One important comorbid condition, congestive heart failure, was specifically studied in a University of Texas analysis [36] of CMS patients entering dialysis from 1995 to 1997. The prevalence of this condition at dialysis initiation was 33%. Mortality outcome favored hemodialysis, with a relative risk of 1.3 for peritoneal dialysis patients.

Only one group of investigators [37] has attempted a randomized, controlled trial of the two dialysis modalities. Not surprisingly, the trial was stopped after only 38 patients were enrolled in 3 years due to a low participation rate of eligible subjects. A survival benefit at 5 years appeared to favor peritoneal dialysis patients, but the number of subjects was far too low to draw reliable conclusions. At present, it is reasonable to advise prospective dialysis candidates that there is not a preponderance of evidence favoring one modality over the other.

Home hemodialysis as a variation of hemodialysis delivery, particularly when provided nocturnally, has enjoyed a resurged interest in recent years in the nephrology community. Numerous reasons have been cited to consider this modality, including improved blood pressure and volume control [38,39], enhanced quality of life [40–42], cost-effective health care delivery [39,43], and possibly, a survival advantage [44–48]. The purported benefits have yet to be confirmed in a prospective, randomized comparison to in-center hemodialysis. Nonetheless, it is sensible to discuss home hemodialysis in pre-ESRD modality counseling. Most hemodialysis patients will start with in-center therapy prior to tackling the training period necessary for home therapy.

Certain comorbidities or patient characteristics may suggest a relative or absolute contraindication to a specific dialysis modality. These features are highlighted in Table 35.1. Patients should be counseled in this regard and guided towards more suitable therapy when such barriers are encountered. Patients should also understand that no care plan is completely inflexible, and modality switching can and should occur if an initial choice is deemed less than optimal by the patient and kidney care team. The initial choice of therapy, however, should be followed by a plan for vascular or peritoneal access preparation.

Table 35.1 Contraindications to specific dialysis modalities.

Hemodialysis
   Relative contraindications
      • Difficult vascular access
        – Severe peripheral arterial vascular disease
        – Central vein stenoses or occlusion
      • Desired home dialysis with lack of appropriate home environment or partner

Peritoneal dialysis
   Absolute contraindications
      • Extensive abdominal adhesions
      • Hydrothorax or diaphragmatic defects
      • Loss of peritoneal membrane function (ultrafiltration, solute clearance)

   Relative contraindications
      • Morbid obesity
      • Severe protein calorie malnutrition
      • Loss of residual renal function
      • Bowel disease
        – Ischemic
        – Chronic inflammatory
        – Diverticulosis or diverticulitis

Vascular access planning for hemodialysis

Evidence for primary arteriovenous fistula first

Vascular access remains the Achilles' heel of hemodialysis therapy. To be sure, the greatest source of complication or substandard treatment is suboptimal vascular access. The native arteriovenous fistula (AVF), either of the classic Brescia-Cimino variety [49] or of the upper arm, remains the best and most durable of the potential choices. Construction of a native fistula requires sufficient lead time for maturation. Furthermore, it has become clear that many native AVFs that fail to develop can be salvaged with aggressive monitoring and intervention [50,51]. Additional time may be needed for revision and satisfactory development. Consequently, although an excellent AVF may mature and be cannulated within 4–8 weeks of creation, the initial attempt at creation of the native AVF should occur at least 6 months before ESRD is anticipated. The maturing fistula should be examined 4–6 weeks after creation [52] and at CKD visit intervals thereafter. Evidence of insufficient development should prompt further evaluation and intervention [51].

Although there have been no specific studies dedicated to the adequacy of vein preservation for a native AVF, it has long been recommended that the nondominant arm should be avoided for needle puncture. Antecedent venous injury may impair the development or function of an AVF. Referral to an experienced surgeon is often accompanied by Doppler assessment of arm veins to select the most suitable site [53,54]. Historically, the initial choice of the AVF site has been the distal upper extremity, thereby allowing preservation of proximal sites as needed for later vascular access attempts. Although sonographic study has improved the number of successful AVF creations in general, success rates remain suboptimal in women, diabetic patients, and the elderly. Miller *et al.* [55] have advocated consideration of upper arm sites as the first choice in these groups. Salvage procedures have been useful in these patients [50,51,56]. Konnor *et al.* [57] achieved superb results, even in high-risk groups, with a combination of careful preoperative examination, ultrasonographic study, use of a variety of AVF locations, and an experienced operator. Under these conditions, primary access survival ranged from 51 to 75% (depending upon gender and diabetes status) for 2 years, and assisted access survival was 75–96% for the same period.

The preference for the native AVF is supported by abundant outcome literature over the past decade. Mortality is clearly influenced by type of vascular access in large cohorts, including the CHOICE study [58], DMMS Wave I [9], and the ESRD Network 6 [10] analysis. In all such studies using AVF patients as the reference group, mortality risk increased in a graded fashion for prosthetic arteriovenous grafts (AVG) and cuffed, tunneled catheters. The increase in mortality is largely attributable to infection. High rates of bacteremia have been described with use of tunneled catheters in particular: 5.5 episodes/1000 catheter–days were reported by Saad [59]. In his study, over 50% of bacteremias were gram-positive cocci, 26.7% were gram-negative rods, and 20.9% were polymicrobial. Endocarditis occurred in 3.5% of patients. Oliver *et al.* [60] found a graded increase in the risk of sepsis from "early" AVF creation, >4 months prior to ESRD, compared to creation 1–4 months prior to ESRD and creation <1 month prior to or after ESRD. This association was presumably due to the need to use catheters as a bridge towards a functioning AVF.

In selected patients, native AVF creation is not feasible due to unsuitability of vessels. The second choice of vascular access is the prosthetic AVG with polytetrafluoroethylene or polyethaneurea. Although these access options do not achieve the long-term durability of the native AVF, primary patency rates are comparable [61–63]. Polytetrafluoroethylene AVG are not cannulated for at least 14 days to allow tissue ingrowth into the graft, but polyethaneurea AVG can be successfully cannulated sooner [64]. Prosthetic AVG typically require repeated intervention for thromboses and stenoses after 2–3 years in order to extend access longevity. Interestingly, although native AVF use has been highly prevalent outside the USA for many years, AVG use within the USA exceeded AVF use into the late 1990s [65–67]. These reports and others spurred the 2000 NKF K/DOQI targets to be at least 50% incident and 40% prevalent native AVF use for hemodialysis patients [68]. Progress towards these goals appeared to be improving in the DOPPS II study [69], with 31% prevalent AVF use, but was still not to target. More recent developments have included the CMS Fistula First initiative [70], which touted achievement of the prevalence target in August 2005 and has extended the goal to a 66% AVF prevalence by June 2009.

Use of tunneled cuffed cannulas

When dialysis need is imminent and vascular access has not otherwise been prepared, the intervention of choice is the placement of a cuffed, tunneled central venous access catheter for hemodialysis. The internal jugular vein, ipsilateral to the dominant arm, is the preferred site. A number of investigators have demonstrated an unacceptably high incidence of subclavian vein stenosis when this vein has been used for dialysis vascular access catheters [71–74]. The subclavian vein should be avoided. Femoral vein catheters are sometimes used when internal jugular sites are not accessible, but this is uncommon in the new ESRD patient. Catheters convey the advantage of immediate use and short-term durability but carry the previously described infection risks and potential for permanent vessel injury through the development of stenoses, thrombosis, or occlusion. Use of catheters remains high even among hemodialysis patients with existing AV fistulae or grafts. Danese *et al.* [75] recently reported a catheter insertion rate of 44/100 patient–years, representing 57% of all Medicare patients incident to hemodialysis from 1996 to 2001. Reasons for catheter use included insufficient AVF maturation or revision, thrombosis, or failure of the permanent AV access.

Late stage 3 and stage 4 CKD patients who are being prepared for hemodialysis therapy are best served by timely referral for a native AVF. It should be noted that inadequate development of the AVF in the pre-ESRD patient might prompt consideration of invasive vascular access imaging to identify potential avenues for salvage, such as angioplasty or venous collateral ligation or coiling. Until recently, the field was evolving to increased use of gadolinium as the contrast agent of choice due to the increased risk of acute kidney injury with iodinated contrast exposure in advanced CKD. However, in the USA, the Food and Drug Administration has recently issued an alert [76] advising caution in the use of gadolinium, at least for CKD stage 5. Concern was prompted by reports of nephrogenic systemic fibrosis and nephrogenic fibrosing dermopathy associated with the use of this agent in patients with very low glomerular filtration rates [77]. In stage 4 CKD patients, at least, a recent report suggested that judicious use (i.e. volumes of <10 mL) of a nonionic, low-osmolarity iodinated contrast agent for fistulography was associated with only a small incidence (4.6%) of contrast-induced nephropathy [78]. None required immediate dialysis.

Peritoneal access planning for peritoneal dialysis

The timing of peritoneal catheter placement for peritoneal dialysis therapy typically occurs much closer to anticipated dialysis initiation, often at early stage 5 of CKD, than vascular access creation for hemodialysis therapy. There are no specific studies or trials published which have addressed the optimal timing of peritoneal catheter placement. Observational experience suggests that peritoneal catheters require at least 2 weeks for satisfactory healing

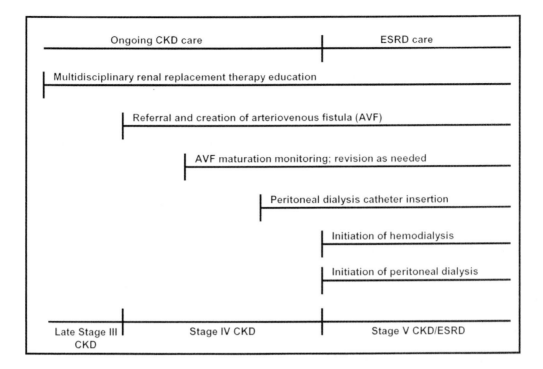

Figure 35.3 Timeline for preparation for dialysis.

and avoidance of peritoneal fluid leakage. They are occasionally used sooner in select circumstances. Nonetheless, referral for evaluation and placement of peritoneal catheters should be done in a fashion that avoids precipitous need to start dialysis and minimizes infection risks.

A variety of catheter types are potentially available, as reviewed elsewhere in this textbook. The most commonly used catheters are made of silicone rubber or polyurethane. A dual-cuffed silicone rubber catheter, the Tenckhoff catheter, is most frequently used. Double-cuffed catheters have been reported to have better longevity and reduced infection risks in several studies [79–82]. However, this was not corroborated in a prospective, randomized, controlled trial of single-cuff versus double-cuff Tenckhoff catheters [83]. Local practice expertise probably is the best benchmark of catheter choice and insertion technique.

Exit site infections and peritonitis have the greatest influence on catheter longevity, and therefore, impact longitudinal success of peritoneal dialysis in general. Successful measures to reduce the incidence of infection at the time of insertion and in the early postoperative period include perioperative antibiotic use [84–86] and immobilization of the external portion of the catheter in an undisturbed fashion (i.e. minimal dressing changes) during the first 1–2 weeks after surgery [87]. Moncrief *et al.* [88] introduced a technique for burying the exterior portion of the catheter subcutaneously for the first 3–5 weeks after surgery, followed by exteriorization. Peritonitis rates appeared to be reduced with this technique compared to historical controls [89]. A subsequent prospective, randomized study [90] of 60 incident peritoneal dialysis patients

did not confirm an advantage for this technique over traditional catheter placement, however. Neither exit site infection nor peritonitis rates differed during the first 24 months of dialysis.

Peritoneal dialysis training by appropriate dialysis personnel usually occurs commensurate with the need to initiate and maintain chronic dialysis therapy. In most circumstances, patients can be taught basic techniques for manual dialysate exchanges within a few days, and subsequent consideration of cycler therapy is tailored to individual situations as detailed in chapters 43–45.

Summary

Successful preparation of the CKD patient for dialysis requires early involvement of the nephrologist. A timeline for subsequent pre-ESRD interventions is summarized in Figure 35.3. Multidisciplinary assessment and education by the kidney care team allows psychological adjustment and an informed modality choice to be made by the patient with the enhanced potential for positive ESRD outcomes. Timely referral for vascular access preparation for potential hemodialysis patients is essential to increase the likelihood of successful creation and maturation of a native AVF. Vascular access catheters are to be avoided, if at all possible, due to a clear association with increased ESRD morbidity and mortality, although there continues to be a subset of patients who require this form of access due to a precipitous need for dialysis or inadequate arteriovenous access. Peritoneal access planning and intervention fall later in the CKD timeline, with greater proximity to ESRD. However, this form of dialysis preparation is also dependent upon appropriate timing and technique considerations in order to maximize the potential for successful ESRD outcomes. Systematic renal replacement therapy planning has been convincingly demonstrated to influence ESRD morbidity and mortality and is the key to a successful transition from CKD to ESRD.

References

1 National Kidney Foundation. *K/DOQI Clinical Practice Guidelines for Chronic Kidney Disease: Executive Summary.* National Kidney Foundation, New York, 2002.

2 Coresh J, Astor BC, Greene T, Eknoyan G, Levey AS. Prevalence of chronic kidney disease and decreased kidney function in the adult US population. Third National Health and Nutrition Examination Survey. *Am J Kidney Dis* 2003; **41:** 1–12.

3 Ratcliffe PJ, Phillips RE, Oliver DO. Late referral for maintenance dialysis. *Br Med J* (Clin Res Ed) 1984; **288:** 441–443.

4 Ellis PA, Reddy V, Bari N, Cairns HS. Late referral of end-stage renal failure. *QJM* 1998; **91:** 727–732.

5 Kessler M, Frimat L, Panescu V, Briancon S. Impact of nephrology referral on early and midterm outcomes in ESRD. EPidemiologie de l'Insuffisance REnale chronique terminale en Lorraine (EPIREL): results of a 2-year, prospective, community-based study. *Am J Kidney Dis* 2003; **42:** 474–485.

6 Kinchen KS, Sadler J, Fink N, Brookmeyer R, Klag MG, Levey AS et al. The timing of specialist evaluation in chronic kidney disease and mortality. *Ann Intern Med* 2002; **137:** 479–486.

7 Stack AG. Impact of timing of nephrology referral and pre-ESRD care on mortality risk among new ESRD patients in the United States. *Am J Kidney Dis* 2003; **41:** 310–318.

8 Khan SS, Xue JL, Kazmi WH, Gilbertson DT, Obrador GT, Pereira BJ et al. Does predialysis nephrology care influence patient survival after initiation of dialysis? *Kidney Int* 2005; **67:** 1038–1046.

9 Dhingra RK, Young EW, Hulbert-Shearon TE, Leavey SF, Port FK. Type of vascular access and mortality in U.S. hemodialysis patients. *Kidney Int* 2001; **60:** 1443–1451.

10 Pastan S, Soucie JM, McClellan WM. Vascular access and increased risk of death among hemodialysis patients. *Kidney Int* 2002; **62:** 620–626.

11 Astor BC, Eustace JA, Powe NR, Klag MJ, Sadler JH, Fink NE et al. Timing of nephrologist referral and arteriovenous access use: the CHOICE Study. *Am J Kidney Dis* 2001; **38:** 494–501.

12 Arora P, Obrador GT, Ruthazer R, Kausz AT, Meyer KB, Jenuleson CS et al. Prevalence, predictors, and consequences of late nephrology referral at a tertiary care center. *J Am Soc Nephrol* 1999; **10:** 1281–1286.

13 Winkelmayer WC, Owen WF, Jr., Levin R, Avorn J. A propensity analysis of late versus early nephrologist referral and mortality on dialysis. *J Am Soc Nephrol* 2003; **14:** 486–492.

14 McLaughlin K, Manns B, Culleton B, Donaldson C, Taub K. An economic evaluation of early versus late referral of patients with progressive renal insufficiency. *Am J Kidney Dis* 2001; **38:** 1122–1128.

15 Mange KC, Joffe MM, Feldman HI. Effect of the use or nonuse of long-term dialysis on the subsequent survival of renal transplants from living donors. *N Engl J Med* 2001; **344:** 726–731.

16 Gaston RS, Basadonna G, Cosio FG, Davis CL, Kasiske BL, Larsen J et al. Transplantation in the diabetic patient with advanced chronic kidney disease: a task force report. *Am J Kidney Dis* 2004; **44:** 529–542.

17 Wolfe RA, Ashby VB, Milford EL, Ojo AO, Ettenger RE, Agodoa LY et al. Comparison of mortality in all patients on dialysis, patients on dialysis awaiting transplantation, and recipients of a first cadaveric transplant. *N Engl J Med* 1999; **341:** 1725–1730.

18 Gomez CG, Valido P, Celadilla O, Bernaldo de Quiros AG, Mojon M. Validity of a standard information protocol provided to end-stage renal disease patients and its effect on treatment selection. *Perit Dial Int* 1999; **19:** 471–477.

19 Marron B, Martinez Ocana JC, Salgueira M, Barril G, Lamas JM, Martin M et al. Analysis of patient flow into dialysis: role of education in choice of dialysis modality. *Perit Dial Int* 2005; **25(Suppl 3):** S56–S59.

20 Devins GM, Mendelssohn DC, Barre PE, Binik YM. Predialysis psychoeducational intervention and coping styles influence time to dialysis in chronic kidney disease. *Am J Kidney Dis* 2003; **42:** 693–703.

21 Devins GM, Mendelssohn DC, Barre PE, Taub K, Binik YM. Predialysis psychoeducational intervention extends survival in CKD: a 20-year follow-up. *Am J Kidney Dis* 2005; **46:** 1088–1098.

22 Curtis BM, Ravani P, Malberti F, Kennett F, Taylor PA, Djurdjev O et al. The short- and long-term impact of multi-disciplinary clinics in addition to standard nephrology care on patient outcomes. *Nephrol Dial Transplant* 2005; **20:** 147–154.

23 Goldstein M, Yassa T, Dacouris N, McFarlane P. Multidisciplinary pre-dialysis care and morbidity and mortality of patients on dialysis. *Am J Kidney Dis* 2004; **44:** 706–714.

24 Fenton SS, Schaubel DE, Desmeules M, Morrison HI, Mao Y, Copleston P et al. Hemodialysis versus peritoneal dialysis: a comparison of adjusted mortality rates. *Am J Kidney Dis* 1997; **30:** 334–342.

25 Collins AJ, Hao W, Xia H, Ebben JP, Everson SE, Constantini EG et al. Mortality risks of peritoneal dialysis and hemodialysis. *Am J Kidney Dis* 1999; **34:** 1065–1074.

26 Heaf JG, Lokkegaard H, Madsen M. Initial survival advantage of peritoneal dialysis relative to haemodialysis. *Nephrol Dial Transplant* 2002; **17:** 112–117.

27 Termorshuizen F, Korevaar JC, Dekker FW, Van Manen JG, Boeschoten EW, Krediet RT et al. Hemodialysis and peritoneal dialysis: comparison of adjusted mortality rates according to the duration of dialysis: analysis of The Netherlands Cooperative Study on the Adequacy of Dialysis 2. *J Am Soc Nephrol* 2003; **14:** 2851–2860.

28 Locatelli F, Marcelli D, Conte F, D'Amico M, Del Vecchio L, Limido A et al. Survival and development of cardiovascular disease by modality of treatment in patients with end-stage renal disease. *J Am Soc Nephrol* 2001; **12:** 2411–2417.

29 Vonesh EF, Moran J. Mortality in end-stage renal disease: a reassessment of differences between patients treated with hemodialysis and peritoneal dialysis. *J Am Soc Nephrol* 1999; **10:** 354–365.

30 Foley RN, Parfrey PS, Harnett JD, Kent GM, O'Dea R, Murray DC et al. Mode of dialysis therapy and mortality in end-stage renal disease. *J Am Soc Nephrol* 1998; **9:** 267–276.

31 Jaar BG, Coresh J, Plantinga LC, Fink NE, Klag MJ, Levey AS et al. Comparing the risk for death with peritoneal dialysis and hemodialysis in a national cohort of patients with chronic kidney disease. *Ann Intern Med* 2005; **143:** 174–183.

32 Xue JL, Everson SE, Constantini EG, Ebben JP, Chen SC, Agodoa LY et al. Peritoneal and hemodialysis. II. Mortality risk associated with initial patient characteristics. *Kidney Int* 2002; **61:** 741–746.

33 Vonesh EF, Snyder JJ, Foley RN, Collins AJ. The differential impact of risk factors on mortality in hemodialysis and peritoneal dialysis. *Kidney Int* 2004; **66:** 2389–2401.

34 Murphy SW, Foley RN, Barrett BJ, Kent GM, Morgan J, Barre P *et al.* Comparative mortality of hemodialysis and peritoneal dialysis in Canada. *Kidney Int* 2000; **57:** 1720–1726.

35 Miskulin DC, Meyer KB, Athienites NV, Martin AA, Terrin N, Marsh JV *et al.* Comorbidity and other factors associated with modality selection in incident dialysis patients: the CHOICE Study. Choices for Healthy Outcomes in Caring for End-Stage Renal Disease. *Am J Kidney Dis* 2002; **39:** 324–336.

36 Stack AG, Molony DA, Rahman NS, Dosekun A, Murthy B. Impact of dialysis modality on survival of new ESRD patients with congestive heart failure in the United States. *Kidney Int* 2003; **64:** 1071–1079.

37 Korevaar JC, Feith GW, Dekker FW, van Manen JG, Boeschoten EW, Bossuyt PM *et al.* Effect of starting with hemodialysis compared with peritoneal dialysis in patients new on dialysis treatment: a randomized controlled trial. *Kidney Int* 2003; **64:** 2222–2228.

38 Pierratos A. Nocturnal home haemodialysis: an update on a 5-year experience. *Nephrol Dial Transplant* 1999; **14:** 2835–2840.

39 McGregor DO, Buttimore AL, Lynn KL, Nicholls MG, Jardine DL. A comparative study of blood pressure control with short in-center versus long home hemodialysis. *Blood Purif* 2001; **19:** 293–300.

40 Evans RW, Manninen DL, Garrison LP, Jr., Hart LG, Blagg CR, Gutman RA *et al.* The quality of life of patients with end-stage renal disease. *N Engl J Med* 1985; **312:** 553–559.

41 McPhatter LL, Lockridge RS, Jr., Albert J, Anderson H, Craft V, Jennings FM *et al.* Nightly home hemodialysis: improvement in nutrition and quality of life. *Adv Ren Replace Ther* 1999; **6:** 358–365.

42 Mohr PE, Neumann PJ, Franco SJ, Marinen J, Lockridge R, Ting G. The case for daily dialysis: its impact on costs and quality of life. *Am J Kidney Dis* 2001; **37:** 777–789.

43 Winkelmayer WC, Weinstein MC, Mittleman MA, Glynn RJ, Pliskin JS. Health economic evaluations: the special case of end-stage renal disease treatment. *Med Decis Making* 2002; **22:** 417–430.

44 Woods JD, Port FK, Stannard D, Blagg CR, Held PJ. Comparison of mortality with home hemodialysis and center hemodialysis: a national study. *Kidney Int* 1996; **49:** 1464–1470.

45 Delano BG. Home hemodialysis offers excellent survival. *Adv Ren Replace Ther* 1996; **3:** 106–111.

46 Mailloux LU, Kapikian N, Napolitano B, Mossey RT, Bellucci AG, Wilkes BM *et al.* Home hemodialysis: patient outcomes during a 24-year period of time from 1970 through 1993. *Adv Ren Replace Ther* 1996; **3:** 112–119.

47 Arkouche W, Traeger J, Delawari E, Sibai-Galland R, Abdullah E, Galland R *et al.* Twenty-five years of experience with out-center hemodialysis. *Kidney Int* 1999; **56:** 2269–2275.

48 McGregor DO, Buttimore AL, Lynn KL. Home hemodialysis: excellent survival at less cost, but still underutilized. *Kidney Int* 2000; **57:** 2654–2655.

49 Brescia MJ, Cimino JE, Appel K, Hurwich BJ. Chronic hemodialysis using venipuncture and a surgically created arteriovenous fistula. *N Engl J Med* 1966; **275:** 1089–1092.

50 Beathard GA, Arnold P, Jackson J, Litchfield T, Physician Operators Forum of RMS Lifeline. Aggressive treatment of early fistula failure. *Kidney Int* 2003; **64:** 1487–1494.

51 Beathard GA, Settle SM, Shields MW. Salvage of the nonfunctioning arteriovenous fistula. *Am J Kidney Dis* 1999; **33:** 910–916.

52 Beathard GA. An algorithm for the physical examination of early fistula failure. *Semin Dial* 2005; **18:** 331–335.

53 Allon M, Lockhart ME, Lilly RZ, Gallichio MH, Young CJ, Barker J *et al.* Effect of preoperative sonographic mapping on vascular access outcomes in hemodialysis patients. *Kidney Int* 2001; **60:** 2013–2020.

54 Robbin ML, Gallichio MH, Deierhoi MH, Young CJ, Weber TM, Allon M. US vascular mapping before hemodialysis access placement. *Radiology* 2000; **217:** 83–88.

55 Miller PE, Tolwani A, Luscy CP, Deierhoi MH, Bailey R, Redden DT *et al.* Predictors of adequacy of arteriovenous fistulas in hemodialysis patients. *Kidney Int* 1999; **56:** 275–280.

56 Miller CD, Robbin ML, Allon M. Gender differences in outcomes of arteriovenous fistulas in hemodialysis patients. *Kidney Int* 2003; **63:** 346–352.

57 Konner K, Hulbert-Shearon TE, Roys EC, Port FK. Tailoring the initial vascular access for dialysis patients. *Kidney Int* 2002; **62:** 329–338.

58 Astor BC, Eustace JA, Powe NR, Klag MJ, Fink NE, Coresh J *et al.* Type of vascular access and survival among incident hemodialysis patients: the Choices for Healthy Outcomes in Caring for ESRD (CHOICE) study. *J Am Soc Nephrol* 2005; **16:** 1449–1455.

59 Saad TF. Bacteremia associated with tunneled, cuffed hemodialysis catheters. *Am J Kidney Dis* 1999; **34:** 1114–1124.

60 Oliver MJ, Rothwell DM, Fung K, Hux JE, Lok CE. Late creation of vascular access for hemodialysis and increased risk of sepsis. *J Am Soc Nephrol* 2004; **15:** 1936–1942.

61 Hodges TC, Fillinger MF, Zwolak RM, Walsh DB, Bech F, Cronenwett JL. Longitudinal comparison of dialysis access methods: risk factors for failure. *J Vasc Surg* 1997; **26:** 1009–1019.

62 Palder SB, Kirkman RL, Whittemore AD, Hakim RM, Lazarus JM, Tilney NL. Vascular access for hemodialysis. Patency rates and results of revision. *Ann Surg* 1985; **202:** 235–239.

63 Kherlakian GM, Roedersheimer LR, Arbaugh JJ, Newmark KJ, King LR. Comparison of autogenous fistula versus expanded polytetrafluoroethylene graft fistula for angioaccess in hemodialysis. *Am J Surg* 1986; **152:** 238–243.

64 Glickman MH, Stokes GK, Ross JR, Schuman ED, Sternbergh WC, III, Lindberg JS *et al.* Multicenter evaluation of a polytetrafluoroethylene vascular access graft as compared with the expanded polytetrafluoroethylene vascular access graft in hemodialysis applications. *J Vasc Surg* 2001; **34:** 465–472.

65 Hirth RA, Turenne MN, Woods JD, Young EW, Port FK, Pauly MV *et al.* Predictors of type of vascular access in hemodialysis patients. *JAMA* 1996; **276:** 1303–1308.

66 Reddan D, Klassen P, Frankenfield DL, Szczech L, Schwab S, Colodonato J *et al.* National profile of practice patterns for hemodialysis vascular access in the United States. *J Am Soc Nephrol* 2002; **13:** 2117–2124.

67 Young EW, Dykstra DM, Goodkin DA, Mapes DL, Wolfe RA, Held PJ. Hemodialysis vascular access preferences and outcomes in the Dialysis Outcomes and Practice Patterns Study (DOPPS). *Kidney Int* 2002; **61:** 2266–2271.

68 NKF. K/DOQI clinical practice guidelines for vascular access: update 2000. *Am J Kidney Dis* 2000; **37:** S137–S181.

69 Port FK, Pisoni RL, Bommer J, Locatelli F, Jadoul M, Eknoyan G *et al.* Improving outcomes for dialysis patients in the International Dialysis Outcomes and Practice Patterns study. *Clin J Am Soc Nephrol* 2006; **1:** 246–255.

70 FistulaFirst National Vascular Access Improvement Initiative. Centers for Medicare and Medicaid Services and the Department of Health and Human Services, 2006.

71 Schwab SJ, Quarles LD, Middleton JP, Cohan RH, Saeed M, Dennis VW. Hemodialysis-associated subclavian vein stenosis. *Kidney Int* 1988; **33:** 1156–1159.

72 Cimochowski GE, Worley E, Rutherford WE, Sartain J, Blondin J, Harter H. Superiority of the internal jugular over the subclavian access for temporary dialysis. *Nephron* 1990; **54:** 154–161.

73 Schillinger F, Schillinger D, Montagnac R, Milcent T. Post catheterisation vein stenosis in haemodialysis: comparative angiographic study of 50 subclavian and 50 internal jugular accesses. *Nephrol Dial Transplant* 1991; **6:** 722–724.

74 Hernandez D, Diaz F, Rufino M, Lorenzo V, Perez T, Rodriguez A *et al.* Subclavian vascular access stenosis in dialysis patients: natural history and risk factors. *J Am Soc Nephrol* 1998; **9:** 1507–1510.

75 Danese MD, Liu Z, Griffiths RI, Dylan M, Yu HT, Dubois R *et al.* Catheter use is high even among hemodialysis patients with a fistula or graft. *Kidney Int* 2006; **70:** 1482–1485.

76 US. Food and Drug Administration. FDA Alert (06/2006): development of serious and sometimes fatal nephrogenic systemic fibrosis/nephrogenic fibrosing dermopathy. US FDA, 2006.

77 Grobner T. Gadolinium: a specific trigger for the development of nephrogenic fibrosing dermopathy and nephrogenic systemic fibrosis? *Nephrol Dial Transplant* 2006; **21:** 1104–1108.

78 Kian K, Wyatt C, Schon D, Packer J, Vassalotti J, Mishler R. Safety of low-dose radiocontrast for interventional AV fistula salvage in stage 4 chronic kidney disease patients. *Kidney Int* 2006; **69:** 1444–1449.

79 Flanigan MJ, Ngheim DD, Schulak JA, Ullrich GE, Freeman RM. The use and complications of three peritoneal dialysis catheter designs. A retrospective analysis. *ASAIO Trans* 1987; **33:** 33–38.

80 Favazza A, Petri R, Montanaro D, Boscutti G, Bresadola F, Mioni G. Insertion of a straight peritoneal catheter in an arcuate subcutaneous tunnel by a tunneler: long-term experience. *Perit Dial Int* 1995; **15:** 357–362.

81 Lewis MA, Smith T, Postlethwaite RJ, Webb NJ. A comparison of double-cuffed with single-cuffed Tenckhoff catheters in the prevention of infection in pediatric patients. *Adv Perit Dial* 1997; **13:** 274–276.

82 Warady BA, Sullivan EK, Alexander SR. Lessons from the peritoneal dialysis patient database: a report of the North American Pediatric Renal Transplant Cooperative study. *Kidney Int Suppl* 1996; **53:** S68–S71.

83 Eklund B, Honkanen E, Kyllonen L, Salmela K, Kala AR. Peritoneal dialysis access: prospective randomized comparison of single-cuff and double-cuff straight Tenckhoff catheters. *Nephrol Dial Transplant* 1997; **12:** 2664–2666.

84 Wikdahl AM, Engman U, Stegmayr BG, Sorenssen JG. One-dose cefuroxime i.v. and i.p. reduces microbial growth in PD patients after catheter insertion. *Nephrol Dial Transplant* 1997; **12:** 157–160.

85 Gadallah MF, Ramdeen G, Mignone J, Patel D, Mitchell L, Tatro S. Role of preoperative antibiotic prophylaxis in preventing postoperative peritonitis in newly placed peritoneal dialysis catheters. *Am J Kidney Dis* 2000; **36:** 1014–1019.

86 Katyal A, Mahale A, Khanna R. Antibiotic prophylaxis before peritoneal dialysis catheter insertion. *Adv Perit Dial* 2002; **18:** 112–115.

87 Gokal R, Alexander S, Ash S, Chen TW, Danielson A, Holmes C *et al.* Peritoneal catheters and exit-site practices toward optimum peritoneal access: 1998 update. (Official report from the International Society for Peritoneal Dialysis). *Perit Dial Int* 1998; **18:** 11–33.

88 Moncrief JW, Popovich RP, Simmons E, Moncrief BA, Dasgupta MK, Costerton JW. Peritoneal access technology. *Perit Dial Int* 1993; **13(Suppl 2):** S121–S123.

89 Moncrief JW, Popovich RP, Dasgupta M, Costerton JW, Simmons E, Moncrief R. Reduction in peritonitis incidence in continuous ambulatory peritoneal dialysis with a new catheter and implantation technique. *Perit Dial Int* 1993; **13(Suppl 2):** S329–S331.

90 Danielsson A, Blohme L, Tranaeus A, Hylander B. A prospective randomized study of the effect of a subcutaneously "buried" peritoneal dialysis catheter technique versus standard technique on the incidence of peritonitis and exit-site infection. *Perit Dial Int* 2002; **22:** 211–219.

6 Chronic Kidney Disease Stage 5: Hemodialysis

36   When to Start Dialysis and Whether the First Treatment Should Be Extracorporeal Therapy or Peritoneal Dialysis

Raymond T. Krediet

Division of Nephrology, Department of Medicine, Academic Medical Center, University of Amsterdam, Amsterdam, The Netherlands

When to start dialysis

Introduction

The issue of timing of initiation of dialysis was first raised by Bonomini *et al.* in the 1970s [1,2]. They reported the highest survival rate in hemodialysis (HD) patients with a residual creatinine clearance between 15 and 21 mL/min. However, criteria for the selection of patients based on residual renal function were not provided. The issue of an "earlier" start, which means with a higher glomerular filtration rate (GFR) than usual, reappeared again in the last decade when the process of developing guidelines for dialysis was started.

Early start or timely referral

A distinction should be made between the timing of referral to a nephrologist and the timing of the start of dialysis treatment. Failure to make this distinction has confused the discussion. It should be emphasized that all studies on late referral to a nephrologist are either retrospective, based on surveys, or prospective cohort studies. Nevertheless, the results are strikingly similar. Late referral for maintenance dialysis is associated with increased mortality [3–11] and decreased quality of life [12,13]. The excess mortality associated with late referral was independent of demographic characteristics, socio-economic status, and comorbidity. Moreover, late referral influenced the dialysis modality choice; patients who obtained predialysis care had a stronger preference for peritoneal dialysis (PD) than patients who did not (late referrals) [14]. In addition, patients who were referred late and started with PD were more likely to switch to HD during the first 6 months compared with patients who were referred in a more timely manner [15]. Despite all the evidence pointing to a beneficial effect of timely referral to a nephrologist, almost one-fourth of patients were referred less than 1 month before the start of dialysis in a survey of eight different European countries [16].

Guidelines and studies

The timing of initiation of dialysis has been the subject of many opinion-based guidelines in the last decade. The US National Kidney Foundation Dialysis Outcomes Quality Initiative (K/DOQI) Workgroup on Peritoneal Dialysis published an opinion-based guideline on the initiation of chronic dialysis treatment [17]. The work group advised that dialysis should be initiated when renal K_t/V_{urea} had fallen to 2.0/week. For a 70-kg man this equals a urea clearance of 8 mL/min, a GFR of 10 mL/min, and a creatinine clearance of 12 mL/min. A lower K_t/V_{urea} would only be acceptable when the normalized protein equivalent of nitrogen appearance, an index of protein intake in stable patients, was at least 0.8 g/kg of body weight/day and the patient was in a good nutritional state. These recommendations were retained in the update, published in 2001. The clinical practice guidelines of the Canadian Society of Nephrology for treatment of patients with chronic kidney disease, published in 1999, were not significantly different from the US guidelines but set the target for the start of dialysis at a GFR of 12 mL/min when symptoms were present, but with an absolute minimum GFR of 6 mL/min [18]. The European Best Practice Guidelines for peritoneal dialysis recommend consideration of initiation of dialysis when the GFR is below 15 mL/min in combination with evidence of poorly controlled conservative treatment. An absolute minimum value was set at 6 mL/min [19].

At the time these guidelines were published many patients typically started dialysis at much lower clearances. In one study from the UK the mean urea clearance was 3.9 mL/min [20]. A study from the USA reported that 63% of the patients had an estimated GFR between 5 and 10 mL/min/1.73 m^2, and 23% had an estimated value below 5 [21]. Although the above guidelines are not evidence based and are far from current practice, they have caused a trend towards earlier initiation of dialysis treatment [22,23].

Currently, no randomized controlled study on the initiation of dialysis is available. The cohort studies do not point to a real benefit for an early start [24,27–30]. The Netherlands Cooperative Study on the Adequacy of Dialysis (NECOSAD) is a multicenter prospective cohort study in which all new dialysis patients are

Evidence-based Nephrology. Edited by Donald Molony and Jonathan Craig
© 2009 Blackwell Publishing, ISBN: 978-1-4051-3975-5.

included and followed at 6-month intervals. GFR is measured as the mean of creatinine and urea clearance at the start of dialysis and thereafter. An analysis of 253 patients showed that 37% started dialysis treatment later than the K/DOQI recommendations (late starters) [24]. The others were defined as timely starters. The adjusted difference in estimated survival time after 3 years on dialysis treatment was small: a benefit of 2.5 months (95% confidence interval, 1.1–4.0) in favor of timely starters. However, this is likely to be explained by lead time bias. Lead time may have an effect on the observed lower mortality risk, and thus longer survival time, in patients classified as timely starters and may be simply a reflection of initiating dialysis at an earlier stage of disease. The lead time could not be measured in the NECOSAD analysis, but taking the normal decline of GFR into account [25,26], it could be estimated as a period of about 6 months. Consequently, the apparent gain in survival from a timely start was presumably due to lead time, instead of an actual improvement in the course of the disease. All patients, timely and late starters, showed a marked improvement in quality of life during the first 6 months after the start of dialysis treatment [27]. Patients who commenced dialysis in time had a significantly better quality of life at initiation of treatment than the late starters. However, these differences disappeared after 1 year on dialysis, and both groups reported a similar quality of life at that time.

A retrospective analysis of a small single-center cohort of new, mainly HD patients from Austria showed no difference in creatinine clearance at the start of dialysis between patients who survived less than 1 year compared with those who survived more than 1 year on dialysis [28]. An analysis of the electronic patient records at the Glasgow Royal Infirmary made it possible to identify patients with an estimated creatinine clearance (Cockcroft-Gault formula) of less than 20 mL/min and who could be followed before the initiation of dialysis and during dialysis with exclusion of late referrals [29]. The date from which a creatinine clearance of 20 mL/min was calculated was used to determine survival time. Patients were divided into an early or late start group by the median creatinine clearance, which was 8.3 mL/min. The authors found no benefit in patient survival from an earlier start of PD. Instead, patients who started dialysis with a lower creatinine clearance tended to survive longer. Although not investigated in this study, the effect may have been due to the well-known fact that dialysis is often started earlier in sicker patients and those with more comorbidity.

An analysis of the Dialysis Morbidity Study Wave II, which is part of the US Renal Data System (USRDS), demonstrated essentially the same finding [30]. Patients with a higher estimated GFR at the start of dialysis had a higher mortality than those with lower values, with a hazard ratio of 1.14 in multivariate analysis.

Conclusions on the start of dialysis

In the absence of randomized controlled studies, the bulk of evidence has shown that late referral to a nephrologist is associated with increased morbidity and mortality. No retrospective or prospective cohort study has shown a benefit of an early start of dialysis on mortality, whereas the effects on quality of life were

only temporary. A randomized controlled trial is currently being performed in Australia and New Zealand (the IDEAL study), but given the present evidence, it is unlikely that the results will be different from the evidence that is currently available.

PD or HD as initial renal replacement therapy

Both PD and HD have positive and negative features. Consequently, these options have to be weighed in individual patients according to their needs, with the aim of providing a patient-tailored renal replacement therapy. The only randomized controlled trial comparing PD and HD as initial renal replacement therapy was underpowered but showed a survival advantage for PD in a cohort of 38 incident ESRD patients in the Netherlands, with unadjusted or age and comorbidity adjusted hazard ratios for death over 5 years for patients randomized to HD vs. PD of 3.8 (95% confidence interval [CI], 1.1–12.6) and 3.6 (95% CI, 0.8–15.4), respectively [31]. The primary outcome of this study, quality of life, showed a trend favoring HD in the first 2 years. Given the effort that was invested to obtain a sufficient number of patients, it is unlikely that more randomized controlled trials on this subject will be performed.

A number of retrospective or prospective studies, performed with cohorts or by using registries, have shown a number of advantages of PD that are especially marked in the first years of treatment. Besides patient survival, these include higher hemoglobin levels [32], better preservation of residual GFR [33–38], and better results after kidney transplantation with regard to delayed graft function [39–41]. Furthermore, when a patient has to be transferred to HD, vascular access surgery can be planned in a timely fashion.

Studies comparing patient survival according to dialysis modality have given divergent results, that is, no difference between HD and PD, better results for HD, or better results for PD. This may be due to differences in study design, study populations, sample size, data collection, and availability of relevant data [42]. Additionally, differences between countries that influence outcomes can be present that are not explained by the above, such as access to health care and the health care system. The CANUSA study showed that the relative risk of death for incident PD patients in the USA was 1.95 compared to those in Canada [43], showing that results of studies on comparisons of survival between PD and HD were different when performed in the USA or in Canada and western Europe.

A retrospective multicenter study performed in the USA with 939 incident patients was published in 1990 [44]. A nonsignificant tendency for better survival for PD patients was found. In contrast, an analysis of a large sample of incident patients from the USRDS found no difference in survival between HD and PD patients, except among diabetic patients, who had a higher relative risk of death when treated with PD [45]. A USRDS analysis of prevalent patients showed that patients treated with PD had a 19% higher adjusted mortality risk than those treated with HD [46], particularly in patients over 55 years, those with diabetes mellitus,

Table 36.1 Comparison of mortality between HD and PD patients: studies from North America.

Study [reference]	No. of patients		Relative risk of death (HD = 1)	
	HD	PD	Nondiabetic	Diabetic
Serkes 1990 [44][a]	342	325	0.62, $P = 0.08$	0.9, NS
Held 1994 [45][b]	3376	681	0.84, NS	1.26, $P = 0.03$
Bloembergen 1995 [46][c]	170,700 pt–yrs (1987–1989 cohort)		1.11, $P < 0.001$	1.38, $P < 0.001$
Fenton 1997 [57][d]	7792	2841	Patients 0–64 yrs	
			0.92, NS	0.92, NS
Vonesh 1999 [47][b]	298,425 pt–yrs (1990–1992 cohort)		1.04, NS	1.11, $P < 0.001$
Collins 1999 [48][e]	99,048 (1994–1996 cohort)	18,110	0.72–0.87, sign	0.86–1.21, sign
Vonesh 2004 [49][e]	352,706 (1995–2000 cohort)	46,234	Patients 45–64 yrs	
			No comorbidity, 0.89, $P < 0.01$	No comorbidity, 1.09, $P < 0.05$
			With comorbidity, 0.99, NS	With comorbidity, 1.22, $P < 0.001$
Jaar 2005 [53][f]	763	274	2.78, sign	1.23, NS

Abbreviations: NS, not significant.
[a] Retrospective multicenter study.
[b] USRDS registry, incident patients.
[c] USRDS registry, prevalent patients.
[d] Canadian organ replacement register, incident patients.
[e] Medicare, incident patients.
[f] Prospective multicenter cohort study.

and in women. However, another analysis of incident USRDS patients showed no differences between survival on PD and HD in various 2-year cohorts from 1982 up to 1993, with the exception of female diabetic patients, who did worse with PD [47]. Another study, however, performed in the same period in the USA reported better survival for PD patients [48].

A more recent analysis by Vonesh *et al.* in 398,940 incident dialysis patients (11.6% PD) identified three factors that influenced the relative risk of death in HD and PD patients: 1) the cause of end-stage renal failure (diabetic vs. nondiabetic patients), 2) age, and 3) the presence or absence of comorbidity at initiation of dialysis [49]. In these analyses HD was associated with an increased risk of death in nondiabetic and young diabetic patients, with no reported baseline comorbidity. When comorbidity was present, no difference in the relative risk of death was found between HD and PD. Their findings differ from the findings of Ganesh *et al.* and Stack *et al.*, who reported an association of increased mortality with PD in certain segments of this same US incident dialysis cohort based on somewhat different analytical methods [50,51,52]. Of potential clinical relevance, Stack *et al.* evaluated the impact of modality choice on survival in individuals with congestive heart failure and separately in patients with very high body mass indices. They reported a survival advantage with HD for patients with CHF and very large body habitus. Whether an age effect, as suggested by the analysis of Vonesh *et al.*, might have accounted for some

of the reported advantage of HD over PD in the latter analyses was not determined. A recently published multicenter prospective cohort study in the USA (CHOICE; 81 dialysis units, 1041 incident patients, 26% PD) reported no difference in adjusted mortality rates between PD and HD patients during the first year of treatment for their entire cohort of incident dialysis patients [53]. However, after the second year, the risk of death was significantly higher in PD patients. This study can be criticized because not all participating dialysis centers provided both dialysis modalities. Furthermore, the as-treated analyses were influenced by the lower technique survival of PD compared with HD.

Results of studies performed in Canada and western Europe are different from those in the USA. The first study comparing continuous ambulatory PD (CAPD) with HD in incident patients was performed in the UK. Using Kaplan-Meier analyses, the patient survival was not different after up to 3 years of follow-up [54]. A similar study from Spain also found no differences in mortality between CAPD and HD [55]. Also, a multicenter comparison between 480 PD and 373 HD patients in Italy showed similar 7-year survival rates for both dialysis modalities after adjustment for differences in case mix [56]. For patients older than 54 years, the risk of death was significantly higher in HD than in CAPD patients. An analysis of the Canadian Organ Replacement Register among 11,970 ESRD patients showed a relative risk of death of 0.73 in PD patients compared with HD. The difference was especially evident

Table 36.2 Comparison of mortality between HD and PD patients: studies from Europe.

Study [reference]	No. of patients		% of patients with diabetes mellitus		Relative risk of death[a] (HD = 1)
	HD	PD	HD	PD	
Gokal 1987 [54][b]	329	610	4	14	NS
Gentil 1991 [55][b]	842	272	2	29	1.18, NS
Maiorca 1991 [56][b]	373	480	7	20	1.35, NS
Van Biesen 2000 [59][c]	223	194	16	27	1.13, NS
Davies 2001 [63][c]	392	205	NA	NA	0.63, P < 0.001
Jager 2001 [60][b]	132	118	17	20	1.15, NS
Locatelli 2001 [61][d]	2772	1292	21	16	1.06, NS
Heaf 2002 [64][d]	4020	2208	18	22	0.86, P < 0.001
Termorshuizen 2003 [62][b]	742	480	23	18	NS
Liem 2007 [65][d]	10,841	5802	15	16	0.43, P < 0.001

Abbreviations: NA, not available; NS, not significant.

[a] Intention to treat analysis; relative risk after adjustment for age and comorbidity.

[b] Multicenter study, incident patients.

[c] Single-center study.

[d] Registry study.

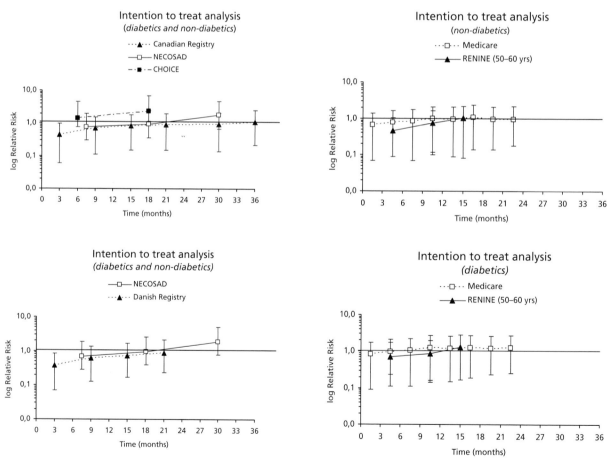

Figure 36.1 Effect of duration of dialysis on relative risk of death of incident PD patients compared with HD (relative risk for HD is 1), plotted on a logarithmic scale. The vertical lines depicts the 95% CI of the relative risk. Left panels show aggregated data for diabetic and nondiabetic patients from the Canadian registry [57], NECOSAD [62], CHOICE [53], and the Danish registry [64]. Right panels show separate analyses for diabetic and nondiabetic patients from the Medicare registry [48] and RENINE, the Dutch registry [65]. For the latter, only results for patients aged 50–60 years are included.

during the first 2 years on PD [57]. A prospective observational cohort study from Canada in 822 incident patients (34% PD), using a scoring system for comorbidity, reported no significant difference in adjusted mortality risks [58].

More recent studies reported either no differences in survival between PD and HD patients [59–62] or a reduced relative risk of death in PD compared to HD [63–65]. The results of the various studies are summarized in Tables 36.1 and 36.2. Large registry studies from Denmark [64] and the Netherlands [65] established better survival rates for incident PD patients in Europe, especially during the first years on treatment. The relative risks of death according to the duration of PD are given in Figure 36.1.

All the studies discussed above are either analyses from registry data or results obtained in prospective cohort studies. Differences in case mix or in determinants of the choice for either dialysis modality cannot be excluded with certainty. This would require a randomized controlled trial. Such a trial would be extremely difficult to perform due to difficulties in patient recruitment, as was the experience with the single randomized controlled trial performed to date [31]. In light of the difficulty in performing such a clinical trial, a targeted randomized controlled trial in patients with diabetes mellitus and/or CHF or a large body habitus might be informative. One small randomized controlled trial in a European population has been published [31]. Although underpowered because of the above reasons, patient survival, a secondary outcome of this study, was better in the PD group than in those randomized to HD after 2 years.

The current state of evidence, that is, the potential benefits of PD, as mentioned in the beginning of this section on PD versus HD as initial renal replacement therapy, combined with the better survival on PD during the first 2 years reported in some observational studies, provides support for the recommendation that PD be considered as initial renal replacement therapy in patients who agree to this and in whom no major contraindications are present, where the definition of the latter may change as new evidence emerges from ongoing analyses of registry data and other observational studies. As elaborated in section 8 of this textbook, to confer the greatest survival and quality of life benefit, a timely transfer to HD should be considered when patients develop severe problems on PD, such as recurrent peritonitis or ultrafiltration failure. This concept of integrative care was first developed by Van Biesen et al., as they showed in a retrospective analysis of their center that patients who started PD and were subsequently transferred to HD had a better survival than those who were treated with HD for the total duration of follow-up [59]. Patients should be informed of the potential benefits of this integrated approach as part of their modality education in the predialysis period.

References

1 Bonomini V, Albertazzi A, Vangelista A, Bortolotti GC, Stefoni S, Scolari MP. Residual renal function and effective rehabilitation in chronic dialysis. *Nephron* 1976; **16**: 89–99.

2 Bonomini V, Feletti C, Scolari MP, Stefoni S. Benfits of early initiation of dialysis. *Kidney Int* 1985; **28(Suppl 17)**: S57–S59.

3 Ratcliffe PJ, Phillips RE, Oliver DO. Late referral for maintenance dialysis. *Brit Med J* 1984; **288**: 441–443.

4 Campbell JD, Ewigman B, Hosokawa M, Van Stone JC. The timing of referral of patients with end-stage renal disease. *Dial Transplant* 1989; **18**: 660–668.

5 Innes A, Rowe PA, Burden RP, Morgan AG. Early deaths on renal replacement therapy: the need for an early nephrological referral. *Nephrol Dial Transplant* 1992; **7**: 467–471.

6 Jungers P, Zingraff J, Albouze G, Chauveau P, Page B, Hannedouche T et al. Late referral to maintenance dialysis: detrimental consequences. *Nephrol Dial Transplant* 1993; **8**: 1089–1093.

7 Khan IH, Catto GRD, Edward N, MacLeod AM. Death during the first 90 days of dialysis: a case-control study. *Am J Kidney Dis* 1995; **25**: 276–280.

8 Sesso R, Belusco AG. Late diagnosis of chronic renal failure and mortality on maintenance dialysis. *Nephrol Dial Transplant* 1996; **11**: 2417–2420.

9 Kinchen KS, Sadler J, Fink N, Brookmeyer R, Klag KJ, Levey AS et al. The timing of specialist evaluation in chronic kidney disease and mortality. *Ann Intern Med* 2002; **137**: 479–486.

10 Khan SS, Xue JL, Kazmi WH, Gilbertson DT, Obrador GT, Pereira BJG et al. Does predialysis nephrology care influence patient survival after initiation of dialysis? *Kidney Int* 2005; **67**: 1038–1046.

11 Dogan E, Erkoc R, Sayarlioglu H, Durmus A, Topal C. Effects of late referral to a nephrologist in patients with chronic renal failure. *Nephrology* 2005; **10**: 516–519.

12 Sesso R, Yoshihiro MM. Time of diagnosis of chronic renal failure and assessment of quality of life in haemodialysis patients. *Nephrol Dial Transplant* 1997; **12**: 2111–2116.

13 Caskey FJ, Wordsworth S, Ben T, de Charro FT, Delcroix C, Dobronravov V et al. Early referral and planned initiation of dialysis: what impact on quality of life? *Nephrol Dial Transplant* 2003; **18**: 1330–1338.

14 Jager KJ, Korevaar JC, Dekker FW, Krediet RT, Boeschoten EW. The effect of contraindications and patient preference on dialysis modality selection in ESRD patients in The Netherlands. *Am J Kidney Dis* 2004; **43**: 891–899.

15 Owen WF, Jr. Patterns of care for patients with chronic kidney disease in the United States: dying for improvement. *J Am Soc Nephrol* 2003; **14(Suppl 2)**: S76–S80.

16 Lameire N, van Biesen W, Dombros N, Dratwa M, Faller B, Gahl M et al. The referral pattern of patients with ESRD is a determinant in the choice of dialysis modality. *Perit Dial Int* 1997; **17(Suppl 3)**: S161–S166.

17 NKF. K/DOQI clinical practice guidelines for hemodialysis and peritoneal dialysis adequacy. *Am J Kidney Dis* 1997; **30(Suppl 2)**: S67–S136.

18 Churchill DN, Blake PG, Goldstein MB, Jindal KK, Toffelmire EB. Clinical practice guidelines of the Canadian Society of Nephrology for treatment of patients with chronic renal failure. *J Am Soc Nephrol* 1999; **10(Suppl 13)**: S287–S321.

19 EBPG Expert Group on Peritoneal Dialysis. European best practice guidelines for peritoneal dialysis. *Nephrol Dial Transplant* 2005; **20(Suppl 9)**: ix3–ix7.

20 Tattersall J, Greenwood R, Farrington K. Urea kinetics and when to commence dialysis. *Am J Nephrol* 1995; **15**: 283–289.

21 Obrador GT, Arora P, Kausz AT, Ruthazer R, Pereira BJG, Levey AS. Level of renal function at the initiation of dialysis in the US end-stage population. *Kidney Int* 1999; **56**: 2227–2235.

22 Obrador GT, Pereira BJ. Early referral to the nephrologist and timely initiation of renal replacement therapy: a paradigm shift in the management

of patients with chronic renal failure. *Am J Kidney Dis* 1998; **31:** 348–417.

23 Termorshuizen F, Korevaar JC, Dekker FW, Jager KJ, van Manen J, Boeschoten EW *et al.* Time trends in initiation and dose of dialysis in end-stage renal disease patients in The Netherlands. *Nephrol Dial Transplant* 2003; **18:** 552–558.

24 Korevaar JC, Jansen MA, Dekker FW, Jager KJ, Boeschoten EW, Krediet RT *et al.* When to initiate dialysis: effect of proposed US guidelines on survival. *Lancet* 2001; **358:** 1046–1050.

25 Hunsicker LG, Adler S, Caggiula A, England BK, Greene T, Kusek JW *et al.* Predictors of the progression of renal disease in the modification of diet in renal disease study. *Kidney Int* 1997; **51:** 1908–1919.

26 Samuelsson O, Attman PO, Knight-Gibson C, Larsson R, Mulec H, Weiss L *et al.* Complex apolipoprotein B-containing lipoprotein particles are associated with a higher rate of progression of human chronic renal insufficiency. *J Am Soc Nephrol* 1998; **9:** 1482–1488.

27 Korevaar JC, Jansen MA, Dekker FW, Boeschoten EW, Bossuyt PMM, Krediet RT *et al.* Evaluation of DOQI guidelines: early start of dialysis treatment is not associated with better health-related quality of life. *Am J Kidney Dis* 2002; **39:** 108–115.

28 Biesenbach G, Hubmann K, Janko O, Schmekal B, Eichbauer-Sturm G. Predialysis management and predictors for early mortality in uremic patients who die within one year after initiation of dialysis therapy. *Ren Fail* 2002; **24:** 197–205.

29 Traynor JP, Simpson K, Geddes CC, Deighan CJ, Fox JG. Early initiation of dialysis fails to prolong survival in patients with end-stage renal failure. *J Am Soc Nephrol* 2002; **13:** 2125–2132.

30 Beddhu S, Samore MH, Roberts MS, Stoddard GJ, Ramhumar N, Pappas LM *et al.* Impact of timing of initiation of dialysis on mortality. *J Am Soc Nephrol* 2003; **14:** 2305–2312.

31 Korevaar JC, Feith GW, Dekker FW, van Manen JG, Boeschoten EW, Bossuyt PMM *et al.* Effect of starting with hemodialysis compared with peritoneal dialysis in patients new on dialysis treatment: a randomized controlled trial. *Kidney Int* 2003; **64:** 2222–2228.

32 Zappacosta AR, Caro Erstes A. Normalization of hematocrit in patients with end stage renal disease on continuous ambulatory peritoneal dialysis. The role of erythropoietin. *Am J Med* 1982; **72:** 53–57.

33 Rottembourg J, Issad B, Gallego JL, Degoulet P, Aime F, Gueffat B *et al.* Evaluation of residual renal function in patients undergoing maintenance haemodialysis or continuous ambulatory peritoneal dialysis. Proc EDTA 1982; **19:** 397–403.

34 Cancarini GC, Brunori G, Camerini C, Brasa S, Manili L, Maiorca R. Renal function recovery and maintenance of residual diuresis in CAPD and hemodialysis. *Perit Dial Int Bull* 1986; **6:** 77–79.

35 Lysaght MJ, Vonesh EF, Gotch F, Ibels L, Keen M, Lindholm B *et al.* The influence of dialysis treatment modality on the decline of remaining renal function. *ASAIO Trans* 1991; **37:** 598–604.

36 Moist LM, Port FK, Orol SM, Young EW, Ostbye T, Wolfe RA. Predictors of loss of residual renal function among new dialysis patients. *J Am Soc Nephrol* 2000; **11:** 556–564.

37 Misra M, Vonesh E, van Stone JC, Moore HL, Prowant B, Nolph KD. Effect of cause and time of dropout on the residual GFR: a comparative analysis of the decline of GFR on dialysis. *Kidney Int* 2001; **59:** 754–763.

38 Jansen MAM, Hart AAM, Korevaar JC, Dekker FW, Boeschoten EW, Krediet RT *et al.* Predictors of the rate of decline of residual renal function in incident dialysis patients. *Kidney Int* 2002; **62:** 1046–1053.

39 Fontan M, Rodriguez-Carmona A, Falcon T, Moncalian J, Oliver J, Valdes F. Renal transplantation in patients undergoing chronic peritoneal dialysis. *Perit Dial Int* 1996; **16:** 48–51.

40 Vanholder R, Heerin P, Loo AV, Biesen WV, Lambert MC, Hesse U *et al.* Reduced incidence of acute renal graft failure in patients treated with peritoneal dialysis, compared to hemodialysis. *Am J Kidney Dis* 1999; **33:** 934–940.

41 Van Biesen W, Vanholder R, Van Loo A, van der Vennet M, Lameire N. Peritoneal dialysis favorably influences early graft function after renal transplantation compared to hemodialysis. *Transplantation* 2000; **69:** 508–514.

42 Port FK, Wolfe RA, Bloembergen WE, Held PJ, Young EW. The study of outcomes for CAPD versus hemodialysis patients. *Perit Dial Int* 1996; **16:** 628–633.

43 Churchill DN, Taylor DW, Keshaviah PR, Canada-USA Peritoneal Dialysis Study Group. Adequacy of dialysis and nutrition in continuous peritoneal dialysis: association with clinical outcomes. *J Am Soc Nephrol* 1996; **7:** 198–207.

44 Serkes KD, Blagg CR, Nolph KD, Vonesh EF, Shapiro F. Comparison of patient and technique survival in continuous ambulatory peritoneal dialysis (CAPD) and hemodialysis: a multicenter study. *Perit Dial Int* 1990; **10:** 15–19.

45 Held PJ, Port FK, Turenne MN, Gaylin DS, Hamburger RJ, Wolfe RA. Continuous ambulatory peritoneal dialysis and hemodialysis: comparison of patient mortality with adjustment for comorbid conditions. *Kidney Int* 1994; **45:** 1163–1169.

46 Bloembergen WE, Port FK, Mauger EA, Wolfe RA. A comparison of mortality between patients treated with hemodialysis and peritoneal dialysis. *J Am Soc Nephrol* 1995; **6:** 177–183.

47 Vonesh EF, Moran J. Mortality in end-stage renal disease: a reassessment of differences between patients treated with hemodialysis and peritoneal dialysis. *J Am Soc Nephrol* 1999; **10:** 354–365.

48 Collins AJ, Hao W, Xia H, Ebben JP, Everson SE, Constantini EG *et al.* Mortality risks of peritoneal dialysis and hemodialysis. *Am J Kidney Dis* 1999; **34:** 1065–1074.

49 Vonesh EF, Snyder JJ, Foley RN, Collins AJ. The differential impact of risk factors on mortality in hemodialysis and peritoneal dialysis. *Kidney Int* 2004; **66:** 2389–2401.

50 Ganesh SK, Hulbert-Shearon T, Port FK, Eagle K, Stack AG. Mortality differences by dialysis modality among incident ESRD patients with and without coronary artery disease. *J Am Soc Nephrol* 2003; **14:** 415–424.

51 Stack AG, Molony DA, Rahman NS, Dosekun A, Murthy B. Impact of dialysis modality on survival of new ESRD patients with congestive heart failure in the United States. *Kidney Int* 2003; **64:** 1071–1079.

52 Stack AG, Murthy BVR, Molony DA. Survival differences between peritoneal dialysis and hemodialysis among "large" ESRD patients in the United States. *Kidney Int* 2004; **65:** 2398–2408.

53 Jaar BG, Coresh J, Plantinga LC, Fink NE, Klag MJ, Levey AS *et al.* Comparing the risk for death with peritoneal dialysis and hemodialysis in a national cohort of patients with chronic kidney disease. *Ann Intern Med* 2005; **143:** 174–183.

54 Gokal R, Jakubowski C, King J, Hunt L, Bogle S, Baillord R *et al.* Outcome in patients on continuous ambulatory peritoneal dialysis and haemodialysis: a 4-year analysis of a prospective multicentre study. *Lancet* 1987; **ii:** 1105–1108.

55 Gentil MA, Carriazo A, Pavon MI, Rosado M, Castillo D, Ramos B *et al.* Comparison of survival in continuous ambulatory peritoneal dial-

ysis and hospital haemodialysis: a multicentre study. *Nephrol Dial Transplant* 1991; **6:** 444–451.

56 Maiorca R, Vonesh EF, Cavalli PL, De Vechi A, Giangrande A, La Greco G *et al.* A multicenter, selection-adjusted comparison of patient and technique survivals on CAPD and hemodialysis. *Perit Dial Int* 19991; **11:** 118–127.

57 Fenton SSA, Schaubel DE, Desmeules M, Morrison HI, Mao Y, Copleston P *et al.* Hemodialysis versus peritoneal dialysis: a comparison of adjusted mortality rates. *Am J Kidney Dis* 1997; **30:** 334–342.

58 Murphy SW, Foley RN, Barrett BJ, Kent GM, Morgan J, Barré P *et al.* Comparative mortality of hemodialysis and peritoneal dialysis in Canada. *Kidney Int* 2000; **57:** 1720–1726.

59 Van Biesen W, Vanholder RC, Veys N, Dhondt A, Lameire N. An evaluation of an integrative care approach for end-stage renal disease patients. *J Am Soc Nephrol* 2000; **11:** 116–125.

60 Jager KJ, Merkus MP, Boeschoten EW, Dekker FW, Tijssen JCP, Krediet RT *et al.* What happens to patients starting dialysis in The Netherlands? *Neth J Med* 2001; **58:** 163–173.

61 Locatelli F, Marcello D, Conte F, D'Amico M, Del Vecchio L, Limido A *et al.* Survival and development of cardiovascular disease by modality of treatment in patients with end-stage renal disease. *Am J Soc Nephrol* 2001; **12:** 2411–2417.

62 Termorshuizen F, Koreveaar JC, Dekker FW, van Manen JG, Boeschoten EW, Krediet RT *et al.* Hemodialysis and peritoneal dialysis: comparison of adjusted mortality rates according to the duration of dialysis: analysis of the Netherlands Cooperative Study on the Adequacy of Dialysis 2. *J Am Soc Nephrol* 2003; **14:** 2851–2860.

63 Davies SJ, van Biesen W, Nicholas J, Lameire N. Integrated care. *Perit Dial Int* 2001; **21(Suppl 3):** S269–S274.

64 Heaf JG, Løkkegaard H, Madson M. Initial survival advantage of peritoneal dialysis relative to haemodialysis. *Nephrol Dial Transplant* 2002; **17:** 112–117.

65 Liem YS, Wong JB, Hunnik MGM, De Charro FTh, Winkelmayer WC. Comparison of hemodialysis and peritoneal dialysis survival in The Netherlands. *Kidney Int* 2007; **72:** 153–158.

37 Modalities of Extracorporeal Therapy: Hemodialysis, Hemofiltration, and Hemodiafiltration

Kannaiyan S. Rabindranath[1] & Norman Muirhead[2]

[1]Renal Unit, Churchill Hospital, Oxford, UK
[2]Division of Nephrology, University of Western Ontario, London, Ontario, Canada

Introduction

The removal of fluids and solutes in humans with kidney failure by an extracorporeal dialysis circuit was first accomplished by George Haas in Germany in 1924. Initial attempts at chronic hemodialysis were unsuccessful, mainly owing to problems with the dialysis membranes and the lack of definitive and convenient arterio-venous access. Conventional chronic hemodialysis became possible with the development of the Scribner shunt and the Brescio-Cimino fistula in the 1960s. Dialysis technology has advanced considerably, and multiple different modalities of extracorporeal renal replacement therapy (RRT) are currently available, including hemodialysis (HD), hemofiltration (HF), hemodiafiltration (HDF), and acetate-free biofiltration (AFB). HD remains the most common form of RRT for end-stage renal disease (ESRD), although there is significant regional variation in practice. In Austria, Belgium, and Germany, 7, 14, and 12.4% of the chronic dialysis population is on HDF, respectively [1,2]. For HF, this proportion is 1.1% in Germany and 1% in Greece [1–3].

Principles of extracorporeal RRT modalities

Extracorporeal RRT involves withdrawing a patient's blood and passing it through a dialysis filter. Within this filter, fluids and solutes are removed from the blood compartment across a semipermeable membrane referred to in the literature as the dialysis membrane or sometimes simply as the membrane or dialyzer. In HD, HDF, and AFB there is passage of dialysis fluid (dialysate) through the dialysis filter on the opposite side of the membrane from the patient's blood in a direction counter to that of the blood flow, whereas HF does not involve the use of a dialysate. The movement of fluid and solutes across the dialysis membrane depends on their molecular weight, hydration radius, and charge, the osmotic gradient across the membrane, the electrochemical gradient across the membrane, the size of pores in the dialysis filter, and the charge on the dialysis membrane.

Fluid is removed principally by ultrafiltration, which is achieved by creating a difference in the transmembrane pressure such that the hydrostatic pressure is greater in the blood compartment than in the dialysate compartment. Solutes can be removed by diffusion or convection. In diffusion, solute removal is driven by the electrochemical transmembrane gradients. In convection, solute removal is by solvent drag, that is, when fluid is removed, solutes passively follow the fluid. The biophysical principles that underlie solute and fluid transfer across a membrane determine the unique properties of each of the modalities discussed in this chapter. A detailed description of the biophysical and mechanical principles of dialysis are beyond the scope of this chapter. Rather, this chapter will address the evidence of how each of these modalities might impact clinical outcomes and the clinical trials evidence that might inform the choice of which modality to select for each clinical indication.

The expected clinical outcomes with each RRT prescription are determined importantly by the biophysical properties of the dialyzer membrane materials. These help determine the water and solute flux characteristics and the biocompatibility of the dialyzer membrane. Dialyzer membranes are composed of two main categories of material, cellulose-based or synthetic. With substituted cellulose membranes, acetyl groups are substituted for hydroxyl groups. By varying the degree of substitution, cellulose acetate, cellulose diacetate, and cellulose triacetate membranes are manufactured. Cellulose-based membranes made by the cuprammonium process (Cuprophane) are hydrophilic and have high porosity but low permeability to solutes. Substituted cellulose membranes, however, are more hydrophobic and have greater solute permeability. Cellulose membranes are relatively inexpensive, are sometimes "recycled," and are therefore the most commonly used membranes worldwide. Synthetic dialysis membranes are composed of a variety of materials, including polyamide, polyacrylonitrile, polysulfone, and polymethylmethacrylate. These membranes are hydrophobic and have larger pore sizes and higher hydraulic permeabilities and solute clearances.

Evidence-based Nephrology. Edited by Donald Molony and Jonathan Craig
© 2009 Blackwell Publishing, ISBN: 978-1-4051-3975-5.

The two main characteristics of dialysis membranes that most affect patient outcomes are their biocompatibility and their flux characteristics. Membranes can be biocompatible or bioincompatible and have high-, mid-, or low-flux characteristics.

Biocompatibility refers to the ability of a material to contact human tissues and blood without inciting a clinically significant inflammatory response. Bioincompatible dialysis membranes typically elicit a brisk inflammatory response, whereas biocompatible membranes elicit little or no clinically apparent inflammatory response. Dialyzer membranes have been shown to cause a variety of inflammatory responses, including activation of the alternate complement pathway, production of chemokines and adhesion molecules, activation of platelets and leukocytes, and induction of a decreased responsiveness of neutrophils and monocytes [4–6]. Such inflammatory responses are thought to have important consequences for the patient, and several adverse patient outcomes have been attributed to them. These include hypoxemia, "dialyzer reactions" (flu-like symptoms, pruritus, nausea, vomiting, headache, and hypotension), and increased production of β_2-microglobulin and its consequent deposition in the tissues, eventually resulting in dialysis-related amyloid arthropathy, increased susceptibility to infection, and increased protein catabolism [7–11]. Given that inflammation is a well-known atherogenic factor, the use of bioincompatible membranes could contribute to the cardiovascular mortality and morbidity in the hemodialysis population. To date, this specific question has not been addressed by either a randomized controlled trial (RCT) or a well-designed observational study.

Flux (classified as high, mid, and low) refers to the permeability characteristics of the dialysis membranes. Hydraulic permeability is measured by the dialyzer ultrafiltration coefficient (kUF), which is defined as the volume of ultrafiltrate formed per hour per millimeter of Hg transmembrane pressure, as determined at a blood flow of 200 mL/min. Membranes with a kUF of >12 mL/h/mmHg or β_2-microglobulin clearance of >20 mL/min are classified as high flux, and those with a kUF of <12 mL/h/mmHg or β_2-microglobulin clearance of <10 mL/min are classified as low flux. These criteria are derived from the HEMO study [12] and the US Food and Drug Administration dialyzer flux criteria [13].

In general, unsubstituted cellulose membranes are bioincompatible and low flux, whereas substituted cellulose membranes are more biocompatible and typically allow for mid- or high-flux characteristics. Synthetic membranes are considered the most biocompatible and can be manufactured to have either low-, mid-, or high-flux characteristics.

The newer RRT modalities, HF, HDF, and AFB, involve convection as the predominant solute clearance modality. All such modalities require high-flux dialysis membranes. In HF, a hemofilter replaces the traditional dialysis filter and no dialysate is used. Fluid is continuously ultrafiltered in excess of the actual fluid removal targets. In a typical HF session, this may involve the generation and removal of 30–40 L of ultrafiltrate. This excess removed ultrafiltrate is replaced by infusion of a suitable replacement fluid either prior to the membrane filter (predilution) or after the fil-

Table 37.1 Current guidelines on membrane characteristics and RRT modality usage.

Guideline	Country	Year	Recommendation
Biocompatibility			
K/DOQI	USA	2006	Avoid use of unsubstituted cellulosic membranes in favor of synthetic dialysis membranes
Renal Association (UK)	UK	2007	Use modified/substituted cellulose and low-flux synthetic membranes over unsubstituted cellulose membranes
CARI	Australia	2005	No recommendation
European Best Practice Guidelines	Europe	2002	Biocompatible high-flux membranes should be preferred
Membrane flux			
K/DOQI	USA	2006	No recommendation
Renal Association (UK)	UK	2007	Use of high-flux dialysis membranes for patients likely to remain on HD for several years and prevalent patients who have been on dialysis for longer than 3.7 yrs
CARI	Australia	2005	No recommendation
European Best Practice Guidelines	Europe	2002	Use of biocompatible high-flux membranes
RRT modality			
K/DOQI	USA	2006	No recommendation
Renal Association (UK)	UK	2007	Use of HDF or high-flux dialysis in patients who are likely to be on dialysis for several years or in prevalent patients who have been on dialysis for greater than 3.7 yrs
CARI	Australia	2005	No recommendation
European Best Practice Guidelines	Europe	2002	No recommendation

ter (along with the venous return; postdilution). HF may be less effective than other methods in removing small solutes, such as urea [14]. HDF is a hybrid system that includes both convection and diffusion [15]. In HD and HDF, the dialysate is buffered either with acetate or bicarbonate buffers. Currently, bicarbonate is the preferred buffer for both HD and HDF, as acetate has been shown to depress myocardial contractility and may, therefore, cause intradialytic hemodynamic instability [16]. AFB, an HDF technique, was introduced in 1985 to avoid the use of acetate in the dialysate. In this technique a hypertonic sodium bicarbonate solution is infused postdilution to manage treatment-related acidosis [17].

Biocompatibility, dialysis membrane flux, and the dialysis technologies themselves have been considered to have major impacts on patient outcomes. Current clinical practice guidelines with respect to these dialysis technology-related factors (Table 37.1) and the available evidence from systematic reviews and randomized controlled trials are reviewed below.

Review of current clinical practice guidelines

Biocompatibility

The Caring for Australians with Renal Impairment (CARI) guidelines [18] make no recommendations regarding dialysis membrane biocompatibility. The National Kidney Foundation's Kidney Diseases Outcomes Quality Initiative (K/DOQI) guidelines recommend avoiding the use of unsubstituted cellulose membranes in favor of synthetic dialysis membranes [19]. The Renal Association (UK) recommends the use of modified or substituted cellulose and low-flux synthetic membranes over unsubstituted cellulose membranes [20]. The European Best Practice Guidelines (EBPG) state that biocompatible high-flux dialyzers are preferred [21]. These differing recommendations result in considerable regional variations in dialyzer membrane utilization patterns.

Membrane flux

No recommendations on optimal membrane flux have been made by CARI or K/DOQI [18,19]. The Renal Association (UK) recommends the use of high-flux dialysis membranes for incident patients likely to remain on HD for several years and prevalent patients who have been on dialysis for longer than 3.7 years [20]. The EBPG state that biocompatible high-flux dialyzers are preferred [21].

RRT modality

CARI, EBPG, and K/DOQI do not recommend the use of any specific extracorporeal RRT modality [18,19,21]. The Renal Association (UK) recommends the use of high-flux HD or HDF in patients likely to remain on HD for several years and prevalent patients who have been on dialysis for longer than 3.7 years [20].

Availability of evidence

There have been a number nonrandomized studies, randomized studies, and systematic reviews reporting patient outcomes based on membrane composition and RRT modality. Apart from the systematic review comparing low- and high-flux dialysis membranes (published in abstract form), the other such reviews that are referred to below have been published in the Cochrane Library. Although these reviews have evaluated several outcomes, we have summarized the results only for the most important clinical outcomes for each of the comparisons mentioned above.

Evidence from nonrandomized studies

Epidemiological studies have generally reported favorable outcomes for biocompatible high-flux membranes compared with unsubstituted cellulose membranes. Woods and Nandakumar used historical controls and found that 463 patients treated with high-flux polysulfone membranes had a 30% improvement in 5-year survival rate (high-flux group, 90%, vs. low-flux group, 60%; $P = 0.029$) [22]. Another retrospective study comparing 107 patients on high-flux HD with 146 on low-flux HD found a significant reduction in relative risk for mortality for patients on high-flux HD (relative risk [RR], 0.24; 95% confidence interval [CI], 0.12–0.49) [23]. Hakim *et al.* in their analysis of 2410 patients from the US Renal Data System (USRDS) reported that the RR for mortality for patients dialyzed with more biocompatible modified cellulose or synthetic membranes was 20% lower than in patients treated using unsubstituted cellulose membranes. In a retrospective cohort study ($n = 12,791$) Port *et al.* [24] reported that those patients dialyzed with synthetic membranes had a significantly lower mortality than patients dialyzed with cellulose-based membranes (RR, 0.82; 95% CI, 0.72–0.93; $P = 0.002$) and that among the synthetic membranes, use of low-flux compared to high-flux membranes was associated with a significantly higher mortality risk (RR, 1.24; 95% CI, 1.02–1.52; $P = 0.04$) [25]. An analysis of 6440 patients in the Lombardy Registry in Italy between 1983 and 1995 found that patients on HF or HDF had a significantly lower risk for carpal tunnel syndrome surgery, a surrogate marker for dialysis-associated amyloidosis (RR, 0.58; 95% CI, 0.35–0.95; $P = 0.03$) compared with those on low-flux HD, but mortality rates were not different (RR, 0.90; 95% CI, 0.76–1.06; $P > 0.05$) [26]. In contrast, Koda *et al.* in a retrospective study of 248 patients reported that patients dialyzed with high-flux membranes had a significantly lower risk of carpal tunnel syndrome (RR, 0.50; 95% CI, 0.25–0.96; $P = 0.03$) as well as a lower mortality (RR, 0.61; 95% CI, 0.40–0.91; $P = 0.02$) [27]. Chanard [28] reported that patients on high-flux HD had less hypotension and other dialysis-related symptoms than those on HD with low-flux cellulose membranes. A study of 15 patients that used a crossover design (online predilution HF to high-flux HD to online predilution HF) reported that patients during the HF phases had significantly fewer intradialytic hypotension episodes per patient per month ($P < 0.04$), significantly fewer muscle cramp episodes, and less need for saline and plasma expanders [29] compared to HD.

Evidence from systematic reviews of RCTs

In the systematic reviews discussed below, comparative data on treatment effects of each extracorporeal RRT method are summarized either as RRs with 95% CIs for dichotomous outcomes or as weighted mean differences (WMD) with 95% CIs for continuous outcomes. These data inform the clinical questions regarding the impact of RRT modality, membrane biocompatibility differences,

Table 37.2 Patient characteristics and interventions in RCTs included in a systematic review comparing cellulose-based and synthetic dialysis membranes.

Study ID[a] [reference]	No. of patients	Mean age (yrs)	Gender (% male)	DM (%)	Interventions compared Synthetic	Cellulose	Follow-up
Aakhus 1995 [31]	8	NR[b]	50	12.5	AN69	Cuprophane	1 session
Bergamo 1991 [32]	328	56.4	50.8	5.5	Polysulfone	Cuprophane	1 session
Blakestijn 1995* [50]	28	NR	35.7	0	Polysulfone	Cuprophane	6 wks
Bonomini 1996 [83]	10	53.4	70	NR	PMMA	Cellulose acetate	3 wks
Caramelo 1994* [84]	22	50	59	0	PAN/polysulfone	Cuprophan	9 mos
Collins 1993 [33]	40	52.5	27.5	42.5	Polyacrylonitrile	Cuprophane	6 mos
Danielson 1986 [34]	7	51	NR	NR	Polycarbonate	Cuprophane	4 wks
Ferreira 2001 [85]	40	60	79.4	NR	AN69	Cellulose acetate and diacetate	1–6.5 yrs
Gardinali 1994* [44]	36	NR	63.9	0	Polyacrylonitrile	Cuprophane	3 mos
Girndt 2000 [86]	21	NR	NR	0	Polyamide	Cuprophane	12 sessions
Goldberg 1996 [87]	29	NR	NR	NR	Polysulfone	Cellulose acetate	8 wks
Grooteman1995 [88]	31	NR	48.3	3.2	Polysulfone	Cellulose triacetate	3 wks
Hakim 1996 [45]	159	52.5	49.5	46	PMMA	Cellulosic	18 mos
Hartmann 1997* [35]	20	51.5	30	0	Polysulfone	Cellulose acetate	1 yr
Hosokawa 1991 [46]	200	53.1	50	NR	PMMA	Cuprophane	1 yr
Lang 2001 [40]	30	44	63.3	13.3	Polysulfone	Cuprophane	2 yrs
Levin 1993 [36]	37	54	62.1	NR	Several	Several	2 wks
Locatelli 1996 [39]	105	54.8	71.4	5.7	Polysulfone	Cuprophane	2 yrs
Locatelli 2000 [47]	84	64.5	64.5	7	PMMA	Cellulose	12 wks
Ottosson 2001 [89]	42	69.1	57.1	14.3	Polyacrylonitrile	Cellulose diacetate	12 wks
Parker 1996 [51]	159	52.5	50	NR	PMMA	Cellulose	18 mos
Quereda 1998* [37]	8	58	25	0	Polyacrylonitrile	Cuprophan	48 sessions
Richardson 2003 [52]	90	61.5	63	NR	Polysulfone	Cellulose triacetate	7 mos
Schaefer 1993 [90]	10	57	70	NR	Polysulfone/AN69	Cuprophane	3 sessions
Schiffl 1995 [48]	24	51	60	0	Polysulfone	Cuprophane	6 yrs
Sklar 1998 [91]	21	61	56.2	43.7	PMMA	Cuprophane	1 wk
Skroeder 1994* [41]	20	61	80	0	Polyamide	Hemophane/cuprophane	36 sessions
Skroeder 1993* [38]	20	59	80	0	Polyamide	Cuprophane	88 sessions
Van Tellingen 2002 [43]	74	66	54	NR	Polysulfone	Cellulose Triacetate	12 wks
Van Tellingen 2004 [92]	10	NA	40	10	Polysulfone	Cellulose triacetate	12 wks
Vanholder 1992 [42]	15	NA	NA	NA	Polysulfone	Cuprophane	12 wks
Ward 1993 [93]	21	50.6	62	NA	AN69	Hemophan/cuprophan	2 wks
Ward 1997 [49]	37	55.6	77	NA	PMMA/Polycarbonate	Cuprophane/cellulose acetate	2 wks

Abbreviations: DM, diabetes mellitus; PAN, polyacrylonitrile; PMMA, polymethylmethacrylate.

[a] Asterisk indicates a study which excluded diabetic, populations.

[b] NR, not reported; data not available from the study report.

and flux rates on clinical outcomes and will be described separately below.

Biocompatibility

There were 32 RCTs included in a systematic review comparing cellulose-based membranes (unsubstituted and substituted or modified cellulose) with synthetic membranes (Tables 37.2–37.3) [30]. This review allows one to compare the risks for each of the major side effects attributable to differences in bioincompatibility of each dialyzer membrane type, more specifically, to evaluate the risk for hypotension, dialysis-associated symptoms, infection, β_2-microglobulin accumulation, hypoalbuminemia, increased protein catabolic rate, and mortality.

Hypotension

In this review, eight studies [31–38] reported data on dialysis-associated symptomatic hypotension or hypotension requiring treatment, but only one study [32] reported data that were suitable for meta-analysis. This study of 328 patients assessed the occurrence of intradialytic symptoms over one dialysis session in which the patient and the medical staff were blinded to the type of dialysis membrane. This RCT did not reveal any difference between patient groups. Similarly, none of the other seven studies reported a decrease in incidence of dialysis-related hypotension with the more biocompatible membranes. In one study that reported the composite occurrence of hypotension requiring treatment, symptomatic hypotension, and asymptomatic hypotension [39], there

Table 37.3 Results of the meta-analysis of RCTs comparing cellulose-based and synthetic membranes.

Outcome analyzed	No. of studies	No. of patients	Results RR (95% CI)	WMD (95% CI)
Dialysis sessions with symptomatic hypotension	1	328	1.22 (0.81–1.84)	
Patients with infections	1	15	0.16 (0.01–2.66)	
Mortality	3	468	1.63 (0.67–3.99)	
Kt/V (substituted cellulose vs. synthetic membranes)	1	20		0.20 (0.11–0.29)[a]
Kt/V (unsubstituted cellulose vs. synthetic membranes)	2	243		−0.10(−0.16 to −0.04)[b]
Predialysis β_2-microglobulin	4	407		−14.67(−33.40 to 4.05)
Total cholesterol (substituted cellulose vs. synthetic membranes)	1	39	–	0.60(−0.04 to 1.24)
Total cholesterol (unsubstituted cellulose vs. synthetic membranes)	1	28	–	−0.49(−1.07 to 0.09)
HDL cholesterol (substituted cellulose vs. synthetic membranes)	1	39	–	0.11 (−0.41 to 0.63)
HDL cholesterol (unsubstituted cellulose vs. synthetic membranes)	1	28	–	0.07 (−0.06 to 0.20)
Triglycerides (substituted cellulose vs. synthetic membranes)	1	39	–	−0.03(−0.43 to 0.37)
Triglycerides (substituted cellulose vs. synthetic membranes)	1	28	–	−0.06(−1.18 to −0.14)
Residual renal function at end of study period	1	30	–	1.10 (0.80 to 1.40)[b]
Average rate of loss of residual renal function	1	20	–	−0.13(−0.17 to −0.19)[b]

Abbreviation: HDL, high-density lipoprotein.

[a] Difference for this outcome significantly in favor of cellulose-based membranes ($P < 0.05$).

[b] Difference for this outcome significantly in favor of synthetric membranes ($P < 0.05$).

was no difference between those dialyzed with Cuprophane membranes and those dialyzed with either low- or high-flux polysulfone membranes. Similarly, another study reported intradialytic hypotension after 10% of treatments with cellulose compared to 11% with polysulfone membranes [40].

Dialysis-associated symptoms

Four trials [33,34,36,41] reported data on the occurrence of dialysis-associated symptoms, including headache, nausea and vomiting, and pruritus. All of these studies were of a crossover design. None reported significant differences between cellulose-based and synthetic membranes for dialysis-associated symptoms.

Infection

One study (15 patients) reported that 3 of 8 patients in the cellulose-based membrane group had infectious episodes compared with 0 of 7 patients in the synthetic membrane group [42]. Another study reported that 9 of 74 patients allotted to either polysulfone or cellulose triacetate membranes developed infections during a study period of 2 weeks [43], but it did not report to which treatment group the patients belonged or whether the between-group incidence of infection was significantly different.

β_2-Microglobulin

Seven trials measured predialysis β_2-microglobulin at the beginning and end of their studies [39,44–49]. The data from the four studies that could be combined by meta-analysis showed that the use of synthetic membranes was not associated with a significantly lower predialysis β_2-microglobulin level in comparison with cellulose membranes (WMD, −14.67, 95% CI, −33.10 to 4.05). There was evidence of significant heterogeneity between these four studies. Neither Hakim's nor Locatelli's team could demonstrate that β_2-microglobulin levels were lower with the use of a low-flux synthetic membrane compared with cellulose membranes [39,45]. However, in six of the seven studies the β_2-microglobulin values rose during the trials when cellulose membranes were used [44–49].

Serum albumin

Data from four trials [39,47,50,51] showed no difference in serum albumin levels between synthetic and cellulose membrane groups (WMD, 0.04; 95% CI −0.13 to 0.21). Parker showed a significantly higher mean serum albumin level in patients treated with synthetic membranes but only after 10 months of the study [51]; by study termination at 18 months there were no differences observed.

Protein catabolic rate

Three studies have reported data on protein catabolic rate as an outcome [39,47,52]. A meta-analysis that included two of these studies [39,47] showed no significant difference attributable to the membrane used (WMD, 0.10; 95% CI, −0.15 to 0.35). One study did not provide the means and standard deviations for the different membrane types but stated that no difference was found ($P = 0.94$) [52].

Mortality

None of the studies reported to date has been sufficiently powered to detect differences in mortality. Three studies that lasted more

Table 37.4 Patient characteristics and interventions in RCTs included in systematic review comparing high- and low-flux dialysis membranes.

Study ID [reference][a]	No. of patients	Mean age (yrs)	Gender (% males)	DM (%)	HTN (%)	Time on Dialysis (mean)	Interventions compared High-flux membrane	Low-flux membrane	Follow-up
Ayli 2004 [94]	48	59.1	54.2	22.9	10.4	46 mos	6 months	Polysulfone	6 mos
Bergamo 1991 [32]	328	56.4	50.8	5.5	NR[b]	78 mos	Polysulfone	Cuprophane	1 session
Blakestijn 1995 [50]*	28	NR	35.7	0 excluded	7.1	NR	Polysulfone	Cuprophane	6 wks
Bonomini 1996 [83]	10	53.4	70	NA	NR	NR	PMMA	Cellulose acetate	3 wks
Churchill 1992 [95]	30	52	59.1	9.1	22.7	3.9 yrs	Cellulose acetate	Cellulose Acetate	8 mos
Collins 1003 [33]	40	52.5	27.5	42.5	NR	NR	Polyacrylonitrile	Cuprophane	6 mos
Eknoyan 2002 [12]	1846	58	43.8	44.7	97.1	3.7 yrs	Several types	Several types	1–6.5 yrs
Gardinali 1994 [44]*	36	NR	63.9	0/NR	0/NR	77 mos	Polyacrylonitrile	Cuprophane	3 mos
Goldberg 1996 [87]	29	NR	NR	NR	NR	NR	Polysulfone	Cellulose Acetate	8 wks
Hartmann 1997 [35]*	20	51.5	30	0 excluded	0 excluded	NR	Polysulfone	Cellulose Acetate	1 yr
House 2000 [96]*	48	56.2	68.8	0 excluded	NA	9.5 mos	Polysulfone	Polysulfone	3 mos
Kuchle 1996 [54]	24	51	60	0	8.3	41 mos	Polysulfone	Cuprophane	6 yrs
Lang 2001 [40]	30	44	63.3	13.3	NR	NR	Polysulfone	Cuprophane	2 yrs
Locatelli 1996 [39]	105	54.8	71.4	5.7	NR	NR	Polysulfone	Cuprophane Polysulfone	2 yrs
Locatelli 2000 [47]	84	64.5	64.5	7	NR	3.8 yrs	PMMA	Cellulose	12 wks
Munger [97]	10	64.7	100	20	20	3.1 yrs	Polysulfone	Cuprammonium	8 sessions
Opatrny 2002 [98]*	25	70	52	0 excluded	NR	24 mos	Polysulfone	Polysulfone	16 wks
Ottosson 2001 [89]	42	69.1	57.1	14.3	NR	18.5 mos	Polyacrylonitrile	Cellulose diacetate	12 wks
Simon 1993 [53]	54	NR	50	NR	NR	NA	Polyacrylonitrile	Cuprophane	1 yr
Sirolli 2000 [99]	8	62.7	50	NR	NR	33.5 mos	PMMA	Cellulose diacetate	18 sessions
Skroeder 1994 [41]	20	61	80	0 excluded	NR	1.7 yrs	Polyamide	Hemophane Cuprophane	36 sessions

Abbreviation: DM, diabetes mellitus; HTN, hypertension; PMMA, polymethylmethacrylate.

[a] An asterisk after a study indicates diabetic population(s) was excluded.

[b] NR, not reported; data not available from the study report.

than 1 year, however, did report mortality [39,40,51]. All compared unsubstituted cellulose versus synthetic membranes, and none of these reported a difference in overall or cardiovascular mortality (overall mortality RR, 1.18; 95% CI, 0.63–2.22).

Membrane flux

A total of 22 RCTs were identified for a systematic review that forms the basis of the discussion in this section, comparing high-flux with low-flux HD (unpublished data) (Tables 37.4 and 37.5). The patient characteristics and interventions in the included RCTs are summarized in Table 37.4, and the results of the meta-analysis are in Table 37.5. This review excluded RCTs comparing HD with HF, HDF, or AFB, as these have been the subject of a separate review. Of these 22 RCTs, only the HEMO study was designed to assess the effect of dialysis membrane flux on mortality (Figure 37.1). This study had a two-by-two factorial design, comparing high-flux versus low-flux dialysis membranes and also conventional dialysis dose (equilibrated Kt/V, −1.05; single-pool Kt/V, −1.25) versus high dialysis dose (equilibrated Kt/V, −1.45; single-pool Kt/V, −1.65).

Mortality

At the end of the trial period in the HEMO study, 429 of 921 patients in the high-flux-group and 442 of 925 patients in the

low-flux group had died [12]. Although no significant difference in all-cause mortality between the patient groups was observed for the entire study period, use of high-flux dialysis membranes was found to reduce cardiovascular mortality and all-cause mortality significantly in patients who had been on dialysis for more than 3.7 years. In the systematic review (Table 37.4), the results from six trials that reported mortality data with a follow-up of 1 year or longer were analyzed. There was a trend toward a difference between high- and low-flux membrane groups even when the analysis was repeated, excluding the HEMO study (RR, 0.89; 95% CI, 0.71–1.13). A meta-analysis of two studies [12,53] showed no significant difference between patient groups for cardiovascular mortality (RR, 0.84; 95% CI, 0.69–1.02).

β$_2$-Microglobulin and dialysis amyloid-associated complications

High-flux HD has consistently been shown in randomized studies to achieve significantly lower predialysis β$_2$-microglobulin concentrations than low-flux dialysis (WMD, −13.50; 95% CI, −15.91 to −10.19). One randomized study of 20 patients followed for over 4 years showed that patients on high-flux dialysis had a significantly lower risk of developing dialysis-related arthropathy (0/10 in the high-flux group vs. 8/10 in the low-flux group; RR, 0.10; 95% CI, 0.00–0.90), but these results may reflect, in part,

Table 37.5 Results of meta-analysis of RCTs comparing high- and low-flux membranes.

Outcome analyzed	No. of studies	No. of patients	Results RR (95% CI)	WMD (95% CI)
All-cause mortality	6	2079	0.89 (0.71–1.13)	
Cardiovascular mortality	2	1900	0.84 (0.69–1.02)	
Infection-related mortality	2	1900	0.92 (0.71–1.19)	
Patients hospitalized	2	74	0.80 (0.52–1.23)	
Patients developing dialysis-related amyloid complications	1	20	0.06 (0.00–0.90)	
Patients experiencing hypotensive episodes during dialysis	2	412	1.24 (0.82–1.87	
Hospital admissions/year/patient	1	105		−2.00 (−12.68 to 8.68)
Predialysis β_2-microglobulin	4	199		−15.91 to −10.19)[a]
β_2- Microglobulin clearance rate (mL/min)	1	1846		30.40 (29.53 to 31.27)[a]
Urea reduction ratio	4	102		−0.03 (−3.18 to 3.13)
Kt/V	3	135		0.08 (−0.08 to 0.24)
Total cholesterol (mmol/L)	4	124		−0.16 (−0.59 to 0.27)
HDL cholesterol	3	109		0.09 (−0.25 to 0.43)
LDL cholesterol	3	109		0.09 (−0.25 to 0.43)
Triglycerides	3	79		−0.30 (−0.57 to −0.02)[a]

Abbreviations: HDL, high-density lipoprotein; LDL, low-density lipoprotein.
[a] Difference for this outcome significantly in favor of high-flux membranes ($P < 0.05$).

the higher-than-expected rate of arthropathy in the conventional dialysis group [54].

Lipid profile
High-flux dialyzers have been reported to have favorable effects on lipid profiles. Meta-analysis of four RCTs showed that high-flux HD resulted in a significant lowering of triglyceride levels alone compared with low-flux HD (Table 37.5). The clinical importance of this observation is not known.

Quality of life
Data from the HEMO study [55] showed that quality of life as measured using three validated tools, the Index of Well-Being, the

Kidney Diseases Quality of Life Long-Form Questionnaire, and the Short Form-36 Questionnaire, was not significantly different between patients on high-flux versus low-flux dialysis.

Extracorporeal RRT modalities

A Cochrane Systematic Review compared HD, HF, HDF, and AFB and identified 20 RCTs reporting clinically relevant outcomes [56] (Table 37.6). We have summarized below the results from this Cochrane Review for mortality, hypotension, β_2-microglobulin, dialysis-related amyloidosis, and quality of life. All results are shown in Table 37.7.

Review: High-Flux Versus Low-Flux membranes for end-stage disease (Versuib 06)
Comparison: 01 High-Flux Versus Low-Flux
Outcome: 01 Morality

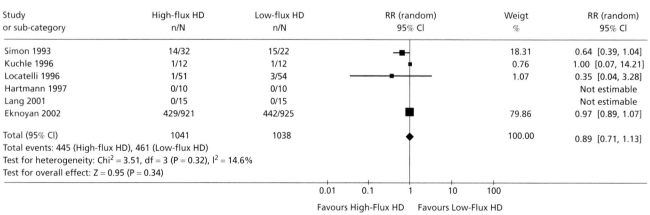

Study or sub-category	High-flux HD n/N	Low-flux HD n/N	RR (random) 95% CI	Weigt %	RR (random) 95% CI
Simon 1993	14/32	15/22		18.31	0.64 [0.39, 1.04]
Kuchle 1996	1/12	1/12		0.76	1.00 [0.07, 14.21]
Locatelli 1996	1/51	3/54		1.07	0.35 [0.04, 3.28]
Hartmann 1997	0/10	0/10			Not estimable
Lang 2001	0/15	0/15			Not estimable
Eknoyan 2002	429/921	442/925		79.86	0.97 [0.89, 1.07]
Total (95% CI)	1041	1038		100.00	0.89 [0.71, 1.13]

Total events: 445 (High-flux HD), 461 (Low-flux HD)
Test for heterogeneity: Chi^2 = 3.51, df = 3 (P = 0.32), I^2 = 14.6%
Test for overall effect: Z = 0.95 (P = 0.34)

0.01 0.1 1 10 100
Favours High-Flux HD   Favours Low-Flux HD

Figure 37.1 Effects of dialysis membrane flux on mortality.

Table 37.6 Patient characteristics and interventions in RCTs included in systematic review comparing the various extracorporeal RRT modalities.

Comparison	Study ID [reference]	No. of patients	Mean age (yrs)	Mean time on dialysis (mos)	Gender (% males)	DM (%)	Follow-up
HF vs. HD	Beerenhout 2005 [57]	40	58.5	28.5	75	NR	12 mos
	Fox 1993 [58]	9	63	54	100	NR	1 session
	Schiffl 1992 [59]	32	NR	NR	NR	NR	48 mos
HDF vs. HD	Bammens 2004 [60]	14	66.6	24.8	71.4	NR	2 wks
	Lin 2001 [61]	57	54	112.5	73.6	12.2	15 mos
	Locatelli 1996 [39]	205	52	NR	72.2	NR	24 mos
	Lornoy 2000 [62]	8	68	81	NA	NR	1 session
	Teo 1987 [63]	13	36.5	NR	40.3	NR	8 mos
	Tuccillo 2002 [64]	12	53	NR	58.3	NR	3 mos
	Ward 2000 [65]	50	56.5	57.5	58	13.3	12 mos
	Wizemann 2000 [66]	44	60.5	NR	56.8	18.2	24 mos
AFB vs. HD	Basile 2001 [67]	11	59.9	53.2	60	NR	12 mos
	Eiselt 2000 [68]	20	42.5	47.5	NA	NR	12 mos
	Noris 1998 [69]	5	57.6	NR	NA	NR	1 wk
	Schrander 1999 [70]	24	65	5.7	70	NR	12 mos
	Todeschini 2002 [71]	9	63.6	NR	33.3	22.2	3 sessions
	Verzetti 1998 [72]	41	60	25	41.4	100	12 mos
AFB vs. HDF	Ding 2002 [73]	12	49.7	83.5	66.6	NR	12 mos
	Movilli 1996 [74]	12	76	18	58.3	NR	6 mos
HF vs. HDF	Altieri 2004 [75]	39	58.4	NR	33.3	NR	1 yr

Abbreviations: DM, diabetes mellitus; NR, not reported (data not available from the study).

Table 37.7 Results of meta-analysis of RCTs comparing the various extracorporeal RRT modalities.

Comparison	Outcome analyzed	No. of studies	No. of patients	Results RR (95% CI)	Results WMD (95% CI)
HDF vs. HD	Mortality	3	316	1.68 (0.23–12.13)	
	Hospital admissions/patient/year	1	45		0.20 (−0.07 to 0.47)
	Hospitalization days	1	45		2.30 (−1.69 to 6.29)
	Predialysis β_2-microglobulin (HDF vs. low-flux HD)	4	407		−14.67(−33.40 to 4.05)[a]
	Predialysis β_2-microglobulin (HDF vs. low-flux HD)	1	39		0.60 (-0.04 to 1.24)
	Kt/V	1	28		−0.49(−1.07 to 0.09)
	Urea reduction ratio	1	39		0.11 (−0.41 to 0.63)
	Intradialytic blood pressure	1	28		0.07 (−0.06 to 0.20)[a]
	Maximal drop in blood pressure	1	39		−0.03(−0.43 to 0.37)[a]
	Triglycerides (substituted cellulose vs. synthetic membranes)	1	28		−0.06(−1.18 to −0.14)
AFB vs. HD	Mortality	2	40	Not estimable, as no event during study period	1.10 (0.80 to 1.40)
	Dialysis sessions complicated by hypotension (%)	1	20		−5.40(−23.71 to 12.91)
	Kt/V	1	20		0.12 (−0.09 to 0.33)
	Mean arterial pressure during dialysis	1	20		1.60 (−12.63 to 15.83)

[a] Difference for this outcome significantly in favor of HDF ($P < 0.05$).

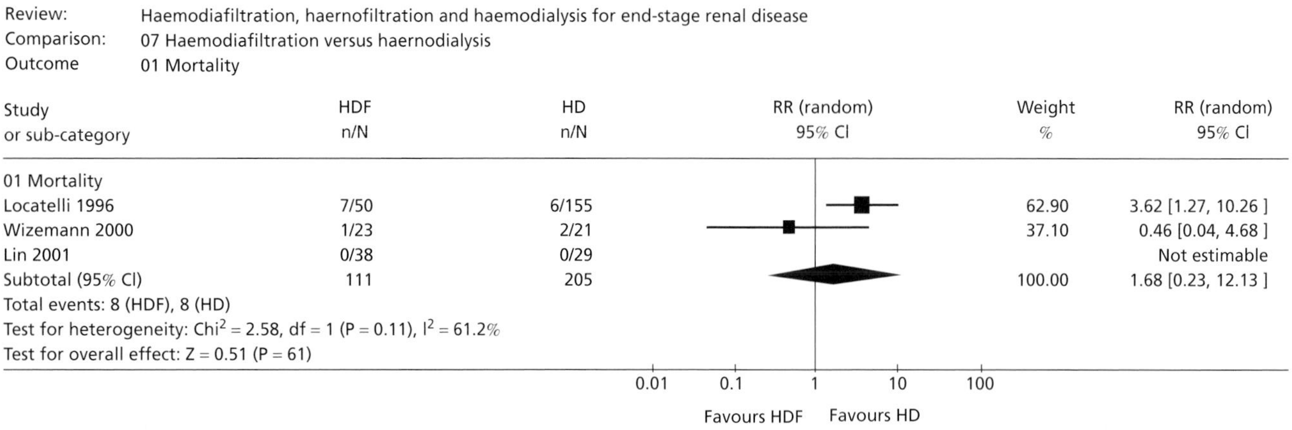

Review: Haemodiafiltration, haernofiltration and haemodialysis for end-stage renal disease
Comparison: 07 Haemodiafiltration versus haernodialysis
Outcome   01 Mortality

Study or sub-category	HDF n/N	HD n/N	RR (random) 95% CI	Weight %	RR (random) 95% CI
01 Mortality					
Locatelli 1996	7/50	6/155		62.90	3.62 [1.27, 10.26]
Wizemann 2000	1/23	2/21		37.10	0.46 [0.04, 4.68]
Lin 2001	0/38	0/29			Not estimable
Subtotal (95% CI)	111	205		100.00	1.68 [0.23, 12.13]

Total events: 8 (HDF), 8 (HD)
Test for heterogeneity: Chi^2 = 2.58, df = 1 (P = 0.11), I^2 = 61.2%
Test for overall effect: Z = 0.51 (P = 61)

0.01   0.1   1   10   100

Favours HDF   Favours HD

Figure 37.2 Effects of RRT modality on mortality (HDF vs. HD).

HF versus HD

Three RCTs compared HF with HD [57–59]. One study of 32 patients (24 HD vs. 8 HF) followed for 4 years reported no deaths [59]. Furthermore, there was no difference in the number of episodes of hypotension between patient groups in one crossover study of nine patients [58]. This study's duration, however, was only one dialysis session. In the study by Schiffl et al. HF was associated with significantly higher β_2-microglobulin levels in the ultrafiltrate compared with high-flux HD, and there was virtually no β_2-microglobulin detected in the dialysate of patients on low-flux HD when Cuprophane membranes were used [59]. The implications of these findings for clinically important outcomes, especially in light of current practices, are unknown.

HDF versus HD

Eight RCTs compared HDF with HD [39,60–66]. Mortality data were obtained from three studies [39,61,66]. A meta-analysis of these studies showed no difference between patient groups (RR, 1.68; 95% CI, 0.23–12.13) (Figure 37.2). The largest RCT [39] comparing HD with HDF had four treatment arms. Mortality was not different when any of the three HD arms was compared separately with HDF; a comparison of the three combined HD groups with the HDF group indicated a higher mortality with HDF (6/155 in the HD group vs. 7/50 in the HDF group; RR, 3.62; 95% CI, 1.27–10.26); this result should be interpreted with caution, as this study was not designed to assess mortality [39]. None of the studies assessed the incidence of symptomatic hypotension, but one study reported that the intradialytic blood pressure was significantly higher and the maximal drop in intradialytic blood pressure lower in patients on HDF [61]. Based on data from two studies, HDF was reported to be associated with significantly lower predialysis β_2-microglobulin values compared with low-flux but not with high-flux HD [39,66]. None of the studies reported data on the incidence of dialysis-related amyloid arthropathy. Two further studies [61,65] reported quality of life results. One study [65] used a validated tool, the Kidney Diseases Questionnaire, and the other used a nonvalidated tool, the Patient Well-Being Score [61].

Patients on HDF had significantly higher end-of-treatment Patient Well-Being scores, whereas no significant difference was found when quality of life was assessed with the Kidney Diseases Questionnaire, with the exception of the physical symptoms component of this tool, which showed that quality of life improved equally with either modality during the course of the study.

AFB versus HD

Six RCTs compared HD versus AFB [67–72]. Data from two studies of 12 months or greater in duration did not report any patient deaths in either RRT group [68,70]. One study of 20 patients found no significant difference in the number of hypotensive episodes in patients undergoing either of these RRT modalities [70]. The remaining studies had crossover designs and hence did not provide mortality data for analysis. None of the studies reported any data on β_2-microglobulin levels.

AFB versus HDF

Two RCTs assessed AFB versus HDF in a total of 24 patients [73,74]. Both were crossover trials and hence the data could only be summarized in a narrative fashion. There was no difference in the number of dialysis sessions for patients reported to have hypotension between patient groups (HDF, 10/72 sessions, vs. AFB, 9/72 sessions). Data on mortality could not be analyzed from these crossover studies. No data on β_2-microglobulin levels were reported.

HF versus HDF

A comparison of HF versus HDF was performed in one RCT [75]. Patients on HF experienced significantly fewer episodes of hypotension per patient per month (HF, 0.5 vs. HDF, 1.1; $P = 0.017$) if they were randomized to start on HDF and crossed over to HF. Predialysis β_2-microglobulin values were also not significantly different between patient groups. Long-term clinical outcomes, such as mortality and cardiovascular morbidity, could not be assessed in this crossover design trial.

Critique of the evidence and guidelines

There are considerable data from observational studies indicating that biocompatible high-flux HD and convective technologies, compared with HD with low-flux cellulose-based membranes, are associated with significant reductions in adverse outcomes, the most important of which are mortality, dialysis-associated amyloid complications, and dialysis-related side effects such as hypotension. The data from RCTs, however, are less compelling.

Of all the RCTS conducted in this area, only the HEMO study was designed with sufficient statistical power to evaluate differences in mortality outcomes for high- and low-flux and high- and low-efficiency dialysis prescriptions. This study did not show any statistically significant differences in mortality between groups. It has, however, been criticized for several reasons, including the use of prevalent rather than incident patients, exclusion of patients over 100 kg in weight, dialyzer reuse, and overrepresentation of women and blacks (both over 60% of the study population). There remains uncertainty, therefore, over the impact of membrane type and flux characteristics on outcomes in HD.

Although cellulose-based membranes elicit more of an inflammatory response than synthetic membranes and therefore could theoretically cause more dialysis-related side effects, none of the RCTs that have examined this question has shown a consistent difference in dialysis-related symptoms with the different membrane types. Thus, an increase in dialysis membrane-related inflammatory responses does not result in predictable adverse clinical symptoms in the short term, nor is it associated with long-term increases in mortality. Whether such inflammation is injurious in the long term remains unknown.

Convective technologies when compared to HD appear in observational studies to result in lower rates of dialysis-related hypotension. Importantly, however, this has not been demonstrated in any of the RCTs that have compared convective technologies to HD. One recent RCT, published after the Cochrane Review, showed that when HD is performed under optimal conditions the hemodynamic parameters and the incidence of hypotension are the same as in HDF [76]. A review of the effects of extracorporeal techniques on blood pressure-related outcomes reached the same conclusion [77]; the authors emphasized that future trials comparing HF and HDF with HD must ensure standardized treatment conditions so that comparisons of the outcomes of the various treatment modalities will be valid.

Even less information is available regarding the impact of membrane type on dialysis-associated amyloidosis. The few published studies were small and generally of too short a duration to draw firm conclusions regarding an outcome that is both uncommon (5–10% of patients at 5 years, 15–30% of patients at 10 years) [78,79] and develops slowly over a period too long for most clinical trials. Although further large observational studies may clarify some of these residual questions, the quality of such evidence is poorer than that which arises from RCTs and will undoubtedly leave uncertainty.

Although some clinical practice guidelines continue to prefer the use of biocompatible membranes, such recommendations are based mostly on opinion rather than RCT evidence. For high-flux membranes, the EBPG [21] recommend their use in all patients whereas the Renal Association (UK) recommends their use in incident patients likely to be on dialysis for several years or prevalent patients who have been on dialysis for more than 3.7 years [20]. The Renal Association (UK) guidelines suggest that HF or HDF may also be beneficial in patients likely to be on dialysis for several years or for long-term prevalent patients, because of improved middle-molecule clearance with these techniques [20]. However, RCTs have not shown HDF to be superior to HD, especially in comparison to high-flux HD. Although HDF may be better than HD in reducing predialysis β_2-microglobulin levels, it is not superior to high-flux HD in this regard. None of the RCTs has shown a significant reduction in dialysis-related hypotension or other symptoms with HDF versus HD.

Conclusions

Despite more than 40 years of experience with RRT, it is surprising and disappointing that the evidence base on which important clinical decisions hinge is not more solid. Several studies have important design flaws, are of insufficient statistical power, or have not addressed appropriate clinical end points. There is a clear need for additional clinical trials that lack these limitations to provide unambiguous guidance for decision making. Future studies must also address important clinical end points, such as mortality, morbidity, and quality of life, and should ideally include rigorous economic evaluations, given the expense of extracorporeal therapies.

At present there are a number of large studies under way that may help to address some of the current deficiencies. The Membranes Permeability Outcomes study is a multicenter study evaluating high- versus low-flux membranes in 600 incident patients (<2 months on RRT) [80]. The CONTRAST study will compare HDF versus low-flux HD in 800 patients and will include a detailed economic evaluation [81]. Another RCT will assess cardiovascular stability and blood pressure control in 246 patients assigned to either HDF or HF compared to low-flux HD [82]. It is hoped that the results of such studies will provide more solid evidence to inform best clinical practices.

References

1 ERA-EDTA Registry. 2003 Annual Report. Academic Medical Center, Amsterdam, the Netherlands, May 2005. http://www.era-edta-reg.org/files/annualreports/pdf/AnnRep2003.pdf.

2 Frei U, Schober-Halstenberg H-J. *Renal Replacement Therapy in Germany*. Annual report 2003/2004. http://quasi-niere.de/english/report/03/world.html.

3 Frei U, Schober-Halstenberg H-J. *Renal Replacement Therapy in Germany.* Annual report 2001/2002. http://www.quasi-niere.de/english/download/reports/Report_2001_2002.pdf.

4 Craddock PR, Fehr J, Dalmasso AP, Brighan KL, Jacob HS. Hemodialysis leukopenia. Pulmonary vascular leukostasis resulting from complement activation by dialyzer cellophane membranes. *J Clin Invest* 1977; **59:** 879–888.

5 Hakim R, Fearon D, Lazarus J. Biocompatibility of dialysis membranes: effects of chronic complement activation. *Kidney Int* 1984; **26:** 194–200.

6 Lonnenman G, Haubitz M, Schindler R. Hemodialysis-associated induction of cytokines. *Blood Purif* 1990; **8:** 214–222.

7 Himmelfarb J, Hakim RM. Biocompatibility and risk of infection in hemodialysis patients. *Nephrol Dial Transplant* 1994; **9(Suppl 2):** S138–S144.

8 De Broe ME. Hemodialysis induced hypoxemia. *Nephrol Dial Transplant* 1994; **9(Suppl 2):** 173–175.

9 Vanholder R, Ringoir S, Dhondt A, Hakim R. Phagocytosis in uremic and hemodialysis patients: a prospective and crossover study. *Kidney Int* 1991; **39:** 320–327.

10 Descamps-Latscha B, Herbelin A. Long-term dialysis and cellular immunity: a critical survey. *Kidney Int Suppl* 1993; **41:** S135–S142.

11 Horl WH, Riegel W, Steinhauer HB, Wanner C, Schollmeyer P, Schaefer R *et al.* Plasma levels of granulocytic components during hemodialysis. *Contrib Nephrol* 1987; **59:** 35–43.

12 Eknoyan G, Beck GJ, Cheung AK, Daugirdas JT, Greene T, Kusek JW *et al.* Effect of dialysis dose and membrane flux in maintenance hemodialysis. *N Eng J Med* 2002; **347(25):** 2010.

13 US Food and Drug Administration. Guidance for the content of premarket notifications for conventional and high permeability hemodialyzers. http://www.fda.gov/cdrh/ode/80.html.

14 Locatelli F, Di Filippo S, Manzoni C. Removal of small and middle molecules by convective techniques. *Nephrol Dial Transplant* 2000; **15(Suppl 2):** 37–44.

15 Schmidt M. Haemodiafiltration. In: *Haemofiltration.* Springer, Berlin, 1986; 265–271.

16 Daugirdas JT. Dialysis hypotension: a hemodynamic analysis. *Kidney Int* 1991; **39(2):** 233–246.

17 Zucchelli P, Santoro A, Ferrari G, Spongano M. Acetate-free biofiltration: hemodiafiltration with base-free dialysate. *Blood Purif* 1990; **8(1):** 14–22.

18 Caring for Australians with Renal Impairment (CARI). Guidelines: Dialysis Membranes. http://www.cari.org.au/dialysis_membranes_jul-2005.pdf.

19 National Kidney Foundation. Kidney Diseases Quality Outcomes Initiative guidelines: dialyzer membrane and reuse. http://www.kidney.org/professionals/KDOQI /guideline_upHD_PD_VA/hd_rec5.htm.

20 Renal Association (UK). Guidelines: Haemodialysis membranes. http://www.renal.org /guidelines/module3a.html#Membranes.

21 European Best Practice Guidelines for haemodialysis, part 1. *Nephrol Dial Transplant* 2002; **17(Suppl 7):** 34–37.

22 Woods HF, Nandakumar M. Improved outcomes for haemodialysis patients treated with high-flux membranes. *Nephrol Dial Transplant* 2001; **15(Suppl 1):** 36–42.

23 Hornberger JC, Chernew M, Petersen J, Garber AM. A multivariate analysis of mortality and hospital admissions with high-flux dialysis. *J Am Soc Nephrol* 1992; **3:** 1227–1237.

24 Hakim RM, Held PJ, Stannard DC, Wolfe RA, Port FK, Daugirdas JT *et al.* Effect of the dialysis membrane on mortality of chronic hemodialysis patients. *Kidney Int* 1996; **50(2):** 566–570.

25 Port FK, Wolfe RA, Hulbert-Shearon TE, Daugirdas JT, Agodoa LYC, Jones C *et al.* Mortality risk by hemodialyzer reuse practice and dialyzer membrane characteristics: results from the USRDS Dialysis Morbidity and Mortality Study. *Am J Kidney Dis* 2001; **37(2):** 276–286.

26 Locatelli F, Marcelli D, Conte F, Limido A, Malberti F, Spotti D. Comparison of mortality in ESRD patients on convective and diffusive extracorporeal treatments. *Kidney Int* 1999; **55(1):** 286–293.

27 Koda Y, Nishi S-I, Miyazaki S, Haginoshita S, Sakurabayashi T, Suzuki M *et al.* Switch from conventional to high-flux membrane reduces the risk of carpal tunnel syndrome and mortality of hemodialysis patients. *Kidney Int* 1997; **52(4):** 1096–1101.

28 Chanard J, Brunois JP, Melin JP, Lavaud S. Long-term results of dialysis therapy with a highly permeable membrane. *Artif Organs* 1982; **6(3):** 261–266.

29 Altieri P, Sorba G, Bolasco P, Asproni E, Ledebo I, Cossu M *et al.* Predilution haemofiltration: the Second Sardinian Multicentre Study. Comparisons between haemofiltration and haemodialysis during identical Kt/V and session times in a long-term cross-over study. *Nephrol Dial Transplant* 2001; **16(6):** 1207–1213.

30 MacLeod AM, Campbell M, Cody JD, Daly C, Donaldson C, Grant A *et al.* Cellulose, modified cellulose and synthetic membranes in the haemodialysis of patients with end-stage renal disease. *Cochrane Database Syst Rev* 2005; **3:** CD003234.

31 Aakhus S, Bjoernstad K, Jorstad S. Systemic cardiovascular response in hemodialysis without and with ultrafiltration with membranes of high and low biocompatibility. *Blood Purif* 1995; **13(5):** 229–240.

32 Bergamo Coopertaive Dialysis Study. Acute intradialytic well-being: results of a clinical trial comparing polysulfone with cuprophan. *Kidney Int* 1991; **40(4):** 714–719.

33 Collins DM, Lambert MB, Tannenbaum JS, Oliverio M, Schwab SJ. Tolerance of hemodialysis: a randomized prospective trial of high-flux versus conventional high-efficiency hemodialysis. *J Am Soc Nephrol* 1993; **4(2):** 148–154.

34 Danielson BG, Hallgren R, Venge P. Patient reactions and granulocyte degranulation during hemodialysis with cuprophane and polycarbonate membranes. A double-blind study. *Blood Purif* 1986; **4(1–3):** 147–150.

35 Hartmann J, Fricke H, Schiffl H. Biocompatible membranes preserve residual renal function in patients undergoing regular hemodialysis. *Am J Kidney Dis* 1997; **30(3):** 366–373.

36 Levin NW, Zasuwa G. Relationship between dialyser type and signs and symptoms. *Nephrol Dial Transplant* 1993; **8(Suppl 2):** 30–39.

37 Quereda C, Orofino L, Marcen R, Sabater J, Matesanz R, Ortuno J. Influence of dialysate and membrane biocompatibility on hemodynamic stability in hemodialysis. *Int J Artif Organs* 1988; **11(4):** 259–264.

38 Skroeder NR, Jacobson SH, Holmquist B, Kjellstrand P, Kjellstrand CM. Beta 2-microglobulin generation and removal in long slow and short fast hemodialysis. *Am J Kidney Dis* 1993; **21(5):** 519–526.

39 Locatelli F, Mastrangelo F, Redaelli B, Ronco C, Marcelli D, LaGreca G *et al.* Effects of different membranes and dialysis technologies on patient treatment tolerance and nutritional parameters. The Italian Cooperative Dialysis Study Group. *Kidney Int* 1996; **50(4):** 1293–1302.

40 Lang SM, Bergner A, Topfer M, Schiffl H. Preservation of residual renal function in dialysis patients: effects of dialysis-technique-related factors. *Perit Dial Int* 2001; **21:** 52–57.

41 Skroeder NR, Jacobson SH, Lins LE, Kjellstrand CM. Acute symptoms during and between hemodialysis: the relative role of speed, duration, and biocompatibility of dialysis. *Artif Organs* 1994; **18:** 880–887.

42 Vanholder R, Van Landschoot N, Waterloos MA, Delanghe J, Van Maele G, Ringoir S. Phagocyte metabolic activity during hemodialysis with different dialyzers not affecting the number of circulating phagocytes. *Int J Artif Organs* 1992; **15(2):** 89–92.

43 Van Tellingen A, Grooteman MPC, Schoorl M, Bartels PCM, Schoorl M, van der Ploeg T *et al.* Intercurrent clinical events are predictive of plasma C-reactive protein levels in hemodialysis patients. *Kidney Int* 2002; **62(2):** 632–638.

44 Gardinali M, Calcagno A, Conciato L, Agostoni A, Rosti A, Cori P *et al.* Complement activation in dialysis: effects on cytokines, lymphocyte activation and beta 2 microglobulin. *Int J Artif Organs* 1994; **17(6):** 337–344.

45 Hakim RM, Wingard RL, Husni L, Parker RA, Parker TF. The effect of membrane biocompatibility on plasma beta 2-microglobulin levels in chronic hemodialysis patients. *J Am Soc Nephrol* 1996; **7(3):** 472–478.

46 Hosokawa S, Yoshida O. Removal of silicon, aluminum and beta

47 microglobulin in chronic haemodialysis patients. *Int Urol Nephrol* 1991; **23(3):** 281–284.

48 Locatelli F, Andrulli S, Pecchini F, Pedrini L, Agliata S, Lucchi L *et al.* Effect of high-flux dialysis on the anaemia of haemodialysis patients. *Nephrol Dial Transplant* 2000; **15(9):** 1399–1409.

49 Schiffl H, Kuchle C, Held E. Beta-2-microglobulin removal by different hemodialysis membranes. *Contrib Nephrol* 1995; **112:** 156–163.

50 Ward RA, Buscaroli A, Schmidt B, Stefoni S, Gurland HJ, Klinkman H. A comparison of dialysers with low-flux membranes: significant differences in spite of many similarities. *Nephrol Dial Transplant* 1997; **12(5):** 965–972.

51 Blankestijn PJ, Vos PF, Rabelink TJ, Van Rijn HJM, Jansen H, Koomans HA. High-flux dialysis membranes improve lipid profile in chronic hemodialysis patients. *J Am Soc Nephrol* 1995; **5(9):** 1703–1708.

52 Parker TF, III, Wingard RL, Husni L, Ikizler A, Parker RA, Hakim RM. Effect of the membrane biocompatibility on nutritional parameters in chronic hemodialysis patients. *Kidney Int* 1996; **49(2):** 551–556.

53 Richardson D, Lindley EJ, Bartlett C, Will EJ. A randomized, controlled study of the consequences of hemodialysis membrane composition on erythropoeitic response. *Am J Kidney Dis* 2003; **42(3):** 551–560.

54 Simon P, Ang KS, Cam G, Benziane A, Bonn F. Indices of adequate dialysis in patients hemolyzed with AN 69 membrane. *Kidney Int* 1993; **43(Suppl 41):** S291–S295.

55 Kuchle C, Fricke H, Held E, Schiffl H. High-flux hemodialysis postpones clinical manifestation of dialysis associated amyloidosis. *Am J Nephrol* 1996; **16(6):** 484–488.

56 Unruh M, Benz R, Greene T, Yan G, Beddhu S, DeVita M *et al.* Effects of hemodialysis dose and membrane flux on health-related quality of life in the HEMO Study. *Kidney Int* 2004; **66:** 355–366.

57 Rabindranath KS, Strippoli GF, Daly C, Roderick PJ, Wallace S, MacLeod AM. Haemodiafiltration, haemofiltration and haemodialysis for end-stage kidney disease. *Cochrane Database Syst Rev* 2006; **4:** CD006258.

58 Beerenhout CH, Luik AJ, Jeuken-Mertens SG, Bekers O, Menheere P, Hover L *et al.* Pre-dilution on-line haemofiltration vs low-flux haemodialysis: a randomized prospective study. *Nephrol Dial Transplant* 2005; **20(6):** 1155–1163.

59 Fox SD, Henderson LW. Cardiovascular response during hemodialysis and hemofiltration: thermal, membrane and catecholamine influences. *Blood Purif* 1993; **11(4):** 224–236.

60 Schiffl H, D'Agostini B, Held E. Removal of beta-2 microglobulin by hemodialysis and hemofiltration: a four year follow-up. *Biomat Artif Cells Immobilization Biotechnol* 1992; **20(5):** 1223–1232.

61 Bammens B, Evenepoel P, Verbeke K, Vanrenterghem Y. Removal of the protein-bound solute p-cresol by convective transport: a randomized crossover study. *Am J Kidney Dis* 2004; **44(2):** 278–285.

62 Lin CL, Huang CC, Chang CT, Wu MS, Hung CC, Chien CC *et al.* Clinical improvement by increased frequency of on-line hemodiafiltration. *Ren Fail* 2001; **23(2):** 193–206.

63 Lornoy W, Becaus I, Billiouw JM, Sierens L, Van Malderen P, D'Haenens P. On-line haemodiafiltration: remarkable removal of β2-microglobulin. Long-term clinical observations. *Nephrol Dial Transplant* 2000; **15(Suppl 1):** 49–54.

64 Teo KK, Basile C, Ulan RA, Hetherington MD, Kappagoda T. Effects of hemodialysis and hypertonic hemodiafiltration on cardiac function compared. *Kidney Int* 1987; **32(3):** 399–407.

65 Tuccillo S, Bellizzi V, Catapano F, Di Iorio B, Esposito L, Giannattasio P *et al.* Acute and chronic effects of standard hemodialysis and soft hemodiafiltration on interdialytic serum phosphate levels. *G Ital Nefrol* 2002; **49(4):** 439–445.

66 Ward RA, Schmidt B, Hullin J, Hillebrand GF, Samtleben W. A comparison of on-line hemodiafiltration and high-flux hemodialysis: a prospective clinical study. *J Am Soc Nephrol* 2000; **11(12):** 2344–2350.

67 Wizemann V, Lotz C, Techert F, Uthoff S. On-line haemodiafiltration versus low-flux haemodialysis. A prospective randomized study. *Nephrol Dial Transplant* 2000; **15(Suppl 1):** 43–48.

68 Basile C, Giordano R, Montanaro A, De Maio PD, De Padova FD, Marangi AL *et al.* Effect of acetate-free biofiltration on the anaemia of haemodialysis patients: a prospective cross-over study. *Nephrol Dial Transplant* 2001; **16(9):** 1914–1919.

69 Eiselt J, Racek J, Opatrny K, Jr. The effect of hemodialysis and acetate-free biofiltration on anemia. *Int J Artif Organs* 2000; **23(3):** 173–180.

70 Noris M, Todeschini M, Casiraghi F, Roccatello D, Martina G, Minetti L *et al.* Effect of acetate, bicarbonate dialysis and acetate free biofiltration on nitric oxide synthesis: implications for dialysis hypotension. *Am J Kidney Dis* 1998; **32(1):** 115–124.

71 Schrander-vd Meer AM, ter Wee PM, Kan G, Donker AJ, van Dorp WT. Improved cardiovascular variables during acetate free biofiltration. *Clin Nephrol* 1999; **51(5):** 304–309.

72 Todeschini M, Macconi D, Fernandez NG, Ghilardi M, Anabaya A, Binda E *et al.* Effect of acetate-free biofiltration and bicarbonate hemodialysis on neutrophil activation. *Am J Kidney Dis* 2002; **40(4):** 783–793.

73 Verzetti G, Navino C, Bolzani R, Galli G, Panzetta G. Acetate-free biofiltration versus bicarbonate haemodialysis in the treatment of patients with diabetic nephropathy: a cross-over multicentric study. *Nephrol Dial Transplant* 1998; **13(4):** 955–961.

74 Ding F, Ahrenholz P, Winkler RE, Ramlow W, Tiess M, Michelsen A *et al.* Online hemodiafiltration versus acetate-free biofiltration: a prospective crossover study. *Artif Organs* 2002; **26(2):** 169–180.

75 Movilli E, Camerini C, Zein H, D'Avolio G, Sandrini M, Strada A *et al.* A prospective comparison of bicarbonate dialysis, hemodiafiltration, and acetate-free biofiltration in the elderly. *Am J Kidney Dis* 1996; **27(4):** 541–547.

76 Altieri P, Sorba G, Bolasco P, Ledebo I, Ganadu M, Ferrara R *et al.* Comparison between hemofiltration and hemodiafiltration in a long-term prospective cross-over study. *J Nephrol* 2004; **17(3):** 414–422.

77 Karamperis N, Sloth E, Jensen JD. Predilution hemodiafiltration displays no hemodynamic advantage over low-flux hemodialysis under matched conditions. *Kidney Int* 2005; **67:** 1601–1608.

78 Maggiore Q, Pizzarelli F, Dattolo P, Maggiore U, Cerrai T. Cardio-vascular stability during haemodialysis, haemofiltration and haemodi-afiltration. *Nephrol Dial Transplant* 2000; **15(Suppl 1):** 68–73.

79 Charra B, Calemard E, Laurent G. Chronic renal failure treatment du-ration and mode: their relevance to the late dialysis periarticular syn-drome. *Blood Purif* 1988; **6:** 1117–1124.

80 Schwarz A, Keller F, Seyfert S, Poll W, Molzahn M, Distler A. Carpal tunnel syndrome: a major complication in long-term hemodialysis pa-tients. *Clin Nephrol* 1984; **22:** 133–137.

81 Locatelli F, Hannadouche T, Jacobson T, La Greca G, Loureiro A, Martin-Malo A *et al.* The effect of membrane permeability on ESRD: de-sign of a prospective randomised multicentre trial. *J Nephrol* 1999; **12:** 85–88.

82 Lars Penne E, Blankestijn PJ, Bots ML, van den Dorpel MA, Grooteman MPC, Nubé MJ, ter Wee PM *et al.* Resolving controversies regarding hemodiafiltration versus hemodialysis: the Dutch Convective Transport Study. *Semin Dial* 2005; **18(1):** 47–51.

83 Bolasco P, Alteiri P, Andrulli S, Basile C, Di Filippo S, Feriani M *et al.* Convection versus diffusion in dialysis: an Italian prospective multicen-tre study. *Nephrol Dial Transplant* 2003; **18(Suppl 7):** vii50–vii54.

84 Bonomini M, Fiederling B, Bucciarelli T, Manfrini V, Di Ilio C, Alber-tazzi A. A new polymethylmethacrylate membrane for hemodialysis. *Int J Artif Organs* 1996; **19(4):** 232–239.

85 Caramelo C, Alcazar R, Gallar P, Teruel JL, Velo M, Ortego O *et al.* Choice of dialysis membrane does not influence the outcome of residual renal function in haemodialysis patients. *Nephrol Dial Transplant* 1994; **9(6):** 675–677.

86 Ferreira A, Ghazali A, Galvao J, Souberbielle JC, Jehle PM, Mohan S *et al.* Effect of type of dialysis membrane on bone in haemodialysis patients. *Nephrol Dial Transplant* 2001; **16(6):** 1230–1238.

87 Girndt M, Lengler S, Kaul H, Sester U, Sester M, Kohler H. Prospective crossover trial of the influence of vitamin E-coated dialyzer membranes on T-cell activation and cytokine induction. *Am J Kidney Dis* 2000; **35(1):** 95–104.

88 Goldberg IJ, Kaufman AM, Lavaris VA, Vanni-Reyes T, Levin NW. High flux dialysis membranes improve plasma lipoprotein profiles in patients with end-stage renal disease. *Nephrol Dial Transplant* 1996; **11(Suppl 2):** 104–107.

89 Grooteman MP, Nube MJ, van Limbeek J, van Houte AJ, Daha MR, van Geelen JA. Biocompatibility and performance of a modified cellulosic and a synthetic high flux dialyzer. A randomized crossover comparison between cellulose triacetate and polysulphon. *ASAIO J* 1995; **41(2):** 215–220.

90 Ottosson P, Attman PO, Knight C, Samuelsson O, Weiss L, Alaupovic P. Do high-flux dialysis membranes affect renal dyslipidemia? *ASAIO J* 2001; **47(3):** 229–234.

91 Schaefer RM, Fink E, Schaefer L, Barkhausen R, Kulzer P, Heidland A. Role of bradykinin in anaphylactoid reactions during hemodialysis with AN69 dialyzers. *Am J Nephrol* 1993; **13(6):** 473–477.

92 Sklar AH, Beezhold DH, Newman N, Hendrickson T, Dreisbach AW. Postdialysis fatigue: lack of effect of a biocompatible membrane. *Am J Kidney Dis* 1998; **31(6):** 1007–1010.

93 Van Tellingen A, Grooteman MPC, Schoorl M, ter Wee PM, Bartels PCM, Schoorl M *et al.* Enhanced long-term reduction of plasma leptin concentrations by super-flux polysulfone dialysers. *Nephrol Dial Trans-plant* 2004; **19(5):** 1198–1203.

94 Ward RA, Schaefer RM, Falkenhagen D, Joshua MS, Heidland A, Klinkmann H *et al.* Biocompatibility of a new high-permeability mod-ified cellulose membrane for haemodialysis. *Nephrol Dial Transplant* 1993; **8(1):** 47–53.

95 Ayli D, Ayli M, Azak A, Yuksel C, Kosmaz GP, Atilgan G *et al.* The effect of high-flux hemodialysis on renal anemia. *J Nephrol* 2004; **17:** 701–706.

96 Churchill DN, Bird DR, Taylor DW, Beecroft ML, Gorman J, Wallace JE. Effect of high-flux hemodialysis on quality of life and neuropsycho-logical function in chronic hemodialysis patients. *Am J Nephrol* 1992; **12:** 412–418.

97 House AA, Wells GA, Donnelly JG, Nadler SP, Hebert PC. Randomized trial of high-flux vs low-flux haemodialysis: effects on homocysteine and lipids. *Nephrol Dial Transplant* 2000; **15:** 1029–1034.

98 Munger MA, Ateshkadi A, Cheung AK, Flaharty KK, Stoddard GJ, Mar-shall EH, Cardiopulmonary events during hemodialysis: effects of dialy-sis membranes and dialysate buffers. *Am J Kidney Dis* 2000; **36:** 130–139.

99 Opatrny K, Jr., Reischig T, Vienken J, Eiselt J, Vit L, Opatrna S *et al.* Does treatment modality have an impact on anemia in patients with chronic renal failure? Effect of low- and high-flux biocompatible dialysis. *Artif Organs* 2002; **26:** 181–188.

100 Sirolli V, Di Sante S, Stuard S, Di Liberato L, Amoroso L, Cappelli P *et al.* Biocompatibility and functional performance of a polyethylene glycol acid-grafted cellulosic membrane for hemodialysis. *Int J Artif Organs* 2000; **23:** 356–364.

38 Dialysis Delivery and Adequacy

Peter Kotanko,[1,2] **Nathan W. Levin,**[2] **& Frank Gotch**[2]

[1] Krankenhaus der Barmherzigen Brüder, Department of Internal Medicine, Graz, Austria
[2] Renal Research Institute, New York, USA

Introduction

It is generally accepted that the delivery of "adequate" or optimal dialysis is associated with improved survival, where adequacy is sometimes defined as that intensity of dialysis that results in the generally most favorable mortality and morbidity outcomes. Findings that have emerged from observational studies and epidemiologic comparisons between countries have suggested that some of the differences in mortality rates observed between countries may be attributable to country-specific differences in customary prescriptions for dialysis dose. These observations have led to a consensus opinion that is reflected in US, UK, European, Canadian, and Australian guidelines that dialysis dose be measured and an adequate dose of dialysis be targeted in all patients on chronic hemodialysis. Kinetic modeling has proven a powerful tool to define the parameters of adequate dialysis, to compare dialysis dosing from one study to the next, and to identify those aspects of the dialysis treatment and the clinical characteristics of the individual patient that might interfere with delivery of the targeted dialysis dose. In this chapter, we shall describe the biophysical basis for kinetic modeling of dialysis and its utility in describing the clinical biochemical impact of chronic dialysis for the individual patient. We shall evaluate observational and randomized clinical trials evidence with regard to competing measures of dialysis adequacy and the impact of observed strata of levels of achieved dialysis clearance on morbidity and mortality that have emerged from these trials.

Kinetic modeling

Kinetic modeling is a widely used analytic process for examining all aspects of the dialysis prescription and its delivery. It is a powerful technique because it describes a system from mass balance. It requires that all model parameters be rigorously defined,

since the validity of the model can be directly determined from the mass balance in the system. It provides a logical system for understanding the clinical problem of adequacy of dialysis. All the stages involved in its analysis must be highly disciplined, because a precise mathematical definition is required for each parameter. Unlike the approximations that are used commonly to evaluate dialysis dose, the relative effect of each parameter can be quantitatively assessed.

The major practical goal of modeling in dialysis is to be able to prescribe and deliver a predetermined dose that is reproducible primarily for urea but analogously for other solutes. The uremic syndrome is only partly responsive to current methods of dialysis therapy, and much morbidity continues to be present and to progress even in well-dialyzed patients. The high mortality rate characteristic among dialysis patients is strongly dependent on background cardiovascular disease and propensity for infection. In addition, since fluid removal is not part of the kinetic model prescription, ultrafiltration time may determine dialysis time in excess of the model. Because even a fully "adequate" dose of dialysis does not directly affect these comorbidities and clinical problems, the dose cannot be determined by clinical symptoms. The current dosing recommendations have evolved from being based largely on data from observational studies to a greater reliance on data from the limited number of randomized controlled trials that have examined this question rigorously. However, uncertainty still exists as to the dialysis dose needed for smaller individuals and for women. Dialysis is almost universally given three times per week. With increasing knowledge of daily short or nocturnal long dialysis, the current approach to dose may need to be changed as evidence emerges from new randomized controlled trials currently in progress.

Calculation of the dose of dialysis is also quite complicated both conceptually and with respect to practical details. While the adequacy of dialysis using urea kinetic modeling (UKM) has been initially defined by observational studies, more recently the evidence derived from randomized trials has provided information that has been formalized in practice guidelines to guide dialysis prescription.

Evidence-based Nephrology. Edited by Donald Molony and Jonathan Craig
© 2009 Blackwell Publishing, ISBN: 978-1-4051-3975-5.

Dialysis delivery

The concept of prescribing the dose of dialysis as Kt/V grew out of examination of the outcomes of the National Cooperative Dialysis Study (NCDS) in the USA [1,2]. The NCDS was designed to study two levels of predialysis blood urea nitrogen (BUN; 70 and 110 mg/dL) and was controlled by UKM. UKM is based on the law of conservation of mass and the concept of urea mass balance, which requires that the amount of urea removed during a dialysis session must equal the amount generated between sessions [3,4]. Removal of urea at any instant is determined by the product of dialyzer urea clearance and plasma urea concentration, whereas urea generation (Gu) is determined by the net rate of protein breakdown or protein catabolic rate (PCR), which in turn, in the absence of acute illness, is determined by the dietary protein intake. Urea generation is normally constant, but removal varies from zero between dialyses to very high rates at the beginning of each individual dialysis session, when the BUN is high, to very low rates at the end, when the BUN has fallen maximally. UKM is derived from mathematical modeling of urea removal and urea generation in dialysis therapy and is used to calculate Gu and to determine the volume of distribution of urea in the body (Vu) from the BUN profile and the dialyzer clearance, treatment time, and frequency of dialyses. In the NCDS, UKM was used to calculate Gu, that is, PCR and Vu, and from these values the magnitude of dialyzer clearance and treatment time required to achieve the targeted predialysis BUN levels in thrice-weekly therapy could be calculated. A further step is necessary to calculate the blood and dialysate flow rates required to achieve optimal dialyzer urea clearance. This is accomplished with use of the dialyzer overall permeability (Ko) and area (A) product or (KoA), which has a specific value for each dialyzer and depends on its membrane area and flow geometry [4,5]. From the KoA, the required blood and dialysate flows can be calculated to effect the desired clearance. These computations are readily available in PC kinetic modeling programs.

Poor clinical outcome (a global clinical composite outcome of *de novo* uremic symptoms, hospitalization, and death during follow-up) in the NCDS could not be predicted from the predialysis BUN alone as anticipated [1]. The NCDS recommended empirically a normalized PCR (nPCR) of 0.8 g/kg/day. When NPCR was ≥0.8 g/kg/day, the high BUN did predict poorer outcome, but when NPCR was <0.8 g/kg/day the global composite clinical outcome was poor irrespective of predialysis BUN. Kinetic analysis showed that outcome could be predicted in all groups when dose was expressed as the product of dialyzer urea clearance and treatment time divided by the urea distribution volume, or Kt/V. In patients with very low nPCR and Gu, very low levels of Kt/V were required to maintain the BUN at target, and these low levels of Kt/V correlated significantly with the global composite clinical outcome failure of the therapy. This relationship was consistent with the concept that urea per se is not the critical toxin, but that it could serve as a surrogate for all low-molecular-weight toxins when the therapy dose is expressed as Kt/V, a relationship which would apply to other low-molecular-weight toxins also. Consequently, UKM no longer aims to reach a specific urea concentration but provides a rational method for prescribing the dose of dialysis, defined as Kt/V, and to monitor dietary protein intake from a determination of Gu. Because all errors in delivery of the dose appear in the calculated value for Vu, when an aberrant Vu is calculated it can be concluded that the dose has not been delivered [3,4].

eKt/V and spKt/V

The calculated Kt/V is proportional to the decrease in BUN during a dialysis session. The single-pool Kt/V (spKt/V) is calculated from the predialysis BUN and the postdialysis BUN obtained 15 s after the end of dialysis. This delay is included to circumvent any access recirculation that might be present, which would lower the BUN and result in an erroneous increase in spKt/V [3,4].

Equally important is the concept of urea "rebound." At the end of the dialysis session the concentration of BUN is lower in the blood and extracellular fluid than in cells [3,4,6]. It requires 30–40 min of urea diffusion between the compartments until there is a uniform concentration (diffusion equilibrium). The difference between the two BUN levels is the rebound. Therefore, the spKt/V calculated using the end-dialysis BUN will be higher than an equilibrated Kt/V (eKt/V), which is calculated from the BUN after postdialysis equilibration. It is the eKt/V that more accurately reflects the effective dose of dialysis. If one accepts that Kt/V represents an accurate picture of dialysis dose with respect to urea and water removal, it should be apparent that one should wait until equilibration is completed to determine Kt/V so that the clinical values used to compute the Kt/V are accurate and errors in prescription are avoided.

The rebound phenomenon and effects on Kt/V and nPCR are illustrated in Figure 38.1. The BUN at the end of dialysis is used to calculate the equilibrated BUN value using validated equations in UKM programs, such as in the Fresenius Medical Care North America (FMCNA) system, rather than by keeping the patient for 30–60 min after termination of dialysis to take the final blood sample. The magnitude of rebound is determined almost entirely by the rate at which the dialysis dose is delivered. The rate of dialysis is defined by spKt/V divided by the treatment time (t), which equals K/V (K is the delivered clearance and V is the volume of distribution of urea equivalent to the total body water). The greater the K/V, the greater the rebound. Because most patients are treated at about the same blood flow (300–400 mL/min) and with the same dialyzer urea clearance (K), the smallest patients (with small V values) will tend to have the highest K/V ratios and the highest rebounds. For example, if a small patient is given the same dose of spKt/V over the same time as a larger patient, the rebound will be identical. That, however, happens infrequently in clinical therapy, and smaller patients are usually treated at higher rates and have more rebound.

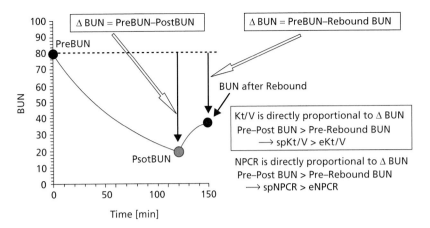

Figure 38.1 The Kt/V and nPCR are both calculated from the magnitude of BUN decrease during dialysis. The apparent drop in BUN will always be larger before rebound occurs. Because spKt/V and spnPCR are calculated from predialysis BUN minus the postdialysis BUN, while eKt/V and e-nPCR are calculated from the predialysis BUN minus the rebound BUN, spKt/V and spNPCR will always be larger than eKt/V and eNPCR.

Dialysis dosing target

The spKt/V obtained from blood urea measurements immediately before and immediately after the completion of dialysis does not account for the change in urea from any rebound and therefore provides a value of dialysis clearance that overestimates the true dialysis urea clearance as determined by the eKt/V by a percentage that is influenced by the magnitude of the rebound. A comparison of the consequences of different dialysis prescriptions on achievement of the customary target measures of adequacy using either spKt/V or eKt/V illustrates some factors that could influence achievement of adequate dialysis and the potential consequences and limitations of protocols that use spKt/V as the measure of achieving true adequacy. The relationship between spKt/V and eKt/V is illustrated in Figure 38.2A, in which the ratios of eKt/V and spKt/V are each plotted as functions of treatment time, t. The Tattersall equation [6] was used to calculate eKt/V over a spKt/V range of 1.3–1.7 and independently of volume, dialyzer clearance, and Gu, with treatment times fixed at six levels ranging from 2.0 to 4.5 h. The lower limit of 1.3 is the lower limit recommended in the National Kidney Foundation Kidney Disease Outcomes Quality Initiative guidelines, and it permits an appropriate dose of dialysis with a reserve in case of delivery problems. The upper limit of 1.7 was chosen because there is no evidence of a benefit with higher spKt/V. Over the ranges calculated, eKt/V is a highly linear function of spKt/V when time is held constant, so a family of six lines is seen (Figure 38.2A). The eKt/V dose target of 1.2 is depicted as a horizontal line on the y axis and the spKt/V dose target of 1.4 as a vertical line on the x axis. The regression lines for the different dialysis times are depicted as solid lines for all segments with eKt/V of ≥1.20 and dashed lines for all segments where eKt/V is <1.20. Note that the two adequacy targets agree only in the left lower portion of the plot, where eKt/V is <1.20 and spKt/V is <1.40. Here they define a domain of inadequacy common to both criteria. Some of the regression lines for spKt/V of >1.4 pass through the inadequate zone because of their high rebound with shorter dialysis times.

The required spKt/V to achieve an eKt/V of 1.20 is shown for each treatment time (Figure 38.2B) by a vertical arrow to the x axis at the point that each regression line reaches the minimum level for adequate dialysis, defined by eKt/V of 1.20. It can be seen that the spKt/V necessary to provide an adequate Kt/V can range from 1.32

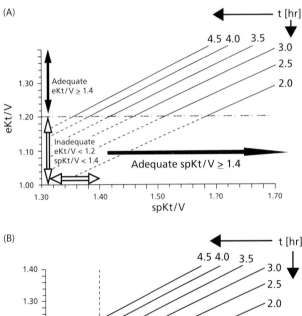

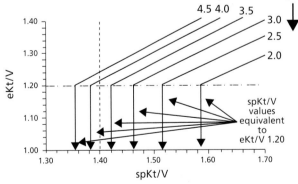

Figure 38.2 (A) Two definitions of adequate dialysis: eKt/V of ≥1.20 and spKt/V of ≥1.40. Note that a substantial number of adequate doses by the criterion of a spKt/V of ≥1.40 are inadequate by the eKt/V ≥1.20 criterion. (B) When treatment time (t) varies in the patient population, there must be a family of spKt/V values ranging from 1.35 to 1.58 to ensure all doses are equivalent to an eKt/V of 1.20.

to 1.58 over a range of dialysis times to provide an eKt/V of 1.20. Therefore, an eKt/V can be associated with several spKt/V values, depending on the dialysis time. In contrast, a single target eKt/V of 1.20 permits determination of the optimal time and spKt/V for each patient in the population.

The nPCR is calculated from the amount of urea removed, which is considered equal to the Gu based on the PCR [4]. As noted above, the postdialysis BUN is artificially low, so if it is used for calculation of nPCR, the urea removal will be overestimated, because it is the difference between this BUN concentration and the predialysis BUN of the next treatment that is used. The nPCR will therefore behave like the Kt/Vs (as above).

Impact of residual renal urea clearance on eKt/V and estimated nPCR

Intermittent hemodialysis is very inefficient. With thrice-weekly hemodialysis of 3–4 h/HD session, urea is being cleared for only 5–7% of the total weekly time while urea and other solutes are generated continuously throughout the week. Consequently, high dialyzer urea clearances are used, which result in an exponential drop in BUN and very inefficient removal of urea and other solutes in the later part of dialysis. A low continuous clearance is far more efficient because the BUN does not fall to very low levels, which is the reason that a lower total clearance is required in continuous ambulatory peritoneal dialysis (CAPD) and potentially with prolonged daily hemodialysis prescriptions as yet to be determined [7]. A weekly Kt/V$_{CAPD}$ of 2.00 with CAPD is equivalent to an eKt/V of 1.2 with thrice-weekly hemodialysis. Recent clinical trials suggest that even this dose of CAPD might be higher than required for optimal outcomes. These data are reviewed in section 8 of this textbook. The standard Kt/V (stdKt/V) calculation [4,7] quantifies the effects of both intermittent and continuous dialysis, giving a dose that applies to all dialysis frequencies and intensities ranging from CAPD, short and long daily HD, to twice-weekly HD. However, in the specific case of thrice-weekly hemodialysis, the residual renal function can be directly expressed as a quantity of eKt/V (abbreviated as eKrt/V) in accordance with the equation eKrt/V = 4.5 × Kru/V (with V in liters and Kru in mL/min, the units of the coefficient 4.5 are liters per milliliter per min Kru per dialysis).

Assuming a V of 30 L, a Kru of 1 mL/min contributes an additional equivalent of 4.5 L of urea clearance per dialysis session, which translates into a gain of eKt/V of 0.15 (4.5/30). If a patient has a Kru of 3 mL/min, it will add 3 × 0.15, or 0.45 to the eKt/V provided by hemodialysis (abbreviated as eKdt/V), a highly significant addition. With this Kru being present, the total equilibrated dialysis dose (eKdrt/V) is simply the sum of eKdt/V and eKrt/V, so that a Kru of 3 mL/min raises an eKt/V of 1.2 to 1.65.

The impact of Kru on total eKdrt/V and estimated nPCR (e-nPCR) is illustrated in Figure 38.3A and B. In Figure 38.3A the Kdrt/V is plotted as a function of Kru for an average-size patient and four levels of eKdt/V (0.40, 0.60, 0.80, and 1.00; these are

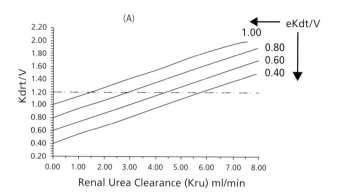

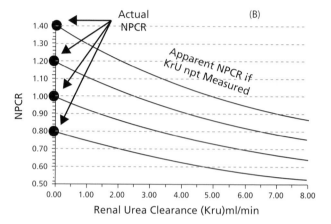

Figure 38.3 (A) Solution for eKdrt/V as a function of Kru for average patient volume (V) of 30 L. As shown, in the average-sized patient, each milliliter of Kru increases eKdrt/V by about 0.15 units of eKt/V. (B) Solutions for "apparent" nPCR if residual Kru is not included in UKM. The presence of Kru lowers the predialysis BUN, which will result in spurious lowering of the nPCR calculated if Kru is not included in the modeling equations. The error introduced will be about −4% for each milliliter per minute of Kru in the average-sized patient.

the y axis values shown when Kru is 0). As discussed above, eKrt/V is additive to eKdt/V. The UKM program in the FMCNA system can calculate the Kdrt/V for thrice-weekly and also twice-weekly dialysis.

In Figure 38.3B the impact of Kru on nPCR is illustrated. Using the UKM, nPCR values of 0.8, 1.0, 1.2, and 1.4 are shown with Kru increasing from 0 to 8 mL/min. The "apparent" e-nPCR values that would be calculated if Kru were present but not measured and assumed to be zero are depicted. For example, if the nPCR were 1.0 and an unmeasured Kru of 3 mL/min were present, the apparent e-nPCR calculated would fall to 0.80 and would be interpreted as a marginal protein intake. Thus, residual renal function (when measured and applied) can have a marked impact on eKt/V and e-nPCR and will further exaggerate the differences between the single-pool and equilibrated measures.

Standard Kt/V

The calculation of standard Kt/V based on the relationship between urea generation and the mean predialysis BUN level makes

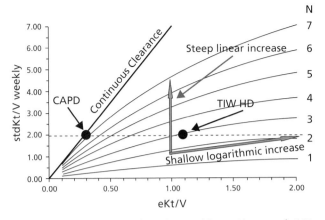

Figure 38.4 Results of solution of the stdKt/V model over wide ranges of eKt/V and weekly dialysis frequency (N). Note that by inspection stdKt/V can be seen to increase linearly as N increases and logarithmically with eKt/V. The doses of adequate continuous ambulatory peritoneal dialysis and thrice-weekly hemodialysis are the same with this model, the weekly stdKt/V of 2.

it possible to compare different doses at different treatment frequencies from one to seven times per week (Figure 38.4).

Use of approximation equations

A number of attempts have been made to greatly simplify urea kinetic calculations [6,8–14]. None of these approximations calculate the urea distribution volume, which is essential to assess therapy delivery and to quantify the dietary protein intake based on PCR. Also, it is not possible to prescribe a desired dose of dialysis (spKt/V) without calculation of V and without prescription calculation routines. The Daugirdas equation [9] is the only reliable equation to estimate spKt/V, but it will not detect errors in therapy delivery because the individual components defining a particular Kt/V (e.g. treatment time, blood flow, residual renal function, and V) are not computed by a kinetic model but lumped together instead, so that a prescription based on the individual components cannot be accurately determined. A volume change with formal UKM suggests that the prescription has not been delivered or that blood drawing errors have occurred.

The most rigorous equation to estimate eKt/V is the Smye equation [13], but this equation is very sensitive to small BUN errors. The most usefully rigorous equation is the Tatersall equation [6] to calculate eKt/V. The Depner-Daugirdas equation [10] provides a reasonable estimate of nPCR but cannot be used to estimate PCR and errors in delivery cannot be identified, for the same reasons as with the Daugirdas equation.

The urea reduction ratio (URR) [12] is widely used to judge adequacy of dialysis dose. It is a very crude estimate of dose but very inexpensive and easy to obtain and therefore widely used. It is probably reasonably suitable for analysis of populations on dialysis but is of limited usefulness for individual patients because a URR cannot be prescribed. The URR is quite sensitive to the magnitude of ultrafiltration, will not identify errors in delivery, and cannot be used to monitor the nutritional status of the patient.

The NCDS and HEMO studies

The utilization of UKM and the Kt/V methodology may have been in part responsible for decreasing hemodialysis times and concomitant increases in mortality observed in dialysis populations in the USA during the 1980s and 1990s. UKM became widely applied after the results of the NCDS were published [1,2]. The NCDS was a landmark study, as it was the first prospective randomized trial for dialysis. A total of 160 chronic dialysis patients undergoing thrice-weekly hemodialysis were observed over a minimum of 6 months and randomly allocated to four treatment arms. Dialysis doses were randomly distributed over a very wide range, with a spKt/V between 0.42 and 1.45. The primary end point in the NCDS was the probability of failure, which was a global clinical composite of *de novo* uremic symptoms, hospitalization, and death during follow-up. The NCDS found that a Kt/V urea above 0.9 with thrice-weekly treatment provided an adequate dialysis prescription in that the patient failure rate of 13% was substantially below that in patients with a lower Kt/V. Although the NCDS included no diabetic patients or those with other important comorbid conditions, a Kt/V of 1.0 was widely accepted after publication of the study results as representing adequate dialysis.

Subsequent observational data from Tassin, France (with an spKt/V of >1.6) [15] and Minnesota (spKt/V of >1.3) [16] reported improved survival with increased spKt/V, and this improvement in survival occurred despite a striking increase in comorbidity, which should have resulted in an overall decreased survival. Using the URR as a measure of dialysis adequacy, it was shown that survival was significantly reduced at URR below 60% [12]. Observational data also suggested that more intensive dialysis leads to improved survival. In one study, increasing the mean spKt/V from 0.82 (pre-1988) to 1.33 led to a reduction in the gross mortality rate from 22.8 to 9.1%/year [17]. It is important to note that an increased spKt/V was only one of multiple parameters that improved from the first period to the second period in these analyses. During this same period the magnitude of inflammatory response induced by dialysis presumably improved with the introduction of more biocompatible dialysis membranes, the observed nPCR increased and plasma albumin concentrations rose. Thus, enhanced nutrition and possibly fewer inflammatory problems might have contributed significantly to if not entirely to the observed improvement in survival. A national sample in the dialysis population in the USA suggested a 7% reduction in mortality for each 0.1 unit increase in spKt/V [18].

It is of note that some studies observed an increased relative risk (RR) of death among patients with high spKt/V values (>1.6) or URR between 75 and 79%, possibly reflecting a subset of the population with disease or malnutrition-imposed reduction in body mass or reflecting errors in postdialysis blood collection leading to artificially low blood urea values [19]. These results were, however, corroborated by data showing that a spKt/V greater than 1.68 was associated with lower survival compared to a range of spKt/V values between 1.23 and 1.68 [20]. Therefore, based upon these observational studies, the optimal dose of hemodialysis remained undefined.

The Hemodialysis (HEMO) study, begun in 1995, aimed to clarify this issue [21]. It was a multicenter clinical trial of hemodialysis prescriptions for patients on thrice-weekly hemodialysis treatment. During the pilot phase of the HEMO study the proposed dose in the standard arm of the study was a spKt/V of 1.1–1.2. However, by the time the final protocol was written, the practice in the USA was to provide doses close to a spKt/V of 1.40, which precluded any investigation of the equivalent dose ranges used in the NCDS. Ultimately, participants (1037 men, 809 women) from over 65 US dialysis facilities were randomized in a two-by-two factorial design to dialysis prescriptions targeted to a standard dose (eKt/V of 1.05, which is equivalent to a URR of 65% or a spKt/V of 1.25) or a high dose (eKt/V of 1.45, which is equivalent to a URR of 75% or a spKt/V of 1.65) and to either low-flux membrane (mean β_2-microglobulin clearance of <10 mL/min) or high-flux membrane (mean β_2-microglobulin clearance of >20 mL/min and ultrafiltration coefficient of >14 mL/h/mmHg).

Despite important exclusion criteria, such as severe congestive heart failure and serum albumin of <2.6 g/dL at baseline, the HEMO study population was representative of the majority of chronic hemodialysis patients. The primary outcome was death from any cause, whereas the main secondary outcomes were the rate of hospitalization and the composite outcomes of first hospitalization for a cardiac problem or death from any cause, first hospitalization for an infectious cause or death, and first decline of greater than 15% of serum albumin from baseline value or death. Mean follow-up was 4.5 years.

The risk of death from any cause (the primary outcome) was the same in the high-dose and standard-dose groups (RR of 0.96 for high versus standard dose, 95% confidence interval [CI], 0.84–1.10). Similarly, there was no difference in all-cause mortality between the high-flux and the low-flux groups (RR, 0.92; 95% CI, 0.81–1.05). The risk of the main secondary outcomes was also the same for both dialysis doses. The prespecified subgroup (unadjusted) analysis revealed a possible interaction between survival and gender, that is, a benefit for women receiving a high dialysis dose (19% lower risk of death than for women in the standard dose group) and, conversely, an increased risk of death for men receiving high-dose dialysis that was 16% higher than that for men receiving standard-dose dialysis in the unadjusted analysis [22].

Post hoc analysis of the HEMO study [23] data showed that the high-flux intervention seemed to be associated with reduced risks of specific cardiac-related events, such as cardiac death (RR for the high-flux arm, 0.80; 95% CI, 0.60–0.99) and the composite of first cardiac hospitalization or cardiac death (RR, 0.87; 95%

CI, 0.76–1.00). Dialysis vintage may interact with the effects of high-flux dialysis on outcomes. In the subgroup that had been on dialysis for >3.7 years before study entry (median time of dialysis for the entire study population), randomization to high-flux dialysis was associated with lower risks of all-cause mortality (RR, 0.68; 95% CI, 0.53–0.86) and cardiac deaths (RR, 0.63; 95% CI, 0.43–0.92) during the time on the study. This apparent benefit seemed to be attenuated when the time before entry was included in the analysis of morbidity. For the subgroup of patients with <3.7 years of dialysis before the study, assignment to high-flux dialysis had no significant effect on any of the examined clinical outcomes.

Originally, the HEMO study was analyzed on an intention-to-treat basis. A subsequent as-treated analysis showed that each 0.10 reduction in achieved eKt/V below the group median was associated with a mortality risk increase of 58% in the standard-dose group and 37% in the high-dose group [24]. Patients in the highest quintile of the standard-dose group had better survival than those in the lowest quintile of the high-dose group. The discrepancies between the results of the intention-to-treat and the as-treated analyses could reflect extraneous factors that were associated with both increased mortality and lower achieved eKt/V, and they provide another concrete example of the problems inherent in relying principally on findings from observational studies, which tend to overestimate the benefits of any therapy, rather than on data from rigorous randomized controlled trials when informing clinical practice decisions. In the HEMO study, factors associated with lower achieved eKt/V were larger anthropometric volume, black race, and comorbidity at baseline, and follow-up factors included use of catheters and grafts (both versus fistula), hospitalization rate, and declining serum albumin levels. Additionally, data from the HEMO study also revealed a coefficient of variation within patients of ~0.1 spKt/V units. In order to provide 95% confidence that the dose will not decrease to less than 1.2 per dialysis for any individual dialysis session, the target dose has to be increased to a spKt/V of 1.4 per dialysis.

Dialysis adequacy: current recommendations

The optimal dose for adequacy of an individual hemodialysis treatment to produce the lowest rate of morbidity and mortality when hemodialysis is administered thrice weekly remains uncertain. The NCDS suggested that there was some minimum level of clearance below which patients would predictably do less well. This finding is relatively intuitive. The HEMO study suggests that this threshold might differ for patients with different baseline characteristics and comorbidities. On the basis of the totality of evidence, however limited the randomized controlled trial evidence might be, several national and international bodies have issued recommendations for hemodialysis adequacy, and these are listed in Table 38.1.

Table 38.1 Recommendations from various countries for adequate thrice-weekly hemodialysis.

Country or region (year recommendation issued)	Recommended minimum (target)[a] values		
	spKt/V	eKt/V	URR (%)
Canada (1999)	1.2		65
Australia (2005)	1.2 (1.4)		65 (70)
Europe (2002)	1.4	1.2	65
UK (2006)	1.3	1.2 (1.4)	65 (70)
USA (2006)	1.2 (1.4)		65 (70)

Source: KDIGO; http://www.kdigo.org/welcome.htm.

[a] The target value (shown in parentheses) to achieve the minimum dose with 95% confidence.

The Frequent Hemodialysis Network trial

Observational studies have suggested improvements with frequent hemodialysis, but its true efficacy and safety remain uncertain. The multicenter, randomized controlled Frequent Hemodialysis Network (FHN) trial aims to compare nocturnal home dialysis (six times per week; 125 patients) with conventional in-center dialysis (125 patients) and short daily in-center dialysis (six times per week; 125 patients) with conventional thrice-weekly hemodialysis (125 patients). The trial will be performed with high-flux dialyzers.

Patient enrollment commenced for the FHN trial in early 2006. Each patient was to be treated and followed for 12 months. Daily HD was to be delivered for 1.5–2.75 h, 6 days/week. The dialysis prescriptions target an eKt/V of 0.9 at each of the six weekly dialysis sessions. Patients assigned to the six-times-per-week nocturnal dialysis followed any dialysis prescription, provided their prescribed weekly stdKt/V was at least 4.0 and treatment time was at least 6.0 h, six times per week. In the conventional hemodialysis group, subjects remained on their usual dialysis prescriptions, subject to a minimum prescribed eKt/V of 1.1. The composite of mortality with the 12-month change in left ventricular mass index (by magnetic resonance imaging) and SF-36 RAND Physical Health Composite are specified as coprimary outcomes. Trial feasibility will be assessed during the first 12 months of enrollment (Vanguard phase). The FHN trials will help to elucidate whether more frequent hemodialysis might improve outcomes in chronic hemodialysis patients. The trial will have important implications for dialysis therapy in the next decades.

References

1 Gotch FA, Sargent JA. A mechanistic analysis of the National Cooperative Dialysis Study (NCDS). *Kidney Int* 1985; **28(3):** 526–534.

2 Lowrie EG, Laird NM, Parker TF, Sargent JA. Effect of the hemodialysis prescription on patient morbidity: report from the National Cooperative Dialysis Study. *N Engl J Med* 1981; **305:** 1176–1181.

3 Gotch F, Keen M. Kinetic modeling in hemodialysis. In: Nissenson AR, Fine RA, editors, *Clinical Dialysis*, 4th edn. McGraw-Hill, New York, 2005;153–203.

4 Sargent J, Gotch F. Principles and biophysics of dialysis. In: Jacobs C, Kjellstrand C, Koch K, Winchester J, editors, *Replacement of Renal Function by Dialysis*, 4th edn. Kluwer Academic Publishers, Dordrecht, the Netherlands, 1996; 34–103.

5 Michaels AS. Operating parameters and performance criteria for hemodialyzers and other membrane-separation devices. *Trans Am Soc Artif Intern Organs* 1966; **12:** 387–392.

6 Tattersall JE, DeTakats D, Chamney P, Greenwood RN, Farrington K. The post-hemodialysis rebound: predicting and quantifying its effect on Kt/V. *Kidney Int* 1996; **50(6):** 2094–2102.

7 Gotch F, Keen M. Kinetic modeling in peritoneal dialysis. In: Nissenson AR, Fine RA, editors, *Clinical Dialysis*, 4th edn. McGraw-Hill, New York, 2005; 385–421.

8 Barth RH. Urea modeling and Kt/V: a critical appraisal. *Kidney Int Suppl* 1993; **41:** S252–S260.

9 Daugirdas JT. Second generation logarithmic estimates of single-pool variable volume Kt/V: an analysis of error. *J Am Soc Nephrol* 1993; **4(5):** 1205–1213.

10 Depner TA, Daugirdas JT. Equations for normalized protein catabolic rate based on two-point modeling of hemodialysis urea kinetics. *J Am Soc Nephrol* 1996; **7(5):** 780–785.

11 Jindal KK, Manuel A, Goldstein MB. Percent reduction in blood urea concentration during hemodialysis (PRU). A simple and accurate method to estimate Kt/V urea. *ASAIO Trans* 1987; **33(3):** 286–288.

12 Owen WF, Jr., Lew NL, Liu Y, Lowrie EG, Lazarus JM. The urea reduction ratio and serum albumin concentration as predictors of mortality in patients undergoing hemodialysis. *N Engl J Med* 1993; **329(14):** 1001–1006.

13 Smye SW, Evans JH, Will E, Brocklebank JT. Paediatric haemodialysis: estimation of treatment efficiency in the presence of urea rebound. *Clin Phys Physiol Meas* 1992; **13(1):** 51–62.

14 Kovacic V, Roguljich IJ. Comparison of methods for hemodialysis dose calculations. *Dial Transplant* 2003; **32:** 170.

15 Charra B, Calemard E, Ruffet M, Chazot C, Terrat JC, Vanel T *et al.* Survival as an index of adequacy of dialysis. *Kidney Int* 1992; **41(5):** 1286–1291.

16 Collins AJ, Ma JZ, Umen A, Keshaviah P. Urea index and other predictors of hemodialysis patient survival. *Am J Kidney Dis* 1994; **23(2):** 272–282.

17 Hakim RM, Breyer J, Ismail N, Schulman G. Effects of dose of dialysis on morbidity and mortality. *Am J Kidney Dis* 1994; **23(5):** 661–669.

18 Held PJ, Port FK, Wolfe RA, Stannard DC, Carroll CE, Daugirdos JT *et al.* The dose of hemodialysis and patient mortality. *Kidney Int* 1996; **50(2):** 550–556.

19 Chertow GM, Owen WF, Lazarus JM, Lew NL, Lowrie EG. Exploring the reverse J-shaped curve between urea reduction ratio and mortality. *Kidney Int* 1999; **56(5):** 1872–1878.

20 Salahudeen AK, Dykes P, May W. Risk factors for higher mortality at the highest levels of spKt/V in haemodialysis patients. *Nephrol Dial Transplant* 2003; **18(7):** 1339–1344.

21 Greene T, Beck GJ, Gassman JJ, Gotch FA, Kusek JW, Levey AS *et al.* Design and statistical issues of the hemodialysis (HEMO) study. *Control Clin Trials* 2000; **21(5):** 502–525.

22 Eknoyan G, Beck GJ, Cheung AK, Daugirdas JT, Greene T, Kusek JW *et al.* Effect of dialysis dose and membrane flux in maintenance hemodialysis. *N Engl J Med* 2002; **347(25):** 2010–2019.

23 Cheung AK, Levin NW, Greene T, Agodoa L, Bailey J, Beck G *et al.* Effects of high-flux hemodialysis on clinical outcomes: results of the HEMO study. *J Am Soc Nephrol* 2003; **14(12):** 3251–3263.

24 Greene T, Daugirdas J, Depner T, Allon M, Beck G, Chumlea C *et al.* Association of achieved dialysis dose with mortality in the hemodialysis study: an example of "dose-targeting bias." *J Am Soc Nephrol* 2005; **16(11):** 3371–3380.

39 General Management of the Hemodialysis Patient

Robert Mactier[1] & David C. Wheeler[2]

[1]NHS Greater Glasgow & Clyde, Scotland, UK
[2]Royal Free and University College Medical School, London, UK

Introduction

In the past, the provision of hemodialysis has focused on achieving prespecified standards of small solute clearance (chapter 44), with little attention given to the more general clinical and laboratory indices of hemodialysis adequacy. A holistic, multidisciplinary approach to the optimal care of the hemodialysis patient should include maintenance of satisfactory nutritional status, correction of metabolic disturbances (including disordered lipid metabolism, predialysis hyperkalemia, and metabolic acidosis), and control of high blood pressure (while avoiding hypotension). These aspects of care should be addressed in addition to the management of anemia (chapter 31), renal bone disease (chapter 34), infection (chapter 40), and vascular access (chapter 42). Despite a paucity of robust clinical data, monitoring and management of the more general aspects of hemodialysis are considered an important component of good practice and have been addressed in clinical practice guidelines developed in Australasia [1], Canada [2], Europe [3–6], the UK [6,7], and the USA [8,9]. Where data from randomized controlled trials are lacking, these guidelines have defined ranges of relevant parameters associated with optimum outcomes reported in large observational studies [10], or when such data are lacking, have used biological plausibility expressed as expert opinion. Such indices typically relate to patients receiving thrice-weekly hemodialysis, although there is no intuitive reason to believe that they should not be applicable to those receiving alternative hemodialysis regimens or hemodiafiltration. This chapter sets out to summarize the available evidence relevant to these more general aspects of the management of the hemodialysis patient as it relates to chronic hemodialysis treatment.

Hyperkalemia

Hyperkalemia is a common indication for emergency hemodialysis and accounts for between 3 and 5% of deaths among dialysis patients [11]. Noncompliance with the dialysis prescription and diet are thought to be the most common contributory factors, although medications such as angiotensin converting enzyme inhibitors, angiotensin receptor blockers, nonsteroidal anti-inflammatory drugs, beta-blockers, and potassium supplements may be implicated. The general principles of the assessment and treatment of disorders of potassium metabolism (hypo- and hyperkalemia) are detailed in chapter 10.3 of this textbook. The specific problem of potassium as it relates to patients on hemodialysic is discussed below.

Treatment of hyperkalemia

Hemodialysis is the most appropriate emergency treatment for hyperkalemia in the dialysis patients. In the chronic dialysis patient with a working vascular access, hemodialysis can be initiated quickly. Serum potassium levels usually fall by 1 mmol/L during the first hour of treatment and by a further 1 mmol/L over the next 2 h [12]. The rate of potassium removal may be enhanced further by increasing the dialyzer blood flow rate or by either raising the bicarbonate or lowering the potassium concentration of the dialysate [13]. An urgent electrocardiogram is of proven value in guiding management of non-hemodialysis-dependent patients with a serum potassium above 6 mmol/L [14] and can be used to dictate which patients should receive additional emergent interventions, such as the administration of intravenous calcium chloride. The results of a Cochrane meta-analysis of controlled trials of nondialytic emergency interventions for hyperkalemia, which was not limited to dialysis patients, can be extrapolated in the absence of better evidence cautiously to the dialysis patient with hyperkalemia. The authors of the Cochrane review concluded that intravenous glucose with insulin and nebulized or inhaled salbutamol were effective in reducing serum potassium levels, but studies were limited by the absence of data on cardiac

Evidence-based Nephrology. Edited by Donald Molony and Jonathan Craig
© 2009 Blackwell Publishing, ISBN: 978-1-4051-3975-5.

arrhythmias and mortality rates [13]. The evidence for efficacy of intravenous bicarbonate and potassium exchange resins in dialysis patients is equivocal, and neither can be recommended as sole therapy in severely hyperkalemic hemodialysis patients [13], especially in light of the effectiveness of hemodialysis in reducing total body potassium burden.

Hypokalemia occurring towards the end or immediately after hemodialysis is common, may increase the risk of cardiac arrhythmias, and can be corrected by increasing the dialysate potassium concentration [15,16]. Table 39.1 shows recommendations for predialysis blood potassium concentrations taken from the available English language clinical practice guidelines.

Metabolic acidosis

Metabolic acidosis is usually detected in dialysis patients by measurement of serum bicarbonate concentrations, although assessment of severity may require analysis of arterial blood pH and gases. In stable hemodialysis patients, the main contributory factors for metabolic acidosis appear to be inadequate dialysis delivery, excessive intake of animal proteins, and high interdialysis weight gain [17,18]. In sick patients, increased protein catabolism, increased lactate production (induced by hypotension or hypoxia), and bicarbonate losses (associated with comorbid illness) may exacerbate the problem [17]. Adverse consequences of a metabolic acidosis include an increase in protein catabolism, there being a well-established association between metabolic acidosis and markers of poor nutritional status [18]. Other adverse associations include a negative inotropic effect, loss of bone mineral, insulin resistance, growth retardation in children, reduced thyroxine levels, altered triglyceride metabolism, hyperkalemia, low serum leptin levels, and enhanced accumulation of β_2-microglobulin [18].

In a large cohort study, predialysis venous blood bicarbonate values between 17.5 and 20 mmol/L were associated with the lowest risk of death among 13,535 hemodialysis patients, whereas the relative risk was increased threefold if the predialysis venous bicarbonate was less than 15 mmol/L [9]. Among more than 7000 unselected hemodialysis patients in the Dialysis Outcomes and Practice Patterns study, the corrected midweek blood bicarbonate concentration averaged 21.9 mmol/L and correlated inversely with the normalized protein catabolic rate (nPCR) and serum albumin [19]. In this observational study, moderate predialysis midweek acidosis was associated with a better nutritional status (nPCR, albumin, PO4) and a lower risk of death and hospitalization compared to patients with severe acidosis (serum bicarbonate levels of less than 16 mmol/L) or a sodium bicarbonate 24 mmol/L greater than [19].

Correction of metabolic acidosis

Several small crossover studies have suggested short-term benefits associated with correcting predialysis acidosis from below 19 mmol/L to above 24 mmol/L, either by increasing the dialysate bicarbonate concentration [20–23] or by the addition of oral bicarbonate supplements [24]. Correction of acidosis reduced whole body protein degradation [20], increased the sensitivity of the parathyroid glands to serum calcium [21,22], improved nutritional status (assessed by measurement of triceps skin fold thickness) [23], and increased serum albumin after 3 months without changes in body weight, Kt/V, or nPCR [24]. However, other studies have shown no increase in serum albumin after correction of acidosis [25]. Furthermore, these studies have not demonstrated any direct impact on mortality or significant morbidities in the long term.

Complete correction of predialysis metabolic acidosis in hemodialysis patients could theoretically contribute to an increased risk of postdialysis metabolic alkalosis with hypoventilation, phosphate transfer into cells, and a higher risk of soft tissue and vascular calcification. Furthermore, the prerequisite sodium load associated with the additional oral or dialysate bicarbonate

Table 39.1 Guidelines for predialysis serum potassium and bicarbonate concentrations in hemodialysis patients.

Clinical practice guideline [reference]	Date of update	Recommendation for predialysis serum potassium concentration	Recommendation for predialysis serum bicarbonate concentration[a]
Caring for Australasians with Renal Impairment [1]	2005	Reduce dietary potassium if >5.5mmol/L	Increase to 23–24 mmol/L
Canadian Society of Nephrology [2]		No recommendation	No recommendation
European Best Practice Guidelines [5]	2007	Reduce dietary potassium if >6 mmol/L	Midweek predialysis target, 20–22 mmol/L
UK Renal Association [7]	2007	3.5–6.5 mmol/L	Target range, 20–26 mmol/L
NKF K/DOQI [8]	2003	No recommendation	Aim for >22mmol/L

[a] Predialysis serum bicarbonate concentration should be measured in a fully filled sample bottle with minimum delay after venipuncture without using a tourniquet.

requirement may contribute to fluid retention and hypertension. In one recent randomized crossover study, the use of standardized bicarbonate bath concentration (32 mmol/L) resulted in more frequent hypotensive episodes despite the greater potential sodium load when compared in the same patients to the use of a low bicarbonate bath concentration (26 mmol/L) [26]. A summary of the recommended targets for predialysis blood bicarbonate levels in hemodialysis patients taken from clinical practice guidelines is shown in Table 39.1 and indicates that a mild degree of predialysis acidosis is generally accepted to minimize the risk of adverse events based on this limited trials evidence.

Hypertension

Although hypertension has been established as an important risk factor for the development of cardiovascular disease in the general population, whether such an association exists in hemodialysis patients, what the actual clinical impact of hypertension treatment is in this population, and what the optimal target for achieved blood pressure should be are all less clear for patients on hemodialysis [27]. A recent systematic review of the available literature showed an association between predialysis hypertension and total mortality in incident cohorts of hemodialysis patients and between better control of predialysis blood pressure and higher patient survival rates [28]. In an observational study of 16,059 incident hemodialysis patients in the USA, baseline systolic blood pressure above or equal to 150 mmHg was associated with a higher risk of death in patients who had survived for at least 3 years, whereas baseline systolic blood pressure below 120 mmHg was associated with a higher risk of death during the first 2 years of dialysis [29]. Systolic blood pressure records obtained outside the dialysis unit were stronger predictors of left ventricular hypertrophy than blood pressure measurements taken while patients were attending for dialysis [30].

Control of blood pressure
Given the association of the highest blood pressure levels with poorer outcomes, the above observations led to the conclusion that control of hypertension is beneficial in the hemodialysis population and more recently to the conclusion that excessive control might be harmful. However, evidence-based target ranges and the optimum timing and method of measurement of blood pressure in hemodialysis patients have not been rigorously defined. Nevertheless, in view of the high cardiovascular morbidity and mortality, clinical practice guidelines recommend tight blood pressure control. For example, the authors of the US Kidney Disease Outcomes Quality Initiative (K/DOQI) extrapolated treatment recommendations from blood pressure control in the general population and advocated a target predialysis blood pressure below 140/90 mmHg and postdialysis blood pressure below 130/80 mmHg [31].

Control of hypertension is facilitated by maintaining a patient at their "dry" body weight, and this is more likely to be achieved with longer-duration or more frequent hemodialysis treatments [31].

Very low mortality rates were observed in a cohort of patients treated with long-duration thrice-weekly hemodialysis, among whom survival was independently associated with improved blood pressure control [32]. Furthermore, lower cardiovascular mortality was related to better long-term optimization of dry body weight [32]. Conversely high-efficiency, short-duration, thrice-weekly hemodialysis has been associated with poor blood pressure control [33]. Retrospective data from a large Japanese cohort showed that patient survival improved with increments in dialysis duration up to 5.5 h beyond baseline after adjusting for dialysis dose [34]. Despite a lack of strong supporting evidence, some clinical practice guidelines recommend that dietary sodium intake not exceed 100 mmol/day in order to facilitate control of hypertension while reducing thirst and minimizing interdialytic weight gains [6,31].

Dialysis-related hypotension

Hypotension is the most frequent complication of hemodialysis and can shorten treatment times, thus reducing the delivered dialysis dose [35]. Dialysis-related hypotension is an independent predictor of poor patient survival [36]. Patients experiencing frequent episodes are at higher risk of death [37], probably because low blood pressure during dialysis can be a marker of severe cardiac disease [38]. The frequency of dialysis-related hypotension is, therefore, an important indicator of the quality of dialysis.

Preventing dialysis-related hypotension
Adjustment of the rate of fluid removal, dialysate sodium concentration, and dialysate temperature (or combinations thereof) minimize the likelihood of hypotension during dialysis [39–42]. Dialysate sodium modelling, or "ramping," can reduce intradialysis cramps and hypotension but may increase thirst, weight gain, and hypertension between dialysis sessions [43]. A recent randomized trial of intradialytic blood volume monitoring demonstrated no difference in weight, blood pressure, or frequency of dialysis-related complications, although hospitalization and mortality rates were higher than in a control group assigned to conventional monitoring [44]. This result was unexpected and might be explained by the unusually low hospitalization and mortality rates in the control group compared with local prevalent hemodialysis patient population. A recent systematic review of 22 studies concluded that a reduction in dialysate temperature is effective in decreasing the incidence of intradialytic hypotension without affecting dialysis adequacy [45].

Nutrition

Malnutrition may develop in hemodialysis patients despite the delivery of an adequate dialysis dose and protein intake [46] and is prevalent in up to 72% of adult hemodialysis patients [47,48]. Nutritional status may start to decline before a patient reaches end-stage kidney disease and should influence the clinician's decision to initiate renal replacement therapy [49]. Chronic inflammation and cardiovascular disease are commonly associated, leading to the concept of the malnutrition–inflammation–atherosclerosis syndrome [50]. It is generally considered that malnutrition and a decline in nutritional status over time are associated with adverse outcomes in hemodialysis patients [51,52], although this has not been confirmed by all studies [53]. Such discrepancies may result from the use of different nutritional markers and reflect a general lack of agreement as to how best to assess nutritional status in hemodialysis populations.

Assessment of nutritional status

Clinical practice guidelines developed in Australasia [1] Canada [2], Europe [5], the UK [6,7], and USA [8,54] make specific recommendations with respect to the assessment of nutritional status in hemodialysis patients (Table 39.2). Although these guidelines differ in terms of which nutritional indices they endorse, they all agree that no single measure alone can be used to assess

nutritional status and that a combination of the measures outlined below should be used. Canadian, UK, and US guidelines clearly state criteria for the diagnosis of malnutrition based on these measurements.

Subjective global assessment

The use of subjective global assessment (SGA) is recommended by all five guidelines and comprises an evaluation of gastrointestinal symptoms (appetite, anorexia, nausea, vomiting, diarrhea), a recording of weight change over time, an estimation of functional impairment, and a subjective visual quantification of subcutaneous tissue and muscle mass [55]. SGA has the advantages of being readily available, cheap, and easy to perform [56]. However, it has not been adequately validated as a measure of malnutrition. While this tool may distinguish those with severe malnutrition from those who are adequately nourished [57], and predicts poor outcomes for those identified by this measure as most severely malnourished [56]. When it does not reliably assess protein malnutrition in dialysis patients compared with more complex methods [57].

Table 39.2 Recommended tools for nutritional assessment and criteria for malnutrition based on current guidelines in hemodialysis patients.

Guideline [reference]	Date updated	Recommended tools for assessment of malnutrition	Criteria for malnutrition
Caring for Australasians with Renal Impairment [1]	2005	Measure of nutritional intake (dietary evaluation, PCR) Long-term measures of nutritional adequacy (total body nitrogen, DEXA, BIA) nPNA, Albumin Urea and creatinine Edema-free body weight SGA	No criteria stated
Canadian Society of Nephrology [2]	1999	Serum albumin nPNA Dietary energy intake SGA Edema-free lean body mass	Albumin <30 g/L Lean body mass <70% (men) or <60% (women)
European Best Practice Guidelines [5]	2006	Dietary assessment, BMI, SGA, anthropometry, nPNA, albumin, prealbumin, cholesterol, technical investigations	No criteria stated
UK Renal Association [7]	2002	SGA Height and weight (BMI) Serum albumin	Unintentional fall in edema-free weight (>10% in last 6 mos). Unintentional fall in BMI, or BMI <18.5 kg/m^2 SGA score less than 5 (on 7-point scale)
K/DOQI [54]	2003	Predialysis serum albumin Percentage of usual body weight Percentage of standard body weight, SGA Dietary interviews and diaries nPNA	Albumin >4 g/dL Prealbumin <30 mg/dL Predialysis creatinine <10 mg/dL

Abbreviations: BMI, body mass index; PCR, protein catabolic rate; DEXA, dual-energy X-ray absorptionetry; nPNA, normalized protein nitrogen appearance; SGA, subjective global assessment.

Markers of visceral protein stores

Like SGA, all five guidelines recommend the use of measurements that reflect visceral protein stores, for example, serum albumin. However, a low serum albumin is strongly correlated with inflammation and is influenced by other factors, such as hydration status [58]. Other readily measurable blood markers of nutritional status include creatinine and thyroid binding protein (prealbumin or more correctly transthyretin). Plasma creatinine concentrations reflect muscle mass, somatic stores, dietary protein intake, residual kidney function, and dialysis dose, but may nonetheless be of value as a marker of nutritional status [59]. Blood transthyretin levels change rapidly when hepatic protein production is impaired and provide useful prognostic information independent of albumin levels in hemodialysis patients [60].

Dietary protein intake

In addition to SGA and markers of visceral protein stores, a measure of dietary protein intake is recommended in the Australasian [1], Canadian [2], European [5], and US [54] guidelines. This generally involves the patient keeping a diary or recalling their recent food intake. A simpler method is to evaluate protein nitrogen appearance (PNA), which is mathematically identical to protein catabolic rate (PCR) and roughly equivalent to protein intake [61]. Under steady-state conditions, nitrogen intake roughly equals total nitrogen loss (total nitrogen appearance) [62]. Thus, PNA can be calculated from total nitrogen appearance (the sum of dialysis, urine, and fecal nitrogen losses) and should be normalized (nPNA) to fat-free, edema-free standardized body weight. Because of the difficulty in measuring nitrogen in stool, equations have been derived to estimate PNA from nitrogen in serum, urine, and dialysate, although these are more accurate in peritoneal dialysis patients, in whom dialysate urea concentrations can be measured directly rather than estimated [54].

Assessment of changes in lean body mass

Another approach is to monitor lean body mass over time. This is best done in practice by using anthropometrics, multifrequency bioimpedance assay (BIA), and dual-energy X-ray absorptiometry (DEXA). BIA parameters indicative of poor nutritional status predicts mortality in dialysis patients [63], and although sequential DEXA measurements are reproducible [64], they have not been validated as outcomes measures. Hand grip strength can also be used as a readily measurable marker of muscle mass and predicts clinical events in men but not women receiving hemodialysis [56].

Management of malnutrition

Regardless of the cause, ongoing provision of an adequate nutritional intake is generally recommended for the prevention and treatment of malnutrition in adults receiving hemodialysis. Although intensive nutritional support undoubtedly improves markers of poor nutritional status, there is currently insufficient evidence to suggest that either the administration of oral supplements [65] or intradialytic parenteral nutrition [66] improves clinical outcomes among such individuals. This should be kept in mind when evaluating the various randomized controlled trials that have used nutritional markers, such as albumin, as a surrogate for clinical benefit [67–75]. These studies, which have examined the value of various dietary interventions and intradialytic parenteral nutrition, are summarized in Table 39.3.

Despite the lack of evidence of benefit, proactive management of malnourished hemodialysis patients is generally recommended [1,2,6–8,54]. The general principles are to ensure that the patient is receiving an adequate dialysis dose and that reversible factors such as inflammation are corrected [76]. In a stepwise approach to nutritional support, attempts should be made initially to increase intake of ordinary foods with the addition of oral supplements as necessary [77]. However, when these strategies fail and assuming that the gastrointestinal tract is functional, enteral feeding should be considered [78], either by nasogastric tube or percutaneous endoscopic gastrostomy. Patients in whom oral nutrition is not feasible or poorly tolerated should be considered for either intradialytic parenteral nutrition or total parenteral nutrition [79]. The benefits of these more aggressive interventions on mortality and morbidity outcomes in either moderately or severely malnourished hemodialysis patients have not been determined in randomized controlled clinical trials.

Dyslipidemia

Pattern and prevalence of dyslipidemia

Hemodialysis patients exhibit a dyslipidemia characterized by elevated plasma triglyceride levels, reflecting the accumulation of chylomicrons [80] and non-high-density triglyceride-rich lipoprotein particles [81]. This results from both an increase in the rate of synthesis and decreased clearance [82]. High-density lipoprotein (HDL) levels are generally reduced, and the distribution of HDL subfractions is abnormal. Whereas low-density lipoprotein (LDL) levels are usually normal, LDL particles tend to be small and of increased density [83], which are characteristics associated with enhanced atherogenicity [84] in the general population.

Clinical practice guidelines developed in Europe [4], the UK [6,7], and USA [85] recommend desirable limits for plasma lipid concentrations in hemodialysis patients (Table 39.4), based largely on ranges felt to be optimal in the general population. For example, the US K/DOQI guidelines use threshold values for LDL, HDL, and triglycerides recommended by the US National Cholesterol Education Program Expert Panel on Detection, Evaluation and Treatment of High Blood Cholesterol in Adults. Using these criteria, only 20.2% of 1047 hemodialysis patients in the Dialysis Morbidity and Mortality Study had normal plasma lipid values, and 61.1% qualified for treatment [85]. The above pattern of dyslipidemia is seen across a wide spectrum of chronic kidney disease and the evidence supporting specific steps in management of these dyslipidemias is reviewed in detail in chapter 32. This chapter will focus on these issues as they relate to hemodialysis patients.

Table 39.3 Published randomized trials assessing the impact of nutritional interventions in hemodialysis patients.

Study author [reference]	Population	Intervention	Outcome marker	Follow-up	Outcome
Cano [67]	26 malnourished HD patients	Peridialytic parenteral nutrition 3× weekly vs. no treatment	Albumin, prealbumin transferrin, body weight, arm circumference	3 mos	Intervention associated with improved serum albumin, prealbumin, body weight, and arm circumference
Cockram [68]	79 normally nourished HD patients	Standard formula vs. two disease-specific supplements (as sole source of nutrition)	Gastrointestinal symptoms, urea kinetics, nPCR	2 wks	No differences in GI symptoms; compared to standard formula; lower phosphorus on disease-specific products
Hiroshige [69]	28 malnourished elderly HD patients	Oral branched-chain amino acids (12 g/day) vs. placebo (crossover)	Serum albumin, anthropometric indices	6 mos	Supplementation increased albumin and improved anthropometric parameters
Kloppenburg [70]	50 HD patients	High-protein diet (and increased dialysis dose)	Protein intake (total nitrogen appearance), food diaries, serum albumin, lean body mass	10 wks	Protein intake increased on high-protein diet but no change in albumin or lean body mass
Kuhlmann [71]	18 malnourished HD patients	Group A: 45 kcal/kg/day with 1.5 g protein/kg/day; Group B: 35 kcal/kg/day with 1.2g protein/kg/day; Group C: usual diet supplemented with 10% protein intake	Serum albumin, prealbumin, dietary intake, and body weight	3 mos	Serum albumin increased in group A only; weight change correlated with mean dietary protein intake
Leon [72]	83 HD patients	Dietician-directed interventions vs. usual care	Change in albumin	6 mos	Dietetic intervention improved albumin levels
Sharma [73]	40 nondiabetic HD patients with BMI <20, albumin <4 g/dL	Disease-specific or standard enteral nutritional supplements vs. usual care	BMI, albumin, functional status	1 mo	Increase in BMI, serum albumin, and functional status among patients receiving supplements
Tietze [74]	19 HD patients	Fish protein vs. placebo (crossover)	Serum proteins, anthropometrics	6 mos	Body weight and arm muscle circumference but not albumin or other anthropometric markers improved during active treatment
Toigo [75]	21 HD patients	Essential amino acids vs. standard amino acid supplement (control)	Biochemisty, anthropometrics, PCR	6 mos	PCR increased more and albumin decreased in those receiving standard amino acids compared to essential amino acids group

Abbreviations: HD, hemodialysis; nPCR, normalized protein catabolic rate; PCR, protein catabolic rate.

Dyslipidemia and cardiovascular disease

Because dialysis patients are at high risk of vascular events, dyslipidemia represents a potentially attractive target for therapeutic intervention. However, although in the general population high blood LDL and low HDL concentrations are associated with increased cardiovascular risk [86], epidemiological studies have failed to demonstrate these relationships in hemodialysis populations [87]. This may be due to the confounding effects of malnutrition and inflammation, because the expected relationships are partly restored when these factors are taken into account [88]. Whether other markers (which might more clearly define the extent of disturbed lipoprotein metabolism) perform better than cholesterol in predicting cardiovascular outcomes in hemodialysis patients remains to be established.

Management of dyslipidemia

Recommendations relating to the management of dyslipidemia usually start with therapeutic life-style changes. Low-fat, low-cholesterol diets [89] and exercise programs [90] favorably modify blood LDL and HDL concentrations in the general population, and at least one small randomized controlled trial has suggested that exercise lowers triglyceride levels in dialysis patients [91]. Fibrates are generally recommended for lowering blood triglyceride concentrations and raising HDL, although use of these agents in hemodialysis patients may be associated with an increased risk of myositis and rhabdomyolysis [85], and benefits have not been properly assessed in outcomes studies.

Statins reduce adverse vascular events in a wide range of populations, particularly in patients with (or those at high risk of

Table 39.4 Current guidelines on targets for lipid reduction in hemodialysis patients.

Guideline	Date updated	Recommendation	Notes
Caring for Australasians with Renal Impairment [1]		No recommendation	
Canadian Society of Nephrology [2]		No recommendation	
European Best Practice Guidelines [4]	2002	LDL cholesterol <100 mg/dL, triglycerides <180 mg/dL, non-HDL cholesterol <130 mg/dL	Blood collected in fasting state
UK Renal Association [7]	2002	Primary prevention: Total cholesterol <195 mg/dL or 30% reduction from baseline	
K/DOQI [85]	2003	LDL cholesterol <100 mg/dL; triglycerides <200 mg/dL; non-HDL cholesterol <130 mg/dL	Bloods collected in fasting state if feasible

developing) cardiovascular disease there is no threshold below which a lower LDL level is not associated with clinical benefit [92]. Whether such benefits apply to hemodialysis patients is less clear. A recent Cochrane review [93] identified six randomized controlled trials that assessed the efficacy of statins in lowering blood lipid levels in hemodialysis populations [94–96] or in populations that included hemodialysis patients [97–99]. These trials are listed in Table 39.5. The authors of the review concluded that when patients were treated for 12 weeks, statins decreased blood cholesterol as effectively as in the general population, although based on these short-term studies they were unable to comment on safety and outcome benefits [93]. A large retrospective study including 3716 incident dialysis patients showed a 36% reduction in cardiovascular events in patients prescribed statins at baseline [100], suggesting that such patients may gain benefit from these agents. However, the

only published prospective randomized controlled trial examining the impact of statin therapy on outcomes among hemodialysis patients has not supported these observational data. In Die Deutsche Diabetes Dialyse (4D) study, 1255 patients with type 2 diabetes receiving hemodialysis were randomized to receive atrovastatin at 20 mg/day or placebo [101]. Active therapy was associated with a 42% reduction in LDL cholesterol levels but made no difference to the primary composite end point of fatal cardiovascular events, nonfatal myocardial infarction, and nonfatal stroke.

Two ongoing studies, the Study of Heart and Renal Protection (SHARP, with simvastatin at 20 mg and ezetimibe at 10 mg versus placebo) [102] and AURORA (A study to evaluate the Use of Rosuvastatin in subjects On Regular hemodialysis: an Assessment) of survival and cardiovascular events; using rosuvastatin at 10 mg versus placebo [103] will provide additional outcome data in

Table 39.5 Randomized trials evaluating the impact of statins on blood lipid levels in hemodialysis patients.

Study author [reference]	Patients	Treatment	% Change compared to baseline or placebo[a]			
			Cholesterol	LDL	HDL	TG
Fiorini [94]	12 HD	Atorvastatin, 10 mg titrating to 40 mg, vs. placebo	−26*	−36*		
Lins [95]	42 HD	Atrovastatin, 10–40 mg	−33*	−43*		
Diepeveen [96]	23 HD, 25 PD	2×2 factorial, Atrovastatin, 40 mg, and alpha-tocopherol 800 IU daily	−34 +1.9	−43 +4.4	−1.9 +4.8	−34 −4.2
PERFECT [97]	107 on HD or PD	2×2 factorial, simvastatin, 10 mg, and enalapril	−13*	−17*		−12*
Saltissi [98]	34 HD, 23 CAPD	Simvastatin, 5–20 mg, vs. placebo, both with dietary intervention	−21 −12	−25 −14	−6 −3	−18 −14
Chang [99]	62 HD	Simvastatin vs. placebo	−16 +2	−41 +3	+3 −3	−17 +2

Abbreviations: HD, hemodialysis; PD, peritoneal dialysis.
[a]*, treatment group significantly different from placebo or control.

hemodialysis populations consisting of predominantly nondiabetic patients. In the interim, the benefits of lipid-lowering therapy in such patients remains uncertain.

Conclusion

Optimal management of the hemodialysis patient should include attention to the more general aspects of care outlined in this chapter and requires a multidisciplinary approach. Failure to address specific aspects such as predialysis hyperkalemia can result rapidly in adverse events, whereas correction of complications such as hypertension and dyslipidemia may have long-term clinical outcome benefits. Despite a lack of robust clinical data, management of these general aspects of care of the hemodialysis patient is considered to be sufficiently important to justify inclusion of target ranges in most clinical practice guidelines. These targets are likely to need revision in the future as the results of outcomes trials become available.

References

1 CARI (Caring for Australians with Renal Impairment) CARI Guidelines Part 1: Dialysis Guidelines. In: Knight J, Vimalachandra D, editors, *Excerpta Medica Communications*, 2000; www.kidney.org.au/cari/.

2 Canadian Society of Nephrology Clinical Practice Guidelines. J Am Soc Nephrol 1999; **10(Suppl 13):** S289–S321.

3 European Best Practice Guidelines for hemodialysis. Part 1. *Nephrol Dial Transplant* 2002; **17(Suppl 7):** S1–S111.

4 European Best Practice Guidelines for hemodialysis. Part 2. *Nephrol Dial Transplant* 2005; **20(Suppl 5):** 148–155.

5 European Best Practice Guidelines. EBPG on nutrition. *Nephrol Dial Transplant* 2007; **22(Suppl 2):** ii45–ii87.

6 Renal Association Standards and Audit Subcommittee. *Treatment of Adults & Children with Renal Failure: Standards and Audit Measures*, 3rd edn. Royal College of Physicians, London, 2002.

7 The Renal Association Clinical Guidelines Committee. *Clinical Practice Guidelines*, 4th edn. The Renal Association, Hampshire, England, 2007, www.renal.org/guidelines.

8 National Kidney Foundation. K/DOQI clinical practice guidelines for hemodialysis adequacy: update 2000. *Am J Kidney Dis* 2000; **37(Suppl 1):** S7–S64.

9 National Kidney Foundation. K/DOQI clinical practice guidelines for hemodialysis adequacy, update 2006. *Am J Kidney Dis*, 2006; **(suppl 1):** S1–S322.

10 Lowrie EG, Lew NL. Death risk in hemodialysis patients: the predictive value of commonly measured variables and an evaluation of death rate differences between facilities. *Am J Kidney Dis* 1990; **15:** 458–482.

11 Morduchowicz G, Winkler J, Derazne E, Van Dyk DJ, Wittenberg C, Zabludowski JR *et al.* Causes of death in patients with end-stage renal disease treated by dialysis in a center in Israel. *Isr J Med Sci* 1992; **28:** 776–779.

12 Ahmed J, Weisberg LS. Hyperkalemia in dialysis patients. *Semin Dial* 2001; **14:** 348–356.

13 Mahoney BA, Smith WA, Lo DS, Tsoi K, Tonelli M, Clase CM. Emergency interventions for hyperkalaemia. *Cochrane Database Syst Rev* 2005: CD003235.

14 Alfonzo AV, Isles C, Geddes C, Deighan C. Potassium disorders: clinical spectrum and emergency management. *Resuscitation* 2006; **70:** 10–25.

15 Wiegand CF, Davin TD, Raij L, Kjellstard CM. Severe hypokalemia induced by hemodialysis. *Arch Int Med* 1981; **141:** 167–170.

16 Bleyer AJ, Hartman J, Brannon PC, Reeves-Daniel A, Satko SG, Russell G. Characteristics of sudden death in hemodialysis patients. *Kidney Int* 2006; **69:** 2268–2273.

17 Mioni R, Gropuzzo M, Messa M, Boscutti G, D'Angelo A, Cruciatti A *et al.* Acid production and base balance in patients on chronic haemodialysis. *Clin Sci* 2001; **101:** 329–337.

18 Kopple JD, Kalanter-Zadeh K, Mehrotra R. Risks of chronic metabolic acidosis in patients with chronic kidney disease. *Kidney Int* 2005; **95(Suppl):** S21–S27.

19 Bommer J, Locatelli F, Satayathum S, Keen ML, Goodkin DA, Saito A *et al.* Association of predialysis serum bicarbonate levels with risk of mortality and hospitalization in the Dialysis Outcomes and Practice Patterns Study (DOPPS). *Am J Kidney Dis* 2004; **44:** 661–671.

20 Graham KA, Reaich D, Channon SM, Downie S, Goodship TH. Correction of acidosis in hemodialysis decreases whole-body protein degradation. *J Am Soc Nephrol* 1997; **8:** 632–637.

21 Lefebvre A, de Vernejoul MC, Gueris J, Goldfarb B, Graulet AM, Morieux C. Optimal correction of acidosis changes progression of dialysis osteodystrophy. *Kidney Int* 1989; **36:** 1112–1118.

22 Graham KA, Hoenich NA, Tarbit M, Ward MK, Goodship TH. Correction of acidosis in hemodialysis patients increases the sensitivity of the parathyroid glands to calcium. *J Am Soc Nephrol* 1997; **8:** 627–631.

23 Williams AJ, Dittmer ID, McArley A, Clarke J. High bicarbonate dialysate in hemodialysis patients: effects on acidosis and nutritional status. *Nephrol Dial Transplant* 1997; **12:** 2633–2637.

24 Movilli E, Zani R, Carli O, Sangalli L, Pola A, Camerini C *et al.* Correction of metabolic acidosis increases serum albumin concentrations and decreases kinetically evaluated protein intake in hemodialysis patients: a prospective study. *Nephrol Dial Transplant* 1998; **13:** 1719–1722.

25 Brady JP, Hasbargen JA. Correction of metabolic acidosis and its effect on albumin in chronic hemodialysis patients. *Am J Kidney Dis* 1998; **31:** 35–40.

26 Gabutti L, Ferrari N, Giudici G, Mombelli G, Marone C. Unexpected hemodynamic instability associated with standard bicarbonate hemodialysis. *Nephrol Dial Transplant* 2003; **18:** 2369–2376.

27 Birchem JA, Fraley MA, Senkottaiyan N, Alpert MA. Influence of hypertension on cardiovascular outcomes in hemodialysis patients. *Semin Dial* 2005; **18:** 391–395.

28 Agarawal R. Hypertension and survival in chronic hemodialysis patients- past lessons and future opportunities. *Kidney Int* 2005; **67:** 1–13.

29 Stidley CA, Hunt WC, Tentori F, Schmidt D, Rohrscheib M, Paine S *et al.* Changing relationship of blood pressure with mortality over time among hemodialysis patients. *J Am Soc Nephrol* 2006; **17:** 513–520.

30 Agarawal R, Brim NJ, Mahenthiran J, Andersen MJ, Saha C. Out-of-hemodialysis-unit blood pressure is a superior determinant of left ventricular hypertrophy. *Hypertension* 2006; **47:** 62–68.

31 National Kidney Foundation. K/DOQI clinical practice guidelines for cardiovascular disease in dialysis patients. *Am J Kidney Dis* 2005; **45:** S1–S153.

32 Charra B, Calemard E, Ruffet M, Chazot C, Terrat JC, Vanel T *et al.* Survival as an index of adequacy of dialysis. *Kidney Int* 1992; **41**: 1286–1291.

33 Rahman M, Dixit A, Donley V, Gupta S, Hanslik T, Lacson E *et al.* Factors associated with inadequate blood pressure control in hypertensive hemodialysis patients. *Am J Kidney Dis* 1999; **33**: 498–506.

34 Shinzato T, Nakal S, Akiba T, Yamazaki C, Sasaki R, Kitaoka T *et al.* Survival in long-term hemodialysis patients: results from the annual survey of the Japanese Society of Dialysis Therapy. *Nephrol Dial Transplant* 1997; **12**: 884–888.

35 Ronco C, Brendolan A, Milan M, Rodeghiero MP, Zanella M, La Greca G. Impact of biofeedback-induced cardiovascular stability on hemodialysis tolerance and efficiency. *Kidney Int* 2000; **58**: 800–808.

36 Shoji T, Tsubakihara Y, Fujii M, Imai E. Hemodialysis-associated hypotension as an independent risk factor for two-year mortality in hemodialysis patients. *Kidney Int* 2004; **66**: 1212–1220.

37 Daugirdas JT. Dialysis hypotension: a hemodynamic analysis. *Kidney Int* 1991; **39**: 233–246.

38 Koch M, Thomas B, Tschope W, Ritz E. Survival and predictors of death in dialysed diabetic patients. *Diabetologia* 1993; **36**: 1113–1117.

39 Poldermans D, Man in 't Veld AJ, Rambaldi R, van den Meiracker AH, van den Dorpel MA, Rocchi G *et al.* Cardiac evaluation in hypotension-prone and hypotension-resistant hemodialysis patients. *Kidney Int* 1999; **56**: 1905–1911.

40 Dheenan S, Henrich WL. Preventing dialysis hypotension: A comparison of usual protective maneuvres. *Kidney Int* 2001; **59**: 1175–1181.

41 Sang GL, Kovithavongs C, Ulan R, Kjellstrand CM. Sodium ramping in hemodialysis: a study of beneficial and adverse effects. *Am J Kidney Dis* 1997; **29**: 669–677.

42 Yu AW, Ing TS, Zabaneh RI, Daugirdas JT. Effect of dialysate temperature on central hemodynamics and urea kinetics. *Kidney Int* 1995; **48**: 237–243.

43 Maggiore Q, Pizzarelli F, Santoro A, Panzetta G, Bonforte G, Hannedouche T *et al.* The effects of control of thermal balance on vascular stability in hemodialysis patients: results of the European randomized clinical trial. *Am J Kidney Dis* 2002; **40**: 280–290.

44 Reddan DN, Szczech LA, Hasselblad V, Lowrie EG, Lindsay RM, Himmelfarb J *et al.* Intradialytic blood volume monitoring in ambulatory hemodialysis patients: a randomized trial. *J Am Soc Nephrol* 2005; **16**: 2162–2169.

45 Selby NM, McIntyre CW. A systematic review of the clinical effects of reducing dialysate fluid temperature. *Nephrol Dial Transplant* 2006; **21**: 1883–1898.

46 Chazot C, Laurent G, Charra B, Blanc C, VoVan C, Jean G *et al.* Malnutrition in long-term hemodialysis survivors. *Nephrol Dial Transplant* 2001; **16**: 61–69.

47 Kopple JD. McCollum Award Lecture 1996: Protein-energy malnutrition in maintenance dialysis patients. *Am J Clin Nutr* 1997; **65**: 1544–1557.

48 Stratton RJ, Green CJ, Elia M, editors. *Disease-Related Malnutrition: an Evidence-Based Approach to Treatment.* CABI, Wallingford, UK, 2003; 35–92.

49 Ikizler TA, Greene JH, Wingard RL, Parker RA, Hakim RM. Spontaneous dietary protein intake during progression of chronic renal failure. *J Am Soc Nephrol* 1995; **6**: 1386–1391.

50 Stenvinkel P, Heimburger O, Paultre F, Diczfalusy U, Wang T, Berglund L *et al.* Strong association between malnutrition, inflammation, and atherosclerosis in chronic renal failure. *Kidney Int* 1999; **55**: 1899–1911.

51 Keane WF, Collins AJ. Influence of co-morbidity on mortality and morbidity in patients treated with hemodialysis. *Am J Kidney Dis* 1994; **24**: 1010–1018.

52 Fung F, Sherrard DJ, Gillen DL, Wong C, Kestenbaum B, Seliger S *et al.* Increased risk for cardiovascular mortality among malnourished end-stage renal disease patients. *Am J Kidney Dis* 2002; **40**: 307–314.

53 Beddhu S, Pappas LM, Ramkumar N, Samore MH. Malnutrition and atherosclerosis in dialysis patients. *J Am Soc Nephrol* 2004; **15**: 733–742.

54 National Kidney Foundation. K/DOQI clinical practice guidelines for nutrition of chronic renal failure. *Am J Kidney Dis* 2001; **37(Suppl 2)**: S66–S70.

55 Enia G, Sicuso C, Alati G, Zoccali C. Subjective global assessment of nutrition in dialysis patients.*Nephrol Dial Transplant* 1993; **8**: 1094–1098.

56 Stenvinkel P, Barany P, Chung SH, Lindholm B, Heimburger O. A comparative analysis of nutritional parameters as predictors of outcome in male and female ESRD patients. *Nephrol Dial Transplant* 2002; **17**: 1266–1274.

57 Cooper BA, Bartlett LH, Aslani A, Allen BJ, Ibels LS, Pollock CA. Validity of subjective global assessment as a nutritional marker in end-stage renal disease. *Am J Kidney Dis* 2002; **40**: 126–132.

58 Jones CH, Akbani H, Croft DC, Worth DP. The relationship between serum albumin and hydration status in hemodialysis patients. *J Ren Nutr* 2002; **12**: 209–212.

59 Cano NJ. Metabolism and clinical interest of serum transthyretin (prealbumin) in dialysis patients. *Clin Chem Lab Med* 2002; **40**: 1313–1319.

60 Chertow GM, Ackert K, Lew NL, Lazarus JM, Lowrie EG. Prealbumin is as important as albumin in the nutritional assessment of hemodialysis patients. *Kidney Int* 2000; **58**: 2512–2517.

61 Peterson S, Sigman-Grant M, Eissenstat B, Kris-Etherton P. Impact of adopting lower-fat food choices on energy and nutrient intakes of American adults. *J Am Diet Assoc* 1999; **99**: 177–183.

62 Kloppenburg WD, Stegeman CA, de Jong PE, Huisman RM. Relating protein intake to nutritional status in hemodialysis patients: how to normalize the protein equivalent of total nitrogen appearance (PNA)? *Nephrol Dial Transplant* 1999; **14**: 2165–2172.

63 Chertow GM, Jacobs DO, Lazarus JM, Lew NL, Lowrie EG. Phase angle predicts survival in hemodialysis patients. *J Ren Nutr* 1997; **7**: 204–207.

64 Kerr PG, Strauss BJ, Atkins RC. Assessment of the nutritional state of dialysis patients. *Blood Purif* 1996; **14**: 382–387.

65 Stratton RJ, Bircher G, Fouque D, Stenvinkel P, de Mutsert R, Engfer M *et al.* Multinutrient oral supplements and tube feeding in maintenance dialysis: a systematic review and meta-analysis. *Am J Kidney Dis* 2005; **46**: 387–405.

66 Cano N. Intradialytic parenteral nutrition: where do we go from here? *J Ren Nutr* 2004; **14**: 3–5.

67 Cano N, Labastie-Coeyrehourq J, Lacombe P, Stroumza P, di Constanzo-Dufetel J, Durbec JP *et al.* Perdialytic parenteral nutrition with lipids and amino acids in malnourished hemodialysis patients. *Am J Clin Nutr* 1990; **52**: 726–730.

68 Cockram DB, Hensley MK, Rodriguez M, Agarwal G, Wennberg A, Ruey P *et al.* Safety and tolerance of medical nutritional products as sole sources of nutrition in people on hemodialysis.*J Ren Nutr* 1998; **8**: 25–33.

69 Hiroshige K, Sonta T, Suda T, Kanegae K, Ohtani A. Oral supplementation of branched-chain amino acid improves nutritional status in elderly patients on chronic haemodialysic. *Nephrol Dial Transplant* 2001; **16**: 1856–1862.

70 Kloppenburg WD, Stegeman CA, Kremer Hovinga TK, Vastenburg G, Vos P, de Jong PE et al. Effect of prescribing a high protein diet and increasing the dose of dialysis on nutrition in stable chronic hemodialysis patients: a randomized controlled trial. *Nephrol Dial Transplant* 2004; **19**: 1212–1223.

71 Kuhlmann MK, Schmidt F, Kohler H. High protein/energy vs. standard protein/energy nutritional regimen in the treatment of malnourished hemodialysis patients. *Miner Electrolyte Metab* 1999; **25**: 306–310.

72 Leon JB, Majerle AD, Soinski JA, Kushner I, Ohri-Vachaspati P, Sehgal AR. Can a nutrition intervention improve albumin levels among hemodialysis patients? A pilot study. *J Ren Nutr* 2001; **11**: 9–15.

73 Sharma M, Rao M, Jacob S, Jacob CK. A controlled trial of intermittent enteral nutrient supplementation in maintenance hemodialysis patients. *J Ren Nutr* 2002; **12**: 229–237.

74 Tietze IN, Pedersen EB. Effect of fish protein supplementation on amino acid profile and nutritional staus in hemodialysis patients. *Nephrol Dial Transplant* 1991; **6**: 948–954.

75 Toigo G, Situlin R, Tamaro G, Del Bianco A, Giuliani V, Dardi F et al. Effect of intravenous supplementation of a new essential amino acid formulation in hemodialysis patients. *Kidney Int Suppl* 1989; **1989**: S278–S281.

76 Fouque D. Nutritional requirements in maintenance hemodialysis. *Adv Ren Replace Ther* 2003; **10**: 183–193.

77 Bossola M, Muscaritoli M, Tazza L, Giungi S, Tortorelli A, Fanelli FR et al. Malnutrition in hemodialysis patients: what therapy? *Am J Kidney Dis* 2005; **46**: 371–386.

78 Holley JL, Kirk J. Enteral tube feeding in a cohort of chronic hemodialysis patients. *J Ren Nutr* 2002; **12**: 177–182.

79 Foulks CJ. Intradialytic parenteral nutrition treatment. *Am J Kidney Dis* 1999; **33**: 1202.

80 Cattran DC, Fenton SS, Wilson DR, Steiner G. Defective triglyceride removal in lipemia associated with peritoneal dialysis and hemodialysis. *Ann Intern Med* 1976; **85**: 29–33.

81 Liu J, Rosner MH. Lipid abnormalities associated with end-stage renal disease. *Semin Dial* 2006; **19**: 32–40.

82 Batista MC, Welty FK, Diffenderfer MR, Sarnak MJ, Schaefer EJ, Lamon-Fava S et al. Apolipoprotein A-I, B-100, and B-48 metabolism in subjects with chronic kidney disease, obesity, and the metabolic syndrome. *Metabolism* 2004; **53**: 1255–1261.

83 Rajman I, Harper L, McPake D, Kendall MJ, Wheeler DC. Low-density lipoprotein subfraction profiles in chronic renal failure. *Nephrol Dial Transplant* 1998; **13**: 2281–2287.

84 Austin MA, King MC, Vranizan KM, Krauss RM. Atherogenic lipoprotein phenotype. A proposed genetic marker for coronary heart disease risk. *Circulation* 1990; **82**: 495–506.

85 National Kidney Foundation. K/DOQI clinical practice guidelines for management of dyslipidemias in patients with kidney disease. *Am J Kidney Dis* 2003; **41(Suppl 3)**: S1–S91.

86 Castelli WP. Lipids, risk factors and ischaemic heart disease. *Atherosclerosis* 1996; **124(Suppl)**: S1–S9.

87 Kalantar-Zadeh K, Block G, Humphreys MH, Kopple JD. Reverse epidemiology of cardiovascular risk factors in maintenance dialysis patients. *Kidney Int* 2003; **63**: 793–808.

88 Liu Y, Coresh J, Eustance JA, Longenecker JC, Jaar B, Fink NE et al. Association between cholesterol level and mortality in dialysis patients: role of inflammation and malnutrition. *JAMA* 2004; **291**: 451–459.

89 Yu-Poth S, Zhao G, Etherton T, Naglak M, Jonnalagadda S, Kris-Etherton PM. Effects of the National Cholesterol Education Program's Step I and Step II dietary intervention programs on cardiovascular disease risk factors: a meta-analysis. *Am J Clin Nutr* 1999; **69**: 632–646.

90 Halbert JA, Silagy CA, Finucane P, Withers RT, Hamdorf PA. Exercise training and blood lipids in hyperlipidemic and normolipidemic adults: a meta-analysis of randomized, controlled trials. *Eur J Clin Nutr* 1999; **53**: 514–522.

91 Goldberg AP, Geltman EM, Hagberg JM, Gavin JR, Delmez JA, Carney RM et al. Therapeutic benefits of exercise training for hemodialysis patients. *Kidney Int* 1983; **16(Suppl)**: S303–S309.

92 Baigent C, Keech A, Kearney PM, Blackwell L, Buck G, Pollicino C et al. Efficacy and safety of cholesterol-lowering treatment: prospective meta-analysis of data from 90,056 participants in 14 randomised trials of statins. *Lancet* 2005; **366**: 1267–1278.

93 Navaneethan SD, Shrivastava R. HMG CoA reductase inhibitors (statins) for dialysis patients. *Cochrane Database Syst Rev* 2004; **18**: CD004289.

94 Fiorini F, Patrone E, Castelluccio A. Clinical investigation on the hypolipidemic effect of simvastatin versus probucol in hemodialyis patients. *Clin Ter* 1994; **145**: 213–217.

95 Lins RL, Matthys KE, Billiouw JM, Dratwa M, Dupont P, Lameire NH et al. Lipid and apoprotein changes during atorvastatin up-titration in hemodialysis patients with hypercholesterolemia: a placebo-controlled study. *Clin Nephrol* 2004; **62**: 287–294.

96 Diepeveen SH, Verhoeven GW, van der Palen J, Dikkeschei LD, van Tits LJ, Kolsters G et al. Effects of atorvastatin and vitamin E on lipoproteins and oxidative stress in dialysis patients: a randomised-controlled trial. *J Intern Med* 2005; **257**: 438–445.

97 Robson R, Collins J, Johnson R, Kitching R, Searle M, Walker R et al. Effects of simvastatin and enalapril on serum lipoprotein concentrations and left ventricular mass in patients on dialysis. The Perfect Study Collaborative Group. *J Nephrol* 1997; **10**: 33–40.

98 Saltissi D, Morgan C, Rigby RJ, Westhuyzen J. Safety and efficacy of simvastatin in hypercholesterolemic patients undergoing chronic renal dialysis. *Am J Kidney Dis* 2002; **39**: 283–290.

99 Chang JW, Yang WS, Min WK, Lee SK, Park JS, Kim SB. Effects of simvastatin on high-sensitivity C-reactive protein and serum albumin in hemodialysis patients. *Am J Kidney Dis* 2002; **39**: 1213–1217.

100 Seliger SL, Weiss NS, Gillen DL, Kestenbaum B, Ball A, Sherrard DJ et al. HMG-CoA reductase inhibitors are associated with reduced mortality in ESRD patients. *Kidney Int* 2002; **61**: 297–304.

101 Wanner C, Krane V, Marz W, Olschewski M, Mann JF, Ruf G et al. Atorvastatin in patients with type 2 diabetes mellitus undergoing hemodialysis. *N Engl J Med* 2005; **353**: 238–248.

102 Baigent C, Landry M. Study of Heart and Renal Protection (SHARP). *Kidney Int* 2003; **(Suppl 84)**: S207–S210.

103 Fellstrom B, Zannad F, Schmieder R, Holdaas H, Jardine A, Rose H et al. Effect of rosuvastatin on outcomes in chronic hemodialysis patients: design and rationale of the AURORA study. *Curr Control Trials Cardiovasc Med* 2005; **6**: 9.

40 Infections in Hemodialysis

Behdad Afzali & David J. A. Goldsmith

Department of Nephrology and Transplantation, Guy's Hospital, London, UK

Introduction

The number of patients referred for consideration of management of end-stage renal disease (ESRD) with renal replacement therapy (RRT) has continued to grow inexorably over the last 3 decades. This has arisen because of a large, mostly unreferred population who meet the criteria for chronic kidney disease (CKD) [1–4], together with increasing societal longevity, prosperity, and willingness to offer expensive medical therapies such as RRT [5,6].

Survival on RRT is markedly compromised by a combination of factors that include cardiovascular disease, malignancy, and infectious diseases. Infection is the second most common cause of death in this cohort and a very frequent cause of patient morbidity [7,8]. It thus constitutes a significant economic outlay [9]. In comparison to the general population, patients on hemodialysis (HD) are much more likely to die of infectious diseases [10], which is the result not only of a higher frequency of infections but also of greater severity of infections in these subjects [10].

Although this phenomenon can be partly explained by negative selection, that is, that healthier HD patients are selected for transplantation, there is nevertheless a very real susceptibility to infection in patients on HD, the etiology of which is multifactorial and includes a state of acquired immunodeficiency, immunocompromise, and increased risk of exposure to pathogenic microorganisms.

It is our intention in this chapter to describe the reasons for the increased risk for blood-borne bacterial infections in HD patients and to explore the evidence for prophylaxis, intervention, and treatment in this complex clinical situation as it relates specifically to infections of the dialysis access catheters. The epidemiology and etiology of non-access-related nosocomial infections that are nevertheless related to the dialysis procedure and the current guidelines for their prevention and management will be discussed in the next chapter.

Susceptibility to infection in patients receiving HD: immunodeficiency

Immunodeficiency can be acquired as part of the process of uremia and is demonstrated by the observation that responses to vaccinations in patients with CKD are poorer than in the general population [11–13] and become less pronounced as CKD progresses [14]. Defects in most components of the immune system have been described and include failure of T-cell costimulation [15,16], altered cytokine production [17], immune deviation toward Th1 responses [18,19], with consequent defective B-cell activity, dysregulation in innate immune mechanisms, defective phagocytosis [20], oxidative stress [21], and inhibition of cellular responses with iron therapy or iron overload [22–25]. In addition, immunodeficiency can arise as a direct result of the underlying cause of the renal failure (e.g. leukopenia in association with multiple myeloma [26] or HIV [27]) or as part of its treatment (e.g. immunosuppression for vasculitis [28]). These many predispositions are further exacerbated by contributory factors such as the marked trends in RRT populations towards increasing age and an increasing proportion of RRT patients whose ESRD has arisen secondary to diabetes mellitus [29]. Malnutrition is common in RRT populations [30] and is yet another factor strongly correlated with increased risk of infections.

Patients on HD are thus immunocompromised in many significant and complementary ways. In addition, there is another highly significant risk factor for infection in HD patients, the presence of plastic lines (dialysis catheters and pacemaker wires) and dialysis needles which circumvent immunological barriers (the skin) and provide ready access for microorganisms to reach the bloodstream. Not surprisingly, the presence of artificial vascular access for HD is the leading risk factor for the development of bacteremia in chronic HD patients [31]. Indwelling plastic materials and wires (as well as polytetrafluoroethylene used in arteriovenous grafts)

Evidence-based Nephrology. Edited by Donald Molony and Jonathan Craig
© 2009 Blackwell Publishing, ISBN: 978-1-4051-3975-5.

also act as niduses of microbiological colonization and subsequent infection, including endovascular infections such as endocarditis, inhibiting normal eradication of microorganisms by immune cells and antibiotics [32].

In-hospital HD exposes patients to hospital-acquired microorganisms, which are generally more fastidious and resistant to antibiotics than their community-acquired counterparts (although this pattern is slowly changing, with the emergence of more resistant organisms in the community [33,34]). Replacement of the endogenous flora with those from the hospital environment is therefore likely and is driven by repeated hospitalization and by the common use of broad-spectrum antibiotics. Many of the above factors also explain the increased incidence of *Clostridium difficile* in CKD and RRT populations. Not surprisingly, the repeated use of broad-spectrum antibiotics in this cohort of individuals has led to a selection in favor of the growth of resistant species, such as methicillin-resistant *Staphylococcus aureus* (MRSA), vancomycin-resistant *Staphylococcus aureus*, vancomycin-resistant enterococcus, and others [35,36]. Nasal carriage of *S. aureus* is not only a prevalent finding in patients on HD (and in HD unit caregivers) but also a strong risk factor for bacteremic episodes [37–39]. A formal measure of prevalence of MRSA carriage in patients on HD in any specific country has not been published, but estimates in patients on peritoneal dialysis stipulate a carriage rate of around 16% [40]. Carriage rates are potentially higher among in-center HD patients, for whom the opportunity for colonization may be higher due to thrice-weekly close proximity to other recently hospitalized patients. Current recommendations in the USA do not require isolation of MRSA patients in free-standing dialysis units beyond universal precautions.

Additionally, HD patients can acquire infectious agents from a number of other sources, including exposure to intravenous substances (such as blood-borne viruses or translocation of skin organisms into the bloodstream during transfusions), dialysis water that may contain killed bacteria or bacterial products, such as endotoxin (fortunately, the occurrence of this in practice is very rare [41] and is reviewed in the next chapter). There are some risks associated with newer trends in HD practice, including bicarbonate-containing dialysate fluid, high-flux dialyzers, and dialyzer reuse, each of which may increase the threat of endotoxin transfer [42,43]. These risks are reviewed in the next chapter. Finally, "holiday dialysis" places the patient in contact with hospital organisms of the receiving institution (risking transport of potentially resistant bacteria between units [44]) and exposure to environmental pathogens, such as malaria-causing *Plasmodium* spp. and hepatitis A virus in certain parts of the world.

Infectious diseases in HD recipients can be divided into those that are related to vascular access and those that are not related to vascular access. Patients with non-vascular access-related infections are usually treated like patients without end-stage kidney failure, although the morbidity and mortality in HD patients presenting with septicemia or bacteremia are generally significantly higher, as these patients present by definition with at least one organ failure (ESRD) and typically multiorgan failure, e.g. cardiac failure or cardiovascular disease.

The remainder of this chapter is focused on septic diseases related to vascular access in HD patients.

Infections related to vascular access

Dialysis-related infections (those that result from vascular access for HD) account for the significant majority of all infections in HD patients and can take a number of forms that will reflect the type of dialysis access *in situ*. Infection can be local or systemic, simple or complicated.

Local infections, as the name implies, are localized to catheter exit site and/or tunnel and may present as purulent drainage from the exit site or as cellulitis of the skin overlying a surgical access site (arteriovenous fistula [AVF] or graft [AVG]) or tunneled dialysis line. Systemic infections arise from infected dialysis lines or surgical access and show features of systemic sepsis, sepsis syndrome, or septic shock. Complicated infections are those in which the access infection results in the following: 1) loss of access because of access thrombosis or surgical excision necessitated for treatment of sepsis [45,46]; 2) metastatic infection from the infected access to distant sites resulting in infective endocarditis [49,50], osteomyelitis or septic arthritis [51], septic pulmonary emboli [52], intervertebral discitis [53,54], and spinal epidural abscess [55] (Table 40.1); and 3) sepsis syndrome and/or death. Infection arising within a thrombosis of a graft [47,48] is also considered a complicated infection.

The overall incidence of access-related infections reported by most studies is on the order of 5 episodes/1000 catheter days [56,57], but it varies according to access type (Table 40.2). As illustrated in Table 40.2, the lowest risk for infection is observed in patients with primary AVF. The risk with AVF is lower roughly by a factor of 4 compared to the risk with AVG, and the risk with AVG is an order of magnitude lower than the risk with tunneled catheters. The data in Table 40.2 have remained consistent in comparisons from country to country and over time. Tunneled cuffed dialysis catheters have a lower risk of infection than their "untunneled" counterparts [58–60].

Table 40.1 Incidence of complications of HD catheter-associated bacteremic episodes.

Complication	Incidence (%)
Sepsis syndrome	6.9–12
Endocarditis	5.8–9.8
Osteomyelitis	2.3
Septic arthritis	2.3
Septic pulmonary emboli	Not known
Spinal epidural abscesses	1.2
Death	12–25.9

Source: Reproduced from Saxena and Panhotra 2005 [156] with kind permission.

Table 40.2 Incidence of bacteremic episodes according to form of dialysis access.

Vascular access type	Infection rate (no. of episodes/ 1000 catheter days)
Untunneled central venous catheters	5.0 (range, 3.8–6.5)
Femoral	7.6 (>10% after 1 wk)
Internal jugular	5.6 (>10% after 2–3 wks)
Subclavian	2.7 (>10% after 4 wks)
Tunneled cuffed central venous catheters	3.5 (range, 1.6–5.5)
Polytetrafluoroethylene arteriovenous graft	0.2 episodes/patient-year
Primary arteriovenous fistula	0.05 episodes/patient-year

Source: Reproduced from Saxena and Panhotra 2005 [156] with permission.

Table 40.3 Bacteria associated with HD catheter-related infections.

Organism	% of isolates[a]
Gram-positive cocci	52–70
Staphylococcus aureus	21.9–60
Staphylococcus epidermidis	8.8–12.6
MRSA	6.0–8.0
Enterococcus faecalis	2.4–8.0
Gram-negative bacilli	24–26.7
Pseudomonas aeruginosa	2.3–15.2
Escherichia coli	10.4
Acinetobacter species	12.8
Serratia marcescens	1.2–2.3
Klebsiella pneumoniae	6.4
Enterobacter cloacae	8.8
Polymicrobial	16.2–20

Source: Reproduced from Saxena and Panhotra 2005 [156] with permission.

[a] Figures are composites from a number of studies and therefore do not add up to 100%.

The higher risk associated with central venous catheters (CVCs), tunneled or not, may be mostly attributable to the formation of a highly organized bacterial biofilm, that is, a hydrated polymeric matrix containing bacteria in which individual bacteria live in specific "microniches" [61] on plastic surfaces [62], which excludes penetration by antibiotics [63], especially glycopeptides [64], and antibodies and which frustrates phagocytosis [32]. Episodic release of planktonic bacteria from the biofilm, which may be a programmed event [61], appears to precede bacteremia and septic symptoms [65]. Indeed, the majority of patients developing metastatic complications of dialysis-related infections are dialyzed via CVCs [66]. In the case of right-sided endocarditis, this may be, at least in part, due to the proximity of internal jugular CVCs to cardiac valves. This propensity for infection might account for the recently reported observations from epidemiological studies that consistently show higher mortality rates among patients dialyzing via a CVC or AVG compared with an AVF [67]. In one recent study, the adjusted relative hazard ratios for death were 1.5 and 1.2 for CVC and AVG, respectively, compared to AVF [67]. This may not be entirely attributable to increased infection rates, as there are likely to be several potential confounding factors; for example, patients referred late to dialysis services who have a higher mortality rate than early referrals [68–70] are more likely to commence dialysis via a CVC than are planned RRT starters. Additionally, patients with diffuse vascular disease ("vasculopaths"), who are generally older, more frail, and possess a greater background cardiovascular morbidity, are more likely to be dialyzed using CVCs. Furthermore, patients dialyzed via fistulae obtain higher blood flow rates on dialysis and obtain a greater effective dialysis dose per session. Vasculopaths, with probable concomitant coronary vessel disease, are more likely to be dialyzed via CVCs than are more fit subjects, who are often younger and in whom an AVF is more likely to mature and be employed successfully.

There are two distinct but overlapping time points for vascular access-related infections: primary infection, occurring at the time of access insertion, or secondary infection, which occurs later and is temporally related to use. In the case of CVCs, microbial infection can occur through the extraluminal or intraluminal routes, referring, respectively, to migration of bacteria from a contaminated catheter exit site down the catheter to the bloodstream or by translocation of bacteria from catheter hubs contaminated during manipulation [71–73]. The former occurs early (typically within less than 10 days [74]), whereas the latter occurs late (generally after 10 days [75]) after catheter insertion and is associated with the extent of and care in handling of the catheter.

The most frequent bacterial microorganisms associated with CVC-related infections are similar to the bacteria associated with infections of AVGs and AVFs (Table 40.3). Although these relative frequencies will differ from center to center, it is nevertheless the case that approximately two-thirds of all infections are caused by gram-positive organisms, whereas the remaining third are accounted for by gram-negative bacteria. Anaerobic, mycobacterial, and fungal infections are rare. The pathological determinants of infection relating to a CVC include the interaction between the material of which the catheter is constructed (some catheters, such as polyurethane, Teflon, and silicone elastomer, are more resistant to infection than polyethylene or polyvinyl chloride [76,77]), its thrombogenicity [78,79], and the virulence factors of local microorganisms. Not surprisingly, organisms with a predilection for skin colonization and biofilm formation are the most frequent causes of catheter-associated infection, and *S. aureus* (methicillin sensitive or resistant) heads the list [80]. Specific pathogenic mechanisms, such as adherence to host adhesion molecules on endothelial cells [81], extracellular matrix [82], platelets [83], and red blood cells [84], confer additional advantages to *S. aureus* in causing invasive and metastatic infections in this setting.

Management of access-related infections in HD

Management of access-related infections can be divided into measures aimed at prevention and those pertaining to treatment once infection has occurred. It is important to stress that although there have been a number of publications looking at the epidemiology of access-related infections and their associated mortality and morbidity, there have been no large-scale controlled trials of interventions aimed at prevention or treatment. Therefore, most guidelines and recommendations are not based on level A evidence.

Prevention of access-related infection
Insertion
Needless to say, primary catheter and surgical access infections can be significantly reduced by good aseptic barrier technique during insertion [85] and use of antiseptic solutions. There have been some suggestions from observational studies that chlorhexidine-based solutions (e.g. 2% in 70% isopropyl alcohol) may be superior to povidone–iodine [86,87]. With whatever cleansing solution is chosen, care is needed to ensure that the substance of the vascular catheter is not adversely affected (e.g. handling that leads to line splitting or disintegration). Polyethylene-based or polyvinyl chloride-based catheters should be avoided in favor of catheters based on polyurethane, Teflon, or silicone elastomer, as the former may be more prone to infection [76,77]. The site of catheter insertion may or may not alter the risk of infection. The evidence comparing the subclavian, jugular, and femoral sites is conflicting but suggests septic episodes are reduced if the subclavian route is selected [88–90]; nevertheless, most tunneled catheters for dialysis are inserted into an internal jugular vein, as the risk of subsequent venous stenosis is significantly higher when a catheters is placed in the subclavian location compared to the internal jugular vein.

Exit site cleansing and skin care
Application of dry gauze rather than transparent film dressings probably has little advantage in prevention of exit site colonization [91,92]. There may be a benefit in treatment of catheter exit sites with mupirocin ointment [93], although there also is a potential risk of damage to polyurethane- or silicone-based catheters from mupirocin [94–96] as well as a potential for development of mupirocin resistance [97]. There is likely, also, to be benefit from topical antiseptic agents, such as chlorhexidine and povidone–iodine [98,99] or other agents such as antibiotic and iodophor ointments [100,101], at the risk of favoring colonization of fungal species [100,101]. There is also evidence from a randomized controlled trial that topical application of honey to exit sites may be effective in reducing catheter-associated infections in hemodialysis patients, although this study was limited by a small number of subjects studied [102]. The maintenance of nursing staff experienced in the care of intravascular catheters [103,104] at adequate levels [105] is paramount. It follows from the evidence that ma-

nipulation of HD catheters and changes of HD catheter dressings should only be performed by trained dialysis staff.

Dialysis cannula characteristics
Given that colonization and subsequent infection are the result of interactions between the catheter material and virulence factors of local microorganisms, a number of catheters are now available which are impregnated with antiseptic or antimicrobial agents. Although there is some evidence demonstrating effectiveness in reducing line-associated infections, one must acknowledge the caveat that the trials have almost exclusively involved the use of triple-lumen uncuffed lines *in situ* for short periods of time (typically less than 30 days). How these results extrapolate to dialysis lines maintained for much more prolonged periods is unknown. Broadly speaking, available impregnated lines include those manufactured with a covering of chlorhexidine and silver sulfadiazine either on the external surface [74,106] or on both the internal and external luminal surfaces [107]. Minocycline and rifampin [108,109], in addition to platinum silver [110], have also been tried, as has silver on the cuff alone [111]. The first two may offer short-term antimicrobial protection, directed mainly against *Staphylococcus epidermidis*, although the evidence is conflicting [74,106,108,109,112,113]. There are concerns about the possibility of selection in favor of resistant organisms [74], and there is an additional risk of anaphylaxis with catheters coated with chlorhexidine and silver sulfadiazine [114] with little evidence in favor of these agents [110,111,115,116]. There are some reports regarding the use of silver-impregnated lines in HD of humans and animals, but the studies have, in general, been small and largely inconclusive due to low event rates (reviewed in reference 117). The antibacterial properties of covalently linked heparin [118] and electrically charged catheters [119] require additional study, and the use of these strategies cannot be supported with the current evidence.

Antibacterial lumen locks
In recent years, some interest has focused on the utility of antimicrobial locks in vascular catheters. Three studies in neutropenic cancer patients compared the use of heparin versus heparin plus vancomycin [120,121] or heparin versus heparin plus vancomycin and ciprofloxacin [122], with encouraging results. In each case, the rate of bacteremia (with vancomycin-sensitive organisms) was lower with the antibiotic-containing locks than with heparin alone, and the time to develop bacteremia was longer. Nevertheless, these were small studies in cohorts that differed significantly from patients on HD, such that the findings may not easily translate to the HD setting. Small-scale randomized controlled studies in patients on HD evaluating gentamicin locks (with citrate or heparin as the anticoagulant) in comparison to heparin alone have shown a reduced incidence of bacteremia and longer catheter survival in the antibiotic treatment arm [123,124]. However, the number of patients recruited was and the duration of these trials was short; therefore, the long-term effects of this approach, namely, long-term efficacy, gentamicin ototoxicity [125,126], and emergence of antibiotic resistance, cannot be properly gauged. Similarly, a

citrate–taurolidine–containing lock solution has been reported to confer an advantage over heparin locking alone in the prevention of dialysis catheter-related sepsis, although this study barely reached statistical significance and the event rate over 90 days of follow-up (four infections vs. none) was small [127]. Given the uncertainties noted above regarding an optimal locking solution, whatever locking solution chosen, vascular access-related infection should be the subject of regular and continuing audit loops to ensure that any changes in clinical practice confer the expected benefits in morbidity reduction.

Because most studies have consistently shown *S. aureus* to be a major pathogen in dialysis-related infections and to be associated frequently with complicated sepsis, the development of vaccines against *S. aureus* has been an important goal in the prevention of dialysis-related infections. The first efficacy trial of a vaccine against *S. aureus* (against serotypes 5 and 8, which account for 85% of all clinical isolates [128]) at a high dose in patients on HD demonstrated an approximately 80% response rate by 2 weeks (i.e. in 80% of subjects an antibody response of at least 80 µg/mL, the minimum protective level, was elicited), which then fell to 26% by the end of the study period (54 weeks). Nevertheless, 11 of 892 versus 26 of 906 subjects developed *S. aureus* bacteremia in the vaccine and control arms, respectively [129]. Unfortunately, the promise of this intervention has not yet been fulfilled. The possibility of developing a "working" staphylococcal vaccine for the dialysis population should not be discounted at this time. However, consideration should be given to inoculating patients at a time before they reach ESRD in order to maximize the immune response to the vaccine, in much the same way as is currently recommended with the hepatitis B and pneumococcal vaccines. Attempts at eliminating nasal carriage of *S. aureus* by topical application of mupirocin ointment [130,131] or oral rifampin [132] are fraught with the potential for the emergence of resistance [131,133] and recolonization after discontinuation of the antibiotics [132] and are, therefore, not likely to be viable long-term solutions.

Despite the measures described above to reduce the incidence of dialysis access-related infections and the potential for future prophylactic regimens, it is clear that the most important method of minimizing infections from dialysis is to reduce the number of patients dialyzed via CVCs in favor of surgically fashioned access, preferably AVFs. Nevertheless, the worldwide trend accompanying the growth of the ESRD population has been an increase in the number of patients dialyzed via tunneled cuffed CVCs and AVGs in preference to AVFs [134]. With the "Fistula First" campaign in North America and many other regional and national initiatives has come the good news that AVF rates are now climbing again: in the UK (based on data from the UK Renal Registry 2005 Report [see chapter 6]), less than 70% of established HD patients were being dialyzed using definitive vascular access and less than 50% of patients known to renal care units started HD with definitive access. Staphylococcal blood infection rates averaged 13/year/100 patients, with 4 cases/year/100 patients being MRSA. It was estimated that about 8–10% of the national UK MRSA burden came from renal dialysis patients. This scandalous state of affairs has

prompted much effort at vascular access service process redesign and numerous initiatives to reduce infections. This is not merely a reflection of limitations imposed by surgical theater time and surgical availability but a very real indication of increasing numbers of patients referred late to renal services who commence dialysis as hospital inpatients via plastic lines [68–70,135] and of patients who have already exhausted all other options for dialysis access.

Treatment of access-related infections

Correct treatment of access-related infection in patients on HD relies critically on early diagnosis and the clinical acumen and experience of the relevant clinicians. Excessive tardiness in removal of infected lines risks complications that include increased mortality and prolonged hospitalization, while overzealous line removal exposes the patient to unnecessary procedures which themselves carry an associated mortality and morbidity. In addition, many patients dialyzed through long-term tunneled lines have already exhausted other forms of access, thereby making line removal precarious. It is certainly in some cases a complex and difficult decision, and there have been no randomized controlled clinical trials or high-quality observational studies to help inform this decision.

The diagnostic criteria for HD catheter-related infections, as defined by the US Centers for Disease Control and Prevention [136,137], are summarized in Table 40.4, although there is some disagreement in the literature [138–140]. Unfortunately, while the diagnostic criteria are formulaic, in practice positive cultures are not always obtained, and when they are interpretation is problematic, as the positive predictive values of catheter and peripheral blood cultures are only 63% and 73%, respectively [141]. Clinical findings are not always reliable; fever, for example, has poor specificity, while encrustment or inflammation of an exit site has poor sensitivity. Furthermore, judgment plays an important role in the diagnosis and management of line-associated infections. Nevertheless, patients on HD who have a fever should have at least two sets of blood cultures sent to the laboratory before commencement of empirical antibiotic treatment.

In general, broad-spectrum antibiotics for common organisms are administered in the hope of eradicating the infection and decolonizing the line. Vancomycin and gentamicin offer coverage against most gram-positive organisms, including the increasingly prevalent MRSA and gram-negative organisms, and are the first-line choice for empirical treatment in many hemodialysis units (Renal Association Clinical Practice Guidelines 2007; http://www.renal.org/guidelines/module3b.html). However, these recommendations are tempered by concerns that overzealous use of vancomycin contributes potentially to the emergence of vancomycin-resistant bacterial species and that the use of gentamicin might contribute to a more rapid decline in residual renal function where preservation of the latter is associated in observational studies with some improvement in long-term outcomes and survival. Thus, whenever possible the antibiotic choice should be modified by initial response to empiric therapy and culture

Table 40.4 Diagnostic criteria for CDC definitions of HD catheter-related infections.

Infection type and criteria[a]

Catheter exit site infection
Erythema, tenderness, induration, or purulence within 2 cm of the skin at exit site of catheter

Positive culture of drainage material (if present)*

Catheter tunnel infection
Erythema, tenderness, induration, or purulence >2 cm of the skin at exit site of catheter

Positive culture of the drainage material (if present)*

Catheter colonization
No clinical symptoms or signs of infection

Positive culture from proximal or distal catheter segment

>1000 CFU on quantitative culture

≥ 15 CFU on semiquantitative culture (e.g. roll-plate method)

Catheter-related bloodstream infection
Clinical symptoms and signs of sepsis

Isolation of same organism from quantitative or semiquantitative culture of distal segment of catheter and from blood[†]

No other source of infection

Source: Summarized from references 136 and 137.
Abbreviations: CDC, Centers for Disease Control and Prevention; CFU, colony-forming units.
Note: Quantitative and semi-quantitative catheter culture methods are preferable over qualitative methods in which a single contaminating microbe can lead to false positive results (71;157).
[a] Symbols: *, laboratory confirmation is not a necessary requirement; [†], in the absence of laboratory confirmation, resolution of fever after removal of a vascular catheter suspected of infection can be considered indirect evidence of catheter-related bloodstream infection.

Table 40.5 NKF K/DOQI suggested indications for removal of infected HD catheters.

Type of infection and indication(s) for HD catheter removal

Catheter exit site infections[a]
Failure of infection to respond to antibiotic therapy

Catheter-related bacteremia[a]
Persistence of symptoms despite more than 36 h of appropriate antibiotic treatment
Any clinically unstable patient

Source: National Kidney Foundation 2000 [142].
[a] New permanent access should not be inserted until blood cultures, performed after cessation of antibiotic treatment, have been negative for at least 48 h.

results when these become available. The length of antibiotic treatment reasonably depends on severity of sepsis, presence or absence of complications (osteomyelitis, for instance, frequently requires long-term antibiotic treatment), and the microorganism and its sensitivity.

Although patients with mild line-associated infections do not usually require line removal, more severe infections usually necessitate prompt removal of the septic focus; in most cases this is the dialysis catheter. Similarly, single positive blood cultures in an otherwise-well patient usually require repetition rather than hasty administration of antibiotics or line removal. The National Kidney Foundation Dialysis Outcomes Quality Initiative's (K/DOQI) guidelines suggested indications for removal of infected HD lines [142] are summarized in Table 40.5. These guidelines are based principally on expert opinion and some observational data. To these, one should perhaps add that unless there are good reasons not to, lines should be removed where there is severe catheter tun-

nel infection unresponsive to antibiotics or in the presence of septic complications, especially endocarditis and septic embolization.

Although many of these end points seem indisputable, there are suggestions, from small studies, that some lines may be salvaged by antibiotic administration alone. The study of Marr *et al.*, for example, showed a 32% salvage rate of infected catheters through antibiotic treatment in a cohort of 38 bacteremic patients [51]. This approach is not entirely risk-free, and the potential for serious complications is appreciable [55]. Similarly, the K/DOQI guidelines advocate that at least 3 weeks of antibiotic treatment are required to eradicate catheter-associated bacteremia (although there is little compelling evidence for this value) and that blood cultures should be negative for at least 48 h before a new tunneled access is inserted [143]. An alternative approach is to replace the existing, infected catheter by exchange over a guidewire while covering the procedure with appropriate antibiotics, the theory being that exchange removes the biofilm as well as the catheter. This approach has met with some success in the small number of small-scale studies in the published literature. Some of these studies reported an almost 90% treatment success rate [144,145]; however, a high incidence of septic complications has also been demonstrated [146], calling into question the safety and utility of this approach.

Exclusion of antibiotics from bacteria growing in biofilms is a common cause of antibiotic failure in line-associated infections. Indeed, antibiotic concentrations must be several orders of magnitude higher (up to 1000 times) in order to kill bacteria in biofilms [147,148]. A number of investigators have, therefore, studied the efficacy of antibiotic locks for the eradication of colonization from infected lines. These have included vancomycin, gentamicin, amikacin, and ciprofloxacin. In general, the reports have been quite encouraging, with several authors demonstrating an almost negligible incidence of bacteremic episodes with this approach [149–151]. Nevertheless, this approach is far from commonplace at present, rarely works for fungal organisms [152], and would be inappropriate for the management of extraluminal infections.

It is important when considering the management of access-related infections in dialysis patients to actively look for the presence of complications, particularly when high-risk organisms are encountered. *S. aureus* and *Candida* species, when presenting as causative organisms of line-related infections, are more likely than other organisms to be associated with complications [153]. *Candida albicans*, in particular, carries a risk of endophthalmitis [154], so attention to visual acuity and ophthalmoscopy should be mandatory in such cases. Persistent positive cultures for any organism (particularly after line removal) should prompt a search for new niduses of infection other than the line, in particular, cardiac valve vegetations and bone involvement [155].

Conclusions

The current risk of infection for HD patients remains unacceptably high. This clinical problem has largely remained unchanged over the situation seen when HD first emerged as a chronic therapy for ESRD and, as such, this is gravely disappointing. There are many competing and interacting reasons for the marked increase in infection in HD patients. These include the compromised immune systems of these patients consequent upon chronic uremia and dialysis-specific risks. The excessive use of CVCs is one of the most important potentially remediable infection risks in HD populations. Thus, no effort must go unspared in the timely formation of definitive vascular access (AVF). Recognition of the very strong patient benefits that result when HD is performed via an AVF has resulted in the "Fistula First" program as a priority for the US Centers for Medicare & Medicaid Services and US ESRD programs. Meticulous care to avoid microbiological contamination (whether using a CVC, graft, or AVF) in HD units is also of the greatest importance. Even with these precautions, the use of prophylactic procedures, such as exit site antimicrobial treatments, attempts to decolonize patients colonized with methicillin-sensitive or -resistant *S. aureus*, and CVC line locks should be seriously considered. Unfortunately, and disappointingly, there is very little high-quality evidence evaluating the effectiveness of any of these interventions in HD populations. This is a truly shocking state of affairs in the fourth successive decade of RRT, which has involved more than 2,000,000 subjects to date. Above all, detection and prevention of infection in this vulnerable patient group must be accorded the very highest priority by all responsible dialysis practitioners.

References

1 John R, Webb M, Young A, Stevens PE. Unreferred chronic kidney disease: a longitudinal study. *Am J Kidney Dis* 2004; **43(5):** 825–835.

2 Coresh J, Astor BC, Greene T, Eknoyan G, Levey AS. Prevalence of chronic kidney disease and decreased kidney function in the adult US population: Third National Health and Nutrition Examination Survey. *Am J Kidney Dis* 2003; **41(1):** 1–12.

3 McGill JB, Brown WW, Chen SC, Collins AJ, Gannon MR. Kidney Early Evaluation Program (KEEP). Findings from a community screening program. *Diabetes Educ* 2004; **30(2):** 196–192, 206.

4 Chadban SJ, Briganti EM, Kerr PG, Dunstan DW, Welborn TA, Zimmet PZ *et al.* Prevalence of kidney damage in Australian adults: the AusDiab kidney study. *J Am Soc Nephrol* 2003; **14(7 Suppl 2):** S131–S138.

5 Carpenter GI. Aging in the United Kingdom and Europe: a snapshot of the future? *J Am Geriatr Soc* 2005; **53(9 Suppl):** S310–S313.

6 Xue JL, Ma JZ, Louis TA, Collins AJ. Forecast of the number of patients with end-stage renal disease in the United States to the year 2010. *J Am Soc Nephrol* 2001; **12(12):** 2753–2758.

7 US Renal Data System. Causes of death. *Am J Kidney Dis* 1997; **30(2 Suppl 1):** S107–S117.

8 Mailloux LU, Bellucci AG, Wilkes BM, Napolitano B, Mossey RT, Lesser M *et al.* Mortality in dialysis patients: analysis of the causes of death. *Am J Kidney Dis* 1991; **18(3):** 326–335.

9 Nissenson AR, Dylan ML, Griffiths RI, Yu HT, Dean BB, Danese MD *et al.* Clinical and economic outcomes of Staphylococcus aureus septicemia in ESRD patients receiving hemodialysis. *Am J Kidney Dis* 2005; **46(2):** 301–308.

10 Sarnak MJ, Jaber BL. Mortality caused by sepsis in patients with end-stage renal disease compared with the general population. *Kidney Int* 2000; **58(4):** 1758–1764.

11 Rautenberg P, Proppe D, Schutte A, Ullmann U. Influenza subtype-specific immunoglobulin A and G responses after booster versus one double-dose vaccination in hemodialysis patients. *Eur J Clin Microbiol Infect Dis* 1989; **8(10):** 897–900.

12 Girndt M, Pietsch M, Kohler H. Tetanus immunization and its association to hepatitis B vaccination in patients with chronic renal failure. *Am J Kidney Dis* 1995; **26(3):** 454–460.

13 Kreft B, Klouche M, Kreft R, Kirchner H, Sack K. Low efficiency of active immunization against diphtheria in chronic hemodialysis patients. *Kidney Int* 1997; **52(1):** 212–216.

14 DaRoza G, Loewen A, Djurdjev O, Love J, Kempston C, Burnett S *et al.* Stage of chronic kidney disease predicts seroconversion after hepatitis B immunization: earlier is better. *Am J Kidney Dis* 2003; **42(6):** 1184–1192.

15 Girndt M, Sester M, Sester U, Kaul H, Kohler H. Defective expression of B7-2 (CD86) on monocytes of dialysis patients correlates to the uremia-associated immune defect. *Kidney Int* 2001; **59(4):** 1382–1389.

16 Girndt M, Kohler H, Schiedhelm-Weick E, Meyer zum Buschenfelde KH, Fleischer B. T cell activation defect in hemodialysis patients: evidence for a role of the B7/CD28 pathway. *Kidney Int* 1993; **44(2):** 359–365.

17 Meuer SC, Hauer M, Kurz P, Meyer zum Buschenfelde KH, Kohler H. Selective blockade of the antigen-receptor-mediated pathway of T cell activation in patients with impaired primary immune responses. *J Clin Invest* 1987; **80(3):** 743–749.

18 Sester U, Sester M, Hauk M, Kaul H, Kohler H, Girndt M. T-cell activation follows Th1 rather than Th2 pattern in haemodialysis patients. *Nephrol Dial Transplant* 2000; **15(8):** 1217–1223.

19 Girndt M, Sester U, Kaul H, Kohler H. Production of proinflammatory and regulatory monokines in hemodialysis patients shown at a single-cell level. *J Am Soc Nephrol* 1998; **9(9):** 1689–1696.

20 Vanholder R, Ringoir S. Infectious morbidity and defects of phagocytic function in end-stage renal disease: a review. *J Am Soc Nephrol* 1993; **3(9):** 1541–1554.

21 Scamps-Latscha B, Jungers P, Witko-Sarsat V. Immune system dysregulation in uremia: role of oxidative stress. *Blood Purif* 2002; **20(5):** 481–484.

22 Patruta SI, Edlinger R, Sunder-Plassmann G, Horl WH. Neutrophil impairment associated with iron therapy in hemodialysis patients

with functional iron deficiency. *J Am Soc Nephrol* 1998; **9(4):** 655–663.

23 Hoen B, Kessler M, Hestin D, Mayeux D. Risk factors for bacterial infections in chronic haemodialysis adult patients: a multicentre prospective survey. *Nephrol Dial Transplant* 1995; **10(3):** 377–381.

24 Seifert A, von HD, Schaefer K. Iron overload, but not treatment with desferrioxamine favours the development of septicemia in patients on maintenance hemodialysis. *Q J Med* 1987; **65(248):** 1015–1024.

25 Flament J, Goldman M, Waterlot Y, Dupont E, Wybran J, Vanherweghem JL. Impairment of phagocyte oxidative metabolism in hemodialyzed patients with iron overload. *Clin Nephrol* 1986; **25(5):** 227–230.

26 Bataille R, Harousseau JL. Multiple myeloma. *N Engl J Med* 1997; **336(23):** 1657–1664.

27 Douek DC, Picker LJ, Koup RA. T cell dynamics in HIV-1 infection. *Annu Rev Immunol* 2003; **21:** 265–304.

28 Lode HM, Schmidt-Ioanas M. Vasculitis and infection: effects of immunosuppressive therapy. *Clin Nephrol* 2005; **64(6):** 475–479.

29 Powe NR, Jaar B, Furth SL, Hermann J, Briggs W. Septicemia in dialysis patients: incidence, risk factors, and prognosis. *Kidney Int* 1999; **55(3):** 1081–1090.

30 Kalantar-Zadeh K, Ikizler TA, Block G, Avram MM, Kopple JD. Malnutrition-inflammation complex syndrome in dialysis patients: causes and consequences. *Am J Kidney Dis* 2003; **42(5):** 864–881.

31 Hoen B, Paul-Dauphin A, Hestin D, Kessler M. EPIBACDIAL: a multicenter prospective study of risk factors for bacteremia in chronic hemodialysis patients. *J Am Soc Nephrol* 1998; **9(5):** 869–876.

32 Costerton JW, Stewart PS, Greenberg EP. Bacterial biofilms: a common cause of persistent infections. *Science* 1999; **284(5418):** 1318–1322.

33 Kanaya AM, Glidden DV, Chambers HF. Identifying pulmonary tuberculosis in patients with negative sputum smear results. *Chest* 2001; **120(2):** 349–355.

34 Groom AV, Wolsey DH, Naimi TS, Smith K, Johnson S, Boxrud D *et al.* Community-acquired methicillin-resistant Staphylococcus aureus in a rural American Indian community. *JAMA* 2001; **286(10):** 1201–1205.

35 Levy SB, FitzGerald GB, Macone AB. Changes in intestinal flora of farm personnel after introduction of a tetracycline-supplemented feed on a farm. *N Engl J Med* 1976; **295(11):** 583–588.

36 Crossley K, Landesman B, Zaske D. An outbreak of infections caused by strains of Staphylococcus aureus resistant to methicillin and aminoglycosides. II. Epidemiologic studies. *J Infect Dis* 1979; **139(3):** 280–287.

37 Yu VL, Goetz A, Wagener M, Smith PB, Rihs JD, Hanchett J *et al.* Staphylococcus aureus nasal carriage and infection in patients on hemodialysis. Efficacy of antibiotic prophylaxis. *N Engl J Med* 1986; **315(2):** 91–96.

38 Saxena AK, Panhotra BR, Venkateshappa CK, Sundaram DS, Naguib M, Uzzaman W *et al.* The impact of nasal carriage of methicillin-resistant and methicillin-susceptible Staphylococcus a ureus (MRSA & MSSA) on vascular access-related septicemia among patients with type-II diabetes on dialysis. *Ren Fail* 2002; **24(6):** 763–777.

39 Kaplowitz LG, Comstock JA, Landwehr DM, Dalton HP, Mayhall CG. Prospective study of microbial colonization of the nose and skin and infection of the vascular access site in hemodialysis patients. *J Clin Microbiol* 1988; **26(7):** 1257–1262.

40 Lye WC, Leong SO, Lee EJ. Methicillin-resistant Staphylococcus aureus nasal carriage and infections in CAPD. *Kidney Int* 1993; **43(6):** 1357–1362.

41 Kumano K, Yokota S, Nanbu M, Sakai T. Do cytokine-inducing substances penetrate through dialysis membranes and stimulate monocytes? *Kidney Int Suppl* 1993; **41:** S205–S208.

42 Lufft V, Mahiout A, Shaldon S, Koch KM, Schindler R. Retention of cytokine-inducing substances inside high-flux dialyzers. *Blood Purif* 1996; **14(1):** 26–34.

43 Pereira BJ, Snodgrass BR, Hogan PJ, King AJ. Diffusive and convective transfer of cytokine-inducing bacterial products across hemodialysis membranes. *Kidney Int* 1995; **47(2):** 603–610.

44 Landman D, Quale JM, Mayorga D, Adedeji A, Vangala K, Ravishankar J *et al.* Citywide clonal outbreak of multiresistant Acinetobacter baumannii and Pseudomonas aeruginosa in Brooklyn, NY: the preantibiotic era has returned. *Arch Intern Med* 2002; **162(13):** 1515–1520.

45 Bhat DJ, Tellis VA, Kohlberg WI, Driscoll B, Veith FJ. Management of sepsis involving expanded polytetrafluoroethylene grafts for hemodialysis access. *Surgery* 1980; **87(4):** 445–450.

46 Raju S. PTFE grafts for hemodialysis access. Techniques for insertion and management of complications. *Ann Surg* 1987; **206(5):** 666–673.

47 Ayus JC, Sheikh-Hamad D. Silent infection in clotted hemodialysis access grafts. *J Am Soc Nephrol* 1998; **9(7):** 1314–1317.

48 Nassar GM, Fishbane S, Ayus JC. Occult infection of old nonfunctioning arteriovenous grafts: a novel cause of erythropoietin resistance and chronic inflammation in hemodialysis patients. *Kidney Int Suppl* 2002; **80:** 49–54.

49 Doulton T, Sabharwal N, Cairns HS, Schelenz S, Eykyn S, O'Donnell P *et al.* Infective endocarditis in dialysis patients: new challenges and old. *Kidney Int* 2003; **64(2):** 720–727.

50 McCarthy JT, Steckelberg JM. Infective endocarditis in patients receiving long-term hemodialysis. *Mayo Clin Proc* 2000; **75(10):** 1008–1014.

51 Marr KA, Sexton DJ, Conlon PJ, Corey GR, Schwab SJ, Kirkland KB. Catheter-related bacteremia and outcome of attempted catheter salvage in patients undergoing hemodialysis. *Ann Intern Med* 1997; **127(4):** 275–280.

52 Dittmer ID, Tomson CR. Pulmonary abscess complicating central venous hemodialysis catheter infection. *Clin Nephrol* 1998; **49(1):** 66.

53 Tanaka N, Kasahara H, Yoshie T, Hora K, Kiyosawa K. Back pain out of the blue in a haemodialysis patient. *Nephrol Dial Transplant* 1999; **14(7):** 1792–1794.

54 Tsuchiya K, Yamaoka K, Tanaka K, Sasaki T. Bacterial spondylodiscitis in the patients with hemodialysis. *Spine* 2004; **29(22):** 2533–2537.

55 Kovalik EC, Raymond JR, Albers FJ, Berkoben M, Butterly DW, Montella B *et al.* A clustering of epidural abscesses in chronic hemodialysis patients: risks of salvaging access catheters in cases of infection. *J Am Soc Nephrol* 1996; **7(10):** 2264–2267.

56 Saad TF. Bacteremia associated with tunneled, cuffed hemodialysis catheters. *Am J Kidney Dis* 1999; **34(6):** 1114–1124.

57 Krishnasami Z, Carlton D, Bimbo L, Taylor ME, Balkovetz DF, Barker J *et al.* Management of hemodialysis catheter-related bacteremia with an adjunctive antibiotic lock solution. *Kidney Int* 2002; **61(3):** 1136–1142.

58 Butterly DW, Schwab SJ. Dialysis access infections. *Curr Opin Nephrol Hypertens* 2000; **9(6):** 631–635.

59 Kairaitis LK, Gottlieb T. Outcome and complications of temporary haemodialysis catheters. *Nephrol Dial Transplant* 1999; **14(7):** 1710–1714.

60 Oliver MJ, Callery SM, Thorpe KE, Schwab SJ, Churchill DN. Risk of bacteremia from temporary hemodialysis catheters by site of insertion and duration of use: a prospective study. *Kidney Int* 2000; **58(6):** 2543–2545.

61 Costerton JW, Lewandowski Z, Caldwell DE, Korber DR, Lappin-Scott HM. Microbial biofilms. *Annu Rev Microbiol* 1995; **49:** 711–745.

62 Lawrence JR, Korber DR, Hoyle BD, Costerton JW, Caldwell DE. Optical sectioning of microbial biofilms. *J Bacteriol* 1991; **173(20)**: 6558–6567.

63 Hoyle BD, Alcantara J, Costerton JW. *Pseudomonas aeruginosa* biofilm as a diffusion barrier to piperacillin. *Antimicrob Agents Chemother* 1992; **36(9)**: 2054–2056.

64 Jefferson KK, Goldmann DA, Pier GB. Use of confocal microscopy to analyze the rate of vancomycin penetration through *Staphylococcus aureus* biofilms. *Antimicrob Agents Chemother* 2005; **49(6)**: 2467–2473.

65 Dittmer ID, Sharp D, McNulty CA, Williams AJ, Banks RA. A prospective study of central venous hemodialysis catheter colonization and peripheral bacteremia. *Clin Nephrol* 1999; **51(1)**: 34–39.

66 Marr KA, Kong L, Fowler VG, Gopal A, Sexton DJ, Conlon PJ *et al.* Incidence and outcome of Staphylococcus aureus bacteremia in hemodialysis patients. *Kidney Int* 1998; **54(5)**: 1684–1689.

67 Astor BC, Eustace JA, Powe NR, Klag MJ, Fink NE, Coresh J. Type of vascular access and survival among incident hemodialysis patients: the Choices for Healthy Outcomes in Caring for ESRD (CHOICE) Study. *J Am Soc Nephrol* 2005; **16(5)**: 1449–1455.

68 Winkelmayer WC, Owen WF, Jr., Levin R, Avorn J. A propensity analysis of late versus early nephrologist referral and mortality on dialysis. *J Am Soc Nephrol* 2003; **14(2)**: 486–492.

69 Ritz E, Koch M, Fliser D, Schwenger V. How can we improve prognosis in diabetic patients with end-stage renal disease? *Diabetes Care* 1999; **22(Suppl 2)**: B80–B83.

70 Innes A, Rowe PA, Burden RP, Morgan AG. Early deaths on renal replacement therapy: the need for early nephrological referral. *Nephrol Dial Transplant* 1992; **7(6)**: 467–471.

71 Maki DG, Weise CE, Sarafin HW. A semiquantitative culture method for identifying intravenous-catheter-related infection. *N Engl J Med* 1977; **296(23)**: 1305–1309.

72 Raad I, Costerton W, Sabharwal U, Sacilowski M, Anaissie E, Bodey GP. Ultrastructural analysis of indwelling vascular catheters: a quantitative relationship between luminal colonization and duration of placement. *J Infect Dis* 1993; **168(2)**: 400–407.

73 Cheesbrough JS, Finch RG, Burden RP. A prospective study of the mechanisms of infection associated with hemodialysis catheters. *J Infect Dis* 1986; **154(4)**: 579–589.

74 Maki DG, Stolz SM, Wheeler S, Mermel LA. Prevention of central venous catheter-related bloodstream infection by use of an antiseptic-impregnated catheter. A randomized, controlled trial. *Ann Intern Med* 1997; **127(4)**: 257–266.

75 Linares J, Sitges-Serra A, Garau J, Perez JL, Martin R. Pathogenesis of catheter sepsis: a prospective study with quantitative and semiquantitative cultures of catheter hub and segments. *J Clin Microbiol* 1985; **21(3)**: 357–360.

76 Sheth NK, Franson TR, Rose HD, Buckmire FL, Cooper JA, Sohnle PG. Colonization of bacteria on polyvinyl chloride and Teflon intravascular catheters in hospitalized patients. *J Clin Microbiol* 1983; **18(5)**: 1061–1063.

77 Ashkenazi S, Weiss E, Drucker MM. Bacterial adherence to intravenous catheters and needles and its influence by cannula type and bacterial surface hydrophobicity. *J Lab Clin Med* 1986; **107(2)**: 136–140.

78 Nachnani GH, Lessin LS, Motomiya T, Jensen WN. Scanning electron microscopy of thrombogenesis on vascular catheter surfaces. *N Engl J Med* 1972; **286(3)**: 139–140.

79 Stillman RM, Soliman F, Garcia L, Sawyer PN. Etiology of catheter-associated sepsis. Correlation with thrombogenicity. *Arch Surg* 1977; **112(12)**: 1497–1499.

80 Fan PY, Schwab SJ. Vascular access: concepts for the 1990s. *J Am Soc Nephrol* 1992; **3(1)**: 1–11.

81 Peacock SJ, Foster TJ, Cameron BJ, Berendt AR. Bacterial fibronectin-binding proteins and endothelial cell surface fibronectin mediate adherence of Staphylococcus aureus to resting human endothelial cells. *Microbiology* 1999; **145**: 3477–3486.

82 Patti JM, Allen BL, McGavin MJ, Hook M. MSCRAMM-mediated adherence of microorganisms to host tissues. *Annu Rev Microbiol* 1994; **48**: 585–617.

83 O'Brien L, Kerrigan SW, Kaw G, Hogan M, Penades J, Litt D *et al.* Multiple mechanisms for the activation of human platelet aggregation by Staphylococcus aureus: roles for the clumping factors ClfA and ClfB, the serine-aspartate repeat protein SdrE and protein A. *Mol Microbiol* 2002; **44(4)**: 1033–1044.

84 Shin PK, Pawar P, Konstantopoulos K, Ross JM. Characteristics of new Staphylococcus aureus-RBC adhesion mechanism independent of fibrinogen and IgG under hydrodynamic shear conditions. *Am J Physiol Cell Physiol* 2005; **289(3)**: C727–C734.

85 Raad II, Hohn DC, Gilbreath BJ, Suleiman N, Hill LA, Bruso PA *et al.* Prevention of central venous catheter-related infections by using maximal sterile barrier precautions during insertion. *Infect Control Hosp Epidemiol* 1994; **15(4 Pt 1)**: 231–238.

86 Maki DG, Ringer M, Alvarado CJ. Prospective randomised trial of povidone-iodine, alcohol, and chlorhexidine for prevention of infection associated with central venous and arterial catheters. *Lancet* 1991; **338(8763)**: 339–343.

87 Chaiyakunapruk N, Veenstra DL, Lipsky BA, Saint S. Chlorhexidine compared with povidone-iodine solution for vascular catheter-site care: a meta-analysis. *Ann Intern Med* 2002; **136(11)**: 792–801.

88 Deshpande KS, Hatem C, Ulrich HL, Currie BP, Aldrich TK, Bryan-Brown CW *et al.* The incidence of infectious complications of central venous catheters at the subclavian, internal jugular, and femoral sites in an intensive care unit population. *Crit Care Med* 2005; **33(1)**: 13–20.

89 Lorente L, Henry C, Martin MM, Jimenez A, Mora ML. Central venous catheter-related infection in a prospective and observational study of 2,595 catheters. *Crit Care* 2005; **9(6)**: R631–R635.

90 Collignon P, Soni N, Pearson I, Sorrell T, Woods P. Sepsis associated with central vein catheters in critically ill patients. *Intensive Care Med* 1988; **14(3)**: 227–231.

91 Maki DG, Ringer M. Evaluation of dressing regimens for prevention of infection with peripheral intravenous catheters. Gauze, a transparent polyurethane dressing, and an iodophor-transparent dressing. *JAMA* 1987; **258(17)**: 2396–2403.

92 Gillies D, O'Riordan L, Carr D, Frost J, Gunning R, O'Brien I. Gauze and tape and transparent polyurethane dressings for central venous catheters. *Cochrane Database Syst Rev* 2003; **4**: CD003827.

93 Johnson DW, MacGinley R, Kay TD, Hawley CM, Campbell SB, Isbel NM *et al.* A randomized controlled trial of topical exit site mupirocin application in patients with tunnelled, cuffed haemodialysis catheters. *Nephrol Dial Transplant* 2002; **17(10)**: 1802–1807.

94 Riu S, Ruiz CG, Martinez-Vea A, Peralta C, Oliver JA. Spontaneous rupture of polyurethane peritoneal catheter. A possible deleterious effect of mupirocin ointment. *Nephrol Dial Transplant* 1998; **13(7)**: 1870–1871.

95 Rao SP, Oreopoulos DG. Unusual complications of a polyurethane PD catheter. *Perit Dial Int* 1997; **17(4)**: 410–412.

96 Khandelwal M, Bailey S, Izatt S, Chu M, Vas S, Bargman J *et al.* Structural changes in silicon rubber peritoneal dialysis catheters in patients

using mupirocin at the exit site. *Int J Artif Organs* 2003; **26**(**10**): 913–917.

97 Zakrzewska-Bode A, Muytjens HL, Liem KD, Hoogkamp-Korstanje JA. Mupirocin resistance in coagulase-negative staphylococci, after topical prophylaxis for the reduction of colonization of central venous catheters. *J Hosp Infect* 1995; **31**(**3**): 189–193.

98 Garland JS, Alex CP, Mueller CD, Otten D, Shivpuri C, Harris MC *et al.* A randomized trial comparing povidone-iodine to a chlorhexidine gluconate-impregnated dressing for prevention of central venous catheter infections in neonates. *Pediatrics* 2001; **107**(**6**): 1431–1436.

99 Levin A, Mason AJ, Jindal KK, Fong IW, Goldstein MB. Prevention of hemodialysis subclavian vein catheter infections by topical povidone-iodine. *Kidney Int* 1991; **40**(**5**): 934–938.

100 Zinner SH, Denny-Brown BC, Braun P, Burke JP, Toala P, Kass EH. Risk of infection with intravenous indwelling catheters: effect of application of antibiotic ointment. *J Infect Dis* 1969; **120**(**5**): 616–619.

101 Maki DG, Band JD. A comparative study of polyantibiotic and iodophor ointments in prevention of vascular catheter-related infection. *Am J Med* 1981; **70**(**3**): 739–744.

102 Johnson DW, van EC, Mudge DW, Wiggins KJ, Armstrong K, Hawley CM *et al.* Randomized, controlled trial of topical exit-site application of honey (Medihoney) versus mupirocin for the prevention of catheter-associated infections in hemodialysis patients. *J Am Soc Nephrol* 2005; **16**(**5**): 1456–1462.

103 Soifer NE, Borzak S, Edlin BR, Weinstein RA. Prevention of peripheral venous catheter complications with an intravenous therapy team: a randomized controlled trial. *Arch Intern Med* 1998; **158**(**5**): 473–477.

104 Vanherweghem JL, Dhaene M, Goldman M, Stolear JC, Sabot JP, Waterlot Y *et al.* Infections associated with subclavian dialysis catheters: the key role of nurse training. *Nephron* 1986; **42**(**2**): 116–119.

105 Fridkin SK, Pear SM, Williamson TH, Galgiani JN, Jarvis WR. The role of understaffing in central venous catheter-associated bloodstream infections. *Infect Control Hosp Epidemiol* 1996; **17**(**3**): 150–158.

106 Veenstra DL, Saint S, Saha S, Lumley T, Sullivan SD. Efficacy of antiseptic-impregnated central venous catheters in preventing catheter-related bloodstream infection: a meta-analysis. *JAMA* 1999; **281**(**3**): 261–267.

107 Bassetti S, Hu J, D'Agostino RB, Jr., Sherertz RJ. Prolonged antimicrobial activity of a catheter containing chlorhexidine-silver sulfadiazine extends protection against catheter infections in vivo. *Antimicrob Agents Chemother* 2001; **45**(**5**): 1535–1538.

108 Raad I, Darouiche R, Hachem R, Mansouri M, Bodey GP. The broad-spectrum activity and efficacy of catheters coated with minocycline and rifampin. *J Infect Dis* 1996; **173**(**2**): 418–424.

109 Darouiche RO, Raad II, Heard SO, Thornby JI, Wenker OC, Gabrielli A *et al.* A comparison of two antimicrobial-impregnated central venous catheters. Catheter Study Group. *N Engl J Med* 1999; **340**(**1**): 1–8.

110 Fraenkel D, Rickard C, Thomas P, Faoagali J, George N, Ware R. A prospective, randomized trial of rifampicin-minocycline-coated and silver-platinum-carbon-impregnated central venous catheters. *Crit Care Med* 2006; **34**(**3**): 668–675.

111 Maki DG, Cobb L, Garman JK, Shapiro JM, Ringer M, Helgerson RB. An attachable silver-impregnated cuff for prevention of infection with central venous catheters: a prospective randomized multicenter trial. *Am J Med* 1988; **85**(**3**): 307–314.

112 Ciresi DL, Albrecht RM, Volkers PA, Scholten DJ. Failure of antiseptic bonding to prevent central venous catheter-related infection and sepsis. *Am Surg* 1996; **62**(**8**): 641–646.

113 Heard SO, Wagle M, Vijayakumar E, McLean S, Brueggemann A, Napolitano LM *et al.* Influence of triple-lumen central venous catheters coated with chlorhexidine and silver sulfadiazine on the incidence of catheter-related bacteremia. *Arch Intern Med* 1998; **158**(**1**): 81–87.

114 Oda T, Hamasaki J, Kanda N, Mikami K. Anaphylactic shock induced by an antiseptic-coated central venous catheter. *Anesthesiology* 1997; **87**(**5**): 1242–1244.

115 Dahlberg PJ, Agger WA, Singer JR, Yutuc WR, Newcomer KL, Schaper A *et al.* Subclavian hemodialysis catheter infections: a prospective, randomized trial of an attachable silver-impregnated cuff for prevention of catheter-related infections. *Infect Control Hosp Epidemiol* 1995; **16**(**9**): 506–511.

116 Groeger JS, Lucas AB, Coit D, LaQuaglia M, Brown AE, Turnbull A *et al.* A prospective, randomized evaluation of the effect of silver impregnated subcutaneous cuffs for preventing tunneled chronic venous access catheter infections in cancer patients. *Ann Surg* 1993; **218**(**2**): 206–210.

117 Bambauer R, Latza R, Bambauer S, Tobin E. Large bore catheters with surface treatments versus untreated catheters for vascular access in hemodialysis. *Artif Organs* 2004; **28**(**7**): 604–610.

118 Appelgren P, Ransjo U, Bindslev L, Espersen F, Larm O. Surface heparinization of central venous catheters reduces microbial colonization in vitro and in vivo: results from a prospective, randomized trial. *Crit Care Med* 1996; **24**(**9**): 1482–1489.

119 Liu WK, Tebbs SE, Byrne PO, Elliott TS. The effects of electric current on bacteria colonising intravenous catheters. *J Infect* 1993; **27**(**3**): 261–269.

120 Henrickson KJ, Axtell RA, Hoover SM, Kuhn SM, Pritchett J, Kehl SC *et al.* Prevention of central venous catheter-related infections and thrombotic events in immunocompromised children by the use of vancomycin/ciprofloxacin/heparin flush solution: a randomized, multicenter, double-blind trial. *J Clin Oncol* 2000; **18**(**6**): 1269–1278.

121 Carratala J, Niubo J, Fernandez-Sevilla A, Juve E, Castellsague X, Berlanga J *et al.* Randomized, double-blind trial of an antibiotic-lock technique for prevention of gram-positive central venous catheter-related infection in neutropenic patients with cancer. *Antimicrob Agents Chemother* 1999; **43**(**9**): 2200–2204.

122 Schwartz C, Henrickson KJ, Roghmann K, Powell K. Prevention of bacteremia attributed to luminal colonization of tunneled central venous catheters with vancomycin-susceptible organisms. *J Clin Oncol* 1990; **8**(**9**): 1591–1597.

123 McIntyre CW, Hulme LJ, Taal M, Fluck RJ. Locking of tunneled hemodialysis catheters with gentamicin and heparin. *Kidney Int* 2004; **66**(**2**): 801–805.

124 Dogra GK, Herson H, Hutchison B, Irish AB, Heath CH, Golledge C *et al.* Prevention of tunneled hemodialysis catheter-related infections using catheter-restricted filling with gentamicin and citrate: a randomized controlled study. *J Am Soc Nephrol* 2002; **13**(**8**): 2133–2139.

125 Saxena AK, Panhotra BR, Naguib M. Sudden irreversible sensory-neural hearing loss in a patient with diabetes receiving amikacin as an antibiotic-heparin lock. *Pharmacotherapy* 2002; **22**(**1**): 105–108.

126 Saxena AK. Characteristics of ototoxicity of aminoglycosides "locked" to prevent hemodialysis catheter-related infections. *Hemodial Int* 2006; **10**(**1**): 94.

127 Betjes MG, van Agteren M. Prevention of dialysis catheter-related sepsis with a citrate-taurolidine-containing lock solution. *Nephrol Dial Transplant* 2004; **19**(**6**): 1546–1551.

128 Arbeit RD, Karakawa WW, Vann WF, Robbins JB. Predominance of two newly described capsular polysaccharide types among clinical isolates of Staphylococcus aureus. *Diagn Microbiol Infect Dis* 1984; **2**(**2**): 85–91.

129 Shinefield H, Black S, Fattom A, Horwith G, Rasgon S, Ordonez J *et al.* Use of a Staphylococcus aureus conjugate vaccine in patients receiving hemodialysis. *N Engl J Med* 2002; **346(7):** 491–496.

130 Kluytmans JA, Manders MJ, van Bommel E, Verbrugh H. Elimination of nasal carriage of Staphylococcus aureus in hemodialysis patients. *Infect Control Hosp Epidemiol* 1996; **17(12):** 793–797.

131 Boelaert JR, Van Landuyt HW, Godard CA, Daneels RF, Schurgers ML, Matthys EG *et al.* Nasal mupirocin ointment decreases the incidence of Staphylococcus aureus bacteraemias in haemodialysis patients. *Nephrol Dial Transplant* 1993; **8(3):** 235–239.

132 McAnally TP, Lewis MR, Brown DR. Effect of rifampin and bacitracin on nasal carriers of *Staphylococcus aureus*. *Antimicrob Agents Chemother* 1984; **25(4):** 422–426.

133 Miller MA, Dascal A, Portnoy J, Mendelson J. Development of mupirocin resistance among methicillin-resistant Staphylococcus aureus after widespread use of nasal mupirocin ointment. *Infect Control Hosp Epidemiol* 1996; **17(12):** 811–813.

134 Mendelssohn DC, Ethier J, Elder SJ, Saran R, Port FK, Pisoni RL. Haemodialysis vascular access problems in Canada: results from the Dialysis Outcomes and Practice Patterns Study (DOPPS II). *Nephrol Dial Transplant* 2006; **21(3):** 721–728.

135 Hood SA, Schillo B, Beane GE, Rozas V, Sondheimer JH. An analysis of the adequacy of preparation for end-stage renal disease care in Michigan. Michigan Renal Plan Task Force. *ASAIO J* 1995; **41(3):** M422–M426.

136 Garner JS, Jarvis WR, Emori TG, Horan TC, Hughes JM. CDC definitions for nosocomial infections, 1988. *Am J Infect Control* 1988; **16(3):** 128–140.

137 Pearson ML. Guideline for prevention of intravascular device-related infections. Part I. Intravascular device-related infections: an overview. The Hospital Infection Control Practices Advisory Committee. *Am J Infect Control* 1996; **24(4):** 262–277.

138 Mermel LA. Defining intravascular catheter-related infections: a plea for uniformity. *Nutrition* 1997; **13(4 Suppl):** 2S–4S.

139 Charalambous C, Swoboda SM, Dick J, Perl T, Lipsett PA. Risk factors and clinical impact of central line infections in the surgical intensive care unit. *Arch Surg* 1998; **133(11):** 1241–1246.

140 Raad I. Intravascular-catheter-related infections. *Lancet* 1998; **351(9106):** 893–898.

141 DesJardin JA, Falagas ME, Ruthazer R, Griffith J, Wawrose D, Schenkein D *et al.* Clinical utility of blood cultures drawn from indwelling central venous catheters in hospitalized patients with cancer. *Ann Intern Med* 1999; **131(9):** 641–647.

142 NKF. K/DOQI clinical practice guidelines for vascular access: update 2000. *Am J Kidney Dis* 2001; **37(1 Suppl 1):** S137–S181.

143 NKF. DOQI clinical practice guidelines for vascular access. *Am J Kidney Dis* 1997; **30(4 Suppl 3):** S150–S191.

144 Shaffer D. Catheter-related sepsis complicating long-term, tunnelled central venous dialysis catheters: management by guidewire exchange. *Am J Kidney Dis* 1995; **25(4):** 593–596.

145 Beathard GA. Management of bacteremia associated with tunneled-cuffed hemodialysis catheters. *J Am Soc Nephrol* 1999; **10(5):** 1045–1049.

146 Tanriover B, Carlton D, Saddekni S, Hamrick K, Oser R, Westfall AO *et al.* Bacteremia associated with tunneled dialysis catheters: comparison of two treatment strategies. *Kidney Int* 2000; **57(5):** 2151–2155.

147 de Ramirez AE, Pascual A, Martinez-Martinez L, Perea EJ. Activity of eight antibacterial agents on Staphylococcus epidermidis attached to Teflon catheters. *J Med Microbiol* 1994; **40(1):** 43–47.

148 Kropec A, Huebner J, Wursthorn M, Daschner FD. In vitro activity of vancomycin and teicoplanin against Staphylococcus aureus and Staphylococcus epidermidis colonizing catheters. *Eur J Clin Microbiol Infect Dis* 1993; **12(7):** 545–548.

149 Messing B, Man F, Colimon R, Thuillier F, Beliah M. Antibiotic-lock technique is an effective treatment of bacterial catheter-related sepsis during parenteral nutrition. *Clin Nutr* 1990; **9(4):** 220–225.

150 Messing B, Peitra-Cohen S, Debure A, Beliah M, Bernier JJ. Antibiotic-lock technique: a new approach to optimal therapy for catheter-related sepsis in home-parenteral nutrition patients. *J Parenter Enteral Nutr* 1988; **12(2):** 185–189.

151 Capdevila JA, Segarra A, Planes AM, Ramirez-Arellano M, Pahissa A, Piera L *et al.* Successful treatment of haemodialysis catheter-related sepsis without catheter removal. *Nephrol Dial Transplant* 1993; **8(3):** 231–234.

152 Benoit JL, Carandang G, Sitrin M, Arnow PM. Intraluminal antibiotic treatment of central venous catheter infections in patients receiving parenteral nutrition at home. *Clin Infect Dis* 1995; **21(5):** 1286–1288.

153 Arnow PM, Quimosing EM, Beach M. Consequences of intravascular catheter sepsis. *Clin Infect Dis* 1993; **16(6):** 778–784.

154 Klotz SA, Penn CC, Negvesky GJ, Butrus SI. Fungal and parasitic infections of the eye. *Clin Microbiol Rev* 2000; **13(4):** 662–685.

155 Haemodialysis-associated infection. *Nephrol Dial Transplant* 2002; **17(Suppl 7):** 72–87.

156 Saxena AK, Panhotra BR. Haemodialysis catheter-related bloodstream infections: current treatment options and strategies for prevention. *Swiss Med Wkly* 2005; **135(9–10):** 127–138.

157 Brun-Buisson C, Abrouk F, Legrand P, Huet Y, Larabi S, Rapin M. Diagnosis of central venous catheter-related sepsis. Critical level of quantitative tip cultures. *Arch Intern Med* 1987; **147(5):** 873–877.

41 Non-Access-Related Nosocomial Infections in Hemodialysis

Brett W. Stephens & Donald A. Molony

Division of Renal Diseases & Hypertension, University of Texas Medical School, Houston, USA

Introduction

Infection is the second most common cause of death among dialysis patients, trailing only cardiovascular disease [1]. Although a significant focus has been placed on access- and catheter-related infections in hemodialysis patients, nosocomial outbreaks and the consequent potential transmission of infection to those on dialysis remains a significant issue. Patients on dialysis are at an increased risk of blood-borne viruses and bacterial infection from contamination [2]. The goal of this chapter is to review nosocomial, non-catheter-related infections that occur on dialysis as well as current guidelines on their prevention, with emphasis on dialysis quality control. Catheter-related infections will be covered in chapter 40.

Background

Several factors account for the pathogenesis of nosocomial infections in dialysis patients, including impaired host immunity, bacterial virulence factors, and exposure created by the dialysis procedure itself (Figure 41.1).

Neutrophils and cell-mediated immunity are both affected by uremia. Impaired chemotaxis, phagocytic activity, and apoptosis are all demonstrated by neutrophils, and decreased lymphocyte proliferation and immunoglobulin levels have been observed. Factors thought to contribute to these findings include malnutrition, iron deficiency or overload, hyperparathyroidism, element deficiencies, and uremia itself.

Increased virulence of bacteria is enhanced by protease, superoxide dismutase, catalase, polysaccharide biofilms, and adherence factors [3]. These patterns of resistance are amplified in nosocomial settings, where resistance is common.

Evidence-based Nephrology. Edited by Donald Molony and Jonathan Craig

The patient's skin, the water system, dialysate, dialyzer, medication vials, prior patients, and staff are all potential sources of contamination [3,4]. Strategies for prevention and management of these nosocomial infections are based on an understanding of their dialysis center-specific epidemiology.

Epidemiology

Several prior observational studies have shown sepsis rates to be around 11% among end-stage renal disease (ESRD) patients within the first several years of dialysis initiation [5]. A study of 393,451 dialysis patients from 1991 to 1999 showed hospitalization rates for sepsis within the first year of hemodialysis to range from 11 to 17% [5]. Septicemia accounts for more than 75% of infectious deaths, with annual death rates from pneumonia and septicemia significantly higher in dialysis patients than in the general population, from 10- to 100-fold higher in the 65- to 75-year-old age group [3]. The risk factors for increased incidence of infection and mortality among ESRD patients are summarized in Table 41.1 [1,3]. Hospitalization for septicemia in ESRD patients is associated with an increased risk of stroke, congestive heart failure, myocardial infarction, and peripheral vascular disease, both in the short term and up to 5 years after the event [3,6].

The recent HEMO trial by Allon and colleagues found an infectious etiology in 23.1% of all deaths, with an annual infection-related death rate of 3.8%. The annual rate of infection-related hospitalizations was 35%, with 77% of the cases being non-access-related [1]. In one study of 433 dialysis patients followed over a 9-year period, the infection rate was found to be 5.7 episodes/1000 days of dialysis, with 18% of the infections being nosocomial [7]. These were not, however, divided into catheter-related versus non-catheter-related infections in this specific study. No study to date has demonstrated the true incidence of nosocomial infections related to the dialysis procedure itself, but this likely remains an important potential source for infections.

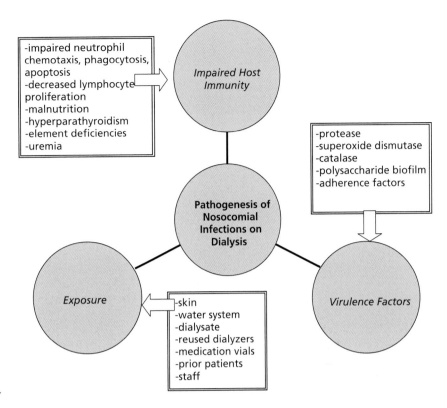

Figure 41.1 Pathogenesis of nosocomial infections [3].

Dialysis-related infections

Bacterial infections

Outbreaks of bloodstream infections in dialysis centers are usually related to contamination of the water treatment and distribution systems, reprocessed dialyzers, or improper setup procedures. Most of our insights into these infections have come from epidemiologic investigations into nosocomial infection outbreaks. One report in Canada showed nine patients in whom *Enterobacter* bacteremia was diagnosed, which was traced to infected, incompetent one-way waste-handling valves. When the dialysis machine was primed, the arterial line was attached to the waste-handling option drain port to discard the saline. After priming, the line was detached from the port and attached to the patient's access. Disinfectants were run through the drain port per the protocol, but the

Table 41.1 Risk factors for increased incidence of infections and mortality in ESRD patients.

Risk factor
Diabetes
Older age
Hypoalbuminemia
Use of temporary dialysis catheters

Sources: Allon *et al.* [1] and Jaber [3].

valves were not checked for competency, possibly allowing backflow of fluid. Cultured bacteria from the case patients and from valves showed identical genomic patterns, which were different from the sink cultures outside the room [8]. Three other similar outbreaks were reported in the USA, UK, and Israel in 1997 due to improperly functioning drain valves [9,10].

Another outbreak also reported during this time in Chicago included 29 episodes of bloodstream infections, with 21 hospitalizations for an average stay of 7 days. Again, the etiology was traced to improper handling of connections and faulty valves [4]. In 1996 the Centers for Disease Control and Prevention (CDC) and Gambro Healthcare surveyed 595 dialysis centers to characterize methods used to disinfect the machines and methods established for quality control. Responses showed that 62% were not disinfecting the sampling ports as often as recommended and only 14% performed the recommended daily quality control of the drain valves [9]. These findings underscore the importance of proper training and quality control measures.

In 1999, an outbreak of *Serratia* bloodstream infections and pyrogenic reactions was traced to contaminated single-use erythropoietin vials that had undergone repeated puncture [2]. Several case reports have also shown infection outbreaks attributed to improper sterilization of reusable dialysis filters [11].

Viral infections

Of particular concern for chronic dialysis patients is the transmission of viral hepatitis B and C, as well as HIV. In England in the late 1960s, there were 12 reported outbreaks of hepatitis B virus (HBV) in dialysis centers that affected more than 300 patients and staff, with a reported mortality rate of 5% [12]. In the USA in 1974, the incidence of HBV was 6.2% for all dialysis patients. This number decreased to 0.06% in 1999 as a result of infection control, vaccination, screening of blood products, and identification and isolation of hepatitis B-positive patients on dialysis [2]. In other parts of the world, such as Africa and the Asia-Pacific region, the prevalence is reported to be as high as 20% [12]. HBV is transmitted by percutaneous or permucosal exposure to contaminated blood. It is a relatively stable virus that can remain viable at room temperature on environmental surfaces for up to 7 days. It may be present on equipment without any evidence of visible blood. Thus, outbreaks still occur when contaminated surfaces are touched by health care workers and spread to others. Other reports have shown transmission from infection control lapses, such as contamination of multidose medication vials [2,13].

Hepatitis C virus (HCV) has been reported to have an incidence of 0.73–3% per patient–year in hemodialysis patients in the USA, with prevalence rates varying from 8% to 59% worldwide [2,12]. Risk factors associated with HCV infection include a history of blood transfusions, the volume of blood transfused, and the number of years on dialysis [2]. In 2001 in France, an outbreak of 22 HCV infections in a single dialysis unit over a 9-month period was reported. No common risk factor or exposure could be found among the patients [14]. Nosocomial HCV transmission has been demonstrated in other dialysis centers, but the exact modes of transmission remain unclear. Studies have demonstrated that patient-to-patient transmission occurs via equipment, devices, multidose vials, and between patients on the same shift who do not share equipment [15]. Reuse of dialyzers has been implicated, and recent studies suggest that patients sharing machines may be at increased risk [2,12,13,15], although the CDC currently does not recommend isolation of HCV-positive patients [16]. Other viral hepatotropic viruses, such as hepatitis GB virus C, hepatitis G virus, and TT virus, have unknown clinical significance in hemodialysis patients [12].

HIV is transmitted by blood and bodily fluids that contain blood. No patient-to-patient transmissions have been reported in dialysis centers in the USA, but there have been case reports of needle stick transmission from patients to staff [2].

Other viral transmissions have been reported, including one case report of possible transmission of West Nile virus. In October 2003, the Georgia Division of Public Health was notified of two patients diagnosed with West Nile virus, both having been dialyzed on the same dialysis machine. They were the only two reported cases of West Nile virus in that Georgia county in 2003 [17], but other modes of transmission not related to dialysis could not be entirely excluded.

Water quality

Every week, dialysis patients are exposed to approximately 400 L of water used in the production of dialysis fluids. This water must meet certain quality standards, which are often stricter than municipal water standards. Municipal drinking water must satisfy standards of turbidity and contamination, all based on the assumption of limited intake of approximately 2 L/day/person. In addition, drinking water has the benefit of being filtered by the gastrointestinal mucosa, unlike dialysate. Thus, tap water must be thoroughly processed before dialysis. Water in the dialysis unit is not only used for dialysate production, but also it may be used for dialyzer rinsing and reuse [18].

Municipal water can contain a variety of chemical and microbiological contaminants. Mineral salts, agricultural products (fertilizers, nitrates, and pesticides) and discarded medications contaminating reservoirs and groundwater sources, heavy metals from pipes, and added agents from a processing plant (iron, aluminum, chlorine, fluoride) may all be present in low levels in drinking water. These amounts become significant when presented in large volumes of dialysate over time, and they have been found to cause acute and chronic poisoning syndromes (Table 41.2) [18]. Specific symptoms include nausea and vomiting, muscular asthenia, acidosis, hypotension or hypertension, hemolysis, anemia, encephalopathy, neurologic problems, fever, and bone alterations [19]. Microbiological contaminants include bacteria, endotoxins, and peptidoglycans, and rarely fungi, viruses, and protozoa. Most of the problems encountered with microbiologic contamination

Table 41.2 Maximum allowable contaminant levels in water.

Contaminant	EPA maximum contaminant level for drinking water (mg/L)	AAMI maximum contaminant level for dialysis (mg/L)	Lowest concentration associated with dialysis toxicity (mg/L)
Sodium	Not regulated	70	300
Potassium	Not regulated	8	
Calcium	Not regulated	2	88
Magnesium	Not regulated	4	
Fluoride	4	0.2	1.0
Chlorine	4	0.5	
Chloramine	4	0.1	0.25
Nitrate	10	2	21
Sulfate	400	100	200
Copper	1.3	0.1	0.49
Barium	2	0.1	
Zinc	5	0.1	0.2
Aluminum	0.2	0.01	0.06
Arsenic	0.05	0.010	
Lead	0.015	0.005	
Silver	0.10	0.005	
Cadmium	0.005	0.001	
Chromium	0.10	0.014	
Mercury	0.002	0.0002	
Selenium	0.05	0.09	
Beryllium	0.004	0.0004	

Sources: Pontoriero *et al.* [18] and AAMI [20].

in dialysate are related to the characteristics and maintenance of water treatment and distribution systems within the dialysis unit [18].

Many dialysis centers use an initial pretreatment of tap water with filters of different porosities to remove suspended particles. These filters also decrease the hardness of the water through sodium exchange cationic resins. Activated carbon filters then remove chlorine and other organic products. These filters, however, can serve as a medium for bacterial growth. Water is then processed by reverse osmosis, a process that involves bulk transport of water under pressure through a semipermeable membrane. This removes 95–98% of dissolved salts, bacteria, endotoxins, and substances with molecular masses of >200 Da [18]. Some centers use two reverse osmosis systems in series, and many combine another purification technique of deionization using ion exchange resins. Water is then distributed under hydraulic pressure to the machines. Reserve tanks are avoided, with the goal of continuous circulation and lack of stagnant zones. Sterilization of the entire system must be conducted at regular intervals [18]. The Association for the Advancement of Medical Instrumentation (AAMI) [20] and the European Pharmacopea [21] have established guidelines for the purity of water (discussed below).

Several studies over the last decade showed that 7.4–35% of all dialysis centers tested did not comply with the AAMI standards, and only 28% performed monthly disinfection procedures [18].

Many *in vitro* and clinical studies have evaluated differences in standard and sterile (ultrapure) dialysate. *In vitro* studies show that transfer of bacterial and endotoxin fragments across dialysis membranes is dependent on both the concentration of endotoxin and the type of membrane used [22]. Cuprophan membranes have the highest permeability to endotoxin [22]. Notably, only high concentrations of endotoxin typically transverse polysulfone or polyamide membranes [22]. Clinical studies have shown that patients dialyzed with ultrapure dialysate, compared to those dialyzed with standard dialysate, have slightly lower levels of C-reactive protein (in both groups, however, the C-reactive protein levels were within the normal reference range), $\beta 2$-microglobulin levels, and incidence of carpal tunnel syndrome. These studies, however, have not demonstrated significant differences in such hard outcomes as mortality or cardiovascular events [23]. Studies have also shown some decrease in pyrogenic reactions with high-flux membranes when ultrapure dialysate is used [24]. Again, these differences were small and no convincing data have been reported to date that ultrapure dialysate reduces the generation of proinflammatory cytokines in patients [22]. Thus, there is currently no good clinical trials evidence that shows that ultrapure dialysate improves morbidity and mortality outcomes.

Dialyzer reuse

Since the early experimental years of dialysis, dialyzers have been reused and processed by various methods. Approximately 63% of centers in the USA reuse dialyzers for some of their patients. Japan currently prohibits reprocessing of dialyzers, and reuse practices vary widely from country to country in Europe [11]. Cleaning and sterilizing methods have changed over the last century. The most common cleaning agents have been hypochlorite and hydrogen peroxide, and the most common sterilizing agents have been formaldehyde and peracetic acid. Heat sterilization has recently come into favor in combination with the above agents. Currently, a majority of centers in the USA use peracetic acid instead of formaldehyde, owing to the lower toxicity, easy removal from stored dialyzers, and decreased environmental problems. Its disadvantages include degradation by heavy metals and organic material at high temperature. Glutaraldehyde is also occasionally used as a sterilizing agent [11].

In 2002, the US Food and Drug Administration approved a new personal hemodialysis machine for home usage (Personal Hemodialysis System, PHD, Aksys, Ltd., Lincolnshire, IL). The machine reuses the dialyzer and lines so that they do not need to be changed more often than once monthly. The machine checks dialyzer performance and prepares ultrapure, infusion-quality dialysis solution. Prior to each dialysis, the entire system is filled with reverse osmosis water, heated to 85°C, and circulated for 1 h, sterilizing the entire system [11].

The advantages of reuse include potential cost savings and a potential for reduced frequency of first-use dialyzer reactions. The first use of dialyzers has rarely been associated with symptoms of respiratory distress, malaise, back pain, chills, or fever. This constellation of symptoms, termed the "new dialyzer syndrome," is thought to be due to traces of substances that remain from the membrane production processes [23], including possibly ethylene oxide, glycerol, alcohols, copper, cyanates, and polyurethane. Reprocessing of these filters causes leaching of these substances [11]. A study by Flemming *et al.* showed that the mean number of symptoms per patient was significantly higher with new dialyzers than with reprocessed ones [23]. New production and sterilization methods and changes in preuse dialyzer preparation within the dialysis unit have almost eliminated this new dialyzer syndrome.

Disadvantages of dialyzer reuse include allergic reactions to disinfecting solutions, residual chemical infusion, pyrogen reaction, inadequate concentration of disinfectant allowing for bacterial contamination, and changes in membrane integrity [23]. Allergic reactions have been seen with formaldehyde and glutaraldehyde exposure, and some association has been found between adverse reactions, angiotensin converting enzyme inhibitors, and reprocessed dialyzers [23]. Several infection outbreaks have been reported following insufficient concentration of sterilizing solutions [11,23,25]. Although some studies have reported an increased incidence of pyrogenic reactions with reuse, other studies have demonstrated the pyrogenic reactions are more strongly associated with dialysate contamination than with dialyzer reuse [23].

Other concerns with reuse include changes in membrane integrity and clearance. Studies in the 1980s showed that a 20% reduction in fiber bundle volume decreased clearance by only 4–11% [23]. Subsequent studies have shown that clearance of both

Study	No. of patients	Study design	Follow-up (years)	Outcome on mortality
Collins *et al.* 1998 [35]	34,348	Retrospective	2–3	No difference
Port *et al.* 2001 [26]	12,791	Retrospective	1–2	No difference
Collins *et al.* 2004 [27]	49,273	Retrospective	1–2	No difference
Lowrie *et al.* 2004 [25]	71,122	Retrospective	1	Mortality lower in those switched from reused to single-use dialyzer
Fan *et al.* 2005 [28]	75,831	Retrospective	1–2	No difference

Table 41.3 Studies on the association between mortality and reused versus single-use dialyzers.

Source: The studies reported in references 23–31 were reviewed.

large and small substances were maintained for up to 30 uses. Even high-flux dialyzers with blood flows of 400 mL/min and 80% fiber bundle volume maintain measured Kt/V values. These optimistic results are not uniformly observed. Thus, studies have shown conflicting results between various lots of the same dialyzers [23]. Additionally, studies have shown decreased Kt/V values with formaldehyde usage, with lower blood flows that result from fiber bundle volume loss and with increased numbers of reprocessing [23]. Thus, the National Kidney Foundation Task Force on Reuse of Dialyzers recommends at least monthly Kt/V or urea reduction ratio determinations to assess dialyzer performance [23].

Dialyzer reuse and mortality have also been examined in several large retrospective studies over the last decade (Table 41.3) [25–31]. Studies prior to this time were conflicting and were confounded by differing practice patterns, reuse procedures, dialyzer membranes, and patient characteristics. A large study of over 12,000 patients in the mid-1990s showed no discernible difference in mortality between single use and reuse and even demonstrated decreased mortality in reuse of high-flux membranes reprocessed with bleach [26]. A subsequent study in the late 1990s of over 49,000 patients confirmed no difference in mortality or first hospitalization between the single-use and reuse groups [27]. Medicare data in 2001 also showed no advantage to single-use dialyzers [28], but a recent study did show a survival advantage in patients who were switched from reuse to single use dialyzers [25]. There have been no high-quality prospective, randomized controlled studies to date to address this issue.

Current National Kidney Foundation Kidney Disease Outcomes Quality Initiative guidelines recommend that dialysis centers reusing dialyzers do so in accordance with AAMI standards while monitoring for delivered dialysis dose [29].

Guidelines and recommendations

Immunizations

Immunization of health care workers with the hepatitis B vaccines has been shown to reduce HBV events, and it should be routinely implemented for all health care and dialysis staff. A 2005 Cochrane systematic review of 21 trials showed that plasma-derived and recombinant vaccines are equally effective in eliciting antibody

levels, with the deltoid intramuscular site preferred. The standard vaccination schedule (0, 1, and 6 months) elicited a better antibody response than the rapid vaccination schedule (0, 1, and 2 months), but it is unclear if booster vaccinations to nonresponders enhance seroconversion [32].

Given the occasional outbreaks of hepatitis in dialysis centers, hepatitis B vaccination should be considered for all ESRD patients. A 2004 Cochrane systematic review of chronic kidney failure patients and hemodialysis patients receiving hepatitis B vaccine did not, however, demonstrate any difference between immunized patients and the placebo group in HBV infection rates [33]. The studies did not show any adverse events secondary to vaccination, however, and so additional randomized trials need to be conducted to provide more sound clinical guidance on this question. The Advisory Committee on Immunization Practices currently recommends that adult dialysis patients receive the hepatitis B vaccine series, pneumococcal vaccine, yearly influenza vaccinations, tetanus-diphtheria toxoids, and varicella vaccine, if susceptible. Antibody levels for HBV should be checked annually and boosters considered if levels are below protective levels [34].

Isolation

Isolation practices for HBV were first implemented in 1977 after factors for transmission were identified. The US CDC recommends routine serologic surveillance of patients and staff, separate isolation rooms for HBV-positive patients, assignment of designated staff and equipment to HBV-positive patients and not to susceptible patients during the same shift, routine cleaning and disinfection of nondisposable items and surfaces, and glove changes between each patient (Table 41.4). With the implementation of these recommendations, a 70–80% reduction in transmission of HBV in hemodialysis facilities has been seen, with occasional outbreaks occurring when there has been a breakdown in one of the above guidelines [6,16].

HCV transmission has been attributed in various studies to contaminated hands of staff members, shared multidose vials of parenteral medications, and inadequate sterilization of dialyzers and machines. No conclusive evidence has shown that HCV is transmitted through sharing of the same machine when proper infection control measures are used, but no studies have proven the contrary [13–15,35]. Recent studies, however, have found

Table 41.4 CDC infection control guidelines for dialysis centers.

Topic	Recommendation(s)
Infection control precautions	Use gloves when touching patient equipment
	Wash/cleanse hands between patients
	Use dedicated supplies at each station
	Prepare all medication in a separate clean area
	Deliver medication individually without common medication carts
Disinfection	Clean environmental surfaces (chair, countertops, external control panel of dialysis machine) after each patient treatment
Cleaning of areas	Designate separate clean areas for storage and preparation of medications; keep contaminated products out of the clean area
Routine serologic screening	Determine HBV surface antigen (HBsAg) level on admission and monthly in HBV-susceptible patients
	Determine anti-HBs antibody titer yearly in those with established protection to evaluate need for booster
	Determine anti-HCV antibody titer semiannually in HCV-susceptible patients
Vaccinations	Vaccinate all susceptible hemodialysis patients and staff
Isolation	HBV-positive patients should be in a separate room.
	HBV-immune patients can be a buffer between the isolation room and HBV-susceptible patients
	Staff should not be assigned to both HBV-positive patients and susceptible patients during the same shift
	HCV-positive patients require no special isolation

Source: Alter *et al.* [16].

associations with transmission and machine usage, and trials of isolation of HCV-positive patients have reported decreased transmission rates [15,36]. The CDC does not, however, recommend isolation of HCV patients. They have concluded that evidence of sufficient strength does not exist to justify these measures [16] beyond universal infection control procedures.

Universal infection control procedures recommended by the CDC include using gloves when touching equipment, washing hands between patients, dedication of supplies to each dialysis station or disinfection before returning to a common area, preparing medications in a separate clean area, keeping contaminated products out of the clean area, and avoiding common medication carts (Table 41.4) [6].

No special isolation precautions have been recommended to date for HIV-infected dialysis patients [16].

Water control

AAMI guidelines [20] state that water used in dialysate production should contain a total microbial count of less than 200 colony-forming units (CFU)/mL and an endotoxin concentration of less than 2 endotoxin units (EU)/mL. At levels of 50 CFU/mL and 1 EU/mL, respectively, AAMI standards require that actions be taken, such as disinfection of the components of the water purification and processing system and dialysate preparation and storage reservoirs where indicated by the culture results. After disinfection of the system, retesting is required by AAMI standards to confirm

improvement in levels and to prevent levels from reaching unacceptable ranges. Microbiologic monitoring should be performed at least monthly, and chemical contaminant monitoring should be done yearly if reverse osmosis and deionization are used. Guidelines for levels of residual sterilization chemicals (Table 41.5) and recommended features of purification systems have also been established. The AAMI has also set guidelines for maximum allowable levels of contaminants. The European Pharmacopoeia has set slightly stricter standards for microbiologic content, with a microbial count of less than 100 CFU/mL and endotoxin concentration of less than 0.25 EU/mL [20].

Dialyzer reuse

AAMI guidelines state that dialyzers used on HBV-positive patients should not be reprocessed. Otherwise, the decision to reprocess dialyzers is left to the physician, and informed consent must be

Table 41.5 Limits on disinfectant residues.

Disinfectant	AAMI recommended limit (mg/L)
Formaldehyde	<5
Peracetic acid	<3[a]
Glutaraldehyde	<3[a]
Sodium hypochlorite (bleach)	<0.5[a]

Source: AAMI [20].
[a] Limit based on dialyzer manufacturer's suggestion.

obtained from the patients. The AAMI guidelines allow for a 10% variance of urea clearance after processing but recommend that the dialysis prescription account for these changes. Fiber bundle volume should be at least 80% of the original volume. Various recommended concentrations and contact times for the sterilizing agents used in cleaning and storage of reprocessed dialyzers have been established and depend on the properties of the sterilizing agents used [20].

Summary

Nosocomial infections related to the dialysis process, although uncommon, continue to occur. An understanding of their etiology and strategies for their prevention have emerged largely from observational studies and evaluations of nosocomial infection outbreaks. These observations have led to the current guidelines that govern the technical aspects of handling of water purification, production and delivery of dialysate, cleansing of equipment, handling of medications, and infection precautions as they relate to patients and staff. Reprocessing of dialyzers introduces additional opportunities for transmission of infection. The benefits and risks of dialyzer reprocessing and optimal therapeutic strategies to minimize risk have not been rigorously investigated with randomized controlled clinical trials. Rigorously conducted clinical trials are needed to address unambiguously the contributions of reuse, if any, to the transmission of bacterial, viral, and fungal infections, to the incitement of an inflammatory cascade that could result in a further deterioration in the immunocompentency of ESRD patients, to the induction of pyrogenic reactions from allergic or chemical exposures or endotoxins, and to overall morbidity and mortality.

References

1 Allon M, Depner TA, Radeva MA, Bailey J, Beddhu S, Butterly D et al. Impact of dialysis dose and membrane on infection-related hospitalization and death: results of the HEMO study. *J Am Soc Nephrol* 2003; **14**: 1863–1870.

2 Tokars J, Arduino MJ, Alter MJ. Infection control in hemodialysis units. *Infect Dis Clin North Am* 2001; **15(3)**: 797–812.

3 Jaber B. Bacterial infection in hemodialysis patients: pathogenesis and prevention. *Kidney Int* 2005; **67**: 2508–2519.

4 Arnow PM, Garcia-Houchins S, Neagle MB, Boya JL, Dillon JJ, Chou T. An outbreak of bloodstream infections from hemodialysis equipment. *J Infect Dis* 1998; **178**: 783–791.

5 Foley R, Guo H, Snyder JJ, Gilbertson DT, Collins AJ. Septicemia in the United States dialysis population, 1991 to 1999. *J Am Soc Nephrol* 2004; **15**: 1038–1045.

6 Yanai M, Uehara Y, Takahashi S. Surveillance of infection control procedures in dialysis units in Japan: a preliminary study. *Ther Apher Dial* 2006; **10(1)**: 78–86.

7 Berman S, Johnson EW, Nakatsu C, Alkan M, Chen R, LeDuc J. Burden of infection in patients with end-stage renal disease requiring long-term dialysis. *Clin Infect Dis* 2004; **39**: 1747–1753.

8 Jochimsen EM, Frenette C, Delorme M, Arduino M, Aguero S, Carson L et al. A cluster of bloodstream infections and pyrogenic reactions among hemodialysis patients traced to dialysis machine waste-handling option units. *Am J Nephrol* 1998; **18**: 485–489.

9 Frenette C, Grillo FG, Dwyer DM, Block C, Backenroth R, Shapiro M et al. Outbreaks of gram-negative bacterial bloodstream infections traced to probable contamination of hemodialysis machines—Canada, 1995; Unites States 1997; and Israel, 1997. *MMWR Morbid Mortal Wkly Rep* 1998; **47(03)**: 55–58.

10 Oliver WJ, Webster OC, Clements H, Weston V, Boswell T. Two cases of *Enterococcus faecalis* bacteremia associated with a hemodialysis machine. *J Infect Dis* 1999; **179**: 1312.

11 Twardowski Z. Dialyzer reuse. Part I. Historical perspective. *Semin Dial* 2006; **19(1)**: 41–53.

12 Tang S, Lai KN. Chronic viral hepatitis in hemodialysis patients. *Hemodial Int* 2005; **9**: 169–179.

13 Froio N, Nicastri E, Comandini UV, Cherubini C, Felicioni R, Solmone M et al. Contamination by hepatitis B and C viruses in the dialysis setting. *Am J Kidney Dis* 2003; **42(3)**: 546–550.

14 Savey A, Simon F, Izopet J, Lepoutre A, Fabry J, Desenclos JC. A large nosocomial outbreak of hepatitis C virus infections at a hemodialysis center. *Infect Control Hosp Epidemiol* 2005; **26(9)**: 752–760.

15 Sartor C, Brunet P, Simon S, Tamealet C, Berland Y, Drancourt M. Transmission of hepatitis C virus between hemodialysis patients sharing the same machine. *Infect Control Hosp Epidemiol* 2004; **25(7)**: 609–611.

16 Alter MJ, Tokars JI, Agodoa LYC, Neuland CY. Recommendations for preventing transmission among chronic hemodialysis patients. *MMWR Morb Mortal Wkly Rep* 2001; **50**: 1–43.

17 Smith CE, Jenkins JM, Staib D, Newell PJ, Mertz KJ, Lance-Parker S et al. Possible dialysis-related West Nile virus transmission—Georgia, 2003. *MMWR Morb Mortal Wkly Rep* 2004; **53(32)**: 738–739.

18 Pontoriero G, Pozzoni P, Andrulli S, Locatelli F. The quality of dialysis water. *Nephrol Dial Transplant* 2003; **18(Suppl 7)**: vii21–vii25.

19 Cappelli G, Perrone S, Ciuffreda A. Water quality for on-line haemodiafiltration. *Nephrol Dial Transplant* 1998; **13(Suppl 5)**: 12–16.

20 Association for the Advancement of Medical Instrumentation (AAMI). 2003. Hemodialysis system. ANSI/AAMI RD_2003

21 Water treatment system: recommendations of the European Pharmacopoeia. *Nephrol Dial Transplant* 2002; **17(Suppl 7)**: 45–46.

22 Bommer J, Jaber BL. Ultrapure dialysate: facts and myths. *Semin Dial* 2006; **19(2)**: 115–119.

23 Twardowski Z. Dialyzer reuse. Part II. Advantages and disadvantages. *Semin Dial* 2006; **19(3)**: 217–226.

24 Bommer J. Sterile filtration of dialysate: is it really of no use? *Nephrol Dial Transplant* 2001; **16**: 1992–1994.

25 Lowrie G, Li Z, Ofsthun N, Lazarus JM. Reprocessing dialysers for multiple uses: recent analysis of death risks for patients. *Nephrol Dial Transplant* 2004; **19**: 2823–2830.

26 Port FK, Wolfe RA, Hulbert-Shearon TE, Daugirdas JT, Agodoa LY, Jones C et al. Mortality risk by hemodialyzer reuse practice and dialyzer membrane characteristics: results for the USRDS Dialysis Morbidity and Mortality Study. *Am J Kidney Dis* 2001; **37(2)**: 276–286.

27 Collins J, Liu J, Ebben JP. Dialyser reuse-associated mortality and hospitalization risk in incident medicare haemodialysis patients, 1998-1999. *Nephrol Dial Transplant* 2004; **19**: 1245–1251.

28 Fan Q, Liu J, Ebben JP, Collins AJ. Reuse-associated mortality in incident hemodialysis patients in the United States, 2000-2001. *Am J Kidney Dis* 2005; **46(4)**: 661–668.

29 *NKF KDOQI Guidelines for Hemodialysis Adequacy.* National Kidney Foundation, New York; 2006.

30 Collins AJ, Ma JZ, Constantini EG, Everson SE. Dialysis unit and patient characteristics associated with reuse practices and mortality: 1989-1993. *J Am Soc Nephrol* 1998; **9(11)**: 2108–2117.

31 Robinson BM, Feldman HI. Dialyzer reuse and patient outcomes: what do we know now? *Semin Dialy* 2005; **18(3)**: 175–179.

32 Chen W, Gluud C. Vaccines for preventing hepatitis B in health-care workers. *Cochrane Database Syst Rev* 2007; **3**: CD000100.

33 Jefferson T, Demicheli V, Deeks J, MacMillan A, Sassi F, Pratt M. Vaccines for preventing hepatitis B in health-care workers. *Cochrane Database Syst Rev* 2000; **2**: CD000100.

34 Rangel MC, Coronado VG, Euler GL, Strikas RA. Vaccine recommendations for patients on chronic dialysis. *Semin Dial* 2000; **13(2)**: 101–107.

35 Baldessar MZ, Bettiol J, Foppa F, Oliveira LH. Hepatitis C risk factor for patients submitted to dialysis. *Brazil J Infect Dis* 2007; **11(1)**: 12–15.

36 Shamshiraz AA, Kamgar M, Bekheirnia MR, Ayazi F, Hashemi SR, Bouzari N *et al.* The role of hemodialysis machine dedication in reducing hepatitis C transmission in the dialysis setting in Iran: a multicenter prospective interventional study. *BMC Nephrol* 2004; **5**: 13.

42 Vascular Access for Hemodialysis

Kevan R. Polkinghorne

Department of Nephrology, Monash Medical Centre, Melbourne, Victoria, Australia

Introduction

Hemodialysis is the dominant form of therapy for patients with end-stage renal disease and requires repetitive, complication-free access to the peripheral blood circulation. Hence, the establishment and maintenance of vascular access is pivotal and has long been labeled the "Achilles' heel" of hemodialysis due to its vital role in the delivery of dialysis [1].

Vascular access for hemodialysis can be achieved in three ways: the native arteriovenous fistula (AVF), the arteriovenous graft (AVG; usually polytetrafluoroethylene), or the cuffed (or uncuffed) central venous catheter (CVC). The main role of the cuffed CVC is as a bridge until either an AVF or an AVG can be constructed or as permanent access in the patient who has exhausted all other vascular access possibilities.

It is well-established that the vascular access of first choice is the AVF [2–4]. This stems from both superior patency rates [2,3], lower infection risk [5], lower costs [6,7], and a lower mortality risk compared with either AVG or CVC [8,9]. Clinical practice guidelines for the USA [3], Canada 4], and Australasia [2] all indicate that AVF is the vascular access of first choice for hemodialysis patients.

Recent randomized controlled trials (RCTs) have focused on the maintenance of vascular access and can be divided into three broad areas: first, the use of vascular access surveillance in prolonging vascular access survival; second, pharmacological approaches to preventing AVF and AVG failure; finally, therapies for preventing cuffed CVC-related bacteremia (CRB). In this review I will summarize the results of RCTs in these three broad areas.

Screening and vascular access survival

Once vascular access has been established, the major clinical goal is to prevent complications, principally, vascular stenosis resulting

Evidence-based Nephrology. Edited by Donald Molony and Jonathan Craig
© 2009 Blackwell Publishing, ISBN: 978-1-4051-3975-5.

in failure (thrombosis) of the AVF or AVG. Screening tests must be efficient at detecting the presence of an underlying significant stenosis, and any correction of a stenosis thus detected should result in a reduction in access thrombosis rates and prolonged access survival. The ability to prevent AVF and AVG failure is an important clinical goal, as early elective repair can avoid interruption to dialysis. Several methods have been advocated as screening for access stenosis, including dynamic venous pressure (DVP) and static venous pressure (SVP), Doppler ultrasound (DU) screening, and the measurement of vascular access blood flow (Qa) 3,4].

Blood flow screening: RCTs

Vascular access blood flow can be measured by indicator dilution techniques or by estimating Qa using either DU or magnetic resonance angiography [3]. Prospective studies including one RCT [10] have sought an association between Qa and the risk of thrombosis and/or the presence of stenosis [10–15]. AVGs are at risk of thrombosis at higher flows (cutoffs of 500–750 mL/min) [12,13] and AVFs are at risk with lower flows (300–500 mL/min), which makes comparisons difficult [15]. All RCTs reporting the effect of Qa surveillance on vascular access survival or thrombosis rates have used ultrasound dilution to measure Qa, and the principles of this method have been well-described [16,17] and reviewed [18–21].

Five RCTs have examined the effect of Qa surveillance and preemptive repair (angioplasty in the majority of studies) on vascular access thrombosis rates and long-term access patency [22–26] (Table 42.1). All studies were small, of variable quality, and used different monitoring frequencies and flow thresholds for the triggering of investigation.

The three studies on AVGs failed to demonstrate a benefit of Qa surveillance despite significantly higher intervention rates in the surveillance groups [23–25]. In one study the Qa group had a significantly higher thrombosis rate than the control group, this being driven largely by multiple thromboses in three AVGs [24]. The positive result in the smallest study was largely driven by an abnormally high thrombosis rate in the control group [22]. Finally, in the study by Smits *et al.* [23], 21 of the 42 thrombotic episodes

Table 42.1 RCTs assessing effects of access blood flow surveillance on access thrombosis rate.

Study type and author [reference]	No. of patients	Controls	Surveillance	Qa threshold[a]	Blinding	ITT	Intervention	Thrombosis rate[b]	Follow-up
AVG studies									
Sands 1999 [22]	35	Nil[c]	SVP + Qa[c]	<750	NS	NS	PCTA	246.7 vs. 23.2*	6 mos
Smits 2001 [23]	53	DVP	Qa	<600	NS	No	PCTA[d]	0.19 vs. 0.24	37.8 pt-yrs
	72	DVP	DVP + Qa	<600	NS	No	PCTA[d]	0.32 vs. 0.28	42.7 pt-yrs
Ram 2003[e] [24]	101	Clinical + DVP	Qa	<600	Yes	Yes	PCTA	0.68 vs. 0.91*	2 yrs
Moist 2003 [25]	112	Clinical + DVP	Clinical + Qa	<650 or 20%↓	Yes	Yes	PCTA	0.41 vs. 0.51	1 yr
AVF studies									
Sands 1999. [22]	68	Nil[b]	SVP + Qa[b]	<750	NS	NS	PCTA	27.1 vs.16.8*	6 ms
Tessitore 2004 [26]	79	Clinical	Qa	<750 or 25%↓	No	Yes	PCTA[d]	HR 3.93**[f]	5 yrs

Abbreviations: PCTA, percutaneous transluminal angioplasty; NS, not stated; ITT, analysis by intention to treat.

[a] Values are in milliliters per minute, all measured monthly except for the Smits *et al.* trial, with 8 weekly measurements, and the Tessitore *et al.* study, with 3 monthly measurements.

[b] Control versus treatment. *, $P < 0.05$; **, $P < 0.01$.

[c] DU was performed every 6 months in all patients.

[d] Further surgical intervention required in 10%.

[e] Results here for the Qa arm versus control.

[f] Overall failure including thrombosis and abandonment HR for control versus treatment (95% CI, 1.42–10.93).

occurred after a positive screening test but before intervention and were excluded from the analysis, reducing the power of the study. Despite this, no difference was seen in thrombosis rates in the Qa surveillance group compared with the control DVP groups.

In the above three negative studies, there were more interventions performed in the Qa surveillance groups, suggesting that more stenoses had been detected, particularly in the two more recent studies [24,25]. Furthermore, in these two studies preemptive angioplasty was performed in all patients, and in the study by Smits *et al.* over 90% of the interventions included angioplasty [23]. The efficacy of the angioplasty procedure in the Qa group is thus in doubt. An increase in Qa immediately postangioplasty, and not necessarily with radiological success (reduction in the stenosis diameter), has been shown to predict outcome postangioplasty [27,28]. However, Qa was not measured immediately postangioplasty in these studies, although Moist *et al.* reported no difference in the postangioplasty Qa rise between the two groups, suggesting that the angioplasty procedures in both groups were equivalent. Whether elective surgical revision of the AVG stenosis would have resulted in an improved outcome has not been studied in any RCT. However, there is evidence that surgical revision may be superior to angioplasty in the treatment of AVG thrombosis [29].

Both studies of AVF demonstrated a significant reduction in thrombosis rate with Qa surveillance. One [22], while positive, had a unusually high background thrombosis rate in the control arm (27.1% in 6 months). There were some methodological flaws in the Tessitore group's study of stenotic AVF [26]. Randomization was by coin toss, and there was no blinding of surveillance allocation. Patency of the AVF in the Qa group lasted significantly longer

than the control group; the specific thrombosis rates in each group, however, were not reported. In addition, a third study that randomized functioning stenotic AVF to angioplasty or no treatment demonstrated a significantly improved AVF survival with angioplasty [30]. These three small studies thus suggest possible benefits of Qa surveillance on AVF survival. However, before definitive recommendations can be made, a larger multicenter study is required. Assuming an annual AVF thrombosis and revision rate of 12–15%/year [31], at least 300 subjects would be needed in each arm to detect a reduction of 30% (relative risk [RR], 0.70; 90% power) in AVF thrombosis and revision rates as a result of Qa screening [10]. Such an RCT is also required to determine whether AVF screening is cost-effective [32].

DU stenosis screening: RCTs

DU screening is a noninvasive procedure that in addition to the measurement of Qa can provide anatomic information on the vascular access. As such, it has been advocated as a screening technique to identify access that is at risk of thrombosis by identifying the anatomic presence of a significant stenosis. It requires, however, specialized equipment and skill and is expensive. A discussion of the technical aspects of DU is beyond the scope of this review, but these issues have been recently summarized by Lockhart and Robbin [33].

Six RCTs [24,34–38] assessing the effect of DU screening for stenosis of AVGs combined with either angioplasty or surgical repair on access thrombosis and survival have been performed (Table 42.2). One study was published in abstract form only [36]. All trials excluded AVF. Two [36,37] of the six studies demonstrated a

Table 42.2 RCTs assessing effects of ultrasound stenosis screening on AVG patency or thrombosis.

Study [reference]	No. of patients	Control	Surveillance	Blinding	ITT	Intervention	Patency[a]	Follow-up
Mayer 1993 [34]	70	Clinical	3 monthly USS	No	Yes	Surgery	80% vs. 62%	2 yrs
Lumsden 1997 [35]	64	No intervention	3 monthly USS	No	Yes	PCTA	51% vs. 47%	2 yrs
Sands 1997 [36]	55	Examination	USS			PCTA	126 vs. 19[b]*	NS
Ram 2003[c] [24]	101	Clinical + DVP	3 monthly USS	Yes	Yes	PCTA	34% vs. 36%[d]	2 yrs
Malik 2005 [37]	192	Clinical/DVP/Qa	3 monthly USS + clinical/DVP/Qa	No	NS	PCTA	RR control, 3.75[e]**	2 yrs
Robbin 2006 [38]	126	Clinical	4 monthly USS	No	Yes	PCTA/Surgery	38 vs. 37 mos[f]	23 mos

Abbreviations: ITT, intention-to-treat analysis; PCTA, percutaneous angioplasty; USS, DU screening; NS, not stated.

[a] Treatment versus control data for 12-month patency unless otherwise stated. *, $P < 0.05$; **, $P < 0.001$.

[b] Rate is per 100 patient-years.

[c] Results shown are for the USS arm versus control.

[d] Patency defined as thrombosis or need for preemptive PCTA.

[e] Patency data were not presented in the study report; unadjusted relative risk of access failure in control was 3.75 (95% CI, 1.7–8.1).

[f] Cumulative survival.

significant increase in patency rates with DU screening and preemptive angioplasty, whereas another study [34] demonstrated a significant reduction at 6 but not at 12 months follow-up. In addition a subanalysis of the study by Lumsden et al. assessing only new AVGs ($n = 21$) [39] demonstrated a significant prolongation of AVG patency ($P = 0.035$) and a reduction in thrombosis rate in the treatment group (0.10 vs. 0.44 thrombosis/patient–dialysis year). The DU arm in another study [24] had the highest preemptive angioplasty rate and a longer thrombosis-free survival, although this outcome did not reach statistical significance ($P = 0.10$). However, neither event-free survival nor 2-year AVG survival (62 vs. 64%) was significantly better in the ultrasound group. The authors have subsequently argued that DU screening, whereas not prolonging AVG survival, reduces morbidity and costs through the reduction in thromboses and less interruption to the hemodialysis treatment [40]. In the most recent study [38], while the frequency of preemptive graft angioplasty was 64% higher in the ultrasound group (1.05 vs. 0.64 events/patient–year; $P < 0.001$) due to an increase in the detection of AVG stenosis, the cumulative graft survival was similar (median survival, 38 vs. 37 months for the DU and control groups, respectively; $P = 0.93$). The thrombosis rates also did not differ (0.67 vs. 0.78/patient–year in DU and control groups, respectively; $P = 0.37$). As with the surveillance studies (Table 42.1), the largely negative results of these trials raise questions on the efficacy of angioplasty to correct the underlying stenosis. However the only study to use surgery also failed to demonstrate any conclusive benefit [34] from DU-based surveillance.

Other screening techniques: RCTs

Numerous other techniques have been advocated, including physical examination and the measurement of access recirculation (AR), dynamic, and/or static venous pressures. Physical examination of the access plays an important role, and some have suggested that this element has been largely ignored [41,42]. Physical findings suggesting a significant venous stenosis include edema of the access extremity, prolonged bleeding postvenipuncture, and changes in the physical characteristics of the pulse or thrill.

AR resulting in reduced dialysis efficiency occurs when the dialyzed blood, returning via the venous needle of the extracorporeal circuit, is taken up again through the arterial needle, bypassing the systemic circulation. It occurs, within the AVG or AVF, when Qa is less than the dialyzer blood flow (Qb) [43]. Thus, the presence of AR signifies a reduced Qa resulting from the presence of a hemodynamically significant stenosis. The clinical usefulness of AR measurements in AVG surveillance is limited because the risk of thrombosis in AVG is high once Qa is reduced to 500–800 mL/min, a range of blood flow which is too high to cause AR [3]. Unlike AVG, AVF blood flow can be decreased to below prescribed dialyzer blood flow and still maintain patency. Thus, the measurement of AR can be a useful tool to detect AVF stenosis, although there have been no RCTs performed to date to evaluate this approach. The measurement of AR using saline dilution failed to detect a significant number of patients with documented low AVF blood flow and thus does not indicate any extra benefit to Qa monitoring [14,44,45].

Pressure within AVGs and AVFs can be considered as a surrogate of blood flow, but the relationship between pressure and flow differs between them (reviewed in reference 46). Pressure is measured either at the venous drip chamber during dialysis (DVP) or with the blood pump stopped (SVP). The standardized methods for measuring both DVP and SVP are outlined in the latest National Kidney Foundation Kidney Disease Outcomes Quality Initiative (K/DOQI) guidelines [3]. Schwab et al. [47] first described an association between raised DVP and the presence of AVG stenosis at the venous anastomosis and subsequently developed a screening and monitoring protocol [48]. Serial measurements should be performed with the trend being more important than single values, remembering that any lesions within the body of an AVG will not be detected if proximal to the venous needle [45]. Given the problems associated with measuring venous drip chamber pressure;

Besarab *et al.* suggested the measurement of intra-access pressure [45,49]. While they demonstrated a reduction in the thrombosis rate using historical controls [49], at present no RCT of either dynamic or intra-access pressure measurements in AVG or AVF has been performed. An RCT of SVP monitoring versus clinical evidence of access dysfunction in AVG [50] showed screening using SVP with angioplasty did not prolong AVG survival, with a trend to a poorer outcome in the SVP group (hazard ratio [HR], 1.75, 95% confidence interval [CI], 0.80–3.83; $P = 0.16$). After adjustment for gender, diabetes, PVD, and access location, the SVP group had a significantly greater risk of access abandonment (HR, 2.91; 95% CI, 1.17–7.20; $P = 0.02$) despite a significantly higher intervention rate. While venous pressure monitoring is widely practiced, the evidence that the detection and treatment of a significant stenosis in AVG prolongs graft survival is of poor quality and requires further study. Since the presence of collaterals prevents the rise in venous pressure consequent to a reduction in Qa due to a stenosis, K/DOQI has not recommended DVP to detect significant stenoses in AVF [3]. Furthermore, normalized venous segment pressures do not correlate with the presence of significant AVF stenosis [45].

Pharmacological approaches to preventing AVF and AVG failure: RCTs

The use of antiplatelet or anticoagulant agents or other drugs to prevent AVF and AVG failure was first discussed in 1967 [51], with a number of studies performed from the mid-1970s using antiplatelet agents [52–55]. Subsequently, with the increased morbidity associated with AVG thrombosis, a number of larger RCTs have recently been performed [56–58]. In addition there are at least two large multicenter studies under way, one with clopidogrel in AVF [59] and one using dipyridamole plus aspirin in AVG [60].

Nine RCTs have been performed, with the majority of the studies using antiplatelet agents [52–56,61] (Table 42.3). One study assessed low-dose warfarin [57] and one evaluated fish oil [58]. In addition, a Cochrane systematic review was published in 2003 [62] that included studies published up to October 2002.

All four RCTs for AVF have assessed the effect of aspirin or ticlopidine on early AVF failure (at 1 month) [52,54,55,61]. One of the study end points was AVF patency rather than its successful use for dialysis. Two of the three smaller studies demonstrated a significant reduction in thrombosis rates in the treatment group [52,55]. However, a subsequent larger study, underpowered due to slow recruitment and a lower-than-expected event rate, failed to confirm this [61].

Four studies assessed thrombosis in AVG at different follow-up times [56–58,63]. Sreedhara *et al.* [63] compared aspirin alone, dipyridamole alone, and dipyridamole plus aspirin with placebo in AVG. Thrombosis rates in the dipyridamole group were significantly lower compared with placebo, while aspirin was associated with a nonsignificant increased thrombosis rate. The combination of aspirin and dipyridamole gave a nonsignificant reduction compared with placebo. The study comparing the combination of

Table 42.3 RCTs of pharmacotherapy for vascular access thrombosis.

Study [reference]	Access type	No. of patients	Intervention	Control	Blinding	ITT	Outcome, follow-up	Result (treatment vs. placebo)
Andrassay 1974 [52]	AVF	92	Aspirin, 500 mg	Placebo	Double	NS	Thrombosis, 1 mo	OR 0.15 (0.03–0.73)[a]
Kobayashi 1980 [53]	AVG/shunt	107	Ticlopidine, 200 mg bid	Placebo	Double	NS	Thrombosis, 3 mos	↓Thrombectomy***
Fiskerstrand 1985 [54]	AVF	18	Ticlopidine 250 mg bid	Placebo	Double	No	Thrombosis, 1 mo	OR 0.40 (0.05–3.42)[a]
Grontoft 1985 [55]	AVF	36	Ticlopidine 250 mg bid	Placebo	Double	Yes	Thrombosis, 1 mo	OR 0.13 (0.02–0.76)[a]
			Dipyridamole 75 mg tds	Placebo	Double	NS	Thrombosis, 18 mos	21 vs. 42%*[c,d]
Sreedhara 1994[63]	AVG[b]	84	Aspirin 325 od	Placebo				80 vs. 42%[c,e]
			Dipyridamole + Aspirin	Placebo				25 vs. 42%[c,f]
Grontoft 1998 [61]	AVF	261	Ticlopidine 250 mg bid	Placebo	Double	Yes	Thrombosis, 1 mo	OR 0.60 (0.30–1.18)[a]
Schmitz 2002[58]	AVG	24	Fish Oil 4000 mg	Placebo	Double	Yes	Thrombosis, 12 mos	24.4% vs. 85.1%***
Crowther 2002[57]	AVG	107	Warfarin (INR 1.4–1.9)	Placebo	Double	Yes	Thrombosis, 24 mos	HR1.76 (0.72–4.34)
Kaufman 2003[g] [56]	AVG	200	Clopidogrel + Aspirin	Placebo	Double	Yes	Thrombosis, 7 mos	HR 0.81 (0.47–1.40)

Abbreviations: ITT, intention-to-treat analysis; NS, not stated; bid, twice a day; tds, XX; od, once a day.

Symbols: ***, $P < 0.05$.

[a] Results taken from the systematic review by Da Silva *et al.* 2003 [62].

[b] New AVG only.

[c] Cumulative thrombosis rates at 18 months.

[d] RR, 0.35 (CI, 0.15–0.80).

[e] RR, 1.99 (CI, 0.88–4.48).

[f] RR for this comparison was not given in the paper.

[g] This study was stopped early during recruitment due to adverse effects (see text).

aspirin and clopidogrel with placebo was stopped early due to a twofold increase in the incidence of bleeding events in the treatment group [56]. Overall there was no difference between the two groups in terms of thrombosis rates (HR, 0.81; 95% CI, 0.47–1.40; $P = 0.41$). Thus, at present the evidence that antiplatelet agents prevent thrombosis in AVG is weak, and the combination of agents may cause harm with increased bleeding risks.

The use of low-dose warfarin (international normalized ratio [INR], 1.4–1.9) compared with placebo was addressed in a well-designed study with blinding of both patients and physicians by using central warfarin monitoring and sham INR values [57]. Treatment with warfarin did not reduce the thrombosis rate; rather, there was a nonsignificant increase in thrombosis rate (HR, 1.76; 95% CI, 0.72–4.34; $P = 0.21$). In addition six major bleeding events occurred in the warfarin group compared with none in the placebo group ($P = 0.03$). Finally, Schmitz *et al.* [58] performed a small RCT assessing fish oil (80% ω-3 fatty acid ethyl esters) versus a control oil (corn oil). Fish oil produced a significant reduction in the thrombosis rate, 24.4 versus 85.1% in the control group at 1 year ($P < 0.05$). Given the small sample size, a confirmatory trial

with a larger sample size is needed to confirm not just the efficacy but also the safety of this treatment before fish oil treatment can be recommended.

Preventing cuffed CRB: RCTs

With the increasing use of cuffed CVC, the prevention of complications related to their use has become a major focus [64]. Commencement of dialysis with a CVC is associated with a higher risk of infectious and all-cause mortality [9], and different strategies to prevent CRB have been the subject of a number of RCTs in the last 5 years. Here I will focus solely on RCTs primarily assessing interventions aimed at reducing cuffed (tunneled) CRB, given that they are the predominant CVC used in chronic hemodialysis patients.

Such trials can be divided into two broad groups; those where the intervention is administered at the exit site to reduce skin bacteria and subsequent catheter colonization, and those where antibiotic catheter lock solutions are instilled to limit the formation

Table 42.4 RCTs of prophylaxis of cuffed (tunneled) CRB in hemodialysis patients.

Prophylaxis group and study [reference]	No. of patients	Intervention	Control	Blinding	ITT	Follow-up[a]	Result (treatment vs. control)[b]
Silver-coated catheters							
Trerotola 1998 [65]	92	Silver catheter	Normal catheter	No	No	92	1.8 vs. 1.1
Lock solutions							
Dogra 2002 [71]	108	Gentamicin/citrate	Heparin	Double	Yes	40	0.3 vs. 4.2**
Pervez 2002 [72]	55	Gentamicin/citrate	Heparin	No	NS	NS[d]	0.62 vs. 2.11
		Sterile Hub bag	Heparin	No	NS		3.05 vs. 2.11
McIntyre 2004 [68]	50	Gentamicin/heparin	Heparin	No	Yes	120	0.3 vs. 4.0*
Betjes 2004[c] [66]	76	Citrate/taurolidine	Heparin	No	NS		0 vs. 2.1*
Bleyer 2005[c] [67]	60	Monocycline-EDTA	Heparin	Double	Yes	78	8.3% vs. 0%[e]
Weijmer 2005[c] [70]	291	Trisodium citrate	Heparin	Double	Yes	NS[f]	1.1 vs. 4.1***
Saxena 2006 [69]	119	Cefotaxime/heparin	Heparin	Double	Yes	NS[g]	1.67 vs. 3.60**
Nori 2006 [73]	62	Minocycline-EDTA	Heparin	No	Yes	NS[h]	0.4 vs. 4*
		Gentamicin/tricitrate	Heparin	No	Yes		0 vs. 4**
Exit site ointment							
Johnson 2002 [77]	50	Mupirocin	No mupirocin	No	Yes	NS	1.6 vs. 10.5**
Lok 2003 [76]	169	Polysporin	Placebo	Double	Yes	NS[i]	0.63 vs. 2.48***
Johnson 2005 [78].	101	Honey	Mupirocin	No	Yes	95	0.97 vs. 0.85

Abbreviations: EDTA, ethylenediaminetetraacetic acid; NS, not stated; ITT, intention-to-treat analysis.
[a] Median or mean catheter days
[b] Rates of CRB/1000 catheter days. *, $P < 0.05$; **, $P < 0.01$; ***, $P < 0.001$.
[c] Study included both cuffed and uncuffed catheters.
[d] Total of 4805 catheter days analyzed.
[e] Rates not stated.
[f] Total of 16,547 catheter days analyzed.
[g] Total of 43,435 catheter days analyzed.
[h] Total of 6189 catheter days analyzed.
[i] Overall follow-up was 6 months.

of a biofilm, which can act as a nidus for CRB. In addition, one study compared silver-coated CVC to standard CVC and did not demonstrate any benefit [65].

All eight studies of catheter lock solutions [66–73] demonstrated a reduction in CRB; although the reduction was not statistically significant in two studies [67,72]. Two other studies demonstrated a significantly lower CRB-related mortality in the antibiotic lock group [69,70]. There are, however, concerns regarding gentamicin-induced ototoxicity [71], the use of high-dose citrate potentially causing fatal arrhythmias [74], and the emergence of antibiotic resistance [75]. Therefore, the optimal antibiotic lock solution has yet to be determined [75].

Three studies have investigated the use of exit site ointment on CRB; two compared an antibiotic ointment to placebo or no ointment [76,77], and a third compared mupirocin with honey [78] (Table 42.4). Both mupirocin [77] and polysorin ointment [76] significantly reduced the incidence of CRB compared with placebo or no treatment although in the mupirocin study the CRB rate in the control group was unusually high. Johnson *et al.* then compared honey with mupirocin [78], given the concerns regarding the emergence of mupirocin resistance [79]. This novel study did not demonstrate any difference in CRB rates between the two interventions, but the study was small. The use of honey would avoid the emergence of antibiotic resistance and is worth further investigation. Whether antibiotic lock solutions are more effective than exit site ointment is currently unknown; the rates of CRB seem similar across the studies, but no RCT has compared them directly.

Conclusions

The establishment and maintenance of vascular access for hemodialysis are major components in the treatment of end-stage renal disease patients. An AVF is the first-choice vascular access for hemodialysis, and attempts to increase the prevalence of AVF have been a major focus of care [2–4]. In addition a large number of recent RCTs have assessing different strategies aimed at maintaining vascular access survival. Further large trials are needed to assess possible cost and benefits of access surveillance and pharmacological interventions to prevent access thrombosis, especially in patients with AVF. Catheters will continue to have a role, and further studies are needed to determine the most effective and safe methods of preventing CRB.

References

1 Kjellstrand CM. The Achilles' heel of the hemodialysis patient. *Arch Intern Med* 1978; **138:** 1063–1064.

2 *The CARI Guidelines: Vascular Access.* 2003. (www.kidney.org.au/cari/drafts/bvascular.html)

3 NKF. KDOQI clinical practice guidelines and clinical practice recommendations for 2006 updates: hemodialysis adequacy, peritoneal dialysis adequacy and vascular access. *Am J Kidney Dis* 2006; **48:** S1–S322.

4 Jindal K, Chan CT, Deziel C, Hirsch D, Soroka SD, Tonelli M *et al.* Hemodialysis clinical practice guidelines for the Canadian Society of Nephrology. *J Am Soc Nephrol* 2006; **17:** S1–27.

5 Nassar GM, Ayus JC. Infectious complications of the hemodialysis access. *Kidney Int* 2001; **60:** 1–13.

6 Lee H, Manns B, Taub K, Ghali WA, Dean S, Johnson D *et al.* Cost analysis of ongoing care of patients with end-stage renal disease: the impact of dialysis modality and dialysis access. *Am J Kidney Dis* 2002; **40:** 611–622.

7 Manns B, Tonelli M, Yilmaz S, Lee H, Laupland K, Klarenbach S *et al.* Establishment and maintenance of vascular access in incident hemodialysis patients: a prospective cost analysis. *J Am Soc Nephrol* 2005; **16:** 201–209.

8 Dhingra RK, Young EW, Hulbert-Shearon TE, Leavey SF, Port FK. Type of vascular access and mortality in U.S. hemodialysis patients. *Kidney Int* 2001; **60:** 1443–1451.

9 Polkinghorne KR, McDonald SP, Atkins RC, Kerr PG. Vascular access and all-cause mortality: a propensity score analysis. *J Am Soc Nephrol* 2004; **15:** 477–486.

10 Polkinghorne KR, Lau KK, Saunder A, Atkins RC, Kerr PG. Does monthly native arteriovenous fistula blood-flow surveillance detect significant stenosis: a randomized controlled trial. *Nephrol Dial Transplant* 2006; **21:** 2498–2506.

11 Strauch BS, O'Connell RS, Geoly KL, Grundlehner M, Yakub YN, Tietjen DP. Forecasting thrombosis of vascular access with Doppler color flow imaging. *Am J Kidney Dis* 1992; **19:** 554–557.

12 Bosman PJ, Boereboom FT, Eikelboom BC, Koomans HA, Blankestijn PJ. Graft flow as a predictor of thrombosis in hemodialysis grafts. *Kidney Int* 1998; **54:** 1726–1730.

13 Neyra NR, Ikizler TA, May RE, Himmelfarb J, Schulman G, Shyr Y *et al.* Change in access blood flow over time predicts vascular access thrombosis. *Kidney Int* 1998; **54:** 1714–1719.

14 Tonelli M, Jindal K, Hirsch D, Taylor S, Kane C, Henbrey S. Screening for subclinical stenosis in native vessel arteriovenous fistulae. *J Am Soc Nephrol* 2001; **12:** 1729–1733.

15 Tonelli M, Jhangri GS, Hirsch DJ, Marryatt J, Mossop P, Wile C *et al.* Best threshold for diagnosis of stenosis or thrombosis within six months of access flow measurement in arteriovenous fistulae. *J Am Soc Nephrol* 2003; **14:** 3264–3269.

16 Krivitski NM. Theory and validation of access flow measurement by dilution technique during hemodialysis. *Kidney Int* 1995; **48:** 244–250.

17 Depner TA, Krivitski NM. Clinical measurement of blood flow in hemodialysis access fistulae and grafts by ultrasound dilution. *ASAIO J* 1995; **41:** M745–M749.

18 Paulson WD. Blood flow surveillance of hemodialysis grafts and the dysfunction hypothesis. *Semin Dial* 2001; **14:** 175–180.

19 Leypoldt JK. Diagnostic methods for vascular access: access flow measurements. *Contrib Nephrol* 2002; **137:** 31–37.

20 Leypoldt JK. Standards for reproducible access flow measurements. *Blood Purif* 2002; **20:** 20–25.

21 Krivitski N, Schneditz D. Arteriovenous vascular access flow measurement: accuracy and clinical implications. *Contrib Nephrol* 2004; **142:** 269–284.

22 Sands JJ, Jabyac PA, Miranda CL, Kapsick BJ. Intervention based on monthly monitoring decreases hemodialysis access thrombosis. *ASAIO J* 1999; **45:** 147–150.

23 Smits JH, van der Linden J, Hagen EC, Modderkolk-Cammeraat EC, Feith GW, Koomans HA *et al.* Graft surveillance: venous pressure, access flow, or the combination? *Kidney Int* 2001; **59:** 1551–1558.

24 Ram SJ, Work J, Caldito GC, Eason JM, Pervez A, Paulson WD. A randomized controlled trial of blood flow and stenosis surveillance of hemodialysis grafts. *Kidney Int* 2003l **64:** 272–280.

25 Moist LM, Churchill DN, House AA, Millward SF, Elliott JE, Kribs SW *et al*. Regular monitoring of access flow compared with monitoring of venous pressure fails to improve graft survival. *J Am Soc Nephrol* 2003; **14:** 2645–2653.

26 Tessitore N, Lipari G, Poli A, Bedogna V, Baggio E, Loschiavo C *et al*. Can blood flow surveillance and pre-emptive repair of subclinical stenosis prolong the useful life of arteriovenous fistulae? A randomized controlled study. *Nephrol Dial Transplant* 2004; **19:** 2325–2333.

27 Ahya SN, Windus DW, Vesely TM. Flow in hemodialysis grafts after angioplasty: Do radiologic criteria predict success? *Kidney Int* 2001; **59:** 1974–1978.

28 van der Linden J, Smits JH, Assink JH, Wolterbeek DW, Zijlstra JJ, de Jong GH *et al*. Short- and long-term functional effects of percutaneous transluminal angioplasty in hemodialysis vascular access. *J Am Soc Nephrol* 2002; **13:** 715–720.

29 Green LD, Lee DS, Kucey DS. A metaanalysis comparing surgical thrombectomy, mechanical thrombectomy, and pharmacomechanical thrombolysis for thrombosed dialysis grafts. *J Vasc Surg* 2002; **36:** 939–945.

30 Tessitore N, Mansueto G, Bedogna V, Lipari G, Poli A, Gammaro L *et al*. A prospective controlled trial on effect of percutaneous transluminal angioplasty on functioning arteriovenous fistulae survival. *J Am Soc Nephrol* 2003; **14:** 1623–1627.

31 Polkinghorne KR, Kerr PG. Vascular access. In: Russ GR, editor, *ANZDATA Registry Report 2002*. Australia and New Zealand Dialysis and Transplant Registry, Adelaide, 2003; 102–107.

32 Tonelli M, Klaarenbach S, Jindal K, Manns B. Economic implications of screening strategies in arteriovenous fistulae. *Kidney Int* 2006; **69:** 2219–2226.

33 Lockhart ME, Robbin ML. Hemodialysis access ultrasound. *Ultrasound Q* 2001; **17:** 157–167.

34 Mayer DA, Zingale RG, Tsapogas MJ. Duplex scanning of expanded polytetrafluroethylene dialysis shunts: impact on patient management and graft survival. *Vasc Surg* 1993; **27:** 647–658.

35 Lumsden AB, MacDonald MJ, Kikeri DK, Harker LA, Allen RC. Hemodialysis access graft stenosis: percutaneous transluminal angioplasty. *J. Surg. Res.* 1997; **68:** 181–185.

36 Sands J, Gandy D, Finn M, Johnson A, Burrows S, Miranda C. Ultrasound-angioplasty program decreases thrombosis rate and cost of PTFE graft maintenance. *J Am Soc Nephrol* 1997; **8:** 171A.

37 Malik J, Slavikova M, Svobodova J, Tuka V. Regular ultrasonographic screening significantly prolongs patency of PTFE grafts. *Kidney Int* 2005; **67:** 1554–1558.

38 Robbin ML, Oser RF, Lee JY, Heudebert GR, Mennemeyer ST, Allon M. Randomized comparison of ultrasound surveillance and clinical monitoring on arteriovenous graft outcomes. *Kidney Int* 2006; **69:** 730–735.

39 Martin LG, MacDonald MJ, Kikeri D, Cotsonis GA, Harker LA, Lumsden AB. Prophylactic angioplasty reduces thrombosis in virgin ePTFE arteriovenous dialysis grafts with greater than 50% stenosis: subset analysis of a prospectively randomized study. *J Vasc Interv Radiol* 1999; **10:** 389–396.

40 Dossabhoy NR, Ram SJ, Nassar R, Work J, Eason JM, Paulson WD. Stenosis surveillance of hemodialysis grafts by duplex ultrasound reduces hospitalizations and cost of care. *Semin Dial* 2005; **18:** 550–557.

41 Beathard GA. Physical examination of the dialysis vascular access. *Semin Dial* 1998; **11:** 231–236.

42 Paulson WD, Ram SJ, Zibari GB. Vascular access: anatomy, examination, management. *Semin Nephrol* 2002; **22:** 183–194.

43 Besarab A, Sherman R. The relationship of recirculation to access blood flow. *Am J Kidney Dis* 1997; **29:** 223–229.

44 Besarab A, Lubkowski T, Frinak S, Ramanathan S, Escobar F. Detecting vascular access dysfunction. *ASAIO J* 1997; **43:** M539–M543.

45 Besarab A, Lubkowski T, Frinak S, Ramanathan S, Escobar F. Detection of access strictures and outlet stenoses in vascular accesses. Which test is best? *ASAIO J* 1997; **43:** M543–M547.

46 Besarab A, Frinak S. Strategies for the prospective detection of access dysfunction. In: Conlon P, Schwab S, Nicholson M, editors, *Hemodialysis Vascular Access: Practice and Problems*. Oxford University Press, Oxford, 2000; 157–182.

47 Schwab SJ, Saeed M, Sussman SK, McCann RL, Stickel DL. Transluminal angioplasty of venous stenoses in polytetrafluoroethylene vascular access grafts. *Kidney Int* 1987; **32:** 395–398.

48 Schwab SJ, Raymond JR, Saeed M, Newman GE, Dennis PA, Bollinger RR. Prevention of hemodialysis fistula thrombosis. Early detection of venous stenoses. *Kidney Int* 1989; **36:** 707–711.

49 Besarab A, Sullivan KL, Ross RP, Moritz MJ. Utility of intra-access pressure monitoring in detecting and correcting venous outlet stenoses prior to thrombosis. *Kidney Int* 1995; **47:** 1364–1373.

50 Dember LM, Holmberg EF, Kaufman JS. Randomized controlled trial of prophylactic repair of hemodialysis arteriovenous graft stenosis. *Kidney Int* 2004; **66:** 390–398.

51 Wing AJ, Curtis JR, De Wardener HE. Reduction of clotting in Scribner shunts by long-term anticoagulation. *Br Med J* 1967; **3:** 143–145.

52 Andrassy K, Malluche H, Bornefeld H, Comberg M, Ritz E, Jesdinsky H *et al*. Prevention of p.o. clotting of av. cimino fistulae with acetylsalicyl acid. Results of a prospective double blind study. *Klin Wochenschr* 1974; **52:** 348–349.

53 Kobayashi K, Maeda K, Koshikawa S, Kawaguchi Y, Shimizu N, Naito C. Antithrombotic therapy with ticlopidine in chronic renal failure patients on maintenance hemodialysis: a multicenter collaborative double blind study. *Thromb Res* 1980; **20:** 255–261.

54 Fiskerstrand CE, Thompson IW, Burnet ME, Williams P, Anderton JL. Double-blind randomized trial of the effect of ticlopidine in arteriovenous fistulas for hemodialysis. *Artif Organs* 1985; **9:** 61–63.

55 Grontoft KC, Mulec H, Gutierrez A, Olander R. Thromboprophylactic effect of ticlopidine in arteriovenous fistulas for haemodialysis. *Scand J Urol Nephrol* 1985; **19:** 55–57.

56 Kaufman JS, O'Connor TZ, Zhang JH, Cronin RE, Fiore LD, Ganz MB *et al*. Randomized controlled trial of clopidogrel plus aspirin to prevent hemodialysis access graft thrombosis. *J Am Soc Nephrol* 2003; **14:** 2313–2321.

57 Crowther MA, Clase CM, Margetts PJ, Julian J, Lambert K, Sneath D *et al*. Low-intensity warfarin is ineffective for the prevention of PTFE graft failure in patients on hemodialysis: a randomized controlled trial. *J Am Soc Nephrol* 2002; **13:** 2331–2337.

58 Schmitz PG, McCloud LK, Reikes ST, Leonard CL, Gellens ME. Prophylaxis of hemodialysis graft thrombosis with fish oil: double-blind, randomized, prospective trial. *J Am Soc Nephrol* 2002; **13:** 184–190.

59 Dember LM, Kaufman JS, Beck GJ, Dixon BS, Gassman JJ, Greene T *et al*. Design of the Dialysis Access Consortium (DAC) clopidogrel prevention of early AV fistula thrombosis trial. *Clin Trials* 2005; **2:** 413–422.

60 Dixon BS, Beck GJ, Dember LM, Depner TA, Gassman JJ, Greene T *et al.* Design of the Dialysis Access Consortium (DAC) aggrenox prevention of access stenosis trial. *Clin Trials* 2005; **2:** 400–412.

61 Grontoft KC, Larsson R, Mulec H, Weiss LG, Dickinson JP. Effects of ticlopidine in AV-fistula surgery in uremia. Fistula Study Group. *Scand J Urol Nephrol* 1998; **32:** 276–283.

62 da Silva AF, Escofet X, Rutherford PA. Medical adjuvant treatment to increase patency of arteriovenous fistulae and grafts. *Cochrane Database Syst Rev* 2003; **2:** CD002786.

63 Sreedhara R, Himmelfarb J, Lazarus JM, Hakim RM. Anti-platelet therapy in graft thrombosis: results of a prospective, randomized, double-blind study. *Kidney Int* 1994; **45:** 1477–1483.

64 Allon M. Dialysis catheter-related bacteremia: treatment and prophylaxis. *Am J Kidney Dis* 2004; **44:** 779–791.

65 Trerotola SO, Johnson MS, Shah H, Kraus MA, McKusky MA, Ambrosius WT *et al.* Tunneled hemodialysis catheters: use of a silver-coated catheter for prevention of infection: a randomized study. *Radiology* 1998; **207:** 491–496.

66 Betjes MG, van Agteren M. Prevention of dialysis catheter-related sepsis with a citrate-taurolidine-containing lock solution. *Nephrol Dial Transplant* 2004; **19:** 1546–1551.

67 Bleyer AJ, Mason L, Russell G, Raad, II, Sherertz RJ. A randomized, controlled trial of a new vascular catheter flush solution (minocycline-EDTA) in temporary hemodialysis access. *Infect Control Hosp Epidemiol* 2005; **26:** 520–524.

68 McIntyre CW, Hulme LJ, Taal M, Fluck RJ. Locking of tunneled hemodialysis catheters with gentamicin and heparin. *Kidney Int* 2004; **66:** 801–805.

69 Saxena AK, Panhotra BR, Sundaram DS, Naguib M, Morsy F, Al-Arabi Al-Ghamdi AM. Enhancing the survival of tunneled haemodialysis catheters usinf an antibiotic lock in the elderly: a randomised, double blind clinical trial. *Nephrology* 2006; **11:** 299–305.

70 Weijmer MC, van den Dorpel MA, Van de Ven PJ, ter Wee PM, van Geelen JA, Groeneveld JO *et al.* Randomized, clinical trial comparison of trisodium citrate 30% and heparin as catheter-locking solution in hemodialysis patients. *J Am Soc Nephrol* 2005; **16:** 2769–2777.

71 Dogra GK, Herson H, Hutchison B, Irish AB, Heath CH, Golledge C *et al.* Prevention of tunneled hemodialysis catheter-related infections using catheter-restricted filling with gentamicin and citrate: a randomized controlled study. *J Am Soc Nephrol* 2002; **13:** 2133–2139.

72 Pervez A, Ahmed S, Ram S, Torres J, Work J, Zaman F *et al.* Antibiotic lock technique for prevention of cuffed tunnel catheter associated bacteremia. *J Vasc Access* 2002; **3:** 108–113.

73 Nori US, Manoharan A, Yee J, Besarab A. Comparison of low-dose gentamicin with minocycline as catheter lock solutions in the prevention of catheter-related bacteremia. *Am J Kidney Dis* 2006; **48:** 596–605.

74 US Food and Drug Administration. FDA Issues Warning on Tricitrasol Dialysis Catheter Anticoagulant, 2000. (http://www.fda.gov/bbs/topics/ANSWERS/ ANS01009.html)

75 Dogra GK. Preventing catheter-related infections with antibiotic lock solutions: are we spoilt for choice? *Nephrology* 2006; **11:** 297–298.

76 Lok CE, Stanley KE, Hux JE, Richardson R, Tobe SW, Conly J. Hemodialysis infection prevention with polysporin ointment. *J Am Soc Nephrol* 2003; **14:** 169–179.

77 Johnson DW, MacGinley R, Kay TD, Hawley CM, Campbell SB, Isbel NM *et al.* A randomized controlled trial of topical exit site mupirocin application in patients with tunnelled, cuffed haemodialysis catheters. *Nephrol Dial Transplant* 2002; **17:** 1802–1807.

78 Johnson DW, van Eps C, Mudge DW, Wiggins KJ, Armstrong K, Hawley CM *et al.* Randomized, controlled trial of topical exit-site application of honey (Medihoney) versus mupirocin for the prevention of catheter-associated infections in hemodialysis patients. *J Am Soc Nephrol* 2005; **16:** 1456–1462.

79 Cookson BD, Lacey RW, Noble WC, Reeves DS, Wise R, Redhead RJ. Mupirocin-resistant Staphylococcus aureus. *Lancet* 1990; **335:** 1095–1096.

7 Chronic Kidney Disease Stage 5: Peritoneal Dialysis

43 Selection of Peritoneal Dialysis as Renal Replacement Therapy

Norbert Lameire, Raymond Vanholder, & Wim Van Biesen

Renal Division, Department of Internal Medicine, University Hospital Ghent, Ghent, Belgium.

Introduction

Patients with end-stage renal dysfunction (chronic kidney disease [CKD] stage 5) will need replacement of their failed kidney function to maintain homeostasis and remain alive.

This renal replacement therapy (RRT) has to comply with some basic objectives: 1) prolong the survival of the patient as much as possible; 2) improve the quality of life (QoL) of the patient as much as possible; 3) be affordable for all patients and societies. There are three major RRT modalities that can be offered to the patient with CKD stage 5: peritoneal dialysis (PD), hemodialysis (HD), and transplantation. Maximal conservative treatment should also be considered, especially in the elderly or in severely disabled patients.

A recent Cochrane review [1] demonstrated the lack of strong evidence to support preferences of one dialysis modality (PD vs. HD) over the other. This review suggested that a randomized controlled trial (RCT) should be performed on this topic. Until now, only one RCT to compare outcomes between HD and PD patients has been conducted [2], but it was terminated prematurely because of problems with patient recruitment, showing that such a randomized trial is not feasible in clinical practice. In addition, there is evidence indicating that a succession of modalities in a flow chart model rather than a "conflictive" (one vs. the other) model should be the preferred methodology to describe and analyze RRT modalities and their outcomes [3]. Indeed, instead of considering HD and PD as competitive methods, it makes more sense to consider them as synergetic methods, in view of the probabilities of technique failure of both modalities [4]. This view holds true for transplantation also, as a transplant kidney will not be immediately available for everybody, thereby necessitating a period on either PD or HD. Technique failure is also a common outcome of transplantation, resulting in patients having to switch back to PD or HD. This model of integrated care (Figure 43.1), in which pa-

tients are offered the three different modalities in a predefined way, according to the needs of the moment, is therefore suggested as the optimal model to maximize survival of patients with end-stage renal disease (ESRD) [5].

Factors driving modality selection

It is clear that modality selection is driven by both medical and nonmedical factors.

Nonmedical factors

Nonmedical factors are far more important in the decision making process for RRT modality selection than previously thought [6–8]. Some important nonmedical factors are the referral pattern of the patient [9,10], the patient education process [11,12], the reimbursement of the different modalities [13,14], and experience of the treating team with PD [8,15].

All epidemiological studies have unequivocally demonstrated that patients who have been referred to a nephrology center less than 3 months before start of RRT are unlikely to start with PD [9]. Some studies indicate that merely "early" referral is not enough to increase the likelihood of patients starting on PD but that a structured education program about the different RRT modalities is necessary [16–20]. This type of pre-ESRD education has a beneficial impact on the overall outcome for the patient, both for life expectancy and QoL. PD patients are more likely to be transplanted in the first year of RRT, which is probably also related to their better preparation [20,21].

There is evidence that it is less costly to treat a patient on PD, compared with HD, even when transfers from PD to HD have been included [22]. HD has a greater labor and "hardware" cost, compared to PD, whereas the biggest costs for PD are the disposable materials [14]. PD also has some hidden economical advantages: no need for patient transport, reduced erythropoetin requirement [23], and fewer investigations, especially for biochemistry and radiology. Given these data, as expected, PD is used more frequently than HD in otherwise-comparable situations and countries with a

Evidence-based Nephrology. Edited by Donald Molony and Jonathan Craig
© 2009 Blackwell Publishing, ISBN: 978-1-4051-3975-5.

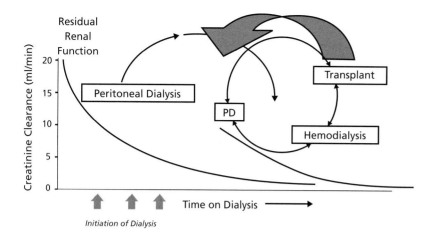

Figure 43.1 Schematic representation of the integrated care concept. Patients with a GFR below a certain threshold should be timely informed about the different treatment options for renal replacement therapy (PD, HD, and TX), taking into account eventual medical contraindications. As a patient's residual renal function declines, renal replacement therapy is started at a level where there is beginning to be uremic damage (e.g. decline of nutritional parameters, incipient fluid overload, etc). Eventual transfers between modalities are planned in function of development of eventual side effects of these modalities.

public-based versus a private-based organization of ESRD health care [24].

Medical factors

Patient survival
Modality choice should be based on relative survival. As transplantation is not an option for many patients, most studies have tried to compare HD and PD as opposite modalities (Table 43.1). There are major differences in statistical and epidemiological approaches in these studies, resulting in apparently conflicting results [25,26]. Some studies evaluated "modality survival," the survival on one single modality with patients being censored at their transfer to another modality. Other studies have used an intention-to-treat principle, where patients were assigned to the modality they started

Table 43.1 Overview of studies comparing outcomes on PD and HD since 1995.

Reference	Prevalent patients	Modality survival	Intention-to-treat survival	No. of HD patients	No. of PD patients	Patient category
[90]	No	No	Yes	767	274	All
[91]						All
[47]	No	No	Yes			All
[92]						All
[46]	No	Yes	Yes			All
[45]	No	Yes	Yes	4568	2443	All
[85]						All
[69]	No	Yes	Yes	93,900	14,022	Congestive heart failure
[93]	No	Yes	Yes	117,213	17,514	Large patients
[41]	No	Yes	Yes	132	167	Single center
[5]	No	Yes	Yes	223	194	Single center
[94]	Yes	Yes	No			All
[85]	No	Yes	Yes	5190	647	Pretransplant
[86]	No	Yes	Yes			Pretransplant
[88]	No	Yes	Yes	39	21	Failed transplant
[68]	No	Yes	Yes			Coronary heart disease
[32]	No	Yes	Yes			Pretransplant
[37]	Yes	Yes	Yes	96	78	Elderly
[45]	No	Yes	Yes	1271	598	All
[2]	No	Yes	Yes	18	20	Prospective, randomized trial
[54]	No	Yes	Yes	2772	1292	All
[95]	No	Yes	Yes	411	411	All
[96]	No	Yes	Yes	742	480	All
[27]	No	Yes	Yes			All
[79]	No	Yes	Yes			Elderly
[78]	Yes	Yes	Yes			Elderly

RRT on, even if they transferred to another modality. Large differences in outcome and interpretation might also arise with the choice to select prevalent (patients already on RRT) or incident (only patients starting newly on RRT) patients, or a mixture [27]. All these studies are confounded by differences in patient mix, differences in experience with one of the two modalities, and differences in technique survival of the two modalities. The difference in technique survival is especially important, as most patients on PD will be transferred to HD during the course of their treatment, or they will be transplanted. Therefore, the question should not be which single RRT modality should be used but which flow chart or succession of RRT modalities will result in the most optimal patient survival: the integrated care approach [5].

There are several theoretical arguments why PD should be a good modality to start RRT: preservation of residual renal function [28,29], avoidance of blood-borne infections [30], better outcome after transplantation [31–35], lower cost [22], and better QoL [2,36,37]. However, with time there might be deterioration of the peritoneal membrane [38] and of residual renal function [39], making adequate PD more difficult and leading to technique failure. In the landmark paper on integrated care, it had already been reported that patients who were maintained on PD too long had a worse survival than those transferred in a timely manner onto HD. Other studies have found an increased mortality in the year after transfer from PD to HD [40,41], a sign that these patients have probably been maintained too long on PD. A timely transfer should be encouraged in such circumstances. In contrast, other patients can be maintained on PD for years, without any change in peritoneal membrane function [42,43]. Differences in genetic makeup [44] and comorbidities probably play an important role in the rate of decline of the peritoneal membrane.

There is also compelling clinical and epidemiological evidence that PD has advantages as the first RRT modality [45–47]. The single randomized trial of PD and HD suggested that PD may have improved survival compared with HD [2]. Evidence coming from large registries and other observational studies also supports the idea that survival is optimized by starting patients on PD and transferring them to HD (Table 43.1).

Quality of life and socio-economical considerations

QoL is an important, but sometimes neglected, issue in RRT. Depression, detected by a simple question on the mood of the patient, was the single best predictor of outcome on RRT [48]. Comparison of QoL with different treatments is difficult, especially in a heterogeneous population like the ESRD population, where different comorbid conditions might have a larger impact on the QoL than the RRT modality per se. Generally, most studies show that QoL is better in PD than in HD patients, certainly in the first year of treatment [49]. Some authors found no difference in QoL between the modalities after 1 year, but that may have occurred if lower QoL domains were falsely attributed to comorbid conditions such as anemia when they should have been more properly considered an effect of the modality itself [50]. Several studies have pointed to a higher employment rate in PD patients [51,52], but this might be

attributable to the differences in case mix. There appears to be a beneficial effect of patient education programs [49] on QoL and patient satisfaction, and some advocate that the higher QoL and satisfaction in PD patients is attributable to this better education rather than the modality. It is conceivable, but data are lacking, that the sense of self-determinism felt by PD patients and having their treatment under their control invokes positive feelings early, but that the constant strain that this responsibility brings, and the increasing complexity of the exchange schedule with declining residual renal function, ultimately leads to burnout.

PD in special patient groups

Diabetics

The outcome for diabetic patients with ESRD is severely compromised by the presence of multiple comorbidities leading to increased cardiovascular risk. Diabetic ESRD patients have mortality rates twice that of nondiabetic patients. Comparisons of outcomes of diabetic patients on HD versus PD are conflicting. In the USA, the PD/HD death rate varies with age and gender [53]. For male patients, there is no difference in outcome between PD and HD. For patients younger than 50 years, there is a definite survival advantage with PD. For female patients older than 50 years, there is an increased mortality risk on PD. In Europe and Canada, in contrast, outcomes of PD and HD patients with diabetes appear to be comparable [47,54]. There is thus no clear reason to withhold PD from diabetic patients, with the exception of older, female diabetic patients.

Anuric patients

Because of the importance of residual renal function (RRF) on survival of PD patients, the use of PD in anuric patients has been discouraged [55]. However, RRF is also an important predictor of outcome in HD patients. Due to the intermittent character of HD treatment, the absence of RRF might be even more dangerous if dietary restrictions are discarded, as suggested by higher mortality in HD patients after a weekend [56,57]. Meanwhile, several large studies have demonstrated that PD in anuric patients is feasible [58,59] and leads to acceptable outcomes. However, to our knowledge, no comparative trials of PD versus HD for anuric patients are available.

It is uncertain whether adequacy standards are achievable in anuric patients, especially those with a higher body mass [58]. Ademex and EAPOS confirm that small-solute clearance is not an important predictor of outcome [58,60]. In EAPOS, ultrafiltration of more than 750 mL/day and nutritional status were related to survival [58]. Therefore, if patients do well clinically on PD and maintain a good nutritional and volume status, there should be no reason to transfer them to HD if they become anuric. Vigilance for overhydration, uremic symptoms, and deterioration of nutritional status should be high in these patients. Because of the importance of maintaining volume status and minimizing glucose load, icodextrin should be used in anuric patients [61,62].

Cardiac patients

Given that uremia is a risk factor for cardiovascular disease [63], there is no evidence that PD provokes more *de novo* heart disease than HD [54]. The emergence of hypertension and left ventricular hypertrophy in PD patients is related to their capacity to maintain an optimal fluid status, i.e. to their residual renal function [64] and their ultrafiltration capacity, although some recent studies have found that the prevalence of left ventricular hypertrophy in ESRD might be overestimated [65]. The use of icodextrin is a useful tool to help maintain adequate ultrafiltration, especially in patients with a more permeable membrane (fast transporters) [61,62], but dietary sodium restriction should also be emphasized, in view of its substantial impact on outcome [66,67].

In patients with preexisting coronary heart disease, it has been suggested that there is a higher mortality on PD than HD [68]. In patients with preexisting congestive heart failure, a poorer outcome was reported for PD than HD patients in one study [69], although another study on the same study population found a higher incidence of *de novo* heart failure in HD patients [70]. Both these studies were large but were retrospective and nonrandomized. As recently reviewed, these studies have some particular sources of bias which mean that the results cannot be generalized [71]. In short, there was a large difference in experience with HD and PD, with about 90% of patients being treated by HD. In addition, the exclusion of patients who died in the first 3 months of treatment biased in favor of HD. Also, both studies only evaluated US Renal Data System (USRDS) PD patients, who had no opportunity to be treated with icodextrin, which could have had an impact on mortality, especially in the patients with congestive heart failure.

In some single-center nonrandomized studies in patients with congestive heart failure, PD has been shown to have a beneficial effect on hospitalization, functional status, and QoL compared to medical treatment alone [72–76]. There is not a higher incidence of stroke between HD and PD patients when there is adjustment for cardiovascular risk factors and blood pressure control [77].

Elderly

Globally, the ESRD population is growing exponentially, and a majority of this increase is among elderly patients. PD has some advantages in these frail patients, such as the continuous, more stable nature of the treatment, in contrast with the fluctuating effects of HD, and home-based care. In addition, the metabolism and muscle mass of older patients is generally low, so that lower fill volumes and/or reduced numbers of exchanges are often sufficient to obtain efficient clearance. Outcome studies of PD in the elderly report acceptable results, comparable with those obtained with HD [17,78], although in the USA a higher mortality has been reported on PD [79].

Some elderly patients are not capable of self-treatment, and so PD may require intensive home-based nursing [80]. Others may prefer the social contact of the dialysis unit and its nursing staff and fellow patients and so opt for HD.

Large or heavy patients

Because of the caloric load inherent in glucose-based PD solutions and the difficulty of achieving standard adequacy measures of small-solute clearance in large or heavy patients, PD has been discouraged in overweight and obese patients. A large observational study [81] found that overweight patients were less likely to start on PD, but if they did, their survival was superior to their smaller counterparts. Abbott *et al.* [82] could not confirm a survival advantage for heavier patients in their analysis, although there probably was some overlap in the populations between the two studies. A large Australian observational study [83] found an increased mortality risk in overweight patients. All these studies are hampered by the lack of a reliable definition of "overweight," as body mass index (BMI) does not discriminate between fat and muscle mass, which have opposite effects on outcomes [84]. This is suggested because of the observation that BMI is positively related to outcome in African Americans (who had a higher muscle mass as the cause of their higher body mass) and negatively related to outcome in females (in whom body mass was mostly increased because of an increase in body fat content). As a general rule, in large, muscular patients where the BMI is mainly fat-free body mass, there is no contraindication for PD. In patients with a high BMI and a high fat mass, data are conflicting. In patients with a large abdominal girth, the abdominal fat mass precludes the use of large intraperitoneal volumes and the choice of PD should probably be discouraged [84].

PD before transplantation and in failed transplant patients

Failed kidney transplantation is one of the increasingly common reasons to start RRT. Assuming the integrated care concept, the impact of the pretransplant RRT modality on the longevity of transplant and patient survival should be considered, as well as whether PD is a suitable modality after transplantation. Here again, available data are from registries and single-center case series, as no RCTs are available.

It was previously thought that PD might have some detrimental impact on transplant survival, but it is now clear that transplant and patient survival after renal transplantation are at least equal to [85,86] or even better [31,32,34] in patients transferring from PD compared with HD. There is no reason why PD should not be started in patients on the waiting list for kidney transplantation.

For the question of whether PD is a suitable therapy after failed transplant, the evidence is even more scarce. From the Australian–New Zealand Registry [87], it is apparent that the survival in new patients starting on PD is comparable to those who start PD after a failed transplant. Some single-center studies [88,89] have shown that survival of patients with failed kidney transplant might be comparable on HD and PD. For the important question of whether it is better to maintain immunosuppression, to preserve RRF as long as possible, or to withdraw it, to avoid infections and other complications, there is no evidence and a randomized trial is warranted.

In conclusion, there is no evidence that PD cannot be advocated in specific patient groups, such as diabetic patients, anuric patients, cardiovascularly compromised patients, patients with failed transplants, or large patients. The evidence seems to indicate that the quality of care and the experience of the center are more important in the determination of outcome than the modality choice by itself.

References

1 Vale L, Cody J, Wallace S, Daly C, Campbell M, Grant A *et al.* Continuous ambulatory peritoneal dialysis (CAPD) versus hospital or home haemodialysis for end-stage renal disease in adults. *Cochrane Database Syst Rev* 2004; **4**: CD003963.

2 Korevaar JC, Feith GW, Dekker FW, van Manen JG, Boeschoten EW, Bossuyt PM *et al.* Effect of starting with hemodialysis compared with peritoneal dialysis in patients new on dialysis treatment: a randomized controlled trial. *Kidney Int* 2003; **64(6)**: 2222–2228.

3 Van Biesen W, Vanholder R, Lameire N. The role of peritoneal dialysis as the first-line renal replacement modality. *Perit Dial Int* 2000; **20(4)**: 375–383.

4 Van Biesen W, Dequidt C, Vijt D, Vanholder R, Lameire N. Analysis of the reasons for transfers between hemodialysis and peritoneal dialysis and their effect on survivals. *Adv Perit Dial* 1998; **14**: 90–94.

5 Van Biesen W, Vanholder RC, Veys N, Dhondt A, Lameire NH. An evaluation of an integrative care approach for end-stage renal disease patients. *J Am Soc Nephrol* 2000; **11(1)**: 116–125.

6 Nissenson AR, Prichard SS, Cheng IK, Gokal R, Kubota M, Maiorca R *et al.* Non-medical factors that impact on ESRD modality selection. *Kidney Int Suppl* 1993; **40**: S120–S127.

7 Blake PG. The complex economics of modality selection. *Perit Dial Int* 2004; **24(6)**: 509–511.

8 Venkataraman V, Nolph KD. Socioeconomic aspects of peritoneal dialysis in North America: role of non medical factors in the choice of dialysis.*Perit Dial Int* 1999; **19(Suppl 2)**: S419–S422.

9 Lameire N, Van Biesen W, Dombros N, Dratwa M, Faller B, Gahl GM *et al.* The referral pattern of patients with ESRD is a determinant in the choice of dialysis modality. *Perit Dial Int* 1997; **17(Suppl 2)**: S161–S166.

10 Diaz-Buxo JA. Early referral and selection of peritoneal dialysis as a treatment modality. *Nephrol Dial Transplant* 2000; **15(2)**: 147–149.

11 Mendelssohn DC. Empowerment of patient preference in dialysis modality selection. *Am J Kidney Dis* 2004; **43(5)**: 930–932.

12 Prichard SS. Treatment modality selection in 150 consecutive patients starting ESRD therapy.*Perit Dial Int* 1996; **16(1)**: 69–72.

13 Prichard SS. Socioeconomic and health-care policies and peritoneal dialysis. *Perit Dial Int* 1996; **16(Suppl 1)**: S378–S380.

14 De Vecchi AF, Dratwa M, Wiedemann ME. Healthcare systems and end-stage renal disease (ESRD) therapies: an international review: costs and reimbursement/funding of ESRD therapies. *Nephrol Dial Transplant* 1999; **14(Suppl 6)**: 31–41.

15 Kendix M. Dialysis modality selection among patients attending free-standing dialysis facilities. *Health Care Financ Rev* 1997; **18(4)**: 3–21.

16 Little J, Irwin A, Marshall T, Rayner H, Smith S. Predicting a patient's choice of dialysis modality: experience in a United Kingdom renal department. *Am J Kidney Dis* 2001; **37(5)**: 981–986.

17 Wuerth DB, Finkelstein SH, Schwetz O, Carey H, Kliger AS, Finkelstein FO. Patients' descriptions of specific factors leading to modality selection of chronic peritoneal dialysis or hemodialysis. *Perit Dial Int* 2002; **22(2)**: 184–190.

18 Ravani P, Marinangeli G, Stacchiotti L, Malberti F. Structured pre-dialysis programs: more than just timely referral? *J Nephrol* 2003; **16(6)**: 862–869.

19 Goovaerts T, Jadoul M, Goffin E. Influence of a pre-dialysis education programme (PDEP) on the mode of renal replacement therapy. *Nephrol Dial Transplant* 2005; **20(9)**: 1842–1847.

20 Curtis BM, Ravani P, Malberti F, Kennett F, Taylor PA, Djurdjev O *et al.* The short- and long-term impact of multi-disciplinary clinics in addition to standard nephrology care on patient outcomes. *Nephrol Dial Transplant* 2005; **20(1)**: 147–154.

21 Stack AG. Impact of timing of nephrology referral and pre-ESRD care on mortality risk among new ESRD patients in the United States. *Am J Kidney Dis* 2003; **41(2)**: 310–318.

22 Shih YC, Guo A, Just PM, Mujais S. Impact of initial dialysis modality and modality switches on Medicare expenditures of end-stage renal disease patients. *Kidney Int* 2005; **68(1)**: 319–329.

23 Coronel F, Herrero JA, Montenegro J, Fernandez C, Gandara A, Conesa J *et al.* Erythropoietin requirements: a comparative multicenter study between peritoneal dialysis and hemodialysis. *J Nephrol* 2003; **16(5)**: 697–702.

24 Van Biesen W, Wiedemann M, Lameire N. End-stage renal disease treatment: a European perspective. *J Am Soc Nephrol* 1998; **9(12 Suppl)**: S55–S62.

25 Van Biesen W, Vanholder R, Debacquer D, De Backer G, Lameire N. Comparison of survival on CAPD and haemodialysis: statistical pitfalls. *Nephrol Dial Transplant* 2000; **15(3)**: 307–311.

26 Vonesh EF. Relative risks can be risky. *Perit Dial Int* 1993; **13(1)**: 5–9.

27 Vonesh EF, Moran J. Mortality in end-stage renal disease: a reassessment of differences between patients treated with hemodialysis and peritoneal dialysis. *J Am Soc Nephrol* 1999; **10(2)**: 354–365.

28 Moist LM, Port FK, Orzol SM, Young EW, Ostbye T, Wolfe RA *et al.* Predictors of loss of residual renal function among new dialysis patients. *J Am Soc Nephrol* 2000; **11(3)**: 556–564.

29 Misra M, Vonesh E, Van Stone JC, Moore HL, Prowant B, Nolph KD. Effect of cause and time of dropout on the residual GFR: a comparative analysis of the decline of GFR on dialysis. *Kidney Int* 2001; **59(2)**: 754–763.

30 Pereira BJ, Levey AS. Hepatitis C virus infection in dialysis and renal transplantation. *Kidney Int* 1997; **51(4)**: 981–999.

31 Van Biesen W, Vanholder R, Van Loo A, Van Der Vennet M, Lameire N. Peritoneal dialysis favorably influences early graft function after renal transplantation compared to hemodialysis. *Transplantation* 2000; **69(4)**: 508–514.

32 Goldfarb-Rumyantzev AS, Hurdle JF, Scandling JD, Baird BC, Cheung AK. The role of pretransplantation renal replacement therapy modality in kidney allograft and recipient survival. *Am J Kidney Dis* 2005; **46(3)**: 537–549.

33 Kim RD, Oreopoulos DG, Qiu K, McGilvray ID, Greig PD, Wright E *et al.* Impact of mode of dialysis on intra-abdominal infection after simultaneous pancreas-kidney transplantation. *Transplantation* 2005; **80(3)**: 339–343.

34 Perez FM, Rodriguez-Carmona A. A comparison of transplant outcomes in peritoneal and hemodialysis patients. *Kidney Int* 2003; **63(5)**: 1956–1957.

35 Snyder JJ, Kasiske BL, Gilbertson DT, Collins AJ. A comparison of transplant outcomes in peritoneal and hemodialysis patients. *Kidney Int* 2002; **62(4)**: 1423–1430.

36 Wu AW, Fink NE, Marsh-Manzi JV, Meyer KB, Finkelstein FO, Chapman MM et al. Changes in quality of life during hemodialysis and peritoneal dialysis treatment: generic and disease specific measures. *J Am Soc Nephrol* 2004; **15**(3): 743–753.

37 Harris SA, Lamping DL, Brown EA, Constantinovici N. Clinical outcomes and quality of life in elderly patients on peritoneal dialysis versus hemodialysis. *Perit Dial Int* 2002; **22**(4): 463–470.

38 Williams JD, Craig KJ, Von Ruhland C, Topley N, Williams GT. The natural course of peritoneal membrane biology during peritoneal dialysis. *Kidney Int Suppl* 2003; **88**: S43–S49.

39 Van Biesen W, Lameire NH. Residual renal function in automated peritoneal dialysis. *Contrib Nephrol* 1999; **129**: 229–246.

40 Fried LF, Bernardini J, Johnston JR, Piraino B. Peritonitis influences mortality in peritoneal dialysis patients. *J Am Soc Nephrol* 1996; **7**(10): 2176–2182.

41 Panagoutsos S, Kantartzi K, Passadakis P, Yannatos E, Mourvati E, Theodoridis M et al. Timely transfer of peritoneal dialysis patients to hemodialysis improves survival rates. *Clin Nephrol* 2006; **65**(1): 43–47.

42 Davies SJ, Phillips L, Naish PF, Russell GI. Peritoneal glucose exposure and changes in membrane solute transport with time on peritoneal dialysis. *J Am Soc Nephrol* 2001; **12**(5): 1046–1051.

43 Sherif A, Nakayama M, Maruyama Y, Yoshida H, Yamamoto H, Yokoyama K et al. Quantitative assessment of the peritoneal vessel density and vasculopathy in CAPD patients. *Nephrol Dial Transplant* 2006; **21**: 1675–1681.

44 Gillerot G, Goffin E, Michel C, Evenepoel P, Biesen WV, Tintillier M et al. Genetic and clinical factors influence the baseline permeability of the peritoneal membrane. *Kidney Int* 2005; **67**(6): 2477–2487.

45 Heaf JG, Lokkegaard H, Madsen M. Initial survival advantage of peritoneal dialysis relative to haemodialysis. *Nephrol Dial Transplant* 2002; **17**(1): 112–117.

46 Foley RN, Parfrey PS, Harnett JD, Kent GM, O'Dea R, Murray DC et al. Mode of dialysis therapy and mortality in end-stage renal disease. *J Am Soc Nephrol* 1998; **9**(2): 267–276.

47 Fenton SS, Schaubel DE, Desmeules M, Morrison HI, Mao Y, Copleston P et al. Hemodialysis versus peritoneal dialysis: a comparison of adjusted mortality rates. *Am J Kidney Dis* 1997; **30**(3): 334–342.

48 Lopes AA, Bragg J, Young E, Goodkin D, Mapes D, Combe C et al. Depression as a predictor of mortality and hospitalization among hemodialysis patients in the United States and Europe. *Kidney Int* 2002; **62**(1): 199–207.

49 Rubin HR, Fink NE, Plantinga LC, Sadler JH, Kliger AS, Powe NR. Patient ratings of dialysis care with peritoneal dialysis vs hemodialysis. *JAMA* 2004; **291**(6): 697–703.

50 Merkus MP, Jager KJ, Dekker FW, De Haan RJ, Boeschoten EW, Krediet RT. Quality of life over time in dialysis: the Netherlands Cooperative Study on the Adequacy of Dialysis. NECOSAD Study Group. *Kidney Int* 1999; **56**(2): 720–728.

51 Merkus MP, Jager KJ, Dekker FW, Boeschoten EW, Stevens P, Krediet RT. Quality of life in patients on chronic dialysis: self-assessment 3 months after the start of treatment. The Necosad Study Group. *Am J Kidney Dis* 1997; **29**(4): 584–592.

52 Julius M, Kneisley JD, Carpentier-Alting P, Hawthorne VM, Wolfe RA, Port FK. A comparison of employment rates of patients treated with continuous ambulatory peritoneal dialysis vs in-center hemodialysis (Michigan End-Stage Renal Disease Study). *Arch Intern Med* 1989; **149**(4): 839–842.

53 Vonesh EF, Snyder JJ, Foley RN, Collins AJ. The differential impact of risk factors on mortality in hemodialysis and peritoneal dialysis. *Kidney Int* 2004; **66**(6): 2389–2401.

54 Locatelli F, Marcelli D, Conte F, D'Amico M, Del Vecchio L, Limido A et al. Survival and development of cardiovascular disease by modality of treatment in patients with end-stage renal disease. *J Am Soc Nephrol* 2001; **12**(11): 2411–2417.

55 Van Biesen W, Vanholder R, Veys N, Lameire N. Peritoneal dialysis in anuric patients: concerns and cautions. *Semin Dial* 2002; **15**(5): 305–310.

56 Bleyer AJ, Russell GB, Satko SG. Sudden and cardiac death rates in hemodialysis patients. *Kidney Int* 1999; **55**(4): 1553–1559.

57 Bleyer AJ, Hartman J, Brannon PC, Reeves-Daniel A, Satko SG, Russell G. Characteristics of sudden death in hemodialysis patients. *Kidney Int* 2006; **69**(12): 2268–2273.

58 Brown EA, Davies SJ, Rutherford P, Meeus F, Borras M, Riegel W et al. Survival of functionally anuric patients on automated peritoneal dialysis: the European APD Outcome Study. *J Am Soc Nephrol* 2003; **14**(11): 2948–2957.

59 Szeto CC, Wong TY, Chow KM, Leung CB, Law MC, Wang AY et al. Impact of dialysis adequacy on the mortality and morbidity of anuric Chinese patients receiving continuous ambulatory peritoneal dialysis. *J Am Soc Nephrol* 2001; **12**(2): 355–360.

60 Paniagua R, Amato D, Vonesh E, Correa-Rotter R, Ramos A, Moran J et al. Effects of increased peritoneal clearances on mortality rates in peritoneal dialysis: ADEMEX, a prospective, randomized, controlled trial. *J Am Soc Nephrol* 2002; **13**(5): 1307–1320.

61 Konings CJ, Kooman JP, Schonck M, Gladziwa U, Wirtz J, van den Wall Bake AW et al. Effect of icodextrin on volume status, blood pressure and echocardiographic parameters: a randomized study. *Kidney Int* 2003; **63**(4): 1556–1563.

62 Davies SJ, Woodrow G, Donovan K, Plum J, Williams P, Johansson AC et al. Icodextrin improves the fluid status of peritoneal dialysis patients: results of a double-blind randomized controlled trial. *J Am Soc Nephrol* 2003; **14**(9): 2338–2344.

63 Vanholder R, Massy Z, Argiles A, Spasovski G, Verbeke F, Lameire N. Chronic kidney disease as cause of cardiovascular morbidity and mortality. *Nephrol Dial Transplant* 2005; **20**: 1048–1056.

64 Lameire N, Bernaert P, Lambert MC, Vijt D. Cardiovascular risk factors and their management in patients on continuous ambulatory peritoneal dialysis. *Kidney Int Suppl* 1994; **48**: S31–S38.

65 Stewart GA, Foster J, Cowan M, Rooney E, McDonagh T, Dargie HJ et al. Echocardiography overestimates left ventricular mass in hemodialysis patients relative to magnetic resonance imaging. *Kidney Int* 1999; **56**(6): 2248–2253.

66 Ates K, Nergizoglu G, Keven K, Sen A, Kutlay S, Erturk S et al. Effect of fluid and sodium removal on mortality in peritoneal dialysis patients. *Kidney Int* 2001; **60**(2): 767–776.

67 Gunal AI, Karaca I, Aygen B, Yavuzkir M, Dogukan A, Celiker H. Strict fluid volume control and left ventricular hypertrophy in hypertensive patients on chronic haemodialysis: a cross-sectional study. *J Int Med Res* 2004; **32**(1): 70–77.

68 Ganesh SK, Hulbert-Shearon T, Port FK, Eagle K, Stack AG. Mortality differences by dialysis modality among incident ESRD patients with and without coronary artery disease. *J Am Soc Nephrol* 2003; **14**(2): 415–424.

69 Stack AG, Molony DA, Rahman NS, Dosekun A, Murthy B. Impact of dialysis modality on survival of new ESRD patients with congestive heart failure in the United States. *Kidney Int* 2003; **64**(3): 1071–1079.

70 Trespalacios FC, Taylor AJ, Agodoa LY, Bakris GL, Abbott KC. Heart failure as a cause for hospitalization in chronic dialysis patients. *Am J Kidney Dis* 2003; **41**(6): 1267–1277.

71 Van Biesen W, Vanholder R, Verbeke F, Lameire N. Is peritoneal dialysis associated with increased cardiovascular morbidity and mortality? *Perit Dial Int* 2006; **26(4)**: 429–434.

72 Gotloib L, Fudin R. The impact of peritoneal dialysis upon quality of life and mortality of patients with end-stage congestive heart failure. *Contrib Nephrol* 2006; **150**: 247–253.

73 Stegmayr BG, Banga R, Lundberg L, Wikdahl AM, Plum-Wirell M. PD treatment for severe congestive heart failure. *Perit Dial Int* 1996; **16(Suppl 1)**: S231–S235.

74 Hebert MJ, Falardeau M, Pichette V, Houde M, Nolin L, Cardinal J *et al.* Continuous ambulatory peritoneal dialysis for patients with severe left ventricular systolic dysfunction and end-stage renal disease. *Am J Kidney Dis* 1995; **25(5)**: 761–768.

75 DiLeo M, Pacitti A, Bergerone S, Pozzi R, Tognarelli G, Segoloni G *et al.* Ultrafiltration in the treatment of refractory congestive heart failure. *Clin Cardiol* 1988; **11(7)**: 449–452.

76 Rubin J, Ball R. Continuous ambulatory peritoneal dialysis as treatment of severe congestive heart failure in the face of chronic renal failure. Report of eight cases. *Arch Intern Med* 1986; **146(8)**: 1533–1535.

77 Seliger SL, Gillen DL, Tirschwell D, Wasse H, Kestenbaum BR, Stehman-Breen CO. Risk factors for incident stroke among patients with end-stage renal disease. *J Am Soc Nephrol* 2003; **14(10)**: 2623–2631.

78 Lamping DL, Constantinovici N, Roderick P, Normand C, Henderson L, Harris S *et al.* Clinical outcomes, quality of life, and costs in the North Thames Dialysis Study of elderly people on dialysis: a prospective cohort study. *Lancet* 2000; **356(9241)**: 1543–1550.

79 Winkelmayer WC, Glynn RJ, Mittleman MA, Levin R, Pliskin JS, Avorn J. Comparing mortality of elderly patients on hemodialysis versus peritoneal dialysis: a propensity score approach. *J Am Soc Nephrol* 2002; **13(9)**: 2353–2362.

80 Baek MY, Kwon TH, Kim YL, Cho DK. CAPD, an acceptable form of therapy in elderly ESRD patients: a comparative study. *Adv Perit Dial* 1997; **13**: 158–161.

81 Snyder JJ, Foley RN, Gilbertson DT, Vonesh EF, Collins AJ. Body size and outcomes on peritoneal dialysis in the United States. *Kidney Int* 2003; **64(5)**: 1838–1844.

82 Abbott KC, Glanton CW, Trespalacios FC, Oliver DK, Ortiz MI, Agodoa LY *et al.* Body mass index, dialysis modality, and survival: analysis of the United States Renal Data System Dialysis Morbidity and Mortality Wave II Study. *Kidney Int* 2004; **65(2)**: 597–605.

83 McDonald SP, Collins JF, Johnson DW. Obesity is associated with worse peritoneal dialysis outcomes in the Australia and New Zealand patient populations. *J Am Soc Nephrol* 2003; **14(11)**: 2894–2901.

84 Ramkumar N, Pappas LM, Beddhu S. Effect of body size and body composition on survival in peritoneal dialysis patients. *Perit Dial Int* 2005; **25(5)**: 461–469.

85 Chalem Y, Ryckelynck JP, Tuppin P, Verger C, Chauve S, Glotz D. Access to, and outcome of, renal transplantation according to treatment modality of end-stage renal disease in France. *Kidney Int* 2005; **67(6)**: 2448–2453.

86 Cosio FG, Alamir A, Yim S, Pesavento TE, Falkenhain ME, Henry ML *et al.* Patient survival after renal transplantation. I. The impact of dialysis pre-transplant. *Kidney Int* 1998; **53(3)**: 767–772.

87 Badve SV, Hawley CM, McDonald SP, Mudge DW, Rosman JB, Brown FG *et al.* Effect of previously failed kidney transplantation on peritoneal dialysis outcomes in the Australian and New Zealand patient populations. *Nephrol Dial Transplant* 2006; **21(3)**: 776–783.

88 de Jonge H, Bammens B, Lemahieu W, Maes BD, Vanrenterghem Y. Comparison of peritoneal dialysis and haemodialysis after renal transplant failure. *Nephrol Dial Transplant* 2006; **21(6)**: 1669–1674.

89 Davies SJ. Peritoneal dialysis in the patient with a failing renal allograft. *Perit Dial Int* 2001; **21(Suppl 3)**: S280–S284.

90 Jaar BG, Coresh J, Plantinga LC, Fink NE, Klag MJ, Levey AS *et al.* Comparing the risk for death with peritoneal dialysis and hemodialysis in a national cohort of patients with chronic kidney disease. *Ann Intern Med* 2005; **143(3)**: 174–183.

91 Maiorca R, Cancarini GC, Zubani R, Camerini C, Manili L, Brunori G *et al.* CAPD viability: a long-term comparison with hemodialysis. *Perit Dial Int* 1996; **16(3)**: 276–287.

92 Mallick NP, Jones E, Selwood N. The European (European Dialysis and Transplantation Association-European Renal Association) Registry. *Am J Kidney Dis* 1995; **25(1)**: 176–187.

93 Stack AG, Murthy BV, Molony DA. Survival differences between peritoneal dialysis and hemodialysis among "large" ESRD patients in the United States. *Kidney Int* 2004; **65(6)**: 2398–2408.

94 Bloembergen WE, Port FK, Mauger EA, Wolfe RA. A comparison of mortality between patients treated with hemodialysis and peritoneal dialysis. *J Am Soc Nephrol* 1995; **6(2)**: 177–183.

95 Murphy SW, Foley RN, Barrett BJ, Kent GM, Morgan J, Barre P *et al.* Comparative mortality of hemodialysis and peritoneal dialysis in Canada. *Kidney Int* 2000; **57(4)**: 1720–1726.

96 Termorshuizen F, Korevaar JC, Dekker FW, van Manen JG, Boeschoten EW, Krediet RT. Hemodialysis and peritoneal dialysis: comparison of adjusted mortality rates according to the duration of dialysis: analysis of The Netherlands Cooperative Study on the Adequacy of Dialysis 2. *J Am Soc Nephrol* 2003; **14(11)**: 2851–2860.

Small Solute Clearance in Peritoneal Dialysis

Sharon J. Nessim & Joanne M. Bargman
Department of Medicine, Division of Nephrology, University of Toronto, Toronto, Canada

Introduction

The ideal method for assessing the adequacy of peritoneal dialysis (PD) has yet to be determined. Early studies attempting to quantify dialysis dose in hemodialysis patients used urea as a putative low-molecular-weight uremic toxin, eventually leading to the establishment of Kt/V_{urea} as a useful proxy for small solute clearance [1,2]. This term, Kt/V_{urea}, factored in several important parameters, including clearance of urea (K), time on dialysis (t), and the urea distribution volume, or total body water (V). At approximately the same time as the studies on Kt/V_{urea} were emerging in the hemodialysis literature, there was a relative paucity of data on quantification of dose of PD, with only one group addressing kinetic modeling of peritoneal transport [3,4]. The data on Kt/V_{urea} in hemodialysis were therefore extrapolated to PD, with the addition of creatinine clearance (CrCl) as an additional proxy. While the current approach to PD adequacy hinges on these measures of small solute clearance, little attention has been paid to clearance of higher-molecular-weight uremic toxins, the so-called middle molecules.

Investigations of the impact of PD dose have largely focused on patient survival, but they have also looked at several other outcomes, including technique survival, hospitalization, nutritional status, and quality of life. In this chapter, we will focus on the existing evidence with respect to the impact of peritoneal solute clearance and residual renal function (RRF) on patient survival, as well as evidence for the targets that are currently in use. We will also discuss strategies to optimize peritoneal solute clearance and preserve RRF, providing evidence when available.

Assessment of small solute clearance

Our understanding of the impact of small solute clearance on patient survival in PD has evolved over time. Early studies suggested

Evidence-based Nephrology. Edited by Donald Molony and Jonathan Craig
© 2009 Blackwell Publishing, ISBN: 978-1-4051-3975-5.

a beneficial effect of small solute clearance as assessed by Kt/V_{urea} and CrCl on survival. The largest of these early studies was the CANUSA study, which evaluated the association between adequacy of PD and patient survival among 680 incident continuous ambulatory peritoneal dialysis (CAPD) patients over 2 years [5]. In this study, total (renal and peritoneal) small solute clearance was found to be an independent predictor of patient survival. Based on a fitted model, there was a 5% decrement in expected patient survival for every 0.1 decrease in total weekly Kt/V_{urea} for values between 1.5 and 2.3 and a 7% decrement in expected survival for every 5 L/week/1.73 m^2 decrease in CrCl. The assumption was that peritoneal and renal contributions to small solute clearance were equal and therefore additive. Improved patient survival with higher clearance was also noted in a 3-year prospective study of 68 CAPD patients reported by Maiorca *et al.* [6]. In that study, a weekly total Kt/V_{urea} of >1.96 was an independent predictor of better patient survival. In a retrospective study by Genestier *et al.*, 201 incident CAPD patients were divided into three groups according to achieved Kt/V_{urea}, either <1.7, 1.7–2.2, or >2.2 [7]. After a mean of 2 years, a Kt/V_{urea} of <1.7 was independently predictive of a higher mortality, with a relative risk (RR) of 1.69. Four additional studies, using univariate models, reported improved survival with weekly Kt/V_{urea} values of at least 1.5, 1.89, 2.0, and 2.0 [8–11].

Based on these data, in 1997, the Kidney Disease Outcomes Quality Initiative (K/DOQI) of the National Kidney Foundation in the USA published guidelines for clearance targets [12]. The guidelines suggested that for CAPD patients, the delivered PD dose should be a total Kt/V_{urea} of at least 2.0 per week and a total CrCl of at least 60 L/week/1.73 m^2. Recognizing that this CrCl target was difficult to achieve in patients with slow peritoneal transport status in the absence of RRF, in 1999 the Canadian Society of Nephrology suggested that two CrCl targets be provided, depending on the patient's peritoneal membrane characteristics [13]. Specifically, the CrCl target remained 60 L/week/1.73 m^2 in high and high-average transporters but was lowered to 50 L/wk/1.73 m^2 in low and low-average transporters. This recommendation was later adopted in the 2000 iteration of the K/DOQI guidelines [14]. In patients on automated PD (APD), although no data were available relating delivered dose of dialysis to patient outcomes, the guidelines recommended slightly higher targets based on the more intermittent nature of APD. For continuous cycling peritoneal dialysis (CCPD), the predominant form of APD, the suggested delivered dose was a total Kt/V_{urea} of at least 2.1 and a total CrCl of at least 63 L/week/1.73 m^2. For nocturnal intermittent peritoneal dialysis (NIPD), the suggested delivered PD dose was a total Kt/V_{urea} of at least 2.2 and a total CrCl of at least 66 L/week/1.73 m^2.

Since the initial studies on which the 1997 and 2000 K/DOQI guidelines were based, several new and important studies have led to the reevaluation of the impact of small solute clearance on outcomes. In 2002, the ADEMEX trial was published [15], representing the largest randomized controlled study published in the PD literature. Its purpose was to assess the effect of small solute clearance on survival. In this study, 965 incident and prevalent PD patients were randomized to a standard CAPD regimen of 2-L exchanges four times daily or a modified dialysis prescription to achieve a peritoneal CrCl of >60 L/week/1.73 m^2. In order to achieve this, individual dwell volumes were increased, followed by the addition of a fifth dwell if the target was not reached by 2 months. Patients were followed for a minimum of 2 years, with a primary end point of death. The mean age of patients enrolled was approximately 47 years, with an incidence of preexisting ischemic heart disease that was low in both groups (<5%) and not different between the two. Whereas the intervention group had significantly higher peritoneal Kt/V_{urea} (2.13 vs. 1.62) and peritoneal CrCl (57 vs. 46 L/week/1.73 m^2) than the control group, there was no difference in patient survival (69.3% vs. 68.3% at 2 years). The major cause of death in both groups was ischemic heart disease. In the control group, a higher death rate due to congestive heart failure and a combination of uremia, hyperkalemia, and acidosis was reported. It should be noted that hyperkalemia and acidosis are complications that rarely occur in PD patients, and it is especially rare to be severe enough to cause death. Because a composite end point of death due to uremia/hyperkalemia/acidosis was used, it is possible that uremia accounted for the majority of the difference between the groups. It is also reported that more patients in the control group withdrew from the study because of uremia. Unfortunately, uremia was not specifically defined, and because the study was not blinded, this may have introduced a significant bias. Knowing which patients were receiving a lower dialysis dose may have led physicians to attribute nonspecific symptoms or death in the control group to uremia. With regard to the higher mortality related to congestive heart failure in the control group, this is not necessarily attributable to underdialysis. Rather, it can be explained by a difference in ultrafiltration attributable to the use of an additional exchange in 22% of patients in the intervention group. In fact, the intervention group had approximately 100 mL/day more ultrafiltration on average than the control group. In contrast to peritoneal clearance in this study, renal Kt/V_{urea} and renal CrCl did emerge as predictors of improved outcome, with an RR of 0.89 per 10-L/week/1.73 m^2 increase in CrCl and 0.94 per 0.1 increase in Kt/V_{urea}.

A second randomized, controlled trial by Lo *et al.* confirmed the lack of survival benefit with increased peritoneal clearance [16]. In this study, 320 incident CAPD patients were randomly assigned to one of three groups: Kt/V_{urea} of 1.5–1.7, 1.7–2.0, or >2.0, and followed over 2 years. Patients with an initial renal Kt/V_{urea} of >1.0 were excluded. Renal Kt/V_{urea} in the study patients was not significantly different between the groups, so that the difference in Kt/V_{urea} was accounted for by differences in peritoneal clearance. Overall 2-year patient survival was 84.9%. After adjustment for age and diabetes, total Kt/V_{urea} did not affect survival in patients with Kt/V_{urea} of >2.0 versus 1.7–2.0, although there was a trend toward better survival in patients with Kt/V_{urea} of 1.7–2.0 versus 1.5–1.7 ($P = 0.054$).

Several observational studies have supported the findings from these randomized trials. The largest study was by Diaz-Buxo *et al.*, who retrospectively analyzed a cohort of 1603 prevalent PD patients for factors associated with a higher mortality over 1 year [17]. Although RRF was strongly correlated with patient survival, peritoneal clearance was not. Rocco *et al.* performed a prospective study in which a cohort of 873 prevalent PD patients followed for 7 months [18]. Again, while the peritoneal clearance achieved was not predictive of outcome, residual renal CrCl and renal Kt/V_{urea} were associated with improved patient survival. A subsequent reanalysis of the CANUSA data, focusing on the relative contributions of renal and peritoneal clearances, provided further supportive data for the impact of RRF on survival [19]. For each 5-L/week/1.73 m^2 increase in renal CrCl there was a 12% decrease in the RR of death. Furthermore, each 250-mL increment in urine volume was associated with a 36% decrease in the RR of death. Neither peritoneal CrCl nor peritoneal ultrafiltration was associated with patient survival. Several other prospective [20–22] and retrospective [23–25] studies have demonstrated a survival benefit with increased renal clearance, with two exceptions [26,27].

Other studies have also demonstrated a lack of survival benefit of increased peritoneal small solute clearance [26,28]. In a study by Jager *et al.*, peritoneal clearance was found to be an independent predictor of outcome, but this was only significant when solute removal was assessed by dialysate urea and creatinine appearance and not when measured by Kt/V_{urea} or CrCl [29]. Unfortunately, interpretation of dialysate urea and creatinine appearance can be problematic, because they are proportional to protein intake and muscle mass, respectively, and well-nourished patients would be expected to have a more favorable outcome. Only three prospective studies using Kt/V_{urea} and/or CrCl have shown a statistically significant beneficial effect of peritoneal clearance on survival, and these have all been in patients with little or no RRF [20,30,31]. The first study to show a positive effect of peritoneal clearance was reported by Szeto *et al.* and involved 140 anuric CAPD patients followed for 22 months [30]. In this group, there was a 6% decrease in the RR of death with an increase in Kt/V_{urea} of 0.1 U/week and a 12% decrease in the RR of death for each 5-L/week/1.73 m^2 increase in peritoneal CrCl. The same investigators subsequently evaluated 5-year follow-up of 270 incident and prevalent CAPD patients with a median residual glomerular filtration rate of

0.82 mL/min [20]. Whereas higher peritoneal Kt/V_{urea} was associated with improved survival generally, this was only the case for prevalent CAPD patients, a group with minimal RRF. A more recent study by Jansen *et al.* followed a cohort of 130 anuric CAPD patients over 2 years [31]. In these patients, peritoneal Kt/V_{urea} and CrCl were not associated with survival when analyzed as continuous variables, but when the results were analyzed dichotomously, a weekly Kt/V_{urea} of <1.5 and a weekly CrCl <40 L/1.73 m^2 were associated with an increased RR for death. Another study to address the issue of solute clearance and survival in anuric patients was published by Bhaskaran *et al.* [32]. In this retrospective cohort study of 122 CAPD and APD patients, after a median of 19.5 months of follow-up, there was a trend towards decreased mortality in those with a peritoneal Kt/V_{urea} of ≥1.85, although the results did not reach statistical significance (RR of death, 0.54; $P = 0.10$). Patients in these studies were mostly or entirely dependent on peritoneal clearance, suggesting that the beneficial effect of higher peritoneal clearance might be more apparent in those lacking RRF. Although the latter four studies suggest a possible benefit of greater peritoneal small solute clearance in anuric patients, there are some data to suggest that this may not be the case. In a prospective study involving a cohort of 177 anuric APD patients followed over 2 years, CrCl was not found to be a predictor of patient survival [33]. Furthermore, in a subgroup analysis of the ADEMEX trial, there was no difference in mortality when patients were stratified for anuria [15]. The studies assessing the effect of small solute clearance on patient survival are summarized in Table 44.1, while those studies specifically addressing clearance in anuric patients are summarized in Table 44.2.

Overall, there is now evidence from two randomized trials and several supporting observational studies that although total clearance is important, improved patient survival is related to renal clearance and not to peritoneal clearance. The basis for the survival advantage associated with RRF is unclear, with several possible contributors. First, the presence of residual urine output facilitates volume management, which may have a favorable effect on blood pressure control and subsequent left ventricular remodeling. Both hypertension and left ventricular hypertrophy are associated with loss of RRF [34,35] and are known to be independent predictors of mortality in PD patients [36]. Secondly, RRF allows for clearance not only of small solutes but also middle molecules [37–39]. The latter are not as easily removed across the peritoneal membrane due to the time dependence of their diffusion and the limited permeability of the peritoneal membrane. Finally, patients with preserved RRF may represent a population who are intrinsically healthier, and thus more likely to survive.

Recommended targets and monitoring of PD adequacy

Although increasing peritoneal clearance does not appear to provide benefit within the dose ranges studied, it is likely that there is a minimum total clearance below which outcomes are affected

[7,8,16,31]. We therefore recommend a *minimum* total Kt/V_{urea} of at least 1.7 per week in all PD patients. The most recent K/DOQI guidelines and International Society of Peritoneal Dialysis guidelines have not included a peritoneal CrCl target [40,41], but the European guidelines consider CrCl to provide added predictive value and continue to recommend a CrCl target of at least 50 L/week/1.73m^2 [42]. It is important to point out that although these minimum targets do not differentiate between renal and peritoneal contributions, it is clear that renal and peritoneal clearance are not simply additive, in that any small solute clearance provided by residual renal function is accompanied by improved clearance of middle molecules and better salt and water control.

Because of the limitations of our current techniques to assess clearance, a patient's clinical status must always be taken into account when trying to determine the adequacy of dialysis. The outcome of interest in the studies discussed has principally been survival. There are no rigorous studies prospectively examining dose of PD and health outcomes other than death. Therefore, the guidelines all suggest that the dose be increased as a trial in the patient not doing well for reasons not explained by comorbidity, regardless of their current prescription.

In order to ensure a minimum total delivered Kt/V_{urea} of at least 1.7, solute clearances can be followed with the use of 24-h collections of dialysate and urine. While data on frequency of measurements are sparse, we would recommend the following schedule. The first measurement of peritoneal and renal Kt/V_{urea} should be performed approximately 1 month after initiation of PD. Subsequent monitoring of peritoneal clearance is somewhat controversial. Although the K/DOQI guidelines recommend checking peritoneal clearance at least once every 4 months, the peritoneal Kt/V_{urea} is unlikely to change in patients with a stable PD prescription. Therefore, an alternative approach would be to remeasure peritoneal clearance only if changes are made to the PD prescription or if there is deterioration in the patient's clinical status. In the event of an episode of peritonitis, peritoneal clearance measurements should not be made until at least 1 month after resolution of the peritonitis. If a patient has >100 mL/day of residual urine output and achieving a total weekly Kt/V_{urea} of at least 1.7 is dependent on the renal contribution, a 24-h urine collection to assess renal Kt/V_{urea} and urine volume should be performed at least every 2 months in order to avoid missing a decline in RRF.

Strategies for optimizing peritoneal solute clearance

The routine measurement of small solute clearance serves to screen patients for evidence of underdialysis. If a patient is not meeting the minimum recommended PD dose, the reason for this should be determined. Before assuming that a given PD prescription is inadequate, patient-related causes of failure, such as noncompliance, lack of understanding, or sampling and collection errors, should be sought. If none of these potential causes is found, several

Table 44.1 Summary of studies assessing effects of small solute clearance on survival in PD patients.

Study	Study design	No. of patients	F/U (mos)	Predictor	Outcome (clearance) Renal	Peritoneal	Total
Paniagua 2002	RCT	965	22	Kt/V ↑ 0.1 U/wk	RR 0.94 ($P = 0.005$)	RR 1 ($P =$ NS)	
Lo 2003	RCT	320	24	Kt/V ↑ 0.1 U/wk			RR 0.94 ($P =$ NS)
Lo 2001	Prospective cohort	937	24	rGFR ↑ 1 ml/min/1.73 m^2 pCrCl ↑ 1 L/wk/1.73 m^2	RR 0.87 ($P =$ NS)	RR 0.99 ($P =$ NS)	
Rocco 2000	Prospective cohort	873	7	Kt/V ↑ 0.1 U/wk	OR 0.88 ($P = 0.003$)	OR 1.0 ($P =$ NS)	OR $= 0.6$ ($P = 0.08$)
Bargman 2001	Prospective cohort	601	24	rGFR ↑ 5 L/wk/1.73 m^2 pCrCl ↑ 5 L/wk/1.73 m^2	RR 0.88 ($P < 0.05$)	RR 1.0 ($P =$ NS)	
Termoshuizen 2003	Prospective cohort	413	36	rGFR ↑ 1 mL/min/1.73 m^2 pCrCl ↑ 1 mL/min/1.73 m^2	RR 0.88 ($P = 0.04$)	RR 0.91 ($P =$ NS)	
Szeto 2004	Prospective cohort	270	35	rGFR ↑ 1 mL/min/1.73 m^2 Kt/V ↑ 0.1 U/wk	RR 0.80 ($P = 0.0001$)	RR 0.94 ($P = 0.03$)	
Szeto 2000	Prospective cohort	270	22	rGFR ↑ 1 mL/min/1.73 m^2 Kt/V ↑ 0.1 U/wk	RR 0.48 ($P < 0.05$)		RR 0.96 ($P < 0.05$)
Wang 2004	Prospective cohort	231	30	RRF vs. no RRF	No RRF: ↑ mortality ($P < 0.005$)		
Davies 1998	Prospective cohort	210	6	Kt/V			RR 0.17 ($P = 0.004$)
Brown 2003	Prospective cohort	177	24	Time-averaged total CrCl		RR 1.01 ($P =$ NS)	
Szeto 2001	Prospective cohort	140	22	Kt/V ↑ 0.1 U/wk		RR 0.94 ($P < 0.05$)	
Jansen 2005	Prospective cohort	130	24	Kt/V/wk < 1.5 CrCl < 40 L/wk/1.73 m^2		RR 3.28 ($P = 0.02$) RR 3.26 ($P = 0.02$)	
Jager 1999	Prospective cohort	118	25	Kt/V ↑ 0.1 U/wk CrCl ↑ 5 L/wk/1.73 m^2 Creatinine appearance (↑ 1 mmol/wk/1.73 m^2)	RR 0.96 ($P =$ NS) RR 0.97 ($P =$ NS) RR 0.95 ($P < 0.01$)	RR 0.95 ($P =$ NS) RR 0.96 ($P =$ NS) RR 0.93 ($P < 0.01$)	RR 0.93 ($P =$ NS) RR 0.96 ($P =$ NS) RR 0.95 ($P < 0.01$)
Chung 2003	Prospective cohort	82	14	rGFR ↑ 1 mL/min/1.73 m^2 Kt/V ↑ 0.1 U/wk	RR 0.79 ($P =$ NS)		RR 1.09 ($P =$ NS)
Maiorca 1995	Prospective cohort	68	36	Kt/V/wk >1.96 vs. <1.96			$P < 0.001$
Perez 2000	Prospective cohort	44	13	Kt/V ↑ 0.1 U/wk			RR 1.02 ($P =$ NS)
Diaz-Buxo 1999	Retrospective	1603	12	CrCl ↑ 10 L/wk/1.73 m^2	OR 0.88 ($P < 0.001$)	OR=1.01 ($P =$ NS)	OR 0.89 ($P =$ NS)
Rocco 2002	Retrospective	1219	12	Kt/V/wk 0.00–0.14 Kt/V/wk 0.15–0.40 Kt/V/wk 0.41–0.77	HR 2.13 ($P < 0.01$) HR 1.67 ($P < 0.01$) HR 1.35 ($P =$ NS)		
Park 2001	Retrospective	212	36–84	Kt/V/wk >2.1 vs. <2.1			$P =$ NS
Genestier 1995	Retrospective	201	24	Kt/V/wk <1.7 vs. >1.7 CrCl <50 vs. >50L/wk			RR 1.69 ($P = 0.09$) RR 4.88 ($P = 0.0005$)
Ates 2001	Retrospective	125	31	rGFR ↑ 1 mL/min/1.73 m^2	RR 0.53 ($P < 0.05$)		
Bhaskaran 2000	Retrospective	122	27	pKt/V/wk >1.85 vs. <1.85		RR 0.54 ($P =$ NS)	
Chung 2003	Retrospective	117	20	RRF 1 mL/min	RR 0.79 ($P = 0.04$)		
Aslam 2000	Retrospective	90	12	Kt/V/wk >2 vs. <2			$P =$ NS

Abbreviations: F/U, follow-up; RCT, randomized controlled trial; GFR, glomerular filtration rate; OR, odds ratio; HR, hazard ratio.

strategies can be employed to optimize a patient's PD prescription in order to improve peritoneal solute clearance. Common interventions include increasing the individual dwell volumes, increasing the frequency of daily exchanges, or increasing peritoneal ultrafiltration [43,44]. Whereas the focus of these interventions is often to increase peritoneal small solute clearance, the importance of middle molecule clearance must also be considered, especially in patients with little or no RRF.

Table 44.2 Summary of studies assessing effects of small solute clearance on survival in anuric PD patients.

Study	Study design	No. of patients	F/U (mos)	Predictor	Outcome
Paniagua 2002	RCT (subgroup analysis)	527	22	Kt/V ↑ 0.1 U/wk	$P = $ NS
Szeto 2001	Prospective	140	22	Kt/V ↑ 0.1 U/wk	RR 0.94 ($P < 0.05$)
Jansen 2005	Prospective	130	24	Kt/V/wk < 1.5 CrCl < 40 L/wk/1.73m^2	RR 3.28 ($P = 0.02$) RR 3.26 ($P = 0.02$)
Brown 2003	Prospective	177	24	Time-averaged total CrCl	RR 1.01 ($P = $ NS)
Bhaskaran 2000	Retrospective	122	27	pKt/V/wk > 1.85 vs. < 1.85	RR 0.54 ($P = $ NS)

Abbreviations: F/U, follow-up; RCT, randomized controlled trial; NS, not significant.

Increasing dwell volumes is an effective means by which peritoneal small solute clearance can be increased in both CAPD and APD patients [45]. The increase in Kt/V$_{urea}$ and CrCl is due to both an increased plasma-to-dialysate concentration gradient [46] and an increased effective peritoneal surface area [47]. Whereas increasing dwell volumes is often effective, this strategy leads to increased intra-abdominal pressure, which may lead to back pain and a higher risk of abdominal wall leaks and hernias [48], although this has not been borne out in some studies [49,50]. The lower intra-abdominal pressure in the supine position [51] may make increasing dwell volumes easier during the overnight exchange in CAPD patients or during the night exchanges in APD patients. An additional concern is that increasing exchange volumes may limit peritoneal ultrafiltration by increasing intra-abdominal pressure [52], but the greater persistence of the osmotic gradient is likely to offset this.

Another commonly used strategy is to increase the frequency of exchanges. In patients on CAPD, this may require increasing from three to four or from four to five exchanges daily. Potential disadvantages include the burden an additional manual exchange places on the patient and a decrease in middle molecule clearance due to a greater proportion of time spent draining and filling with less time for dialysate to dwell in the peritoneal cavity. In patients on cycler-based therapy, we advise against the use of NIPD unless a large amount of RRF remains or other special mitigating circumstances exist. An excellent method of increasing clearance in patients on NIPD is to add a day dwell. Maximizing the time spent with dialysate in the peritoneal cavity, especially with the use of a long dwell, is an important strategy because this leads to improvement in clearance of both small and larger solutes. Although increasing the frequency of night-time cycles can also augment peritoneal small solute clearance by maximizing the concentration gradient between blood and dialysate [53], there are some concerns with this strategy. First, if the cycles become too short, especially with larger dwell volumes, solute clearance will diminish owing to the "lost time" during draining and filling [54]. In addition, rapid cycling can lead to reduced net sodium removal due to sodium sieving [55]. For these reasons, we do not recommend routinely increasing frequency of cycles on APD to optimize peritoneal clearance.

Increasing peritoneal ultrafiltration is another method of increasing peritoneal clearance. Raising the gradient for diffusion with the use of hypertonic glucose or icodextrin is the primary means by which ultrafiltration can be increased [56,57], with the additional fluid removal leading to increased clearance via convective transport. However, use of long-term hypertonic glucose as a method to optimize peritoneal clearance is not generally recommended given the potential deleterious effects on the peritoneal membrane [58]. Icodextrin is a viable option for the long dwell in patients in whom poor ultrafiltration is an issue [59], but it is not generally recommended for the sole purpose of increasing clearance.

Ultimately, the decision about which strategy should be used to optimize peritoneal solute clearance will depend on the individual patient. Factors to consider include peritoneal membrane characteristics, the potential impact of increasing intra-abdominal pressure, and the patient's abilities and preferences. In general, attention should be focused on maximizing the time with dialysate in the peritoneal cavity.

Strategies for preserving RRF

Because of the impact of RRF on the outcome of patients on PD, its preservation is of utmost importance. Strategies to preserve RRF include use of medications that might slow the decline in RRF and avoidance of agents known to have deleterious effects. Because of the paucity of data, many of our current practices are extrapolated from patients with chronic kidney disease.

The only renal protective strategy for which there is evidence in PD patients involves use of agents that block the renin–angiotensin system (Table 44.3). Although this strategy is known to be effective in both hypertensive and normotensive patients with many forms of chronic kidney disease, the data for patients on dialysis are not as robust. Two randomized controlled studies have assessed the effect of renin–angiotensin system blockade on RRF, one using an angiotensin converting enzyme inhibitor (ACEi) and the other using an angiotensin receptor blocker (ARB). Li *et al.* randomly assigned 60 hypertensive PD patients to receive either ramipril at

Table 44.3 Summary of studies assessing effects of ACEi and ARBs on RRF in PD patients.

Study	Study design	No. of patients	F/U (mos)	Intervention	Outcome	Results
Li 2003	RCT	60	12	Ramipril vs. other antihypertensive	GFR change (mL/min)	−2.07 vs. −3.00 ($P = 0.03$)
Suzuki 2004	RCT	34	24	Valsartan vs. other antihypertensive	RRF change (mL/min)	+1.1 vs. −3.1 ($P < 0.01$)
Singhal 2000	Prospective	242	27	ACEi vs. no ACEi	Slope of GFR change	−0.14 vs. −0.16 ($P = $ NS)
Johnson 2003	Prospective	146	21	ACEi vs. no ACEi	Slope of RRF decline	HR 0.81 ($P = $ NS)
Moist 2000	Retrospective	1032	18	ACEi vs. no ACEi	Urine volume >200 vs. <200 mL/day	OR 0.70 ($P = 0.02$)

Abbreviations: F/U, follow-up; RCT, randomized controlled trial; GFR, glomerular filtration rate; NS, not significant; HR, hazard ratio; OR, odds ratio.

5 mg daily or no treatment [60]. Over the 12 months of the study, the mean RRF decline was approximately 1 mL/min less in the patients treated with ramipril despite similar blood pressure control in both groups. Furthermore, at 12 months, fewer patients in the ramipril group were anuric. A smaller study by Suzuki *et al.* randomized 34 hypertensive CAPD patients to receive either valsartan or placebo and assessed the effect on RRF [61]. Similar to the Li study, use of valsartan was associated with a slower decline in RRF despite similar blood pressure control in the groups. A large retrospective analysis of 1032 PD patients also demonstrated favorable results, with use of an ACEi being associated with an adjusted odds ratio of RRF decline of 0.70 [62]. These results are in contrast to findings reported for two prospective cohort studies that assessed risk factors for decline in RRF [63,64]. Both studies found that the use of an ACEi was not an independent predictor of the rate of decline in RRF. Based on the above data, we would recommend the use of ACEis or ARBs in hypertensive patients and consider their use even in normotensive patients to preserve RRF.

Aminoglycosides are frequently used to treat peritonitis in PD patients because of their effectiveness as bactericidal agents and the ease of intraperitoneal administration. They are, however, also nephrotoxic. Several prospective cohort studies and one random-ized controlled trial have assessed the effect of aminoglycosides on RRF (Table 44.4). Shemin *et al.* assessed the rate of decline in RRF in 72 PD patients followed for 4 years [65]. Patients who had peritonitis episodes treated with intraperitoneal or intravenous aminoglycosides had more rapid decline in renal creatinine clear-ance and residual urine volume than either those who had never had a peritonitis episode or those who had peritonitis treated with other nonnephrotoxic antibiotics. In another study analyzing the risk factors associated with a faster rate of decline, use of amino-glycosides was found to be an independent predictor of a more rapid loss of RRF [64]. In contrast to the findings in the above studies, Baker *et al.*, using a prospective cohort design with a his-torical control, did not find an accelerated decline in RRF with the use of aminoglycosides to treat peritonitis [66]. Most recently, a prospective, randomized, controlled trial compared the use of cefazolin and ceftazidime with cefazolin and netilmicin for the em-piric treatment of peritonitis in 50 PD patients with RRF [67]. In both groups there was a significant decline in RRF at 2 weeks that returned to near baseline by 6 weeks, but there was no significant difference in RRF between the groups. Although this represents the only randomized study of aminoglycosides and RRF, the follow-up period was short and some of the patients in the aminoglycoside

Table 44.4 Summary of studies assessing effects of aminoglycosides on RRF in PD patients.

Study	Study design	No. of patients	F/U	Intervention	Outcome	Results
Lui, 2005	RCT	50	6 wks	Netilmicin vs. ceftazidime	GFR decline (mL/min) Urine output change (mL/day)	+0.09 vs. −0.10 ($P = $ NS) −96 vs. −96 ($P = $ NS)
Singhal, 2000	Prospective	242	27 mos	Aminoglycoside >5 days vs. none	Slope of GFR decline	$P = 0.0006$
Baker, 2003	Prospective	205	<6 mos	Gentamicin vs. none	GFR change (mL/min/mo) Urine output change (mL/day/mo)	−0.08 vs. −0.017 ($P = $ NS) −8.8 vs. −34.7 ($P = $ NS)
Shemin, 1999	Prospective	72	14 mos	Aminoglycoside >3 days vs. none	CrCl change (mL/min/mo) Urine output change (mL/day/mo)	−0.66 vs. −0.21 (p<0.01) −74 vs. −15 ($P < 0.01$)

Abbreviations: F/U, follow-up; RCT, randomized controlled trial; GFR, glomerular filtration rate; NS, not significant.

Table 44.5 Overall evidence ratings and recommendations for small solute clearance target and renoprotective strategies.

Intervention	Overall evidence rating			Comment	Recommendation[a]			Comment
	High	Moderate	Low		I	II	III	
Minimum total Kt/V > 1.7		X		2 RCTs and several corroborating prospective studies	X			Recommend minimum Kt/V > 1.7
RAS blockade to preserve RRF								Recommend ACEi or ARB in hypertensive patients, consider use in normotensive patients
Hypertensive patients		X		2 RCTs, but small number of patients	X			
Normotensive patients		X		No RCTs, extrapolated from CKD literature		X		
Avoidance of aminoglycosides to preserve RRF			X	Conflicting data		X		Suggest avoidance based on other effective alternatives

Abbreviations: RAS, renin–angiotensin system; RCT, randomized controlled trial.

[a] Recommendations based on quality of evidence. I, recommend; II, suggest; III, no recommendation possible.

group were exposed to only a few days of netilmicin. In summary, although the data are conflicting, we would suggest avoidance of aminoglycosides when possible in patients with RRF, given the availability of equally efficacious alternatives in the treatment of most cases of PD peritonitis.

Until recently, there were no data on the effect of radiocontrast media on RRF in dialysis patients. Within the past year, two small, prospective studies have addressed this issue [68,69]. Although one of the studies demonstrated a temporary decline in RRF 6 days after radiocontrast administration [68], neither study showed a lasting decline in renal clearance. Nevertheless, given the small numbers of patients in these dialysis studies and the clear data in patients with chronic kidney disease, it would be prudent to avoid using radiocontrast media if other acceptable alternatives exist. If use of radiocontrast dye is required, volume contraction should be avoided, and the smallest volume of the least toxic dye should be used. Where there are conflicting data on the use of N-acetylcysteine in chronic kidney disease [70] and there are no data for dialysis patients, its use could be considered based on the fact that it is relative safe and inexpensive. Despite the lack of evidence in dialysis patients, we would also recommend avoidance of nonsteroidal anti-inflammatory drugs or any other known nephrotoxins in patients with RRF.

If there is a significant decline in RRF that cannot be explained, consideration should always be given to the possibilities of volume depletion or obstruction, as these are easily correctable causes of loss of RRF.

Conclusions

Our understanding of the effect of PD adequacy on outcomes is subject to the limitations of the existing literature. In the absence of a gold standard for assessing adequacy, all studies to date have

focused on small solute clearance. This has led to a relative neglect of the impact of middle molecule clearance on outcome. The data presented in this chapter highlight the relative contributions of renal and peritoneal clearance to PD adequacy, demonstrating that maintenance of residual renal clearance is critically important to patient survival. It is not yet clear if RRF is causally related to the survival advantage as a result of improved volume management and middle molecule clearance, or if it is merely an association, with RRF serving a marker of a healthier population.

While the existing data suggest that peritoneal clearance does not significantly impact patient survival, we cannot exclude the possibility that the dose ranges used in the studies assessing the effect of peritoneal clearance are too narrow to detect a difference. Further exploration of this possibility depends on the development of techniques that would allow achievement of much higher peritoneal solute clearance. Furthermore, it is possible that patient selection has had an impact on the results of some of the major studies discussed above. It is well-known that dialysis patients with several comorbidities tend to do poorly, so that increasing peritoneal clearance in these patients may not impact favorably on outcome. In contrast, the healthiest dialysis patients with few or no comorbidities are likely to do well over the relatively short duration of follow-up included in most studies, regardless of changes in peritoneal clearance. Thus, inclusion of these two extremes of patient groups could potentially dilute the impact of increasing clearance in a population at moderate risk. Studies particularly targeting this moderate risk population would therefore be informative.

Based on the available evidence, our recommendations (summarized in Table 44.5) include the following. In the absence of a better clearance marker, we recommend a minimum total Kt/V_{urea} target of 1.7. Peritoneal and renal clearances should be followed serially to ensure that this target is met, with equal attention paid to the patient's clinical status for signs and symptoms of underdialysis. Efforts to improve peritoneal clearance must shift from a focus on small solute clearance to one that includes middle molecule clearance. Furthermore, the true adequacy of PD as a form of renal replacement therapy depends not only on successful clearance of uremic toxins, but also on adequate volume management through a combination of peritoneal ultrafiltration and residual urine volume. Finally, given the survival advantage that is associated with renal clearance, every effort should be made to preserve RRF with the avoidance of potential nephrotoxins, the use of agents with potentially protective effects, and a search for reversible etiologies when a decline in RRF is noted.

References

1 Lowrie E, Laird N, Parker T, Sargent JA. Effect of the hemodialysis prescription on patient morbidity: report from the National Cooperative Dialysis Study (NCDS). *N Engl J Med* 1981; **305:** 1176–1181.

2 Gotch FA, Sargent J. A mechanistic analysis of the National Cooperative Dialysis Study (NCDS). *Kidney Int* 1985; **28:** 526–534.

3 Popovich RP, Moncrief JW, Nolph KD, Ghods AJ, Twardowski ZJ, Pyle WK. Continuous ambulatory peritoneal dialysis. *Ann Intern Med* 1978; **88(4):** 449–456.

4 Popovich RP, Moncrief J. Kinetic modeling of peritoneal transport. *Contrib Nephrol* 1979; **17:** 59–72.

5 CANUSA Peritoneal Dialysis Study Group. Adequacy of dialysis and nutrition in continuous peritoneal dialysis: association with clinical outcomes. *J Am Soc Nephrol* 1996; **7:** 198–207.

6 Maiorca R, Brunori G, Zubani R, Cancarini GC, Manili L, Camerini C et al. Predictive value of dialysis adequacy and nutritional indices for mortality and morbidity in CAPD and HD patients. A longitudinal study. *Nephrol Dial Transplant* 1995; **10:** 2295–2305.

7 Genestier S, Hedelin G, Schaffer P, Faller B. Prognostic factors in CAPD patients: a retrospective study of a 10-year period. *Nephrol Dial Transplant* 1995; **10:** 1905–1911.

8 Blake PG, Balaskas E, Blake R, Oreopoulos DG. Urea kinetics has limited relevance in assessing adequacy of dialysis in CAPD. *Adv Perit Dial* 1992; **8:** 65–70.

9 Teehan BP, Schleifer CR, Brown J. Urea kinetic modeling is an appropriate assessment of adequacy. *Semin Dial* 1992; **5:** 189–192.

10 De Alvaro F, Bajo MA, Alvarez-Ude F, Vigil A, Molina A, Coronel F et al. Adequacy of peritoneal dialysis: does Kt/V have the same predictive value as in HD? A multicenter study. *Adv Perit Dial* 1992; **8:** 93–97.

11 Lameire NH, Vanholder R, Veyt D, Lambert MC, Rignoir S. A longitudinal, five year survey of urea kinetic parameters in CAPD patients. *Kidney Int* 1992; **42:** 426–432.

12 National Kidney Foundation. NKF-DOQI clinical practice guidelines for peritoneal dialysis adequacy. *Am J Kidney Dis* 1997; **30(3 Suppl 2):** S67–S136.

13 Bargman JM, Bick J, Cartier P, Dasgupta MK, Fine A, Lavoie SD et al. Guidelines for adequacy and nutrition in peritoneal dialysis. Canadian Society of Nephrology. *J Am Soc Nephrol* 1999; **10(Suppl 13):** S311–S321.

14 National Kidney Foundation. NKF-K/DOQI clinical practice guidelines for peritoneal dialysis adequacy: update 2000. *Am J Kidney Dis* 2001; **37(1 Suppl 1):** S65–S136.

15 Paniagua R, Amato D, Vonesh E, Correa-Rotter R, Ramos A, Moran J et al. Effects of increased peritoneal clearances on mortality rates in peritoneal dialysis: ADEMEX, a prospective, randomized, controlled trial. *J Am Soc Nephrol* 2002; **13(5):** 1307–1320.

16 Lo WK, Ho YW, Li CS, Wong KS, Chan TM, Yu AW et al. Effect of Kt/V on survival and clinical outcome in CAPD patients in a randomized, prospective study. *Kidney Int* 2003; **64(2):** 649–656.

17 Diaz-Buxo JA, Lowrie EG, Lew NL, Zhang SM, Zhu X, Lazarus JM. Associates of mortality among peritoneal dialysis patients with special reference to peritoneal transport rates and solute clearance. *Am J Kidney Dis* 1999; **33(3):** 523–534.

18 Rocco M, Soucie JM, Pastan S, McClellan WM. Peritoneal dialysis adequacy and risk of death. *Kidney Int* 2000; **58(1):** 446–457.

19 Bargman JM, Thorpe KE, Churchill DN. Relative contribution of residual renal function and peritoneal clearance to adequacy of dialysis: a reanalysis of the CANUSA study. *J Am Soc Nephrol* 2001; **12(10):** 2158–2162.

20 Szeto CC, Wong TY, Chow KM, Leung B, Law MC, Li PK. Independent effects of renal and peritoneal creatinine clearances on the mortality of peritoneal dialysis patients. *Perit Dial Int* 2004; **24(1):** 58–64.

21 Szeto CC, Wong TY, Leung CB, Wang AY, Law MC, Lui SF et al. Importance of dialysis adequacy in mortality and morbidity of Chinese CAPD patients. *Kidney Int* 2000; **58(1):** 400–407.

22 Wang AY, Wang M, Woo J, Lam CW, Lui SF, Li PK et al. Inflammation, residual kidney function, and cardiac hypertrophy are interrelated and combine adversely to enhance mortality and cardiovascular death risk of peritoneal dialysis patients. *J Am Soc Nephrol* 2004; **15(8):** 2186–2194.

23 Rocco MV, Frankenfield DL, Prowant B, Frederick P, Flanigan MJ, et al. Risk factors for early mortality in U.S. peritoneal dialysis patients: impact of residual renal function. *Perit Dial Int* 2002; **22(3):** 371–379.

24 Chung SH, Heimburger O, Stenvinkel P, Qureshi AR, Lindholm B. Association between residual renal function, inflammation and patient survival in new peritoneal dialysis patients. *Nephrol Dial Transplant* 2003; **18(3):** 590–597.

25 Ates K, Nergizolglu G, Keven K, Sen A, Kutlay S, Erturk S et al. Effect of fluid and sodium removal on mortality in peritoneal dialysis patients. *Kidney Int* 2001; **60(2):** 767–776.

26 Lo WK, Tong KL, Li CS, Chan TM, Wong AK, Ho YW et al. Relationship between adequacy of dialysis and nutritional status, and their impact on patient survival on CAPD in Hong Kong. *Perit Dial Int.* 2001; **21(5):** 441–447.

27 Chung SH, Heimburger O, Stenvinkel P, Wang T, Lindholm B. Influence of peritoneal transport rate, inflammation, and fluid removal on nutritional status and clinical outcome in prevalent peritoneal dialysis patients. *Perit Dial Int* 2003; **23(2):** 174–183.

28 Termorshuizen F, Korevaar JC, Dekker FW, van Manen JG, Boeschoten EW, Krediet EW et al. The relative importance of residual renal function compared peritoneal clearance for patient survival and quality of life: an analysis of the Netherlands Cooperative Study on the Adequacy of Dialysis (NECOSAD)-2. *Am J Kidney Dis* 2003; **41(6):** 1293–1302.

29 Jager KJ, Merkus MP, Dekker FW, Boeschoten EW, Tijssen JG, Stevens JG et al. Mortality and technique failure in patients starting chronic peritoneal dialysis: results of the Netherlands Cooperative Study on the Adequacy of Dialysis (NECOSAD). *Kidney Int.* 1999; **55(4):** 1476–1485.

30 Szeto CC, Wong TY, Chow KM, Leung CB, Law MC, Wang AY et al. Impact of dialysis adequacy on the mortality and morbidity of anuric Chinese patients receiving continuous ambulatory peritoneal dialysis. *J Am Soc Nephrol* 2001; **12(2):** 355–360.

31 Jansen MA, Termoshuizen F, Korevaar JC, Dekker FW, Boeschoten E, Krediet RT et al. Predictors of survival in anuric peritoneal dialysis patients. *Kidney Int* 2005; **68(3):** 1199–1205.

32 Bhaskaran S, Schaubel DE, Jassal SV, Thodis E, Singhal MK, Bargman JM *et al.* The effect of small solute clearances on survival of anuric peritoneal dialysis patients. *Perit Dial Int* 2000; **20(2):** 181–187.

33 Brown EA, Davies SJ, Rutherford P, Meeus F, Borras M, Riegel W *et al.* Survival of functionally anuric patients on automated peritoneal dialysis: the European APD Outcome Study. *J Am Soc Nephrol* 2003; **14:** 2948–2957.

34 Menon MK, Naimark DM, Bargman JM, Vas SI, Oreopoulos DG. Long-term blood pressure control in a cohort of peritoneal dialysis patients and its association with residual renal function. *Nephrol Dial Transplant* 2001; **16:** 2207–2213.

35 Wang AY, Wang M, Woo J, Law MC, Chow KM, Li PK *et al.* A novel association between residual renal function and left ventricular hypertrophy in peritoneal dialysis patients. *Kidney Int* 2002; **62:** 639–647.

36 Wang AY, Wang M, Woo J, Lam CW, Lui SF, Li PK *et al.* Inflammation, residual kidney function, and cardiac hypertrophy are interrelated and combine adversely to enhance mortality and cardiovascular death risk of peritoneal dialysis patients. *J Am Soc Nephrol* 2004; **15(8):** 2186–2194.

37 Bammens B, Evenepoel P, Verbeke K, Vanrenterghem Y. Removal of middle molecules and protein bound solutes by peritoneal dialysis and relation with uremic symptoms. *Kidney Int* 2003; **64(6):** 2238–2243.

38 Bammens B, Evenepoel P, Verbeke K, Vanrenterghem Y. Time profiles of peritoneal and renal clearances of different uremic solutes in incident peritoneal dialysis patients. *Am J Kidney Dis* 2005; **46(3):** 512–519.

39 Monitini G, Amici G, Milan S, Mussap M, Naturale M, Ratsch IM *et al.* Middle molecule and small protein removal in children on peritoneal dialysis. *Kidney Int* 2002; **61(3):** 1153–1159.

40 K/DOQI guidelines. *Am J Kidney Dis* 2006; in press.

41 ISPD guidelines. *Perit Dial Int* 2006; in press.

42 Dombros N, Dratwa M, Feriani M, Gokal R, Heimburger O, Krediet R *et al.* European best practice guidelines for peritoneal dialysis: adequacy of peritoneal dialysis. *Nephrol Dial Transplant* 2005; **20(Suppl 9):** ix24–ix27.

43 Krediet RT, Douma CE, van Olden RW, Ho-dac-Pannekeet MM, Struijk DG. Augmenting solute clearance in peritoneal dialysis. *Kidney Int* 1998; **54:** 2218–2225.

44 Blake P, Burkart JM, Churchill DN, Daugirdas J, Depner T, Hamburger RJ *et al.* Recommended clinical practices for maximizing peritoneal dialysis clearances. *Perit Dial Int* 1996; **16:** 448–456.

45 Krediet RT, Boeschoten EW, Struijk DG, Arisz L. Differences in the peritoneal transport of water, solutes and proteins between dialysis with two- and with three-litre exchanges. *Nephrol Dial Transplant* 1988; **2:** 198–204.

46 Wang T, Heimbürger O, Cheng HH, Waniewski J, Bergstrom J, Lindholm B. Effect of increased dialysate fill volume on peritoneal fluid and solute transport. *Kidney Int* 1997; **52:** 1068–1076.

47 Chagnac A, Herskovitz P, Ori Y, Weinstein T, Hirsh J, Katz M *et al.* Effect of increased dialysate volume on peritoneal surface area among peritoneal dialysis patients. *J Am Soc Nephrol* 2002; **13(10):** 2554–2559.

48 Aranda RA, Romao JE, Jr., Kakehashi E, Domingos W, Sabbaga E, Marcondes M *et al.* Intraperitoneal pressure and hernias in children on peritoneal dialysis. *Pediatr Nephrol* 2000; **14(1):** 22–24.

49 Hussain SI, Bernardini J, Piraino B. The risk of hernia with large exchange volumes. *Adv Perit Dial* 1998; **14:** 105–107.

50 Del Peso G, Bajo MA, Costero O, Hevia C, Gil F, Diaz C *et al.* Risk factors for abdominal wall complications in peritoneal dialysis patients. *Perit Dial Int* 2003; **23(3):** 249–254.

51 Twardowski ZJ, Khanna R, Nolph KD, Scalamogna A, Metzler MH, Schneider TW *et al.* Intraabdominal pressures during natural activities in patients treated with continuous ambulatory peritoneal dialysis. *Nephron* 1986; **44(2):** 129–135.

52 Imholz A, Koomen G, Struijk D, Arisz L, Krediet RT. Effect of an increased intraperitoneal pressure on fluid and solute transport during CAPD. *Kidney Int* 1993; **44:** 1078–1085.

53 Juergensen PH, Murphy AL, Kliger AS, Finkelstein FO. Increasing the dialysis volume and frequency in a fixed period of time in CPD patients: the effect on Kpt/V and creatinine clearance. *Perit Dial Int* 2002; **22(6):** 693–697.

54 Boen S. Kinetics of peritoneal dialysis. *Medicine* 1961; **40:** 243–287.

55 Rodriguez-Carmona A, Perez Fontan M. Sodium removal in patients undergoing CAPD and automated peritoneal dialysis. *Perit Dial Int* 2002; **22(6):** 705–712.

56 Imholz A, Koomen G, Struijk D, Arisz L, Krediet RT. Effect of dialysate osmolarity on the transport of low-molecular weight solutes and proteins during CAPD. *Kidney Int* 1993; **43:** 1339–1346.

57 Ho-Dac-Panekeet MM, Schouten N, Langedijk MJ, Hiralall JK, de Waart DR, Strujik DG *et al.* Peritoneal transport characteristics with glucose polymer based dialysate. *Kidney Int* 1996; **50:** 979–986.

58 Davies SJ, Phillips L, Naish PF, Russell GI. Peritoneal glucose exposure and changes in membrane solute transport with time on peritoneal dialysis. *J Am Soc Nephrol* 2001; **12:** 1046–1051.

59 Davies SJ, Woodrow G, Donovan K, Plum J, Williams P, Johansson AC *et al.* Icodextrin improves the fluid status of peritoneal dialysis patients: results of a double-blind randomized controlled trial. *J Am Soc Nephrol* 2003; **14(9):** 2338–2344.

60 Li PK, Chow KM, Wong TY, Leung CB, Szeto CC. Effect of an angiotensin-converting enzyme inhibitor on residual renal function in patients receiving peritoneal dialysis. A randomized, controlled study. *Ann Intern Med* 2003; **139(2):** 105–112.

61 Suzuki, H, Kanno, Y, Sugahara, S, Okada H, Nakamoto H. Effects of an angiotensin II receptor blocker, valsartan, on residual renal function in patients on CAPD. *Am J Kidney Dis* 2004; **43(6):** 1056–1064.

62 Moist LM, Port FK, Orzol SM, Young EW, Ostbye T, Wolfe RA *et al.* Predictors of loss of residual renal function among new dialysis patients. *J Am Soc Nephrol* 2000; **11(3):** 556–564.

63 Johnson DW, Mudge DW, Sturtevant JM, Hawley CM, Campbell SB, Isbel NM *et al.* Predictors of decline in residual renal function in new peritoneal dialysis patients. *Perit Dial Int* 2003; **23(3):** 276–283.

64 Singhal MK, Bhaskaran S, Vidgen E, Barman JM, Vas SI, Oreopoulos DG. Rate of decline of residual renal function in patients on peritoneal dialysis and the factors affecting it. *Perit Dial Int* 2000; **20(4):** 429–438.

65 Shemin D, Maaz D, St. Pierre D, Kahn SI, Chazan JA. Effect of aminoglycoside use of residual renal function in peritoneal dialysis patients. *Am J Kidney Dis* 1999; **34(1):** 14–20.

66 Baker RJ, Senior H, Clemenger M, Brown EA. Empirical aminoglycosides for peritonitis do not affect residual renal function. *Am J Kidney Dis* 2003; **41(3):** 670–675.

67 Lui SL, Cheng SW, Ng F, Ng SY, Wan KM, Yip T *et al.* Cefazolin plus netil-imicin versus cefazolin plus ceftazidime for treating CAPD peritonitis: effect on residual renal function. *Kidney Int* 2005; **68(5):** 2375–2380.

68 Dittrich E, Puttinger H, Schillinger M, Lang I, Stefenelli T, Horl WH *et al.* Effect of radio contrast media on residual renal function in peritoneal dialysis patients: a prospective study. *Nephrol Dial Transplant* 2006; **21:** 1334–1339.

69 Moranne O, Willoteaux S, Pagniez D, Dequeidt P, Boulanger E. Effect of iodinated contrast agents on residual renal function in PD patients. *Nephrol Dial Transplant* 2006; **21:** 1040–1045.

70 Kshirsagar AV, Poole C, Mottl A, Shoham D, Franceschini N, Tudor G *et al.* N-acetylcysteine for the prevention of radiocontrast-induced nephropathy: a meta-analysis of prospective controlled trials. *J Am Soc Nephrol* 2004; **15:** 761–769.

45 Salt and Water Balance in Peritoneal Dialysis

Cheuk-Chun Szeto & Philip Kam-Tao Li

Department of Medicine & Therapeutics, Prince of Wales Hospital, The Chinese University of Hong Kong, Shatin, Hong Kong, China

Influence of salt and water removal

It is now recognized that cardiovascular disease is the most significant comorbidity among peritoneal dialysis (PD) patients [1], and there is increasing evidence that suboptimal fluid management is associated with cardiovascular risk and overall mortality [2].

PD patients are generally volume expanded when compared with hemodialysis (HD) patients [3]. Recently, Konings *et al.* [4] showed that extracellular fluid (ECF) volume significantly correlated with diastolic blood pressure and left ventricular end diastolic diameter in PD patients. In addition, continuous ambulatory PD (CAPD) patients with suboptimal blood pressure control have more expanded ECF volumes and a higher prevalence of left ventricular hypertrophy compared with those with well-controlled blood pressure [5]. Several studies in the 1990s showed that a higher peritoneal solute transport was associated with improved technique and patient survival [6–9]. In addition, observational studies showed that a higher peritoneal salt and water removal was associated with better patient survival [10,11]. For example, in the European APD Outcome Study (EAPOS), anuric patients on automated PD (APD) had worse survival if their baseline daily ultrafiltration (UF) was below 750 mL [11,12]. More recently, Chung *et al.* [13] showed that low total fluid removal on PD is associated with higher serum C-reactive protein levels, indicating systemic inflammation, as well as markers of poor nutrition. It is, however, possible that sodium and fluid removal in this study were simply a marker for a healthier, better-nourished patient who eats and drinks more [14].

Assessment and monitoring of salt and water balance

Monitoring of weight, course of residual renal function, and achieved UF with current dialysis prescription should be done in all PD patients [15]. This approach will allow for early detection of and correction of problems. The volume status of patients on PD should be used as a core indicator of dialysis adequacy [15]. Constant reevaluation, by physicians and nurses, of the patient's target weight in the light of blood pressure and other indicators of fluid overload is required. Blood pressure should be normalized by fluid removal alone, without antihypertensive drugs, until it is proven that this strategy is not adequate. Routine performance of peritoneal function tests, described in the next section, should also be done, to identify patients with problems of peritoneal transport in whom monitoring of fluid status is particularly critical [15].

Tests of peritoneal transport

A patient's peritoneal membrane transport status should be evaluated in order to find an appropriate PD modality and prescription. Because both elimination of uremic toxins and UF account for adequacy, a test method should reliably evaluate both small solute and water permeability.

Peritoneal equilibration test

Numerous techniques for measuring peritoneal transport are available, of which the most widely used is the peritoneal equilibration test (PET) [16]. The PET was the first method to quantify individual peritoneal membrane characteristics, and it is highly reproducible. The procedure is summarized in Table 45.1. Based on population studies, patients are categorized as low, low-average, high-average, or high transporters. A problem with conventional PET is that it primarily measures small solute clearance and does not directly evaluate causes of UF problems (see below). The procedural steps in the PET may actually overestimate peritoneal membrane transport and underestimate the variation in peritoneal transport that may occur under actual clinical conditions [17]. PET alone does not give an assessment of dialysis adequacy.

Evidence-based Nephrology. Edited by Donald Molony and Jonathan Craig
© 2009 Blackwell Publishing, ISBN: 978-1-4051-3975-5.

Table 45.1 PET procedure[a].

1) After an overnight exchange of an 8- to12-h dwell, 2 L of a 2.5% glucose concentration solution is instilled and allowed to dwell for 4 h.
2) Several times during the dwell, the patient is requested to roll from side to side.
3) Dialysate urea, glucose, sodium, and creatinine are measured at 0, 2, and 4 h.
4) A blood sample is taken after 2 h.
5) The drain bag is measured to assess both drain and net UF volume.
6) Dialysate-to-plasma ratios (D/P) are calculated for creatinine, urea, and sodium at 0, 2, and 4 h.
7) The ratio of glucose at drain time to the dialysate glucose concentration at time zero (Dt/D0) is measured.

[a] Adapted from Twardowski *et al.* 1987 [15].

Other tests of peritoneal function

Fast PET

Because the PET is labor-intensive, the fast PET [18] provides a simpler alternative by requiring only one dialysate sample. After draining the overnight dwell, the patient starts an exchange at home and arrives at the center in time for drainage of this 4-h dwell. A blood sample is taken at the end of the exchange. The analysis of the fast PET is identical to that for the standard PET, but only two reliable measures of peritoneal membrane permeability are determined, the dialysate-to-plasma ratio (D/P) for creatinine and dialysate glucose, after 4 h. If these two measures give contradictory results, it may be difficult to accurately interpret the test.

Short PET

The original PET was standardized for a long overnight exchange, but recent data have shown that this is unnecessary. For clinical purposes, the short PET [19] was introduced, accepting any dwell time between 3 and 12 h for the prior exchange.

Peritoneal function test

The peritoneal function test (PFT) has been extensively used and validated [20,21]. It measures the peritoneal mass transfer area coefficient during routine exchanges instead of under the highly controlled conditions required for the PET. This test also allows the clinician to assess total delivered dose of dialysis as well as protein and calorie nutrition. The PFT requires 24-h dialysate and urinary collection, and a specific computerized kinetic modeling program is used for calculations.

PD capacity program

The PD capacity (PDC) program is based on the three-pore model [22,23] and describes the peritoneal membrane characteristics using three parameters:

1) The area parameter, which determines the diffusion of small solutes

2) The final reabsorption rate of fluid when the glucose gradient has dissipated

3) The large-pore fluid flux, which determines the loss of protein.

Patients are asked to perform five exchanges. Data are combined with a computerized mathematical approach employing the three-pore model to estimate the parameters of membrane function.

Dialysis adequacy and transport test

The dailysis adequacy and transport test (DATT) was introduced by Rocco *et al.* [24,25]. For this test, the patients are asked to perform their exchanges as usual. Only a serum sample and a 10-mL aliquot from a pooled, well-mixed 24-h dialysate are required, and the 24-h D/P is calculated. DATT has only been validated for patients on a fixed CAPD schedule of three or four 2-L exchanges [26,27].

Accelerated peritoneal examination

The accelerated peritoneal examination (APEX) test has the same regimen as the PET, but it summarizes, in a single number, the peritoneal permeability for both glucose and urea [28] and represents the time at which glucose and urea equilibration curves cross. Generally, the APEX may be shorter than a PET, because most patients exhibit a crossing of the curves before 2 h. The shorter the APEX time, the higher the peritoneal permeability; the longer the time, the lower the peritoneal permeability. The APEX time may identify the optimum contact time between the functional peritoneal membrane surface area and the dialysate for the individual patient. If UF is the major goal, short dwell times should be used. If solute clearance is the major goal, longer dwell times should be used.

Standard peritoneal permeability analysis

The standard peritoneal permeability analysis (SPA) uses intraperitoneally administered dextran 70 to study fluid kinetics during a 4-h dwell [29]. The test was originally developed using the lowest glucose concentration. In the SPA, the mass transfer area coefficient (MTAC) of small solutes, the proportion of glucose absorbed, and the peritoneal clearances of serum protein are calculated. The PET parameters can be calculated from the SPA parameters. Conversely, the D/P creatinine and the Dt/D0 glucose values can be used with the drained volume to calculate the MTAC of creatinine and the proportion of glucose absorbed. Using SPA, with the highest glucose concentration, provides more valid data on UF, because the larger drained volume reduces measurement error and the sodium sieving phenomenon associated with a hypertonic glucose solution provides an assessment of aquaporin-mediated water transport. The magnitude of the dip in D/P sodium is a rough estimate of the water channel function.

Timing and frequency of the test

Peritoneal transport characteristics change significantly within the first month of PD, and so the results of the tests described above need to be considered in the context of how long an individual patient has been on PD. Peritoneal function tests performed during the first month of PD should be interpreted as preliminary and confirmed by an additional test 4 weeks later [30]. Like all tests, peritoneal membrane function tests, both in terms of solute clearance or UF, are subject to measurement error. Several exchanges within 24 h can be used to reduce this error, as with the PFT or PDC, as well as repeated testing over time. Because most creatinine assays based on the Jaffé method are also sensitive to glucose, dialysate creatinine concentrations are falsely high and need to be corrected for high dialysate glucose concentrations.

It is unclear how often peritoneal function should be assessed. The National Kidney Foundation Dialysis Outcomes Quality Initiatives guidelines recommend a measurement every 4 months [31]. The recommendation, however, may not be practical, because the tests are time-consuming for both patients and nurses.

Pediatric patients

A full discussion on peritoneal function tests in pediatric patients is beyond the scope of this chapter. Differences in peritoneal transport between children and adults have been postulated, but a recent study from Bouts *et al.* [32] did not confirm this theory. In general, all the tests described here are also applicable in children but, for most pediatric nephrologists, the standard PET is probably the test most commonly used.

Classification, diagnosis, and management of UF failure

The International Society for Peritoneal Dialysis Ad Hoc Committee on Ultrafiltration Management in Peritoneal Dialysis has published a comprehensive guideline in this area [15]. Patients presenting with the clinical syndrome of inability to maintain target weight and an edema-free state need to be carefully evaluated before being labeled "ultrafiltration failure" [15]. The clinical approach to PD patients with fluid overload and possible UF failure is outlined in Figure 45.1.

In general, reversible causes, such as dietary noncompliance, problems in the PD prescription, and mechanical problems, should be considered and may account for a large proportion of cases of fluid overload. Two groups of PD-related mechanical complications warrant more detailed discussion:

Dialysate leaks

Dialysate leaks from the abdominal cavity decrease drain volumes and net fluid removal. Net fluid removal from leaks into the abdominal wall or pleural space is decreased because of reabsorption

from the interstitial spaces or sequestration in the pleural space. Leaks into the interstitial space are commonly accompanied by abdominal wall edema with or without genital edema. Leaks can occur at any time but are often seen after being on PD for several months. They usually occur at the catheter insertion site but can occur at an abdominal wall hernia site or after abdominal surgery [33–35]. Diagnosis is confirmed by using radiographic techniques that include intraperitoneal infusion of a dialysis solution to which contrast has been added, followed by computed tomography (the so-called "CT peritoneogram"), or by the intraperitoneal infusion of radioisotope with peritoneal scintigraphy [33,34,36–42]. Leaks associated with hernias usually require surgical repair and a temporary transfer to HD. Leaks occurring in the absence of a hernia usually represent a tear in the parietal peritoneum. Small leaks may respond to peritoneal rest with HD support or the use of intermittent PD without the need for surgical repair. Recurrence may require surgical repair [35].

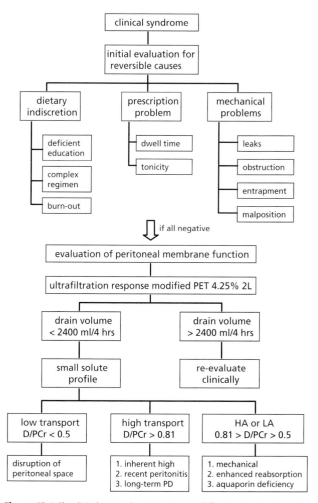

Figure 45.1 The clinical approach to PD patients with fluid overload and possible UF failure. HA, high-average transporter; LA, low-average transporter; D/PCr, dialysate-to-plasma creatinine ratio at 4 h. (Adapted from Mujais *et al.*, *Perit Dial Int* 2000 [15].)

Catheter problems

Catheter-related problems contributing to poor drain volumes include obstruction, entrapment, or malposition. Constipation is a also a common and readily reversible cause. Catheter obstruction, either partial or complete, often results from fibrin plugs within the catheter lumen but can be due to omentum obstructing the catheter ports or to a kinked catheter. The diagnosis is usually by exclusion, because radiographic evaluation is generally not helpful except in identifying kinked catheters. Treatment consists of aggressive flushing of the catheter with a dialysate-filled syringe or the use of fibrinolytic agents when fibrin-related occlusion is suspected. If the intra-abdominal portion of the catheter is entrapped in a compartment formed by adhesions, surgical lysis of the adhesions can be considered if the adhesions are not too extensive. If the adhesions are extensive, conversion to long-term HD is necessary.

Further evaluation of peritoneal function

If the initial workup does not identify a reversible cause, evaluation of the peritoneal membrane function is needed (Figure 45.1). Traditionally, peritoneal membrane function has been assessed by the PET, but this test has been standardized to classify membrane function [16] primarily in terms of small solute clearance and not for problems with UF. A modification of the standard PET introduced by Krediet *et al.* [43] offers a convenient alternative. The procedure of the modified PET is summarized in Table 45.2. Briefly, it consists of replacing the 2.5% dextrose solution of the standard PET with a 4.25% dextrose solution, thereby satisfying the criterion of maximal osmotic drive required for proper evaluation of UF capacity. A value of less than 400 mL net UF in a 4-h dwell correlates well with clinical behavior and avoids false-positive results [15]. The peritoneal conditions that would result in a drain volume of less than 2400 mL in 4 h can be separated by

examination of the small solute characteristics (i.e. D/P creatinine ratio at 4 h).

Low drain volume and high transport

Patients with a low drain volume and D/P creatinine greater than 0.81 represent the largest group of patients with inadequate filtration due to peritoneal membrane problem. These patients fall into three groups:

1) Patients with an inherent high small solute transport profile at initiation of dialysis
2) Patients with current or recent peritonitis
3) Patients who develop a high transport profile in the course of long-term PD.

These patients tend to have adequate low-molecular-weight solute transport but have poor UF due to rapid absorption of glucose and dissipation of the osmotic gradient.

Inherent high transport

Around 10% of patients starting PD display an inherent high transport profile. Patients in this group have very efficient membranes for small solute clearance but difficulty in UF, particularly in long dwell cycles. These patients are at risk of high protein losses in the peritoneum. High levels of technique failure and mortality have been reported in this group [7,44,45]. These patients typically do well on CAPD until residual renal volume decreases, at which time it may become difficult to maintain euvolemia and blood pressure control on standard CAPD. APD and icodextrin for the long dwell are recommended therapeutic approaches.

Recent peritonitis

Fluid retention is common during episodes of peritonitis [46–48]. During peritonitis, there is an increase in the D/P ratio for creatinine, an increase in protein losses, and a decrease in net

Table 45.2 Modified PET procedure (4.25% dextrose)[a].

---

1) On the evening prior to the test, the patient should perform a standard CAPD 8- to 12-h overnight dwell.

2) With the patient upright, drain the overnight dwell over 20 min and note the volume drained. Save the sample for creatinine and glucose measurements to allow for determination of residual volume.

3) With the patient supine, infuse 2.0 L of 4.25% dialysis solution over 10 min. The patient should roll from side to side after each 400 mL of solution is infused.

4) Note the time the infusion is complete: this is the "zero hour" dwell time.

5) At 0-h, 1-h, and 2-h dwell times:
   - Drain 200 mL of effluent into bag
   - Mix bag by inverting 2–3 times
   - Using aseptic technique, draw a 10-mL sample from medication port
   - Reinfuse the 190 mL of effluent into the patient
   - Transfer the 10-mL sample to red-top tube and label appropriately

6) At 2-h dwell time, draw blood sample for creatinine, sodium, and glucose measurements

7) At 4-h dwell time:
   - With patient upright, drain exchange over 20 min
   - Mix bag by inverting 2–3 times
   - Using aseptic technique, draw a 10-mL sample from medication port
   - Measure and record volume drained
   - Transfer 10-mL sample to red-top tube and label appropriately

8) Send all effluent samples and one blood sample to laboratory for creatinine, sodium, and glucose measurements

---

[a] Adapted from Mujais *et al.* 2000 [14].

UF—changes that are usually reversible. We have shown previously that the change of D/P, followed up for over 2 years, had no significant correlation with the total number of peritonitis episodes, but after severe peritonitis, patients had a greater change of D/P than patients who experienced no severe infection [49]. Previous studies suggested that reduced UF during peritonitis can be satisfactorily managed with the use of icodextrin [50].

High transport during long-term PD

The natural history of peritoneal membrane transport has been debated [51–57]. The emerging picture is that some increase in D/P creatinine does occur due to an increase in peritoneal membrane functional surface area [52,59–62]. A history of recurrent peritonitis and extensive use of hypertonic exchanges has been observed in some, but not all, studies. In contrast to the situation seen with peritonitis, the changes of solute transport in this group tend to be permanent, but it is often easy to maintain total solute clearance despite a tendency toward clinical volume overload.

In general, for patients with UF failure and a high transport profile of small solute clearance, APD and icodextrin for the long dwell are the recommended therapeutic approaches. Icodextrin solutions have been shown to be superior to glucose-based solutions in achieving net UF during long dwells in most patients, particularly in high transporters [63–69]. Icodextrin has also been shown to be effective during peritonitis [50]. In areas of the world where icodextrin dialysis solutions are not available, shortening dwell time is the preferred approach. In CAPD patients, this can be achieved with the use of an automated nighttime exchange device, which will shorten dwell time and has the additional benefit of improving small solute clearance with little impact on patient lifestyle. In patients on APD, omitting the daytime exchange and optimizing the nighttime regimen may be sufficient. If small solute clearance is inadequate, a short daytime exchange with midday drainage will improve solute clearance without compromising UF. In a few patients, adjunctive, temporary, or permanent HD may be required.

Low drain volume and low transport

The combination of low drain volume and low small solute transport is rare and reflects a major disruption of the peritoneal membrane or intraperitoneal fluid distribution [70]. It is usually due to adhesions, and the functional consequences may be related to fluid trapping in small spaces. Peritoneography may be helpful in making the diagnosis by identifying sequestered spaces. Poor UF in association with low transport is reported to occur in advanced stages of sclerosing peritonitis [70,71], but a high transport rate has also been described in the same setting [70–72]. Because this condition results in both inadequate volume and solute removal, transfer to HD is generally required unless patients have some degree of residual renal function [73]. Patients with a low transport rate, leaks, mechanical problems, or high lymphatic reabsorption also present with low drain volume and low small solute transport. These conditions need exclusion before low transport should be determined to be the reason for UF failure.

Low drain volume and high-average or low-average transport

In general, a low drain volume coupled with high-average or low-average transport can result from four possible etiologies [15]:
1) Mechanical problems
2) Lymphatic reabsorption
3) Tissue reabsorption
4) Aquaporin deficiency.

Mechanical problems

The possibility of mechanical problems needs to be reconsidered, particularly if the initial evaluation has not been thorough.

Lymphatic reabsorption and/or tissue reabsorption

These two conditions often coexist. Definitive proof of the condition requires identification of high macromolecule clearance from the peritoneal cavity [74,75]. Measurement of lymphatic flow is uncommon in clinical practice due to the complexity of the procedure. In the absence of such a test, the diagnosis is made by exclusion of mechanical catheter problems, aquaporin deficiency, and increased hydraulic conductance. Management encompasses all interventions that maximize UF, such as short dwell time and high-tonicity dialysate [76]. Use of pharmacological reduction of lymphatic absorption [77], intraperitoneal administration of phosphatidylcholine [78–80], and bethanechol chloride (a parasympatho-mimetic drug) [81] have been reported in small studies.

Aquaporin deficiency

Aquaporin deficiency is a rare condition, and only a small number of definite cases have been reported [82]. Various indirect methods can be applied in clinical practice to estimate the magnitude of aquaporin-mediated water transport. The so-called sieving of Na^+ is the simplest one [82–86]. Another simple way to assess aquaporin-mediated transport is to calculate the difference in net UF obtained after a 4-h dwell with 1.5% glucose and with 4.25% glucose dialysate [15]. Patients with aquaporin deficiency continue to have significant UF via nonaquaporin pathways, which can be enhanced by the use of icodextrin in long dwells, allowing for sustained fluid removal [66,69,87,88]. For glucose-based exchanges, short dwells are also preferable as in patients with a high transport profile.

Measures augmenting salt and water removal in PD patients

Dietary intake

It is generally accepted that dietary restrictions are more liberal in PD patients because of the continuous nature of the dialysis modality and the better preservation of residual diuresis. Tzamaloukas *et al.* [89], however, found that lack of dietary sodium restriction was a major independent risk factor for symptomatic fluid retention. Education on salt restriction resulted in weight reduction, blood pressure reduction, and decreased cardiothoracic index (an indirect measure of left ventricular overload) [90]. Dietary counseling to reduce salt and water intake is therefore important [15] to maintain desired weight and reduce cardiovascular risk.

Hyperglycemia control

In diabetic patients, hyperglycemia can adversely affect the maintenance of an osmotic gradient across the peritoneal membrane [15]. Control of hyperglycemia may increase UF without the need to use hypertonic glucose solutions. Because glucose control is mostly self-monitored and managed, patients should be educated about the importance of glucose control for PD adequacy.

Increase urinary excretion

In patients with residual renal function, salt excretion can be increased by diuretics, particularly loop diuretics. Van Olden et al. [91] demonstrated that the effect varies with dose and degree of residual renal function. A single dose of 2 g of frusemide resulted in a median increase in urine volume of 400 mL and a mean extra sodium removal of 54 mmol/L [91]. In this short-term study, diuretics did not affect the residual creatinine clearance, and there were no alterations in peritoneal transport of solutes or water. The long-term effect over 1 year of frusemide in PD was evaluated by Medcalf et al. [92] using a dose of 250 mg/day versus placebo. In the group receiving frusemide, diuresis and sodium excretion were more preserved, but the rate of deterioration of residual renal function was no different between the groups. Maintenance of residual renal function is important in PD patients, as there is a clear relation with survival. Nephrotoxic drugs and contrast media should be avoided as much as possible. We have previously demonstrated the use of ramipril can slow the decline in residual renal function [93], and this was later supported by a study using an angiotensin receptor blocker [94]. The administration of biocompatible PD solution with low glucose degradation product also showed a beneficial effect on residual renal function [95].

Salt removal by PD

Considering UF to be equivalent to sodium removal is a dangerous paradigm [96]. During the initial period of a PD dwell, there is a considerable sodium sieving, resulting in almost pure water removal, without sodium. Short, hypertonic dwells, such as those applied during APD, result in a removal of hypotonic water, leaving the patient's plasma hypertonic, and thirst results.

Data from an uncontrolled study suggested that sodium removal during APD was lower than during CAPD [97]. However, two open-label randomized controlled trials did not show a significant difference in UF between APD and CAPD (Table 45.3) [98,99].

When used as the osmotic agent, the glucose polymer icodextrin facilitates the convective transport of sodium across the peritoneal membrane. A number of studies have demonstrated better UF and improvement in fluid status after the introduction of icodextrin for the long dwell for both APD and CAPD (Table 45.4) [100–108].

It has been suggested that sodium removal could be improved by enhancing the sodium gradient between plasma and dialysate with a low sodium dialysate. Such a low sodium solution has, however, a lower total osmolarity, necessitating a higher glucose concentration to achieve enough osmotic capacity. The results of two short-term studies were inconsistent (Table 45.5), probably due to the difference in actual sodium concentration of the solutions tested [109,110].

A number of intraperitoneal agents have also been tested (Table 45.6) [111–116]. Although many of these agents appeared to improve peritoneal clearance of small solute or water, all published trials were short term and small. The long-term efficacy and safety of these agents remain to be proved.

Preservation of peritoneal membrane function

The acute (and possibly chronic) impact of peritonitis on membrane function was discussed in the previous section. Minimization of damage to the peritoneal membrane by implementation of strategies to decrease the peritonitis rate should be universally applied, including the use of improved connectology systems [117].

The use of more biocompatible solutions may also influence membrane preservation. A retrospective observational study that compared incident PD patients treated with conventional PD solution to those treated with the new pH neutral lactate buffer solution, found a significant survival advantage with the new solution [118]. Available controlled studies show that the effect of biocompatible solution depends on the actual composition of the product (Table 45.7) [119–124]. In general, amino acid-based PD solution does not affect UF or sodium removal [119–121]. The

Table 45.3 Randomized controlled trials on the effects of automated PD versus CAPD.

Study [reference]	No. of subjects	Design	Treatment group	Duration (mos)	Effects
Bro et al. [98]	34	Open label	APD	6	Peritoneal transport and UF not described
Rodriguez et al. [99]	45	Open label	TPD, CCPD	2	Better peritoneal clearance of urea and creatinine; UF not described

Abbreviations: TPD, tidal peritoneal dialysis; CCPD, continuous cyclic peritoneal dialysis.

Table 45.4 Published trials on the effects of icodextrin PD solution on UF.

Study [reference]	No. of subjects	Dialysis type	Design[a]	Treatment group	Control group	Duration	Effects
Konings et al. [100]	40	CAPD	Open label	7.5% icodextrin	Standard glucose	4 mos	Better UF, 1670 ± 1038 vs. 744 ± 767 mL
Posthuma et al. [101]	38	APD	Open label	7.5% icodextrin	Standard glucose	2 yrs	Increasec UF by at least 261 mL
Davies et al. [102]	50	CAPD	Multicenter double blind	7.5% icodextrin	2.27% glucose	6 mos	Improved UF by 258.6 mL (control group: worse UF by −141.8 mL); also improved sodium removal
Wolfson et al. [103]	175	CAPD	Double blind	7.5% icodextrin	2.5% dextrose	52 wks	Better UF, 587.2 vs. 346.2 mL
Plum et al. [104]	39	APD	Multicenter double blind	7.5% icodextrin	2.27% glucose	16 wks	Better UF, 278 ± 43 vs. -138 ± 81 mL
Mistry et al. [105]	209	CAPD	Open label	7.5% icodextrin	1.36% and 3.86% glucose	6 mos	Better UF than 1.36% glucose at 8 h (527 ± 44 vs. 101 ± 48 mL); no difference from 3.86% glucose
Finkelstein et al. [106]	92	APD	Multicenter double blind	7.5% icodextrin	4.25% dextrose	2 wks	Improved UF 141.6 ± 75.4 to 540.2 ± 46.8 ml; no change in UF in control group
Posthuman et al. [107]	23	APD	Open label	7.5% icodextrin	4.25% dextrose	12 mos	Better UF, 218 ± 57 vs. 36 ± 115 mL; result was insignificant at 12 mos
Dallas et al. [108]	8	Both CAPD and APD	Randomized	7.5% icodextrin, 1.36% glucose	7.5% icodextrin	4 wks	Improved UF, 750 (650–828) to 1000 (889–1100) mL

[a] All studies were parallel, randomized controlled trials, except the one by Dallas et al. [108], which was a crossover study.

Table 45.5 Published studies on the effects of low-sodium PD solution[a].

Study [reference]	No. of subjects	Treatment group	Control group	Effect
Leypoldt et al. [109]	10	Na 105 mmol/L	Na 132 mmol/L	Low-sodium solution had better sodium and water removal
Amici et al. [110]	10	Na 126 mmol/L	Na 132 mmol/L	No difference in sodium or water removal

[a] Both studies focused on acute effects and used a crossover design.

Table 45.6 Published trials on effects of intraperitoneal agents on peritoneal transport.

Study [reference]	No. of subjects	Design[a]	Agents	Duration	Effect
Sjoland et al. [111]	21	Double blind	Tinzaparin	3 mos each	Reduced D/P creatinine, increased UF volume
Moberly et al. [112]	13	Open label	Hyaluronan	Single exchange	Marginal increase in UF volume, no change in creatinine clearance
el-Sherif et al. [113]	21	Open label	Minoxidil	Single exchange	Increase in UF volume
Hasbargen et al. [114]	7	Open label	Neostigmine	Single exchange	No effect
Kalra et al. [115]	25	Double blind	Sodium nitroprusside, chlorpromazine	Single exchange	Increased urea and creatinine clearance
Favazza et al. [116]	9	Open label	Clonidine, enalapril, nifedipine	2 weeks each	Increased creatinine and β2-microglobulin clearance by enalapril and nifedipine

[a] All studies entailed a crossover design.

Table 45.7 Published trials on the use of biocompatible PD solutions.

Study [reference]	No. of subjects	Design[a]	Treatment group	Duration	Effect(s)
van Biesen *et al.* [119]	10	Multicenter RCT	0.6% amino acid, 1.4% glycerol	3 mos	Improved PDE CA125 level; no difference in UF or nutritional parameters
Li *et al.* [120]	60	RCT	1.1% amino acid	3 yrs	Better NPNA, no difference in UF
Plum *et al.* [121]	10	Crossover	1% amino acid Bicarbonate buffered	1 day	No difference in UF
Schmitt *et al.* [122]	25[#]	Crossover	pH neutral, bicarbonate buffered	1 day	No change in peritoneal surface area
Williams *et al.* [123]	86	Multicenter crossover	pH neutral, lactate buffered, low GDP	12 wks each	Improved PDE markers of peritoneal membrane integrity and reduced circulating AGE, possibly better residual renal function
Tranaeus [124]	106	RCT	25 mmol/L bicarbonate + 15 mmol/L lactate	12 mos	Better UF of about 150 mL/day

Abbreviations: RCT, randomized controlled trila; GDP, glucose degradation product; PDE, PD effluent; AGE, advanced glucation end product; NPNA, normalized protein nitrogen appearance.

[a] All trials entailed an open-label design.

[b] Paediatric cases.

effects of neutral pH and/or bicarbonate-buffered solution have been inconsistent [122–124].

Temporary cessation of PD (the so-called peritoneal rest) has been used in a few patients with high small solute transport characteristics with some success and may be a reasonable option to consider if other approaches are unsuccessful [125–127]. Alternatively, reduction in exposure of the peritoneal membrane to glucose may lead to some improvement in transport parameters [128].

Acknowledgments

This study was supported in part by the Chinese University of Hong Kong Research Grant Account 6900570.

References

1 Li PKT, Chow KM. The clinical and epidemiological aspects of vascular mortality in chronic peritoneal dialysis patients. *Perit Dial Int* 2005; **25(S3):** S80–S83.

2 McCormick BB, Bargman JM. The implications of the ADEMEX study for the peritoneal dialysis prescription: the role of small solute clearance versus salt and water removal. *Curr Opin Nephrol Hypertens* 2003; **12:** 581–585.

3 Enia G, Mallamaci F, Benedetto FA, Panuccio V, Parlongo S, Cutrupi S *et al.* Long-term CAPD patients are volume expanded and display more severe left ventricular hypertrophy than haemodialysis patients. *Nephrol Dial Transplant* 2001; **16:** 1459–1464.

4 Konings CJAM, Kooman JP, Schonck M, Dammers R, Cheriex E, Palmans Meulemans AP *et al.* Fluid status, blood pressure, and

cardiovascular abnormalities in patients on peritoneal dialysis. *Perit Dial Int* 2002; **22:** 477–487.

5 Koc M, Toprak A, Tezcan H, Bihorac A, Akoglu E, Ozener IC. Uncontrolled hypertension due to volume overload contributes to higher left ventricular mass index in CAPD patients. *Nephrol Dial Transplant* 2002; **17:** 1661–1666.

6 Churchill DN, Thorpe KE, Nolph KD, Keshaviah PR, Oreopoulos DG, Page D. Increased peritoneal membrane transport is associated with decreased patient and technique survival for continuous peritoneal dialysis patients. *J Am Soc Nephrol* 1998; **9:** 1285–1292.

7 Wang T, Heimburger O, Waniewski J, Bergstrom J, Lindholm B. Increased peritoneal permeability is associated with decreased fluid and small-solute removal and higher mortality in CAPD patients. *Nephrol Dial Transplant* 1998; **13:** 1242–1249.

8 Szeto CC, Law MC, Wong TY, Leung CB, Li PKT. Peritoneal transport status correlates with morbidity but not longitudinal change of nutritional status of continuous ambulatory peritoneal dialysis patients: a 2-year prospective study. *Am J Kidney Dis* 2001; **37:** 329–336.

9 Cueto-Manzano AM, Correa-Rotter R. Is high peritoneal transport rate an independent risk factor for CAPD mortality? *Kidney Int* 2000; **57:** 314–320.

10 Paniagua R, Amato D, Vonesh E, Correa-Rotter R, Ramos A, Moran J *et al.* Effects of increased peritoneal clearances on mortality rates in peritoneal dialysis: ADEMEX, a prospective, randomized, controlled trial. *J Am Soc Nephrol* 2002; **13:** 1307–1320.

11 Brown EA, Davies SJ, Rutherford P, Meeus F, Borras M, Riegel W *et al.* Survival of functionally anuric patients on automated peritoneal dialysis: the European APD Outcome Study. *J Am Soc Nephrol* 2003; **14:** 2948–2957.

12 Ates K, Nergizoglu G, Keven K, Sen A, Kutlay S, Erturk S *et al.* Effect of fluid and sodium removal on mortality in peritoneal dialysis patients. *Kidney Int* 2001; **60:** 767–776.

13 Chung SH, Heimburger O, Stenvinkel P, Wang T, Lindholm B. Influence of peritoneal transport rate, inflammation, and fluid removal on

nutritional status and clinical outcome in prevalent peritoneal dialysis patients. *Perit Dial Int* 2003; **23:** 174–183.

14 Sharma AP, Blake PG. Should 'fluid removal' be used as an adequacy target in peritoneal dialysis? *Perit Dial Int* 2003; **23:** 107–108.

15 Mujais S, Nolph K, Gokal R, Blake P, Burkart J, Coles G *et al.* Evaluation and management of ultrafiltration problems in peritoneal dialysis. *Perit Dial Int* 2000; **20(Suppl 4):** S5–S21.

16 Twardowski ZJ, Nolph K, Khanna R, Prowant B, Ryan L, Moore H *et al.* Peritoneal equilibration test. *Perit Dial Bull* 1987; **7:** 138–147.

17 Gotch F, Schoenfeld PY, Gentile DE. The peritoneal equilibration test (PET) is not a realistic measure of peritoneal clearance (PC). *J Am Soc Nephrol* 1991; **2:** 361. (Abstract.)

18 Twardowski ZJ. PET: a simpler approach for determining prescriptions for adequate dialysis therapy. *Adv Perit Dial* 1990; **6:** 186–191.

19 Twardowski ZJ, Prowant BF, Moore HL, Lou LC, White E, Farris K. Short peritoneal equilibration test: impact of preceding dwell time. *Adv Perit Dial* 2003; **19:** 53–58.

20 Gotch FA, Keen ML. Kinetic modelling in peritoneal dialysis. In: Nissenson AR, Fine RN, Gentile DE, editors. *Clinical Dialysis*, 3rd edn. Appleton & Lange, Norwalk, CT, 1995; 343–375.

21 Gotch FA, Lipps BJ, Keen ML, Panlilio F. Computerized urea kinetic modeling to prescribe and monitor delivered Kt/V (pKt/V, dKt/V) in peritoneal dialysis. *Adv Perit Dial* 1996; **12:** 43–45.

22 Haraldsson B. Assessing the peritoneal dialysis capacities of individual patients. *Kidney Int* 1995; **47:** 1187–1198.

23 Rippe B, Stelin G, Haraldsson B. Computer simulations of peritoneal fluid transport in CAPD. *Kidney Int* 1991; **40:** 315–325.

24 Rocco MV, Jordan JR, Burkart JM. Determination of peritoneal transport characteristics with 24-hour dialysate collections: dialysis adequacy and transport test. *J Am Soc Nephrol* 1994; **5:** 1333–1338.

25 Rocco MV, Jordan JR, Burkart JM. 24-hour dialysate collection for determination of peritoneal membrane transport characteristics: Longitudinal follow-up data for the dialysis adequacy and transport test (DATT). *Perit Dial Int* 1996; **16:** 590–593.

26 Paniagua R, Amato D, Correa-Rotter R, Ramos A, Vonesh EF, Mujais SK. Correlation between peritoneal equilabration test and dialysis adequacy and transport test, for peritoneal transport type characterization. *Perit Dial Int* 2000; **20:** 53–59.

27 Szeto CC, Wong TY, Chow KM, Leung CB, Li PKT. Dialysis adequacy and transport test for characterization of peritoneal transport type in Chinese peritoneal dialysis patients receiving three daily exchanges. *Am J Kidney Dis* 2002; **39:** 1287–1299.

28 Verger C, Larpent L, Veniez G, Brunetot N, Corvaisier B. L'APEX: description et utilisation. *Perit Dial Bull* 1991; **1:** 36–40.

29 Smit W, Langedijk MJ, Schouten N, van den Berg N, Struijk DG, Krediet RT. A comparison between 1.36% and 3.86% glucose dialysis solution for the assessment of peritoneal membrane function. *Perit Dial Int* 2000; **20:** 734–741.

30 Johnson DW, Mudge DW, Blizzard S, Arndt M, O'Shea A, Watt R *et al.* A comparison of peritoneal equilibration tests performed 1 and 4 weeks after PD commencement. *Perit Dial Int* 2004; **24:** 460–465.

31 National Kidney Foundation. K/DOQI clinical practice guidelines for peritoneal dialysis adequacy, 2000. *Am J Kidney Dis* 2001; **37(Suppl 1):** S65–S136.

32 Bouts AH, Davin JC, Groothoff JW, Van Amstel SP, Zweers MM, Krediet RT. Standard peritoneal permeability analysis in children. *J Am Soc Nephrol* 2000; **11:** 943–950.

33 Litherland J, Gibson M, Sambrook P, Lupton E, Beaman M, Ackrill P. Investigation and treatment of poor drains of dialysate fluid associated with anterior abdominal wall leaks in patients on chronic ambulatory peritoneal dialysis. *Nephrol Dial Transplant* 1992; **7:** 1030–1034.

34 Litherland J, Lupton EW, Ackrill PA, Venning M, Sambrook P. Computed tomographic peritoneography: CT manifestations in the investigation of leaks and abnormal collections in patients on CAPD. *Nephrol Dial Transplant* 1994; **9:** 1449–1452.

35 Tzamaloukas A, Gibel L, Eisenberg B, Goldman R, Kanig S, Zager P *et al.* Early and late peritoneal leaks in patients on CAPD. *Adv Perit Dial* 1990; **6:** 64–71.

36 Scanziani R, Dozio B, Caimi F, De Rossi N, Magfri F, Surian M. Peritoneography and peritoneal computerized tomography: a new approach to noninfectious complications of CAPD. *Nephrol Dial Transplant* 1992; **7:** 1035–1038.

37 Cochran ST, Do HM, Ronaghi A, Nissenson AR, Kadell BM. Complications of peritoneal dialysis: evaluation with CT peritoneography. *Radiographics* 1997; **17:** 869–878.

38 Twardowski ZJ, Tully R, Nichols W. Computerized tomography CT in the diagnosis of subcutaneous leak sites during continuous ambulatory peritoneal dialysis (CAPD). *Perit Dial Bull* 1984; **4:** 163–166.

39 Schultz S, Harmon T, Nachtnebel K. Computerized tomographic scanning with intraperitoneal contrast enhancement in a CAPD patient with localized edema. *Perit Dial Bull* 1984; **4:** 253–254.

40 Wankowicz Z, Pietrzak B, Przedlacki J. Colloid peritoneoscintigraphy in complications of CAPD. *Perit Dial Bull* 1988; **4:** 138–143.

41 Kopecky R, Frymoyer P, Witanowski L, Thomas F, Wojtaszek J, Reinitz E. Prospective peritoneal scintigraphy in patients beginning continuous ambulatory peritoneal dialysis. *Am J Kidney Dis* 1990; **15:** 228–236.

42 Pannekeet MM, Imholz AL, Struijk DG, Koomen GC, Langedijk MJ, Schouten N *et al.* The standard peritoneal permeability analysis: a tool for the assessment of peritoneal permeability characteristics in CAPD patients. *Kidney Int* 1995; **48:** 866–875.

43 Ho-dac-Pannekeet MM, Atasever B, Struijk DG, Krediet RT. Analysis of ultrafiltration failure in peritoneal dialysis patients by means of standard peritoneal permeability analysis. *Perit Dial Int* 1997; **17:** 144–150.

44 Davies SJ, Phillips L, Russel GI. Peritoneal solute transport predicts survival on CAPD independently of residual renal function. *Nephrol Dial Transplant* 1998; **13:** 962–968.

45 Churchill DN, Thorpe KE, Nolph KD, Keshaviah PR, Pagé D, Oreopoulos DG. Increased peritoneal transport is associated with decreased CAPD technique and patient survival. *J Am Soc Nephrol* 1997; **8:** 189A.

46 Krediet RT, Zuyderhoudt FMJ, Boeschoten EW, Arisz L. Alterations in the peritoneal transport of water and solutes during peritonitis in continuous ambulatory peritoneal dialysis patients. *Eur J Clin Invest* 1987; **17:** 43–52.

47 Gotloib L, Shostak A, Bar-Shella P, Cohen R. Continuous mesothelial injury and regeneration during long-term peritoneal dialysis. *Perit Dial Bull* 1987; **7:** 148–155.

48 Hagmolen W, Ho-dac-Pannekeet MM, Struijk DG, Krediet RT. Mesothelial regeneration after peritonitis in dialysis patients. *J Am Soc Nephrol* 1997; **8:** 180A.

49 Wong TY, Szeto CC, Lai KB, Lai KN, Li PKT. Longitudinal study of peritoneal membrane function in CAPD: relationship with peritonitis and fibrosing factors. *Perit Dial Int* 2000; **20:** 679–686

50 Posthuma N, ter Wee PM, Donker AJM, Peers EM, Oe PL, Verbrugh HA. Icodextrin use in CCPD patients during peritonitis: ultrafiltration and serum disaccharide concentrations. *Nephrol Dial Transplant* 1998; **13:** 2341–2344.

51 Selgas R, Bajo MA, Paiva A, Del Peso G, Diaz C, Aguilera A *et al.* Stability of the peritoneal membrane in long-term peritoneal dialysis patients. *Adv Ren Replace Ther* 1998; **5:** 168–178.

52 Wideroë FE, Smeby LC, Mjøland S, Dahl K, Berg KJ, Aas TW. Long-term changes in transperitoneal water transport during continuous ambulatory peritoneal dialysis. *Nephron* 1984; **38:** 238–247.

53 Selgas R, Fernandez-Reyes MJ, Bosque E, Bajo M-A, Borrego F, Jimenez C *et al.* Functional longevity of the human peritoneum: how long is continuous peritoneal dialysis possible? Results of a prospective medium long-term study. *Am J Kidney Dis* 1994; **23:** 64–73.

54 Davies SJ, Bryan J, Phillips L, Russel GI. Longitudinal changes in peritoneal kinetics: the effects of peritoneal dialysis and peritonitis. *Nephrol Dial Transplant* 1996; **11:** 448–456.

55 Lameire N, Vanholder R, Veys D, Lambert MC, Ringoir S. A longitudinal, five year survey of urea kinetic parameters in CAPD patients. *Kidney Int* 1992; **42:** 426–433.

56 Struijk DG, Krediet RT, Koomen GCM, Boeschoten EW, Hoek FJ, Arisz L. A prospective study of peritoneal transport in CAPD patients. *Kidney Int* 1994; **45:** 1739–1744.

57 Faller B, Lameire N. Evolution of clinical parameters and peritoneal function in a cohort of CAPD patients followed over 7 years. *Nephrol Dial Transplant* 1994; **9:** 280–286.

58 Krediet RT, Boeschoten EW, Zuyderhoudt FMJ, Arisz L. Peritoneal transport characteristics of water, low molecular weight solutes and proteins during long-term continuous ambulatory peritoneal dialysis. *Perit Dial Bull* 1986; **6:** 61–65.

59 Krediet RT, Zemel D, Imholz ALT, Koomen GCM, Struijk DG, Arisz L. Indices of peritoneal permeability and surface area. *Perit Dial Int* 1993; **13(Suppl 2):** S31–S34.

60 Krediet RT, Zemel D, Imholz ALT, Struijk DG. Impact of surface area and permeability on solute clearances. *Perit Dial Int* 1994; **14(Suppl 3):** S70–S77.

61 Krediet RT. Prevention and treatment of peritoneal dialysis membrane failure. *Adv Ren Replace Ther* 1998; **5:** 212.

62 Ho-dac-Pannekeet MM, Hiralall JK, Struijk DG, Krediet RT. Longitudinal follow-up of CA 125 in peritoneal effluent. *Kidney Int* 1997; **51:** 888–893.

63 Imholz ALT, Brown CB, Koomen GCM, Arisz L, Krediet RT. The effect of glucose polymers on water removal and protein clearances during CAPD. *Adv Perit Dial* 1993; **9:** 25–30.

64 Ho-dac-Pannekeet MM, Schouten N, Langendijk MJ, Hiralall JK, de Waart DR, Struijk DG *et al.* Peritoneal transport characteristics with glucose polymer based dialysate. *Kidney Int* 1996; **50:** 979–986.

65 Peers E, Gokal R. Icodextrin: overview of clinical experience. *Perit Dial Int* 1997; **17:** 22–26.

66 Peers E, Gokal R. Icodextrin provides long dwell peritoneal dialysis and maintenance of intraperitoneal volume. *Artif Organs* 1998; **22:** 8–12.

67 Posthuma N, ter Wee PM, Verbrugh HA, Oe PL, Peers E, Sayers J *et al.* Icodextrin instead of glucose during the daytime dwell in CCPD increases ultrafiltration and 24-h dialysis creatinine clearance. *Nephrol Dial Transplant* 1997; **12(Suppl 1):** 550–553.

68 Woodrow G, Stables G, Oldroyd R, Gibson J, Turney JH, Brownjohn AM. Comparison of icodextrin and glucose solutions for the daytime dwell in automated peritoneal dialysis. *Nephrol Dial Transplant* 1999; **14:** 1530–1535.

69 Wilkie ME, Plant MJ, Edwards L, Brown CB. Icodextrin 7.5% dialysate solution (glucose polymer) in patients with ultrafiltration failure: extension of technique survival. *Perit Dial Int* 1997; **17:** 84–87.

70 Krediet RT, Struijk DG, Boeschoten EW, Koomen GCM, Stouthard JML, Hock FJ *et al.* The time course of peritoneal transport kinetics in continuous ambulatory peritoneal dialysis patients who develop sclerosing peritonitis. *Am J Kidney Dis* 1989; **13:** 299–307.

71 Hendriks PM, Ho-dac-Pannekeet MM, van Gulik TM, Struijk DG, Phoa SS, Sie L *et al.* Peritoneal sclerosis in chronic peritoneal dialysis patients: analysis of clinical presentation, risk factors and peritoneal transport kinetics. *Perit Dial Int* 1997; **17:** 136–143.

72 Campbell S, Clarke P, Hawley C, Wigan M, Kerlin P, Butler J *et al.* Sclerosing peritonitis: identification of diagnostic, clinical and radiological features. *Am J Kidney Dis* 1994; **24:** 819–825.

73 Mactier RA. Investigation and management of ultrafiltration failure in CAPD. *Adv Perit Dial* 1991; **7:** 57–62.

74 Abensur H, Romao J, Prado E, Kakehashi E, Sabbaga E, Marcondes M. Use of dextran 70 to estimate peritoneal lymphatic absorption rate in CAPD. *Adv Perit Dial* 1992; **8:** 3–6.

75 Krediet RT, Struijk DG, Koomen GCM, Arisz L. Peritoneal fluid kinetics during CAPD measured with intraperitoneal dextran 70. *ASAIO Trans* 1991; **37:** 662–667.

76 Mujais S. Ultrafiltration management in automated peritoneal dialysis. *Contrib Nephrol* 1999; **129:** 255–266.

77 Mactier RA, Khanna R, Moore H, Twardowski ZJ, Nolph KD. Pharmacological reduction of lymphatic absorption from the peritoneal cavity increases net ultrafiltration and solute clearances in peritoneal dialysis. *Nephron* 1988; **50:** 229–232.

78 Chan PC, Tam SC, Robinson JD, Yu L, Ip MS, Chan CY *et al.* Effect of phosphatidylcholine on ultrafiltration in patients on continuous ambulatory peritoneal dialysis. *Nephron* 1991; **59:** 100–103.

79 Mactier RA, Khanna R, Twardowski ZJ, Moore H, Nolph KD. Influence of phosphatidylcholine on lymphatic absorption during peritoneal dialysis in the rat. *Perit Dial Int* 1988; **8:** 179–186.

80 Struijk DG, van der Reijden HJ, Krediet RT, Koomen GCM, Arisz L. Effect of phosphatidylcholine on peritoneal transport and lymphatic absorption in a CAPD patient with sclerosing peritonitis. *Nephron* 1989; **51:** 577–578.

81 Baranowska-Daca E, Torneli J, Popovich RP, Moncrief JW. Use of bethanechol chloride to increase available ultrafiltration in CAPD. *Adv Perit Dial* 1995; **11:** 69–72.

82 Monquil MC, Imholz AL, Struijk DJ, Krediet R. Does impaired transcellular water transport contribute to net ultrafiltration failure during CAPD? *Perit Dial Int* 1995; **15:** 42–48.

83 Nolph KD, Twardowski ZJ, Popovich RP, Rubin J. Equilibration of peritoneal dialysis solutions during long-dwell exchanges. *J Lab Clin Med* 1979; **93:** 246–256.

84 Chen TW, Khanna R, Moore H, Twardowski ZJ, Nolph KD. Sieving and reflection coefficients for sodium salts and glucose during peritoneal dialysis. *J Am Soc Nephrol* 1991; **2:** 1092–1100.

85 Waniewski J, Heimbürger O, Werynski A, Lindholm B. Aqueous solute concentrations and evaluation of mass transport coefficients in peritoneal dialysis. *Nephrol Dial Transplant* 1992; **7:** 50–56.

86 Zweers MM, Struijk DG, Krediet RT. Correcting sodium sieving for diffusion from the circulation (Abstract). *Perit Dial Int* 1999; **19(Suppl 1):** S12.

87 Krediet R, Ho-dac-Pannekeet MM, Imholz AL, Struijk DG. Icodextrin's effects on peritoneal transport. *Perit Dial Int* 1997; **17:** 35–41.

88 Rippe B, Zakaria ER, Carlsson O. Theoretical analysis of osmotic agents in peritoneal dialysis: what size is an ideal osmotic agent? *Perit Dial Int* 1996; **16(Suppl 1):** S97–S103.

89 Tzamaloukas AH, Saddler MC, Murata GH, Malhotra D, Sena P, Simon D *et al.* Symptomatic fluid retention in patients on continuous peritoneal dialysis. *J Am Soc Nephrol* 1995; **6:** 198–206

90 Gunal AI, Duman S, Ozkahya M, Toz H, Asci G, Akcicek F *et al.* Strict volume control normalizes hypertension in peritoneal dialysis patients. *Am J Kidney Dis* 2001; **37:** 588–593.

91 van Olden RW, Guchelaar HJ, Struijk DG, Krediet RT, Arisz L. Acute effects of high-dose furosemide on residual renal function in CAPD patients. *Perit Dial Int* 2003; **23:** 339–347.

92 Medcalf JF, Harris KP, Walls J. Role of diuretics in the preservation of residual renal function in patients on CAPD. *Kidney Int* 2001; **59:** 1128–1133.

93 Li PKT, Chow KM, Wong TY, Leung CB, Szeto CC. Effects of an angiotensin converting enzyme inhibitor on residual renal function in patients receiving peritoneal dialysis: a prospective randomized study. *Ann Intern Med* 2003; **139:** 105–112.

94 Suzuki H, Kanno Y, Sugahara S, Okada H, Nakamoto H. Effects of an angiotensin II receptor blocker, valsartan, on residual renal function in patients on CAPD. *Am J Kidney Dis* 2004; **43:** 1056–1064.

95 Williams JD, Topley N, Craig KJ, Mackenzie RK, Pischetsrieder M, Lage C *et al.* The Euro-Balance Trial: the effect of a new biocompatible peritoneal dialysis fluid (balance) on the peritoneal membrane. *Kidney Int* 2004; **66:** 408–418.

96 Van Biesen W, Vanholder R, Veys N, Lameire N. Improving salt balance in peritoneal dialysis patients. *Perit Dial Int* 2005; **25(Suppl 3):** S73–S75.

97 Rodriguez-Carmona A, Perez-Fontan M, Garca-Naveiro R, Villaverde P, Peteiro J. Compared time profiles of ultrafiltration, sodium removal, and renal function in incident CAPD and automated peritoneal dialysis patients. *Am J Kidney Dis* 2004; **44:** 132–145.

98 Bro S, Bjorner JB, Tofte-Jensen P, Klem S, Almtoft B, Danielsen H *et al.* A prospective, randomized multicenter study comparing APD and CAPD treatment. *Perit Dial Int* 1999; **19:** 526–533.

99 Rodriguez AM, Diaz NV, Cubillo LP, Plana JT, Riscos MA, Delgado RM *et al.* Automated peritoneal dialysis: a Spanish multicentre study. *Nephrol Dial Transplant* 1998; **13:** 2335–2340.

100 Konings CJ, Kooman JP, Schonck M, Gladziwa U, Wirtz J, van den Wall Bake AW *et al.* Effect of icodextrin on volume status, blood pressure and echocardiographic parameters: a randomized study. *Kidney Int* 2003; **63:** 1556–1563.

101 Posthuma N, ter Wee PM, Donker AJ, Oe PL, Peers EM, Verbrugh HA. Assessment of the effectiveness, safety, and biocompatibility of icodextrin in automated peritoneal dialysis. The Dextrin in APD in Amsterdam (DIANA) Group. *Perit Dial Int* 2000; **20(Suppl 2):** S106–S113.

102 Davies SJ, Woodrow G, Donovan K, Plum J, Williams P, Johansson AC *et al.* Icodextrin improves the fluid status of peritoneal dialysis patients: results of a double-blind randomized controlled trial. *J Am Soc Nephrol* 2003; **14:** 2338–2344.

103 Wolfson M, Piraino B, Hamburger RJ, Morton AR, Icodextrin Study Group. A randomized controlled trial to evaluate the efficacy and safety of icodextrin in peritoneal dialysis. *Am J Kidney Dis* 2002; **40:** 1055–1065.

104 Plum J, Gentile S, Verger C, Brunkhorst R, Bahner U, Faller B *et al.* Efficacy and safety of a 7.5% icodextrin peritoneal dialysis solution in patients treated with automated peritoneal dialysis. *Am J Kidney Dis* 2002; **39:** 862–871.

105 Mistry CD, Gokal R, Peers E. A randomized multicenter clinical trial comparing isosmolar icodextrin with hyperosmolar glucose solutions

in CAPD. MIDAS Study Group. Multicenter Investigation of Icodextrin in Ambulatory Peritoneal Dialysis. *Kidney Int* 1994; **46:** 496–503.

106 Finkelstein F, Healy H, Abu-Alfa A, Ahmad S, Brown F, Gehr T *et al.* Superiority of icodextrin compared with 4.25% dextrose for peritoneal ultrafiltration. *J Am Soc Nephrol* 2005; **16:** 546–554.

107 Posthuma N, ter Wee PM, Verbrugh HA, Oe PL, Peers E, Sayers J *et al.* Icodextrin instead of glucose during the daytime dwell in CCPD increases ultrafiltration and 24-h dialysate creatinine clearance. *Nephrol Dial Transplant* 1997; **12:** 550–553.

108 Dallas F, Jenkins SB, Wilkie ME. Enhanced ultrafiltration using 7.5% icodextrin/1.36% glucose combination dialysate: a pilot study. *Perit Dial Int* 2004; **24:** 542–546.

109 Leypoldt JK, Charney DI, Cheung AK, Naprestek CL, Akin BH, Shockley TR. Ultrafiltration and solute kinetics using low sodium peritoneal dialysate. *Kidney Int* 1995; **48:** 1959–1966.

110 Amici G, Virga G, Da Rin G, Teodori T, Calzavara P, Bocci C. Low sodium concentration solution in normohydrated CAPD patients. *Adv Perit Dial* 1995; **11:** 78–82.

111 Sjoland JA, Smith Pedersen R, Jespersen J, Gram J. Intraperitoneal heparin reduces peritoneal permeability and increases ultrafiltration in peritoneal dialysis patients. *Nephrol Dial Transplant* 2004; **19:** 1264–1268.

112 Moberly JB, Sorkin M, Kucharski A, Ogle K, Mongoven J, Skoufos L *et al.* Effects of intraperitoneal hyaluronan on peritoneal fluid and solute transport in peritoneal dialysis patients. *Perit Dial Int* 2003; **23:** 63–73.

113 el-Sherif AK, Rizkalla NH, Essawy MH, el-Gohary AM. Minoxidil selectively improves peritoneal ultrafiltration. *Perit Dial Int* 1996; **16(Suppl 1):** S91–S94.

114 Hasbargen JA, Hasbargen BJ, Fortenbery EJ. Effect of intraperitoneal neostigmine on peritoneal transport characteristics in CAPD. *Kidney Int* 1992; **42:** 1398–1400.

115 Kalra OP, Aggarwal HK, Mahajan SK, Seth RK. Effect of vasodilator and surface active drugs on the efficacy of peritoneal dialysis. *J Assoc Physicians India* 1992; **40:** 233–236.

116 Favazza A, Motanaro D, Messa P, Antonucci F, Gropuzzo M, Mioni G. Peritoneal clearances in hypertensive CAPD patients after oral administration of clonidine, enalapril, and nifedipine. *Perit Dial Int* 1992; **12:** 287–291.

117 Li PKT, Law MC, Chow KM, Chan WK, Szeto CC, Cheng YL *et al.* Comparison of clinical outcome and ease of handling in two double-bag systems in continuous ambulatory peritoneal dialysis: a prospective randomized controlled multi-center study. *Am J Kidney Dis* 2002; **40:** 373–380.

118 Lee HY, Park HC, Seo BJ, Do JY, Yun SR, Song HY *et al.* Superior patient survival for continuous ambulatory peritoneal dialysis patients treated with a peritoneal dialysis fluid with neutral pH and low glucose degradation product concentration (balance). *Perit Dial Int* 2005; **25:** 248–255.

119 Van Biesen W, Boer W, De Greve B, Dequidt C, Vijt D, Faict D *et al.* A randomized clinical trial with a 0.6% amino acid/1.4% glycerol peritoneal dialysis solution. *Perit Dial Int* 2004; **24:** 222–230.

120 Li FK, Chan LY, Woo JC, Ho SK, Lo WK, Lai KN *et al.* A 3-year, prospective, randomized, controlled study on amino acid dialysate in patients on CAPD. *Am J Kidney Dis* 2003; **42:** 173–183.

121 Plum J, Erren C, Fieseler C, Kirchgessner J, Passlick-Deetjen J, Grabensee B. An amino acid-based peritoneal dialysis fluid buffered with bicarbonate versus glucose/bicarbonate and glucose/lactate solutions:

an intraindividual randomized study. *Perit Dial Int* 1999; **19**: 418–428.

122 Schmitt CP, Haraldsson B, Doetschmann R, Zimmering M, Greiner C, Boswald M *et al.* Effects of pH-neutral, bicarbonate-buffered dialysis fluid on peritoneal transport kinetics in children. *Kidney Int* 2002; **61**: 1527–1536.

123 Williams JD, Topley N, Craig KJ, Mackenzie RK, Pischetsrieder M, Lage C *et al.* The Euro-Balance Trial: the effect of a new biocompatible peritoneal dialysis fluid (balance) on the peritoneal membrane. *Kidney Int* 2004; **66**: 408–418.

124 Tranaeus A. A long-term study of a bicarbonate/lactate-based peritoneal dialysis solution–clinical benefits. The Bicarbonate/Lactate Study Group. *Perit Dial Int* 2000; **20**: 516–523.

125 Miranda B, Selgas R, Celadilla O, Munoz J, Sanchez Sicilia L. Peritoneal resting and heparinization as an effective treatment for ultrafiltration failure in patients on CAPD. *Contrib Nephrol* 1991; **89**: 199–204.

126 De Alvaro F, Castro MJ, Dapena F, Bajo MA, Fernandez-Reyes MJ, Romero JR *et al.* Peritoneal resting is beneficial in peritoneal hyperpermeability and ultrafiltration failure. *Adv Perit Dial* 1993; **9**: 56–61.

127 Burkhart J, Stallard R. Result of peritoneal membrane (PM) resting (R) on dialysate (d) CA125 levels and PET results. *Perit Dial Int* 1997; **17(Suppl 1)**: S5. (Abstract.)

128 Ho-dac-Pannekeet MM, Struijk DG, Krediet R. Improvement of transcellular water transport by treatment with glucose free dialysate in patients with ultrafiltration failure. *Nephrol Dial Transplant* 1996; **11**: 255.

46 Impact of Peritoneal Dialysis Solutions on Outcomes

David W. Johnson[1] & John D. Williams[2]

[1]Department of Renal Medicine, University of Queensland at Princess Alexandra Hospital, Brisbane, Australia
[2]Department of Nephrology, Cardiff University, Heath Park, Cardiff, United Kingdom

Introduction

Over the past 25 years, peritoneal dialysis (PD) has become an established and successful form of renal replacement therapy for patients with stage 5 (end-stage) chronic kidney disease. Most published cohort studies suggest that the medium-term survival (up to 3–4 years) of patients treated with PD is at least comparable [1,2], and possibly superior [3,4], to that of patients receiving hemodialysis (HD). PD also potentially offers a number of other important clinical advantages over HD, including better preservation of residual renal function, reduced erythropoietic stimulatory agent and blood transfusion requirements, decreased risk of blood-borne infections (such as hepatitis B and C), improved quality of life, enhanced treatment satisfaction, preservation of vascular access sites, and improved subsequent renal allograft function [5,6].

However, the major drawback of PD is its limited technique survival. According to the Australian and New Zealand Dialysis and Transplant (ANZDATA) Registry, the crude technique failure rate for PD is 21.7/100 patient-years and only 4% of patients experience at least 5 years of continuous PD [7]. Even after censoring for kidney transplantation, the median technique survival on peritoneal dialysis is 2.5 years. Approximately half of all technique failure episodes are due to either peritonitis (27%) or peritoneal membrane failure culminating in inadequate small solute clearance and/or impaired ultrafiltration (23%) [7]. A large body of basic research in animal models and peritoneal cell culture systems has suggested that a major contributor to the high technique failure rate is the bioincompatible nature of conventional PD fluid. Such fluids may have a negative impact on host defense as well as having a profibrotic effect on the peritoneal membrane [8–10]. Conventional PD fluids are considered "unphysiological," based on their acidic pH (5.0–5.8), high lactate concentrations (30–40 mmol/L), high osmolality (320–520 mOsm/kg), high glucose concentrations (31–236 mmol/L), and contamination by glucose degradation products (GDP) generated during the heat sterilization process [11]. Such solutions reduce the viability and growth of peritoneal mesothelial cells and fibroblasts in vitro, alter the turnover of structural collagen, and modify the homeostatic balance of cytokines and growth factors [10,12,13]. The viability and function of peritoneal phagocytic cells, such as macrophages, are also impaired by standard peritoneal fluids [11,12]. Moreover, experimental and clinical exposure of the peritoneal membrane to conventional PD solutions causes significant histopathological changes over time, including loss of the surface mesothelial cell layer, thickening of the submesothelial compact zone, and the development of a progressive vasculopathy [14,15]. Most of these adverse effects of dialysate on the peritoneal membrane appear to be accounted for by acidic pH and high concentrations of GDPs, because they were largely avoided in in vivo studies by the use of neutral-buffered, low-GDP fluids [10,11,16,17]. In addition to their direct cytotoxicity and stimulation of inflammatory cytokine production, GDPs promote the formation and deposition of advanced glycation end products (AGEs) in the peritoneal membrane, which in turn correlates with peritoneal membrane fibrosis and histopathology [18,19].

Recently, manufacturers of PD fluids have developed more biocompatible solutions, consisting of neutral pH, low-GDP, bicarbonate- or lactate-buffered solutions, in order to reduce membrane damage associated with PD. These fluids have consistently been shown in both in vitro and in vivo animal studies to better preserve peritoneal membrane structure and function compared with the less expensive, traditional fluids [10–12,20]. These fluids may also offer additional systemic benefits by reducing inflammation, lowering circulating AGE, and preserving residual renal function. However, whether these experimental benefits translate into improved outcomes for patients on PD needs to be demonstrated to justify the additional costs of the newer solutions. In addition to these biocompatible solutions, manufacturers have also developed "glucose alternative" solutions to improve PD as a therapy. So far, the available evidence indicates that fluid status, body composition, and diabetic control can be manipulated.

Additional peritoneal membrane benefits may be realized as a result of avoidance of glucose and AGEs.

The aim of this chapter is to review the impact of the newer PD solutions on clinical outcomes, based on the currently available randomized controlled trials.

Neutral pH, lactate-buffered, low-GDP fluids

The development of multicompartment bag systems, in which alkaline and acidic fluid compartments are kept separate, has permitted the sterilization of glucose at very low pH with greatly reduced GDP formation but the formation of neutral or near-neutral pH final dialysis solutions following mixing of the compartments prior to instilling into the peritoneal cavity. A summary of the randomized controlled clinical trials involving neutral pH, lactate-buffered, low-GDP, multichambered PD fluids is provided in Table 46.1.

Williams *et al.* [21] conducted a multicenter, open-label, randomized crossover study of conventional, acidic, lactate-buffered fluid (Stay-safe; Fresenius Medical Care, Bad Homburg, Germany) with neutral pH, lactate-buffered, low-GDP fluid (Balance; Fresenius Medical Care, Bad Homburg, Germany) in 86 prevalent continuous ambulatory PD (CAPD) patients from 22 centers in 11 European countries. The participants underwent a 4-week run-in phase on conventional fluid after which they were randomized in a

Table 46.1 Characteristics of the populations and interventions in the randomized trials of biocompatible solutions in PD.

Study ID [reference]	Interventions	No. of patients	Follow-up
Neutral pH, lactate-buffered, low-GDP vs. acidic pH, lactate-buffered, high-GDP fluids			
Williams [21]	Balance vs. Stay-safe	86 CAPD	24 wks
Rippe [22]	Gambrosol-Trio vs. Gamrosol	80 CAPD	2 yrs
Zeier [23]	Gambrosol-Trio vs. Gamrosol	21 CAPD	16 wks
Neutral pH, bicarbonate (± lactate)-buffered, low-GDP vs. acidic pH, lactate-buffered, high-GDP fluids			
Cooker [29]	Physioneal (25 mmol/L bicarbonate/15 mmol/L lactate) vs. Dianeal	92 CAPD	6 mos
Jones [30]	Physioneal (25 mmol/L bicarbonate/15 mmol/L lactate) vs. Dianeal	106 CAPD	6 mos
Fuesshoeller [31]	Physioneal (25 mmol/L bicarbonate/15 mmol/L lactate) vs. Dianeal	14 APD	12 mos
Mactier [33]	Bicarbonate/lactate (25/15 mmol/L) vs. bicarbonate (38 mmol/L) vs. Dianeal	18 CAPD	3 days
Tranaeus [35]	Physioneal (25 mmol/L bicarbonate/15 mmol/L lactate) vs. Dianeal	106 CAPD	12 mos
Carrasco [36]	Bicarbonate/lactate (25/15 mmol/L) vs. lactate (35 mmol/L)	31 CAPD	3 mos
Coles [39]	Bicarbonate/lactate (25/15 mmol/L) vs. bicarbonate (38 mmol/L) vs. lactate (40 mmol/L)	59 CAPD	2 mos
Feriani [38]	Bicavera (bicarbonate 34 mmol/L) vs. lactate (35 mmol/L)	123 CAPD	6 mos
Haas [32]	Bicavera (bicarbonate 34 mmol/L) vs. lactate (35 mmol/L)	28 APD	24 wks
Icodextrin vs. glucose exchanges			
Mistry [47]	7.5% Icodextrin vs. 1.36% or 3.86% glucose	209 CAPD	6 mos
Posthuma [48]	7.5% Icodextrin vs. variable glucose strengths	23 APD	6 mos
Plum [49]	7.5% Icodextrin vs. 2.27% glucose	39 APD	12 wks
Wolfson [50]	7.5% Icodextrin vs. 2.5% glucose	175 CAPD/APD	1 yr
Gokal [55]	7.5% Icodextrin vs. 1.36% or 3.86% glucose	23 CAPD	6 mos
Konings [58]	7.5% Icodextrin vs. 1.36% glucose	40 CAPD/APD	4 mos
Davies [59]	7.5% Icodextrin vs. 2.27% glucose	50 CAPD/APD	6 mos
Finkelstein [54]	7.5% Icodextrin vs. 4.25% dextrose	92	2 weeks
Selby [81]	7.5% Icodextrin vs. 1.36% glucose	8	2 days
Guo [62]	7.5% Icodextrin vs. 2.5% glucose	93	13 weeks
Posthuma [73]	7.5% Icodextrin vs. 2.5% glucose	38 CCPD	2 years
Ota [56]	7.5% Icodextrin vs. 1.36% glucose	18 CAPD	6 weeks
Amino acid dialysates versus glucose exchanges			
Qamar [79]	1.1% amino acids vs. 1.36% glucose (1 exchange daily)	7 CAPD	3 months
Misra [76]	1.1% amino acids vs. 1.36% glucose (1 exchange daily)	18 CAPD	6 months
Jones .(77)	1.1% amino acids vs. glucose (1 exchange daily)	134 CAPD	3 months
Qamar [80]	1.1% amino acids vs. glucose (1 exchange daily)	7 CCPD	3 months
Li [75]	1.1% amino acids vs. glucose (1 exchange daily)	60 CAPD	3 years
Tjiong [78]	1.1% amino acids vs. variable (1.36–3.86%) glucose	8 APD	7 days
Van Biesen [82]	0.6% amino acids/1.4% glycerol vs. variable glucose (1 exchange daily)	10 CAPD	3 months
Glucose-sparing regimens			
Le Poole [37]	1 x Nutrineal, 1 x Extraneal, 2 x Physioneal (NEPP) vs 4 x Dianeal	63 CAPD	30 weeks

1:1 ratio to the control versus intervention groups. After 12 weeks of monitoring in this first treatment phase, the groups switched therapies and were observed for a further 12 weeks. The method of allocation concealment was not explicitly stated. A total of 71 patients with complete measurements were included in the per protocol analysis (18% dropout rate). The primary outcome measure was the concentration of CA125, a possible marker of mesothelial cell mass and/or viability, in the dialysate effluent at 12 weeks and was significantly higher in the low-GDP fluid group. This was accompanied by higher effluent levels of procollagen peptide, lower levels of hyaluronan, and unchanged levels of vascular endothelial growth factor and tumor necrosis factor-α. Patients exposed to low-GDP fluids were also observed to have falls in circulating GDP (carboxymethyl-lysine and imidazoline) levels. Clinical measurements demonstrated increases in renal urea and creatinine clearances, increases in Kt/V, increases in urine volumes, and decreases in peritoneal ultrafiltration volumes (associated with an increased dialysate/plasma creatinine ratio). Peritonitis incidence was comparable in both groups, although the study was inadequately powered to detect a difference in this or other clinical end points. The study was significantly limited by its short duration, small sample size, use of surrogate markers, the possibility of co-intervention bias in view of the open-label nature of the study, and the potential for informative censoring as a result of the 18% dropout rate over 24 weeks.

Similar findings were reported in an open-label, parallel design, randomized controlled trial of conventional, acidic, lactate-buffered fluid (Gambrosol; Gambro, Lund, Sweden) with pH 6.5, lactate-buffered, low-GDP fluid (Gambrosol-Trio; Gambro, Lund, Sweden) in 80 CAPD patients followed for 2 years [22]. Although only 13 patients completed the 2-year study (84% dropout), the principal findings were that patients receiving low-GDP fluid treatment exhibited significantly higher dialysate CA 125, procollagen-1-C-terminal peptide, and procollagen-3-N-terminal peptide and significantly lower concentrations of hyaluronon in the overnight effluent. The new fluid did not significantly influence either the frequency of peritonitis or peritoneal transport characteristics compared with conventional fluid, but the study was not adequately powered for these end points, and baseline data were limited. Zeier *et al.* [23] also conducted a randomized crossover trial of Gambrosol versus Gambrosol-Trio over two consecutive observation periods of 8 weeks each in 21 stable, prevalent CAPD patients. They reported a significant 3.5-fold increase in dialysate effluent CA125 concentrations within 4 weeks of Gambrosol-Trio exposure.

To date, there have been no randomized controlled trials of neutral pH, lactate-buffered, low-GDP fluids versus conventional fluids that have been adequately powered to assess "hard" or patient-level clinical end points. A recent, large, retrospective, observational cohort study in Korea described superior survival in 611 patients treated with Balance compared with 551 patients using standard Stay-safe solution (74% vs. 62% at 28 months; $P = 0.032$) [24]. The hazard ratio for mortality was 0.75 (95% confidence interval, 0.56–0.99) in the Balance group, after adjust-

ment for age, gender, and diabetes mellitus in a multivariate Cox proportional hazards model analysis. A follow-up report of 1909 incident PD patients, in which prescription of low-GDP solutions reached between 70 and 80% by the year 2003, also demonstrated superior patient survival in patients treated with low-GDP fluids [25]. The major limitations of this study were the lack of stratification or statistical adjustment for cardiovascular disease, hypertension, and socio-economic status and potential selection bias with residual confounding. This is probable given that patients treated with low-GDP solutions were significantly more likely to be younger and treated at large PD centers than those patients who received standard PD solutions. There may also have been a center effect bias, given that 25 centers exclusively contributed Balance patients, 25 exclusively contributed conventional fluid patients, and the remaining 33 contributed a mixture of Balance and Staysafe patients. An open-label, multicenter, phase IV, randomized controlled trial of Gambrosol Trio ($n = 43$) versus Gambrosol ($n = 26$) was recently presented (Diurest study) [26]. Although not yet published, the investigators reported a significantly slower rate of residual renal function decline in those treated with Gambrosol Trio. However, this study was potentially confounded by a substantially higher glucose usage, higher initial weight loss, and appreciable initial blood pressure drop in the control group, raising the possibility that factors other than the type of fluid used (e.g. volume depletion) may have accounted for the differential decline in renal function between the two study groups. In contrast, Fan *et al.* [27] recently presented an abstract reporting results of a controlled trial of 120 incident PD patients randomized to receive Balance or conventional fluid (Stay-safe) for a mean follow-up period of 11.3 months. No differences were observed between the two groups in residual renal function, peritonitis, peritoneal transport characteristics, or the primary composite end point of time to death or transfer to HD. A large, multicenter, prospective, randomized controlled trial of Balance versus Staysafe in 420 incident PD patients followed for 2 years is currently underway in Australia, New Zealand, and Singapore (balANZ trial) [28]. The primary outcome measure will be rate of decline of residual renal function (analysis of covariance), with secondary analysis of time to anuria, patient survival, technique survival, peritoneal transport characteristics, measures of dialysis adequacy, and ultrafiltration. In the meantime, there is insufficient clinical evidence to draw conclusions about the relative efficacy and safety of neutral pH, lactate-buffered, low-GDP fluids compared with conventional PD fluids.

Neutral pH, bicarbonate ($\pm$ lactate)-buffered, low-GDP fluids

As with the lactate-buffered, low-GDP solutions, many clinical trials involving bicarbonate-buffered, reduced-GDP fluids have been small, short term, and primarily focused on unvalidated surrogate end points of dialysate effluent markers. Cooker *et al.* [29] demonstrated significant reductions in dialysate effluent concentrations of interleukin-6 and vascular endothelial growth factor within 3 months in 61 patients randomly allocated to neutral pH, bicarbonate/lactate-buffered, reduced-GDP fluid (Physioneal; Baxter Healthcare) compared with 31 patients receiving conventional PD fluid (Dianeal; Baxter Healthcare). Similar results have also been described from other studies [30–32].

The most consistent clinical benefit demonstrated for bicarbonate-buffered fluids is a reduction of inflow pain [31,33–35]. Mactier *et al.* [33] conducted a double-blind, randomized, crossover trial to determine the effects of bicarbonate (38 mM)-containing and bicarbonate (25 mM)-lactate (15 mM)-containing PD solutions on infusion pain in patients who experienced inflow pain with conventional lactate (40 mM) solution. For all pain variables assessed, the bicarbonate-lactate solution was more effective than the bicarbonate solution in alleviating pain. Similar findings have been reported in open-label studies [31,34,35].

In some studies, bicarbonate/lactate-buffered solutions have also been found to be associated with better control of metabolic acidosis compared with lactate-buffered solutions [36,37]. Carrasco *et al.* [36] reported a significant increase in venous plasma bicarbonate concentration by 3.1 mmol/L (95% confidence interval, 1.6–4.8) from a baseline level of 23.0 mmol/L during treatment with the bicarbonate-lactate solution. The number of acidotic patients (venous plasma bicarbonate of <24 mmol/L) was statistically significantly reduced at every treatment period visit in the bicarbonate-lactate group ($P < 0.05$). Similarly, a prospective crossover study of 74 patients allocated to four daily exchanges of standard PD solution (Dianeal) versus a glucose-sparing regimen (two exchanges Physioneal, one exchange Extraneal, and one exchange Nutrineal) observed that the latter regimen was associated with significantly higher plasma bicarbonate levels [37]. In contrast, three other randomized controlled trials did not find any significant differences in acid–base status between patients treated with bicarbonate-lactate solutions versus conventional fluids [35,38,39].

Conflicting results have also been reported for peritoneal ultrafiltration, with two studies (different fluids) observing increased drainage volumes with bicarbonate-lactate solutions [35,40] while other investigations found no alteration in ultrafiltration [32,36–39].

None of the trials to date have had sufficient samples sizes or follow-up times to evaluate the impact of bicarbonate/lactate-buffered, low-GDP solutions on peritonitis rates, residual renal function decline, technique survival, or patient survival. A prospective registry analysis of PD patients treated with alternative PD solutions in 12 countries observed that bicarbonate/lactate solutions were associated with decreased peritonitis duration and rate compared with standard PD fluids [9]. However, these results were likely to have been significantly influenced by selection bias.

The relative importance of the buffer (lactate versus bicarbonate) to peritoneal membrane biocompatibility has not yet been addressed by randomized controlled trials. A prospective, nonrandomized trial of 34 mmol/L bicarbonate-buffered versus 35 mmol/L lactate-buffered PD fluid in 36 patients over 12 months showed comparable peritoneal clearances and correction of metabolic acidosis between the two groups but better preservation of residual renal function in the patients receiving bicarbonate-buffered fluid [41]. However, this trial may have been confounded by selection bias since patients nonrandomly allocated to the bicarbonate group were significantly more likely to be female and have lower peritoneal ultrafiltration values at baseline. There is currently a randomized controlled study under way in which 60 pediatric PD patients will be randomly assigned to receive either lactate-containing Balance solution or the bicarbonate-buffered Bicavera solution for a period of 10 months to determine whether these fluids evoke any differences in preservation of peritoneal transport characteristics [13].

Icodextrin

Icodextrin is a starch-derived, high-molecular-weight glucose polymer that was first used as an osmotic alternative to glucose for PD in the 1980s [42]. Since that time, there has been increasing interest in the use of icodextrin-containing PD solutions because of their demonstrated ability to induce sustained peritoneal ultrafiltration. Fluid removal is achieved by colloidal, rather than crystalline, osmotic pressure and is most pronounced over prolonged (12–16 h) dwells [43]. There is also emerging evidence that this iso-osmotic solution may be less damaging to the peritoneal membrane than glucose-based dialysates (reviewed in references 44 to 46).

To date, there have been a number of open-label, randomized controlled trials of the glucose polymer, which have demonstrated that icodextrin is comparable to hypertonic (3.86%) glucose for net peritoneal ultrafiltration and small solute clearance during long (8–16 h) dwells (Table 46.1). The first of these investigations was the Multicentre Investigation of Icodextrin in Ambulatory Peritoneal Dialysis Study (MIDAS) [47]. In this multicenter trial, 209 stable patients from 11 centers (representing approximately 5% of the UK CAPD population) were randomly allocated to receive an overnight exchange with either 7.5% icodextrin ($n = 106$) or conventional (1.36 or 3.86%) glucose solutions. A total of 138 patients completed the 6-month study (67 icodextrin, 71 control). An intention-to-treat analysis demonstrated that the mean overnight peritoneal ultrafiltration achieved with icodextrin was equivalent to that of 3.86% glucose at 8 h (510 ± 48 vs. 448 ± 60 mL; $P = 0.44$). Following a 12-h dwell, icodextrin tended to promote a greater degree of fluid removal (552 ± 44 vs. 414 ± 78 mL), but the difference just failed to achieve statistical significance ($P = 0.06$). There were no reported adverse clinical effects over the period of the study. A second, smaller, single-center, randomized controlled trial in continuous cycling PD (CCPD) patients compared the ultrafiltration potential of icodextrin ($n = 23$) with that of variable glucose strengths ($n = 19$) during the daytime dwell (14–15 h) [48]. Daytime ultrafiltration volumes were significantly higher in icodextrin-treated than glucose-treated patients at 3 months (168 ± 57 vs. 42 ± 139 mL, respectively; $P < 0.05$), 6 months (218 ± 57 vs. 36 ± 115 mL; $P < 0.05$), and 9 months (224 ± 71 vs. -30 ± 87 mL; $P < 0.05$). Two other randomized controlled trials demonstrated that icodextrin promoted significantly higher ultrafiltration volumes than 2.5% glucose [49,50]. A subsequent, short-duration, randomized, sequential study of 2.27% glucose, 3.86% glucose, and 7.5% icodextrin during the long daytime dwell (13.8–15.5 h) in 17 CCPD patients confirmed that median ultrafiltration volumes were comparable between icodextrin and 3.86% glucose (260 vs. 100 mL; P not significant) but were significantly greater than 2.27% glucose (-190 mL; $P < 0.005$) [51]. Importantly, the difference in daytime ultrafiltration between icodextrin and 3.86% glucose was positively correlated with the dialysate/plasma creatinine ratio, suggesting that icodextrin may achieve superior fluid removal compared with glucose-based dialysates in subjects with higher peritoneal membrane transport characteristics. This finding was supported by several other transport studies [52,53]. A recent randomized controlled trial demonstrated that icodextrin was superior to 4.25% glucose for long dwell fluid removal in high and high-average transporters [54].

Several randomized controlled trials have also demonstrated that icodextrin offers an ultrafiltration advantage compared with glucose-based dialysates in patients with enhanced membrane permeability due to acute peritonitis. In the MIDAS study [55], 23 patients in the glucose group and 22 patients in the icodextrin group experienced CAPD-associated peritonitis. During these infective episodes, mean overnight ultrafiltration volumes decreased slightly from 218 ± 354 mL to 185 ± 218 mL in the glucose group (P not significant) but significantly increased in the icodextrin group, from 570 ± 146 mL to 723 ± 218 mL ($P < 0.01$). Similar findings have been reported by Ota *et al.* [56]. A randomized study in CCPD patients [57] found that mean daytime and total 24-h ultrafiltration fell significantly during peritonitis episodes by approximately 600 mL but were well-maintained in icodextrin-treated patients. The mean differences in daytime and 24-h fluid removal between the two groups exceeded 1000 mL.

Although augmented peritoneal fluid removal by icodextrin should intuitively help to correct fluid overload in PD patients, this outcome has been poorly studied. Konings *et al.* [58] randomly allocated 40 PD patients to icodextrin or 1.36% glucose during the long dwell. The use of icodextrin was associated with a significant reduction in extracellular water and left ventricular mass. Davies *et al.* [59] also reported significant improvements in fluid status in high transporters treated with icodextrin compared with 2.27% glucose. These findings, together with those of Finkelstein *et al.* [54], support the recommendations of the ISPD Ad Hoc Committee on Ultrafiltration Management in Peritoneal Dialysis that icodextrin be used for the long dwell in high transporter patients with a net peritoneal ultrafiltration of less than 400 mL/4 h [60].

Clinical experience with icodextrin in children is extremely limited. The best available study is a sequential trial by de Boer and colleagues [61] in which 11 children underwent peritoneal dwells with 1.36% glucose, 7.5% icodextrin, or 3.86% glucose for 12 h. The ultrafiltration achieved with icodextrin was comparable with that of 3.86% glucose but significantly greater than with 1.36%

glucose. No significant adverse effects were observed over a subsequent 6-week period of polyglucose administration.

Apart from the well-documented effects of icodextrin on peritoneal ultrafiltration, polyglucose solution has also been shown in one randomized controlled trial to promote clinically important improvements in quality of life scores within 13 weeks of treatment commencement compared with glucose solutions [62]. Although there are nonrandomized studies suggesting that polyglucose may additionally prolong PD technique survival [63–65], there is no high-level clinical evidence to support this.

Several *in vitro* and *ex vivo* studies have suggested that icodextrin may offer improved peritoneal membrane biocompatibility compared with conventional glucose-based dialysates by virtue of decreased glucose exposure, iso-osmolarity, and reduced carbonyl stress [66,67]. Short-term clinical studies involving generally small numbers of patients have demonstrated that dialytic small solute clearances and peritoneal transport characteristics remain well-preserved on icodextrin therapy for up to 24 months of follow-up [47,48,68–72]. Moreover, a prospective, open-label, randomized controlled trial of 38 CCPD patients in two centers showed that dialysate effluent concentrations of a variety of peritoneal membrane markers (CA125, interleukin-8, carboxy-terminal propeptide of type I procollagen, and amino-terminal propeptide of type III procollagen) did not differ between glucose- and icodextrin-treated patients over a 2-year period [73]. However, there have been no longer-term clinical studies comparing the relative effects of icodextrin and glucose on peritoneal membrane structure or function. Icodextrin use is associated with an increased incidence of rash, mild hyponatremia, mild elevations of plasma alkaline phosphatase levels, and elevation of plasma oligosaccharide concentrations, leading to overestimation of blood sugar measurements based on the glucose deshydrogenase pyrroloquinolenequinone method [50,74].

Amino acid dialysates

Dialysates using amino acids as an alternative osmotic agent to glucose may be more biocompatible by virtue of their more physiological pH (6.7), relatively low osmolality (365 mOsm/kg), and avoidance of glucose and GDPs. However, most available studies have not been of sufficient size or duration to demonstrate any clinically important effects on peritonitis rates, peritoneal transport characteristics, technique survival, or patient survival (Table 46.1). The largest trial to date involved 60 malnourished CAPD patients randomly allocated to replace one exchange daily with amino acid dialysate (Nutrineal; Baxter Healthcare) or to continue with dextrose dialysate (Dianeal; Baxter Healthcare) over a 3-year follow-up period [75]. The composite nutritional indices, daily ultrafiltration volumes, small solute clearances, and survival rates did not differ significantly between the two groups.

Some studies have suggested that malnourished PD patients may derive modest nutritional benefit from such solutions [76–78]. However, other randomized controlled trials have failed to

Table 46.2 Evidence ratings and recommendations for dialysate solutions in PD.

Intervention	Existing systematic reviews[a]	Overall evidence rating[b]			Very low	Comment	Recommendation[c]			Comment
		High	Moderate	Low			I	II	III	
Neutral pH, lactate-buffered, low-GDP vs. acidic pH, lactate-buffered, high-GDP fluids	None			?		Few RCTs, small sample size, short duration, suboptimal methodological quality, surrogate outcomes of questionable clinical relevance			?	Further trials with patient-level outcomes required
Neutral pH, bicarbonate (±lactate)-buffered, low-GDP vs. acidic pH, lactate-buffered, high-GDP fluids	None			?		Few RCTs, small sample size, short duration, suboptimal methodological quality, mostly surrogate outcomes of questionable clinical relevance		?		Neutral pH, bicarbonate (±lactate)-buffered, low-GDP fluids appear useful for ameliorating infusion pain; further trials required to examine impact on other patient-level outcomes (peritonitis, peritoneal transport characteristics, technique survival, patient survival)
Icodextrin vs. glucose exchanges	None		?			Moderate number of RCTs, small to moderate sample sizes, suboptimal methodological quality, consistent findings	?			Icodextrin promotes superior fluid removal compared with glucose exchanges, especially in high and high-average transporters; further trials required to examine impact on other patient-level outcomes (peritonitis, peritoneal transport characteristics, technique survival, patient survival)
Amino acid dialysates vs. glucose exchanges	None			?		Few RCTs, small sample size, short duration, suboptimal methodological quality, surrogate outcomes of questionable clinical relevance, inconsistent findings			?	Further trials with patient-level outcomes required
Glucose-sparing regimens vs, glucose exchanges	None			?		1 RCT, suboptimal methodological quality, surrogate outcomes			?	Further trials with patient-level outcomes required

[a] If no existing systematic review, overall evidence rating will start at moderate.

[b] Domains that are considered include study design, study quality, and consistency and directness of findings.

[c] Domains that are considered include trade-offs between benefits and harms, translation into clinical practice, uncertainty about baseline risk of population of interest, and quality of evidence. I, recommend; II, suggest; III, no recommendation possible.

demonstrate any significant nutritional benefit of amino acid dialysates [75,79,80]. The ultrafiltration effect is comparable to that achieved with 1.5% glucose.

Conclusions

The published studies of newer, "biocompatible" fluids have to date been limited by small sample sizes, relatively short durations, suboptimal methodologic quality, and a predominant focus on surrogate markers of questionable clinical importance (such as dialysate effluent concentrations of CA125) (Table 46.2). In spite of these limitations, there is reasonable evidence to recommend the use of neutral pH, bicarbonate-buffered or lactate-buffered, low-GDP fluids in patients with clinically significant infusion pain, and the use of icodextrin in the long dwell to enhance fluid removal in PD patients, particularly in high and high-average transporters. There is scant, conflicting evidence that amino acid dialysates may confer modest benefits to surrogate nutritional markers in malnourished PD patients. However, there is insufficient evidence to date to permit conclusions to be drawn about the impact of any of these biocompatible solutions relative to cheaper, conventional PD fluids based on "hard," clinical end points, such as peritoneal transport characteristics, peritonitis rates, residual renal function preservation, technique survival, or patient survival. Large, well-designed, adequately powered, randomized controlled trials are eagerly awaited.

References

1 Serkes KD, Blagg CR, Nolph KD, Vonesh EF, Shapiro F. Comparison of patient and technique survival in continuous ambulatory peritoneal dialysis (CAPD) and hemodialysis: a multicenter study. *Perit Dial Int* 1990; **10:** 15–19.

2 Vonesh EF, Moran J. Mortality in end-stage renal disease: a reassessment of differences between patients treated with hemodialysis and peritoneal dialysis. *J Am Soc Nephrol* 1999; **10:** 354–365.

3 Fenton SS, Schaubel DE, Desmeules M, Morrison HI, Mao Y, Copleston P et al. Hemodialysis versus peritoneal dialysis: a comparison of adjusted mortality rates. *Am J Kidney Dis* 1997; **30:** 334–342.

4 Tanna MM, Vonesh EF, Korbet SM. Patient survival among incident peritoneal dialysis and hemodialysis patients in an urban setting. *Am J Kidney Dis* 2000; **36:** 1175–1182.

5 Blake PG. Integrated end-stage renal disease care: the role of peritoneal dialysis. *Nephrol Dial Transplant* 2001; **16(Suppl 5):** 61–66.

6 Davies SJ, Van Biesen W, Nicholas J, Lameire N. Integrated care. *Perit Dial Int* 2001; **21(Suppl 3):** S269–S274.

7 Johnson DW, McDonald SP, Excell L, Livingston B, Shtangey V. Peritoneal dialysis. In: McDonald SP, Excell L, editors, ANZDATA Registry Report 2005. Australia and New Zealand Dialysis and Transplant Registry, Adelaide, South Australie, 2006; 84–100.

8 Topley N. Membrane longevity in peritoneal dialysis: impact of infection and bio-incompatible solutions. *Adv Ren Replace Ther* 1998; **5:** 179–184.

9 Pecoits-Filho R, Stenvinkel P, Heimburger O, Lindholm B. Beyond the membrane: the role of new PD solutions in enhancing global biocompatibility. *Kidney Int Suppl* 2003; **2003:** S124–S132.

10 Witowski J, Jorres A. Effects of peritoneal dialysis solutions on the peritoneal membrane: clinical consequences. *Perit Dial Int* 2005; **25(Suppl 3):** S31–S34.

11 Topley N. In vitro biocompatibility of bicarbonate-based peritoneal dialysis solutions. *Perit Dial Int* 1997; **17:** 42–47.

12 Schambye HT. Effect of different buffers on the biocompatibility of CAPD solutions. *Perit Dial Int* 1996; **16(Suppl 1):** S130–S136.

13 Nau B, Schmitt CP, Almeida M, Arbeiter K, Ardissino G, Bonzel KE et al. BIOKID: randomized controlled trial comparing bicarbonate and lactate buffer in biocompatible peritoneal dialysis solutions in children. *BMC Nephrol* 2004; **5:** 14.

14 Williams JD, Craig KJ, Topley N, Von Ruhland C, Fallon M, Newman GR et al. Morphologic changes in the peritoneal membrane of patients with renal disease. *J Am Soc Nephrol* 2002; **13:** 470–479.

15 Dobbie JW, Anderson JD, Hind C. Long-term effects of peritoneal dialysis on peritoneal morphology. *Perit Dial Int* 1994; **14(Suppl 3):** S16–S20.

16 Mortier S, Faict D, Schalkwijk CG, Lameire NH, De Vriese AS. Long-term exposure to new peritoneal dialysis solutions: Effects on the peritoneal membrane. *Kidney Int* 2004; **66:** 1257–1265.

17 Mortier S, Faict D, Lameire NH, De Vriese AS. Benefits of switching from a conventional to a low-GDP bicarbonate/lactate-buffered dialysis solution in a rat model. *Kidney Int* 2005; **67:** 1559–1565.

18 Nakayama M, Kawaguchi Y, Yamada K, Hasegawa T, Takazoe K, Katoh N et al. Immunohistochemical detection of advanced glycosylation end-products in the peritoneum and its possible pathophysiological role in CAPD. *Kidney Int* 1997; **51:** 182–186.

19 Honda K, Nitta K, Horita S, Yumura W, Nihei H, Nagai R et al. Accumulation of advanced glycation end products in the peritoneal vasculature of continuous ambulatory peritoneal dialysis patients with low ultrafiltration. *Nephrol Dial Transplant* 1999; **14:** 1541–1549.

20 Jorres A, Gahl GM, Topley N, Neubauer A, Ludat K, Muller C et al. In-vitro biocompatibility of alternative CAPD fluids; comparison of bicarbonate-buffered and glucose-polymer-based solutions. *Nephrol Dial Transplant* 1994; **9:** 785–790.

21 Williams JD, Topley N, Craig KJ, Mackenzie RK, Pischetsrieder M, Lage C et al. The Euro-Balance Trial: the effect of a new biocompatible peritoneal dialysis fluid (balance) on the peritoneal membrane. *Kidney Int* 2004; **66:** 408–418.

22 Rippe B, Simonsen O, Heimburger O, Christensson A, Haraldsson B, Stelin G et al. Long-term clinical effects of a peritoneal dialysis fluid with less glucose degradation products. *Kidney Int* 2001; **59:** 348–357.

23 Zeier M, Schwenger V, Deppisch R, Haug U, Weigel K, Bahner U et al. Glucose degradation products in PD fluids: do they disappear from the peritoneal cavity and enter the systemic circulation? *Kidney Int* 2003; **63:** 298–305.

24 Lee HY, Park HC, Seo BJ, Do JY, Yun SR, Song HY et al. Superior patient survival for continuous ambulatory peritoneal dialysis patients treated with a peritoneal dialysis fluid with neutral pH and low glucose degradation product concentration (Balance). *Perit Dial Int* 2005; **25:** 248–255.

25 Lee HY, Choi HY, Park HC, Seo BJ, Do JY, Yun SR et al. Changing prescribing practice in CAPD patients in Korea: increased utilization of low GDP solutions improves patient outcome. *Nephrol Dial Transplant* 2006; **21:** 2893–2899.

26 Haag-Weber M, Haug U, Weislander A, Nabut J, Deppish R. Decline of residual renal function in peritoneal dialysis patients depends on uptake of carbonyl compounds from the peritoneal cavity: first data of a prospective clinical trial. *J Am Soc Nephrol* 2003; **14:** 476A.

27 Fan SLS, Pile T, Punzalan S, Raftery M, Yaqoob MM. Prospective randomised controlled trial of biocompatible PD solutions in incident PD patients: interim analysis. *J Am Soc Nephrol* 2006; **17**: 279A.

28 Brown F, Johnson DW. A randomized controlled trial to determine whether treatment with at neutral pH, low glucose degradation product dialysate (balance) prolongs residual renal function in peritoneal dialysis patients. *Perit Dial Int* 2006; **26**: 112–113.

29 Cooker LA, Luneburg P, Holmes CJ, Jones S, Topley N. Interleukin-6 levels decrease in effluent from patients dialyzed with bicarbonate/lactate-based peritoneal dialysis solutions. *Perit Dial Int* 2001; **21(Suppl 3)**: S102–S107.

30 Jones S, Holmes CJ, Krediet RT, Mackenzie R, Faict D, Tranaeus A et al. Bicarbonate/lactate-based peritoneal dialysis solution increases cancer antigen 125 and decreases hyaluronic acid levels. *Kidney Int* 2001; **59**: 1529–1538.

31 Fusshoeller A, Plail M, Grabensee B, Plum J. Biocompatibility pattern of a bicarbonate/lactate-buffered peritoneal dialysis fluid in APD: a prospective, randomized study. *Nephrol Dial Transplant* 2004; **19**: 2101–2106.

32 Haas S, Schmitt CP, Arbeiter K, Bonzel KE, Fischbach M, John U et al. Improved acidosis correction and recovery of mesothelial cell mass with neutral-pH bicarbonate dialysis solution among children undergoing automated peritoneal dialysis. *J Am Soc Nephrol* 2003; **14**: 2632–2638.

33 Mactier RA, Sprosen TS, Gokal R, Williams PF, Lindbergh M, Naik RB et al. Bicarbonate and bicarbonate/lactate peritoneal dialysis solutions for the treatment of infusion pain. *Kidney Int* 1998; **53**: 1061–1067.

34 Rippe B, Simonsen O, Wieslander A, Landgren C. Clinical and physiological effects of a new, less toxic and less acidic fluid for peritoneal dialysis. *Perit Dial Int* 1997; **17**: 27–34.

35 Tranaeus A. A long-term study of a bicarbonate/lactate-based peritoneal dialysis solution: clinical benefits. The Bicarbonate/Lactate Study Group. *Perit Dial Int* 2000; **20**: 516–523.

36 Carrasco AM, Rubio MA, Sanchez Tommero JA, Fernandez GF, Gonzalez RM, del Peso GG et al. Acidosis correction with a new 25 mmol/l bicarbonate/15 mmol/l lactate peritoneal dialysis solution. *Perit Dial Int* 2001; **21**: 546–553.

37 le Poole CY, van Ittersum FJ, Weijmer MC, Valentijn RM, ter Wee PM. Clinical effects of a peritoneal dialysis regimen low in glucose in new peritoneal dialysis patients: a randomized crossover study. *Adv Perit Dial* 2004; **20**: 170–176.

38 Feriani M, Kirchgessner J, La Greca G, Passlick-Deetjen J. Randomized long-term evaluation of bicarbonate-buffered CAPD solution. *Kidney Int* 1998; **54**: 1731–1738.

39 Coles GA, O'Donoghue DJ, Pritchard N, Ogg CS, Jani FM, Gokal R et al. A controlled trial of two bicarbonate-containing dialysis fluids for CAPD: final report. *Nephrol Dial Transplant* 1998; **13**: 3165–3171.

40 Simonsen O, Sterner G, Carlsson O, Wieslander A, Rippe B. Improvement of peritoneal ultrafiltration with peritoneal dialysis solution buffered with bicarbonate/lactate mixture. *Perit Dial Int* 2006; **26**: 353–359.

41 Montenegro J, Saracho RM, Martinez IM, Munoz RI, Ocharan JJ, Valladares E. Long-term clinical experience with pure bicarbonate peritoneal dialysis solutions. *Perit Dial Int* 2006; **26**: 89–94.

42 Rubin J, Klein E, Jones Q, Planch A, Bower J. Evaluation of a polymer dialysate. *Trans Am Soc Artif Intern Organs* 1983; **29**: 62–66.

43 Peers E, Gokal R. Icodextrin provides long dwell peritoneal dialysis and maintenance of intraperitoneal volume. *Artif Organs* 1998; **22**: 8–12.

44 Coles GA. Biocompatibility and new fluids. *Perit Dial Int* 1999; **19(Suppl 2)**: S267–S270.

45 Garcia-Lopez E, Lindholm B, Tranaeus A. Biocompatibility of new peritoneal dialysis solutions: clinical experience. *Perit Dial Int* 2000; **20(Suppl 5)**: S48–S56.

46 Chung SH, Stenvinkel P, Bergstrom J, Lindholm B. Biocompatibility of new peritoneal dialysis solutions: what can we hope to achieve? *Perit Dial Int* 2000; **20(Suppl 5)**: S57–S67.

47 Mistry CD, Gokal R, Peers E. A randomized multicenter clinical trial comparing isosmolar icodextrin with hyperosmolar glucose solutions in CAPD. MIDAS Study Group. Multicenter Investigation of Icodextrin in Ambulatory Peritoneal Dialysis. *Kidney Int* 1994; **46**: 496–503.

48 Posthuma N, ter Weel PM, Verbrugh HA, Oe PL, Peers E, Sayers J et al. Icodextrin instead of glucose during the daytime dwell in CCPD increases ultrafiltration and 24-h dialysate creatinine clearance. *Nephrol Dial Transplant* 1997; **12**: 550–553.

49 Plum J, Gentile S, Verger C, Brunkhorst R, Bahner U, Faller B et al. Efficacy and safety of a 7.5% icodextrin peritoneal dialysis solution in patients treated with automated peritoneal dialysis. *Am J Kidney Dis* 2002; **39**: 862–871.

50 Wolfson M, Piraino B, Hamburger RJ, Morton AR. A randomized controlled trial to evaluate the efficacy and safety of icodextrin in peritoneal dialysis. *Am J Kidney Dis* 2002; **40**: 1055–1065.

51 Woodrow G, Stables G, Oldroyd B, Gibson J, Turney JH, Brownjohn AM. Comparison of icodextrin and glucose solutions for the daytime dwell in automated peritoneal dialysis. *Nephrol Dial Transplant* 1999; **14**: 1530–1535.

52 Ho-dac-Pannekeet MM, Schouten N, Langendijk MJ, Hiralall JK, de Waart DR, Struijk DG et al. Peritoneal transport characteristics with glucose polymer based dialysate. *Kidney Int* 1996; **50**: 979–986.

53 Wiggins KJ, Rumpsfeld M, Blizzard S, Johnson DW. Predictors of a favourable response to icodextrin in peritoneal dialysis patients with ultrafiltration failure. *Nephrology* (Carlton) 2005; **10**: 33–36.

54 Finkelstein F, Healy H, Abu-Alfa A, Ahmad S, Brown F, Gehr T et al. Superiority of icodextrin compared with 4.25% dextrose for peritoneal ultrafiltration. *J Am Soc Nephrol* 2005; **16**: 546–554.

55 Gokal R, Mistry CD, Peers EM. Peritonitis occurrence in a multicenter study of icodextrin and glucose in CAPD. MIDAS Study Group. Multicenter Investigation of Icodextrin in Ambulatory Dialysis. *Perit Dial Int* 1995; **15**: 226–230.

56 Ota K, Akiba T, Nakao T, Nakayama M, Maeba T, Park MS et al. Peritoneal ultrafiltration and serum icodextrin concentration during dialysis with 7.5% icodextrin solution in Japanese patients. *Perit Dial Int* 2003; **23**: 356–361.

57 Posthuma N, ter Weel PM, Donker AJ, Peers EM, Oe PL, Verbrugh HA. Icodextrin use in CCPD patients during peritonitis: ultrafiltration and serum disaccharide concentrations. *Nephrol Dial Transplant* 1998; **13**: 2341–2344.

58 Konings CJ, Kooman JP, Schonck M, Gladziwa U, Wirtz J, van den Wall Bake AW et al. Effect of icodextrin on volume status, blood pressure and echocardiographic parameters: a randomized study. *Kidney Int* 2003; **63**: 1556–1563.

59 Davies SJ, Woodrow G, Donovan K, Plum J, Williams P, Johansson AC et al. Icodextrin improves the fluid status of peritoneal dialysis patients: results of a double-blind randomized controlled trial. *J Am Soc Nephrol* 2003; **14**: 2338–2344.

60 Mujais S, Nolph K, Gokal R, Blake P, Burkart J, Coles G et al. Evaluation and management of ultrafiltration problems in peritoneal dialysis. International Society for Peritoneal Dialysis Ad Hoc Committee on

Ultrafiltration Management in Peritoneal Dialysis. *Perit Dial Int* 2000; **20(Suppl 4):** S5–S21.

61 de Boer AW, Schroder CH, van Vliet R, Willems JL, Monnens LA. Clinical experience with icodextrin in children: ultrafiltration profiles and metabolism. *Pediatr Nephrol* 2000; **15:** 21–24.

62 Guo A, Wolfson M, Holt R. Early quality of life benefits of icodextrin in peritoneal dialysis. *Kidney Int Suppl* 2002; **2002:** S72–S79.

63 Johnson DW, Arndt M, O'Shea A, Watt R, Hamilton J, Vincent K. Icodextrin as salvage therapy for peritoneal dialysis patients with refractory fluid overload. *BMC Nephrol* 2002; **2002:** 2.

64 Wilkie ME, Plant MJ, Edwards L, Brown CB. Icodextrin 7.5% dialysate solution (glucose polymer) in patients with ultrafiltration failure: extension of CAPD technique survival. *Perit Dial Int* 1997; **17:** 84–87.

65 Peers EM, Scrimgeour AC, Haycox AR. Cost-containment in CAPD patients with ultrafiltration failure. *Clin Drug Invest* 1995; **10:** 53–58.

66 Dawnay AB, Millar DJ. Glycation and advanced glycation end-product formation with icodextrin and dextrose. *Perit Dial Int* 1997; **17:** 52–58.

67 de Fijter CW, Verbrugh HA, Oe LP, Heezius E, Donker AJ, Verhoef J *et al.* Biocompatibility of a glucose-polymer-containing peritoneal dialysis fluid. *Am J Kidney Dis* 1993; **21:** 411–418.

68 Krediet RT, Douma CE, Ho dac Pannekeet MM, Imholz AL, Zemel D, Zweers MM *et al.* Impact of different dialysis solutions on solute and water transport. *Perit Dial Int* 1997; **17(Suppl 2):** S17–S26.

69 Krediet RT, Ho-dac-Pannekeet MM, Imholz AL, Struijk DG. Icodextrin's effects on peritoneal transport. *Perit Dial Int* 1997; **17:** 35–41.

70 Posthuma N, ter Wee P, Donker AJ, Dekker HA, Oe PL, Verbrugh HA. Peritoneal defense using icodextrin or glucose for daytime dwell in CCPD patients. *Perit Dial Int* 1999; **19:** 334–342.

71 Woodrow G, Oldroyd B, Stables G, Gibson J, Turney JH, Brownjohn AM. Effects of icodextrin in automated peritoneal dialysis on blood pressure and bioelectrical impedance analysis. *Nephrol Dial Transplant* 2000; **15:** 862–866.

72 Posthuma N, Verbrugh HA, Donker AJ, van Dorp W, Dekker HA, Peers EM *et al.* Peritoneal kinetics and mesothelial markers in CCPD using icodextrin for daytime dwell for two years. *Perit Dial Int* 2000; **20:** 174–180.

73 Posthuma N, ter Wee PM, Donker AJ, Oe PL, Peers EM, Verbrugh HA. Assessment of the effectiveness, safety, and biocompatibility of icodextrin in automated peritoneal dialysis. The Dextrin in APD in Amsterdam (DIANA) Group. *Perit Dial Int* 2000; **20(Suppl 2):** S106–S113.

74 Wens R, Taminne M, Devriendt J, Collart F, Broeders N, Mestrez F *et al.* A previously undescribed side effect of icodextrin: overestimation of glycemia by glucose analyzer. *Perit Dial Int* 1998; **18:** 603–609.

75 Li FK, Chan LY, Woo JC, Ho SK, Lo WK, Lai KN *et al.* A 3-year, prospective, randomized, controlled study on amino acid dialysate in patients on CAPD. *Am J Kidney Dis* 2003; **42:** 173–183.

76 Misra M, Ashworth J, Reaveley DA, Muller B, Brown EA. Nutritional effects of amino acid dialysate (Nutrineal) in CAPD patients. *Adv Perit Dial* 1996; **12:** 311–314.

77 Jones M, Hagen T, Boyle CA, Vonesh E, Hamburger R, Charytan C *et al.* Treatment of malnutrition with 1.1% amino acid peritoneal dialysis solution: results of a multicenter outpatient study. *Am J Kidney Dis* 1998; **32:** 761–769.

78 Tjiong HL, van den Berg JW, Wattimena JL, Rietveld T, van Dijk LJ, van der Wiel AM *et al.* Dialysate as food: combined amino acid and glucose dialysate improves protein anabolism in renal failure patients on automated peritoneal dialysis. *J Am Soc Nephrol* 2005; **16:** 1486–1493.

79 Qamar IU, Levin L, Balfe JW, Balfe JA, Secker D, Zlotkin S. Effects of 3-month amino acid dialysis compared to dextrose dialysis in children on continuous ambulatory peritoneal dialysis. *Perit Dial Int* 1994; **14:** 34–41.

80 Qamar IU, Secker D, Levin L, Balfe JA, Zlotkin S, Balfe JW. Effects of amino acid dialysis compared to dextrose dialysis in children on continuous cycling peritoneal dialysis. *Perit Dial Int* 1999; **19:** 237–247.

81 Selby NM, Fonseca S, Hulme L, Fluck RJ, Taal MW, McIntyre CW. Hypertonic glucose-based peritoneal dialysate is associated with higher blood pressure and adverse haemodynamics as compared with icodextrin. *Nephrol Dial Transplant* 2005; **20:** 1848–1853.

82 Van Biesen W, Boer W, De Greve B, Dequidt C, Vijt D, Faict D *et al.* A randomized clinical trial with a 0.6% amino acid/1.4% glycerol peritoneal dialysis solution. *Perit Dial Int* 2004; **24:** 222–230.

47 Prevention and Treatment of Peritoneal Dialysis-Related Infections

Giovanni F. M. Strippoli,[1] Kathryn J. Wiggins,[2] David W. Johnson,[3] Sankar Navaneethan,[4] Giovanni Cancarini,[5] & Jonathan C. Craig[1]

[1] NHMRC Centre for Clinical Research Excellence in renal medicine, Cochrane Renal Group, University of Sydney, School of Public Health, Australia

[2] The University of Melbourne Department of Medicine at St. Vincent's Hospital, Melbourne, Australia

[3] Department of Renal Medicine, University of Queensland at Princess Alexandra Hospital, Woolloongabba, Brisbane, Australia

[4] Department of Medicine, Unity Health System, Rochester, New York, USA

[5] Section and Division of Nephrology, Department of Experimental and Applied Medicine, University and Spedali Civili, Brescia, Italy

Introduction

Peritoneal dialysis (PD) is an effective and widely used form of renal replacement therapy and accounts for 15–50% of renal replacement therapy for patients with end-stage renal disease (ESRD). The longevity of PD and its broader uptake are reduced by the risk of PD-related infections [1]. The overall incidence of peritonitis is about one episode for every 19 patient months on PD [2], although this figure ranges from 1 in every 9.1 to 1 in every 27.9 patient– months [3–5]. Peritonitis tends to be recurrent, with a very high rate of relapse (approximately 0.5 episodes/patient/year) [6]. Risk factors for developing peritonitis include advancing age [7,8], some ethnic groups [9,10], comorbidities such as diabetes and obesity [11], tropical climates [12,13], depression [14], nasal carriage of *Staphylococcus aureus* [15,16], and presence of exit site infections. Catheter design, implantation technique, and connection methodology also modulate the risk of peritonitis. It is unclear whether PD modality (continuous ambulatory PD [CAPD] or automated PD [APD]) affects peritonitis rates [17,18].

PD-related infections may also require hospitalization [19] and result in adverse effects from the required antibiotic treatment. Peritonitis, particularly due to *S. aureus*, is a major cause of catheter removal and subsequent technique failure in patients receiving PD [20]. Peritonitis is also associated with an increased mortality risk in some patient groups [21]. Longer-term consequences of peritonitis include the development of ultrafiltration failure [22] and an increased likelihood of developing encapsulating sclerosing peritonitis [23,24].

The ultimate goal for PD-related infections is prevention. To date, this has primarily focused on antimicrobial prophylaxis and modifications of the PD catheter and connection system. Antimicrobial interventions include oral and topical antibiotics [25], topical disinfectants, and prophylactic treatment of *S. aureus* nasal carriage [26]. All of these strategies, particularly cleansing and disinfection of the exit site, are widely accepted, but practice patterns are variable and trials results are conflicting [27–30]. Catheter-related intervention strategies that have been studied include modifications of catheter design, implantation technique, connection methodology, and PD modality [15,16].

When infection does occur, early and effective management is important to reduce complications such as progression from exit site infection to peritonitis and relapse of peritonitis. The mainstay of management of peritonitis is antimicrobial therapy, although adjunctive treatments such as fibrinolytic agents [31,32], peritoneal lavage [33], and intraperitoneal immunoglobulin administration [34] have been used. Peritonitis antibiotic regimens vary in the class of antimicrobial agent(s) used, route of administration, dosing frequency, and total duration of therapy. Center-specific factors such as patterns of antimicrobial resistance and regional isolation also play a role in making treatment decisions [35].

In this chapter we review current evidence about the prevention and treatment of PD-related infections.

Definitions

Definitions of exit site infections, tunnel infections, and peritonitis have varied in clinical trials, particularly regarding the time frame in which a second episode defines relapsed peritonitis rather than a new episode. Definitions have become more uniform in recent studies. Current guidelines on prevention and treatment of

Evidence-based Nephrology. Edited by Donald Molony and Jonathan Craig
© 2009 Blackwell Publishing, ISBN: 978-1-4051-3975-5.

peritonitis [3,36] are based on similar definitions, which are summarized below.

Exit site and tunnel infections

An exit site infection is present when there is purulent drainage from the exit site. This may be accompanied by pericatheter swelling, erythema, and tenderness. Erythema or serous discharge alone may or may not represent infection. A positive culture from a swab in the absence of clinical signs may represent bacterial colonization but not infection. Tunnel infections in the absence of concomitant exit site infection are rare. There may be signs of inflammation (erythema, edema, and or tenderness) over the subcutaneous tunnel, but some tunnel infections may be clinically occult and require sonographic studies for detection.

Peritonitis

Peritonitis may be directly related to the PD procedure (PD-associated peritonitis) or mybe independent of the PD catheter and related to intra-abdominal events, such as perforated viscera. General criteria for diagnosis are discussed more extensively in the chapter, but definitions of different types of peritonitis are listed here:
• *Refractory peritonitis:* persistence of clinical symptoms and signs beyond day 4 or 5 of therapy
• *Relapsing peritonitis:* an episode that occurs within 4 weeks of completion of therapy of a prior episode with the same organism or one sterile episode
• *Repeat peritonitis:* an episode that occurs more than 4 weeks after completion of therapy of a prior episode with the same organism
• *Recurrent peritonitis:* an episode that occurs within 4 weeks of completion of therapy for a prior episode but with a different organism.

Diagnosis of peritonitis

Appearance of cloudy effluent suggests a diagnosis of peritonitis, but confirmation is required and is defined by the presence of two of three of the following findings:
1) Cloudy effluent fluid with leukocyte count over 100/mm^3, with more than 50% neutrophils
2) Abdominal pain
3) Positive culture or Gram stain of peritoneal effluent.

The patient suffering from peritonitis often satisfies all these criteria. However, not all centers can perform a Gram stain, and culture becomes positive many hours and sometimes days after admission. Decision on treatment is therefore often based on the two first criteria. Clinical history, occurrence of fever, increased peripheral blood leukocyte count, and other typical symptoms of infection may be suggestive of the diagnosis.

Cloudy effluent

The sign of cloudy effluent requires confirmation by a differential cell count from the peritoneal effluent; a finding of >50%

neutrophils is equally important as the total white blood cell count of 100 cells/μl. Because an increase in white blood cell count can be delayed in some cases, a cell count lower than 100/μl does not rule out the diagnosis of peritonitis. A repeat count on the effluent following an exchange often shows a cell count increase. Leukocyte esterase reagent strips are used in many centers to enable the patient to check the effluent at home, thereby reducing the time to diagnosis and confirming an increased white blood cell count as the cause of nonclear effluent. Sensitivity and specificity of the leukocyte esterase test are comparable to those with visual assessment and light microscopy.

A cloudy peritoneal effluent can also appear in conditions other than infectious peritonitis. A mild hemoperitoneum, due to capillary rupture, ovulation, or retrograde menstruation is not infrequent; the effluent has a characteristic red discoloration and only a few white blood cells are seen on microscopy. Cloudy effluent with an increased number of eosinophils can simulate infectious peritonitis. Peritoneal eosinophilia is arbitrarily defined as an absolute eosinophil count of >100/μl, or eosinophils >10% of total effluent leukocytes if the eosinophil count is >40/μl. It is considered to be due to an allergic reaction occurring after catheter implantation or from dialysate additives, air introduced into the peritoneal cavity, the PD catheter, plasticizers from the dialysis bag or tubing, or even mechanical trauma from a fill volume that is too large. Increased eosinophil counts have been reported with one brand of vancomycin and with fungal and parasitic infections.

Chylous effluent, due to a breach of lymphatic vessels, has an opaline appearance. This often increases after a meal and has a higher number of lymphocytes and measurable amounts of triglycerides. A cloudy effluent with an increased white blood cell count, mimicking infectious peritonitis, can also occur during chemical peritonitis due to accidental introduction of disinfectants into the peritoneal cavity; the differential diagnosis is based on clinical history, negative culture, and rapid spontaneous improvement. Peritoneal diffusion of malignancy can also cause cloudy effluent, but this is a rare event. Finally, a cloudy fluid often appears in the first bag exchange after a period of empty abdomen ("dry abdomen") and is due to the accumulation of cells in the peritoneal cavity. Clear effluent is typically observed when dialysis fluid is constantly present and regularly exchanged in the peritoneal cavity. Inappropriate suspicion of peritonitis in patients undergoing intermittent PD or APD may occur, as the first exchange is often cloudy in these patients. To obviate the risk, one should infuse 1 L of peritoneal dialysis fluid and permit it to dwell for a minimum of 1–2 h before draining and examining for turbidity and for cell count; alternatively, a rapid flushing of the peritoneal cavity with 1–2 L of dialysis fluid can precede that maneuver.

Abdominal pain

The symptom of abdominal pain is not unique to infectious peritonitis. In peritonitis, abdominal pain is typically generalized and is often associated with rebound tenderness. The first site of pain in PD-related infectious peritonitis is often the epigastric region, which then spreads to the whole abdomen. The intensity of pain is very variable and may not correlate with the degree of cloudy effluent; some patients have a frank cloudy effluent with little pain, and others complain of severe pain but have relatively clear effluent. Different causative microorganisms cause different pain severities; streptococcal peritonitis, for example, is generally associated with severe pain. Peritonitis occurring in PD patients may also be secondary to primary disease in abdominal organs, and other abdominal conditions may mimic the pain of peritonitis. This differentiation is critical for therapy. Diverticulitis should be suspected when pain is localized to the left iliac fossa. Appendicitis should be ruled out when the first localized pain is in the right iliac fossa, and pain in the right hypochondrium necessitates consideration of cholecystitis.

Gram stain and culture

Gram stain is positive in up to 40% cases and is concordant with culture results. Despite the substantial false-negative rate, because it has a high specificity, when positive the Gram stain may provide early identification of the likely causative organism and so can guide empiric therapy. A positive culture confirms the clinical diagnosis of infectious peritonitis, often within 24–48 h after empiric therapy has commenced. Causative microorganisms include gram-negative and gram-positive bacteria, fungi, yeasts, and typical and atypical mycobacteria. The possibility of a viral peritonitis cannot be excluded, but literature on this topic is only anecdotal. Culture is negative in 10–20% of cases of clinically diagnosed infectious peritonitis. The low concentration of microorganisms in the effluent accounts for negative culture results, but other causes have been reported, including insufficient volume of the effluent sample, concurrent use of antibiotics, inadequate culture technique, and failure to concentrate by centrifugation. Other causes are endotoxins or contaminants of either the dialysis fluid or medications introduced in the peritoneal cavity.

Other signs and symptoms may also be present in peritonitis, including:

1) Pneumoperitoneum: appearance of a small amount of air in the peritoneal cavity is easily diagnosed by chest X-ray, and very small amounts can be detected by computed tomography. Pneumoperitoneum suggests bowel perforation but can also be due to accidental introduction of air during an exchange.

2) Amylase concentration in peritoneal fluid amylase is less than 100 U/L in PD patients with primary infectious peritonitis and higher during either pancreatitis or infections of other abdominal organs.

3) When peritonitis is suspected, the physical examination should include a careful inspection of the exit site and tunnel of the catheter, because peritonitis could be secondary to the peritoneal spread of bacteria from this site. Any drainage from the exit site should be cultured, along with the effluent. If the exit site is culture positive for the same organism as the peritoneal effluent, then it is very likely that the origin of peritonitis is the catheter.

4) Peripheral cell counts including a differential count. Infectious peritonitis is generally associated with an increase in the white blood cell count.

5) Fever and loss of appetite are also frequent. Chills, vomiting, lack of bowel sounds, tachycardia, and hypotension occur in the most severe cases. In some patients (e.g. the elderly or those on immunosuppressive therapy), these signs may be less severe.

Available guidelines for prevention and treatment of exit site and tunnel infection and peritonitis

Prevention of exit site and tunnel infections and peritonitis

The International Society for Peritoneal Dialysis (ISPD) [36], Australian and New Zealand Society of Nephrology (Caring for Australians with Renal Impairment [CARI]) [3], and the British Renal Association (BRA) have issued guidelines regarding use of antimicrobial agents for peritonitis prevention. All three recommend use of topical antibiotic agents to reduce the risk of S. aureus exit site and tunnel infections. The BRA guidelines recommend mupirocin applied to exit sites, whereas CARI and ISPD suggest both intranasal and exit site mupirocin administration. The ISPD also lists exit site gentamicin as a potential prophylactic agent. Further strategies recommended by both CARI and ISPD are prophylactic use of nystatin during antibiotic therapy to reduce the incidence of fungal peritonitis and prophylactic antibiotic administration at the time of catheter placement. CARI recommends use of a first-generation cephalosporin for this purpose.

With regard to catheter-related interventions, there is consensus among all three guidelines that no single type of catheter is superior in reducing infection rates. ISPD guidelines state that a downward-placed catheter may reduce infection rates. No other recommendations regarding catheter placement have been issued.

Treatment of exit site and tunnel infections

ISPD guidelines recommend prompt and aggressive treatment of exit site infections, particularly those due to S. aureus and *Pseudomonas aeruginosa*, as these organisms frequently lead to peritonitis. The guidelines state that treatment with oral antibiotics is as effective as intraperitoneal therapy, with the exception of infections due to multidrug-resistant S. aureus. CARI suggestions for clinical care indicate that antibiotic therapy should match the likely local pathogens but that no antibiotic regimen has proven to be superior.

Treatment of peritonitis

ISPD and CARI guidelines both state that empirical therapy with antibiotics that will cover both gram-negative and gram-positive organisms should be initiated at the time a diagnosis of peritonitis is suspected. Specific antibiotic agents are not recommended, but the ISPD guidelines suggest that local patterns of causative organisms and bacterial resistance should be taken into consideration by each center. Following identification of a specific organism targeted therapy should commence. The suggested duration of therapy in the ISPD guidelines is 2 weeks in most cases but 3 weeks for severe infections, such as infection due to *Staphylococcus* or *Pseudomonas* species.

In addition to antimicrobial agents, ISPD recommends catheter removal for refractory and relapsing peritonitis and fungal peritonitis. CARI makes no recommendation about timing of catheter removal, due to lack of evidence, but does state that catheter removal is superior to urokinase.

Available evidence for prevention and treatment of exit site and tunnel infections and peritonitis

Systematic reviews of randomized trials of interventions to prevent and treat PD-related infections have been carried out. Specifically, there is one Cochrane Review covering the area of antimicrobial agents [37] and two covering catheter-related interventions to prevent PD-related infection [38,39]; there is also a published protocol of treatment for PD peritonitis [40], and preliminary results have been presented in abstract form [41]. Since completion of these reviews, one additional randomized controlled trial (RCT) has been published [42]. The characteristics of populations and interventions in the trials included in these Cochrane reviews (Tables 47.1 to 47.3) and their major findings (Tables 47.4 to 47.6) are provided at the end of the chapter.

Antimicrobial agents for prevention of PD-associated infections

Oral antibiotic prophylaxis has not been shown to prevent PD-related infections (Figure 47.1). The two interventions that have been shown to be effective in preventing PD-related infections are administration of intranasal mupirocin to PD patients colonized with *S. aureus* and preoperative intravenous antibiotic prophylaxis. In one trial, nasal mupirocin compared with placebo significantly reduced the exit site and tunnel infection rate and *S. aureus* nasal carriage, but no significant effect of mupirocin on peritonitis rates was observed [37] (Figure 47.2). These findings support the ISPD and CARI recommendations indicating that topical nasal therapy should be used. The benefit of mupirocin was only observed for the outcome measure of rates of exit site and tunnel infections, and not for the proportion of patients with these infections. This means that mupirocin may only reduce the risk of exit site and tunnel infections in patients who are frequent relapsers, or it is possible that these results simply demonstrate the trials are more likely to find an effect when event rates occur more commonly (episodes of infection rather than number of patients with exit site and tunnel infections). The greatest concern regarding routine use of topical mupirocin is the risk of emergence of mupirocin-resistant bacteria, although this remains a theoretical risk to date. The trial of nasal mupirocin, which has the longest follow-up duration available to date, had a follow-up period of only 18 months and was inadequate to assess the development of resistance [43].

The recommendation by CARI and BRA to apply mupirocin to the exit site is not supported by current evidence. There have been no reported RCTs which have assessed the effectiveness of application of mupirocin to the catheter exit site or to PD patients other than those with nasal colonization by *S. aureus*. However, this intervention is widely used and unlikely to cause harm.

Two other topical antimicrobial therapies are available in addition to mupirocin. Bernardini *et al.* prospectively compared topical application of mupirocin and gentamicin to the exit site in a randomized, controlled, blinded trial [42]. They found that topical gentamicin was associated with a reduction in the rate of catheter infections, time to first catheter infection, and catheter infections due to *Pseudomonas aeruginosa*. All-cause and gram-negative peritonitis rates were reduced in the gentamicin group when the results were analyzed according to treatment received, but there were no differences on intention to treat analysis (0.56/year with mupirocin vs. 0.30/year for gentamicin; $P = 0.08$). There were no reports of gentamicin ototoxicity. Although the results of this study appear favorable, the median follow-up in this study was 8 months, and long-term data on the development of gentamicin-resistant microorganisms will be important.

Medihoney has antimicrobial properties and may be associated with a lower risk of facilitating the development of multidrug-resistant microorganisms than antibiotics. Noninferiority of Medihoney with topical mupirocin has been demonstrated in the prevention of hemodialysis catheter-associated sepsis [44], but there are no published trials of Medihoney use in PD.

The use of perioperative intravenous antibiotic prophylaxis compared with no treatment has been shown to reduce the risk of early (<1 month postinsertion) peritonitis considerably but not the risk of exit site and tunnel infection [37] (Figure 47.3). There was no significant difference in the risk of peritonitis more than 1 month after catheter insertion. Postoperative infection rates in the control arms of each of the evaluated trials were high, ranging from 12–46%, and the applicability of these data to PD units with lower infection rates following PD catheter insertion is unclear. Current CARI guidelines suggest use of first-generation cephalosporins in this setting, based on extrapolations from the results of preoperative antibiotic trials in patients without ESRD [3], but the evidence supporting the use of first-generation cephalosporins in PD patients undergoing Tenckhoff catheter insertion is sparse. Four RCTs of different preoperative antibiotic prophylaxis regimens were identified in a systematic review [45–48]. These included parenteral gentamicin, vancomycin, cephazolin, and cefuroxime, with only two evaluating a first-generation cephalosporin. One small trial involving 27 PD patients found that cephazolin and gentamicin were ineffective compared with no treatment [45], and the largest of the meta-analyses (221 patients) observed that cephazolin was inferior to vancomycin with respect to preventing postoperative catheter-associated infections (7% vs. 1%; $P < 0.05$) [46]. The recommendation of a first-generation cephalosporin in preference to vancomycin may be a reasonable compromise because of the risk of vancomycin-resistant *Enterococcus* spp. and *S. aureus*. The ISPD guidelines address this issue by recommending

Table 47.1 Characteristics of populations and interventions in randomized trials of antimicrobial agents for prevention of peritonitis in PD.[a]

Study ID	% of patients that were diabetic	Interventions	No. of patients	Follow-up (mos)
Oral antibiotics vs. placebo/no treatment				
Blowey 1994[b]	NA	Rifampin (20 mg/kg/day) in 2 doses for 5 days + bacitracin (nasal) 2 times/day × 7 days	15	1
Churchill 1988	NA	Trimethoprim (160 mg/day)-sulfamethoxazole (800 mg/day) × 12 mos	105	12
Low 1980	NA	Cefalexin 500 mg × 2/day	50	2–3
Sesso 1994[c]	23	Ofloxacin 200 mg/day × 5 days	22	7
Swartz 1991	34	Trimethoprim-sulfamethoxazole ("low dose") or cephalexin (250 mg) or clindamycin (300 mg)	59	12
Zimmerman 1991	41	Rifampin 300 mg × 2/day × 5 days, every 3 months	64	18
Nasal antibiotics vs. placebo/no treatment				
Mupirocin SG 1996	20	Mupirocin (2%) nasal ointment b.i.d. × 5 days, every 1 month	267	18
Sesso 1994[c]	23	Sodium fusidate (2%) nasal ointment twice daily × 5 days	22	7
Oral antifungal agents vs. placebo/no treatment				
Wai-Kei Lo 1996[d]	17	Nystatin 500,000 U × 4/day (whenever other antibiotics were administered)	397	24
Topical disinfectants vs. placebo/no treatment				
Luzar 1990[e]	22	Povidone iodine (20 g/L) and nonocclusive dressing 2–3 times/week	127	9
Waite 1997	33	Povidone iodine (10%) ointment 3.5 g at every dressing change	117	14
Wilson 1997	NA	Povidone iodine (2.5%) dry powder spray at every dressing change	149	10
Germicidal devices vs. placebo/no treatment				
Nolph 1985	20	Ultraviolet germicidal chamber for bag outlet port	167	36
Vaccines vs. placebo/no treatment				
Poole-Warren 1991	17	Staphypan Berna	124	12
Perioperative intravenous prophylaxis vs. placebo/no treatment				
Bennett-Jones 1988	0	Gentamicin (i.v.) 1.5 mg/kg at time of catheter placement	27	1
Gadallah 2000[c, f]	23	Vancomycin (i.v.) 1000 mg 12 h before catheter placement	221	0.5
Lye 1992	40	Cefazolin (i.v.) 500 mg or gentamicin (i.v.) 80 mg 1 h before catheter placement	50	3
Wikdahl 1997	34	Cefuroxime (i.v.) 1.5 g at time of catheter placement + 250 mg i.p. in first dialysis bag	38	0.3
Nasal antibiotics vs. oral or nasal antibiotic				
Bernardini 1996	34	Mupirocin (2%) nasal ointment, daily applications vs. rifampin (oral) 300 mg × 2/day × 5 days, every 3 mos	82	25
Perez-Fontan 1992	16	Mupirocin (2%) nasal ointment t.i.d. × 7 days vs. neomycin sulfate (0.1%) nasal ointment t.i.d. × 7 days	32	3
Perioperative intravenous prophylaxis				
Lye 1992	60	Cefazolin (i.v.) 500 mg before catheter placement vs. gentamicin (i.v.) 80 mg <60 min before catheter placement	50	2

Abbreviations: NA, not applicable or not available; b.i.d., twice a day; t.i.d., three times a day; i.v., intravenous; i.p., intraperitoneal.

[a] Results of either placebo or no-treatment controlled trials or head-to-head trials of different antimicrobial regimens. Trials are grouped in alphabetical order and by type of intervention. Mean age ranged from 40–60 years for all trials with the exception of one pediatric trial.

[b] Pediatric trial.

[c] Trial with three arms.

[d] This trial focused on prophylaxis of *Candida* peritonitis in patients receiving treatment for bacterial peritonitis.

[e] The control group for this trial was soap and water.

[f] The control group for this trial was either no treatment or cefazolin (i.v.), 1000 mg, 3 h before catheter placement, or no treatment.

Table 47.2 Characteristics of populations and interventions in RCTs of catheter-related interventions for prevention of peritonitis in PD.[a]

Study ID [reference]	% of patients that were diabetic	Interventions	No. of patients	Follow-up (mos)
Surgical catheter insertion technique				
Gadallah 1999[17]	36	Laparoscopy vs. standard laparotomy	148	36
Tsimoyiannis 2000 [18]	NA	Laparoscopy vs. standard laparotomy	50	21
Wright 1999 [19]	NA	Laparoscopy vs. standard laparotomy	50	24
Danielsson 2002 [20]	28	Subcutaneous buried vs. standard insertion	60	24
Moncrief-Popovich 1998 [21]	NA	Subcutaneous buried vs. standard insertion	113	NA
Park 1998 [22]	43	Subcutaneous buried vs. standard insertion	60	24
Ejlersen 1990 [23]	NA	Midline vs. lateral	37	3
Rubin 1990[b] [24]	24	Midline vs. lateral	83	NA
Straight vs. coiled catheter				
Akyol 1990 [25]	12	Tenckhoff (straight) vs. Tenckhoff (curled) catheter	40	13
Dasgupta 2000 [26]	NA	Tenckhoff (straight) vs. Moncrief-Popovich (curled) catheter	41	NA
Eklund 1994 [27]	13	Single-cuff straight Tenckhoff vs. one bubble slanted flange single-cuff Swan Neck (coiled) catheter	40	NA
Eklund 1995 [28]	16	Two-cuff straight Tenckhoff catheter vs. two-cuff Swan neck (coiled) catheter	40	NA
Lye 1996 [29]	35	Double cuffed Swan-neck (coiled) vs. double-cuffed Tenckhoff (straight) catheter	40	12
Nielsen 1995 [30]	18	Tenckhoff (straight) vs. permanently bent Swan neck (curled) catheter	72	6
Rubin 1990[b] [24]	24	Straight vs. coiled catheter	83	NA
Scott 1994[c] [31]	NA	Double cuffed Tenckhoff (straight) vs. Toronto Western (curled) vs. standard coiled Oreopoulos	89	12
Y-set vs. conventional spike catheter or modified Y-set				
Cheng 1994 [32]	15	O-set versus conventional spike vs. UVXD[d]	100	>12
Churchill 1989 [33]	NA	Y-set plus sodium hypochlorite vs. standard system	124	12
Dryden 1992 [34]	15	Y-set (Freeline solo) vs. standard system	80	3–36
Li 1996 [35]	20	Y-set (Ultraset) vs. conventional spike	40	12
Lindholm 1988 [36]	28	5F take-off system vs. conventional	58	9
Maiorca 1983 [37]	NA	Y-set plus sodium hypochlorite vs. standard system	62	18–24
Owen 1992 [38]	NA	O-set vs. standard	60	>12
Rottembourg 1987 [39]	22	Y-set (Y-set or O-set or 5F safe-lock) vs. conventional	55	33
Viglino 1989 [40]	1	Y-set vs. Travenol Advanced Bystem	60	13
Viglino 1993 [41]	20	Y-set vs. T-set	122	15
Y-set vs. double bag				
Harris 1996 [42]	15	Y-set (standard) vs. double bag (Freeline solo)	66	18
Kiernan 1995 [43]	25	Ultra Y-set vs. Ultra Twin Bag	83	4.5
Li 1999 [44]	24	Y-set (Ultraset) vs. double bag (Ultrabag) system	120	16
Monteon 1998[c] [45]	50	Y-set vs. double bag vs. straight spike	147	12
Miscellaneous				
De Fijter 1991 [46]	NA	Y-set CAPD vs. CCPD	56	18
Bro 1999 [47]	4	Y-set CAPD vs. APD (NIPD or CCPD)	34	6
Eklund 1997 [48]	26	Single cuff vs. double cuff Tenckhoff catheter	60	20
Li 2002 [49]	38	Ultrabag vs. Stay-safe	102	>12
Pommer 1998 [50]	20	Silver ring vs. none	195	4.5
Trooskin 1990 [51]	NA	Antibiotic treated catheter vs. none	86	NA
Turner 1992[c] [52]	20	Immobilizer device vs. tape vs. no immobilization	66	0.25–15

Abbreviations: NA, not available; CCPD, continuous cycling PD; NIPD, nocturnal intermittent PD.

[a] Trials were all in adult populations. Trials are grouped in alphabetical order and by type of intervention.

[b] Trial with four arms.

[c] Trial with three arms.

[d] Ultraviolet irradiation connection box machine.

Table 47.3 Characteristics of populations and interventions in RCTs of interventions for treatment of peritonitis in PD.[a]

Study ID	% of patients that were diabetic	Interventions	No. of patients	Follow-up (days)
Same antibiotic IV vs. IP				
Bailie 1987	NA	Vancomycin 1g IP LD then 25 mg/L IP qid vs. vancomycin 1 g IV LD then 25 mg/L IP qid; 14-day course	20	NA
Bennet-Jones 1990	NA	Vancomycin 20 mg/L IP qid + tobramycin 4 mg/L IP qid vs. vancomyin 0.5–1 g IV days 1 & 6 + tobramycin 1 mg/kg IV LD then 20–60 mg IV according to levels; PO antibiotics at day 4; 10-day course	75	14
Same antibiotic oral vs. IP				
Boeschoten 1985	NA	Cephradine 500 mg IP LD then 250 mg IP qid vs. cephradine 500 mg PO LD then 250 mg PO qid; treatment until 1 week after dialysate cleared	39	14
Cheng 1993	NA	Ciprofloxacin 200 mg IP LD then 25 mg/L IP qid vs. ciprofloxacin 750 mg PO bd; 10-day course	48	28
Cheng 1997	NA	Ofloxacin 100 mg/L IP LD then 25 mg/L IP qid vs. ofloxacin 400 mg PO LD then 300 mg PO od; 10-day course	35	28
Different antibiotic oral vs. IP				
Bennet-Jones 1987	NA	Vancomycin 25 mg/L qid IP + gentamicin 8 mg/L qid IP 48 h then 4 mg/L qid vs. ciprofloxacin 750 mg PO td for 24 h then 750 mg PO bd; 10-day course	48	28
Chan 1990	NA	Cephalothin 250 mg/L IP qid + tobramycin 8 mg/L qid vs. ofloxacin 400 mg PO LD then 300 mg PO od ± rifampin 300 mg PO od; 10-day course	106	28
Cheng 1991	NA	Vancomycin 500 mg IP LD then 30 mg/L IP qid + aztreonam 500 mg/L IP LD then 250 mg/L IP qid vs. ofloxacin 400 mg PO LD then 300 mg PO od; 10-day course	45	28
Cheng 1998	NA	Vancomycin 1–2 g IP days 1 & 7 + netromycin 20 mg/L IP od vs. vancomycin 1–2 g IP days 1 & 7 + levofloxacin 300 mg PO od; 10-day course	100	28[b]
Gucek 1994	NA	Cephazolin 100 mg IP LD then 250 mg IP qid + netilmycin 80–120 mg LD then 40 mg IP daily vs. ofloxacin 300 mg PO LD then 200 mg PO od + netilmycin 80–120 mg LD then 40 mg IP daily; 10-day course	38	NA
Lye 1993	NA	Gentamicin 80 mg IP LD then 15 mg/2 L IP qid + vancomycin 1 g IP day 1 vs. pefloxacin 400 mg PO bd + vancomycin 1 g IP day 1; 14-day course	60	14
Tapson 1990	NA	Vancomycin 30 mg IP qid + netilmycin 30 mg IP to alternate exchanges vs. ciprofloxcain 500 mg PO qid; 10-day course	50	28
Continuous vs. intermittent IP antibiotics				
Boyce 1988	NA	Vancomycin 1 g IP LD then 30 mg/L qid vs. vancomycin 30 mg/kg days 1 and 8, treatment until 5 days after dialysate cleared	51	28
Lye 1995	NA	Gentamicin 10mg/ L IP qid + vancomycin 1g IP day 1 vs gentamicin 40 mg IP od + vancomycin 1 g IP day 1; 14-day course	100	28
Schaeffer 1999	NA	Vancomycin 15 mg/kg body wt LD then 30 mg/L qid + ceftazidime 250 mg/L LD then 125 mg/L qid vs. vancomycin 30 mg/kg IP days 1& 7 + ceftazidime 500 mg/L IP LD then 250 mg/L IP od ; OR Teicolpanin 7.5 mg/kg body wt LD then 20 mg/L qid + ceftazidime 250 mg/L LD then 125 mg/L qid vs. teicoplanin 15 mg/kg IP days 1 & 7 + ceftazidime 500 mg/L IP LD then 250 mg/L IP od; 10-day course (all treatment arms)	93	NA
Velasquez-Jones 1995	NA	Vancomycin 500 mg/L IP LD then 15 mg/L IP qid vs. vancomycin 30 mg/kg IP days 1 & 7; 10-day course	21	28
Different antibiotic IP				
Anwar 1995	NA	Vancomycin 250 mg IP LD then 25 mg IP bd + netilmycin 30–50 mg IP LD then 20–25 mg IP bd vs. imipenem 1 g IP bd; treatment until 5 days after dialysate cleared	56	NA
Bowley 1998	NA	Vancomycin 50 mg IP qid for 48 h then 25 mg IP qid vs. teicoplanin 50 mg IP qid for 48 h then 25 mg IP qid; 7-day course	12	5
De Fijter 2001	22	Cephradine 250 mg/L IP qid vs. ciprofloxacin 50 mg/L IP qid + rifampin 50 mg/L qid; 14-day course	98	14
Flanigan 1991	50	Vancomycin 25 mg/L IP vs. cephazolin 50 mg/L IP; 14-day course	263	14
Friedland 1990	28	Vancomycin 12.5 mg/L IP qid + gentamicin 4 mg/L bd vs. ciprofloxacin 20 mg/L IP qid; 10-day course	40	10

(continued)

Table 47.3 (continued)

Study ID	% of patients that were diabetic	No. of Interventions	Follow-up patients	(days)
Gucek 1997	NA	Vancomycin 2 g IP every 5–7 days + ceftazidime 1 g IP LD then 250 mg IP qid vs. cephazolin 500 mg IP LD then 250 mg qid + netilmicin 80–120 mg IP LD then 40 mg IP od; 14- to 28-day course	52	NA
Jimenez 1996	NA	Vancomycin IP + tobramycin IP vs. vancomycin IP + cefotaxime IP	47	NA
Khairullah 2002	NA	Vancomycin 1 g/L IP day 1 & day 5 or 8 + gentamicin 40 mg IP od vs. cephazolin 1 g IP LD then 125 mg/L qid + gentamicin 40 mg IP od; 14- to 21-day course	42	14–21
Lui 2005	NA	Cefazolin 1 g IP od + netilmycin 0.6 mg/kg IP od vs. cefazolin 1 g IP od + ceftazidime 1 g IP od; 14-day course	102	42
Leung 2005	39	Cefazolin 1 g IP LD then 250 mg IP qid + ceftazidime 1 g IP LD then 50 mg IP qid vs. imipenem 500 mg IP LD then 100 mg IP qid,	102	
Lupo 1997	NA	Cephalothin 2 g IV then 500 mg IP bd + tobramycin 120 mg IM LD then 10 mg IP qid vs. teicoplanin 400 mg IV LD then 40 mg IP qid + tobramycin 120 mg IM LD then 10 mg IP qid; 21-day course	65	NA
Wale 1992	NA	Teicoplanin 20 mg/L IP qid + aztreonam 250 mg/L IP qid vs. cefuroxime 125 mg/L IP qid; minimum 10-day course (at least 5 days from when dialysate cleared)	60	> 10 + 5[c]
Were 1992	NA	Vancomycin 50 mg IP bd + netilmicin 50 mg IP LD then 25 mg IP bd vs. cefuroxime 40 mg/L IP qid; treatment until 5 days after dialysate cleared	20	5[c]
Wong 2001	NA	Vancomycin 1 g IP days 1 & 7 + netilmicin 80 mg IP LD then 40 mg IP od vs. cefepime 2 g IP LD then 1 g IP daily; 10-day course	60	10
Antibiotic vs. nonantimicrobial procedure or nonantimicrobial procedure vs. placebo or other nonantimicrobial procedure				
Coban 2004	NA	Ampicillin-sulbactam 1 g IP tds + netilmycin 150 mg IP LD then 50 mg IP od vs. 320 mg IgG IP qid + antibiotics		
Eljersen 1991	NA	Vancomycin IP + netilmicin IP vs. rapid peritoneal lavage for 24 h + IP antibiotics	36	30[d]
Gadallah 2000	NA	Vancomycin-gentamicin vs. urokinase 5000 IU in 2.5 mL normal saline + antibiotics	80	
Innes 1993	NA	Placebo vs. urokinase	25	
Tong 2005	28	Cephazolin-netilmycin IP + placebo (20 mL normal saline) vs. cephazolin-netilmycin IP + urokinase 60,000 IU IP diluted in 20 mL of normal saline	88	28
Williams 1989	NA	Catheter removal and replacement vs. urokinase 5000 IU in 2 mL	37	90–360

Abbreviations: NA, not available; IP, intraperitoneal; PO, per oral; IV, intravenous, IM, intramuscular; od, once a day; bd, twice a day; qid, four times a day; IgG, immunoglobulin G; LD.

[a] Trials are grouped in alphabetical order and by type of interventions.

[b] Number of days from effluent clearing.

[c] Beyond total clearing of dialysate and a decrease in the dialysate white blood cell count $<100/mm^3$.

[d] After cessation of antibiotic treatment.

that each program weigh the benefits of vancomycin with the risk of emergence of resistant microorganisms.

Nystatin significantly reduced the risk of *Candida* spp. peritonitis in PD patients. The applicability of this finding is limited, given the relatively high occurrence rate reported in the control arm of the one large trial identified (8.5% over 2 years) [49]. However, in light of the high disease burden associated with fungal peritonitis and absence of adverse effects of nystatin, implementation of this practice, as recommended by the ISPD guidelines, appears to be of net clinical benefit.

Topical antiseptic agents were recommended in the previous version of the ISPD guidelines, but not in the current edition. Variations of this practice, along with use of other antimicrobial interventions, are not supported by any evidence, or else they have not been the subject of clinical trials. A meta-analysis of three RCTs

of topical povidone–iodine or powder sprays showed no benefit compared with nondisinfectant soap and water [37]. Moreover, although side effects were generally inadequately reported, one study observed that skin rashes occurred in 6% of patients following povidone–iodine application [50]. There is no evidence to support regular topical exit site disinfection with antibacterial soap or a medical antiseptic to keep the exit site clean and to diminish resident bacteria. Trials of UV germicidal chambers around the connection device [51] and anti-staphylococcal vaccine [52] also showed no significant effects of the intervention. There have been no controlled trials evaluating the effects of antibacterial soap.

Overall, although a number of trials have assessed the benefits of different antimicrobial interventions to prevent peritonitis in PD, the majority of trials enrolled few patients over relatively short

Table 47.4 Effects of antimicrobial agents in preventing peritonitis, exit site and tunnel infection, catheter removal or replacement, and all-cause mortality in PD.

Intervention[a]	Peritonitis		Peritonitis rate		Exit site and tunnel infection trials		Exit site and tunnel infection rate		Catheter removal or replacement		All-cause mortality	
	No. of trials (no. of patients)	RR (95% CI)	No. of trials (no. of patient-mos)	RR (95% CI)	No. of trials (no. of patients)	RR (95% CI)	No. of trials (no. of patient-mos)	RR (95% CI)	No. of trials (no. of patients)	RR (95% CI)	No. of trials (no. of patients)	RR (95% CI)
Oral antibiotics (cotrimoxazole, cephalexin, ofloxacin, rifampin)	4 (235)	0.76 (0.38–1.53)	2 (670)	0.74 (0.39–1.37)	2 (31)	0.29 (0.09–0.97)			4 (235)	0.73 (0.39–1.38)	4 (195)	0.84 (0.39–1.79)
Nasal antibiotics (mupirocin)	2 (282)	0.94 (0.67–1.33)	1 (2626)	0.84 (0.44–1.60)	2 (282)	0.97 (0.64–1.49)	1 (2716)	0.58 (0.40–0.85)	2 (282)	0.44 (0.44–1.79)		
Oral antifungal agents (nystatin)	1 (397)	0.10 (0.03–0.31)										
Topical disinfectants (povidone-iodine)	3 (382)	0.72 (0.46–1.11)			3 (381)	0.71 (0.49–1.03)			2 (266)	0.73 (0.34–1.55)	2 (266)	1.24 (0.54–2.84)
Germicidal devices			1 (167)	1.04 (0.71–1.53)								
Vaccines			1 (124)	0.89 (0.58–1.37)	1 (1099)	1.02 (0.70–1.48)						
Perioperative i.v. antibiotics (gentamicin, vancomycin, cefazolin, cefuroxime)	4 (335)	0.44 (0.13–1.54)			2 (114)	0.34 (0.02–6.49)						

Abbreviations: RR, relative risk; CI, confidence interval; i.v., intravenous.
[a] All trials had a placebo/no treatment controlled arm.

Table 47.5 Effects of catheter-related interventions for preventing peritonitis, exit site and tunnel infection, catheter removal or replacement, and all-cause mortality in PD.

Experimental Intervention	Control	Peritonitis		Peritonitis rate		Exit site and tunnel infection		Exit site and tunnel infection rate		Catheter removal or replacement		All-cause mortality	
		No. of trials (no. of patients)	RR (95% CI)	No. of trials (no. of patient-mos)	RR (95% CI)	No. of trials (no. of patients)	RR (95% CI)	No. of trials (no. of patient-mos)	RR (95% CI)	No. of trials (no. of patients)	RR (95% CI)	No. of trials (no. of patients)	RR (95% CI)
Laparoscopy	Laparotomy	3 (238)	0.68 (0.41–1.15)	1 (375)	0.89 (0.39–2.07)	1 (148)	0.11 (0.01–1.92)					2 (193)	1.08 (0.52–2.26)
Standard insertion	Resting but no subcutaneous burying			2 (2511)	1.16 (0.37–3.60)			2 (2511)	1.15 (0.39–3.42)			2 (119)	0.90 (0.39–2.08)
Midline insertion	Lateral insertion	2 (120)	0.65 (0.32–1.33)			2 (120)	0.56 (0.12–2.58)			1 (83)	0.57 (0.33–0.98)	1 (37)	8.50 (0.50–143.32)
Straight catheter	Coiled catheter	5 (324)	1.14 (0.73–1.79)	4 (2589)	0.89 (0.63–1.26)	6 (332)	1.26 (0.91–1.73)	3 (1933)	1.04 (0.73–1.47)	5 (275)	1.11 (0.53–2.31)	4 (209)	0.26 (0.07–0.99)
Y-set system	Standard spike system	7 (485)	0.64 (0.53–0.77)	8 (7417)	0.49 (0.40–0.61)	3 (226)	1.0 (0.70–1.43)	2 (2841)	1.24 (0.91–1.79)	2 (126)	0.80 (0.40–1.63)	5 (386)	0.96 (0.47–1.95)
Double bag system	Y-set system	3 (292)	0.59 (0.35–1.01)	4 (4139)	0.90 (0.49–1.66)			2 (2139)	1.04 (0.52–2.06)	3 (321)	0.83 (0.40–1.73)	2 (174)	1.58 (0.48–5.26)

Abbreviations: RR, relative risk; CI, confidence interval.

Table 47.6 Effects of interventions to treat PD-related infections.

Experimental intervention	Control intervention	Treatment failure		Relapse		Catheter removal or replacement		All-cause mortality	
		No. of trials (no. of patients)	RR (95% CI)	No. of trials (no. of patients)	RR (95% CI)	No. of trials (no. of patients)	RR (95% CI)	No. of trials (no. of patients)	RR (95% CI)
Antimicrobial treatments									
Intravenous	Intraperitoneal	1 (95)	3.52 (1.26–9.81)						
Drug A oral	Drug A intraperitoneal	2 (83)	1.66 (0.98–2.83)	2 (83)	3.38 (0.74–15.35)	1 (48)	2.00 (0.19–20.61)		
Regimen A oral	Regimen B intraperitoneal	7 (451)	1.17 (0.86–1.59)	5 (303)	1.17 (0.63–2.14)	2 (170)	1.18 (0.49–2.87)	1 (46)	0.36 (0.02–8.46)
Low dose	High dose	1 (28)	4.00 (1.17–13.66)	1 (28)	12.00 (1.60–90.23)				
Intermittent	Continuous	5 (338)	0.69 (0.37–1.30)	4 (324)	0.93 (0.63–1.39)				
First-generation cephalosporin	Glycopeptide	3 (370)	1.84 (0.95–3.58)	3 (350)	1.68 (0.84–3.36)	2 (365)	0.92 (0.36–2.33)		
Teicoplanin	Vancomycin	2 (178)	1.08 (0.37–3.12)	2 (178)	0.93 (0.53–1.64)				
Oral regimen A	Oral regimen B	1 (74)	0.88 (0.35–2.17)			1 (74)	2.00 (0.19–21.11)		
Other interventions									
Peritoneal lavage	Standard therapy	1 (36)	2.50 (0.56–11.25)						
Urokinase	Catheter removal and replacement	1 (37)	2.35 (1.13–4.91)	1 (37)	2.35 (1.13–4.91)				
Urokinase	Placebo	2 (113)	0.60 (0.32–1.14)	2 (168)	0.89 (0.35–2.22)	2 (168)	0.70 (0.37–1.30)	1 (88)	1.00 (0.21–4.69)

Abbreviations: RR, relative risk; CI, confidence interval.

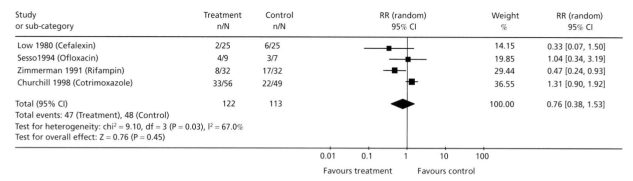

Figure 47.1 Effects of oral antibiotics on number of patients who develop peritonitis (one or more episodes) on PD.

periods of follow-up, did not adequately assess harms, and did not fulfill widely accepted quality standards for reporting. Almost all trials evaluated in the systematic reviews failed to specify whether randomization allocation was concealed, outcome assessors were blinded, or data were analyzed on an intention-to-treat basis. These issues, together with the small sample sizes of all but three trials, reduce the strength of the conclusions that may be drawn at present. The possibility of a type 2 statistical error for some of the less frequently observed outcome measures (e.g. catheter

loss) cannot be excluded; almost all analyses were consistent with both clinically important benefits and harms from the intervention, such was the imprecision of the estimates. The absence of statistical significance in the overall risk estimates provided by many trials means that we do not know whether the intervention is effective or that an intervention is definitely ineffective. Some studies, such as those involving prophylactic oral antibiotics, date back to the 1980s, when peritonitis rates were much higher than those observed more recently. Thus, the generalizability of

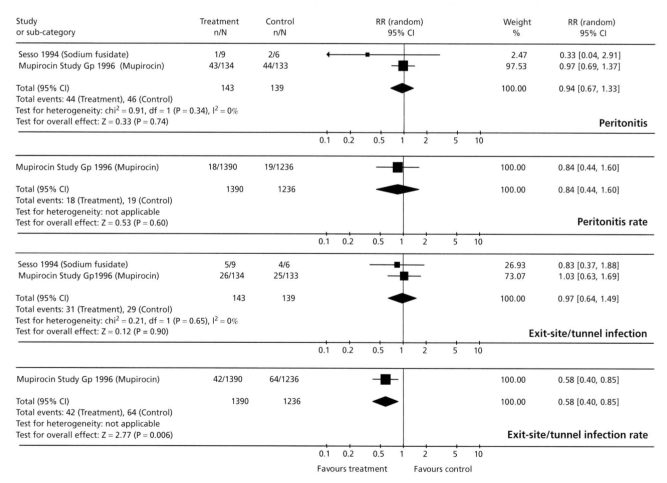

Figure 47.2 Effects of nasal antibiotics on number of patients who develop peritonitis (one or more episodes), the peritonitis rate, number of patients who develop exit site or tunnel infection (one or more episodes), and the exit site or tunnel infection rate in PD.

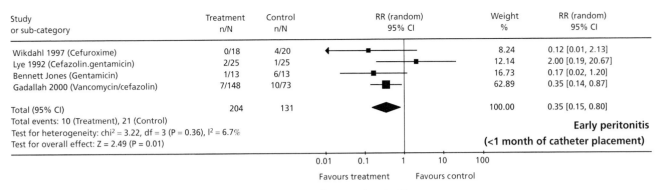

Study or sub-category	Treatment n/N	Control n/N	RR (random) 95% CI	Weight %	RR (random) 95% CI
Wikdahl 1997 (Cefuroxime)	0/18	4/20		8.24	0.12 [0.01, 2.13]
Lye 1992 (Cefazolin.gentamicin)	2/25	1/25		12.14	2.00 [0.19, 20.67]
Bennett Jones (Gentamicin)	1/13	6/13		16.73	0.17 [0.02, 1.20]
Gadallah 2000 (Vancomycin/cefazolin)	7/148	10/73		62.89	0.35 [0.14, 0.87]
Total (95% CI)	204	131		100.00	0.35 [0.15, 0.80]

Total events: 10 (Treatment), 21 (Control)
Test for heterogeneity: chi² = 3.22, df = 3 (P = 0.36), I² = 6.7%
Test for overall effect: Z = 2.49 (P = 0.01)

Early peritonitis (<1 month of catheter placement)

0.01　0.1　1　10　100
Favours treatment　Favours control

Figure 47.3 Intravenous antibiotic prophylaxis versus placebo or not treatment: effects on early peritonitis.

these studies to contemporary practice is questionable, although the likelihood that further trials will be carried out is low. Items that need to be considered when making a recommendation or suggestion about these interventions include the size and estimate of the effect, the likelihood that, if further studies were to be conducted, they would find different effects than those already published, and the trade-offs between potential benefits and harms. Table 47.7, below, presents a grading of the available evidence with relevant recommendations and suggestions for clinical care.

Table 47.7 Evidence ratings and recommendations for catheter-related interventions to prevent peritonitis and exit site and tunnel infection in PD.

Intervention	Existing systematic reviews[a]	Overall evidence rating[b] High	Moderate	Low	Comment	Recommendation[c] I[a]	II[b]	III[c]	Comment
Laparoscopy vs. laparotomy	●			●	3 RCTs, no heterogeneity, poor methodological quality		●		Moderate/imprecise effect size, low evidence base, no excess harms documented, higher likelihood of acceptance by patients
Standard insertion (resting and subcutaneous burying) vs. resting but no subcutaneous burying	●			●	3 RCTs, high heterogeneity, poor methodological quality		●		Moderate/imprecise effect size, low evidence base, no excess harms documented
Midline insertion vs. lateral insertion	●			●	2 RCTs, no heterogeneity, poor methodological quality		●		Moderate/imprecise effect size, low evidence base, no excess harms documented
Straight catheter vs. coiled catheter	●		●		8 RCTs no heterogeneity, 4 RCTs poor methodological quality			●	Undetermined effect, moderate evidence base, potential for increased harm
Y-set system vs. standard spike	●		●		10 RCTs little heterogeneity, 5 RCTs poor methodological quality	●			Large effect size, moderate evidence base, no excess harms documented, Y-set standard practice in several countries
Double bag systems vs. Y-set	●		●		4 RCTs high heterogeneity, 2 RCTs poor methodological quality		●		Moderate/imprecise effect size, moderate evidence base, no excess harms documented, double-bag standard practice in several countries

[a] If no existing systematic review, overall evidence rating will start at moderate.
[b] Evidence rating based on number of trials, study design, study quality, and consistency of results.
[c] Recommendations based on efficacy, trade-offs between benefits and harms, quality of evidence, and availability of medication. I, recommend; II, suggest; III, no recommendation possible.

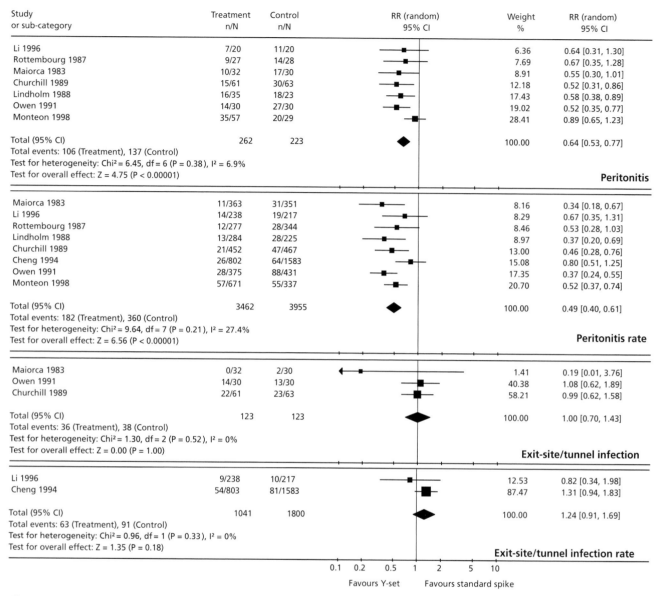

Figure 47.4 Y-set versus standard spike catheters: effects on peritonitis, peritonitis rate, and exit site or tunnel infection rate.

Catheter-related interventions for prevention of peritonitis

The only catheter-related measure that has been shown to reduce peritonitis rates in a systematic review is the use of disconnect systems rather than conventional spike systems [39]. The use of the Y-set compared to standard spike systems was associated with a significantly lower risk of peritonitis and peritonitis rate, but no differences in the risk and rates of exit site and tunnel infection, catheter removal or replacement, or all-cause mortality were found (Figure 47.4). One trial of 60 patients also showed a significant increase in the risk of technique failure with the Y-set [53]. These results support the recommendations of the BRA and CARI guidelines against the use of conventional spike connection systems. Although the ISPD and National Kidney Foundation Kidney

Disease Outcomes Quality Initiative (K/DOQI) clinical practice guidelines make no specific recommendations about connection methodology, spike and luer lock connect system usage has generally been declining in recent years. In the UK, the use of connect PD systems decreased from 22% in 1998 to less than 1% in 2002 [54]. A similar experience has been reported in Australia and New Zealand [55]. The double-bag systems are associated with a reduction in the risk of peritonitis compared to Y-set systems, although statistical significance has not been attained (Figure 47.5).

Other catheter-related interventions that have been the subject of RCTs and included in systematic reviews are surgical approaches (laparoscopy vs. laparotomy, standard insertion and resting vs. implantation and subcutaneous burying, and midline vs. lateral insertion), type of PD catheter (straight vs. coiled, single vs. double

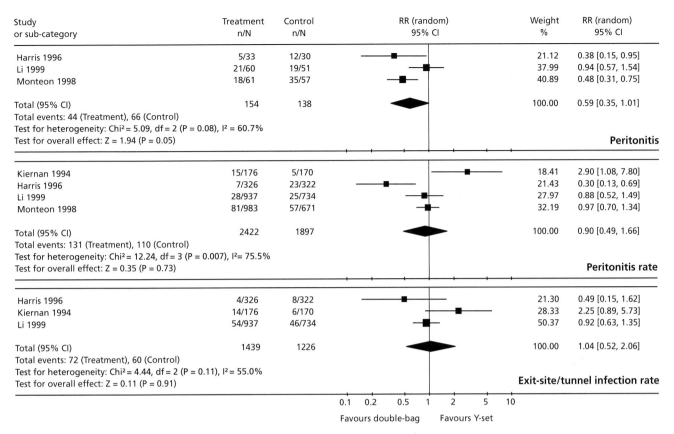

Figure 47.5 Double bag versus Y-systems: effects on peritonitis, peritonitis rate, and exit site or tunnel infection rate.

cuffed, antibiotic impregnated vs. standard catheters), use of silver rings, immobilization devices, and use of the Ultrabag versus the Stay-safe set. None of these has been shown to significantly affect the rates of exit site and tunnel infections or peritonitis, but wide point estimates around the comparison of laparoscopy vs. laparotomy for insertion of PD catheters demonstrate a lack of statistical power [39]. Further trials in these areas should be encouraged.

A meta-analysis of eight RCTs comparing straight versus coiled catheters demonstrated a reduction in all-cause mortality associated with straight catheters. This result was largely unexplained, particularly in view of the similar rates of peritonitis, exit site and tunnel infections, and catheter removal or replacement observed with the two catheter types. Causes of death were not reported to clarify the reason for the result. Potential alternative explanations include a type 1 statistical error (most likely) or inadequate randomization, possibly due to suboptimal allocation concealment. This result should be interpreted with caution and may warrant further studies.

Several retrospective, observational studies have suggested that APD is associated with a reduced risk of peritonitis compared with CAPD and have speculated that this may reflect the reduced number of connections (and therefore opportunities for intra-luminal contamination) involved with APD. However, interpretation of these findings is potentially confounded by the possibility of selection and recall biases. In the available Cochrane Review, only

two small, relatively short-duration RCTs of APD versus CAPD were identified and no differences in PD outcomes were observed, but the possibility of a type 2 statistical error could not be excluded [56,57].

As with antimicrobial preventative interventions, there is a relative paucity of quality RCTs in this area, and trial methodology has been generally poor. Many studies are small and often short in duration, so that the possibility of a type 2 statistical error for some of the less frequently observed outcome measures (e.g. catheter loss) cannot not be excluded. Moreover, evidence of trial heterogeneity was found in some analyses of peritonitis rates (such as for laparoscopy vs. laparotomy and twin bag vs. Y-set), which most likely reflected significant intertrial variability in duration of follow-up. These issues reduce the strength of the conclusions that may be drawn. However, the likelihood that further trials will be carried out in this area is relatively low, so clinicians need to make decisions based on these data alone. Table 47.8 presents a grading of the available evidence with relevant recommendations and suggestions.

Treatment of exit site and tunnel infections

Two trials comparing antibiotic regimens for treatment of exit site and tunnel infections have been conducted. In one, intraperitoneal vancomycin–oral rifampin were found to be equally effective as intraperitoneal vancomycin–oral trimethoprim-sulfamethoxa-

Table 47.8 Evidence ratings and recommendations for antimicrobial interventions to prevent peritonitis and exit site or tunnel infection in PD.

Intervention	Existing systematic reviews[a]	Overall evidence rating[b]			Comment	Recommendation[c]			Comment
		High	Moderate	Low		I[a]	II[b]	III[c]	
Oral antibiotics vs. placebo/no treatment	•		•		6 RCTs high heterogeneity, 4 RCTs poor methodological quality	•			Moderate/imprecise effect size, moderate evidence base, potential for development of antibiotic resistance, no other excess harm documented
Nasal antibiotics (mupirocin) vs. placebo	•	•			3 RCTs no heterogeneity, 2 RCTs poor methodological quality	•			Large effect size, high evidence base, potential for development of antibiotic resistance, no other excess harm documented
Oral antifungal agents (nistatin) vs. placebo/no treatment	•	•			1 RCT, large sample size	•			Large effect size, high evidence base, no excess harm documented
Topical disinfectants (povidone-iodine) vs. placebo/no treatment	•		•		3 RCTs no heterogeneity, poor methodological quality	•			Moderate/imprecise effect size, moderate evidence base, low likelihood that intervention may cause harms, topical disinfection of catheter exit site represents standard practice in many countries
Germicidal devices for connectology	•		•		1 RCT, small sample size, poor methodological quality			•	Small/imprecise effect size, moderate evidence base
Vaccines vs. placebo/no treatment	•		•		1 RCT, small sample size, poor methodological quality			•	Small/imprecise effect size, moderate evidence, low biological plausibility of effect
Perioperative i.v. antibiotics vs. placebo	•		•		5 RCTs low heterogeneity, 3 RCTs poor methodological quality	•			Large effect size, moderate evidence, no excess harms documented and unlikely to cause harm
Nasal or topical mupirocin vs. placebo	•			•	1 RCT, small sample size, poor methodological quality			•	Small/imprecise effect size, low evidence

Abbreviation: i.v., intravenous.

[a] If no existing systematic review, overall evidence rating will start at moderate.

[b] Evidence rating based on number of trials, study design, study quality, and consistency of results.

[c] Recommendations based on efficacy, trade-offs between benefits and harms, quality of evidence, and availability of medication. I, recommend; II, suggest; III, no recommendation possible.

zole (cure rates of 86% vs. 89%, respectively) [58]. Concerns about multidrug-resistant organisms limit widespread application of either of these regimens. The second trial found intraperitoneal clindamycin to be superior to oral clindamycin; however, this trial was conducted in the early 1990s, again limiting applicability to current practice [59].

Treatment of peritonitis

A large number of antibiotic regimens used in the treatment of peritonitis have been evaluated in RCTs. Only two antibiotic regimens were found to be superior in a systematic review [41]; however, in both cases the applicability to current practice was low. Meta-analysis of two trials comparing cephazolin and vancomycin found the latter to be superior at reducing treatment failure and relapse. This finding was strongly influenced by a large number of patients in one trial in which a low dose of cephazolin (25 mg/L) was used [60]. The other trial included in the meta-analysis used a cephazolin dose of 125 mg/L, as is recommended in the ISPD guidelines, and found the two agents to be equivalent [61]. Further, when all glycopeptide-based regimens were compared to first-generation cephalosporin-based regimens, no difference was found (Figure 47.6). Intraperitoneal

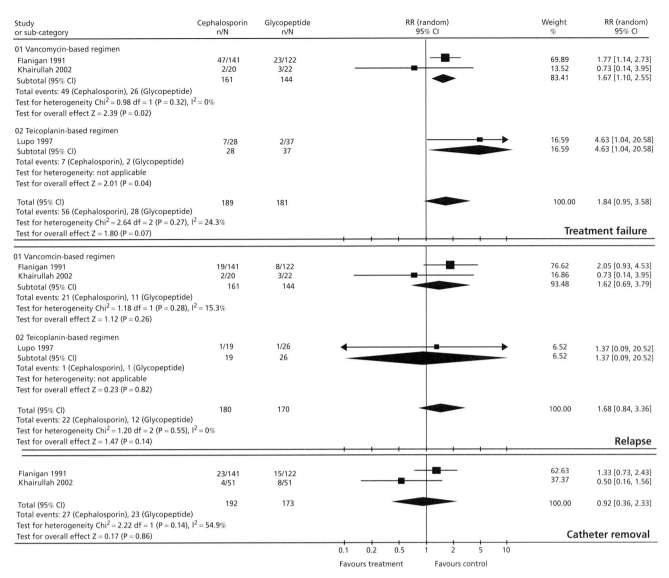

Study or sub-category	Cephalosporin n/N	Glycopeptide n/N	RR (random) 95% CI	Weight %	RR (random) 95% CI
01 Vancomycin-based regimen					
Flanigan 1991	47/141	23/122		69.89	1.77 [1.14, 2.73]
Khairullah 2002	2/20	3/22		13.52	0.73 [0.14, 3.95]
Subtotal (95% CI)	161	144		83.41	1.67 [1.10, 2.55]
Total events: 49 (Cephalosporin), 26 (Glycopeptide)					
Test for heterogeneity Chi² = 0.98 df = 1 (P = 0.32), I² = 0%					
Test for overall effect Z = 2.39 (P = 0.02)					
02 Teicoplanin-based regimen					
Lupo 1997	7/28	2/37		16.59	4.63 [1.04, 20.58]
Subtotal (95% CI)	28	37		16.59	4.63 [1.04, 20.58]
Total events: 7 (Cephalosporin), 2 (Glycopeptide)					
Test for heterogeneity: not applicable					
Test for overall effect Z = 2.01 (P = 0.04)					
Total (95% CI)	189	181		100.00	1.84 [0.95, 3.58]
Total events: 56 (Cephalosporin), 28 (Glycopeptide)					
Test for heterogeneity Chi² = 2.64 df = 2 (P = 0.27), I² = 24.3%					
Test for overall effect Z = 1.80 (P = 0.07)				**Treatment failure**	

Study or sub-category	Cephalosporin n/N	Glycopeptide n/N	RR (random) 95% CI	Weight %	RR (random) 95% CI
01 Vancomcin-based regimen					
Flanigan 1991	19/141	8/122		76.62	2.05 [0.93, 4.53]
Khairullah 2002	2/20	3/22		16.86	0.73 [0.14, 3.95]
Subtotal (95% CI)	161	144		93.48	1.62 [0.69, 3.79]
Total events: 21 (Cephalosporin), 11 (Glycopeptide)					
Test for heterogeneity Chi² = 1.18 df = 1 (P = 0.28), I² = 15.3%					
Test for overall effect Z = 1.12 (P = 0.26)					
02 Teicoplanin-based regimen					
Lupo 1997	1/19	1/26		6.52	1.37 [0.09, 20.52]
Subtotal (95% CI)	19	26		6.52	1.37 [0.09, 20.52]
Total events: 1 (Cephalosporin), 1 (Glycopeptide)					
Test for heterogeneity: not applicable					
Test for overall effect Z = 0.23 (P = 0.82)					
Total (95% CI)	180	170		100.00	1.68 [0.84, 3.36]
Total events: 22 (Cephalosporin), 12 (Glycopeptide)					
Test for heterogeneity Chi² = 1.20 df = 2 (P = 0.55), I² = 0%					
Test for overall effect Z = 1.47 (P = 0.14)				**Relapse**	

Study or sub-category	Cephalosporin n/N	Glycopeptide n/N	RR (random) 95% CI	Weight %	RR (random) 95% CI
Flanigan 1991	23/141	15/122		62.63	1.33 [0.73, 2.43]
Khairullah 2002	4/51	8/51		37.37	0.50 [0.16, 1.56]
Total (95% CI)	192	173		100.00	0.92 [0.36, 2.33]
Total events: 27 (Cephalosporin), 23 (Glycopeptide)					
Test for heterogeneity Chi² = 2.22 df = 1 (P = 0.14), I² = 54.9%					
Test for overall effect Z = 0.17 (P = 0.86)				**Catheter removal**	

0.1 0.2 0.5 1 2 5 10
Favours treatment   Favours control

Figure 47.6 Glycopeptide versus first-generation cephalosporin-based intraperitoneal antibiotic regimens: effects on treatment failure, relapse, and catheter removal.

ciprofloxacin–rifampin was found to be superior to intraperitoneal cephradine in one trial [35]. The usefulness of this finding is limited by the use of monotherapy with a first-generation cephalosporin in one treatment arm, without any broad gram-negative cover, a practice which is now uncommon. Similarly, first-line use of ciprofloxacin and rifampin is restricted in many centers due to concern regarding the risk of emergence of multidrug-resistant organisms. Details on other antibiotic regimens tested in RCTs are reported in Table 47.6.

No currently available guidelines recommend specific antibiotic regimens, reflecting the paucity of available evidence; however, information regarding factors requiring consideration when selecting antibiotics has been provided in the guidelines. ISPD guidelines recommend that there should be center-specific selection of an agent(s) according to local causative microorganism and resistance patterns [36]. The impact of local microbial resistance on peritonitis outcomes was apparent in two trials comparing oral and intraperitoneal quinolone use. In both studies, response rates were low for both treatment arms (41.7% and 55.6% in the per oral group and 66.7% and 70.6% in the intraperitoneal group, respectively) [62]. Microorganism resistance to quinolones was the major cause of treatment failure, and previous exposure to quinolones was a risk factor for infection with resistant microorganisms. Similarly, the emergence of vancomycin-resistant enterococci is associated with use of broad-spectrum antibiotics [63,64]. CARI suggests avoidance of aminoglycosides where possible to avoid ototoxicity and nephrotoxicity. Decline in residual renal function with an aminoglycoside-based antibiotic regimens was assessed in one trial of 102 patients with peritonitis [65]. In this study there was no increased loss of residual renal function with a netilmycin-based regimen compared to ceftazidime use for gram-negative cover. Few trials evaluated ototoxicity, despite the

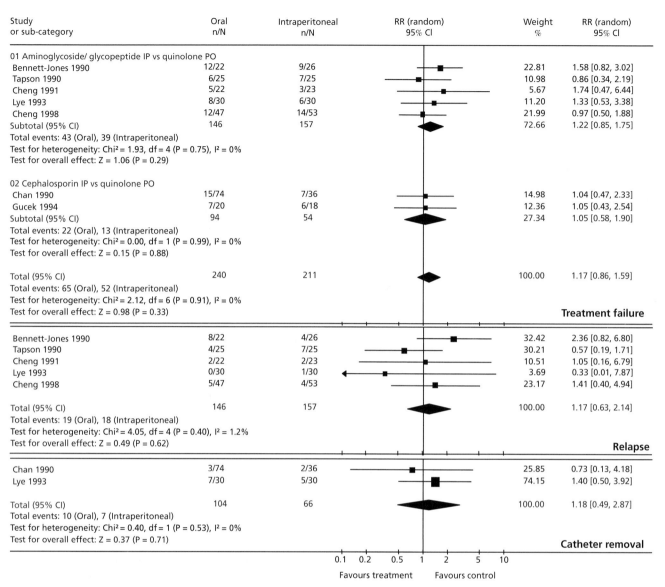

Study or sub-category	Oral n/N	Intraperitoneal n/N	RR (random) 95% CI	Weight %	RR (random) 95% CI
01 Aminoglycoside/ glycopeptide IP vs quinolone PO					
Bennett-Jones 1990	12/22	9/26		22.81	1.58 [0.82, 3.02]
Tapson 1990	6/25	7/25		10.98	0.86 [0.34, 2.19]
Cheng 1991	5/22	3/23		5.67	1.74 [0.47, 6.44]
Lye 1993	8/30	6/30		11.20	1.33 [0.53, 3.38]
Cheng 1998	12/47	14/53		21.99	0.97 [0.50, 1.88]
Subtotal (95% CI)	146	157		72.66	1.22 [0.85, 1.75]
Total events: 43 (Oral), 39 (Intraperitoneal)					
Test for heterogeneity: Chi² = 1.93, df = 4 (P = 0.75), I² = 0%					
Test for overall effect: Z = 1.06 (P = 0.29)					
02 Cephalosporin IP vs quinolone PO					
Chan 1990	15/74	7/36		14.98	1.04 [0.47, 2.33]
Gucek 1994	7/20	6/18		12.36	1.05 [0.43, 2.54]
Subtotal (95% CI)	94	54		27.34	1.05 [0.58, 1.90]
Total events: 22 (Oral), 13 (Intraperitoneal)					
Test for heterogeneity: Chi² = 0.00, df = 1 (P = 0.99), I² = 0%					
Test for overall effect: Z = 0.15 (P = 0.88)					
Total (95% CI)	240	211		100.00	1.17 [0.86, 1.59]
Total events: 65 (Oral), 52 (Intraperitoneal)					
Test for heterogeneity: Chi² = 2.12, df = 6 (P = 0.91), I² = 0%					
Test for overall effect: Z = 0.98 (P = 0.33)				**Treatment failure**	
Bennett-Jones 1990	8/22	4/26		32.42	2.36 [0.82, 6.80]
Tapson 1990	4/25	7/25		30.21	0.57 [0.19, 1.71]
Cheng 1991	2/22	2/23		10.51	1.05 [0.16, 6.79]
Lye 1993	0/30	1/30		3.69	0.33 [0.01, 7.87]
Cheng 1998	5/47	4/53		23.17	1.41 [0.40, 4.94]
Total (95% CI)	146	157		100.00	1.17 [0.63, 2.14]
Total events: 19 (Oral), 18 (Intraperitoneal)					
Test for heterogeneity: Chi² = 4.05, df = 4 (P = 0.40), I² = 1.2%					
Test for overall effect: Z = 0.49 (P = 0.62)				**Relapse**	
Chan 1990	3/74	2/36		25.85	0.73 [0.13, 4.18]
Lye 1993	7/30	5/30		74.15	1.40 [0.50, 3.92]
Total (95% CI)	104	66		100.00	1.18 [0.49, 2.87]
Total events: 10 (Oral), 7 (Intraperitoneal)					
Test for heterogeneity: Chi² = 0.40, df = 1 (P = 0.53), I² = 0%					
Test for overall effect: Z = 0.37 (P = 0.71)				**Catheter removal**	

0.1   0.2   0.5   1   2   5   10
Favours treatment   Favours control

Figure 47.7 Intraperitoneal versus oral antibiotics: effects on treatment failure, relapse, and catheter removal.

fact that this is a clinically relevant and frequently encountered complication.

The optimal route of antibiotic administration has been addressed in trials comparing oral and intraperitoneal administration [62,66–72] and comparing intravenous and intraperitoneal dosing [73]. One trial found intraperitoneal therapy to be superior to a regimen where the initial antibiotics were given intravenously, followed by oral antibiotics at day 4 if considered appropriate. This finding may relate to achievement of higher intraperitoneal antibiotic concentrations with intraperitoneal versus systemic dosing and early use of oral therapy; however, a meta-analysis of 10 trials found that oral dosing was equivalent to intraperitoneal dosing (Figure 47.7). This was demonstrated when the same drug was administered intraperitoneally and orally [62,67,74] and when oral

quinolone monotherapy was compared to intraperitoneal combination therapy.

The ISPD guidelines recommend adjustment of some drug doses in patients with residual renal function and high transporters to compensate for increased urinary and peritoneal clearance, respectively. RCTs performed to date have not compared different dosing regimens or stratified patients according to residual renal function. Small pharmacokinetic studies found no difference in drug levels or clearances in patients stratified according to glomerular filtration rate; however, there were very small patient numbers [75,76]. Further evaluation in this area is required.

Intermittent dosing (daily or less frequent) was equivalent to continuous dosing (with each exchange) in four trials [77–79] (Figure 47.8). The applicability of results from trials of intermittent

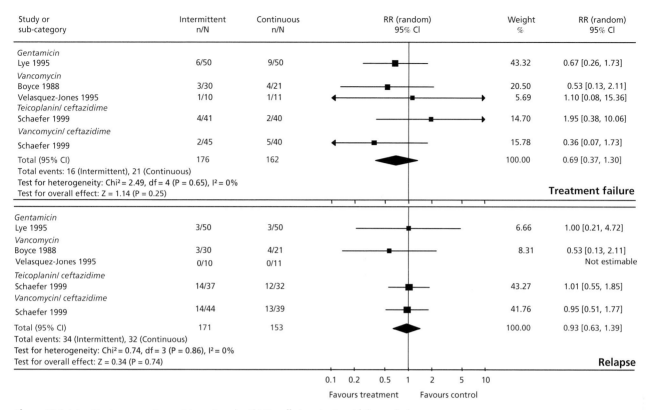

Study or sub-category	Intermittent n/N	Continuous n/N	RR (random) 95% CI	Weight %	RR (random) 95% CI
Gentamicin					
Lye 1995	6/50	9/50		43.32	0.67 [0.26, 1.73]
Vancomycin					
Boyce 1988	3/30	4/21		20.50	0.53 [0.13, 2.11]
Velasquez-Jones 1995	1/10	1/11		5.69	1.10 [0.08, 15.36]
Teicoplanin/ ceftazidime					
Schaefer 1999	4/41	2/40		14.70	1.95 [0.38, 10.06]
Vancomycin/ ceftazidime					
Schaefer 1999	2/45	5/40		15.78	0.36 [0.07, 1.73]
Total (95% CI)	176	162		100.00	0.69 [0.37, 1.30]
Total events: 16 (Intermittent), 21 (Continuous)					
Test for heterogeneity: Chi² = 2.49, df = 4 (P = 0.65), I² = 0%					
Test for overall effect: Z = 1.14 (P = 0.25)					**Treatment failure**
Gentamicin					
Lye 1995	3/50	3/50		6.66	1.00 [0.21, 4.72]
Vancomycin					
Boyce 1988	3/30	4/21		8.31	0.53 [0.13, 2.11]
Velasquez-Jones 1995	0/10	0/11			Not estimable
Teicoplanin/ ceftazidime					
Schaefer 1999	14/37	12/32		43.27	1.01 [0.55, 1.85]
Vancomycin/ ceftazidime					
Schaefer 1999	14/44	13/39		41.76	0.95 [0.51, 1.77]
Total (95% CI)	171	153		100.00	0.93 [0.63, 1.39]
Total events: 34 (Intermittent), 32 (Continuous)					
Test for heterogeneity: Chi² = 0.74, df = 3 (P = 0.86), I² = 0%					
Test for overall effect: Z = 0.34 (P = 0.74)					**Relapse**

0.1 0.2   0.5   1   2   5   10
Favours treatment   Favours control

Figure 47.8 Intermittent versus continuous intraperitoneal antibiotics: effects on treatment failure and relapse.

drug therapy in CAPD to APD is unclear. Drug half-lives are greater and clearance is more rapid in cycler dwells compared to noncycler dwells [80]. Pharmacokinetic studies of intraperitoneal antibiotic dosing suggest that therapeutic drug levels are achieved during 6-h dwells [75,76]; therefore, it is likely that a patient can remain on APD as long as there is at least a 6-h daytime dwell during which antibiotics can be administered.

Peritoneal lavage in conjunction with antibiotic treatment provided no additional benefit in one trial, and it appears to have no routine place in peritonitis treatment [33]. Urokinase had no

advantages over placebo in improving response rates or reducing relapse [32,81,82] and, when compared to early catheter removal, urokinase was clearly inferior [83] (Figure 47.9). Overall, urokinase appears to have no role in standard treatment regimens. One study of intraperitoneal immunoglobulin administration in conjunction with antibiotics found that the treatment group achieved biochemical and clinical parameters of improvement sooner and that the duration of antibiotic therapy was shorter [34]. However, the response rate was 100% in both groups with no relapses during a 3-month follow-up period, suggesting that use

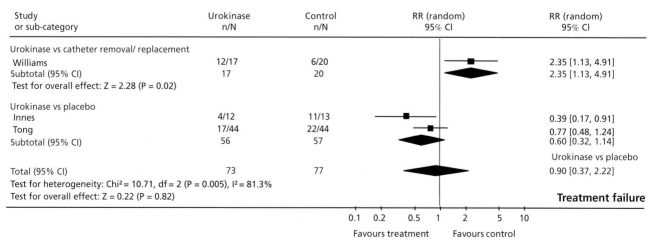

Study or sub-category	Urokinase n/N	Control n/N	RR (random) 95% CI	RR (random) 95% CI
Urokinase vs catheter removal/ replacement				
Williams	12/17	6/20		2.35 [1.13, 4.91]
Subtotal (95% CI)	17	20		2.35 [1.13, 4.91]
Test for overall effect: Z = 2.28 (P = 0.02)				
Urokinase vs placebo				
Innes	4/12	11/13		0.39 [0.17, 0.91]
Tong	17/44	22/44		0.77 [0.48, 1.24]
Subtotal (95% CI)	56	57		0.60 [0.32, 1.14]
				Urokinase vs placebo
Total (95% CI)	73	77		0.90 [0.37, 2.22]
Test for heterogeneity: Chi² = 10.71, df = 2 (P = 0.005), I² = 81.3%				
Test for overall effect: Z = 0.22 (P = 0.82)				**Treatment failure**

0.1 0.2   0.5   1   2   5   10
Favours treatment   Favours control

Figure 47.9 Urokinase treatment versus catheter removal or replacement versus placebo: effects on treatment failure.

Table 47.9 Evidence ratings and recommendations for interventions to treat PD-related infections.

Intervention	Existing systematic reviews[a]	Overall evidence rating[b]			Comment	Recommendation[c]			Comment
		High	Moderate	Low		I[a]	II[b]	III[c]	
Intravenous vs. intraperitoneal antibiotics	•		•		2 RCTs, small sample size, 1 RCT poor methodological quality	•			Moderate effect size, low evidence base, no harm demonstrated, likely to be more acceptable to patients, facilitates outpatient management
Oral vs. intraperitoneal antibiotics	•		•		10 RCTs, low heterogeneity, 5 RCTs poor methodological quality		•		Undetermined effect, large evidence base, high risk of resistant microorganisms with oral antibiotic regimens used
High-dose vs. low-dose antibiotics	•			•	Subset of 1 RCT, small sample size			•	Large effect size, low evidence base, moderate likelihood of harm
Intermittent vs. continuous intraperitoneal antibiotics	•		•		4 RCTs, low heterogeneity, 2 RCTs poor methodological quality		•		Undetermined effect, moderate evidence base, no harm demonstrated, greater acceptance by patients likely, applicability to APD and antibiotics with different pharmacokinetic properties unclear
Regimen A vs. regimen B intraperitoneal antibiotics	•		•		14 RCTs, small sample sizes, 9 RCTs poor methodological quality			•	Small, imprecise effect size, small evidence base, low applicability to current practice, no harm demonstrated
Regimen A vs. regimen B oral antibiotics	•		•		1 RCT, small sample size, poor methodological quality			•	Undetermined effect, low evidence base, no harm demonstrated
Peritoneal lavage vs. standard therapy	•			•	1 RCT, small sample size, poor methodological quality			•	Undetermined effect, low evidence base, no harm demonstrated
Urokinase vs. placebo or routine catheter removal/ replacement	•		•		4 RCTs, high heterogeneity, 1 RCT poor methodological quality	•			Large effect size for catheter removal or replacement, moderate evidence base, no harm demonstrated
Intraperitoneal immunoglobulin vs. standard therapy	•			•	1 RCT, small sample size			•	Large effect size on laboratory parameters but no effect on clinical outcomes, no harm, biologically plausible

[a] If no existing systematic review, overall evidence rating will start at moderate.

[b] Evidence rating based on number of trials, study design, study quality. and consistency of results.

[c] Recommendation based on efficacy, trade-offs between benefits and harms, quality of evidence, and availability of medication. I, recommend; II, suggest; III, no recommendation possible.

of immunoglobulin does not change overall patient outcomes. This, together with the expense and limited availability of immunoglobulin therapy, reduces the feasibility of this treatment as part of routine therapy at the present time.

There have been no clinical trials evaluating the role of routine early catheter removal in refractory peritonitis or of temporary transfer of patients from APD to CAPD. In the latter case the question of when to safely recommence APD has also not been addressed.

Surgical peritonitis refers to cases in which peritonitis arises from intra-abdominal pathology. This may manifest as polymicrobial peritonitis. Such cases are usually treated by laparotomy and catheter removal at the same time as the underlying pathology is addressed, followed by a course of broad-spectrum intravenous antibiotics. There have been no trials addressing the treatment of this situation, and such trials are unlikely to be performed.

As with infection prevention trials, systematic reviews of peritonitis treatment trials are limited by the suboptimal methodological quality of many trials, in particular, inadequate randomization and concealment methods were common. Definitions of peritonitis, successful treatment, and relapse varied between trials, thereby reducing their comparability. Similarly, antibiotic doses were not consistent across studies. The follow-up period of most included trials was 28 days or less, meaning that several long-term outcomes of peritonitis treatment, such as technique failure and longer-term mortality, were not evaluated. Studies tended to focus on choice and route of antibiotic without consideration of other variables, such as total duration of therapy or drug dose. To date, there have been no RCTs of treatment for fungal peritonitis, a condition that is associated with almost 100% catheter loss and high levels of mortality. Reported trials often predate the current era of lower peritonitis rates, newer antibiotic therapies, and increased awareness of multidrug-resistant organisms, thereby potentially reducing the applicability of our meta-analyses or the individual trials' results. These aspects all need to be considered when making a decision about recommending or suggesting adoption of these interventions.

Conclusions

There is evidence from clinical trials to support a small number of effective interventions in prevention and treatment of PD-related infections and some evidence that other interventions, which are in current use, are not likely to be studied further nor to cause substantial harm. The recommendations and suggestions for clinical care that can be made based on currently available evidence are summarized in Table 47.7 to 47.9, below. Eradication of nasal *S. aureus* carriage with topical mupirocin reduces the risk of exit site and tunnel infections (but not peritonitis), and intravenous antibiotic administration prior to PD catheter insertion prevents the risk of early postoperative peritonitis. These strategies can be recommended. Concomitant use of oral nystatin with antibiotic therapy to reduce the occurrence of *Candida* peritonitis isrecommended. Disconnect (twin bag and Y-set) systems are clearly superior to conventional spike systems for the prevention of peritonitis and should be recommended; however, there is no clear advantage of twin bag over Y-set systems, different catheter designs, implantation techniques, or APD.

Treatment of peritonitis should consist of antimicrobial therapy, but most antibiotic regimens for empiric treatment are similar in efficacy, so no specific regimen can be recommended. Available evidence shows intraperitoneal administration of antibiotics to be superior to intravenous administration, the intraperitoneal route is more likely to be acceptable to patients, and this mode of administration is therefore recommended. Oral quinolones and intraperitoneal regimens have equal levels of efficacy, but due to a general increase in community levels of quinolone-resistant

microorganisms, this therapy is not recommended. Intermittent therapy appears to be equivalent to continuous therapy; however, further trials involving patients on APD are required, and thus this therapy can be suggested but not recommended. In relapsing or resistant peritonitis, catheter removal, and not urokinase, is recommended. There are insufficient trial data to make recommendations about peritoneal lavage, intraperitoneal immunoglobulin, or different dosing regimens.

There remains a need in this area for well-designed, randomized controlled studies. The design of such studies should focus on adequate allocation concealment and blinding of outcome assessors. In many cases, blinding of participants and investigators is difficult due to overt differences in interventions; however, when possible this should occur. Blinded measurements of outcomes are always possible. Preventative strategies that would be particularly worth investigating are trials of laparoscopy versus laparotomy for catheter insertion, exploring effects on early peritonitis (less than 1 month from catheter insertion), and of straight versus coiled catheters. Current data for both of these have suggested possible differences that require substantiation. Trials in these areas should be adequately powered to detect relevant outcomes. Studies of topical Medihoney application to reduce infection rates would be valuable, as this is a readily available treatment that is likely to be associated with minimal harm. Further studies of peritonitis treatment should be designed with follow-up periods sufficient to allow evaluation of outcomes, such as ultrafiltration failure, technique failure, and all-cause mortality. Specific interventions to be addressed include duration of antibiotic therapy and intraperitoneal courses versus combined intraperitoneal–per oral courses. Stratification of patients into CAPD and APD would be beneficial given the increasing number of patients on the latter therapy.

References

1 Heaf J. Underutilization of peritoneal dialysis. *JAMA* 2004; **291(6):** 740–742.

2 Kavanagh D, Prescott GJ, Mactier RA. Peritoneal dialysis-associated peritonitis in Scotland (1999-2002). *Nephrol Dial Transplant* 2004; **19(10):** 2584–2591.

3 CARI Guidelines (Caring for Australians with Renal Impairment). *Nephrology* (Carlton) 2005; **9(Suppl 3):** S1–S106.

4 Grunberg J, Verocay MC, Rebori A, Ramela V, Amaral C, Hekimian G *et al.* Twenty years' pediatric chronic peritoneal dialysis in Uruguay: patient and technique survival. *Pediatr Nephrol* 2005; **20(9):** 1315–1319.

5 Katz IJ, Sofianou L, Hopley M. An African community-based chronic ambulatory peritoneal dialysis programme. *Nephrol Dial Transplant* 2001; **16(12):** 2395–2400.

6 Vas S, Oreopoulos DG. Infections in patients undergoing peritoneal dialysis. *Infect Dis Clin North Am* 2001; **15(3):** 743–774.

7 Oxton LL, Zimmerman SW, Roecker EB, Wakeen M. Risk factors for peritoneal dialysis-related infections. *Perit Dial Int* 1994; **14(2):** 137–144.

8 Salusky I, Holloway M. Selection of peritoneal dialysis for pediatric patients. *Perit Dial Int* 1994; **17(3):** S35–S37.

9 Juergensen PH, Gorban-Brennan N, Troidle L, Finkelstein FO. Racial differences and peritonitis in an urban peritoneal dialysis center. *Adv Perit Dial* 2002; **18**: 117–118.

10 Lim WH, Johnson DW, McDonald SP. Higher rate and earlier peritonitis in Aboriginal patients compared to non-Aboriginal patients with end-stage renal failure maintained on peritoneal dialysis in Australia: analysis of ANZDATA. *Nephrology* (Carlton) 2005; **10(2)**: 192–197.

11 McDonald SP, Collins JF, Rumpsfeld M, Johnson DW. Obesity is a risk factor for peritonitis in the Australian and New Zealand peritoneal dialysis patient populations. *Perit Dial Int* 2004; **24(4)**: 340–346.

12 Alves FR, Dantas RC, Lugon JR. Higher incidence of catheter-related infections in a tropical climate. *Adv Perit Dial* 1993; **9**: 244–247.

13 Szeto CC, Chow KM, Wong TY, Leung CB, Li PK. Influence of climate on the incidence of peritoneal dialysis-related peritonitis. *Perit Dial Int* 2003; **23(6)**: 580–586.

14 Troidle L, Watnick S, Wuerth DB, Gorban-Brennan N, Kliger AS, Finkelstein FO. Depression and its association with peritonitis in long-term peritoneal dialysis patients. *Am J Kidney Dis* 2003; **42(2)**: 350–354.

15 Golper TA, Brier ME, Bunke M, Schreiber MJ, Bartlett DK, Hamilton RW *et al*. Risk factors for peritonitis in long-term peritoneal dialysis: the Network 9 peritonitis and catheter survival studies. Academic Subcommittee of the Steering Committee of the Network 9 Peritonitis and Catheter Survival Studies. *Am J Kidney Dis* 1996; **28(3)**: 428–436.

16 Schaefer F. Management of peritonitis in children receiving chronic peritoneal dialysis. *Paediatr Drugs* 2003; **5(5)**: 315–325.

17 Huang JW, Hung KY, Yen CJ, Wu KD, Tsai TJ. Comparison of infectious complications in peritoneal dialysis patients using either a twin-bag system or automated peritoneal dialysis. *Nephrol Dial Transplant* 2001; **16(3)**: 604–607.

18 Oo TN, Roberts TL, Collins AJ. A comparison of peritonitis rates from the United States Renal Data System database: CAPD versus continuous cycling peritoneal dialysis patients. *Am J Kidney Dis* 2005; **45(2)**: 372–380.

19 Churchill DN, Thorpe KE, Vonesh EF, Keshaviah PR. Lower probability of patient survival with continuous peritoneal dialysis in the United States compared with Canada. Canada-USA (CANUSA) Peritoneal Dialysis Study Group. *J Am Soc Nephrol* 1997; **8(6)**: 965–971.

20 Piraino B. Staphylococcus aureus infections in dialysis patients: focus on prevention. *ASAIO J* 2000; **46(6)**: S13–S17.

21 Fried LF, Bernardini J, Johnston JR, Piraino B. Peritonitis influences mortality in peritoneal dialysis patients. *J Am Soc Nephrol* 1996; **7(10)**: 2176–2182.

22 Davies SJ, Bryan J, Phillips L, Russell GI. Longitudinal changes in peritoneal kinetics: the effects of peritoneal dialysis and peritonitis. *Nephrol Dial Transplant* 1996; **11(3)**: 498–506.

23 Kawanishi H, Watanabe H, Moriishi M, Tsuchiya S. Successful surgical management of encapsulating peritoneal sclerosis. *Perit Dial Int* 2005; **25(Suppl 4)**: S39–S47.

24 Rigby RJ, Hawley CM. Sclerosing peritonitis: the experience in Australia. *Nephrol Dial Transplant* 1998; **13(1)**: 154–159.

25 Thodis E, Passadakis P, Panagoutsos S, Bacharaki D, Euthimiadou A, Vargemezis V. The effectiveness of mupirocin preventing Staphylococcus aureus in catheter-related infections in peritoneal dialysis. *Adv Perit Dial* 2000; **16**: 257–261.

26 Piraino B. ADEMEX: how should it change our practice? Adequacy of Peritoneal Dialysis in Mexico. *Perit Dial Int* 2002; **22(5)**: 552–554.

27 Burkart JM. Recommendations for clinical practice and research needs directed at reducing morbidity and mortality in peritoneal dialysis. *Perit Dial Int* 1997; **17(Suppl 3)**: S6–S8.

28 Luzar MA, Brown CB, Balf D, Hill L, Issad B, Monnier B *et al*. Exit-site care and exit-site infection in continuous ambulatory peritoneal dialysis (CAPD): results of a randomized multicenter trial. *Perit Dial Int* 1990; **10(1)**: 25–29.

29 Peacock SJ, Mandal S, Bowler IC. Preventing Staphylococcus aureus infection in the renal unit. *QJM* 2002; **95(6)**: 405–410.

30 Piraino B. Infectious complications of peritoneal dialysis. *Perit Dial Int* 1997; **17(Suppl 3)**: S15–S18.

31 Pickering SJ, Fleming SJ, Bowley JA, Sissons P, Oppenheim BA, Burnie J *et al*. Urokinase: a treatment for relapsing peritonitis due to coagulase-negative staphylococci. *Nephrol Dial Transplant* 1989; **4(1)**: 62–65.

32 Innes A, Burden RP, Finch RG, Morgan AG. Treatment of resistant peritonitis in continuous ambulatory peritoneal dialysis with intraperitoneal urokinase: a double-blind clinical trial. *Nephrol Dial Transplant* 1994; **9(7)**: 797–799.

33 Ejlersen E, Brandi L, Lokkegaard H, Ladefoged J, Kopp R, Haarh P. Is initial (24 hours) lavage necessary in treatment of CAPD peritonitis? *Perit Dial Int* 1991; **11(1)**: 38–42.

34 Coban E, Ozdogan M, Tuncer M, Bozcuk H, Ersoy F. The value of low-dose intraperitoneal immunoglobulin administration in the treatment of peritoneal dialysis-related peritonitis. *J Nephrol* 2004; **17(3)**: 427–430.

35 Kan GW, Thomas MA, Heath CH. A 12-month review of peritoneal dialysis-related peritonitis in Western Australia: is empiric vancomycin still indicated for some patients? *Perit Dial Int* 2003; **23(5)**: 465–468.

36 Piraino B, Bailie GR, Bernardini J, Boeschoten E, Gupta A, Holmes C *et al*. Peritoneal dialysis-related infections recommendations: 2005 update. *Perit Dial Int* 2005; **25(2)**: 107–131.

37 Strippoli GF, Tong A, Johnson D, Schena FP, Craig JC. Antimicrobial agents to prevent peritonitis in peritoneal dialysis: a systematic review of randomized controlled trials. *Am J Kidney Dis* 2004; **44(4)**: 591–603.

38 Daly CD, Campbell MK, MacLeod AM, Cody DJ, Vale LD, Grant AM *et al*. Do the Y-set and double-bag systems reduce the incidence of CAPD peritonitis? A systematic review of randomized controlled trials. *Nephrol Dial Transplant* 2001; **16(2)**: 341–347.

39 Strippoli GF, Tong A, Johnson D, Schena FP, Craig JC. Catheter-related interventions to prevent peritonitis in peritoneal dialysis: a systematic review of randomized, controlled trials. *J Am Soc Nephrol* 2004; **15(10)**: 2735–2746.

40 Wiggins K, Craig J, Johnson D, Strippoli G. Treatment for Peritoneal Dialysis-Associated Peritonitis. John Wiley & Sons, Ltd., New York, 2005.

41 Wiggins K, Johnson D, Craig J, Strippoli G. A systematic review of trials of peritoneal dialysis-associated treatment (abstract). Annual Scientific Meeting of American Society of Nephrology. Philadelphia, 2005.

42 Bernardini J, Bender F, Florio T, Sloand J, Palmmontalbano L, Fried L *et al*. Randomized, double-blind trial of antibiotic exit site cream for prevention of exit site infection in peritoneal dialysis patients. *J Am Soc Nephrol* 2005; **16(2)**: 539–545.

43 Davey P, Craig AM, Hau C, Malek M. Cost-effectiveness of prophylactic nasal mupirocin in patients undergoing peritoneal dialysis based on a randomized, placebo-controlled trial. *J Antimicrob Chemother* 1999; **43(1)**: 105–112.

44 Johnson DW, van Eps C, Mudge DW, Wiggins KJ, Armstrong K, Hawley CM *et al*. Randomized, controlled trial of topical exit-site application of honey (Medihoney) versus mupirocin for the prevention of catheter-associated infections in hemodialysis patients. *J Am Soc Nephrol* 2005; **16(5)**: 1456–1462.

45 Bennet-Jones D, Martin J, Barratt A, Duffy T, Naish P, Aber G. Prophylactic gentamicin in the prevention of early exit-site infections and peritonitis in CAPD. *Adv Perit Dial* 1998; **4**: 147–150.

46 Gadallah MF, Ramdeen G, Torres C, Mignone J, Patel D, Mitchell L *et al.* Preoperative vancomycin prophylaxis for newly placed peritoneal dialysis catheters prevents postoperative peritonitis. *Adv Perit Dial* 2000; **16**: 199–203.

47 Lye WC, Lee EJ, Tan CC. Prophylactic antibiotics in the insertion of Tenckhoff catheters. *Scand J Urol Nephrol* 1992; **26(2)**: 177–180.

48 Wikdahl AM, Engman U, Stegmayr BG, Sorenssen JG. One-dose cefuroxime i.v. and i.p. reduces microbial growth in PD patients after catheter insertion. *Nephrol Dial Transplant* 1997; **12(1)**: 157–160.

49 Lo WK, Chan CY, Cheng SW, Poon JF, Chan DT, Cheng IK. A prospective randomized control study of oral nystatin prophylaxis for Candida peritonitis complicating continuous ambulatory peritoneal dialysis. *Am J Kidney Dis* 1996; **28(4)**: 549–552.

50 Wilson AP, Lewis C, O'Sullivan H, Shetty N, Neild GH, Mansell M. The use of povidone iodine in exit site care for patients undergoing continuous peritoneal dialysis (CAPD). *J Hosp Infect* 1997; **35(4)**: 287–293.

51 Nolph K, Prowant B, Serkes K, *et al.* A randomized multicenter clinical trial to evaluate the effects of an ultraviolet germicidal system on peritonitis rate in continuous ambulatory peritoneal dialysis. *Perit Dial Bull* 1985; **1**: 19–24.

52 Poole-Warren LA, Hallett MD, Hone PW, Burden SH, Farrell PC. Vaccination for prevention of CAPD associated staphylococcal infection: results of a prospective multicentre clinical trial. *Clin Nephrol* 1991; **35(5)**: 198–206.

53 Owen JE, Walker RG, Lemon J, Brett L, Mitrou D, Becker GJ. Randomized study of peritonitis with conventional versus O-set techniques in continuous ambulatory peritoneal dialysis. *Perit Dial Int* 1992; **12(2)**: 216–220.

54 Ansell D, Feest T. UK Renal Registry Report 1998. Bristol, United Kingdom, 1998.

55 Johnson D. Peritoneal dialysis. In: McDonald S, Russ G, editors, *ANZDATA Registry Report 2003*. Adelaide, 1998; 39–54.

56 Bro S, Bjorner JB, Tofte-Jensen P, Klem S, Almtoft B, Danielsen H *et al.* A prospective, randomized multicenter study comparing APD and CAPD treatment. *Perit Dial Int* 1999; **19(6)**: 526–533.

57 De Fijter C, Oe P, Nauta JJ, van der Meulen J, ter Wee PM, Snoek FJ *et al.* A prospective randomised trial comparing the peritonitis incidence of CAPD and Y-connector (CAPD-Y) with continuous cyclic peritoneal dialysis (CCPD). *Adv Perit Dial* 1991; **7**: 186–189.

58 Flanigan MJ, Hochstetler LA, Langholdt D, Lim VS. Continuous ambulatory peritoneal dialysis catheter infections: diagnosis and management. *Perit Dial Int* 1994; **14(3)**: 248–254.

59 Plum J, Artik S, Busch T, Sahin K, Grabensee B. Oral versus intraperitoneal application of clindamycin in tunnel infections: a prospective, randomised study in CAPD patients. *Perit Dial Int* 1997; **17**: 486–492.

60 Flanigan MJ, Lim VS. Initial treatment of dialysis associated peritonitis: a controlled trial of vancomycin versus cefazolin. *Perit Dial Int* 1991; **11(1)**: 31–37.

61 Khairullah Q, Provenzano R, Tayeb J, Ahmad A, Balakrishnan R, Morrison L. Comparison of vancomycin versus cefazolin as initial therapy for peritonitis in peritoneal dialysis patients. *Perit Dial Int* 2002; **22(3)**: 339–344.

62 Cheng IK, Chan CY, Wong WT, Cheng SW, Ritchie CW, Cheung WC *et al.* A randomized prospective comparison of oral versus intraperitoneal ciprofloxacin as the primary treatment of peritonitis complicating continuous ambulatory peritoneal dialysis. *Perit Dial Int* 1993; **13(Suppl 2)**: S351–S354.

63 Carmeli Y, Eliopoulos GM, Samore MH. Antecedent treatment with different antibiotic agents as a risk factor for vancomycin-resistant Enterococcus. *Emerg Infect Dis* 2002; **8(8)**: 802–807.

64 Oprea SF, Zaidi N, Donabedian SM, Balasubramaniam M, Hershberger E, Zervos MJ. Molecular and clinical epidemiology of vancomycin-resistant Enterococcus faecalis. *J Antimicrob Chemother* 2004; **53(4)**: 626–630.

65 Lui SL, Cheng SW, Ng F, Ng SY, Wan KM, Yip T *et al.* Cefazolin plus netilmicin versus cefazolin plus ceftazidime for treating CAPD peritonitis: effect on residual renal function. *Kidney Int* 2005; **68(5)**: 2375–2380.

66 Bennett-Jones DN, Russell GI, Barrett A. A comparison between oral ciprofloxacin and intra-peritoneal vancomycin and gentamicin in the treatment of CAPD peritonitis. *J Antimicrob Chemother* 1990; **26(Suppl F)**: 73–76.

67 Boeschoten EW, Rietra PJ, Krediet RT, Visser MJ, Arisz L. CAPD peritonitis: a prospective randomized trial of oral versus intraperitoneal treatment with cephradine. *J Antimicrob Chemother* 1985; **16(6)**: 789–797.

68 Chan MK, Cheng IK, Ng WS. A randomized prospective trial of three different regimens of treatment of peritonitis in patients on continuous ambulatory peritoneal dialysis. *Am J Kidney Dis* 1990; **15(2)**: 155–159.

69 Cheng IK, Chan CY, Wong WT. A randomised prospective comparison of oral ofloxacin and intraperitoneal vancomycin plus aztreonam in the treatment of bacterial peritonitis complicating continuous ambulatory peritoneal dialysis (CAPD). *Perit Dial Int* 1991; **11(1)**: 27–30.

70 Gucek A, Bren AF, Lindic J, Hergouth V, Mlinsek D. Is monotherapy with cefazolin or ofloxacin an adequate treatment for peritonitis in CAPD patients? *Adv Perit Dial* 1994; **10**: 144–146.

71 Lye WC, Lee EJ, van der Straaten J. Intraperitoneal vancomycin/oral pefloxacin versus intraperitoneal vancomycin/gentamicin in the treatment of continuous ambulatory peritoneal dialysis peritonitis. *Perit Dial Int* 1993; **13(Suppl 2)**: S348–S350.

72 Tapson JS, Orr KE, George JC, Stansfield E, Bint AJ, Ward MK. A comparison between oral ciprofloxacin and intraperitoneal vancomycin and netilmicin in CAPD peritonitis. *J Antimicrob Chemother* 1990; **26(Suppl F)**: 63–71.

73 Bailie GR, Morton R, Ganguli L, Keaney M, Waldek S. Intravenous or intraperitoneal vancomycin for the treatment of continuous ambulatory peritoneal dialysis associated gram-positive peritonitis? *Nephron* 1987; **46(3)**: 316–318.

74 Cheng I, Lui S, Fang G, Chau P, Cheng S, Chiu F *et al.* A randomised prospective comparison of oral versus intraperitoneal ofloxacin as the primary treatment of CAPD peritonitis. *Nephrology* 1997; **3**: 431–435.

75 Grabe DW, Bailie GR, Eisele G, Frye RF. Pharmacokinetics of intermittent intraperitoneal ceftazidime. *Am J Kidney Dis* 1999; **33(1)**: 111–117.

76 Manley HJ, Bailie GR, Asher RD, Eisele G, Frye RF. Pharmacokinetics of intermittent intraperitoneal cefazolin in continuous ambulatory peritoneal dialysis patients. *Perit Dial Int* 1999; **19(1)**: 65–70.

77 Boyce NW, Wood C, Thomson NM, Kerr P, Atkins RC. Intraperitoneal (IP) vancomycin therapy for CAPD peritonitis: a prospective, randomized comparison of intermittent v continuous therapy. *Am J Kidney Dis* 1988; **12(4)**: 304–306.

78 Lye WC, Wong PL, van der Straaten JC, Leong SO, Lee EJ. A prospective randomized comparison of single versus multidose gentamicin in the treatment of CAPD peritonitis. *Adv Perit Dial* 1995; **11**: 179–181.

79 Schaefer F, Klaus G, Muller-Wiefel DE, Mehls O. Intermittent versus continuous intraperitoneal glycopeptide/ceftazidime treatment in children

with peritoneal dialysis-associated peritonitis. The Mid-European Pediatric Peritoneal Dialysis Study Group (MEPPS). *J Am Soc Nephrol* 1999; **10(1):** 136–145.

80 Manley HJ, Bailie GR. Treatment of peritonitis in APD: pharmacokinetic principles. *Semin Dial* 2002; **15(6):** 418–421.

81 Gadallah MF, Tamayo A, Sandborn M, Ramdeen G, Moles K. Role of intraperitoneal urokinase in acute peritonitis and prevention of catheter loss in peritoneal dialysis patients. *Adv Perit Dial* 2000; **16:** 233–236.

82 Tong MK, Leung KT, Siu YP, Lee KF, Lee HK, Yung CY *et al.* Use of intraperitoneal urokinase for resistant bacterial peritonitis in continuous ambulatory peritoneal dialysis. *J Nephrol* 2005; **18(2):** 204–208.

83 Williams AJ, Boletis I, Johnson BF, Raftery AT, Cohen GL, Moorhead PJ *et al.* Tenckhoff catheter replacement or intraperitoneal urokinase: a randomised trial in the management of recurrent continuous ambulatory peritoneal dialysis (CAPD) peritonitis. *Perit Dial Int* 1989; **9(1):** 65–67.

8   Transplantation

48 Evaluation and Selection of the Kidney Transplant Candidate

Bryce Kiberd

Dalhouise University, Halifax, Nova Scotia, Canada

Introduction

Kidney transplantation improves quality of life and length of life and costs less than dialysis (Table 48.1) [1–4]. However, comparing outcomes for transplanted patients to the general dialysis or wait-listed population is not ideal, because there are survival and selection biases [5–7]. Less than half of patients on dialysis are considered for transplantation; <3% of dialysis patients more than 70 years old are on the transplant waiting list [6], and most older patients who are on the list will either die or be removed from the list before receiving a transplant [8]. The process of selection is an essential but problematic activity. Most guidelines have focused on evaluation, leaving patient selection to a center's discretion [9–13].

Organ allocation policies recognize the need to find a balance between conflicting goals [11–14]. Goals of selection include the following: 1) maximize patient and graft survival, 2) minimize disparities in waiting time, 3) minimize deaths while waiting, and 4) maximize opportunity. Achieving equality may reduce utility. Attempts to minimize deaths on the list by performing transplants in the elderly will limit the ability to maximize survival by transplanting in younger patients. These competing goals are the root of the difficulty in defining selection criteria. One compromise is to limit transplantation to patients with reasonable life expectancies who are likely to live beyond current waiting times [12].

Cardiovascular disease

Recommendations

All patients should undergo cardiac evaluation by history, physical, electrocardiogram, and chest radiograph. Further testing should be based on the initial assessment. Contraindications to transplantation include progressive angina, recent myocardial infarction (<6 months), and diffuse coronary artery or valve disease that is not correctable.

Evidence

Because cardiac disease is prevalent and the major cause of excess mortality, evaluating the extent of the disease and implementing preventive strategies is reasonable [15]. Congestive heart failure and ischemic heart disease occur in 27% and 29% of incident dialysis patients, respectively, and both are associated with reduced likelihood of transplantation [16].

Potential transplant recipients with cardiac symptoms or active disease deserve further evaluation, as in the general population [17]. Many uremic patients are sedentary or have symptoms that are ascribed to anemia or poor general health. Screening the high-risk asymptomatic recipient may be useful. Because the transplant procedure meets the criteria for high risk, as it involves vascular surgery and fluid shifts, and most patients have at least intermediate clinical risk factors (diabetes mellitus, renal impairment, ischemic heart disease), further evaluation is within accepted guidelines [18]. There are data supporting routine evaluation in asymptomatic potential kidney transplant patients. A relatively old study in a small group of high-risk diabetic uremic patients showed that there were a greater number of cardiac end points in the medical treatment arm (calcium channel blockers and aspirin) than in the intervention arm (angioplasty or bypass surgery) [19]. The extent of routine revascularization in asymptomatic pretransplant patients undergoing preparation for listing has not been quantified well in the nondiabetic population or in a larger diabetic population. A major reason for uncertainty is that a large trial ($n = 510$) in nontransplant patients found preoperative invasive treatment did not improve survival after noncardiovascular surgery [20].

Patients older than 45 years or with diabetes mellitus, prior cardiac history, or other multiple risk factors may benefit from noninvasive testing. In a meta-analysis, noninvasive tests did predict later cardiac events and death with reasonable accuracy [21]. There is no consensus on what is the best noninvasive test. A number of studies have examined the accuracy of tests to detect coronary

Evidence-based Nephrology. Edited by Donald Molony and Jonathan Craig

Table 48.1 Survival advantages of kidney transplantation.

Age at transplantation (yrs)	gained with kidney transplantation (vs. dialysis)[a]		
	USRDS 2004 [3]	Gill *et al* [2][b]	Wolfe *et al.* [1][b]
0–14	29.5	17.2 (0–19 yrs old)	13.0 (0–19 yrs old)
15–19	22.1		
20–24	21.0	14.8 (20–39 yrs old)	17.0 (20–39 yrs old)
25–29	19.4		
30–34	17.6		
35–39	14.7		
40–44	13.8	9.4 (40–59 yrs old)	11.0 (40–59 yrs old)
45–49	12.1		
50–54	10.5		
55–59	9.0		
60–64	7.5	6.2	4.0 (60–74 yrs old)
65–69	6.3	5.3	
70–74	5.2	3.7 (70–79 yrs old)	
75–79	4.7		

[a] Methods for calculating survival advantages differed for each study.

[b] For the Gill *et al.* and Wolfe *et al.* studies, some wider age ranges were evaluated than in the USRDS study.

artery disease (Table 48.2) [11, 21–30]. Because of the high pretest likelihood, some have argued cardiac catheterization is the best approach [31]. Routine cardiac catheterization in high-risk patients is performed in only a minority of US centers [32]. Given that the availability of tests varies among centers and that not all tests are appropriate for any one patient, the local cardiologist should guide test selection. Patients with advanced disease, low functional capacity, or who do not have circumscribed arterial lesions that are amenable to treatment are likely do poorly with, or without, a transplant. Multivessel disease was an exclusion criterion in 88% of centers in a recent European survey [33]. Preoperative invasive therapy is likely to be of limited value in patients

with asymptomatic single- or double-vessel disease that is not a proximal left anterior descending lesion and not associated with impaired ventricular function. Discussions of further indications for corrective surgery and the evidence in asymptomatic patients are beyond the scope of this article.

Guidelines recommend periodic reevaluation [34,35], but cardiac evaluation in asymptomatic patients after listing is not routinely practiced and subsequent invasive therapy is unlikely. Kasiske reported intervention (angioplasty or bypass surgery) in only 9% of patients screened, with similar rates in the rescreened [36]. In a preliminary medical decision analysis, rescreening diabetic patients would be cost-effective if screening identified a

Table 48.2 Noninvasive screening for coronary artery disease.

Study [reference]	Population	n	Test	Criterion (% extent of stenosis)	Sensitivity (%)
Reis [24]	Pretransplant	97	DSE	>75	92
Vandanberg [22]	Diabetes mellitus, pretransplant	41	Pharmacologic thallium	>75	62
Vandanberg [22]	Diabetes mellitus, pretransplant	35	Exercise thallium	>75	50
Herzog [23]	Pretransplant	50	DSE	>75	75
De Lima [30]	Pretransplant	89	DSE	>70	44
De Lima [30]	Pretransplant	102	Pharmacologic SPECT	>70	64
West [28]	Pretransplant	33	DSE	>70	92
Boudreau [25]	Diabetes mellitus, pretransplant	80	Pharmacologic thallium	>70	86
Marwick [26]	Pretransplant	45	Pharmacologic thallium	>70	75
Worthley [27]	Pretransplant	50	Tachycardic Stress	>70	87

Abbreviations: DSE, dobutamine stress echocardiogram; SPECT, single photon emission computed tomography.

significant proportion with covert disease who subsequently received invasive therapy that allowed them to remain listed and where covert disease was associated with higher mortality rates [37]. What studies do not report is the extent to which evaluation results in appropriate delisting decisions.

There is a trend away from preoperative surgery and toward the use of medical interventions to prevent cardiovascular disease [38,39], although use of medications, even in high-risk wait list patients, is low [40]. Although a recent randomized controlled trial failed to show the benefits of statin therapy in diabetic hemodialysis patients [41], many study subjects were unlikely to be transplant candidates, and another randomized control trial demonstrated the benefit of statins posttransplantation in this subgroup in a post hoc analysis [41,42]. Without evidence of harm, it seems reasonable to consider greater use of cardiovascular disease risk-reducing medications in patients waiting for kidney transplantation.

Patients with symptomatic cardiac valve heart disease should be treated as these patients are in the general population. Patients denied appropriate surgical correction because of reduced life expectancy or excessive risk should not be considered for kidney transplantation (unless done in conjunction with cardiac transplantation). Isolated uremic cardiomyopathy is not an absolute contraindication to transplantation [43,44].

Cerebral vascular disease

Recommendation

Ancillary testing for cerebral vascular disease may be required based on history. A stroke or transient ischemic attack (TIA) within 3 months is an absolute contraindication to transplantation.

Evidence

Stroke mortality is the third (8%) most common cause of death posttransplantation [45,46]. Mortality after a stroke is 50% at 3 months [46].

Patients with a stroke or TIA should be treated with control of blood pressure, antithrombotic therapy for atrial fibrillation, and antiplatelet therapy [47]. Statins may also lower the incidence of stroke [48]. The optimal waiting time to allow recovery from injury is unknown, but waiting 2–3 months [49], the period in which there is the highest risk of recurrence is recommended. The short-term stroke risk is 11% after a TIA, and so a patient with a TIA should be considered at the same risk as a patient with a completed stroke [50]. Guidelines for patients with symptomatic or asymptomatic carotid disease who might benefit from endarterectomy are available elsewhere [51].

Screening for cerebral aneurysms in autosomal dominant polycystic kidney disease is controversial because it is uncertain whether screening and treatment confers net clinical benefit compared with treatment of only symptomatic patients [52]. The prevalence of aneurysms is likely to be higher in patients with a family history of stroke [53]. Younger patients with asymptomatic aneurysms of >10 mm should be considered for intervention [54].

Peripheral vascular disease

Recommendations

Ancillary testing for peripheral vascular disease should be based on history or physical findings. Large uncorrected aortic aneurysm, severe occlusive iliac disease, active gangrene, or recent atheroembolic events are contraindications to listing.

Evidence

Peripheral vascular disease is present in about 15% of incident dialysis patients and is associated with increased mortality (hazard ratio, 2.4) [55]. The prevalence of peripheral vascular disease at the time of transplantation is about 5–6% and is also associated with reduced survival [2,56].

Recent practice guidelines recommend screening for abdominal aneurysms in men between 65 and 75 years of age who have smoked, with uncertainty about similarly aged men who have never smoked [57]. Large abdominal aneurysms of 5–5.9 cm have rupture rates ranging from 4 to 14%/year and those of >6.0 cm have rupture rates of greater than 20%/year with high subsequent mortality [58]. Patients who are not considered candidates for repair because of high comorbidity are not likely to be transplant candidates. Patients with severe vascular disease in the iliac arterial system should be identified in order to prevent inadequate flow to the newly transplanted kidney.

Pulmonary disease

Recommendations

All patients should undergo a history, physical, and chest radiograph. Ancillary testing may be required in symptomatic patients or those with an abnormal chest radiograph. Advanced irreversible pulmonary disease or frequent lower tract infections are contraindications to transplantation.

Evidence

Uncontrolled asthma, severe chronic obstructive pulmonary disease and/or pulmonary fibrosis or restrictive disease with a low forced expiratory volume in 1 s (FEV1) of <25% of predicted value, low PO_2 (<60 mmHg) on room air, or with exercise desaturation (SaO_2) of <90% were acknowledged by consensus to be absolute contraindications [10]. Patients with less respiratory compromise but likely to progress and those with frequent infections (>4 lower respiratory infections in the last year) were also felt to be noncandidates. Patients with these disorders, typically with a best FEV1 of <40% of normal, have high mortality rates, with 50% survival at about 6 years. Patients with a FEV1 of <25% of predicted have an even lower survival [59], and patients requiring home oxygen therapy have a 5-year survival as low as 30% [60]. The incidence and case fatality rate of pneumonia have decreased over time [61], but patients with frequent infections prior

Target organ	Test	Test frequency	Age (yrs) at screening
Bladder	Cytoscopy	Not routine	>50 and high risk
Breast	Mammography	Every 1–2 yrs	>40
Colorectal[a]	FOBT	Annually (FOBT)	>50
	Sigmoidoscopy	Every 5 yrs	
	Colonoscopy	Every 10 yrs	
Kaposi sarcoma	Physical	Once	All
	HHV-8		High risk
Leukemia	CBC	Every year	All
Liver	Ultrasound or CT	Once	High risk, annually
Lung	CXR	Once	All
Lymphoma	Physical	Every year	All
	EBV status		
Melanoma	Physical	Once	ALL
Myeloma	Immunoelectropheresis	Once	>50
Prostate	Digital rectal	Every year	>50
	Prostate-specific antigen		
Kidney	Ultrasound or CT	Once	>50
Skin	Physical	Once	All
Testicular	Physical	Once	All men
Uterine cervix	PAP smear	1–3 yrs	>20 or sexually active
	Pelvic exam		

Source: Kasiske *et al.* 2001 [11].

Abbreviations: FOBT, fecal occult blood test; HHV-8, human herpesvirus 8; CBC, complete blood cell count; CT, computerized tomography; CXR, chest X-ray.

[a] Abnormalities detected by screening require additional tests.

to transplantation, in the absence of immunosuppression therapy, should be considered high risk.

Cancer

Recommendations

Selected patients should undergo cancer screening prior to transplantation. Patients with a past history of cancer will need further testing and an observation period for recurrence, and the advice of an oncologist prior to transplantation should be considered. Patients with advanced-stage cancers are not candidates for transplantation.

Evidence

Cancer is more common in end-stage renal disease patients than the general population [62]. Some cancers have mortality rates that exceed the dialysis mortality rate [63]. Transplanting patients with a high risk of cancer-associated mortality is not likely to improve outcomes.

The US Preventive Services Task Force has provided recommendations for screening specific cancers in men and woman in the general population [57]. Overall, colorectal, cervical, and breast cancer screening have the highest evidence. Other strategies, such as prostate cancer screening, are inconclusive although widely practiced. It is possible that detecting cancers through screening may do more harm to patients who might otherwise receive a transplant promptly. Table 48.3 gives a list of potential screening strategies. The evidence for referral to screening in the general population is different for screening to determine transplant eligibility. Avoiding transplantation in a cancer patient with limited life expectancy concerns more the prudent use of a scarce resource than a strategy to improve life expectancy.

In general, about 50% of cancers recur within <2 years, 33% between 2 and 5 years, and about 15% more than 5 years after the first cancer [11]. Published cancer recurrence rates are inaccurate due to selection bias. Data from the Israel Penn International Tumor Transplant Registry do not have a reliable denominator to accurately calculate rates [64]. Table 48.4 gives a list of the cancers and recommended waiting times, taking into account the evidence.

Table 48.4 Recommended transplantation wait times for specific cancers.

Cancer site or type	Wait time (yrs)
Breast	>5 (>2 for early disease)
Bladder	>2
Colorectal	>5 (>2 for Dukes stage A or B1)
Kaposi sarcoma	>2
Leukemia	>2 (limited data to make recommendation)
Liver	Unable to give recommendation
Lung	>2
Lymphoma	>2
Melanoma	>5 (>2 melanoma *in situ*)
Myeloma	Unable to give recommendation
Prostate	>2 (localized disease possibly shorter wait)
Renal/Wilm's tumor	>2 (>5 for large cancers; no wait for incidental of <5 cm)
Skin (non-melanoma)	0–2 (no wait for basal cell)
Testicular	>2
Thyroid	>2
Uterine or cervix	>2

Sources: Kasiske *et al.* 2001 [11] and European Best Practices Guidelines 2000 [13].

Published guidelines give more details on individual cancers [11–13].

Infections

Recommendations

Ideally, patients should be free of all active infections at the time of transplantation. Patients should be tested for immunity to varicella-zoster virus, Epstein-Barr virus (EBV), cytomegalovirus (CMV), and HIV. HIV-infected patients may be considered for kidney transplantation if they meet certain criteria.

Evidence

All guidelines recommend that patients be free of active infection. Infection is the second most common cause of death (21%) within the first year after transplantation [65]. Given that the early transplant period is the time of intense immunosuppression, the recommendations are reasonable and are unlikely to be tested in a clinical trial.

The prevalence of treatable occult dental disease, detected with routine screening by panoramic radiographs, and the consequences avoided compared with treating symptomatic patients have not been systematically evaluated. It is reasonable to refer patients with symptoms or obvious disease. In a European survey, 61% of centers referred all patients for dental consultation [33].

Mycobacterial infections may be more common in the end-stage renal disease population than in the general population [66]. Patients on dialysis may be anergic, and testing may underestimate true exposure. Administering two-step tuberculin skin testing may improve detection [67]. The risks and benefits of pretransplant

prophylaxis, early posttransplant prophylaxis, or watchful waiting are all acceptable but may depend on other risk factors [66].

Patients seronegative for varicella-zoster virus should be considered for vaccination pretransplantation, because this infection can be fatal in a transplant recipient [68]. Although donor–recipient CMV matching is not routinely performed, knowledge of donor and recipient status predicts posttransplant CMV infection. CMV disease is a potentially fatal infection, and chemoprophylaxis is very effective [69]. Evidence for screening for EBV is not as effective. Seroprevalence of EBV is high in adults, and donor–recipient matching is not performed. Naïve recipients are at greater risk for infection and posttransplant lymphoproliferative disease [70]. Surveillance strategies for EBV are under evaluation.

Patients with HIV have received solid organ transplants with success, and outcomes appear to be equivalent to the general transplant population, but HIV-infected patients who have received transplants are a selected group. Prospective studies are underway to better define which HIV-infected patients should be transplanted. Excellent results have been demonstrated in patients with undetectable plasma HIV viral loads for 3 months, a CD4+ T-cell count of more than 200 cells/μL for 6 months, and no history of opportunistic infection or neoplasm [71].

Liver disease

Recommendations

Patients should be screened for liver disease. Patients with overt liver disease or positive for hepatitis B or C virus should be referred to a hepatologist for assessment of the extent of disease, a discussion of prognosis, ongoing monitoring, and candidacy for specific treatment.

Evidence

The prevalence of hepatitis C-positive kidney transplant recipients in the USA is 6.8% [72], and the prevalence of hepatitis B surface antigen in the US dialysis population is <1% [73]. Liver failure is a significant cause of morbidity and mortality in hepatitis B and C patients. In a pooled analysis, hepatitis C antibody was a significant risk factor for death and graft failure (relative risk [RR], 1.8 and 1.6, respectively) [74], but in a recent UNOS registry analysis, hepatitis C patients had an increase in adjusted mortality of only 1.2 ($P = 0.04$) [75]. Patients that were hepatitis C positive had many characteristics associated with inferior survival, including higher rates of regrafts, cadaver donors, and longer duration of dialysis. Differences in patient selection for transplantation and treatment will more than likely change the natural history of these infections [76].

Because biochemical tests may not reflect the extent of disease, a liver biopsy is recommended in those without portal hypertension [77]. The biopsy results may direct therapy. Hepatitis C patients with chronic hepatitis can be considered for a course of pegylated interferon [78]. Hepatitis B patients with active viral replication can be considered for a course of lamivudine [79]. All of the antiviral studies are small and lack hard end points. It is not clear whether patients with compensated cirrhosis are candidates for kidney-alone transplantation. At issue is whether kidney transplantation confers a survival advantage over the risk of progressive liver disease. Patients with decompensated disease can be considered for combined kidney–liver transplantation.

Gastrointestinal disease

Recommendations
Patients with a recent history or symptoms of gastrointestinal bleeding, peptic ulcer disease, biliary disease, or diverticulitis should be investigated and treated pretransplant. Patients without symptoms should not be screened.

Evidence
In a European survey, active peptic ulcer disease was a criterion for exclusion from transplantation in 57% of centers [33]. The incidence of early posttransplant gastroduodenal disease with prophylaxis is low, at about 3% [80]. *Helicobacter pylori* screening has not been recommended, since the association with adverse outcomes is weak.

The prevalence of asymptomatic cholelithiasis in the transplant population ranges between 5 and 10% [81]. Although the cumulative risk of symptomatic disease, morbidity, and mortality in the asymptomatic transplant candidate is unclear, there is no evidence that patients need to be screened or require surgery.

Complications of diverticular disease, such as perforation and obstruction, have high mortality rates but occur infrequently [82]. Asymptomatic disease is common, and guidelines do not recommend routine screening, but they do recommend surgical correction in immunocompromised patients even after a single episode of diverticulitis [83,84].

Systemic disease

Recommendations
Most systemic diseases should be quiescent prior to transplantation. Selected patients with primary hyperoxaluria can be considered for transplantation.

Evidence
All systemic diseases can recur. The major issues are measuring disease activity and the optimal timing of transplantation. Balancing the benefits of transplantation, the harms of ongoing dialysis, and risks of recurrence are difficult, especially in a recipient with a potential live donor.

Patients with primary hyperoxaluria have a poor prognosis, and many centers avoid transplantation in such patients [33]. A combined liver–kidney transplant potentially provides sufficient enzyme to correct disease and prevent recurrence [85], but studies have not shown a clear benefit for a combined procedure versus

kidney transplantation alone, which may reflect selection biases. Patients with large systemic oxalate burdens are at high risk of early graft loss and may do poorly with either of these options. Patients with a preemptive kidney transplant, or who are transplanted soon after dialysis is initiated, do well without a liver transplant.

Anti-glomerular basement membrane (anti-GBM) disease recurs in <10% of patients and has been associated with circulating antibodies at the time of transplantation [13,86]. Several guidelines recommend waiting until anti-GBM antibodies are undetectable and patients are off therapy for at least 6 months [11–13]. It is not likely that prospective information on the negative and positive predictive values of antibody levels for disease recurrence will be available.

Systemic lupus erythematosus recurs in <10% of transplant patients but may be higher if histopathological criteria are used, although graft loss is uncommon and outcomes are comparable to those in the general transplant population [87,88]. Practice guidelines recommend waiting until the disease is clinically and immunologically quiescent [11–13]. The evidence requiring a long delay prior to transplantation is limited and anecdotal.

ANCA-positive vasculitis patients have modest (up to 20%) recurrence rates posttransplantation [89]. Graft loss due to recurrent disease occurs in <10% and may occur late posttransplantation. ANCA levels do not predict disease recurrence posttransplantation. Most of the available data are from cases series, with little information from large registry analyses. Many practice guidelines recommend a period of observation off cytotoxic therapy. The length of wait has not been clearly established, and the time on dialysis does not impact disease recurrence [89].

Hemolytic uremic syndrome (HUS) recurrence rates may be high and overall survival reduced [90]. Risk of recurrence with epidemic HUS (toxigenic *Escherichia coli*) is uncommon. Nonepidemic HUS is associated with higher recurrence rates (>20%) [91]. Other proposed risk factors, including living donor, use of calcineurin inhibitors, older age, and shorter interval between onset and transplantation, have not been consistently reported. Up to 40% of familial cases and 20% of sporadic cases are linked to mutations in the factor H gene [92], but genetic screening is not readily available and is of uncertain value for predicting recurrence. The utility of repeated transplantation in this group needs to be demonstrated, as recurrence with graft loss is high [93].

Recurrent disease

Recommendations
Patients that lose their first transplant from recurrent focal segmental glomerulosclerosis and patients with Alport syndrome losing a transplant from *de novo* anti-GBM disease are at high risk of recurrence that may preclude retransplantation.

Evidence
No cause of primary kidney disease precludes kidney transplantation absolutely, and in most conditions a second transplant is

reasonable. However, focal segmental glomerulosclerosis has relatively high recurrence rates (20–50%) with subsequent graft loss [94]. The rate of progression of the primary disease, duration of pretransplant dialysis, and younger age may be risk factors, but their clinical predictive accuracy has not been quantified and is not likely to be used to deny kidney transplantation. Measuring recipient disease activity by permeability bioassay is not useful [95]. There are insufficient data to support pre- or posttransplant plasmapheresis prophylaxis [96]. Waiting until the patient is anuric or free of nephrotic-range proteinuria or proceeding by performing bilateral nephrectomy has also not been tested. The use of genetic testing is also currently unproven [97]. Retransplantation may be precluded in patients with early recurrence and a rapid rate of graft loss, because the disease may have a high rate of recurrence in subsequent transplants.

Alport syndrome is a hereditary deficiency of basement membrane collagen, and recurrence of disease is neither expected nor found. However, the disease is associated with an aggressive posttransplant anti-GBM disease in approximately 5% of patients which almost always results in graft loss [98]. Recurrence is high and may preclude a second attempt despite aggressive treatment.

Urological issues

Recommendations

A dysfunctional bladder or urinary diversion is not a contraindication to transplantation.

Evidence

Patients with known bladder problems or symptoms should be referred for urologic evaluation. Pretransplant correction of reflux reduces posttransplant urinary tract infections in children, but urinary tract infection is uncommon and so the clinical benefit of this intervention is uncertain [99]. All patients should have an adequate urinary reservoir to permit storage at a low pressure and a patent passageway with a reliable method of achieving complete evacuation [100]. There are a number of different urinary diversion procedures, but all have significant risk of recurrent infection [101]. Bladder augmentation has also been used in contracted and neuropathic bladders. Successful management with intermittent self-catheterization is an option. Newer modalities to treat hyperreflexive bladders are being investigated [102]. Overall patient and graft survival do not appear to be adversely affected, and therefore corrected urinary problems should not limit eligibility [103,104].

Obesity

Recommendations

Obesity is not an absolute contraindication to transplantation.

Evidence

Although obesity is associated with some adverse outcomes, reporting has been inconsistent [11,105–107]. Patients with very high body mass indices (>36 kg/m^2) are at higher risk of death (RR, 1.34) and graft loss (RR, 1.39) [105]. Not all surgeons are willing to transplant the very obese, and this may be a limiting factor. There is no evidence that weight loss prior to surgery improves outcomes.

Compliance and adherence

Recommendations

Patients must understand the risks and benefits of transplantation and demonstrate adherence to therapy.

Evidence

Noncompliance is the second (28%) most common medical reason for patient exclusion [108] and was a definite exclusion in 61% of European centers surveyed [33]. In a US survey, 83% of clinicians assess compliance based on dialysis attendance [32]. Most centers have a policy on drug abuse. The period of abstinence required before eligibility varies considerably. Smoking, although discouraged, has not limited eligibility in most centers. Unfortunately, measuring and predicting noncompliance and sustained drug abstinence with accuracy is difficult, leaving centers to decide by local consensus.

References

1 Wolfe RA, Ashby VB, Milford EL, Ojo AO, Ettenger RE, Agodoa LY *et al.* Comparison of mortality in all patients on dialysis, patients on dialysis awaiting transplantation, and recipients of a first cadaveric transplant. *N Engl J Med* 1999; **341:** 1725–1730.

2 Gill JS, Tonelli M, Johnson N, Kiberd B, Landsberg D, Pereira BJ. The impact of waiting time and comorbid conditions on the survival benefit of kidney transplantation. *Kidney Int* 2005; **68:** 2345–2351.

3 US Renal Data System. *USRDS 2005 Annual Data Report: Atlas of End-Stage Renal Disease in the United States.* National Institutes of Health, National Institute of Diabetes and Digestive and Kidney Diseases, Bethesda, 2005.

4 Laupacis A, Keown P, Pus N, Krueger H, Ferguson B, Wong C *et al.* A study of the quality of life and cost-utility of renal transplantation. *Kidney Int* 1996; **50:** 235–242.

5 Gill JS, Tonelli M, Landsberg D, Pereira BJG. Factors not incorporated in the organ allocation scheme influence the likelihood of kidney transplantation. *Am J Transplant* 2005; **5(Suppl 11):** 261A.

6 Vianello A, Spinello M, Palminteri G, Brunello A, Calconi G, Maresca MC. Are the baseline chances of survival comparable between the candidates for kidney transplantation who actually receive a graft and those who never get one? *Nephrol Dial Transplant* 2002; **17:** 1093–1098.

7 UNOS website. http://www.unos.org/.

8 Danovitch GM, Cohen DJ, Weir MR, Stock PG, Bennett WM, Christensen LL *et al.* AJT Annual report. Current status of kidney and

pancreas transplantation in the United States, 1994-2003. *Am J Transplant* 2005; **5**: 904–915.

9 Steinman TI, Becker BN, Frost AE, Olthoff KM, Smart FW, Suki WN *et al*. Guidelines for the referral and management of patients eligible for solid organ transplantation. *Transplantation* 2001; **71**: 1189–1204.

10 Epstein AM, Ayanian JZ, Keogh JH, Noonan SJ, Armistead N, Cleary PD *et al*. Racial disparities in access to renal transplantation: clinically appropriate or due to underuse or overuse? *N Engl J Med* 2000; **343**: 1537–1544.

11 Kasiske BL, Cangro CB, Hariharan S, Hricik DE, Kerman RH, Roth D *et al*. The evaluation of renal transplantation candidates: clinical practice guidelines. *Am J Transplant* 2001; **1**(**Suppl 2**): 3–95.

12 Knoll G, Cockfield S, Blydt-Hansen T, Baran D, Kiberd D, Landsberg D *et al*. Canadian Society of Transplantation consensus guidelines on eligibility for kidney transplantation. *CMAJ* 2005; **173**: 1181–1184.

13 European Expert Group on Renal Transplantation, European Renal Association, European Society for Organ Transplantation. European Best Practice guidelines for renal transplantation. Part 1. *Nephrol Dial Transplant* 2000; **15**(**Suppl 7**): 1–85.

14 UNOS. http://www.unos.org/news/newsDetail.asp?id=147.

15 Foley RN, Parfrey PS, Sarnak MJ. Clinical epidemiology of cardiovascular disease in chronic renal disease. *Am J Kidney Dis* 1998; **32**(**5 Suppl 3**): S112–S119.

16 Satayathum S, Pisoni RL, McCullough KP, Merion RM, Wikstrom B, Levin N *et al*. Kidney transplantation and wait-listing rates from the international Dialysis Outcomes and Practice Patterns Study (DOPPS). *Kidney Int* 2005; **68**: 330–337.

17 Klocke FJ, Baird MG, Lorell BH, Bateman TM, Messer JV, Berman DS *et al*. ACC/AHA/ASNC guidelines for the clinical use of cardiac radionuclide imaging. Executive summary: a report of the American College of Cardiology/American Heart Association Task Force on Practice Guidelines. *Circulation* 2003; **108**: 1404–1418.

18 Eagle KA, Berger PB, Calkins H, Chaitman BR, Ewy GA, Fleischmann KE *et al*. ACC/AHA guideline update for perioperative cardiovascular evaluation for noncardiac surgery. Executive summary: a report of the American College of Cardiology/American Heart Association Task Force on Practice Guidelines. *Circulation* 2002; **105**: 1257–1267.

19 Manske CL, Wang Y, Rector T, Wilson RF, White CW. Coronary revascularisation in insulin-dependent diabetic patients with chronic renal failure. *Lancet* 1992; **340**: 998–1002.

20 McFalls EO, Ward HB, Moritz TE, Goldman S, Krupski WC, Littooy F *et al*. Coronary-artery revascularization before elective major vascular surgery. *N Engl J Med* 2004; **351**: 2795–2804.

21 Rabbat CG, Treleaven DJ, Russell JD, Ludwin D, Cook DJ. Prognostic value of myocardial perfusion studies in patients with end-stage renal disease assessed for kidney or kidney-pancreas transplantation: a meta-analysis. *J Am Soc Nephrol* 2003; **14**: 431–439.

22 Vandenberg BF, Rossen JD, Grover-McKay M, Shammas NW, Burns TL, Rezai K. Evaluation of diabetic patients for renal and pancreas transplantation: noninvasive screening for coronary artery disease using radionuclide methods. *Transplantation* 1996; **62**: 1230–1235

23 Herzog CA, Marwick TH, Pheley AM, White CW, Rao VK, Dick CD. Dobutamine stress echocardiography for the detection of significant coronary artery disease in renal transplant candidates. *Am J Kidney Dis* 1999; **33**: 1080–1090.

24 Reis G, Marcovitz PA, Leichtman AB, Merion RM, Fay WP, Wens SW *et al*. Usefulness of dobutamine stress echocardiography in detecting coronary artery disease in end-stage renal disease. *Am J Cardiol* 1995; **75**: 707–710.

25 Boudreau RJ, Strony JT, duCret RP, Kuni CC, Wang Y, Wilson RF *et al*. Perfusion thallium imaging of type I diabetes patients with end-stage renal disease: comparison of oral and intravenous dipyridamole administration. *Radiology* 1990; **175**: 103–105.

26 Marwick TH, Steinmuller DR, Underwood DA, Hobbs RE, Go RT, Swift C *et al*. Ineffectiveness of dipyridamole SPECT thallium imaging as a screening technique for coronary artery disease in patients with end-stage renal failure. *Transplantation* 1990; **49**: 100–103.

27 Worthley MI, Unger SA, Mathew TH, Russ GR, Horowitz JD. Usefulness of tachycardic-stress perfusion imaging to predict coronary artery disease in high-risk patients with chronic renal failure. *Am J Cardiol* 2003; **92**: 1318–1320.

28 West JC, Napoliello DA, Costello JM, Nassef LA, Butcher RJ, Hartle JE *et al*. Preoperative dobutamine stress echocardiography versus cardiac arteriography for risk assessment prior to renal transplantation. *Transpl Int* 2000; **139**(**Suppl 1**): S27–S30.

29 Schmidt A, Stefenelli T, Schuster E, Mayer G. Informational contribution of noninvasive screening tests for coronary artery disease in patients on chronic renal replacement therapy. *Am J Kidney Dis*. 2001; **37**: 56–63.

30 De Lima JJ, Sabbaga E, Vieira ML, de Paula FJ, Ianhez LE, Krieger EM *et al*. Coronary angiography is the best predictor of events in renal transplant candidates compared with noninvasive testing. *Hypertension* 2003; **42**: 263–268.

31 Fishbane S. Cardiovascular risk evaluation before kidney transplantation. *J Am Soc Nephrol* 2005; **16**: 843–845.

32 Ramos EL, Kasiske BL, Alexander SR, Danovitch GM, Harmon WE, Kahana L *et al*. The evaluation of candidates for renal transplantation. The current practice of U.S. transplant centers. *Transplantation* 1994; **57**: 490–497.

33 Fritsche L, Vanrenterghem Y, Nordal KP, Grinyo JM, Moreso F, Budde K *et al*. Practice variations in the evaluation of adult candidates for cadaveric kidney transplantation: a survey of the European Transplant Centers. *Transplantation* 2000; **70**: 1492–1497.

34 Matas AJ, Kasiske B, Miller L. Proposed guidelines for re-evaluation of patients on the waiting list for renal cadaver transplantation. *Transplantation* 2002; **73**: 811–812.

35 Danovitch GM, Hariharan S, Pirsch JD, Rush D, Roth D, Ramos E *et al*. Management of the waiting list for cadaveric kidney transplants: report of a survey and recommendations by the Clinical Practice Guidelines Committee of the American Society of Transplantation. *J Am Soc Nephrol* 2002; **13**: 528–535.

36 Kasiske BL, Malik MA, Herzog CA. Risk-stratified screening for ischemic heart disease in kidney transplant candidates. *Transplantation* 2005; **80**: 815–820.

37 Kiberd BA, Dipchand C, Keough-Ryan T. Cardiovascular re-evaluation for patients with diabetes mellitus in the kidney wait list. *J Am Soc Nephrol* 2003; **14**: 438A.

38 Grayburn PA, Hillis LD. Cardiac events in patients undergoing noncardiac surgery: shifting the paradigm from noninvasive risk stratification to therapy. *Ann Intern Med* 2003; **138**: 506–511.

39 Devereaux PJ, Goldman L, Yusuf S, Gilbert K, Leslie K, Guyatt GH. Surveillance and prevention of major perioperative ischemic cardiac events in patients undergoing noncardiac surgery: a review. *CMAJ* 2005; **73**: 779–788.

40 Gill JS, Ma I, Landsberg D, Johnson N, Levin A. Cardiovascular events and investigation in patients who are awaiting cadaveric kidney transplantation. *J Am Soc Nephrol* 2005; **16:** 808–816.

41 Wanner C, Krane V, Marz W, Olschewski M, Mann JF, Ruf G *et al.* Atorvastatin in patients with type 2 diabetes mellitus undergoing hemodialysis. *N Engl J Med* 2005; **353:** 238–248.

42 Jardine AG, Holdaas H, Fellstrom B, Cole E, Nyberg G, Gronhagen-Riska C *et al.* Fluvastatin prevents cardiac death and myocardial infarction in renal transplant recipients: post-hoc subgroup analyses of the ALERT Study. *Am J Transplant* 2004; **4:** 988–995.

43 Parfrey PS, Harnett JD, Foley RN, Kent GM, Murray DC, Barre PE *et al.* Impact of renal transplantation on uremic cardiomyopathy. *Transplantation* 1995; **60:** 908–914.

44 Wali RK, Wang GS, Gottlieb SS, Bellumkonda L, Hansalia R, Ramos E *et al.* Effect of kidney transplantation on left ventricular systolic dysfunction and congestive heart failure in patients with end-stage renal disease. *J Am Coll Cardiol* 2005; **45:** 1051–1060.

45 Ojo AO, Hanson JA, Wolfe RA, Leichtman AB, Agodoa LY, Port FK. Long-term survival in renal transplant recipients with graft function. *Kidney Int* 2000; **57:** 307–313.

46 Oliveras A, Roquer J, Puig JM, Rodriguez A, Mir M, Orfila MA *et al.* Stroke in renal transplant recipients: epidemiology, predictive risk factors and outcome. *Clin Transplant* 2003; **17:** 1–8.

47 Strauss SE, Majumdar SR, McAlister FA. New evidence for stroke prevention: scientific review. *JAMA* 2002; **288:** 1388–1395.

48 Law MR, Wald NJ, Rudnicka AR. Quantifying effect of statins on low density lipoprotein cholesterol, ischaemic heart disease, and stroke: systematic review and meta-analysis. *BMJ* 2003; **326:** 1423.

49 Lefevre F, Woolger JM. Surgery in the patient with neurologic disease. *Med Clin North Am* 2003; **87:** 257–271.

50 Johnston SC. Transient ischemic attack. *N Engl J Med* 2003; **347:** 1687.

51 Hart RG, Bailey RD. An assessment of guidelines for prevention of ischemic stroke. *Neurology* 2002; **59(7):** 977–982.

52 Mariani L, Bianchetti MG, Schroth G, Seiler RW. Cerebral aneurysms in patients with autosomal dominant polycystic kidney disease: to screen, to clip, to coil? *Nephrol Dial Transplant* 1999; **14:** 2319–2322.

53 Belz MM, Hughes RL, Kaehny WD, Johnson AM, Fick-Brosnahan GM, Earnest MP *et al.* Familial clustering of ruptured intracranial aneurysms in autosomal dominant polycystic kidney disease. *Am J Kidney Dis* 2001; **38:** 770–776.

54 Bederson JB, Awad IA, Wiebers DO, Piepgras D, Haley EC, Jr., Brott T *et al.* Recommendations for the management of patients with unruptured intracranial aneurysms: a statement for healthcare professionals from the Stroke Council of the American Heart Association. *Stroke* 2000; **31:** 2742–2750.

55 Chua BSY, Szczech A, Frankenfield DL, *et al.* Peripheral vascular disease (PVD): is it a risk factor for mortality in end-stage renal disease (ESRD)? *J Am Soc Nephrol* 2003; **14:** 262A.

56 Kasiske BL, Snyder JJ, Maclean JR. Peripheral vascular disease in the United States kidney transplant and wait listing population, 1995-2001. *Am J Transplant* 2005; **5(Suppl 11):** 553A.

57 US Preventive Services Task Force. http://www.ahrq.gov/clinic/uspstfix.htm.

58 Brown PM, Sobolev B, Zelt DT. Selective management of abdominal aortic aneurysms smaller than 5.0 cm in a prospective sizing program with gender-specific analysis. *J Vasc Surg* 2003; **37:** 280–284.

59 Hansen EF, Phanareth K, Laursen LC, Kok-Jensen A, Dirksen A. Reversible and irreversible airflow obstruction as predictor of overall mortality in asthma and chronic obstructive pulmonary disease. *Am J Respir Crit Care Med.* 1999; **159(4 Pt 1):** 1267–1271.

60 Chailleux E, Fauroux B, Binet F, Dautzenberg B, Polu JM. Predictors of survival in patients receiving domiciliary oxygen therapy or mechanical ventilation. A 10-year analysis of ANTADIR Observatory. *Chest* 1996; **109:** 741–749.

61 Sileri P, Pursell KJ, Coady NT, Giacomoni A, Berliti S, Tzoracoleftherakis E *et al.* A standardized protocol for the treatment of severe pneumonia in kidney transplant recipients. *Clin Transplant* 2002; **16:** 450–454.

62 Maisonneuve P, Agodoa L, Gellert R, Stewart JH, Buccianti G, Lowenfels AB *et al.* Cancer in patients on dialysis for end-stage renal disease: an international collaborative study. *Lancet* 1999; **354:** 93–99.

63 Ries LAG, Eisner MP, Kosary CL, *et al.* (editors). *SEER Cancer Statistics Review, 1975-2002.* National Cancer Institute, Bethesda, MD.

64 Israel Penn International Transplant Tumor Registry. http://www.ipittr.uc.edu/Publications/public.cfm.

65 Gill JS, Pereira BJ. Death in the first year after kidney transplantation: implications for patients on the transplant waiting list. *Transplantation* 2003; **75:** 113–117.

66 Rubin RH. Management of tuberculosis in the transplant recipient. *Am J Transplant* 2005; **5:** 2599–2600.

67 Dogan E, Erkoc R, Sayarlioglu H, Uzun K. Tuberculin skin test results and the booster phenomenon in two-step tuberculin skin testing in hemodialysis patients. *Ren Fail* 2005; **27:** 425–428.

68 Olson AD, Shope TC, Flynn JT. Pretransplant varicella vaccination is cost-effective in pediatric renal transplantation. *Pediatr Transplant* 2001; **5:** 44–50.

69 Kalil AC, Levitsky J, Lyden E, Stoner J, Freifeld AG. Meta-analysis: the efficacy of strategies to prevent organ disease by cytomegalovirus in solid organ transplant recipients. *Ann Intern Med* 2005; **143:** 870–880.

70 Allen UD, Farkas G, Hebert D, Weitzman S, Stephens D, Petric M *et al.* Risk factors for post-transplant lymphoproliferative disorder in pediatric patients: a case-control study. *Pediatr Transplant* 2005; **9:** 450–455.

71 Stock PG, Roland ME, Carlson L, Freise CE, Roberts JP, Hirose R *et al.* Kidney and liver transplantation in human immunodeficiency virus-infected patients: a pilot safety and efficacy study. *Transplantation* 2003; **76:** 370–375.

72 Abbott KC, Bucci JR, Matsumoto CS, Swanson SJ, Agodoa LY, Holtzmuller KC *et al.* Hepatitis C and renal transplantation in the era of modern immunosuppression. *J Am Soc Nephrol* 2003; **14:** 2908–2918.

73 Tokars JI, Finelli L, Alter MJ, Arduino MJ. National surveillance of dialysis-associated diseases in the United States, 2001. *Semin Dial* 2004; **17:** 310–319.

74 Fabrizi F, Martin P, Dixit V, Bunnapradist S, Dulai G. Hepatitis C virus antibody status and survival after renal transplantation: meta-analysis of observational studies. *Am J Transplant* 2005; **5:** 1452–1461.

75 Batty DS, Jr., Swanson SJ, Kirk AD, Ko CW, Agodoa LY, Abbott KC. Hepatitis C virus seropositivity at the time of renal transplantation in the United States: associated factors and patient survival. *Am J Transplant* 2001; **1:** 179–184.

76 Fong TL, Bunnapradist S, Jordan SC, Cho YW. Impact of hepatitis B core antibody status on outcomes of cadaveric renal transplantation: analysis of United network of organ sharing database between 1994 and 1999. *Transplantation* 2002; **73:** 85–89.

77 Gane E, Pilmore H. Management of chronic viral hepatitis before and after renal transplantation. *Transplantation* 2002; **74:** 427–437.

78 Gonzalez-Roncero F, Gentil MA, Valdivia MA, Algarra G, Pereira P, Toro J *et al.* Outcome of kidney transplant in chronic hepatitis C virus

patients: effect of pretransplantation interferon-α2b monotherapy. *Transplant Proc* 2003; **35:** 1745–1747.

79 Fabrizi F, Dulai G, Dixit V, Bunnapradist S, Martin P. Lamivudine for the treatment of hepatitis B virus-related liver disease after renal transplantation: meta-analysis of clinical trials. *Transplantation* 2004; **77:** 859–864.

80 Sarkio S, Halme L, Kyllonen L, Salmela K. Severe gastrointestinal complications after 1,515 adult kidney transplantations. *Transpl Int* 2004; **17:** 505–510.

81 Greenstein SM, Katz S, Sun S, Glicklich D, Schechner R, Kutcher R *et al.* Prevalence of asymptomatic cholelithiasis and risk of acute cholecystitis after kidney transplantation. *Transplantation* 1997; **63:** 1030–1032.

82 Lederman ED, Conti DJ, Lempert N, Singh TP, Lee EC. Complicated diverticulitis following renal transplantation. *Dis Colon Rectum* 1998; **41:** 613–618.

83 Stollman NH, Raskin JB. Diverticular disease of the colon. *Lancet* 2004; **363:** 631–639.

84 Stollman NH, Raskin JB. Diagnosis and management of diverticular disease of the colon in adults: Ad Hoc Practice Parameters Committee of the American College of Gastroenterology. *Am J Gastroenterol* 1999; **94:** 3110–3121.

85 Monico CG, Milliner DS. Combined liver-kidney and kidney-alone transplantation in primary hyperoxaluria. *Liver Transplant* 2001; **7:** 954–963.

86 Netzer KO, Merkel F, Weber M. Goodpasture syndrome and end-stage renal failure: to transplant or not to transplant? *Nephrol Dial Transplant* 1998; **13:** 1346–1348.

87 Bartosh SM, Fine RN, Sullivan EK. Outcome after transplantation of young patients with systemic lupus erythematosus: a report of the North American Pediatric Renal Transplant Cooperative Study. *Transplantation* 2001; **72:** 973–978.

88 Moroni G, Tantardini F, Gallelli B, Quaglini S, Banfi G, Poli F *et al.* The long-term prognosis of renal transplantation in patients with lupus nephritis. *Am J Kidney Dis* 2005; **45:** 903–11.

89 Nachman PH, Segelmark M, Westman K, Hogan SL, Satterly KK, Jennette JC *et al.* Recurrent ANCA-associated small vessel vasculitis after transplantation: a pooled analysis. *Kidney Int* 1999; **56:** 1544–1550.

90 Ducloux D, Rebibou JM, Semhoun-Ducloux S, Jamali M, Fournier V, Bresson-Vautrin C *et al.* Recurrence of hemolytic-uremic syndrome in renal transplant recipients: a meta-analysis. *Transplantation* 1998; **65:** 1405–1407.

91 Loirat C, Niaudet P. The risk of recurrence of hemolytic uremic syndrome after renal transplantation in children. *Pediatr Nephrol* 2003; **18:** 1095–1101.

92 Noris M, Remuzzi G. Hemolytic uremic syndrome. Disease of the month. *J Am Soc Nephrol* 2005; **16:** 1035–1050.

93 Artz MA, Steenbergen EJ, Hoitsma AJ, Monnens LA, Wetzels JF. Renal transplantation in patients with hemolytic uremic syndrome: high rate of recurrence and increased incidence of acute rejections. *Transplantation* 2003; **76:** 821–826.

94 Briganti EM, Russ GR, McNeil JJ, Atkins RC, Chadban SJ. Risk of renal allograft loss from recurrent glomerulonephritis. *N Engl J Med* 2002; **347:** 103–109.

95 Ghiggeri GM, Artero M, Carraro M, Candiano G, Musante L, Bruschi M *et al.* Glomerular albumin permeability as an in vitro model for characterizing the mechanism of focal glomerulosclerosis and predicting post-transplant recurrence. *Pediatr Transplant* 2004; **8:** 339–343.

96 Gohh RY, Yango AF, Morrissey PE, Monaco AP, Gautam A, Sharma M *et al.* Preemptive plasmapheresis and recurrence of FSGS in high-risk renal transplant recipients. *Am J Transplant* 2005; **5:** 2907–2912.

97 Vincenti F, Ghiggeri GM. New insights into the pathogenesis and the therapy of recurrent focal glomerulosclerosis. *Am J Transplant* 2005; **5:** 1179–1185.

98 Browne G, Brown PA, Tomson CR, Fleming S, Allen A, Herriot R *et al.* Retransplantation in Alport post-transplant anti-GBM disease. *Kidney Int* 2004; **65:** 675–681.

99 Erturk E, Burzon DT, Orloff M, Rabinowitz R. Outcome of patients with vesicoureteral reflux after renal transplantation: the effect of pretransplantation surgery on posttransplant urinary tract infections. *Urology* 1998; **51:** 27–30.

100 Churchill BM, Jayanthi RV, McLorie GA, Khoury AE. Paediatric renal transplantation into the abnormal urinary tract. *Pediatr Nephrol* 1996; **10:** 113–120.

101 Falagas ME, Vergidis PI. Urinary tract infections in patients with urinary diversion. *Am J Kidney Dis* 2005; **46:** 1030–1037.

102 Schulte-Baukloh H, Michael T, Sturzebecher B, Knispel HH. Botulinum: a toxin detrusor injection as a novel approach in the treatment of bladder spasticity in children with neurogenic bladder. *Eur Urol* 2003; **44:** 139–143.

103 Capizzi A, Zanon GF, Zacchello G, Rigamonti W. Kidney transplantation in children with reconstructed bladder. *Transplantation* 2004; **77:** 1113–1116.

104 Rigamonti W, Capizzi A, Zacchello G, Capizzi V, Zanon GF, Montini G *et al.* Kidney transplantation into bladder augmentation or urinary diversion: long-term results. *Transplantation* 2005; **80:** 1435–1440.

105 Meier-Kriesche H-U, Arndorfer JA, Kaplan B. The impact of body mass index on renal transplant outcomes: a significant independent risk factor for graft failure and patient death. *Transplantation* 2002; **73:** 70–74.

106 Johnson DW, Isbel NM, Brown AM, Kay TD, Franzen K, Hawley CM *et al.* The effect of obesity on renal transplant outcomes. *Transplantation* 2002; **74:** 675–680.

107 Howard RJ, Thal VB, Patton PR, Hemming AW, Reed AI, Van der Weft WJ *et al.* Obesity does not portend a bad outcome for kidney transplant recipients. *Transplantation* 2002; **73:** 53–55.

108 Holley JL, Monaghan J, Byer B, Bronsther O. An examination of the renal transplant evaluation process focusing on cost and the reasons for patient exclusion. *Am J Kidney Dis* 1998; **32:** 567–574.

49 Evaluation and Selection of the Living Kidney Donor

Connie L. Davis

Division of Nephrology, Department of Medicine, University of Washington School of Medicine, Seattle, USA

Introduction

Transplantation with a living kidney donor is the treatment of choice for end-stage renal disease (ESRD). Although the focus is often on the recipient regaining health, an equally important goal is making sure that the living donor will be able to maintain their own health after donation. Medical evaluation of the donor is aimed to detect medical abnormalities that would put them at risk for donor surgery or to develop ESRD. The evaluation also should exclude diseases (infection, malignancy) that may be transmitted to the recipient. Finally, the evaluation attempts to identify conditions where the removal of one kidney could increase the risk of disease progression or limit the delivery of optimal care. There have been no randomized controlled trials in the living donor population; all data are from single-center, retrospective, or more recently, prospective cohort trials. Few studies have included control groups, and those that did usually recruited control subjects from the general population, which may not be the most appropriate for comparison, as living donors should represent the healthiest members of society.

The overall evaluation process

Evaluation of the living donor starts with education about the donation process and a screening history by the living donor coordinator. Often the prospective donor will be asked to supply a copy of their most recent history and physical and laboratory examinations to the transplant center. Early in the evaluation process, the donor's blood type is ascertained to determine compatibility with the recipient. If this information, plus the screening interview, do not exclude donation, then the prospective donor undergoes a complete history and physical examination, laboratory testing, cross-matching, and finally renal imaging [1,2]. The

Evidence-based Nephrology. Edited by Donald Molony and Jonathan Craig
© 2009 Blackwell Publishing, ISBN: 978-1-4051-3975-5.

donor evaluation is completed with visits to the transplant social worker, psychologist, or psychiatrist (Table 49.1).

Medical evaluation of the living donor has been standardized based on two large conferences with broad representation from the transplant community [3]. However, some testing issues (e.g. type of urinary protein measurement, method of glomerular filtration rate [GFR] determination, anatomic testing method) remain to be established (http://www.bts.org.uk/) [3].

Immediate surgical risk: assessment of cardiopulmonary and coagulation systems

Cardiopulmonary disease

Cardiac evaluations include medical history, physical examination, electrocardiogram, and chest X-ray [4,5]. If these suggest ischemia, then a stress test (exercise or pharmacologic) should be performed. An individual with myocardial dysfunction should not donate, as kidney dysfunction is a common accompaniment to heart failure [6–8]. Coronary lesions requiring intervention should be treated and stable prior to donation. Careful assessment for renovascular disease is needed in those with coronary artery disease [9,10].

Valvular integrity is ascertained by questioning about past rheumatic fever, use of fenfluramine or phentermine, prosthetic valve placement, dyspnea, and cough. The possibility of valvular abnormalities should be particularly considered in family members of those with autosomal-dominant polycystic kidney disease [11,12]. Absolute contraindications to donation are symptomatic valvular disease, severe valvular disease even if asymptomatic, and valvular disease with abnormal cardiac function and/or ischemia [13]. Relative contraindications are the presence of a prosthetic valve and moderate regurgitant valvular disease with otherwise-normal echocardiographic findings.

Postoperative pulmonary complications are as prevalent as cardiac complications and contribute similarly to morbidity, mortality, and length of stay after noncardiac surgery. The probability of pulmonary disease should be determined through a history (cough, smoking, dyspnea), physical examination, and a chest

Table 49.1 Donor evaluation.

History: Look for/ask about
  Hypertension
  Diabetes
  General state – weight loss/gain, strength, sweats
  Findings from prior medical evaluations
  NSAIDs/medications
  Family history
    Diabetes
    Cardiovascular disease
    Autoimmune diseases
    Kidney disease
    Cancer
    Thromboembolic disease
    Degenerative neurological diseases
  Their birth weight
  Obstetric history
  Smoking, drug, or alcohol use
  Infections
    Prior jaundice
    Blood product administration
    Travel abroad
    Malaria
    Exposure to tuberculosis
    Intravenous drug use
    Sexual history
  Nephrolithiasis
  Travel abroad
  Thromboembolic disease
  Vascular – exercise tolerance, claudication, chest pain
  Vocation/avocation
  Willingness to donate
Physical exam: evaluate/look for
  Blood pressure
  Weight/height
  Arthritis
  Autoimmunity
  Cancer:
    Prostate
    Breast
    Colorectal
    Lymph nodes
  Cardiovascular disease
Laboratory
  Urinalysis
  Electrolytes, liver panel
  Fasting blood glucose, lipid profile
  CBC with platelets, coagulation screen
  24-h urine, creatinine clearance, protein excretion or GFR (iothalamate clearance) and protein determination (or protein/creatinine ratio and urine albumin determination)
  Antiviral screening: HCV, HBV, HIV, EBV, CMV, HSV
  PPD (controversial in nonendemic areas), RPR
  EKG, chest X-ray
  PAP, prostate exam
  Age/family history determined
    ETT, ECHO
    Colonoscopy, ultrasound
    Mammogram/PSA
Anatomic evaluation per local expertise
    CT angiogram
    Multislice CT (96% accuracy compared to operative findings)
    MRI angiogram
    Standard arteriogram
    Digital subtraction angiography

radiograph [14]. If indicated by history and examination, pulmonary function testing, echocardiogram, and/or sleep studies should be performed [15]. In all cases, donors should be encouraged to cease smoking for at least 4–8 weeks before surgery to minimize the risk for pneumonia and wound complications [16,17]. Pulmonary contraindications to donation include cystic fibrosis, sarcoidosis, interstitial lung disease with fixed pulmonary hypertension and persistent hypoxemia, primary and secondary pulmonary hypertension, severe sleep apnea, severe chronic obstructive pulmonary disease, asthma complicated with status asthmaticus, and α_1-antitrypsin deficiency. Relative contraindications to donation are mild sleep apnea without a history of pulmonary hypertension, chronic hypoxia, or arrhythmias on bilevel or continuous positive airway pressure therapy [15,18].

Coagulation abnormalities

A history of venous thromboembolism should be ascertained. Only if present should a comprehensive coagulation profile be done, as these tests are expensive and are unlikely to change management [19–21]. Oral contraceptives and hormone replacement therapy are commonly used in the general population and may increase the risk for postoperative venous thrombosis [22,23]. In general it is advised that hormone replacement be withheld for at least 1 month prior to an elective surgery, although not all current data or reviews support this practice [22–27].

Mortality

Postoperative

Only recently has the United Network for Organ Sharing (UNOS) begun collecting information about short-term donor outcomes (Table 49.2). The mortality rate for living donor nephrectomy using a laparoscopic technique is 0.03% from surveys and single-center sources. Data from UNOS and the Social Security Death Master File on donors from October 1999 to October 2004 reveal a 0.04% 30-day mortality and a 0.09% 1-year mortality for kidney donors (Organ Procurement and Transplantation Network [OPTN] data as of April 2005). Several deaths have been due to failure of the clips placed on the remnant donor renal artery, resulting in massive hemorrhage, rather than an impaired cardiovascular state of the donor [28].

Long term

The underlying premise of living kidney donation is that the removal of one kidney does not impair survival or long-term kidney function in the donor. Reports of relatively homogenous northern European populations after nephrectomy by Narkun-Burgess (for trauma), Fehrman-Ekholm (for kidney donation), and Najarian (for kidney donation) suggest that live kidney donation is safe (Figure 49.1) [29–33]. A meta-analysis of outcomes in 3124 subjects with reduced kidney mass mostly due to kidney donation (60.5%) showed a 17.1 mL/min average decrease in GFR after nephrectomy but no progressive decline in renal function with time [34].

Table 49.2 Operative mortality in living kidney donors.

Study author [reference]	Data source	No. of donors	% Mortality
Kok 2006 [173]	Trial of randomized open vs. laparoscopic donation in two Norwegian programs	100	0
UNOS/OPTN 2005 [183]	UNOS/OPTN database, USA, 10/99–10/04	30,716	0.04 (at 30 days)
UNOS/OPTN 2005 [183]	UNOS/OPTN database, USA, 10/99–10/04	30,716	0.09 (at 1 yr)
Pietrabissa 2004 [175]	Survey of Italian programs	401	0
Matas 2003 [174]	Survey of US programs	10,828	0.02
Hartmann 2003 [54]	Single program plus Norwegian Registry	1800	0

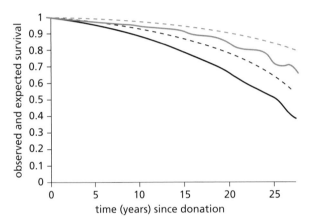

Figure 49.1 Survival of Swedish kidney donors compared to general Swedish population. The donors demonstrated superior survival [30].

However, the profile of donors has changed over time to include those with isolated medical abnormalities, such as essential hypertension, an increased body mass index (BMI), isolated hematuria, dyslipidemia, and stone disease. Follow-up has not been long enough to be confident that these various comorbid conditions will not adversely influence survival (Table 49.3). Furthermore, the UNOS/OPTN data combined with those of the Social Security Death Master File for those donating between October 1999 and

October 2004 reveals a 0.18% donor mortality rate (www.optn.org; OPTN data as of April 2005). Although cause of death is generally listed as unknown, one category of death is concerning: death due to accident, homicide, or suicide (OPTN/UNOS data as of April 2005). In particular, younger donors seem to be at increased risk for this outcome and need to be carefully evaluated psychologically for the risk of self-destructive behavior following donation [35,36] (National Center for Health Statistics 2003; www.cdc.gov/nchs/datawh/statab/unpubd/mortabs/gmwk210_10.htm).

Renal evaluation

GFR

Establishing baseline renal function is critical. Although serum/plasma creatinine, 24-h creatinine clearance and calculated clearances based upon the plasma creatinine have been used to determine GFR, they are not accurate enough for the purposes of living donation (http://www.bts.org.uk/) [37–39]. Similarly, although changes in cystatin C levels may be more predictive of changes in renal function than the serum creatinine, cystatin C is also not sufficiently accurate for estimating renal function in people with normal GFR [40–42]. Measuring the clearance of compounds such as ^{51}Cr-EDTA, [^{125}I]iothalamate, and

Table 49.3 Long-term donor mortality.

Study author [reference]	No. died/total donors	No. with death caused by:		
		Cardiovascular	Cancer	Liver disease
Gossmann 2005 [57]	7/152	2	5	
Rizvi 2005 [64]	5/133	3	1	1
Ramcharan 2002 [147]	84/464	NA	NA	NA
Najarian 1992 [33]	15/78	7	6	NA
Williams 1986 [65]	4/50	NA	2	1

Abbreviations: NA, not available.

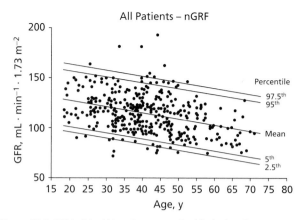

Figure 49.2 GFR in living kidney donors normalized for body surface area, shown by age (both men and women are included) [37].

Table 49.4 Age-associated GFR in living donor candidates.

Age (yrs)	Normalized GFR (mL/min/1.73 m^2) in healthy donors, by percentile			
	2.5th	5th	Mean	95th
20	87	91	111	136
25	84	88	109	133
30	81	85	107	131
35	79	83	104	128
40	77	81	102	126
45	74	78	99	123
50	72	76	97	121
55	70	73	94	119
60	67	71	92	116
65	65	69	89	113
70	62	66	87	111
75	60	64	84	109

Source: Rule *et al.* 2004 [37].

^{99}mTc-diethylenetriaminepenta-acetic acid (DTPA), or nonradiolabeled iohexol or iothalamate provides more accurate measurements of GFR [43–46]. Whatever measurement is used, the GFR must be interpreted in the context of age, gender, and body size and corrected for body surface area.

The threshold of normal kidney function has seemingly declined with time. Inulin clearance studies in 1950 reported the normal GFR was 130 mL/min/1.73 m^2 for young men and 120 mL/min/1.73 m^2 for young women [47,48]. An age-related decline in renal function of 10 mL/min/1.73 m^2 was noted after age 40, such that the GFR at age 80 was half that at age 40. More current studies have been performed using ^{125}I-labeled or cold iothalamate [37,47,49]. Gonwa *et al.* reported a slightly lower GFR of 102 ± 15 mL/min/1.73 m^2 for men and 114 ± 17 mL/min/1.73 m^2 for women age 21–30 years old, compared to data from earlier studies [49]. The GFR for men and women ages 51–60 was 84 ± 13 and 79 ± 15 mL/min/1.73 m^2, respectively. Rule *et al.* recently reported on the GFR of 365 potential kidney donors and found similar results to Gonwa's study (Figure 49.2) [37]. In general, living donors should be required to have a GFR that is average for their age (Table 49.4). Furthermore, because GFR declines with age, a donor's projected GFR at age 80 should be ≥40–50 mL/min/1.73 m^2 [50]. Most centers have chosen a GFR of 80 mL/min/1.73 m^2 to be the lower limit for donation [1-3] (see http://www.bts.org.uk/.).

Following donation, the average renal function has been shown to decrease by 27% compared to the predonation value (Table 49.5) [51]. The limitations of these studies include being single-center data, loss to follow-up (only about 50–60% of the original cohort), and that the ethnicity of those studied was almost uniformly white individuals. Furthermore, few studies report on the development of ESRD in prior living donors and again, usually only from white populations (Table 49.6). The concern is that ESRD may develop more frequently in those of other than northern European heritage. Additionally, donor characteristics are changing from what they were several decades ago. For instance, the average weight of the living donor has increased, concurrently with that of the general population [52]. Further study is needed in order to determine the true incidence and risks for renal function decline with a preeminent focus on hyperfiltration and components of metabolic syndrome [53].

ESRD

Hartmann *et al.* reported that 7 of 1800 (0.4%) living donors developed ESRD [54] (Tables 49.6 and 49.7). More recent published data suggest that between 0.2–0.4% of donors of Northern European descent have developed ESRD (32). Ojo and Davis performed a preliminary evaluation of the Scientific Registry of Transplant Recipients (SRTR) and Centers for Medicare and Medicaid Services ESRD databases (OPTN/SRTR as of March 2005). The maximum incidence of ESRD was estimated to be 0.10% in white donors and 0.52% in black donors. The most recent data from UNOS/OPTN reports 121 living donors listed for kidney transplant: 35.5% female, 64.5% male (compared to 42% of all donors), 43% white, 42.1% black (compared to 13% of all donors), and 10% Hispanic (based upon OPTN data as of May 2006). Age at donation was between 18 and 34 years in 66.3%, 35–49 years in 27.6%, and 50–64 years in 6.1%. Duration between listing for transplant and donation and the age at donation varied (Table 49.7). The cause of ESRD was glomerular disease in 24.8%, diabetes in 10.7%, hypertension in 19%, vascular disease in 6.6%, tubular/interstitial disease in 5.8%, other in 5.8%, transplant failure in 5.8%, neoplasm in 4.1%, not reported in 0.8%, and unknown in 17.4%. When evaluating only those donating since 1994 and who had been placed on the kidney transplant wait list since 1996, the rate of ESRD over 12 years appears to be 0.02%. Again, 45% of donors who developed ESRD were black. In summary, most donors who developed ESRD were young at donation, more often black, and male. The length between donation and kidney failure is usually over 15 years, and conditions associated with metabolic syndrome appear to provide significant risk.

Ahmed *et al.* reported on 34 African American donors and compared the results to those of 23 Caucasian donors [55]. Although

Table 49.5 Kidney function after donation.

Study author [reference]	Mean duration (yrs) of follow-up (range)	Completeness of follow-up (% of donors) (n)	Study method	Creatinine clearance, mL/min (avg ± SD) At donation	At follow-up
Ramcharan 2002 [147]	20–37	14	Natural history	NA	NA; serum creatinine 1.2 ± 0.04 mg/dL
Goldfarb 2001 [176]	25 (20–32)	39 (180)	Natural history	NA	72% of predonation value
Fehrman-Ekholm 2001 [31]	12 ± 8	87	Natural history/ population control		
Gossman 2005 [57]	11 ± 7 (1–28)	93 (152)	Natural history	119 ± 30	99 ± 30
Rizvi 2005 [64]	3 ± 3.2 (0.5–18)	56.5 (734)	Natural history	101 ± 28	87 ± 20
Gracida 2002 [177]	6.7 ± 2.7 (0.6–9.5)	100 (628)	Natural history	116 ± 39.5	77.9 ±17.6
Haberal 1998 [178]	10.2 (0.8–22)	12.2	Randomly selected donors	108.4	96.8
Toronyi 1998 [179]	8.9	38	Natural history	NA	98[a]
Najarian 1992 [33]	23.7 (21–29)	42	Cohort compared to siblings	103 ± 4	82 ± 2
Liounis 1988 [180] Women Men	1–11	90	Natural history	94 103	80 98
ODonnell 1986 [181]	5.8 (3–18)	36 (33)	Case–control	107.9 ± 15.5	99.6 ± 22.3
Williams 1986 [65]	12.6 (10–18)	68	Cohort compared to siblings	101 ± 5	78 ± 6
Vincenti 1983 [58]	15.8 ± 0.3 (14.5–18.5)	31 (20)	Natural history	103 ± 4	80 ± 4

Abbreviation: NA, not available.
[a] By Tc-99mMAG-3 scintigraphy.

Table 49.6 Development of ESRD in living donors.

Study author [reference]	Follow-up (% of donors)	No. with ESRD/total no. at risk (%)	ESRD (%) by race Caucasian	African American
UNOS/OPTN 2005 [183]	UNOS/OPTN[a]	104/68,623 (0.15)	0.1	0.52
Ellison 2002 [79]	Donated after 1988 listed for transplant	20/48,278 (0.04)	NR	NR
Hartmann 2003 [54]	100	7/1800 (0.38)	NR	NR
Gossman 2005 [57]	93	0/157 (0)	NR	NR
Rizvi 2005 [64]	56.5	1/734 (0.14)	NR	NR
Ramcharan 2002 [147]	60	5/464 (1.1)	NR	NR
Fehrman-Ekholm 2001 [31]	87	2/401 (0.49)	NR	NR
Goldfarb 2001 [176]	39	2/180 (1.1)	NR	NR
Williams 1986 [65]	89	0/50 (0)	NR	NR

Abbreviation: NR, not reported.
[a] Data are from the USRDS and UNOS/OPTN as of April 2005 for donors on dialysis or on the transplant waiting list.

Table 49.7 ESRD among kidney donors.

Age at donation	No. of donors (%) in age group who developed ESRD by the indicated time postdonation (yrs)						Total no. of patients in age group
	Not reported	0–5	6–10	11–15	16–25	≥26	
Not reported	23 (100)						23
18–34		6 (9.2)	9 (13.8)	10 (15.4)	26 (40)	14 (21.5)	65
35–49		4 (14.8)	2 (7.4)	2 (7.4)	15 (55.6)	4 (14.8)	27
50–64			3 (50)	3 (50)			6
Total	23 (19)	10 (8.3)	14 (11.6)	15 (12.4)	41 (33.9)	18 (14.9)	121

Source: Based upon OPTN data, as of May 2006.

the serum creatinine was not different at donation between black and white donors, the number of donors with a serum creatinine that increased over 50% was higher in African American donors. Given that the risk of ESRD after donation appears higher than previously recognized (even if the absolute numbers are small), renal evaluation, especially of African American donors, needs to be undertaken with special care.

Proteinuria screening

Urine protein (β_2-microglobulin, immunoglobulin G [IgG]) and albumin excretion after nephrectomy was studied by Strandgaard *et al.* [56,57]. The fractional clearances of β_2-microglobulin, IgG, and albumin increased markedly immediately after nephrectomy and peaked within 3 days. By 2 weeks the excretion of albumin and IgG was normal, but that of β_2-microglobulin remained increased. In the long term, although a significant number of living donors

excreted more than 150 mg/day of total protein, most of the protein was not albumin (Table 49.8) [57,58].

Urine protein excretion is associated with the development of ESRD and cardiovascular disease [59–63]. Even minimal albuminuria is associated with vascular disease development [61,62]. Interestingly, proteinuria in living donor studies has not generally been associated with decreased renal function, hypertension, or obesity [51,57,58,64,65]. However, studies have not been long enough in duration, nor large enough, to confidently exclude such associations. Additionally, the relationship between microalbuminuria and cardiovascular morbidity and mortality has not been investigated in donors (Table 49.9) [57]. Until these studies are completed it is prudent to measure both total protein and albumin excretion in living donors.

Urine collection should be timed to provide an accurate representation of albumin excretion. Urinary albumin excretion is higher during the day and with exercise, acute febrile illnesses,

Table 49.8 Proteinuria in living donors.

Study author [reference]	Follow-up (yrs)	Completeness of follow-up (% of donors)	% of donors with proteinuria (>150 mg/day)		% with excessive proteinuria
			Predonation	Postdonation[a]	
Ramcharan 2002 [147]	20–37	14.6	0	10 (dipstick)	
Goldfarb 2001 [176]	25	39	0	19	7 (>0.8 g/day)
Fehrman-Ekholm 2001 [31]	12 ± 8	87	0	10	
Gossmann 2005 [57]	11 ± 7	93	0	56	
Rizvi 2005 [64]	3 ± 3.2	56.5	0	24.3	
Haberal 1998 [178]	10.2	12.2	0	4 (>100 mg/day)	1 (>0.7 g/day)
Borchhardt 1996 [77]	6.4 ± 2	19	4.5	14	
Najarian 1992 [33]	>20	39		23	7.6 (>300 mg/day)
Liounis 1988 []	1–11	90	2.4	7.3	0
O'Donnell 1986 [181]	5.8	36	0	6	0
Williams 1986 [65]	12.6	68	0	50 (for <30 yrs old at donation); 25 (for >30 yrs at donation)	No nephritic-range proteinuria
Vincenti 1983 [58]	15.8 ± 0.3	31	0	141 ± 20	10 (>200 mg/day)

[a] When postdonation proteinuria was based on a measure other than the 150 mg/day cutoff, the method is indicated in parentheses.

Table 49.9 Albuminuria in living donors.

Study author [reference]	Duration of follow-up (yrs)	Completeness of follow-up (% of donors)	% of donors with albuminuria	
			Predonation	Postdonation
Gossmann 2005 [57]	11 ± 7	93	NA	10
Schostak 2004 [182]	7	52		23
Goldfarb 2001 [176]	25	39	NA	36
Borchhardt 1996 [77]	6.4 ± 2	19	NA	22
Najarian 1992 [33]	23.7	39	NA	6
Vincenti 1983 [58]	15.8 ± 0.3	31	NA	5

Abbreviation: NA, not applicable.

excessive water consumption, and menstruation [66]. At least two first-morning specimens collected on different days, free of these confounders, should be obtained for protein and albumin creatinine ratios [67].

Routine donor kidney biopsy

Donor kidney biopsies have rarely been performed or correlated with donor outcome. Goecke *et al.* reported on donors who were biopsied at donation and clinically evaluated more than 10 years after nephrectomy [68]. Biopsies from 29 donors showed normal pathology in 13, chronic ischemic glomerular changes in 9, thick glomerular basement membrane in 2, thin glomerular basement membrane in 1, and IgA nephropathy in 4. Urinary sediment was abnormal at follow-up in 11 donors (9 with microhematuria). There was no association between the biopsy results and subsequent creatinine clearance or proteinuria. These results suggest that kidney biopsy at donation is not beneficial from the donor's perspective.

Hypertension

Hypertension is associated with microalbuminuria, kidney failure, and cardiovascular disease [69–71]. This relationship is particularly pronounced in those with mild kidney dysfunction (GFR <60 mL/min), a level of kidney dysfunction seen in some living donors in the years following surgery [72]. Although controversy surrounds the direct causal relationship between hypertension and kidney disease, the link is strong enough to consider hypertension as a risk for living kidney donors.

The Third National Health and Nutrition Examination Survey (NHANES III) evaluated the association between blood pressure and albuminuria in 9462 people without hypertension (BP of >140/90 mmHg) or diabetes. In this study those with high-normal blood pressure (130–139/85–89 mmHg) had a significantly increased odds of microalbuminuria compared to those with optimal blood pressure (<120/80; odds ratio, 2.13; 95% confidence interval [CI], 1.51–3.01) [73]. African Americans had the highest risk for microalbuminuria (OR, 1.30; CI, 1.04–1.64) compared to Mexican Americans and non-Hispanic whites. This finding was also illustrated in a longitudinal 15-year study of young (age 18–30 years at onset) adult blacks and whites where increases in blood pressure within the normal range were associated with albuminuria many years later, especially in Blacks [74].

Blood pressure at the time of living donation has usually been normal, defined as ≤140/90 mmHg without antihypertensive treatment, rising to 10–40% postdonation (Table 49.10). However, even normotensive donors after nephrectomy may have decreased nocturnal blood pressure decline [75,76], secondary to a decline in renal function following surgery. Comparing the rates of hypertension in living donors to that of their nondonor siblings revealed similar degrees of hypertension [33]. Likewise, the prevalence of hypertension in living donors has been reported to be less than, the same as, or slightly increased compared to the general age-matched population [33,51,77].

A recent meta-analysis of all studies of more than 10 living donors in whom blood pressure was assessed at least 1 year after donation was recently reported [78]. Donors were compared with control groups of similar age, gender, and ethnicity. Although the authors reported significant limitations of the analysis, the conclusion of the study was that kidney donors may have a 5-mmHg increase in blood pressure within 5–10 years after donation over that anticipated with normal aging, consistent with the findings of an earlier meta-analysis by Kasiske *et al.* [51]. Finally, Saxen *et al.* compared blood pressure change in normotensive individuals who underwent unilateral nephrectomy for kidney donation (*n* = 25) or removal of renal cell carcinoma (*n* = 7) to binephric healthy controls [53]. Young kidney donors (average age, 35 years, range, 21–48) demonstrated a 7-mmHg increase in mean arterial pressure compared to the binephric control group. Older subjects (>55 years old) did not have increased blood pressure compared to control subjects over 55 years old.

Although there is no proven association between a predonation blood pressure and the development of ESRD, many of the donors who have reached ESRD have been reported to do so because of hypertension [79]. Furthermore, the prevalence of hypertension is increasing. The NHANES study found that hypertension was identified in 7.8% of individuals 18–39 years old, 30.6% of those 40–59 years old, and 64.5% of those ≥60 years old [80]. Thus, the evaluation for hypertension remains important, although the degree of risk for donors with hypertension and no abnormal urine microscopy, albuminuria, or decreased renal function has not been established [81].

Table 49.10 Development of hypertension after living kidney donation.

Study autor [reference]	Completeness of follow-up (% of donors)	Duration of follow-up (yrs), avg $\pm$ SD	Avg BP (mmHg)		% of donors hypertensive
			Predonation	Postdonation	
Ramcharan 2002 [147]	12	20–37	NA	NA	36
Fehrman-Ekholm 2001 [31]	87	12 $\pm$ 8	NA	NA	38
Goldfarb 2001 [176]	36	25	123 $\pm$ 12/79 $\pm$ 7	136 $\pm$ 19/79 $\pm$ 9	48
Gossmann 2005 [57]	93	11 $\pm$ 7	125 $\pm$ 15/79 $\pm$ 11	134 $\pm$ 19/ 81 $\pm$ 9	30
Rizvi 2005 [64]	56.5	3 $\pm$ 3.2	126 $\pm$ 13/79 $\pm$ 9	123 $\pm$ 15/81 $\pm$ 10	10
Sansalone 2006 [148]	100	7.9	NA	NA	8.7
Schostak 2004 [182]	52	7	NA	NA	36
Najarian 1992 [33]	46	23.7	118 $\pm$ 2/76 $\pm$ 1	134 $\pm$ 2/80 $\pm$ 1	32
Haberal 1998 [178]	12.2	10.2	131.7 $\pm$ 21.2[a]	139.6 $\pm$ 20.9[a]	8.8
Toronyi 1998 [179]	38	8.9	NA	NA	17
O'Donnell 1986 [181]	36	5.8	80.4 $\pm$ 11.7[b]	83.1 $\pm$7.3[b]	12
Borchhardt 1996 [77]	19	6.4 $\pm$ 2	NA	NA	23
Williams 1986 [65]	68	12.6	NA	NA	47
Vincenti 1983 [58]	31	15.8 $\pm$ 0.3	124 $\pm$ 3/78 $\pm$ 2	122 $\pm$ 4/77 $\pm$ 2	15

Abbreviations: BP, blood pressure; NA, not available.

[a] Systolic blood pressure.

[b] Diastolic pressure.

At the Mayo Clinic, hypertensive donors were not found to have increased short-term morbidity [76], but these donors were all over age 50, Caucasian, had controlled blood pressure with an angiotensin converting enzyme inhibitor and hydrochlorathiazide, a normal GFR (by iothalamate clearance) for age, and no microalbuminuria at donation [76,82]. A study from India likewise found no short-term morbidity in 18 hypertensive donors, with a median follow-up of 30 months, except the need to increase antihypertensive treatment in two of the donors [83]. These and other studies of hypertensive donors also need to investigate the long-term implication of a blood pressure pattern that does not dip at night [84,85]. When living donors with hypertension are accepted, the estimated increase in transplantation is only about 2% [86].

The living donor evaluation should include blood pressure measurements by experienced health care providers on three separate occasions; verification of elevated levels should be undertaken with ambulatory blood pressure monitoring, as about 10–20% may be found to have normal blood pressure [1,76,87,88]. If elevated blood pressures are detected and the prospective donor is still under consideration, then in addition to the standard donor evaluation, an ECHO and ophthalmologic evaluation should be performed to look for secondary consequences of hypertension.

Hematuria

Isolated hematuria in a prospective donor necessitates consideration of thin glomerular basement membrane disease (TBMD) and glomerulonephritis (especially IgA nephropathy) as well as urinary tract infection, malignancy, renal cystic disease and nephrolithiasis [89,90]. Microscopic hematuria is a relatively common problem,

as demonstrated in a mass screening study in Japan, where 4% of adult men and 10% of adult women had microscopic hematuria [91]. Persistent microscopic hematuria was seen in approximately 20–40% of these individuals, with an overall risk of malignancy of approximately 4.8%, which increased with age and was more common in men [89,90]. TBMD accounts for approximately one-third of the hematuria in those without malignancy or other structural abnormality [92–94]. TBMD has been found in up to 5–9% of unselected (deceased) donor kidney transplant biopsies [95,96]. IgA nephropathy also accounts for approximately one-third of glomerular-derived microscopic hematuria [92–94]. Suzuki *et al.* found latent mesangial IgA deposition in 16% (82/510) of living donor allografts biopsied at implantation; one had proteinuria [97]. Hematuria was more pronounced in those with IgA deposition but not detected in all. Koushik *et al.* reported the evaluation of 14 kidney donors with persistent hematuria (>1/hpf) [98]. This represented 2.7% (14/512) of their prospective donors. Ten underwent biopsy. Two biopsies were normal, one had IgA nephropathy, four had TBMD, one had glomerulosclerosis, one had nonhomogenous basement membrane abnormalities, and one had TBMD with early hypertensive changes. Two donor candidates had normal biopsies, and two with TBMD donated.

The real question in those with hematuria is, what is the long-term risk for kidney failure? How often do IgA deposition and TBMD indicate a risk for progressive renal disease? Unfortunately, Suzuki *et al.* did not have outcome data on the living donors with IgA deposition, some of whom had diffuse proliferative lesions (personal communication). Koushik *et al.* have 15-month follow-up on the two donors with TBMD; at the last report, these donors had not developed hypertension, proteinuria, or azotemia [98].

Isolated hematuria, however, is not necessarily benign. Nieuwhof *et al.* reported on a subset of subjects with greater than 6 months of microscopic hematuria but without extrarenal symptoms or anatomic abnormalities [92–94]. IgA deposition was found in 27, TBMD in 19, and 24 had normal histology. All were normotensive with normal renal function. Over a median of 12 years of follow-up (range, 9–15 years), the incidence of hypertension in those with TBMD exceeded that of healthy controls (35% vs. 8%). Renal function (inulin clearance) at follow-up was reduced in three of seven normotensive subjects with TBMD. Others have reported the development of ESRD in individuals with isolated TBMD including a kidney donor [99–103].

IgA deposition in the same study was associated, after a median follow-up of 11 years, with a higher rate of hypertension compared to controls [92,94]. Two of 27 went into histologic remission, and 12 showed disease progression, of whom 3 developed renal failure. Initial proteinuria over 1 g/day was associated with a high activity score and progression. IgA deposition may occur with TBMD, but without hearing or ocular alterations, and has an increasingly evident familial predisposition [104–106].

The investigation of hematuria in prospective donors includes urine culture, repeated urinalyses, urine protein and albumin measurement, and anatomical studies to determine the presence of cysts, nephrolithiasis, tumor, or vascular lesions. If the studies continue to reveal only hematuria, and if the donor accepts the risk and still wishes to proceed with donation, then a renal biopsy is indicated. If IgA nephropathy (proliferation, mesangial expansion) is discovered, the individual should forgo donation. However, the implications of isolated mesangial IgA without other manifestations of nephropathy are not known and this requires further study. Donation should be decided upon in the context of family history, absolute renal function, the presence of interstitial disease, and age. If TBMD is discovered, then it could be argued that only those over age 50 should donate, as they should have already manifested the risk for progressive kidney failure. Such donors, however, should have normal GFR for age, no albuminuria, and have a predictable family history of disease progression. Further research is needed before fully informed decisions can be made about accepting donors with TBMD [107,108].

Polycystic kidney disease

Testing prospective donors at risk for polycystic kidney disease (PCKD) must be 100% accurate. Ultrasound is 100% reliable for ruling out PCKD in individuals at risk who are age 30 or older, but the sensitivity is less in those under 30 years [109]. The resolution of computed tomography (CT) and magnetic resonance imaging (MRI) for small cystic structures is better than for ultrasound [110,111]. On average, ultrasound can detect cysts of 1.0 cm, CT with intravenous contrast can detect cysts of 0.5 cm, and heavily T2-weighted MRI can detect cysts of 0.3 cm in diameter. Therefore, wherever possible, linkage analysis should be performed in prospective donors at risk who are under age 30, but if genetic testing is not a possibility, CT and/or MRI may provide better sensitivity than ultrasound [112,113]. In the near future, more specific gene tests for the diagnosis of PCKD will be available [114–118].

Nephrolithiasis

Nephrolithiasis is a relative contraindication for live kidney donation with urinary tract obstruction in a single kidney [1,2]. Those with a history of bilateral stones or stones demonstrating high rates of recurrence (cystine or struvite stones) should not donate [119]. Additionally, those with systemic disorders leading to high rates of recurrence, such as primary or enteric hyperoxaluria, distal renal tubular acidosis, sarcoidosis, inflammatory bowel disease, or other conditions causing nephrocalcinosis, etc., should not donate. However, an asymptomatic potential donor with a current single stone may be suitable if the donor does not have a high risk of recurrence, the current stone is less than 1.5 cm in size, and it is potentially removable during transplant [120]. One report of 10 such donors showed no recurrent stone formation over an average of 36.4 months of follow-up [121]. The evaluation of an asymptomatic donor with a single prior episode of nephrolithiasis should include measurement of serum calcium, creatinine, albumin, and parathyroid hormone, spot urine for cystine, a urinalysis and urine culture, a helical CT, stone analysis if possible, and a 24-h sample urine for oxalate and creatinine.

Other testing

Psychological evaluation

There has not been any standardization of the predonation psychological evaluation. Usually, the evaluation is completed by the transplant program social worker, but ideally, programs should also have a psychologist. All prospective donors should be queried about their concerns regarding coercion, transplant success, recipient survival, their reasons for donation [122,123], and their expectations of the donor experience. More detailed psychological evaluation is required for people inquiring about altruistic donation, because of high rates of depression and other psychiatric illness [124–126]. Because UNOS data show an increase in suicide and accidental death in young donors compared to the general population, young donor candidates should be evaluated for suicidal ideation and excessive risk-taking behaviors (UNOS data as of April 2005; National Center for Health Statistics).

Anatomic evaluation

The angiogram has been supplanted by the CT angiogram or magnetic resonance angiogram [127]. The overall accuracy of multirow detector CT angiogram to detect renal arterial anatomy compared to surgical findings is between 93 and 100% depending upon the number of channels used [128–130]. The overall accuracy of the magnetic resonance angiogram compared to angiography or surgically determined anatomy is 80–100% [131–133]. Venous anatomy has been confirmed to correlate with surgical findings in 95–100% with either technique ([129,130,132].

Other issues

Obesity

Obesity is associated with diabetes, cardiovascular disease, hyperfiltration, hypertension, nephrolithiasis, renal cell cancer, proteinuria, and chronic kidney disease [134–139]. Obese donors have a larger glomerular planar surface area, which correlates with donor weight and microalbumin excretion [140]. Obese donors also have more tubular dilatation and a trend toward more arterial hyalinosis. Further evidence for the association between obesity and kidney failure is demonstrated by the decrease in glomerular hyperfiltration, excessive renal plasma flow, and albuminuria with weight reduction [141].

Praga *et al.* described 73 subjects from Spain who underwent unilateral nephrectomy without known disease in the contralateral kidney [142]. Those with a BMI over 30 kg/m^2 at the time of surgery were found to develop proteinuria and kidney failure 10–20 years later. The average BMI in the obese group at nephrectomy was 31.6 kg/m^2, compared to 24.3 kg/m^2 in the nonobese group.

Of concern for the health of future kidney donors is that albuminuria has been demonstrated in up to 5.8% of obese teenagers (BMI, >35 kg/m^2), especially in association with hyperinsulinemia, impaired glucose tolerance, and hypertension [143,144]. Future donors may have a longer exposure to the metabolic syndrome than donors from previous eras and so may develop more renal and cardiovascular disease, nephrolithiasis, and cancer. Careful instruction about possible future health risks needs to be given to donors who are obese (or smoke). Education on healthier life choices and weight reduction programs should also be included in the plan for donation. In the future, selection of the donor may be aided by noting the distribution of fat in an obese donor candidate, because visceral adiposity is associated with harmful cytokine levels which may contribute to future renal disease [145].

Even with the apparent risks of obesity, many programs are accepting obese living donors. Heimbach *et al.* has prospectively evaluated obese donors over 12 months [52]. To date, the accepted obese donor has been found to have a higher baseline blood pressure, glucose level, and lipid levels than nonobese donors, although the levels are still within the high-normal range. So far, the obese donors have not had lower GFRs (by iothalamate clearance) or higher protein excretion rates compared to the normal BMI donors. The Swiss donor registry has likewise not yet noted a change in albuminuria in obese donors over 5 years from donation, although one donor has developed diabetes, hypertension, proteinuria, and kidney failure [146].

The risk of diabetes must be carefully considered in obese donors. Rizvi *et al.* reported the development of diabetes in 3.6% of 734 donors followed for 3 years on average (maximum follow-up, 18 years) [64]. Obesity was associated with the development of diabetes and hypertension. Ramcharan and Matas reported that 7.6% (19/250) of donors responding to their survey had developed diabetes over 20–37 years after donation [147]. Sansalone

et al. noted 1.2% of 162 donors developed type 2 diabetes within 4.5–11 years of donation [148].

Obesity increases the future risk of diabetes substantially. Even without overt obesity, those with a family history of diabetes or other associated risk factors should be concerned about their risk of developing the disease. As diabetes is a contraindication to live kidney donation, all prospective donors should be evaluated with a fasting blood sugar, and a 75-g 2-h oral glucose tolerance test should be performed if they have a fasting glucose between 5.55–6.66 mmol/L, a first-degree relative with diabetes, a history of gestational diabetes or delivery of babies over 4 Kgs, a blood pressure over 149/90, fasting triglyceride levels of 2.8 mmol/L, a BMI over 30 kg/m^2, a high-density lipoprotein level of 0.9 mmol/L, are less than 40 years old, or have a second-degree relative with diabetes.

Age

Age is associated with declines in GFR and increases in proteinuria and blood pressure. Older donors have been defined variably as those over the age of 50–60 years. No matter the age threshold, older donors have a lower GFR and higher blood pressure compared to younger donors [76,149,150]. However, as have all donors, they have been selected for a lack of proteinuria.

The rate of acceptance of older donors varies worldwide. In the USA, the number of living kidney donors over age 65 has been between 41 and 64/year since 1997 [83,151–153]. There has, however, been a steady increase in US donors between the ages of 50 and 64 (based upon OPTN data as of August 25, 2006).

Surgical complications, including death, have been rare in elderly living donors, with either open or laparoscopic procedures [151–157]. Following donation, the serum creatinine may be somewhat higher and GFR lower for older versus younger donors [152,157,158]. However, the single-kidney GFR in older donors increases by the same proportion (10–40%) as in younger donors [53,83,150,154,155,159]. Furthermore, no deterioration in renal function of elderly donors has been found for up to 7 years follow-up [155,156]. To date, based upon limited numbers and duration of follow-up, there has not been an increased risk of ESRD or cardiovascular mortality in older donors. In one report, 1 of 112 elderly donors died of pneumonia, 1 of a motor vehicle accident, and 1 of suicide [155]. In another report, 2 of 26 donors developed coronary artery disease 3 and 5 years after donation but were still alive [156]. How this compares to what they would have experienced without donation is unknown.

Renal vascular disease

Renovascular disease has been found in up to 10% of those undergoing donor evaluation [160]. Fibromuscular dysplasia (FMD) is found in about 2–4% of prospective donors [160–162]. In a study of 1862 renal angiograms performed in potential living donors, 71 demonstrated FMD [161]. The average age of the donor candidates with FMD was 50.8 years, and 75% were women. Thirty candidates who did not undergo nephrectomy were followed over a mean of 7.5 years, and 8 (26.6%) developed hypertension. Nineteen who donated were followed for a mean of 4.4 years and 5 (26.3%) developed hypertension. This compared to 3 of 49 (6.1%) control subjects selected from the group of healthy age- and sex-matched controls without FMD who developed hypertension over 7.1 years of follow-up. Indudhara et al. followed 19 living donors who had FMD [163]. A total of 37 individuals with FMD had been considered for donation but 18 were rejected due to disease severity or the availability of another donor. Donors were older than those who did not donate (50.5 vs. 44.7 years) and had less severe disease; only one had bilateral disease. At a median follow-up of 4.5 years (range, 2 months–12 years), none of the donors had hypertension or increased serum creatinine levels. Of the 18 patients not undergoing nephrectomy, 11 were contacted and none had developed hypertension, proteinuria, or an abnormal serum creatinine. This study concluded that an evaluation for bilateral and distal branch disease should be performed prior to donor nephrectomy in an individual with FMD, and donors with severe and diffuse disease should not be selected for donation. The age of the prospective donor should also be considered, with the outcome in donors over age 50 more predictable and benign than in younger donors. Similar conclusions were drawn by authors of a paper reporting on three donors with FMD, none of whom developed hypertension within 21–115 months of follow-up [164]. However, given these sparse data, a donor with FMD may still progress and so require blood pressure monitoring and vascular imaging postnephrectomy. Recently, there was a report of a 41-year-old female donor who had such mild disease that it was not detected by spiral CT predonation, but within 1 year of nephrectomy she developed severe renal artery stenosis complicated by accelerated hypertension [165].

Atherosclerotic renal vascular disease should be considered a relative contraindication for living donation [166]. If renal atherosclerosis is present, the donor should be normotensive, have normal renal function, and have only unilateral disease [164,167]. Careful evaluation for coronary disease should be undertaken, given the significant correlation of renal atherosclerosis with coronary artery disease [10,168]. Likewise, investigations to determine the presence of peripheral vascular disease should be undertaken [169]. Donors with renal atherosclerosis should have regularly scheduled visits to assess blood pressure and vascular integrity following donation.

Malignancy and infection

A prior history of the following malignancies usually excludes live kidney donation: melanoma, testicular cancer, renal cell carcinoma, choriocarcinoma, hematological malignancy, bronchial cancer, breast cancer, or monoclonal gammopathy [3]. A prior history of malignancy may only be acceptable for donation if prior treatment of the malignancy does not decrease renal reserve or place the donor at increased risk for ESRD, does not increase the operative risk of nephrectomy, and if the specific cancer is curable and transmission of the cancer can reasonably be excluded. Consultation with an oncologist may be required.

An individual with an active infection that requires nephrotoxic treatments or which may be complicated by renal disease should not be a living donor. Some of these infections include HIV, hepatitis C, hepatitis B, recurrent urinary tract infections, endocarditis, and malaria [3]. Tuberculosis can cause renal dysfunction through obstruction. Transmission of the infection may also be fatal to the recipient. It is uncertain whether donors should be screened for tuberculosis using a tuberculin skin test. Recently, a paper from Mexico reported that if the potential living donor ($n = 217$) had a negative chest X-ray, urinalysis, and excretory urography, isoniazid treatment of the donor did not change the risk of transmission of tuberculosis or change the donor's rate of developing active tuberculosis [170]. This study should be validated by studies in other countries, but it does raise the question about the need for routine tuberculosis skin testing for living kidney donors.

Consent

During the medical evaluation there is an ongoing dialogue between the prospective donor and transplant team to ensure continued comfort with the decision to donate. Conversations are held to determine whether the donor understands the social and health implications of donation and whether there is evidence of coercion. This dialogue is the foundation of informed consent. The components of informed consent discussed with the donor include the impact of donation on their social and financial wellbeing, the short-term morbidity and mortality directly related to the surgery, the future risk of renal insufficiency and failure, the risk of de novo medical problems on kidney and overall health (i.e. hypertension, diabetes), and the risk of allograft failure in the recipient due to rejection, technical problems, recurrent disease, and/or comorbid medical problems [171,172].

References

1 Gabolde M, Herve C, Moulin AM. Evaluation, selection, and follow-up of live kidney donors: a review of current practice in French renal transplant centres. *Nephrol Dial Transplant* 2001; **16(10):** 2048–2052.

2 Bia MJ, Ramos EL, Danovitch GM, Gaston RS, Harmon WE, Leichtman AB et al. Evaluation of living renal donors. The current practice of US transplant centers. *Transplantation* 1995; **60(4):** 322–327.

3 Delmonico FL. A report of the Amsterdam forum on the care of the live kidney donor: data and medical guidelines. *Transplantation* 2005; **79(6 Suppl):** S53–S66.

4 Chassot PG, Delabays A, Spahn DR. Preoperative evaluation of patients with, or at risk of, coronary artery disease undergoing non-cardiac surgery. *Br J Anaesth* 2002; **89(5):** 747–759.

5 Devereaux PJ, Goldman L, Cook DJ, Gilbert K, Leslie K, Guyatt GH. Perioperative cardiac events in patients undergoing noncardiac surgery: a review of the magnitude of the problem, the pathophysiology of the events and methods to estimate and communicate risk. *CMAJ* 2005; **173(6):** 627–634.

6 De Santo NG, Cirillo M, Perna A, Pollastro RM, Frangiosa A, Di Stazio E et al. The kidney in heart failure. *Semin Nephrol* 2005; **25(6):** 404–407.

7 Go AS, Yang J, Ackerson LM, Lepper K, Robbins S, Massie BM *et al.* Hemoglobin level, chronic kidney disease, and the risks of death and hospitalization in adults with chronic heart failure: the Anemia in Chronic Heart Failure: Outcomes and Resource Utilization (ANCHOR) Study. *Circulation* 2006; **113(23)**: 2713–2723.

8 Smith GL, Lichtman JH, Bracken MB, Shlipak MG, Phillips CO, DiCapua P *et al.* Renal impairment and outcomes in heart failure: systematic review and meta-analysis. *J Am Coll Cardiol* 2006; **47(10)**: 1987–1996.

9 Cohen MG, Pascua JA, Garcia-Ben M, Rojas-Matas CA Gabay JM, Berrocal DH *et al.* A simple prediction rule for significant renal artery stenosis in patients undergoing cardiac catheterization. *Am Heart J* 2005; **150(6)**: 1204–1211.

10 Edwards MS, Hansen KJ, Craven TE, Bleyer AJ, Burke GL, Levy PJ *et al.* Associations between renovascular disease and prevalent cardiovascular disease in the elderly: a population-based study. *Vasc Endovascular Surg* 2004; **38(1)**: 25–35.

11 Ivy DD, Shaffer EM, Johnson AM, Kimberling WJ, Dobin A, Gabow PA. Cardiovascular abnormalities in children with autosomal dominant polycystic kidney disease. *J Am Soc Nephrol* 1995; **5(12)**: 2032–2036.

12 Hossack KF, Leddy CL, Johnson AM, Schrier RW, Gabow PA. Echocardiographic findings in autosomal dominant polycystic kidney disease. *N Engl J Med* 1988; **319(14)**: 907–912.

13 Fahy BG, Hasnain JU, Flowers JL, Plotkin JS, Odonkor P, Ferguson MK. Transesophageal echocardiographic detection of gas embolism and cardiac valvular dysfunction during laparoscopic nephrectomy. *Anesth Analg* 1999; **88(3)**: 500–504.

14 Qaseem A, Snow V, Fitterman N, Hornbake ER, Lawrence VA, Smetana GW *et al.* Risk assessment for and strategies to reduce perioperative pulmonary complications for patients undergoing noncardiothoracic surgery: a guideline from the American College of Physicians. *Ann Intern Med* 2006; **144(8)**: 575–580.

15 Kinebuchi S, Kazama JJ, Satoh M, Sakai K, Nakayama H, Yoshizawa H *et al.* Short-term use of continuous positive airway pressure ameliorates glomerular hyperfiltration in patients with obstructive sleep apnoea syndrome. *Clin Sci* (London) 2004; **107(3)**: 317–322.

16 Lawrence VA, Cornell JE, Smetana GW. Strategies to reduce postoperative pulmonary complications after noncardiothoracic surgery: systematic review for the American College of Physicians. *Ann Intern Med* 2006; **144(8)**: 596–608.

17 Moller A, Villebro N. Interventions for preoperative smoking cessation. *Cochrane Database Syst Rev* 2005; **3**: CD002294.

18 Krishna J, Shah ZA, Merchant M, Klein JB, Gozal D. Urinary protein expression patterns in children with sleep-disordered breathing: preliminary findings. *Sleep Med* 2006; **7(3)**: 221–227.

19 Wahlander K, Larson G, Lindahl TL, Andersson C, Frison L, Gustafsson D *et al.* Factor V Leiden (G1691A and prothrombin gene G20210A mutations as potential risk factors for venous thromboembolism after total hip or total knee replacement surgery. *Thromb Haemost* 2002; **87(4)**: 580–585.

20 De Stefano V, Martinelli I, Mannucci PM, Paclaroni K, Chisulo P, Casorelli I *et al.* The risk of recurrent deep venous thrombosis among heterozygous carriers of both factor V Leiden and the G20210A prothrombin mutation. *N Engl J Med* 1999; **341(11)**: 801–806.

21 Abbasi S, Khan FA. Effect of pre-operative coagulation testing on intraoperative transfusion requirements in surgical patients. *J Coll Physicians Surg Pak* 2005; **15(6)**: 319–322.

22 Robinson GE, Burren T, Mackie IJ, Bounds W, Walshe K, Faint R *et al.* Changes in haemostasis after stopping the combined contraceptive pill: implications for major surgery. *BMJ* 1991; **302(6771)**: 269–271.

23 Grady D, Wenger NK, Herrington D, Khan S, Hunninghake D, Vittinghoff E *et al.* Postmenopausal hormone therapy increases risk for venous thromboembolic disease. The Heart and Estrogen/progestin Replacement Study. *Ann Intern Med* 2000; **132(9)**: 689–696.

24 Wu O. Postmenopausal hormone replacement therapy and venous thromboembolism. *Gend Med* 2005; **2(Suppl A)**: S18–S27.

25 Hurbanek JG, Jaffer AK, Morra N, Karafa M, Brotman DJ. Postmenopausal hormone replacement and venous thromboembolism following hip and knee arthroplasty. *Thromb Haemost* 2004; **92(2)**: 337–343.

26 Shackelford DP, Lalikos JF. Estrogen replacement therapy and the surgeon. *Am J Surg* 2000; **179(4)**: 333–336.

27 Edmonds MJ, Crichton TJ, Runciman WB, Pradhan M. Evidence-based risk factors for postoperative deep vein thrombosis. *Aust N Z J Surg* 2004; **74(12)**: 1082–1097.

28 Friedman AL, Peters TG, Jones KW, Boulware LE, Ratner LE. Fatal and nonfatal hemorrhagic complications of living kidney donation. *Ann Surg* 2006; **243(1)**: 126–130.

29 Narkun-Burgess DM, Nolan CR, Norman JE, Page WF, Miller PL, Meyer TW. Forty-five year follow-up after uninephrectomy. *Kidney Int* 1993; **43(5)**: 1110–1115.

30 Fehrman-Ekholm I, Elinder CG, Stenbeck M, Tyden G, Groth CG. Kidney donors live longer. *Transplantation* 1997; **64(7)**: 976–978.

31 Fehrman-Ekholm I, Duner F, Brink B, Tyden G, Elinder CG. No evidence of accelerated loss of kidney function iin living kidney donors: results from a cross-sectional follow-up. *Transplantation* 2001; **72(3)**: 444–449.

32 Fehrman-Ekholm I, Thiel GT. *Long-term Risks after Kidney Donation.* Taylor & Francis, London, 2005.

33 Najarian JS, Chavers BM, McHugh LE, Matas AJ. 20 years or more of follow-up of living kidney donors. *Lancet* 1992; **340(8823)**: 807–810.

34 Kasiske BL, Bia MJ. The evaluation and selection of living kidney donors. *Am J Kidney Dis* 1995; **26(2)**: 387–398.

35 Jordan J, Sann U, Janton A, Gossman J, Kramer W, Kachel HG *et al.* Living kidney donors' long-term psychological status and health behavior after nephrectomy: a retrospective study. *J Nephrol* 2004; **17(5)**: 728–735.

36 Corley MC, Elswick RK, Sargeant CC, Scott S. Attitude, self-image, and quality of life of living kidney donors. *Nephrol Nurs J* 2000; **27(1)**: 43–50.

37 Rule AD, Gussak HM, Pond GR, Bergstrath EJ, Stegall MD, Cosio FG *et al.* Measured and estimated GFR in healthy potential kidney donors. *Am J Kidney Dis* 2004; **43(1)**: 112–119.

38 Bertolatus JA, Goddard L. Evaluation of renal function in potential living kidney donors. *Transplantation* 2001; **71(2)**: 256–260.

39 LIn J, Knight EL, Hogan ML, Singh AK. A comparison of prediction equations for estimating glomerular filtration rate in adults without kidney disease. *J Am Soc Nephrol* 2003; **14**: 2573–2580.

40 John GT, Fleming JJ, Talaulikar GS, Selvakumar R, Thomas PP, Jacob CK. Measurement of renla function in kidney donors using serum cystatin C and beta(2)-microglobulin. *Ann Clin Biochem* 2003; **40(6)**: 656–658.

41 Rule AD, Bergstralh EJ, Slezak JM, Bergert J, Larson TS. Glomerular filtration rate estimated by cystatin C among different clinical presentations. *Kidney Int* 2006; **69(2)**: 399–405.

42 Perkins BA, Nelson RG, Ostander BE, Blouch KL, Krolewski AS, Myers BD et al. Detection of renal function decline in patients with diabetes and normal or elevated GFR by serial measurments of serum cystatin C concentration: results of a 4-year follow-up study. *J Am Soc Nephrol* 2005; **16(5)**: 1404–1412.

43 Perrone RD, Steinman TI, Beck GJ, Skibinski CI, Royal HD, Lawlor M et al. Utility of radioisotopic filtration markers in chronic renal insufficiency: simultaneous comparison of ^{125}I-iothalamate, [169]Yb-DTPA, [99]mTc-DTPA, and inulin. The Modification of Diet in Renal Disease Study. *Am J Kidney Dis* 1990; **16(3)**: 224–235.

44 Notghi A, Merrick MV, Ferrington C, Anderton JL. A comparison of simplified and standard methods for the measurement of glomerular filtration rate and renal tubular function. *Br J Radiol* 1986; **59(697)**: 35–39.

45 Durand E, Prigent A. The basics of renal imaging and function studies. *Q J Nucl Med* 2002; **46(4)**: 249–267.

46 Moore AE, Park-Holohan SJ, Blake GM, Fogelman I. Conventional measurements of GFR using 51Cr-EDTA overestimate true renal clearance by 10 percent. *Eur J Nucl Med Mol Imaging* 2003; **30(1)**: 4–8.

47 Piepsz A, Pintelon H, Ham HR. Estimation of normal chromium-51 ethylenediamine tetraacetic acid clearance in children. *Eur J Nucl Med* 1994; **21**: 12–16.

48 Davies DF, Shock MW. Age changes in glomerular filtrations rate, effective renal plasma flow and tubular excretory capacity in adult males. *J Clin Invest* 1950; **29**: 496–507.

49 Gonwa TA, Atkins C, Zhang YA, Parker TF, Hunt JM, Lu CY et al. Glomerular filtration rates in persons evaluated as living-related donors: are our standards too high? *Transplantation* 1993; **55(5)**: 983–985.

50 Fehrman-Ekholm I, Skeppholm L. Renal function in the elderly (>70 years old) measured by means of iohexol clearance, serum creatinine, serum urea and estimated clearance. *Scand J Urol Nephrol* 2004; **38(1)**: 73–77.

51 Kasiske BL, Ma JZ, Louis TA, Swan SK. Long-term effects of reduced renal mass in humans. *Kidney Int* 1995; **48(3)**: 814–819.

52 Heimbach JK, Taler SJ, Prieto M, Cosio FG, Textor SC, Kudva YC et al. Obesity in living kidney donors: clinical characteristics and outcomes in the era of laparoscopic donor nephrectomy. *Am J Transplant* 2005; **5(5)**: 1057–1064.

53 Saxena AB, Myers BD, Derby G, Blouch RL, Yan J, Ho B et al. Adaptive hyperfiltration in the aging kidney after contralateral nephrectomy. *Am J Physiol Renal Physiol* 2006; **291(3)**: F629–F634.

54 Hartmann A, Fauchald P, Westlie L, Brekke IB, Holdaas H. The risk of living kidney donation. *Nephrol Dial Transplant* 2003; **18(5)**: 871–873.

55 Ahmed J, Shah V, Malinzak L, et al. Comparison of the increase in serum creatinine post kidney donation between African American and Caucasian donors. *Am J Transplant* 2005; **5(Suppl 11)**: A416.

56 Strandgaard S, Kamper A, Skaarup P, Holstein-Rathlou NH, Leyssac PP, Munck O. Changes in glomerular filtration rate, lithium clearance and plasma protein clearances in the early phase after unilateral nephrectomy in living healthy renal transplant donors. *Clin Sci* (London) 1988; **75(6)**: 655–659.

57 Gossmann J, Wilhelm A, Kachel HG, Jordan J, Sann U, Geiger H et al. Long-term consequences of live kidney donation follow-up in 93% of living kidney donors in a single transplant center. *Am J Transplant* 2005; **5(10)**: 2417–2424.

58 Vincenti F, Amend WJ, Jr., Kaysen G, Feduska N, Birnbaum J, Duca R et al. Long-term renal function in kidney donors. Sustained compensatory hyperfiltration with no adverse effects. *Transplantation* 1983; **36(6)**: 626–629.

59 Iseki K, Ikemiya Y, Iseki C, Takishita S. Proteinuria and the risk of developing end-stage renal disease. *Kidney Int* 2003; **63(4)**: 1468–1474.

60 Yuyun MF, Khaw KT, Luben R, Welch A, Bingham S, Day NE et al. Microalbuminuria, cardiovascular risk factors and cardiovascular morbidity in a British population: the EPIC-Norfolk population-based study. *Eur J Cardiovasc Prev Rehabil* 2004; **11(3)**: 207–213.

61 Yuyun MF, Khaw KT, Luben R, Welch A, Bingham S, Day NE et al. A prospective study of microalbuminuria and incident coronary heart disease and its prognostic significance in a British population: the EPIC-Norfolk study. *Am J Epidemiol* 2004; **159(3)**: 284–293.

62 Yuyun MF, Khaw KT, Luben R, Welch A, Bingham S, Day NE et al. Microalbuminuria and stroke in a British population: the European Prospective Investigation into Cancer in Norfolk (EPIC-Norfolk) population study. *J Intern Med* 2004; **255(2)**: 247–256.

63 Wang Z, Hoy WE. Albuminuria and incident coronary heart disease in Australian Aboriginal people. *Kidney Int* 2005; **68(3)**: 1289–1293.

64 Rizvi SA, Naqvi SA, Jawad F, Ahmed E, Asghar A, Zafar MN et al. Living kidney donor follow-up in a dedicated clinic. *Transplantation* 2005; **79(9)**: 1247–1251.

65 Williams SL, Oler J, Jorkasky DK. Long-term renal function in kidney donors: a comparison of donors and their siblings. *Ann Intern Med* 1986; **105(1)**: 1–8.

66 Mogensen CE, Vestbo E, Poulsen PL, Christiansen C, Damsgaard EM, Eiskjaer H et al. Microalbuminuria and potential confounders. A review and some observations on variability of urinary albumin excretion. *Diabetes Care* 1995; **18(4)**: 572–581.

67 Gansevoort RT, Verhave JC, Hillege HL, Burgerhof JG, Bakker SJ, de Zeeuw D et al. The validity of screening based on spot morning urine samples to detect subjects with microalbuminuria in the general population. *Kidney Int Suppl* 2005 **94**: S28–S35.

68 Goecke H, Ortiz AM, Troncoso P, Martinez L, Jara A, Valdes G et al. Influence of the kidney histology at the time of donation on long term kidney function in living kidney donors. *Transplant Proc* 2005; **37(8)**: 3351–3353.

69 Dell'omo G, Giorgi D, Di Bello V, Mariani M, Pedrinelli R. Blood pressure independent association of microalbuminuria and left ventricular hypertrophy in hypertensive men. *J Intern Med* 2003; **254(1)**: 76–84.

70 Dell'Omo G, Penno G, Giorgi D, Di Bello V, Mariani M, Pedrinelli R. Association between high-normal albuminuria and risk factors for cardiovascular and renal disease in essential hypertensive men. *Am J Kidney Dis* 2002; **40(1)**: 1–8.

71 Pedrinelli R, Dell'Omo G, Penno G, Di Bello V, Giorgi D, Pellegrini G et al. Microalbuminuria, a parameter independent of metabolic influences in hypertensive men. *J Hypertens* 2003; **21(6)**: 1163–1169.

72 Leoncini G, Viazzi F, Parodi D, Vettoretti S, Ratto E, Ravera M et al. Mild renal dysfunction and subclinical cardiovascular damage in primary hypertension. *Hypertension* 2003; **42(1)**: 14–18.

73 Knight EL, Kramer HM, Curhan GC. High-normal blood pressure and microalbuminuria. *Am J Kidney Dis* 2003; **41(3)**: 588–595.

74 Murtaugh MA, Jacobs DR, Jr., Yu X, Gross MD, Steffes M. Correlates of urinary albumin excretion in young adult blacks and whites: the Coronary Artery Risk Development in Young Adults Study. *Am J Epidemiol* 2003; **158(7)**: 676–686.

75 Goto N, Uchida K, Morozumi K, Ueki T, Matsuoka S, Katayama A et al. Circadian blood pressure rhythm is disturbed by nephrectomy. *Hypertens Res* 2005; **28(4)**: 301–306.

76 Textor SC, Taler SJ, Driscoll N, Larson TS, Gloor J, Griffin M et al. Blood pressure and renal function after kidney donation from hypertensive living donors. *Transplantation* 2004; **78**(2): 276–282.

77 Borchhardt KA, Yilmaz N, Haas M, Mayer G. Renal function and glomerular permselectivity late after living related donor transplantation. *Transplantation* 1996; **62**(1): 47–51.

78 Boudville N, Prasad GV, Knoll G, Muirhead N, Thiessen-Philbrook H, Yang RC et al. Meta-analysis: risk for hypertension in living kidney donors. *Ann Intern Med* 2006; **145**(3): 185–196.

79 Ellison MD, McBride MA, Taranto SE, Delmonico FL, Kauffman HM. Living kidney donors in need of kidney transplants: a report from the organ procurement and transplantation network. *Transplantation* 2002; **74**(9): 1349–1351.

80 Wang YY, Wang QJ. The prevalence of prehypertension and hypertension among US adults according to the New Joint National Committee Guidelines: new challenges of the old problem. *Arch Intern Med* 2004; **164**(19): 2126–2134.

81 Steiner RW, Gert B. A technique for presenting risk and outcome data to potential living renal transplant donors. *Transplantation* 2001; **71**(8): 1056–1057.

82 Textor SC, Taler SJ, Prieto M, et al. Hypertensive living renal donors have lower blood pressures and urinary microalbumin one year after nephrectomey. *Am J Transplant* 2003; **3**(Suppl 5): A192.

83 Srivastava A, Sinha T, Varma PP, Karan SC, Sandhu AS, Sethi GS et al. Experience with marginal living related kidney donors: are they becoming routine or are there still any doubts? *Urology* 2005; **66**(5): 971–975.

84 Cuspidi C, Michev I, Meani S, Severgnini B, Fusi V, Corti C et al. Reduced nocturnal fall in blood pressure, assessed by two ambulatory blood pressure monitorings and cardiac alterations in early phases of untreated essential hypertension. *J Hum Hypertens* 2003; **17**(4): 245–251.

85 Marinakis AG, Vyssoulis GP, Michaelides AP, Karpanou EA, Cokkinos DV, Toutouzas PK. Impact of abnormal nocturnal blood pressure fall on vascular function. *Am J Hypertens* 2003; **16**(3): 209–213.

86 Karpinski M, Knoll G, Cohn A, Yang R, Garg A, Storsley L. The impact of accepting living kidney donors with mild hypertension or proteinuria on transplantation rates. *Am J Kidney Dis* 2006; **47**(2): 317–323.

87 Ozdemir N, Guz G, Muderrisoglu H, Demirag A, Arat Z, Pekkara O et al. Ambulatory blood pressure monitoring in potential renal transplant donors. *Transplant Proc* 1999; **31**(8): 3369–3370.

88 Textor SC, S.J. T, Larson TS, Prieto M, Griffin M, Gloor J et al. Blood pressure evaluation among older living kidney donors. *J Am Soc Nephrol* 2003; **14**: 2159–2167.

89 Jaffe JS, Ginsberg PC, Gill R, Harkaway RC. A new diagnostic algorithm for the evaluation of microscopic hematuria. *Urology* 2001; **57**(5): 889–894.

90 Edwards TJ, Dickinson AJ, Natale S, Gosling J, McGrath JS. A prospective analysis of the diagnostic yield resulting from the attendance of 4020 patients at a protocol-driven haematuria clinic. *BJU Int* 2006; **97**(2): 301–305.

91 Iseki K. The Okinawa screening program. *J Am Soc Nephrol* 2003; **14**(7 Suppl 2): S127–S130.

92 Nieuwhof C, Doorenbos C, Grave W, de Heer F, de Leeuw P, Zeppenfeldt E et al. A prospective study of the natural history of idiopathic nonproteinuric hematuria. *Kidney Int* 1996; **49**(1): 222–225.

93 Nieuwhof CM, de Heer F, de Leeuw P, van Breda Vriesman PJ. Thin GBM nephropathy: premature glomerular obsolescence is associated with hypertension and late onset renal failure. *Kidney Int* 1997; **51**(5): 1596–1601.

94 Nieuwhof C, Kruytzer M, Frederiks P, van Breda Vriesman PJ. Chronicity index and mesangial IgG deposition are risk factors for hypertension and renal failure in early IgA nephropathy. *Am J Kidney Dis* 1998; **31**(6): 962–970.

95 Dische FE, Anderson VE, Keane SJ, Taube D, Bewick M, Parsons V. Incidence of thin membrane nephropathy: morphometric investigation of a population sample. *J Clin Pathol* 1990; **43**(6): 457–460.

96 Dische FE. Measurement of glomerular basement membrane thickness and its application to the diagnosis of thin-membrane nephropathy. *Arch Pathol Lab Med* 1992; **116**(1): 43–49.

97 Suzuki K, Honda K, Tanabe K, Toma H, Nihei H, Yamaguchi Y. Incidence of latent mesangial IgA deposition in renal allograft donors in Japan. *Kidney Int* 2003; **63**(6): 2286–2294.

98 Koushik R, Garvey C, Manivel JC, Matas AJ, Kasiske BL. Persistent, asymptomatic, microscopic hematuria in prospective kidney donors. *Transplantation* 2005; **80**(10): 1425–1429.

99 Liapis H, Gokden N, Hmiel P, Miner JH. Histopathology, ultrastructure, and clinical phenotypes in thin glomerular basement membrane disease variants. *Hum Pathol* 2002; **33**(8): 836–845.

100 Gandhi S, Kalantar-Zadeh K, Don BR. Thin-glomerular-basement-membrane nephropathy: is it a benign cause of isolated hematuria? *South Med J* 2002; **95**(7): 768–771.

101 Auwardt R, Savige J, Wilson D. A comparison of the clinical and laboratory features of thin basement membrane disease (TBMD) and IgA glomerulonephritis (IgA GN). *Clin Nephrol* 1999; **52**(1): 1–4.

102 Savige J, Rana K, Tonna S, Buzza M, Dagher H, Wang YY. Thin basement membrane nephropathy. *Kidney Int* 2003; **64**(4): 1169–1178.

103 van Paassen P, van Breda Vriesman PJ, van Rie H, Tervaert JW. Signs and symptoms of thin basement membrane nephropathy: a prospective regional study on primary glomerular disease. The Limburg Renal Registry. *Kidney Int* 2004; **66**(3): 909–913.

104 Schena FP, Cerullo G, Torres DD, Scolari F, Foramitti M, Amoroso A et al. The IgA nephropathy Biobank. An important starting point for the genetic dissection of a complex trait. *BMC Nephrol* 2005; **6**: 14.

105 Chow KM, Wong TY, Li PK. Genetics of common progressive renal disease. *Kidney Int Suppl* 2005; **94**: S41–S45.

106 Frasca GM, Soverini L, Gharavi AG, Lifton RP, Canova C, Preda P et al. Thin basement membrane disease in patients with familial IgA nephropathy. *J Nephrol* 2004; **17**(6): 778–785.

107 Hudson BG, Tryggvason K, Sundaramoorthy M, Neilson EG. Alport's syndrome, Goodpasture's syndrome, and type IV collagen. *N Engl J Med* 2003; **348**(25): 2543–2556.

108 Rana K, Wang YY, Buzza M, Tonna S, Zhang KW, Lin T et al. The genetics of thin basement membrane nephropathy. *Semin Nephrol* 2005; **25**(3): 163–170.

109 Nicolau C, Torra R, Badenas C, Vilana R, Bianchi L, Gilabert R et al. Autosomal dominant polycystic kidney disease type 1 and 2: Assessment of US sensitivity for diagnosis. *Radiology* 1999; **213**: 273–276.

110 Zand MS, Strang J, Dumlao M, Rubens D, Erturk E, Bronsther O. Screening a living kidney donor for polycystic kidney disease using heavily T2 weighted MRI. *Am J Kidney Dis* 2001; **37**(2): 612–619.

111 Cassart M, Massez A, Metens T, Rypens F, Lambot MA, Hall M et al. Complementary role of MRI after sonography in assessing bilateral urinary tract anomalies in the fetus. *Am J Roentgenol* 2004; **182**(3): 689–695.

112 Chapman AB, Guay-Woodford LM, Grantham JJ, Torres VE, Bae KT, Baumgarten DA et al. Renal structure in early autosomal-dominant polycystic kidney disease (ADPKD): the Consortium for Radiologic

Imaging Studies of Polycystic Kidney Disease (CRISP) cohort. *Kidney Int* 2003; **64(3):** 1035–1045.

113 Zand MS, Strang J, Dumlao M, Rubens D, Erturk E, Bronsther O. Screening a living kidney donor for polycystic kidney disease using heavily T2-weighted MRI. *Am J Kidney Dis* 2001; **37(3):** 612–619.

114 Rossetti S, Chauveau D, Walker D, Saggar-Malik A, Winearls CG, Torres VE *et al.* A complete mutation screen of the ADPKD genes by DHPLC. *Kidney Int* 2002; **61(5):** 1588–1599.

115 Rossetti S, Chauveau D, Kubly V, Slezak JM, Saggar-Malik AK, Pei Y *et al.* Association of mutation position in polycystic kidney disease 1 (PKD1) gene and development of a vascular phenotype. *Lancet* 2003; **361(9376):** 2196–2201.

116 Rossetti S, Torra R, Coto E, Consugar M, Kubly V, Malaga S *et al.* A complete mutation screen of PKHD1 in autosomal-recessive polycystic kidney disease (ARPKD) pedigrees. *Kidney Int* 2003; **64(2):** 391–403.

117 Magistroni R, He N, Wang K, Andrew R, Johnson A, Gabow P *et al.* Genotype-renal function correlation in type 2 autosomal dominant polycystic kidney disease. *J Am Soc Nephrol* 2003; **14(5):** 1164–1174.

118 Phakdeekitcharoen B, Watnick TJ, Germino GG. Mutation analysis of the entire replicated portion of PKD1 using genomic DNA samples. *J Am Soc Nephrol* 2001; **12(5):** 955–963.

119 Lee YH, Huang WC, Chang LS, Chen MT, Yang YF, Huang JK. The long-term stone recurrence rate and renal function change in unilateral nephrectomy urolithiasis patients. *J Urol* 1994; **152:** 1386–1388.

120 Delmonico FL. The consensus statement of the Amsterdam Forum on the care of the live kidney donor. *Transplantation* 2004; **78(4):** 491–492.

121 Rashid MG, Konnak JW, Wolf JS, Jr., Punch JD, Magee JC, Arenas JD *et al.* Ex vivo ureteroscopic treatment of calculi in donor kidneys at renal transplantation. *J Urol* 2004; **171(1):** 58–60.

122 Adams P, Cohen DJ, Danovitch GM, Edington RM, Gaston RS, Jacobs CL *et al.* The nondirected live-kidney donor: ethical considerations and practice guidelines: a national conference report. *Transplantation* 2002; **74(4):** 582–589.

123 Wright L, Faith K, Richardson R, Grant D. Ethical guidelines for the evaluation of living organ donors. *Can J Surg* 2004; **47(6):** 408–413.

124 Jacobs CL, Roman D, Garvey C, Kahn J, Matas AJ. Twenty-two nondirected kidney donors: an update on a single center's experience. *Am J Transplant* 2004; **4(7):** 1110–1116.

125 Jendrisak MD, Hong B, Shenoy S, Lowell J, Desai N, Chapman W *et al.* Altruistic living donors: evaluation for nondirected kidney or liver donation. *Am J Transplant* 2006; **6(1):** 115–120.

126 Ku JH. Health-related quality of life of living kidney donors: review of the short form 36-health questionnaire survey. *Transplant Int* 2005; **18(12):** 1309–1317.

127 Kawamoto S, Fishman EK. MDCT angiography of living laparoscopic renal donors. *Abdom Imag* 2006; **31(3):** 361–373.

128 Hanninen EL, Denecke T, Stelter L, Pech M, Podrabsky P, Pratschke J *et al.* Preoperative evaluation of living kidney donors using multirow detector computed tomography: comparison with digital subtraction angiography and intraoperative findings. *Transplant Int* 2005; **18(10):** 1134–1141.

129 Raman SS, Pojchamarnwiputh S, Muangsomboon K, Schulam PG, Gritsch HA, Lu DS. Utility of 16-MDCT angiography for comprehensive preoperative vascular evaluation of laparoscopic renal donors. *Am J Roentgenol* 2006; **186(6):** 1630–1638.

130 Rastogi N, Sahani DV, Blake MA, Ko DC, Mueller PR. Evaluation of living renal donors: accuracy of three-dimensional 16-section CT. *Radiology* 2006; **240(1):** 136–144.

131 Prosst RL, Fernandez ED, Neff W, Braun C, Neufang T, Post S. Evaluation of MR-angiography for pre-operative assessment of living kidney donors. *Clin Transplant* 2005; **19(4):** 522–526.

132 Hodgson DJ, Jan W, Rankin S, Koffman G, Khan MS. Magnetic resonance renal angiography and venography: an analysis of 111 consecutive scans before donor nephrectomy. *BJU Int* 2006; **97(3):** 584–586.

133 Al-Saeed O, Ismail M, Sheikh M, Al-Moosawi M, Al-Khawari H. Contrast-enhanced three-dimensional fast-spoiled gradient magnetic resonance angiography of the renal arteries for potential living renal transplant donors: a comparative study with digital subtraction angiography. *Australas Radiol* 2005; **49(3):** 214–217.

134 Ejerblad E, Fored CM, Lindblad P, Fryzek J, McLaughlin JK, Nyren O. Obesity and risk for chronic renal failure. *J Am Soc Nephrol* 2006; **17(6):** 1695–1702.

135 Tanaka H, Shiohira Y, Uezu Y, Higa A, Iseki K. Metabolic syndrome and chronic kidney disease in Okinawa, Japan. *Kidney Int* 2006; **69(2):** 369–374.

136 Tozawa M, Iseki K, Iseki C, Oshiro S, Ikemiya Y, Takishita S. Influence of smoking and obesity on the development of proteinuria. *Kidney Int* 2002; **62(3):** 956–962.

137 Hsu C, McCulloch CE, Iribarren C, Darbinian J, Go AS. Body mass index and risk for end-stage renal disease. *Ann Intern Med* 2006;144(1): 21-8.

138 Iseki K, Ikemiya Y, Kinjo K, Inoue T, Iseki C, Takishita S. Body mass index and the risk of development of end-stage renal disease in a screened cohort. *Kidney Int* 2004; **65(5):** 1870–1876.

139 Hallan SI, de Mutsert R, Carlsen S, Dekker FW, Aasarod K, Holmen J. Obesity, smoking and physical inactivity as risk factors for chronic kidney disease; are men more vulnerable. *Am J Kidney Dis* 2006; **47(3):** 396–405.

140 Rea DJ, Heimbach JK, Grande JP, Textor SC, Taler SJ, Prieto M *et al.* Glomerular volume and renal histology in obese and non-obese living kidney donors. *Kidney Int* 2006; **70:** 1636–1641.

141 Chagnac A, Weinstein T, Herman M, Hirsh J, Gafter U, Ori Y. The effects of weight loss on renal function in patients with severe obesity. *J Am Soc Nephrol* 2003; **14(6):** 1480–1486.

142 Praga M, Hernandez E, Herrero JC, Morales E, Revilla Y, Diaz-Gonzalez R *et al.* Influence of obesity on the appearance of proteinuria and renal insufficiency after unilateral nephrectomy. *Kidney Int* 2000; **58(5):** 2111–2118.

143 Csernus K, Lanyi E, Erhardt E, Molnar D. Effect of childhood obesity and obesity-related cardiovascular risk factors on glomerular and tubular protein excretion. *Eur J Pediatr* 2005; **164:** 44–49.

144 Ferris ME, Hogan SL, Ray S, *et al.* Albuminuria and obesity in health young adults: results from the Add Health Wave III Study. *J Am Soc Nephrol* 2004; **15:** 142A.

145 Sibley SD, Zhau L, Ibrahim HN. Urinary TGFB-1 is related to body fat distribution. *J Am Soc Nephrol* 2004; **15:** 708A.

146 Thiel GT, Nolte C, Tsinalis D. Living kidney donors with isolated medical abnormalities: the SOL-DHR experience. In: Gaston RS, Wadstrom J, editors. *Living Donor Kidney Transplantation.* Taylor & Francis, London, 2005; 55–73.

147 Ramcharan T, Matas AJ. Long-term (20-37 years) follow-up of living kidney donors. *Am J Transplant* 2002; **2(10):** 959–964.

148 Sansalone CV, Maione G, Aseni P, Rossetti O, Mangoni I, Soldano S *et al.* Early and late residual renal function and surgical complications in living donors: a 15-year experience at a single institution. *Transplant Proc* 2006; **38(4):** 994–995.

149 Johnson SR, Khwaja K, Pavlakis M, Monaco AP, Hanto DW. Older living donors provide excellent quality kidneys: a single center experience (older living donors). *Clin Transplant* 2005; **19(5):** 600–606.

150 De La Vega LS, Torres A, Bohorquez HE, Heimbach JK, Gloor JM, Schwab TR *et al.* Patient and graft outcomes from older living kidney donors are similar to those from younger donors despite lower GFR. *Kidney Int* 2004; **66(4):** 1654–1661.

151 Kostakis AJ, Kyriakidis S, Garbis S, Diles K, Sotirchos G, Koutsogiorgas P *et al.* The fate of renal transplants from elderly living related donors. *Transplant Proc* 1990; **22(4):** 1432–1433.

152 Hayashi T, Koga S, Higashi Y, Ohtomo Y, Satomura K, Mannami M. Living-related renal transplantation from elderly donors (older than 66 years of age). *Transplant Proc* 1995; **27(1):** 984–985.

153 Berardinelli L. Living donor transplantations with marginal kidneys. *Transplant Proc* 2003; **35(3):** 941–943.

154 Kumar A, Mandhani A, Verma BS, Srivastava A, Gupta A, Sharma RK *et al.* Expanding the living related donor pool in renal transplantation: use of marginal donors. *J Urol* 2000; **163(1):** 33–36.

155 Kumar A, Verma BS, Srivastava A, Bhandari M, Gupta A, Sharma RK. Long-term followup of elderly donors in a live related renal transplant program. *J Urol* 2000; **163(6):** 1654–1658.

156 Ivanovski N, Popov Z, Kolevski P, Cakalaroski K, Stojkovski L, Spasovski G *et al.* Living related renal transplantation–the use of advanced age donors. *Clin Nephrol* 2001; **55(4):** 309–312.

157 Jacobs SC, Ramey JR, Sklar GN, Bartlett ST. Laparoscopic kidney donation from patients older than 60 years. *J Am Coll Surg* 2004; **198(6):** 892–897.

158 Sesso R, Whelton PK, Klag MJ. Effect of age and gender on kidney function in renal transplant donors: a prospective study. *Clin Nephrol* 1993; **40(1):** 31–37.

159 Velosa JA, Offord KP, Schroeder DR. Effect of age, sex, and glomerular filtration rate on renal function outcome of living kidney donors. *Transplantation* 1995; **60(12):** 1618–1621.

160 Neymark E, LaBerge JM, Hirose R, Metzer SS, Kerlan RK, Jr., Wilson MW *et al.* Arteriographic detection of renovascular disease in potential renal donors: incidence and effect on donor surgery. *Radiology* 2000; **214(3):** 755–760.

161 Cragg AH, Smith TP, Thompson BH, Maroney TP, Stanson AW, Shaw GT *et al.* Incidental fibromuscular dysplasia in potential renal donors: Long-term clinical follow-up. *Radiology* 1989; **172(1):** 145–147.

162 Andreoni KA, Weeks SM, Gerber DA, Fair JH, Mauro MA, McCoy L *et al.* Incidence of donor renal fibromuscular dysplasia: does it justify routine angiography? *Transplantation* 2002; **73(7):** 1112–1116.

163 Indudhara R, Kenney, Bueschen AJ, Burns JR. Live donor nephrectomy in patients with fibromuscular dysplasia of the renal arteries. *J Urol* 1999; **162(3 Pt 1):** 678–681.

164 Nahas WC, Lucon AM, Mazzucchi E, Scafuri AG, Neto ED, Ianhez LE *et al.* Kidney transplantation: the use of living donors with renal artery lesions. *J Urol* 1998; **160(4):** 1244–1247.

165 Parasuraman R, Attallah N, Venkat KK, Yoshida A, Abouljoud M, Khanal S *et al.* Rapid progression of native renal artery fibromuscular dysplasia following kidney donation. *Am J Transplant* 2004; **4(11):** 1910–1914.

166 Serrano DP, Flechner SM, Modlin CS, Streem SB, Goldfarb DA, Novick AC. The use of kidneys from living donors with renal vascular disease: expanding the donor pool. *J Urol* 1997; **157(5):** 1587–1591.

167 Zierler RE, Bergelin RO, Davidson RC, Cantwell-Gab K, Polissar NL, Strandness DE, Jr. A prospective study of disease progression in patients with atherosclerotic renal artery stenosis. *Am J Hypertens* 1996; **9(11):** 1055–1061.

168 Pillay WR, Kan YM, Crinnion JN, Wolfe JH. Prospective multicentre study of the natural history of atherosclerotic renal artery stenosis in patients with peripheral vascular disease. *Br J Surg* 2002; **89(6):** 737–740.

169 Zierler RE, Bergelin RO, Polissar NL, Beach KW, Caps MT, Cantwell-Gab K *et al.* Carotid and lower extremity arterial disease in patients with renal artery atherosclerosis. *Arch Intern Med* 1998; **158(7):** 761–767.

170 Hernandez-Hernandez E, Alberu J, Gonzalez-Michaca L, Bobadilla-del Valle M, Correa-Rotter R, Sifuentes-Osornio J. Screening for tuberculosis in the study of the living renal donor in a developing country. *Transplantation* 2006; **81(2):** 290–292.

171 Boulware LE, Ratner LE, Sosa JA, Tu AH, Nagula S, Simpkins CE *et al.* The general public's concerns about clinical risk in live kidney donation. *Am J Transplant* 2002; **2(2):** 186–193.

172 Delmonico FL, Harmon WE. The use of a minor as a live kidney donor. *Am J Transplant* 2002; **2(4):** 333–336.

173 Kok NF, Alwayn IP, Lind MY, Tran KT, Weimar W, JN IJ. Donor nephrectomy: mini-incision muscle-splitting open approach versus laparoscopy. *Transplantation* 2006; **81(6):** 881–887.

174 Matas AJ, Bartlett ST, Leichtman AB, Delmonico FL. Morbidity and mortality after living kidney donation, 1999-2001: survey of United States transplant centers. *Am J Transplant* 2003; **3(7):** 830–834.

175 Pietrabissa A, Boggi U, Vistoli F, Moretto C, Ghilli M, Mosca F. Laparoscopic living donor nephrectomy in Italy: a national profile. *Transplant Proc* 2004; **36(3):** 460–463.

176 Goldfarb DA, Matin SF, Braun WE, Schreiber MJ, Mastroianni B, Papajcik D *et al.* Renal outcome 25 years after donor nephrectomy. *J Urol* 2001; **166(6):** 2043–2047.

177 Gracida C, Melchor JL, Espinoza R, Cedillo U, Cancino J. Experience in a single transplant center with 421 living donors: follow-up of 9 years. *Transplant Proc* 2002; **34(7):** 2535–2536.

178 Haberal M, Karakayali H, Moray G, Demirag A, Yildirim S, Bilgin N. Long-term follow-up of 102 living kidney donors. *Clin Nephrol* 1998; **50(4):** 232–235.

179 Toronyi E, Alfoldy F, Jaray J, Remport A, Hidvegi M, Dabasi G *et al.* Evaluation of the state of health of living related kidney transplantation donors. *Transplant Int* 1998; **11(Suppl 1):** S57–S59.

180 Liounis B, Roy LP, Thompson JF, May J, Sheil AG. The living, related kidney donor: a follow-up study. *Med J Aust* 1988; **148(9):** 436–437.

181 O'Donnell D, Seggie J, Levinson I, et al. Renal function after nephrectomy for donor organs. *S Afr Med J* 1986; **69(3):** 177–179.

182 Schostak M, Wloch H, Muller M, Schrader M, Offermann G, Miller K. Optimizing open live-donor nephrectomy - long-term donor outcome. *Clin Transplant* 2004; **18(3):** 301–305.

183 UNOS/OPTN Annual Report 2005 http://www.ustransplant.org/annual_reports/archives/2005/default.htm

50 Predictors of Transplant Outcomes

Krista L. Lentine[1], Robert M. Perkins[2], & Kevin C. Abbott[3]

[1] Saint Louis University Medical Centre, St. Louis, Missouri, USA
[2] Medigan Army Medical Center, Ft. Lewis, WA, USA
[3] Walter Reed Army Medical Center, Washington, DC, USA

Introduction

Graft and patient survival after kidney transplantation have traditionally been the outcomes reported. Detailed data from the USA are available in annual reports of the United Network for Organ Sharing [1] and the United States Renal Data System (USRDS) [2]. European data are available from the European Renal Association/European Dialysis and Transplant Association [3]. Recently, USRDS also listed incidence rates for cardiovascular disease after kidney transplantation. Two key outcomes form the assumption underlying kidney transplantation. Namely, kidney transplantation is associated with improved survival and quality of life compared to dialysis. Until recently, a survival advantage of kidney transplantation had not been widely accepted, and kidney transplantation was advocated primarily for improved quality of life. The first part of this chapter will review studies that have compared mortality between kidney transplantation and dialysis in general and among specific subgroups of patients. This survival advantage appears to be due to the reduced incidence of cardiovascular disease. In contrast, the incidence rates of infections and malignancies are not reduced and may even be higher after transplantation compared to dialysis.

Although short-term patient and graft survival rates have improved significantly in recent years, no comparable improvement in long-term survival rates has occurred, suggesting allograft rejection is not a valid useful surrogate outcome in clinical trials, and this highlights the importance of emerging infections, such as BK virus.

The importance of individual predictors of transplant outcomes has also changed over time. The importance of HLA matching has declined, and it is now recognized that HLA matching has different implications for black and white organ recipients. Some recent reports advocate deemphasizing HLA matching as a way to reduce racial disparities in organ allocation [4]. Given the increasing mismatch between donor supply and demand, organs from older and higher-risk donors (extended criteria donors [ECD]) are being offered more frequently, particularly to older recipients, resulting in survival benefits to the recipient.

In contrast to the dialysis population, no large randomized trials comparing different interventions or the "dose" of therapy (as measured primarily by donor/recipient nephron mass) have been performed for kidney transplantation. Because almost all outcome data are observational, many of the selection criteria recommended for randomized clinical trials do not apply. Once a particular finding has been reported in registry data, follow-up reports are generally lacking. Therefore, identifying and pooling studies, a common practice among randomized clinical trials, does not apply as much to these observational studies. Additionally, some of the statistical methods commonly used in the studies, especially survival analysis and its many variations, may not be as familiar to clinicians and other health care providers as are the methods used in randomized clinical trials.

Definitions

To assess the major outcomes associated with kidney transplantation, the following questions were examined:
- Is kidney transplantation associated with reduced mortality compared to its alternative therapies, that is, hemodialysis and peritoneal dialysis?
- In what specific subgroups has a survival advantage of kidney transplantation over dialysis been shown?
- Are long-term outcomes associated with kidney transplantation improving?
- How reliable are surrogate outcomes for graft loss, such as allograft rejection or posttransplant serum creatinine levels?
- Have the predictive values of certain factors for graft loss, such as HLA matching or duration of dialysis prior to transplant, changed over time?

Evidence-based Nephrology. Edited by Donald Molony and Jonathan Craig
© 2009 Blackwell Publishing, ISBN: 978-1-4051-3975-5.

The quality checklist for observational trials is quite different and more extensive than for randomized controlled trials [5] and has not been used extensively in previous reviews.

Survival benefit of kidney transplantation

Three studies have compared adjusted mortality after kidney transplantation compared to remaining on the kidney transplant waiting list, that is, patients presumed to be of comparable health status. In the first and largest study, Wolfe *et al.* [6] estimated that the projected life remaining was 10 years for those on dialysis and 20 years for those who received kidney transplants, with a reduction in mortality of 68% for kidney transplant recipients compared to dialysis. This risk varied by time after transplant; early after transplant, mortality risk was actually increased (due to perioperative mortality, especially from cardiovascular disease and infections). Thereafter, mortality slowly declined; at 106 days incident risk was equal, and by 244 days cumulative survival was equal. The greatest relative improvement in survival was for patients with diabetes as a cause of end-stage kidney disease.

Studies in other countries (Canada [7] and Scotland [8]) have shown similar results, including the increased early risk of mortality after transplant and gradual lowering of mortality. The study from Scotland adjusted for comorbidities more completely.

Other studies showed a relative survival benefit of kidney transplantation for every subgroup identified, including patients with hepatitis C [9] or who were obese [10,11]. Still other studies showed that patients with presumed diabetes had improved survival with simultaneous kidney and pancreas transplant, compared to cadaveric kidney transplant alone; survival with a solitary living donor kidney was comparable to that of receiving a kidney and pancreas transplant [12]. Use of ECD kidneys, primarily from older donors and donors with certain high-risk characteristics defined as those associated with a relative risk of graft loss of ≥1.7 compared to "standard" kidneys, was also associated with improved mortality for elderly recipients [13]. A more recent study confirmed this finding and identified those subgroups most likely to benefit from ECD kidneys, namely, those with prolonged expected waiting times on dialysis, those with diabetes, and those over 40 years old [14].

Is long-term kidney allograft survival improving?

Short-term graft survival after kidney transplantation has increased progressively from 1988 to 1996 [15], but from 1995 to 2000 there was not a comparable increase in graft survival beyond 2 years [16] (Figure 50.1). The same authors compared actual Kaplan-Meier renal allograft half-lives to the projected half-lives from the same year and documented substantial disparities between projected and actual allograft half-lives [17]. Two other studies assessed change in serum creatinine and estimated glomerular filtration rate (eGFR) and concluded that the rate of decline in allograft function after transplantation has improved [18,19]. A different study demonstrated the relatively poor predictive value of serum creatinine in predicting allograft loss after transplantation [20]. Another study from the same group showed that, recently,

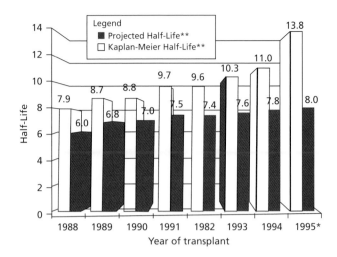

* Kaplan-Meier half-life based on time to 51.0% survial
** as published in NEJM (March, 2000).

Figure 50.1 Projected Half-Lives (white bars) of deceased donors kidney transplants (including re-transplants) vs. actual Half-Lives (dark bars).

rates of death attributed to cardiovascular disease and infection have decreased among wait-listed dialysis and transplant patients, whereas rates of death attributed to malignancy have not [21]. Thus, available observational data suggest that long-term kidney allograft and patient survival rates are improving.

Are traditional predictors of transplant outcomes becoming less reliable?

The results of national sharing of fully HLA-matched kidneys were reported in 2000 [22]. The UNOS allocation program has changed over time from an initial "six-antigen match" to any donor who had no HLA-A, -B, or -DR antigens that were not also detected in the recipient (referred to as no mismatches). That is, the recipient was matched for these HLA antigens, but may still have had antigens that were not present in the donor. Ten-year graft survival was 52% for HLA-matched kidneys versus 37% for non-HLA-matched kidneys (including any degree of HLA mismatch). The authors found that, apart from zero-mismatch kidneys, HLA matching had diminishing importance over time.

Another report did not show improved graft survival in transported organs that were fully HLA matched, but rather a significantly higher risk of graft failure in these organs compared with locally transplanted kidneys [23]. Yet another study showed that over four successive years (1994–1998), HLA had progressively less significant association with graft survival after kidney transplant than nonimmunologic factors [24].

If it is true that HLA matching now has little effect on outcomes, then removing HLA-B matching as a priority for the allocation of cadaveric kidneys could reduce existing racial imbalances by increasing the number of transplants in non-white patients, with only a small increase in the rate of graft loss [25]. Recipient race, especially being black, has been an independent predictor of increased risk of graft loss in US [26], but not European, transplant

Two Major Pathways to Allograft Failure

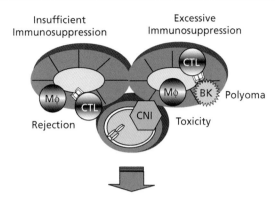

Figure 50.2 The three general pathways to allograft deterioration: allograft rejection (acute and chronic), infection (with BK/polyomavirus specifically affecting the allograft), and calcineurin inhibitor toxicity. (From Rush 2006 [29], reproduced with permission.)

populations [27]. Whether recipient race is truly an independent risk factor for graft outcomes or this observation is confounded by socio-economic factors or other differences between populations and/or transplant practices between US and European centers is uncertain. Of note, the Veterans Administration Health Affairs System, in which most medications are provided without cost, similar in many ways to European health systems, found that for black recipients race was still an independent risk factor for graft outcome.

In summary, HLA matching is decreasing in relative importance as a predictor of outcomes, and its use in organ allocation is rapidly evolving.

Which surrogate or composite outcomes should be used in kidney transplantation?

The dwindling frequency and predictive usefulness of allograft rejection in kidney transplantation pose a vexing dilemma. One potential explanation for the lack of improvement in long-term outcomes despite reduction in allograft rejection rates could be due to a higher proportion of more severe, antibody-mediated rejection causing a disproportionate impact in the minority of allograft recipients it affects [28]. Another possibility is that enhanced immunosuppression has led to increased risk of calcineurin inhibitor-related nephrotoxicity and opportunistic infections, of which BK virus nephropathy in particular may lead to graft failure. Recent reviews suggest the two extremes of immunosuppression should both be given equal emphasis given their risks (Figure 50.2) [29]. This unfortunately would greatly reduce the utility of allograft rejection in clinical trials. The limited usefulness of serum creatinine or eGFR, or even renal histology, in predicting allograft failure has increased attention on other surrogate or composite markers for allograft survival, although there is no current agreement on which combination of markers should be used [30], a dilemma not unique to transplantation [31].

Conclusions

It will never be ethical or feasible to perform randomized, controlled trials comparing kidney transplantation versus dialysis. Prior to the publication of the seminal article of Wolfe *et al.*, transplant professionals could counsel prospective patients that they were likely to have an improved quality of life after kidney transplantation. A potential survival advantage was regarded as unproven, because previous studies had not adjusted for the considerable selection bias of deciding which dialysis patients should be enrolled on the kidney transplant waiting list. Dialysis patients enrolled on the waiting list have significantly lower risk of mortality, even when adjusted for other factors, compared to dialysis patients not selected for enrollment. This research group's use of wait-listed dialysis patients as the control group, in addition to their ability to study the entire population of US wait-listed patients and follow those who received kidney transplants for many years, provided convincing data for the medical community. Table 50.1 summarizes the findings from studies of patients on kidney transplant waiting lists.

Nevertheless, there remain important differences between wait-listed patients and those who receive kidney transplants, which was shown by the Scottish study and from the study of obese wait-listed patients. However, adjustment for these comorbid factors in that study actually strengthened the association of kidney transplantation with reduced mortality.

Current immunosuppressive practices after kidney transplantation have largely succeeded in reducing the incidence of the typical target end point, renal allograft rejection. The dilemma now is that reduced allograft rejection rates do not seem to correlate with improved long-term renal allograft survival. This may be due to the changing nature of renal allograft rejection itself, or to a greater frequency of infectious complications which may directly impact graft function. Given the difficulties in showing improvements in short-term renal allograft function, the future dilemma will be to determine which surrogate outcomes, or combination of surrogate outcomes, are appropriate to use in clinical trials. No consensus currently exists.

Infections after kidney transplantation

In this section we will focus on major infectious complications, namely, cytomegalovirus (CMV) and urinary tract infections (UTIs), that may affect patient and allograft survival after kidney transplantation, with attention to risk factors and proven management strategies. BK virus nephropathy is discussed in detail in chapter 26.

CMV

CMV is a DNA virus of the herpesvirus family (human herpesvirus 5). It is the most common viral infection complicating solid organ transplantation. Various incidence rates have been reported, depending on the definitions used (asymptomatic infection versus clinical CMV disease), the patient populations (CMV serologic

Table 50.1 Studies of patients on kidney transplant waiting lists.

Study [reference]	Methods	Participants	Follow-up (yrs)	Study period	Outcome(s)	Notes	Handling of missing values	Statistical analysis	Generalizability
Wolfe 1999 [6]	Retrospective cohort study of USRDS	46,164 patients on maintenance dialysis enrolled on kidney transplant waiting list, USA	1–7	1991–1997	Death (rate per 100 person-years): wait list, 6.3; transplant, 3.8; RR death after transplant, 0.32 (95% CI, 0.30–0.35)	No assessment of comorbidity other than cause of ESRD, assumed since all were wait-listed that health status was comparable	Not stated (other than exclusion)	Yes	Yes
Rabbat 2000 [7]	Retrospective cohort study	1156 patients on maintenance dialysis enrolled on waiting list in Ontario Province, Canada	1–5	1990–1995	Death: wait list, 5%; transplant, 3.4%; RR death after transplant, 0.25 (95% CI, 0.14–0.42)		Not stated	Yes	Yes
Oniscu *et al.* 2005 [8]	Retrospective cohort study	1732 patients enrolled on kidney transplant waiting list in Scotland	3	1989–1999	Death (rate per 100 person-years): wait list, 9.02; transplant, 4.13; RR death after transplant, 0.28 (95% CI, 0.20–0.39)	Comorbidity data accounted for	Not stated	Yes	Yes
Pereira 1998 [9]	Retrospective cohort study of New England Organ Bank	573 HCV$^+$ and matched HCV$^-$ patients on dialysis waiting list		1990–1995	Death	Selection bias in those who had HCV status determined, considerable numbers missing	Yes	Yes	Yes
Glanton 2003 [10]	Retrospective cohort study of USRDS	7521 ESRD patients with BMI $\geq$30 kg/m^2	1–5	1995–1999	Death	BMI crude indicator of body fat	Yes	Yes	Yes
Ojo 2001 [12]	Retrospective cohort study of USRDS	13,467 patients with type I diabetes on maintenance dialysis enrolled on kidney transplant waiting list	1–7	1992–1998	Death (rate per 100 person-years): SPK, 4.0; LD, 4.1; CAD, 5.9; RR death after transplant: SPK, 0.40; LD, 0.45; CAD, 0.75	Type 1 diabetes assumed from age, not confirmed	Not stated (other than exclusion)	Yes	Yes
Ojo 2001 [13]	Retrospective cohort study of USRDS	122,175 patients on maintenance dialysis enrolled on kidney transplant waiting list	1–7	1992–1998	Death (annual rate): wait list, 6.3%; marginal donor kidneys, 4.7%; ideal donor kidneys, 3.3%; RR marginal donor 0.75, RR ideal donor kidney 0.52		Yes	Yes	
Merion 2005 [14]	Retrospective cohort study of USRDS	109,127 patients on maintenance dialysis enrolled on kidney transplant waiting list	1–9	1995–2002	Death		Yes	Yes	

Study	Design	Population		Years	Outcome			
Hariharan 2000 [15]	Retrospective cohort study of USRDS	93,934 renal transplant recipients	1–7	1988–1996	Graft failure		Yes	Yes
Meier-Kriesche 2004 [16]	Retrospective cohort study of USRDS	62,103 kidney transplant recipients	1–7	1995–2000	Graft loss		Yes	Yes
Meier-Kriesche 2004 [17]	Retrospective cohort study of USRDS	77,937 renal transplant recipients	1–15	1988–1995	Graft survival		Yes	Yes
Kasiske et al. 2005 [18]	Retrospective multicenter study	9515 renal transplant patients at five US centers	Up to 12	1984–2002	MDRD eGFR		Yes	Yes
Keith et al. 2005 [19]	Retrospective study of UNOS	40,164 renal transplant recipients	Up to 4[a]	1991–2000	MDRD eGFR		Yes	Yes
Meier-Kriesche 2001 [21]	Retrospective cohort study of USRDS	104,000 patients on maintenance dialysis enrolled on kidney transplant waiting list	1–7	1988–1996	Death		Yes	Yes
Takemoto 2000 [22]	Retrospective cohort study of UNOS	88,978 patients on maintenance dialysis enrolled on kidney transplant waiting list	10	1987–1999	Death		Yes	Yes
Mange 2001 [23]	Retrospective cohort study of UNOS	5446 kidney pairs (10,892 allografts)	1–4	1992–1998	Graft failure: preemptive, 3.8%; conventional, 5.8%		Yes	Yes
Su 2004 [24]	Retrospective cohort study of USRDS	33,443 kidney transplant recipients	1–7	1994–1998	Death		Yes	Yes
Robert 2004 [25]	Retrospective cohort study of USRDS	71,595 patients on maintenance dialysis enrolled on kidney transplant waiting list	1–7	1994–1997	Rates of transplantation, graft failure		Yes	Yes
Chakkera 2005 [26]	Retrospective cohort study of VA and Medicare transplant recipients	79,361 transplant recipients	1–7	1991–2000	Rates of graft failure		Yes	Yes
Pallet 2005 [27]	Retrospective single-center study, France	1092 living donor transplant recipients	1–7	1994–1997	Rates of transplantation, graft failure	Did not specify or apparently adjust for donor type (cadaveric vs. living)	Yes	Yes

Note: Data are presented only from studies for which results could readily be presented in tabular form.
Abbreviations: RR, relative risk; CI, confidence interval; ESRD, end-stage renal disease; HCV, hepatitis C virus; BMI, body mass index.

Table 50.2 Allograft and patient outcomes by CMV serostatus, CMV infection, and CMV disease.

Topic	Allograft outcome	Reference	Patient outcome	Reference
CMV serostatus[a]				
R+ vs. R−	DGF RR, +13.6%; graft loss RR, −9.3%	Schnitzler 2003 [36]		
R+ vs. R−			RR CMV disease at 1 yr, −39.0%	Schnitzler 2003 [36]
D+/R−	Acute rejection OR. 2.28 (95% CI, 1.26–4.11)	McLaughlin 2002 [37]		
D+/R− vs. D−/R−	Graft loss RR, +21.4%	Schnitzler 2003 [36]	RR CMV disease at 1 yr, 63.0%	Schnitzler 2003 [36]
D+/R+ vs. D−/R+			RR CMV disease at 1 yr, 73.1%	Schnitzler 2003 [36]
CMV infection	Acute rejection RR, 1.6 (95% CI, 1.1–2.5)	Sagedal 2002 [38]	RR death, 2.90 (95% CI, 1.61–5.22)	Sagedal 2004 [35]
CMV disease	Acute rejection RR, 2.5 (95% CI, 1.2–5.1)	Sagedal 2002 [38]	RR death, 2.50 (95% CI, 1.31–4.79)	Sagedal KI [35]

Note: All studies are observational.

Abbreviations: RR, relative risk; OR, odds ratio; CI, confidence interval; DGF, Delayed Graft function.

[a] The serostatuses of the donor (D) and recipient (R) are indicated (+ and −).

status of donor and recipient pretransplant), the induction and maintenance immunosuppressive regimens, and the use of prophylactic medications. Reported rates range from 8 to 63% [32–35]. The period from 1 to 6 months after transplantation, correlating with the most intense period of immunosuppression, is the highest risk period for CMV infection and disease.

Risk factors for posttransplantation CMV disease include CMV-seropositive donor status, use of antilymphocyte agents as induction therapy, and with more uncertainty, the use of mycophenolate mofetil (compared with azathioprine) as maintenance immunosuppression [36].

Allograft and patient outcomes by CMV serostatus, episodes of CMV infection, and episodes of CMV disease are outlined in Table 50.2. Based upon the results of several large retrospective cohort studies, donor seropositivity and donor and recipient sero-mismatching (D+/R−) reduce graft outcomes. Increased recipient mortality has been associated with CMV donor seropositivity as well as CMV infection.

Recommendations

Based on two meta-analyses, we recommend a prophylactic rather than preemptive antiviral strategy in recipients of kidney transplants for protection against CMV-related morbidity and mortality [39, 40]. Lack of evidence precludes designating a specific treatment after transplantation.

UTIs

UTIs are the most common form of bacterial infection following kidney transplantation and may affect allograft and patient outcomes directly with the infection itself and indirectly by possibly activating the rejection process [41].

In kidney transplant recipients not receiving prophylaxis, UTIs occur in 35–50%, predominantly in the first 6 months after transplantation [42]. Variability in rates reported may be explained by differences in the definition of UTI, methods of urine sampling, and the use or absence of perioperative and postoperative antibiotic prophylaxis [43]. Prophylactic therapy is associated with a

reduction of early UTI incidence of greater than 50%, although over half of all female recipients (and nearly half of male recipients) will still develop a UTI (as defined by medical claims) within 3 years after transplantation [44].

Although data are very weak, UTIs, regardless of timing of occurrence posttransplant, may negatively impact allograft and patient outcomes. Rice *et al.* recently reported in a prospective cohort study of kidney transplant patients with UTI that renal allograft injury (defined as a 20% or greater rise from baseline in peak serum creatinine within 24–48 h of positive urine culture) was significantly associated with P fimbriated *Escherichia coli* isolates (62% vs. 29%; $P = 0.03$) [45]. Although this study did not follow patients until graft failure or death, it suggests that a unique pattern of uropathogenic serotypes and adherence factors may contribute to allograft injury in kidney transplant patients with UTI in a manner quite unlikely to be influenced by other comorbid illnesses or other potential confounders. Muller *et al.* identified UTIs as a risk factor for chronic renal allograft rejection in a single-center, retrospective cohort analysis [46]. In a larger retrospective cohort study, Abbott *et al.* examined graft and patient survival after late-onset UTI (greater than 6 months posttransplant) [14]. The results of this study suggest that late-onset UTIs are not benign. However, both studies are retrospective and observational in nature and subject to ascertainment bias, in that urine cultures may be ordered more often in patients who are not doing well from any cause. The details and results of both of these studies are outlined in Tables 50.3 and 50.4.

Antibiotic prophylaxis for prevention of UTI is the topic of a Cochrane systematic review [47]. Few studies have been carried out using a randomized, double-blinded methodology, and none has yet shown whether antibiotic prophylaxis improves renal allograft survival or patient survival.

Management strategies

Given the morbidity and mortality associated with UTIs in the kidney transplant population, prevention is the primary management strategy. Prophylactic therapy (with either trimethoprim or

Table 50.3 UTI studies: study descriptions.

Study [reference]	Population	Design	Intervention	Primary outcome	Secondary outcome
Muller *et al.* 1998 [46]	All adult kidney transplant recipients, 1972–1991, single European center (*n* = 576)	Retrospective cohort study; those with biopsy-proven chronic rejection within 5 yrs posttransplant vs. those without clinical suspicion of rejection	None	UTI rates	
Abbott *et al.* 2004 [44]	All Medicare (US) primary renal transplant recipients, 1996–2000 (*n* = 28,942)	Retrospective cohort study examining impact of UTI occurring later than 6 mos posttransplant	None	All-cause death; graft loss	Time to first Medicare claim for UTI

an oral fluoroquinolone) significantly reduces the incidence of UTIs.

Cardiovascular disease and posttransplantation outcomes

Rationale for cardiovascular risk assessment among transplant candidates and recipients
Given the high incidence and adverse effects of posttransplantation cardiovascular disease, the National Kidney Foundation Kidney Disease Outcomes Quality Initiative (K/DOQI) workgroup on chronic kidney disease concluded that kidney transplant recipients should be considered to be in the highest risk group for cardiovascular events, that is, coronary heart disease equivalent [48]. Although this emphasizes the severity of the problem, it does not reflect the heterogeneity of risk among the more than 115,000 patients currently living with kidney transplants in the USA [2] as well as those in other countries. Between 100,000 and 150,000 persons will be registered on the kidney transplant waiting list by 2010, and they will have unique cardiovascular risk management issues dictated by their need to maintain preparedness for transplant surgery [49]. Applying the most intensive screening and therapeutic strategies to all these patients is impractical, given limited health care resources, and may produce costs and treatment-related risks that outweigh benefits. This may be especially true

Table 50.4 UTI studies: results.

Study [reference]	Results
Muller *et al.* 1998 [46]	Significantly higher rates of UTI (after 3 yrs posttransplant) in patients with biopsy-proven chronic rejection
Abbott *et al.* 2004 [44]	Late UTI associated with death (AHR, 2.93; 95% CI, 2.22–3.85; *P* < 0.001) and graft loss (AHR, 1.85; 95% CI, 1.29–2.64, *P* < 0.05) Cumulative incidence of UTI at 3 yrs was 60% for women and 47% for men

Abbreviations: AHR, adjusted hazard ration; CI, confidence interval.

in subgroups of patients that are unlikely to have cardiovascular events. Methods for individualizing cardiovascular risk assessment among transplant recipients are needed.

Pretransplantation cardiac screening
Pretransplantation cardiovascular disease is a strong predictor of posttransplantation cardiac events [50–52]. It has been proposed that serial cardiac surveillance of transplant candidates on the waiting list may improve outcomes after transplantation. Consensus-based guidelines were developed that incorporate diabetes status, ischemic heart disease, peripheral vascular disease, results of non-invasive stress tests, and revascularization into an algorithm for suggested frequency of cardiac surveillance by stress echocardiography or combined resting echocardiography and nuclear stress imaging [53,54].

Clinical risk scores
Clinical prediction tools translate patient risk profiles into estimates of the absolute risk of an event during an observation interval and are useful for prognostication and for guiding the intensity of risk management. The most widely used tool for cardiac risk prediction in the general population, the Framingham Heart Score (FHS), estimates 10-year risk of new-onset coronary heart disease in stable persons based on age, cholesterol level, blood pressure, smoking history. and diabetes status [55]. Many FHS risk factors are prevalent among transplant recipients [50,56], suggesting that the FHS may predict coronary heart disease events after transplantation.

Performance of risk assessment strategies
Pretransplant cardiac screening
A recent American Transplantation Society survey reported wide variability among centers in the practice of cardiac surveillance of patients on the waiting list [49]. Few studies have examined outcomes associated with adherence to screening recommendations. Recently, a prospective, observational study of 604 transplant candidates in British Columbia found that surveillance based on ongoing clinical assessment resulted in fewer investigations (*n* = 171) than suggested by guidelines (*n* = 503) over a mean period of follow-up of 3.7 ± 1.8 years [57]. There was no difference in total

Study [reference]	Kasiske *et al.* 2000 [58]	Ducloux *et al.* 2004 [59]
Methods	Historical cohort	Historical cohort
Participants	1124 KTR at a single center	344 KTR at a single center
Years of transplant	1963–1997	NA
Sampling criteria	Allograft functional and free of heart disease at 1 yr after transplant	Serum creatinine ≤4.5 mg/dL and free of heart disease at 1 yr after transplant
Outcome measures	MI, coronary revascularization, or death due to IHD	MI, coronary revascularization, or angina with abnormal coronary arteriography
Observation interval	1 yr after transplant to death, loss to follow-up, or end of study (date not specified)	1 yr after transplant to death, loss to follow-up, or end of study (date not specified)
Performance of FHS	Underestimation of risk due to increased observed risk conferred by diabetes (HR in men 2.8, CI 1.7–4.5 vs. 1.5 in FHS; HR in women 5.4, CI 2.7–11 vs. 1.8 in FHS) and to lesser extent, age and smoking	Underestimation of risk; prediction of 16/27 (59%) observed coronary events
Level of evidence	4	4

Abbreviations: IHD, ischemic heart disease; KTR, kidney transplant recipient; NA, not available or not applicable; MI, myocardial infarction; HR, hazard ratio; CI, confidence interval.

cardiovascular event rates after listing among subsets who did receive the recommended frequency of investigations (99 per 1000 person-years) and those who did not (67 per 1000 person-years), but potential selection biases in a retrospective study make it difficult to draw firm conclusions.

FHS and nontraditional factors

The FHS was developed for risk stratification of stable outpatients and has limited applicability in the prediction of peritransplantation coronary disease events precipitated by surgical stress. Several studies have shown limitations of the FHS even among stable kidney transplant recipients [58,59] (Table 50.5). Whereas individual Framingham factors are significantly associated with coronary risk among renal allograft recipients, effect sizes are altered such that risk estimates from the traditional algorithm are generally lower than the observed risk in this population. Features of this miscalibration include largest errors among those at highest risk, driven in part by underappreciation of diabetes-related risk.

A number of nontraditional risk factors and elements unique to kidney disease and transplantation have been linked with cardiovascular risk after transplantation, including C-reactive protein [59], hyperhomocysteinemia [59], duration of pretransplant dialysis [60], donor comorbidities [56], immunosuppressive drug regimen [61], viral infections [62], acute rejection [63], new-onset diabetes [64], and the quality and persistence of allograft function [51,52,65–71]. These factors are important considerations for the development of transplant-specific risk indices, but current clinical applications for risk stratification are uncertain. However, the

relationship of the quality and maintenance of allograft function to cardiovascular risk is also important, because strategies for preservation of renal function may also reduce cardiovascular risk. A summary of the incidence and prognosis of congestive heart failure after kidney transplantation is provided in Table 50.6.

Recommendations

Kidney transplant recipients should be evaluated for traditional Framingham risk factors. These factors are markers of increased risk, but quantitative estimations of coronary risk after transplant are not possible using the general population FHS. Patients with graft dysfunction, and especially those with graft failure, should be considered at increased risk for diverse presentations of cardiovascular disease including ischemic heart disease, congestive heart failure, and arrhythmias.

Interventions for cardiovascular risk reduction
Dyslipidemia

Hyperlipidemia is a common and potentially modifiable metabolic abnormality among kidney transplant recipients [72]. Lipid-lowering therapy with HMG-CoA reductase inhibitors (statins) has repeatedly been shown to decrease cardiovascular events and mortality in the general population [73,74], suggesting that statin therapy may improve outcomes after kidney transplantation. The Assessment of Lescol in Renal Transplantation (ALERT) study is the only randomized controlled trial of an intervention designed to expressly target cardiovascular disease outcomes after kidney transplantation [75]. In this study, 2101 stable kidney transplant

Table 50.6 Incidence and prognosis of congestive heart failure after kidney transplantation.

Study [reference]	Rigatto *et al.* 2002 [63]	Abbott *et al.* 2002 [69]	Lentine *et al.* 2005 [52]
Methods	Historical cohort	Historical cohort	Historical cohort
Participants	638 adult KTR from two Canadian centers	33,479 KTR recorded in the USRDS	27,011 adult KTR recorded in the USRDS
Period (yrs) of transplants evaluated	1969–1999	June 1994–June 1997	1995–2001
Sampling criteria	Allograft functional and free of heart disease at 1 yr after transplant		First transplant; Medicare as primary payer; no evidence of CHF prior to transplant in the registry
Outcome measures	First clinical indication of CHF based on reported dyspnea plus supporting examination or radiographic signs	First hospitalization with primary discharge diagnosis of CHF	First CHF diagnosis, defined as 1 Medicare inpatient claim with diagnosis for CHF or 2 outpatient/physician supplier claims
Observation interval	1 yr after transplant to graft failure, death, loss to follow-up, or end of study (date not specified)	Transplant to death, loss to follow-up, 3 yrs posttransplant, or end of study (July 1997)	Transplant to death, loss to follow-up, 3 yrs posttransplant, or end of study (December 2001)
Incidence of cardiovascular events	3.6% (CI 2.0-5.2%) at 5 yrs; 12.1% (CI 8.6–16%) at 10 yrs; 13/1000 PY	12/1000 PY	7.8% (CI 7.6–8.3%) at 6 mos; 18.3% (17.8–18.9%) at 3 yrs; 78/1000 PY
Mortality implications	AHR 1.5 (CI 1.1–2.1)[a]	AHR 3.7 (CI 2.2-6.1)[a]	AHR 2.6 (CI 2.4–2.9)[a]
Graft implications	NA (censored at graft loss)	NA	AHR 2.7 (CI 2.4–3.0) for death-censored loss[a]
Level of evidence	4	4	4

Abbreviations: CHF, congestive heart failure; KTR, kidney transplant recipient; CI, confidence interval; AHR, adjusted hazard ratio; PY, person-year; NA, not available.
[a] Analyzed as time-varying outcome predictor.

recipients were randomly assigned to fluvastatin or placebo. Details of the trial and its findings are shown in Table 50.7. Statin therapy lowered lower-density lipoprotein cholesterol (average difference of 38 mg/dL), and there was a trend towards a reduction in the primary composite outcome, but this did not reach statistical significance. Secondary analyses suggest that fluvastatin may be associated with significantly fewer cardiac deaths or nonfatal myocardial infarctions [76], particularly when initiated early after transplant [77], and an open-label extension trial detected a significant reduction in the primary end point in the fluvastatin group by intention-to-treat analysis [78] (Table 50.7). Notably, there were no significant differences in patient or graft survival in the ALERT extension trial, suggesting a possible redistribution in causes of death.

Immunosuppressive regimen choice

Many immunosuppressive medications are associated with adverse effects on traditional cardiovascular risk factors, such as lipid levels, blood pressure, and glycemic control. Thus, modification of the immunosuppression regimen is frequently proposed as a strategy for cardiovascular risk reduction after transplant. The effect of immunosuppressive regimen on cardiovascular end points (except for all-cause mortality) has not been directly assessed in a clinical trial. A number of small studies have examined effects of drug conversion and withdrawal strategies on surrogates of cardiovascular risk, including blood pressure, lipid levels, and glycemic control,

but the actions of specific agents on individual surrogate end points preclude extrapolation to cardiovascular events.

Several studies have attempted to improve our understanding of differences in net cardiovascular risk conferred by calcineurin inhibitor choice using the FHS as a composite of surrogate factors. For example, an open-label comparison of tacrolimus versus cyclosporine, randomly allocated at transplantation with concomitant azathioprine and corticosteroids, found higher time-averaged glucose levels but lower total cholesterol and blood pressure in the tacrolimus arm over 6 months of observation; FHS was lower only among tacrolimus-treated men [61]. Late, open-label conversion of cyclosporine to tacrolimus in patients taking corticosteroids with or without an antimetabolite has been shown to reduce FHS (5.7± 4.3 to 4.8 ± 5.3 at 24 months postrandomization) [79], although early benefit was not present in statin-treated patients [80]. These analyses should be interpreted cautiously, given the aforementioned limitations of the FHS in kidney transplant recipients, in particular, underestimation of risk associated with diabetes [58] may bias the FHS in favor of tacrolimus, which is more likely to cause hyperglycemia and posttransplant diabetes [61,81].

Recommendations

Based on suggestive findings from the ALERT study, along with convincing studies of statin therapy in the general population, several national groups, including the NKF K-DOQI, recommend use of statins in transplant recipients with hypercholesterolemia

Table 50.7 Evidence on efficacy of statin therapy for cardiovascular risk reduction after kidney transplantation: data from the ALERT trial, its extension study, and secondary analyses.

Study [reference]	Holdaas *et al.* 2003 [75] (ALERT)	Jardine *et al.* 2004 [84]	Holdaas *et al.* 2005 [77]	Holdaas *et al.* 2005 [78]
Methods	Placebo-controlled, double-blinded RCT	Historical cohort, secondary analysis of RCT	Historical cohort, secondary analysis of RCT	Open-label continuation trial
Participants	2102 adult KTR recruited from 84 centers in Europe and Canada	Participants in ALERT	Participants in ALERT	1652 patients who completed ALERT (*n* = 1787) and consented to open-label drug, continued monitoring, and/or data collection
Enrollment period sampling criteria	June 1996–October 1997 At least 6 mos posttransplant; stable graft function; cyclosporine-based immunosuppression; total cholesterol 154–347 mg/dL	As in ALERT As in ALERT	As in ALERT As in ALERT	As in ALERT ALERT participants who consented to participation
Intervention or exposure measure	Random assignment to fluvastatin 40 mg/day or placebo	Random assignment to fluvastatin 40 mg/day or placebo	Fluvastatin vs. placebo, according to time elapsed from transplant to enrollment	All participants were offered fluvastatin 80 mg/day, regardless of initial assignment Outcomes were analyzed according to treatment allocation in the core study
Outcome measures	MACE composite, defined as cardiac death, nonfatal MI, or revascularization	Cardiac death or nonfatal MI (alternative to primary end point in the core trial)	Cardiac death or nonfatal MI	MACE composite, cardiac death or nonfatal MI, all-cause mortality
Observation interval	Mean 5.1 ± 1.1 yrs after enrollment	As in ALERT	As in ALERT	Enrollment to 2 yrs after final visit of ALERT (mean, 6.7 yrs)
Risk relationship	AHR 0.83 (CI 0.64–1.06; *P* = 0.14)	AHR 0.65 (CI 0.48–0.88)	AHR 0.41 (CI 0.18–0.92) for patients initiating therapy at 0–2 yrs vs. >6 yrs posttransplant	AHR for MACE, 0.79 (CI, 0.63–0.99) among those randomized to fluvastatin in core study; cardiac death or nonfatal MI also reduced No difference in total mortality
Level of evidence	1	4	4	3

Abbreviations: RCT, randomized clinical trial; KTR, kidney transplant recipient; MI, myocardial infarction; AHR, adjusted hazard ratio; CI, confidence interval; MACE, major adverse cardiac events.

[72]. In parallel with recommendations of the Adult Treatment Panel III (ATP III) for high-risk members of the general population, the NKF suggests treatment to achieve a goal lower-density lipoprotein cholesterol of less than 100 mg/dL [82]. However, the ATP III and NKF guidelines were published before availability of newer lipid-lowering data, which suggest even lower levels may be beneficial in high-risk patients without kidney disease [83]. Additional studies are warranted to determine if aggressive lipid lowering may be beneficial for reduction of cardiovascular risk after kidney transplantation.

At present, there is insufficient evidence with respect to clinical outcomes to recommend adoption of particular immunosuppressive strategies for cardiovascular risk reduction. The immunosuppressive regimen should be individualized to manage competing risks of rejection versus drug side effect profiles, considering patient history and characteristics. Studies of the cardiovascular consequences of immunosuppression should consider the possibility of effect modification by cardiovascular drugs such as statins.

Summary

Observational data now strongly support the view that kidney transplantation offers a survival advantage for patients with chronic kidney disease in comparison with remaining on long-term dialysis. This advantage applies to all subgroups that have so far been investigated. This advantage in survival appears mainly related to reduction in cardiovascular disease, whereas infectious complications may not be reduced. Because of immunosuppression, kidney transplant recipients are at risk for infections not often seen in the general population. Emergent infections, such as BK virus infections, have become widely recognized and have had a substantial impact on graft loss in the modern era, although no generally accepted guidelines for diagnosis and management have yet been published and no FDA accepted treatments are yet available. Infections generally assumed to have been relegated to the past, such as CMV and UTI, remain serious problems after kidney transplantation. Finally, although cardiovascular disease is less common after kidney transplantation than among long-term dialysis patients, cardiovascular disease is still more common than in the general population and remains the leading cause of death with graft function.

References

1 http://www.ustransplant.org/csi/current/nationalviewer.espx?v=k1

2 United States Renal Data System Annual Data Report, 2005. http://www.usrds.org.

3 Association ERA-EDTA 2006 report page 62. http://www.era-edta-reg.org/index.jsp

4 Bryan CF, Harrell KM, Mitchell SI, Warady BA, Aeder MI, Luger AM *et al.* HLA points assigned in cadaveric kidney allocation should be revisited: an analysis of HLA class II molecularly typed patients and donors. *Am J Transplant* 2003; **3(4):** 459–464.

5 Tooth L, Ware R, Bain C, Purdie DM, Dobson A. Quality of reporting of observational longitudinal research. *Am J Epidemiol* 2005; **161(3):** 280–288.

6 Wolfe RA, Ashby VB, Milford EL, Ojo AO, Ettenger RE, Agodoa LY *et al.* Comparison of mortality in all patients on dialysis, patients on dialysis awaiting transplantation, and recipients of a first cadaveric transplant. *N Engl J Med* 1999; **341(23):** 1725–1730.

7 Rabbat CG, Thorpe KE, Russell JD, Churchill DN. Comparison of mortality risk for dialysis patients and cadaveric first renal transplant recipients in Ontario, Canada. *J Am Soc Nephrol* 2000; **11(5):** 917–922.

8 Oniscu GC, Brown H, Forsythe JL. Impact of cadaveric renal transplantation on survival in patients listed for transplantation. *J Am Soc Nephrol* 2005; **16(6):** 1859–1865.

9 Pereira BJ, Natov SN, Bouthot BA, Murthy BV, Ruthazer R, Schmid CH *et al.* Effects of hepatitis C infection and renal transplantation on survival in end-stage renal disease. The New England Organ Bank Hepatitis C Study Group. *Kidney Int* 1998; **53(5):** 1374–1381.

10 Glanton CW, Kao TC, Cruess D, Agodoa LY, Abbott KC. Impact of renal transplantation on survival in end-stage renal disease patients with elevated body mass index. *Kidney Int* 2003; **63(2):** 647–653.

11 Pelletier SJ, Maraschio MA, Schaubel DE, Dykstra DM, Punch JD, Wolfe RA *et al.* Survival benefit of kidney and liver transplantation for obese patients on the waiting list. *Clin Transplant* 2003; **2003:** 77–88.

12 Ojo AO, Meier-Kriesche HU, Hanson JA, Leichtman A, Magee JC, Cibrik D *et al.* The impact of simultaneous pancreas-kidney transplantation on long-term patient survival. *Transplantation* 2001; **71(1):** 82–90.

13 Ojo AO, Hanson JA, Meier-Kriesche H, Okechukwu CN, Wolfe RA, Leichtman AB *et al.* Survival in recipients of marginal cadaveric donor kidneys compared with other recipients and wait-listed transplant candidates. *J Am Soc Nephrol* 2001; **12(3):** 589–597.

14 Merion RM, Ashby VB, Wolfe RA, Distant DA, Hulbert-Shearon TE, Metzger RA *et al.* Deceased-donor characteristics and the survival benefit of kidney transplantation. *JAMA* 2005; **294(21):** 2726–2733.

15 Hariharan S, Johnson CP, Bresnahan BA, Taranto SE, McIntosh MJ, Stablein D. Improved graft survival after renal transplantation in the United States, 1988 to 1996. *N Engl J Med* 2000; **342(9):** 605–612.

16 Meier-Kriesche HU, Schold JD, Srinivas TR, Kaplan B. Lack of improvement in renal allograft survival despite a marked decrease in acute rejection rates over the most recent era. *Am J Transplant* 2004; **4(3):** 378–383.

17 Meier-Kriesche HU, Schold JD, Kaplan B. Long-term renal allograft survival: have we made significant progress or is it time to rethink our analytic and therapeutic strategies? *Am J Transplant* 2004; **4(8):** 1289–1295.

18 Kasiske BL, Gaston RS, Gourishankar S, Halloran PF, Matas AJ, Jeffery J *et al.* Long-term deterioration of kidney allograft function. *Am J Transplant* 2005; **5(6):** 1405–1414.

19 Keith DS, DeMattos A, Golconda M, Prather J, Cantarovich M, Paraskevas S *et al.* Factors associated with improvement in deceased donor renal allograft function in the 1990s. *J Am Soc Nephrol* 2005; **16(5):** 1512–1521.

20 Kaplan B, Schold J, Meier-Kriesche HU. Poor predictive value of serum creatinine for renal allograft loss. *Am J Transplant* 2003; **3(12):** 1560–1565.

21 Meier-Kriesche HU, Ojo AO, Port FK, Arndorfer JA, Cibrik DM, Kaplan B. Survival improvement among patients with end-stage renal disease: trends over time for transplant recipients and wait-listed patients. *J Am Soc Nephrol* 2001; **12(6):** 1293–1296.

22 Takemoto SK, Terasaki PI, Gjertson DW, Cecka JM. Twelve years' experience with national sharing of HLA-matched cadaveric kidneys for transplantation. *N Engl J Med* 2000; **343(15):** 1078–1084.

23 Mange KC, Cherikh WS, Maghirang J, Bloom RD. A comparison of the survival of shipped and locally transplanted cadaveric renal allografts. *N Engl J Med* 2001; **345(17):** 1237–1242.

24 Su X, Zenios SA, Chakkera H, Milford EL, Chertow GM. Diminishing significance of HLA matching in kidney transplantation. *Am J Transplant* 2004; **4(9):** 1501–1508.

25 Roberts JP, Wolfe RA, Bragg-Gresham JL, Rush SH, Wynn JJ, Distant DA *et al.* Effect of changing the priority for HLA matching on the rates and outcomes of kidney transplantation in minority groups. *N Engl J Med* 2004; **350(6):** 545–551.

26 Chakkera HA, O'Hare AM, Johansen KL, Hynes D, Stroupe K, Colin PM *et al.* Influence of race on kidney transplant outcomes within and outside the Department of Veterans Affairs. *J Am Soc Nephrol* 2005; **16(1):** 269–277.

27 Pallet N, Thervet E, Alberti C, Emal-Aglae V, Bedrossian J, Martinez F *et al.* Kidney transplant in black recipients: are African Europeans different from African Americans? *Am J Transplant* 2005; **5(11):** 2682–2687.

28 Takemoto SK, Zeevi A, Feng s *et al.* National conference to ussers antibody-mediated rejection in solid organ transplantation. *Am J Transplant* 2004; **4:** 1033–41.

29 Rush D. Protocol transplant biopsies: an underutilized tool in kidney transplantation. *Clin J Am Soc Nephrol* 2006; **1:** 138–143.

30 Hariharan S, Kasiske B, Matas A, Cohen A, Harmon W, Rabb H. Surrogate markers for long-term renal allograft survival. *Am J Transplant* 2004; **4(7):** 1179–1183.

31 Manns B, Owen WF Jr, WinRelmayer WC, Devereanx PJ, Tonelth M. Sirnoqale markers in clinical studies: problems solved or created? *Am J Kidney Dis* 2006; **48:** 159–66.

32 Brennan DC, Flavin K, Lowell JA, Howard TK, Shenoy S, Burgess S *et al.* A randomized, double-blinded comparison of thymoglobulin versus Atgam for induction immunosuppressive therapy in adult renal transplant recipients. *Transplantation* 1999; **67(7):** 1011–1018.

33 Sia IG, Patel R. New strategies for prevention and therapy of cytomegalovirus infection and disease in solid-organ transplant recipients. *Clin Microbiol Rev* 2000; **13**(1): 83–121.

34 Paya FN, Razonable RR. *Cytomegalovirus Infection after Organ Transplantation.* Lippincott, Williams & Wilkins, Philadelphia, 2003.

35 Sagedal S, Hartmann A, Nordal KP, Osnes K, Leivestad T, Foss A *et al.* Impact of early cytomegalovirus infection and disease on long-term recipient and kidney graft survival. *Kidney Int* 2004; **66**(1): 329–337.

36 Schnitzler MA, Lowell JA, Hardinger KL, Boxerman SB, Bailey TC, Brennan DC. The association of cytomegalovirus sero-pairing with outcomes and costs following cadaveric renal transplantation prior to the introduction of oral ganciclovir CMV prophylaxis. *Am J Transplant* 2003; **3**(4): 445–451.

37 McLaughlin K, Wu C, Fick G, Muirhead N, Hollomby D, Jevnikar A. Cytomegalovirus seromismatching increases the risk of acute renal allograft rejection. *Transplantation* 2002; **74**(6): 813–816.

38 Sageda S, Nordal KP, Hartmann A, Sund S, Scott H, Degre M *et al.* The impact of cytomegalovirus infection and disease on rejection episodes in renal allograft recipients. *Am J Transplant* 2002; **2**(9): 850–856.

39 Hodson EM, Craig JC, Strippoli GFM, Webster AC. Antiviral medications for preventing cytomegalovirus disease in solid organ transplant recipients. *Cochrane Database of Systematic Reviews* 2008.

40 Strippoli GF, Hodson EM, Jones CJ, Craig JC. Pre-emptive treatment for cytomegalovirus viraemia to prevent cytomegalovirus disease in solid organ transplant recipients. *Cochrane Database of Systematic Reviews* 2006.

41 Schmaldienst S, Dittrich E, Horl WH. Urinary tract infections after renal transplantation. *Curr Opin Urol* 2002; **12**(2): 125–130.

42 Hibberd PL, Tolkoff-Rubin NE, Doran M, Delvecchio A, Cosimi AB, Delmonico FL *et al.* Trimethoprim-sulfamethoxazole compared with ciprofloxacin for the prevention of urinary tract infection in renal transplant recipients. A double-blind, randomized controlled trial. *Online J Curr Clin Trials* 1992 Aug 11; 15.

43 Franz M, Schmaldienst S, Horl WH. *Renal Infections.* Lippincott Williams & Wilkins, Philadelphia, 2001.

44 Abbott KC, Swanson SJ, Richter ER, Bohen EM, Agodoa LY, Peters TG *et al.* Late urinary tract infection after renal transplantation in the United States. *Am J Kidney Dis* 2004; **44**(2): 353–362.

45 Rice JC, Peng T, Kuo YF, Pendyala S, Simmons L, Boughton J *et al.* Renal allograft injury is associated with urinary tract infection caused by Escherichia coli bearing adherence factors. *Am J Transplant* 2006; **6**: 2375–2383.

46 Muller V, Becker G, Delfs M, Albrecht KH, Philipp T, Heemann U. Do urinary tract infections trigger chronic kidney transplant rejection in man? *J Urol* 1998; **159**(6): 1826–1829.

47 Alkatheri A. Antibiotics for preventing urinary tract infections in kidney transplant recipients. *Cochrane Syst Database Rev* 2008; **2**: CD006026.

48 Levey AS, Beto JA, Coronado BE, Eknoyan G, Foley RN, Kasiske BL *et al.* Controlling the epidemic of cardiovascular disease in chronic renal disease: what do we know? What do we need to learn? Where do we go from here? National Kidney Foundation Task Force on Cardiovascular Disease. *Am J Kidney Dis* 1998; **32**(5): 853–906.

49 Danovitch GM, Hariharan S, Pirsch JD, Rush D, Roth D, Ramos E *et al.* Management of the waiting list for cadaveric kidney transplants: report of a survey and recommendations by the Clinical Practice Guidelines

Committee of the American Society of Transplantation. *J Am Soc Nephrol* 2002; **13**(2): 528–535.

50 Kasiske BL. Risk factors for accelerated atherosclerosis in renal transplant recipients. *Am J Med* 1988; **84**(6): 985–992.

51 Lentine KL, Brennan DC, Schnitzler MA. Incidence and predictors of myocardial infarction after kidney transplantation. *J Am Soc Nephrol* 2005; **16**(2): 496–506.

52 Lentine KL, Schnitzler MA, Abbott KC, Li L, Burroughs TE, Irish W *et al.* De novo congestive heart failure after kidney transplantation: a common condition with poor prognostic implications. *Am J Kidney Dis* 2005; **46**(4): 720–733.

53 Matas AJ, Kasiske B, Miller L. Proposed guidelines for re-evaluation of patients on the waiting list for renal cadaver transplantation. *Transplantation* 2002; **73**(5): 811–812.

54 Gaston RS, Danovitch GM, Adams PL, Wynn JJ, Merion RM, Deierhoi MH *et al.* The report of a national conference on the wait list for kidney transplantation. *Am J Transplant* 2003; **3**(7): 775–785.

55 Wilson PW, D'Agostino RB, Levy D, Belanger AM, Silbershatz H, Kannel WB. Prediction of coronary heart disease using risk factor categories. *Circulation* 1998; **97**(18): 1837–1847.

56 Kasiske BL, Guijarro C, Massy ZA, Wiederkehr MR, Ma JZ. Cardiovascular disease after renal transplantation. *J Am Soc Nephrol* 1996; **7**(1): 158–165.

57 Gill JS, Ma I, Landsberg D, Johnson N, Levin A. Cardiovascular events and investigation in patients who are awaiting cadaveric kidney transplantation. *J Am Soc Nephrol* 2005; **16**(3): 808–816.

58 Kasiske BL, Chakkera HA, Roel J. Explained and unexplained ischemic heart disease risk after renal transplantation. *J Am Soc Nephrol* 2000; **11**(9): 1735–1743.

59 Ducloux D, Kazory A, Chalopin JM. Predicting coronary heart disease in renal transplant recipients: a prospective study. *Kidney Int* 2004; **66**(1): 441–447.

60 Ponticelli C, Villa M, Cesana B, Montagnino G, Tarantino A. Risk factors for late kidney allograft failure. *Kidney Int* 2002; **62**(5): 1848–1854.

61 Kramer BK, Zulke C, Kammerl MC, Schmidt C, Hengstenberg C, Fischereder M *et al.* Cardiovascular risk factors and estimated risk for CAD in a randomized trial comparing calcineurin inhibitors in renal transplantation. *Am J Transplant* 2003; **3**(8): 982–987.

62 Diaz JM, Sainz Z, Guirado LL, Ortiz-Herbener F, Picazo M, Garcia-Camin R *et al.* Risk factors for cardiovascular disease after renal transplantation. *Transplant Proc* 2003; **35**(5): 1722–1724.

63 Rigatto C, Parfrey P, Foley R, Negrijn C, Tribula C, Jeffery J. Congestive heart failure in renal transplant recipients: risk factors, outcomes, and relationship with ischemic heart disease. *J Am Soc Nephrol* 2002; **13**(4): 1084–1090.

64 Cosio FG, Pesavento TE, Kim S, Osei K, Henry M, Ferguson RM. Patient survival after renal transplantation. IV. Impact of post-transplant diabetes. *Kidney Int* 2002; **62**(4): 1440–1446.

65 Abbott KC, Yuan CM, Taylor AJ, Cruess DF, Agodoa LY. Early renal insufficiency and hospitalized heart disease after renal transplantation in the era of modern immunosuppression. *J Am Soc Nephrol* 2003; **14**(9): 2358–1265.

66 Meier-Kriesche HU, Baliga R, Kaplan B. Decreased renal function is a strong risk factor for cardiovascular death after renal transplantation. *Transplantation* 2003; **75**(8): 1291–1295.

67 Fellstrom B, Jardine AG, Soveri I, Cole E, Neumayer HH, Maes B *et al.* Renal dysfunction is a strong and independent risk factor for mortality and

cardiovascular complications in renal transplantation. *Am J Transplant* 2005; **5(8):** 1986–1991.

68 Abbott KC, Bucci JR, Cruess D, Taylor AJ, Agodoa LY. Graft loss and acute coronary syndromes after renal transplantation in the United States. *J Am Soc Nephrol* 2002; **13(10):** 2560–2569.

69 Abbott KC, Hypolite IO, Hshieh P, Cruess D, Taylor AJ, Agodoa LY. Hospitalized congestive heart failure after renal transplantation in the United States. *Ann Epidemiol* 2002; **12(2):** 115–122.

70 Meier-Kriesche HU, Schold JD, Srinivas TR, Reed A, Kaplan B. Kidney transplantation halts cardiovascular disease progression in patients with end-stage renal disease. *Am J Transplant* 2004; **4(10):** 1662–1668.

71 Lentine KL, Schnitzler MA, Abbott KC, Li L, Xiao H, Burroughs TE *et al.* Incidence, predictors, and associated outcomes of atrial fibrillation after kidney transplantation. *Clin J Am Soc Nephrol* 2006; **1:** 288–296.

72 Kasiske B, Cosio FG, Beto J, Bolton K, Chavers BM, Grimm R, Jr *et al.* Clinical practice guidelines for managing dyslipidemias in kidney transplant patients: a report from the Managing Dyslipidemias in Chronic Kidney Disease Work Group of the National Kidney Foundation Kidney Disease Outcomes Quality Initiative. *Am J Transplant* 2004; **4(Suppl 7):** 13–53.

73 Hebert PR, Gaziano JM, Chan KS, Hennekens CH. Cholesterol lowering with statin drugs, risk of stroke, and total mortality. An overview of randomized trials. *JAMA* 1997; **278(4):** 313–321.

74 Di Mascio R, Marchioli R, Tognoni G. Cholesterol reduction and stroke occurrence: an overview of randomized clinical trials. *Cerebrovasc Dis* 2000; **10(2):** 85–92.

75 Holdaas H, Fellstrom B, Jardine AG, Holme I, Nyberg G, Fauchald P *et al.* Effect of fluvastatin on cardiac outcomes in renal transplant recipients: a multicentre, randomised, placebo-controlled trial. *Lancet* 2003; **361(9374):** 2024–2031.

76 Jardine AG, Fellstrom B, Logan JO, Cole E, Nyberg G, Gronhagen-Riska C *et al.* Cardiovascular risk and renal transplantation: post hoc analyses of the Assessment of Lescol in Renal Transplantation (ALERT) study. *Am J Kidney Dis* 2005; **46(3):** 529–536.

77 Holdaas H, Fellstrom B, Jardine AG, Nyberg G, Gronhagen-Riska C, Madsen S *et al.* Beneficial effect of early initiation of lipid-lowering therapy following renal transplantation. *Nephrol Dial Transplant* 2005; **20(5):** 974–980.

78 Holdaas H, Fellstrom B, Cole E, Nyberg G, Olsson AG, Pedersen TR *et al.* Long-term cardiac outcomes in renal transplant recipients receiving fluvastatin: the ALERT extension study. *Am J Transplant* 2005; **5(12):** 2929–2936.

79 Artz MA, Boots JM, Ligtenberg G, Roodnat JI, Christiaans MH, Vos PF *et al.* Conversion from cyclosporine to tacrolimus improves quality-of-life indices, renal graft function and cardiovascular risk profile. *Am J Transplant* 2004; **4(6):** 937–945.

80 Artz MA, Boots JM, Ligtenberg G, Roodnat JI, Christiaans MH, Vos PF *et al.* Improved cardiovascular risk profile and renal function in renal transplant patients after randomized conversion from cyclosporine to tacrolimus. *J Am Soc Nephrol* 2003; **14(7):** 1880–1888.

81 Kasiske BL, Snyder JJ, Gilbertson D, Matas AJ. Diabetes mellitus after kidney transplantation in the United States. *Am J Transplant* 2003; **3(2):** 178–185.

82 Executive Summary of the Third Report of the National Cholesterol Education Program (NCEP) Expert Panel on Detection, Evaluation, and Treatment of High Blood Cholesterol in Adults (Adult Treatment Panel III). *JAMA* 2001; **285(19):** 2486–2497.

83 Grundy SM, Cleeman JI, Merz CN, Brewer HB, Jr., Clark LT, Hunninghake DB *et al.* Implications of recent clinical trials for the National Cholesterol Education Program Adult Treatment Panel III guidelines. *Circulation* 2004; **110(2):** 227–239.

84 Jardine AG, Holdaas H, Fellstrom B, Cole E, Nyberg G, Gronhagen-Riska C *et al.* Fluvastatin prevents cardiac death and myocardial infarction in renal transplant recipients: post-hoc subgroup analyses of the ALERT Study. *Am J Transplant* 2004; **4(6):** 988–995.

51 The Early Course: Induction, Delayed Function, and Rejection

Paul A. Keown

Departments of Medicine and Pathology and Laboratory Medicine, University of British Columbia, Vancouver, BC, Canada

Introduction

The success of kidney transplantation has increased dramatically, driven by innovations in biology, medicine, and surgery. Almost 40% of patients with chronic kidney disease in Canada and Australia and 30% of those in the USA are now maintained with a functioning transplant [1–3], although other developed countries such as Germany and Japan have lower transplantation rates (1 and 10%, respectively) due to societal, logistical, or economic factors [3,4]. Understanding of biological processes of graft injury and selective inhibition of key molecular steps in alloantigen response has been critical in this evolution [5–7]. Patient and graft survival now exceed 95% and 90%, respectively, during the first year, and over 80% of patients remain free from acute rejection [1–3]. Complications have diminished in frequency and severity; life-threatening bacterial, fungal, and viral infections are now uncommon; and there has been a corresponding improvement in both quality of life and overall cost-effectiveness [8–11].

The first 3 months posttransplant remain a critical period during which the graft is at risk of physiological and immunological injury, which may reduce long-term success [2]. Optimal care requires precise estimation of recipient risk, appropriate prophylaxis, accurate diagnosis, and speedy intervention to prevent graft injury. Potent biological immunosuppression is often used to complement conventional pharmacological maintenance immunosuppression to minimize the risks of delayed graft function (DGF) and rejection, whereas plasma exchange may be employed to remove antibodies against donor HLA antigens and mitigate severe humoral injury [12]. It is challenging to define optimal strategies for early transplant care, because formal randomized clinical trials are often lacking or do not explore all potential treatment options or therapeutic combinations. This chapter therefore summarizes the principal issues of induction therapy, DGF, and rejection; it documents the current treatment guidelines and reviews the emerging evidence in each of these areas.

Definitions

Induction therapy

Induction refers to the use of potent immunosuppression administered around the time of transplantation to reduce the risk of acute rejection, minimize delayed graft function, and decrease subsequent renal toxicity by permitting a reduction in calcineurin inhibitors during the critical posttransplant period [12]. Induction therapy most commonly consists of a short course of polyclonal or monoclonal antibodies directed against discrete epitopes on the lymphocyte surface. It is normally administered in addition to routine maintenance therapy, which may be reduced, or individual agents may be withheld during this time to minimize specific drug toxicity or global immunosuppression.

DGF (Delayed Graft Function)

DGF is frequently defined as the requirement for dialysis in the first 7 days posttransplant, although this lacks both sensitivity (missing subjects with mild impairment not requiring dialysis) and specificity (including subjects requiring dialysis for other reasons, such as accelerated rejection) [13]. A more precise definition includes a urine output of less than 1200 mL/day, decline of serum creatinine of less than 10% in the first 2 days, or achievement of a functional threshold (e.g. serum creatinine less than 220 μmol/L or estimated glomerular filtration rate above 10 mL/min). However, calculation of creatinine elimination kinetics perhaps provides the most objective measure of early function [14].

Rejection

Graft rejection is classically divided into three categories. Hyperacute rejection usually presents within the first hours following graft implantation and is characterized by endothelial injury, vascular occlusion, and microvascular thrombosis of the graft [15]. It is now uncommon, occurring in <1% of patients, is caused by

Evidence-based Nephrology. Edited by Donald Molony and Jonathan Craig
© 2009 Blackwell Publishing, ISBN: 978-1-4051-3975-5.

preformed antibodies to donor transplantation antigens, and is resistant to conventional therapy, often leading to graft loss. Acute rejection occurs in around 10% of patients reported to the US Renal Data System (USRDS) [2] and typically presents from day 3 to 90 posttransplant, although it may occur later if immunosuppression is decreased due to comorbidity or noncompliance. Acute rejection may comprise both cell-mediated and antibody-mediated injury [15]; the former typically responds readily to conventional therapy, whereas antibody-mediated rejection is more resistant or refractory. Chronic rejection usually presents after the first year and has often been included in the confusing term "chronic allograft nephropathy," which is now discouraged [16]. The diagnostic features include specific histological changes in the glomeruli, interstitium, tubules, and vessels, diffuse C4d deposition, and circulating donor-specific antibody (DSA). Chronic rejection responds poorly to therapy.

Guidelines

Induction therapy

The European Best Practice Guidelines [15] provide recommendations for the use of induction therapy based on level A evidence (systematic reviews of randomized trials). These state that prophylactic immunosuppression with antibody may be administered to kidney transplant recipients as an optional initial therapy to reduce the number and severity of rejections during the first 3–6 months after transplantation, although benefits must be balanced against the risks of overimmunosuppression with increased susceptibility to opportunistic viral infection and posttransplant lymphoproliferative disease. They emphasize that induction therapy with polyclonal (ALG or ATG) or monoclonal (OKT3) antibodies administered during the perioperative period for a limited time (1–3 weeks) does not consistently improve graft survival at 3 years posttransplant in unselected recipients. Recipients with DGF, or recipients with low and high panel-reactive antibodies directed to HLA antigens may benefit from classical induction therapy with ALG, ATG, or monoclonal antibodies (OKT3), and these agents show equivalent efficacy. Finally, they noted that safe and effective prophylaxis has been achieved with high-affinity humanized or chimeric monoclonal antibodies (daclizumab and basiliximab, respectively), which target the interleukin-2 (IL-2) receptor.

DGF

Guidelines provide recommendations for the management of the donor and recipient during the perioperative phase to maximize organ quality and recipient volume status based on level B or C (observational) evidence .[15,17–19]. Central components of these include recommendations that management of the donor should be similar to normal intensive care, but the objectives are to support future function of renal, cardiac, and pulmonary grafts. A simplified goal for managing the donor may be to maintain a central venous pressure of 10 cm water, a systemic blood pressure of 100 mm/Hg, and a urine output of 100 mL/h. Preoperative dialysis

should not be performed routinely except for patients with heart failure or hyperkalemia, and preoperative hypovolemia should be avoided to prevent DGF. Caution should be used with marginal donors, including the elderly (>60 years), particularly those with prior hypertension, diabetes, or intrinsic renal disease, who have a calculated glomerular filtration rate of <60 mL/min. Such organs should preferentially be offered to older recipients (over 60 years) with a limited life expectancy and who provide informed consent to receipt of such an organ. The recipient should not be dialyzed routinely pretransplant, except for those with heart failure or hyperkalemia, and hypovolemia should be avoided to prevent DGF. Graft function should be monitored closely in patients with delayed function, vascular, and urological complications, drug toxicity and infection should be also excluded as causes, and surveillance biopsies should be considered [15].

Rejection

Formal guidelines provide recommendations for the detection of donor-specific anti-HLA antibodies, histological diagnosis, and treatment of rejection based on level B or C evidence [15,19–22]. A cross-match test must be performed pretransplantation on current serum using at least one method that detects complement-dependent antibodies, and a positive immunoglobulin G (IgG) cross-match is considered an absolute preclusion to transplant. Historical sera should also be tested, and a positive historical cross-match may increase the risk of rejection and indicate a need for more intensive immunosuppression [22] or be a contraindication in patients receiving a repeat transplant and in those with high panel-reactive antibodies [15]. Flow cytometry may be used to increase the sensitivity of antibody detection, although guidelines differ regarding the implication of a positive flow cross-match [15,19,22]. Posttransplant monitoring of DSA may be of value in the diagnosis or prognosis of rejection and should be monitored if possible, particularly at the time of biopsy [15,22].

Histological diagnosis and categorization of rejection is standardized in the Banff criteria, which are updated following each biennial meeting [16,21,23]. Criteria for hyperacute or accelerated acute antibody-mediated rejection and grades I–III acute rejection are defined in the 1997 criteria [23], whereas the characteristics of chronic rejection have been clarified and distinguished from other forms of chronic graft injury in the 2005 criteria [16]. Patients should be monitored routinely for evidence of graft dysfunction [15,19,22,24]. Acute rejection should be considered in patients with a rapid rise in serum creatinine of 10–25% over baseline, with or without a decline in urine output; graft biopsy should be performed to confirm rejection, and reporting should be standardized according to an internationally agreed-upon scheme [15]. High-dose intravenous methylprednisolone is recommended for treatment of the first acute rejection episode, and ATG is preferred to OKT3 for subsequent or severe episodes in light of their respective toxicities [15]. Alteration in baseline therapy and the use of plasmapheresis with or without intravenous immunoglobulin (IVIG) may be required in refractory cases [15,22]. Subsequent deterioration in graft function or new proteinuria should be investigated fully to determine the cause, including chronic rejection, although no guidelines yet exist for therapy of proven benefit [19,22,25].

Available evidence

Not all key aspects of care in the early posttransplant period have been subject to appropriately powered and designed randomized clinical trials. Several systematic reviews and meta-analyses addressed those randomized controlled trials that have evaluated the use of induction therapy and the management of DGF and rejection, and many smaller high-quality studies have provided additional insight and guidance into these aspects of care. The key information derived from these studies is reviewed in the sections below.

Induction therapy

Systematic reviews of induction therapy performed by Gaston, Hardinger, Chapman, Kirk, Nashan, and colleagues chronicle the changing role of this therapy during the past decade [6,12,26–28]. In prior years, induction was employed principally for patients at high risk of immunological or physiological graft injury due to its cost, toxicity, and paucity of high-level evidence for benefit and cost-effectiveness in low-risk subjects [29–32]. However, it has experienced a resurgence with the availability of more consistent, safe, and effective biological preparations, and accumulating data show that induction therapy offers a significant reduction in the incidence of acute graft rejection following living or cadaver donor transplantation (Figure 51.1) [32].

The principal polyclonal antibodies employed today are equine-derived ATGAM, and rabbit-derived ATG-Fresenius and Thymoglobulin [33]. The last of these is the most widely used in

North America, particularly in subjects who are sensitized, who are undergoing retransplantation, or who have DGF [31]. These agents have composite molecular actions, including ligation of surface epitopes, T- and B-lymphocyte deletion via tumor necrosis factor/Fas-mediated apoptosis, selective downregulation of gene expression, and the induction of CD4$^+$ CD25$^+$ FoxP3 regulatory cells [34–36]. Administration has varied from 1 to 10 days, although treatment for 5–10 days is now most common. Reported efficacy varies according to the product and the target population, so that evaluation of relative risk or benefit is complex. Studies have shown that Thymoglobulin is superior to ATGAM [37] in reducing the cumulative probability of acute graft rejection ($P = 0.001$–0.004). However, it did not improve graft or patient survival and significantly increased the risk of cytomegalovirus (CMV) and other viral infections, leukopenia, and other hematological complications compared with pharmacological immunosuppression ($P = 0.001$–0.05).

Two recent randomized studies suggest that ATG exerts a positive effect in low-risk kidney transplant recipients when calcineurin inhibitor therapy is delayed [38,39]. In the first study of 309 deceased donor graft recipients, patients randomized to receive ATG for 10 days followed by tacrolimus had significantly fewer biopsy-confirmed acute rejection episodes (15% vs. 30%; $P = 0.001$) than those treated with tacrolimus from the time of transplantation. However, patient and graft survival, DGF, and graft function 1 year posttransplant were similar between the groups, and viral and other infections were more common in the ATG group. The second study involved 555 deceased donor graft recipients. Patients randomized to receive ATG for 10 days followed by tacrolimus had a lower incidence of biopsy-proven rejection than those receiving ATG followed by cyclosporine or those commencing tacrolimus from the time of transplant (15% vs. 21.2% vs. 25%; $P = 0.004$ and 0.177) [39]. Again, cumulative

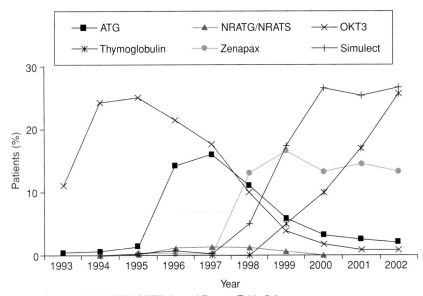

Source: 2003 OPTN/SRTR Annual Report, Table 5.6a

Figure 51.1 Trends in kidney transplant induction immunosuppression. (From Kaufmann *et al.* 2004 [45].)

patient and graft survival and mean serum creatinine levels were similar among the groups, and hematological and viral complications were higher in the ATG groups. The elevated risk in the cyclosporine-treated group may reflect imbalances in the number of patients with a prior transplant or increased PRA in this group [39].

The prophylactic use of Muromonab (OKT3) has declined substantially during the same period due to substantial toxicity and lack of demonstrable benefit [40,41]. Large-scale national and international studies show that the relative risk of posttransplant lymphoproliferative disease is increased by 1.5- to 2-fold in patients receiving Muromonab compared with no induction therapy [30,42–44]. Muromonab is now used in less than 1% of patients [45] and has been largely replaced by ATG in high-risk subjects or anti-CD25 antibodies in low-risk patients [32,46], although data showing differences in graft or patient survival are lacking [47]. Novel anti-CD3 molecules with differing isotypes or epitope specificities [48] are under investigation, but their benefit/toxicity ratio remains unproven.

Alemtuzumab (Campath-1H) is a humanized monoclonal antibody to CD52 that causes long-lasting depletion of human B and T cells. Alemtuzumab offers potential practical benefits over polyclonal depleting antibodies, with lower cost and simplicity of intravenous access. A systematic review by Morris *et al.* showed that despite increasing use, the level of evidence for its role in transplantation is limited [49]. Preliminary noncontrolled studies indicate that graft rejection, graft loss, mortality rates, and infectious complications are comparable or perhaps superior to patients receiving anti-CD25 monoclonals and conventional triple or quadruple therapy. The expectation of patient and graft survival exceeds 95% at 500 days [50], and steroid avoidance and minimization of long-term maintenance immunosuppression may be possible [51,52–55]. Two small randomized controlled trials confirmed that the incidence of acute rejection is not different from control therapy, although steroid-free and calcineurin-sparing protocols are possible [56,57]. Although there is a profound and long-lasting T-cell lymphopenia after administration of alemtuzumab, there is no apparent increase in infection, posttransplantation lymphoproliferative disease, or other side effects other than perhaps autoimmune disease. However, the limited studies available at present do not support early hopes of immune accommodation permitting withdrawal of maintenance therapy.

Basiliximab and daclizumab (anti-CD25) are monoclonal antibodies to the IL-2 receptor that bind selectively to the CD25 molecule, inhibiting high-affinity IL-2 binding to this structure and inhibiting the proliferative signals critical for lymphocyte activation. Basiliximab is a chimeric molecule that includes the complete variable region of the original anti-CD25 molecule, and it is normally administered on two occasions within the first posttransplant week. Daclizumab, a humanized molecule that includes only the hypervariable region of the murine antibody whereas the remainder is of human origin, exhibits slightly lower binding affinity and is given more frequently throughout the first 2 months [12,13]. Both have long terminal half-lives (2 weeks) and deplete CD25 expression for an average of 45 and 90 days, respectively.

A number of meta-analyses have examined the efficacy and toxicity of these drugs [8,58]. The most extensive has been completed by Webster and colleagues, who included 38 current studies of anti-CD25 antibody use comprising 4893 subjects [59] (Table 51.1). The antibody was compared to placebo or no therapy in 16 studies (2682 subjects) and to another monoclonal or polyclonal antibody in 14 studies (1108 subjects). Two studies compared the antibodies directly, and the remaining studies examined other treatment comparisons or dosing strategies. Cyclosporine A was employed as maintenance immunosuppression in 32 studies, and tacrolimus was used in the remainder. Results were homogeneous among all studies with no discernable difference between the two anti-CD25 antibodies. Anti-CD25 therapy reduced the incidence of clinical acute rejection in the first 6 months by 34% (relative risk [RR], (Figure 51.2), 0.66, 95% confidence interval [CI], 0.59–0.74), biopsy-proven rejection by 36%, and steroid-resistant rejection by 49% (RR, 0.51; CI, 0.38–0.67). Graft loss (RR, 0.84; CI, 0.64–1.10) (Figure 51.3) and CMV infection (RR, 0.82; CI, 0.65–1.03) were also reduced at 1 year in patients receiving anti-CD25 therapy, although these did not reach statistical significance. On this basis, for every 100 subjects treated with these agents, 14 would be expected to avoid acute rejection and 8 to avoid steroid-resistant rejection [59].

Anti-CD25 antibodies were comparable in efficacy to other monoclonal or polyclonal antibodies, and no significant differences were evident for graft rejection or loss, CMV infection, mortality, or other principal outcomes [59] (Figure 51.4). Fever, leukopenia, thrombocytopenia, and overall adverse reactions were significantly lower in subjects receiving anti-CD25 therapy than other induction therapies. Basiliximab and daclizumab were compared directly in only two small studies comprising 82 subjects. Despite the limitations in sample size and study design, there was no difference in reduction of rejection risk between the two agents (RR, 0.67 [CI, 0.59–0.77] vs. RR, 0.66 [CI, 0.53–0.82]).

DGF

DGF occurs in approximately 4% of live donor recipients and 23% of deceased donor graft recipients (overall reported range, 2–50%) [2,13] and varies from mild impairment with slow recovery to persistent oliguric renal failure and graft loss [13,17,18]. DGF may result both from donor factors, which include donor source, age, renal function, comorbidity, clinical support, and surgical technique, and recipient factors, including surgical implantation, vascular competency, volume status, immunological sensitization, and immunosuppressive therapy [13]. Careful management of all of these is required to reduce immediate injury and ensure long-term success.

The European Expert Group has defined the ideal deceased (cadaver) donor as a previously healthy individual, aged 10–55 years, brain dead due to trauma or intracerebral bleeding, with no ongoing infection and excellent organ function [17]. However, the majority of donors no longer fulfill these criteria, and

Table 51.1 Clinical trials of anti-CD25 monoclonal antibodies following kidney transplantation.

Trial	n	% Cadaveric donor	% 1st transplant	IL2RA (n)	Comparator (n)	Calcineurin inhibitor (initial dose, mg/kg/day: trough, ng/mL)	Antiproliferative agent (Aza in mg/kg/day, MMF in g/day)	Follow-up (yrs)
Il2Ra vs placebo/no treatment								
Ahsan 2002	100	70	100	Daclizumab (50)	None (50)	T (0.16–0.2: 10–15)	MMF (1)	1
Baczkowska 2002	32	NS	NS	Daclizumab (16)	None (16)	Cy (5–10: NS)	MMF (2)	0.3[b]
Daclizumab double 1999	275	100	100	Daclizumab (141)	Placebo (134)	Cy (10: NS)	—	3
Daclizumab triple 1998	260	100	100	Daclizumab (126)	Placebo (134)	Cy (NS: NS)	Aza (NS)	3
Davies/Lawen 2000	123	76	89	Basiliximab (59)	Placebo (64)	Cy (8–10: 100–400)	MMF (2–3)	1
de Boccardo 2002	310	45	NS	Basiliximab (NS)	Placebo (NS)	Cy (10: NS)	Aza (1–2)	0.5[b]
Folkmane 2001	71	100	NS	Basiliximab (23)	None (23/25)	Cy (NS: 150–300)	Aza (1–2) or MMF (2)	1
Kahan 1999	346	70	100	Basiliximab (173)	Placebo (173)	Cy (NS: 150–450)	—	1
Kirkman 1991	80	NS	100	Anti-TAC (40)	None (40)	Cy (4–8: NS)	Aza (2)	1
Kirkman 1989	21	100	100	Anti-TAC (12)	None (9)	Cy (8–12: NS)	— or Aza (2)	1
Kyllonen 2002[c]	104	100	ns	Basiliximab (52)	None (52)	Cy (5: NS)	Aza or MMF (NS)	1
Nashan 1997	376	100	100	Basiliximab (190)	Placebo (186)	Cy (NS: 150–450)	—	1
Pisani 2001	32	NS	81	Basiliximab (10/9)	None (13)	Cy (8: 350–400)	MMF (1.5)	0.5[b]
Ponticelli 2001	340	83	93	Basiliximab (168)	Placebo (172)	Cy (10: 150–300)	Aza (1–2)	1
Sandrini 2002	156	NS	100	Basiliximab (79)	Placebo (77)	Cy (NS: NS)	Aza (NS)	1[b]
Sheashaa 2003	100	0	100	Basiliximab (50)	None (50)	Cy (8: 125–150)	Aza (1)	3
van Gelder 1996	60	78	100	BT563 (30)	Placebo (30)	Cy (8: 300)	—	3
Il2Ra vs. other antibody								
Brennan 2002	212	100	NS	Basiliximab (106)	ATG (106)	Cy (12–16: NS)	MMF (2)	0.5[b]
Flechner 2000	45	NS	NS	Basiliximab (23)	OKT3 (22)	Cy (NS: NS)	MMF (2)	0.5[b]

Hourmant 1994	40	NS	33B3.1 (20)	ATG (20)	Cy (8: 150–250)	Aza (2)	1
Kriaa 1993	40	100	Lo-tact-1 (20)	ALG (20)	Cy (8: NS)	Aza (1)	1
Kyllonen 2002[c]	104	100	Basiliximab (52)	ATG (52)	Cy (5: NS)	Aza or MMF (NS)	1
Lacha 2001	28	NS	Daclizumab (14)	OKT3 (14)	Cy (8: NS)	MMF (2)	0.5
Lebranchu 2002	103	100	Basiliximab (52)	ATG (51)	Cy (6–8: 150–200)	MMF (2)	1
Mourad 2002	89	98.5	Basiliximab (46)	ATG (43)	Cy (6: NS)	MMF (2)	0.5[b]
Philosophe 2002	50	NS	Daclizumab (26)	OKT3 (24)	T (NS: NS)	MMF (NS)	1[b]
Poufarziani 2003	25	0	Daclizumab (11)	ALG (14)	Cy (NS: NS)	MMF (NS)	1[b]
Shidban 2000	42	100	Basiliximab (22)	OKT3 (20)	Cy (NS: NS)	MMF (NS)	0.5[b]
Shidban 2003	75	100	Basiliximab (25)	ATG (50)	Cy (NS: NS)	MMF (NS)	0.5[b]
Sollinger 2001	135	62	Basiliximab (70)	ATG (65)	Cy (6–10: NS)	MMF (2–3)	1
Soulillou 1990	100	100	33B3.1 (50)	33B3.1 (50)	Cy (8: 300–600)	Aza (2)	1
Tullius 2003	124	100	Basiliximab (62)	ATG (62)	T (0.2: 10)	—	1
IL2Ra vs. other agents							
Garcia 2002	49	0	Daclizumab, MMF(23)	T, Aza, (26)	T (0.1–0.15: NS)	MMF (2–3), Aza (2)	0.5[b]
Khan 2000	59	NS	Basiliximab (29)	Daclizumab (30)	T or Cy (NS: NS)	MMF (NS) or Aza (NS)	0.25
ATLAS 2003	457	NS	Basiliximab (153)	MMF (151) ; MMF/P (147)	T (0.2: 5–15)	MMF (2)	0.5[b]
Kumar 2002	27	NS	High basiliximab, low P (17)	Basiliximab, normal P (10)	Cy (NS: NS)	MMF (NS)	1
Matl 2001	202	100	Basiliximab (102) standard	Basiliximab (100) 1 x high	Cy (10: NS)	Aza (1–2)	1
Nair 2001	23	26	Basiliximab (10)	Daclizumab (13)	Cy (7: NS)	MMF (2)	0.5[b]
van Riemsdijk 2002	130	NS	Daclizumab, no P (64)	P (66)	T (NS: NS)	MMF (NS)	0.5[b]

Source: Webster *et al.* 2004 [59].

Abbreviations: NS, not stated; T, tacrolimus; Aza, azathioprine; MMF, mycophenolate mofetil; P, steroid; Cy, cyclosporine; —, no agent used.

[a] Additional immunosuppressive agents. All trials (except for van Riemsdijk 2002 and ATLAS 2003) also used steroid therapy in all arms.

[b] Trials are ongoing.

[c] Kyllonen 2002 (156 participants) has three arms comparing IL2Ra with either no treatment or with ATG and so appears in both comparisons.

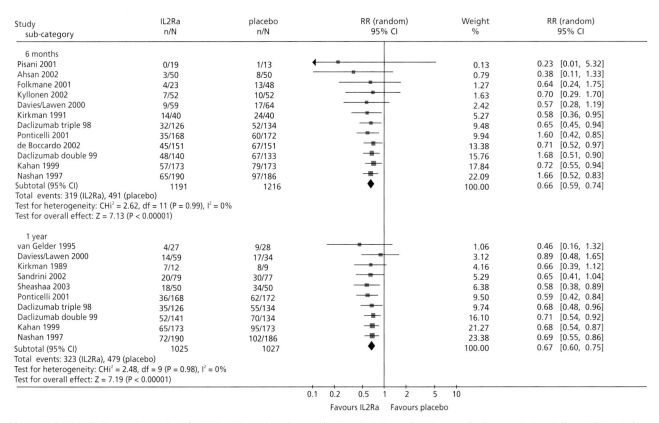

Study sub-category	IL2Ra n/N	placebo n/N	RR (random) 95% CI	Weight %	RR (random) 95% CI
6 months					
Pisani 2001	0/19	1/13		0.13	0.23 [0.01, 5.32]
Ahsan 2002	3/50	8/50		0.79	0.38 [0.11, 1.33]
Folkmane 2001	4/23	13/48		1.27	0.64 [0.24, 1.75]
Kyllonen 2002	7/52	10/52		1.63	0.70 [0.29, 1.70]
Davies/Lawen 2000	9/59	17/64		2.42	0.57 [0.28, 1.19]
Kirkman 1991	14/40	24/40		5.27	0.58 [0.36, 0.95]
Daclizumab triple 98	32/126	52/134		9.48	0.65 [0.45, 0.94]
Ponticelli 2001	35/168	60/172		9.94	1.60 [0.42, 0.85]
de Boccardo 2002	45/151	67/151		13.38	0.71 [0.52, 0.97]
Daclizumab double 99	48/140	67/133		15.76	1.68 [0.51, 0.90]
Kahan 1999	57/173	79/173		17.84	0.72 [0.55, 0.94]
Nashan 1997	65/190	97/186		22.09	1.66 [0.52, 0.83]
Subtotal (95% CI)	1191	1216		100.00	0.66 [0.59, 0.74]
Total events: 319 (IL2Ra), 491 (placebo)					
Test for heterogeneity: CHi² = 2.62, df = 11 (P = 0.99), I² = 0%					
Test for overall effect: Z = 7.13 (P < 0.00001)					
1 year					
van Gelder 1995	4/27	9/28		1.06	0.46 [0.16, 1.32]
Daviess/Lawen 2000	14/59	17/34		3.12	0.89 [0.48, 1.65]
Kirkman 1989	7/12	8/9		4.16	0.66 [0.39, 1.12]
Sandrini 2002	20/79	30/77		5.29	0.65 [0.41, 1.04]
Sheashaa 2003	18/50	34/50		6.38	0.58 [0.38, 0.89]
Ponticelli 2001	36/168	62/172		9.50	0.59 [0.42, 0.84]
Daclizumab triple 98	35/126	55/134		9.74	0.68 [0.48, 0.96]
Daclizumab double 99	52/141	70/134		16.10	0.71 [0.54, 0.92]
Kahan 1999	65/173	95/173		21.27	0.68 [0.54, 0.87]
Nashan 1997	72/190	102/186		23.38	0.69 [0.55, 0.86]
Subtotal (95% CI)	1025	1027		100.00	0.67 [0.60, 0.75]
Total events: 323 (IL2Ra), 479 (placebo)					
Test for heterogeneity: CHi² = 2.48, df = 9 (P = 0.98), I² = 0%					
Test for overall effect: Z = 7.19 (P < 0.00001)					

0.1 0.2 0.5 1 2 5 10
Favours IL2Ra   Favours placebo

Figure 51.2 Clinically diagnosed acute allograft rejection at 6 months and 1 year after transplantation: anti-CD25 versus placebo or no treatment. (From Webster *et al.* 2004 [59].)

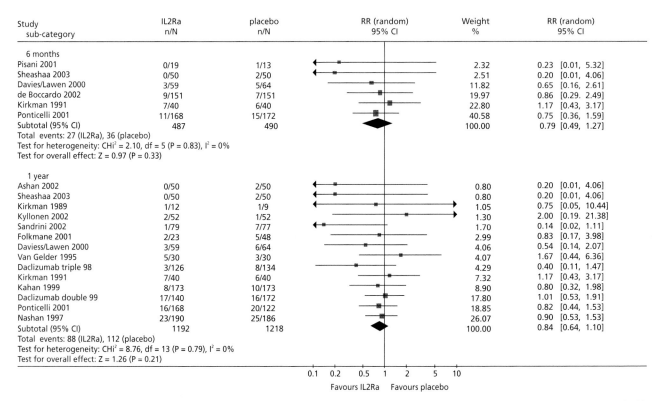

Study sub-category	IL2Ra n/N	placebo n/N	RR (random) 95% CI	Weight %	RR (random) 95% CI
6 months					
Pisani 2001	0/19	1/13		2.32	0.23 [0.01, 5.32]
Sheashaa 2003	0/50	2/50		2.51	0.20 [0.01, 4.06]
Davies/Lawen 2000	3/59	5/64		11.82	0.65 [0.16, 2.61]
de Boccardo 2002	9/151	7/151		19.97	0.86 [0.29, 2.49]
Kirkman 1991	7/40	6/40		22.80	1.17 [0.43, 3.17]
Ponticelli 2001	11/168	15/172		40.58	0.75 [0.36, 1.59]
Subtotal (95% CI)	487	490		100.00	0.79 [0.49, 1.27]
Total events: 27 (IL2Ra), 36 (placebo)					
Test for heterogeneity: CHi² = 2.10, df = 5 (P = 0.83), I² = 0%					
Test for overall effect: Z = 0.97 (P = 0.33)					
1 year					
Ashan 2002	0/50	2/50		0.80	0.20 [0.01, 4.06]
Sheashaa 2003	0/50	2/50		0.80	0.20 [0.01, 4.06]
Kirkman 1989	1/12	1/9		1.05	0.75 [0.05, 10.44]
Kyllonen 2002	2/52	1/52		1.30	2.00 [0.19, 21.38]
Sandrini 2002	1/79	7/77		1.70	0.14 [0.02, 1.11]
Folkmane 2001	2/23	5/48		2.99	0.83 [0.17, 3.98]
Daviess/Lawen 2000	3/59	6/64		4.06	0.54 [0.14, 2.07]
Van Gelder 1995	5/30	3/30		4.07	1.67 [0.44, 6.36]
Daclizumab triple 98	3/126	8/134		4.29	0.40 [0.11, 1.47]
Kirkman 1991	7/40	6/40		7.32	1.17 [0.43, 3.17]
Kahan 1999	8/173	10/173		8.90	0.80 [0.32, 1.98]
Daclizumab double 99	17/140	16/172		17.80	1.01 [0.53, 1.91]
Ponticelli 2001	16/168	20/122		18.85	0.82 [0.44, 1.53]
Nashan 1997	23/190	25/186		26.07	0.90 [0.53, 1.53]
Subtotal (95% CI)	1192	1218		100.00	0.84 [0.64, 1.10]
Total events: 88 (IL2Ra), 112 (placebo)					
Test for heterogeneity: CHi² = 8.76, df = 13 (P = 0.79), I² = 0%					
Test for overall effect: Z = 1.26 (P = 0.21)					

0.1 0.2 0.5 1 2 5 10
Favours IL2Ra   Favours placebo

Figure 51.3 Graft loss censored for death at 6 months and 1 year after transplantation, with anti-CD25 versus placebo or no treatment. (From Webster *et al.* 2004 [59].)

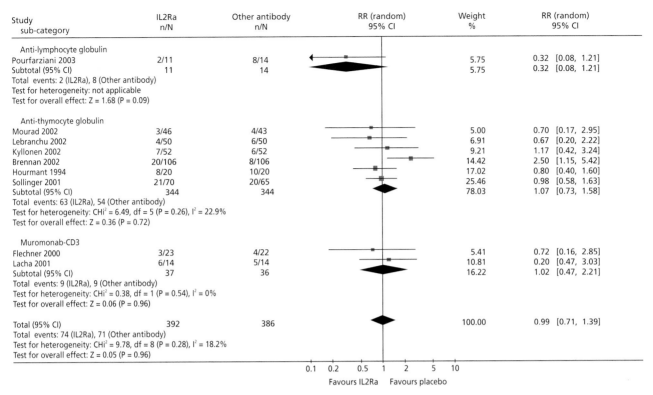

Study sub-category	IL2Ra n/N	Other antibody n/N	RR (random) 95% CI	Weight %	RR (random) 95% CI
Anti-lymphocyte globulin					
Pourfarziani 2003	2/11	8/14		5.75	0.32 [0.08, 1.21]
Subtotal (95% CI)	11	14		5.75	0.32 [0.08, 1.21]
Total events: 2 (IL2Ra), 8 (Other antibody)					
Test for heterogeneity: not applicable					
Test for overall effect: Z = 1.68 (P = 0.09)					
Anti-thymocyte globulin					
Mourad 2002	3/46	4/43		5.00	0.70 [0.17, 2.95]
Lebranchu 2002	4/50	6/50		6.91	0.67 [0.20, 2.22]
Kyllonen 2002	7/52	6/52		9.21	1.17 [0.42, 3.24]
Brennan 2002	20/106	8/106		14.42	2.50 [1.15, 5.42]
Hourmant 1994	8/20	10/20		17.02	0.80 [0.40, 1.60]
Sollinger 2001	21/70	20/65		25.46	0.98 [0.58, 1.63]
Subtotal (95% CI)	344	344		78.03	1.07 [0.73, 1.58]
Total events: 63 (IL2Ra), 54 (Other antibody)					
Test for heterogeneity: CHi² = 6.49, df = 5 (P = 0.26), I² = 22.9%					
Test for overall effect: Z = 0.36 (P = 0.72)					
Muromonab-CD3					
Flechner 2000	3/23	4/22		5.41	0.72 [0.16, 2.85]
Lacha 2001	6/14	5/14		10.81	0.20 [0.47, 3.03]
Subtotal (95% CI)	37	36		16.22	1.02 [0.47, 2.21]
Total events: 9 (IL2Ra), 9 (Other antibody)					
Test for heterogeneity: CHi² = 0.38, df = 1 (P = 0.54), I² = 0%					
Test for overall effect: Z = 0.06 (P = 0.96)					
Total (95% CI)	392	386		100.00	0.99 [0.71, 1.39]
Total events: 74 (IL2Ra), 71 (Other antibody)					
Test for heterogeneity: CHi² = 9.78, df = 8 (P = 0.28), I² = 18.2%					
Test for overall effect: Z = 0.05 (P = 0.96)					

0.1   0.2   0.5   1   2   5   10
Favours IL2Ra   Favours placebo

Figure 51.4 Clinically diagnosed acute allograft rejection at 6 months after transplantation: anti-CD25 versus other monoclonal or polyclonal antibodies, stratified by antibody class. (From Webster *et al.* 2004 [59].)

the pressing shortage of deceased donor organs has expanded the sources and criteria for donor acceptance [60–62]. Cadaver donors now frequently include the elderly and those with vascular disease, long-term insulin-dependent diabetes, hypertension, or other risk factors that may impair renal function [17]. Non-heart-

Table 51.2 Proposed strategies to prevent ischemia–reperfusion injury and DGF.

Recipient fluid management
- Volume expansion with colloid or crystalloid
- Mannitol or furosemide

Vasodilatory agents
- Calcium channel blockers
- Prostacyclin
- Atrial natriuretic peptide
- Selective and nonselective endothelin receptor antagonists

Antioxidants
- *N*-Acetylcysteine
- Propionyl-l-carnitine
- Inhibitors of inducible nitric oxide synthetase

Biological agents
- Monoclonal antibodies to ICAM-I, LFA-1, and tumor necsrosis factor-α
- CTLA4 fusion protein
- Insulin-like growth factor 1

Source: Adapted from Perico *et al.* 2004 [13].

beating cadaver donors are used in centers equipped for this service [17], and expanded-criteria living donors are now being accepted in an increasing number of centers. There is good evidence that expanded-criteria donors with an adequate pretransplant kidney biopsy should be utilized but that the risk of physiological injury to the transplanted organ is increased and the probability of delayed or impaired function is increased [13,63].

There is little evidence that recipient dialysis modalities confer different risks for DGF, although there are trends towards superior function in patients receiving peritoneal dialysis and inferior outcome in those on home nocturnal dialysis [64,65]. These studies need to be confirmed but have potential importance only in cases where transplantation is imminent. Similarly, although immunological sensitization increases the risk of DGF, there is no evidence that desensitization techniques reduce this probability. Minimization of warm and cold ischemia times are critical in reducing ischemia–reperfusion injury (Table 51.2), and retrospective studies suggest that pulsatile perfusion may significantly reduce the risks of DGF, but the benefit if any remains to be proven in appropriately designed prospective studies [66].

Posttransplant initiatives to minimize DGF have been reviewed by Perico *et al.* [13]. Recipient hypovolemia or hypotension can affect the early function of the graft, and intensive support with crystalloid, colloid, or dopamine may be required [18]. Mannitol given just prior to reperfusion may improve early function by virtue of its antioxidant properties, but whether furosemide enhances glomerular filtration or simply increases urine volume is

Table 51.3 Banff diagnostic categories for renal allograft biopsies, 2005 update. (Solez et al, Am J. Transplant, 7, 518–526, 2007, table 2)

1. Normal

2. Antbody-mediated rejection

Due to documented anti-donor antibody ('suspicious for' if antibody not demonstrated; (may coincide with categories 3–61)

Acute antibody-mediated rejection

Type (grade)

   i. ATN-like-C4d+, minimal inflammation

   ii. Capillary-margination and/or thromboses, C4d+

   iii. Arterial-v3, C4d+

Chronic active antibody-mediated rejection[1]

Glomerular double contours and/or particular capillary basement membrane multilsyering and/or interstitial fibrosis/tubular atrophy and/or fibrous intimal thickening in arteriea, C4d+

3. Borderline changes: 'suspicious' for acute T-cell-mediated rejection

The category is used when no intimal arteritis is present, but there are foci of tubultis It1, t2 or t3 with i0 or iIl although the t2 t2 threshold for rejection diagnosis is not met (may coincide with categories 2, 5 and 6)

4. T-cell-mediated rejection[1] (may coincide with categories 2, 5 and 6)

Acute T-cell-mediated rejection

Type (grade)

   IA. Cases with significant interstitial infliltration t > 25% of parendhyma affected, i2 or i3 and foci of moderate tubulitis (i2)

   IB. Cases with significant interstitial infiltration t > 25% of parenchyma affected, i2 or i3 and foci of severe tututlis (t3)

   IIA. Cases with mild to moderate intimal arteritis (v1)

   IIB. Cases with severe intimal arteritis comprising >25% of the lumical area (v2)

   III. Cases with 'transmural' arteritis and/or arterial fibrinoid change and necrosis of medial smooth muscle cells with accompanying hymphocytic inflammation (v3)

Chronic active T-cell-mediated rejection[1]

'Chronic alongraft arteriopathy' tarterial intimal fibrosis with mononuclear cell infiltration in fibrosis, formation of neo-intimal

5. Interstitial fibrosis and tubular atrophy, no evidence of any specific eticlogy[1]

Grade

   i. Mild interstitial fibrosis and tubular atrophy I < 25% of cortical areal

   ii. Moderate interstitial fibrosis and tubular atrophy 126–50% of cortical areal

   iii. Severe interstitial fibrosis and tubular atrophyloss I > 50% of cortical area)

(may include nor-specific vascular and glomerular aclerosis, but severity graded by tubulointerctitial features)

6. Other: Changes not considered to be due to rejection-acute and/or chronic the dagnosis given in Table 1); may coincide with categories 2–5

[1] Indicates changes in the updated Bani CE schema.

unclear. Randomized studies have shown that pretreatment of the donor or recipient with calcium channel blockers prior to grafting, or administration of these into the graft artery, may improve initial function. Evidence regarding the use of atrial natruretic peptide or its synthetic forms is conflicting, and additional studies are required. Similarly, although inhibition of free radical mediated injury by *N*-acetylcysteine or inhibitors of inducible nitric oxide synthetase is appealing, these approaches remain in the experimental domain [13]. Finally, neither modulation of key cell surface products, such as ICAM by enlimomab or of LFA-1 by odulimonab, or use of the growth factor insulin-like growth factor 1 have proven successful in this setting [13,67].

Two important changes in immunosuppression designed to optimize initial function include the increasing use of induction therapy and the transient or permanent avoidance of calcineurin inhibitors. These approaches are often employed in subjects at risk or in those with established graft dysfunction, although absolute evidence of benefit is still lacking. Small randomized studies have shown that the use of ATG is associated with improved early graft function [68], whereas the effect of anti-CD25 therapy remains uncertain, particularly since subjects at greatest risk of delayed function are often those at high immunological risk [13]. Calcineurin inhibitors may be withheld for the first 7–10 days [38,39,69] or replaced by nonnephrotoxic agents, such as mycophenolate mofetil or sirolimus [70]. Knight and colleagues suggested that the combination of ATG and sirolimus in high-risk patients and basiliximab and sirolimus in low-risk subjects is an effective combination for minimizing both DGF and acute rejection [71]. However, other reports indicate that sirolimus itself may cause direct renal tubular toxicity and promote or prolong delayed function of the graft, particularly when used in combination with a calcineurin inhibitor [72,73]. The most common therapeutic approach at present is therefore the use of an induction agent in combination with mycophenolate mofetil and the delayed introduction of a calcineurin inhibitor if this is to be employed for long-tern therapy until graft function is established.

Graft rejection

The Banff system (Table 51.3), first introduced in 1993 [74], provides a universal system for histological categorization of graft injury ranging from cellular infiltration to fibrosis and scarring, and attempts to incorporate new diagnostic and mechanistic understandings in order to provide a common framework for scientific and clinical evaluation. During the past decade, the focus has gradually shifted from cellular injury to mixed patterns or pure antibody-mediated rejection [20,21]. This is now recognized as perhaps the most important immunological threat to graft success [22,75–77] and is characterized by the combination of circulating donor-specific anti-HLA antibody, the deposition of C4d in the graft, and evidence of histologic injury and physiological dysfunction [22]. Innovations in management of graft rejection have been directed principally to the reversal and prevention of humoral injury.

Numerous treatments have been employed for graft rejection, depending on the time of presentation, clinical severity, histology, and comorbidity. Their efficacy may depend on the expression of antibody-mediated rejection across the spectrum from predominant cellular injury to mixed antibody-mediated rejection with high DSA titers to finally pure T-cell-poor antibody-mediated rejection [76]. For example, Banff type I tubulo-interstitial cellular injury within the first 6 months of transplant usually responds to intravenous steroids and increased maintenance immuno-suppression, whereas Banff type II transplant endarteritis that is C4d negative often requires antilymphocyte antibody treatment [76]. Mixed patterns with C4d deposition are most commonly treated with a full course of depleting antilymphocyte agents, such as ATG, which can clear both cellular and humoral components.

A meta-analysis by Webster and colleagues examined the use of polyclonal or monoclonal antibodies for treatment or graft rejection [78]. This analysis revealed a total of 21 trials in 49 reports, although only 2 of these were conducted within the last decade (Table 51.4). Most were small, incompletely reported especially for potential harm, and did not define outcome measures adequately (Table 51.5). Fourteen of these trials encompassing 965 patients compared therapies for first rejection episodes. Eight of these compared antilymphocyte antibodies against steroids, two against other antibodies, and four against other therapies. Meta-analysis indicated that antibody was superior to steroid in reversing rejection (RR, 0.57; CI, 0.38–0.87) and preventing graft loss (death-censored RR, 0.74; CI, 0.58–0.95) (Figures 51.5 and 51.6) but there was no difference in preventing subsequent rejection (RR, 0.67; CI, 0.43–1.04) or death (RR, 1.16; CI, 0.57–2.33) at 1 year. Seven trials encompassing 422 patients investigated treatment of steroid-resistant rejection. There was no benefit of Muromonab CD3 over ATG (Table 51.6) or ALG in reversing rejection (RR, 1.32; CI, 0.33–5.28) (Figure 51.7), preventing subsequent rejection (RR, 0.99; CI, 0.61–1.59), or preventing graft loss (RR, 1.80; CI, 0.29–11.23) or death (RR, 0.39; CI, 0.09–1.65). However, Sun and colleagues have shown that mixed cellular and antibody-mediated rejection with circulating DSA and C4d deposition can also be reversed by intravenous steroids followed by conversion from cyclosporine to tacrolimus, or by an increase in the tacrolimus dose for those already on this medication, without ATG use [79]. More stringent studies are therefore required in this field.

The treatment of predominantly antibody-mediated rejection episodes with high-titer DSA and positive C4d, typically recognized as "pure or dominant antibody-mediated rejection" and associated with rapid deterioration in graft function, is extremely challenging. It increasingly incorporates the use of antibody removal with plasmapheresis and inhibition of new antibody formation via the use of IVIG acting through the Fc feedback loop [80,81]. Anti-CD20 (rituximab) monoclonal antibody may be used simultaneously to inhibit antibody formation systemically or within the graft [81], although few randomized studies are available to demonstrate the utility and safety of these procedures and no systematic or meta-analyses have thus far been published.

The AHG-CDC assay currently used to measure recipient sensitization and to define antibody specificity [22,82] lacks sensitivity, and the flow cytometry cross-match (FCXM) assay [83], which is more sensitive for detecting low levels of antilymphocyte antibodies [83–88], is widely employed as a key measure of sensitization. A

positive FCXM has been proposed as a valid rationale to withhold transplantation, to augment immunosuppression, or to employ innovative strategies to reduce sensitization [22,82,89], but the prognostic value remains unclear [82]. Many reports have suggested that recipients with a positive FCXM, especially those at high immunological risk, experienced a greater incidence of acute rejection and early graft loss [20,90–93]. In contrast, other studies have shown negative results or indicated little incremental advantage of FCXM in terms of reducing acute rejection episodes and graft loss [20,94–96]. Prospective and blinded evaluation shows that the FCXM has little independent incremental predictive value compared with AHG-CDC, and positive and negative post-test probabilities for acute rejection or graft loss are low [97], perhaps reflecting the recognized lack of analytical specificity. Newer high-resolution solid-phase technologies using HLA antigens bound to microparticles offer both specificity and sensitivity [98] and may be a superior tool for both pretransplant screening and posttransplant monitoring [99].

Two principal methods have been employed for reducing DSA pre- or posttransplant, but comparison is difficult because of differences in diagnostic methodologies, degrees of sensitization, and patient risk factors [100]. The first employs high-dose IVIG to treat patients previously screened for responsiveness using an *in vitro* CDC assay with a panel of normal controls under conditions resembling those of the normal cross-match [101]. Patients in a randomized prospective placebo controlled study received 2 g/kg IVIG (or placebo) monthly for 4 months pretransplant and for a further 4 months after transplant. Panel reactive antibocties (PRA) levels declined by approximately 20% in the IVIG group by 4 months of treatment ($P = 0.0007$) and rose slowly thereafter to prior levels. The number of patients who could be transplanted was twice as high in the IVIG group ($P = 0.048$), time to transplant was significantly shortened ($P = 0.049$), and the number of repeat transplants performed was also increased. Graft failure occurred in 25% of IVIG recipients compared with 38% of controls, although the incidence of acute rejection was higher in the IVIG group ($P = 0.042$) [101]. Side effects were few and not sustained.

The second protocol employs four daily plasmapheresis sessions with low-dose IVIG for antibody reduction, often with rituximab [102]. In the comparative study, anti-HLA antibodies were determined by AHG-CDC, FCXM, and solid-phase single-antigen assays. The success of desensitization correlated with the baseline antibody level in each group: all patients with PRA titers of <1:4 had a negative cross-match compared with either protocols, while only 10% of those with titers of >1:32 achieved a negative cross-match. Overall, 38% of those receiving high-dose IVIG achieved a negative cross-match but 80% had acute rejection, whereas 84–88% of those receiving plasmapheresis and low-dose IVIG achieved a negative cross-match and 29–37% experienced rejection [102]. At the present time, it therefore appears that desensitization is possible in patients with antibody titers of <1:16 and that a combination of IVIG and plasma exchange achieves

Table 51.4 Use of antibodies for treatment of graft rejection: characteristics of patients, randomized treatments, and baseline immunosuppressive therapy.

Trial name	Antibody intervention (dose, duration)	Randomized comparator (dose, duration)	n	% Deceased donor	% 1st transplant	Background immunosuppression (initial; maintenance dose)	Follow-up (months)
Trials of antibodies for treatment of first rejection episode							
Antibody vs. steroid							
Sheild 1979	ATG (15 mg/kg, 14 days)	MP (1 g/day, 5 days)	20	0	ns	Aza (2–3 mg/kg/day), Pred (2 mg/kg/day; 10–20)	26
Filo 1980	ATG (10 mg/kg, 15 days), irradiation (450 rada)	Pred (15 mg/kg/day, 10 days), irradiation (450 rads)	114	100	100	Aza (2 mg/kg/day), MP (30 mg/kg; 0.5 mg/kg)	36
Hoitsma 1982	ATG (2–7 mg/kg, 21 days)	Pred (200, 30-day taper)	40	100	85	Aza (1.5–3 mg/kg/day), Pred (100; 25)	6
Glass 1983	ALG (30 mg/kg, 14 days) or ATG (15 mg/kg, 14 days)	Pred (3 mg/kg, 21 days)	62	NS	NS	Aza (150), Pred (30–120; 30)	12
Streem 1983	ALG (15–20 mg/kg, 10 days)	MP (1 g/day, 6 days)	23	100	100	ALG (15–30 mg/kg/day, 14 days, Aza (1.5–2 mg/kg/day), Pred (intervention 30, control 2 mg/kg/day)	20
Goldstein 1985	Muromonab CD3 (5 mg/day, 14 days)	MP (500 mg/day, 3 days)	123	100	87	Aza (100–150), Pred (2 mg/kg/day; 0.5 mg/kg/day)	24
Hilbrands 1996	ATG (100 mg/dY, 10 days)	MP (1 g/day, 3 days)	26	100	100	Cy (NS), Pred (NS)	>16
Theodorakis 1998	ATG (4 mg/kg, 7 days)	MP (750 mg/day, 3 days)	50	100	ns	Cy (50–150), MP (4–8 mg/day; attempt withdrawal)	48
Antibody and steroid vs. steroid alone							
Birkeland 1975	ALG (20 mg/kg, 21 days), Pred (30 mg/kg, 10 days)	Pred (30 mg/kg, 10 days)	30	NS	NS	Aza (0–3 mg/kg/day), Pred (50; 10)	77
Antibody vs. other antibody							
Baldi 2000	Muromonab CD3 (5 mg/day, 10 days)	ATG (4 mg/kg, 10 days)	56	NS	NS	ALG (1 mL/kg, 14days), Cy (8–10 mg/kg/day; NS), Aza (1 mg.kg), Pred (0.7 mg/kg, 0.1 mg/kg)	127
Waid 1992	Muromonab CD3 (5 mg/day, 7 days) then Cy (200)	T10B9.1A31 (12 mg/day, 7 days) then Cy (200)	178	NS	37	Aza (1.5–2 mg/kg/d) Pred (60; 30)	48
Formulation comparisons							
Johnson 1989	ATS rabbit (NS)	ATG horse (NS)	128	NS	NS	NS	12

Study	Treatment 1	Treatment 2				Concomitant therapy	
Antibody vs. other treatment							
Hourmant 1985	ALG (NS)	Cy (250–700), Pred (5 mg/kg/day, 5 days)	58	92	97	ALG (NS, 21 days), Aza (2–3 mg/kg/day), Pred (60; 15)	18
Howard 1977	ALG (20 mg/day, 10 days), radiation (150 rads)	IVIG (20 mg/dy, 10 days), radiation (150 rads)	57	39	100	Aza (NS), Pred (2 mg/kg/day; 0.5 mg/kg/day)	
Trials of treatment of resistant acute rejection							
Hesse 1990	Muromonab CD3 (5 mg/day, 10 days)	ALG (0.5 mL/kg, 10 days)	60	NS	NS	ALG (0.5 mL/kg, 2–7 days), Aza (1–3 mg/kg/day, 2–7 days), then Cy (300–400; 300–400), Pred (100; 7.5)	
Barenbrock 1994	Muromonab CD3 (5 mg/day, 10 days)	ATG (5 mg/kg, 10 days)	38	100	NS	Cy (5–10 mg/kg/day), Aza (150), Pred (100; 20)	
Mariat 1998	Muromonab CD3 (5 mg/day, 10 days)	ATG (1.5 mg/kg/day, 10 days)	60	NS	93	Cy (NS; NS), Aza (NS), Pred (NS)	
Midtvedt 2003	Muromonab CD3 (2.5 mg/kg, as per T-cell count, 10 days)	ATG (1–2 mg/kg, as per T-cell count, 10 days)	55	58	NS	Cy (140–300;70–150), Aza (NS), Pred (80;10)	
Different formulations of antibody							
Gaber 1998	ATG rabbit (1.5 mg/kg/day, 7–10 days)	ATG horse (15 mg/kg/day, 7–10 days)	163	66	94	Cy (NS), Aza (NS), Pred (NS)	
Different doses of same antibody							
Midvedt 1996	Muromonab CD3 (2.5 mg/day, 10 days)	Muromonab CD3 (5 mg/day, 10 days)	23	65	100	Cy (140–300; 140–300), Aza (NS), Pred (NS)	
Antibody vs. other treatment							
Casadei 1998	Muromonab-CD3 (5 mg/day, 14 days)	IVIG (500 mg/kg/day, 7 days)	23	65	100	Cy (400; 150–200), Aza (2 mg/kg/day), Pred (1.5 mg/kg/day; 0.1 mg/kg/day)	

Source: Webster *et al.* 2004 [59].

Abbreviations: NS, not stated; ATG, antithymocyte globulin; ATS, antithymocyte serum; ALG, antilymphocyte globulin; MP, methylprednisone; Pred, oral prednisolone in milligrams per day unless otherwise stated; Cy, cyclosporine 12 h post-dose nadir blood level, in nanograms per milliliter unless otherwise stated; Aza, azathioprine (in milligrams per day) unless otherwise stated

Table 51.5 Summary of relative effects of antibody versus steroid alone for treatment of first rejection episode stratified by antibody comparator, within 12 months of treatment.

Outcome	No. of trials	No. of participants	Relative risk (95% confidence interval)[a]	Heterogeneity	
				P[b]	I^2 (%)
Failure of rejection reversal	6	334	0.57 (0.38–0.87)	0.234	11.7
Muromonab CD3	1	120	0.31 (0.14–0.68)		
ATG	3	139	0.50 (0.26–0.96)	0.94	0
ALG	2	85	0.96 (0.52–1.75)	0.71	0
Further treatment required	3	83	0.59 (0.27–1.29)	0.72	0
ATG	2	60	0.64 (0.29–1.43)	0.69	0
ALG	1	23	0.59 (0.27–1.29)		
Graft loss or death with functioning graft	7	380	0.82 (0.67–1.00)	0.84	0
Muromonab CD3	1	120	0.84 (0.65–1.10)		
ATG	3	155	0.71 (0.48–1.04)	0.76	0
ALG	2	85	0.93 (0.56–1.54)	0.52	0
Death	6	318	1.16 (0.57–2.33)	0.78	0
Muromonab CD3	1	120	1.40 (0.53–3.70)		
ATG	3	113	0.73 (0.12–4.43)	0.48	0
ALG	2	85	1.05 (0.31–3.60)	0.46	0
Infection as cause of death	3	164	0.74 (0.21–2.63)	0.83	0
Infection (all cause)	4	206	0.88 (0.59–1.31)	0.14	44.8
Muromonab CD3	1	123	1.05 (0.82–1.35)		
ATG	20	6	1.46 (0.11–18.53)	0.07	70.1
ALG	1	23	0.82 (0.42–1.60)		
CMV infection	3	83	0.65 (0.09–4.71)	0.17	47.8
ATG	2	60	1.25 (0.39–3.99)		
ALG	1	13	0.15 (0.01–2.70)		
Fever, chills, malaise following drug administration	3	185	45.97 (9.31–227.09)	0.29	18.8
Muromonab CD3	1	125	91.55 (5.77–1453.49)		
ATG	2	60	23.00 (3.27–161.87)	0.27	18.1

Source: Webster *et al.* 2004 [59].

[a] Relative risk values of <1 favor treatment with antibody.

[b] P value for Cochran Q ?[2] test for heterogeneity.

this most effectively and may enable transplantation for patients otherwise denied this treatment.

Conclusion

A growing evidence base is now available to guide the management of patients during the critical first 3 months posttransplant. However, the numerous therapeutic options, treatment combinations, and dosing regimens remain challenging for clinicians, and the relatively limited number of high-quality and appropriately powered randomized and blinded clinical trials do not provide adequate evidence for all key decisions.

It now appears apparent that biologic induction immunosuppression increases the freedom from acute rejection and is increasingly employed for this purpose, particularly in North America. Selection between polyclonal and monoclonal agents remains difficult but may be determined by safety and side effects. In general, for patients at low immunological risk, anti-CD25 antibodies offer an equivalent reduction in rejection risk to ATG but with a lower incidence of infection and adverse effects. Although the evidence is not clear for patients at high immunological risk, most centers will select ATG in preference to anti-CD25 agents for these subjects in order to maximize immunosuppression.

DGF remains problematic, particularly in sensitized recipients of grafts from extended criteria donors. In this setting, evidence suggests that biologic induction with delay in introduction of calcineurin inhibitors offers the greatest opportunity for early establishment of function, although the evidence base is not adequate to support this with a high degree of confidence. New approaches in which potent biological induction with depleting antibodies are

Study or sub-category	Antibody n/N	steroid n/N	RR (random) 95% CI	Weight %	RR (random) 95% CI
muromonab-CD3 versus steroid					
Goldstein 1985	38/58	33/45		24.47	0.89 [0.69, 1.15]
Subtotal (95% CI)	58	45		24.47	0.89 [0.69, 1.15]
Total events: 38 (Antibody), 33 (steroid)					
Test for heterogeneity: not applicable					
Test for overall effect: Z = 0.86 (P = 0.39)					
ATG v steroid					
Shield 1979	1/10	5/10		4.20	0.20 [0.03, 1.42]
Hibrands 1996	3/19	8/17		9.34	0.34 [0.20, 1.06]
Hoitsma 1982	6/20	6/20		11.86	1.00 [0.39, 2.58]
Theodorakis 1998	4/25	18/25		12.09	0.22 [0.09, 0.56]
Filo 1980	16/36	15/43		18.83	1.27 [0.74, 1.20]
Subtotal (95% CI)	110	115		56.32	0.52 [0.22, 1.21]
Total events: 30 (Antibody), 52 (steroid)					
Test for heterogeneity: CHi² = 14.77, df = 4 (P = 0.005), I² = 72.9%					
Test for overall effect: Z = 1.52 (P = 0.13)					
ALG v steroid					
Glass 1983	2/35	2/27		4.44	0.77 [0.12, 5.13]
Streem 1983	5/11	9/12		14.77	0.68 [0.32, 1.46]
Subtotal (95% CI)	46	39		19.21	0.69 [0.34, 1.41]
Total events: 7 (Antibody), 10 (steroid)					
Test for heterogeneity: CHi² = 0.02, df = 1 (P = 0.90), I² = 0%					
Test for overall effect: Z = 1.02 (P = 0.31)					
Total (95% CI)	214	199		100.00	0.67 [0.43, 1.04]
Total events: 75 (Antibody), 95 (steroid)					
Test for heterogeneity: CHi² = 16.58, df = 7 (P = 0.02), I² = 57.8%					
Test for overall effect: Z = 1.80 (P = 0.07)					

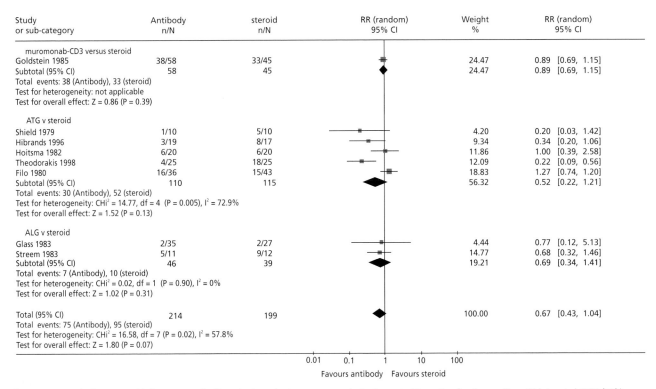

0.01 0.1 1 10 100
Favours antibody   Favours steroid

Figure 51.5 Antibodies vs. steroids for treatment for first rejection episodes: recurrence of rejection up to 12 months after therapy. (From Webster *et al.* 2004 [59].)

Study or sub-category	Antibody n/N	steroid n/N	RR (random) 95% CI	Weight %	RR (random) 95% CI
muromonab-CD3 versus steroid					
Goldstein 1985	28/62	33/58		49.84	0.75 [0.53, 1.06]
Subtotal (95% CI)	62	58		49.84	0.75 [0.53, 1.06]
Total events: 28 (antibody), 35 (steroid)					
Test for heterogeneity: not applicable					
Test for overall effect: Z = 1.65 (P = 0.10)					
ATG v versus steroid					
Shield 1979	1/10	0/10		0.62	3.00 [0.14, 65.90]
Hibrands 1996	3/19	6/17		3.97	0.45 [0.13, 1.52]
Hoitsma 1982	6/20	6/20		6.60	1.00 [0.39, 2.58]
Filo 1980	14/36	25/43		25.51	0.67 [0.41, 1.08]
Subtotal (95% CI)	85	90		36.70	0.71 [0.47, 1.06]
Total events: 24 (antibody), 37 (steroid)					
Test for heterogeneity: CHi² = 1.95, df = 3 (P = 0.58), I² = 0%					
Test for overall effect: Z = 1.70 (P = 0.09)					
ALG versus steroid					
Streem 1983	1/11	2/12		1.16	0.55 [0.06, 5.21]
Glass 1983	11/35	10/27		12.30	0.85 [0.42, 1.70]
Subtotal (95% CI)	46	39		13.46	0.82 [0.42, 1.59]
Total events: 12 (antibody), 12 (steroid)					
Test for heterogeneity: CHi² = 0.14, df = 1 (P = 0.71), I² = 0%					
Test for overall effect: Z = 0.60 (P = 0.55)					
Total (95% CI)	193	187		100.00	0.74 [0.58, 0.95]
Total events: 64 (antibody), 84 (steroid)					
Test for heterogeneity: CHi² = 2.22, df = 6 (P = 0.90), I² = 0%					
Test for overall effect: Z = 2.41 (P = 0.02)					

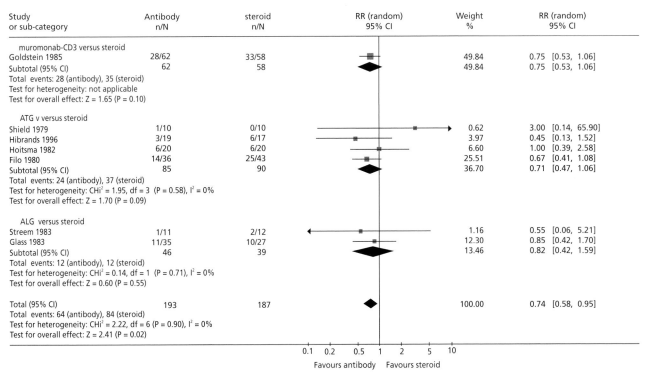

0.1 0.2 0.5 1 2 5 10
Favours antibody   Favours steroid

Figure 51.6 Antibodies vs. steroids for treatment for first rejection episodes: graft loss (censored for death with a functioning graft) within 18 months after therapy. (From Webster *et al.* 2004 [59].)

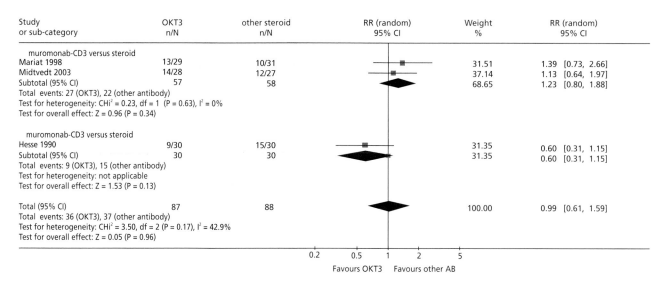

Figure 51.7 Treatment of acute steroid-resistant rejection with Muromonab versus other antibodies: recurrent rejection up to 12 months posttreatment. (From Webster *et al.* 2004 [59].)

used to permit the complete elimination of calcineurin inhibitors may provide an option to optimize early and long-term graft function, but such studies are still under way.

The incidence of classical acute rejection is declining with improved immunosuppression, and such rejection responds promptly to simple therapy with steroids or to secondary treatment with ATG. Strategies to reduce pretransplant sensitization to donor HLA antigens and to avoid the risk of hyperacute or accelerated rejection permit transplantation in settings previously considered impossible. The risks of severe antibody-mediated rejection following transplantation remain high in this setting, however, and may be treated with the same techniques of biological immunosuppression, intravenous immunoglobulin and plasmapheresis. The availability of new monoclonals directed at the B lymphocyte may play an important role in this setting and further reduce the risks of antibody-mediated rejection, which is currently one of the most important immunological barriers to successful transplantation.

Table 51.6 Summary of relative effects of Muromonab versus other antibodies for treatment of resistant rejection, within 12 months of treatment.

| Outcome | No of trials | No. of participants | Relative risk (95% confidence interval)[a] | Heterogeneity | |
				P[b]	I^2 %
Failure of acute rejection reversal	3	136	1.32 (0.33, 5.28)	0.35	5.4
Graft loss (death censored)	3	136	1.80 (0.29, 11.12)	0.17	43.6
Graft loss or death with a functioning graft	3	136	1.08 (0.38, 3.10)	0.26	26.3
Death	3	175	0.39 (0.09, 1.65)	0.97	0
Infection as a cause of death	2	76	0.68 (0.17, 2.65)	0.77	0
CMV	3	175	0.88 (0.60, 1.28)	0.51	0
Malignancy	2	115	2.09 (0.28, 15.66)	0.40	0
Fever , chills, malaise following drug administration	2	81	3.21 (1.34, 7.70)		
Serum creatinine (μmol/L)	3	120	10.04[c] (−16.68, 36.77)	0.35	4.6

Source: Webster *et al.* 2004 [59].

[a] Relative risk values of <1 (or WMD of <0) favor treatment with Muromonab CD3.

[b] *P* value for Cochran Q ?^{2} test for heterogeneity.

[c] Value for serum creatinine is the weighted mean difference (and confidence interval).

References

1 Australia and New Zealand Dialysis and Transplant Registry A. ANZ-DATA Registry Report 2006. Australia and New Zealand Dialysis and Transplant Registry, Adelaide, South Australia, 2006.

2 US Renal Data System. Annual Data Report: Atlas of End-Stage Renal Disease in the United States. National Institutes of Health, National Institute of Diabetes and Digestive and Kidney Diseases, Bethesda, 2006.

3 Canadian Organ Replacement Register. Treatment of End-Sage Organ Failure in Canada 1995 to 2004. Canadian Institute for Health Information, Ottawa, Ontario, 2006.

4 Van Dijk P. Renal replacement therapy in Europe. The results of a collaborative effort by the ERA-EDTA and six national or regional registries. *Nephrol Dial Transplant* 2001; **16:** 1120–1129.

5 Yang H. Maintenance immunosuppression regimens: conversion, minimization, withdrawal, and avoidance. *Am J Kidney Dis* 2006; **47(4 Suppl 2):** S37–S51.

6 Gaston R. Current and evolving immunosuppressive regimens in kidney transplantation. *Am J Kidney Dis* 2006; **47:** S3–21.

7 Zand M. Immunosuppression and immune monitoring after renal transplantation. *Semin Dial* 2005; **18:** 511–519.

8 Keown P, Balshaw R, Khorasheh S, Chong M, Marra C, Kalo Z et al. Meta-analysis of basiliximab for immunoprophylaxis in renal transplantation. *BioDrugs* 2003; **17:** 271–279.

9 Yao G, Albon E, Adi Y, Milford D, Bayliss S, Ready A et al. A systematic review and economic model of the clinical and cost-effectiveness of immunosuppressive therapy for renal transplantation in children. *Health Technol Assess* 2006; **10(49):** 1–157.

10 Winkelmayer W, Weinstein M, Mittleman M, Glynn RJ, Pliskin JS. Health economic evaluations: the special case of end-stage renal disease treatment. *Med Decis Making* 2002; **22:** 417–430.

11 Parasuraman R, Yee J, Karthikeyan V, del Busto R. Infectious complications in renal transplant recipients. *Adv Chronic Kidney Dis* 2006; **13:** 280–294.

12 Kirk A. Induction immunosuppression. *Transplantation* 2006; **82:** 593–602.

13 Perico N, Cattaneo D, Sayegh M, Remuzzi G. Delayed graft function in kidney transplantation. *Lancet* 2004; **364:** 1814–1827.

14 Shackleton C, Keown P, McLoughlin MG, Scudamore CH, Schechter MT, Cameron EC et al. The quality of initial function following renal transplantation determined by creatinine elimination kinetics. Comparison of Minnesota antilymphocyte globulin and cyclosporine induction immunosuppression. *Transplantation* 1991; **52:** 1008–1013.

15 European Expert Group on Renal Transplantation E. European Best Practice guidelines for renal transplantation (part 1). Section III: the transplant recipient from initial transplant hospitalization to 1 year post transplant. *Nephrol Dial Transplant* 2000; **15:** 52–85.

16 Solez K, Colvin R, Racusen L, Sis B, Halloran PF, Birk PE et al. Banff '05 Meeting Report: differential diagnosis of chronic allograft injury and elimination of chronic allograft nephropathy ("CAN"). *Am J Transplant* 2007; **7:** 518–526.

17 European Expert Group on Renal Transplantation E. European Best Practice guidelines for renal transplantation (part 1). Section II: evaluation and selection of donors. *Nephrol Dial Transplant* 2000; **15:** 39–51.

18 Schnuelle P, Johannes van der Woude F. Perioperative fluid management in renal transplantation: a narrative review of the literature. *Transplant Int* 2006; **19:** 947–959.

19 Kalble T, Lucan M, Nicita G, Sells R, Burgos Revilla FJ, Wiesel M et al. EAU guidelines on renal transplantation. *Eur Urol* 2005; **47:** 156–166.

20 Racusen L, Colvin R, Solez K, Mihatsch MJ, Halloran PF, Campbell PM et al. Antibody-mediated rejection criteria: an addition to the Banff 97 classification of renal allograft rejection. *Am J Transplant* 2003; **3:** 708–714.

21 Racusen L, Halloran P, Solez K. Banff 2003 meeting report: new diagnostic insights and standards. *Am J Transplant* 2004; **4:** 1562–1566.

22 Takemoto S, Zeevi A, Feng S, Colvin RB, Jordan S, Kobashigawa J et al. National conference to assess antibody-mediated rejection in solid organ transplantation. *Am J Transplant* 2004; **4:** 1033–1041.

23 Racusen L, Solez K, Colvin R, Bonsib SM, Castro MC, Cavallo T et al. The Banff 97 working classification of renal allograft pathology. *Kidney Int* 1999; **55:** 713–723.

24 Kasiske B, Vazquez M, Harmon W, Brown RS, Danovitch GM, Gaston RS et al. Recommendations for the outpatient surveillance of renal transplant recipients. American Society of Transplantation. *J Am Soc Nephrol* 2000; **11:** S1–S86.

25 European Expert Group on Renal Transplantation E. European Best Practice guidelines for renal transplantation. Section IV: long-term management of the transplant recipient. IV.2.1. Differential diagnosis of chronic graft dysfunction. *Nephrol Dial Transplant* 2002; **17:** 4–8.

26 Hardinger K. Rabbit antithymocyte globulin induction therapy in adult renal transplantation. *Pharmacotherapy* 2006; **26:** 1771–1783.

27 Chapman T, Keating G. Basiliximab: a review of its use as induction therapy in renal transplantation. *Drugs* 2003; **63:** 2803–2835.

28 Nashan B. Antibody induction therapy in renal transplant patients receiving calcineurin-inhibitor immunosuppressive regimens: a comparative review. *BioDrugs* 2005; **19:** 39–46.

29 Kasiske B, Johnson H, Goerdt P, Heim-Duthoy KL, Rao VK, Dahl DC et al. A randomized trial comparing cyclosporine induction with sequential therapy in renal transplant recipients. *Am J Kidney Dis* 1997; **30:** 639–645.

30 Cherikh W, Kauffman H, McBride M, Maghirang J, Swinnen LJ, Hanto DW. Association of the type of induction immunosuppression with posttransplant lymphoproliferative disorder, graft survival, and patient survival after primary kidney transplantation. *Transplantation* 2003; **76:** 1289–1292.

31 Bunnapradist S, Takemoto S. Multivariate analyses of antibody induction therapies. *Clin Transplant* 2003; **2003:** 405–417.

32 Bunnapradist S, Daswani A, Takemoto S. Patterns of administration of antibody induction therapy and their associated outcomes. *Clin Transplant* 2002; **2002:** 351–358.

33 Nashan B. Antibody induction therapy in renal transplant patients receiving calcineurin-inhibitor immunosuppressive regimens: a comparative review. *BioDrugs* 2005; **19:** 39–46.

34 Lopez M, Clarkson M, Albin M, Sayegh MH, Najafian N. A novel mechanism of action for anti-thymocyte globulin: induction of $CD4^+CD25^+Foxp3^+$ regulatory T cells. *J Am Soc Nephrol* 2006; **17:** 2844–2853.

35 Dubey S, Nityanand S. Involvement of Fas and TNF pathways in the induction of apoptosis of T cells by antithymocyte globulin. *Ann Hematol* 2003; **82:** 496–499.

36 Simon T, Opelz G, Weimer R, Feustel A, Ott RC, Susal C. The effect of ATG on cytokine and cytotoxic T-lymphocyte gene expression in renal allograft recipients during the early post-transplant period. *Clin Transplant* 2003; **17:** 217–224.

37 Brennan D, Flavin K, Lowell J, Howark TK, Shenoy S, Burgess S *et al.* A randomized, double-blinded comparison of Thymoglobulin versus Atgam for induction immunosuppressive therapy in adult renal transplant recipients. *Transplantation* 1999; **67**: 1011–1018.

38 Mourad G, Garrigue V, Squifflet J, Besse T, Berthoux F, Alamartine E *et al.* Induction versus noninduction in renal transplant recipients with tacrolimus-based immunosuppression. *Transplantation* 2001; **72**: 1050–1055.

39 Charpentier B, Rostaing L, Berthoux F, Lang P, Civati G, Touraine JL *et al.* A three-arm study comparing immediate tacrolimus therapy with antithymocyte globulin induction therapy followed by tacrolimus or cyclosporine A in adult renal transplant recipients. *Transplantation* 2003; **75**: 844–851.

40 Benfield M, Tejani A, Harmon W, McDonald R, Stablein DM, McIntosh M *et al.* A randomized multicenter trial of OKT3 mAbs induction compared with intravenous cyclosporine in pediatric renal transplantation *Pediatr Transplant* 2005; **9**: 282–292.

41 Vincenti F. A drug of the past, a lesson for the future. *Pediatr Transplant* 2005; **9**: 267–268.

42 Opelz G. Efficacy of rejection prophylaxis with OKT3 in renal transplantation. Collaborative Transplant Study. *Transplantation* 1995; **60**: 1220–1224.

43 Caillard S, Dharnidharka V, Agodoa L, Bohen E, Abbott K. Posttransplant lymphoproliferative disorders after renal transplantation in the United States in era of modern immunosuppression. *Transplantation* 2005; **80**: 1233–1243.

44 Bustami R, Ojo A, Wolfe R, Merion RM, Bennett WM, McDiarmid SV *et al.* Immunosuppression and the risk of post-transplant malignancy among cadaveric first kidney transplant recipients. *Am J Transplant* 2004; **4**: 87–93.

45 Kaufman D, Shapiro R, Lucey M, Cherikh WS, Bustami R, Dyke DB. Immunosuppression: practice and trends. *Am J Transplant* 2004; **4**: 38–53.

46 USOPTN. 2004 annual report of the US Organ Procurement and Transplantation Network and the Scientific Registry of Transplant Recipients: Transplant Data 1994-2003. Department of Health and Human Services, Health Resources and Services Administration, Healthcare Systems Bureau, Division of Transplantation, Rockville, MD, 2005

47 Hardinger K. Rabbit antithymocyte globulin induction therapy in adult renal transplantation. *Pharmacotherapy* 2006; **26**: 1771–1783.

48 Norman D, Vincenti F, de Mattos A, Barry JM, Levitt DJ, Wedel NI *et al.* Phase I trial of HuM291, a humanized anti-CD3 antibody, in patients receiving renal allografts from living donors. *Transplantation* 2000; **70**: 1707–1712.

49 Morris P, Russell N. Alemtuzumab (Campath-¹H): a systematic review in organ transplantation. *Transplantation* 2006; **81**: 1361–1367.

50 Tan H, Kaczorowski D, Basu A, Unruh M, McCauley J, Wu C *et al.* Living donor renal transplantation using alemtuzumab induction and tacrolimus monotherapy. *Am J Transplant* 2006; **6**: 2409–2417.

51 Ciancio G, Burke G, Gaynor J, Mattiazzi A, Roohipour R, Carreno MR *et al.* The use of Campath-1H as induction therapy in renal transplantation: preliminary results. *Transplantation* 2004; **78**: 426–433.

52 Magliocca J, Knechtle S. The evolving role of alemtuzumab (Campath-1H) for immunosuppressive therapy in organ transplantation. *Transplant Int* 2006; **19**: 705–714.

53 Barth R, Janus C, Lillesand C, Radke NA, Pirsch JD, Becker BN *et al.* Outcomes at 3 years of a prospective pilot study of Campath-1H and sirolimus immunosuppression for renal transplantation. *Transplant Int* 2006; **19**: 885–892.

54 Kaufman D, Leventhal J, Axelrod D, Gallon LG, Stuart FP. Alemtuzumab induction and prednisone-free maintenance immunotherapy in kidney transplantation: comparison with basiliximab induction–long-term results. *Am J Transplant* 2005; **5**: 2539–2548.

55 Watson C, Bradley J, Friend P, Firth T, Taylor CJ, Bradley JR *et al.* Alemtuzumab (CAMPATH 1H) induction therapy in cadaveric kidney transplantation: efficacy and safety at five years. *Am J Transplant* 2005; **5**: 1347–1353.

56 Vathsala A, Ona E, Tan S, Suresh S, Lou HX, Casacola CB *et al.* Randomized trial of Alemtuzumab for prevention of graft rejection and preservation of renal function after kidney transplantation. *Transplantation* 2005; **80**: 765–774.

57 Ciancio G, Burke G, Gaynor J, Carreno MR, Cirocco RE, Mathew JM *et al.* A randomized trial of three renal transplant induction antibodies: early comparison of tacrolimus, mycophenolate mofetil, and steroid dosing, and newer immune-monitoring. *Transplantation* 2005; **80**: 457–465.

58 Adu D, Cockwell P, Ives N, Shaw J, Wheatley K. Interleukin-2 receptor monoclonal antibodies in renal transplantation: meta-analysis of randomised trials. *BMJ* 2003; **326(7393)**: 789.

59 Webster A, Playford E, Higgins G, Chapman JR, Craig JC. Interleukin 2 receptor antagonists for renal transplant recipients: a meta-analysis of randomized trials. *Transplantation* 2004; **77**: 166–176.

60 Andreoni K, Brayman K, Guidinger M, Sommers CM, Sung RS. Kidney and pancreas transplantation in the United States, 1996-2005. *Am J Transplant* 2007; **7**: 1359–1375.

61 O'Connor K, Delmonico F. Increasing the supply of kidneys for transplantation. *Semin Dial* 2005; **18**: 460–462.

62 Delmonico F, Sheehy E, Marks WH, Baliga P, McGowan JJ, Magee JC. Organ donation and utilization in the United States, 2004. *Am J Transplant* 2005; **5**: 862–873.

63 Perico N, Ruggenenti P, Scalamogna M, Remuzzi G. Tackling the shortage of donor kidneys: how to use the best that we have. *Am J Nephrol* 2003; **23**: 245–259.

64 Snyder J, Kasiske B, Gilbertson D, Collins AJ. A comparison of transplant outcomes in peritoneal and hemodialysis patients. *Kidney Int* 2002; **62**: 1423–1430.

65 McCormick B, Pierratos A, Fenton S, Jain V, Zaltzman J, Chan CT. Review of clinical outcomes in nocturnal haemodialysis patients after renal transplantation. *Nephrol Dial Transplant* 2004; **19**: 714–719.

66 Matsuoka L, Shah T, Aswad S, Bunnapradist S, Cho Y, Mendez RG *et al.* Pulsatile perfusion reduces the incidence of delayed graft function in expanded criteria donor kidney transplantation. *Am J Transplant* 2006; **6**: 1473–1478.

67 Hladunewich M, Corrigan G, Derby G, Ramaswamy D, Kambham N, Scandling JD *et al.* A randomized, placebo-controlled trial of IGF-1 for delayed graft function: a human model to study postischemic ARF. *Kidney Int* 2003; **64**: 593–602.

68 Goggins W, Pascual M, Powelson J, Magee C, Tolkoff-Rubin N, Farrell ML *et al.* A prospective, randomized, clinical trial of intraoperative versus postoperative Thymoglobulin in adult cadaveric renal transplant recipients. *Transplantation* 2003; **76**: 798–802.

69 Shaffer D, Langone A, Nylander W, Goral S, Kizilisik AT, Helderman JH. A pilot protocol of a calcineurin-inhibitor free regimen for kidney transplant recipients of marginal donor kidneys or with delayed graft function. *Clin Transplant* 2003; **17**: 31–34.

70 Knight R, Kahan B. The place of sirolimus in kidney transplantation: can we reduce calcineurin inhibitor renal toxicity? *Kidney Int* 2006; **70**: 994–999.

71 Knight R, Kerman R, Schoenberg L, Podder H, Van Buren CT, Katz S et al. The selective use of basiliximab versus thymoglobulin in combination with sirolimus for cadaveric renal transplant recipients at low risk versus high risk for delayed graft function. *Transplantation* 2004; **78**: 904–910.

72 McTaggart R, Tomlanovich S, Bostrom A, Roberts JP, Feng S. Comparison of outcomes after delayed graft function: sirolimus-based versus other calcineurin-inhibitor sparing induction immunosuppression regimens. *Transplantation* 2004; **78**: 475–480.

73 Smith K, Wrenshall L, Nicosia R, Pichler R, Marsh CL, Alpers CE et al. Delayed graft function and cast nephropathy associated with tacrolimus plus rapamycin use. *J Am Soc Nephrol* 2003; **14**: 1037–1045.

74 Solez K, Axelsen R, Benediktsson H, Burdick JF, Cohen AH, Colvin RB et al. International standardization of criteria for the histologic diagnosis of renal allograft rejection: the Banff working classification of kidney transplant pathology. *Kidney Int* 1993; **44**: 411–422.

75 Terasaki P, Cai J. Humoral theory of transplantation: further evidence. *Curr Opin Immunol* 2005; **17**: 541–545.

76 Nickeleit V, Andreoni K. The classification and treatment of antibody-mediated renal allograft injury: where do we stand? *Kidney Int* 2007; **71**: 7–11.

77 Moll S, Pascual M. Humoral rejection of organ allografts. *Am J Transplant* 2005; **5**: 2611–2618.

78 Webster A, Pankhurst T, Rinaldi F, Chapman JR, Craig JC. Monoclonal and polyclonal antibody therapy for treating acute rejection in kidney transplant recipients: a systematic review of randomized trial data. *Transplantation* 2006; **81**: 953–965.

79 Sun Q, Liu Z, Cheng Z, Ji S, Zeng C, Li LS. Treatment of early mixed cellular and humoral renal allograft rejection with tacrolimus and mycophenolate mofetil. *Kidney Int* 2007; **71**: 24–30.

80 Montgomery R, Zachary A, Racusen L, Leffell MS, King KE, Burdick J et al. Plasmapheresis and intravenous immune globulin provides effective rescue therapy for refractory humoral rejection and allows kidneys to be successfully transplanted into cross-match-positive recipients. *Transplantation* 2000; **70**: 887–895.

81 Jordan S, Vo A, Tyan D, Nast CC, Toyoda M. Current approaches to treatment of antibody-mediated rejection. *Pediatr Transplant* 2005; **9**: 408–415.

82 Gebel H, Bray R, Nickerson P. Pre-transplant assessment of donor-reactive, HLA-specific antibodies in renal transplantation: contraindication vs. risk. *Am J Transplant* 2003; **3**: 1488–1500.

83 Garovoy MG, Rheinschmidt MA, Bigos M, Perkins H, Colombe B, Feduska N et al. Flow cytometry analysis: a high technology crossmatch technique facilitating transplantation. *Transplant Proc* 1983; **15**: 1939–1944.

84 Leenaerts PL, De Ruysscher D, Vandeputte M, Waer M. Measurement of alloantibody by flow cytometry. *J Immunol Methods* 1990; **130**: 73.

85 Scornik JC, Brunson ME, Schaub B, Howard RJ, Pfaff WW. The crossmatch in renal transplantation. *Transplantation* 1994; **57**: 621–625.

86 Cook DJ, Fettouh HI, Gjertson DW, Cecka JM. Flow cytometry crossmatching (FCXM) in the UNOS Kidney Transplant Registry. *Clin Transplant* 1998; **1998**: 413–419.

87 Bray R, Nolen J, Larsen C, Pearson T, Newell KA, Kokko K et al. Transplanting the highly sensitized patient: the Emory algorithm. *Am J Transplant* 2006; **6**: 2307.

88 Harmer AW. Utilization of crossmatch techniques for renal transplantation. *Curr Opin Nephrol Hypertens* 1998; **7**: 687–690.

89 Fuggle S, Martin S. Toward performing transplantation in highly sensitized patients. *Transplantation* 2004; **78**: 186–189.

90 O'Rourke R, Osorio R, Freise C, Lou CD, Garovoy MR, Bacchetti P et al. Flow cytometry crossmatching as a predictor of acute rejection in sensitized recipients of cadaveric renal transplants. *Clin Transplant* 2000; **14**: 167–173.

91 Karpinski M, Rush D, Jeffery J, Exner M, Regele H, Dancea S et al. Flow cytometric crossmatching in primary renal transplant recipients with a negative anti-human globulin enhanced cytotoxicity crossmatch. *J Am Soc Nephrol* 2001; **12**: 2807–2814.

92 Utzig MJ, Blumke M, Wolff-Vorbeck G, Lang H, Kirste G. Flow cytometry cross-match: a method for predicting graft rejection. *Transplant Proc* 1997; **63**: 551.

93 Ogura K, Terasaki P, Johnson C, Mendez R, Rosenthal JT, Ettenger R et al. The significance of a positive flow cytometry crossmatch test in primary kidney transplantation. *Transplantation* 1993; **56**: 294–298.

94 Christiaans MHL, Overhof R, ten Haaft A, Nieman F, van Hooff JP, van den Berg-Loonen EM et al. No advantage of flow cytometry crossmatch over complement-dependent cytotoxicity in immunologically well-documented renal allograft recipients. *Transplant Proc* 1996; **62**: 1341.

95 Henry M, Pelletier R, Elkhammas E, Bumgardner GL, Davies EA, Ferguson RM. A randomized prospective trial of OKT3 induction in the current immunosuppression era. *Clin Transplant* 2001; **15**: 410–414.

96 Evans PR, Lane AC, Lambert CM, Reynolds WM, Wilson PJ, Harris KR et al. Lack of correlation between IgG T-lymphocyte flow cytometric crossmatches with primary renal allograft outcome. *Transplant Int* 1992; **5**: S609–S612.

97 Wen R, Wu V, Dmitrienko S, Yu A, Balshaw R, Keown PA et al. Biomarkers in transplantation: prospective, blinded measurement of predictive value for the flow cytometry crossmatch after negative antiglobulin crossmatch in kidney transplantation. *Kidney Int* 2006; **70**: 1474–1481.

98 Gibney E, Cagle L, Freed B, Warnell SE, Chan L, Wiseman AC. Detection of donor-specific antibodies using HLA-coated microspheres: another tool for kidney transplant risk stratification. *Nephrol Dial Transplant* 2006; **21**: 2625–2629.

99 Vasilescu E, Ho E, Colovai A, Vlad G, Foca-Rodi A, Markowitz GS et al. Alloantibodies and the outcome of cadaver kidney allografts. *Hum Immunol* 2006; **67**: 597–604.

100 Jordan S, Vo A, Peng A, Toyoda A, Tyan D. Intravenous gammaglobulin (IVIG): a novel approach to improve transplant rates and outcomes in highly HLA-sensitized patients. *Am J Transplant* 2006; **6**: 459–466.

101 Jordan S, Tyan D, Stablein D, McIntosh M, Rose S, Vo A et al. Evaluation of intravenous immunoglobulin as an agent to lower allosensitization and improve transplantation in highly sensitized adult patients with end-stage renal disease: report of the NIH IG02 trial. *J Am Soc Nephrol* 2004; **15**: 3256–3262.

102 Stegall M, Gloor J, Winters J, Moore SB, Degoey S. A comparison of plasmapheresis versus high-dose IVIG desensitization in renal allograft recipients with high levels of donor specific alloantibody. *Am J Transplant* 2006; **6**: 346–351.

103 Nankivell B, Chapman J. Chronic allograft nephropathy: current concepts and future directions. *Transplantation* 2006; **81**: 643–654.

52 Maintenance Immunosuppression

Yves Vanrenterghem

Department of Nephvosy Gasthuisberg, University of Hospital, Leuven, Belgium

Introduction

In the last decad the number of immunosuppressive agents used in solid organ transplantation has rapidly increased. Their modes of action and their specific nonimmune toxicities have been recently reviewed in detail by Halloran [1]. Because these immunosuppressive drugs interrupt different pathways of the lymphocyte activation cascade, combined use is preferred in order to increase their efficacy (suppressing rejection) and to limit their drug-specific toxicity. At present several new drug combinations have been tested in clinical trials, but often without adequately establishing dosing, efficacy, and safety [2]. This chapter will be limited to a description of the specific immunosuppressive drug combinations that have been evaluated in large-scale clinical trials with long-term follow-up.

When reviewing the literature on maintenance immunosuppressive therapy, several problems emerge. A first problem concerns the lack of a good definition of what exactly constitutes "maintenance" immunosuppression. In an overview of the evolution of immunosuppression between 1994 and 2004, and based on the OPTN/SRTR data, maintenance immunosuppression was defined as the therapy at the time of discharge [3]. In his review, Halloran coined the terms preadaptation maintenance therapy and postadaptation therapy, but without providing a clear definition of either [1]. Although it is common practice to reduce the daily dose of immunosuppressive agents with time after transplantation, very few authors have assessed the optimal maintenance dose in properly designed long-term studies. The concept of tailor-made immunosuppression, aimed at fulfilling the clinical requirements outlined by the individual patient profile, is becoming more popular, but the evidence-based allocation of an optimal protocol to a specific patient category remains limited [4]. In addition, most controlled trials analyzing the efficacy and safety of newer immunosuppressive drugs have had a short follow-up, often limited to 1 year or less. Only a limited number of trials provide long-term follow-up data. Moreover, the study protocols of the latter often allow a change in therapy after the end of the study period, resulting in a substantial number of patients who are no longer on their allocated regimen. In his excellent review on immunosuppression for long-term maintenance of renal allograft function, Offermann correctly stated that most long-term data available in the literature are descriptive, retrospective, nonrandomized, and uncontrolled. He also stressed that, although registry data have the advantage of large numbers and long-term follow-up, with respect to immunosuppressive therapy, selection bias is often present or difficult to identify [5]. For all these reasons the proposed long-term efficacy and safety of maintenance immunosuppressive regimens are not always based on trial evidence.

Tacrolimus–mycophenolate mofetil–corticosteroids: the current standard of maintenance immunosuppression

After the publication of the first results of the European trial comparing cyclosporine A (CsA) with azathioprine (Aza) in combination with corticosteroids [6], most kidney transplant centers progressively switched to CsA and corticosteroids. The second calcineurin inhibitor (CNI), tacrolimus (Tac), was introduced in clinical practice following the publication of the results of the European and US randomized controlled trials comparing Tac with CsA [7,8]. After some initial reluctance to switch from CsA to Tac [9], over the last years Tac has become the CNI of choice in many kidney transplant programs. Based on figures from the 2005 OPTN/SRTR Annual Report, 93% of the renal transplant patients in the USA received CNIs as part of their maintenance therapy, and 72% of them are using Tac [3]. The reason why transplant physicians now prefer Tac is its higher efficacy (lower incidence of acute rejection and improved graft survival), even if compared to the newer microemulsion formulation of CsA, Neoral [10], and its more favorable risk profile. In the Margreiter study, as in previous studies comparing Tac with CsA, similar patient and graft

Evidence-based Nephrology. Edited by Donald Molony and Jonathan Craig
© 2009 Blackwell Publishing, ISBN: 978-1-4051-3975-5.

survival were seen, with a significantly lower incidence of acute rejections in the Tac-treated patients. The incidences of hypertension and hypercholesterolemia were also significantly lower in the Tac-treated patients. In contrast to prior studies, the incidence of diabetes mellitus, defined as the need for insulin for more than 30 consecutive days, was similar in both groups.

The question of whether the better short-term results with Tac also translate into improved late outcomes has to be answered with more caution. Both the US and the European trials comparing CsA and Tac have reported their 5-year results [11,12]. In the US trial the intent-to-treat analysis revealed similar patient and graft survival (79.1% vs. 81.4% and 64.3% vs. 64.6%). The rate of crossover was significantly higher among patients randomized to receive CsA therapy (27.5% vs. 9.3%; $P < 0.001$). Graft survival at 5 years was significantly better in the Tac arm when crossover due to rejection was counted as graft failure (63.8% vs. 53.8%; $P = 0.014$). The latter method of analysis may however have introduced a substantial bias. Tac use was also associated with significantly reduced requirements of antihypertensive and lipid-lowering medications, and Tac-associated insulin dependence was often reversible. In the European trial, patient and graft survival at 5 years were comparable. However, in the Tac-treated patients, the incidence of biopsy-confirmed chronic rejection was significantly lower (6.6% vs. 15.3%; $P < 0.01$) and the projected half-life was 15.8 years for the Tac patients versus 10.8 years for the CsA patients. In a registry analysis of more than 32,000 patients, chronic allograft failure at 4 years was similar for Tac and the microemulsion of CsA, whereas it was significantly higher in the patients treated with the original formulation of CsA [13]. In a subsequent study by the same authors, using a paired kidney analysis of the same SRTR database, a difference in risk for 5-year survival or graft loss could not be demonstrated, but renal function was superior for Tac at all time points [14]. In the single-center randomized trial from Cardiff, the 6-year graft survival was significantly higher in the 115 Tac-treated patients than in the 117 patients receiving CsA microemulsion (81% vs. 60%; $P = 0.0496$) [15].

With the exception of the first CsA European trial [6], the above-mentioned trials have always used CNIs in combination with anti-metabolites and corticosteroids. In the European Tac versus CsA trial, Aza was given for the first 3 months of the study and, where possible, discontinued thereafter. However, no data were provided on the exact number of patients who really stopped Aza [7]. In the US trial, Aza was administered throughout the entire study [8]. In the Margreiter study, Aza was also part of the immunosuppressive therapy in both arms [10]. In the mid-1990s, three randomized double-blind clinical trials compared the efficacy and safety of a triple-drug combination of CsA, mycophenolate mofetil (MMF), and corticosteroids with a combination of either CsA, placebo and corticosteroids, or CsA, Aza, and corticosteroids [16–18]. As summarized in the pooled analysis paper, adding MMF in a daily dose of 2 or 3g significantly reduced the incidence of acute rejection from 40.8% in the placebo–Aza patients to 19.8% and 16.5% for the MMF 2-g and the MMF 3-g groups, respectively [19]. Due to the higher number of side effects in the 3-g

group, a preferred daily dose of 2-g was subsequently proposed. This favorable effect of MMF on acute rejection was also seen when MMF was added to Tac-based immunosuppressive regimens [20,21]. Whereas in the European trial a significant reduction of the incidence of rejection was also seen in the 1-g MMF arm, this effect could only be demonstrated in the 2-g MMF arm in the US study. There has been no good explanation for these different findings. The three pivotal trials showing the superiority of MMF over Aza were conducted with the old formulation of CsA. More recently, Remuzzi et al. conducted a multicenter, randomized trial comparing Aza and MMF in association with the new microemulsion formulation Neoral [22]. In this trial no advantage of MMF over Aza in terms of prevention of acute rejection could be found, but there was no change in clinical practice in most transplant centers [23]. Several analyses of large transplant registries have indeed indicated that the use of MMF decreases the risk of developing chronic allograft nephropathy [24], slows the decline of glomerular filtration rate [25], and improves long-term outcome even in immunologically high-risk patients, such as African Americans [26].

Maintenance immunosuppression without corticosteroids

Based on the well-known corticosteroid-sparing effect of CsA, soon after its more widespread use, several attempts were made to completely withdraw corticosteroids from maintenance immunosuppression. The proponents of withdrawal stressed the benefits of corticosteroid discontinuation, such as improved control of hypertension [27] and hyperlipidemia [28,29], the lower incidence of de novo diabetes mellitus [30], less frequent cataracts [31], better control of body weight [32], and better preservation of bone mineral density [33]. The opponents considered that the potential benefits, which seemed to be not sustainable [34], did not outweigh the increased risk of acute rejection. The latter conclusion was further strengthened by the results of a meta-analysis by Kasiske published in 2000 [35]. In the nine prednisone withdrawal trials ($n = 1461$), the proportion of patients with acute rejection was increased by 0.14 ($P < 0.001$) and the relative risk (RR) of graft failure was also increased (RR, 1.4). In seven of the nine trials CsA and Aza were used.

In two more recent prednisone withdrawal trials, MMF was used, but the difference in acute rejection between withdrawal and control groups was not different compared with the trials that did not use MMF. In the US study, in which corticosteroids were discontinued at 3 months, enrollment was stopped after 266 patients were randomized, because of excess rejection in the corticosteroid withdrawal group (21% vs. 4.4%) [36]. In the European trial, the withdrawal group not only stopped corticosteroids but also received only 50% of the corticosteroid dose during the first 3 months compared to the control group [29]. The greatest difference in the occurrence of acute rejection was seen in the first two posttransplant weeks. In the 3 months after withdrawal of corticosteriods, only 4% of the patients without corticosteroids developed an acute rejection, versus 0.4% in the group maintained on corticosteroids. In addition, no difference in the incidence of rejection was seen in the subgroup of patients who had received induction with antithymocyte globulin (ATG). In a large European randomized study of patients treated with Tac–MMF–corticosteroids, a low incidence of acute rejection (6%) was seen after corticosteroids were stopped at 3 months [37]. At least from the two European trials, it can be concluded that withdrawing corticosteroids 3 months after transplantation is associated with a very low risk of acute rejection (4–6%) and that these rejections can easily be controlled. In other words, almost 95% of these patients can be successfully withdrawn from corticosteroids.

As the follow-up of these trials was short, no conclusions can be made whether corticosteroids withdrawal is also safe in the long run. Concerns about the long-term safety are at least partially based on the findings of a Canadian multicenter controlled trial published in 1992 by Sinclair [38]. In this trial, conducted between 1982 and 1985, patients were treated initially with CsA and steroids. At 3 months they were randomized either to stop steroids or to continue dual therapy. Although the early results were very promising, after 5 years the corticosteroid withdrawal patients had significantly worse graft survival ($P = 0.03$). Long-term data from other randomized controlled trials are lacking. In 2005, Opelz published the results of a large study that compared patients prospectively withdrawn from corticosteroids with controls selected from the Collaborative Transplant Study (CTS) registry [39]. Thus, this study was not a randomized trial, and unfortunately both kidney and heart transplant recipients were included. There were 1110 deceased-donor kidney recipients and 450 heart recipients included in the analysis. All patients were immunologically low-risk patients. Corticosteroids were withdrawn no earlier than 6 months posttransplantation. Each patient was matched with three patients from the CTS database. A comparison of 7-year outcome in the kidney transplant recipients (94% receiving cyclosporine; 97% Caucasian) showed a benefit of corticosteroid withdrawal versus corticosteroid continuation for graft survival (81.9% vs. 75.3%; $P = 0.0001$), patient survival (88.8% vs. 84.3%; $P = 0.0016$), and death-censored graft survival (91.8% vs. 87.9%; $P = 0.0091$). A total of 58.6% of the kidney transplant patients never required corticosteroids during follow-up. A 5-year outcome study of 589 kidney transplant recipients (transplanted in Minneapolis) showed comparable results after corticosteroid withdrawal [40]. In contrast to most earlier published studies, patients were already withdrawn from corticosteroids on postoperative day 6. All patients received induction with ATG and were maintained on dual therapy of either CsA–MMF or Tac–MMF.

Based on available evidence, it appears that corticosteroid withdrawal can be safely performed in almost 95% of immunologically low-risk patients. Antibody induction may have a protective role [29]. Whether very early (<7 days) withdrawal of corticosteroids may be even more successful must be confirmed by more studies [40,41].

Maintenance immunosuppression without CNIs

Since the introduction of CsA, it has been observed that kidney function in CsA-treated patients is worse than in patients treated with Aza and steroids [6]. It is now generally accepted that chronic CNI administration causes nephrotoxicity that is clinically and histologically difficult to distinguish from chronic allograft nephropathy, and although the number of studies is low, the same holds true for Tac [42,43]. Therefore, numerous investigators evaluated CsA withdrawal strategies, via a conversion from CsA to Aza or through withdrawal of CsA from an Aza-containing regimen. A constant finding in most of these conversion trials was a trend toward an improvement in renal function. However, the "price" for this was an increased risk for acute rejection. Both in 1993 and in 2000, Kasiske published a meta-analysis of randomized, controlled trials that examined CsA withdrawal [35,44]. The results of the meta-analysis published in 2000 included 13 studies that were completed before 1999 and indicated that CsA withdrawal was associated with a higher incidence of acute rejection (pooled mean difference, 0.11; $P < 0.0001$) but that CsA withdrawal did not adversely affect graft survival, even in studies with long-term follow-up (maximum follow-up, 96 months) [35]. Even after the publication of this meta-analysis, systematic withdrawal of CNIs did not become common practice in most transplant centers, mainly because of concerns about rejection after CNI withdrawal.

Since the more widespread use of MMF instead of Aza, new attempts have been made to withdraw CsA from MMF-based regimens. When CsA was withdrawn 6 months after transplantation, as was performed in two Dutch randomized multicenter trials, an incremental increase in acute rejection was observed, comparable with CsA withdrawal from Aza (e.g. 6.3% and 20.6%) [45,46]. Similar data were found in the French randomized trial in which CsA or MMF withdrawal 3 months after transplantation was compared [47]. Although in this trial all patients received induction with ATG, the probability of acute rejection was 18.5% in the CsA withdrawal group versus 5.6% in the MMF withdrawal arm. This study is one of the few that examined risk factors of acute rejection after CsA withdrawal. Borderline changes in the biopsy before withdrawal as well as a lower area under the curve exposure of mycophenolic acid at the time of withdrawal proved to be significant risk factors for acute rejection after CsA discontinuation. A withdrawal later after transplantation (at least 1 year posttransplantation) resulted in comparable results: the cumulative incidence of acute rejection or graft loss due to rejection 5 years after transplantation was significantly higher in the CsA withdrawal group (19%) versus the group maintained on CsA (5%) ($P = 0.01$) [48].

More recently, CsA withdrawal from regimens containing the mTOR inhibitor SRL has been advocated. Three randomized studies have analyzed the safety of CsA withdrawal from a CsA–SRL–steroid regimen. In the Rapamune Maintenance Regimen Trial, 430 of a total of 525 patients were randomly assigned at 3 months posttransplantation to one of two treatment arms (SRL–CsA–steroids or SRL–steroids) [49]. One of the main early findings was a progressive increase of the calculated creatinine clearance after CsA withdrawal, compared to the group maintained on triple-drug therapy. However, a significant difference in the occurrence of acute rejection after randomization was seen (4.2% and 9.8% for the SRL–CsA–steroid and SRL–steroid arms, respectively; $P = 0.035$). In the 36-month report a trend toward a better graft survival was seen in the CsA withdrawal arm [50], a difference that became significant when analyzing the 48-month results [51]. Protocol biopsies performed at baseline, 12 months, and 36 months confirmed that early CsA withdrawal led to significantly less chronic allograft damage [52]. Apart from the rather high number of patients withdrawn from the study, the long-term conclusions of this study are limited by the fact that it became obvious that a combination of CsA and SRL in standard doses, as were initially used, is indeed nephrotoxic [53] and results in worse graft survival compared to the combination of CsA and MMF [54]. Similar results are seen with the combination of CsA and everolimus [55]. Two smaller CsA elimination trials confirmed the improvement of renal function after CsA withdrawal, but with a smaller risk of acute rejection than in the Rapamune Maintenance Regimen Trial [56,57]. A major limitation of these three SRL–CsA withdrawal trials is that only patients with a low to moderate immunological risk have been included. In addition, more widespread use of SRL has also revealed an increasing number of adverse effects not reported in the early trials [58]. On the other hand, the reduced risk of developing posttransplant *de novo* malignancies on SRL therapy, as recently suggested in an analysis of UNOS registry data, is an intriguing finding [59]. If confirmed in randomized trials, this may be a strong reason for more systematic withdrawal of CNI.

Finally, when trying answer the question of whether CNIs can or should be withdrawn from maintenance immunosuppressive regimens, the following should be kept in mind:

• Although in all studies CNI discontinuation is associated with an amelioration of renal allograft function, this has not resulted in better long-term graft survival. In the study by Abramowicz, graft survival was even worse [48]. Only in the Rapamune Maintenance Regimen Trial was better graft survival seen at 4 years, compared to a group of patients treated with a nephrotoxic maintenance regimen [49]. One of the reasons why improved long-term outcome is not seen may be that follow-up has not yet been long enough to detect a difference. Although it has been shown that 1-year serum creatinine is strongly correlated with long-term renal graft survival [60], the change in serum creatinine after CNI discontinuation is probably too small to have a significant impact on the long-term outcome.

• That chronic administration of CNIs may result in end-stage renal failure has clearly been shown in nonrenal solid organ allograft recipients [62,63]. From these reports it is clear that the development of end-stage renal failure is multifactorial, and the risk factors for developing end-stage renal failure are poorly understood [64]. The question as to what extent pure CNI-mediated nephrotoxicity is responsible for graft loss after kidney transplantation will at least for the moment remain unanswered because of a lack of long-term controlled trials. In Figure 52.1 the long-term

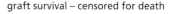

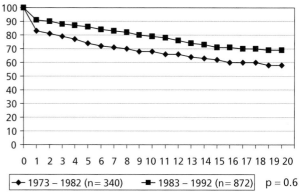

Figure 52.1 Actuarial graft survival (censored for death) in 340 patients transplanted between 1973 and 1982 with ATG-Aza-corticosteroids and in 872 patients transplanted between 1983 and 1992 with a CsA-based immunosuppressive regimen.

graft survival (censored for death) of 340 patients transplanted between 1973 and 1982 with an immunosuppressive protocol consisting of ATG–Aza–steroids in our unit is compared with that of 872 patients transplanted between 1983 and 1992 with a CsA-based immunosuppressive regimen. Although the use of CsA resulted in a significant improvement of the 1-year outcome, the slope of the two curves after the first year is similar, suggesting no deleterious effect of the long-term use of CsA. One of the reason for this finding may be the relatively low doses of CsA that have been used. As shown in Figure 52.2, the mean daily dose of CsA used at the end of the first year after transplantation has progressively decreased over the last 2 decades. The same trend can be seen for the mean daily dose at 10 years. That the dose of CNIs can be safely reduced to 50% of the doses normally used and is associated with improved renal function has been shown by Kuypers *et al.* in a small retrospective study [65]. These findings have now been confirmed by a large multicenter randomized trial [66]. It has also been shown that low doses of CsA in association with MMF lead to similar inhibition of

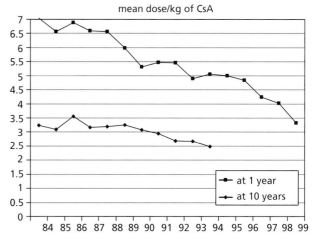

Figure 52.2 Mean daily dose of CsA used at the end of the first year after transplantation and at the end of the 10th year after transplantation.

calcineurin activity and cytokine production as conventional CsA exposure in maintenance immunosuppression [67].

During the last 2 or 3 years, new combinations of drugs, with or without CNIs, have been tested. It is beyond the scope of this chapter to review the results of these trials, because the trials are small, often from a single center, not controlled, and have too short follow-up to allow any conclusion as to their role as maintenance immunosuppression. In a few years maintenance immunosuppression may be become completely different from what we currently consider standard practice in most centers. For example, blocking T-cell activation at the signal 2 level by a selective costimulatory blocker such as Belatacept may be a good candidate [68].

References

1 Halloran PF. Immunosuppressive drugs for kidney transplantation. *N Engl J Med* 2004; **351:** 2715–2729.

2 Matas AJ. What's new and what's hot in transplantation: clinical science ATC 2003. *Am J Transplant* 2003; **3:** 1465–1473.

3 Meier-Kriesche HU, Li S, Gruessner RWG, Fung JJ, Bustami RT, Barr ML *et al*. Immunosuppression: evolution in practice and trends, 1994–2004. *Am J Transplant* 2006; **6:** 1111–1131.

4 Kuypers DRJ, Vanrenterghem YFC. Tailoring immunosuppressive therapy. *Nephrol Dial Transplant* 2002; **17:** 2051–2054.

5 Offermann G. Immunosuppression for long-term maintenance of renal allograft function. *Drugs* 2004; **64:** 1325–1338.

6 European Multicentre Trial Group. Cyclosporin in cadaveric renal transplantation: one-year follow-up of a multicentre trial. *Lancet* 1983; **ii:** 986–989.

7 Mayer AD, Dmitrewski J, Squifflet JP, Besse T, Grabensee B, Klein B *et al*. Multicenter randomized trial comparing tacrolimus (FK506) and cyclosporine in the prevention of renal allograft rejection. *Transplantation* 1997; **64:** 436–443.

8 Pirsch JD, Miller J, Deierhoi MH, Vincenti F, Filo RS, FK506 Kidney Transplant Study Group. A comparison of Tacrolimus (FK506) and cyclosporine for immunosuppression after cadaveric renal transplantation. *Transplantation* 1997; **63:** 977–983.

9 Danovitch GM. Cyclosporin or tacrolimus: which agent to choose? *Nephrol Dial Transplant* 1997; **12:** 1566–1568.

10 Margreiter R, European Tacrolimus vs Ciclosporin Microemulsion Renal Transplantation Study Group. Efficacy and safety of tacrolimus compared with ciclosporin microemulsion in renal transplantation: a randomized multicentre study. *Lancet* 2002; **359:** 741–746.

11 Vincenti F, Jensik SC, Filo RS, Miller J, Pirsch J. A long-term comparison of tacrolimus (FK506) and cyclosporine in kidney transplantation: evidence for improved allograft survival at five years. *Transplantation* 2002; **73:** 775–782.

12 Mayer AD, European Tacrolimus Multicentre Renal Study Group. Chronic rejection and graft half-life: five-year follow-up of the European tacrolimus multicenter renal study. *Transplant Proc* 2002; **34:** 1491–1492.

13 Meier-Kriesche HU, Kaplan B. Cyclosporine emulsion and tacrolimus are associated with decreased chronic allograft failure and improved long-term graft survival as compared with Sandimmune. *Am J Transplant* 2002; **2:** 100–104.

14 Kaplan B, Schold JD, Meier-Kriesche HU. Long-term graft survival with Neoral and Tacrolimus: a paired kidney analysis. *J Am Soc Nephrol* 2003; **14:** 2980–2984.

15 Jurewicz WA. Tacrolimus versus ciclosporin immunosuppression: long-term outcome in renal transplantation. *Nephrol Dial Transplant* 2003; **18(Suppl):** i7–i11.

16 European Mycophenolate Mofetil Cooperative Study Group. Placebo-controlled study of mycophenolate mofetil combined with cyclosporine and corticosteroids for prevention of acute rejection. *Lancet* 1995; **345:** 1321–1325.

17 Sollinger HW, U.S. Renal Transplant Mycophenolate Mofetil Study Group. Mycophenolate mofetil for the prevention of acute rejection in primary cadaveric renal allograft recipients. *Transplantation* 1995; **60:** 225–232.

18 Tricontinental Mycophenolate Mofetil Renal Transplantation Study Group. A blinded randomized clinical trial of mycophenolate mofetil for the prevention of acute rejection in cadaveric renal transplantation. *Transplantation* 1996; **61:** 1029–1037.

19 Halloran P, Mathew T, Tomlanovich S, Groth C, Hooftman L, Barker C *et al*. Mycophenolate mofetil in renal allograft recipients. A pooled efficacy analysis of three randomized, double-blind, clinical studies in prevention of rejection. *Transplantation* 1997; **63:** 39–47.

20 Squifflet JP, Backman L, Claesson K, Dietl KH, Ekberg H, Forsythe JL *et al*. Dose optimization of mycophenolate mofetil when administered with a low dose of tacrolimus in cadaveric renal transplant recipients. *Transplantation* 2001; **72:** 63–69.

21 Miller J, Mendez R, Pirsch JD, Jensik SC, FK506/MMF Dose-Ranging Kidney Transplant Study Group. Safety and efficacy of tacrolimus in combination with mycophenolate mofetil (MMF) in cadaveric renal transplant recipients. *Transplantation* 2000; **69:** 875–880.

22 Remuzzi G, Lesti M, Gotti E, Dimitrov BD, Ene-Lordache B, Gherardi G *et al*. Mycophenolate mofetil versus azathioprine for prevention of acute rejection in renal transplantation 5MYSS): a randomized trial. *Lancet* 2004; **364:** 503–512.

23 Maes B, Vanrenterghem Y. MYSS: should we alter clinical practice? *Lancet* 2004; **364:** 2016–2017 (letter).

24 Ojo AO, Meier-Kriesche HU, Hanson JA, Leichtman AB, Cibrik D, Magee JC *et al*. Mycophenolate mofetil reduces late renal allograft loss independent of acute rejection. *Transplantation* 2000; **69:** 2405–2409.

25 Gill JS, Tonelli M, Mix CH, Johnson N, Pereira BJG. The effect of maintenance immunosuppression medication on the change in kidney allograft function. *Kidney Int* 2004; **65:** 692–699.

26 Meier-Kriesche HU, Ojo AO, Leichtman AB, Punch JD, Hanson JA, Cibrik DM *et al*. Effect of mycophenolate mofetil on long-term outcomes in African American renal transplant recipients. *J Am Soc Nephrol* 2000; **11:** 2366–2370.

27 Hricik DE, Lautman J, Bartucci MR, Moir EJ, Mayes JT, Schulak JA. Variable effects of steroid withdrawal on blood pressure reduction in cyclosporine-treated renal transplant recipients. *Transplantation* 1992; **53:** 1232–1235.

28 Hricik DE, Mayes JT, Schulak JA. Independent effects of cyclosporine and prednisone on posttransplant hypercholesterolemia. *Am J Kidney Dis* 1991; **18:** 353–358.

29 Vanrenterghem Y, Lebranchu Y, Hene R, Oppenheimer F, Ekberg H, Steroid Dosing Study Group. Double-blind comparison of two corticosteroid regimens plus mycophenolate mofetil and cyclosporine for prevention of acute renal allograft rejection. *Transplantation* 2000; **70:** 1352–1359.

30 Hricik DE, Bartucci MR, Moir EJ, Mayes JT, Schulak JA. Effects of steroid withdrawal on posttransplant diabetes mellitus in cyclosporine-treated renal transplant recipients. *Transplantation* 1991; **51**: 374–377.

31 Montagnino G, Tarantino A, Segolini GP, Cambi V, Rizzo G, Altieri P *et al.* Long-term results of a randomized study comparing three immunosuppressive schedules with cyclosporine in cadaveric kidney transplantation. *J Am Soc Nephrol* 2001; **12**: 2163–2169.

32 van den Ham ECH, Kooman JP, Christiaans MHL, Nieman FHM, van Hooff JP. Weight changes after renal transplantation: a comparison between patients on 5-mg maintenance steroid therapy and those on steroid-free immunosuppressive therapy. *Transplant Int* 2003; **16**: 300–306.

33 van den Ham ECH, Kooman JP, Christiaans MHL, van Hooff JP. The influence of early steroid withdrawal on body composition and bone mineral density in renal Transplantation patients. *Transplant Int* 2003; **16**: 82–87.

34 Sivaraman P, Nussbaumer G, Landsberg D. Lack of long-term benefits of steroid withdrawal in renal transplant recipients. *Am J Kidney Dis* 2001; **37**: 1162–1169.

35 Kasiske BL, Chakkera HA, Louis TA, Ma JZ. A meta-analysis of immunosuppression withdrawal in renal transplantation. *J Am Soc Nephrol* 2000; **11**: 1910–1917.

36 Ahsan N, Hricik D, Matas A, Rose S, Tomlanovich S, Wilkinson A *et al.* Prednisone withdrawal in kidney transplant recipients on cyclosporine and mycophenolate mofetil: a prospective randomized study. *Transplantation* 1999; **68**: 1865–1874.

37 Vanrenterghem Y, van Hooff JP, Squifflet JP, Salmela K, Rigotto P, Jindal RM *et al.* Minimization of immunosuppressive therapy after renal transplantation: Results of a randomized controlled trial. *Am J Transplant* 2005; **5**: 87–95.

38 Sinclair NR, Canadian Multicentre Transplant Study Group. Low-dose steroid therapy in cyclosporine-treated renal transplant recipients with well-functioning grafts. *Can Med Assoc J* 1992; **147**: 645–657.

39 Opelz G, Döhler B, Laux G, Collaborative Transplant Study. Long-term prospective study of steroid withdrawal in kidney and heart transplant recipients. *Am J Transplant* 2005; **5**: 720–728.

40 Matas AJ, Kandaswamy R, Gillingham KJ, McHugh L, Ibrahim H, Kasiske B *et al.* Prednisone-free maintenance immunosuppression: a 5-year experience. *Am J Transplant* 2005; **5**: 2473–2478.

41 Vincenti F, Monaco A, Grinyo J, Kinkhabwala M, Roza A. Multicenter randomized prospectice trial of steroid withdrawal in renal transplant recipients receiving Basiliximab, cyclosporine microemulsion and mycophenolate mofetil. *Am J Transplant* 2003; **3**: 306–311.

42 Bennett WM, DeMattis A, Meyer MM, Andoh T, Barry JM. Chronic cyclosporine nephropathy: the Achilles' heel of immunosuppressive therapy. *Kidney Int* 1996; **50**: 1089–1100.

43 Nankivell BJ, Borrows RJ, Fung CL, O'Connell J, Allen RDM, Chapman JR. The natural history of chronic allograft nephropathy. *N Engl J Med* 2003; **349**: 2326–2333.

44 Kasiske BL, Heim-Duthoy K, Ma JZ. Elective cyclosporine withdrawal after renal transplantation: a meta-analysis. *JAMA* 1993; **269**: 395–400.

45 Schuelle P, van der Heide JH, Tegzess A, Verburgh CA, Paul LC, van der Woude FJ *et al.* Open randomized trial comparing early withdrawal of either cyclosporine or mycophenolate mofetil in stable renal transplant recipients initially treated with a triple drug regimen. *J Am Soc Nephrol* 2002; **13**: 536–543.

46 Smak Gregoor PJH, de Sévaux RGL, Ligtenberg G, Hoitsma AJ, Hené RJ, Weimar W *et al.* Withdrawal of cyclosporine or prednisone six months after kidney transplantation in patients on triple drug therapy: a randomized, prospective, multicenter study. *J Am Soc Nephrol* 2002; **13**: 1365–1373.

47 Hazzan M, Labalette M, Copin MC, Glowacki F, Provôt F, Pruv FR *et al.* Predictive factors of acute rejection after early cyclosporine withdrawal in renal transplant recipients who receive mycophenolate mofetil: results from a prospective randomized trial. *J Am Soc Nephrol* 2005; **16**: 2509–2516.

48 Abramowicz D, del Carmen Rial M, Vitko S, del Castillo D, Manas D, Lao M *et al.* Cyclosporine withdrawal from a mycophenolate mofetil-containing immunosuppressive regimen: results of a five-year, prospective, randomized study. *J Am Soc Nephrol* 2005; **16**: 2234–2240.

49 Johnson RWG, Kreis H, Oberbauer R, Brattstrom C, Claesson K, Eris J. Sirolimus allows early cyclosporine withdrawal in renal transplantation resulting in improved renal function and lower blood pressure. *Transplantation* 2001; **72**: 777–786.

50 Kreis H, Oberbauer R, Campistol JM, Mathew T, Daloze P, Schena FP *et al.* Long-term benefits with sirolimus-based therapy after early cyclosporine withdrawal. *J Am Soc Nephrol* 2004; **15**: 809–817.

51 Oberbauer R, Segoloni G, Campistol JM, Kreis H, Mota A, Lawen J *et al.* Early cyclosporine withdrawal from a sirolimlus-based regimen results in better renal allograft survival and renal function at 48 months after transplantation. *Transplant Int* 2005; **18**: 22–28.

52 Mota A, Arias M, Taskinen E, Paavonen T, Brault Y, Legendre C *et al.* Sirolimus-based therapy following early cyclosporine withdrawal provides significantly improved renal histology and function at 3 years. *Am J Transplant* 2004; **4(6)**: 953–961.

53 Chueh SJ, Kahan BD. Clinical application of sirolimus in renal transplantation: un update. *Transplant Int* 2005; **18**: 261–277.

54 Meier-Kriesche HU, Steffen BJ, Chu AH, Loveland JJ, Gordon RD, Morris JA *et al.* Sirolimus with Neoral versus mycophenolate mofetil with Neoral is associated with decreased renal allograft survival. *Am J Transplant* 2004; **4**: 2058–2066.

55 Lorber MI, Mulgaonkar S, Butt KM, Elkhammas E, Mendez R, Rajagopalan PR *et al.* Everolimus versus mycophenolate mofetil in the prevention of rejection in de novo renal transplant recipients: a 3-year randomized, multicenter, phase III study. *Transplantation* 2005; **80**: 244–252.

56 Gonwa TA, Hricik DE, Brinker K, Grinyo JM, Schena FP, Sirolimus Renal Function Study Group. Improved renal function in sirolimus-treated renal transplant patients after early cyclosporine elimination. *Transplantation* 2002; **74**: 1561–1567.

57 Baboolal K. A phase III prospective, randomized study to evaluate concentration-controlled sirolimus (rapamune) with cyclosporine dose minimization or elimination at six months in de novo renal allograft recipients. *Transplantation* 2003; **75**: 1404–1408.

58 Kuypers DRJ. Benefit-risk assessment of sirolimus in renal transplantation. *Drug Safety* 2005; **28**: 153–181.

59 Kauffman HM, Cherikh WS, Cheng Y, Hanto DW, Kahan BD. Maintenance immunosuppression with target-of-rapamycin inhibitors is associated with a reduced incidence of de novo malignancies. *Transplantation* 2005; **80**: 883–889.

60 Hariharan S, McBride MA, Cherikh WS, Tolleris CB, Bresnahan BA, Johnson CP. Post-transplant renal function in the first year predicts long-term kidney transplant survival. *Kidney Int* 2002; **62**: 311–318.

61 Myers BD, Roos J, Newton L, Luetscher J, Perloth M. Cyclosporine-associated chronic nephropathy. *N Engl J Med* 1984; **311**: 699–705.

62 Parry G, Meiser B, Rabago G. The clinical impact of cyclosporine nephrotoxicity in heart transplantation. *Transplantation* 2000; **69(Suppl 12):** S23–S26.

63 Fisher N, Mlalag M, Gonzalez-Pinto I. The clinical impact of cyclosporine nephrotoxicity in liver transplantation. *Transplantation* 2000; **69(Suppl 12):** S18–S22.

64 Lynn M, Abreo K, Zibari G, McDonald J. End-stage renal disease in liver transplants. *Clin Transplant* 2001; **15(Suppl 6):** 66–69.

65 Kuypers DRJ, Evenepoel P, Maes B, Coosemans W, Pirenne J, Vanrenterghem Y. The use of anti-CD25 monoclonal antibody and mycophenolate mofetil enables to use a low-dose tacrolimus and early withdrawal of steroids in renal transplant recipients. *Clin Transplant* 2003; **17:** 234–241.

66 Nashan B, Ekberg H, Grinyo J, Vanrenterghem Y, Vincenti F, Calleja E *et al.* Cyclosporine sparing with mycophenolate mofetil, daclizumab and corticosteroids in renal allograft recipients: the Caesar study, 36 months results. WTC Boston, 2006; abstr. 1096.

67 Grinyo JM, Cruzado JM, Millan O, Caldes A, Sabaté I, Gil-Vernet S *et al.* Low-dose cyclosporine with mycophenolate mofetil induces similar calcineurin activity and cytokine inhibition as does tandard-dose cyclosporine in stable renal allografts. *Transplantation* 2004; **78:** 1400–1403.

68 Vincenti F, Larsen C, Durrbach A, Wekerle T, Nashan B, Blancho G *et al.* Costimulation blockade with Belatacept in renal transplantation. *N Engl J Med* 2005; **353:** 770–781.

53 Chronic Allograft Nephropathy

Bengt C. Fellström,[1] Alan Jardine,[2] & Hallvard Holdaas[3]

[1]Department of Medicine, Renal Unit, University Hospital, Uppsala, Sweden
[2]Nephrology & Transplantation, BHF Cardiovascular Research Centre, University of Glasgow, Glasgow G12 8TA, UK
[3]Department of Nephrology, Rikshospitalet, Oslo, Norway

Chronic allograft nephropathy (CAN) is the major preventable cause of late graft loss in kidney transplantation. Overall, death ("death with a functioning graft") constitutes about 50% of "graft failures," whereas CAN and recurrence of the primary kidney disease account for the remainder [1–3]. Graft loss due to premature cardiovascular death and CAN may be linked due to shared risk factors in kidney transplant recipients. Although short-term outcomes in kidney transplantation have improved over time, a significant proportion of grafts develop progressive dysfunction and fail within 10 years [1,2], and the balance of evidence is that long-term graft survival has not improved despite advances in immunosuppressive therapy [4–7]. Graft failure has major human and economic sequelae. In the USA, approximately 4700 patients with failed transplants restarted dialysis in 2002, representing about 5% of the total number of patients starting dialysis [7] and 2–3% of the transplant population. In our own experience in maintenance kidney transplant patients, there has been an annual rate of (death-censored) graft loss of 2.2%, of which 82% was considered to be due to CAN [3,8].

Definition

Historically, CAN has been defined as a combination of histological features that includes interstitial fibrosis, tubular atrophy, vascular intimal hyperplasia, fibrosis or hyalinosis, and transplant glomerulopathy. The histological changes are generally associated with variably reduced renal transplant function, although histological changes usually precede functional deterioration, and with hyperfiltration in the remaining nephrons [2]. The pathophysiological processes underlying CAN include both immunologically driven chronic rejection and nonimmune processes, such as hypertension and chronic calcineurin inhibitor (CNI) toxicity. Recurrence of native kidney diseases, such as certain types of glomerulonephritis (immunoglobulin A nephropathy, membranous nephropathy, and focal segmental glomerulosclerosis) or recurrence of diabetes nephropathy, are usually excluded from the diagnosis of CAN. Recent seminal studies from Australia, in which protocol biopsies were performed in patients who received kidney–pancreas transplants after a 10-year posttransplant follow-up, reported the prospective development of histopathological changes [9,10]. These reports demonstrated that chronic interstitial fibrosis and tubular atrophy emerge very early following transplantation and precede both arteriolar hyalinosis and fibrointimal thickening, as well as chronic glomerulopathy. The occurrence of CNI nephrotoxicity was also assessed and found in almost 90–100% at 10 years after transplantation in CNI-treated patients [9,10]. The authors concluded that CAN is a sequential multifactorial process in which clinical and subclinical rejection in the early stages contribute to interstitial fibrosis, tubular atrophy, and nephron loss that together constitute CAN. Later damage appeared to be predominantly associated with a histological pattern suggestive of CNI toxicity, defined as striped cortical fibrosis or new onset of arteriolar hyalinosis together with tubular microcalcification. It should be pointed out that, despite the progressive histological changes during the 10-year follow-up, there was only a 10–15% reduction in renal function in this series

The course of CAN

When describing the course and development of CAN, it is important to separate the early injury and its impact on early graft function from the subsequent deterioration of renal graft function [2,7,9]. Several factors determine early transplant function, including injury due to acute rejection (AR) episodes, ischemia and reperfusion damage, and preformed structural changes of the kidney related to donor age (and premorbid conditions, such as hypertension), plus thrombotic and other vascular damage in the perioperative period [7,9,10]. The donor source also influences the onset of function, where recipients of transplants from living donors exhibit better early function compared to recipients

Evidence-based Nephrology. Edited by Donald Molony and Jonathan Craig
© 2009 Blackwell Publishing, ISBN: 978-1-4051-3975-5.

from cadaveric donors. In the longer term many additional factors play an important role, determining the fate of renal transplant function. Such progression factors include the level of transplant function achieved in the early posttransplant period, hypertension, proteinuria, hyperlipidemia, cigarette smoking, and viral infections [2].

Immunological injury

Acute rejection episodes

A great number of studies have demonstrated that acute rejection episodes influence the future development of CAN, specifically, the features of chronic rejection. Thus, kidney transplant recipients without prior clinical acute rejection have a substantially longer graft half-life than patients with previous acute rejection [11]. The association between AR episodes and CAN appears strongest for acute vascular rejection, rather than tubulo-interstitial rejection episodes [12]. AR episodes followed by loss of graft function have a stronger negative impact on long-term outcome than those with functional recovery [13]. In our own long-term outcome study, treatment for previous AR episodes was a significant risk factor for graft loss in a univariate analysis, but poor graft function (a result of early AR, among other factors) was the dominant risk factor [8].

Subclinical rejection

Recently, a great deal of attention has also been paid to subclinical rejection and its impact on the future development of CAN [14–16]. Subclinical rejection is defined as lymphocyte or monocyte infiltration in the graft without functional deterioration. This form of rejection damages the kidney through low-grade inflammation, which leads to gradual injury and destruction and remodeling of the functional unit of the kidney. Randomized treatment of subclinical rejection is reported to lead to improved long-term graft function [14].

Antibody-mediated rejection

In addition to T-cell-mediated rejection—and its influence on the future development of CAN—it has been recognized that the presence of HLA antibodies has a strong adverse impact on the development of CAN [17,18]. Posttransplant antibodies are significantly more common in CAN patients, their presence being associated with subsequent renal dysfunction and graft loss from chronic rejection [19]. Thus, anti-HLA antibodies both prior to and after transplantation are associated with development of CAN. Furthermore, C4d deposition (a marker of humoral rejection) has been found in more than one-third of late allograft biopsies [20], in particular localized to the peritubular capillaries and in cases with transplant glomerulopathy. Antibodies against non-HLA antigens, such as endothelial cell antigens, have been described in both kidney transplant recipients and recipients of cardiac allografts complicated by CAN or transplant arteriosclerosis, respectively [21–23] (Figure 53.1).

Another interesting aspect from a pathophysiological viewpoint is the relationship between oxidative stress-induced accelerated aging and cellular "exhaustion" and graft loss (replicative senescence). Many different types of injury, including oxidative

	Allo-immune response (HLA-MM; presensitization)	Innate immune response	Nonimmune reactivity
Primary Injury	• Acute cellular rejection • Humoral acute rejection (HLA-Ab)	• Donor brain death • Ischemia-reperfusion injury • Hyperglycemia	• Preformed graft injury - poor quality of graft - old donor age
Secondary Injury	• Sub-acute cellular rejection • De novo formation of HLA-Ab (CHR)	• Non-HLA-Abformation (CHR) • Hyperlipidemia • Proteinuria • BK-virus nephropathy • ROS-excess & senescence	• Chronic CNI toxicity and other nephrotoxic agents • Hypertension
	C H R O N I C A L L O G R A F T N E P H R O P A T H Y		

Figure 53.1 Allo- and innate immune reactivity and nonimmune factors contributing to primary and secondary injuries leading to chronic allograft nephropathy in kidney transplant patients.

stress and aging, target the telomere, resulting in loss of telomere length and altered function of telomere binding proteins. In both experimental animals and explanted human kidneys, CAN is associated with telomere shortening, the determinants of which include donor age, perioperative ischemia–reperfusion injury, and posttransplant oxidative stresses, including acute rejection [24–26]. Pretransplant measurement of telomere length may provide a useful objective predictor for the subsequent development of CAN.

Clinical factors and progression of CAN

Ongoing pathophysiological stressors, such as hyperfiltration, proteinuria, hypertension, cigarette smoking, hyperlipidemia, and reactive oxidative species (ROS) production, have long been suggested as mediators of CAN, based upon circumstantial evidence. All are biologically plausible and have been reported individually to be related to future deterioration of transplant function and eventually graft loss. In the ALERT trial of 2102 long-term kidney transplant recipients, renal dysfunction and proteinuria were the two strongest, independent risk factors for future graft loss [3,8] and confirmed the findings from previous studies that proteinuria is a strong risk factor for CAN and future graft loss [27] (Figure 53.2). Proteinuria is a powerful risk factor for renal dysfunction in general and is dependent upon both glomerular leakage and impaired tubular reabsorption. Reabsorbed filtered protein is known to lead to an increase in interstitial chemoattractants, cytokines, and monocyte infiltration, which may cause additional interstitial and tubular damage and may contribute to CAN [28]. The tubular cell is both a focus of injury in CAN and a potential source of factors that contribute to interstitial cellular infiltration and fibrosis. Thus, uncontrolled ROS production from tubular cell mitochondria may also contribute to continued tubular injury and apoptosis, and both interstitial nitrothyrosine and ROS production are increased in CAN [29].

BK virus nephropathy

Polyoma virus infection is increasingly recognized as a complication in renal transplant recipients (RTR) [30–33]. Polyoma virus is widely prevalent in nature, and most people are exposed by adulthood. The BK virus by itself, in the background population, has low morbidity, long latency, and asymptomatic reactivation [34]. BK virus allograft nephropathy (BKVAN) emerged as a cause of renal allograft dysfunction in the mid-1990s, when more powerful immunosuppression was introduced. In recent years, routine posttransplant protocol biopsies have also detected BKVAN in the absence of serum creatinine elevation [16,35]. Virus replicates within tubules and forms intranuclear inclusions with focal interstitial mononuclear inflammatory cell infiltrates and tubulitis.

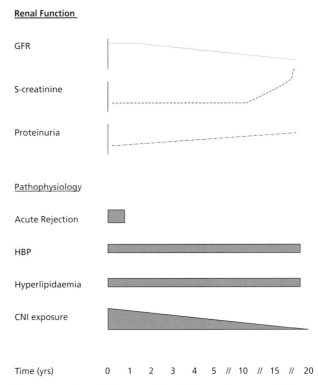

Figure 53.2 Schematic of the time relationship between factors contributing to development of CAN, renal function, and proteinuria in kidney transplantation.

BKVAN-induced nephropathy may lead to chronic graft dysfunction [30–35]. Renal interstitial inflammation with BKVAN cannot always be differentiated from acute rejection. Moreover, the final stage of chronic tubulo-interstitial scarring and atrophic tubules may resemble a nonspecific pattern of fibrosis and tubular atrophy. Thus, BKVAN-induced nephropathy may lead to chronic graft dysfunction.

CNI nephrotoxicity

Reports of Cyclosporine A (CsA) and tacrolimus (Tac) nephrotoxicity are increasingly common late after transplantation [9] and cannot be distinguished from each other based upon histology. CNI nephrotoxicity lesions include arteriolar hyalinosis, striped fibrosis, and tubular vacuolizations. Cyclosporine A-induced arteriolopathy is characterized by vacuolation and necrosis of smooth muscle and endothelial cells with hyaline deposits, considered to be the most characteristic marker of CNI nephrotoxicity [36–38]. Progressive arteriolar hyalinosis causes vascular narrowing and ischemic injury. Striped fibrosis of the cortex is usually regarded as the most pathognomonic sign of CNI nephrotoxicity [39], but tubular vacuolization may also occur as part of CNI nephrotoxicity. The progressive character of CNI nephrotoxicity is the reason for trials focusing on reduction or withdrawal of CNI in kidney transplant subjects with signs of CNI nephrotoxicity with or without deterioration of kidney transplant function.

Table 53.1 Prevention modalities in CAN: hypothetical, indicative, and evidence based.

Target	Action	Evidence[a]	Reference(s)
Primary Prevention			
Ischemia–reperfusion injury	Reduce ischemia time	I	40
	Antioxidant drugs, protective genes	H	41
Acute cellular rejection	Immunosuppressive treatment to prevent acute rejection	E	44, 45
	Prevention vs. acute rejection per se		
Humoral rejection	Pretreatment	I	43
(HLA and non-HLA Ab)	Removal of Ab by PP or immune absorption		
	Prevention neoformation of Ab		
	C IVIG		
	Rituximab		
	Cyclophosphamide		
Secondary prevention			
CNI toxicity (CONVERT, TRANCEPT, REFERENCE,	Selection of CNI	H/I/N	47, 48/49, 50/51, 52
and MODIFY studies)	Reduction or withdrawal of CNI ± mTORi	H/I	53–55, 58/56, 57, 69
	Reduction of withdrawal of CNI ± introduction of MMF	/I/	/49, 59–65/67, 68
Subclinical rejection	Corticosteroid treatment		
	Other rejection treatment		
de novo formation of HLA- or non-HLA Ab (CHR)	Removal of Ab	H	43
	Prevention of continued formation of Ab (IVIG, Rituximab, cytostatics)	H	43
Tertiary prevention (progression factors)			
Proteinuria	ACEi, ARB introduction	H/N	75–78/79
Hypertension	CCB; ACEi		
Hyperlipidemia	Statins	N	3
BK virus	Reduction or change of immunosuppression	H	70
	Leflunomide	H	71, 72
	Cidofovir		
Stressors and ROS excess (senescence)	Reduce stressors		
	Antioxidative measures		
	Remove nephrotoxic agents		

Abbreviations: Ab, antibody; IVIG, intravenous immunoglobulin; CCB, calcium channel blocker; PP, plasma pheresis
[a] Evidence categories: H, hypothetical; I, indicative (inadequate small clinical studies); E, solid evidence based upon controlled randomized trials; N, no effect.

Prevention and treatment

There is no specific intervention to prevent or treat CAN. The primary aim is to minimize exposure to risk factors for development of CAN. When CAN is established, the aim of disease management is to minimize exposure to risk factors for progression, including modification of immunosuppressive treatment, and to commence interventions for specific progression factors, such as proteinuria and hypertension. Lately, the focus has been on the differential effects of immunosuppressive agents with regard to nephrotoxicity, specifically, the reduction or withdrawal of CNI and their replacement with nonnephrotoxic agents, to limit the risk of AR (Table 53.1).

Primary prevention

Preventive measures include minimization of ischemia–reperfusion damage, prevention of AR episodes by optimal immunosuppressive treatment, and pretreatment of recipients with HLA antibodies. Registry studies have shown that delayed graft function, which is strongly related to the length of warm and cold ischemia preceding reperfusion, has a clear association with later development of CAN and subsequent graft loss [40]. Hence, there is a general consensus that shorter ischemia–reperfusion times lead to better long-term graft survival. With regard to drugs used for reduction of ischemia–reperfusion damage, very little has been achieved in clinical transplantation, although a number of compounds efficiently reduce the effects of prolonged ischemic injury in experimental animal models. One topical approach is the use of gene transfer to upregulate protective genes [41].

Additional preventive measures include the pretransplant identification of sensitized patients and pretreatment of sensitized recipients, because of the strong association between presensitization and subsequent development of CAN or humoral-driven chronic rejection [42]. Various modalities have been used for pretreatment of sensitized patients, including either plasmapheresis combined with intravenous immunoglobulins or rituximab [43]. These treatment modalities have been shown to reduce the occurrence of acute antibody-mediated rejection episodes. The extent to which the frequency of chronic antibody-mediated rejection becomes attenuated by these treatment modalities remains to be seen, but early results are encouraging and long-term graft survival does appear to improve [42,43].

The most important means of prevention is effective immunosuppressive treatment to prevent acute cellular rejection. This can be considered as not only a preventive strategy but also as part of the long-term management of CAN, given that different immunosuppressive protocols affect the development of CAN via their contribution to nephrotoxic injury. In contrast with secondary treatment of CAN based upon diagnostic evidence (e.g. SWITCH studies, which will be covered below), studies that target early AR provide evidence on the effect of reduced AR on subsequent development of histological CAN and its functional sequelae [44,45]: the rate of decline of glomerular filtration rate (GFR) and/or differences in the development of CNI nephrotoxicity. Because CNI nephrotoxicity is an important component of CAN, many primary prevention studies have focused on reduction of CNI nephrotoxicity and reduction of early and late posttransplant graft dysfunction.

First, the choice of CNI, Tacrolimus or Cyclosporine A, together with the monitoring strategy (trough levels vs. blood levels at a given time point) have been examined in a number of clinical studies. Most of these studies were powered only to compare AR rates, and the effects on other end points, including graft function, rate of deterioration of GFR, or long-term graft survival must be viewed with this caveat. The impact of CNI choice has recently been reviewed [46]. The balance of evidence is that Tacrolimus is associated with lower rates of AR than Cyclosporine A (with conventional trough monitoring), although AR rates when C2 monitoring is used approach those of Tacrolimus. Given our understanding of the impact of AR on CAN, one would predict that Tacrolimus would be associated with less CAN. In one randomized trial [47], an increase in interstitial fibrosis was demonstrated with Cyclosporine A compared to Tacrolimus. In another small randomized study renal function was significantly better and the degree of interstitial fibrosis less in Tacrolimus-treated patients than in those treated with Cyclosporine A, and there was also an advantage with regard to graft survival [48]. Renal function should be considered a surrogate end point, but it is also one of the strongest predictors of future graft loss [2,8]. There are a few studies that have compared graft function in Tacrolimus-treated versus Cyclosporine A-treated patients. The findings from the recent SYM-PHONY and DIRECT studies [49,50], which compared various therapeutic regimens containing Tacrolimus and Cyclosporine A, do tend to support the notion that Tacrolimus use leads to better early graft function, particularly when Tacrolimus is used with mycophenolate mofetil (MMF) and when low trough levels (3–7 nmol/L) are targeted. But these are all relatively small studies with short follow-up, provide little data on the long-term impact on CAN, and neither registry studies [51] nor biopsy-based studies [52] provide consistent support for one or the other CNI.

Another recent primary prevention approach has been to compare the use of CNI with mTOR inhibitors (sirolimus [SRL] or everolimus [EVL]), which are potent immunosuppressive and antiproliferative agents but without direct nephrotoxic effects. This class of compounds also seems to be useful in prevention of scarring processes and the development of intimal hyperplasia in blood vessels. Studies comparing SRL and Cyclosporine A as primary immunosuppressive agent [53–55] have demonstrated lower serum creatinine and higher GFR in SRL-treated patients. To what extent this would translate into a lower propensity for development of CAN is not known, but similar findings were made in another primary prevention study that compared renal transplant function in patients treated with Cyclosporine A and SRL, where Cyclosporine A was withdrawn after 3 months in a randomized fashion combined with increased doses of SRL [56]. Histological evaluation of biopsies taken during follow-up in a subgroup of this study also showed less interstitial damage or CAN in patients who withdrew from Cyclosporine A [57]. However, the interpretation of these data is clouded by the early combination of SRL with Cyclosporine A, a combination that is known to potentiate the nephrotoxicity of Cyclosporine A. Similar findings have been observed with EVL. Compared with Cyclosporine A alone, EVL alone or in combination with low-dose Cyclosporine A (40% of original dose) had beneficial effects on renal function [58]. Short-term reports have shown better renal function with "high-dose" EVL or moderate doses of EVL combined with a low dose of Cyclosporine A, compared to Cyclosporine A alone. However, there are no long-term data available at the present time.

Secondary prevention

The risk of AR decreases with time after transplantation. This observation provides an alternative two-phase strategy to limit AR by the early use of CNI followed by CNI minimization or withdrawal (to limit CNI nephrotoxicity and its contribution to CAN) by the introduction (or dose increase) of nonnephrotoxic agents, such as MMF or mTOR inhibitors. There is debate whether such a strategy should be part of the treatment protocol, at 3–6 months after transplantation, and preempt the development of histological or functional CAN. The latter approach has been studied in clinical trials. When MMF was used to allow CNI minimization or withdrawal in patients with declining renal function and biopsy-proven CAN, there was an improvement in renal function [59]. Subsequently, several other small studies demonstrated similar findings with improved renal transplant function upon reduction or withdrawal of Cyclosporine A, facilitated by substitution by, or concomitant treatment with, MMF [60–65]. Most of these studies have been small, open studies. Also, there is a complex pharmacokinetic interaction between Cyclosporine A and MMF such that that high-dose Cyclosporine A reduces the exposure of MMF, whereas reduced Cyclosporine A increases the exposure to MMF and thereby the risk of MMF-related side effects. This is true to a lesser extent in the combination of Tacrolimus and MMF [66].

Withdrawal of CNI in stable maintenance renal transplant patients receiving CNI together with MMF and glucocorticoids improved renal transplant function, albeit with a slight increase in modest acute rejection [67].

Switch studies

An ongoing observational study (TRANCEPT) is capturing data in patients with declining renal function, with or without biopsy-proven CAN, for whom CNI have been reduced or withdrawn in parallel with introduction of MMF. An interim report made at the WTC 2006 [68] demonstrated a significant change in the slope of the calculated GFR at the time of the switch.

Other switch studies have been conducted in patients switched from CNI-based therapy to SRL (CONVERT trial). In the CONVERT trial, preconversion biopsies were made and transplant biopsies will also be performed by the end of the study. A total of 800 patients were recruited, but the group with low GFR (<40 mL/min) had to be stopped after only 70–80 patients, due to adverse side effects. A 1-year, interim analysis in patients who had preserved renal function (GFR, 40–70 mL/min) at inclusion reported potential benefits on renal function, provided that proteinuria was low, whereas patients with GFR below 40 mL/min that were converted to SRL experienced a high frequency of side effects without any improvement in kidney transplant function [69].

Combining mTOR inhibitors and CNI may lead to an enhanced form of nephrotoxicity unless the Cyclosporine A or Tacrolimus dose is reduced substantially (tentatively by two-thirds), apparently due to increased formation of ROS causing renal injury (unpublished data).

Another (ongoing) switch study is the ASCERTAIN study, in which stable RTR patients with GFR of 30–70 mL/min were randomized (total of 450 patients; three groups) to EVL with CNI minimization or elimination, or conventional CNI-based therapy. The study is targeting transplant function, biopsy scoring of CAN, and carotid intima media thickness. To date just over half the study population has been recruited; the study will be reported in 2008–2009.

Treatment of BK virus infection

The treatment of manifest BK virus nephropathy is problematic. The options are reduced immunosuppressive medication (with the associated risk of acute rejection), with or without concomitant virus therapy [34]. In a recent report, leflunomide was used as antiviral therapy, together with a reduction in immunosuppression, mycophenalate was discontinued, and Tacrolimus was given in a reduced dose. Marked reductions in viremia and viruria were observed. However, the seemingly beneficial effect of leflunomide

might have been secondary to reduced immunosuppression [70]. Cidofovir has also been used in the treatment of BKVAN, with mixed results [71,72]. Overall, the treatment modalities for BK virus nephropathy are hampered by a lack of randomized controlled studies, and the precise place of BKVAN as a component of CAN or as a separate entity remains to be resolved.

Treatment with nonimmunosuppressive agents

Since hypertension, both systemic and intraglomerular, is implicated in CAN, the use of angiotensin converting enzyme inhibitors (ACEi) and angiotensin II receptor blockers (ARB) is a logical therapeutic approach. These agents slow the decline in renal function in patients with diabetic and nondiabetic renal disease [73,74], and their beneficial effects on blood pressure and proteinuria in renal transplant recipients have been well-described [75–78]. Lin and colleagues demonstrated that patients treated with ACEi or ARB had a lower incidence and slower progression of renal insufficiency, together with a significant decrease in the combined end point of graft failure or death in patients receiving the ACEi or ARB. Campistol and colleagues found that patients with documented CAN had higher levels of transforming growth factor-β than a control group of 15 kidney transplant recipients with normal renal function and without CAN. Treatment with losartan caused a decrease in the transforming growth factor-β levels, which reached those of the control transplant recipients without CAN. However, the same study group recently presented the results of a randomized placebo-controlled study with losartan, which failed to shown any clinical benefit of losartan on CAN (AALOGRAFT) [79].

Statin treatment

The similarities between the pathophysiological processes underlying glomerulosclerosis and atherosclerosis suggest that statin therapy (and lipid lowering in general) may be a useful strategy. However, in the ALERT study, effective lipid lowering with fluvastatin, with 5–7 years follow-up in 2100 patients, had no impact on graft survival, rate of decline of function, or proteinuria. Thus, as monotherapy at least, statin treatment has no effect on CAN [3].

Overall impact of CAN

Although we have focused on the effects of CAN on the graft, there are additional considerations. Graft failure is associated with major increments in cardiovascular and all-cause mortality risks, reflecting the reverse of the published survival benefits of transplantation over dialysis (e.g. Wolfe) [80,81]. Thus, patients in the ALERT study who experienced graft loss had an overall doubling of cardiovascular and noncardiovascular event rates. In a mathematical modeling study by McLean and Jardine [82], graft failure was associated with a threefold increase in overall risk. The potential impacts of CAN and future reduction in CAN can only really be estimated. At the present time approximately 3% of all patients with functioning transplants return to dialysis per annum, representing about 5% of all those patients starting dialysis each year.

Slowing the rate of graft failure would increase the number of patients with functioning grafts and also the proportion of patients who die with a functioning graft. Those patients who return to dialysis will tend to be older and have a corresponding adverse impact on survival on the dialysis population. Thus, the overall benefit of reducing graft loss due to CAN is predicted to be an increase the proportion of patients with end-stage renal disease living with a functioning graft and a reduction in the proportion of patients on maintenance dialysis.

Summary and conclusion

CAN is a clinical diagnosis, the components of which are progressive deterioration in graft function, premature graft failure, and proteinuria, associated with histological changes of interstitial fibrosis, tubular loss and atrophy, and vascular and glomerular changes. It has two broad determinants, immunological, specifically the occurrence and severity of rejection episodes, and non-immunological, specifically hypertension, proteinuria, hyperlipidemia, and the nephrotoxic effects of immunosuppressive drugs. Despite our improved understanding of the mechanisms and natural history of CAN, therapeutic strategies have not been established. As a consequence of reluctance to change immunosuppression in patients with stable graft function, there are few data to support changing immunosuppression to prevent CAN; although CNI reduction or withdrawal under cover of increased MMF has proven benefits, these are marginal. The emerging importance of CAN is a reflection of the success in preventing AR and should now become the focus of clinical trials in transplantation.

References

1 Paul LC. Chronic allograft nephropathy: an update. *Kidney Int* 1999; **56(3):** 783–793.

2 Joosten SA, Sijpkens YWJ, van Kooten C, Paul CL. Chronic allograft rejection: Pathophysiologic considerations. *Kidney Int* 2005; **68(1):** 1–13.

3 Fellstrom B, Holdaas H, Jardine AG, Holme I, Nyberg G, Fauchald P *et al.* Effect of fluvastatin on renal end points in the Assessment of Lescol in Renal Transplant (ALERT) trial. *Kidney Int* 2004; **66(4):** 1549–1555.

4 Hariharan S, Johnson CP, Bresnahan BA, Taranto SE, McIntosh MJ, Stablein D. Improved graft survival after renal transplantation in the United States, 1988 to 1996. *N Engl J Med* 2000; **342(9):** 605–612.

5 Meier-Kriesche HU, Schold JD, Kaplan B. Long-term renal allograft survival: have we made significant progress or is it time to rethink our analytic and therapeutic strategies? *Am J Transplant* 2004; **4(8):** 1289–1295.

6 US Renal Data System. *USRDS 2004 Annual Report: Atlas of End-Stage Renal Disease in the United States.* National Institutes of Health, National Institute of Diabetes and Digestive and Kidney Diseases, Bethesda, 2004.

7 Meyers CM, Kirk AD. Workshop on late renal allograft dysfunction. *Am J Transplant* 2005; **5(7):** 1600–1605.

8 Fellström B, Jardine AG, Soveri I, Cole E, Grönhagen-Riska C, Neumayer HH *et al.* Renal dysfunction as a risk factor for mortality and cardiovascular disease in renal transplantation: experience from the assessment of Lescol in renal transplantation trial. *Transplantation* 2005; **79(9):** 1160–1163.

9 Nankivell BJ, Borrows RJ, Fung CL-S, O'Connell PJ, Allen RDM, Chapman JR. The natural history of chronic allograft nephropathy. *N Engl J Med* 2003; **349(24):** 2326–2333.

10 Nankivell BJ, Chapman JR. Chronic allograft nephropathy: current concepts and future directions. *Transplantation* 2006; **81(5):** 643–654.

11 Lindholm A, Ohlman S, Albrechtsen D, Tufveson G, Persson H, Persson NH. The impact of acute rejection episodes on long-term graft function and outcome in 1347 primary renal transplants treated by 3 cyclosporine regimens. *Transplantation* 1993; **56(2):** 307–315.

12 van Saase JL, van der Woude FJ, Thorogood J, Hollander AA, van Es LA, Weening JJ *et al.* The relation between acute vascular and interstitial renal allograft rejection and subsequent chronic rejection. *Transplantation* 1995; **59(9):** 1280–1285.

13 Madden RL, Mulhern JG, Benedetto BJ, O'Shea MH, Germain MJ, Braden GL *et al.* Completely reversed acute rejection is not a significant risk factor for the development of chronic rejection in renal allograft recipients. *Transplant Int* 2000; **13(5):** 344–350.

14 Rush D, Nickerson P, Gough J, McKenna R, Grimm P, Cheang M *et al.* Beneficial effects of treatment of early subclinical rejection: a randomized study. *J Am Soc Nephrol* 1998; **9(11):** 2129–2134.

15 Rush DN, Karpinski ME, Nickerson P, Dancea S, Birk P, Jeffery JR. Does subclinical rejection ctongribute to chronic rejection in renal transplant patients? *Clin Transplant* 1999; **13(6):** 441–446.

16 Nankivell BJ, Chapman JR. The significance of subclinical rejection and the value of protocol biopsies. *Am J Transplantation* 2006; **6(1):** 2006–2012.

17 Lee PC, Terasaki PI, Takemoto SK, Lee PH, Hung CJ, Chen YL *et al.* All chronic rejection failures of kidney transplants were preceded by the development of HLA antibodies. *Transplantation* 2002; **74(8):** 1192–1194.

18 Terasaki PI. Humoral theory of transplantation. *Am J Transplant* 2003; **3(6):** 665–673.

19 Piazza A, Poggi E, Borrelli L, Servetti S, Monaco PI, Buonomo O *et al.* Impact of donor-specific antibodies on chronic rejection occurrence and graft loss in renal transplantation: posttransplant analysis using flow cytometric techniques. *Transplantation* 2001; **71(8):** 1106–1112.

20 Regele H, Bohmig GA, Habicht A, Gollowitzer D, Schillinger M, Rockenschaub S *et al.* Capillary deposition of complement split product C4d in renal allografts is associated with basement membrane injury in peritubular and glomerular capillaries: a contribution of humoral immunity to chronic allograft rejection. *J Am Soc Nephrol* 2002; **13(9):** 2371–2380.

21 Ball B, Mousson C, Ratignier C, Guignier F, Glotz D, Rifle G. Antibodies to vascular endothelial cells in chronic rejection of renal allografts. *Transplant Proc* 2000; **32(2):** 353–354.

22 Joosten SA, Sijpkens YW, van Ham V, Trouw LA, van der Vlag J, van den Heuvel B *et al.* Antibody response against the glomerular basement membrane protein agrin in patients with transplant glomerulopathy. *Am J Transplant* 2005; **5(2):** 383–393.

23 Smith JD, Rose M. Detection and clinical relevance of antibodies after transplantation. *Methods Mol Biol* 2006; **333:** 227–246.

24 Halloran PF, Melk A, Barth C. Rethinking chronic allograft nephropathy: the concept of accelerated senescence. *J Am Soc Nephrol* 1999; **10(1):** 167–181.

25 Melk A, Ramassar V, Helms LM, Moore R, Rayner D, Solez K *et al.* Telomere shortening in kidneys with age. *J Am Soc Nephrol* 2000; **11(3):** 444–453.

26 Joosten SA, van Ham V, Nolan CE, Borrias MC, Jardine AG, Shiels PG et al. Telomere shortening and cellular senescence in a model of chronic renal allograft rejection. *Am J Pathol* 2003; **162(4):** 1305–1312.

27 Vathsala A, Verani R, Schoenberg L, Lewis RM, Van Buren CT, Kerman RG et al. Proteinuria in cyclosporine-treated renal transplant recipients. *Transplantation* 1990; **49(1):** 35–41.

28 Zoja C, Benigni A, Remuzzi G. Cellular responses to protein overload: key event in renal disease progression. *Curr Opin Nephrol Hypertens* 2004; **13(1):** 31–37.

29 Albrecht EW, Stegeman CA, Tiebosch AT, Tegzess AM, van Goor H. Expression of inducible and endothelial nitric oxide synthases, formation of peroxynitrite and reactive oxygen species in human chronic renal transplant failure. *Am J Transplant* 2002; **2(5):** 448–453.

30 Nickeleit V, Hirsch HH, Binet IF, Gudat F, Prince O, Dalquen P et al. Polyomavirus infection of renal allograft recipients: from latent infection to manifest disease. *J Am Soc Nephrol* 1999; **10(5):** 1080–1089.

31 Mathur VS, Olson JL, Darragh TM, Yen TSB. Polyomavirus-induced interstitial nephritis in two renal transplant recipients: case reports and review of the literature. *Am J Kidney Dis* 1997; **29(5):** 754–758.

32 Randhawa PS, Finkelstein S, Scantlebury V, Shapiro R, Vivas C, Jordan M et al. Human polyoma virus-associated interstitial nephritis in the allograft kidney. *Transplantation* 1999; **67(1):** 103–109.

33 Nickeleit V, Klimkait T, Binet IF, Dalquen P, Del Zenero V, Thiel G et al. Testing for polyomavirus type BK DNA in plasma to identify renal-allograft recipients with viral nephropathy. *N Engl J Med* 2000; **342(18):** 1309–1315.

34 Hirsch HH, Steiger J. Polyomavirus BK. *Lancet Infect Dis* 2003; **3(10):** 611–623.

35 Hariharan S. BK virus nephritis after renal transplantation. *Kidney Int* 2006; **69(4):** 655–662.

36 Mihatsch MJ, Thiel G, Ryffel B. Histopathology of cyclosporine nephrotoxicity. *Transplant Proc* 1988; **20(3 Suppl 3):** 759–771.

37 Mihatsch MJ, Ryffel B, Gudat F. The differential diagnosis between rejection and cyclosporine toxicity. *Kidney Int* 1995; **52(Suppl):** S63–S69.

38 Davies DR, Bittmann I, Pardo J. Histopathology of calcineurin inhibitor-induced nephrotoxicity. *Transplantation* 2000; **69(12 Suppl):** SS11–SS13.

39 Dell'Antonio G, Randhawa PS. "Striped" pattern of medullary ray fibrosis in allograft biopsies from kidney transplant recipients maintained on tacrolimus. *Transplantation* 1999; **67(3):** 484–486.

40 Gjertson DW. A multi-factor analysis of kidney graft outcomes at one and five years posttransplantation: 1996 UNOS update. *Clin Transplant* 1996; **1996:** 343–360.

41 Hancock WW, Buelow R, Sayegh MH, Turka LA. Antibody-induced transplant arteriosclerosis is prevented by graft expression of anti-oxidant and anti-apoptotic genes. *Nat Med* 1998; **4(12):** 1392–1396.

42 Mauiyyedi S, Pelle PD, Saidman S, Collins AB, Pascual M, Tolkoff-Rubin NE et al. Chronic humoral rejection: identification of antibody-mediated chronic renal allograft rejection by C4d deposits in peritubular capillaries. *J Am Soc Nephrol* 2001; **12(3):** 574–582.

43 Takemoto SK, Zeevi A, Feng S, Colvin RB, Jordan S, Kobashigawa J et al. National conference to assess antibody-mediated rejection in solid organ transplantation. *Am J Transplant* 2004; **4(7):** 1033–1041.

44 Humar A, Payne WD, Sutherland DE, Matas AJ. Clinical determinants of multiple acute rejection episodes in kidney transplant recipients. *Transplantation* 2000; **69(11):** 2357–2360.

45 Sijpkens YW, Doxiadis II, Mallat MJ, de Fijter JW, Bruijn JA, Claas FH et al. Early versus late acute rejection episodes in renal transplantation. *Transplantation* 2003; **75(2):** 204–208.

46 Tanabe K. Calcineurin inhibitors in renal transplantation: what is the best option? *Drugs* 2003; **63(15):** 1535–1548.

47 Murphy GJ, Waller JR, Sandford RS, Furness PH, Nocholson ML. Randomized clinical trial of the effect of microemulsion cyclosporine and tacrolimus on renal allograft fibrosis. *Br J Surg* 2003; **90(6):** 680–686.

48 Jurewicz WA. Tacrolimus versus cyclosporin immunosuppression: long-term outcome in renal transplantation. *Nephrol Dial Transplant* 2003; **18(Suppl 1):** i7–i11.

49 Ekberg H, Tedesco-Silva H, Demirbas H, Vitko S, Nashan B, Gurkan A et al. Reduced exposure to calcineurine inhibitors in renal transplantation, NEJM 2007; **357:** 2562–75.

50 Vincenti F, Friman S, Scheuermann E, Rostaing L, DIRECT Study Group. Results of an international randomised trial comparing glucose metabolism disorders and outcome with cyclosporine versus tacrotimus. Am J Transplant 2007; **7:** 1506–14.

51 Irish W, Sherrill B, Brennann DC, Lowell J, Schnitzler M. Three-year post-transplant graft survival in renal-transplant patients with graft function at 6 months receiving tacrolimus or cyclosporine microemulsion within a triple-drug regimen. *Transplantation* 2003; **76(12):** 1686–1690.

52 Solez K, Vincenti F, Filo RS. Histopathologic findings from 2-year protocol biopsies from a U.S: multicenter kidney transplant trial comparing tacrolimus versus cyclosporine: a report of the FK506 Kidney Transplant Study Group. *Transplantation* 1998; **66(12):** 1736–1740.

53 Kreis H, Cisterne JM, Land W, Wramner L, Squifflet JP, Abramowicz D et al. Sirolimus in association with mycophenolate mofetik induction for the prevention of acute graft rejection in renal allograft recipients. *Transplantation* 2000; **69(7):** 1252–1260.

54 Groth CG, Backman L, Morales JM, Calne R, Kreis H, Lang P et al. Sirolimus (rapamycin)-based therapy in human renal transplantation: similar efficacy and different toxicity compared with cyclosporine. Sirolimus European Renal Transplant Study Group. *Transplantation* 1999; **67(7):** 1036–1042.

55 Flechner SM, Goldfarb D, Modlin C, Feng J, Krishnamurthi V, Mastroianni B et al. Kidney transplantation without calcineurin inhibitor drugs: A prospective, randomized trial of sirolimus versus cyclosporine. *Transplantation* 2002; **74(8):** 1070–1076.

56 Johnson RW, Kreis H, Oberbauer R, Brattstrom C, Claesson K, Eris J. Sirolimus allows early cyclosporine withdrawal in renal transplantation resulting in improved renal function and lower blood pressure. *Transplantation* 2001; **72(5):** 777–786.

57 Stallone G, Di Paolo S, Schena A, Infante B, Grandaliano G, Battaglia M et al. Early withdrawal of cyclosporine A improves 1-year kidney graft structure and function in sirolimus-treated patients. *Transplantation* 2003; **75(7):** 998–1003.

58 Nashan B, Curtis J, Ponticelli C, Mourad G, Jaffe J, Haas T et al. Everolimus and reduced-exposure cyclosporine in de novo renal-transplant recipients: a three-year phase II, randomized, multicenter, open-label study. *Transplantation* 2004; **78(9):** 1332–1340.

59 Weir MR, Ward MT, Blahut SA, Klassen DK, Cangro CB, Bartlett ST et al. Long-term impact of discontinued or reduced calcineurin inhibitor in patients with chronic allograft nephropathy. *Kidney Int* 2001; **59(4):** 1567–1573.

60 Khachatryan N, Wauters JP, Vogel P. Effect of mycophenolate mofetil in combination with standard immunosuppression in chronic transplant nephropathy: 1 year experience. *Transplant Proc* 2002; **34(3):** 807–808.

61 Ducloux D, Motte G, Billerey C, Bresson-Vautrin C, Vautrin P, Rebibou JM et al. Cyclosporin withdrawal with concomitant conversion from

azathiprine to mycophenolate mofetil in renal transplant recipients with chronic allograft nephropathy: a 2-year follow-up. *Transplant Int* 2002; **15(8):** 387–392.

62 Merville P, Berge F, Deminiere C, Morel D, Chong G, Durand D *et al.* Lower incidence of chronic allograft nephropathy at 1 year post-transplantation in patients treated with mycophenolate mofetil. *Am J Transplant* 2004; **4(11):** 1769–1775.

63 Afzali B, Shah S, Chowdhury P, O'Sullivan H, Taylor J, Goldsmith D. Low dose mycophenolate mofetil is effective and safe treatment to permit phased reduction in calcineurin inhibitors in chronic allograft nephropathy. *Transplantation* 2005; **79(3):** 304–309.

64 Kessler M, Frimat L, Cassuto-Viguier E, Charpentier B, Djeffal R, Noel C *et al.* Impact of cyclosporine reduction with MMF in chronic allograft dysfunction: 4-year results of a multicenter randomized controlled study. The "reference" study. Abstr 850, 2006.

65 Pereira LM, de Castro MCR, Ventura CG, Soares PS, Ferreira GF, Saldanha LB *et al.* A prospective, randomized and controlled trial of tacrolimus minimization in renal transplantation: 1-year result of the MoDIFY study. Abstr 53, 2006.

66 Kuriata-Kordek M, Boratynska M, Falkiewicz K, Porazko T, Urbaniak J, Wozniak M *et al.* The influence of calcineurin inhibitors on mycophenolic acid pharmacokinetics. *Transplant Proc* 2003; **35(6):** 2369–2371.

67 Abramowicz D, Manas D, Lao M, Vanrenterghem Y, Del Castillo D, Wijngaard P *et al.* Cyclosporine withdrawal from a mycophenolate mofetil-containing immunosuppressive regimen in stable kidney transplant recipients: A randomized, controlled study. *Transplantation* 2002; **74(12):** 1725–1734.

68 Meier-Kriesche HU, Heemann U, Merville P, Tedesco da Silva H, Mamelok RD, Bernasconi C. TRANCEPT: a prospective observational global clinical study of patients switched to MMF at least 6 months after renal transplantation. Abstr 578, 2006.

69 Schena FP, Vitko S, Wali R, Pascoe MD, Alberu J, del Carmen Rial M *et al.* Efficacy and safety of conversion from calcineurin inhibitors to sirolimus versus continued use of calcineurin inhibitors in renal allograft recipients: 18-month results from a randomized, open-label comparative trial. Abstr 1026 World Transplant Congress, 2006.

70 Williams JW, Javaid B, Kadambi PV, Gillen D, Harland R, Thistlewaite JR *et al.* Leflunomid for polyomavirus type BK nephropathy. *N Engl J Med* 2005; **352(11):** 1157–1158.

71 Vats A, Shapiro R, Singh Randhawa P, Scantlebury V, Tuzuner A, Saxena M *et al.* Quantitative viral load monitoring and cidofovir therapy for the management of BK virus-associated nephropathy with cidofovir. *Transplantation* 2003; **75(1):** 105–112.

72 Kadambi PV, Josephson MA, Williams J, Corey L, Jerome KR, Meehan SM *et al.* Treatment of refractory BK virus-associated nephropathy with cidofovir. *Am J Transplant* 2003; **3(2):** 186–191.

73 Maschio G, Alberti D, Janin G, Locatelli F, Mann JF, Motolese M *et al.* Effect of angiotensin-converting-enzyme inhibitor benazepril on the progression of chronic renal insufficiency. *N Engl J Med* 1996; **334(15):** 939–945.

74 Lewis EJ, Hunsicker LG, Bain RP, Rohde RD. The effect of angiotensin-converting enzyme-inhibition on diabetic nephropathy. *N Engl J Med* 1993; **329(20):** 1456–1462.

75 Stigant CE, Cohen J, Vivera M, Zaltzman JS. ACE inhibitors and angiotensin II antagonists in renal transplantation: an analysis of safety and efficacy. *Am J Kidney Dis* 2000; **35(1):** 58–63.

76 Omoto K, Tanabe K, Tokumoto T, Shimmura H, Ishida H, Toma H. Use of candesartan cilexitil decreases proteinuria in renal transplant patients with chronic allograft dysfunction. *Transplantation* 2003; **76(8):** 1170–1174.

77 Lin J, Valeri AM, Markowitz GS, D'Agati VD, Cohen DJ, Radhakrishnan J. Angiotensin converting enzyme inhibition in chronic allograft nephropathy. *Transplantation* 2002; **73(5):** 783–788.

78 Artz MA, Hilbrands LB, Borm G, Assmann KJ, Wetzels JF. Blockade of the renin-angiotensin system increases graft survival in patients with chronic allograft nephropathy. *Nephrol Dial Transplant* 2004; **19(11):** 2852–2857.

79 Campistol JM, Del Moral RG, Alarcon A, Gonzalez-Molina M, Arias M, Morales JM *et al.* Angiotensin II receptor blockage in kidney transplantation. Design and progress of the AALLOGRAFT study. World Transplant Congress 2006. *Am J Transplant* 2006; **6(Suppl 2):** 238.

80 Fellström B, Jardine AG, Soveri I, Cole E, Neumayer HH, Maes B *et al.* Renal dysfunction as a strong and independent risk factor for mortality and cardiovascular complications in renal transplantation. *Am J Transplant* 2005; **5(8):** 1986–1991.

81 Wolfe RA, Ashby VB, Milford EL, Ojo AO, Ettenger RE, Agodoa LY *et al.* Comparison of mortality in all patients on dialysis, patients on dialysis awaiting transplantation, and recipients of a first cadaveric transplant. *N Engl J Med.* 1999; **341(23):** 1725–1730.

82 McLean DR, Jardine AG. A simulation model to investigate the impact of cardiovascular risk in renal transplantation. *Transplant Proc* 2005; **37(5):** 2135–2143.

9 Disorders of Electrolytes (Acute and Chronic)

54 Overview of Electrolyte and Acid–Base Disorders

L. Lee Hamm & Michael Haderlie

Department of Medicine, Tulane University School of Medicine, New Orleans, USA

Introduction to evidence-based electrolyte disorders section

Electrolyte and acid–base disorders are common. However, seldom has the diagnosis or the treatment of these conditions been evaluated using an evidence-based approach. The reasons for this can be readily discerned. The most common electrolyte and acid–base disorders are secondary to other identifiable underlying conditions or treatments and are not primary disorders. For example, hyponatremia commonly occurs in association with congestive heart failure; hypokalemia occurs with diuretic use, and metabolic acidosis occurs frequently with sepsis and lactic acidosis. The primary electrolyte and acid–base disorders are often of several distinct etiologies. Diagnosis and treatment vary by condition and thus the therapeutic approaches to each of these electrolyte or acid–base disorders cannot necessarily be lumped together. For example, treatment of metabolic acidosis from sepsis-induced lactic acidosis will differ dramatically from treatment for metabolic acidosis associated with chronic kidney disease (CKD). The usual treatment is also frequently directed predominantly at the primary underlying disorder, not the secondary electrolyte abnormality. Therefore, an evidence-based approach to most of the electrolyte and acid–base conditions has not been attempted to any significant extent.

Some electrolyte and acid–base disorders do occur as primary disorders. These are usually the result of renal tubular disorders, because the kidneys and specifically the tubular segments of the nephron are the main regulatory site of the electrolyte and acid–base composition of the body. However, all of these primary electrolyte and acid–base disorders that arise from abnormalities in renal tubular transport properties are unusual or rare (with perhaps a few exceptions), and are therefore also difficult to evaluate with typical evidence-based approaches. Another reason for the limited number of evidence-based studies evaluating the diagnosis and management of electrolyte and acid–base disorders is the widely held view that most clinical electrolyte and acid–base issues are adequately addressed by a solid understanding of their physiologic mechanisms and that this physiologic perspective provides a sufficient basis for determining the optimal strategies for their diagnosis and treatment. Diagnosis of these disorders is frequently simple and straightforward (although diagnosis of the underlying causes may not be); for example, to diagnose hypokalemia, one measures the plasma potassium, and the confidence levels for normal values are assessed routinely by clinical laboratories. Therefore, the electrolyte and acid–base disorders covered in this chapter are selective rather than comprehensive.

This chapter will briefly discuss metabolic acid–base disorders. Because much of the approach to acid–base disorders is covered in standard texts and reviews, the focus here will be on areas where some systematic contemporary evidence-based approaches have been provided. Respiratory disorders will not be covered in any detail here. Subsequent chapters will discuss other electrolyte disorders and renal stone disease.

Normal physiology of acid–base homeostasis

Homeostasis of the body's acid–base balance occurs by mechanisms that maintain the systemic arterial pH between 7.35 and 7.45. These mechanisms include ventilatory control of volatile carbon dioxide (CO_2), regulation of HCO_3^- by the kidneys, and moderation by various buffer systems, particularly blood and tissue proteins, bone, and the CO_2/HCO_3^- buffer system. The CO_2/HCO_3^- buffer system is especially important because its components can be directly adjusted independently in the body by the lungs and kidneys, respectively. The interrelationship of the components of systemic pH can be described by the Henderson–Hasselbalch equation: $pH = 6.1 + \log \frac{HCO_3^-}{PaCO_2 \times 0.03}$.

Normal physiologic processes generate large quantities of CO_2 (which can be considered a volatile acid) that are exhaled by the lungs. Failure of adequate excretion of CO_2, such as with severe

Evidence-based Nephrology. Edited by Donald Molony and Jonathan Craig
© 2009 Blackwell Publishing, ISBN: 978-1-4051-3975-5.

decompensated chronic obstructive pulmonary disease, causes respiratory acidosis. Excess excretion of CO_2, such as with hyperventilation, causes respiratory alkalosis. With normal metabolism, nonvolatile acids are also generated from dietary acids and as a by-product of normal metabolism; nonvolatile acids consume HCO_3, thereby decreasing pH and, thus, will cause metabolic acidosis if not excreted adequately. One role of the kidneys is to excrete this nonvolatile acid and in the process generate new HCO_3, which replaces that consumed by these nonvolatile acids. Under usual circumstances acid production and renal excretion are matched to maintain a plasma HCO_3 concentration of approximately 23–26 mM. The kidneys regulate plasma bicarbonate concentration by three main mechanisms. First, reabsorption of bicarbonate filtered by the glomeruli occurs in several sites along the nephron: the proximal tubule reabsorbs 70–80% of filtered HCO_3^-; the thick ascending limbs reabsorb another 10–15%; the collecting ducts reabsorb most of the remainder such that virtually no bicarbonate appears in the urine under normal circumstances. Second, the kidneys excrete acid into the urine and in the process generate bicarbonate. Finally, ammonium, NH_4^+, excretion into the urine also produces bicarbonate; NH_4^+ is produced in the proximal tubule via deamination of glutamine and is excreted into the urine by complex processes which depend to a significant extent on acidification of the urine. These processes work normally to maintain acid–base homeostasis; however, these same processes can create disturbances under certain conditions.

The lungs and kidneys together under normal circumstances mediate the physiologic compensatory responses to acid–base abnormalities (Table 54.1). Metabolic acid–base disorders can elicit an immediate compensatory response by altering respiration and the excretion of CO_2. Respiratory derangements also elicit a compensatory response with changes in the renal handling of bicarbonate; however, the renal response to respiratory acid–base changes takes several days to complete. Because these compensations are predictable for a given simple acid–base disorder, failure of compensation indicates another coexisting acid–base disorder. Predictable compensations to simple acid–base disorders were investigated many years ago and were used to create nomograms to diagnose acid–base disorders and to create common formulas used to predict their compensation. Such studies represented an initial evidence-based approach but are not detailed here because they are generally accepted.

Diagnosis of acid–base disorders

Acid–base disorders are commonly seen in clinical practice. Although the possibility of an acid–base disorder may be suggested by a patient's history and physical examination, the presence of an acid–base disorder is usually confirmed by abnormalities in arterial blood gas and/or electrolyte values. The calculated HCO_3^- from the arterial blood gas should closely approximate the measured HCO_3^- (or total CO_2) from the electrolyte panel. An abnormally low pH is an acidemia (either metabolic, usually with a low HCO_3^-, or respiratory, with a high pCO_2), and a high pH is an alkalemia. However, because two or more processes may be occurring simultaneously, possibly with opposite effects on pH, identification and recognition of processes in distinction from the pH, per se, are important. In this regard, calculation of the anion gap $[Na^+ - (Cl^- + HCO_3^-)]$, which represents the unmeasured anions in plasma, is also important in diagnosing specific acid–base disorders, even in the absence of changes in plasma HCO_3^- [1]. An elevated anion gap (normal, 6–11 mM in most laboratories) is usually associated with a metabolic acidosis, particularly if the level exceeds 20 mM [2,3]. However, an elevated anion gap may not be a sensitive indicator of lactic acidosis in critically ill patients [4]. In recent years some investigators have proposed a different approach to understanding acid–base disorders, the so-called Stewart approach [5,6], but no clear benefits to this approach have yet been proven.

Metabolic acidosis

There are many well-established causes of metabolic acidosis (Table 54.2). The mechanistic etiologies of metabolic acidoses include large endogenous or exogenous acid loads that consume plasma HCO_3^-, loss of HCO_3^- from the gastrointestinal tract or kidneys, and/or the failure of the kidneys to excrete acids accumulated as the normal by-products of metabolism. Clinically, however, metabolic acidosis is usually approached by first categorizing the condition as either a high anion gap acidosis or a normal anion gap (or hyperchloremic) metabolic acidosis. Those conditions causing a high anion gap metabolic acidosis include kidney failure, ketoacidosis (either diabetic or alcoholic), lactic acidosis, and intoxications. Four intoxications have been associated with

Table 54.1 Response to simple acid–base disorders.

Primary disorder	pH	pCO_2	HCO_3^-	Cl^-	Predicted response
Metabolic acidosis	Low	Low	Low*	↑ or →	$\Delta\,pCO2\,(\downarrow) = 1.0\text{–}1.4 \times \Delta\,HCO_3^-$
Respiratory acidosis	Low	High*	High	↓	Acute $\Delta\,HCO_3^-\,(\uparrow) = 0.1 \times \Delta\,pCO_2$
					Chronic $\Delta\,HCO_3^-\,(\uparrow) = 0.25\text{–}0.55 \times \Delta\,pCO_2$
Metabolic alkalosis	High	High	High*	↓	$\Delta\,pCO2\,(\uparrow) = 0.4\text{–}0.9 \times \Delta\,HCO_3^-$
Respiratory alkalosis	High	Low*	Low	↑	Acute $\Delta\,HCO_3^-\,(\downarrow) = 0.2\text{–}0.25 \times \Delta\,pCO_2$
					Chronic $\Delta\,HCO_3^-\,(\downarrow) = 0.4\text{–}0.5 \times \Delta\,pCO_2$

*Primary abnormality

Table 54.2 Causes of metabolic acidosis.

High anion gap
- Renal failure (severe)
- Lactic acidosis
  – L: tissue hypoxia, tumors
  – D: short bowel syndrome, mental status changes; not measured by routine lab
- Ketoacidosis: diabetic, alcoholic
- Poisonings
  – Salicylate (usually associated with respiratory alkalosis)
  – Ethylene glycol
  – Methanol
  – Acetaminophen-induced 5-oxoprolinuria (pyroglutamic aciduria)

Normal anion gap
- Diarrhea (loss HCO_3)
- Renal tubular acidosis
- Renal failure
- Ureterosigmoidostomy
- Carbonic anhydrase inhibitors (e.g. acetazolamide for glaucoma)
- Dilution with hyperchloremic solutions (e.g. saline)
- Pancreatic or biliary diversion
- Administration of inorganic acid or acid equivalents
- Ketoacidosis, well hydrated or excretion of Na^+ ketones

metabolic acidosis: salicylate, methanol, ethylene glycol, and recently acetaminophen [7,8]. Simple laboratory tests (i.e. serum creatinine, glucose, urine and plasma ketones, lactate, and toxicology screening) can usually distinguish among these possibilities.

Although renal failure and ketoacidosis are classically associated with an elevated anion gap, both conditions may also result in a normal anion gap acidosis. Metabolic acidosis with a normal anion gap often results from gastrointestinal loss of HCO_3^- (from diarrhea or conditions such as ureterosigmoidostomies) but may be secondary to renal tubular acidosis (RTA). RTA represents a group of disorders that present with normal anion gap or hyperchloremic metabolic acidosis with a normal blood urea nitrogen and creatinine. They are classified as proximal (type II) RTA, in which renal bicarbonate excretion is excessive, and distal RTA (types I and IV), in which distal H^+ secretion and/or ammonium ion excretion are impaired. Urine pH is high (more alkaline than is appropriate) in type I RTA but can be appropriately acidic in proximal (type II) RTA and type IV RTA. Both types I and II are rare, particularly in adults, and are usually secondary to some underlying cause that should be identified. Hypokalemia is a typical feature in types I and II and may be more of a clinical issue than the acidosis. In contrast, type IV RTA is characterized by hyperkalemia and also frequently by low renin and aldosterone. Type IV RTA is quite common in patients with moderate renal insufficiency, particularly CKD secondary to diabetic nephropathy. Other causes of normal anion gap metabolic acidosis include carbonic anhydrase inhibitors, dilution with hyperchloremic solutions such as saline, and pancreatic or biliary diversion procedures.

Consequences of severe acute acidemia (blood pH < 7.1–7.2) include predisposition to cardiac arrhythmias, venoconstric-

tion, characteristic increase in ventilation, central nervous system depression, decreased total peripheral vascular resistance, pulmonary edema, decreased blood pressure, reduced hepatic blood flow, and impaired oxygen delivery. Acidemia also suppresses myocardial contractility; however, inotropic function is typically normal because of catecholamine release induced by acidosis. These alterations in organ function can contribute to increased morbidity and mortality; however, the role of acidosis per se is not clear. In fact, some acutely beneficial effects of acidosis have been proposed [5]. Chronic acidosis is associated with bone resorption, growth failure in children, kidney stones from hypocitraturia and hypercalciuria, possibly accelerated renal fibrosis, and muscle wasting from protein catabolism.

Treatment of metabolic acidosis

The mainstay of treatment for metabolic acidosis is correction of the underlying condition [9–11]. An area of interest and some controversy has been whether alkali treatment is beneficial to patients, particularly those with acute acidosis. Acute infusions of sodium bicarbonate have the possible detrimental effects of volume overload, hyperosmolality, decreased ionized calcium, increased cellular production of acids and, paradoxically, decreases in cerebrospinal fluid pH and cellular pH [12,13]. Some specific entities which have received particular attention will be addressed. The controversy regarding the use of bicarbonate therapy in the treatment of severe acidemia centers on three clinical disease states: lactic acidosis, metabolic acidosis and hypercarbia associated with cardiac arrest, and diabetic ketoacidosis [11].

Lactic acidosis

Lactic acidosis is typically caused by tissue hypoxia (type A lactic acidosis) either from inadequate tissue circulatory perfusion or acute hypoxemia. Typical etiologies for inadequate tissue perfusion include sepsis, cardiogenic shock, and hypovolemic shock. Some malignancies, drugs (e.g. metformin and some antiretroviral agents in particular), and hereditary metabolic disorders have also been recognized to cause lactic acidosis. The diagnosis can be confirmed by an elevated lactate level, although the level may not correlate well with either the degree of acidosis or the change in anion gap.

Most patients with lactic acidosis are critically ill with profound acidosis a major component of their condition. Although treatment of the underlying condition is always attempted, treatment of the acidosis per se with alkalinizing agents would seem logical. However, infusion of sodium bicarbonate frequently fails to adequately correct the acidosis. No studies have shown a survival advantage. In addition, two small randomized controlled trials (24 patients total) did not find any hemodynamic improvement in treating lactic acidosis with sodium bicarbonate [14,15]. Dichloroacetate administration was found effective in animals, but a sizable clinical trial failed to show any hemodynamic improvement or survival benefit with this therapy despite an improvement in pH [16]. Other buffers such as Carbicarb (a mixture of sodium bicarbonate and sodium carbonate) and TRAM [Tris(hydroxymethyl)-aminomethane] have been used in animal studies but have not been evaluated in suitable clinical studies in humans [13,17]. Lactic acidosis and acidosis associated with acute renal failure have also been treated in nonrandomized, noncontrolled studies with continuous hemofiltration methods with improvement found in several parameters, but rigorous controlled clinical studies have not been performed [18–22].

Guidelines on cardiopulmonary arrest (in which lactic acidosis is usually present) have progressively restricted the recommendation for sodium bicarbonate based on studies showing lack of benefit in many circumstances [23,24]. Similar to other findings noted above, a systematic review of controlled trials in preterm infants with metabolic acidosis also found insufficient evidence for the use of base infusion in this condition [25]; as in other conditions of acidosis, this indicates a paucity of adequate randomized controlled trials, not a finding that this treatment is not useful.

Acidosis in CKD

CKD with a glomerular filtration rate of less than 20–25% of normal is frequently accompanied by chronic metabolic acidosis. Acidosis is generally mild to moderate in degree, with plasma bicarbonate concentrations ranging from 12 to 22 mEq/L (mmol/L), with values rarely less than 12 mEq/L in the absence of an increased acid load [26]. The degree of acidosis generally correlates with severity of renal failure and usually is more severe at a lower glomerular filtration rate. The metabolic acidosis can be of the high anion gap type, although the anion gap can be normal or only moderately increased, even in patients with stage 4–5 CKD. Long-term adverse consequences have been associated with metabolic acidosis, including muscle wasting, malnutrition, bone disease and demineralization, impaired growth, abnormalities in growth hormone and thyroid hormone secretion, impaired insulin sensitivity, progression of renal failure, and exacerbation of β_2-microglobulin accumulation. In these cases of acidosis, administration of bicarbonate may be warranted; however, base therapy aimed at normalization of plasma bicarbonate concentration might be associated with certain complications, such as volume overload, exacerbation of hypertension, and facilitation of vascular calcifications. Whether normalization of plasma bicarbonate concentrations in all patients with CKD is desirable therefore requires additional study.

At present, although the National Kidney Foundation Kidney Disease Outcomes Quality Initiative (K/DOQI) guidelines recognize the possible negative effects of metabolic acidosis, it is recommended that plasma bicarbonate concentrations in patients with CKD, both before and after the initiation of maintenance dialysis therapy, be increased to 22 mEq/L, but not to completely normal values [27]. Epidemiological studies in hemodialysis patients suggest that normalization of serum bicarbonate levels is associated with a higher mortality rate than when the lower K/DOQI level is targeted. These studies do not permit exclusion of confounding that may account for an apparent favorable survival with mainte-

nance of a mild acidosis in hemodialysis patients. The argument against recommending full normalization of plasma bicarbonate concentrations is currently under further investigation.

Because controlled studies examining the impact of different levels of acidemia are yet to be reported, it is not clear whether complete normalization of plasma bicarbonate concentrations is necessary or desirable. However, compelling studies have shown that even the small acid load resulting from the metabolism of ingested foodstuffs can have a negative impact on bone and muscle metabolism, even when plasma bicarbonate concentrations are within the normal range. A systematic review of the literature on chronic metabolic acidosis in patients with CKD concluded that randomized controlled trials of correcting metabolic acidosis in predialysis patients and in children are lacking [28]; for dialysis patients, three small trials have provided evidence of protein and bone metabolism improvement with treatment of acidosis, but no large robust trials have been reported that have also evaluated the impact of correction of the metabolic acidosis on mortality and morbidity [28].

RTA type IV

Type IV RTA is also called hyperkalemic distal RTA. In this disorder, distal tubule secretion of hydrogen and potassium ions is abnormal. Of the types of RTA, type IV is the most common. It is an acquired disorder and is usually seen in patients with at least some renal insufficiency, often secondary to diabetic nephropathy. Drug-induced type IV RTA (e.g. from cyclosporine, tacrolimus, angiotensin converting enzyme inhibitors, angiotensin receptor blockers, and aldosterone antagonists) is generally seen in patients who already have existing renal insufficiency. Patients who have hypoaldosteronism from pure adrenal abnormalities typically have normal or high renin levels, while patients with disorders associated with CKD typically have low renin levels. In type IV RTA, control of plasma potassium is often more of an issue than the acidosis. All patients should be instructed to maintain a low-potassium diet. In addition, offending drugs that may interfere with aldosterone action should be discontinued if possible. Fludrocortisone is also effective in patients with hyporeninemic hypoaldosteronism. Type IV RTA may respond to fludrocortisone therapy alone [29]; however, administration of a loop diuretic and/or a potassium-binding resin such as Kayexelate and/or oral bicarbonate is usually preferable [30,31], because fludrocortisone will often worsen the volume overload and hypertension that are frequently present in patients with CKD.

Treatment of other causes of metabolic acidosis

In ketoacidosis, similar to other causes of acute acidosis, studies have not shown a clear benefit from sodium bicarbonate administration [24,32,33]. Guidelines for children with diabetic ketoacidosis do not generally recommend bicarbonate, but there are areas where additional studies are needed [34,35]. Despite the lack of clear data in support of bicarbonate usage in acute organic metabolic acidosis, many clinicians (including this author, in cases with adult patients) use relatively slow infusion of iso-osmolar sodium bicarbonate in some cases of severe acidosis [24].

Thiamine administration has been recommended by some, based on theoretical and anecdotal grounds in both the ketoacidosis and the lactic acidosis that arise in the presence of nucleoside analog reverse transcriptase inhibitors [36,37]. L-Carnitine has also been tried for the latter condition [38,39].

In toxin-induced metabolic acidosis of the increased anion gap type, one of the relatively new aspects of treatment is the use of fomepizole for ethylene glycol and methanol intoxications [40,41]. The full benefits of this approach await validation in a large randomized controlled trial.

Metabolic alkalosis

Metabolic alkalosis and alkalemia are common and associated with significant morbidity [42]. The detrimental effects of alkalemia include neuromuscular irritability, arrhythmias, hypokalemia, central nervous system dysfunction, and decreased ventilatory drive. Metabolic alkalosis is usually caused by one of two conditions associated with volume and chloride depletion: 1) loss of gastric contents from vomiting or nasogastric suction, or 2) diuretic use (Table 54.3). In these conditions, the kidneys are unable to excrete the excess HCO_3^- because of the volume and chloride depletion; therefore, treatment with sodium chloride (and often potassium to correct simultaneous potassium deficiency) and/or discontinuation of diuretics is sufficient treatment. These conditions are characterized by, and can be confirmed by, the presence of a low urine chloride (usually less than 20 mEq/L) if diuretics have not been administered recently.

Table 54.3 Metabolic alkalosis: usual causes.

1 Chloride responsive (associated with volume depletion; urinary chloride <20, unless recent diureticse; usually normal or low blood pressure; low K^+; secondary increases in aldosterone)
- Vomiting or nasogastric suction
- Diuretics
- Rarely, congenital chloride diarrhea, cystic fibrosis, chloride-free infant formula

2 Chloride-resistant (associated with excess mineralocorticoids; urinary chloride > 20)
- Hypertension, mineralocorticoid excess (or similar biological action)
  - Secondary hyperaldosteronism (e.g. RAS)
  - Primary hyperaldosteronism (e.g. adenoma or Cushing's)
  - Licorice
  - Genetic forms of hypertension (Liddle's syndrome, etc.)
- Normal or low blood pressure, salt wasting, secondary increase in aldosterone (Bartter's or Gitelman's syndromes)

3 Hypokalemia: usually contributes to categories 1 and 2; severe ↓K^+ alone can rarely cause metabolic alkalosis

4 Posthypercapnic metabolic alkalosis

5 Renal insufficiency with alkali administration (e.g. milk alkali syndrome)

A second category of metabolic alkalosis is associated with elevated urinary chloride (greater than 20 mEq/L) and hypertension; these are frequently associated with syndromes of mineralocorticoid excess, such as in primary hyperaldosteronism or Cushing's syndrome. Little's syndrome (with severe hypertension caused by abnormal sodium channels in the collecting duct) and renal artery stenosis can appear similar. Two conditions, Gitelman's syndrome and Bartter's syndrome, are associated with inherited tubular abnormalities of sodium chloride reabsorption, and patients frequently have metabolic alkalosis, hypokalemia, and elevated aldosterone but have normal or low blood pressure. These conditions mimic diuretic abuse with either thiazide diuretics or loop diuretics, respectively.

Occasionally, metabolic alkalosis can result from severe potassium deficiency alone or from alkali administration in the setting of renal insufficiency; a subcategory of the latter is the milk alkali syndrome. Metabolic alkalosis can also result after chronic hypercapnia (with compensatory increases in plasma HCO_3) has been treated acutely, so-called posthypercapnia metabolic alkalosis.

Treatment of metabolic alkalosis is directed at the primary abnormality, as suggested above. Decreasing acetate administration in parenteral nutrition solutions and decreasing gastric acid removal (when nasogastric suction is ongoing) with proton pump inhibitors or H-2 blockers may be useful adjuncts. Occasionally, administration of acetazolamide, a carbonic anhydrase inhibitor, can be useful in facilitating urinary excretion of HCO_3 [43,44]. Under unusual circumstances, metabolic alkalosis can be treated with acidifying agents or with hemodialysis.

Contemporary evidence-based approaches to either the diagnosis or the treatment of metabolic alkalosis have not been performed.

Summary

Available evidence-based trials of the diagnosis and optimal treatment of acid–base disorders are scarce. Thus, current practice relies almost entirely on an approach based on physiologic reasoning. New evidence from higher-quality observational studies and some small randomized controlled trials evaluating outcomes with treatment of various types of metabolic acidosis with sodium bicarbonate have demonstrated that basing therapeutic recommendations on a physiologically based logic might prove inadequate. Thus, sodium bicarbonate infusion may correct an acid pH without obvious improvements in survival or morbidity. Additional randomized clinical trials are indicated to help determine the optimal mode and magnitude for acid–base treatment strategies. Some of these strategies might involve administration of buffer, and others might be directed at correcting the underlying renal tubular transport abnormalities responsible for generation of the acid–base disorder. In the latter case, an understanding of the renal tubular pathophysiology of these acid–base disorders should lead to the generation of new hypotheses regarding treatment and inform the design of clinical trials.

Similar limitations in the corpus of clinical trials evidence are found when attempting to construct evidence-based recommendations for the diagnosis and management of electrolyte disorders, especially those due to renal tubulopathies. The best evidence that informs the management of disorders of water, sodium, and potassium are reviewed in the next two chapters. Tubular transport disorders also play a key role in abnormalities of renal divalent cation handling and pathogenesis of renal stone disease. An evidence-based approach to the diagnosis and treatment of renal stone disease will be reviewed in chapter 57.

References

1 Kraut JA, Madias NE. Serum anion gap: its uses and limitations in clinical medicine. *Clin J Am Soc Nephrol* 2007; **2**: 162–174.

2 Gabow PA, Kaehny WD, Fennessey PV, Goodman SI, Gross PA, Schrier RW. Diagnostic importance of an increased serum anion gap. *N Engl J Med* 1980; **303**: 854–858.

3 Winter SD, Pearson JR, Gabow PA, Schultz AL, Lepoff RB. The fall of the serum anion gap. *Arch Intern Med* 1990; **150**: 311–313.

4 Levraut J, Bounatirou T, Ichai C, Ciais JF, Jambou P, Hechema R *et al.* Reliability of anion gap as an indicator of blood lactate in critically ill patients. *Intensive Care Med* 1997; **23**: 417–422.

5 Levraut J, Grimaud D. Treatment of metabolic acidosis. *Curr Opin Crit Care* 2003; **9**: 260–265.

6 Ring T, Frische S, Nielsen S. Clinical review: renal tubular acidosis. A physicochemical approach. *Crit Care* 2005; **9**: 573–580.

7 Fenves AZ, Kirkpatrick HM, III, Patel VV, Sweetman L, Emmett M. Increased anion gap metabolic acidosis as a result of 5-oxoproline (pyroglutamic acid): a role for acetaminophen. *Clin J Am Soc Nephrol* 2006; **1**: 441–447.

8 Humphreys BD, Forman JP, Zandi-Nejad K, Bazari H, Seifter J, Magee CC. Acetaminophen-induced anion gap metabolic acidosis and 5-oxoprolinuria (pyroglutamic aciduria) acquired in hospital. *Am J Kidney Dis* 2005; **46**: 143–146.

9 Adrogue HJ. Metabolic acidosis: pathophysiology, diagnosis and management. *J Nephrol* 2006; **19(Suppl 9)**: S62–S69.

10 Adrogue HJ, Madias NE. Management of life-threatening acid-base disorders. First of two parts. *N Engl J Med* 1998; **338**: 26–34.

11 Kraut JA, Kurtz I. Use of base in the treatment of severe acidemic states. *Am J Kidney Dis* 2001; **38**: 703–727.

12 Forsythe SM, Schmidt GA. Sodium bicarbonate for the treatment of lactic acidosis. *Chest* 2000; **117**: 260–267.

13 Gehlbach BK, Schmidt GA. Bench-to-bedside review: treating acid-base abnormalities in the intensive care unit: the role of buffers. *Crit Care* 2004; **8**: 259–265.

14 Cooper DJ, Walley KR, Wiggs BR, Russell JA. Bicarbonate does not improve hemodynamics in critically ill patients who have lactic acidosis. A prospective, controlled clinical study. *Ann Intern Med* 1990; **112**: 492–498.

15 Mathieu D, Neviere R, Billard V, Fleyfel M, Wattel F. Effects of bicarbonate therapy on hemodynamics and tissue oxygenation in patients with lactic acidosis: a prospective, controlled clinical study. *Crit Care Med* 1991; **19**: 1352–1356.

16 Stacpoole PW, Wright EC, Baumgartner TG, Bersin RM, Buchalter S, Curry SH *et al.* A controlled clinical trial of dichloroacetate for treatment

of lactic acidosis in adults. The Dichloroacetate-Lactic Acidosis Study Group. *N Engl J Med* 1992; **327**: 1564–1569.

17 Cariou A, Vinsonneau C, Dhainaut JF. Adjunctive therapies in sepsis: an evidence-based review. *Crit Care Med* 2004; **32**: S562–S570.

18 Hilton PJ, Taylor J, Forni LG, Treacher DF. Bicarbonate-based haemofiltration in the management of acute renal failure with lactic acidosis. *QJM* 1998; **91**: 279–283.

19 Naka T, Bellomo R. Bench-to-bedside review: treating acid-base abnormalities in the intensive care unit: the role of renal replacement therapy. *Crit Care* 2004; **8**: 108–114.

20 Schetz M. Non-renal indications for continuous renal replacement therapy. *Kidney Int Suppl* 1999; **1999**: S88–S94.

21 Schoolwerth AC, Kaneko TM, Sedlacek M, Block CA, Remillard BD. Acid-base disturbances in the intensive care unit: metabolic acidosis. *Semin Dial* 2006; **19**: 492–495.

22 Uchino S, Bellomo R, Ronco C. Intermittent versus continuous renal replacement therapy in the ICU: impact on electrolyte and acid-base balance. *Intensive Care Med* 2001; **27**: 1037–1043.

23 AHA. 2005 American Heart Association guidelines for cardiopulmonary resuscitation (CPR) and emergency cardiovascular care (ECC) of pediatric and neonatal patients: pediatric basic life support. *Pediatrics* 2006; **117**: e989–e1004.

24 Andrade OV, Ihara FO, Troster EJ. Metabolic acidosis in childhood: why, when and how to treat. *J Pediatr* 2007; **83**: S11–S21.

25 Lawn CJ, Weir FJ, McGuire W. Base administration or fluid bolus for preventing morbidity and mortality in preterm infants with metabolic acidosis. *Cochrane Database Syst Rev* 2005; **2**: CD003215.

26 Gauthier P, Simon EE, Lemann J. Acidosis in chronic renal failure. In: Dubose T, Hamm L (editors), *Acid-Base and Electrolyte Disorders*. Saunders, Philadelphia, 2002; 207–216.

27 K/DOQI clinical practice guidelines for bone metabolism and disease in chronic kidney disease. *Am J Kidney Dis* 2003; **42**: S1–S201.

28 Roderick P, Willis NS, Blakeley S, Jones C, Tomson C. Correction of chronic metabolic acidosis for chronic kidney disease patients. *Cochrane Database Syst Rev* 2007; **1**: CD001890.

29 Sebastian A, Schambelan M, Lindenfeld S, Morris RC, Jr. Amelioration of metabolic acidosis with fludrocortisone therapy in hyporeninemic hypoaldosteronism. *N Engl J Med* 1977; **297**: 576–583.

30 Maher T, Schambelan M, Kurtz I, Hulter HN, Jones JW, Sebastian A. Amelioration of metabolic acidosis by dietary potassium restriction in hyperkalemic patients with chronic renal insufficiency. *J Lab Clin Med* 1984; **103**: 432–445.

31 Sebastian A, Schambelan M, Sutton JM. Amelioration of hyperchloremic acidosis with furosemide therapy in patients with chronic renal insufficiency and type 4 renal tubular acidosis. *Am J Nephrol* 1984; **4**: 287–300.

32 Lever E, Jaspan JB. Sodium bicarbonate therapy in severe diabetic ketoacidosis. *Am J Med* 1983; **75**: 263–268.

33 Morris LR, Murphy MB, Kitabchi AE. Bicarbonate therapy in severe diabetic ketoacidosis. *Ann Intern Med* 1986; **105**: 836–840.

34 Dunger DB, Sperling MA, Acerini CL, Bohn DJ, Daneman D, Danne TP *et al.* European Society for Paediatric Endocrinology/Lawson Wilkins Pediatric Endocrine Society consensus statement on diabetic ketoacidosis in children and adolescents. *Pediatrics* 2004; **113**: e133–e140.

35 Wolfsdorf J, Glaser N, Sperling MA. Diabetic ketoacidosis in infants, children, and adolescents: a consensus statement from the American Diabetes Association. *Diabetes Care* 2006; **29**: 1150–1159.

36 Halperin ML, Cherney DZI, Kamel KS. Ketoacidosis. In: Dubose T, Hamm L (editors), *Acid-Base and Electrolyte Disorders*. Saunders, Philadelphia, 2002; 67–82.

37 Schramm C, Wanitschke R, Galle PR. Thiamine for the treatment of nucleoside analogue-induced severe lactic acidosis. *Eur J Anaesthesiol* 1999; **16**: 733–735.

38 Claessens YE, Cariou A, Monchi M, Soufir L, Azoulay E, Rouges P *et al.* Detecting life-threatening lactic acidosis related to nucleoside-analog treatment of human immunodeficiency virus-infected patients, and treatment with L-carnitine. *Crit Care Med* 2003; **31**: 1042–1047.

39 Claessens YE, Chiche JD, Mira JP, Cariou A. Bench-to-bedside review: severe lactic acidosis in HIV patients treated with nucleoside analogue reverse transcriptase inhibitors.*Crit Care* 2003; **7**: 226–232.

40 Brent J, McMartin K, Phillips S, Aaron C, Kulig K. Fomepizole for the treatment of methanol poisoning. *N Engl J Med* 2001; **344**: 424–429.

41 Brent J, McMartin K, Phillips S, Burkhart KK, Donovan JW, Wells M *et al.* Fomepizole for the treatment of ethylene glycol poisoning. Methylpyrazole for Toxic Alcohols Study Group. *N Engl J Med* 1999; **340**: 832–838.

42 Hamm LL. Mixed acid-base disorders. In: Fluids and Electrolytes, 3rd edition. Kokko, JP and Tannen, R (eds.), Saunders, 1996.

43 Berthelsen P. Cardiovascular performance and oxyhemoglobin dissociation after acetazolamide in metabolic alkalosis. *Intensive Care Med* 1982; **8**: 269–274.

44 Moffett BS, Moffett TI, Dickerson HA. Acetazolamide therapy for hypochloremic metabolic alkalosis in pediatric patients with heart disease. *Am J Ther* 2007; **14**: 331–335.

55 Hyponatremia

Chukwuma Eze & Eric E. Simon

Section of Nephrology and Hypertension, Department of Medicine, Tulane University school of Medicine, New Orleans, LA, USA

Introduction

Hyponatremia represents a decrease of blood sodium relative to water. This review will concentrate on disorders in which the serum osmolality is concomitantly reduced (hypotonic hyponatremia) in the adult population. We will concentrate on clinical evidence pertaining to the setting and risk factors for hyponatremia and its treatment. We will not discuss in detail the diagnosis, differential diagnosis, or pathophysiology.

In the vast majority of cases, hyponatremia is causally associated with elevated antidiuretic hormone (ADH) levels and an impaired ability to excrete water. In the case of hypovolemic patients, ADH levels are elevated as a physiologic response to severe intravascular volume depletion. Many of the patients with clinical euvolemia and hyponatremia have the syndrome of inappropriate ADH secretion (SIADH), and others have thiazide diuretic-induced hyponatremia or psychogenic polydipsia (which may also be associated with elevated ADH levels). Those hyponatremic patients with obvious volume expansion include patients with CHF and cirrhosis who also have elevated ADH levels.

Clinical manifestations

Symptoms of hyponatremia are potentially due to two factors: the decrease in osmolality with resulting brain edema and the hyponatremia per se. Symptoms are variable, depending on the blood sodium level, the rate of onset, severity, age, comorbidities, etc. The tolerance of severe levels of hyponatremia, especially when it has developed over days and weeks, is due to brain adaptations. Our knowledge about the consequences and adaptations to hyponatremia are necessarily derived from animal studies and are crucial to understanding the effects of hyponatremia and the

consequences of treatment. With the acute development of hyponatremia, water leaves the extracellular space down its concentration gradient into the intracellular space, causing cell swelling. The brain, encased by the cranium, is particularly prone to the effects of swelling. Because of the constraints of the skull, the brain is limited to about a 10% increase in volume before death from brain herniation ensues [1]. The onset of hyponatremia is countered by brain adaptations, notably, the loss of solutes. The loss of solutes from the intracellular space attenuates the intracellular accumulation of water, limiting cerebral edema. Initially, electrolytes including potassium are lost. In rats, significant electrolyte loss is observed as early as 6 h and is essentially maximal by 24 h after the onset of hyponatremia [2,3]. Within 24 h there is also loss of non-electrolyte osmols, such as myoinositol, which continues for about 48 h. In part because of the loss of these electrolytes and organic molecules, slowly developing hyponatremia is often well-tolerated. At some point, these adaptations are exceeded and overt symptoms ensue. Symptoms referable to hyponatremia include altered sensorium, lethargy, headache, nausea, dizziness, vertigo, falls, and muscle cramps. More severe manifestations include seizures, noncardiogenic pulmonary edema, respiratory arrest, brain stem herniation, and death. The onset of severe symptoms, such as seizures, whether during acute or chronic hyponatremia, signifies critical brain edema and constitutes a medical emergency. With chronic hyponatremia, because the brain has adapted by loss of osmols, rapidly raising the serum sodium concentration back to closer-to-normal levels may have adverse effects, such as central pontine myelinolysis (CPM). It is believed that the loss of brain solutes makes the brain susceptible to intracellular dehydration during rapid correction of hyponatremia. Studies in rats and dogs have demonstrated this phenomenon. On the other hand, complete correction of the blood sodium is not required to alleviate the hyponatremia-induced elevated pressures in the brain to noncritical levels [1]. Thus, the optimal treatment of hyponatremia needs to take into account these experimental observations and theoretical considerations.

Due to brain adaptations, overt symptoms are generally not encountered in patients with chronic hyponatremia until the serum

Evidence-based Nephrology. Edited by Donald Molony and Jonathan Craig
© 2009 Blackwell Publishing, ISBN: 978-1-4051-3975-5.

sodium has fallen below 125 mEq/L, and often lower concentrations are observed in patients without symptoms. However, some patients have overt symptoms with serum sodium concentrations over 120 mmol/L (see, for instance, Figures 2 and 3 in reference 4). Many of these patients with symptoms at higher sodium levels have acute or subacute hyponatremia. In acute hyponatremia, frank cerebral edema has been documented in experimental animals.

Whether patients with chronic hyponatremia and moderately depressed blood sodium levels have truly normal central nervous system (CNS) function is questionable. Patients with psychogenic polydipsia were found to exhibit neurologic deficits when hyponatremic that were not clearly related to the underlying psychosis [5]. Even more convincingly, a recent study in patients with SIADH found neurological abnormalities, including gait disturbances, present even in mild hyponatremia, a symptom that may contribute to the increased incidence of falls observed in the hyponatremic patients [6]. Similarly, correction of hyponatremia with a vasopressin antagonist resulted in an improvement in self-reported changes in sensorium [7].

Incidence, morbidity, and mortality

General hospital setting

Hyponatremia is a common clinical condition. The incidence depends on the clinical setting and the definition of hyponatremia. Normally, serum and plasma sodium levels are identical, with the lower limit of normal defined as 136 mmol/L. Two large prospective studies have helped define the frequency and etiologies responsible for hyponatremia. Anderson *et al.* prospectively examined patients admitted to a university hospital and carefully delineated the incidence of and the likely etiologies for the hyponatremia in this hospital cohort [8]. The incidence and prevalence of hyponatremia, defined as a plasma sodium concentration of less than 130 mEq/L, were 1.0% and 2.5%, respectively. Two-thirds of these patients developed hyponatremia after admission to the hospital. Hyperglycemia, a cause of nonhypotonic hyponatremia, was present in 16%, laboratory error in 5%, and severe kidney failure in 9%. The remainder had hypotonic hyponatremia. Of these, 19% were hypovolemic, 17% had edema, and 34% were clinically normovolemic. Most of the latter group were thought to have SIADH and, overall in those in whom it was measured, 97% of patients with hypotonic hyponatremia exhibited elevated ADH levels. Severe hyponatremia, defined as a plasma sodium concentration of less than 120 mEq/L, was seen in 12% of the hyponatremic patients.

A recent study from Singapore [9] examined plasma samples obtained from both hospital and clinic settings. In the hospital setting, the incidence of serum sodium of <126 mEq/L was 6.2% and for levels <115 mEq/L the incidence was 1.2%. Similar to the Anderson *et al.* study, more than half of the patients who developed severe hyponatremia (serum sodium, <126 mEq/L) did so after hospitalization. The incidence of severe hyponatremia in the hospital was about 20 times that seen in a community care

setting. The prevalence of hyponatremia increased progressively with age, starting at age 40. A retrospective analysis suggested that patients admitted to an intensive care unit have an even higher incidence of hyponatremia of 30% [10].

Mortality associated with hyponatremia may be from associated conditions causing the hyponatremia or the hyponatremia itself via its CNS effects. Mortality varies depending on the setting. Observational studies that have permitted quantification of the mortality risk associated with hyponatremia in various clinical circumstances were summarized by Lee *et al.* [11] and will not be repeated here in detail. Hospitalized patients with a blood sodium of less than 120 mEq/L show a 20–50% mortality. A recent study by Hoorn *et al.* [12] addressed the incidence and causes of hyponatremia in 5437 hospitalized patients. Severe hyponatremia (plasma Na of ≤125 mEq/L) was seen in 3% of patients in whom plasma sodium was measured (54% of total admissions). These patients were followed as a cohort. About equal numbers of these patients had developed severe hyponatremia in the hospital versus presenting with hyponatremia on admission. Symptoms attributable to hyponatremia per se were found in 36% of this cohort (27 patients). Mortality was 19% (76 patients) for patients with severe hyponatremia, a finding that is consistent with the previous studies cited. However, only half of the patients who died were felt to have had symptomatic hyponatremia antemortum. Thus, how much of the morbidity and mortality was attributable to the observed hyponatremia is unknown, but hyponatremia probably played a role in at least 19 patients, including three of the deaths. The risk factors identified in these observational studies for the development of severe hyponatremia in the hospital setting included prescription of thiazide diuretics and ADH-stimulating drugs, surgery, and the administration of hypotonic fluids.

Nursing home patients

A combined retrospective and prospective study of nursing home patients found a high prevalence of hyponatremia (<135 mEq/L) of 18% compared to an age- and gender-matched control population prevalence of 8% [13]. Of the nursing home patients in this study, 53% had at least one episode of hyponatremia during a 1-year period. However, hyponatremia did not confer excess mortality. The high mortality (17%) in the patients exhibiting hyponatremia was no different from normonatremic patients (21%). Thus, it is difficult to assign a precise mortality risk to hyponatremia in such a nursing home population per se versus an increased mortality risk attributable to their underlying diseases. Nevertheless, clinical observations as well as observational studies examining the effects of treatment versus no treatment (albeit not in a controlled manner) are supportive of the view that symptomatic hyponatremia causes death and other adverse outcomes. This causal link will be discussed further in the section on treatment, below.

Psychogenic polydipsia

The entity of hyponatremia in patients with psychiatric illness has been reviewed by de Leon *et al.* [14]. There is a high incidence of psychogenic polydipsia, especially in patients with schizophrenia, which generally precedes episodes of frank hyponatremia. Overall, patients with schizophrenia have a 3–5% incidence of hyponatremia. Those who develop hyponatremia are generally found to have impaired water excretion due to elevated ADH levels despite volume expansion and excessive water loads. The elevated ADH levels are in turn usually attributable either to medications or to the psychosis itself [15]. The hyponatremia and/or its correction may be life-threatening [16] but may also contribute to more persistently impaired CNS function [5].

Postoperative

Arieff presented disturbing clinical vignettes describing young, otherwise-healthy women who underwent surgery and in the subsequent postoperative period were found to have severe hyponatremia and severe neurologic abnormalities [17]. The majority of these patients subsequently experienced respiratory arrest followed by permanent neurologic impairment or death. In the postoperative period, multiple mechanisms impair free water excretion and stimulate ADH, including volume depletion, drugs, and pain. Especially if hypotonic fluids are administered, hyponatremia may result. The true incidence of postoperative hyponatremia is unknown and likely varies between centers depending on the awareness of the anesthesia and surgical staff of the dangers of hypotonic fluid administration (either as dextrose in water [which is effectively water after metabolism of dextrose] or as hypotonic irrigation solutions). The incidence of postoperative hyponatremia (plasma sodium of <130 mEq/L) as reported for 1986 from the University of Colorado was 4.4%, with a mortality rate of 4.2% (two patients); mortality was significantly higher than that for normonatremic surgical patients (0.2%) [18]. However, no symptoms of hyponatremia were present in these two patients. Importantly, 94% of the patients with hyponatremia were given hypotonic fluids. This suggests that this complication is largely preventable.

Over a 14-year period at the Mayo Clinic, 290,815 female patients between 15 and 50 years of age underwent surgery. Eleven (0.004%) patients had metabolic encephalopathy, new-onset seizures, or CPM in association with hyponatremia. None had cardiac arrest, as was reported in the series reported by Arieff. The authors concluded that the incidence of this entity is extremely low though nevertheless important.

Hyponatremia after transurethral resection of the prostate deserves further comment. During the procedure, irrigation with large volumes of fluid commonly containing glycine, but no sodium, has been used routinely in the past. Absorption of this hypotonic fluid results in increased glycine levels and hyponatremia. The use of sodium-containing irrigants is precluded by the electrical conduction of electrolyte solutions during the use of electrocautery. Newer methods should make this practice obsolete [19].

Cerebral salt wasting

Excessive urinary loss of sodium in association with CNS disease resulting in hypovolemia and hyponatremia was first described in

1950s. The recognition of the syndrome of cerebral salt wasting (CSW) has reemerged in recent years [20]. The pathophysiology of CSW is unclear, but elaboration of a natriuretic hormone(s) such as brain natriuretic protein has been proposed. The resulting volume depletion leads to elaboration of ADH and impaired ability to excrete water. The high ADH levels and the difficulty in assessing volume status have often led to the confusion of this entity with SIADH. For instance, uric acid levels, usually high in volume depletion, are low in SIADH because of volume expansion. They are also low in CSW, perhaps due to the elaboration of a natriuretic and uricosuric hormone [21]. Renin and aldosterone levels may also be low in CSW due to decreased neural input to the kidney from the brain. Most of the cases of CSW have been described after subarachnoid hemorrhage, but CSW has been seen in a variety of other CNS diseases and injuries. The existence of this entity has been supported by balance and hemodynamic studies which have tended to rule out SIADH; the true incidence of CSW is not known. As the treatment of hyponatremia in other settings such as SIADH involves water restriction, the distinction between CSW and SIADH is critical: water restriction in CSW would only exacerbate the volume depletion and not address the need for volume repletion.

Marathon runners

Hyponatremia has long been described during prolonged exercise. New studies have defined the incidence and risk factors in marathon runners. Runners have been advised to drink before they are thirsty. A popular method of running marathons is to walk through every water stop for about 1 min, often spaced every mile, and drink plenty of fluids during the walking segments. Marathons have become increasingly more popular in recent years, attracting many slower runners. Almond *et al.* [22] prospectively studied runners in the Boston Marathon. They enrolled 766 runners, although only 488 gave a blood sample at the end. Thirteen percent had serum sodium levels of ≤135 mmol/L, with three at <120 mmol/L (0.6%). Factors that predicted hyponatremia after multivariate analysis were body mass index (BMI; both high and low), longer racing time, and weight change (gain) during the marathon (with a surprising number of runners, both with and without hyponatremia, actually gaining weight). The type of fluid intake did not influence the prevalence of hyponatremia. This and other studies have led to new recommendations for fluid intake during marathons [23]. However, it should be pointed out that not all runners develop hyponatremia. A study of finishers of the 2003 Boston Marathon showed that among those 140 runners who had collapsed, 6% were hyponatremic and 69% were normonatremic, while 25% were actually hypernatremic [24].

HIV/AIDS

Hyponatremia has been found with a high frequency in persons with AIDS and AIDS-related complex. In a 3-month prospective study of 259 admissions with 212 patients, Tang *et al.* [25] noted hyponatremia (serum sodium of <135 mmol/L) during 38% of hospitalizations. Hyponatremia was present on admission in more than half of these episodes. The majority of episodes were in euvolemic patients and were attributed to SIADH, with most of the rest attributable to hypovolemia of a gastrointestinal etiology. Hyponatremia in this setting was associated with longer admissions and increased mortality.

Drugs

Drugs are an important cause of hyponatremia and, as indicated above, contribute to hyponatremia in psychogenic polydipsia. Selective serotonin reuptake inhibitors used for depression are an important class of drugs that produce hyponatremia in a relatively large percentage of patients. A retrospective analysis of 845 patients aged 65 years or over showed an incidence of hyponatremia, defined as a plasma sodium of <130 mmol/L, of approximately 0.5% [26]. More recently a prospective study of 75 patients revealed a 12% incidence of hyponatremia defined as a plasma sodium of <130 mmol/L [27]. Most had no or mild symptoms, such as nausea and fatigue, but one patient became confused. The appearance of hyponatremia was generally seen during the first 2 weeks of treatment and was more common in those with lower baseline plasma sodium levels and lower BMIs.

Thiazide diuretics are associated with hyponatremia. The actual incidence is not clear. Because of the large number of patients treated with diuretics, they are an important cause of hyponatremia. In a series of 1000 consecutive hospitalized patients, severe hyponatremia (plasma sodium of <129 mmol/L) occurred in 9.1% of the patients on diuretics versus 5.7% of those not treated with diuretics [28]. Diuretic-induced hyponatremia is more common with thiazide than loop diuretics and when it occurs it often appears within 2 weeks of starting therapy [29]. Thiazides may cause volume depletion in some patients with stimulation of ADH secretion. However, in others there is apparent SIADH with features of volume expansion, such as low uric acid levels. Stimulation of thirst also appears to be an important component of thiazide-induced hyponatremia. Risk factors for thiazide-induced hyponatremia, analyzed in a case–control study, include advanced age and low BMI [30].

The drug Ecstasy has also been implicated in acute hyponatremia by stimulating ADH levels and thirst [31]. The incidence for this is unknown.

Desmopressin is used to correct bleeding diatheses from von Wildebrand factor deficiency and, as expected, can cause hyponatremia, although the true incidence of desmopressin-induced hyponatremia in this setting is unknown. Larger numbers of adults are treated with desmopressin to treat nocturia. Rembratt *et al.* [32] compiled information on 632 patients from three trials. The incidence of hyponatremia in this population was high, averaging 15%, with 3% of all treated patients having at least one sodium reading of <125 mmol/L. Risk factors for the development of hyponatremia included low body weight, age of ≥65 years, and low basal serum sodium levels [32]. These findings imply that elderly patients with low baseline sodium should not be treated with desmopressin.

Cirrhosis

Hyponatremia in cirrhosis results from neuro-hormonal activation, including a nonosmotic vasopressin release. In the hospitalized cirrhotic patient population, the prevalence of hyponatremia, defined as a serum sodium level of <130 mEq/L, is about 30% [33,34]. There is a near-uniform association with ascites in these series, with infections and diuretic use also contributing. Borroni *et al.* reported a mortality of 26% in the hyponatremia cohort; elevated bilirubin (>2 mg/dL) and serum urea (>43 mg/dL) were independently correlated with mortality [34]. Mortality was even higher (48%) in the group with severe hyponatremia (serum sodium of <125 mmol/L). Studies have not shown an independent association of hyponatremia with adverse clinical outcomes. It is yet to be established whether hyponatremia is an independent risk factor for death rather than a confounder, that is, a comorbid event associated with other independent risk factors for death.

Congestive heart failure

CHF is associated with neuro-hormonal activation with stimulation of the renin–angiotensin system, the sympathetic nervous system, and arginine vasopressin. These result in a defect in water excretion and increase in thirst. Hyponatremia in CHF portends a poor prognosis. In the 1980s Packer and colleagues [35] found that the presence of hyponatremia predicted mortality in patients with CHF. In 203 patients with severe CHF, median survival for those with a normal serum sodium (>137 mmol/L) was 373 days, versus only 164 days for those with hyponatremia [35]. Treatment with angiotensin converting enzyme inhibitors improved the hyponatremia [36,37]. Packer *et al.* also showed in a retrospective analysis that treatment of CHF with angiotensin converting enzyme inhibitors was associated with decreased mortality in the hyponatremic patients [35]. As described below, vasopressin antagonists may also decrease mortality in hyponatremic patients.

Treatment

Before treatment is contemplated, a plasma osmolality measurement is generally needed to verify the presence of hypotonic hyponatremia, although exceptions such as hyponatremia in marathon runners exist. Despite the use of ion-specific electrodes, falsely low serum sodium values are still encountered.

Hyponatremic encephalopathy

The overriding issues regarding the proper treatment of hyponatremia are the rapidity and magnitude of correction of acute and chronic hyponatremia. Unfortunately, there are no randomized, controlled trials (RCTs) that have addressed these issues. Further, many of the studies that evaluated treatment strategies have included both patients with acute and patients with chronic hyponatremia and have at times not distinguished between these two fundamentally different patient groups. Furthermore, these studies have described a variety of methods of correction of hyponatremia (or no correction). Definitions of acute and chronic hyponatremia vary between studies. The studies are typically small. And, most importantly, the methods of correction are usually interrogated without comparisons to a control treatment strategy, making bias very possible. Often the patient undergoing the experimental treatment is compared to historic controls or to contemporary patients who have not been enrolled in an RCT. For instance, patients with severe underlying diseases might not be treated aggressively and may be included in the control group for comparison to patients treated aggressively. The rates of correction are not always comparable between studies, and overall rates may mask periods of treatment in which rates of correction were either faster or slower than the reported mean. Thus, the treatment of hyponatremia remains controversial, with insufficient data from RCTs to fully inform therapy. The controversy can be summarized as follows. If a symptomatic patient is corrected slowly, permanent neurologic sequelae may ensue, and some have argued that rapidly correcting sodium is safe and effective in avoiding these sequelae. On the other hand, it has been argued that slow correction leads to better outcomes and that overly rapid correction also often leads to permanent neurologic sequelae, especially demyelinating lesions, such as CPM or osmotic demyelinating syndrome.

As there are no controlled trials, a careful evaluation of the reported studies (Table 55.1), in conjunction with clinical reasoning dictated by pathophysiologic principles, may allow for reasonable conclusions about treatment in the absence of more robust clinical trials evidence. Some of the studies (mostly retrospective cohorts) have divided patients into arbitrary correction rate groups (expressed either as milliequivalents per liter per hour or as a cumulative magnitude of correction over a time interval, such as 24 h) and then have reported the incidence of complications. Other studies (nested case–control study design) have divided the patients into those with complications versus those without and then compared their rates of correction.

In 1982 Ayus *et al.* [38] presented a case series of seven selected cases of severe hyponatremia who were corrected rapidly and who experienced no neurologic sequelae. Only two of the cases were clearly acute. All were treated at a relatively rapid rate, yet none had neurologic sequelae. The authors reviewed the literature up to that time (case reports and small case series) and suggested that those patients who were treated rapidly (>1 mEq/L/h) generally (11 of 12) recovered without sequelae, whereas those who were treated more gradually (13 patients) all had neurologic sequelae. Similarly, Worthley [39] reported that four of five patients with acute hyponatremia treated rapidly did well. One 47-year-old woman exhibited neurologic sequelae after a seizure in the postoperative period, but effects of treatment could not be ruled out as a cause of her neurologic symptoms. Ashouri [40] presented eight elderly patients with severely symptomatic, diuretic-induced, hyponatremia who were treated with hypertonic saline at a moderately rapid rate. All were said to have recovered without sequelae, although one patient could conceivably have had CPM. It was not stated if these cases were selected or consecutive. None of these three studies examined different rates of correction, and all were small.

In what remains one of the largest series of symptomatic hyponatremia (64 patients), Sterns [41] in a retrospective analysis reported that treatment of 26 patients (25 chronic, 1 acute) with hyponatremia at a rate of <0.55 mmol/L/h to a level of 120 mmol/L resulted in no sequelae. Although none of the 7 patients with acute hyponatremia who were treated at a rate higher than this had sequelae, 7 of 27 with chronic hyponatremia who were treated at the higher rate were reported to have had neurologic sequelae, including CPM. None of these seven were corrected to frankly hypernatremic levels, and most were corrected to hyponatremic levels. However, all seven patients were corrected at a rate of >12 mmol/L/day.

Ayus *et al.* [42] advocated a more aggressive approach to treatment in a combined prospective observational study and retrospective study of cases of CPM and also a literature review. Thirty-three patients, studied prospectively, were treated at a rapid rate and had no neurologic sequelae. The magnitude of correction at 24 h (20 ± 1 mEq/L/h) was higher than the rate reported by Sterns. In those patients who were selected because they had CPM, the magnitude of correction of 37 ± 3 mEq/L at 41 ± 3 h was higher than in those patients who had no sequelae (21 ± 1 mEq/L at 48 h). Similarly, data gleaned from the literature for patients with demyelinating lesions showed a higher magnitude of correction (27 ± 2 mEq/L at 39 ± 4 h) than in patients without sequelae. Both groups with CNS events had a higher magnitude of correction (both $P < 0.01$) at 24 h than those without CNS events, although the actual levels were not stated. The authors concluded that patients could be safely corrected rapidly but only if the magnitude of the correction was kept to less than 25 mEq/L at 48 h. Although 25 mEq/L at 48 h is similar to 12 mEq/L at 24 h, much of the controversy actually stems from this difference. In the study by Ayus *et al.* the magnitude of correction at 24 h was higher than that in Sterns [41] and to an extent that was associated with neurologic sequelae in the Sterns study.

Brunner *et al.* [43] prospectively studied 13 hyponatremic patients admitted from the emergency room. Three of 13 developed CPM. The rate of correction in these patients with CPM was significantly higher than those who had no sequelae. One of the patients with CPM had acute hyponatremia after transurethral resection of the prostate. Although his serum sodium on admission at 133 mmol/L was only mildly decreased, the magnitude of correction was 40 mmol/L in the first 24 h.

Cheng *et al.* [44] examined retrospectively severe hyponatremia in a large psychiatric hospitalized population. The nurses were trained to recognize the potential of psychogenic polydipsia and, when suspected, action was taken promptly. Therefore, the 13 patients with seizures were all considered to have acute hyponatremia. Treatment varied from hypertonic saline to water restriction. (Note that patients with psychogenic polydipsia often have a large spontaneous water diuresis). All recovered uneventfully after a rate of correction averaging 1 mmol/L/h. Tanneau *et al.* [16], however, found complications after treatment of hyponatremia in patients with psychogenic polydipsia. They examined retrospectively 24 separate episodes in 12 patients with hyponatremia and

Table 55.1 Studies examining correction of symptomatic hyponatremia

Study [reference]	Date	Study type	Inclusion	Population	Total Number	Acute	Chronic	Overall rate Correction (mmol/L/h)	Mortality or CNS complications — Slow	Rapid (mmol/L/h)	P	Magnitude 24 h — Low	High (mmol/L/h)	P	Complications — No	Yes	n^a	P
Ayus [38]	1982	Retrospective Consecutive cases			7	2	5	2.4 ± 0.5		0/7[b]					Magnitude corrections at ≤24 h (mmol/L) 28.6 + 3.9 (SE)[c]		0	
Worthley [39]	1986	Cases	<110		5	5	0	2.14 ± 0.49		0/5[b,d]								
Sterns [41]	1987	Retrospective	≤110	General Hospital	62	10	54	0.59 chronic 1.57 acute	<0.55[e] 0/25 0/1	>0.55 7/27 0/7	0.02							
Ayus [42]	1987	Prospective[f]	≤120	General Hospital	33	3	30	1.3 ± 0.2[f2]							Magnitude corrections (mmol/L) 20 ± 1 at 24 h[f3] 0 ; 21 ± 1 at 48 h 0			
		Retrospective Literature			12 17	2	10	1.0 ± 0.2 0.7 ± 0.1								37 ± 3 at 48 h ; 27 ± 2 at 39 h	12 17	<0.001[f4] <0.01[f4]
Brunner [43]	1990	Prospective	<115	ER	13	3[g]	10								Rate correction (mmol/L/h)[g2] 0.74 ± 0.32 (SD) 1.25 ± 0.4 ; Magnitude correction at 24 h (mmol/L) 17.5	30	3 7	0.04
Cheng [44]	1990	Retrospective	≤120	Psychogenic polydipsia with seizures	13[h]	13	0	0.96 ± 0.06[i]	0.4 0/1	≥ 0.7 1/26					Magnitude correction at 24 h (mmol/L) 21.6 ± 1.4 (SE)	0	<0.02	
Sonnenblick [29]	1993	Retrospective diuretics	<115	Diuretic	68		68		<0.6 3/38[k]	>0.6 11/30[k]	0.004	<20 4/37[k]	>20 7/22[k]	0.05				
Tanneau [16]	1994	Retrospective	≤115	Psych	12[l]												5[l2]	
Ellis [45]	1995	Prospective/ Observational	≤120	General Hospital	184	39	145	0.35	<0.4[m] 1/98	>0.4[m] 9/57		<10[m] 1/98	>10[m] 9/57		Magnitude of correction at 24 h (mmol/L) 15.5 ± 5.1 (SD) 21.8 ± 3.9 ; Magnitude of correction at 24h (mmol/L) 8.2	12.1	10	0.0125

(Continued)

Table 55.1 (Continued)

Study [reference]	Date	Study type	Inclusion	Population	Total Number	Acute	Chronic	Overall rate Correction (mmol/L/h)	Mortality or CNS complications Slow	Rapid	P	Magnitude 24 h Low	High	P	Complications No	Yes	n^b	P
									(mmol/L/h)	(mmol/L/h)		(mmol/L/h)	(mmol/L/h)					
Ayus [46]	1999	Prospective/ Observational[n]	<130	Symptomatic Postmenopausal	53		53		0.1 14/14	0.7 0/17 0.8[n3] 14/22		3[f2] 14/14	14[f2] 0/17 22[f2,n3] 14/22 >25 0/17 cpm		Mortality by final [Na] (mmol/L) at 48 h 127 ± 8	118 ± 10		
Nzure [47]	2003	Retrospective	≤ 115	General Hospital	168	138	28	0.8									34	0.0016

a Number with complications.
b All patients considered rapid.
c Derived from Table 1.
d One patient had early seizure and permanent neurologic damage.
e 4 patients who died were excluded from analysis; correction to 120 mEq/L.
f Prospectively looked at patients with follow-up CT; those without CT (excluded patients) had no clinical evidence of neurologic damage. Retrospectively analyzed those with demyelinating lesions on CT or autopsy. Literature review included those with neurologic damage in which rate of correction was described.
f2 Initial correction rates.
f3 All corrected by <25 mmol at 24 h except two with acute hyponatremia.
f4 P vs. prospective group.
g Acute vs. chronic not explicitly stated; we assume those that presented to the hospital were chronic and those that developed hyponatremia in the hospital were acute.
g2 Overall rate at 24 h. During the first 8 h, 1.4 ± 0.8 vs. 2.8 ± 0.72 in those with CPM.
g3 Any persistent CNS complications (excluding 2 patients with preexisting CNS abnormalities)
h 27 episodes of seizures in 13 patients.
i Calculated from 24-h data in Table 55.3; rate in first 12 h was 1.26 ± 0.1 mM/h.
j 68 patients including 14 of the authors' own in whom data on rate of recovery could be determined.
k Death or CPM; includes patients from Ref. 40.
l 24 episodes.
l2 All 5 with complications developed hyponatremia at home and therefore may have not been acute.
m Abstracted from Fig 1, which includes only treated patients. Only 1 was acute (evidently in the rapid treatment group).
n Prospective but selected.
n2 Taken from the means in Table 2.
n3 Patients were treated with sodium chloride only after respiratory insufficiency.

Table 55.2 Evidence ratings and recommendations for treatment of acute symptomatic hyponatremia.

Intervention	Existing systematic reviews[a]	Overall evidence rating[b]				Comment	Recommendation[c]			Comment
		High	Moderate	Low	Very low		I	II	III	
Rapid vs. slow correction	Yes		✓			Prospective and retrospective studies; no RCTs	✓			Controversial; rapid correction until severe symptoms controlled, not to exceed 8–12 mM in first 24 h; avoid overcorrection
Hypertonic saline	No		✓			Prospective and retrospective studies; no RCTs	✓			Current gold standard for severe symptomatic hyponatremia; may combine with diuretics
V-2 receptor antagonists (avoid)	No		✓			No data for acute hyponatremia	✓			Avoid; data for only chronic hyponatremia; rate may be too slow for acute hyponatremia

[a] If no existing systematic reviews, overall evidence rating starts at moderate.

[b] High for RCT with precise estimates, adequate allocation concealment, blinding of participants and investigators, use of intention-to-treat analysis, and loss to follow-up <20%; moderate if RCT but estimates imprecise, potential for type 1 or 2 statistical error, unclear allocation concealment, no intention-to-treat analysis; low in all other cases; judgment also accounts for directness of findings.

[c] Recommendation or suggestion is based upon whether further research is likely to change confidence in estimate of effect; assessment accounts for trade-offs between benefits and harms, translation into clinical practice, uncertainty about baseline risk of population of interest, and quality of evidence. I, recommend; II, suggest; III, no recommendation possible.

Table 55.3 Evidence ratings and recommendations for treatment of chronic symptomatic hyponatremia.

Intervention	Existing systematic reviews[a]	Overall evidence rating[b]					Recommendation[c]			
		High	Moderate	Low	Very low	Comment	I	II	III	Comment
Slow vs. rapid correction	Yes		✓			Retrospective and observational studies; no RCTs		✓		Trend toward more neurologic sequelae with rapid vs. slow correction
Hypertonic saline vs. normal saline	No			✓		No comparative studies		✓		Most studies have used hypertonic saline; avoid normal saline in SIADH
V-2 receptor antagonists (avoid)	No			✓		No studies in symptomatic patients		✓		Avoid; no data available; may be too slow for initial correction
Urea	No			✓		Small uncontrolled trials			✓	Experience too limited to recommend
Water restriction alone (avoid)	No			✓		No controlled studies		✓		Avoid unless spontaneous water diuresis begins; poor outcomes in patients with severe symptoms corrected at very slow rates such as with water restriction alone

[a] If no existing systematic reviews, overall evidence rating starts at moderate.

[b] High for RCT with precise estimates, adequate allocation concealment, blinding of participants and investigators, use of intention-to-treat analysis, and loss to follow-up <20%; moderate if RCT but estimates imprecise, potential for type 1 or 2 statistical error, unclear allocation concealment, no intention-to-treat analysis; low in all other cases; judgment also accounts for directness of findings.

[c] Recommendation or suggestion is based upon whether further research is likely to change confidence in estimate of effect; assessment accounts for trade-offs between benefits and harms, translation into clinical practice, uncertainty about baseline risk of population of interest, and quality of evidence. I, recommend; II, suggest; III, no recommendation possible.

Table 55.4 Evidence ratings and recommendations for treatment of chronic asymptomatic hyponatremia.

Intervention	Existing systematic reviews[a]	Overall evidence rating[b]				Comment	Recommendation[c]			Comment
		High	Moderate	Low	Very low		I	II	III	
Slow vs. rapid correction	No		✓			No systematic studies in asymptomatic patients; ample animal data	✓			If asymptomatic, no role for rapid correction
Water restriction	No		✓			Few RCTs; used as comparison group for vasopressin antagonists		✓		May prevent further decline in serum sodium; usually ineffective in correcting hyponatremia due to increased thirst
V-2 receptor antagonists	No		✓			Several RCTs using vasopressin antagonists		✓		Oral agent (tolvaptan) showed significant sustained improvement in hyponatremia; not yet approved for use
Demeclocycline vs. lithium	No			✓		One small nonrandomized study		✓		Demecocycline is superior to lithium; avoid in liver dysfunction
Urea	No			✓		Small-sized uncontrolled; case reports			✓	Well-tolerated with few side effects; limited clinical experience

[a] If no existing systematic reviews, overall evidence rating starts at moderate.

[b] High for RCT with precise estimates, adequate allocation concealment, blinding of participants and investigators, use of intention-to-treat analysis, and loss to follow-up <20%; moderate if RCT but estimates imprecise, potential for type 1 or 2 statistical error, unclear allocation concealment, no intention-to-treat analysis; low in all other cases; judgment also accounts for directness of findings.

[c] Recommendation or suggestion is based upon whether further research is likely to change confidence in estimate of effect; assessment accounts for trade-offs between benefits and harms, translation into clinical practice, uncertainty about baseline risk of population of interest, and quality of evidence. I, recommend; II, suggest; III, no recommendation possible.

serum sodium concentrations of ≤115 mmol/L. Five patients suffered neurologic sequelae. The overall rate of correction was 1.9 mmol/L/h. In those with no sequelae, the magnitude of correction over the first 24 h was significantly lower than those with adverse events (15.5 ± 5.1 vs. 21.8 ± 3.9 mmol/L). Of note, however, was the finding that all of the patients with sequelae developed hyponatremia at home. Therefore, it is likely that some or all of those with sequelae did not have acute hyponatremia.

Sonnenblick et al. [29] analyzed retrospectively 14 patients with diuretic-induced hyponatremia and sodium levels of <115 mmol/L. Using definitions of rapidity of correction similar to Sterns (less than or greater than 0.6 mmol/L/h), they found that 8% of those in the slower correction rate group had sequelae (death or demyelinating syndrome) versus 37% in the more rapid rate group. Looking at the data by magnitude of correction at 24 h, those with a correction of <20 mmol/L in the first 24 h had an 11% complication rate, compared to a 32% complication rate in those corrected by >20 mmol/L.

In one of the earliest prospectively assembled cohorts, Ellis [45] evaluated a large number of patients (184) with sodium levels of ≤120 mmol/L. Patients who recovered without complications had a rise in sodium of 8.2 mmol/L in the first 24 h, whereas those who developed complications were corrected on average by 12.1 mmol/L. Figure 4 of that paper allowed an evaluation of the effects of magnitude of correction on the complication rate. In those corrected by less than 10 mmol/L at 24 h, 1 of 100 patients had neurologic sequelae attributable to treatment, whereas in those corrected to ≥10 mmol/L, 9 of 58 developed complications. Thus, these studies support an even more cautious approach than that suggested by Sterns. However, as with all of these studies, the patients were not randomized to the different treatment groups. Although the majority of the patients had chronic hyponatremia, the results were not factored for acuity of the baseline hyponatremia. One could postulate that the rate that emerged from the prospective cohort of Ellis was too slow for patients with acute hyponatremia. If the cutoff rate were set at 14 mmol/L/24 h, then 7.7% (1 patient) who were corrected faster than this rate had an adverse neurologic sequela, versus 6.2% of those corrected at a slower rate. Thus, although the author supports a slower rate of correction, alternative interpretations are possible.

Ayus and Arieff [46], in a prospective observational study, examined the outcomes of postmenopausal women with hyponatremia defined as a serum sodium of <130 mmol/L (higher than the other studies cited). Postmenopausal women were studied because they were felt to have a "lower risk" than premenopausal women. All of the patients treated initially with water restriction alone developed complications, whereas none of the cohort corrected at a faster rate (averaging 0.8 mmol/L/h) exhibited neurologic sequelae. The latter group had an average rise in their serum sodium of about 14 mmol/L at 24 h. In those treated with water restriction only, the rise in plasma sodium after 24 h was only about 3 mmol/L. Twenty-two patients were seen by the authors after they had already had a respiratory event. They were then further corrected more rapidly at 0.8 mmol/L/h, but the neurologic sequelae persisted in 14 patients

despite the correction. The authors concluded that prompt treatment at fast rates, prior to a respiratory event, is critical. The data support the view that symptomatic patients represent an emergency that must be corrected with saline, as those who ultimately experienced adverse events had an extremely low rate of correction. However, the data do not adequately address the optimal speed for this rapid correction, as the numbers of patients studied were low and the patients were not randomized.

The most recent study, by Nzerue et al. [47], examined 168 patients admitted to a tertiary care hospital with sodium levels of ≤115 mmol/L. Those with no observed sequelae were corrected at a higher rate than those with complications. The sodium at 48 h was 127 mmol/L in those without complications and 118 mmol/L in those with complications. The authors concluded that rapid correction is better. However, most of the patients in this study had acute hyponatremia (82%), yet the rate of correction in those with sequelae was minimal. This again supports the view that symptomatic hyponatremia should be corrected with saline, but the study did not adequately address the optimal rate of correction.

Based on these studies, general guidelines have been suggested to maximize the potential for recovery while avoiding CPM [48–51]. However, case reports have continued to be presented which describe CPM in patients despite correction at relatively low rates [52–55]. Patients with preexisting malnutrition and/or potassium depletion appear to be at particular risk of CPM [56]. It has been postulated that these patients are unable to reaccumulate brain osmols during correction of hyponatremia, making them particularly vulnerable to brain dehydration.

There are no studies that have examined the specific mode of treatment of acute symptomatic hyponatremia, and guidelines are largely based on theoretical arguments. The studies cited above used a variety of methods of treatment. In the euvolemic symptomatic patient, hypertonic saline is recommended because saline may aggravate hyponatremia, especially in patients with SIADH. The administration of normal saline to patients with SIADH can actually decrease the serum sodium, as the patients may excrete the sodium while reabsorbing the water because of inhibition of aldosterone and elevated levels of ADH. However, there have been no controlled studies comparing directly saline and hypertonic saline. Furosemide has been used to lower urine osmolality, but its role has not been systematically evaluated. Furosemide does not consistently lower urine osmolality below plasma and thus normal saline could theoretically aggravate hyponatremia even in the face of furosemide treatment. Furosemide would of course be useful in the hypervolemic patient to prevent further volume overload. ADH antagonists have no role at this time in the acute treatment of hyponatremia because they have not been studied for this indication and because the studies so far suggest that the rate of correction would be too slow. Urea has been used in symptomatic hyponatremia but experience is limited [57].

Chronic asymptomatic hyponatremia

Patients with chronic hyponatremia, because of physiological compensation, are often relatively asymptomatic from a CNS standpoint despite critically low serum sodium levels. There are no studies that have directly addressed what course of treatment should be undertaken. There is general agreement that such patients should not be treated "aggressively" and that water restriction is the preferred mode of treatment to allow for the slow correction of the serum sodium to a more acceptable range. There is general agreement that saline plays no role in the immediate or long-term treatment of chronic hyponatremia. On the other hand, there are no studies demonstrating that water restriction is actually effective in the long term. Theoretically, all patients should improve with water restriction, but thirst will often overcome the patient's ability to adhere to the prescribed water restriction. One of the few studies that examined the effects of water restriction showed that a 1-L/day restriction in patients with cirrhosis did not improve their hyponatremia (although hyponatremia did not worsen, either) [58]. Alternative therapies to promote water excretion by inhibiting ADH activity have not been systematically evaluated. The toxicity of lithium has made its use problematic. Doxycycline is preferred to lithium because of generally lower toxicity but is not devoid of toxicity, and long-term therapy with doxycycline has not been evaluated. The presence of liver dysfunction has been shown to increase doxycycline toxicity and the risk of kidney failure [59]. Thus, its use in cirrhotic patients with hyponatremia is contraindicated. Urea appears to be safe and effective, but experience is limited to case reports by one group of investigators who have used urea in cases of SIADH [60,61], cirrhosis [62], and psychogenic polydipsia [63]. New ADH antagonists are currently being evaluated.

Prospective randomized trials have now been performed to examine the effects of the treatment of hyponatremia with ADH antagonists in cirrhosis [7,58,64], CHF [7,64,65], and SIADH [7,64,66]. Short-term clinical trials have demonstrated that ADH antagonists are effective in correcting promptly the hyponatremia under these clinical circumstances. In CHF they have also been shown in a retrospective analysis to decrease overall mortality [67]. There have been, however, few long-term studies to evaluate the effectiveness of these antagonists in improving mortality or significant long-term morbidities under these conditions. The efficacy of the oral V2 antagonist tolvaptan has been studied with both short-term and long-term RCTs, and the short-term outcome results are encouraging; the long-term results are more disappointing. In short-term use (6 and 30 days) in patients with heart failure, cirrhosis, and SIADH, the effects were sustained over the month of the study without serious adverse effects. In those patients with severe hyponatremia there was a measurable subjective improvement in CNS symptoms [7]. In only 4 of 225 patients treated with tolvaptan did the rate of correction of the presenting hyponatremia possibly exceed the recommended rate for chronic hyponatremia (>0.5 mmol/L over the fist 24 h). Thus, these agents may ultimately prove to be effective in controlling symptomatic hyponatremia and perhaps may ultimately improve mortality. With regard to this latter outcome, the results of a large RCT with long-term follow-up investigating the use of tolvaptan in patients with CHF were negative. Konstam and coworkers, reporting on the results of the EVEREST trial, an event-driven masked RCT with 4133 patients, observed that treatment of patients hospitalized for CHF with tolvaptan for at least 60 days did not result in significant improvement in long-term morbidity and mortality (median observation period, 9.9 months) [68]. Another somewhat smaller RCT (120 patients each in two arms) evaluating tolvaptan's effects on left ventricular end-diastolic volume in heart failure noted in a post hoc time-to-event analysis that patients assigned to the tolvaptan arm demonstrated improvement long-term outcomes for the composite outcome of mortality and CHF hospitalizations [69]. The long-term effectiveness of tolvaptan in managing the hyponatremia of SIADH and cirrhosis and the potential benefits of tolvaptan treatment on mortality and morbidity attributable to chronic hyponatremia in these disease states have not been unambiguously demonstrated by the currently published clinical RCTs.

Summary of recommendations for various entities

Acute hyponatremia

Acute hyponatremia warrants immediate correction. The studies cited above suggest that if the patient develops hyponatremia rapidly, correction can be rapid without significant sequelae. However, if the time over which hyponatremia has developed is unknown, it seems prudent to be more cautious, as some physiologic adaptation may have already occurred. In this latter case, a relatively rapid rate of correction (1–3 mmol/L/h) for a few hours will decrease brain edema and alleviate the immediate prospect of brain herniation. Then, the rate of correction should be slowed so that the total rise is no greater than 12 mmol in the first 24 h. Protocols for the administration of hypertonic saline can be found elsewhere [50]. It should be noted, however, that the specific recommendations noted here are based exclusively on observational studies and may need to be changed substantially if and when any robust evidence from randomized clinical trials emerges. The investigation of the new ADH antagonists might provide an ideal opportunity to re-examine all aspects of treatment strategies for acute and chronic hyponatremia rigorously using more robust clinical RCT approaches.

The following comments are for some specific settings in which this occurs.

- *Psychogenic polydipsia with hyponatremia:* Even after presenting with severe symptoms attributable to hyponatremia, most patients with psychogenic polydipsia appear to recover uneventfully. Once these patients stop drinking copious quantities of fluids, they usually excrete a relatively dilute urine. If the patient has acute hyponatremia (which usually means the condition has developed under observation in the hospital), it can be corrected quite rapidly without sequelae. However, if the time to development is unknown, the study by Tanneau *et al.* [16] suggests that these patients should be treated as if they have chronic symptomatic hyponatremia and, thus, extremely rapid correction should be avoided.

• *Postoperative hyonatremia:* Reports from Arieff, Ayus, and colleagues [17,70] have provided compelling evidence that the presence of severe hyponatremia with symptoms postoperatively constitutes a medical emergency and requires prompt administration of hypertonic saline at rates suggested above. Again, complete correction may not be desirable, but rather should be tempered to account for any adaptation that may have occurred by the time the entity was discovered.

• *Endurance athletes:* Hyponatremia occurring in marathon runners or in triathletes can all be assumed to be acute. If discovered in the medical tent, hypertonic saline should be rapidly administered (a bolus of 100 ml of 3% saline has been suggested [23]). Such rapid correction should pose no risk based on the acuity. It is likely that complete correction acutely will have no additional adverse consequences, but no studies have addressed this issue.

Chronic hyponatremia

Chronic hyponatremia with symptoms

Patients with severe hyponatremia and symptoms require correction. Of those patients who are volume depleted, there are no studies comparing modes of treatment or rates of correction. Normal saline is considered customary treatment for correction of the volume depletion, but the optimal rate of correction of plasma sodium that might result from administration of normal saline has not been determined. The best available evidence supports the recommendation that a rate of correction similar to that for all patients with chronic symptomatic hyponatremia be used. As pointed out by Adrogue and Madias [50], correction of hypovolemia will inhibit ADH secretion, resulting potentially in a more dilute urine and potentially in correction at too rapid a rate. Thus, some authors have suggested that administration of hypotonic fluids may actually be required to slow the rate of correction in this setting.

In euvolemic patients, hypertonic saline is the preferred method of correction for symptomatic chronic hyponatremia, as many of these patients will have SIADH, and administration of normal saline has been associated in some observational studies with actual initial worsening of the hyponatremia (see above). The data reviewed above do not allow a definitive recommendation of the rate or magnitude of correction. At this time, we would recommend that, in general, a rate of about 0.5 mmol/L/h and no greater than 8 mmol total in the first 24 h. However, if the patient has more severe symptoms, such as seizures, a faster initial rate of 1–2 mmol/L/h for 2–3 h might be indicated, as this rapid initial rate of correction might be more likely to relieve deleterious cerebral edema. The rate might then be slowed so the total correction would not exceed 8 mmol in the first 24 h.

The available literature does not allow a definitive recommendation that would prevent all complications in all patients. We have recommended a rate of about 0.5 mmol/L/h and no greater than 8 mmol total in the first 24 h. This rate might result in neurologic sequelae if the patient subsequently has seizures or respiratory arrest. On the other hand, a more rapid rate would increase the risk of demyelinating disease. Again, guidelines for the administration

of hypertonic saline to achieve these recommended rates of correction can be found elsewhere [50].

In the hypervolemic patient with CNS manifestations, the same considerations apply as for the clinically euvolemic patient. The use of ADH antagonists rather than hypertonic saline would seem especially suited to this group of patients, who already have an increase in extracellular fluid volume. However, the studies to date have not addressed the use of ADH antagonists for treatment of symptomatic hyponatremia. With the current level of experience, the rate of correction is not completely predictable and may be too slow when a patient exhibits CNS symptoms, and thus hypertonic saline with furosemide is currently considered preferable.

Chronic asymptomatic hyponatremia

Many patients with SIADH, cirrhosis, and heart failure are asymptomatic. Current best evidence, in the absence of any clinical RCTs, supports the recommendations that these patients be treated initially with water restriction. Demeclocycline can be considered for patients without liver failure who fail fluid restriction, but long-term toxicity is possible. The use of ADH antagonists will likely prove useful, but no studies to date have addressed their long-term efficacy, safety, and cost.

References

1 Sterns RH. The treatment of hyponatremia: first, do no harm. *Am J Med* 1990; **88:** 557–560.

2 Sterns RH, Thomas DJ, Herndon RM. Brain dehydration and neurologic deterioration after rapid correction of hyponatremia. *Kidney Int* 1989; **35:** 69–75.

3 Lien YH, Shapiro JI, Chan L. Study of brain electrolytes and organic osmolytes during correction of chronic hyponatremia. Implications for the pathogenesis of central pontine myelinolysis. *J Clin Invest* 1991; **88:** 303–309.

4 Chow KM, Kwan BC, Szeto CC. Clinical studies of thiazide-induced hyponatremia. *J Natl Med Assoc* 2004; **96:** 1305–1308.

5 Shutty MS, Jr., Briscoe L, Sautter S, Leadbetter RA. Neuropsychological manifestations of hyponatremia in chronic schizophrenic patients with the syndrome of psychosis, intermittent hyponatremia and polydipsia (PIP). *Schizophr Res* 1993; **10:** 125–130.

6 Renneboog B, Musch W, Vandemergel X, Manto MU, Decaux G. Mild chronic hyponatremia is associated with falls, unsteadiness, and attention deficits. *Am J Med* 2006; **119:** 71–78.

7 Schrier RW, Gross P, Gheorghiade M, Berl T, Verbalis JG, Czerwiec FS *et al.* Tolvaptan, a selective oral vasopressin V2-receptor antagonist, for hyponatremia. *N Engl J Med* 2006; **355:** 2099–2112.

8 Anderson RJ, Chung HM, Kluge R, Schrier RW. Hyponatremia: a prospective analysis of its epidemiology and the pathogenetic role of vasopressin. *Ann Intern Med* 1985; **102:** 164–168.

9 Hawkins RC. Age and gender as risk factors for hyponatremia and hypernatremia. *Clin Chim Acta* 2003; **337:** 169–172.

10 DeVita MV, Gardenswartz MH, Konecky A, Zabetakis PM. Incidence and etiology of hyponatremia in an intensive care unit. *Clin Nephrol* 1990; **34:** 163–166.

11 Lee CT, Guo HR, Chen JB. Hyponatremia in the emergency department. *Am J Emerg Med* 2000; **18:** 264–268.

12 Hoorn EJ, Lindemans J, Zietse R. Development of severe hyponatraemia in hospitalized patients: treatment-related risk factors and inadequate management. *Nephrol Dial Transplant* 2006; **21:** 70–76.

13 Miller M, Morley JE, Rubenstein LZ. Hyponatremia in a nursing home population. *J Am Geriatr Soc* 1995; **43:** 1410–1413.

14 de Leon J, Verghese C, Tracy JI, Josiassen RC, Simpsom GM. Polydipsia and water intoxication in psychiatric patients: a review of the epidemiological literature. *Biol Psychiatry* 1994; **35:** 408–419.

15 Goldman MB, Robertson GL, Luchins DJ, Hedeker D, Pandey GN. Psychotic exacerbations and enhanced vasopressin secretion in schizophrenic patients with hyponatremia and polydipsia. *Arch Gen Psychiatry* 1997; **54:** 443–449.

16 Tanneau RS, Henry A, Rouhart F, Bourbigot B, Garo B, Macoquard Y *et al.* High incidence of neurologic complications following rapid correction of severe hyponatremia in polydipsic patients. *J Clin Psychiatry* 1994; **55:** 349–354.

17 Arieff AI. Hyponatremia, convulsions, respiratory arrest, and permanent brain damage after elective surgery in healthy women. *N Engl J Med* 1986; **314:** 1529–1535.

18 Chung HM, Kluge R, Schrier RW, Anderson RJ. Postoperative hyponatremia. A prospective study. *Arch Intern Med* 1986; **146:** 333–336.

19 Issa MM, Young MR, Bullock AR, Bouet R, Petros JA. Dilutional hyponatremia of TURP syndrome: a historical event in the 21st century. *Urology* 2004; **64:** 298–301.

20 Palmer BF. Hyponatremia in patients with central nervous system disease: SIADH versus CSW. *Trends Endocrinol Metab* 2003; **14:** 182–187.

21 Maesaka JK, Fishbane S. Regulation of renal urate excretion: a critical review. *Am J Kidney Dis* 1998; **32:** 917–933.

22 Almond CS, Shin AY, Fortescue EB, Mannix RC, Wypij D, Binstadt BA *et al.* Hyponatremia among runners in the Boston Marathon. *N Engl J Med* 2005; **352:** 1550–1556.

23 Hew-Butler T, Almond C, Ayus JC, Dugas J, Meeuwisse W, Noakes T *et al.* Consensus statement of the 1st International Exercise-Associated Hyponatremia Consensus Development Conference, Cape Town, South Africa 2005. *Clin J Sport Med* 2005; **15:** 208–213.

24 Kratz A, Siegel AJ, Verbalis JG, Adner MM, Shirey T, Lee-Lewandrowski E *et al.* Sodium status of collapsed marathon runners. *Arch Pathol Lab Med* 2005; **129:** 227–230.

25 Tang WW, Kaptein EM, Feinstein EI, Massry SG. Hyponatremia in hospitalized patients with the acquired immunodeficiency syndrome (AIDS) and the AIDS-related complex. *Am J Med* 1993; **94:** 169–174.

26 Wilkinson TJ, Begg EJ, Winter AC, Sainsbury R. Incidence and risk factors for hyponatraemia following treatment with fluoxetine or paroxetine in elderly people. *Br J Clin Pharmacol* 1999; **47:** 211–217.

27 Fabian TJ, Amico JA, Kroboth PD, Mulsant BH, Corey SE, Begley AE *et al.* Paroxetine-induced hyponatremia in older adults: a 12-week prospective study. *Arch Intern Med* 2004; **164:** 327–332.

28 Byatt CM, Millard PH, Levin GE. Diuretics and electrolyte disturbances in 1000 consecutive geriatric admissions. *J R Soc Med* 1990; **83:** 704–708.

29 Sonnenblick M, Friedlander Y, Rosin AJ. Diuretic-induced severe hyponatremia. Review and analysis of 129 reported patients. *Chest* 1993; **103:** 601–606.

30 Chow KM, Szeto CC, Wong TY, Leung CB, Li PK. Risk factors for thiazide-induced hyponatraemia. *QJM* 2003; **96:** 911–917.

31 Budisavljevic MN, Stewart L, Sahn SA, Ploth DW. Hyponatremia associated with 3,4-methylenedioxymethylamphetamine ("ecstasy") abuse. *Am J Med Sci* 2003; **326:** 89–93.

32 Rembratt A, Riis A, Norgaard JP. Desmopressin treatment in nocturia; an analysis of risk factors for hyponatremia. *Neurourol Urodyn* 2006; **25:** 105–109.

33 Porcel A, Diaz F, Rendon P, Macias M, Martin-Herrera L, Giron-Gonzalez JA. Dilutional hyponatremia in patients with cirrhosis and ascites. *Arch Intern Med* 2002; **162:** 323–328.

34 Borroni G, Maggi A, Sangiovanni A, Cazzaniga M, Salerno F. Clinical relevance of hyponatraemia for the hospital outcome of cirrhotic patients. *Dig Liver Dis* 2000; **32:** 605–610.

35 Lee WH, Packer M. Prognostic importance of serum sodium concentration and its modification by converting-enzyme inhibition in patients with severe chronic heart failure. *Circulation* 1986; **73:** 257–267.

36 Dzau VJ, Hollenberg NK. Renal response to captopril in severe heart failure: role of furosemide in natriuresis and reversal of hyponatremia. *Ann Intern Med* 1984; **100:** 777–782.

37 Packer M, Medina N, Yushak M. Correction of dilutional hyponatremia in severe chronic heart failure by converting-enzyme inhibition. *Ann Intern Med* 1984; **100:** 782–789.

38 Ayus JC, Olivero JJ, Frommer JP. Rapid correction of severe hyponatremia with intravenous hypertonic saline solution. *Am J Med* 1982; **72:** 43–48.

39 Worthley LI, Thomas PD. Treatment of hyponatraemic seizures with intravenous 29.2% saline. *Br Med J* (Clin Res Ed) 1986; **292:** 168–170.

40 Ashouri OS. Severe diuretic-induced hyponatremia in the elderly. A series of eight patients. *Arch Intern Med* 1986; **146:** 1355–1357.

41 Sterns RH. Severe symptomatic hyponatremia: treatment and outcome. A study of 64 cases. *Ann Intern Med* 1987; **107:** 656–664.

42 Ayus JC, Krothapalli RK, Arieff AI. Treatment of symptomatic hyponatremia and its relation to brain damage. A prospective study. *N Engl J Med* 1987; **317:** 1190–1195.

43 Brunner JE, Redmond JM, Haggar AM, Kruger DF, Elias SB. Central pontine myelinolysis and pontine lesions after rapid correction of hyponatremia: a prospective magnetic resonance imaging study. *Ann Neurol* 1990; **27:** 61–66.

44 Cheng JC, Zikos D, Skopicki HA, Peterson DR, Fisher KA. Long-term neurologic outcome in psychogenic water drinkers with severe symptomatic hyponatremia: the effect of rapid correction. *Am J Med* 1990; **88:** 561–566.

45 Ellis SJ. Severe hyponatraemia: complications and treatment. *QJM* 1995; **88:** 905–909.

46 Ayus JC, Arieff AI. Chronic hyponatremic encephalopathy in postmenopausal women: association of therapies with morbidity and mortality. *JAMA* 1999; **281:** 2299–2304.

47 Nzerue CM, Baffoe-Bonnie H, You W, Falana B, Dai S. Predictors of outcome in hospitalized patients with severe hyponatremia. *J Natl Med Assoc* 2003; **95:** 335–343.

48 Sterns RH. Severe hyponatremia: the case for conservative management. *Crit Care Med* 1992; **20:** 534–539.

49 Oh MS, Kim HJ, Carroll HJ. Recommendations for treatment of symptomatic hyponatremia. *Nephron* 1995; **70:** 143–150.

50 Adrogue HJ, Madias NE. Hyponatremia. *N Engl J Med* 2000; **342:** 1581–1589.

51 Decaux G, Soupart A. Treatment of symptomatic hyponatremia. *Am J Med Sci* 2003; **326:** 25–30.

52 Spengos K, Vassilopoulou S, Tsivgoulis G, Dimitrakopoulos A, Toulas P, Vassilapoulos D. Hyponatraemia and central pontine myelinolysis after elective colonoscopy. *Eur J Neurol* 2005; **12:** 322–323.

53 Dellabarca C, Servilla KS, Hart B, Murata GH, Tzamaloukas AH. Osmotic myelinolysis following chronic hyponatremia corrected at an overall rate consistent with current recommendations. *Int Urol Nephrol* 2005; **37:** 171–173.

54 Leens C, Mukendi R, Foret F, Hacourt A, Devuyst O, Colin IM. Central and extrapontine myelinolysis in a patient in spite of a careful correction of hyponatremia. *Clin Nephrol* 2001; **55:** 248–253.

55 Omari A, Kormas N, Field M. Delayed onset of central pontine myelinolysis despite appropriate correction of hyponatraemia. *Intern Med J* 2002; **32:** 273–274.

56 Lohr JW. Osmotic demyelination syndrome following correction of hyponatremia: association with hypokalemia. *Am J Med* 1994; **96:** 408–413.

57 Decaux G, Unger J, Brimioulle S, Mockel J. Hyponatremia in the syndrome of inappropriate secretion of antidiuretic hormone. Rapid correction with urea, sodium chloride, and water restriction therapy. *JAMA* 1982; **247:** 471–474.

58 Gerbes AL, Gulberg V, Gines P, Decaux G, Gross P, Gandjini H *et al.* Therapy of hyponatremia in cirrhosis with a vasopressin receptor antagonist: a randomized double-blind multicenter trial. *Gastroenterology* 2003; **124:** 933–939.

59 Carrilho F, Bosch J, Arroyo V, Mas A, Viver J, Rodes J. Renal failure associated with demeclocycline in cirrhosis. *Ann Intern Med* 1977; **87:** 195–197.

60 Decaux G, Brimioulle S, Genette F, Mockel J. Treatment of the syndrome of inappropriate secretion of antidiuretic hormone by urea. *Am J Med* 1980; **69:** 99–106.

61 Decaux G, Genette F. Urea for long-term treatment of syndrome of inappropriate secretion of antidiuretic hormone. *Br Med J* (Clin Res Ed) 1981; **283:** 1081–1083.

62 Decaux G, Mols P, Cauchie P, Flamion B, Delwiche F. Treatment of hyponatremic cirrhosis with ascites resistant to diuretics by urea. *Nephron* 1986; **44:** 337–343.

63 Verhoeven A, Musch W, Decaux G. Treatment of the polydipsia-hyponatremia syndrome with urea. *J Clin Psychiatry* 2005; **66:** 1372–1375.

64 Wong F, Blei AT, Blendis LM, Thuluvath PJ. A vasopressin receptor antagonist (VPA-985) improves serum sodium concentration in patients with hyponatremia: a multicenter, randomized, placebo-controlled trial. *Hepatology* 2003; **37:** 182–191.

65 Gheorghiade M, Niazi I, Ouyang J, Czerwiec F, Kambayashi J, Zampino M *et al.* Vasopressin V2-receptor blockade with tolvaptan in patients with chronic heart failure: results from a double-blind, randomized trial. *Circulation* 2003; **107:** 2690–2696.

66 Saito T, Ishikawa S, Abe K, Kamoi K, Yamada K, Shimizu K *et al.* Acute aquaresis by the nonpeptide arginine vasopressin (AVP) antagonist OPC-31260 improves hyponatremia in patients with syndrome of inappropriate secretion of antidiuretic hormone (SIADH). *J Clin Endocrinol Metab* 1997; **82:** 1054–1057.

67 Gheorghiade M, Gattis WA, O'Connor CM, Adams KF, Jr., Elkayam U, Barbagelata A *et al.* Effects of tolvaptan, a vasopressin antagonist, in patients hospitalized with worsening heart failure: a randomized controlled trial. *JAMA* 2004; **291:** 1963–1971.

68 Konstam MA, Gheorghiade M, Burnett JC, Jr., Grinfield L, Maggioni AP, Swedberg K *et al.* Effects of oral tolvaptan in patients hospitalized for worsening heart failure: the EVEREST outcome trial. *JAMA* 2007; **297:** 1319–1331.

69 Udelson JE, McGrew FA, Flores E, Ibrahim H, Katz S, Koshkarian G *et al.* Multicenter, randomized, double-blind, placebo-controlled study on the effect of oral tolvaptan on left ventricular dilation and function in patients with heart failure and systolic dysfunction. *J Am Coll Cardiol* 2007; **49:** 2151–2159.

70 Ayus JC, Wheeler JM, Arieff AI. Postoperative hyponatremic encephalopathy in menstruant women. *Ann Intern Med* 1992; **117:** 891–897.

56 Potassium Disorders

John R. Foringer, Christopher Norris, & Kevin W. Finkel

Division of Renal Diseases & Hypertension, University of Texas Medical School, Houston, USA

Introduction

Potassium (K^+) is the major intracellular cation, with 98% of body K^+ being located in cells [1]. It has two major physiological functions. First, it participates in the regulation of metabolic processes such as protein and glycogen synthesis [2]. As a result, disturbances in K^+ concentrations can lead to impaired cellular function. Second, the ratio of intracellular to extracellular K^+ concentration is a major determinant of the resting membrane potential across the cell wall [3]. Therefore, alterations in the K^+ concentration can result in potentially fatal cardiac arrhythmias and muscle paralysis.

The mechanisms of K^+ distribution, absorption, and excretion are tightly regulated, because small changes in the serum concentration of K^+ can be potentially fatal. The various factors that affect K^+ balance are listed in Table 56.1. Knowledge of these variables can be useful in both diagnosis and treatment of K^+ disorders. Although it is intuitively obvious that treatment for K^+ disorders is the administration or enhanced removal of the cation, depending on the presence of hypokalemia or hyperkalemia, respectively, few data are available from controlled clinical trials to inform the safest or most effective treatment regimens. We review the available data here to provide the best-evidence approach to the treatment of K^+ disorders.

Hyperkalemia

Hyperkalemia is a common clinical occurrence in both the inpatient and outpatient settings. Because it is often asymptomatic, life-threatening cardiac arrhythmias or muscle paralysis can be the first manifestation. Management of hyperkalemia requires exclusion of rare causes of pseudohyperkalemia, review of an electrocardio-

gram (ECG) to gauge the cardiac consequences of hyperkalemia, and institution of appropriate therapy.

Clinical features

Clinical signs of hyperkalemia are essentially limited to muscle weakness and cardiac arrhythmias. Muscle weakness has been attributed to reduced resting membrane potential. This change, by inactivating sodium (Na^+) channels, leads to decreased membrane excitability and impaired neuromuscular conduction [4]. Muscle weakness predominates, and ascending paralysis may ensue [5,6]. Usually, trunk and respiratory muscles are spared, so that the paretic effects of hyperkalemia are rarely life-threatening. Muscle weakness usually appears when serum K^+ levels exceed 7 mEq/L. However, in patients with hyperkalemic periodic paralysis, symptoms can occur at much lower concentrations [7].

The most important effect of hyperkalemia is on the myocardium. By lowering the resting membrane potential, hyperkalemia decreases cardiac conduction velocity and increases the rate of repolarization [8]. The progressive disturbance in cardiac conduction can be detected by changes in the ECG as the serum K^+ concentration increases [8–10]. Mild elevations of the serum K^+ concentration produce symmetric peaking of the T wave (tenting), particularly in the precordial leads. More advanced changes include lengthening of the PR interval, widening of the QRS complex, reduction in the P wave amplitude, and eventual atrial arrest. Severe hyperkalemia produces a sine wave pattern due to a greatly widened QRS complex, high T waves, and loss of P waves. Any of these patterns may be signs of impending ventricular fibrillation and sudden cardiac death and should trigger immediate and aggressive treatment.

Neither the serum K^+ concentration nor the ECG pattern is a perfect means of assessing the risk to the patient. The correlation of absolute K^+ levels with ECG findings is dependent on a number of factors, including rate of increase and patient sensitivity. Therefore, progression of hyperkalemia from mild to lethal arrhythmias is unpredictable, and any ECG changes should be treated as a medical emergency.

Evidence-based Nephrology. Edited by Donald Molony and Jonathan Craig
© 2009 Blackwell Publishing, ISBN: 978-1-4051-3975-5.

Table 56.1 Factors affecting K$^+$ concentration.

Cellular distribution
Na$^+$,K$^+$-ATPase
Catecholamines
Insulin
Plasma K$^+$ concentration
Exercise
pH
Cell breakdown
Plasma osmolality
Excretion
Aldosterone
Antidiuretic hormone
Urinary flow
pH
Medications
Nonreabsorbed urinary anions
Colonic function

Causes of hyperkalemia

The differential diagnosis of hyperkalemia can be simplistically expressed as pseudohyperkalemia, excessive input, decreased output, and cellular redistribution, as shown in Table 56.2.

In pseudohyperkalemia, the K$^+$ concentration is artifactually high. Spurious causes of hyperkalemia include marked thrombocytosis (platelet count >1,000,000), severe leukocytosis (white

Table 56.2 Causes of hyperkalemia.

Pseudohyperkalemia
Hemolysis of blood specimen
Thrombocytosis
Extreme leukocytosis
Potassium loading
Hemolysis
Rhabdomyolysis
Crush injury
Transfusions
Potassium infusions
Reduced excretion
Renal failure
Severe volume depletion
Hypoadrenalism
Drugs
   K$^+$-sparing diuretics
   Cyclosporine
   Bactrim
   Converting enzyme inhibitors
   Heparin
   Nonsteroidal agents
Redistribution
Hyperosmolality
Insulin deficiency
β-Blockade
Acidosis

blood cell count >200,000), and hemolysis during blood drawing [1]. When a high K$^+$ level in a patient is reported on the laboratory slip as hemolyzed, it is imperative to check an ECG while awaiting a repeat test to rule out the need for emergent treatment. Patients may experience potentially fatal arrhythmias while awaiting a repeat K$^+$ level because the sample was reported as hemolyzed.

Excessive administration of K$^+$ is a rare cause of hyperkalemia in otherwise-healthy subjects. Because the kidneys are capable of excreting large quantities of K$^+$, hyperkalemia usually results from the presence of an additional factor that interferes with kidney excretion of K$^+$, such as a decreased glomerular filtration rate (GFR), hypoaldosteronism, or medications such as converting enzyme inhibitors or K$^+$-sparing diuretics. Commonly, cell lysis from hemolytic anemia, rhabdomyolysis, tumor lysis syndrome, and crush injuries results in severe hyperkalemia where the quantity of K$^+$ released into the plasma overwhelms the capacity of the kidneys to excrete the load [11,12].

The majority of cases of hyperkalemia are due to a defect in renal K$^+$ excretion in the presence of ongoing unrestricted intake. The impaired renal K$^+$ excretion is typically due to decreased GFR or to aldosterone deficiency. It should be noted that because the kidneys are so efficient at eliminating K$^+$, the GFR should be ≤15 mL/min before renal failure is considered the sole cause of hyperkalemia. Medications such as K$^+$-sparing diuretics, cyclosporine, Bactrim, converting enzyme inhibitors, and nonsteroidal agents also impair the renal excretion of K$^+$. Finally, because K$^+$ excretion is dependent on urinary flow and distal nephron Na$^+$ delivery, severe volume depletion itself can result in hyperkalemia.

Redistribution hyperkalemia is caused by K$^+$ transiently leaving cells, thereby raising the serum K$^+$ concentration. Total body K$^+$ need not be elevated for hyperkalemia to develop. Because the majority of total body K$^+$ is located in the intracellular compartment, relatively small shifts into the extracellular space can cause large increases in the plasma K$^+$ concentration. Insulin deficiency or resistance, by decreasing the activity of the Na$^+$,K$^+$-ATPase, results in K$^+$ efflux from the cell's interior [13,14]. Hyperosmolality may be associated with hyperkalemia [15,16]. The increase in extracellular osmolality leads to cell shrinkage, resulting in an increased intracellular K$^+$ concentration driving K$^+$ exit. β-Adrenergic antagonists, by blocking renin-stimulated angiotensin II production, can also produce hyperkalemia [17].

Metabolic acidosis is often cited as a cause of redistribution hyperkalemia. However, this is a much more prominent effect of mineral acidosis (hydrochloric acid, ammonium chloride) than the more clinically relevant organic acidosis (lactate, ketoacidosis) [18]. Mineral acids are largely dissociated and cause intracellular acidosis by electrogenic proton uptake, resulting in membrane depolarization and a favorable gradient for K$^+$ exit [19]. In contrast, organic acids are incompletely dissociated and relatively permeable across cell membranes, so that their diffusion has minimal effect on the membrane potential [18,20,21]. However, the effect of acidosis on K$^+$ concentration is more complex than simply the type of base. Acidosis stimulates the H$^+$,K$^+$-ATPase in the collecting duct, resulting in increased K$^+$ reabsorption [22]. Renal

Table 56.3 Treatment of hyperkalemia.

Agent	Mechanism	Onset	Duration	Caution(s)	Evidence
Calcium gluconate 10 mL, 10% solution (1 g) i.v., over 5–10 min	Temporarily antagonizes cardiac effects of hyperkalemia	1–3 min	30–60 min	May induce digitalis toxicity; precipitates with bicarbonate	No clinical trials; based on animal data and case series; likely very effective
Regular insulin 10 units i.v. with 50 ml 50% glucose	Temporarily translocates K^+ into cells	10–20 min	4–6 h	Hyperglycemia and hyperosmolality with worsening hyperkalemia	Good evidence based on multiple RCTs
β_2-Agonists (10–20 mg nebulized albuterol)	Temporarily translocates K^+ into cells	30 min	2–4 h	Tachycardia and coronary ischemia	Good evidence based on RCTs; not effective in 20–30% of patients
Sodium polystyrene sulfonate, 60 g p.o. or retention enema	Na^+–K^+ exchange in colonic fluid	1–2 h	4–6 h	Precipitation of fluid overload; colonic necrosis with enema and sorbitol	Little or no evidence of efficacy in acute hyperkalemia beyond that seen with diarrhea from simple cathartics
Sodium bicarbonate 1 ampule (50 mEq) i.v. over 5–10 min	May cause temporary transcellular shift in face of acidosis	Variable	Variable	Hypernatremia; hypocalcemia with seizures; volume overload	Little or no evidence of effectiveness in multiple studies; consider in patients with severe acidosis
Hemodialysis	Diffusive or convective K^+ removal	Immediate	Until dialysis completed	Arrhythmias if removal too rapid	Definitive means of potassium removal; no RCTs

Abbreviations: i.v., intravenous; p.o., per os (by mouth).

secretion of K^+ is also inhibited by acidosis: intracellular acidosis decreases the probability of open collecting duct K^+ channels and ammoniagenesis inhibits K^+ secretion in the collecting duct as well [23,24].

Treatment

Treatment of hyperkalemia is directed by its severity, presence or absence of ECG changes, and underlying cause. Therapies are divided into those that immediately minimize cardiac affects of hyperkalemia, those that transiently reduce plasma K^+ concentration by causing intracellular relocation, and those that remove K^+ from the body.

Although dialysis is the most effective means of removing K^+, it should never be considered as first-line therapy for life-threatening hyperkalemia because it typically entails delays in its application (venous access and equipment or personnel availability). Rather, medical therapy as a temporizing measure is the treatment of choice. However, the medical management of hyperkalemia remains controversial and is based on relatively few clinical trials. As reported in a recent systematic review for the Cochrane Database, no studies on the treatment of clinically relevant hyperkalemia have reported mortality or cardiac arrhythmia outcomes [25]. Reports have focused on serum K^+ levels only and appeared to be studies of convenient patient samples with modest hyperkalemia and some degree of renal impairment. Furthermore, the changes in K^+ concentration were reported in several different ways, limiting the number of studies from which data could be combined

in a systematic review. The evidence for the various treatment options of hyperkalemia are described below and summarized in Table 56.3.

Calcium (Ca^{2+}) gluconate chloride

Intravenous Ca^{2+} administration antagonizes the effects of hyperkalemia on the myocardial conduction system and myocardial repolarization. Administration of Ca^{2+} is the most rapid method for treatment of hyperkalemia and is effective in patients with normal serum Ca^{2+} concentrations [26].

Interestingly, although all modern review articles and chapters on hyperkalemia recommend intravenous Ca^{2+} administration, there are no published clinical trials on the topic. Often, no reference at all is cited for the recommendation. Most data are derived from electrophysiological studies of the canine heart or case reports in humans on the effectiveness of Ca^{2+} administration [27]. This is not to say that Ca^{2+} is not effective or should not be given, because much anecdotal clinical experience demonstrates its usefulness, and withholding treatment for patients with hyperkalemia-induced arrhythmias would be unethical. Rather, it merely demonstrates how clinical practice is often based on experience for which rigorous clinical data are limited.

Insulin

Insulin rapidly stimulates K^+ uptake by cells, primarily hepatocytes and myocytes [28]. Ten units of regular insulin are administered intravenously, usually with glucose to avoid hypoglycemia.

The effect of insulin on serum K^+ levels is seen within 10–20 min and lasts for 4–6 h [29].

In several clinical trials, insulin administration, either alone or in combination with other agents, consistently lowered the plasma K^+ concentration compared to placebo [30,31]. The reduction in K^+ concentration observed was in the range of 0.65–1.0 mEq/L. Delayed hypoglycemia was common (up to 75% of patients) if less than 30 g of glucose was administered with the insulin [32].

β_2-Agonists

Nebulized or inhaled β_2-agonists have been proven effective in the treatment of hyperkalemia in most, but not all, clinical trials [33]. In general, inhaled β_2-agonists are effective within 30 min and the duration of action is 2–4 h. In two studies, however, 20–30% of patients were unresponsive to β_2-agonists [32,34]. Most studies used a 10-mg dose, although one study showed that a 20-mg dose was more effective at 2 h in lowering K^+ [35]. A frequent error when administering β_2-agonists is underdosing with the agent. For hyperkalemia, the dose is close to 10 times the nebulized dose for bronchospasm. In two studies, the combination of β_2-agonists with insulin was more effective than treatment with insulin alone [28,32]. In summary, β_2-agonist administration is an effective method of transiently lowering the serum K^+ level but should always be combined with insulin and/or glucose because of the lack of response seen in some patients.

Bicarbonate

The treatment of hyperkalemia with bicarbonate has typically been studied as part of other multiple interventions. Four studies examined the efficacy of bicarbonate, and all failed to show any reduction in the K^+ concentration at 1 h [36]. In the only randomized trial of it use, bicarbonate had no significant effect on plasma K^+ concentration in the first 60 min after administration [37]. However, these trials did not include patients with severe acidosis and hyperkalemia. Therefore, it may be reasonable to consider bicarbonate administration as an adjunct therapy to both insulin and β_2-agonists when treating hyperkalemia in the face of concomitant metabolic acidosis, but clear clinical trial evidence to support this strategy is lacking. Furthermore, administration of bicarbonate to susceptible patients may potentially cause hypertension, pulmonary edema, hypernatremia, and tetany.

Sodium polystyrene sulfonate (Kayexalate)

Sodium polystyrene sulfonate (Kayexalate) is a resin that exchanges Na^+ for K^+ in the gastrointestinal tract, thereby removing K^+ from the body when the resin is excreted as stool. This is in contradistinction to the mechanism of action of insulin, β_2-agonists, and bicarbonate, which transiently lower the K^+ concentration by promoting cellular uptake without lowering the total body K^+ burden. In general, 1 g of resin removes 1 mEq of K^+ in exchange from 2–3 mEq of Na^+. Therefore, edema, hypertension, and rarely pulmonary edema can occur. Kayexalate can be administered either by mouth or via rectum with a retention enema. Sorbitol is of-ten added to the resin when taken orally to facilitate excretion, but sorbitol should be avoided with enemas because such use has been associated with intestinal necrosis and perforation [38]. Animal models suggest that sorbitol may be the causative agent by precipitating mucosal dehydration.

Resin binders are routinely recommended for treatment or prevention of hyperkalemia, and the reported rate of K^+ removal is slow, requiring almost 4 h for full effect. However, there exist few trials that have actually assessed the efficacy of sodium polystyrene resin [36]. Two reports are commonly cited in support of the use of resins [39,40]. However, in those studies, multiple doses were used, sometimes for a number of days, and the effect on plasma K^+ was noted after 1–5 days. In two studies in healthy subjects, the exchange resin was no better than the cathartics sorbitol or Na^+ sulfate alone [41,42]. Finally, in patients on dialysis, the exchange resin was no more effective in increasing stool K^+ loss and lowering serum K^+ levels than cathartics alone [41].

Hemodialysis

Hemodialysis is the definitive and most effective means of K^+ removal from the body. The plasma K^+ concentration falls rapidly in the first hour of dialysis, and if a low K^+ bath is used, plasma levels can fall by 1.2–1.5 mEq/L/h [31]. Potassium levels may rebound after hemodialysis has finished, and it may take several hours for it to reach its stable postdialysis plateau [43]. Also, temporizing agents such as insulin, β_2-agonists, and bicarbonate by translocating K^+ out of the plasma may decrease the total amount of K^+ removed during dialysis [44]. Hemodialysis is indicated for severe hyperkalemia after temporizing measures have been instituted, although there have been no clinical trials comparing hemodialysis to medical therapy alone. Peritoneal dialysis and continuous venovenous dialysis are effective in chronic hyperkalemic states, but the rate of removal is too slow to recommend their use in severe acute hyperkalemia.

Summary

The standardized treatment of severe hyperkalemia has been described in numerous books and reviews, yet is based on limited clinical data. Based on the limited available evidence we recommend the following for the management of hyperkalemia:

1 An ECG should be obtained and pseudohyperkalemia should be ruled out.

2 Calcium gluconate chloride should be administered intravenously with any ECG changes.

3 Intravenous insulin with glucose is the treatment of choice to transiently lower K^+ concentrations.

4 β_2-Agonists should be given in conjunction with insulin, but never alone.

5 Bicarbonate is likely ineffective in most cases. It may be a consideration in patients with severe metabolic acidosis.

6 Exchange resins do not appear to be reliably effective in lowering serum K^+ levels in acute hyperkalemia and are associated with intestinal necrosis when sorbitol is used in a retention enema. If used, multiple doses are likely necessary and sorbitol should be avoided.

7 Hemodialysis is the definitive method for net K^+ removal from the body.

Hypokalemia

Clinical features

Clinical signs of hypokalemia are similar to those of hyperkalemia, with muscle weakness and arrhythmias predominating. The severity of symptoms tends to correlate with the level and duration of hypokalemia. Typically, there are no symptoms unless the plasma K^+ level is less than 3 mEq/L or there is a sudden drop in the extracellular K^+ concentration. Arrhythmias can develop with plasma K^+ greater than 3 mEq/L when there is another predisposing factor.

Muscle weakness is uncommon if the K^+ level is greater than 2.5 mEq/L as long as the decrease in K^+ concentration has not been sudden [45]. The weakness is ascending in character and can involve the gastrointestinal muscles, leading to ileus, abdominal distention, anorexia, nausea, and vomiting [46]. The respiratory muscles are rarely involved, resulting in respiratory failure and need for mechanical ventilation. Patients may experience cramps, paresthesias, tetany, tenderness, atrophy, and rhabdomyolysis.

Cardiac arrhythmias that can result from hypokalemia include atrial and ventricular premature beats, sinus bradycardia, paroxysmal atrial or junctional tachycardia, atrioventricular blocks, ventricular tachycardia, and ventricular fibrillation [45]. Changes on the ECG associated with hypokalemia are depression of the ST segment, diminished amplitude of the T waves, and increased amplitude of the U waves [47]. Other factors may contribute to the development of arrhythmias, including concomitant use of digoxin, cardiac ischemia, hypomagnesemia, and increased β-adrenergic activity [48,49].

Hypokalemia can adversely affect renal function. Chronic hypokalemia impairs urinary concentration, leading to symptoms of nocturia, polyuria, and polydipsia. Chronic hypokalemia can also cause hypokalemic nephropathy with vacuolar lesions in the proximal tubular epithelium. These changes are initially reversible with potassium repletion, but if persistent, interstitial fibrosis, tubular atrophy, and cyst formation may ensue [50–54].

Causes of hypokalemia

Potassium homeostasis is maintained by potassium intake and excretion or cellular shifts between the extracellular and intracellular fluid compartments. The differential diagnosis of hypokalemia can be separated into spurious hypokalemia, redistribution hypokalemia, renal and extrarenal K^+ loss, and inadequate intake. Hypokalemia due to inadequate intake is rare secondary to the kidney's ability to avidly conserve K^+. Marked leukocytosis (white blood cell count, >100,000) can cause pseudohypokalemia if the sample sits at room temperature and the white blood cells take up

the K^+. Therefore, the differential diagnosis of true hypokalemia primarily involves the loss of K^+ or its redistribution.

Transcellular redistribution of K^+ usually occurs in the face of normal total body K^+ levels. Metabolic alkalosis can result in redistribution as K^+ shifts into cells. It has been suggested that an increase in the pH by 0.1 will decrease the K^+ concentration by 0.3 mEq/L. Respiratory alkalosis has a minor effect on cellular shifts of K^+. Increased Na^+,K^+-ATPase stimulation with medications such as β_2-agonists, theophylline, dobutamine, dopamine, and insulin results in net cellular K^+ uptake and hypokalemia.

Hypokalemia results most commonly from excessive K^+ loss. This loss can be renal or extrarenal, the latter from either the gastrointestinal tract or the skin. Secretory diarrhea causes loss of K^+ with bicarbonate. Nasogastric suction and vomiting lead to hypokalemia by loss of K^+ in gastric contents and renal losses associated with metabolic alkalosis. Associated hyperaldosteronism with volume depletion exacerbates the hypokalemia induced by vomiting. Cutaneous losses of K^+ occur with sweating. Exuberant exercise may produce up to 12 L/day of sweat with a K^+ concentration of approximately 9 mEq/L.

Renal loss of K^+ is the most common reason for hypokalemia. Medications like loop diuretics and penicillin derivatives (nonreabsorbable anions) promote K^+ loss.

Hypomagnesemia can lead to hypokalemia through reduced Na^+ absorption by the thick ascending limb of Henle, resulting in K^+ wasting. Cisplatin is a common cause of magnesium wasting with resultant hypokalemia. Magnesium repletion is essential to the correction of hypokalemia.

Mineralocorticoid excess classically presents with hypokalemia associated with elevated aldosterone levels and hypertension. Primary aldosteronism is generally caused by aldosterone-producing adenomas of the adrenal glands. Liddle's syndrome has features of hyperaldosteronism but aldosterone levels are normal. These findings are attributable to mutations in the epithelial Na^+ channel in the cortical collecting duct that result in increased Na^+ reabsorption causing a hypokalemic metabolic alkalosis with volume expansion and hypertension. Bartter syndrome, on the other hand, is a renal tubulopathy that presents with hypokalemia, metabolic alkalosis, and normal blood pressure secondary to salt wasting and is due to one of several defects that result in impaired salt reabsorption in the thick ascending limb. Hyperreninemia is present with secondary hyperaldosteronism. A more complete list of the causes of hypokalemia is found in Table 56.4.

Treatment

The goal of therapy for hypokalemia is to prevent life-threatening complications. If there is any evidence of muscular weakness or ECG changes, repletion should be instituted immediately. The amount of K^+ given as well as the route of administration is variable and depends on the etiology of the hypokalemia and the clinical situation (Table 56.5). Care must be taken not to give excessive K^+ to a patient with hypokalemia. Therapy should not only

Table 56.4 Causes of hypokalemia.

Pseudohypokalemia
White blood cell count >100,000
Recent insulin injection

Inadequate K$^+$ intake

Redistribution
Alkalosis
Insulin excess
β_2-Adrenergic excess
Hypokalemic periodic paralysis, thyrotoxic periodic paralysis
Theophylline toxicity
Barium poisoning
Chloroquine intoxication
Hypothermia

Excessive sweating

Gastrointestinal losses
Vomiting
Nasogastric suctioning
Diarrhea
Therapy with K$^+$-binding resins

Renal losses
Medications
   Diuretics
   Amphotericin B
   Penicillin derivatives
   Aminoglycosides
   Ifosfamide
   Cisplatin
   Fludrocortisone
   High-dose glucocorticoids
Intrinsic renal disease
   Metabolic Acidosis, Renal Tubular Acidosis (RTA)
   Liddle syndrome
   Bartter syndrome
   Gitelman's syndrome
   Nephrogenic diabetes insipidus
Mineralocorticoid excess
   Primary or secondary hyperaldosteronism
   Licorice ingestion
   Cushing's syndrome
Hyperreninemia
   Renal artery stenosis
Hypomagnesemia
Dialysis, plasmapheresis

---

include the correction of total body K$^+$ depletion but reduction of ongoing K$^+$ losses and correction of the underlying disorder.

Oral K$^+$ replacement

With a K$^+$ concentration of >3.0 mEq/L, treatment with oral K$^+$ is usually sufficient. The plasma K$^+$ concentration will typically increase by 1–1.5 mEq/L after 40–60 mEq of oral K$^+$. This rise is somewhat transient, as most K$^+$ will eventually move into the cell interior [55,56]. A repeat measurement of the plasma K$^+$ concentration 4 h later can determine if further supplementation is necessary.

Replacement with potassium chloride (KCl) is best suited for conditions involving metabolic alkalosis with hypokalemia. Many times there is an associated hypochloremia. The KCl can appropriately replace the deficit, whereas other forms, such as K$^+$ with bicarbonate or citrate, can worsen the alkalosis and thereby accentuate the concomitant renal K$^+$ loss [57,58]. On the other hand, in renal tubular acidosis with hypokalemia, such formulations are better choices. Repletion by increasing consumption of foods high in K$^+$ is generally less effective than oral medicinal K$^+$ replacement for hypokalemia associated with chloride depletion [46].

Intravenous K$^+$ replacement

In patients who cannot take oral K$^+$, are undergoing treatment which will cause rapid intracellular shift of K$^+$, or have life-threatening arrhythmias or weakness, intravenous KCl replacement is used for treatment of hypokalemia. Conventional practice limits intravenous K$^+$ repletion to 10 mEq/h through a peripheral venous catheter or 20 mEq/h through a central venous catheter. The concentration of the KCl replacement solution is limited to 20 mEq/100 mL. The reasons given for this are to avoid infusion pain, sclerosis of the vein used for infusion, and arrhythmias that can result from higher concentrations or rates of infusion of KCl. However, studies have reported successfully giving 40–100 mEq/h of KCl to patients with paralysis or arrhythmia [59–62]. There can be ECG changes consistent with those of hyperkalemia or even complete heart block when giving greater than 80 mEq/h of KCl, so this rate of repletion should be reserved for life-threatening situations [63]. Arrhythmias have been successfully treated with intravenous solutions containing a K$^+$ concentration of 200 mEq/L [62,64,65]. Replacement fluids with such high concentrations are reserved for patients with volume overload.

Potassium-containing replacement fluid is typically made with saline. Dextrose-containing solutions can lead to a transient decrease in the plasma K$^+$ concentration due to an intracellular shift of K$^+$ from dextrose-stimulated insulin release. This is an important consideration in a patient with severe hypokalemia [46,66].

Certain patient groups often develop hypophosphatemia and hypokalemia. These include patients treated for diabetic ketoacidosis with insulin, patients recovering from severe malnutritional states (refeeding syndrome), and patients receiving continuous dialysis treatments. Mild to moderate phosphate deficits (serum phosphate concentration of 1.27–2.48 mg/dL) can be safely corrected with 15 mmol K$^+$ phosphate intravenously. In more severe hypophosphatemia ($\leq$1.24 mg/dL), 30 mmol K$^+$ phosphate has been used safely, although repeated doses were required for normalization of phosphate levels [67].

Magnesium (Mg^{2+}) repletion

Refractory hypokalemia can be a result of hypomagnesemia [68]. Correction of hypokalemia in the face of hypomagnesemia

Table 56.5 Treatment of hypokalemia.

Agent	Indications	Rate, dosage	Caution(s)	Evidence for rate of replacement
Oral K^+	Non-life-threatening hypokalemia; K^+ >3 mEq/L	Based on K^+ deficit and ongoing losses; 40–60 mEq, raise K^+ by 1–1.5 mEq/L	Large doses and sustained release forms can lead to gastric irritation	No randomized trials; based on case studies, likely to be accurate
i.v. K^+	K^+ <3 mEq/L; life-threatening arrhythmia or muscle weakness; inability to take oral medications	10–20 mEq/h, up to 100 mEq/h if life-threatening arrhythmia	Arrhythmia risk if >80 mEq/h; risk of hyperkalemia with overcorrection	No randomized trials; based on cohort and case studies; good evidence to limit to 60 mEq/h for most situations to avoid inducing arrhythmias
Magnesium repletion	Hypokalemia with associated hypomagnesemia	Replete Mg^{2+} prior to K^+ repletion		No randomized trials; based on reviews and *in vitro* data, likely to work
K^+-sparing diuretics	Hypokalemia resistant to treatment	Start with low dose and titrate as needed	Monitor for hyperkalemia if concomitant use of ACE inhibitors or K^+ replacement	No randomized trials; based on cohort and case series, likely to work

Abbreviations: i.v., intravenous; ACE, angiotensin converting enzyme.

requires repletion of Mg^{2+} prior to K^+ repletion for the reasons mentioned above.

K^+-sparing diuretics

In certain conditions, including primary hyperaldosteronism, chronic diuretic therapy, and Gitelman's syndrome, continued urinary loss of K^+ is limited by development of chronic hypokalemia leading to K^+ retention by the kidneys. Repletion of K^+ will paradoxically diminish this renal K^+ retention and result in incomplete correction of hypokalemia. In these conditions, it is often necessary to use a K^+-sparing diuretic in addition to K^+ supplementation [69–71]. The K^+ concentration should be monitored to avoid hyperkalemia in patients on K^+ supplementation, particularly in the presence of diabetes or chronic kidney disease.

Summary

Although a common problem, there are few data from rigorous clinical trials on the appropriate treatment of hypokalemia. Based on this limited evidence, we recommend the following:

1 Rule out spurious or pseudohypokalemia.

2 Review patient's medication list for a causative agent and discontinue if present.

3 Determine if hypokalemia is due to redistribution versus true K^+ loss or depletion.

4 With severe hypokalemia with a $[K^+]$ of <3 mEq/L, life-threatening arrhythmia, or muscle weakness, give intravenous K^+ until $[K^+]$ is >3 or symptoms resolve. Then, continue to replete the K^+ deficit with oral K^+. Hypokalemia due to redistribution requires significantly lower doses of K^+ than does hypokalemia due to loss.

5 Intravenous K^+ should be given at a rate of 10–20 mEq/h in most instances. In the presence of life-threatening arrhythmia due to hypokalemia, 80–200 mEq/h of K^+ can be given. Caution should be taken with rates over 80 mEq/h.

6 With $[K^+]$ of >3 mEq/L, oral K^+ replacement should be used unless the patient is unable to take oral medications.

7 The choice of K^+ preparation should be based on associated conditions, such as acidosis, alkalosis, and hypophosphatemia.

8 Addition of foods high in K^+ to the diet is generally less effective than administration of oral K^+.

9 If concomitant hypomagnesemia is present, give Mg^{2+} to correct the deficit prior to correction of hypokalemia.

10 K^+-sparing diuretics may be added to K^+ supplementation to treat conditions with resistant hypokalemia.

References

1 Brown RS. Extrarenal potassium homeostasis. *Kidney Int* 1986; **30(1)**: 116–127.

2 Knochel JP. Neuromuscular manifestations of electrolyte disorders. *Am J Med* 1982; **72(3)**: 521–535.

3 DeVoe RD, MaloneyPC. Principles of cell homeostasis. In: Mountcastle VB (editor), *Medical Physiology*, 14th edn. Mosby, St. Louis, 1980.

4 Berne RM, Levey M. *Cardiovascular Physiology*, 4th edn. Mosby, St. Louis, 1981; 7–17.

5 Epstein F. Signs and symptoms of electrolyte disorders. In: Maxwell KC (editor), *Clinical Disorders of Fluid and Electrolytes Metabolism*. McGraw-Hill, New York, 1980.

6 Finch CA, Flynn JM. Clinical syndrome of potassium intoxication. *Am J Med* 1946; **1**: 337.

7 Fontaine B, Lapie P, Plassart E, Tabti N, Nicole S, Reboul J *et al.* Periodic paralysis and voltage-gated ion channels. *Kidney Int* 1996; **49(1)**: 9–18.

8 Surawicz B. Relationship between electrocardiogram and electrolytes. *Am Heart J* 1967; **73(6)**: 814–834.

9 Surawicz B, Chlebus H, Mazzoleni A. Hemodynamic and electrocardiographic effects of hyperpotassemia. Differences in response to slow and rapid increases in concentration of plasma K. *Am Heart J* 1967; **73(5)**: 647–664.

10 Sutton PM, Taggart P, Spear DW, Drake HF, Swanton RH, Emanuel RW. Monophasic action potential recordings in response to graded hyperkalemia in dogs. *Am J Physiol* 1989; **256(4 Pt 2)**: H956–H961.

11 Lordon RE, Burton JR. Post-traumatic renal failure in military personnel in Southeast Asia. Experience at Clark USAF hospital, Republic of the Philippines. *Am J Med* 1972; **53(2)**: 137–147.

12 Arseneau JC, Bagley CM, Anderson T, Canellos GP. Hyperkalaemia, a sequel to chemotherapy of Burkitt's lymphoma. *Lancet* 1973; **i(7793)**: 10–14.

13 Adrogue HJ, Lederer ED, Suki WN, Eknoyan G. Determinants of plasma potassium levels in diabetic ketoacidosis. *Medicine* (Baltimore) 1986; **65(3)**: 163–172.

14 DeFronzo RA, Sherwin RS, Dillingham M, Hendler R, Tamborlane WV, Felig P. Influence of basal insulin and glucagon secretion on potassium and sodium metabolism. Studies with somatostatin in normal dogs and in normal and diabetic human beings. *J Clin Invest* 1978; **61(2)**: 472–479.

15 Conte G, Dal Canton A, Imperatore P, De Nicola L, Gigliotti G, Pisanti N *et al*. Acute increase in plasma osmolality as a cause of hyperkalemia in patients with renal failure. *Kidney Int* 1990; **38(2)**: 301–307.

16 Makoff DL, da Silva JA, Rosenbaum BJ, Levy SE, Maxwell MH. Hypertonic expansion: acid-base and electrolyte changes. *Am J Physiol* 1970; **218(4)**: 1201–1207.

17 Rosa RM, Silva P, Young JB, Landsberg L, Brown RS, Rose JW *et al*. Adrenergic modulation of extrarenal potassium disposal. *N Engl J Med* 1980; **302(8)**: 431–434.

18 Adrogue HJ, Madias NE. Changes in plasma potassium concentration during acute acid-base disturbances. *Am J Med* 1981; **71(3)**: 456–467.

19 Magner PO, Robinson L, Halperin RM, Zettle R, Halperin ML. The plasma potassium concentration in metabolic acidosis: a re-evaluation. *Am J Kidney Dis* 1988; **11(3)**: 220–224.

20 Fulop M. Serum potassium in lactic acidosis and ketoacidosis. *N Engl J Med* 1979; **300(19)**: 1087–1089.

21 Graber M. A model of the hyperkalemia produced by metabolic acidosis. *Am J Kidney Dis* 1993; **22(3)**: 436–444.

22 Wingo CS, Armitage FE. Potassium transport in the kidney: regulation and physiological relevance of H^+,K^+-ATPase. *Semin Nephrol* 1993; **13(2)**: 213–224.

23 Wang WH, Schwab A, Giebisch G. Regulation of small-conductance K^+ channel in apical membrane of rat cortical collecting tubule. *Am J Physiol* 1990; **259(3 Pt 2)**: F494–F502.

24 Hamm LL, Gillespie C, Klahr S. NH_4Cl inhibition of transport in the rabbit cortical collecting tubule. *Am J Physiol* 1985; **248(5 Pt 2)**: F631–F637.

25 Mahoney BA, Smith WA, Lo DS, Tsoi K, Tonelli M, Clase CM. Emergency interventions for hyperkalaemia. *Cochrane Database Syst Rev* 2005; **2**: CD003235.

26 Salem MM, Rosa RM, Batlle DC. Extrarenal potassium tolerance in chronic renal failure: implications for the treatment of acute hyperkalemia. *Am J Kidney Dis* 1991; **18(4)**: 421–440.

27 Fisch C. Relation of electrolyte disturbances to cardiac arrhythmias. *Circulation* 1973; **47(2)**: 408–419.

28 Lens XM, Montoliu J, Cases A, Campistol JM, Revert L. Treatment of hyperkalaemia in renal failure: salbutamol v. insulin. *Nephrol Dial Transplant* 1989; **4(3)**: 228–232.

29 Allon M, Shanklin N. Effect of bicarbonate administration on plasma potassium in dialysis patients: interactions with insulin and albuterol. *Am J Kidney Dis* 1996; **28(4)**: 508–514.

30 Kim HJ. Combined effect of bicarbonate and insulin with glucose in acute therapy of hyperkalemia in end-stage renal disease patients. *Nephron* 1996; **72(3)**: 476–482.

31 Blumberg A, Weidmann P, Shaw S, Gnadinger M. Effect of various therapeutic approaches on plasma potassium and major regulating factors in terminal renal failure. *Am J Med* 1988; **85(4)**: 507–512.

32 Allon M, Copkney C. Albuterol and insulin for treatment of hyperkalemia in hemodialysis patients. *Kidney Int* 1990; **38(5)**: 869–872.

33 McClure RJ, Prasad VK, Brocklebank JT. Treatment of hyperkalaemia using intravenous and nebulised salbutamol. *Arch Dis Child* 1994; **70(2)**: 126–128.

34 Noyan A, Anarat A, Pirti M, Yurdakul Z. Treatment of hyperkalemia in children with intravenous salbutamol. *Acta Paediatr Jpn* 1995; **37(3)**: 355–357.

35 Allon M, Dunlay R, Copkney C. Nebulized albuterol for acute hyperkalemia in patients on hemodialysis. *Ann Intern Med* 1989; **110(6)**: 426–429.

36 Ahee P, Crowe AV. The management of hyperkalaemia in the emergency department. *J Accid Emerg Med* 2000; **17(3)**: 188–191.

37 Allon M. Treatment and prevention of hyperkalemia in end-stage renal disease. *Kidney Int* 1993; **43(6)**: 1197–1209.

38 Roy-Chaudhury P, Meisels IS, Freedman S, Steinman TI, Steer M. Combined gastric and ileocecal toxicity (serpiginous ulcers) after oral kayexalate in sorbital therapy. *Am J Kidney Dis* 1997; **30(1)**: 120–122.

39 Flinn RB, Merrill JP, Welzant WR. Treatment of the oliguric patient with a new sodium exchange resin and sorbitol. *N Engl J Med* 1961; **264**: 111–115.

40 Scherr L, Ogden DA, Mead AW, Spritz N, Rubin AL. Management of hyperkalemia with a cation exchange resin. *N Engl J Med* 1961; **264**: 115–119.

41 Gruy-Kapral C, Emmett M, Santa Ana CA, Porter JL, Fordtran JS, Fine KD. Effect of single dose resin-cathartic therapy on serum potassium concentration in patients with end-stage renal disease. *J Am Soc Nephrol* 1998; **9(10)**: 1924–1930.

42 Emmett M, Hootkins RE, Fine KD, Santa Ana CA, Porter JL, Fordtran JS. Effect of three laxatives and a cation exchange resin on fecal sodium and potassium excretion. *Gastroenterology* 1995; **108(3)**: 752–760.

43 Feig PU, Shook A, Sterns RH. Effect of potassium removal during hemodialysis on the plasma potassium concentration. *Nephron* 1981; **27(1)**: 25–30.

44 Allon M. Hyperkalemia in end-stage renal disease: mechanisms and management. *J Am Soc Nephrol* 1995; **6(4)**: 1134–1142.

45 Rose BD, Post TW. *Clinical Physiology of Acid-Base and Electrolyte Disorders*, 5th edn. McGraw-Hill, New York, 2001.

46 Gennari FJ. Hypokalemia. *N Engl J Med* 1998; **339(7)**: 451–458.

47 Cohn JN, Kowey PR, Whelton PK, Prisant LM. New guidelines for potassium replacement in clinical practice: a contemporary review by the National Council on Potassium in Clinical Practice. *Arch Intern Med* 2000; **160(16)**: 2429–2436.

48 Struthers AD, Whitesmith R, Reid JL. Prior thiazide diuretic treatment increases adrenaline-induced hypokalaemia. *Lancet* 1983; **i(8338)**: 1358–1361.

49 Lipworth BJ, McDevitt DG, Struthers AD. Prior treatment with diuretic augments the hypokalemic and electrocardiographic effects of inhaled albuterol. *Am J Med* 1989; **86(6 Pt 1)**: 653–657.

50 Rubini ME. Water excretion in potassium-deficient man. *J Clin Invest* 1961; **40**: 2215–2224.

51 Tizianello A, Garibotto G, Robaudo C, Saffioti S, Pontremoli R, Bruzzone M *et al.* Renal ammoniagenesis in humans with chronic potassium depletion. *Kidney Int* 1991; **40(4)**: 772–778.

52 Capasso, G, Jaeger P, Giebisch G, Guckian V, Malnic G. Renal bicarbonate reabsorption in the rat. II. Distal tubule load dependence and effect of hypokalemia. *J Clin Invest* 1987; **80(2)**: 409–414.

53 Riemenschneider T, Bohle A. Morphologic aspects of low-potassium and low-sodium nephropathy. *Clin Nephrol* 1983; **19(6)**: 271–279.

54 Torres VE, Young WF, Jr., Offord KP, Hattery RR. Association of hypokalemia, aldosteronism, and renal cysts. *N Engl J Med* 1990; **322(6)**: 345–351.

55 Nicolis GL, Kahn T, Sanchez A, Gabrilove JL. Glucose-induced hyperkalemia in diabetic subjects. *Arch Intern Med* 1981; **141(1)**: 49–53.

56 Keith N. Some effects of potassium salts in men. *Ann Intern Med* 1942; **16**: 879.

57 Villamil MF, Deland EC, Henney RP, Maloney JV, Jr. Anion effects on cation movements during correction of potassium depletion. *Am J Physiol* 1975; **229(1)**: 161–166.

58 Schwartz WB, de Van Ypersele S, Kassirer JP. Role of anions in metabolic alkalosis and potassium deficiency. *N Engl J Med* 1968; **279(12)**: 630–639.

59 Pullen H, Doig A, Lambie AT. Intensive intravenous potassium replacement therapy. *Lancet* 1967; **ii(7520)**: 809–811.

60 Seftel HC, Kew MC. Early and intensive potassium replacement in diabetic acidosis. *Diabetes* 1966; **15(9)**: 694–696.

61 Abramson E, Arky R. Diabetic acidosis with initial hypokalemia. Therapeutic implications. *JAMA* 1966; **196(5)**: 401–403.

62 Hamill RJ, Robinson LM, Wexler HR, Moote C. Efficacy and safety of potassium infusion therapy in hypokalemic critically ill patients. *Crit Care Med* 1991; **19(5)**: 694–699.

63 Swales JD. Hypokalaemia and the electrocardiogram. *Lancet* 1964; **ii**: 1365–1316.

64 Clementsen HJ. Potassium therapy. A break with tradition. *Lancet* 1962; **ii**: 175–177.

65 Kruse JA, Carlson RW. Rapid correction of hypokalemia using concentrated intravenous potassium chloride infusions. *Arch Intern Med* 1990; **150(3)**: 613–617.

66 Kunin AS, Surawicz B, Sims EA. Decrease in serum potassium concentrations and appearance of cardiac arrhythmias during infusion of potassium with glucose in potassium-depleted patients. *N Engl J Med* 1962; **266**: 228–233.

67 Perreault MM, Ostrop NJ, Tierney MG. Efficacy and safety of intravenous phosphate replacement in critically ill patients. *Ann Pharmacother* 1997; **31(6)**: 683–688.

68 Whang R, Whang DD, Ryan MP. Refractory potassium repletion. A consequence of magnesium deficiency. *Arch Intern Med* 1992; **152(1)**: 40–45.

69 Griffing GT, Cole AG, Aurecchia SA, Sindler BH, Kamonicky P, Melby JC. Amiloride in primary hyperaldosteronism. *Clin Pharmacol Ther* 1982; **31(1)**: 56–61.

70 Ganguly A, Weinberger MH. Triamterene-thiazide combination: alternative therapy for primary aldosteronism. *Clin Pharmacol Ther* 1981; **30(2)**: 246–250.

71 Ghose RP, Hall PM, Bravo EL. Medical management of aldosterone-producing adenomas. *Ann Intern Med* 1999; **131(2)**: 105–108.

57 Metabolic Evaluation and Prevention of Renal Stone Disease

David S. Goldfarb

Nephrology Section, New York Harbor VA Medical Center; Department of Urology, St. Vincent's Hospital, and New York University School of Medicine, New York, USA

Introduction

The field of kidney stone prevention is marked by a relative paucity of high-grade data suitable for inclusion in a textbook promoting evidence-based medicine. The reasons for this scarcity are not clear, as kidney stones are quite prevalent. For example, stones affect as many as 6–15% of American men and 2–7% of American women [1]; this gender ratio is relatively consistent in other countries. Worldwide data suggest an overall prevalence of 1–5% in Asia, 5–10% in Europe, and as high as 20% in Saudi Arabia. Epidemiologic studies in the USA, Italy, Japan, and elsewhere have suggested an increasing prevalence worldwide [1–3]. The reasons for these increased rates remain speculative, although new epidemiologic data have begun to elucidate possible explanations [4].

This chapter will focus on the evaluation of stone formers and the measures taken to prevent stone recurrence. Topics that will be considered only briefly here are the urologic aspects of stone disease, including the differential diagnosis of renal colic, the management of renal colic, and the surgical management of ureteral stones.

Urologic aspects of stone disease

Many studies have clearly demonstrated the superiority of computerized tomography (CT) without contrast as the preferred diagnostic test in the evaluation of patients with suspected renal colic, repeatedly surpassing intravenous pyelography and ultrasound [5,6]. In a study of 97 patients with renal colic, CT had a sensitivity of 94% and a specificity of 97%; the corresponding

values for intravenous pyelography were 52% and 94%, whereas ultrasound yielded values of 19% and 97% [6].

Microhematuria is neither sensitive nor specific for stones. Using helical CT as the "gold standard" for the presence or absence of stones shows that 33% of patients with stones had ≥5 red blood cells/high-power field (RBC/field) and 11% had none [7]. Of patients without stones, 24% had more than 5 RBC/field and 51% had more than 1 RBC/field.

The differential diagnosis and immediate, urgent management of acute presentation with a renal stone have been reviewed elsewhere [8]. Nonsteroidal anti-inflammatory drugs are generally preferred to opiates in the management of renal colic, as they have been shown more effective for pain relief in randomized controlled trials and cause less sedation and vomiting [9,10]. Several randomized controlled trials have demonstrated the efficacy of tamsulosin in promoting spontaneous passage of ureteral stones [11]. Nifedipine and steroids have also been shown to be effective compared to control therapy [12]. No evidence supports administration of intravenous fluids to patients with renal colic to promote stone passage; fluids are appropriate only to replete extracellular fluid volume deficiencies in patients who have experienced significant volume loss from nausea or vomiting.

The American Urologic Association and the European Association of Urology have promulgated guidelines regarding the management of ureteral stones, although these have not been updated recently [13,14]. The choice between extracorporeal shock wave lithotripsy, ureteroscopy, and percutaneous nephrostolithotomy depends on stone composition, size, location, and the experience of the treating urologist. A recent retrospective study suggested an increased risk of diabetes and hypertension in patients undergoing extracorporeal shock wave lithotripsy in those treated with a brand of lithotriptor, the Dornier HM3, which is used much less commonly today [15]. Confounding that may have accounted for the observed association could not be excluded from this retrospective analysis. Newer lithotriptors are less powerful and may be associated with less damage to the kidney and pancreas, although no prospective data are available to confirm their relative greater safety. Obesity, hypertension, and diabetes have all been associated

Evidence-based Nephrology. Edited by Donald Molony and Jonathan Craig
© 2009 Blackwell Publishing, ISBN: 978-1-4051-3975-5.

with an increased risk of stone formation, so whether lithotripsy truly has a causal effect on these findings through as-yet-unknown mechanisms is questionable.

Guidelines on evaluation and management of stone formers

Two sets of guidelines, one a consensus statement from the National Institutes of Health in the USA and one from the European Association of Urology, regarding medical evaluation and treatment of patients with stones have been issued; neither can be considered up to date, however [14,16]. It is disappointing that the relative scarcity of randomized, controlled trials in the field means that neither set of guidelines is far from current practice. Neither set concentrated on distinguishing superior trials or evaluating varying levels of evidence.

Evaluation of stone formers

Stone disease is highly recurrent. After presenting with renal stones, guidelines recommend that patients undergo an evaluation for any associated conditions and assessment of their risk for stone recurrence [16]. These guidelines are founded on the biological reasoning that for the individual patient, management and prevention of stone recurrence can be based on a solid physiologic understanding of the unique factors in the individual that are responsible for the stone formation. The overall utility of the recommended comprehensive evaluation of the patient with renal stones has not been evaluated with rigorous randomized controlled clinical trials.

Epidemiologic data have consistently shown an association of animal protein intake with more stones [17], and urinary risk factors for stone formation worsen with diets with more animal protein intake and lower quantities of fruits and vegetables [18,19]. Prospective epidemiologic studies have also shown that men and women with the highest dietary calcium ingestion (mostly via dairy products) have the lowest associated prevalence of stones [17,20]. Both obesity and diabetes are now recognized as important risk factors for stones [21,22]. Occupations that expose people to hot environments are associated with stones [23], and stones are more frequent at geographically lower latitudes [1]. Many medications are associated with stones, including poorly soluble drugs like indinivir and high-dose sulfa antibiotics, carbonic anhydrase inhibitors like topiramate and acetazolamide, and contributors to increased urinary calcium, such as calcium supplements and vitamin D [24]. A family history of stones should be sought, as the hereditability of the risk of stones is high, as indicated by a 56% concordance for stones in a study of twins after excluding the influence of a common environment and diet [25]. The genes responsible for the hereditary contribution have not yet been determined. Family history of kidney disease may reveal stone-associated conditions, such as polycystic kidney disease or renal tubular acidosis. Patients

with a variety of bowel diseases that may influence urine mineral, citrate, oxalate, and uric acid composition and patients with gout are affected more frequently by stones [26,27].

The guidelines recommend that stones or fragments be submitted to analysis at least once for each patient for determination of composition by X-ray crystallography or infrared spectroscopy.

Patients should have serum chemistries determined and urinalysis performed. Patients with hypercalcemia (or high-normal serum calcium values) should have primary hyperparathyroidism ruled out by measurement of parathyroid hormone [28]. Sarcoidosis should also be considered in the differential diagnosis. A finding of a high urine pH or pyuria should lead to urine cultures and consideration of struvite stones. Low serum bicarbonate concentrations with a concomitant alkaline urine pH of 6.0 or higher should raise the possibility of renal tubular acidosis (RTA). If imaging of the kidneys has not been obtained, all patients should have at least a renal ultrasound (a sensitive study for screening kidneys for stones, but insensitive for ureteral stones [see above]) to document the presence or absence of additional stones; polycystic kidney disease can simultaneously be eliminated from consideration as well.

Twenty-four-hour urine collections to determine urinary risk factors for stone recurrence and for assignation of preventive treatments are generally reserved for patients with recurrent stones and for children after their first stone episode [16]. One should also consider evaluating patients with large stones or stones requiring urologic intervention. Urine collections are usually performed on patients' *ad libitum* diets. Analytes should include components of stone salts, urine volume, and pH, as well as measures revealing dietary intake of sodium, potassium, and protein. Based on urine composition, supersaturation of crystal-forming phases can be calculated by the laboratory, so that changes in multiple urinary variables can be translated into a single number correlating with stone risk.

Stone composition also correlates with urinary supersaturation. For patients with hypercalciuria, protocols used to classify the etiology of the abnormality and then treat based on the results of this classification are currently not recommended.

Calcium stones

The prevention of calcium stones, whether these stones are predominantly calcium oxalate or phosphate salts, can consist of fluid therapy, as discussed following, manipulation of diet, or pharmacologic therapy. Nonspecific preventive measures, detailed on the next page, are directed at all calcium stone formers, while more specific therapies are directed at specific abnormalities as revealed in the urinary variables determined from a 24-h urine collection. The most common urinary variable abnormality seen in calcium stone formers is hypercalciuria, often defined as >4 mg (0.1 mmol) of calcium/kg body weight/day. However, like blood pressure, urine calcium excretion is a continuous variable, and attempts to define an upper limit of normal may be artificial. Hypercalciuria in most cases remains an idiopathic disorder, with a likely genetic contribution that has not yet been well defined. Hypercalciuria may be exacerbated by increased renal sodium excretion.

Citrate is an inhibitor of calcium crystallization and of crystal aggregation. Hypocitraturia, defined variously as <250–500 mg (1.3–2.6 mmol)/day, is another relatively common abnormality associated with calcium stone formation and is often caused by increased acid loads, such as ingestion of animal protein, diarrhea, or RTA with hypokalemia or with metabolic acidosis of any cause. Hypocitraturia is often idiopathic as well.

Hyperoxaluria is defined as more than 40 mg (about 0.4 mmol) urinary oxalate/day. Both dietary and metabolic components contribute, and the relative proportions appear to vary among individuals. Hyperuricosuria is a risk factor for calcium stones because uric acid causes "salting out" of calcium oxalate. It is most often encountered in patients with greater ingestion of animal protein.

Nonspecific prevention of stone recurrence

The only Cochrane review currently available regarding prevention of stone recurrence examined the benefit of increasing fluid intake [29]. There has been only one randomized, controlled trial in which patients with calcium stones were randomly assigned to two groups, only one of which was told to increase fluid intake [30]. In the increased-fluid group, 12 of 99 patients had a stone recurrence within 5 years, compared to 27 of 100 in the control group ($P = 0.008$). The former group increased 24-h urine volume from 1.1 to 2.6 L at 5 years whereas the control group, with a urine volume on study entry of 1.0 L, did not demonstrate a significant change in urine volume at any point during the study.

The Cochrane review considered this one study inadequate because of small numbers, short follow-up, and some questions about the randomization [29]. The review calls for additional research and states that "no conclusions can be drawn on increased water intake for the primary and secondary prevention of urinary calculi." This is not a practical assessment. It seems very unlikely, given the clear role of fluid intake in lowering urinary supersaturation, as well as the safety, low cost, and experience with the intervention, that additional research will be forthcoming. Whether fluid intake is effective in preventing noncalcium stones has not been tested, although the potential benefit of the therapy that is supported by epidemiological observations can be stressed, especially for patients with cystinuria.

Diet
The evidence that diet contributes to stones is summarized above and elsewhere in other publications [31]. A relative paucity of randomized controlled trials however means that many recommendations are based on epidemiologic data or on measurement of urinary chemistries after dietary manipulation. On the basis of this evidence, prevention regimens should include increased fluid intake and a diet that includes moderate but not low calcium intake and reductions in the intake of salt, oxalate, and animal protein.

Table 57.1 Composition of the "normal" calcium diet for prevention of stone recurrences in patients with hypercalciuria.

Component	Amount
Calcium	1200 mg (30 mmol)
Total protein	93 g
From meat or fish	21 g
From milk or milk products	31 g
From bread, pasta, and vegetables	41 g
Sodium chloride	50 mmol
Oxalate	2.2 mmol
Potassium	120 mmol
Phosphorus	49 mmol
Magnesium	14.5 mmol
Lipids	93 g
Carbohydrates	333 g
Fiber	40 g
Calories	2540 kcal
Water in foods	1550 mL

Source: Borghi et al. [32].

The only positive controlled trial of diet reported to date randomized men with hypercalciuria and recurrent calcium stones to one of two regimens [32]. One consisted of restrictions in calcium intake to 400 mg (10 mmol)/day; the other recommended a "normal" calcium intake of 1200 mg (30 mmol)/day and restricted animal protein (52 g) and salt intake (50 mmol) (details are shown in Table 57.1). Both groups were advised regarding oxalate restriction. At 5 years, the group on the higher-calcium, low-salt, low-animal protein diet had a reduction in stone recurrence by nearly 50% compared to the group on the low-calcium diet (Figure 57.1). The putative effect was attributed to the effect of calcium ingestion in reducing urinary oxalate while sodium restriction limited urinary calcium excretion, although mediation of the observed benefit through protein and salt restriction independent of calcium supplementation could not be excluded. Although bone mineral density was not measured, one would anticipate that the group in this study that had the higher calcium intake would have had less demineralization than the other group. It is worth mentioning that the "normal" 1200-mg calcium intake is higher than many people in Western societies usually ingest. For those who are lactose intolerant and other abstainers from dairy intake, lactose-free products or orange juice fortified with calcium are alternatives.

Given the evidence that obesity and diabetes are associated with stones, one might expect that weight loss would be associated with stone prevention, but this hypothesis has not yet been tested. Increasing ingestion of fruits and vegetables, after reduction of animal protein intake, is associated with increased urinary volume and citrate excretion and reductions in uric acid excretion [19]. It is anticipated that these changes alone might lead to a reduced occurrence of stones. Weight loss should be accomplished via well-rounded calorie-restricted diets and not via high-protein regimens such as the Atkins or South Beach diets [33]. A diet shown

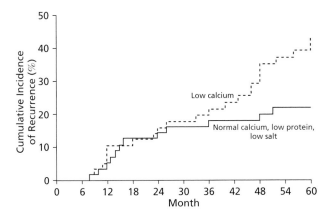

Figure 57.1 Kaplan-Meier estimates of cumulative incidence of recurrent stones, according to assigned diet: low calcium vs "normal" calcium, restricted animal protein, salt, and oxalate [32]. The relative risk of a recurrence in the group assigned to the low-calcium diet was 0.49 (95% confidence interval, 0.24–0.98; $P = 0.04$). Copyright © 2002 Massachusetts Medical Society; all rights reserved.

to be effective in the management of hypertension (from the Dietary Approaches to Stop Hypertension [DASH] study) might be a preferred, albeit untested, method of preventing stones and improving bone health [34].

Medications

Pharmacologic therapies for which randomized controlled trials are available and with demonstrated efficacy for prevention of recurrent calcium stones are thiazides for hypercalciuria, potassium citrate for hypocitraturia, and allopurinol for hyperuricosuria.

Thiazides

Thiazide diuretics have consistently been shown in randomized controlled trials to reduce stone recurrence in patients with hypercalciuria. Their action in the distal tubule is associated with decreased urinary calcium excretion. Table 57.2 summarizes the clinical studies. A meta-analysis of the five studies summarized in Table 57.2 plus one other of short follow-up concluded that thiazides were effective [35]; risk reduction was 21.3% compared with no treatment or placebo. The term "thiazides" here includes the thiazide-like drugs chlorthalidone and indapamide. Thiazides are associated with hypokalemia, which in turn can reduce urinary citrate excretion. Their use is therefore often accompanied by potassium citrate supplements. Triamterene, which is often used to reduce urinary potassium losses when thiazides are used to treat hypertension, is poorly soluble in the tubular fluid of the distal nephron, has been reported to form radiolucent renal stones composed of the medication, and is therefore contraindicated in stone

Table 57.2 Randomized controlled trials[a] of "thiazides" for prevention of stone recurrence.

Study ID [reference]	Drug(s) (dose)	Control	No. of patients	Follow-up (mos)	% Recurrence in controls	% Recurrence in treated group	P value	Comment
Borghi [18]	Indapamide[b] (2.5 mg)	Not treated	50	36	42.8	15.8	<0.02	A third arm with allopurinol and indapamide had no greater effect than indapamide alone
Ettinger [63]	Chlorthalidone (25 or 50 mg)	Placebo	73	36	45	16 (25 mg), 13 (50 mg)	<0.05	"Recurrence" includes stone growth
Laerum [64]	HCTZ (25 mg) + KCl (8.0 mEq b.i.d.)	Placebo	50	36	48	22	0.05	
Ohkawa [65]	Trichlormethiazide (4 mg)	Not treated	175	26	NA	NA	<0.05	Recurrence rates were not given, but rates of stone formation were lower in active thiazide group than in control
Robertson [66]	Bendroflumethiazide (2.5 mg) + KCl (14.8 mEq)	Not treated	22	36–60	NA	NA	<0.05	Small preliminary report; full report not published; recurrence rates not given, but rates of stone formation were lower in active thiazide group compared to control; two other arms, one with allopurinol and one with orthophosphate, had no effects compared to placebo

Abbreviations: HCTZ: hydrochlorothiazide; b.i.d., twice a day; NA, not available.
[a]Studies with less than 2 years of follow-up and those reported only as abstracts are not included.
[b]Indapamide is a nonthiazide diuretic with similar activity.

Table 57.3 Randomized controlled trials of other pharmacologic interventions for prevention of calcium stone recurrence.

Intervention [reference]	Indication	Control (*n*)	Duration (mos)	% Recurrence (intervention vs. control)	Stone formation rate/patient-yr (intervention vs. control)	Statistical significance
Potassium citrate, 30–60 mEq/day (*n* = 18) [36]	Hypocitraturia	Placebo (20)	36	28 vs. 80	0.1 ± 0.2 vs. 1.1 ± 0.3	*P* < 0.001
Potassium/magnesium citrate, 42 mEq; potassium, 21 mEq; magnesium, 63 mEq (*n* = 16) [37]	Calcium stones	Placebo (25)	36	12.9 vs. 63.6	NA	RR reduction, 0.16 (95% CI 0.05–0.46)
Allopurinol, 100 mg t.i.d. (*n* = 29) [38]	Hyperuricosuria (excluding hypercalciuria)	Placebo (31)	24	31.0 vs. 58.1	0.12 vs. 0.26	*P* < 0.05

Abbreviations: t.i.d., three times a day; RR, relative risk; CI, confidence interval.

formers; amiloride or spironolactone are preferred as potassium-sparing diuretics in this population. The thiazides' antihypertensive effects, their long history of efficacy in systolic hypertension, especially in the elderly, and their association with increases in bone mineral density and reduction in fracture rates make thiazides the first-line therapy in patients with stones who are also affected by these other conditions. Young and otherwise-healthy stone formers will also benefit, with minimal reductions in blood pressure in most normotensive individuals. The hypocalciuric effect is greater in patients who succeed in reducing sodium intake.

Citrate

For patients with hypocitraturia, potassium citrate supplementation was shown to prevent stone recurrence in one randomized controlled trial [36] (Table 57.3). A preparation of potassium and magnesium citrate, not commercially available, was also effective for patients with calcium stones, irrespective of urinary citrate excretion [37]. Sodium citrate is associated with increased urinary calcium excretion and should be avoided.

Allopurinol

The effect of uric acid on precipitation of calcium oxalate led to a positive randomized controlled trial of allopurinol for prevention of recurrent calcium stones in patients with hyperuricosuria [38] (Table 57.3). Small and therefore inadequate studies in patients without hyperuricosuria showed no benefit.

Other therapies

A variety of other therapies have been tested in randomized controlled trials, and these have not demonstrated efficacy. Other customary therapies have not been tested in well-designed trials. There is currently no evidence supporting the use of cellulose phosphate, sodium phosphate, or orthophosphate. Magnesium may be effective *in vitro* in preventing crystallization of calcium salts, but no human data exist to show that it is effective *in vivo*; it may, however, be indicated in patients with bowel dis-

ease, who often have hypomagnesiuria. Reduction of urinary oxalate, whether through dietary restriction, calcium supplementation, or other oxalate binders, has not been shown to prevent stone recurrence.

Calcium phosphate stones

The therapies recommended for the prevention of recurrent calcium phosphate stones have not been studied in randomized controlled trials. Calcium phosphate, usually in the form of hydroxyapatite, is frequently a minor component of calcium oxalate stones, but only about 15% of calcium stones are composed of more than 50% calcium phosphate [39]. A major determinant of calcium phosphate crystal formation is higher urine pH.

Two diagnoses should be considered in patients with predominant calcium phosphate stones: RTA and primary hyperparathyroidism. Distal RTA (or type I RTA) is associated with an increase in urine pH, which is the major reason why the associated stone composition is often calcium phosphate. The diagnosis of incomplete RTA is made when serum bicarbonate is normal but urinary pH is high and citrate excretion is low. Although not required for diagnosis, defects in urinary acidification are usually found in response to testing with ammonium chloride. A defect in acidification can also be suspected if the apparent level of ammonium excretion estimated from the urinary anion gap is low. The accompanying metabolic acidosis, with or without decreased serum bicarbonate, is associated with hypocitraturia. Hypercalciuria and osteoporosis are also often present as a result of acidosis-induced stimulation of osteoclast activity and inhibition of renal calcium reabsorption [40]. Nephrocalcinosis is often seen on abdominal radiography or ultrasound. Treatment with bicarbonate or citrate to raise serum bicarbonate and urinary citrate excretion appeared to reduce stone recurrence in uncontrolled observational studies of RTA and incomplete RTA [41,42]. Potassium bicarbonate or citrate preparations are preferred to sodium salts to minimize hypercalciuria. Citrate supplementation is complicated by an ensuing increase in urinary pH which could theoretically worsen calcium phosphate precipitation. Treatment with thiazides to lower urinary calcium excretion might make citrate supplementation safer in patients whose hypercalciuria persists despite successful treatment of acidosis and might contribute to increasing bone mineral density.

The effects of parathyroid hormone (PTH) to increase intestinal absorption of calcium via stimulated synthesis of 1,25-dihydroxy-vitamin D and to mobilize directly both calcium and phosphate from demineralizing bone contribute to calcium phosphate stone formation. Calcium oxalate stones occur as well. The diagnosis should also be suspected in women or patients with a family history of stones or parathyroid disease. PTH should be measured in patients with high-normal or high values of serum calcium; serum ionized calcium is a more sensitive test. As many as one-third of patients with hyperparathyroidism and calcium stones may be normocalciuric, suggesting that other factors may contribute to stone formation. The therapy is surgical parathyroidectomy, although stone recurrence after gland removal is surprisingly high [43]. For those patients in whom surgical therapy is contraindicated due to coexisting morbidities, thiazides may reduce urinary calcium but increase serum calcium concentration. The calcimimetic agent cinacalcet lowered serum PTH levels in a placebo-controlled randomized trial, but a clear beneficial effect on urinary risk factors was not demonstrated [44], and cinacalcet is currently not approved for this indication.

Struvite stones

Struvite stones, constituting 10–15% of all urinary tract stones, result from urinary tract infections with organisms that produce the enzyme urease, which catalyzes the conversion of urea to CO_2 and ammonia [45]. Ammonia alkalinizes the urine, and pH values of 7.5 or more result. Such values are rarely seen, even with renal tubular acidosis or vegetarian diets: high urine pH should always lead to obtaining a urine for bacterial culture. Struvite precipitates at these high pH values; the crystals are composed of calcium phosphate (in the form of carbonate apatite) and magnesium ammonium phosphate (leading to their alternative name of "triple-phosphate" stones). These stones are often large and can form staghorn calculi, stones which extend into multiple calyces of the kidney pelvis. (Staghorn calculi may be composed of any stone-forming crystal: cystine, calcium oxalate, calcium phosphate, and uric acid). Affected patients are often, but not always, those with recurrent infections associated with spinal cord injury such as a neurogenic bladder, chronic bladder dysfunction from other causes such as multiple sclerosis, and other disorders treated with chronic indwelling catheters.

The therapy of struvite stones is surgical removal, either via ureteroscopy or percutaneous nephrostolithotomy [46]. Extracorporeal shock wave lithotripsy should be tried only for relatively small stones in normal urinary tracts. Nonsurgical therapy is associated with sepsis or deterioration of kidney function, which may eventually require treatment by nephrectomy [47], especially in patients with end-stage renal disease in whom a kidney transplant is anticipated. Long-term, low-dose suppressive antibiotics, such as nitrofurantoin or sulfamethoxazole–trimethoprim, may be appropriate when stones have been completely eradicated by surgical therapy, but this strategy has not been the subject of any long-term randomized controlled trials.

Although the urease inhibitor acetohydroxamic acid has been shown to effectively reduce urinary ammonia levels and stone growth, its use should be reserved for patients with significant contraindications to endourologic surgery or who have failed surgical eradication [48–50]. The incidence of side effects reported in the clinical trials was significant, with relatively high proportions of patients taking the drug withdrawing from these studies [50]. These studies predate the current technology of endourology and effective stone removal, so that the relevance of the drug for stone disease management currently is less clear.

Patients with struvite stones and chronic infection often have metabolic abnormalities which may be responsible for causing calcium stones, which in turn contribute to initiation of infection and struvite formation [51]. Metabolic evaluation with 24-h urine collection after complete stone removal is recommended, although whether specific treatment based on the measured metabolic abnormalities will reduce struvite stone recurrence is unknown.

Uric acid stones

Uric acid is the major constituent of about 5–10% of stones; recent evidence demonstrates that uric acid stones make up a much larger proportion of stones among diabetics and obese patients [52,53]. There have been no randomized controlled trials of prevention of uric acid stones. The pathophysiology of uric acid stones and the therapy that arises from an understanding of this pathophysiology are relatively clear and effective, respectively [54]. There are three major factors that account for increases in urinary uric acid supersaturation: low urine volume, hyperuricosuria, and low urine pH [55]. The latter is by far the most important variable affecting uric acid supersaturation. As the pK of uric acid is 5.6, at low urine pH (5.5 or less) most uric acid is in the poorly soluble, protonated form and thus crystalluria and stones may result. At higher urinary pH (6.0 or more) most uric acid is in the dissociated, ionic, and therefore highly soluble form, and crystals will dissolve and stones are therefore unlikely. The amount of uric acid in the urine is much less important: with a low pH, even relatively little uric acid in the urine can result in stones, whereas at higher urine pH even relatively greater degrees of hyperuricosuria are not associated with stone formation.

Because low urine pH is a major cause of uric acid stones, conditions associated with more acidic urine are frequently implicated. Chronic bowel diseases, such as ulcerative colitis, Crohn's disease, chronic diarrhea, and ileostomy are often causative [26]. These bowel disorders may also be associated with low urine volume as the result of stool salt and water losses. Increasing body weight is also associated with decreasing urine pH [56]. Diabetes is associated with a higher prevalence of stones in general [22] and a higher proportion of uric acid stones than seen in the general population [52]. The link between obesity, diabetes, and low urine pH resulting in uric acid stones may be due to a reduction in renal ammoniagenesis associated with insulin resistance.

Hyperuricosuria may be idiopathic or result from excessive ingestion of animal protein (poultry, fish, beef, eggs, lamb, etc). About 20% of patients with gout are overproducers of uric acid and have hyperuricosuria. However, even patients with gout and lesser values for uric acid excretion may have low urine pH, resulting in an increased risk for uric acid stones. These patients' gout-associated uric acid stones may be the result of the low urine pH associated with their higher body mass index or diabetes rather than gout per se, although even after correction for body mass, gout is associated with a greater risk of stones [27]. Less frequently, hyperuricosuria is the result of hematologic disorders, such as polycythemia vera, lymphoproliferative disorders, or abnormalities in uric acid metabolism, such as Lesch-Nyan syndrome. Hyperuricosuria can also arise from uricosuric drugs, such as probenecid or high-dose salicylates.

The major implication for therapy in patients with uric acid stones is that alkalinization of the urine is far more likely to be successful than therapy with the xanthine oxidase inhibitor allopurinol. Significant reductions in uric acid excretion achieved by allopurinol will be associated with continued stone production if urinary pH is not raised. If alkalinization is successful, reduction of uric acid excretion is not very important. Alkalinization is most often achieved with potassium citrate in varying doses, from 20 to 40 mEq once or twice a day. Potassium citrate is preferable to sodium citrate, as the sodium excretion may be associated with increased calciuria, although hypertension and hypervolemia or pulmonary congestion are less likely than with sodium chloride supplementation. Citrate salts may be better tolerated than sodium or potassium bicarbonate, but they do cause gastrointestinal symptoms in some patients, especially elderly patients. Sodium bicarbonate, however, is the cheapest form of alkalinization therapy. Allopurinol is reserved for patients with significant hyperuricosuria (more than 800–900 mg/day) in whom alkalinization is not easily achieved. Such patients may be those who become hypertensive or hypervolemic with sodium salts, hyperkalemic with potassium citrate, or have more marked metabolic acidosis due to chronic diarrheal conditions, such as that seen in some patients with ileostomies. Patients with these bowel disorders have continued intestinal losses of base and may, therefore, exhibit persistently lower serum bicarbonate concentrations that interfere with achieving bicarbonaturia and urinary alkalinization. Alkalinization of the urine throughout the day should be the goal for patients with stones in place, in whom stone dissolution may be possible. Once-a-day, or even every-other-day, orally administered alkalinization is often adequate for purposes of prophylaxis only, as demonstrated in a single anecdotal series [57].

Reduction in animal protein intake may be useful in reducing uricosuria and mitigating the metabolic acid load that contributes to the low urine pH. Increased ingestion of fruits and vegetables can be associated with increases in urine volume and urinary pH as well [19]. However, the benefit of protein restriction may be insignificant in patients with obesity and diabetes. Although specific therapy for such patients has not yet been investigated, such patients may have a lesser impact from protein restriction and might benefit more from weight loss and exercise to prevent the onset of diabetes.

Acetazolamide, a carbonic anhydrase inhibitor, causes diminished reabsorption of bicarbonate in the renal proximal tubule. Urinary alkalinization results and could be associated with dissolution of uric acid stones or prevention of stone recurrence. However, its use is accompanied by metabolic acidosis (superimposed on patients who often already have a degree of acidosis) and hypokalemia, making it less desirable for chronic use. The drug is reserved for patients who have difficulties with potassium and sodium citrate or bicarbonate.

Cystinuria

Cystinuria is responsible for 1% of all stones. There have been no randomized controlled trials of treatment for recurrence of stones in patients with cystinuria. The condition is the result of an autosomal recessive mutation in one of the two components of the proximal tubule's major cystine transporter. There have been advances in the collection of urine and assays for cystine that might change management of the disease. Urine collections for cystine should be alkalinized in order to solubilize precipitated cystine and avoid underestimating the excretion of cystine [58]. A solid-phase assay has recently been developed to avoid interference of thiol drugs with cystine measurements and could yield more accurate measures of cystine excretion and solubility [59]. Validation of the utility of this technique is not yet available.

Prevention of recurrent cystine stones has four components: fluids, diet, urinary alkalinization, and thiol medications. Patients should maintain high urine volumes, at least 1 L/250 mg of cystine (about 1 mmol)/day. The diet should have limited intake of animal protein, which contains methionine, the metabolic precursor of cystine [60], and of salt, the excretion of which is accompanied by more urinary cystine [59]. It should be noted that the experimental literature demonstrating an effect of dietary restriction of protein and salt does not include stones as an end point but does include changes in urinary cystine excretion. Protein restriction may also be useful in causing a degree of urinary alkalinization and reducing the amount of citrate supplementation required to achieve a higher urinary pH. Urinary alkalinization to pH 7.0 or more significantly increases cystine solubility; potassium citrate is preferred to the sodium preparation.

Thiol drugs containing a sulfhydryl group can break the disulfide bridge of cystine and form two molecules of cysteine bound to the drug; cysteine and cysteine-drug complexes are more soluble than cystine. Available drugs include tiopronin (α-mercaptopropionylglycine), D-penicillamine, and a less-effective agent, captopril. The drugs are associated with improvements in cystine solubility, but their efficacies in preventing stones have been demonstrated only in relatively small anecdotal series, rather than in controlled trials [61,62].

References

1 Stamatelou KK, Francis ME, Jones CA, Nyberg LM, Curhan GC. Time trends in reported prevalence of kidney stones in the United States: 1976-1994. *Kidney Int* 2003; **63(5)**: 1817–1823.

2 Trinchieri A, Coppi F, Montanari E, Del Nero A, Zanetti G, Pisani E. Increase in the prevalence of symptomatic upper urinary tract stones during the last ten years. *Eur Urol* 2000; **37(1)**: 23–25.

3 Yoshida O, Terai A, Ohkawa T, Okada Y. National trend of the incidence of urolithiasis in Japan from 1965 to 1995. *Kidney Int* 1999; **56(5)**: 1899–1904.

4 Goldfarb DS. Increasing prevalence of kidney stones in the United States. *Kidney Int* 2003; **63(5)**: 1951–1952.

5 Longo J, Akbar SA, Schaff T, Jafri ZH, Jackson RE. A prospective comparative study of non-contrast helical computed tomography and intravenous urogram for the assessment of renal colic. *Emergency Radiol* 2001; **8(5)**: 285–292.

6 Yilmaz S, Sindel T, Arslan G, Ozkaynak C, Karaali K, Kabaalioglu A *et al.* Renal colic: comparison of spiral CT, US and IVU in the detection of ureteral calculi. *Eur Radiol* 1998; **8(2)**: 212–217.

7 Bove P, Kaplan D, Dalrymple N, Rosenfield AT, Verga M, Anderson K *et al.* Reexamining the value of hematuria testing in patients with acute flank pain. *J Urol* 1999; **162(3 Pt 1)**: 685–687.

8 Portis AJ, Sundaram CP. Diagnosis and initial management of kidney stones. *Am Fam Physician* 2001; **63(7)**: 1329–1338.

9 Holdgate A, Pollock T. Nonsteroidal anti-inflammatory drugs (NSAIDs) versus opioids for acute renal colic. *Cochrane Database Syst Rev* 2005; **2**: CD004137.

10 Larkin GL, Peacock WF, Pearl SM, Blair GA, D'Amico F. Efficacy of ketorolac tromethamine versus meperidine in the ED treatment of acute renal colic. *Am J Emerg Med* 1999; **17(1)**: 6–10.

11 Dellabella M, Milanese G, Muzzonigro G. Randomized trial of the efficacy of tamsulosin, nifedipine and phloroglucinol in medical expulsive therapy for distal ureteral calculi. *J Urol* 2005; **174(1)**: 167–172.

12 Porpiglia F, Destefanis P, Fiori C, Fontana D. Effectiveness of nifedipine and deflazacort in the management of distal ureter stones. *Urology* 2000; **56(4)**: 579–582.

13 Segura JW, Preminger GM, Assimos DG, Dretler SP, Kahn RI, Lingeman JE *et al.* Ureteral Stones Clinical Guidelines Panel summary report on the management of ureteral calculi. The American Urological Association. *J Urol* 1997; **158(5)**: 1915–1921.

14 Tiselius HG, Ackermann D, Alken P, Buck C, Conort P, Gallucci M. Guidelines on urolithiasis. *Eur Urol* 2001; **40(4)**: 362–371.

15 Krambeck AE, Gettman MT, Rohlinger AL, Lohse CM, Patterson DE, Segura JW. Diabetes mellitus and hypertension associated with shock wave lithotripsy of renal and proximal ureteral stones at 19 years of followup. *J Urol* 2006; **175(5)**: 1742–1747.

16 National Institutes of Health Consensus Development Conference on Prevention and Treatment of Kidney Stones. Bethesda, Maryland, March 28–30, 1988. *J Urol* 1989; **141(3 Pt 2)**: 705–808.

17 Curhan GC, Willett WC, Rimm EB, Stampfer MJ. A prospective study of dietary calcium and other nutrients and the risk of symptomatic kidney stones. *N Engl J Med* 1993; **328(12)**: 833–838.

18 Borghi L, Meschi T, Guerra A, Novarini A. Randomized prospective study of a nonthiazide diuretic, indapamide, in preventing calcium stone recurrences. *J Cardiovasc Pharmacol* 1993; **22(Suppl 6)**: S78–S86.

19 Meschi T, Maggiore U, Fiaccadori E, Schianchi T, Bosi S, Adorni G *et al.* The effect of fruits and vegetables on urinary stone risk factors. *Kidney Int* 2004; **66(6)**: 2402–2410.

20 Curhan GC, Willett WC, Speizer FE, Spiegelman D, Stampfer MJ. Comparison of dietary calcium with supplemental calcium and other nutrients as factors affecting the risk for kidney stones in women. *Ann Intern Med* 1997; **126(7)**: 497–504.

21 Taylor EN, Stampfer MJ, Curhan GC. Obesity, weight gain, and the risk of kidney stones. *JAMA* 2005; **293(4)**: 455–462.

22 Taylor EN, Stampfer MJ, Curhan GC. Diabetes mellitus and the risk of nephrolithiasis. *Kidney Int* 2005; **68(3)**: 1230–1235.

23 Borghi L, Meschi T, Amato F, Novarini A, Romanelli A, Cigala F. Hot occupation and nephrolithiasis. *J Urol* 1993; **150(6)**: 1757–1760.

24 Daudon M, Jungers P. Drug-induced renal calculi: epidemiology, prevention and management. *Drugs* 2004; **64(3)**: 245–275.

25 Goldfarb DS, Fischer ME, Keich Y, Goldberg J. A twin study of genetic and dietary influences on nephrolithiasis: a report from the Vietnam Era Twin (VET) Registry. *Kidney Int* 2005; **67(3)**: 1053–1061.

26 Parks JH, Worcester EM, O'Connor RC, Coe FL. Urine stone risk factors in nephrolithiasis patients with and without bowel disease. *Kidney Int* 2003; **63(1)**: 255–265.

27 Kramer HJ, Choi HK, Atkinson K, Stampfer M, Curhan GC. The association between gout and nephrolithiasis in men: The Health Professionals' Follow-Up Study. *Kidney Int* 2003; **64(3)**: 1022–1026.

28 Rodman JS, Mahler RJ. Kidney stones as a manifestation of hypercalcemic disorders. Hyperparathyroidism and sarcoidosis. *Urol Clin North Am* 2000; **27(2)**: 275–285.

29 Qiang W, Ke Z. Water for preventing urinary calculi (Cochrane review). *Cochrane Database Syst Rev* 2004; **3**: CD004292.

30 Borghi L, Meschi T, Amato F, Briganti A, Novarini A, Giannini A. Urinary volume, water and recurrences in idiopathic calcium nephrolithiasis: a 5-year randomized prospective study. *J Urol* 1996; **155(3)**: 839–843.

31 Taylor EN, Curhan GC. Diet and fluid prescription in stone disease. *Kidney Int* 2006; **70(5)**: 835–839.

32 Borghi L, Schianchi T, Meschi T, Guerra A, Allegri F, Maggiore U *et al.* Comparison of two diets for the prevention of recurrent stones in idiopathic hypercalciuria. *N Engl J Med* 2002; **346(2)**: 77–84.

33 Kielb S, Koo HP, Bloom DA, Faerber GJ. Nephrolithiasis associated with the ketogenic diet. *J Urol* 2000; **164(2)**: 464–466.

34 Sacks FM, Svetkey LP, Vollmer WM, Appel LJ, Bray GA, Harsha D *et al.* Effects on blood pressure of reduced dietary sodium and the Dietary Approaches to Stop Hypertension (DASH) diet. DASH-Sodium Collaborative Research Group. *N Engl J Med* 2001; **344(1)**: 3–10.

35 Pearle MS, Roehrborn CG, Pak CY. Meta-analysis of randomized trials for medical prevention of calcium oxalate nephrolithiasis. *J Endourol* 1999; **13(9)**: 679–685.

36 Barcelo P, Wuhl O, Servitge E, Rousaud A, Pak CY. Randomized double-blind study of potassium citrate in idiopathic hypocitraturic calcium nephrolithiasis. *J Urol* 1993; **150(6)**: 1761–1764.

37 Ettinger B, Pak CY, Citron JT, Thomas C, Adams-Huet B, Vangessel A. Potassium-magnesium citrate is an effective prophylaxis against recurrent calcium oxalate nephrolithiasis. *J Urol* 1997; **158(6)**: 2069–2073.

38 Ettinger B, Tang A, Citron JT, Livermore B, Williams T. Randomized trial of allopurinol in the prevention of calcium oxalate calculi. *N Engl J Med* 1986; **315**(22): 1386–1389.

39 Gault MH, Chafe L. Relationship of frequency, age, sex, stone weight and composition in 15,624 stones: comparison of results for 1980 to 1983 and 1995 to 1998. *J Urol* 2000; **164**(2): 302–307.

40 Morris RC, Jr., Sebastian A. Alkali therapy in renal tubular acidosis: who needs it? *J Am Soc Nephrol* 2002; **13**(8): 2186–2188.

41 Caruana RJ, Buckalew VM, Jr. The syndrome of distal (type 1) renal tubular acidosis. Clinical and laboratory findings in 58 cases. *Medicine* (Baltimore) 1988; **67**(2): 84–99.

42 Preminger GM, Sakhaee K, Skurla C, Pak CY. Prevention of recurrent calcium stone formation with potassium citrate therapy in patients with distal renal tubular acidosis. *J Urol* 1985; **134**(1): 20–23.

43 Mollerup CL, Lindewald H. Renal stones and primary hyperparathyroidism: natural history of renal stone disease after successful parathyroidectomy. *World J Surg* 1999; **23**(2): 173–175.

44 Peacock M, Bilezikian JP, Klassen PS, Guo MD, Turner SA, Shoback D. Cinacalcet hydrochloride maintains long-term normocalcemia in patients with primary hyperparathyroidism. *J Clin Endocrinol Metab* 2005; **90**(1): 135–141.

45 Rodman JS. Struvite stones. *Nephron* 1999; **81**(Suppl): 150–159.

46 Preminger GM, Assimos DG, Lingeman JE, Nakada SY, Pearle MS, Wolf JS, Jr. AUA guideline on management of staghorn calculi: diagnosis and treatment recommendations. *J Urol* 2005; **173**(6): 1991–2000.

47 Teichman JM, Long RD, Hulbert JC. Long-term renal fate and prognosis after staghorn calculus management. *J Urol* 1995; **153**(5): 1403–1407.

48 Griffith DP, Khonsari F, Skurnick JH, James KE. A randomized trial of acetohydroxamic acid for the treatment and prevention of infection-induced urinary stones in spinal cord injury patients. *J Urol* 1988; **140**(2): 318–324.

49 Griffith DP, Gleeson MJ, Lee H, Longuet R, Deman E, Earle N. Randomized, double-blind trial of Lithostat (acetohydroxamic acid) in the palliative treatment of infection-induced urinary calculi. *Eur Urol* 1991; **20**(3): 243–247.

50 Williams JJ, Rodman JS, Peterson CM. A randomized double-blind study of acetohydroxamic acid in struvite nephrolithiasis. *N Engl J Med* 1984; **311**(12): 760–764.

51 Kristensen C, Parks JH, Lindheimer M, Coe FL. Reduced glomerular filtration rate and hypercalciuria in primary struvite nephrolithiasis. *Kidney Int* 1987; **32**(5): 749–753.

52 Pak CY, Sakhaee K, Moe O, Preminger GM, Poindexter JR, Peterson RD et al. Biochemical profile of stone-forming patients with diabetes mellitus. *Urology* 2003; **61**(3): 523–527.

53 Ekeruo WO, Tan YH, Young MD, Dahm P, Maloney ME, Mathias BJ et al. Metabolic risk factors and the impact of medical therapy on the management of nephrolithiasis in obese patients. *J Urol* 2004; **172**(1): 159–163.

54 Asplin JR. Uric acid stones. *Semin Nephrol* 1996; **16**(5): 412–424.

55 Maalouf NM, Cameron MA, Moe OW, Sakhaee K. Novel insights into the pathogenesis of uric acid nephrolithiasis. *Curr Opin Nephrol Hypertens* 2004; **13**(2): 181–189.

56 Maalouf NM, Sakhaee K, Parks JH, Coe FL, Adams-Huet B, Pak CY. Association of urinary pH with body weight in nephrolithiasis. *Kidney Int* 2004; **65**(4): 1422–1425.

57 Rodman JS. Prophylaxis of uric acid stones with alternate day doses of alkaline potassium salts. *J Urol* 1991; **145**(1): 97–99.

58 Nakagawa Y, Asplin JR, Goldfarb DS, Parks JH, Coe FL. Clinical use of cystine supersaturation measurements. *J Urol* 2000; **164**(5): 1481–1485.

59 Goldfarb DS, Coe FL, Asplin JR. Urinary cystine excretion and capacity in patients with cystinuria. *Kidney Int* 2006; **69**(6): 1041–1047.

60 Rodman JS, Blackburn P, Williams JJ, Brown A, Pospischil MA, Peterson CM. The effect of dietary protein on cystine excretion in patients with cystinuria. *Clin Nephrol* 1984; **22**(6): 273–278.

61 Dolin D, Asplin JR, Flegel L, Grasso M, Goldfarb DS. Effect of cystine-binding thiol drugs on urinary cystine capacity in patients with cystinuria. *J Endourol* 2005; **19**: 429–432.

62 Pak CY, Fuller C, Sakhaee K, Zerwekh JE, Adams BV. Management of cystine nephrolithiasis with alpha-mercaptopropionylglycine. *J Urol* 1986; **136**(5): 1003–1008.

63 Ettinger B, Citron JT, Livermore B, Dolman LI. Chlorthalidone reduces calcium oxalate calculous recurrence but magnesium hydroxide does not. *J Urol* 1988; **139**(4): 679–684.

64 Laerum E, Larsen S. Thiazide prophylaxis of urolithiasis. A double-blind study in general practice. *Acta Med Scand* 1984; **215**(4): 383–389.

65 Ohkawa M, Tokunaga S, Nakashima T, Orito M, Hisazumi H. Thiazide treatment for calcium urolithiasis in patients with idiopathic hypercalciuria. *Br J Urol* 1992; **69**(6): 571–576.

66 Robertson WG, Peacock M, Selby PL, Williams RE, Clark P, Chisholm CD et al. A multicentre trial to evaluate three treatments for recurrent idiopathic calcium stone disease: a preliminary report. In: Schwille PO, Smith LH, Robertson WG, Vahlensieck W (editors), *Urolithiasis and Related Clinical Research*, Plenum Press, New York, 1985; 1545.

10 Pediatrics

Themes Across Renal Disease and Renal Failure

58 Growth, Nutrition, and Pubertal Development

Lesley Rees

Consultant Paediatric Nephrologist Great Ormond St Hospital for Children NHS Trust, London, UK

Phases of normal growth and influence of renal disease

Normal growth can be divided into four phases: prenatal, infantile, childhood, and pubertal. Each growth phase has different determinants, but growth is most affected during periods when it is the most rapid.

Prenatal phase

Growth *in utero* is more rapid than at any other time; around 30% of final height (FH) is achieved by birth. Intrauterine growth retardation (IUGR) has a profound effect on postnatal growth: children remain small and catch-up is rare. Kidney disease is a risk factor for IUGR. An adverse environment *in utero* impairs kidney development and makes the kidneys more vulnerable to damage from a range of pathological processes [1–5]. An increased incidence of IUGR has also been demonstrated in children with nephrotic syndrome and is associated with increased risk of relapses and steroid resistance [6–8].

Infantile phase

The extremely rapid prenatal rate of growth gradually decreases from >25 cm/year at birth to an average of 18 cm/year at 1 year of age and 10 cm/year at 2 years of age. One-half of adult height is achieved by the age of 2 years. This phase is highly dependent on nutrition: 170 Kcal/day are stored in new tissue in the newborn term infant, falling to 50–60 Kcal/day at 6 months, 30–40 by 1 year, and 20–30 by 2 years. Maintenance of normal growth is very difficult in young children with chronic kidney failure (CKF). Poor feeding and vomiting are common, and urological malformations, the most common cause of CKF in infancy, may result in sepsis, further aggravating the feeding problems or necessitating investigation and treatments with associated periods of fasting [1,9–14].

Childhood phase

Growth during the childhood phase becomes more dependent on the growth hormone (GH)–insulin-like growth factor 1 axis. GH is secreted in pulses, particularly at night, and this secretion is important for its actions. The growth rate decelerates throughout childhood until the onset of sex hormone production. Prolonged slowing of growth, in association with lack of development of secondary sexual characteristics (prepubertal deceleration), often causes concern and is a complication of long-term steroid therapy [15,16]. Growth will not resume until the onset of puberty.

Pubertal phase

Acceleration of growth during puberty is dependent upon the co-ordination of GH and sex steroid production, which, together with nutrition and general health, modify the genetic growth potential. Rising sex steroid concentrations stimulate GH production by increasing the amplitude of GH secretory pulses. Together, they have an anabolic effect on muscle mass, bone mineralization, and body proportions. Rates of growth may reach as high as 12 cm/year. The pubertal growth spurt will not take place until the appearance of secondary sexual characteristics. In girls this occurs early, soon after the onset of breast development; in boys it occurs later, after the onset of penile and pubic hair development and not until the testes have grown to 10–12 mL. Growth rates should therefore be interpreted with knowledge of the corresponding pubertal stage. Pubertal development and growth may be affected by CKF and steroid therapy [15–18].

Prevalence, severity, and natural history of growth disorders in chronic kidney disease

Steroid-sensitive nephrotic syndrome

The main potential impediment to growth in steroid-sensitive nephrotic syndrome is the steroid treatment rather than the disease itself. However, despite multiple courses and sometimes prolonged treatment, the majority of studies have shown little reduction in long-term growth potential. In 1985, the first report

Evidence-based Nephrology. Edited by Donald Molony and Jonathan Craig
© 2009 Blackwell Publishing, ISBN: 978-1-4051-3975-5.

demonstrated that, although growth was suppressed while taking steroids, those who had completed growth had a mean height standard deviation score (HtSDS) of −0.22 [19]. In the most recent report, median final HtSDS was normal, at −0.4 [20]. Although obesity and reduced appendicular lean mass are relatively common, these too resolve by adulthood [20,21].

Use of steroid-sparing agents results in improved growth. Children with severe growth impairment treated with cyclophosphamide demonstrated dramatic catch-up: HtSDS increased from −2.29 to −0.43 [22]. Similar results were shown in 12 children following treatment with alkylating agents: growth rate increased from 4.3 to 8.7 cm/year [23]. Studies of GH secretion have demonstrated that normal pulsatility is lost during steroid treatment [24] and recovers after its cessation [15]. Normal growth has been demonstrated in children prescribed cyclosporine A or tacrolimus [25].

It is likely that children with more severe renal disease have the most growth retardation. The mean duration of prednisone treatment and the average cumulative dose, especially when given for >6 months/year at a dose of >0.2 mg/kg/day, have been shown to be major predictors of poor growth outcome [26,27].

Another factor that may confound accurate interpretation of studies is the age at administration of steroids. Prepubertal growth may be unaffected: 21 prepubertal children grew normally on a mean yearly cumulative doses of prednisone of 6300, 3459, 2677, and 2081 mg/m^2 at the first, second, third, and fourth years, respectively [28]. Children taking steroids during the pubertal phase may have delayed development of secondary sexual characteristics and therefore delayed onset of the growth spurt. This causes a fall in HtSDS, which may be particularly pronounced, especially in those on long-term steroids [29], but growth continues for a longer time and ultimate height may not be affected [15,16]. This effect is greater in boys and in patients treated in the immediate prepubertal period, rather than those who are already established in puberty when steroids are started. Those who were on prednisolone after the age of 9 years in girls and 11 years in boys were at higher risk for height loss [27]. The FH of boys on steroids from 12 to 16 years of age and of girls from 10 to 14 years of age were −2 standard deviations (SD) below target height, but if steroids were withdrawn by the age of 14 years in boys and 12 years in girls, FH was within the normal range [30].

Chronic kidney failure

Prenatal and infantile phases

Many infants are already growth-retarded by the time they are first seen in a pediatric nephrology service, with losses as high as −1.68 SD from birth (−5 SD/year) [31]. HtSDS is below the normal range in most studies [1,9–14]. Approximately one-third of the fall in HtSDS occurs during fetal growth and one-third occurs during the first 3 months of life, accompanied by a similar fall in head circumference [32–34]. Infants who grew well continued with catch-up in early childhood [13,31]. As well as IUGR, a proportion of infants have comorbidities and associated syndromes which may in themselves affect growth. Although one-half of those with a glomerular filtration rate (GFR) of <35 mL/min/1.73 m^2 showed catch-up growth, many that grew poorly had IUGR [1].

Childhood phase

By the childhood phase, many patients with CKF that developed in infancy are growth-retarded, with growth paralleling the percentiles but not catching up [31,34,35]. Growth seems to be affected with even mild CKF, and these observations have changed little since 1996, when mean HtSDS was −1.5 in 1725 patients, to 1998, when HtSDS was −1.4 (with one-third of values greater than −1.88) in 3863 patients, and −1.4 in 2001 with 4666 patients aged <20 years and with GFR of <75 mL/min/1.73 m^2 [36–38]. More severe CKF has a greater effect on HtSDS: 321 children aged 1–10 years with congenital CKF divided according to GFR above versus below 25 mL/min/1.73 m^2 had HtSDS of −1.65 and −2.79, respectively (mean, −2.37) [35]. HtSDS may decline progressively, falling from −1.6 to −2.1 over 3.5 ± 3.3 years in 22 patients aged <14 years with a GFR of 32.6 ± 24.8 mL/min/1.73 m^2 [39]. However, this has not been found in all studies. In one study, improvement of +0.3 SD occurred over 2 years in 99 children with a median GFR of 22 mL/min/1.73 m^2 and HtSDS of −1.73 [40]; a smaller study had similar findings [41].

Pubertal phase

The pubertal phase is a phase of rapid growth and is another period when loss of height potential can occur. Early studies in children with severe CKF demonstrated that puberty was delayed by approximately 2.5 years in both sexes, with an irreversible decline in HtSDS [42], but others have reported normal pubertal progression and growth [31,34,43].

Dialysis

Many studies have combined children of all ages and dialysis modality (peritoneal dialysis [PD] and hemodialysis [HD]): of 651 patients aged <18 years, 266 (41%) had an HtSDS of less than −1.88 [44], and 57% of over 200 on PD had retarded growth [45]. Growth retardation is reported to occur less frequently with continuous ambulatory PD than with continuous cycling PD or HD (changes in HtSDS, −0.55, −1.69, and −1.80, respectively, over 6–12 months) [46], although this effect was most noticeable in older children [47].

Infantile phase

Reports vary considerably, but generally infants with chronic kidney disease either show no improvement or have worsening growth retardation without nutritional support. No change in HtSDS has been reported (−2.51 to −2.74) in 15 children <2 years old treated with continuous ambulatory PD [48]. Deterioration in HtSDS occurred in 17 infants on PD [49], and a decline in HtSDS by −0.29 SD/year has also been reported, along with a significant improvement between the first (−0.50) and the second (−0.23) years, in 22 children starting PD in infancy [50]. Good growth with nutritional support has been reported in some, but not all, studies (Table 58.1).

There are fewer studies of growth in infants on HD. In those ages 0–1 and 2–5 years at the start of HD and/or PD, HtSDS was −1.99 and −2.05, respectively, falling to −2.46 and −2.32 at 1 year and −2.06 and −2.00 at 2 years [51]. There have been two studies of HD, one reporting no change from HtSDS −1.6 in 18 infants on HD for up to 2 years [52], and the other reporting an HtSDS of −3.59 in 10 infants weighing <10 kg, only one of whom showed any improvement in HtSDS over a mean duration of 8.5 months [53].

Childhood phase

Reports on growth in the childhood phase vary, from improvement from −2.13 to −1.66 in 34 patients on PD for 6 months [54], to no change over 1 year [55,56], to a declining HtSDS from −1.71 to −1.86 at 1 year and −2.12 at 2 years in children on PD or HD aged 6–12 years (51).

Pubertal phase

Puberty may be delayed with poor growth [57]. HtSDS fell from −1.97 to −2.36 in 94 adolescents on HD for 3 years [58], from −1.39 to −1.59 at 1 year, and to −1.83 at 2 years in those on PD or HD [51].

Posttransplantation

Mean (range) HtSDS values at the time of transplantation for all ages have been reported to be −2.11 (−5.05 to −0.27), improving to −1.50 (−3.67 to −1.27) at 7 years posttransplant in 85 children [59] and −2.20 improving to −2.0 at 1 year in 64 children but with no further increases in years 2 and 3. Overall, more than 40% had values that remained less than −2 SD [60]. Some, but not all, studies show growth posttransplant to be superior to growth on dialysis, particularly in younger children [47,61,62]. However, comparison is difficult because, as well as age at transplant, growth is influenced by pretransplant height deficit (the greater the height deficit the greater the catch-up), which is in turn influenced by time of diagnosis and duration of dialysis [61]. Several studies have demonstrated the importance of GFR [61,62]: each increase in serum creatinine of 90 μmol/L (1 mg/dL) is associated with −0.17 SD [63]. Immunosuppressive regimens, especially steroid administration, affect growth (see below).

Infantile phase

Children under 2 years old have the greatest improvement in HtSDS, with gains of +1 SD overall [63] and +1.4 SD in six in-fants [64] and −3.2 to −1.6 and −1.4 at 5 and 10 years of age, respectively, in 30 infants [65]. One study showed no change from −1.1 SD over 7 years [66].

Childhood phase

Improvement in growth diminishes throughout childhood: 47% of children <6 years old at the time of transplant and 22% aged >6 years gained 1 SD [63]; height deficit was reduced by one-third in those receiving transplants before 5 years compared to an increase of up to 22% in older children [67]. HtSDS changed from −2.1 to −1.0 at 1 year, to −1.1 at 5 years, and to −0.14 at 10 years in 54 children who received transplants before age 5 years [68]; from −2.0 to −1.8, −1.5, and −1.5 at 1, 2, and 5 years posttransplant in 39 children <6 years of age [69]; and from −1.71 to −1.14 at 1 year and −0.55 at 5 years in 20 children <8.5 years of age [13]. Growth rates improved from 4.9 to 8.0 cm/year (+0.6 SD) within 2 years and increased FH by 1.3 SD [61].

Pubertal phase

Onset of puberty may be delayed but is in accordance with bone age. In 68 patients, mean chronological age and peak height velocity were 14.6 ± 1.9 and 13.3 ± 1.9 years and 6.6 ± 1.6 and 6.5 ± 2.9 cm/year in boys and girls, respectively. Menarche was attained at 15.9 years, and the duration of pubertal development was within normal limits [57]. Steroids may contribute to this delay [17]. HtSDS increased by 1.3 SD and 0.7 SD until FH occurred in children who received transplants before and after the start of puberty, respectively, although pubertal height gain was reduced by 20% [61]. HtSDS increased from −1.8 to −1.6, −1.5, −1.0, −0.7, and −0.6/year over five consecutive years in 54 adolescents [70]. Total pubertal height gain was greater in younger children, in those transplanted before the onset of puberty, and in those with better graft function [61,70].

Obesity posttransplantation

Obesity occurs in up to 13% of children with renal transplants and is associated with young age, male gender, short stature, duration of dialysis, and the number of grafts received [71,72]. Obesity may not be more common than in the normal population and is strongly related to the body mass index (BMI) of the mother [60].

Final height

FH is less than −2 SD in up to 47% of patients [57,61,73–75], with a mean of −2.01 in boys and −1.4 in girls among 60 patients not on recombinant human GH (rhGH) [75]. Conservative management is associated with a better FH than for those on renal replacement therapy (−1.15 vs. -2.1) [75]. FH was not reached until 20.2 ± 1.8 years in boys and 18.8 ± 2 years in girls [57,75], with a gain of +0.87 and +0.3 SD, respectively, after the age of 18 years [75]. Young age at start of dialysis and at transplant, short stature at transplant [60,73], and graft function [60] predict FH.

Table 58.1 Effects of dietary supplementation, specialist input by a dietician, and tube feeding on growth.

Study [reference]	No. of patients	Age (yrs)	GFR (mL/min/1.73 m²)	Diet	No. with nasogastric/ no. with gastrostomy	Duration (mos)	Growth
Improvement in growth							
Ledermann 1999 [11]	26 9	0–2 2–5	29 with GFR of 6–26, 6 on PD	100% EAR calories for CA, 100% RDA protein for Ht age with protein supplement for PD	20/9 8 Nissen	24	WtSDS −3.1 to −1.7 at 1 yr, −1.4 at 2 yrs, HtSDS −2.9 to −2.2 to −2.1; WtSDS −2.3 to −2 at 1 yr, −1.1 at 2 yrs, HtSDS −2.3 to −2.0 to −2.0
Kari 2000 [13]	24 13	0.3–2	<20 PD	100% EAR calories for CA, 100% RDA protein for Ht age with protein supplement for PD	13/17 14 Nissen	≥24	HtSDS −2.34 to −1.93; HtSDS −2.17 to −1.24
Parekh 2002 [14]	17 7	<1	<65, polyuric PD	100–160 cal and 2–2.5 g protein/kg/day, 2–4 mEq sodium, 0.3–0.5cal/mL	Both ? ratio	12–24	ΔHtSDS +1.37 at 1 yr, +1.82 at 2 yrs
Ledermann 2000 [82]	20	<1	PD	100% EAR calories for CA, 100% RDA protein for Ht age with protein supplement for PD	10/8 7 Nissen	1–59	WtSDS −1.6 at start, −0.3 at 1 yr, 0.3 at 2 yrs. HtSDS −1.8 to −1.1 to −0.8
Claris-Appiani 1995 [83]	2 3	<2 >2	CRF	101–115% EAR energy, 75–113% protein	5/0	12	ΔHtSDS +1.56, WtSDS +1.72
Strife 1986 [84]	3	1.7–3.0	20–25	Starting with 50 cal/kg and increasing	3/0	11–16	WtVel from <5% to >95%, HtVel from 5–40% to 80–95%
Norman 2004 [85]	25 21	2–16	51–75, 25–50	Intensive input from dietician and supplementation if EAR energy and RNI micronutrients <80%	0/1	24	All on supplements increased Ht and Wt SDS; No change in HtSDS if GFR >50; HtSDS +0.1 SD, correlation between intake and ΔHtSDS if GFR <50
Guillot 1980 [86]	3	<3		Energy 116% EAR, protein 84%	3/0	4–37	2 improved growth, 1 did not
Brewer 1990 [88]	14	3days to 3.1	PD	>90% RDA for energy for height age, 3–4 g/kg protein	13/0	3–33	Increase in HtSDS and WtSDS in 11
No change in growth rate							
Shroff 2003 [52]	18	0.5–2	HD	100% EAR calories for CA, 100% RDA protein for Ht age with protein supplement for PD	9/8	0.3–26	No change in HtSDS or WtSDS

(Continued)

Table 58.1 (*Continued*)

Study [reference]	No. of patients	Age (yrs)	GFR (mL/min/1.73 m²)	Diet	No. with nasogastric/no. with gastrostomy	Duration (mos)	Growth
Reed 1998 [80]	7	0.6 ± 0.7	Mean 17 (<30)	Energy based on median Wt for CA	7/0	18.6 ± 4.5	HtSDS −0.9 to −1.1, WtSDS −0.4 to −0.2
Coleman 1999 [87]	13	0.2–8.5	PD	5.9 and 3.1 dietician contacts/mo	1/7	36	HtSDS from −1.2 to −1.14 and WtSDS from −1.32 to −0.73
Initial decline then normalization of growth							
Van Dyck 1999 [12]	15	<1	Creatinine > 1mg/dl in 1st yr	1.8–2.2 g protein/kg/day (EAA supplements 20% of protein in first year), energy 120% EAR	0/0	36	Drop in first 3 months, stable after, Ht SDS −1.96, WtSDS-1.37
Abitbol 1993 [78]	12	0.25–2	<70	100% RDA energy, >140% protein	9/3	Up to 24	Ht and WtVel lowest (−2SD) by 6 months and Ht and WtSDS by 12 months of age, then stable at −2SD
Ramage 1999 [81]	8 / 7	<2.5 / >2.5	PD	Aiming for 100% RNI calories or greater if no response	0/12	12	Decline in HtSDS arrested / No change
Deterioration in growth							
Ellis 2001 [79]	137	<5	PD/HD	Not specified	Equal at <2yrs, 29%/57% at 2–5yrs	Until age 6 yrs	WtSDS −0.77 at start, −2.04 at 1 yr, HtSDS −1.75 and −2.89 without supplements, Wt SDS −1.33 and −1.70 and HtSDS −1.76 and −2.88 with supplements respectively

Abbreviations: Vel, velocity; CA, chronological age; EAR, estimated average requirement; RDA, recommended dietary allowance; RNI, recommended nutrient intake; Ht, height; Wt, weight.

Table 58.2 EAA supplements and growth.

Study [reference]	No. of patients	GFR (mL/min/1.73 m^2)	Diet	Duration (mos)	Outcome
Jones 1980 [97]	7	Severe CKF	Protein RDA for Ht age, half as EAAs	6–8	Improved nitrogen balance but no increase in HtSDS
Jureidini 1990 [94]	10	Severe CKF	Low protein and EAAs	36	Increase in Ht and WtVel
Mir 2005 [95]	20	<50	0.6 g/kg protein and ketoacids	30	HtSDS from −1.93 to −1.37
Zachwieja 1994 [96]	10	HD	AAs 0.25 g/kg body weight i.v. with dialysis	2 of 3	No improvement in plasma AAs

Abbreviations: RDA, recommended dietary allowance; Ht, height; i.v., intravenous; Wt, weight; Vel, velocity.

Available guidelines

The National Kidney Foundation's Kidney Disease Outcomes Quality Initiative has published guidelines for the nutritional management of children with kidney disease [76], including methods of assessment of nutritional status, management of acid–base status, role of urea kinetic modeling, interval measurements for assessment of nutritional status, energy, protein, vitamin, and mineral intakes, dietetic input, nutritional supplements, and use of rhGH. British Renal Association standards cover the role of the pediatric dietician and nutritional recommendations for energy, protein, and phosphate [77].

Evidence for benefits of interventions on nutrition and growth

Nutrition
Dietary supplementation, input by a dietician specialist, and nasogastric or gastrostomy feeds
The benefits of supplemental feeds in CKF and dialysis patients have been studied in case series and cohort studies [11–14,52,78–88] (Table 58.1). All but two studies focused on children younger than 2 years of age, who would be expected to benefit most from intensive nutrition. In eight studies there was an improvement in HtSDS [11,13,14,82–86,88], in three studies there was an initial decline followed by normalization of growth [12,78,81], in three studies there was no significant change [52,80,87], and in one study there was a decline in HtSDS [79]. Six studies included older children. Of these six, three showed an improvement in growth [11,83,85], two showed no change [81,87], and one showed a decline in HtSDS [79]. The normal age-related requirements for energy and protein seem to be needed for growth improvement, with an increased protein allowance for children on PD and a smaller supplement for those on HD to allow for losses in dialysate. The benefits of intervention by a dietician were demonstrated in two studies, but it is likely that none of the studies could have been achieved without provision of dietetic input.

Administration of nutritional supplementation was by nasogastric tube or gastrostomy in all but one study. Complications were not specified but are known to occur primarily in children on PD. Postgastrostomy, there is an early risk for peritonitis, but this resolves. There is an increased risk of exit site infection and catheter removal from infection when the gastrostomy tube is inserted after PD has started, a risk that may be reduced if open rather than percutaneous surgery is used. Paraoesophageal hernias have been reported [89,90]. Successful track closure on removal and normal feeding posttransplant are the usual outcomes [91,92].

Essential amino acid supplements
Serum essential amino acids (EAAs) may be low in CKF, particularly during PD [93]. It has been suggested that a low-protein diet supplemented with EAAs might ensure adequate intake and reduce protein toxicity, thereby benefiting growth. The small cohort studies available have been inconclusive [94-97] (Table 58.2).

Amino acids-containing PD solutions
Excessive glucose absorption and also dialysate AA and protein losses contribute to malnutrition during PD. It has been suggested that using an AA dialysate might both decrease glucose load and replace AA losses. However, although AAs are absorbed in proportion to the concentration difference between dialysate and plasma [98,99], there is no evidence for long-term nutritional benefit with the more costly AA-based dialysis solutions than the standard glucose-based solutions [100] (Table 58.3). Equivalent amounts of urea and creatinine are removed by both methods. With AA solutions, normoglycemia is maintained although ultrafiltration is variable [101–103]. It may be that using a combination of glucose and AA solutions increases protein synthesis [104]. There have been no adverse effects reported.

Intradialytic parenteral nutrition
Losses of AAs occur into the dialysate during HD, depending on their plasma concentrations and molecular weights. Studies of intradialytic parenteral nutrition have shown an increase in body weight but not serum albumin. No complications have been

Table 58.3 AA-containing PD solutions and growth.

Study [reference]	No. of patients	Dialysis	Dialysate	Duration	Outcome
Canepa 1990 [98]	7	CAPD	1% AA exchange compared to glucose 1.36%	1 exchange	Rise in plasma AAs proportional to amount of AA in dialysate; amount of AA absorbed 66% after 1 h, 86% after 4 and 6 h; loss of 116 ± 69 µmol/kg body wt with glucose
Hanning RM 1987 [99]	8	CAPD	AA-based dialysate	1 exchange	Absorption of 70–73% of AAs peaking at 1 h and varied with concentration difference; levels at pre-exchange at end of cycle
Canepa 1991 [100]	8	CAPD	First morning exchange of 1% AA dialysate	12–18 mos	No improvement in any plasma or anthropometric parameter of nutrition; plasma urea increased; plasma EAAs improved but intracellular pool did not
Qamar 1994 [102]	7	CAPD	AA or dextrose dialysate	3 mos, crossover	No nutritional benefit from AA dialysis
Qamar 1999 [103]	7	CCPD	AA or dextrose dialysate	3 mos, crossover	During AA, appetite, calorie, and protein intake improved and total body nitrogen increased in one-half of children; plasma albumin did not change; fasting AAs were comparable to baseline; plasma urea was higher
Canepa 2001 [104]	10	CCPD	3:1 ratio of glucose to AA	8 infusions	Glucose absorption was 33.7%, AA 55.2%; plasma AA levels high but plasma urea did not increase

Abbreviations: CAPD, continuous ambulatory PD; CCPD, continuous cycling PD.

reported, but the studies conducted have been very small [105–108] (Table 58.4).

Dialysis adequacy

Increasing dialysis dose might be expected to benefit appetite, nutrition, and growth, and this has been found in some studies [109–111], but it needs to be balanced against increasing dialysate albumin losses during PD [112] and increasing AA losses during HD [113] (Table 58.5). This may be possible with careful attention to diet. PD causes an influx of glucose, which can contribute to obesity. High transporter status was associated negatively with HtSDS and positively with BMISDS in 51 children on PD. Large dialysate volumes also increase BMISDS [114]. For HD it is not clear if there

is a maximum optimum dose. Studies of daily HD, which is likely to offer the most benefit, have been promising [115].

Residual renal function increases clearance and growth. HtSDS improved from −1.78 to −1.64 over 1 year of PD in 12 patients with RRF but declined from −1.37 to −1.90 in 12 patients without residual renal function. Weekly Kt/V was not different, and only the native kidney Kt/V and creatinine clearance correlated with growth, suggesting that clearance obtained by PD cannot be equated with that obtained by native kidneys [116]. Eleven of 20 patients on PD with a minimum Kt/V of 2.1, daily protein intake of 3.25 g/kg/day, and HtSDS of −2.3 improved their HtSDS by 0.55, whereas in the other 9 it declined by −0.50. Variables affecting growth were nitrogen balance and residual Kt/V [117].

Table 58.4 Intradialytic parenteral nutrition and growth.

Study [reference]	No. of patients	Intradialytic (HD) treatment	Outcome
Abitbol 1984 [105]	3	AAs added to dialysate in increasing concentrations	Zero flux of AA nitrogen when 22 mg/100 ml of AA additive in the dialysate; increase in plasma non-EAAs but not of EAAs
Krause 2002 [106]	4, malnourished	8.5% AA solution, 10–15% dextrose, 20% fat emulsion for 7–12 weeks	Oral intake improved; Wt did not improve during treatment, but did subsequently; albumin did not change
Goldstein 2002 [107]	3, malnourished adolescents	70% dextrose, 15% AAs, 20% lipids, 6 weeks	Wt improved but not albumin
Orellana 2005 [108]	9 with >10% Wt loss and <90th percentile of ideal body Wt	Thrice weekly for 3–22 mos	In six patients, BMI and PCR increased, serum albumin did not change

Abbreviations: Wt, weight; PCR, protein catabolic rate.

Table 58.5 Dialysis adequacy and growth.

Study [reference]	No. of patients	Age (yrs)	Duration (mos)	PD/HD	Kt/V	CrCl mL/1.73 m²/URR	Outcome
Holtta 2000 [109]	10	<5	9	CCPD	3.1	59	Catch-up growth in 62%, better than Kt/V 1.7 and CrCl >40 (historical)
	11	>5			3.2	78	
Marsenic 2001 [110]	15	14.5 ± 3.8	38 sessions	HD	<1.3->1.6	URR 85%	nPCR lowest if <1.3, no improvement when >1.6
Tom 1999 [111]	12	0.6–14	4–81	HD	>2.0 and high dietary intake	URR >85%	+0.31 SD/yr, normal pubertal growth
Brem 2000 [112]	23	14.3 ± 3.6	18	HD	Review, noninterventional		No association with albumin; inverse correlation with albumin, particularly if Kt/V >2.75
	30	10.6 ± 4.7		PD			
van Hoeck 2003 [113]	8	2–12	1 week crossover of NIPD ± daytime icodextrin		Kt/V increased from 1.99 to 2.54	CrCl increased from 35 to 65	No change in plasma albumin or PD losses, increased AA losses but no change in plasma AAs

Abbreviations: CCPD, continuous cycling PD, peritoneal dialysis; NIPD, nocturnal intermittent peritoneal dialysis; URR, urea reduction ratio; nPCR, normalized protein catabolic rate.

rhGH

The efficacy of rhGH in CKF and posttransplantation has been the subject of a Cochrane review [118]. Fifteen randomized controlled trials involving 629 children were identified [119–131]. Ten trials compared rhGH with placebo or no treatment [119–127] (Table 58.6). rhGH at 28 IU/m²/week resulted in a significant increase in HtSDS at 1 year (weighted mean difference, 0.78 SDS, 95% confidence interval, 0.52–1.04) and a significant increase in height velocity at 6 months (weighted mean difference, 2.85 cm/6 months; 95% confidence interval, 2.22–3.48) and 1 year (weighted mean difference, 3.80 cm/year; 95% confidence interval, 3.20–4.39) [118]. Results were independent of pubertal stage or treatment modality (CKF, dialysis, or transplant). The frequencies of reported side effects were similar for the rhGH-treated group and the controls. There was no further improvement in subsequent years of treatment. It is not certain whether rhGH therapy improves FH, but data from cohort studies suggest that it does [118]. The remaining five trials compared two different doses of rhGH: four trials compared 28 IU/m²/week with 14 IU/m²/week in CKF [129–131], dialysis [129–131], and posttransplant [130–132] patients. The group treated with 28 IU/m²/week showed a 1.34-cm/year (0.55–2.13) increase in height velocity compared to those given 14 IU/m²/week. However, increasing the dose to 56 IU/m²/week showed no further benefit over 28 IU/m²/week [131].

Alternate-day steroids and steroid withdrawal posttransplantation

Better growth occurs in children on alternate-day versus daily steroids, with no detriment to graft function [133–136] (Table 58.7). However, this may be confounded by selection bias of patients with better graft function to the alternate-day regimen [135,136].

Some have recommended no steroids or steroid withdrawal, and relevant studies have been reviewed recently [137,138]. Steroid withdrawal over 2–12 months was associated with improved growth in six of seven studies [139–145] but again, selection bias applies. The same is true for patients managed with steroid-free immunosuppression [138,146,147].

Deflazacort is derived from prednisolone and is said to have equivalent immunosuppressive effects to prednisolone and prednisone but with less toxicity. It was shown to improve growth and body composition after kidney transplantation when used in an equivalent dose to prednisolone in four studies by the same group [148–151]. However, a blinded controlled trial over 1 year in 40 patients with steroid-sensitive nephrotic syndrome showed no benefit on growth [152].

Effect of height on long-term outcome

Malnutrition and poor growth are associated with increased morbidity and mortality. Patients <18 years of age initiating dialysis with hypoalbuminemia are at a higher risk for death: in 1723 children, each decrease in serum albumin of 10 g/L was associated with a 54% higher risk of death, which was independent of other potential confounding variables [153]. An HtSDS less than −2.5 at dialysis initiation is associated with poor school attendance, more time in the hospital, and a twofold higher risk of death [154,155]. Each decrease in HtSDS or Ht velocity by 1 SD was associated with a 14% or 12% increase in risk for death, respectively. A U-shaped association between BMI and death, with low and high BMIs associated with an increased risk for death, has been demonstrated [156].

Table 58.6 Effects of rhGH on growth versus placebo or no treatment.

Study [reference]	No. of patients	Type of patients	Experimental intervention (rhGH dose)	Control intervention	Ht velocity, cm/yr (SD), with 1 yr of rhGH [treated (T) vs. control (C)]	ΔHtSDS[a] (SD) with 1 yr of rhGH [treated (T) vs. control (C)]
Fine 1994 [119]	82	Predialysis, prepuberty	28 IU/m²/wk s.c. for 24 mos	Placebo injection s.c. for 24 mos	T: 10.7 (3.1); C: 6.5 (2.6)	T: 1.01 (0.94); C: −0.08 (0.96)
Fine 2002 [120]	52	Posttransplant, pre-/early puberty	28 IU/m²/wk s.c. for 12 mos	No treatment	T: 8.59 (2.46); C: 4.23 (1.92)	HtSDS, T: −2.58 (1.04); C: −2.99 (0.88)
Ghio 2002 [121]	21	Posttransplant, prepuberty	30 IU/m²/wk s.c. for 12 mos	No treatment	T: 6.48 (3.44); C: 4.60 (4.46)	
Guest 1998 [122]	85	Posttransplant, pre-/early puberty	30 IU/m²/wk s.c. for 12 mos	No treatment	ΔHt: 3.60 (2.29); velocity: 0.40 (2.46)	T: 0.30 (1.11); C: 0.00 (1.30)
Hokken-Koelega 1991 [123]	16	Predialysis, prepuberty	28 IU/m²/wk s.c. for 6 mos	Placebo injection s.c. for 6 mos	T: 5.2 (1.2); C: 1.5 (0.4) (over 6 mos)	
Hokken-Koelega 1996 [124]	11	Posttransplant, pre-/early puberty	28 IU/m²/wk s.c. for 6 mos	Placebo injection s.c. for 6 mos	T: 1.4 (0.5–2.6); C: 0.8 (0.6–1.8) per 6 mos	T: −3.0 (−7.6 to −1.2); C: −2.6 (−3.6 to −2.1) (per 6 mos)
Kuizon 1998 [125]	14	Dialysis, prepuberty	28 IU/m²/wk s.c. for 6 mos	No treatment	T: 6.30 (2.94); C: 3.60 (1.41)	HtSDS, T: −1.36 (0.59); C: −2.18 (1.05)
Maxwell 1998 (2 trials) [126]	22	Transplant, pre-/early puberty	28 IU/m²/wk s.c. for 12 mos	No treatment	Change in Ht: 4.90 (2.26); velocity: 0.00 (1.85)	T; 0.88 (1.17); C: −0.20 (0.67)
Powell 1997 [127]	69	Predialysis, prepuberty	28 IU/m²/wk s.c. for 12 mos	No treatment	T: 8.00 (2.10); C: 4.80 (1.70)	T: 0.80 (0.50); C: 0.00 (0.30)
Sanchez 2002 [128]	23	Transplant, prepuberty	28 IU/m²/wk s.c. for 12 mos	No treatment		HtSDS, T: −1.09 (1.00); C: −2.80 (1.00)

Abbreviation: s.c., subcutaneous.

[a]For three studies, the HtSDS is shown, rather than the change in HtSDS.

Table 58.7 Effects of alternate-day steroids posttransplantation on growth.

Study [reference]	No. of patients on daily/no. on alt.-day steroids	Steroid regimen	Outcome
Broyer 1992 [133]	18/17	Randomized to daily or alternate day for 1 yr; all on alternate day in second year	1st yr, −0.29 SD on daily, +0.49 SD alternate day; 2nd yr, +0.29 SD and +0.52 SD
Feldhoff 1984 [134]	15/15	15 switched to alternate day matched with 15 on daily	Increase in HtVel in the 2nd but not the 1st yr
Kaiser 1994 [135]	24/31	31 switched to alternate day, but daily group had worse graft function and higher dose	+0.94 SD alternate day, −0.86 SD daily
Jabs 1996 [136]	1664/337	Not known how regimen selected	HtSDS up to 24 mos +0.5 SD on alternate day and +0.1 SD on daily

Abbreviation: Vel, velocity.

Table 58.8 Evidence table for all interventions on growth.

Intervention	SR[a]	Evidence rating[b,c] High	Evidence rating[b,c] Moderate	Evidence rating[b,c] Low	Comment	Recommendation[d] I	Recommendation[d] II	Recommendation[d] III	Comment
rhGH									
rhGH vs placebo or no treatment	+	•			10 RCTs (395 patients); variable quality; consistent results	•			Small benefit; height increase 3.80 (3.13–4.59) cm in 1 yr; harms of daily injections; high cost
rhGH 28 vs 14 IU/m^2/wk	+		•		5 RCTs (129 patients); variable quality; consistent results			•	Height increase 1.34 (0.55–2.13) cm in 1 yr; high cost
Oral nutritional supplements/dietetic input/nasogastric or gastrostomy feeds									
Composite intervention in <2 yrs of age	—			•	10 case series (169 patients); generally consistent results		•		Benefit of improved/stable growth exceeds reported harms
Composite intervention in >2 yrs of age	—			•	9 case series (232 patients); inconsistent results			•	Uncertain benefit; few reported harms
AA supplements/intradialytic parenteral nutrition									
EAA supplements	—			•	4 case series (47 patients); inconsistent results			•	Uncertain benefit; growth reported in 3 of 4 studies; no evidence on harms; expensive
Amino acid vs glucose PD solutions	—			•	6 observational studies (47 patients); inconsistent results			•	No demonstrated benefit; no difference in harms; growth reported in 2 of 6 studies; expensive
Intradialytic parenteral nutrition	—			•	4 case series (19 patients); inconsistent results			•	Uncertain benefit; no difference in harms; growth reported in 3 of 4 studies; expensive
Dialysis adequacy									
Increase in dialysis adequacy	—			•	5 case series (109 patients); consistent results			•	Uncertain benefit; no harms reported; growth reported in 2 of 5 studies
Alternate-day steroids/steroid withdrawal posttransplant									
Alternate-day steroids	—		•		1 RCT (35 patients) and 3 case series (2086 patients); consistent results		•		Increased HtSDS; no increase in harms; patient selection bias
Steroid withdrawal or no-steroid regimen	—			•	7 observational studies (237 patients); consistent results			•	Improved HtSDS; no increase in harms; patient selection bias

[a]Systematic review of randomized controlled trials (RCTs).
[b]Evidence rating based on study design, study quality, consistency, and directness of results. [c]No intervention was rated with a high evidence rating.
[d]Recommendations based on trade-offs between benefits and harms, quality of evidence, translation of evidence into practice in a specific setting including availability of medication, and any uncertainty about the baseline risk of the disease in the population. I, recommend; II, suggest; III, no recommendation possible.

Conclusions

Short stature is common in children of all ages who have renal disease and it has an important influence on outcome. Results of potential interventions to improve growth are summarized in Table 58.8. Adequate nutrition is vital, particularly in the first 2 years of life but also in older children. Feedings often need to be administered by nasogastric or gastrostomy tubes and require dietetic input for prescription adjustment. There is no evidence of benefit from EAAs orally, AA-based PD solutions, or intradialytic parenteral nutrition. Dialysis prescription is likely to affect growth, but the ideal dose is unknown. The use of the lowest possible alternate-day steroid dose offers the best chance of good growth posttransplantation. One year of rhGH may improve growth by 4 cm/year for all treatment modalities and may improve FH. All these interventions have a very low complication rate.

References

1 Rees L, Rigden SP, Ward GM. Chronic renal failure and growth. *Arch Dis Child* 1989; **64**: 573–577.

2 Lackland DT, Bendall HE, Osmond C, Egan BM, Barker DJ. Low birth weights contribute to high rates of early-onset chronic renal failure in the southeastern United States. *Arch Intern Med* 2000; **160**: 1472–1476.

3 Rodriguez-Soriano J, Aguirre M, Oliveros R, Vallo A. Long-term renal follow-up of extremely low birth weight infants. *Pediatr Nephrol* 2005; **20**: 579–584.

4 Simeoni U, Zetterstrom R. Long-term circulatory and renal consequences of intrauterine growth restriction. *Acta Paediatr* 2005; **94**: 819–824.

5 Keijzer-Veen MG, Schrevel M, Finken MJ, Dekker FW, Nauta J, Hille ET *et al.* Microalbuminuria and lower glomerular filtration rate at young adult age in subjects born very premature and after intrauterine growth retardation. *J Am Soc Nephrol* 2005; **16**: 2531–2532.

6 Zidar N, Avgustin Cavic M, Kenda RB, Ferluga D. Unfavorable course of minimal change nephrotic syndrome in children with intrauterine growth retardation. *Kidney Int* 1998; **54**: 1320–1323.

7 Sheu JN, Chen JH. Minimal change nephrotic syndrome in children with intrauterine growth retardation. *Am J Kidney Dis* 2001; **37**: 909–914.

8 Na YW, Yang HJ, Choi JH, Yoo KH, Hong YS, Lee JW *et al.* Effect of intrauterine growth retardation on the progression of nephrotic syndrome. *Am J Nephrol* 2002; **22**: 463–467.

9 Rizzoni G, Basso T, Setari M. Growth in children with chronic renal failure on conservative treatment. *Kidney Int* 1984; **26**: 52–58.

10 Karlberg J, Schaefer F, Hennicke M, Wingen AM, Rigden S, Mehls O. Early age-dependent growth impairment in chronic renal failure. European Study Group for Nutritional Treatment of Chronic Renal Failure in Childhood. *Pediatr Nephrol* 1996; **10**: 283–287.

11 Ledermann SE, Shaw V, Trompeter RS. Long-term enteral nutrition in infants and young children with chronic renal failure. *Pediatr Nephrol* 1999; **13**: 870–5.

12 Van Dyck M, Bilem N, Proesmans W. Conservative treatment for chronic renal failure from birth: a 3-year follow-up study. *Pediatr Nephrol* 1999; **13**: 865–869.

13 Kari JA, Gonzalez C, Ledermann SE, Shaw V, Rees L. Outcome and growth of infants with severe chronic renal failure. *Kidney Int* 2000; **57**: 1681–1687.

14 Parekh RS, Flynn JT, Smoyer WE, Milne JL, Kershaw DB, Bunchman TE *et al.* Improved growth in young children with severe chronic renal insufficiency who use specified nutritional therapy. *J Am Soc Nephrol* 2002; **13**: 1421–1422.

15 Rees L, Greene SA, Adlard P, Jones J, Haycock GB, Rigden SP *et al.* Growth and endocrine function in steroid sensitive nephrotic syndrome. *Arch Dis Child* 1988; **63**: 484–490.

16 Polito C, Di Toro R. Delayed pubertal growth spurt in glomerulopathic boys receiving alternate-day prednisone. *Child Nephrol Urol* 1992; **12**: 202–207.

17 Rees L, Greene SA, Adlard P, Jones J, Haycock GB, Rigden SP *et al.* Growth and endocrine function after renal transplantation. *Arch Dis Child* 1988; **63**: 1326–1332.

18 Wuhl E, Schaefer F. Puberty in chronic renal failure. *Adv Ren Replace Ther* 1999; **6**: 335–343.

19 Foote KD, Brocklebank JT, Meadow SR. Height attainment in children with steroid-responsive nephrotic syndrome. *Lancet* 1985; **ii**: 917–919.

20 Ruth EM, Kemper MJ, Leumann EP, Laube GF, Neuhaus TJ. Children with steroid-sensitive nephrotic syndrome come of age: long-term outcome. *J Pediatr* 2005; **147**: 202–207.

21 Foster BJ, Shults J, Zemel BS, Leonard MB. Interactions between growth and body composition in children treated with high-dose chronic glucocorticoids. *Am J Clin Nutr* 2004; **80**: 1334–1341.

22 Berns JS, Gaudio KM, Krassner LS, Anderson FP, Durante D, McDonald BM, *et al.* Steroid-responsive nephrotic syndrome of childhood: a long-term study of clinical course, histopathology, efficacy of cyclophosphamide therapy, and effects on growth. *Am J Kidney Dis* 1987; **9**: 108–114.

23 Padilla R, Brem AS. Linear growth of children with nephrotic syndrome: effect of alkylating agents. *Pediatrics* 1989; **84**: 495–9.

24 Soliman AT, Madina EH, Abdel Fattah M, el Zalabany MM, Asfour M, Morsi MR. Nocturnal growth hormone (GH) secretion and GH response to clonidine provocation in children before and after long-term prednisone therapy. *J Trop Pediatr* 1995; **41**: 344–347.

25 Sinha MD, Macleod R, Rigby E, Godfrey B, Clark A. Treatment of severe steroid-dependent nephrotic syndrome (SDNS) in children with tacrolimus. *Nephrol Dial Transplant* 2006; **21**: 1761–1763.

26 Tsau YK, Chen CH, Lee PI. Growth in children with nephrotic syndrome. *Taiwan Yi Xue Hui Za Zhi* 1989; **88**: 900–906.

27 Emma F, Sesto A, Rizzoni G. Long-term linear growth of children with severe steroid-responsive nephrotic syndrome. *Pediatr Nephrol* 2003; **18**: 783–788.

28 Saha MT, Laippala P, Lenko HL. Normal growth of prepubertal nephrotic children during long-term treatment with repeated courses of prednisone. *Acta Paediatr* 1998; **87**: 545–548.

29 Donatti TL, Koch VH, Fujimura MD, Okay Y. Growth in steroid-responsive nephrotic syndrome: a study of 85 pediatric patients. *Pediatr Nephrol* 2003; **18**: 789–795.

30 Kitamura M. Growth retardation in children with frequent relapsing nephrotic syndrome on steroid: improvement of height velocity after administration of immunosuppressive agent. *Nippon Jinzo Gakkai Shi* 1992; **34**: 117–124.

31 Kleinknecht C, Broyer M, Huot D, Marti-Henneberg C, Dartois AM. Growth and development of nondialyzed children with chronic renal failure. *Kidney Int Suppl* 1983; **15**: S40–S47.

32 Karlberg J, Schaefer F, Hennicke M, Wingen AM, Rigden S, Mehls O. Early age-dependent growth impairment in chronic renal failure. European Study Group for Nutritional Treatment of Chronic Renal Failure in Childhood. *Pediatr Nephrol* 1996; **10**: 283–287.

33 Van Dyck M, Proesmans W. Head circumference in chronic renal failure from birth. *Clin Nephrol* 2001; **56**: S13–S16.

34 Rizzoni G, Basso T, Setari M. Growth in children with chronic renal failure on conservative treatment. *Kidney Int* 1984; **26**: 52–58.

35 Karlberg J, Schaefer F, Hennicke M, Wingen AM, Rigden S, Mehls O. Early age-dependent growth impairment in chronic renal failure. European Study Group for Nutritional Treatment of Chronic Renal Failure in Childhood. *Pediatr Nephrol* 1996; **10**: 283–287.

36 Fivush BA, Jabs K, Neu AM, Sullivan EK, Feld L, Kohaut E *et al.* Chronic renal insufficiency in children and adolescents: the 1996 annual report of NAPRTCS. North American Pediatric Renal Transplant Cooperative Study. *Pediatr Nephrol* 1998; **12**: 328–337.

37 Lewy JE. Treatment of children in the U.S. with end-stage renal disease (ESRD). *Med Arh* 2001; **55**: 201–202.

38 Seikaly MG, Ho PL, Emmett L, Fine RN, Tejani A. Chronic renal insufficiency in children: the 2001 Annual Report of the NAPRTCS. *Pediatr Nephrol* 2003; **18**: 796–804.

39 Riano Galan I, Rey Galan C, Del Molino Anta A, Santos Rodriguez F, Malaga Guerrero S, Crespo Hernandez M. Chronic renal insufficiency in 22 children: diagnosis and evolution. *An Esp Pediatr* 1989; **30**: 275–278.

40 Waller S, Ledermann S, Trompeter R, van't Hoff W, Ridout D, Rees L. Catch-up growth with normal parathyroid hormone levels in chronic renal failure. *Pediatr Nephrol* 2003; **18**: 1236–1241.

41 Polito C, Greco L, Totino SF, Oporto MR, La Manna A, Strano CG *et al.* Statural growth of children with chronic renal failure on conservative treatment. *Acta Paediatr Scand* 1987; **76**: 97–102.

42 Scharer K. Growth and development of children with chronic renal failure. Study Group on Pubertal Development in Chronic Renal Failure. *Acta Paediatr Scand Suppl* 1990; **366**: 90–92.

43 Polito C, La Manna A, Iovene A, Stabile D. Pubertal growth in children with chronic renal failure on conservative treatment. *Pediatr Nephrol* 1995; **9**: 734–736.

44 Gorman G, Fivush B, Frankenfield D, Warady B, Watkins S, Brem A *et al.* Short stature and growth hormone use in pediatric hemodialysis patients. *Pediatr Nephrol* 2005; **20**: 1794–1800.

45 Schaefer F, Klaus G, Muller-Wiefel DE, Mehls O. Current practice of peritoneal dialysis in children: results of a longitudinal survey. Mid European Pediatric Peritoneal Dialysis Study Group (MEPPS). *Perit Dial Int* 1999; **19**(Suppl 2): S445–S449.

46 Kaiser BA, Polinsky MS, Stover J, Morgenstern BZ, Baluarte HJ. Growth of children following the initiation of dialysis: a comparison of three dialysis modalities. *Pediatr Nephrol* 1994; **8**: 733–738.

47 Turenne MN, Port FK, Strawderman RL, Ettenger RB, Alexander SR, Lewy JE, Jones CA, Agodoa LY, Held PJ. Growth rates in pediatric dialysis patients and renal transplant recipients. *Am J Kidney Dis* 1997; **30**: 193–203.

48 Honda M, Kamiyama Y, Kawamura K, Kawahara K, Shishido S, Nakai H *et al.* Growth, development and nutritional status in Japanese children under 2 years on continuous ambulatory peritoneal dialysis. *Pediatr Nephrol* 1995; **9**: 543–548.

49 Qamar IU, Balfe JW. Experience with chronic peritoneal dialysis in infants. *Child Nephrol Urol* 1991; **11**: 159–164.

50 Verrina E, Zacchello G, Perfumo F, Edefonti A, Sorino P, Bassi S *et al.* Clinical experience in the treatment of infants with chronic peritoneal dialysis. *Adv Perit Dial* 1995; **11**: 281–284.

51 Neu AM, Ho PL, McDonald RA, Warady BA. Chronic dialysis in children and adolescents. The 2001 annual report of the North American Pediatric Renal Transplant Cooperative Study. *Pediatr Nephrol* 2002; **17**: 656–663.

52 Shroff R, Wright E, Ledermann S, Hutchinson C, Rees L. Chronic hemodialysis in infants and children under 2 years of age. *Pediatr Nephrol* 2003; **18**: 378–383.

53 Al-Hermi BE, Al-Saran K, Secker D, Geary DF. Hemodialysis for end-stage renal disease in children weighing less than 10 kg. *Pediatr Nephrol* 1999; **13**: 401–403.

54 Shroff R, Rees L, Trompeter R, Hutchinson C, Ledermann S. Long-term outcome of chronic dialysis in children. *Pediatr Nephrol* 2006; **21**: 257–264.

55 Cansick J, Ridout D, Waller S, Rees L. Growth in and PTH in prepubertal children on long-term dialysis. *Pediatr Nephrol* 2007; **22**: 1349–1354.

56 Holtta TM, Ronnholm KA, Jalanko H, Ala-Houhala M, Antikainen M, Holmberg C. Peritoneal dialysis in children under 5 years of age. *Perit Dial Int* 1997; **17**(6): 573–580.

57 Van Diemen-Steenvoorde R, Donckerwolcke RA. Growth and sexual maturation in paediatric patients treated by dialysis and following kidney transplantation. *Acta Paediatr Scand Suppl* 1988; **343**: 109–117.

58 Neu AM, Bedinger M, Fivush BA, Warady BA, Watkins SL, Friedman AL *et al.* Growth in adolescent hemodialysis patients: data from the Centers for Medicare & Medicaid Services ESRD Clinical Performance Measures Project. *Pediatr Nephrol* 2005; **20**: 1156–1160.

59 Ninik A, McTaggart SJ, Gulati S, Powell HR, Jones CL, Walker RG. Factors influencing growth and final height after renal transplantation. *Pediatr Transplant* 2002; **6**: 219–223.

60 Vester U, Schaefer A, Kranz B, Wingen AM, Nadalin S, Paul A *et al.* Development of growth and body mass index after pediatric renal transplantation. *Pediatr Transplant* 2005; **9**: 445–449.

61 Nissel R, Brazda I, Feneberg R, Wigger M, Greiner C, Querfeld U *et al.* Effect of renal transplantation in childhood on longitudinal growth and adult height. *Kidney Int* 2004; **66**: 792–800.

62 Iitaka K, Hojo M, Moriya S, Sakai T, Endo T. Comparison of growth during continuous ambulatory peritoneal dialysis and renal transplantation using conventional immunosuppressive drugs in children. *Perit Dial Int* 1998; **18**: 395–401.

63 Tejani A, Fine R, Alexander S, Harmon W, Stablein D. Factors predictive of sustained growth in children after renal transplantation. The North American Pediatric Renal Transplant Cooperative Study. *J Pediatr* 1993; **122**: 397–402.

64 So SK, Chang PN, Najarian JS, Mauer SM, Simmons RL, Nevins TE. Growth and development in infants after renal transplantation. *J Pediatr* 1987; **110**: 343–350.

65 Humar A, Arrazola L, Mauer M, Matas AJ, Najarian JS. Kidney transplantation in young children: should there be a minimum age? *Pediatr Nephrol* 2001; **16**: 941–945.

66 Qvist E, Marttinen E, Ronnholm K, Antikainen M, Jalanko H, Sipila I *et al.* Growth after renal transplantation in infancy or early childhood. *Pediatr Nephrol* 2002; **17**: 438–443.

67 Tejani AH, Sullivan EK, Harmon WE, Fine RN, Kohaut E, Emmett L *et al.* Pediatric renal transplantation: the NAPRTCS experience. *Clin Transpl* 1997; **1997**: 87–100.

68 Kari JA, Romagnoli J, Duffy P, Fernando ON, Rees L, Trompeter RS. Renal transplantation in children under 5 years of age. *Pediatr Nephrol* 1999; **13**: 730–736.

69 Dall'Amico R, Ginevri F, Ghio L, Murer L, Perfumo F, Zanon GF et al. Successful renal transplantation in children under 6 years of age. *Pediatr Nephrol* 2001; **16**: 1–7.

70 Maxwell H, Haffner D, Rees L. Catch-up growth occurs after renal transplantation in children of pubertal age. *J Pediatr* 1998; **133**: 435–440.

71 Omoloja A, Stolfi A, Mitsnefes M. Pediatric obesity at renal transplantation: a single center experience. *Pediatr Transplant* 2005; **9**: 770–772.

72 Hanevold CD, Ho PL, Talley L, Mitsnefes MM. Obesity and renal transplant outcome: a report of the North American Pediatric Renal Transplant Cooperative Study. *Pediatrics* 2005; **115**: 352–356.

73 Rodriguez-Soriano J, Vallo A, Quintela MJ, Malaga S, Loris C. Predictors of final adult height after renal transplantation during childhood: a single-center study. *Nephron* 2000; **86**: 266–273.

74 Motoyama O, Hasegawa A, Ohara T, Satoh M, Shishido S, Honda M et al. A prospective trial of steroid withdrawal after renal transplantation treated with cyclosporine and mizoribine in children: results obtained between 1990 and 2003. *Pediatr Transplant* 2005; **9**: 232–238.

75 Andre JL, Bourquard R, Guillemin F, Krier MJ, Briancon S. Final height in children with chronic renal failure who have not received growth hormone. *Pediatr Nephrol* 2003; **18**: 685–691.

76 K/DOQI clinical practice guidelines for nutrition in chronic renal failure. *Am J Kidney Dis* 2000; **35**(Suppl 2): S105–S136.

77 Renal Association. *Treatment of Adults and Children with Renal Failure. Standards and Audit Measures*, 3rd edn. The Renal Association, Hampshire, UK, 2002; 66–68.

78 Abitbol CL, Zilleruelo G, Montane B, Strauss J. Growth of uremic infants on forced feeding regimens. *Pediatr Nephrol*. 1993; **7**(2): 173–177.

79 Ellis EN, Yiu V, Harley F, Donaldson LA, Hand M, Warady BA et al. The impact of supplemental feeding in young children on dialysis: a report of the North American Pediatric Renal Transplant Cooperative Study. *Pediatr Nephrol* 2001; **16**: 404–408.

80 Reed EE, Roy LP, Gaskin KJ, Knight JF. Nutritional intervention and growth in children with chronic renal failure. *J Ren Nutr* 1998; **8**: 122–126.

81 Ramage IJ, Geary DF, Harvey E, Secker DJ, Balfe JA, Balfe JW. Efficacy of gastrostomy feeding in infants and older children receiving chronic peritoneal dialysis. *Perit Dial Int* 1999; **19**: 231–236.

82 Ledermann SE, Scanes ME, Fernando ON, Duffy PG, Madden SJ, Trompeter RS. Long-term outcome of peritoneal dialysis in infants. *J Pediatr* 2000; **136**: 24–29.

83 Claris-Appiani A, Ardissino GL, Dacco V, Funari C, Terzi F. Catch-up growth in children with chronic renal failure treated with long-term enteral nutrition. *J Parenter Enteral Nutr* 1995; **19**: 175–178.

84 Strife CF, Quinlan M, Mears K, Davey ML, Clardy C. Improved growth of three uremic children by nocturnal nasogastric feedings. *Am J Dis Child* 1986; **140**: 438–443.

85 Norman LJ, Macdonald IA, Watson AR. Optimising nutrition in chronic renal insufficiency—growth. *Pediatr Nephrol* 2004; **19**: 1245–1252.

86 Guillot M, Broyer M, Cathelineau L, Boulegue D, Dartois AM, Folio D, Guimbaud P. Continuous enteral feeding in pediatric nephrology. Long-term results in children with congenital nephrotic syndrome, severe cystinosis and renal failure. *Arch Fr Pediatr* 1980; **37**: 497–505.

87 Coleman JE, Norman LJ, Watson AR. Provision of dietetic care in children on chronic peritoneal dialysis. *J Ren Nutr* 1999; **9**: 145–148.

88 Brewer ED. Growth of small children managed with chronic peritoneal dialysis and nasogastric tube feedings: 203-month experience in 14 patients. *Adv Perit Dial* 1990; **6**: 269–272.

89 Ledermann SE, Spitz L, Moloney J, Rees L, Trompeter RS. Gastrostomy feeding in infants and children on peritoneal dialysis. *Pediatr Nephrol* 2002; **17**: 246–250.

90 Ramage IJ, Harvey E, Geary DF, Hebert D, Balfe JA, Balfe JW. Complications of gastrostomy feeding in children receiving peritoneal dialysis. *Pediatr Nephrol* 1999; **13**: 249–252.

91 Davies BW, Watson AR, Coleman JE, Rance CH. Do gastrostomies close spontaneously? A review of the fate of gastrostomies following successful renal transplantation in children. *Pediatr Surg Int* 2001; **17**: 326–328.

92 Coleman JE, Watson AR. Growth posttransplantation in children previously treated with chronic dialysis and gastrostomy feeding. *Adv Perit Dial* 1998; **14**: 269–273.

93 Murakami R, Momota T, Yoshiya K, Yoshikawa N, Nakamura H, Honda M et al. Serum carnitine and nutritional status in children treated with continuous ambulatory peritoneal dialysis. *J Pediatr Gastroenterol Nutr* 1990; **11**: 371–374.

94 Jureidini KF, Hogg RJ, van Renen MJ, Southwood TR, Henning PH, Cobiac L et al. Evaluation of long-term aggressive dietary management of chronic renal failure in children. *Pediatr Nephrol* 1990; **4**: 1–10.

95 Mir S, Ozkayin N, Akgun A. The role of keto acids in the supportive treatment of children with chronic renal failure. *Pediatr Nephrol* 2005; **20**: 950–955.

96 Zachwieja J, Duran M, Joles JA, Allers PJ, van de Hurk D, Frankhuisen JJ et al. Amino acid and carnitine supplementation in haemodialysed children. *Pediatr Nephrol* 1994; **8**: 739–743.

97 Jones RW, Dalton N, Start K, El-Bishti MM, Chantler C. Oral essential amino acid supplements in children with advanced chronic renal failure. *Am J Clin Nutr* 1980; **33**: 1696–1702.

98 Canepa A, Perfumo F, Carrea A, Piccardo MT, Ciardi MR, Cantaluppi A et al. Continuous ambulatory peritoneal dialysis (CAPD) of children with amino acid solutions: technical and metabolic aspects. *Perit Dial Int* 1990; **10**: 215–220.

99 Hanning RM, Balfe JW, Zlotkin SH. Effect of amino acid containing dialysis solutions on plasma amino acid profiles in children with chronic renal failure. *J Pediatr Gastroenterol Nutr* 1987; **6**: 942–947.

100 Canepa A, Perfumo F, Carrea A, Giallongo F, Verrina E, Cantaluppi A et al. Long-term effect of amino-acid dialysis solution in children on continuous ambulatory peritoneal dialysis. *Pediatr Nephrol* 1991; **5**: 215–219.

101 Hanning RM, Balfe JW, Zlotkin SH. Effectiveness and nutritional consequences of amino acid-based vs glucose-based dialysis solutions in infants and children receiving CAPD. *Am J Clin Nutr* 1987; **46**: 22–30.

102 Qamar IU, Levin L, Balfe JW, Balfe JA, Secker D, Zlotkin S. Effects of 3-month amino acid dialysis compared to dextrose dialysis in children on continuous ambulatory peritoneal dialysis. *Perit Dial Int* 1994; **14**: 4–6.

103 Qamar IU, Secker D, Levin L, Balfe JA, Zlotkin S, Balfe JW. Effects of amino acid dialysis compared to dextrose dialysis in children on continuous cycling peritoneal dialysis. *Perit Dial Int* 1999; **19**: 237–247.

104 Canepa A, Carrea A, Menoni S, Verrina E, Trivelli A, Gusmano R et al. Acute effects of simultaneous intraperitoneal infusion of glucose and amino acids. *Kidney Int* 2001; **59**: 1967–1973.

105 Abitbol CL, Mrozinska K, Mandel S, McVicar M, Wapnir RA. Effects of amino acid additives during hemodialysis of children. *J Parenter Enteral Nutr* 1984; **8**: 25–29.

106 Krause I, Shamir R, Davidovits M, Frishman S, Cleper R, Gamzo Z et al. Intradialytic parenteral nutrition in malnourished children treated with hemodialysis. *J Ren Nutr* 2002; **12**: 55–59.

107 Goldstein SL, Baronette S, Gambrell TV, Currier H, Brewer ED. nPCR assessment and IDPN treatment of malnutrition in pediatric hemodialysis patients. *Pediatr Nephrol* 2002; **17**: 531–534.

108 Orellana P, Juarez-Congelosi M, Goldstein SL. Intradialytic parenteral nutrition treatment and biochemical marker assessment for malnutrition in adolescent maintenance hemodialysis patients. *J Ren Nutr* 2005; **15**: 312–317.

109 Holtta T, Ronnholm K, Jalanko H, Holmberg C. Clinical outcome of pediatric patients on peritoneal dialysis under adequacy control. *Pediatr Nephrol* 2000; **14**: 889–897.

110 Marsenic O, Peco-Antic A, Jovanovic O. Effect of dialysis dose on nutritional status of children on chronic hemodialysis. *Nephron* 2001; **88**: 273–275.

111 Tom A, McCauley L, Bell L, Rodd C, Espinosa P, Yu G et al. Growth during maintenance hemodialysis: impact of enhanced nutrition and clearance. *J Pediatr* 1999; **134**: 464–471.

112 Brem AS, Lambert C, Hill C, Kitsen J, Shemin DG. Outcome data on pediatric dialysis patients from the end-stage renal disease clinical indicators project. *Am J Kidney Dis* 2000; **36**: 310–317.

113 van Hoeck KJ, Rusthoven E, Vermeylen L, Vandesompel A, Marescau B, Lilien M et al. Nutritional effects of increasing dialysis dose by adding an icodextrin daytime dwell to nocturnal intermittent peritoneal dialysis (NIPD) in children. *Nephrol Dial Transplant* 2003; **18**: 1383–1387.

114 Schaefer F, Klaus G, Mehls O. Peritoneal transport properties and dialysis dose affect growth and nutritional status in children on chronic peritoneal dialysis. Mid-European Pediatric Peritoneal Dialysis Study Group. *J Am Soc Nephrol* 1999; **10**: 1786–1792.

115 Fischbach M, Terzic J, Menouer S, Dheu C, Soskin S, Helmstetter A et al. Intensified and daily hemodialysis in children might improve statural growth. *Pediatr Nephrol* 2006; **21**: 1746–1752.

116 Chadha V, Blowey DL, Warady BA. Is growth a valid outcome measure of dialysis clearance in children undergoing peritoneal dialysis? *Perit Dial Int* 2001; **21(Suppl 3)**: S179–S184.

117 Cano F, Azocar PM, Marin BV, Rodriguez SE, Delucchi BA, Ratner RR et al. Dialysis dose, nutrition and growth among pediatric patients on peritoneal dialysis. *Rev Med Chil* 2005; **133**: 1455–1464.

118 Vimalachandra D, Hodson EM, Willis NS, Craig JC, Cowell C, Knight JF. Growth hormone for children with chronic kidney disease. *Cochrane Database Syst Rev.* 2006 ; **3**: CD003264.

119 Fine RN, Kohaut EC, Brown D, Perlman AJ. Growth after recombinant human growth hormone treatment in children with chronic renal failure: report of a multicenter randomized double-blind placebo-controlled study. Genentech Cooperative Study Group. *J Pediatrics* 1994; **124**: 374–382.

120 Fine RN, Stablein D, Cohen AH, Tejani A, Kohaut E. Recombinant human growth hormone post-renal transplantation in children: a randomized controlled study of the NAPRTCS. *Kidney Int* 2002; **62**: 688–696.

121 Ghio L, Damiani B, Garavaglia R, Oppizzi G, Taioli E, Edefonti A. Lipid profile during rhGH therapy in pediatric renal transplant patients. *Pediatr Transplant* 2002; **6**: 127–131.

122 Guest G, Berard E, Crosnier H, Chevallier T, Rappaport R, Broyer M. Effects of growth hormone in short children after renal transplantation. *Pediatr Nephrol* 1998; **12**: 437–446.

123 Hokken-Koelega AC, Stijnen T, de Muinck Keizer-Schrama SM, Wit JM, Wolff ED, de Jong MC et al. Placebo-controlled, double-blind, cross-over trial of growth hormone treatment in prepubertal children with chronic renal failure. *Lancet* 1991; **338**: 585–590.

124 Hokken-Koelega AC, Sitjnen T, de Jong RC, Donckerwolcke RA, Groothoff JW, Wolff ED et al. A placebo-controlled, double-blind trial of growth hormone treatment in prepubertal children after renal transplant. *Kidney Int* 1996; **53**: 128–134.

125 Kuizon BD, Goodman WG, Gales B, Juppner H, Salusky IB. Effects of growth hormone on bone and mineral metabolism in dialyzed children. *J Am Soc Nephrol* 1998; **9**: 546–547.

126 Maxwell H, Rees L. Randomised controlled trial of recombinant human growth hormone in prepubertal and pubertal renal transplant recipients. British Association for Pediatric Nephrology. *Arch Dis Child* 1998; **79**: 481–487.

127 Powell DR, Liu F, Baker BK, Hintz RL, Lee PD, Durham SK et al. Modulation of growth factors by growth hormone in children with chronic renal failure. The Southwest Pediatric Nephrology Study Group. *Kidney Int* 1997; **51**: 1970–1979.

128 Sanchez CP, Kuizon BD, Goodman WG, Gales B, Ettenger RB, Inez Boechat M et al. Growth hormone and the skeleton in pediatric renal allograft recipients. *Pediatr Nephrol* 2002; **17**: 322–328.

129 Hertel NT, Holmberg C, Rönnholm KAR, Jacobsen BB, Ølgaard, Meeuwisse GW et al. Recombinant human growth hormone treatment, using two dose regimens in children with chronic renal failure: a report on linear growth and adverse effects. *J Pediatr Endocrinol* 2002; **15(5)**: 577–588.

130 Kitagawa T, Ito K, Ito H, Sakai T, Wada H, Kajiwara N. GH treatment of children with chronic renal insufficiency: a Japanese clinical trial. *Clin Pediatr Endocrinol* 1997; **6(Suppl 10)**: 73–80.

131 Hokken-Koelega AC, Stijnen T, de Jong MC, Donckerwolcke RA, de Muinck Keizer-Schrama SM, Blum WF et al. Double blind trial comparing the effects of two doses of growth hormone in prepubertal patients with chronic renal insufficiency. *J Clin Endocrinol Metab* 1994; **79(4)**: 1185–1190.

132 Ito K, Kawaguchi H. The use of rhGH in growth failure in children with various renal diseases. *Clin Pediatr Endocrinol* 1997; **6(Suppl 9)**: 49–53.

133 Broyer M, Guest G, Gagnadoux MF. Growth rate in children receiving alternate-day corticosteroid treatment after kidney transplantation. *J Pediatr* 1992; **120**: 721–725.

134 Feldhoff C, Goldman AI, Najarian JS, Mauer SM. A comparison of alternate day and daily steroid therapy in children following renal transplantation. *Int J Pediatr Nephrol* 1984; **5**: 11–14.

135 Kaiser BA, Polinsky MS, Palmer JA, Dunn S, Mochon M, Flynn JT et al. Growth after conversion to alternate-day corticosteroids in children with renal transplants: a single-center study. *Pediatr Nephrol* 1994; **8**: 320–325.

136 Jabs K, Sullivan EK, Avner ED, Harmon WE. Alternate-day steroid dosing improves growth without adversely affecting graft survival or long-term graft function. A report of the North American Pediatric Renal Transplant Cooperative Study. *Transplantation* 1996; **61**: 31–36.

137 Tonshoff B, Hocker B, Weber LT. Steroid withdrawal in pediatric and adult renal transplant recipients. *Pediatr Nephrol* 2005; **20**: 409–417.

138 Vidhun JR, Sarwal MM. Corticosteroid avoidance in pediatric renal transplantation. *Pediatr Nephrol* 2005; **20**: 418–426.

139 Guyot C, Karam G, Soulillou JP. Pediatric renal transplantation without maintenance steroids. *Transplant Proc* 1994; **26**: 97.

140 Motoyama O, Hasegawa A, Ohara T, Hattori M, Kawaguchi H, Takahashi K et al. A prospective trial of steroid cessation after renal transplantation in pediatric patients treated with cyclosporine and mizoribine. *Pediatr Transplant* 1997; **1**: 29–36.

141 Aikawa A, Miyagi M, Motoyama O, Shigetomi Y, Ohara T, Hirayama N *et al*. Pathological evaluation of steroid withdrawal in pediatric renal transplant recipients. *Pediatr Transplant* 1999; **3**: 131–138.

142 Reisman L, Lieberman KV, Burrows L, Schanzer H. Follow-up of cyclosporine-treated pediatric renal allograft recipients after cessation of prednisone. *Transplantation* 1990; **49**: 76–80.

143 Ellis D. Growth and renal function after steroid-free tacrolimus-based immunosuppression in children with renal transplants. *Pediatr Nephrol* 2000; **14**: 689–694.

144 Chao SM, Jones CL, Powell HR, Johnstone L, Francis DM, Becker GJ *et al*. Triple immunosuppression with subsequent prednisolone withdrawal: 6 years' experience in paediatric renal allograft recipients. *Pediatr Nephrol* 1994; **8**: 62–69.

145 Hasegawa A, Motoyama O, Shishido S, Ito K, Tsuzuki K, Takahashi K *et al*. A prospective trial of steroid withdrawal after renal transplantation in children: results obtained 1990 and 2002. *Transplant Proc* 2004; **36(2 Suppl)**: 216S–219S.

146 Birkeland SA, Larsen KE, Rohr N. Pediatric renal transplantation without steroids. *Pediatr Nephrol* 1998; **12**: 87–92.

147 Sarwal MM, Vidhun JR, Alexander SR, Satterwhite T, Millan M, Salvatierra O, Jr. Continued superior outcomes with modification and lengthened follow-up of a steroid-avoidance pilot with extended daclizumab induction in pediatric renal transplantation. *Transplantation* 2003; **76**: 1331–1339.

148 Ferraris JR, Day PF, Gutman R, Granillo E, Ramirez J, Ruiz S *et al*. Effect of therapy with a new glucocorticoid, deflazacort, on linear growth and growth hormone secretion after renal transplantation. *J Pediatr* 1992; **121(5 Pt 1)**: 809–813.

149 Ferraris JR, Pasqualini T. Therapy with a new glucocorticoid: effect of deflazacort on linear growth and growth hormone secretion in renal transplantation. *J Rheumatol Suppl* 1993; **37**: 43–46.

150 Ferraris JR, Pennisi P, Pasqualini T, Jasper H. Effects of deflazacort immunosuppression on long-term growth and growth factors after renal transplantation. *Pediatr Nephrol* 1997; **11**: 322–324.

151 Ferraris JR, Pasqualini T, Legal S, Sorroche P, Galich AM, Pennisi P *et al*. Effect of deflazacort versus methylprednisone on growth, body composition, lipid profile, and bone mass after renal transplantation. The Deflazacort Study Group. *Pediatr Nephrol* 2000; **14**: 682–688.

152 Broyer M, Terzi F, Lehnert A, Gagnadoux MF, Guest G, Niaudet P. A controlled study of deflazacort in the treatment of idiopathic nephrotic syndrome. *Pediatr Nephrol* 1997; **11**: 418–422.

153 Wong CS, Hingorani S, Gillen DL, Sherrard DJ, Watkins SL, Brandt JR *et al*. Hypoalbuminemia and risk of death in pediatric patients with end-stage renal disease. *Kidney Int*. 2002; **61(2)**: 630–637.

154 Furth SL, Stablein D, Fine RN, Powe NR, Fivush BA. Adverse clinical outcomes associated with short stature at dialysis initiation: a report of the North American Pediatric Renal Transplant Cooperative Study. *Pediatrics* 2002; **109(5)**: 909–913.

155 Furth SL, Hwang W, Yang C, Neu AM, Fivush BA, Powe NR. Growth failure, risk of hospitalization and death for children with end-stage renal disease. *Pediatr Nephrol* 2002; **17(6)**: 450–455.

156 Wong CS, Gipson DS, Gillen DL, Emerson S, Koepsell T, Sherrard DJ *et al*. Anthropometric measures and risk of death in children with end-stage renal disease. *Am J Kidney Dis* 2000; **36(4)**: 811–819.

59 Hypertension, Cardiovascular Disease, and Lipid Abnormalities in Children with Chronic Kidney Failure

Elke Wühl & Franz Schaefer

Division of Pediatric Nephrology, Center for Pediatric and Adolescent Medicine, University of Heidelberg,
Im Neuenheimer Feld 430, 69120 Heidelberg, Germany

Introduction

Cardiovascular complications are the major cause of the excessive morbidity and mortality observed in adults with chronic kidney disease (CKD). Significant cardiovascular disease (CVD) occurs also in children with CKD and is the leading cause of death in young adults with childhood-onset end-stage renal disease (ESRD) [1,2]. Even in the pediatric age range, where cardiovascular mortality is extremely low, 25% of deaths in ESRD are attributable to CVD [3]. This increased cardiovascular risk appears to be related to increased exposure to general risk factors, such as hypertension and dyslipidemia, as well as to conditions specifically associated with uremia, including abnormal mineral metabolism, chronic inflammation, oxidative stress, and anemia. This section reviews the current strategies to prevent, detect, and treat cardiovascular complications and disease progression in children with CKD.

Hypertension

CKD is the most prevalent cause of arterial hypertension in the pediatric population, accounting for at least three-fourths of cases requiring pharmacological therapy [4]. This is in striking contrast to adults, in whom primary (or essential) hypertension predominates. The fraction of children with secondary hypertension decreases throughout childhood, whereas the prevalence of essential hypertension increases. Within the pediatric CKD population, the prevalence of hypertension is 20–50% in CKD stages II–IV, 50–80% in dialyzed patients, and up to 80% in kidney allograft recipients [5–8].

Multiple factors contribute to the high prevalence of hypertension in this population. Sympathetic hyperactivation is a key feature of CKD, which appears to occur very early in the course of CKD. The renin–angiotensin system (RAS) is activated in most pediatric nephropathies. Salt and fluid overload and functional nitric oxide deficiency due to accumulation of the circulating nitric oxide synthetase inhibitor asymmetric dimethyl-arginine contribute to hypertension in advanced CKD. Hypertensiogenic effects of calcineurin inhibitors and glucocorticoids play a major role in immunosuppressant-dependent nephropathies and after kidney transplantation.

The measurement and interpretation of blood pressure (BP) in pediatric patients is complicated by the marked physiological changes in body dimensions and cardiovascular dynamics that occur across childhood. Hence, the assessment of BP in children and adolescents should follow standardized measurement procedures and use appropriate normative BP data sets.

Measurement of BP in children and selection of appropriate normative data

BP measurements should be performed according to the guidelines of the National High Blood Pressure Education Program Working Group [9] after 5 min of rest, with the child sitting in an upright position (infants supine). An appropriate cuff with an inflatable bladder width of at least 40% of the upper arm circumference and a bladder length of 80–100% of arm circumference should be used. There is still no consensus on the preferred measurement device. Although the automated oscillometric technology is rapidly gaining popularity, the *Fourth Report* [9] still recommends auscultation, reasoning that most available reference values are based on this method and suggesting that oscillometric measurements above the 90th percentile should be repeated with auscultation. For auscultatory measurements, systolic BP is defined by the onset of tapping Korotkoff sounds (K1), and diastolic BP is defined by the disappearance of Korotkoff sounds (K5). However, elevated BP values must be confirmed on repeated visits or by ambulatory BP monitoring (ABPM) before classifying a child as hypertensive [9].

ABPM has become recognized in recent years as a new diagnostic reference standard for the investigation of hypertension in adults and children alike. The large number of BP measurements

Evidence-based Nephrology. Edited by Donald Molony and Jonathan Craig
© 2009 Blackwell Publishing, ISBN: 978-1-4051-3975-5.

obtained outside the office setting largely eliminates the "white coat effect" and also diurnal BP variability [10–13]. ABPM is superior to casual BP measurements in predicting cardiovascular outcomes in adults [14]. Although ABPM is technically feasible in children aged 3 years and older, the major drawbacks of this method are the logistic challenges associated with returning the device after use and the sophisticated biostatistical workup of the readings. Manual home BP monitoring is becoming a popular partial alternative to ABPM, avoiding the "white coat" setting, and a valuable way of actively involving patients in disease management [15]. However, the pediatric use of home BP measurements is hampered by the lack of comprehensive normative data. From a practical viewpoint, the greater sensitivity of BP measurements in the clinic (clinic BP) justifies its use in screening examinations, whereas ambulatory and home measurements show greater specificity and are therefore especially suited to confirm a suspected diagnosis of hypertension [16].

In adults, cardiovascular risk is a function of BP, even below the arbitrary cutoff levels that define hypertension. This has led to a steady lowering of the recommended BP levels in adults over the last few decades [17]. Pediatric studies linking BP to cardiovascular outcomes are lacking. Therefore, the pediatric definition of hypertension is based on the BP distribution in the general pediatric population from birth to age 18 years and is dependent on height, age, and gender. Although early reports regarded children at the 95th BP percentile as high-normal, the most recent guidelines [9], reflecting the trend in adult hypertension research, label BP values between the 90th and 95th percentiles or any value above 120/80 mmHg (whatever BP threshold is lower, irrespective of age) as prehypertensive. Systolic or diastolic BP values exceeding the 95th percentile are labeled as hypertensive (stage 1: systolic or diastolic BP in 95th to 99th percentile +5 mmHg; stage 2: systolic or diastolic BP in >99th percentile +5 mmHg).

The most comprehensive and commonly used pediatric normative data sets for auscultatory casual BP have been published by the National High BP Education Program for North America [9] and by de Man *et al.* for European children [18]. Reference data for casual oscillometric BP measurements are available for North American children [19,20]. For ABPM measurements, normative data have been provided both for oscillatory [21,22] and for auscultatory [23] ABPM measurements. No normative data exist for home BP measurements in children oscillatory normative BP data are available [24].

Efficacies of strategies for prevention and treatment of hypertension in children

In children with mild hypertension or essential hypertension, non-pharmacological treatment (therapeutic life-style modifications, including diet, exercise, and stress reduction) might be successful in lowering BP. Although difficult to achieve, weight loss is effective in lowering BP in overweight children [9,25]. Although restriction of sodium in salt-sensitive adults is beneficial in those with hypertension [26], evidence for a direct relationship between

sodium intake, diet, and BP in children is less conclusive, based on a meta-analysis of 37 pediatric studies [27].

In case of resistance to therapeutic life-style modification, and in most children with secondary hypertension, pharmacological treatment is required. The goal of antihypertensive treatment in children is reduction of BP below the 95th percentile unless concurrent conditions (such as CKD or diabetes) are present, in which case BP should be lowered at least below the 90th percentile (or <120/80 mmHg, whichever BP level is lower). Whether even stricter blood pressure control to levels below the 50th percentile will be of additional benefit in those children is the subject of the current ESCAPE trial [28].

Pharmacological treatment should be initiated with a single agent. Drug classes acceptable for use in children include angiotensin converting enzyme (ACE) inhibitors, angiotensin receptor blockers (ARBs), β-receptor blockers, calcium channel blockers, and diuretics [9]. Although most antihypertensive drugs marketed for adults have been used in children, few drugs have been proven effective and safe in children and received explicit regulatory authority approval for pediatric use to date (US Food and Drug Administration-approved drugs include, by class: ACE inhibitors benazepril, enalapril, fosinopril, and lisinopril; ARBs irbesartan and losartan; the β-receptor blocker propranolol; the Ca channel blocker amlodipine; and diuretics furosemide and hydrochlorothiazide). Recent clinical trials stimulated by the Best Pharmaceuticals for Children Act in the USA and emerging similar legislation in Europe are about to expand the number of drugs with pediatric dosage information.

In dialyzed children, dry weight [29] and dialysis prescription [30] must be frequently adapted to avoid fluid overload-induced hypertension. In pediatric kidney transplant recipients, modification of immunosuppressive medication, including calcineurin inhibitor and steroid withdrawal, may result in improved BP control [31].

The evidence ratings of recommendations for preventive strategies and treatment of hypertension in children with CKD are summarized in Tables 59.1 and 59.4. Because no systematic reviews exist for the treatment of hypertension in children, the overall evidence rating is only moderate. Life-style modification and diet failed to demonstrate a significant beneficial effect on hypertension in children with CKD. Data on steroid withdrawal in children with a transplanted kidney suggest a beneficial effect of steroid-free immunosuppressive regimens on BP. There is evidence that Ca channel blockers, ACE inhibitors, and ARBs are effective and safe in lowering BP in pediatric renal hypertension. Considering their superior side effect profile and in accordance with data in adults, ACE inhibitors and ARBs should be preferred over Ca channel blockers as first-line antihypertensive agents in children with CKD.

CVD in children with CKF

Left ventricular hypertrophy (LVH) is second only to age as the most powerful predictor of cardiovascular events in adults. The best noninvasive assessment of cardiac mass is the estimation of

Table 59.1 Evidence ratings and recommendations for treatment of hypertension in children with CKD.

Intervention	Existing systematic pediatric reviews	Overall evidence rating[a]			Recommendation[b]			
		Moderate	Low	Comment	I	II	III	Comment
Therapeutic life-style modification	No		●	No evidence from pediatric CTs; some evidence from adult RCTs			●	No conclusive data from children with CKD
Reduction of salt intake, dietary intervention	No	●		Pediatric meta-analysis, Cochrane review from adult studies		●		Data from pediatric meta-analysis inconclusive
Efficacy of antihypertensive agents								
β-blockers	No	●		One short-term study in 11 children with CKD; evidence from adult RCTs	●			Consistently effective in lowering BP
Ca^{2+} channel blockers	No	●		Moderate evidence from pediatric CTs (4 trials, 150 CKD patients); evidence from adult RCTs	●			Consistently effective in lowering BP
ACE inhibitors and ARBs	No	●		Good evidence from pediatric CTs (9 trials, >600 CKD patients)	●			Consistently effective in lowering BP and proteinuria
Superiority of RAS antagonists in treating CKD-related hypertension	No	●		High evidence from adult RCTs	●			Equally effective in lowering BP, additional reduction of proteinuria
Other interventions								
Adjustment of dry weight (CKD 5)	No	●		Limited evidence from pediatric CTs; evidence from adult studies	●			Favorable outcome under intensified dialysis regimen and dry weight adjustment
Steroid withdrawal in transplant patients	No	●		Limited evidence from pediatric data; evidence from adult RCTs	●			Pediatric RCT underway

Abbreviations: RCT, randomized controlled trial; CT, clinical trial.

[a]Evidence rating based on study design, study quality, consistency, and directness of results. No intervention was rated with a high or a very low evidence rating.

[b]Recommendations based on trade-offs between benefits and harms, quality of evidence, translation of evidence into practice in a specific setting including availability of medication, and any uncertainty about the baseline risk of the disease in the population. I, recommend; II, suggest; III, no recommendation possible.

left ventricular mass (LVM) by echocardiographic standardized measurements. Age, height, weight, gender, and BP each exert an independent influence on LVM in children [32]. Using the Devereux formula indexed to height (in meters) to the power of 2.7 will partly correct for the influence of body dimensions and age [33–35]. Controversy exists about the cutoff levels of LVM to define LVH in children. The *Fourth Report* [9] suggests using the adult level (i.e. 51 g/m$^{2.7}$), but this is very conservative, because the 95th percentile of LVM in children is approximately 38 g/m$^{2.7}$ and the adult 97th percentile of 51 g/m$^{2.7}$ is far above the 99th pediatric percentile [36]. Although studies linking LVM to CVD in children are lacking, it appears reasonable to define, in analogy to BP limits, any LVM above the 95th percentile as significant LVH to be considered for intensified antihypertensive treatment. An LVM index of 38–51 would indicate mild to moderate LVH, and an index above 51 would indicate severe LVH.

LVH is the most common identifiable cardiac alteration in ESRD, affecting approximately one-third of children with CKD

stages II–IV [36–38] and up to 80% of dialysis patients [2,39–41]. Notably, in children with mild to moderate CKD, LVM is only weakly inversely correlated with glomerular filtration rate (GFR), and LVH is common, even in patients with minimal impairment of renal function. In children after kidney transplantation, LVH often persists despite improved renal function [42,43]. Both concentric and eccentric changes in left ventricular geometry are common, independent of the level of residual renal function [36,40]. The increase of LVM in children with CKD is associated with an impairment of intrinsic left ventricular contractility [44].

The factors associated with LVH are similar to those observed in adults with CKD. Hemoglobin is inversely correlated with LVM [36,40] and LV function [44]. The role of hypertension in LVH in children with CKD is still unclear. BP was correlated with LVM in children with severe LVH on dialysis, but not in a large cohort of children with stage II–IV CKD [36,40]. Hyperparathyroidism is correlated with LVH in adults [45,46] as well as in children [47,48]. Moreover, an association of LVH and abnormal LV geometry with increased C-reactive protein levels has suggested a role of occult inflammation in the pathogenesis of LVH in CKD [36].

An increase in carotid artery intima media thickness (IMT), as measured by high-resolution ultrasound, is considered an early marker of arteriosclerosis and a sensitive predictor of cardiovascular events both in the general population and in adult dialysis patients [49,50]. Increased carotid IMT has also been demonstrated in children who are considered at risk for CVD due to hypertension, obesity, or hyperlipidemia. Increased IMT that develops in the course of CKD is associated with stiffening of the large arteries, an abnormality that is related directly to an increased load to the left ventricle and impaired peripheral blood flow [51]. In children and adolescents with CKD on dialysis and after kidney transplantation significant increases of carotid IMT are detectable. The degree of vascular pathology depends on the level of renal dysfunction and is most marked in patients on dialysis [1,52–54]. The morphological changes are associated with an increased stiffness of large arteries. After correcting for BP, the total duration of dialysis, cumulative intake of calcium-containing phosphate binders, and time-integrated plasma parathyroid hormone levels are predictive of the alterations in carotid IMT and elasticity [47,52], strongly suggesting causative roles of the excessive calcium–phosphate load on dialysis and/or vascular actions of parathyroid hormone in CKD-associated arteriopathy .

Efficacies of strategies for prevention of CVD in children

The multifactorial etiology of CVD in CKD requires a multifaceted preventive strategy. The cardiovascular protective efficacies of individual preventive measures are supported by variable levels of evidence.

Anemia is associated with increased LVM and decreased cardiac function [55]. Thus, in concordance with the National Kidney Foundation Kidney Disease Outcomes Quality Initiative (K/DOQI) guidelines on management of renal anemia in children, maintenance of normal hemoglobin levels should be aimed for by early initiation of erythropoietin and iron therapy [56]. However, correction of anemia does not result in complete regression of LVH in adults, and full correction is associated with increased all-cause mortality [57,58].

In patients on dialysis, optimization of dry weight and reduction of interdialytic weight gain in hemodialysis may reduce volume effects on the cardiovascular system and, in addition, volume-dependent hypertension and activation of the RAS might be lessened.

Hypertension should be controlled adequately (see above), aiming for a BP target below the 90th percentile. A meta-analysis of more than 100 studies in adults yielded a moderately strong relationship between BP reduction and LVM regression [59]. Drug class-specific mechanisms may contribute to LVH regression beyond BP normalization. In a meta-analysis of 80 trials comparing the effects of different classes of antihypertensives on LVM in

adults, ACE inhibitors and ARBs exerted an additional beneficial effect on the prevention or regression of CVD [60].

In children with mild to moderate CKD, complete normalization of BP by ACE inhibition and the addition of other antihypertensive agents, if required, caused regression of LVM into the normal range in the vast majority of patients presenting with LVH (ESCAPE trial, unpublished data), despite the fact that a correlation between BP and LVM has been observed only in children with ESRD but not in stage II–IV CKD [2,36,40].

Calcium–phosphorus ion product and parathyroid hormone levels are correlated with carotid IMT and cumulative calcium-based phosphate binder intake with vascular morphology and function [47,52]. Hence, tight control of calcium–phosphorus metabolism with maintenance of normal calcium and phosphorus balances and prevention or correction of hyperparathyroidism is probably essential to improve the cardiovascular status of children with CKD. In adult dialysis patients the use of calcium-free phosphate binders largely halted coronary artery calcification, whereas progressive calcium deposition was seen in patients receiving calcium-based phosphate binders [61].

Renal function is correlated with carotid IMT, arterial function, and LVH. Uremic toxins and/or the state of microinflammation associated with failing kidney function may play a direct role in morphological and functional changes of the vascular wall and the myocardium. Therefore, renoprotective pharmacotherapy and correction of renal function by kidney transplantation may also be effective measures to prevent cardiovascular disease in CKD patients. Successful kidney transplantation led to partial regression of the CKD-associated carotid arteriopathy in children within 1 year of observation [62].

Progression of CKD toward end-stage renal failure is common and occurs irrespective of the underlying renal disease. There is clear evidence that hypertension and proteinuria are independent risk factors for progressive CKD in adult patients [63–65]. Dietary protein intake did not affect the rate of CKD progression substantially in seven randomized controlled clinical trials of adult nondiabetic nephropathies. However, a recent Cochrane review that combined these trials showed that reduction of protein intake delays the need for renal replacement therapy [66], most likely by reducing the accumulation of nitrogenous waste products. In a randomized controlled trial in children with CKD, prospective institution of a low-protein diet did not affect the rate of GFR loss, but proteinuria and hypertension were independent predictors of disease progression in the secondary data analysis [67].

Blockade of the RAS by ACE inhibitors and more recently, ARBs, has become the pharmacotherapy of first choice in children as in adults with CKD. Besides lowering BP effectively, RAS antagonists substantially reduce proteinuria. Several trials in adults with various acquired nephropathies have confirmed the initial evidence from animal models that RAS antagonists exert a specific renoprotective effect that exceeds the general beneficial effect of BP control [68–73]. The magnitude of the advantage of RAS antagonists over other antihypertensive agents is still under debate [74].

Limited published information is available regarding renoprotection in children with CKD. Small uncontrolled studies showed stable kidney function in children post-hemolytic uremic syndrome during long-term ACE inhibition [75], stable GFR during 2.5 years of losartan treatment in children with proteinuric CKD [76], and attenuated histologic progression in children with immunoglobulin A nephropathy receiving combined RAS blockade [77]. The ongoing ESCAPE trial has demonstrated efficient BP and proteinuria reductions by ramipril in 400 children with CKD [28]. The long-term antiproteinuric and renoprotective efficacies of ACE inhibition will become clear after completion of this 5-year trial in 2008 and analysis of the data.

There is evidence that the RAS is incompletely suppressed by ACE inhibition alone, and the possibility of partial secondary resistance has been suggested ("aldosterone escape," or compensatory upregulation of ACE-independent angiotensin II production) [78,79]. Therefore the combination of an ACE inhibitor and an ARB may be favorable if proteinuria persists or increases despite ACE inhibition at maximally tolerable doses. This concept has been proven in adults [80,81]; however, pediatric data are not available to date.

Aldosterone antagonists also lower BP by RAS suppression. Whereas the use of spironolactone is limited by endocrine side effects, the new aldosterone antagonist eplerenone has minimal affinity for progesterone and androgen receptors. Apart from the risk of hyperkalemia, reported side effects are similar to placebo [82]. Combined therapy of eplerenone and an ACE inhibitor increased patient survival in adults with congestive heart failure [83]. However, combination therapy appears limited in CKD patients due to the potentiated risk of hyperkalemia [84,85].

A summary of the evidence ratings for prevention strategies in CVD in children with CKD is given in Tables 59.2 and 59.4. Data on prevention of pediatric CVD are limited. However, there is evidence from adult studies that normalization of BP (by RAS antagonists), an optimized dialysis regimen, and adequate treatment of CKD-related diseases (anemia, hyperparathyroidism, malnutrition) might prevent CVD in CKD patients. This evidence may be extrapolated to children.

Lipid abnormalities in pediatric kidney disease

Epidemiological studies have identified dyslipidemia as an independent risk factor for CVD. Kidney disorders are often associated with dyslipidemia, and some evidence suggests that dyslipidemia is an independent risk factor not only for CVD but also for progressive chronic kidney failure [86].

Dyslipidemia in adults is defined by total cholesterol of >240 mg/dL (>6.24 mmol/L), low-density lipoprotein (LDL) cholesterol of >160 mg/dL (>4.16 mmol/L), triglyceride levels of >200 mg/dL (>2.28 mmol/L), or high-density lipoprotein (HDL) cholesterol of <40 mg/dL (>1.04 mmol/L) [87]. In contrast, dyslipidemia in children is defined by cholesterol or triglyceride levels exceeding the 95th percentile for age and gender [88].

The dyslipidemic pattern differs between the major renal disease entities [88]. In nephrotic syndrome, marked hypercholesterolemia or combined hyperlipidemia is present in the majority of children and adults with active disease [89–92]. The alterations are mainly caused by lipid transport protein imbalances resulting from urinary protein loss and exaggerated hepatic *de novo* synthesis of lipoproteins. All apolipoprotein B-containing lipoproteins [i.e. VLDL, LDL, and lipoprotein(a), abbreviated Lp(a)] are increased. Persistent hyperlipidemia in nephrotic syndrome has a pro-atherosclerotic effect and contributes to CVD not only in adults [93] but also in children [94]. In CKD the degree of dyslipidemia parallels the degree of renal function impairment. Chronic renal insufficiency commonly progresses to ESRD, and there is relatively little information about the CVD risk associated with chronic renal insufficiency as an entity distinct from ESRD. Underlying mechanisms of uremic dyslipidemia include insulin resistance [95], hyperparathyroidism [96], malnutrition, acidosis [97], and impaired catabolism of triglyceride-rich lipoproteins by decreased activity of lipoprotein lipase and hepatic triglyceride lipase [98,99], whereas lipoprotein synthesis appears to be unaltered. In line with findings in adults, children with CKD have elevated serum triglycerides, whereas total cholesterol is close to normal. Hemodialysis does not seem to alter the pattern of dyslipidemia associated with CKD, whereas peritoneal dialysis contributes to an elevation of total cholesterol with a further increase in hypertriglyceridemia [88], probably due to further increased insulin resistance secondary to continuous glucose absorption from the dialysis fluid. In hemodialysis patients the use of heparins may acutely disturb the action of lipoprotein lipase. Whereas early analyses suggested less marked lipid alterations by low-molecular-weight heparins compared to conventional heparin in dialysis patients [100], this was not confirmed in later studies [101]. Due to the heparin interference, lipid patterns in hemodialysis patients should be assessed prior to a hemodialysis session.

After kidney transplantation, glucocorticoid administration leads to elevated cholesterol and triglyceride levels. Calcineurin inhibitors are associated with increased total cholesterol and apoB-associated cholesterol (including HDL cholesterol), whereas total triglycerides and HDL levels are less affected [102]. The dyslipidemic effect appears less marked in patients receiving tacrolimus compared to cyclosporine. The recently introduced mTOR antagonists dose-dependently induce hypertriglyceridemia and an increase of LDL cholesterol and apoB lipoproteins [103].

Efficacies of strategies for prevention and treatment of lipid abnormalities in children

The broad spectrum of factors influencing lipid metabolism in CKD demands a multifaceted prevention and therapeutic approach. General measures to prevent dyslipidemia in CKD patients include prevention or treatment of malnutrition and correction of metabolic acidosis, hyperparathyroidism, and anemia, all of which may contribute to dyslipidemia [97,104,105]. In addition, extrapolating from evidence in the general population, therapeutic

Table 59.2 Evidence ratings and recommendations for treatment of CVD in children with CKD.

| Intervention | Existing systematic pediatric reviews | Overall evidence rating[b] | | | Recommendation[c] | | | |
		Moderate	Low	Comment	I	II	III	Comment
LVH and vascular alterations[a]								
Normalization of BP	No	●		Limited data from one pediatric RCT; evidence from adult RCTs	●			Adequate BP control recommended in general; BP reduction associated with regression of LVH
Superiority of RAS antagonists	No	●		Limited data from one pediatric RCT; evidence from adult RCTs	●			Extrapolated from findings in adults; pediatric RCTs lacking
Adjustment of dry weight (CKD 5)	No	●		Limited data from pediatric CTs; evidence from adult studies	●			Extrapolated from findings in adults; pediatric RCTs lacking
Optimization of dialysis regimen (CKD 5)	No	●		Limited data from pediatric CTs; evidence from adult studies	●			Extrapolated from findings in adults; pediatric RCTs lacking
Adequate control of hyperparathyroidism	No	●		Limited data from pediatric CTs; evidence from adult studies	●			Extrapolated from findings in adults
Calcium sparing by use of Ca^{2+}-free phosphate binder (Sevelamer)	No	●		No data from pediatric CTs; high evidence from adult RCTs	●			Extrapolated from findings in adults
Correction of anemia	No	●		Limited data from pediatric CTs; evidence from adult RCTs	●			Inconsistent effect of correction of hemoglobin level on LVH
Treatment of malnutrition and hypalbuminemia	No	●		Limited data from pediatric CTs; evidence from adult studies	●			Extrapolated from findings in adults
(Early) kidney transplantation	No	●		Evidence from pediatric and adult studies	●			

Abbreviations: RCT, randomized controlled trial; CT, clinical trial;

[a]LVH is an unvalidated surrogate outcome only, and reversal may not result in improved cardiovascular outcomes.

[b]Evidence rating based on study design, study quality, consistency, and directness of results. No intervention was rated with a high or a very low evidence rating.

[c]Recommendations based on trade-offs between benefits and harms, quality of evidence, translation of evidence into practice in a specific setting including availability of medication, and any uncertainty about the baseline risk of the disease in the population. I, recommend; II, suggest; III, no recommendation possible.

life-style modifications (diet, exercise, weight reduction) are recommended for adults and children with CKD-related dyslipidemia [106]. In children who have received transplants, dietary interventions have lowered lipid levels at least in the short term [107]. However, the lipid-lowering effect of life-style modifications in CKD patients is small. Nonetheless, diet and physical exercise may exert beneficial effects on cardiovascular health independent of those on dyslipidemia. Dietary supplementation of fish oil effectively improved lipid profiles in a small cohort of children receiving renal replacement therapy [108].

In adult patients with nephrotic syndrome, a variety of lipid-lowering drugs has been tested, including statins, fibrates, bile acid-binding resins, and probucol. Simvastatin and lovastatin were effective and well-tolerated in a limited number of children with nephrotic syndrome treated for months to years [109,110]. Triglycerides and cholesterol were reduced by approximately 40% after 6 months of simvastatin treatment in a small cohort of younger children with steroid-resistant nephrotic syndrome in whom dietary advice had influenced lipid levels only marginally [109]. Probucol is also effective in children with nephrotic syndrome, but it caused QT prolongation in 4 of 22 patients in an uncontrolled prospective trial [111].

Because large trials for primary and secondary prevention of CVD in the general adult population provide a clear rationale for treatment of dyslipidemias, especially with statins, this treatment has also been proposed for adults with CKD. Statins effectively lower cholesterol and triglyceride levels in CKD patients by up to 30% [106]. This is suggestive of a beneficial effect on CVD, and most studies have demonstrated significant CVD risk reduction [112–114]. However, a recent large randomized prospective trial in hemodialyzed adults with diabetic nephropathy [112] showed no significant effect of statin therapy on overall patient mortality despite significant reduction of lipid levels. A pooled analysis of 30 completed clinical trials [113] analyzing the efficacy and safety of fluvastatin in adult patients with mild to severe chronic kidney failure suggested a reduction of cardiac death and nonfatal myocardial infarction. However, treatment did not reduce the rate of coronary intervention procedures. Fluvastatin treatment in adult kidney transplant recipients also resulted in a nonsignificant reduction in CVD [114]. However, no conclusive data are available on the overall mortality risk reduction in CKD patients. Future and ongoing trials need to clarify whether statin therapy is beneficial not only to cardiac but also to overall mortality in patients with different stages of CKD and at what stage of disease the initiation of treatment should be recommended.

Statin therapy may have beneficial effects on renal disease progression, not only by their lipid-lowering effects but also by lipid-independent (pleiotropic) effects. Statins inhibit signaling molecules at several points in inflammatory pathways. Anti-inflammatory effects and improved endothelial function are thought to be partially responsible for CVD risk reduction and improved renal function [115]. Furthermore, there is also evidence for synergistic effects of statins and RAS inhibitors on prevention

of kidney disease progression [116]. In younger children statins are used reluctantly, as the impacts of HMG-CoA reductase inhibitors on nutrition, growth, and pubertal maturation have not been fully elucidated yet. Therefore, the K/DOQI recommendations restrict statin treatment to children >10 years old with LDL levels of >160 mg/dL (>4.16 mmol/L) and non-HDL cholesterol of >190 mg/dL (>4.94 mmol/L) while on dialysis [106].

In adolescents statins are safe and effective [109,110,117], and several smaller studies in children with CKD have provided some evidence that statin treatment may be safely used in younger children as well. However, long-term data on efficacy in pediatric patients are still missing, and safety information on use of statins in children is not conclusive. Rhabdomyolysis and hepatic dysfunction appear to be potential side effects and occur in up to 5% of treated children [88,118].

Although bile acid resins are safe to use in children with CKD of all ages without dose adjustment, adherence to therapy is often poor due to a high incidence of adverse effects, including constipation, abdominal discomfort, flatulence, nausea, and vomiting. Moreover, application of bile acid sequestrants may interfere with cyclosporine treatment. Thus, additional information is required before statins or other lipid-lowering agents can be recommended for use in children or adolescents with CKD-related hyperlipidemia.

The evidence ratings for preventive strategies and treatments of dyslipidemia in children with CKD are summarized in Tables 59.3 and 59.4.

Table 59.3 Evidence ratings and recommendations for treatment of dyslipidemia in children with CKD.

Intervention	Existing systematic pediatric reviews	Overall evidence rating[b]		Comment	Recommendation[c]			Comment
		Moderate	Low		I	II	III	
Diet, therapeutic life-style modifications	no	•		some evidence from pediatric data evidence from adult RCTs	•			Recommended for all children with dyslipidemia [112]
Lipid-lowering treatment	no	•		limited data from pediatric CTs evidence from adult RCTs		•		Long-term effect of treatment in adults with CKD inconclusive
Statins	no	•		limited data from pediatric CTs evidence from adult RCTs		• (adolescents)	• (children)	No conclusive data on risks or benefits in children with CKD stages II–IV; recommended for CKD stage V adolescents only
Steroid withdrawal in Tx patients	no	•		evidence from CTs in pediatric Tx; evidence from adult RCTs		•		Pediatric RCT underway

Abbreviations: Tx, transplanted; RCT, randomized controlled trial; CT, clinical trial
[a]If no existing systematic review, overall evidence rating will start at moderate.
[b]Domains that are considered include study design, study quality, consistency, and directness of findings. No studies received an evidence rating of high or very low.
[c]Domains that are considered include trade-offs between benefits and harms, translation into clinical practice, uncertainty about baseline risk of population of interest, and quality of evidence. I, recommend; II, suggest; III, no recommendation possible.

Table 59.4 Summary of pediatric trials on the treatment of hypertension, CVD, and dyslipidemia in children with CKD.

Intervention	Study [reference]	Design	Conclusions and comments
Hypertension			
Reduction of salt intake, dietary intervention	Simons-Morton & Obarzanek 1997 [27]	Pediatric meta-analysis (25 observational studies, 12 intervention studies including 8 RCTs).	Studies with methodological problems included; results from observational studies and RCTs suggest that higher sodium intake is related to higher BP in children and adolescents; overall data not conclusive
Efficacy of antihypertensive agents			
β-blockers	Bachmann 1984 [119]	Prospective, open-label study, propranolol vs. chlorthalidone in 11 hypertensive CKD children treated for 4–6 wks	Propranolol effective in lowering mean BP by 22.3 mmHg
Ca²⁺ channel blockers	Silverstein *et al.* 1999 [120]	Retrospective, cross-over study comparing safety and efficacy of nifedipine vs.amlodipine in 24 pediatric kidney transplant patients	Nifedipine and amlodipine equally effective in lowering BP; nifedipine treatment associated with higher incidence of side effects (headache, flushing, dizziness, gingival hyperplasia; 91.7% of patients)
	Von Vigier *et al.* 2001 [121]	Open-label study in 43 CKD children treated with amlodipine for 16 wks.	Amlodipine effective and rather well-tolerated (BP lowering by 17/10 mmHg; side effects: edema, flushing, or headache; in 6 patients)
	Flynn *et al.* 2004 [122]	Randomized, double-blind, placebo-controlled study in 268 hypertensive children (25% CKD) (4-week dose response, 4-week withdrawal of either placebo or amlodipine.	Amlodipine effective in lowering BP in a dose-dependent manner
	Flynn 2005 [123]	Retrospective evaluation of amlodipine monotherapy > 6 months in 33 children (24 CKD patients)	Small study suggesting good tolerability and efficacy of amlodipine (sustained BP lowering by 8 mmHg)
ACE inhibitors	Mirkin & Newman 1985 [124]	Prospective, open-label clinical trial on efficacy and safety of captopril in 73 children treated for 3–12 months.	ACE inhibition consistently effective in lowering or normalizing BP and lowering proteinuria in children with CKD; effect on renal disease progression remains to be shown
	Callis *et al.* 1986 [125]	Retrospective observational study in 42 children with ESRD treated with captopril for 18–78 mos.	
	Wells *et al.* 2002 [126]	Prospective, randomized, double-blind, placebo-controlled multicenter trial in 110 children (50% CKD); 2-wk dose response, 2-wk either enalapril or placebo withdrawal study	
	Proesmans & Van Dyck 2004 [127]	Retrospective analysis of 10 children with CKD and Alport syndrome.	
	Soergel *et al.* 2000 [128]	Prospective, open-label, clinical trial on antihypertensive and antiproteinuric effects of ramipril monotherapy in 14 hypertensive CKD children treated for 6 mos	
	Seeman *et al.* 2004 [129]	Prospective, open-label, clinical trial in 31 children with CKD, proteinuria or hypertension treated with ramipril for 6 mos	
	Wühl *et al.* 2004 [28]	Multicenter, prospective clinical trial on antihypertensive and antiproteinuric effects of fixed-dose ramipril (6 mg/m²/day) in 400 children with CKD	
AT1 receptor antagonists	Ellis *et al.* 2004 [130]	Prospective, open-label, clinical trial in 52 CKD children with proteinuria (22 proteinuria+hypertension)	Experience with AT1-receptor antagonists in children limited Losartan and irbesartan effective in lowering BP.
	Franscini *et al.* 2002 [131]	Prospective, open-label study on the efficacy and safety of irbesartan in 44 CKD children treated for 18 weeks.	

	Reference	Study description	Results
Steroid withdrawal in kidney transplant patients	Höcker et al. 2004 [31]	Retrospective case-control study on the safety and efficacy of steroid withdrawal in 20 renal transplant children (mean follow-up 46 mo)	Decrease of mean arterial BP SDS by 45%.
LVH, vascular alterations Normalization of BP	ESCAPE trial (unpublished data)	Prospective, randomized, open label study on the effect of intensified BP control on left ventricular hypertrophy and function in CKD children	Normalization of BP resulted in decrease of prevalence of left ventricular hypertrophy in children with CKD stage II-IV.
Optimization of dialysis regimen (CKD 5)	Fischbach et al. 2004 [30]	Prospective, single-center observational, trial on the effect of daily on-line hemodiafiltration (6 x 3 h/week) in 5 children	Intensified dialysis resulted in BP reduction, reduced size and improved function of left ventricle.
Dyslipidemia Diet, therapeutic life-style modification	K/DOQI 2003 [106]	K/DOQI guidelines	
	Goren et al. 1991 [108]	Prospective, open-label study on the effect of 8 weeks of daily oral fish oil supplementation on serum lipid levels in 16 ESRD patients (age 7–8 years).	No change of cholesterol levels, 27% decrease of triglyceride levels, improvement of atherogenic serum lipoprotein profile.
Lipid-lowering treatments Statins	K/DOQI 2003 [106]	K/DOQI guidelines	
	Coleman & Watson 1996 [109]	Single center observational study on the efficacy and tolerability of diet prior to and under statin treatment (mean dose 10mg/d) in 7 children with steroid resistant nephrotic syndrome, aged 1.8 to 16.3 years.	41% reduction of cholesterol, 44% reduction of triglycerides at mo 6, sustained effect at mo 12. No clinical side effects.
	Sanjad et al. 1997 [110]	Single center, prospective, observational study on the effect of statin treatment for 1 to 5 years in 12 infants and children with steroid resistant nephrotic syndrome.	40% reduction of cholesterol, 44% reduction of LDL cholesterol and 33% reduction of triglyceride levels. No side effects reported
	Butani 2005 [132]	Prospective open-label study on the effect of 12-month statin therapy on lipid status in 17 pediatric renal transplant recipients.	Significant decline in total cholesterol, serum triglycerides, LDL- and also HDL-cholesterol. Increase of prevalence of hypercholesterolemia from 31% pretransplant to 0% after 1 year.
	Argent et al. 2003 [133]	Prospective, open-label study in 9 pediatric renal transplant patients on the effect of atorvastatin.	41% reduction of cholesterol and 44% reduction of triglycerides. No adverse side affects on allograft function.
Probucol	Querfeld et al. 1999 [111]	Prospective, open-label, multicenter study on the effect of probucol on hyperlipidemia, proteinuria and glomerular filtration rate in 14 children for 8 to 24 weeks.	Positive effect of probucol on lipid profile (decrease of cholesterol 25%, HDL 24%, VLDL 27%, triglycerides 15%)
Steroid withdrawal in kidney transplant patients	Vidhun & Sarwal 2005 [134]	Review of 20 prospective trials on steroid free immunosuppression in children and adults (7 pediatric studies, 237 children) after renal transplantation.	Advantage on lipid profile in 3 pediatric studies.
	Sarwal et al. 2001 [135]	Prospective, open label study of complete steroid avoidance in 10 pediatric kidney recipients (age 5-21 years) compared to 37 matched historical controls.	No hypertension and no hypercholesterolemia in the steroid free group (significant difference vs. controls).

Life-style modification and diet are generally recommended in adults and children with dyslipidemia, irrespective of the underlying disease. In children who have undergone kidney transplantation a few studies suggest a beneficial effect of steroid-free immunosuppression on dyslipidemia.

Also, there are only a few studies on the efficacy of lipid-lowering drugs in children. There is some evidence that statins are effective in lowering serum lipid levels in children and adolescents with CKD. However, safety data in children are limited and not conclusive. To date, official treatment recommendations (K/DOQI) restrict the use of statins to adolescents with ESRD.

Conclusions

CVD is a common problem in children with CKD, starting as early as in the second decade of life. Therefore, treatment strategies aiming for CVD risk reduction are mandatory and should consider therapeutic life-style modifications (healthy diet, physical activity, maintenance of normal weight, abstinence from smoking) and correction of uremia-related risk factors. BP should be lowered below the 90th percentile using drugs controlling the RAS, proteinuria should be minimized, and renal anemia, metabolic acidosis, and mineral metabolism should be corrected. Whether correction of dyslipidemia results in improved cardiovascular and kidney survival remains to be shown.

Although there is evidence that treatment regimens established in adults are also safe and effective in children, further studies in pediatric patients with CKD are necessary to confirm these findings.

References

1 Oh J, Wunsch R, Turzer M, Bahner M, Raggi P, Querfeld U *et al.* Advanced coronary and carotid arteriopathy in young adults with childhood-onset chronic renal failure. *Circulation* 2002; **106**: 100–105.

2 Gruppen MP, Groothoff JW, Prins M, van der Wouw P, Offringa M, Bos WJ *et al.* Cardiac disease in young adult patients with end-stage renal disease since childhood: a Dutch cohort study. *Kidney Int* 2003; **63**: 1058–1065.

3 Parekh RS, Caroll CE, Wolfe RA, Port FK. Cardiovascular mortality in children and young adults with end-stage kidney disease. *J Pediatr* 2002; **141**: 191–197.

4 Schärer K. Hypertension in children and adolescents. In: Malluche HH, Sawaya BP, Sayegh MH (editors), *Clinical Nephrology, Dialysis and Transplantation: a Continuously Updated Textbook.* Deisenhofen, Dustri-Verlag, Deisenhofen, Germany, 1999; 1–28.

5 Mitsnefes MM, Ho P-L, McEnery PT. Hypertension and progression of chronic renal insufficiency in children: a report of the North American Pediatric Renal Transplant Cooperative Study (NAPRTCS). *J Am Soc Nephrol* 2003; **14**: 2618–2622.

6 Seeman T, Simkova E, Kreisinger J, Vondrak K, Dusek J, Gilik J *et al.* Control of hypertension in children after renal transplantation. *Pediatr Transplant* 2006; **10**: 316–322.

7 Lingens N, Dobos E, Witte K, Busch C, Lemmer B, Klaus G *et al.* Twenty-four-hour ambulatory blood pressure profiles in pediatric patients after renal transplantation. *Pediatr Nephrol* 1997; **11**: 23–26.

8 Schaefer F, Mehls O. Hypertension in chronic kidney disease. In: Portman RJ, Sorof JM, Ingelfinger JR (editors), *Pediatric Hypertension.* Humana Press, Totowa, NJ, 2003.

9 National High Blood Pressure Education Program Working Group on High Blood Pressure in Children and Adolescents. The Fourth Report on the Diagnosis, Evaluation, and Treatment of High Blood Pressure in Children and Adolescents. *Pediatrics* 2004; **114**: 555–576.

10 Sorof JM, Portman RJ. White coat hypertension in children with elevated casual blood pressure. *J Pediatr* 2000; **137**: 493–497.

11 Hadtstein C, Wühl E, Soergel M, Witte K, Schaefer F. Normative values for circadian and ultradian cardiovascular rhythms in childhood. *Hypertension* 2004; **43**: 547–554.

12 Portaluppi F, Montanari L, Ferlini M, Gilli P. Altered circadian rhythms of blood pressure and heart rate in non-hemodialysis chronic renal failure. *Chronobiol Int* 1990; **7**: 321–327.

13 Wühl E, Hadtstein C, Mehls O, Schaefer F, ESCAPE Trial Group. Ultradian but not circadian blood pressure rhythms correlate with renal dysfunction in children with chronic renal failure. *J Am Soc Nephrol* 2005; **16**: 746–754.

14 Verdeccia P. Using out of office blood pressure monitoring in the management of hypertension. *Curr Hypertens Rep* 2001; **3**: 400–405.

15 Ogedegbe G, Schoenthaler A. A systematic review of the effects of home blood pressure monitoring on medication adherence. *J Clin Hypertens* (Greenwich) 2006; **8**: 174–180.

16 Wühl E, Hadtstein C, Mehls O, Schaefer F, ESCAPE Trial Group. Home, clinic, and ambulatory blood pressure monitoring in children with chronic renal failure. *Pediatr Res* 2004; **55**: 492–497.

17 Chobanian AV, Bakris GL, Black DL, Cushman WC, Green LA, Izzo JLJ *et al.* The Seventh Report of the Joint National Committee on Prevention, Detection, Evaluation, and Treatment of High Blood Pressure: the JNC 7 report. *JAMA* 2003; **289**: 2560–2571.

18 de Man SA, André JL, Bachmann HJ, Grobbee DE, Ibsen KK, Laaser U *et al.* Blood pressure in childhood: pooled findings of six European studies. *J Hypertens* 1991; **9**: 109–114.

19 Park MK, Menard SM, Schoolfield J. Oscillometric blood pressure standards for children. *Pediatr Cardiol* 2005; **26**: 601–607.

20 Park MK, Menard SM. Normative oscillometric blood pressure values in the first 5 years in an office setting. *Am J Dis Child* 1989; **143**: 860–864.

21 Soergel M, Kirschstein M, Busch C, Danne T, Gellermann J, Holl R *et al.* Oscillometric twenty-four-hour ambulatory blood pressure values in healthy children and adolescents: a multicenter trial including 1141 subjects. *J Pediatr* 1997; **130**: 178–184.

22 Wühl E, Witte K, Soergel M, Mehls O, Schaefer F, the German Working Group on Pediatric Hypertension. Distribution of 24-h ambulatory blood pressure in children: normalized reference values and role of body dimensions. *J Hypertens* 2002; **20**: 1995–2007.

23 O'Sullivan JJ, Derrick G, Griggs P, Foxall R, Aitkin M, Wren C. Ambulatory blood pressure in schoolchildren. *Arch Dis Child* 1999; **80**: 529–532.

24 Stergiou GS, Yannes NG, Rarra VC, Panagiotakas DB. Home blood pressure normalcy in children and adolescents: the Arsakeion School Study. *J Hypertens* 2007; 25: 1375–9.

25 Clarke WR, Woolson RF, Lauer RM. Changes in ponderosity and blood pressure in childhood: The Muscatine Study. *Am J Epidemiol* 1986; **124**: 195–206.

26 Sacks FM, Svetkey LP, Vollmer WM, Appel LJ, Bray GA, Harsha D *et al.* Effect on blood pressure of reduced dietary sodium and the Dietary Approaches to Stop Hypertension (DASH) diet. *N Engl J Med* 2001; **344**: 3–10.

27 Simons-Morton DG, Obarzanek E. Diet and blood pressure in children and adolescents. *Pediatr Nephrol* 1997; **11**: 244–249.

28 Wühl E, Mehls O, Schaefer F, ESCAPE Trial Group. Antihypertensive and antiproteinuric efficacy of ramipril in children with chronic renal failure. *Kidney Int* 2004; **66**: 768–776.

29 Michael M, Brewer ED, Goldstein SL. Blood volume monitoring to achieve target weight in pediatric hemodialysis patients. *Pediatr Nephrol* 2004; **19**: 432–437.

30 Fischbach M, Terzic J, Laugel V, Dheu C, Menouer S, Helms P *et al.* Daily on-line hemodiafiltration: a pilot trial in children. *Nephrol Dial Transplant* 2004; **19**: 2360–2367.

31 Höcker B, John U, Plank C, Wühl E, Weber LT, Misselwitz J *et al.* Successful withdrawal of steroids in pediatric renal transplant recipients receiving cyclosporine A and mycophenolate mofetil treatment: results after four years. *Transplantation* 2004; **78**: 228–234.

32 Malcolm DD, Burns TL, Mahoney LT, Lauer RM. Factors affecting left ventricular mass in childhood: the Muscatine study. *Pediatrics* 1993; **92**: 703–709.

33 Sahn DJ, DeMaria A, Kisslo J, Weyman A. Recommendations regarding quantitation in M-mode echocardiography: results of a survey of echocardiographic measurements. *Circulation* 1978; **58**: 1072–1083.

34 Devereux RB, Alonso DR, Lutas EM, Gottlieb GJ, Campo E, Sachs I *et al.* Echocardiographic assessment of left ventricular hypertrophy: comparison to necropsy findings. *Am J Cardiol* 1986; **57**: 450–458.

35 de Simone G, Daniels SR, Devereux RB, Meyer RA, Roman MJ, de Divitiis O *et al.* Left ventricular mass and body size in normotensive children and adults: assessment of allometric relations and impact of overweight. *J Am Coll Cardiol* 1992; **20**: 1251–1260.

36 Matteucci MC, Wühl E, Picca S, Mastrostefano A, Rinelli G, Romano C *et al.* Left ventricular geometry in children with mild to moderate chronic renal insufficiency. *J Am Soc Nephrol* 2006; **17**: 218–226.

37 Johnstone LM, Jones CL, Grigg LE, Wilkinson JL, Walker RG, Powell HR. Left ventricular abnormalities in children, adolescents and young adults with renal disease. *Kidney Int* 1996; **50**: 998–1006.

38 Mitsnefes MM, Kimball TR, Witt SA, Glascock BJ, Khoury PR, Daniels SR. Left ventricular mass and systolic performance in pediatric patients with chronic renal failure. *Circulation* 2003; **107**: 864–868.

39 Parfrey PS, Foley RN. The clinical epidemiology of cardiac disease in chronic renal failure. *J Am Soc Nephrol* 1999; **10**: 1606–1615.

40 Mitsnefes MM, Daniels SR, Schwartz SM, Meyer RA, Khoury P, Strife CF. Severe left ventricular hypertrophy in pediatric dialysis: prevalence and predictors. *Pediatr Nephrol* 2000; **14**: 898–902.

41 Longenecker JC, Coresh J, Powe NR, Levey AS, Fink NE, Martin A *et al.* Traditional cardiovascular disease risk factors in dialysis patients compared with the general population: the CHOICE study. *J Am Soc Nephrol* 2002; **13**: 1918–1927.

42 Matteucci MC, Giordano U, Calzolari A, Turchetta A, Santilli A, Rizzoni G. Left ventricular hypertrophy, treadmill tests, and 24-hour blood pressure in pediatric transplant patients. *Kidney Int* 1999; **56**: 1566–1570.

43 Mitsnefes MM, Schwartz SM, Daniels SR, Kimball TR, Khoury P, Strife CF. Changes in left ventricular mass in children and adolescents after renal transplantation. *Pediatr Transplant* 2001; **5**: 279–284.

44 Chinali M, de Simone G, Matteucci MC, Picca S, Mastrostefano A, Anarat A *et al.* Reduced systolic myocardial function in children with chronic renal insufficiency. *J Am Soc Nephrol* 2007; **18**: 593–598.

45 Andersson P, Rydberg E, Willenheimer R. Primary hyperparathyroidism and heart disease: a review. *Eur Heart J* 2004; **25**: 1776–1787.

46 Rostand SG, Drüeke TB. Parathyroid hormone, vitamin D and cardiovascular disease in chronic renal failure. *Kidney Int* 1999; **56**: 383–392.

47 Mitsnefes MM, Kimball TR, Kartal J, Witt SA, Glascock BJ, Khoury PR *et al.* Cardiac and vascular adaptation in pediatric patients with chronic kidney disease: role of calcium-phosphorus metabolism. *J Am Soc Nephrol* 2005; **16**: 2796–2803.

48 Besbas N, Saatci U, Ozkutlu S, Bakkaloglu A, Soylemezoglu O, Ozen S. Effects of secondary hyperparathyroidism on cardiac function in pediatric patients on hemodialysis. *Turk J Pediatr* 1995; **37**: 299–304.

49 Ludwig M, von Petzinger-Kruthoff A, von Buquoy M, Stumpe KO. Intima media thickness of the carotid arteries: early pointer to arteriosclerosis and therapeutic endpoint. *Ultraschall Med* 2003; **24**: 162–174.

50 Guerin AP, London GM, Marchais SJ, Metivier F. Arterial stiffening and vascular calcifications in end-stage renal disease. *Nephrol Dial Transplant* 2000; **15**: 1014–1021.

51 Rubba P, Mercuri M, Faccenda F, Iannuzzi A, Irace C, Strisciuglio P *et al.* Premature carotid arteriosclerosis: does it occur in both familial hypercholesterolemia and homocystinuria? Ultrasound assessment of arterial intima-media thickness and blood flow velocity. *Stroke* 1994; **25**: 943–950.

52 Litwin M, Wühl E, Jourdan C, Trelewicz J, Niemirska A, Fahr K *et al.* Altered morphologic properties of large arteries in children with chronic renal failure and after renal transplantation. *J Am Soc Nephrol* 2005; **16**: 1494–1500.

53 Mitsnefes MM, Kimball TR, Witt SA, Glascock BJ, Khoury MS, Daniels SR. Abnormal carotid artery structure and function in children and adolescents with successful renal transplantation. *Circulation* 2004; **110**: 97–101.

54 Saygili A, Barutcu O, Cengiz N, Tarhan N, Pourbagher A, Niron E *et al.* Carotid intima-media thickness and left ventricular changes in children with end-stage renal disease. *Transplant Proc* 2002; **34**: 2073–2075.

55 Greenbaum LA. Anemia in children with chronic kidney disease. *Adv Chronic Kidney Dis* 2005; **12**: 385–396.

56 NKF. K/DOQI guidelines. III. Clinical practice recommendations for anemia in chronic kidney disease in children. *Am J Kidney Dis* 2006; **47(Suppl 3)**: S86–S108.

57 Locatelli F, Pozzoni P, Del Vecchio L. Anemia and heart failure in chronic kidney disease. *Semin Nephrol* 2005; **25**: 392–396.

58 Sunder-Plassmann G, Horl WH. Effect of erythropoietin on cardiovascular diseases. *Am J Kidney Dis* 2001; **38(Suppl 1)**: S20–S25.

59 Dahlof B, Pennert L, Hansson L. Reversal of left ventricular hypertrophy in hypertensive patients. A metaanalysis of 109 treatment studies. *Am J Hypertens* 1992; **5**: 92–110.

60 Klingbeil AU, Schneider M, Martus P, Messerli FH, Schmieder RE. A meta-analysis of the effects of treatment on left ventricular mass in essential hypertension. *Am J Med* 2003; **115**: 41–46.

61 Chertow GM. Slowing the progression of vascular calcification in hemodialysis. *J Am Soc Nephrol* 2003; **14**: S310–S314.

62 Litwin M, Wühl E, Jourdan C, Niemirska A, Schenk JP, Jobs K *et al.* Evolution of large-vessel arteriopathy in paediatric patients with chronic kidney disease. *Nephrol Dial Transplant* 2008. (Epub ahead of print; posting date 14 March 2008; doi:10.1093/ndt/gfn083.)

63 Klag MJ, Whelton PK, Randall BL, Neaton JD, Brancati FL, Ford CE *et al.* Blood pressure and end-stage renal disease in men. *Hypertension* 1996; **13**: 180–193.

64 Iseki K, Ikemiya Y, Iseki C, Takishita S. Proteinuria and the risk of developing end-stage renal disease. *Kidney Int* 2003; **63**: 1468–1474.

65 Locatelli F, Marcelli D, Comelli M, Alberti D, Graziani G, Buccianti G *et al*. Proteinuria and blood pressure as causal components of progression to end-stage renal failure. Northern Italian Cooperative Study Group. *Nephrol Dial Transplant* 1996; **11**: 461–467.

66 Fouque D, Laville M, Boissel JP. Low-protein diets for chronic kidney disease in non diabetic adults (Cochrane review). In: *The Renal Health Library*, Update Software Ltd., Oxford, 2005.

67 Wingen AM, Fabian-Bach C, Schaefer F, Mehls O. Randomised multicentre study of a low-protein diet on the progression of chronic renal failure in children. European Study Group of Nutritional Treatment of Chronic Renal Failure in Childhood. *Lancet* 1997; **349**: 1117–1123.

68 Maschio G, Alberti D, Janin G, Locatelli F, Mann JF, Motolese M *et al*. Effect of angiotensin-converting-enzme inhibitor benazepril on the progression of chronic renal insufficiency. *N Engl J Med* 1996; **334**: 939–945.

69 The GISEN Group (Gruppo Italiano di Studi Epidemiologici in Nefrologia). Randomised placebo-controlled trial of effect of ramipril on decline in glomerular filtration rate and risk of terminal renal failure in proteinuric, non-diabetic nephroptahy. *Lancet* 1997; **349**: 1857–1863.

70 Parving HH, Andersen AR, Smidt UM, Svendsen PA. Early aggressive antihypertensive treatment reduces rate of decline in kidney function in diabetic nephropathy. *Lancet* 1983; **i**: 1175–1179.

71 Jafar TH, Schmid CH, Landa M, Giatras J, Toto R, Remuzzi G *et al*. Angiotensin-converting enzyme inhibitors and progression of nondiabetic renal disease. A meta-analysis of patient-level data. *Ann Intern Med* 2001; **135**: 73–87.

72 Lewis EJ, Hunsicker LG, Raymond PB, Rohde RD *et al*. The effect of angiotensin-converting-enzyme inhibition on diabetic nephropathy. *N Engl J Med* 1993; **329**: 1456–1462.

73 Kamper AL, Strandgaard S, Leyssac P. Effect of enalapril on the progression of chronic renal failure: a randomized controlled trial. *Am J Hypertens* 1992; **5**: 423–430.

74 Casas JP, Weiliang C, Loukogeorgakis S, Vallance P, Smeeth L, Hingorani AD *et al*. Effect of inhibitors of the renin-angiotensin system and other antihypertensive drugs on renal outcomes: systematic review and meta-analysis. *Lancet* 2005; **366**: 2026–2033.

75 Van Dyck M, Proesmans W. Renoprotection by ACE inhibitors after severe hemolytic uremic syndrome. *Pediatr Nephrol* 2004; **19**: 688–690.

76 Ellis D, Vats A, Moritz ML, Reitz S, Grosso MJ, Janosky JE. Long-term antiproteinuric and renoprotective efficacy and safety of losartan in children with proteinuria. *J Pediatr* 2003; **143**: 89–97.

77 Tanaka H, Suzuki K, Nakahata T, Tsugawa K, Konno Y, Tsuruga K *et al*. Combined therapy of enalapril and losartan attenuates histologic progression in immunoglobulin A nephropathy. *Pediatr Int* 2004; **46**: 576–579.

78 Mooser V, Nussberger J, Juillerat L, Burnier M, Waeber B, Bidiville J *et al*. Reactive hyperreninemia is a major determinant of plasma angiotensin II during ACE inhibition. *J Cardiovasc Pharmacol* 1990; **15**: 276–282.

79 van den Meiracker AH, Man n 't Veld AJ, Admiraal PJ, Ritsema van Eck HJ, Boomsma F, Derkx FH *et al*. Partial escape of agiotensin converting enzyme (ACE) inhibition during prolonged ACE inhibitor treatment: does it exist and does it affect the antihypertensive response? *J Hypertens* 1992; **10**: 803–812.

80 MacKinnon M, Shurraw S, Akbari A, Knoll GA, Jaffey J, Clark HD. Combination therapy with an angiotensin receptor blocker and an ACE inhibitor in proteinuric renal disease: a systematic review of the efficacy and safety data. *Am J Kidney Dis* 2006; **48**: 8–20.

81 Nakao N, Yoshimura A, Morita H, Takada M, Kayano T, Ideura T. Combination treatment of angiotensin-II receptor blocker and angiotensin-converting-enzyme inhibitor in non-diabetic renal disease (COOPERATE): a randomised controlled trial. *Lancet* 2003; **361**: 117–124.

82 White WB, Carr AA, Krause S, Jordan R, Roniker B, Oigman W. Assessment of the novel selective aldosterone blocker eplerenone using ambulatory and clinical blood pressure in patients with systemic hypertension. *Am J Cardiol* 2003; **92**: 38–42.

83 Pitt B, Remme W, Zannad F, Neaton J, Martinez F, Roniker B *et al*. Eplerenone, a selective aldosterone blocker, in patients with left ventricular dysfunction after myocardial infarction. *N Engl J Med* 2003; **348**: 1309–1321.

84 Effectiveness of spironolactone added to an angiotensin-converting enzyme inhibitor and a loop diuretic for severe chronic congestive heart failure (the Randomized Aldactone Evaluation Study [RALES]). *Am J Cardiol* 1996; **78**: 902–907.

85 Sato A, Saruta T, Funder JW. Combination therapy with aldosterone blockade and renin-angiotensin inhibitors confers organ protection. *Hypertens Res* 2006; **29**: 211–216.

86 Muntner P, Coresh J, Clinton Smith J, Eckfeldt J, Klag MJ. Plasma lipids and risk of developing renal dysfunction: the Atherosclerosis Risk in Communities Study. *Kidney Int* 2000; **58**: 293–301.

87 *Third Report of the National Cholesterol Education Programme (NCEP) Expert Panel on Detection, Evaluation, and Treatment of High Blood Cholesterol in Adults* (adult treatment panel III), executive summary. NIH publication 01-3670 2001. NIH, Bethesda, 2001.

88 Saland MJ, Ginsberg H, Fisher EA. Dyslipidemia in pediatric renal disease: epidemiology, pathophysiology, and management. *Curr Opin Pediatr* 2002; **14**: 197–204.

89 Joven J, Villabona C, Vilella E, Masana L, Elberti R, Valles M. Abnormalities of lipoprotein metabolism in patients with the nephrotic syndrome. *N Engl J Med* 1990; **323**: 579–584.

90 Baxter JH, Goodman HC, Havel RJ. Serum lipid and lipoprotein alterations in nephrosis. *J Clin Invest* 1960; **39**: 455–465.

91 Nephrotic syndrome in children: prediction of histopathology from clinical and laboratory characteristics at time of diagnosis. A report of the International Study of Kidney Disease in Children. *Kidney Int* 1978; **13**: 159–165.

92 Querfeld U, Gnasso A, Haberbosch W, Augustin J, Schärer K. Lipoprotein profiles at different stages of the nephrotic syndrome. *Eur J Pediatr* 1988; **147**: 233–238.

93 Ordonez JD, Hiatt RA, Killebrew EJ, Fireman BH. The increased risk of coronary heart disease associated with nephrotic syndrome. *Kidney Int* 1993; **44**: 638–642.

94 Portman R, Hawkins E, Verani R. Premature arteriosclerosis (PA) in pediatric renal patients: report of the Southwest Pediatric Nephrology Study Group. *Pediatr Res* 1991; **29**: 349A.

95 Cheng SC, Chu TS, Huang KY, Chen YM, Chang WK, Tsai TJ *et al*. Association of hypertriglyceridemia and insulin resistance in uremic patients undergoing CAPD. *Perit Dial Int* 2001; **21**: 282–289.

96 Mak RH. 1,25-Dihydroxyvitamin D3 corrects insulin and lipid abnormalities in uremia. *Kidney Int* 1998; **53**: 1353–1357.

97 Mak RH. Effect of metabolic acidosis on hyperlipidemia in uremia. *Pediatr Nephrol* 1999; **13**: 891–893.

98 Chan PC, Persaud J, Varghese Z, Kingstone D, Baillod RA, Moorhead JF. Apolipoprotein B turnover in dialysis patients: its relationship to pathogenesis of hyperlipidemia. *Clin Nephrol* 1989; **31**: 88–95.

99 Horkko S, Huttunen K, Kesaniemi YA. Decreased clearance of low-density lipoproteins in uremic patients under dialysis treatment. *Kidney Int* 1995; **47**: 1732–1740.

100 Wiemer J, Winkler K, Baumstark M, Marz W, Scherberich JE. Influence of low molecular weight heparin compared to conventional heparin for anticoagulation during hemodialysis on low density lipoprotein subclasses. *Nephrol Dial Transplant* 2002; **17**: 2231–2238.

101 Nasstrom B, Stegmayr B, Olivecrona G, Olivecrona T. Lipoprotein lipase in hemodialysis patients: indications that low molecular weight heparine depletes functional stores, despite low plasma levels of the enzyme. *BMC Nephrol* 2004; **3**: 17.

102 Ballantyne CM, Podet EJ, Patsch WP, Harati Y, Appel V, Gotto AMJ *et al.* Effects of cyclosporine therapy on plasma lipoprotein levels. *JAMA* 1989; **262**: 53–56.

103 Andrés V, Castro C, Campistol JM. Potential role of proliferation signal inhibitors on atherosclerosis in renal transplant patients. *Nephrol Dial Transplant* 2006; **21(Suppl 3)**: 14–17.

104 Mak RH. Metabolic effects of erythropoietin in patients on peritoneal dialysis. *Pediatr Nephrol* 1998; **12**: 660–665.

105 Mak RH. Effect of metabolic acidosis on insulin action and secretion in uremia. *Kidney Int* 1998; **54**: 603–607.

106 Kidney Disease Outcomes Quality Initiative (K/DOQI) Group. K/DOQI clinical practice guidelines for management of dyslipidemias in patients with kidney disease. *Am J Kidney Dis* 2003; **41(Suppl 3)**: S1–S91.

107 Delucchi A, Marin V, Trabucco G, Azocar M, Salas P, Gutierrez E *et al.* Dyslipidemia and dietary modification in Chilenian renal pediatric transplantation. *Transplant Proc* 2001; **33**: 2008–2013.

108 Goren A, Stankiewicz H, Goldstein R, Drukker A. Fish oil treatment of hyperlipidemia in children and adolescents receiving renal replacement therapy. *Pediatrics* 1991; **88**: 265–268.

109 Coleman JE, Watson AR. Hyperlipidemia, diet and simvastatin therapy in steroid-resistant nephrotic syndrome of childhood. *Pediatr Nephrol* 1996; **10**: 171–174.

110 Sanjad SA, al-Abbad A, Al-Shorafa S. Management of hyperlipidemia in children with refractory nephrotic syndrome: the effect of statin therapy. *J Pediatr* 1997; **130**: 470–474.

111 Querfeld U, Kohl B, Fiehn W, Minor T, Michalk D, Schärer K *et al.* Probucol for treatment of hyperlipidemia in persistent childhood nephrotic syndrome. Report of a prospective uncontrolled multicenter study. *Pediatr Nephrol* 1999; **13**: 7–12.

112 Wanner C, Krane V. Lessons learnt from the 4D Trial. *Nephrol Ther* 2006; **2**: 3–7.

113 Holdaas H, Wanner C, Abletshauser C, Gimpelewicz C, Isaacsohn J. The effect of fluvastatin on cardiac outcomes in patients with moderate to severe renal insufficiency: a pooled analysis of double-blind, randomized trials. *Int J Cardiol* 2007; **117**: 64–74.

114 Holdaas H, Fellstrom B, Jardine AG, Nyberg G, Gronhagen Riska C, Madsen S *et al.* Beneficial effect of early initiation of lipid lowering therapy following renal transplantation. *Nephrol Dial Transplant* 2005; **20**: 974–980.

115 Epstein M, Campese VM. Pleiotropic effects of 3-hydroxy-3-methylglutaryl coenzyme a reductase inhibitors on renal function. *Am J Kidney Dis* 2005; **45**: 2–14.

116 Zoja C, Corna D, Rottoli D, Cattaneo D, Zanchi C, Tomasoni S *et al.* Effect of combining ACE inhibitor and statin in severe experimental nephropathy. *Kidney Int* 2002; **61**: 1635–1645.

117 Rodenburg J, Vissers MN, Daniels SR, Wiegman A, Kastelein JJ. Lipid lowering medication. *Pediatr Endocrinol Rev* 2004; **2(Suppl 1)**: 171–180.

118 Chin C, Gamberg P, Miller J, Luikart H, Bernstein D. Efficacy and safety of atorvastatin after pediatric heart transplantation. *J Heart Lung Transplant* 2002; **21**: 1213–1217.

119 Bachmann H. Propranolol versus chlorthalidone: a prospective therapeutic trial in children with chronic hypertension. *Helv Paediat Acta* 1984; **39**: 55–61.

120 Silverstein DM, Palmer J, Baluarte HJ, Brass C, Conley SB, Polinsky MS. Use of calcium channel blockers in pediatric renal transplant recipients. *Pediatr Transplant* 1999; **3**: 288–292.

121 von Vigier RO, Franscini LM, Bianda ND, Pfister R, Casaulta Aebischer C, Bianchetti MG. Antihypertensive efficacy of amlodipine in children with chronic kidney disease. *J Hum Hypertens* 2001; **15**: 387–391.

122 Flynn JT, Newburger JW, Daniels SR, Sanders SP, Portman RJ, Hogg RJ *et al.* A randomized-placebo-controlled trial of amlodipine in children with hypertension. *J Pediatr* 2004; **145**: 353–359.

123 Flynn JT. Efficacy and safety of prolonged amlodipine treatment in hypertensive children. *Pediatr Nephrol* 2005; **20**: 631–635.

124 Mirkin BL, Newman TJ. Efficacy and safety of captopril in the treatment of severe childhood hypertension: report of the international collaborative study group. *Pediatrics* 1985; **75**: 1091–1100.

125 Callis L, Vila A, Catala J, Gras X. Long-term treatment with captopril in pediatric patients with severe hypertension and chronic renal failure. *Clin Exp Hypertens* 1986; **8**: 847–851.

126 Wells T, Frame V, Soffer B, Shaw W, Zhang Z, Herrera P *et al.* A double-blind, placebo-controlled dose-response study of the effectiveness and safety of enalapril for children with hypertension. *J Clin Pharmacol* 2002; **42**: 870–880.

127 Proesmans W, Van Dyck M. Enalapril in children with Alport syndrome. *Pediatr Nephrol* 2004; **19**: 271–275.

128 Soergel M, Verho M, Wuhl E, Gellermann J, Teichert L, Scharer K. Effect of ramipril on ambulatory blood pressure and albuminuria in renal hypertension. *Pediatr Nephrol* 2000; **15**: 113–118.

129 Seeman T, Dusek J, Vondrak K, Flogelova H, Geier P, Janda J. Ramipril in the treatment of hypertension and proteinuria in children with chronic kidney disease. *Am J Hypertens* 2004; **17**: 415–420.

130 Ellis D, Vats A, Moritz ML, Reitz S, Grosso MJ, Janosky JE. Long-term antiproteinuric and renoprotective efficacy and safety of losartan in children with proteinuria. *J Pediatr* 2004; **144**: 834–835.

131 Franscini LM, Von Vigier RO, Pfister R, Casaulta-Aebischer C, Fossali E, Bianchetti MG. Effectiveness and safety of the angiotensin II antagonist irbesartan in children with chronic kidney disease. *Am J Hypertens* 2002; **15**: 1057–1063.

132 Butani L. Prospective monitoring of lipid profiles in children receiving pravastatin pre-emptively after renal transplantation. *Pediatr Transplant* 2005; **9**: 746–753.

133 Argent E, Kainer G, Aitken M, Rosenberg AR, Mackie FE. Atorvastatin treatment for hyperlipidemia in pediatric renal transplant recipients. *Pediatr Transplant* 2003; **7**: 38–42.

134 Vidhun JR, Sarwal MM. Corticosteroid avoidance in pediatric renal transplantation. *Pediatr Nephrol* 2005; **20**: 418–426.

135 Sarwal MM, Yorgin PD, Alexander S, Millan MT, Belson A, Belanger N *et al.* Promising early outcomes with a novel, complete steroid avoidance immunosuppressive protocol in pediatric renal transplantation. *Transplantation* 2001; **15**: 13–21.

60 Bones Across Kidney Disease and Kidney Failure

Mary B. Leonard

Department of Pediatrics, The Children's Hospital of Philadelphia, and Department of Biostatistics and Epidemiology, University of Pennsylvania School of Medicine, Philadelphia, USA

Introduction

Renal osteodystrophy is a multifactorial and widespread disorder of bone metabolism in chronic kidney disease (CKD). As renal failure progresses, ensuing abnormal parathyroid hormone (PTH) secretion results in deterioration of trabecular microarchitecture, thinning of cortical bone, and increased cortical porosity [1]. Despite widespread use of phosphate binders and vitamin D therapies, hip fracture rates in young adults on dialysis are 100-fold greater than in healthy controls [2]. Significantly greater vertebral and extremity fracture rates have also been demonstrated in pediatric solid organ transplant recipients compared with healthy controls [3]: the age- and sex-adjusted hazard ratios for vertebral fractures were 61.3 (95% confidence interval [CI], 40.7–92.4) compared with over 200,000 population-based controls.

Throughout childhood and adolescence, normal bone mineral acquisition results in gender-, maturation-, and site-specific increases in bone density and dimensions. Children with CKD have multiple risk factors for impaired bone development, including abnormal mineral metabolism, secondary hyperparathyroidism, poor linear growth, delayed development, malnutrition (including vitamin D insufficiency), decreased weight-bearing activity, and immunosuppressive therapies. The impact of these threats to bone health may be immediate, resulting in fragility fractures, or delayed, due to suboptimal peak bone mass accrual. The signs and symptoms of renal bone disease seen in adults, such as subperiosteal resorption, osteosclerosis, fractures, and muscle weakness, may also complicate CKD in childhood. In addition, the effects of abnormal bone and mineral metabolism on endochondral ossification during growth result in complications in the epiphyseal region that are unique to children with CKD. These complications include linear growth failure, slipped epiphyses, and skeletal deformities resembling vitamin D deficiency rickets.

Histomorphometry of renal osteodystrophy in children

Renal osteodystrophy encompasses a heterogeneous group of disorders. The most common form is high-turnover disease due to secondary hyperparathyroidism, phosphate retention, hypocalcemia, reduced renal 1α-hydroxylation of 25(OH)-vitamin D to generate $1,25(OH)_2$-vitamin D (calcitriol), skeletal resistance to the actions of PTH, and decreased numbers of calcium-sensing receptors and vitamin D receptors in the parathyroid gland [4]. Therapies to increase serum calcium, decrease phosphate, and reduce PTH levels have resulted in decreased severity of hyperparathyroidism; however, these therapies are associated with low-turnover disease (adynamic bone disease) [5]. Table 60.1 summarizes published bone biopsy studies in children on dialysis, illustrating the greater prevalence of adynamic bone in the more recent series. Nonetheless, high-turnover bone diseases (osteitis fibrosa and mild lesions of secondary hyperparathyroidism) still frequently complicate pediatric CKD [6,7].

PTH assays and bone turnover in pediatric CKD

Numerous studies suggest that patients with end-stage renal disease (ESRD) require PTH levels well above the normal range (10–65 pg/mL) to maintain normal bone turnover. This peripheral resistance to the effects of PTH is due, in part, to downregulation of the PTH/PTHrP receptor [8]. The presence of circulating PTH fragments and the potentially antagonistic effects of the 7–84 PTH fragment may also contribute [9]. The prediction of bone turnover based on PTH levels is further complicated by the fact that the state of skeletal resistance to PTH progresses with further declines in renal function. That is, PTH levels that predict normal bone turnover in pediatric patients on dialysis are associated with high-turnover bone disease in patients in the earlier stages of CKD [10].

Evidence-based Nephrology. Edited by Donald Molony and Jonathan Craig
© 2009 Blackwell Publishing, ISBN: 978-1-4051-3975-5.

Table 60.1 Bone histomorphometry and PTH levels in children and adolescents on maintenance dialysis.

Study [reference], country	Year	n	Dialysis	Histomorphometry	PTH levels and bone turnover
Salusky [95], USA	1988	44	PD	• 39% osteitis fibrosa • 25% mild high turnover • 11% adynamic bone • 9% osteomalacia • 16% normal	• Bone formation rates correlated positively with PTH levels and negatively with bone aluminium content
Salusky [12], USA	1994	55	PD	• 50% osteitis fibrosa • 9% mild high turnover • 22% adynamic bone • 19% normal	• Serum PTH >200 pg/mL and calcium <10 mg/dL: 85% sensitive and 100% specific for identifying low-turnover disease • Serum PTH <200 pg/mL: 100% sensitive and 79% specific for identifying high-turnover disease; specificity increases to 92% using combined criteria of PTH <150 pg/mL and calcium >10 ng/dL
Yalcinkaya [7], Turkey	2000	17	PD	• 47% high turnover • 29% adynamic bone • 24% mixed turnover	• Serum PTH >200 pg/mL: 100% sensitive and 66% specific for identifying high-turnover disease • Serum PTH <200 pg/mL: 100% sensitive and 92% specific for identifying low-turnover disease
Ziolkowska [6], Poland	2000	51	PD or HD	• 24% high turnover • 27% adynamic bone • 2% osteomalacia • 10% mixed turnover • 37% normal	• In patients with normal bone turnover, 69% had PTH level of 50–150 pg/mL • Serum PTH <150 pg/mL: 100% sensitive and 33% specific for identifying low-turnover disease • Serum PTH >200 pg/mL: 75% sensitive and 95% specific for identifying high-turnover disease

Abbreivations: PD, peritoneal dialysis; HD, hemodialysis.

PTH levels discriminate moderately well between low- and high-turnover renal osteodystrophy in children and adults on dialysis. Multiple studies have been performed using intact PTH assays to diagnose high-turnover bone disorders and distinguish them from low-turnover disorders in adults [11]. The sensitivity and specificity of PTH levels in the discrimination of biopsy-proven low- and high-turnover disease have been examined in three series of children on maintenance dialysis [6,7,12]; the results are summarized in Table 60.1. The 1994 study by Salusky *et al.* suggested that combined consideration of the serum calcium and serum PTH levels improves the sensitivity and specificity of the assays [12].

PTH is a single-chain polypeptide of 84 amino acids. The studies described above were based on "intact-PTH" sandwich radioimmunometric assays. However, these assays also measure large PTH fragments, namely, 7-84 PTH [13]. These N-terminal-truncated PTH fragments may inhibit the action of PTH by blocking binding to its receptor, PTHR1, in bone cells [14,15]. In contrast, the newer-generation PTH assays only measure the 1-84 molecule [16]; however, the utility of these PTH assays has not been established. In a longitudinal study of 51 pediatric dialysis patients, the intact PTH (1-84 plus 7-84) and 1-84 PTH assay results were highly correlated ($R = 0.98$) [17]; however, there was substantial intra- and interpatient variability in the ratio of the 1-84 frag-

ment to intact PTH level. One study in adults suggested that a 1-84/7-84 PTH ratio of less than 1.0 predicted biopsy-proven low-turnover bone disease [18]. Other investigators have been unable to confirm these findings in adults [19–21]. In children, a bone biopsy study in 33 peritoneal dialysis patients demonstrated that intact PTH and 1-84 PTH levels were highly correlated ($R = 0.89$), and the bioactive 1-84 fragment did not correlate with bone formation any better than conventional intact PTH. Furthermore, the 1-84/7-84 PTH ratio did not distinguish between high- and low-turnover disease. The identification of more specific, non-invasive measures of bone turnover remains an area of active investigation.

Although the advantages of new-generation PTH assays and ratios in predicting bone turnover in children remain unproven, a recent study suggested that the 1-84/7-84 PTH ratio was positively correlated with improvements in height Z-scores [22]. Among 162 children and adolescents with estimated glomerular filtration rates (GFR) of less than 60 mL/min/1.73 m^2, there was no relationship between PTH concentration and change in height Z-score over an average interval of 1 year. However, the 1-84/7-84 PTH ratio was lower in dialyzed patients ($P = 0.003$) and in those with worsening renal function ($P < 0.05$), and there was a positive correlation between the 1-84/7-84 PTH ratio and the change in height Z-scores ($R = 0.2$; $P = 0.01$).

Treatment of renal osteodystrophy in children

Phosphate binders

Diminished phosphorus filtration and excretion result in hyperphosphatemia in the majority of children and adults with CKD, contributing to the progression of secondary hyperparathyroidism and renal osteodystrophy. Recent observational studies in adults have demonstrated an association between hyperphosphatemia and increased cardiovascular morbidity in adult dialysis patients [23–25]. Therefore, adequate control of serum phosphorus is a cornerstone of CKD management. Strategies to reduce serum phosphorus levels include restriction of dietary phosphorus, dialysis, and oral phosphate binders. After the recognition that aluminum hydroxide was associated with encephalopathy and osteomalacia, calcium salts emerged as the primary phosphate binder. Calcium carbonate controls phosphorus; however, its effectiveness may be limited by hypercalcemia, especially when administered with vitamin D. Calcium acetate binds approximately twice the amount of phosphorus per amount of calcium absorbed, compared with calcium carbonate [26]. Concerns regarding the potential role of calcium loading in the progression of cardiovascular calcification have resulted in increased use of noncalcium, nonaluminum phosphate binders. Of note, increased intima media thickness of the carotid arteries has been observed in children and adolescents with CKD and correlated with the mean past serum calcium–phosphorus product, the cumulative dose of calcium-based phosphate binders, and the time-averaged mean calcitriol dose [27]. Other studies have confirmed that the occurrence of vascular calcification in children and young adults with childhood-onset CKD was associated with the cumulative intake of calcium-containing phosphate binders, serum phosphorus levels, and the calcium–phosphorus product [28–30].

Sevelamer hydrochloride is a novel, nonaluminum, noncalcium phosphate-binding polymer. As recently reviewed by Coladonato [31], clinical trials in adults comparing sevelamer with calcium-containing phosphate binders have produced conflicting results. The open-label Treat-to-Goal study demonstrated no differences in the final calcium–phosphorus product; however, sevelamer was associated with attenuation of coronary and aortic calcification [32]. In contrast, the double-blind Calcium Acetate Renagel Evaluation trial showed that calcium acetate more effectively lowered serum phosphorus and calcium–phosphorus product than did sevelamer.

Calcium-containing phosphate binders effectively reduce serum phosphorus levels in children and are the first-line treatment in pediatric CKD [33,34]. However, calcium-containing phosphate binders are also associated with hypercalcemic episodes in children. Two randomized clinical trials comparing sevelamer and calcium-containing phosphate binders have been reported in children [35,36]. The studies are summarized in Table 60.2. Briefly, Pieper *et al.* conducted a multicenter, randomized, open-label, crossover study comparing the efficacy and safety of sevelamer versus calcium acetate in children with CKD [35]. Salusky *et al.*

Table 60.2 Phosphate binders in children and adolescents with CKD.

Study [reference], year	Study design (duration)	Interventions	Primary outcome	n	CKD	Results
Pieper [35], 2006	Randomized open-label, crossover trial (8 wks per arm)	Sevelamer vs. calcium acetate	Serum phosphorus	40 randomized; 18 completed the trial	11 on HD 6 on PD 1 pre-ESRD	• Equivalent reduction in serum phosphorus levels in sevelamer and control groups (-1.5 ± 1.6 vs. -1.7 ± 1.7 mg/dL) • Greater incidence of hypercalcemia ($P < .001$) with calcium acetate • Total cholesterol (-27%; $P < 0.02$) and low-density lipoprotein cholesterol (-34%; $P < 0.005$) decreased significantly with sevelamer
Salusky [35], 2005	2×2 factorial, randomized control trial (8 mos)	Sevelamer vs. calcium carbonate + oral doxercalciferol vs. calcitriol	Bone histology (all patients had high turnover at baseline)	42 randomized; 29 completed	PD	• Equivalent reduction in bone formation rates in sevelamer and control groups ($-53 \pm 11\%$ vs. $-49 \pm 7\%$) • Serum calcium and Ca–P product increased with calcium carbonate ($P < 0.001$) • Hypercalcemic episodes more frequent with calcium carbonate ($P < 0.01$)

Abbreviations: HD, hemodialysis; PD, peritoneal dialysis.

conducted a multicenter, randomized trial comparing sevelamer and calcium carbonate in children on peritoneal dialysis with bone biopsy evidence of secondary hyperparathyroidism [36]. These two trials demonstrated that treatment with either sevelamer or calcium-containing phosphate binders resulted in equivalent control of the biochemical and/or skeletal lesions in CKD. Sevelamer, however, was associated with less hypercalcemia, thereby potentially increasing the safety of treatment with active vitamin D sterols.

Vitamin D

Impaired calcitriol synthesis is one of the major factors that contributes to the pathogenesis of renal osteodystrophy. In adults with moderate CKD, several placebo-controlled trials demonstrated that calcitriol therapy was associated with reduction in PTH levels and improvement in bone biopsy results without compromising renal function [37–39]. Early case series of daily oral calcitriol in children reported reductions in PTH levels with variable healing of skeletal lesions [40,41]. Details for these case series and the studies described below are provided in Table 60.3.

Prospective studies in adults showed that intermittent oral calcitriol was just as effective as daily dosing in reducing PTH levels and bone formation rates [42,43]. A case series of intermittent oral or intraperitoneal (i.p.) calcitriol therapy in 14 children on peritoneal dialysis [44] and a randomized clinical trial comparing intermittent oral versus i.p. calcitriol in 33 children with biopsy-proven high-turnover disease [5] demonstrated improvements in skeletal lesions. However, both studies reported that a substantial proportion of subjects on intermittent therapy developed adynamic bone.

It has been suggested that intermittent calcitriol therapy, combined with calcium-containing phosphate binders, may adversely affect chondrocyte activity in the epiphyseal growth plate, with a consequent reduction in linear growth. Schmitt et al. conducted a randomized study in 24 prepubertal children with CKD, comparing the effect of daily versus twice-weekly oral calcitriol therapy [45]. The degree of growth suppression and change in height Z-scores were comparable between groups; however, growth velocity was positively associated with PTH levels. Similarly, Kuizon et al. examined changes in height Z-scores in 16 children treated with intermittent calcitriol therapy [46]. The largest reductions in height Z-scores were seen in patients who developed adynamic bone lesions. In contrast, a retrospective cohort study of 99 children with CKD (GFR of <41 mL/min/1.32 m^2; median GFR, 22) and an overall mean change in height Z-score of +0.3 indicated that catch-up growth can occur with PTH levels in the high normal range during treatment with 1-α-calcidiol and calcium supplements [47].

In 2005, Greenbaum et al. reported the results of a double-blind, placebo-controlled study of the safety and efficacy of intravenous calcitriol for the treatment of secondary hyperparathyroidism in children on hemodialysis [48]. Although a greater proportion of children in the calcitriol group had substantial reductions in PTH levels compared with the placebo group, the incidences of elevated calcium–phosphorus product, hyperphosphatemia, and hypercalcemia were significantly higher in the calcitriol group.

Therapy with calcitriol is associated with hypercalcemia and hyperphosphatemia, which may limit its use and may contribute to vascular calcification. Milner et al. conducted a retrospective chart review of postmortem evidence of soft tissue and vascular calcification in 120 children with ESRD [49]. Soft tissue calcification was found in 72 patients (60%), and 36% had systemic calcinosis. Vitamin D therapy showed the strongest independent association with calcinosis, and the probability of calcinosis was higher in patients receiving calcitriol compared with dihydrotachysterol and vitamin D$_2$ or D$_3$.

New vitamin D analogs have been developed to minimize intestinal calcium and phosphorus absorption while suppressing PTH levels. These include 22-oxacalcitriol in Japan and 19-nor-1,25-dihydroxyvitamin D$_2$ (paracalcitol) and 1α-hydroxyvitamin D$_2$ (doxercalciferol) in the USA. Prospective comparisons against calcitriol are very limited, and the skeletal response to the new active vitamin D sterols remains to be determined. However, data in adults suggested that 19-nor-1,25-dihydroxyvitamin D$_2$ was associated with greater survival in those on hemodialysis compared with calcitriol [50]. In addition, recent studies of 1α-hydroxyvitamin D$_2$ [51] and 19-nor-1,25-dihydroxyvitamin D$_2$ [52] suggest that these agents lower PTH levels with few episodes of hypercalcemia. Finally, a recent study in 29 children suggests that oral 1α-hydroxyvitamin D$_2$ given thrice weekly is as effective as calcitriol in reducing PTH levels and improving the skeletal lesions of secondary hyperparathyroidism in children treated with peritoneal dialysis [36].

The National Kidney Foundation Kidney Disease Outcomes Quality Initiative (K/DOQI) clinical practice guidelines for bone metabolism and disease in children with chronic kidney disease future [53] provide multiple algorithms for calcitriol therapy, based on CKD stage, serum 25(OH)-vitamin D levels, subject weight, and serum calcium, phosphorus, and PTH levels.

Glucocorticoid-induced osteoporosis in pediatric CKD

Glucocorticoids are widely used in the treatment of kidney disease (e.g. nephrotic syndrome and renal transplantation) and impact bone formation and resorption. Glucocorticoids inhibit osteoblasts, thereby reducing bone formation [54]; the growing skeleton may be especially vulnerable to these effects. Although decreased bone mineral density (BMD) has been described in pediatric disorders requiring glucocorticoids and a population-based study reported increased fracture risk in children requiring repeated courses of glucocorticoids [55], some of the detrimental bone effects attributed to glucocorticoids may be due to the underlying inflammatory disease. For example, inflammatory cytokines that are elevated in chronic disease, such as tumor necrosis factor alpha, suppress bone formation and promote bone resorption through mechanisms similar to glucocorticoid effects [56].

Table 60.3 Vitamin D therapy in children and adolescents with CKD

Study [reference], year	Study design (duration)	Intervention(s)	Primary outcome(s)	n	CKD	Results
Chesney [40], 1978	Case series (up to 26 mos)	Daily oral calcitriol	Serum PTH	6		• Serum PTH levels decreased and lesions of rickets improved
Goodman [41], 1991	Case series (12 mos)	Daily oral calcitriol	Bone histology	33	PD	• Severe osteitis fibrosa failed to improve but lesions of mild secondary hyperparathyroidism improved
Goodman [44], 1994	Case series (12 mos)	Intermittent oral or i.p. calcitriol	Bone histology	14	PD	• Osteitis fibrosa resolved in 10 of 11 cases • Bone formation decreased in all patients • 6 patients developed adynamic bone
Salusky [5], 1998	Randomized controlled trial (12 mos)	Thrice-weekly i.p. vs. oral calcitriol	Bone histology, serum calcium and PTH	46 randomized; 33 completed	PD	• Equivalent improvements in bone histology • 33% developed adynamic bone • Serum calcium levels higher and reductions in PTH greater in subjects treated with i.p. calcitriol (both $P < 0.0001$)
Kuizon [46], 1998	Case series (24 mos)	Intermittent calcitriol over 12 mos vs. daily therapy during prior 12 mos	Growth	16 prepubertal	PD	• Height Z-scores decreased from -1.8 ± 0.32 to -2.0 ± 0.33 ($P < 0.01$) during intermittent calcitriol therapy • Greater growth deficits in children with adynamic bone after 12 mos intermittent treatment • Change in height Z-scores correlated with serum PTH ($r = 0.71$; $P < 0.01$) during intermittent calcitriol therapy
Schmitt [45], 2003	Randomized controlled trial (12 mos)	Daily vs. twice-weekly oral calcitriol	PTH and growth	24	PD	• PTH decreased significantly in both groups; magnitude of change did not differ between treatment arms • Equivalent change in height Z-scores in daily and intermittent groups (-0.18 ± 0.34 vs. -0.05 ± 0.52) • Growth velocity positively associated with PTH levels
Greenbaum [48], 2005	Randomized controlled trial (12 wks)	Thrice-weekly intravenous calcitriol vs. placebo	$\geq 30\%$ decline in PTH from baseline	47	HD	• Greater proportion of patients in calcitriol group had two consecutive $\geq 30\%$ decreases in PTH than placebo group (52% vs. 19%; $P = 0.03$) • Incidences of elevated Ca–P product and hypercalcemia higher in calcitriol group (both $P = 0.01$)
Salusky [36], 2005	2 × 2 factorial, randomized control trial (8 mos)	Thrice-weekly oral doxercalciferol vs. calcitriol + sevelamer vs. calcium carbonate	Bone histology (all patients had high turnover at baseline)	42 randomized; 29 completed	PD	• Doxercalciferol and calcitriol equally effective in reducing PTH levels and improving skeletal lesions of secondary hyperparathyroidism

Abbreviations: PD, peritoneal dialysis; HD, hemodialysis.

Childhood steroid-sensitive nephrotic syndrome (SSNS) provides a clinical model of chronic glucocorticoid therapy in the absence of significant persistent underlying disease activity. The nephrotic state is clinically quiescent as long as high-dose glucocorticoid therapy is continued. Unfortunately, SSNS relapses in the majority of children when the glucocorticoids are reduced, resulting in protracted, repeated courses of glucocorticoids. The standard prednisone dose for relapses is 2 mg/kg/day [57], far exceeding the 5 mg/day considered a risk factor for glucocorticoid-induced osteoporosis in adults [58]. Although SSNS relapses are associated with transient increases in cytokines, these abnormalities promptly resolve with remission [59]. Therefore, SSNS serves as a clinical model without significant sustained systemic inflammatory involvement to examine the effects of glucocorticoids on the growing skeleton.

Leonard *et al.* examined spine and whole-body bone mineral content (BMC) by dual-energy X-ray absorptiometry (DXA) in a cross-sectional study of 60 children and adolescents with established SSNS and 195 healthy controls. The SSNS subjects had received an average of 23,000 mg of glucocorticoids over a 4-year interval. SSNS subjects had significantly decreased height ($P = 0.008$) and increased body mass index (BMI) Z-scores ($P < 0.001$), compared with controls. The prevalence of obesity in the control group was 16%, consistent with the 15.5% prevalence of obesity in children and adolescents nationwide [60]. In contrast, 38% of the subjects with SSNS were obese. Spine BMC, adjusted for bone area, age, sex, Tanner stage, and race, did not differ significantly between patients and controls ($P = 0.51$). The authors documented that obesity, in otherwise-healthy children, was associated with significant increases in whole-body, hip, and spine BMC and bone size [61,62]. Therefore, the models were adjusted for BMI Z-score. In the adjusted model, spine BMC was 4% lower in SSNS subjects than controls (ratio, 0.96; CI, 0.92–0.99; $P = 0.01$). Whole-body BMC, adjusted for height, age, sex, Tanner stage, and race, was 11% higher in SSNS subjects than controls (ratio, 1.11; CI, 1.05–1.18; $P < 0.001$); however, the addition of BMI Z-score to the model eliminated the association with the SSNS (ratio, 0.99; CI, 0.94–1.03; $P = 0.55$). These data suggested that intermittent treatment with high-dose glucocorticoids during growth was not associated with significant bone deficits relative to age, bone size, sex, and maturation in SSNS. Glucocorticoid-induced obesity was associated with increased whole-body BMC and maintenance of spine BMC.

Other studies have examined DXA BMD in SSNS. Gulati *et al.* reported that children in India with nephrotic syndrome had low BMD for age [63]. However, this study included children with steroid-resistant nephrotic syndrome and did not include controls. Furthermore, the DXA reference data used in this study have been shown to overestimate the prevalence of osteoporosis in boys [64], and 80% of the nephrotic syndrome subjects in the Gulati study were boys.

A recent study in the UK examined BMD using DXA and quantitative computed tomography (QCT) in 34 young adults with a history of childhood nephrotic syndrome. The mean height and BMI Z-scores were -0.45 ± 0.92 and 1.62 ± 1.53, respectively. DXA BMD Z-scores in the spine and hip were not reduced compared to controls. There was a significant reduction in QCT distal radial trabecular volumetric BMD (mean Z-score, -0.95 ± 0.99). However, the distal radial total volumetric BMD Z-score (0.00 ± 0.95) was normal. A more recent study using DXA hip structural analyses software [65] demonstrated that childhood SSNS was associated with significantly increased bone dimensions (periosteal circumference) and bone mass in the cortical shaft of the femur [66]. Therefore, one interpretation of these studies is that

trabecular BMD is decreased and cortical bone mass is increased (secondary to obesity) in SSNS. The fracture implications of these alterations are not known.

Finally, Bak *et al.* recently reported the results of a randomized prospective study of the effects and prophylactic role of calcium plus vitamin D treatment on bone metabolism in 40 children with SSNS [67]. All patients received prednisolone treatment (2 mg/kg/day for 4 weeks followed by alternate days at the same dose for 4 weeks). The patients were randomized into treatment (vitamin D at 400 IU plus calcium at 1 g daily) and nontreatment groups. Spine BMD was measured by DXA and decreased significantly during prednisolone therapy in both the treatment and nontreatment groups; however, the percentage decrease in BMD was significantly lower in the treatment group (4.6%) than in the nontreatment group (13.0%). Future studies are needed to determine the long-term effects of calcium and vitamin D in SSNS.

Quantitative assessment of bone status in children

Classification of bone health and relation to fracture risk

DXA is widely accepted as a quantitative measurement technique for assessing skeletal status. In elderly adults, DXA BMD is a sufficiently robust predictor of osteoporotic fractures that it can be used to define the disease. The diagnosis of osteoporosis in adults is based on a T-score, the comparison of a measured BMD result with the average BMD of young adults at the time of peak bone mass [68]. In contrast, children are assessed relative to age or body size, and the results are expressed as a Z-score. Despite the growing body of published normative data utilizing DXA in children, there are no evidence-based guidelines for the definition of osteoporosis in children. Fractures occur commonly in otherwise-healthy children, with a peak incidence during early adolescence, around the time of the pubertal growth spurt [69]. Several studies have compared the DXA BMD of normal children and adolescents with forearm fractures to that of age-matched controls without fractures. Most studies [70–74], but not all [75,76], found that mean DXA BMD was significantly lower in children with forearm fractures than in controls.

DXA has several limitations that can be pronounced in the assessment of children. These include difficulties in scan acquisition due to limitations in the bone edge detection software for children [77,78], difficulties in the interpretation of DXA results in children with variable body size, body composition, and skeletal maturation, and limited reference data [64]. A significant limitation of DXA is the reliance on measurement of areal rather than volumetric BMD. DXA provides an estimate of BMD expressed as grams per anatomical region (e.g. individual vertebrae, whole body, or hip). Dividing the BMC within the defined anatomical region (in grams) by the projected area of the bone (in square centimeters) then produces the "areal BMD" (in grams per square centimeter). This BMD is not a measure of volumetric density (grams per cubic centimeter) because it provides no information about the depth of bone. Bones of larger width and height also tend to be thicker. Because bone thickness is not factored into DXA estimates of BMD, reliance on the areal BMD inherently underestimates the bone density of short people. Despite identical volumetric bone density, a child with smaller bones will appear to have a mineralization disorder (decreased areal BMD). This is clearly an important artifact in children with chronic diseases, such as CKD, that are associated with poor growth [79].

A recent study highlighted the importance of these limitations [80]: among children referred for enrollment in a pediatric osteoporosis protocol based on low DXA spine BMD, 80% had at least one error in interpretation of the DXA scan. Ultimately, only 26% retained the diagnosis of low BMD.

Limitations of DXA in CKD

DXA has additional important limitations in patients with CKD; these limitations were recently reviewed for children undergoing kidney transplantation [81]. Trabecular and cortical bone behave differently in response to increased PTH levels: trabecular bone mass increases and cortical bone mass decreases [1]. The two-dimensional posterior–anterior DXA projection of the spine captures the largely trabecular vertebral body, as well as the superimposed cortical spinous processes. However, the lateral projection allows one to distinguish between the vertebral body and posterior elements. A study in adults with primary hyperparathyroidism illustrated the limitations of DXA in the setting of increased PTH [82]: the mean spine BMD on the posterior–anterior projection

Table 60.4 Evidence ratings and recommendations for interventions to improve bone metabolism in children with CKD.

| Intervention | SR[a] | Evidence rating[b] | | | Recommendation[c] | | | |
		Moderate	Low	Comment	I	II	III	Comment
Phosphate binders								
Calcium carbonate	–		•	2 case series (15 and 63 subjects)	•			Calcium carbonate reduces serum phosphorus in children with CKD
Sevelamer vs. calcium acetate	+	•		1 RCT (40 subjects enrolled, 18 completed the crossover trial)		•		Equivalent reduction in phosphorus levels and Ca–P product in the two groups; calcium acetate associated with more frequent hypercalcemic episodes
Sevelamer vs. calcium carbonate	+	•		1 RCT (42 subjects enrolled, 29 completed the trial)		•		Equivalent reduction in skeletal lesions of secondary hyperparathyroidism in the two groups; calcium carbonate associated with greater calcium, Ca–P product, and more frequent hypercalcemic episodes
Vitamin D therapy								
Oral daily calcitriol	–		•	2 case series (6 children with CKD; 33 children on PD)			•	PTH levels improved; severe osteitis fibrosis persisted or progressed in some subjects
Oral intermittent calcitriol	–		•	2 case series (14 and 16 children on PD)			•	Nearly half developed adynamic bone; may be associated with poor growth
Oral daily vs. oral intermittent calcitriol	+	•		1 RCT in 24 children on PD			•	Comparable growth velocity and decreases in PTH
Intermittent oral vs. intraperitoneal calcitriol	+	•		1 RCT in 46 children on PD		•		Equivalent improvements in bone histology (33% adynamic bone), but calcium levels were higher and reductions in PTH levels were greater in subjects treated with i.p. calcitriol
Intravenous calcitriol vs. placebo	+	•		1 RCT in 47 children on HD		•		Calcitriol reduces PTH levels but is associated with hypercalcemia and hyperphosphatemia
Intermittent oral doxercalciferol vs. calcitriol	+	•		1 RCT (42 subjects enrolled, 29 completed the trial)		•		Doxercalciferol and calcitriol equally effective in reducing PTH levels and improving skeletal lesions of secondary hyperparathyroidism

Abbreviations: RCT, randomized controlled trial; PD, peritoneal dialysis; HD, hemodialysis.

[a]Systematic review of randomized controlled trials.

[b]Evidence rating based on study design, study quality, and consistency and directness of results. No intervention was rated with a high evidence rating.

[c]Recommendations based trade-offs between benefits and harms, quality of evidence, translation of evidence into practice in a specific setting including availability of medication and any uncertainty about the baseline risk of the disease in the population. I, recommend; II, suggest; III, no recommendation possible.

was normal, but the lateral scan revealed increased BMD in the predominantly trabecular vertebral body and decreased BMD in the cortical spinous processes. Clearly, because trabecular and cortical bone behave differently in response to increased parathyroid activity and DXA does not distinguish between renal osteodystrophy effects on the two types of bone, DXA is of limited value in CKD. The conflicting data on DXA-derived measures of BMD in CKD are consistent with these limitations: DXA results have been variable, with mean BMD values that are higher than, the same as, or lower than control subjects [83–90]. Given the limitations of DXA in children with CKD, the National Kidney Foundation clinical practice guidelines do not recommend DXA scans for children with CKD [53].

QCT

QCT provides a cross-sectional image unobscured by overlying structures [91]. In contrast to DXA, this technique describes authentic volumetric BMD (in grams per cubic centimeter), accurately measures bone dimensions, and distinguishes between cortical and trabecular bone. In order to minimize radiation exposure, special high-resolution scanners have been developed for the peripheral skeleton (pQCT). Spine QCT data in CKD confirmed biopsy histomorphometric data: trabecular BMD was increased in high-turnover disease ($+1.6$ standard deviations) and decreased in low-turnover disease (-1.2 standard deviations), relative to age-matched controls [92].

The impact of CKD on BMD during childhood was examined using pQCT in 21 children on peritoneal dialysis [93]. Trabecular BMD was significantly higher ($P < 0.0001$) and cortical BMD was significantly lower ($P < 0.001$) in children with CKD compared with controls. In patients with adynamic bone, trabecular BMD was less than in those with high-turnover lesions ($P < 0.001$). Similarly, cortical BMD was lower in patients with high-turnover lesions than in those with low-turnover lesions ($P < 0.05$).

A recent study by Jamal et al. underscored the advantages of QCT versus DXA in CKD [94]. She reported that DXA in the hip and spine failed to discriminate between patients with and without fractures; in contrast, QCT measures of cortical BMD and thickness discriminated between fractures and nonfractures very well.

Summary

The management of renal osteodystrophy in children should be tailored to optimize rates of bone turnover, bone acquisition, and growth, while avoiding metabolic abnormalities associated with vascular calcifications. The evidence ratings for phosphate binders and vitamin D therapy are summarized in Table 60.4. The paucity of randomized controlled trials and the poor subject retention in some trials reflect the difficulties in conducting these multicenter studies in children with CKD. As detailed in the National Kidney Foundation K/DOQI clinical practice guidelines for bone metabolism and disease in children with chronic kidney disease

future studies [53], studies are needed to address the impact of existing therapies and new vitamin D analogs on bone health, growth, and vascular calcification in children.

References

1 Parfitt AM. A structural approach to renal bone disease. *J Bone Miner Res* 1998; **13(8)**: 1213–1220.

2 Alem AM, Sherrard DJ, Gillen DL, Weiss NS, Beresford SA, Heckbert SR et al. Increased risk of hip fracture among patients with end-stage renal disease. *Kidney Int* 2000; **58(1)**: 396–399.

3 Helenius I, Remes V, Salminen S, Valta H, Makitie O, Holmberg C et al. Incidence and predictors of fractures in children after solid organ transplantation: a 5-year prospective, population-based study. *J Bone Miner Res* 2006; **21(3)**: 380–387.

4 Hendy GN, Hruska KA, Mathew S, Goltzman D. New insights into mineral and skeletal regulation by active forms of vitamin D. *Kidney Int* 2006; **69(2)**: 218–223.

5 Salusky IB, Kuizon BD, Belin TR, Ramirez JA, Gales B, Segre GV et al. Intermittent calcitriol therapy in secondary hyperparathyroidism: a comparison between oral and intraperitoneal administration. *Kidney Int* 1998; **54(3)**: 907–914.

6 Ziolkowska H, Paniczyk-Tomaszewska M, Debinski A, Polowiec Z, Sawicki A, Sieniawska M. Bone biopsy results and serum bone turnover parameters in uremic children. *Acta Paediatr* 2000; **89(6)**: 666–671.

7 Yalcinkaya F, Ince E, Tumer N, Ensari A, Ozkaya N. Spectrum of renal osteodystrophy in children on continuous ambulatory peritoneal dialysis. *Pediatr Int* 2000; **42(1)**: 53–57.

8 Tian J, Smogorzewski M, Kedes L, Massry SG. PTH-PTHrP receptor mRNA is downregulated in chronic renal failure. *Am J Nephrol* 1994; **14(1)**: 41–46.

9 Slatopolsky E, Finch J, Clay P, Martin D, Sicard G, Singer G et al. A novel mechanism for skeletal resistance in uremia. *Kidney Int* 2000; **58(2)**: 753–761.

10 Salusky IB. Are new vitamin D analogues in renal bone disease superior to calcitriol? *Pediatr Nephrol* 2005; **20(3)**: 393–398.

11 NKF. K/DOQI clinical practice guidelines for bone metabolism and disease in chronic kidney disease. *Am J Kidney Dis* 2003; **42(4 Suppl 3)**: S1–S201.

12 Salusky IB, Ramirez JA, Oppenheim W, Gales B, Segre GV, Goodman WG. Biochemical markers of renal osteodystrophy in pediatric patients undergoing CAPD/CCPD. *Kidney Int* 1994; **45(1)**: 253–258.

13 Brossard JH, Cloutier M, Roy L, Lepage R, Gascon-Barre M, D'Amour P. Accumulation of a non-(1-84) molecular form of parathyroid hormone (PTH) detected by intact PTH assay in renal failure: importance in the interpretation of PTH values. *J Clin Endocrinol Metab* 1996; **81(11)**: 3923–3929.

14 Kaji H, Sugimoto T, Kanatani M, Miyauchi A, Kimura T, Sakakibara S et al. Carboxyl-terminal parathyroid hormone fragments stimulate osteoclast-like cell formation and osteoclastic activity. *Endocrinology* 1994; **134(4)**: 1897–1904.

15 Langub MC, Monier-Faugere MC, Wang G, Williams JP, Koszewski NJ, Malluche HH. Administration of PTH-(7-84) antagonizes the effects of PTH-(1-84) on bone in rats with moderate renal failure. *Endocrinology* 2003; **144(4)**: 1135–1138.

16 Gao P, Scheibel S, D'Amour P, John MR, Rao SD, Schmidt-Gayk H et al. Development of a novel immunoradiometric assay exclusively for

biologically active whole parathyroid hormone 1-84: implications for improvement of accurate assessment of parathyroid function. *J Bone Miner Res* 2001; **16**(4): 605–614.

17 Sheth RD, Goldstein SL. Comparison of 1-84 and intact parathyroid hormone assay in pediatric dialysis patients. *Pediatr Nephrol* 2005; **20**(7): 977–981.

18 Monier-Faugere MC, Geng Z, Mawad H, Friedler RM, Gao P, Cantor TL *et al.* Improved assessment of bone turnover by the PTH-(1-84)/large C-PTH fragments ratio in ESRD patients. *Kidney Int* 2001; **60**: 1460–1468.

19 Reichel H, Esser A, Roth HJ, Schmidt-Gayk H. Influence of PTH assay methodology on differential diagnosis of renal bone disease. *Nephrol Dial Transplant* 2003; **18**(4): 759–768.

20 Salusky IB, Goodman WG, Kuizon BD, Lavigne JR, Zahranik RJ, Gales B *et al.* Similar predictive value of bone turnover using first- and second-generation immunometric PTH assays in pediatric patients treated with peritoneal dialysis. *Kidney Int* 2003; **63**(5): 1801–1808.

21 Coen G, Bonucci E, Ballanti P, Balducci A, Calabria S, Nicolai GA *et al.* PTH 1-84 and PTH "7-84" in the noninvasive diagnosis of renal bone disease. *Am J Kidney Dis* 2002; **40**(2): 348–354.

22 Waller SC, Ridout D, Cantor T, Rees L. Parathyroid hormone and growth in children with chronic renal failure. *Kidney Int* 2005; **67**(6): 2338–2345.

23 Block GA, Hulbert-Shearon TE, Levin NW, Port FK. Association of serum phosphorus and calcium x phosphate product with mortality risk in chronic hemodialysis patients: a national study. *Am J Kidney Dis* 1998; **31**(4): 607–617.

24 Block GA, Klassen PS, Lazarus JM, Ofsthun N, Lowrie EG, Chertow GM. Mineral metabolism, mortality, and morbidity in maintenance hemodialysis. *J Am Soc Nephrol* 2004; **15**(8): 2208–2218.

25 Ganesh SK, Stack AG, Levin NW, Hulbert-Shearon T, Port FK. Association of elevated serum PO_4, Ca x PO_4 product, and parathyroid hormone with cardiac mortality risk in chronic hemodialysis patients. *J Am Soc Nephrol* 2001; **12**(10): 2131–2138.

26 Schaefer K, Scheer J, Asmus G, Umlauf E, Hagemann J, von Herrath D. The treatment of uraemic hyperphosphataemia with calcium acetate and calcium carbonate: a comparative study. *Nephrol Dial Transplant* 1991; **6**(3): 170–175.

27 Litwin M, Wuhl E, Jourdan C, Trelewicz J, Niemirska A, Fahr K *et al.* Altered morphologic properties of large arteries in children with chronic renal failure and after renal transplantation. *J Am Soc Nephrol* 2005; **16**(5): 1494–1500.

28 Goodman WG, Goldin J, Kuizon BD, Yoon C, Gales B, Sider D *et al.* Coronary-artery calcification in young adults with end-stage renal disease who are undergoing dialysis. *N Engl J Med* 2000; **342**(20): 1478–1483.

29 Oh J, Wunsch R, Turzer M, Bahner M, Raggi P, Querfeld U *et al.* Advanced coronary and carotid arteriopathy in young adults with childhood-onset chronic renal failure. *Circulation* 2002; **106**(1): 100–105.

30 Chertow GM, Raggi P, Chasan-Taber S, Bommer J, Holzer H, Burke SK. Determinants of progressive vascular calcification in haemodialysis patients. *Nephrol Dial Transplant* 2004; **19**(6): 1489–1496.

31 Coladonato JA. Control of hyperphosphatemia among patients with ESRD. *J Am Soc Nephrol* 2005; **16**(Suppl 2): S107–S114.

32 Chertow GM, Burke SK, Raggi P. Sevelamer attenuates the progression of coronary and aortic calcification in hemodialysis patients. *Kidney Int* 2002; **62**(1): 245–252.

33 Salusky IB, Coburn JW, Foley J, Nelson P, Fine RN. Effects of oral calcium carbonate on control of serum phosphorus and changes in plasma aluminum levels after discontinuation of aluminum-containing gels in children receiving dialysis. *J Pediatr* 1986; **108**(5 Pt 1): 767–770.

34 Clark AG, Oner A, Ward G, Turner C, Rigden SP, Haycock GB *et al.* Safety and efficacy of calcium carbonate in children with chronic renal failure. *Nephrol Dial Transplant* 1989; **4**(6): 539–544.

35 Pieper AK, Haffner D, Hoppe B, Dittrich K, Offner G, Bonzel KE *et al.* A randomized crossover trial comparing sevelamer with calcium acetate in children with CKD. *Am J Kidney Dis* 2006; **47**(4): 625–635.

36 Salusky IB, Goodman WG, Sahney S, Gales B, Perilloux A, Wang HJ *et al.* Sevelamer controls parathyroid hormone-induced bone disease as efficiently as calcium carbonate without increasing serum calcium levels during therapy with active vitamin D sterols. *J Am Soc Nephrol* 2005; **16**(8): 2501–2508.

37 Nordal KP, Dahl E. Low dose calcitriol versus placebo in patients with predialysis chronic renal failure. *J Clin Endocrinol Metab* 1988; **67**(5): 929–936.

38 Coen G, Mazzaferro S, Bonucci E, Ballanti P, Massimetti C, Donato G *et al.* Treatment of secondary hyperparathyroidism of predialysis chronic renal failure with low doses of $1,25(OH)_2D_3$: humoral and histomorphometric results. *Miner Electrolyte Metab* 1986; **12**(5–6): 375–382.

39 Bianchi ML, Colantonio G, Campanini F, Rossi R, Valenti G, Ortolani S *et al.* Calcitriol and calcium carbonate therapy in early chronic renal failure. *Nephrol Dial Transplant* 1994; **9**(11): 1595–1599.

40 Chesney RW, Moorthy AV, Eisman JA, Jax DK, Mazess RB, DeLuca HF. Increased growth after long-term oral $1\alpha,25$-vitamin D_3 in childhood renal osteodystrophy. *N Engl J Med* 1978; **298**(5): 238–242.

41 Goodman WG, Salusky IB. Evolution of secondary hyperparathyroidism during oral calcitriol therapy in pediatric renal osteodystrophy. *Contrib Nephrol* 1991; **90**: 189–195.

42 Quarles LD, Yohay DA, Carroll BA, Spritzer CE, Minda SA, Bartholomay D *et al.* Prospective trial of pulse oral versus intravenous calcitriol treatment of hyperparathyroidism in ESRD. *Kidney Int* 1994; **45**(6): 1710–1721.

43 Levine BS, Song M. Pharmacokinetics and efficacy of pulse oral versus intravenous calcitriol in hemodialysis patients. *J Am Soc Nephrol* 1996; **7**(3): 488–496.

44 Goodman WG, Ramirez JA, Belin TR, Chon Y, Gales B, Segre GV *et al.* Development of adynamic bone in patients with secondary hyperparathyroidism after intermittent calcitriol therapy. *Kidney Int* 1994; **46**(4): 1160–1166.

45 Schmitt CP, Ardissino G, Testa S, Claris-Appiani A, Mehls O. Growth in children with chronic renal failure on intermittent versus daily calcitriol. *Pediatr Nephrol* 2003; **18**(5): 440–444.

46 Kuizon BD, Goodman WG, Juppner H, Boechat I, Nelson P, Gales B *et al.* Diminished linear growth during intermittent calcitriol therapy in children undergoing CCPD. *Kidney Int* 1998; **53**(1): 205–211.

47 Waller S, Ledermann S, Trompeter R, van't Hoff W, Ridout D, Rees L. Catch-up growth with normal parathyroid hormone levels in chronic renal failure. *Pediatr Nephrol* 2003; **18**(12): 1236–1241.

48 Greenbaum LA, Grenda R, Qiu P, Restaino I, Wojtak A, Paredes A *et al.* Intravenous calcitriol for treatment of hyperparathyroidism in children on hemodialysis. *Pediatr Nephrol* 2005; **20**(5): 622–630.

49 Milliner DS, Zinsmeister AR, Lieberman E, Landing B. Soft tissue calcification in pediatric patients with end-stage renal disease. *Kidney Int* 1990; **38**(5): 931–936.

50 Teng M, Wolf M, Lowrie E, Ofsthun N, Lazarus JM, Thadhani R. Survival of patients undergoing hemodialysis with paricalcitol or calcitriol therapy. *N Engl J Med* 2003; **349**(5): 446–456.

51 Coburn JW, Maung HM, Elangovan L, Germain MJ, Lindberg JS, Sprague SM *et al.* Doxercalciferol safely suppresses PTH levels in patients with

secondary hyperparathyroidism associated with chronic kidney disease stages 3 and 4. *Am J Kidney Dis* 2004; **43**(5): 877–890.

52 Sprague SM, Lerma E, McCormmick D, Abraham M, Batlle D. Suppression of parathyroid hormone secretion in hemodialysis patients: comparison of paricalcitol with calcitriol. *Am J Kidney Dis* 2001; **38**(5 **Suppl 5**): S51–S56.

53 K/DOQI Clinical Practice Guidelines for bone metabolism and disease in children with chronic kidney disease. *Am J Kidney Dis* 2005; **46**(**Suppl 1**): S1–S103.

54 Canalis E. Mechanisms of glucocorticoid action in bone. *Curr Osteoporos Rep* 2005; **3**(3): 98–102.

55 van Staa TP, Cooper C, Leufkens HG, Bishop N. Children and the risk of fractures caused by oral corticosteroids. *J Bone Miner Res* 2003; **18**(5): 913–918.

56 Walsh MC, Kim N, Kadono Y, Rho J, Lee SY, Lorenzo J *et al.* Osteoimmunology: interplay between the immune system and bone metabolism. *Annu Rev Immunol* 2006; **24**: 33–63.

57 Brodehl J. The treatment of minimal change nephrotic syndrome: lessons learned from multicentre co-operative studies. *Eur J Pediatr* 1991; **150**(6): 380–387.

58 van Staa TP, Leufkens HG, Cooper C. The epidemiology of corticosteroid-induced osteoporosis: a meta-analysis. *Osteoporos Int* 2002; **13**(10): 777–787.

59 Daniel V, Trautmann Y, Konrad M, Nayir A, Scharer K. T-lymphocyte populations, cytokines and other growth factors in serum and urine of children with idiopathic nephrotic syndrome. *Clin Nephrol* 1997; **47**(5): 289–297.

60 Ogden CL, Flegal KM, Carroll MD, Johnson CL. Prevalence and trends in overweight among US children and adolescents, 1999–2000. *JAMA* 2002; **288**(14): 1728–1732.

61 Petit MA, Beck TJ, Shults J, Zemel BS, Foster BJ, Leonard MB. Proximal femur bone geometry is appropriately adapted to lean mass in overweight children and adolescents. *Bone* 2005; **36**(3): 568–576.

62 Leonard MB, Shults J, Wilson BA, Tershakovec AM, Zemel BS. Obesity during childhood and adolescence augments bone mass and bone dimensions. *Am J Clin Nutr* 2004; **80**(2): 514–523.

63 Gulati S, Godbole M, Singh U, Gulati K, Srivastava A. Are children with idiopathic nephrotic syndrome at risk for metabolic bone disease? *Am J Kidney Dis* 2003; **41**(6): 1163–1169.

64 Leonard MB, Propert KJ, Zemel BS, Stallings VA, Feldman HI. Discrepancies in pediatric bone mineral density reference data: potential for misdiagnosis of osteopenia. *J Pediatr* 1999; **135**(2 Pt 1): 182–188.

65 Beck TJ, Ruff CB, Warden KE, Scott WW, Jr., Rao GU. Predicting femoral neck strength from bone mineral data. A structural approach. *Invest Radiol* 1990; **25**(1): 6–18.

66 Burnham JM, Shults J, Petit MA, Semeao E, Beck TJ, Zemel BS *et al.* Alterations in proximal femur geometry in children treated with glucocorticoids for Crohn disease or nephrotic syndrome: impact of the underlying disease. *J Bone Miner Res* 2007; **22**(4): 551–559.

67 Bak M, Serdaroglu E, Guclu R. Prophylactic calcium and vitamin D treatments in steroid-treated children with nephrotic syndrome. *Pediatr Nephrol* 2006; **21**(3): 350–354.

68 WHO. The WHO Study Group: assessment of fracture risk and its application to screening for postmenopausal osteoporosis. Geneva, Switzerland, 1994.

69 Khosla S, Melton LJ, III, Dekutoski MB, Achenbach SJ, Oberg AL, Riggs BL. Incidence of childhood distal forearm fractures over 30 years: a population-based study. *JAMA* 2003; **290**(11): 1479–1485.

70 Chan GM, Hess M, Hollis J, Book LS. Bone mineral status in childhood accidental fractures. *Am J Dis Child* 1984; **138**(6): 569–570.

71 Goulding A, Cannan R, Williams SM, Gold EJ, Taylor RW, Lewis-Barned NJ. Bone mineral density in girls with forearm fractures. *J Bone Miner Res* 1998; **13**(1): 143–148.

72 Goulding A, Jones IE, Taylor RW, Williams SM, Manning PJ. Bone mineral density and body composition in boys with distal forearm fractures: a dual-energy X-ray absorptiometry study. *J Pediatr* 2001; **139**(4): 509–515.

73 Goulding A, Jones IE, Taylor RW, Manning PJ, Williams SM. More broken bones: a 4-year double cohort study of young girls with and without distal forearm fractures. *J Bone Miner Res* 2000; **15**(10): 2011–2018.

74 Ma D, Jones G. The association between bone mineral density, metacarpal morphometry, and upper limb fractures in children: a population-based case-control study. *J Clin Endocrinol Metab* 2003; **88**(4): 1486–1491.

75 Ma DQ, Jones G. Clinical risk factors but not bone density are associated with prevalent fractures in prepubertal children. *J Paediatr Child Health* 2002; **38**(5): 497–500.

76 Cook SD, Harding AF, Morgan EL, Doucet HJ, Bennett JT, O'Brien M *et al.* Association of bone mineral density and pediatric fractures. *J Pediatr Orthop* 1987; **7**(4): 424–427.

77 Leonard MB, Feldman HI, Zemel BS, Berlin JA, Barden EM, Stallings VA. Evaluation of low density spine software for the assessment of bone mineral density in children. *J Bone Miner Res* 1998; **13**(11): 1687–1690.

78 Shypailo RJ, Ellis KJ. Bone assessment in children: comparison of fan-beam DXA analysis. *J Clin Densitom* 2005; **8**(4): 445–453.

79 Stephens M, Batres LA, Ng D, Baldassano R. Growth failure in the child with inflammatory bowel disease. *Semin Gastrointest Dis* 2001; **12**(4): 253–262.

80 Gafni RI, Baron J. Overdiagnosis of osteoporosis in children due to misinterpretation of dual-energy X-ray absorptiometry (DEXA). *J Pediatr* 2004; **144**(2): 253–257.

81 Leonard MB. Assessment of bone mass following renal transplantation in children. *Pediatr Nephrol* 2005; **20**(3): 360–367.

82 Miller MA, Chin J, Miller SC, Fox J. Disparate effects of mild, moderate, and severe secondary hyperparathyroidism on cancellous and cortical bone in rats with chronic renal insufficiency. *Bone* 1998; **23**: 257–266.

83 Kim H, Chang K, Lee T, Kwon J, Park S. Bone mineral density after renal transplantation. *Transplant Proc* 1998; **30**(7): 3029–3030.

84 Hurst G, Alloway R, Hathaway D, Somerville T, Hughes T, Gaber A. Stabilization of bone mass after renal transplant with preemptive care. *Transplant Proc* 1998; **30**(4): 1327–1328.

85 Aroldi A, Tarantino A, Montagnino G, Cesana B, Cocucci C, Ponticelli C. Effects of three immunosuppressive regimens on vertebral bone density in renal transplant recipients: a prospective study. *Transplantation* 1997; **63**(3): 380–386.

86 Pichette V, Bonnardeaux A, Prudhomme L, Gagne M, Cardinal J, Ouimet D. Long-term bone loss in kidney transplant recipients: a cross-sectional and longitudinal study. *Am J Kidney Dis* 1996; **28**(1): 105–114.

87 Setterberg L, Sandberg J, Elinder CG, Nordenstrom J. Bone demineralization after renal transplantation: contribution of secondary hyperparathyroidism manifested by hypercalcaemia. *Nephrol Dial Transplant* 1996; **11**(9): 1825–1828.

88 Yazawa K, Ishikawa T, Ichikawa Y, Shin J, Usui Y, Hanafusa T *et al.* Positive effects of kidney transplantation on bone mass. *Transplant Proc* 1998; **30**(7): 3031–3033.

89 Klaus G, Paschen C, Wuster C, Kovacs GT, Barden J, Mehls O *et al.* Weight-/height-related bone mineral density is not reduced after renal transplantation. *Pediatr Nephrol* 1998; **12(5)**: 343–348.

90 Faugere M-C, Qi Q, Mawad H, Friedler RM, Malluche HH. High prevalence of low bone turnover and delayed mineralization in patients after kidney transplantation. *J Am Soc Nephrol* 1999; **10**: A3823.

91 Gilsanz V. Bone density in children: a review of the available techniques and indications. *Eur J Radiol* 1998; **26(2)**: 177–182.

92 Torres A, Lorenzo V, Gonzalez-Posada JM. Comparison of histomorphometry and computerized tomography of the spine in quantitating trabecular bone in renal osteodystrophy. *Nephron* 1986; **44(4)**: 282–287.

93 Lima EM, Goodman WG, Kuizon BD, Gales B, Emerick A, Goldin J *et al.* Bone density measurements in pediatric patients with renal osteodystrophy. *Pediatr Nephrol* 2003; **18(6)**: 554–559.

94 Jamal SA, Gilbert J, Gordon C, Bauer DC. Cortical pQCT measures are associated with fractures in dialysis patients. *J Bone Miner Res* 2006; **21(4)**: 543–548.

95 Salusky IB, Coburn JW, Brill J, Foley J, Slatopolsky E, Fine RN *et al.* Bone disease in pediatric patients undergoing dialysis with CAPD or CCPD. *Kidney Int* 1988; **33(5)**: 975–982.

61 Anemia

Susan Furth[1] & Sandra Amaral[2]

[1]Johns Hopkins University, Baltimore, USA
[2]Emory University and Children's Healthcare of Atlanta, Atlanta, USA

Introduction: causes of anemia in chronic kidney disease

Anemia is a common problem in children and adolescents with chronic and end-stage kidney disease. A recent cross-sectional study of 366 children and adolescents with chronic kidney disease (CKD) stages 1–5 revealed anemia, defined as any medical treatment for anemia or hemoglobin (Hb) of <12 mg/dL, in 36.6%, which varied from 31% at stage 1 to 93.3% at stages 4 and 5 CKD [1]. Similarly, in a report by the North American Pediatric Renal Transplant Cooperative Study of children with an estimated glomerular filtration rate (GFR) of <75 mL/min/1.73 m², 30% (of 1725) had anemia, as defined by a hematocrit of <30% [2]. Compared to adults on chronic dialysis in the USA, pediatric patients more often have mean annual Hb levels of <11 g/dL, with 54% versus 39.8% in pediatric versus adult hemodialysis (HD) patients and 69.5% versus 55.1% pediatric versus adult peritoneal dialysis patients [3]. Anemia remains a problem even after kidney transplantation. The prevalence of anemia posttransplant in one single-center study of 231 pediatric patients was 25.5% at 1 year posttransplantation [4].

A number of factors contribute to the development of anemia in children and adults with kidney disease. As kidney function declines, affected individuals experience a decrease in circulating red blood cell mass, indicated by low blood Hb concentration. The kidney plays a central role in regulating red blood cell mass through the production of erythropoietin and the regulation of plasma volume through excretion of salt and water. It has been proposed that the kidney functions as a "critmeter" by sensing oxygen tension and extracellular volume and translating a measure of plasma volume as tissue oxygen pressure in order to regulate erythropoietin production [5]. Effective circulating red blood cell mass is controlled by specialized interstitial cells in the kidney cortex that are exquisitely sensitive to small changes in tissue oxygenation. If tissue oxygenation decreases because of anemia or other causes, these specialized interstitial cells in the kidney cortex sense hypoxia and produce erythropoietin. Surface receptors on erythroid colony-forming units, the progenitors of red blood cells, bind erythropoietin, thus preventing apoptosis. If erythropoietin production is impaired in kidney disease, there is no inhibition of apoptosis and erythrocyte progenitor cells experience cell death. Also, nutritional problems during CKD and end-stage renal disease (ESRD) can lead to folate and vitamin B_{12} deficiency, leading to disordered DNA synthesis, maturation arrest, and ineffective erythropoiesis. Iron deficiency can also slow synthesis of heme and globin and further impair erythropoiesis. Inflammation, another common problem in CKD, impairs both erythropoiesis and the utilization of iron in red blood cell production. Inflammatory cytokines inhibit erythropoietin production, impair the growth of red blood cell progenitors, and stimulate hepatic release of hepciden, which blocks iron absorption in the gut [5].

Definitions and guidelines

Recently in the USA, the National Kidney Foundation Kidney Disease Outcomes Quality Initiative (K/DOQI) published clinical practice guidelines for anemia in CKD based on an evidence-based review. In the production of the guidelines, a systematic literature review was performed of Hb thresholds for initiating therapy, Hb level therapeutic goals, iron status goals, and efficacy of adjuvants in achieving Hb goals. When the quality of evidence was considered high or moderately high, clinical practice guidelines were presented based on the evidence. When the quality of the evidence was low, very low, or missing, the workgroups presented clinical practice recommendations. For the pediatric population, clinical practice recommendations were presented. As stated by the committee, "the only evidence of sufficient strength to support evidence based guidelines are available from studies of the adult population" [6]. The K/DOQI pediatric workgroup defined anemia in a child as a reduction in Hb level to less than the fifth percentile for their age and sex, with the caveat that adjustment in normal levels should be done for children living at higher altitudes. The normative values

Evidence-based Nephrology. Edited by Donald Molony and Jonathan Craig
© 2009 Blackwell Publishing, ISBN: 978-1-4051-3975-5.

Table 61.1 Definitions of anemia in children with CKD.

Age group (yrs)	5th percentile Hb level (g/dL)	
	Boys	Girls
1–2	10.7	10.8
3–5	11.2	11.1
6–8	11.5	11.5
9–11	12.0	11.9
12–14	12.4	11.7
15–19	13.5	11.5

Source: Adapted from the K/DOQI recommendations [6].

for children older than 1 year of age published in the K/DOQI guidelines were adapted from data from the National Health and Nutrition Evaluation Survey III reference data [6] (Table 61.1), whereas the values for children from birth to 1 year of age were derived from the textbook *Hematology of Infancy and Childhood* [7]. The workgroup included clinical practice recommendations on evaluation of anemia in CKD (Table 61.2), target Hb range (>11 g/dL), use of erythropoiesis-stimulating agents (ESAs) and iron agents, as well as adjuvants, transfusion indications, and evaluation of persistent failure to reach or maintain intended Hb level. The conclusions of the K/DOQI pediatric workgroup on each of these topics are presented throughout this chapter.

Other national guidelines groups, including the Caring for Australians with Renal Impairment (CARI) group [8], have reviewed the issue of anemia in CKD in pediatrics. With regard to anemia and growth in children, the CARI group systematically reviewed the evidence and determined that no evidence-based recommendations were possible based on level I or II evidence in 2005. In suggestions for clinical care, they stated that there was no evidence to support that treatment of anemia improves growth in pediatric CKD cases; however, correction of anemia is indicated to improve quality of life (QoL) and cardiac performance (Table 61.3). In 2003, the European Pediatric Peritoneal Dialysis Working Group published guidelines on the management of anemia in pediatric peritoneal dialysis patients. These guidelines stated that after a thorough diagnostic workup, anemia treatment should aim for a target Hb concentration of at least 11 g/dL through administration of erythropoietin and iron preparations.

Table 61.2 Recommendations for anemia evaluation in pediatric CKD.

Recommendations for anemia evaluation in pediatric CKD

CBC, including MCH, MCV, MCHC, WBC with differential and platelet counts
Absolute reticulocyte count
Serum ferritin
Transferrin saturation

Source: Adapted from the K/DOQI recommendations [6].
Abbreviations: CBC, complete blood count; MCH, mean corpuscular Hb; MCV, mean corpuscular volume; MCHC, mean corpuscular Hb concentration, WBC, white blood cells.

Table 61.3 Published clinical practice recommendations on anemia in pediatric CKD.

Guideline or CPR	Source	Year	Reference
National Kidney Foundation K/DOQI clinical practice recommendations for anemia in chronic kidney disease in children	U.S. NKF KDOQI	2006	[6]
The CARI guidelines: nutrition and growth in kidney disease	Australia CARI	2005	[8]
Management of anemia in pediatric peritoneal dialysis patients	European Pediatric Peritoneal Dialysis Working Group	2003	[9]

Abbreviations: CPR, clinical practice recommendation.

Iron should preferably be prescribed as an oral preparation, and there is no place for carnitine supplementation in the treatment of anemia in pediatric peritoneal dialysis patients (Table 61.4) [9].

Sequelae of anemia in CKD

Risk of death

Studies in adults with ESRD have consistently demonstrated reduced risk of death and hospitalization when Hb levels are ≥11 g/dL, but the upper limit of target Hb is more controversial [10–12]. In 2004, the Cochrane Renal Group performed a meta-analysis of randomized clinical trials (RCTs) to evaluate the harms and benefits of different Hb targets in adult patients with CKD; they found lower risk of all-cause mortality with Hb of <12 versus >13 g/dL (relative risk [RR], 0.84; 95% confidence interval [CI], 0.71–1.00) [13]. This Cochrane review was updated in August 2006, included 22 RCTs, and had similar results [14]. The authors indicated the need for more adequately powered and better-designed trials. In November 2006, two additional RCTs investigating optimal target Hb were published [15,16]. Drueke *et al.* randomly assigned 603 patients with estimated GFRs of 15–35 mL/min/1.73 m^2 and Hb of 11–12.5 g/dL to a target Hb of 13–15 g/dL versus Hb of 10.5–11.5 g/dL. Over 3 years, they found that early complete correction of anemia did not reduce risk of cardiovascular events in patients with CKD.

Singh *et al.* conducted an open-label trial of 1432 patients with CKD assigned to receive epoetin alfa to either a target Hb of 13.5 g/dL or Hb of 11.3 g/dL [16]. In this study, the use of target Hb of 13.5 g/dL versus 11.3 g/dL was associated with an increased risk of death, myocardial infarction, hospitalization for congestive heart failure, and stroke. In children, there is less systematic evidence concerning the risks of anemia in CKD. The NKF K/DOQI practice guidelines for anemia management were primarily based on adult studies. In the pediatric population, Warady and Ho demonstrated an association between baseline hematocrit of <33% at 30 days post-initiation of dialysis and increased risk of

Table 61.4 Anemia treatment clinical practice recommendations from K/DOQI.

Parameter	ESAs	Iron agents
Frequency of monitoring	Hb monitored monthly: target, >11 g/dL	Iron status tests every month with initial ESA treatment, then every 3 months Goals: serum ferritin >100 ng/mL, TSAT >20%; if ferritin >500 ng/mL, assess clinical status
Dosing	Determined by Hb level, target level, and observed rate of increase	Related to iron preparation chosen
Contraindications	Hypertension, vascular access occlusion, inadequate dialysis, history of seizures, or compromised nutritional status *are not* contraindications	Risk of acute adverse events: hypotension, anaphylactoid reactions
Route of administration	Determined by clinical conditions; convenience favors s.c. in non-HD and i.v. administration in HD CKD	Prefer i.v. in patient with HD CKD, i.v. or oral in for nondialysis CKD or PD CKD
Frequency	Determined by treatment stage, setting, efficacy considerations, and class of ESA; convenience favors less frequent administration, particularly in non-HD CKD	Related to selected iron preparation

Source: Adapted from the K/DOQI recommendations [6].
Abbreviations: s.c., subcutaneous; TSAT, transferrin saturation.

prolonged hospitalization and death in incident ESRD patients less than 18 years of age from the NAPRTCS registry [17]. Using data from the US Centers for Medicare and Medicaid Services' ESRD Clinical Performance Measures Project (Oct–Dec 1999 and 2000) linked with the US Renal Data System hospitalization and mortality records, Amaral *et al.* assessed whether achieving target Hb levels of >11 g/dL in 677 adolescents on HD was associated with decreased risk of death. In this retrospective cohort study, 11.7% with Hb of <11 g/dL at study entry died compared to 5% of those with initial Hb of ≥11 g/dL ($P < 0.0001$) [18]. In a multivariate analysis, Hb of ≥11 g/dL was associated with decreased risk of death (hazard ratio [HR], 0.38; 95% CI, 0.20–0.72). When Hb was recategorized into Hb levels of <10, ≥10 to <11, ≥11 to ≤12, and >12 g/dL, risk of mortality declined as Hb level increased. At Hb levels of 11 to ≤12 g/dL versus <10 g/dL, mortality risk decreased by 70% (HR, 0.30; 95% CI, 0.19–0.74). Risk of mortality was similar for Hb levels of 11–12 g/dL and >12 g/dL. Hb of >12 g/dL remained strongly associated with decreased risk of mortality (HR, 0.20; 95% CI, 0.07–0.56) [18]. This observational study's findings are consistent with literature on adults, showing decreased mortality in ESRD patients who meet Hb targets of >11 g/dL for adolescents on HD.

There are currently no pediatric data to support an Hb target above the current target of 11 g/dL; furthermore, no pediatric study to date has weighed the cost of increased use of ESAs with the benefits of achieving a normalized Hb. Future studies in the form of RCTs are needed to assess optimal Hb levels for all adolescents with CKD and ESRD. To this end, the pediatric workgroup of the K/DOQI committee recommended the lower limit of Hb as 11 g/dL or greater, but in the opinion of the workgroup, there was insufficient evidence to recommend an upper limit of Hb. These guidelines were formulated prior to the two recent RCTs in adults, which were consistent with higher mortality with higher Hb levels,

and the FDA Black Box warning (issued in February 2007), which advised about the increased risk of death with higher Hb targets. An upper limit of 12 g/dL is reasonable in this context.

Risk of CKD progression

A number of studies have suggested that anemia may accelerate decline in kidney function through decreased oxygen delivery to tissues, accelerating ischemic changes and increasing endothelial injury. It has been proposed that hypoxia of renal tubule cells may stimulate extracellular matrix production and release of profibrotic cytokines, thereby accelerating kidney disease progression. Several clinical trials in adults have suggested that erythropoietin treatment and correction of anemia may ameliorate the progression of CKD [19]. In children, a recent prospective cohort study by Furth *et al.* demonstrated an association between anemia and accelerated progression of CKD in children, independent of GFR [20]. However, at the time of this writing, there is insufficient evidence to suggest that treatment of anemia slows progression of CKD in the pediatric population.

Anemia, QoL, and cognitive function

Anemia associated with CKD has long been associated with a negative impact on QoL. Several studies have revealed that the treatment of anemia in CKD improves QoL in adults with CKD and ESRD [21–24]. One single, blind, placebo-controlled crossover study in 11 children with ESRD showed improvement in exercise tolerance, physical performance, and health and better school attendance with correction of anemia [25]. Decreasing anemia using recombinant human erythropoietin in a multicenter pediatric study of 44 children with chronic kidney failure undergoing HD also showed marked improvement in QoL, particularly in activity levels [26]. Another cross-sectional study, by Gerson *et al.*, examined the link between QoL and anemia in a cross-section of 116 adolescents with renal insufficiency on dialysis and post-kidney transplantation. The authors found that anemia was associated with poorer QoL [27]. By caregiver assessment, adolescents with kidney disease and anemia (defined as hematocrit of <36%) were less satisfied with their health, participated less in activities at school and with friends, and were less physically active. These findings mirrored findings of studies examining the correlation between anemia and QoL in adults with CKD.

Regarding cognitive function, one multicenter trial of subcutaneous erythropoietin showed increased Wechsler intelligence scores in 11 children with chronic kidney failure who were treated for anemia over a 12-month period [28]. In the literature on adults, several studies have demonstrated significant improvement in electrophysiological markers of cognitive function with improvement of anemia in patients with chronic and end-stage renal disease [29–34]. Further study in the pediatric population is needed.

Cardiac function

In adults, observational evidence in CKD has shown an association between anemia and left ventricular hypertrophy (LVH) [35,36]. Optimal Hb levels to prevent LVH and cardiovascular events are not clear, based on the current body of evidence [37,38]; some studies have suggested increased risk at higher Hb levels. In 1998, Besarab et al. halted an RCT in adults with cardiac disease on HD who were receiving Epoetin to achieve a hematocrit of 42% versus 30%. The group with a higher hematocrit experienced decreased event-free survival [39]. More recently, Volkova and Arab performed an evidence-based literature review of the relationship between Hb and/or hematocrit and mortality in dialysis patients. They included five trials and 13 observational studies. They showed either no effect or a benefit of Hb level target higher than 11 g/dL in a general dialysis population and increased mortality associated with greater Hb concentration in cardiac patients [40]. They concluded that "most observational studies supported the increased mortality associated with Hb levels less than the reference range of Hb 11–12 g/dL (110–120 g/L)"... and that "evidence of risks or benefits of Hb levels greater than 11–12 g/dL (110–120 g/L) is variable" [40].

Evidence supporting cardiac benefits associated with the treatment of anemia in children with CKD is more limited, although cardiac-related events and LV remodeling have been reported in pediatric CKD and ESRD populations, including children post-kidney transplantation [41–43]. According to the K/DOQI reviews, a single blinded crossover trial of 11 children aged 2–12 years on dialysis demonstrated an improvement in cardiac index by 6 months and significant reduction in LV mass by 12 months in those treated with ESAs [44]. Two additional observational studies of patients with severe LVH demonstrated that children with lower Hb levels had more severe LVH and lower LV compliance [45,46].

Treatment

Anemia therapy in patients with CKD requires the effective use of ESAs and iron agents to achieve and maintain target Hb levels. In 1989, recombinant human erythropoietin was first introduced to stimulate bone marrow production of red blood cells. Since then, other forms of ESAs have been developed. The term ESA refers to any agent used to enhance erythropoiesis by acting directly or indirectly on the erythropoietin receptor. Currently available ESAs include the Epoetins (Epoetin alpha and beta) and darbopoetin, the hyperglycosolated EPO analog [47]. Epoetins are short-acting and are generally dosed 1–3 times per week. Darbopoetin is long-acting and can be dosed once every 2 weeks. A summary of the clinical practice recommendations of the pediatric workgroup of the K/DOQI treatment guidelines is included in Table 61.4. There is little available evidence in the form of RCTs to assess differential efficacy between ESAs in children or adults with CKD (Tables 61.5 and 61.6). Warady et al. randomized 124 children on stable recombinant human erythropoietin to either continue on recombinant human erythropoietin or convert to darbopoetin. The authors detected no statistically significant difference in mean change in Hb between the two groups [48]. Thus, because there are some data in pediatrics supporting the adult findings and no data supporting differing recommendations, the current practice recommendations have been adapted from the evidence-based recommendations in adults. In general, it is recommended that Hb be monitored monthly, with closer monitoring at 1- to 2-week intervals when initiating and/or making significant changes to the ESA dose. Initial doses and dose adjustments vary widely in pediatrics. All pediatric providers are advised to carefully evaluate the individual patient's response and to adjust dosing regimens and frequency of monitoring accordingly. For short-acting ESAs administered in the dialysis population, reports suggest that peritoneal dialysis patients require approximately 225 U/kg/week compared to 300 U/kg/week for HD patients. Younger patients <1 year old require an average of 350 U/kg/week. For the nondialysis population, fewer reports are available, but doses of 150–450 U/kg/week have been used. Fewer data are available on dose requirements for long-acting ESAs (darbopoetin alfa) in either dialysis or nondialysis populations. There is a wide range of recommended dosing, 0.25–0.75 µg/kg/week, and most frequently 0.45 µg/kg/week is recommended [6]. Reports on acceptable rates of increases of Hb levels in pediatric CKD vary widely. The European Pediatric Peritoneal Dialysis workgroup recommended an increase of approximately 0.66 g/dL/month as a minimally acceptable level [9].

In children with CKD, as in adults with CKD, the most common reason for poor response to ESA therapy is iron deficiency. Iron repletion in CKD requires either intravenous (i.v.) or oral iron therapy. Current i.v. forms of iron supplementation include iron dextran, sodium ferric gluconate, and iron sucrose. There are currently no adequately powered trials comparing i.v. agents for adults or children [49]. Several studies comparing i.v. versus oral iron in adult HD and CKD patients demonstrated superior efficacy of i.v. forms of iron in repleting iron stores and minimizing ESA dosing [50–52]. RCT evidence comparing i.v. versus oral iron in adult CKD, including nondialysis, HD, and peritoneal dialysis patients, is presented in Table 61.6. In 2005, Gillespie and Wolf published a meta-analysis that combined clinical data on i.v. iron use in

Table 61.5 Pediatric studies examining efficacy of erythropoiesis stimulating agents (ESAs) in anemia of CKD and ESRD for pediatric patients.

Reference*	Type	Population	Intervention	Sample Size	Follow-up	Outcome
Sinai-Trieman et al, 1989	Prospective cohort	Transfusion-dependent PD pts	Subcutaneous (SC) recombinant human erythropoietin (rHuEpo): initial dose 150 units/kg thrice weekly	5 children, 12-18 yrs old	8 mos	All pts had increase in Hemoglobin (Hb) and reticulocyte count and none required further transfusions.
Offner et al, 1990	Prospective cohort	CAPD and CCPD	300 units/kg IV rHuEpo once weekly	14 children, 6–22 yrs old	One year	Mean Hematocrit (HCT) and retic. count increased within one month. Dosage was decreased after 3 mos to keep HCT >30%.
Campos and Garin, 1992	Prospective cohort	HD	IV rHuEpo: thrice weekly	11 children, 6 mos-20 yrs old	9 mos	HCT rose after 8 wks from 20.3% (mean) to 31.7%.
Reddingius et al, 1992	Prospective cohort	CAPD	Intraperitoneal (IP) rHuEpo: initial dose 300 units/kg/week	16 children	8 mos	Mean Hb increased. No pts required blood transfusions after initiation of therapy.
Montini et al, 1993	Prospective cohort	PD	SC rHuEPO: initial dose 25 IU/kg twice weekly	24 children	24 wks	6 pts censored, 18 remaining pts all had increased Hb.
Brandt et al, 1999	Prospective randomized study	CKD, PD and HD pts	IV or SC rHuEPO: low-dose (150 units/kg/week) vs. high-dose (450 units/kg/week) divided thrice weekly	44 children <21 yrs old: 25 pre-dialysis, 10 PD, 9 HD	12 wks or until "target" Hb was attained	82% pts reached "target" Hb by 8 wks; 95% pts in high-dose group reached target vs. 66% in low-dose group. HD pts required higher doses.
De Palo et al, 2004	Prospective cohort	HD pts previously on epoietin alfa	Darbepoetin 1.59 ± 1.19 mcg/kg/week	7 children	6 mos	Increase of >1g/dL Hb in first month. By 2nd month, dose reduced. Mean Hb at 3 mos 11.8 ± 1.4 g/dL and mean darbepoietin dose 0.51 ± 0.51 mcg/kg/week.
Geary et al, 2005	Prospective cohort	CKD with GFR <30 cc/min/1.73 m², HD and PD pts	Darbepoetin alfa 0.45 mcg/kg/week	23 children	28 wks	73% of pts were receiving darbepoetin less than once weekly by 12 wks and 87% by 28 wks to maintain Hb 10–12.5 g/dL.
Durkan et al, 2006	Prospective cohort	Infants with CKD <8 kg	Darbepoetin 0.5 mcg/kg/week	6 infants	20 wks	For 3 pts, mean darbepoietin dose was decreased and dosing interval increased to 3–4 wks. 3 pts required increase in weekly dose.
Warady et al, 2006	Randomized open-label, non-inferiority study	CKD with GFR <30 cc/min/1.73m², HD and PD pts who were receiving stable rHuEpo treatment	Subjects randomized (1:2) to either continue rHuEpo or convert to darbepoetin alfa	124 children, aged 1–18 yrs, receiving stable rHuEpo	28 wks	Adjusted mean change in Hb between baseline and evaluation period for rHuEpo vs. darbepoetin groups was not statistically different. Darbopoetin was found to be non-inferior to rHuEpo.

*References listed in reference section.[57–62]

children on HD [53]. They included nine studies that included eight cohort studies and one prospective trial with historical controls, and they showed increased Hb, ferritin, and transferrin saturation levels and reduced use of ESAs with i.v. iron use. In 2006, Warady *et al.* performed an RCT to examine the preferential route of iron administration for children. The authors prospectively randomized 35 iron-replete children <20 years old with ESRD on HD to receive either i.v. iron dextran with each dialysis session (*n* = 18) or oral iron daily (*n* = 17) for up to 16 weeks. In both groups the Hb was stable, but the i.v. iron group experienced a

Table 61.6 Erythropoiesis stimulating agents. Evidence-based recommendations.

Intervention	Systematic review	Evidence rating[a]	Comment on rating	Recommendation[b]	Comment on recommendation
rHuEpo once weekly vs. twice weekly in dialysis pts	Cochrane Review, 2005[63]: 11 RCT of 719 pts	Moderate	The duration and frequency of the studies differed and there were small nos. of participants.	There is insufficient evidence to recommend one regimen of frequency of rHuEpo dosing.	There was no significant difference between once weekly vs. twice weekly dosing. Large RCTs with longer duration and greater nos. of subjects are needed.
ESA vs. placebo in HD and PD pts	12 RCT, including one pediatric*	Moderate	The duration, dosing frequency and outcomes of the studies differed.	The current body of evidence is insufficient to recommend one ESA agent or dosing pattern and potential benefits and risk must be weighed for each patient.	ESAs are effective for reducing the requirement for blood transfusions in ESRD pts. ESRD pts on ESA therapy may have improved quality of life. Use of ESAs may be associated with increased blood pressure and lower Kt/V. It is difficult to assess the separate impact of ESAs from improved Hb and HCT.
rHuEpo in pre-dialysis pts vs. no treatment or placebo	Cochrane Review, 2005[64]: 15 trials, including 461 pts	High for reduction in anemia. Moderate for improved quality of life and exercise capacity. Low for impact on progression of CKD.	rHuEpo was shown to correct anemia and reduce need for blood transfusion. Quality of life and exercise capacity also improved in the treatment group.	rHuEpo may be used to reduce anemia for people with chronic kidney disease who do not yet require dialysis.	Further study is needed to assess whether rHuEpo use can slow the progression of CKD.
Epoetin vs. Darbopoetin (short-acting vs. long-acting ESAs)	1 RCT[65] of 522 HD and PD pts, 1 cross-over study[66] of 524 pts with CKD	Low	There is only one RCT currently published which compares darbopoetin and Epoetin in the form of RCT. This study shows no statistically significant difference between the two types of ESA. For the cross-over study, there was no control group.	There is insufficient evidence to recommend one ESA agent's use over another's.	Darbopoetin alfa was found to maintain Hb as effectively as rHuEpo but with a reduced dose frequency for up to 52 weeks in both studies.

*Data adapted from "Clinical Practice Recommendations for Adults 2.1:Hb Range" Am J Kidney Dis 2006; 47:S33-S53

Table 61.7 Iron supplements. Evidence-based recommendations for CKD, including Nondialysis, Hemodialysis and Peritoneal Dialysis[a]. *Data adapted from "Clinical Practice Recommendations for Adults 3.2: Using Iron Agents" Am J Kidney Dis 2006; 47:S58-S70.

Intervention: IV vs. PO iron	Systematic review	Evidence rating[b]	Comment on rating	Recommendation[c]	Comment on recommendation
IV iron dextran vs. oral iron[d]	3 RCTs: 2 HD pts, 1 ND pts (2 RCT included placebo arm, 1 RCT included PD)	Moderately high to high for HD pts. Moderately high for ND and PD pts.	Some inconsistencies for studies which examined ND-CKD pts. Studies in HD pts were reasonably consistent. No RCTs with PD pts only.	The preferred route of iron administration is IV in pts with HD-CKD. The route of iron administration may be either IV or PO for ND-CKD and PD-CKD pts.	Final mean Hb ranged higher 0.9-4.5 g/dL (90-450 g/dL) in IV arms vs. PO for HD pts. Mean final ESA dose was lower in IV arms in studies with HD pts. No significant difference in ESA dosing was found in nondialysis pts on IV vs PO iron.
IV iron sucrose vs. oral iron[d]	3 RCTs: ND pts				
IV iron sodium gluconate vs. oral iron[d]	1 RCT: HD pts				

[a] Nondialysis (ND), Hemodialysis (HD), Peritoneal Dialysis (PD).
[b] Evidence rating based on study design, study quality, consistency and directness of results.
[c] Recommendation based on assessment of risks and benefits, quality of evidence, translation of evidence into practice.
[d] oral iron = ferrous sulfate or iron polysaccharide.

significant increase in serum ferritin and the oral iron group did not. There was no statistically significant difference in ESA dosing detected between the two groups [54]. Thus, further study is needed to compare various methods of iron administration for children. For iron agents and iron dosing, the K/DOQI pediatric group stated goals of avoiding storage iron depletion, preventing iron-deficient erythropoiesis, and achieving and maintaining target Hb levels, as outlined in Table 61.4. Hyporesponse to ESAs and iron therapy is defined as "a significant increase in the erythropoiesis stimulating agent dose requirement to maintain a certain Hb level or a significant decrease in Hb levels at a constant erythropoiesis stimulating agent dose, or a failure to increase the Hb level to greater than 11 g/dL (110 g/L) despite an erythropoiesis stimulating agent dose equivalent to epoeitin greater than 500 IU/kg/week."

In addition to iron deficiency, there are a few readily reversible factors that contribute to ESA hyporesponsiveness. Some evidence suggests that younger children, those with hyperparathyroidism, and those with more evidence of inflammation are at increased risk of hyporesponsiveness. Although several pharmacological and nonpharmacological agents have been studied as potential adjuvants to ESA and iron treatment for CKD in children, in the opinion of the K/DOQI workgroup there is insufficient evidence to recommend the use of either L-carnitine or vitamin C in the management of anemia in children with CKD. Additionally, as in adults, androgens should not be used as an adjuvant to ESA treatment in anemic patients with CKD. Red blood cell transfusion should be used cautiously in patients with CKD because of the potential for development of sensitivity that would adversely affect future kidney transplantation. There is no evidence to suggest that a single Hb concentration justifies or requires transfusion.

In summary, anemia is a prevalent and serious problem among children with CKD. At all stages of CKD, low Hb has been associated with increased risk of hospitalization and death, more rapid decline in GFR, lower cognitive function, increased LVH, and decreased LV compliance. Guidelines for clinical management of anemia in children with CKD are primarily based on adult data. Although the majority of existing pediatric studies do support the current adult guidelines, more pediatric-based research in the form of multicentered RCTs is needed to establish valid pediatric-specific treatment goals. At this time, for children with CKD, the treatment goal for anemia management should be a target Hb of ≥11g/dL and <12 g/dL, using ESAs and iron as necessary adjuncts to achieve this target.

References

1 Wong H, Mylrea K, Feber S, Drukker A, Filler G. Prevalence of complications in children with chronic kidney disease according to KDOQI. *Kidney Int* 2006; **70**: 585–590.

2 Fivush BA, Jabs K, Neu AM, Sullivan EK, Feld L, Kohaut E *et al.* Chronic renal insufficiency in children and adolescents: the 1996 annual report of NAPRTCS. North American Pediatric Renal Transplant Cooperative Study. *Pediatr Nephrol* 1998; **12**(4): 328–337.

3 Chavers KI, Roberts TL, Herzog CA, Collins AJ, St. Peter WL. Prevalence of anemia in erythropoietin-treated pediatric as compared to adult chronic dialysis patients. *Kidney Int* 2004; **65**: 266–273.

4 Mitsnefes M, Subat-Dezulovic M, Khoary PR, Goebel J, Strite CF. Increasing incidence of post kidney transplant anemia in children. *Am J Kidney Transplant* 2005; **5**: 1713–1718.

5 Donnelly S. Why is erythropoietin made in the kidney? The kidney functions as a "critmeter." *Adv Exp Med Biol* 2003; **543**: 73–87.

6 NKF. KDOQI clinical practice recommendations for anemia in chronic kidney disease in children. *Am J Kidney Dis* 2006; **47**(5 Suppl 3): S86–S108.

7 Nathan DG, Orkin SH, Ginsburg D, Look AT, Oski FA. Appendix 11. Normal hematologic values in children. *Nathan and Oski's Hematology of Infancy and Childhood*. Saunders, Philadelphia, 2003; 1841.

8 Pollock C, Voss D, Hodson E, Crompton C, Caring for Australasians with Renal Impairment (CARI). The CARI guidelines. Nutrition and growth in kidney disease. *Nephrology* (Carlton) 2005; **10(Suppl 5)**: S177–S230.

9 Schroder CH, European Pediatric Peritoneal Dialysis Working Group. The management of anemia in pediatric peritoneal dialysis patients. Guidelines by an ad hoc European committee. *Pediatr Nephrol* 2003; **18(8)**: 805–809.

10 Foley RN, Parfrey PS, Harnett JD, Kent GM, Murray DC, Barre PE. The impact of anemia on cardiomyopathy, morbidity and mortality in end-stage renal disease. *Am J Kidney Dis* 1996; **28(1)**: 53–61.

11 Ofsthun N, Labrecque J, Lacson E, Keen M, Lazarus JM. The effects of higher Hb levels on mortality and hospitalization in hemodialysis patients. *Kidney Int* 2003; **63(5)**: 1908–1914.

12 Xia H, Ebben J, Ma JZ, Collins AJ. Hematocrit levels and hospitalization risks in hemodialysis patients. *J Am Soc Nephrol* 1999; **10(6)**: 1309–1316.

13 Strippoli GF, Craig JC, Manno C, Schena FP. Hb targets for the anemia of chronic kidney disease: a meta-analysis of randomized, controlled trials. *J Am Soc Nephrol* 2004; **15(12)**: 3154–3165.

14 Strippoli GF, Navaneethan SD, Craig JC. Haemoglobin and haematocrit targets for the anaemia of chronic kidney disease. *Cochrane Database Syst Rev* 2006; **4**: CD003967.

15 Drueke T, Locatelli F, Clyne N, Eckardt, K, MacDougall I, Tsakiris D *et al*. Normalization of hemoglobin level in patients with chronic kidney disease and anemia. *N Engl J Med* 2006; **355**: 2071–2084.

16 Singh A, Szczech L, Tang K, Barnhart H, Sapp S, Wolfson M *et al*. Correction of anemia with epoetin alfa in chronic kidney disease. *N Engl J Med* 2006; **355**: 2085–2098.

17 Warady BA, Ho M. Morbidity and mortality in children with anemia at initiation of dialysis. *Pediatr Nephrol* 2003; **18**: 1055–1062.

18 Amaral S, Hwang W, Fivush B, Neu A, Frankenfeld D, Furth S. Association of mortality and hospitalization with achievement of adult hemoglobin targets in adolescents who are on hemodialysis. *J Am Soc Nephrol* 2006; **17(10)**: 2878–2885.

19 Rossert J, Levin A, Roger SD, Horl WH, Fouqueray B, Gassmann-Mayer C *et al*. Effect of early correction of anemia on progression of CKD. *Am J Kidney Dis* 2006; **47**: 738–750.

20 Furth SL, Cole SR, Fadrowski JJ, Gerson A, Pierce CB, Chandra M *et al*. The association of anemia and hypoalbuminemia with accelerated decline in GFR among adolescents with chronic kidney disease. *Pediatr Nephrol* 2007; **22**: 265–271.

21 Moreno F, Sanz-Guajardo D, López-Gómez JM, Jofre R, Valderrábano F. Increasing the hematocrit has a beneficial effect on quality of life and is safe in selected hemodialysis patients. *J Am Soc Nephrol* 2000; **11**: 335–342.

22 Beusterien KM, Nissenson AR, Port FK, Kelly M, Steinwald B, Ware JE, Jr. The effects of recombinant human erythropoietin on functional health and well-being in chronic dialysis patients. *J Am Soc Nephrol* 1996; **7**: 763–773.

23 Moreno F, Aracil FJ, Pérez R, Valderrábano F. Controlled study on the improvement of quality of life of elderly hemodialysis patients after correcting end-stage renal disease-related anemia with erythropoietin. *Am J Kidney Dis* 1996; **27(4)**: 548–556.

24 Bárány P, Petterson E, Konarski-Svensson JK. Long-term effects on quality of life in hemodialysis patients of correction of anaemia with erythropoietin. *Nephrol Dial Transplant* 1993; **8**: 426–432.

25 Morris K, Sharp J, Watson S, Coulthard M. Non-cardiac benefits of human recombinant erythropoietin in end stage renal failure and anemia. *Arch Dis Child* 1993; **69(5)**: 580–586.

26 Van Damme-Lombaerts R, Broyer M, Businger J, Baldauf C, Stocker H. A study of recombinant human erythropoietin in the treatment of anemia of chronic renal failure in children on hemodialysis. *Pediatr Nephrol* 1994; **8**: 338–342.

27 Gerson A, Hwang W, Fiorenza J, Barth K, Kaskel F, Weiss L *et al*. Anemia and health-related quality of life in adolescents with chronic kidney disease. *Am J Kidney Dis* 2004; **44(6)**: 1017–1023.

28 Burke J. Low-dose subcutaneous recombinant erythropoietin in children with chronic renal failure. *Pediatr Nephrol* 1995; **9(5)**: 558–561.

29 Singh N, Sahni V, Wadhwa A, Garg S, Bajaj S, Kohli R *et al*. Effect of improvement in anemia on electroneurophysiological markers (P300) of cognitive dysfunction in chronic kidney disease. *Hemodial Int* 2006; **10(3)**: 267–273.

30 Pickett J, Theberge D, Brown W. Normalizing hematocrit in dialysis patients improves brain function. *Am J Kidney Dis* 1999; **33**: 1122–1130.

31 Marsh J, Brown W, Woicott D. rHuEPO treatment improves brain and cognitive function of anemic dialysis patients. *Kidney Int* 1991; **39**: 155–163.

32 Grimm G, Stockenhuber F, Schneeweiss B. Improvement of brain function in hemodialyis patients treated with erythropoietin. *Kidney Int* 1990; **38**: 480–486.

33 Sagales T, Gimeno V, Planella J. Effects of rHuEPO on Q-EEG and event-related potentials in chronic renal failure. *Kidney Int* 1993; **44**: 1109–1115.

34 Metry G, Wikstrom B, Valind S, Sandhagen B. Effect of normalization of hematocrit on brain circulation and metabolism in hemodialysis patients. *J Am Soc Nephrol* 1999; **10**: 854–863.

35 Levin A, Thompson CR, Ethier J, Carlisle EJ, Tobe S, Mendelssohn D *et al*. Left ventricular mass index increase in early renal disease: impact of decline in hemoglobin. *Am J Kidney Dis* 1999; **34(1)**: 125–134.

36 Levin A, Djurdjev O, Thompson C, Barrett B, Ethier J, Carlisle E *et al*. Canadian randomized trial of hemoglobin maintenance to prevent or delay left ventricular mass growth in patients with CKD. *Am J Kidney Dis* 2005; **46(5)**: 799–811.

37 Roger SD, McMahon LP, Clarkson A, Disney A, Harris D, Hawley C *et al*. Effects of early and late intervention with epoetin alpha on left ventricular mass among patients with chronic kidney disease (stage 3 or 4): results of a randomized clinical trial. *J Am Soc Nephrol* 2004; **15(1)**: 148–146.

38 Griffith T, Reddan DN, Klassen PS, Owen WF. Left ventricular hypertrophy: a surrogate end point or correlate of cardiovascular events in kidney disease? *Nephrol Dial Transplant* 2003; **18**: 2479–2482.

39 Besarab A, Bolton WK, Browne JK, Egrie JC, Nissenson AR, Okamoto DM *et al*. The effects of normal as compared with low hematocrit values in patients with cardiac disease who are receiving hemodialysis and epoetin. *N Engl J Med* 1998; **339**: 584–590.

40 Volkova N, Arab L. Evidence-based systematic literature review of hemoglobin/hematocrit and all-cause mortality in dialysis patients. *Am J Kidney Dis* 2006; **47**: 24–36.

41 Chavers B, Li S, Collins AJ, Herzog CA. Cardiovascular disease in pediatric chronic dialysis patients. *Kidney Int* 2002; **62**: 648–653.

42 Matteucci MC, Wuhl E, Picca S, Mastrostefano A, Rinelli G, Romano C *et al*. Left ventricular geometry in children with mild to moderate chronic renal insufficiency. J Am Soc Nephrol 2006; **17(1)**: 218–226.

43 El Husseini AA, Sheashaa HA, Hassan NA, El-Demerdash FM, Sobh MA, Ghoneim MA. Echocardiographic changes and risk factors for left

ventricular hypertrophy in children and adolescents after renal transplantation. *Pediatr Transplant* 2004; **8**(3): 249–254.

44 Morris KP, Skinner JR, Hunter S, Coulthard MG. Short term correction of anaemia with recombinant human erythropoietin and reduction of cardiac output in end stage renal failure. *Arch Dis Child* 1993; **68**(5): 644–648.

45 Mitsnefes MM, Daniels SR, Schwartz SM, Meyer RA, Khoury P, Strife CF. Severe left ventricular hypertorophy in pediatric dialysis: prevalence and predictors. *Pediatr Nephrol* 2003; **14**: 898–902.

46 Mitsnefes MM, Kimball TR, Border WL, Witt SA, Glascock BJ, Khoury PR *et al*. Impaired left ventricular diastolic function in children with chronic renal failure. *Kidney Int* 2004; **65**:1461–1466.

47 Deicher R, Horl W. Differentiating factors between erythropoiesis-stimulating agents. Drugs 2004; **64**(5): 499–509.

48 Warady BA, Arar MY, Lerner G, Nakanishi AM, Stehman-Breen C. Darbepoetin alfa for the treatment of anemia in pediatric patients with chronic kidney disease. *Pediatr Nephrol* 2006; **21**(8): 1144–1152.

49 NKF. KDOQI clinical practice recommendations for anemia in chronic kidney disease in adults. *Am J Kidney Dis* 2006; **47**(5 **Suppl 3**): S58–S78.

50 Fishbane S, Frei GL, Maesaka J. Reduction in recombinant human erythropoietin doses by the use of chronic intravenous iron supplementation. *Am J Kidney Dis* 1995; **26**: 41–46.

51 MacDougall IC, Tucker B, Thompson J, Tomson CR, Baker LR, Raine AE. A randomized controlled study of iron supplementation in patients treated with erythropoietin. *Kidney Int* 1996; **50**: 1694–1699.

52 Agarwal R, Rizkala AR, Bastani B, Kaskas MO, Leehey DJ, Besarab A. A randomized controlled trial of oral versus intravenous iron in chronic kidney disease. *Am J Nephrol* 2006; **26**(5): 445–454.

53 Gillespie R, Wolf F. Intravenous iron therapy in pediatric hemodialysis patients: a meta-analysis.*Pediatr Nephrol* 2004; **19**: 662–666.

54 Warady B, Kausz A, Lerner G, Brewer E, Chadha V, Brugnara C *et al*. Iron therapy in the pediatric hemodialysis population. *Pediatr Nephrol* 2004; **19**: 655–661.

55 Sinai-Trieman L, Salusky IB, Fine RN. Use of subcutaneous recombinant human erythropoietin in children undergoing continuous cycling peritoneal dialysis. *J Pediatr* 1989; **114**: 550–554.

56 Offner G, Hoyer PF, Latta K, Winkler L, Brodehl J, Scigalla P. One year's experience with recombinant erythropoietin in children undergoing continuous ambulatory or cycling peritoneal dialysis. *Pediatr Nephrol* 1990; **4**: 498–500.

57 Campos A, Garin EH. Therapy of renal anemia in children and adolescents with recombinant human erythropoietin (rHuEPO). *Clin Pediatr* 1992; **31**: 94–99.

58 Reddingius RE, Schroder CH, Monnens LA. Intraperitoneal administration of recombinant human erythropoietin in children on continuous ambulatory peritoneal dialysis. *Eur J Pediatr* 1992: 151(7): 540–542.

59 Montini G, Zacchello G, Perfumo F, Edefonti A, Bassi S, Cantaluppi A *et al*. Pharmacokinetics and hematologic response to subcutaneous administration of recombinant human erythropoietin in children undergoing long-term peritoneal dialysis: a multicenter study. *J Pediatr* 1993; **122**: 297–302.

60 Brandt JR, Avner ED, Hickman RO, Watkins SL. Safety and efficacy of erythropoietin in children with chronic renal failure. *Pediatr Nephrol* 1999; **13**: 143–147.

61 De Palo T, Giordano M, Palumbo F, Bellantuono R, Messina G, Colella V *et al*. Clinical experience with darbepoietin alfa (NESP) in children undergoing hemodialysis. *Pediatr Nephrol* 2004; **19**: 337–340.

62 Geary DF, Keating LE, Vigneux A, Stephens D, Hebert D, Harvey EA. Darbepoetin alfa (Aranesp) in children with chronic renal failure. *Kidney Int* 2005; **68**: 1759–1765.

63 Durkan AM, Keating LE, Vigneux A, Geary DF. The use of darbpoetin in infants with chronic renal impairment. *Pediatr Nephrol* 2006; **21**(5): 694–697.

64 Cody J, Daly C, Campbell M, Donaldson C, Khan I, Vale L *et al*. Frequency of administration of recombinant human erythropoietin for anaemia of end-stage renal disease in dialysis patients. *Cochrane Database Syst Rev* 2005; **3**: CD003895.

65 Cody J, Daly C, Campbell M, Donaldson C, Khan I, Rabindranath K *et al*. Recombinant human erythropoietin for chronic renal failure anaemia in pre-dialysis patients. *Cochrane Database Syst Rev* 2005; **3**: CD003266.

66 Vanrenterghem Y, Barany P, Mann JF, Kerr PG, Wilson J, Baker NF *et al*. Randomized trial of darbepoetin alfa for treatment of renal anemia at a reduced dose frequency compared with rHuEPO in dialysis patients. *Kidney Int* 2002; **62**: 2167–2175.

67 Hertel J, Locay H, Scarlata D, Jackson L, Prathikanti R, Audhya P. Darbepoetin alfa administered every other week maintains hemoglobin levels over 52 weeks in patients with chronic kidney disease converting from once-weekly recombinant human erythropoietin: results from simplify the treatment of anemia with Aranesp (STAAR). *Am J Nephrol* 2006; **26**: 149–156.

Management of Renal Failure/Transplants

62 Renal Transplantation

Pierre Cochat & Justine Bacchetta

Centre de Référence des Maladies Rénales Rares, & Inserm UMRS-820, Hôpital Femme mère enfant, Bron, France,
Hospices Civils de Lyon & Université de Lyon, Lyon, France

Successful kidney transplantation has been shown to be associated with less disability and greater well-being compared with either in-center hemodialysis or continuous ambulatory peritoneal dialysis in adults [1]e. Despite major advances in pediatric dialysis strategies, kidney transplantation remains the treatment of choice for children with end-stage renal disease (ESRD) [2,3]e. Indications for pediatric renal transplantation include the following: 1) symptoms of uremia not responsive to conservative therapy; 2) failure to thrive due to limitations in total caloric intake; 3) delayed psychomotor development; 4) uncontrolled hypervolemia; 5) uncontrolled hyperkalemia; and 6) metabolic bone disease due to renal osteodystrophy. Preemptive transplantation should be performed whenever it is available, using either living or deceased donors. Transplantation care of pediatric patients must be provided by a multidisciplinary team of pediatric health care professionals.

In order to improve standards and results of pediatric kidney transplantation, several issues should be specifically addressed, such as patient selection, choice of study end points, standardized definitions and classification of histopathology, qualification and quantification of acute and chronic graft dysfunction, strategies for limiting the number of patients, investigation of surrogate markers, and new approaches to statistical analysis and decision making [4]. The CONSORT (Consolidated Standards of Reporting Trials) and QUOROM (Quality of Reporting of Meta-analyses) criteria should be integrated in the process of any design and analysis of further clinical trials, but randomized controlled clinical trials in pediatrics are scarce. To date, most information about kidney transplantation in children comes from experience in adults, but a substantial number of problems are specific to the pediatric age group [5]e.

Note: Throughout this chapter, reference numbers corresponding to systematic reviews and meta-analyses for adult populations are followed by a superscript "a," pediatric study references are followed by "p," combined adult and pediatric study references

are followed by "c," reference numbers corresponding to randomized controlled trials (RCTs) are followed by "r," and reference numbers for literature reviews and expert opinions are followed by "e."

Epidemiology and outcomes for patient and graft

Trends in pediatric renal transplantation have been changing during the last decade [6], with remarkable improvement in the rates of acute rejection, rejection reversal, short- and long-term survival, and quality of life. In addition, 1-year graft survival has become comparable between recipients of deceased donor and living donor transplants, as well as in infants compared to other age groups. However, some problems remain, such as nonadherence in adolescents, chronic rejection, and the adverse effects of immunosuppression.

Patient and graft survival

North American and French reports from 2004 on pediatric transplant activity are summarized in Table 62.1 [7,8]. The North American Pediatric Renal Transplant Cooperative Study (NAPRTCS) is a voluntary registry, and the French registry includes all children with ESRD. Causes of graft failure are listed in Table 62.2, and causes of death are listed in Table 62.3 [8]. Patient survival in North America is shown on Table 62.4 [8].

Short- and middle-term outcomes

From most recent series in children, 1-, 3-, and 5-year graft survival rates are 91–95%, 83–87%, and 80–85% for living donor recipients and 83–92%, 71–75%, and 65–74% for deceased donor recipients, respectively [8,9]. Current transplantation strategies have brought the short-term graft survival of deceased donor transplantation very close to that of living donor transplantation. Even in two series of 68 and 45 high-risk infant recipients 15 kg or smaller, graft survival was excellent, with 92% at 1 year and 85% at 5 and

Evidence-based Nephrology. Edited by Donald Molony and Jonathan Craig
© 2009 Blackwell Publishing, ISBN: 978-1-4051-3975-5.

Table 62.1 Summary of the North American (2005) and French (2004) reports.

Patient characteristic	% of patients with indicated characteristic	
	France (90 patients)[a]	North America (8435 patients)[b]
Primary diagnosis		
Glomerulonephritis	25.6	24.8
Malformation	25.6	34.1
Inherited renal disease	16.7	13.5
Chronic tubulo-interstitial nephritis	18.8	7.0
Vascular disease	2.2	4.4
Other/unknown	11.1	16.2
Recipient age (years)		
0–2	6.2	5.3
2–10	43.2	35.6
11–15	46.9	31.3
>16	3.7	23.7
Recipient gender		
Male	51.9	59.4
Female	48.1	40.6
No. of transplant		
Primary transplant	95.1	82.3
Repeat transplant	4.9	17.7
Preemptive transplantation	22.0	24.6
Type of donor		
Living	19.8	52.0
Deceased	80.2	48.0
Donor (cadaver) age (years)		
0–2	0	1.6
2–10	19.8	20.0
11–15	37.0	15.6
16–29	22.2	30.0
>30	21.0	32.8
Graft survival (years)		
1	92.8 (LD + DD)	94.8 (LD), 91.7 (DD)
5	82.9 (LD + DD)	85.0 (LD), 74.2 (DD)

Sources: Agence de la Biomedicne [7] and NAPRTCS [8].
Abbreviations: LD, living donor; DD, deceased donor.
[a]: annual report
[b]: cumulative report

10 years in one series [10] and 100% at 2 years and 89.6% at 8 years in the other series [11].

Long-term data

The current overall half-life of kidney transplants is 19–20 years [12], but there have been few long-term studies in children. Offner *et al.* reported a 25-year actuarial survival of 81% for patients and 31% for the first graft, with best results with a living donor, preemptive transplant, and with immunosuppression using cyclosporine A [13].

Table 62.2 Causes of graft failure among pediatric kidney transplant recipients in North America[a].

Cause of graft failure	% of all graft failures
Chronic rejection	33.6
Acute rejection	13.1
Vascular thrombosis	10.6
Death with functioning graft	9.2
Recurrence of primary disease	6.9
Patient discontinued medication	4.4
Primary non function	2.2
Bacterial or viral infection	1.8
Accelerated acute rejection	1.7
Other technical	1.3
Malignancy	1.2
Hyperacute rejection	0.7
Renal artery stenosis	0.6
Cyclosporine toxicity	0.4
de novo kidney disease	0.4
Other/unknown	11.9

[a] In the NAPRTCS 2005 report [8], a total of 2414 graft failures among 9243 transplants (26.1%) were reported.

Table 62.3 Causes of death among pediatric kidney transplant recipients in North America.

Cause of death	% of all deaths
Cardiopulmonary	15.4
Bacterial infection	12.9
Cancer or malignancy	11.1
Viral infection	8.5
Other infection	7.9
Hemorrhage	6.7
Dialysis-related complication	2.8
Disease recurrence	1.6
Other	24.4
Unknown	8.7

[a] In the NAPRTCS 2005 report [8], a total of 495 deaths among 8420 patients have been reported.

Table 62.4 Three-year kidney transplant patient survival in North America.

Recipient age (years)	% Survival at 3 years (mean ± SE)	
	Living donor (*n* = 4801)	Cadaver donor (*n* = 4427)
0–1	91.90 ± 1.54	81.30 ± 4.00
2–5	96.90 ± 0.70	91.70 ± 1.27
6–12	97.60 ± 0.42	96.10 ± 0.56
>12	97.10 ± 0.43	97.50 ± 0.55
All ages	96.80 ± 0.26	95.90 ± 0.39

Source: NAPRTCS [8].

Estimation of graft function

As well as patient and graft survival, pediatric renal transplant outcomes can be evaluated using surrogate markers, such as glomerular filtration rate (GFR) and kidney biopsy. GFR closely correlates with disease progression and interstitial fibrosis, but the ideal test for GFR assessment remains to be determined. In transplant patients, GFR is most commonly estimated using inulin clearance, [^{125}I]iothalamate, EDTA-^{51}Cr, and cystatin-C [14]. In addition, both surveillance and clinically indicated kidney biopsies provide relevant information for the care of children with transplants and can be performed with minimal risk. In the NAPRTCS experience of 212 biopsies from 21 centers, 9 (4.2%) biopsy-related adverse events were reported (gross hematuria in 6, perinephric hematoma in 1, and intraperitoneal graft bleeding requiring transfusions and surgical exploration in 2) [15].

Other outcomes of pediatric renal transplant

Organ transplantation has been shown to produce improvements in physical functioning, mental health and cognitive status, social functioning, and overall quality of life perceptions [16]^c. Compared to other renal replacement therapies in adults, successful renal transplantation results in less disability and greater well-being [1]. In addition, a randomized trial showed that exercise training after kidney transplantation resulted in higher levels of measured physical functioning (with measurement of peak oxygen uptake and isokinetic muscle testing for muscle strength) and self-reported physical functioning (via the SF-36 Health Status Questionnaire); however, exercise alone did not affect body composition as assessed by dual-energy X-ray absorptiometry [17]^r.

Growth is a major issue in children posttransplant. Several studies have evaluated the safety and efficacy of recombinant human growth hormone (rhGH) after pediatric renal transplantation, with a small number of placebo-controlled randomized trials published. One showed a significant improvement in height velocity without any acceleration in bone maturation, increase in acute rejection rate, or change in GFR [18]^r. In an open-label randomized crossover multicenter trial (rhGH vs. no rhGH), growth velocity was significantly increased (7.7 cm versus 4.6 cm during the first year of treatment), although an increased risk of rejection was reported in patients with a previous history of more than one acute rejection episode [19]^r. In contrast, another study with comparable design found no significant change in the incidence of acute rejection [20]^r. Most of these trials were small and gave conflicting results, particularly for final height. The largest multicenter experience is from the NAPRTCS (randomized controlled study of 68 children), which concluded that rhGH is safe and effective in relation to growth velocity without an associated increase in adverse events, including rejection episodes [21]^r. Regardless of their treatment status (chronic renal insufficiency, maintenance dialysis, or posttransplant), the use of rhGH is recommended at a dose of 1.4 mg/m^2 per day (0.05 mg/kg/day), which provides a significant increase in growth velocity at least for the first 2 years of treatment [20,22]. Regarding bone structure, rhGH has been shown to maintain bone mass but is unable to increase bone for-

mation rate [23]. The use of oral alfacalcidol (0.25 µg/day) in children with low bone mineral density (BMD) as measured by dual-energy X-ray absorptiometry seemed to be safe and efficient, as BMD increased from –2.1 to –0.6 g/cm^2 ($P < 0.001$) in a RCT of 30 children [24]^r.

These favorable results for growth and nutrition in pediatric kidney transplant patients were in part independent of rhGH and due to other interventions, such as volunteer bias, steroid-sparing regiment, optimization of protein and energy intake, and correction of metabolic acidosis.

Donor and recipient factors affecting outcome

Donor factors

Living kidney donation is an important source of organs for children with ESRD, and there has been a major trend to laparoscopic donor nephrectomy during the last decade. There is limited RCT evidence supporting this practice, but it is likely to become the standard method for donor nephrectomy due to greater donor satisfaction, less morbidity, and equivalent graft outcome [25,26].

Due to organ shortage, kidneys from non-heart-beating donors have been used increasingly in selected centers during the last decade. From a case series in adults (72 non-heart-beating donors vs. 192 heart-beating donors), the 5-year survival was 73% and 65%, respectively (not statistically significant), suggesting that kidneys from non-heart-beating donors are a useful source of organs for transplantation [27]. The current experience with non-heart-beating donors in pediatric recipients is very limited, but such donors may be considered in the near future for pediatric recipients.

Recipient factors

The use of kidney-protecting agents to prevent acute tubular necrosis has been investigated in adults and was summarized in a large literature review [28]^e that concluded that despite the large number of potentially beneficial drugs (frusemide, dopamine, theophylline, mannitol, β2-adrenergic receptor agonists, cardiac glycosides, natriuretic peptides, prostaglandins, and nitric oxide), volume loading and maintenance of renal perfusion pressure with pressor agents (catecholamines) appear to be the only reliable protectors of kidney function in critically ill patients with ischemic injury to the tubule. High-dose calcium antagonists may have a benefit following kidney transplantation in adults [29,30].

Evidence for efficacy of primary immunosuppression regimens for both induction and maintenance

Induction therapy

Induction therapy is used for prophylaxis against acute rejection in kidney transplant recipients. A systematic review of RCTs found that interleukin-2 receptor antagonists were as effective as other antibody therapies but provided significant fewer side effects; there was no apparent difference between basiliximab and daclizumab [31].

In a multicenter randomized trial in children, OKT3 was compared to intravenous cyclosporine A. Maintenance immunosuppression included oral cyclosporine A (an oil-based preparation and a microemulsion were randomized, 1:1), methylprednisolone–prednisone, and either azathioprine or mycophenolate mofetil [32][r]. Graft failure after 4 years appeared to be more frequent with OKT3, but results were not significant (27% vs. 19%; $P = 0.15$), and the incidence of acute rejection was not improved by OKT3 induction therapy compared with intravenous cyclosporine A induction.

Trials of induction therapy are associated with different concomitant medications, so that recommendations for pediatric use may be questionable. Generally, the use of OKT3 is now limited to patients with steroid-resistant acute rejection. Induction therapy with basiliximab or daclizumab is still under investigation in the pediatric population and may help in steroid and calcineurin inhibitor sparing. Available data about induction therapies in pediatric renal transplantation are summarized in Table 62.7, [32–41].

Maintenance immunosuppression

Most standard protocols in current use include three drugs from different pharmacological groups, each directed to a site in the T-cell activation and proliferation cascade: a calcineurin inhibitor (cyclosporine A or tacrolimus), an antiproliferative agent (mycophenolate mofetil or azathioprine), and steroids (prednisolone or prednisone). It is still unclear whether new regimens are more specific or simply provide more adequate immunosuppression.

When used as primary immunosuppression in adults, tacrolimus is superior to cyclosporine A microemulsion for both graft function and graft survival, as shown in an RCT with a 2-year follow-up that aimed at blood level targets of 10–20 and 5–15 ng/mL for tacrolimus and 100–400 and 100–200 ng/mL for cyclosporine A during months 0–3 and 4–6, respectively [42]. Such conclusions have been confirmed by systematic reviews, but the rates of posttransplant diabetes and neurological and gastrointestinal side effects are increased with tacrolimus [43]. From the same review, there was insufficient information to assess the cost and quality of life of tacrolimus versus cyclosporine A. A randomized multicenter trial in children that compared tacrolimus and cyclosporine A microemulsion found a lower incidence of acute rejection (36.9 vs. 59.1%, respectively; $P = 0.003$) and a lower incidence of steroid-resistant acute rejection episodes (7.8 vs. 25.8%, respectively; $P = 0.001$) with tacrolimus. At 1 year, patient survival was similar (96.1% vs. 96.6%), and the mean GFR (estimated using the Schwartz formula) was significantly higher in the tacrolimus group (62 ± 20 vs. 56 ± 21 mL/min/1.73 m^2) [44][r]. At 4 years, patient survival was similar but graft survival and renal function were significantly better in the tacrolimus group [45][r]. There was no difference in the incidence of serious adverse events (posttransplant lymphoproliferative disease [PTLD], life-threatening infections, etc.).

The use of tacrolimus in children may be associated with some specific problems (gastrointestinal disturbances, food allergy, incidence of PTLD, diabetes, or incidence of BK virus nephropathy), and these have not been investigated sufficiently in this age group. The use of calcineurin inhibitors could therefore be based on cyclosporine A initially with a later switch to tacrolimus using lower trough blood concentrations (5–10 ng/mL instead of 10–20 ng/mL). Transplant recipients could be switched from cyclosporine A to tacrolimus in those at higher risk for chronic renal allograft failure. In a RCT of 186 adult patients, conversion resulted in improved renal function and lipid profiles and significantly fewer cardiovascular events, with no differences in the incidence of acute rejection or new-onset hyperglycemia [46]. In children, there have been no RCTs evaluating treatment conversion from cyclosporine A to tacrolimus.

The experience with sirolimus is still limited in children, and most information has come from trials in adult recipients [47][a]. In a long-term RCT of tacrolimus–sirolimus (group A) versus tacrolimus–mycophenolate mofetil (group B) versus cyclosporine A–sirolimus (group C), the 3-year interim analysis showed the following: 1) patient and graft survival were not significantly different; 2) group B had a lower rate of biopsy-proven acute rejection episodes (10, vs. 26% in group A and 20% in group C); 3) there was a trend for better GFR in groups A (72.8 ± 4.3 mL/min) and B (721.1 ± 4.1 mL/min) vs. group C (61.8 ± 3.8 mL/min); and 4) there was less *de novo* development of posttransplant diabetes mellitus and lipid disorders in group B compared to group A and group C. A combination of tacrolimus and mycophenolate mofetil seemed, therefore, superior to other combinations, including sirolimus [48][r]. Everolimus was also compared to mycophenolate mofetil in a 3-year randomized, multicenter study, with comparable efficacy but more adverse events with everolimus [49][r].

Because maintenance therapy with calcineurin inhibitors is responsible for some graft nephrotoxicity, various calcineurin inhibitor-sparing schedules have been proposed. The use of sirolimus maintenance therapy instead of cyclosporine A may be an option [50][r], but withdrawal of cyclosporine A from a mycophenolate mofetil-containing regimen results in an increased risk of acute rejection and graft loss despite better 1- and 5-year posttransplant GFR [51][r].

The question of steroid withdrawal is very relevant to children because of the growth, bone, and cosmetic complications of long-term steroid use. A meta-analysis of six trials (four with cyclosporine A and two with tacrolimus, all with initiation of steroid withdrawal at 3–6 months posttransplantation) in both adult and pediatric patients on triple therapy with a calcineurin inhibitor and mycophenolate mofetil showed a low but significant risk of acute rejection after steroid withdrawal (relative risk [RR], 2.28; 95% confidence interval [CI], 1.65–3.16). However, the risk of subsequent early graft failure was not increased (RR, 0.73; CI, 0.42–1.25) in either the short- or medium-term follow-up [52][a,c]. Further reports have been published, including a randomized trial comparing a combination of daclizumab, tacrolimus, and mycophenolate mofetil (group A, $n = 260$) versus tacrolimus, mycophenolate mofetil, and steroids (group B, $n = 278$) at 6 months posttransplant [53][a]; 88.8% of patients in group A remained free from steroids, the incidences of biopsy-proven acute rejection (16.5% in both groups) and renal function (median serum creatinine of 125 μmol/L [1.39 mg/dL] in group A vs. 131 [1.46 mg/dL] in group B) were comparable, and the overall safety profile was similar in both groups. In group A, the incidence of new-onset insulin-dependent diabetes mellitus was significantly reduced (5.4% vs. 0.4%), and the mean total cholesterol concentration was lower. A comparable study aimed at avoiding steroids has been designed recently for the pediatric population and is currently under way. In a randomized study of 27 prepubertal patients, deflazacort was shown to be superior to methylprednisolone for the outcomes of height loss, bone loss, fat accumulation, and lipoprotein profile [54][r]. However, deflazacort is not widely available, and confirmatory studies are needed before deflazacort can be recommended as the steroid of choice in children.

Available data about maintenance therapy in pediatric renal transplantation are summarized in Table 62.7, [44,45,55–80] .

Evidence for efficacy of treatment of acute rejection

The evidence base for the treatment of acute rejection in children is very limited, so that it is not discussed further in this chapter.

Epidemiology, outcomes, and management of chronic rejection and allograft nephropathy

Chronic rejection is responsible for one-third of all graft failure in North America [8] (Table 62.2). There has been no pediatric study on the effects of fish oil supplementation on kidney transplantation, but there have been several RCTs in adults. It has been concluded that there is no significant change in either 1-year rejection rate (RR, 0.91; CI, 0.74–1.10) or overall graft survival (RR, 1.00; CI, 0.96–1.05); there was only a slight benefit on triglyceride levels [81][a].

Epidemiology, outcomes, and management of infectious diseases

Cytomegalovirus

Cytomegalovirus (CMV) infection is associated with substantial morbidity and mortality in solid organ transplant recipients, mainly during the first 6 months after transplantation. Antiviral drugs against CMV include acyclovir, ganciclovir, valacyclovir, and valganciclovir. Compared to placebo or no therapy, both universal prophylaxis (odds ratio [OR], 0.20; CI, 0.13–0.31) and preemptive strategies (OR, 0.28; CI, 0.11–0.69) reduce CMV organ disease

in solid organ transplant recipients [82][a]. In kidney transplant recipients, prophylactic treatment using acyclovir and/or ganciclovir in 100 patients would avoid 18 patients developing CMV disease and 19 developing CMV infection [83,84][c]. Oral versus intravenous preemptive treatment showed no significant difference for the outcomes of CMV disease or all-cause mortality [84][c]. The risk of acute rejection is reduced by both preemptive and prophylactic treatment [82][a,c], and there is no significant difference in the relative effects of either treatment [84][a,c]. All-cause mortality is comparable between preemptive treatment and prophylaxis, but confidence intervals are wide, and head-to-head trials are required to determine the relative benefits and harms of preemptive and prophylaxis therapy [84][a,c]. The benefit of prophylactic strategies has been reported in high-risk organ transplant recipients (i.e. donors with positive CMV serostatus and recipients with negative CMV serostatus with or without antibody induction) in reducing CMV organ disease [82][a]. However, two Cochrane reviews did not find any difference in benefit between high-risk patients (i.e. CMV-positive recipients and CMV-negative recipients of CMV-positive organ donors) and other patients [83,84][a,c]. In the Cochrane meta-analysis, ganciclovir was more effective than acyclovir in preventing CMV disease (RR, 0.37; 95% CI, 0.23–0.60); valganciclovir and intravenous ganciclovir were as effective as oral ganciclovir [83][a]. Overall, there is a much stronger evidence base for routine use than preemptive use of antiviral medications. There are considerably more and larger trials, and some important outcomes have been demonstrated for routine use—reduction in graft loss and all-cause mortality—which have not been shown in preemptive trials. Also, benefit has been shown in all donor groups, except in the uncommon scenario of a CMV-negative recipient of CMV-negative donor, in which the risk is very low.

Many meta-analyses and RCTs have included transplantations of all organs and all recipient ages, which limits conclusions for pediatric renal transplantation, and the specific profile of serological status in children is rarely considered separately. In addition, several studies did not provide information to discriminate between CMV organ disease and CMV syndrome or data about the timing of CMV organ disease.

Other viruses

Most PTLD cases are associated with Epstein–Barr virus (EBV) infection. EBV infection is a major issue in pediatric solid organ transplantation, because many recipients are EBV negative and many donors are EBV positive, resulting in a high risk of primary infection (and a relatively low risk of reactivation compared with adults). The risk of incidence of PTLD is significantly higher in pediatric kidney recipients, 1.2–10.1%, compared to 1.0–2.3% in adults [85][e]. PTLD is related to the total burden of immunosuppression. Its treatment includes a reduction in immunosuppression, anti-B-cell antibodies (rituximab), and sometimes chemotherapy. There is no evidence-based information on the most appropriate management, including prophylactic, preemptive, versus curative treatments for children or adults [85][e].

BK virus represents a growing cause of chronic graft dysfunction and graft loss. In the general healthy adult population, seroprevalence is 65–90%. In adults after transplantation, 30–60% of patients develop viruria, 10–20% viremia, and 5–10% BK-associated nephropathy [86][r]. Up to 50% of patients with BK-associated nephropathy have premature graft loss. A retrospective study in 100 children found a 70% seroprevalence for BK virus before transplantation, a 26% prevalence for viruria, 5% for viremia, and 3% for BK virus-associated nephropathy [87]. Recipient seronegativity is a risk factor for BK virus-associated nephropathy. When BK virus-associated nephropathy occurs, viremia and viruria findings are positive [88]. There is no consensus for treatment of BK virus infection; a decrease in immunosuppression, particularly calcineurin inhibitors, is often proposed. Small series have evaluated cidofovir, leflunomide, intravenous immunoglobulins, and fluoroquinolones; however, further evaluation with prospective controlled studies is warranted [89][c].

Despite their frequency in transplant patients, there is no available evidence on the treatment of warts. A systematic review of studies in nonimmunocompromised patients (only 2 trials are classified as high-quality among 50 trials) has shown that topical treatments containing salicylic acid have a therapeutic effect and there is some evidence for the efficacy of dinitrochlorobenzene; less evidence was found for the efficacy of other treatments, including cryotherapy [90][a,c].

Fungal infections

Invasive fungal infections may cause morbidity and mortality in solid organ transplant recipients. However, unlike liver transplant recipients, neither fluconazole nor clotrimazole significantly reduce invasive fungal infection in renal transplant recipients [91][c].

Available data about CMV, EBV, and antifungal therapy in pediatric renal transplantation are summarized in Table 62.7, [92–99].

Epidemiology, outcomes, and management of disease recurrence

The posttransplant recurrence rates of primary diseases are listed in Table 62.5. Recurrence of the primary disease is responsible for about 7% of all graft failures in North America [8] (Table 62.2). This proportion has increased during the last decade, relative to other causes of graft failure, because of improvements in treatment for acute rejection during the first months posttransplantation. Because recurrence of individual diseases is relatively infrequent, management is mainly based on information obtained from nonrandomized and uncontrolled case series.

Steroid-resistant nephrotic syndrome

Steroid-resistant nephrotic syndrome is the cause of 10–12% of ESRD in children and is one of the most challenging recurrent diseases to treat posttransplantation. It recurs in about

Table 62.5 Recurrence rates of primary diseases in children and adults after renal transplantation.

Primary disease	Recurrence rate (%)
Steroid-resistant nephrotic syndrome (FSGS)	20–65
FSGS in case of retransplantation	80–100
IgA nephropathy (Berger disease and HSP)	50–60
MPGN type 1	20–80
MPGN type 2	80–100
Atypical HUS	30–80
Systemic lupus erythematosus	30–40
Primary hyperoxaluria type 1	90–100

Abbreviation: HSP, Henoch-Schönlein purpura.
FSGS: Focal segmental glomerulosclerosis
MPGN: membrano-proliferative glomerulonephritis

one-third of recipients with primary focal segmental glomerulosclerosis (FSGS), and graft loss occurs in about one-third. The overall graft survival is 50–55% 6 years after transplantation (Table 62.5) [100,101][e]. The presence of a circulating factor(s) and also T-cell activation have been implicated, so that recurrence usually occurs immediately after transplantation. Risk factors for recurrence have been reported [100,101][e] and include the following: aggressive clinical course of primary FSGS with a time interval from diagnosis to ESRD of less than 3 years, age at onset of nephrotic syndrome between 6 and 15 years, histopathology of the native kidney consistent with diffuse mesangial proliferation, Caucasian background, and first graft failure after recurrence. The influence of genetic factors (e.g. podocin mutation) is still under investigation [100,101][e]. There is no association between duration of dialysis prior to transplantation, HLA-DR matching, type of donor, or pretransplant nephrectomy and risk of recurrence [100,101][e]. Several case series reported the efficacy of either high-dose cyclosporine A (oral dose to maintain a trough level of 200–300 ng/mL) and plasmapheresis–protein adsorption (5–30 sessions) with or without cyclophosphamide instead of azathioprine or mycophenolate mofetil [100,101].[e] There is no clear benefit of protein adsorption over plasmapheresis, and cyclosporine A seems to be more effective than tacrolimus. There is no evidence on the optimal duration of these two therapeutic options, and no randomized trial has been published. Nevertheless, on the basis of the current available literature, the use of early plasmapheresis (1–3 days following the onset of posttransplant nephrotic syndrome) may be recommended for renal transplant patients with recurrent steroid-resistant nephrotic syndrome [101–103][e]. The use of preemptive plasmapheresis in high-risk patients (rapid progression to renal failure or previous recurrence posttransplantation) was evaluated in a prospective nonrandomized study. Ten adult patients underwent a course of eight plasmaphereses in the perioperative period. Seven patients were free of recurrence (238–1258 days of follow-up) [104]. A retrospective pediatric study found similar results [105]. However, larger randomized and controlled studies are warranted for the evaluation of preemptive plasmapheresis. The use of living donors is debated, because there has been no graft survival benefit demonstrated in large series from collaborative studies [106], whereas it may benefit individual patients, provided that it is associated with pretransplantation cyclosporine A therapy [101][e].

Other recurrent diseases

The risk of histopathologic recurrence of immunoglobulin A (IgA) nephropathy (Berger disease and Henoch-Schönlein purpura) is 50–60% and seems to be increased for living donor transplantation (Table 62.5), but graft loss from recurrence is below 5% and no specific treatment has been investigated [101][e].

The risk of histopathologic recurrence of membrano-proliferative glomerulonephritis (MPGN) type 1 is 20–80% in a first graft (Table 62.6), often leading to progressive graft failure and recurrence in further grafts. Graft survival after recurrence of proteinuria averages 40 months, and no immunological intervention, including plasmapheresis, has been successful [101][e]. MPGN type 2 has a very high risk of histopathologic recurrence (Table 62.5) but a relatively low rate of graft loss due to recurrence; no treatment can reasonably be recommended.

Atypical hemolytic uremic syndrome (HUS) is associated with variable risk of recurrence according to its pathophysiology, but time to recurrence is usually less than 1 month (Table 62.5). There is a 40–80% risk of recurrence and subsequent graft failure in patients with abnormal complement alternative pathway proteins (factor H deficiency, presence of anti-factor H autoantibodies, factor I deficiency, or abnormal MCP/CD46 ratio) [101][e]; the management of such a recurrence is rather challenging, and combined liver (factor H source) and kidney (target organ) transplantation has been attempted with variable outcomes. In the absence of available protein substitution (with factor H-enriched plasma fraction, recombinant factor H, end-pathway complement inhibitors, liver transplantation, or gene therapy), retransplantation of such patients should be avoided. In contrast, the management of ESRD patients with HUS due to von Willebrand factor deficiency (ADAMTS 13) is easier in case of recurrence, because fresh frozen plasma (10 mL/kg every 2–4 weeks) is able to provide enough replacement enzyme protein, and recombinant ADAMTS 13 will be available in the future. The use of cyclosporine A has no effect on outcome or HUS recurrence, but some immunological events, such as CMV infec-tion, allograft rejection, and bacterial infection, may trigger HUS recurrence [101][e].

Available data about disease recurrence in pediatric renal transplantation are summarized in Table 62.7 [101,105,107–113].

Epidemiology, outcomes, and management of malignancy

Due to ongoing evolution of immunosuppression strategies, both long-term graft survival and risk of malignancy have increased, without any improvements in overall patient survival [8]. Changes in risks of malignancies are shown in Table 62.6.

Evidence for effects of treatment adherence on graft outcome

Adherence to medical regimens after kidney transplantation is a major issue regarding the functional status of the transplanted organ [114]. Nonadherence with medication, medical procedures, and/or diet is one of the main causes of chronic allograft nephropathy, graft loss, and mortality. The risk of nonadherence is increased by distance to the treatment center, economic difficulties, degree of social support, psychological distress, family functioning, and physiological side effects of drugs. The transition from childhood to adulthood may be challenging for patients with kidney transplants because of low self-esteem, social adjustment difficulties, depression, and behavioral disturbances. However, independent of the immunological rationale and favorable results associated with treatment adherence, there is no available evidence to correlate adherence and graft and patient outcomes.

Conclusions

Pediatric kidney transplantation is characterized by specific primary diseases (urinary tract malformations, renal dysplasia or hypoplasia, focal segmental glomerular diseases, inherited renal diseases, etc.) associated with specific problems posttransplantation. In addition, kidney transplantation requires special surgical and postoperative care in small children and special education for adolescents due to adherence issues. Moreover, due to specific serological and pharmacokinetic profiles, there are many differences between adult and pediatric kidney transplantation. Table 62.8 summarizes the evidence rating and recommendations for interventions in pediatric renal transplant recipients. High evidence data in pediatric renal transplantation are missing (e.g. use of mTor inhibitors or corticoid withdrawal, management of acute rejection, CMV prophylaxis and recurrence, etc.). We are still far from evidence-based recommendations for all aspects of managing the pediatric kidney transplant recipient, and so many further trials are required.

Table 62.6 Posttransplant malignancy rates in North America.

Time period (no. of transplants during period)	% Malignancy rate (mean $\pm$ SE) at:	
	1 year	3 years
1987–1991 (2689)	0.62 ± 0.16	0.96 ± 0.21
1992–1995 (2530)	1.30 ± 0.24	2.00 ± 0.30
1996–2004 (4024)	2.00 ± 0.25	3.14 ± 0.34

[a] In the NAPRTCS 2005 report [8], a total of 232 malignancies (179 lymphoproliferative diseases and 43 nonlymphoproliferative neoplasias) were reported.

Table 62.7 Summary of pediatric studies in renal transplantation[a].

Therapy group and intervention	Reference(s)	Design and results, including adverse effects	Conclusions and comments
Induction therapy			
Antibody therapy: OKT-3	Benfield 2005 [32]	Multicenter RCT, open label, parallel groups 287 patients, 147 OKT3, 140 iv cyclosporine	The incidence of acute rejection and graft failure in pediatric patients is not improved by OKT3 induction therapy relative to cyclosporine induction.
		OKT3: 2.5 mg/kg (for <30 kg body weight) or 5 mg/kg (>30 kg). First perioperative dose, then daily i.v. infusion; 10 doses	
		Cyclosporine: 165 mg/m^2 (<6 yrs) or 4.5 mg/kg (>6 yrs), intraoperatively, as continuous infusion over 24-h period; i.v. administration for first 3 days after transplantation.	OKT3 graft survival is inferior in children under 6 yrs ($P = 0.05$, unadjusted for multiple comparisons).
		Maintenance therapy: second randomization to receive either oral cyclosporine (Sandimmune or Neoral), 500 mg/m^2 (<6 yrs) or 15 mg/kg (>6 yrs). Full dose on day 3 in the i.v. cyclosporine group and low dose (250 mg/m^2) from day 3–10 then full dose in OKT3 group. Other immunosuppressive drugs: CS and azathioprine (2 mg/kg/day) or MMF (600 mg/m^2 twice daily).	The use of OKT3 as induction therapy should be abandoned.
		Results: 1 yr same graft survival and renal function; 4 yr, no significant difference for graft loss (27% in OKT3 group vs 19%; $P = 0.154$), incidence of rejections and incidence of steroid-resistant rejections.	
		In multivariate analysis, OKT3 seems to have a numerically inferior graft survival, but confidence intervals are wide (RR 1.4, CI 0.8–2.2; $P = 0.22$).	
		No differences for PTLD, infections, or patient survival.	
Antibody therapy: ATG-ALG	Acott 2001 [33]	Retrospective study with historic group control, comparing induction ATG/ALG and basiliximab.	No RCTs about ATG-ALG are available in pediatric renal transplant recipients.
		50 patients (27 ATG/ALG and 23 basiliximab)	
		Results: 3 yr similar graft survival (94%)	
		Side effects: unexplained fever (52% ATG-ALG vs 0% basiliximab group), lymphopenia in both groups. Pulmonary edema, fluid retention, and thrombocytopenia with ATG-ALG. EBV and CMV infections more frequent in ATG-ALG group.	
		Basiliximab seems to be superior to ATG-ALG for induction therapy for pediatric renal transplantation.	
	Khositseth 2005 [34]	Historical cohort study to compare efficacy and safety of ATGAM vs thymoglobulin, as polyclonal antibody induction. 198 patients.	
		Results: Significantly lower incidence of acute rejection with thymoglobulin. Significantly higher incidence of EBV infection with thymoglobulin. No differences for patient and graft survival, CAN, PTLD, and other infections.	
	Dharnidharka 2005 [35]	Retrospective study to estimate risk for PTLD after polyclonal antibody induction.	
		87 cases of PTLD among 5238 kidney transplant recipients. In an analysis restricted to pediatric recipients, equine ATG was associated with a higher adjusted relative risk for PTLD compared with rATG and ALG.	
	Kamel 2005 and 2006 [36,37]	1) Prospective open controlled trial in parallel groups, evaluating rATG as induction therapy for pediatric deceased donor kidney transplantation.	
		120 consecutive kidney transplants in 95 patients.	
		Results: actuarial graft survival in group receiving rATG significantly better than control group. Significant difference in incidence of graft loss secondary to acute rejection. No difference in infectious complications. No PTLD.	
		2) Retrospective study to evaluate efficacy of rATG in preventing graft thrombosis. 95 patients receiving 120 kidney transplants.	
		rATG use reduced the risk of graft thrombosis in multivariate analysis; classic risks of graft thrombosis were similar in both groups.	
	Shapiro 2006 [38]	Prospective open noncontrolled trial, evaluating antilymphocyte antibody induction and tacrolimus monotherapy.	
		17 patients; two groups: ATG ($n = 8$) and alemtuzumab ($n = 9$). Results: acute rejection seems to be more frequent with ATG induction, but difference in efficacy is small.	
		Side effects: no systemic infectious complications, no PTLD, two diabetes mellitus cases. Data were not recorded for BK virus.	

	Study	Description / Results	Comments
	Ault 2002 [39]	Retrospective study, evaluating short-term outcome of rATG induction; 17 patients. Results: 1-yr patient and graft survival 100 and 93%, respectively. No symptomatic CMV or EBV infections. No PTLD.	
	Hastings 2006 [40]	Retrospective study, evaluating long-term outcome of rATG induction. First results described by Ault (2002); 33 patients. Results: 3-yr graft survival 73%; no PTLD, no malignancy. One case symptomatic CMV disease. None of the patients experienced an infusion reaction.	
IL-2 receptor blockers	Grenda 2006 [41]	Multicenter RCT, open label, parallel groups. 192 patients; 93 tacrolimus + azathioprine + CS; 99 patients tacrolimus + azathioprine + CS + 2 doses of basiliximab (10 mg for body weight <40 kg, and 20 mg for >40 kg; day 0 and day 4) Target serum levels of tacrolimus: 10–20 ng/mL from day 0–21 and 5–15 ng/mL after day 21. Initial dose of tacrolimus 0.3 mg/kg per day, in two equal oral doses. Results at 6 months: no difference in incidence of acute rejection or steroid-resistant acute rejection, graft survival, patient survival, and renal function. Two side effects significantly more frequent in basiliximab group: toxic nephropathy (increase of serum creatinine >10% above baseline posttransplant with undesired increase in tacrolimus whole-blood trough levels and resolving after tacrolimus dose reduction) and abdominal pain. No differences for diabetes mellitus, antihypertensive use, cholesterol levels, infections, and malignancies.	Adding basiliximab to a tacrolimus-based regimen is safe in pediatric patients; however, it does not improve clinical efficacy at 6 months.
Maintenance therapy			
Antiproliferative agents	Bunchman 2001, 2005 [55,56]	Prospective, multicenter, open-label, single-arm study. Evaluation of MMF as primary immunosuppression. 100 patients. Results, 1yrs: patient and graft survival 98 and 93%, respectively. 49% of patients experienced side effects resulting in MMF reduction or cessation. Trend toward more frequent diarrhea, leukopenia, sepsis, and anemia in children under 6 yrs. Results, 3 yrs: side effects accounted for 12% of premature withdrawals of MMF. At least one rejection episode occurred in 30% of patients. Creatinine clearance remained stable during the 3-yr follow-up period for patients who did not lose their graft. Side effects: 25% hematological disturbances (leukopenia) and 16% diarrhea; more often in youngest age group (<6 yrs). 57 recipients experienced at least one opportunistic infection: 22 CMV viremia, 1 CMV infection, 4 CMV tissue invasions, 1 Aspergillus, 1 PTLD.	No RCT with MMF are available. Since some MMF-related side effects occur more frequently with high MMF exposure and since rejection episodes are conversely more frequent with low MMF exposure, therapeutic drug monitoring of MMF may be useful to enhance the efficacy and safety of MMF therapy in the pediatric renal transplantation population. This hypothesis is currently being tested in an ongoing RCT, in both adult and pediatric kidney transplant recipients.
	Virji 2001 [57]	Retrospective single-center study. Evaluation of MMF as primary immunosuppression or rescue. 24 patients. Side effects: diarrhea, abdominal pain, leukopenia, thrombocytopenia, symptomatic CMV infection. No malignancy.	
	Jungraithmayr 2003 [58]	Evaluation of MMF as primary immunosuppression. 86 patients. Historic group control ($n = 54$). At 3 yrs, patient and graft survivals favorable to MMF compared to azathioprine. Infection rates similar to those reported in adults.	
	Ojogho 2003, Ojogho 2002 [59,60]	Retrospective study. Controlled to historic cohort to examine use of MMF in immunosuppressive strategy avoiding antibody induction. 43 patients, 30 historic control patients. Results, 1 yr: no differences for renal function, graft and patient survival, urinary tract infections, and PTLD. MMF seemed to result in fewer CMV infections, but results not statistically significant.	

(continued)

Table 62.7 (*continued*).

Therapy group and intervention	Reference(s)	Design and results, including adverse effects	Conclusions and comments
	Ojogho 2005 [61]	Retrospective single-center study to evaluate use of MMF in immunosuppressive strategy avoiding antibody induction vs induction with basiliximab. 41 patients (25 no induction, 16 induction with basiliximab) Results, 6 months: no differences for incidence of acute rejection, graft and patient survival, urinary infections, and CMV infection. Results, 1 yr: no difference for graft and patient survival	
	Cransberg 2005 [62]	Evaluation of MMF as primary immunosuppression. 96 patients. Historic group control (*n* = 207). Graft loss, incidence of acute rejection, and CMV infections significantly decreased with MMF. No differences for malignancies. Bronchiectasis described as a new complication of MMF treatment.	
	Ferraris 2005 [63]	Evaluation of MMF as primary immunosuppression. 29 patients. Historic group control. Significant improvement of linear growth (reduction in dose of steroids) and renal function at 5 yrs in MMF group. Significant decrease in incidence of acute rejection.	
	Otukesh 2005 [64]	Retrospective controlled single-center evaluation of MMF as primary immunosuppression or as rescue treatment in CAN. 216 patients, 100 MMF and 116 azathioprine. Results: significantly fewer graft failures in MMF group. Patients who received MMF as primary immunosuppression experienced significantly fewer graft loss and acute rejection episodes in first 3 months. Patients who received MMF at the time of diagnosis of CAN had significant better graft survival than those receiving azathioprine.	
	Henne 2003 [65]	Evaluation of MMF in CAN. Noncontrolled open trial. 36 patients. Promising results at 1 yr.	
	Benz 2006 [66]	Retrospective evaluation of MMF in addition with cyclosporine A in CAN. 17 patients. Results: after introduction of MMF, stabilization of GFR; after cyclosporine A reduction, improvement of GFR. 1 acute rejection episode.	
Steroid withdrawal	Chakrabarti 2000 [67]	Withdrawal of CS, retrospective study, 80 patients receiving tacrolimus-based immunosuppression. 1-, 3-, and 5-year actuarial patient survival rates in withdrawal group were 100, 98, and 96% and the actuarial graft survival rates were 100, 95, and 82%. 22.5% of patients restarted on CS.	In 1994, a systematic review of published pediatric studies showed that under maintenance with cyclosporine A monotherapy or dual therapy with cyclosporine A and azathioprine, steroid withdrawal was associated with a significant risk of acute transplant rejection [115]. CS withdrawal or avoidance in children on newer immunosuppressive therapies: evidence rating of these studies does not allow clinicians to determine whether CS can be withdrawn safely. An RCT is under way in pediatric patients.
	Höcker 2004 [68]	Withdrawal of CS, retrospective case control study. 40 patients. CS withdrawal was not systematic (*n* = 20). After CS withdrawal, graft function remained stable, and prepubertal and pubertal patients exhibited significant catch-up growth; mean arterial blood pressure and use of antihypertensive drugs decreased. In conclusion, late steroid withdrawal seems to be safe and successful in stable patients under immunosuppressive maintenance therapy with cyclosporine A and MMF.	

	Oberholzer 2005 [69]	Early withdrawal of CS, retrospective case–control study with age-matched historic controls. 13 patients and 13 historic controls. No difference for graft and patient survival. Significantly higher creatinine clearance at 6 and 12 months, lower delta BMI, higher delta height Z-score, less hyperlipidemia and need for antihypertensive drugs in withdrawal group.	The incidence of BK virus-associated nephropathy and food allergy has not been studied. These problems have not been investigated enough in the pediatric population.
	Birkeland 1998 [70]	Avoidance of CS: retrospective study. 14 patients receiving initial course of ALG, cyclosporine A w/ or w/o MMF. Same levels of long-term graft survival and renal function as data reported in registries of pediatric renal transplant recipients.	The beneficial effect on lipid profiles of tacrolimus may be of particular importance for cardiovascular disease prevention.
	Sarwal 2003 [71]	Avoidance of CS; pilot steroid-free protocol, controlled to matched cohort. 57 patients. Daclizumab induction, tacrolimus and MMF. Results, 1 yr: steroid-free recipients showed significant improvement for acute rejection, graft function, hypertension, and growth. No increased infectious complications.	
Calcineurin inhibitors	Trompeter 2002, 2005 [44,45]	Multicenter RCT, open label, parallel groups. 196 patients (103 tacrolimus, 93 cyclosporine A). Tacrolimus: 0.15 mg/kg b.i.d; target serum levels 10–20 ng/mL from day 0–30 and 5–10 ng/mL after day 30. Cyclosporine: 150 mg/m² b.i.d; target serum levels 150–250 ng/mL during the first 6 weeks, 100–200 ng/mL after the sixth week posttransplant.	
		Results, 1 yr: significantly lower incidence acute rejections and steroid-resistant acute rejections, better renal function (Schwartz) in tacrolimus group. Hypomagnesemia and diarrhea significantly more frequent with tacrolimus, whereas hypertrichosis and flu syndrome more frequent with cyclosporine. No differences for hypertension, urinary tract infections, diabetes mellitus, and PTLD.	
		Results, 4 yrs: significantly better graft survival (86 vs 69%; $P = 0.025$) and renal function (71.5 ± 22.9 vs 53 ± 21.6 mL/min/1.73 m²; $P = 0.0001$) in tacrolimus group. No differences for patient survival (90–95%), PTLD, use of antihypertensives, or diabetes mellitus. Significantly higher cholesterol level in cyclosporine group.	
Sirolimus and everolimus	Vester 2002 [72]	Open, prospective, multicenter, nonrandomized trial to study efficacy, tolerability, and safety of everolimus as primary treatment in combination with CS and Neoral in 10 patients.	No RCT available.
		Results, 3 months: no acute rejection, no graft failure, no death.	Heavy proteinuria has been described in pediatric renal transplant patients receiving sirolimus [116]; two hypotheses are discussed (toxic effect of sirolimus and/or lower CNI exposure). Early detection of proteinuria may be helpful.
		Severe side effects observed in 4 patients: lymphocele, urinary tract infections, dyslipidemia, lymphocele abscess, fever, and unexplained increased creatinine. Neither CMV disease nor pneumocystosis (systematic cotrimoxazole prophylaxis).	Another side effect of sirolimus has been described: gastrointestinal leukocytoclastic vasculitis, which disappeared after sirolimus discontinuation [117].
			Overall, side effects appear to be important with mTor inhibitors.
			Further larger studies are necessary to assess the impact of side events in pediatric transplant population receiving sirolimus and to evaluate the full potential of sirolimus as initial immunosuppression and/or as a rescue drug in CAN.

(continued)

Table 62.7 (continued).

Therapy group and intervention	Reference(s)	Design and results, including adverse effects	Conclusions and comments
	Vilalta 2003 [73]	Open, prospective, nonrandomized, noncontrolled trial to study efficacy and safety of sirolimus (1.15 mg/m²/day) as primary treatment. 6 patients.	
		Results, 1 yr: all patients show normal creatinine levels and lead normal lives. No adverse effects or opportunistic infections observed. After cyclosporine withdrawal, sirolimus doses were increased by mean 40%.	
	Filler 2005 [74]	Retrospective single-center study to evaluate retrospectively sirolimus efficacy as rescue agent in patients with CAN and receiving tacrolimus-based immunosuppression. 8 patients.	
		Results: when adding sirolimus, a significant decrease in tacrolimus dose observed; tacrolimus blood levels should be monitored frequently in this situation.	
	Hymes 2005 [75]	Monocenter, open, prospective, nonrandomized, noncontrolled trial to evaluate sirolimus efficacy and safety as a primary treatment. 66 patients.	
		Results, 6 months: patient and graft survival 100 and 98%, acute rejection 11%, acute steroid-resistant rejection 0%, mean serum creatinine 0.9 ± 0.4 mg/dL.	
		Side effects described: EBV, PTLD, CMV, surgical wound dehiscence, noninfectious pneumonitis, nephrotic syndrome, diabetes mellitus, perinephric abscess, and serum cholesterol levels higher than 200 mg/dL.	
	Ibanez 2005 [76]	Retrospective study of 18 patients to evaluate retrospectively sirolimus efficacy and safety as a rescue agent.	
		Results, 3 months: significant improvement in renal function. Steroid-sensitive acute rejection episode occurred early after conversion. No differences for proteinuria, serum cholesterol, triglycerides, and platelet counts.	
		Three serious side effects: central nervous system relapse of EBV-related B-cell lymphoma, sepsis in course of acute pyelonephritis, and asymptomatic pancreatic pseudocyst. Other side effects: HSV infections (oral acyclovir, no need to change immunosuppression), leg lymphedema. No need to discontinue sirolimus.	
	Höcker 2006 [77]	Single-center case–control study, 10 patients sirolimus, MMF, CS, CNI withdrawal vs 9 patients CNI minimization, MMF, CS. Patients with chronic CNI toxicity.	
		Results, 1yr: no acute rejection, significant improvement in renal function in both groups. Absolute and relative gains of GFR in the two groups not significantly different.	
		Side effects: no differences between the two groups for hypertension, infectious episodes, or white blood cell count. Hypercholesterolemia in 70% of patients receiving sirolimus.	
	Garcia 2006 [78]	Retrospective study, 16 patients, to evaluate retrospectively sirolimus efficacy and safety as a rescue agent. Different immunosuppressive regimens.	
		Side effects: nephrotic proteinuria, anemia (25% of patients needed erythropoietin therapy), hypercholesterolemia requiring statins in 5 children, and mucosal ulceration. Heterogenous patients; a favorable evolution was observed in 11 patients.	
	Falger 2006 [118]	Monocenter, open, prospective, nonrandomized, noncontrolled trial to evaluate effects of conversion protocol (from CNI to sirolimus) in CAN. 8 patients.	
		Results, 1 yr: significant stabilization of GFR, no graft loss, no discontinuation of sirolimus.	
		Side effects: initial increase of triglycerides and serum cholesterol that both decreased towards initial values at 1 yr. Acne, bacterial pneumonia, CMV-pneumonitis, HSV labialis, diarrhea.	
	Harmon 2006 [80]	Pilot trial of CNI avoidance after living donor kidney transplantation. 34 patients.	
		Results: two graft losses (1 CAN, 1 PTLD). Patient survival 100%. Acute rejection at 6 and 12 months, 21.8 and 31.5%, respectively. Side effects: 2 PTLD	

Anti-infective therapy

CMV therapy	Flynn 1997 [92]	CMV prophylaxis treatment. Prospective open study, evaluating efficacy of i.v. immunoglobulins as prophylaxis to CMV-negative children who received CMV-positive allografts. Historic controls. Results: prophylactic treatment significantly decreased incidence of CMV disease posttransplantation. CMV diseases also occured significantly later than in untreated children. Infections seem to be less severe with prophylaxis.	Few trials are available in children.
	Bock 1997 [93]	CMV prophylaxis treatment. NAPRTCS registry, patients hospitalized for CMV infections during the first post-renal transplant year ($n = 142$). Retrospective case–control study. Results: prophylaxis with anti-CMV IgG significantly reduced risk of CMV hospitalization. Prophylactic use of antiviral agents was associated with significantly decreased risk of major organ involvement during CMV infection. Among patients with CMV, the 3-yr graft survival was significantly better for those who received any form of prophylaxis than for those who received none.	No RCTs available.
	Filler 1998 [94]	CMV prophylaxis treatment. Prospective pharmacokinetic study of oral ganciclovir. 14 patients, CMV serenegative who received a graft from a CMV-seropositive donor. Results: no CMV disease developed in any of the patients during oral ganciclovir. One patient presented with positive CMV viremia 5 weeks after discontinuation of ganciclovir. No particular side effects	
	Rubik 2006 [95]	CMV prophylaxis treatment. Prospective open noncontrolled evaluation of pharmacokinetics of valganciclovir oral suspension. 10 patients. Results: no episode of drug toxicity or withdrawal. Data about efficacy not reported.	
	Melgosa-Hijosa 2004 [96]	CMV preemptive treatment. Open, noncontrolled prospective study. 42 patients all receiving i.v. ganciclovir prophylaxis for CMV posttransplant. CMV viremia in 22 children, 5 were symptomatic. Asymptomatic patients received oral ganciclovir. Symptomatic patients received i.v. ganciclovir. Results: no CMV disease, ganciclovir resistance, acute renal rejection, or renal dysfunction. GFR at 1 yr similar to that of uninfected children.	
EBV therapy	Srivastava 1999 [97]	Retrospective monocenter study. 84 renal transplant recipients, 6 PTLD. All positive EBV serology and PCR at time of diagnosis of PTLD. Treatment consisted of reduced immunosuppression and ganciclovir/acyclovir in all patients. Results: PTLD resolved in all patients and all patients are alive 2–54 months after PTLD diagnosis.	Treatments of both EBV infection and PTLD remain controversial in adults. Very few trials are available in children. No RCTs are available. Surveillance of EBV viremia may be useful to promptly reduce immunosuppression [119]. Data about the benefit of antiviral agents in positive EBV viremia without PTLD remain uncertain; however, many centers seem to use prophylactic antiviral agents during the first 3/6 months after transplantation [119]. Many treatments have been proposed for established PTLD: immunosuppressive drug reduction is used in over 90% of cases. Rituximab, interferon alpha, chemotherapy, radiotherapy, and surgery have been proposed [85].

(continued)

Table 62.7 (continued).

Therapy group and intervention	Reference(s)	Design and results, including adverse effects	Conclusions and comments
	Shroff 2002 [98]	Prospective EBV surveillance post-transplant. 43 patients. Aim of study was to detect EBV viremia as early as possible and thereby attempt to avoid PTLD by reduction of immunosuppression. Results: higher incidence of EBV disease in children receiving quadruple therapy and tacrolimus compared with those given cyclosporine-based immunosuppression. After positive EBV viremia, immunosuppression was reduced and all patients remained asymptomatic.	No RCTs are available in children.
Fungal	Playford 2004 [99]	No specific data for pediatric patients.	Cochrane systematic review: in renal transplant recipients, neither ketoconazole nor clotrimazole significantly reduced invasive infections.
Disease recurrence			
FSGS	Seikaly 2004, Newstead 2003, Dall'Amico 1999, Salomon 2003, Ohta 2001, Dantal 1994 [101,105,107–110]	Different therapeutic options have been reported. Plasmapheresis (PP): Ohta found prophylactic PP may be valuable. retrospective analysis of 21 allografts, receiving either prophylactic PP (n = 15) or curative PP (n = 6) revealed 5 recurrences in the prophylactic group vs 4 recurrences in nonprophylactic group. D'All Amico found PP after recurrence seemed to provide remission. In open noncontrolled trial, proteinuria decreased in 9 of 11 patients treated with PP and cyclophosphamide after recurrence of FSGS; in 7 persistent remission was obtained. Cyclophosphamide (see above) Cyclosporine: uncontrolled clinical studies are not conclusive. i.v. cyclosporine (3 mg/kg/day with target blood level 250–350 ng/mL) induced remission of recurrence of FSGS in 14 of 17 patients. Persistent remission observed in 11 children. Plasma protein absorption: efficacy of this modality therapy is not encouraging. ACEi, indomethacin: reported to partially reduce proteinuria without affecting graft survival	No RCTs are available; management of recurrence of FSGS posttransplant is still controversial. There are only nonblinded, noncontrolled case series. Multicenter international RCTs are lacking.
HUS	Seikaly 2004, Quan 2001, Loirat 2003 [101,111,112]	NAPRTCS report: of 68 renal allografts, HUS recurred in 6 allografts. Poor outcome (83% graft loss) despite treatment with fresh-frozen plasma or PP. Cyclosporine had no effect on outcome or HUS recurrence. French report: risk of recurrence different, according to D+HUS (0.8%) or D-HUS (21%). Cyclosporine and tacrolimus may cause thrombotic microangiopathy; however, avoidance of CNI does not seem to prevent recurrence of HUS in children D-HUS.	No RCT available. Apart from the exceptional situation of deficiency of Von Willebrand factor-cleaving protease, there is currently no effective treatment of HUS after transplantation.
MPGN	Seikaly 2004 [101]	Anecdotal responses to PP have been reported in adults. Treatment of recurrent MPGN type 2 with PP induced remission in a single pediatric patient.	Very few data are available; there are no RCTs. Clinical recurrence is often characterized as asymptomatic proteinuria and low complement 3 levels.
IgA/HSP	Seikaly 2004 and Ponticelli 2004 [101,113]	Symptoms are often minor and could include hematuria and proteinuria. No pediatric data. Probable interest in ACEi in adults in decreasing proteinuria.	After recurrence of nephropathy, incidence of graft loss seems to be different in IgA nephropathy (3%) and in Henoch-Schönlein purpura (22%). Moreover, recurrence is more frequent with living, related donor than cadaveric donor in both diseases.

Abbreviations: CAD/LD: cadaveric donor/living donor; CNI, calcineurin inhibitors; CAN, chronic allograft nephropathy; ALG, antilymphocyte globulin; rATG, rabbit polyclonal antithymocyte globulin; CS, corticosteroids; MMF, mycophenolate mofetil; PP, plasmapheresis; HSV, herpes simplex virus; D+HUS/D-HUS, HUS with/without diarrhea; IgA/HSP, IgA nephropathy and Henoch-Schönlein purpura; WBC, white blood cell count. ACE: ansiotensiu converting enzyme inhibitors

a When RCTs were available, other studies have not been included. Only pediatric trials or reports about renal transplantation have been taken into account.

Table 62.8 Evidence ratings and recommendations for interventions in renal transplant recipients[a].

Intervention [reference(s)]	SR[b]	Evidence rating[c]				Recommendation[d]			Comment
		High	Moderate	Low	Comment	I	II	III	
Induction with IL-2 receptor blockers (Il2-Ra) [41,120]	C–A+	•A		•C	Systematic review in adults (Cochrane), 4893 patients 1 RCT, 192 children Consistent results		•		In adults, compared with placebo, no differences for graft loss at 1 and 3 yrs (RR 0.88, 95% CI 0.64–1.22). Incidence of acute rejections decreased at 1 yr (RR 0.67, 95% CI 0.6–0.75). No differences for malignancies and CMV infections at 1 yr. Compared with other antibody induction, no significant difference for efficacy, but adverse effects favored Il2Ra. High evidence. In children, adding basiliximab to a tacrolimus-based regimen is safe; however, it does not improve clinical efficacy at 6 months. Moderate evidence. Need more data on long-term efficacy.
OKT3 vs i.v. cyclosporine [32]	C–		•		1 RCT, 287 children Consistent results	•			Use of OKT3 induction therapy should be avoided. Moderate evidence.
Polyclonal and monoclonal antibodies for treating acute rejection [31]	C–A+		•		Systematic review in adults (Cochrane), 1387 patients			•	In reversing first rejection any antibody is better than steroids (RR 0.74, 95% CI 0.58–0.95). In reversing steroid-resistant rejection, effects of different antibodies not significantly different. Moderate to high evidence. Need more pediatric data.
Tacrolimus vs cyclosporine [43,45]	C–A+	•A		•C	Systematic review in adults (Cochrane), 4102 patients 1 RCT, 196 children Consistent results		•		In adults, tacrolimus is superior to cyclosporine in improving graft survival (at 6 months, RR 0.56, 9% CI 0.36–0.86) and preventing acute rejection (at 1 yr, RR 0.69, 95% CI 0.6–0.79), but more diabetes mellitus (RR 1.86, 95% CI 1.11–3.09) and gastrointestinal side effects are described. No differences in infections or malignancies. High evidence. In children, tacrolimus seems more effective than cyclosporine. Moderate evidence. Need more data on harms.
Sirolimus [47,121]	C–A+		•A	•C	Systematic review in adults (Cochrane) for primary immunosuppression (7114 patients) Systematic review in adults (Mulay) for conversion from CNI to sirolimus in CAN (1040 patients) At least 9 case series in children (176 patients)			•	Need more data for primary immunosuppression and rescue treatment, for both efficacy and safety. Moderate to low evidence for children. Side effects. Need more data on benefits and harms in children.
Mycophenolate vs azathioprine [122]	C–A+		•A	•C	Systematic review in adults, 8457 patients for efficacy and 6387 for safety At least 3 case series in children (429 patients) 1 ongoing RCT in children		•		MMF more efficient than azathioprine in reducing incidence of acute rejections but associated with an increase in gastrointestinal, hematological, and infectious (CMV infections) side effects. No confidence intervals available. Moderate evidence. Need more data on benefits and harms in children.

(continued)

Table 62.8 (continued).

Intervention [reference(s)]	Evidence rating[c]					Recommendation[d]			
	SR[b]	High	Moderate	Low	Comment	I	II	III	Comment
Steroid withdrawal [52,123]	C– A+	• A		C	Systematic reviews in adults, 1519 patients and 1681 patients. At least 5 case series in children (204 patients) 1 ongoing RCT in children			•	Pascual: Renal allograft recipients on triple therapy with calcineurin inhibitor, MMF, and steroids are at low but significant risk of acute rejection after steroid withdrawal (RR 2.28, 95% CI 1.65–3.16) but do not present an increased risk of early graft failure (RR 0.73, 95% CI 0.42–1.28). Tan: Similar results for acute rejection. Steroid withdrawal reduces incidence of opportunistic and urinary tract infections (RR 0.8, 95% CI 0.64–1 and RR 0.74, 95% CI 0.6–0.92, respectively) High evidence in adults. Need more data on benefits and harms in children.
Anti-CMV therapy [83,84]	C– A+	• A		C	Systematic review in adults (Cochrane). At least 5 case series in children (208 patients)		•		Prophylaxis with antiviral therapy reduces risk of CMV disease (RR 0.42, 95% CI 0.34–0.52), CMV infection (RR 0.61, 95% CI 0.48–0.77) and all-cause mortality (RR 0.63, 95% CI 0.43–0.92) in solid organ transplant recipients. No conclusion for preemptive therapy vs prophylaxis. Moderate to high evidence. Need more pediatric data.
Treatment for FSGS recurrence	C– A			• A, C	Only case series in adults and children.			•	Low evidence. Need more data.
Treatment for HUS recurrence	C– A			• A, C	Only case series in adults and children.			•	Low evidence. Need more data.
Treatment with GH [22]	C+			• C	Systematic review in children (629 patients with CKD)	•			1 yr of 28 IU/m²/wk rhGH in children with CKD resulted in 3.8 cm/yr increase in height velocity above that of untreated patients (95% CI 3.2–4.39). Trials too short to determine if continuing treatment resulted in increase in final adult height. High evidence. Moderate benefit. Harms of daily injections. High cost.

Abbreviations: CNI, calcineurin inhibitor; MMF, mycophenolate mofetil; CAN, chronic allograft nephropathy; CKD, chronic kidney disease.

[a] RCTs in children have been taken into account. There are no systematic reviews in for pediatric renal transplantation, except for GH therapy. Where no pediatric data were available, systematic reviews in adults are listed.

[b] Systematic review of RCTs. C, children; A, adults; –, no systematic review; +, systematic review of RCT.

[c] Evidence rating based on study design, study quality, consistency, and directness of results. No intervention was rated with a high evidence rating.

[d] Recommendations based on trade-offs between benefits and harms, quality of evidence, and translation of evidence into practice in a specific setting, including availability of medication and any uncertainty about baseline risk of disease in the population. I, recommend to give or not to give; II, suggest to give or not to give; III, no recommendation possible.

References

1 Cameron JI, Whiteside C, Katz J, Devins GM. Differences in quality of life across renal replacement therapies: a meta-analytic comparison. *Am J Kidney Dis* 2000; **35(4)**: 629–637.

2 Cochat P, Offner G. European Best Practice guidelines for renal transplantation. Part 2. Paediatrics (specific problems). *Nephrol Dial Transplant* 2002; **17(Suppl 4)**: 55–58.

3 Davis ID, Bunchman TE, Grimm PC, Benfield MR, Briscoe DM, Harmon WE *et al.* Pediatric renal transplantation: indications and special considerations. A position paper from the Pediatric Committee of the American Society of Transplant Physicians. *Pediatr Transplant* 1998; **2(2)**: 117–129.

4 Landais P, Daures JP. Clinical trials, immunosuppression and renal transplantation: new trends in design and analysis. *Pediatr Nephrol* 2002; **17(8)**: 573–584.

5 Filler G. Evidence-based immunosuppression after pediatric renal transplantation—a dream? *Transplant Proc* 2003; **35(6)**: 2125–2127.

6 Benfield MR, McDonald RA, Bartosh S, Ho PL, Harmon W. Changing trends in pediatric transplantation: 2001 Annual Report of the North American Pediatric Renal Transplant Cooperative Study. *Pediatr Transplant* 2003; **7(4)**: 321–335.

7 Agence de la Biomédecine. Rapport d'activité 2004. http://www.efg.sante.fr/fr /index.asp.

8 North American Pediatric Renal Transplant Cooperative Study (NAPRTCS). Annual report 2005. https://web.emmes.com/study/ped/annlrpt/anlrpt.2005.pdf.

9 Seikaly M, Ho PL, Emmett L, Tejani A. The 12th Annual Report of the North American Pediatric Renal Transplant Cooperative Study: renal transplantation from 1987 through 1998. *Pediatr Transplant* 2001; **5(3)**: 215–231.

10 Neipp M, Offner G, Luck R, Latta K, Strehlau J, Schlitt HJ *et al.* Kidney transplant in children weighing less than 15 kg: donor selection and technical considerations. *Transplantation* 2002; **73(3)**: 409–416.

11 Millan MT, Sarwal MM, Lemley KV, Yorgin P, Orlandi P, So S *et al.* A 100% 2-year graft survival can be attained in high-risk 15-kg or smaller infant recipients of kidney allografts. *Arch Surg* 2000; **135(9)**: 1063–1068.

12 Collaborative Transplant Study 2006. http://www.ctstransplant.org.

13 Offner G, Latta K, Hoyer PF, Baum HJ, Ehrich JH, Pichlmayr R *et al.* Kidney transplanted children come of age. *Kidney Int* 1999; **55(4)**: 1509–1517.

14 Filler G, Browne R, Seikaly MG. Glomerular filtration rate as a putative "surrogate end-point" for renal transplant clinical trials in children. *Pediatr Transplant* 2003; **7(1)**: 18–24.

15 Benfield MR, Herrin J, Feld L, Rose S, Stablein D, Tejani A. Safety of kidney biopsy in pediatric transplantation: a report of the Controlled Clinical Trials in Pediatric Transplantation Trial of Induction Therapy Study Group. *Transplantation* 1999; **67(4)**: 544–547.

16 Dew MA, Switzer GE, Goycoolea JM, Allen AS, DiMartini A, Kormos RL *et al.* Does transplantation produce quality of life benefits? A quantitative analysis of the literature. *Transplantation* 1997; **64(9)**: 1261–1273.

17 Painter PL, Hector L, Ray K, Lynes L, Dibble S, Paul SM *et al.* A randomized trial of exercise training after renal transplantation. *Transplantation* 2002; **74(1)**: 42–48.

18 Hokken-Koelega AC, Stijnen T, de Jong RC, Donckerwolcke RA, Groothoff JW, Wolff ED *et al.* A placebo-controlled, double-blind trial of growth hormone treatment in prepubertal children after renal transplant. *Kidney Int Suppl* 1996; **53**: S128–S134.

19 Guest G, Berard E, Crosnier H, Chevallier T, Rappaport R, Broyer M. Effects of growth hormone in short children after renal transplantation. French Society of Pediatric Nephrology. *Pediatr Nephrol* 1998; **12(6)**: 437–446.

20 Maxwell H, Rees L. Randomised controlled trial of recombinant human growth hormone in prepubertal and pubertal renal transplant recipients. British Association for Pediatric Nephrology. *Arch Dis Child* 1998; **79(6)**: 481–487.

21 Fine RN, Stablein D, Cohen AH, Tejani A, Kohaut E. Recombinant human growth hormone post-renal transplantation in children: a randomized controlled study of the NAPRTCS. *Kidney Int* 2002; **62(2)**: 688–696.

22 Vimalachandra D, Hodson EM, Willis NS, Craig JC, Cowell C, Knight JF. Growth hormone for children with chronic kidney disease. *Cochrane Database Syst Rev* 2006; **3**: CD003264.

23 Sanchez CP, Kuizon BD, Goodman WG, Gales B, Ettenger RB, Boechat MI *et al.* Growth hormone and the skeleton in pediatric renal allograft recipients. *Pediatr Nephrol* 2002; **17(5)**: 322–328.

24 El-Husseini AA, El-Agroudy AE, El-Sayed M, Sobh MA, Ghoneim MA. A prospective randomized study for the treatment of bone loss with vitamin D during kidney transplantation in children and adolescents. *Am J Transplant* 2004; **4(12)**: 2052–2057.

25 Handschin AE, Weber M, Demartines N, Clavien PA. Laparoscopic donor nephrectomy. *Br J Surg* 2003; **90(11)**: 1323–1332.

26 Simforoosh N, Basiri A, Tabibi A, Shakhssalim N, Hosseini Moghaddam SM. Comparison of laparoscopic and open donor nephrectomy: a randomized controlled trial. *BJU Int* 2005; **95(6)**: 851–855.

27 Metcalfe MS, Butterworth PC, White SA, Saunders RN, Murphy GJ, Taub N *et al.* A case-control comparison of the results of renal transplantation from heart-beating and non-heart-beating donors. *Transplantation* 2001; **71(11)**: 1556–1559.

28 Duke GJ. Renal protective agents: a review. *Crit Care Resusc* 1999; **1(3)**: 265–275.

29 van Riemsdijk IC, Mulder PG, de Fijter JW, Bruijn JA, van Hooff JP, Hoitsma AJ *et al.* Addition of isradipine (Lomir) results in a better renal function after kidney transplantation: a double-blind, randomized, placebo-controlled, multi-center study. *Transplantation* 2000; **70(1)**: 122–126.

30 Wagner K, Albrecht S, Neumayer HH. Prevention of posttransplant acute tubular necrosis by the calcium antagonist diltiazem: a prospective randomized study. *Am J Nephrol* 1987; **7(4)**: 287–291.

31 Webster A, Pankhurst T, Rinaldi F, Chapman JR, Craig JC. Polyclonal and monoclonal antibodies for treating acute rejection episodes in kidney transplant recipients. *Cochrane Database Syst Rev* 2006; **2**: CD004756.

32 Benfield MR, Tejani A, Harmon WE, McDonald R, Stablein DM, McIntosh M *et al.* A randomized multicenter trial of OKT3 mAbs induction compared with intravenous cyclosporine in pediatric renal transplantation. *Pediatr Transplant* 2005; **9(3)**: 282–292.

33 Acott PD, Lawen J, Lee S, Crocker JF. Basiliximab versus ATG/ALG induction in pediatric renal transplants: comparison of herpes virus profile and rejection rates. *Transplant Proc* 2001; **33(7–8)**: 3180–3183.

34 Khositseth S, Matas A, Cook ME, Gillingham KJ, Chavers BM. Thymoglobulin versus ATGAM induction therapy in pediatric kidney transplant recipients: a single-center report. *Transplantation* 2005; **79(8)**: 958–963.

35 Dharnidharka VR, Stevens G. Risk for post-transplant lymphoproliferative disorder after polyclonal antibody induction in kidney transplantation. *Pediatr Transplant* 2005; **9**(5): 622–626.

36 Kamel MH, Mohan P, Little DM, Awan A, Hickey DP. Rabbit antithymocyte globulin as induction immunotherapy for pediatric deceased donor kidney transplantation. *J Urol* 2005; **174**(2): 703–707.

37 Kamel MH, Mohan P, Conlon PJ, Little DM, O'Kelly P, Hickey DP. Rabbit antithymocyte globulin related decrease in platelet count reduced risk of pediatric renal transplant graft thrombosis. *Pediatr Transplant* 2006; **10**(7): 816–821.

38 Shapiro R, Ellis D, Tan HP, Moritz ML, Basu A, Vats AN *et al.* Antilymphoid antibody preconditioning and tacrolimus monotherapy for pediatric kidney transplantation. *J Pediatr* 2006; **148**(6): 813–818.

39 Ault BH, Honaker MR, Osama Gaber A, Jones DP, Duhart BT, Jr, Powell SL *et al.* Short-term outcomes of thymoglobulin induction in pediatric renal transplant recipients. *Pediatr Nephrol* 2002; **17**(10): 815–818.

40 Colleen Hastings M, Wyatt RJ, Lau KK, Jones DP, Powell SL, Hays DW *et al.* Five years' experience with thymoglobulin induction in a pediatric renal transplant population. *Pediatr Transplant* 2006; **10**(7): 805–810.

41 Grenda R, Watson A, Vondrak K, Webb NJ, Beattie J, Fitzpatrick M *et al.* A prospective, randomized, multicenter trial of tacrolimus-based therapy with or without basiliximab in pediatric renal transplantation. *Am J Transplant* 2006; **6**(7): 1666–1672.

42 Kramer BK, Montagnino G, Del Castillo D, Margreiter R, Sperschneider H, Olbricht CJ *et al.* Efficacy and safety of tacrolimus compared with cyclosporin A microemulsion in renal transplantation: 2 year follow-up results. *Nephrol Dial Transplant* 2005; **20**(5): 968–973.

43 Webster A, Woodroffe RC, Taylor RS, Chapman JR, Craig JC. Tacrolimus versus cyclosporin as primary immunosuppression for kidney transplant recipients. *Cochrane Database Syst Rev* 2005; **4**: CD003961.

44 Trompeter R, Filler G, Webb NJ, Watson AR, Milford DV, Tyden G *et al.* Randomized trial of tacrolimus versus cyclosporin microemulsion in renal transplantation. *Pediatr Nephrol* 2002; **17**(3): 141–149.

45 Filler G, Webb NJ, Milford DV, Watson AR, Gellermann J, Tyden G *et al.* Four-year data after pediatric renal transplantation: a randomized trial of tacrolimus vs. cyclosporin microemulsion. *Pediatr Transplant* 2005; **9**(4): 498–503.

46 Waid T. Tacrolimus as secondary intervention vs. cyclosporine continuation in patients at risk for chronic renal allograft failure. *Clin Transplant* 2005; **19**(5): 573–580.

47 Webster AC, Lee VW, Chapman JR, Craig JC. Target of rapamycin inhibitors (TOR-I; sirolimus and everolimus) for primary immunosuppression in kidney transplant recipients. *Cochrane Database Syst Rev* 2006; **2**: CD004290.

48 Ciancio G, Burke GW, Gaynor JJ, Ruiz P, Roth D, Kupin W *et al.* A randomized long-term trial of tacrolimus/sirolimus versus tacrolimums/mycophenolate versus cyclosporine/sirolimus in renal transplantation: three-year analysis. *Transplantation* 2006; **81**(6): 845–852.

49 Lorber MI, Mulgaonkar S, Butt KM, Elkhammas E, Mendez R, Rajagopalan PR *et al.* Everolimus versus mycophenolate mofetil in the prevention of rejection in de novo renal transplant recipients: a 3-year randomized, multicenter, phase III study. *Transplantation* 2005; **80**(2): 244–252.

50 Russ G, Segoloni G, Oberbauer R, Legendre C, Mota A, Eris J *et al.* Superior outcomes in renal transplantation after early cyclosporine withdrawal and sirolimus maintenance therapy, regardless of baseline renal function. *Transplantation* 2005; **80**(9): 1204–1211.

51 Abramowicz D, Del Carmen Rial M, Vitko S, del Castillo D, Manas D, Lao M *et al.* Cyclosporine withdrawal from a mycophenolate mofetil-

containing immunosuppressive regimen: results of a five-year, prospective, randomized study. *J Am Soc Nephrol* 2005; **16**(7): 2234–2240.

52 Pascual J, Quereda C, Zamora J, Hernandez D. Steroid withdrawal in renal transplant patients on triple therapy with a calcineurin inhibitor and mycophenolate mofetil: a meta-analysis of randomized, controlled trials. *Transplantation* 2004; **78**(10): 1548–1556.

53 Rostaing L, Cantarovich D, Mourad G, Budde K, Rigotti P, Mariat C *et al.* Corticosteroid-free immunosuppression with tacrolimus, mycophenolate mofetil, and daclizumab induction in renal transplantation. *Transplantation* 2005; **79**(7): 807–814.

54 Ferraris JR, Pasqualini T, Legal S, Sorroche P, Galich AM, Pennisi P *et al.* Effect of deflazacort versus methylprednisone on growth, body composition, lipid profile, and bone mass after renal transplantation. The Deflazacort Study Group. *Pediatr Nephrol* 2000; **14**(7): 682–688.

55 Bunchman T, Navarro M, Broyer M, Sherbotie J, Chavers B, Tonshoff B *et al.* The use of mycophenolate mofetil suspension in pediatric renal allograft recipients. *Pediatr Nephrol* 2001; **16**(12): 978–984.

56 Hocker B, Weber LT, Bunchman T, Rashford M, Tonshoff B. Mycophenolate mofetil suspension in pediatric renal transplantation: three-year data from the tricontinental trial. *Pediatr Transplant* 2005; **9**(4): 504–511.

57 Virji M, Carter JE, Lirenman DS. Single-center experience with mycophenolate mofetil in pediatric renal transplant recipients. *Pediatr Transplant* 2001; **5**(4): 293–296.

58 Jungraithmayr T, Staskewitz A, Kirste G, Boswald M, Bulla M, Burghard R *et al.* Pediatric renal transplantation with mycophenolate mofetil-based immunosuppression without induction: results after three years. *Transplantation* 2003; **75**(4): 454–461.

59 Ojogho ON, Sahney S, Cutler D, Baron PW, Abdelhalim FM, Hasan SM *et al.* Mycophenolate mofetil without antibody induction in pediatric renal transplantation. *Transplant Proc* 2002; **34**(5): 1953–1954.

60 Ojogho O, Sahney S, Cutler D, Baron PW, Abdelhalim FM, Hasan SM *et al.* Mycophenolate mofetil without antibody induction in cadaver vs. living donor pediatric renal transplantation. *Pediatr Transplant* 2003; **7**(2): 137–141.

61 Ojogho O, Sahney S, Cutler D, Baron PW, Abdelhalim FM, James S *et al.* Mycophenolate mofetil in pediatric renal transplantation: non-induction vs. induction with basiliximab. *Pediatr Transplant* 2005; **9**(1): 80–83.

62 Cransberg K, Marlies Cornelissen EA, Davin JC, Van Hoeck KJ, Lilien MR, Stijnen T *et al.* Improved outcome of pediatric kidney transplantations in the Netherlands—effect of the introduction of mycophenolate mofetil? *Pediatr Transplant* 2005; **9**(1): 104–111.

63 Ferraris JR, Ghezzi LF, Vallejo G, Piantanida JJ, Araujo JL, Sojo ET. Improved long-term allograft function in pediatric renal transplantation with mycophenolate mofetil. *Pediatr Transplant* 2005; **9**(2): 178–182.

64 Otukesh H, Sharifian M, Basiri A, Simfroosh N, Hoseini R, Sedigh N *et al.* Mycophenolate mofetil in pediatric renal transplantation. *Transplant Proc* 2005; **37**(7): 3012–3015.

65 Henne T, Latta K, Strehlau J, Pape L, Ehrich JH, Offner G. Mycophenolate mofetil-induced reversal of glomerular filtration loss in children with chronic allograft nephropathy. *Transplantation* 2003; **76**(9): 1326–1330.

66 Benz K, Plank C, Griebel M, Montoya C, Dotsch J, Klare B. Mycophenolate mofetil introduction stabilizes and subsequent cyclosporine A reduction slightly improves kidney function in pediatric renal transplant patients: a retrospective analysis. *Pediatr Transplant* 2006; **10**(3): 331–336.

67 Chakrabarti P, Wong HY, Scantlebury VP, Jordan ML, Vivas C, Ellis D *et al.* Outcome after steroid withdrawal in pediatric renal transplant patients receiving tacrolimus-based immunosuppression. *Transplantation* 2000; **70(5)**: 760–764.

68 Hocker B, John U, Plank C, Wuhl E, Weber LT, Misselwitz J *et al.* Successful withdrawal of steroids in pediatric renal transplant recipients receiving cyclosporine A and mycophenolate mofetil treatment: results after four years. *Transplantation* 2004; **78(2)**: 228–234.

69 Oberholzer J, John E, Lumpaopong A, Testa G, Sankary HN, Briars L *et al.* Early discontinuation of steroids is safe and effective in pediatric kidney transplant recipients. *Pediatr Transplant* 2005; **9(4)**: 456–463.

70 Birkeland SA, Larsen KE, Rohr N. Pediatric renal transplantation without steroids. *Pediatr Nephrol* 1998; **12(2)**: 87–92.

71 Sarwal MM, Vidhun JR, Alexander SR, Satterwhite T, Millan M, Salvatierra O, Jr. Continued superior outcomes with modification and lengthened follow-up of a steroid-avoidance pilot with extended daclizumab induction in pediatric renal transplantation. *Transplantation* 2003; **76(9)**: 1331–1339.

72 Vester U, Kranz B, Wehr S, Boger R, Hoyer PF. Everolimus (Certican) in combination with neoral in pediatric renal transplant recipients: interim analysis after 3 months. *Transplant Proc* 2002; **34(6)**: 2209–2210.

73 Vilalta R, Vila A, Nieto J, Callis L. Rapamycin use and rapid withdrawal of calcineurin inhibitors in pediatric renal transplantation. *Transplant Proc* 2003; **35(2)**: 703–704.

74 Filler G, Womiloju T, Feber J, Lepage N, Christians U. Adding sirolimus to tacrolimus-based immunosuppression in pediatric renal transplant recipients reduces tacrolimus exposure. *Am J Transplant* 2005; **5(8)**: 2005–2010.

75 Hymes LC, Warshaw BL. Sirolimus in pediatric patients: results in the first 6 months post-renal transplant. *Pediatr Transplant* 2005; **9(4)**: 520–522.

76 Ibanez JP, Monteverde ML, Goldberg J, Diaz MA, Turconi A. Sirolimus in pediatric renal transplantation. *Transplant Proc* 2005; **37(2)**: 682–684.

77 Hocker B, Feneberg R, Kopf S, Weber LT, Waldherr R, Wuhl E *et al.* SRL-based immunosuppression vs. CNI minimization in pediatric renal transplant recipients with chronic CNI nephrotoxicity. *Pediatr Transplant* 2006; **10(5)**: 593–601.

78 Garcia CD, Bittencourt VB, Alves AB, Garcia VD, Tumelero A, Antonello JS *et al.* Conversion to sirolimus in pediatric renal transplantation recipients. *Transplant Proc* 2006; **38(6)**: 1901–1903.

79 Falger JC, Mueller T, Arbeiter K, Boehm M, Regele H, Balzar E *et al.* Conversion from calcineurin inhibitor to sirolimus in pediatric chronic allograft nephropathy. *Pediatr Transplant* 2006; **10(5)**: 565–569.

80 Harmon W, Meyers K, Ingelfinger J, McDonald R, McIntosh M, Ho M *et al.* Safety and efficacy of a calcineurin inhibitor avoidance regimen in pediatric renal transplantation. *J Am Soc Nephrol* 2006; **17(6)**: 1735–1745.

81 Tatsioni A, Chung M, Sun Y, Kupelnick B, Lichtenstein AH, Perrone R *et al.* Effects of fish oil supplementation on kidney transplantation: a systematic review and meta-analysis of randomized, controlled trials. *J Am Soc Nephrol* 2005; **16(8)**: 2462–2470.

82 Kalil AC, Levitsky J, Lyden E, Stoner J, Freifeld AG. Meta-analysis: the efficacy of strategies to prevent organ disease by cytomegalovirus in solid organ transplant recipients. *Ann Intern Med* 2005; **143(12)**: 870–880.

83 Hodson EM, Barclay PG, Craig JC, Jones C, Kable K, Strippoli GF *et al.* Antiviral medications for preventing cytomegalovirus disease in solid organ transplant recipients. *Cochrane Database Syst Rev* 2005; **4**: CD003774.

84 Strippoli GF, Hodson EM, Jones CJ, Craig JC. Pre-emptive treatment for cytomegalovirus viraemia to prevent cytomegalovirus disease in solid organ transplant recipients. *Cochrane Database Syst Rev* 2006; **1**: CD005133.

85 Taylor AL, Marcus R, Bradley JA. Post-transplant lymphoproliferative disorders (PTLD) after solid organ transplantation. *Crit Rev Oncol Hematol* 2005; **56(1)**: 155–167.

86 Brennan DC, Agha I, Bohl DL, Schnitzler MA, Hardinger KL, Lockwood M *et al.* Incidence of BK with tacrolimus versus cyclosporine and impact of preemptive immunosuppression reduction. *Am J Transplant* 2005; **5(3)**: 582–594.

87 Ginevri F, De Santis R, Comoli P, Pastorino N, Rossi C, Botti G *et al.* Polyomavirus BK infection in pediatric kidney-allograft recipients: a single-center analysis of incidence, risk factors, and novel therapeutic approaches. *Transplantation* 2003; **75(8)**: 1266–1270.

88 Smith JM, McDonald RA, Finn LS, Healey PJ, Davis CL, Limaye AP. Polyomavirus nephropathy in pediatric kidney transplant recipients. *Am J Transplant* 2004; **4(12)**: 2109–2117.

89 Trofe J, Hirsch HH, Ramos E. Polyomavirus-associated nephropathy: update of clinical management in kidney transplant patients. *Transpl Infect Dis* 2006; **8(2)**: 76–85.

90 Gibbs S, Harvey I, Sterling J, Stark R. Local treatments for cutaneous warts: systematic review. *BMJ* 2002; **325(7362)**: 461.

91 Playford EG, Webster AC, Sorrell TC, Craig JC. Antifungal agents for preventing fungal infections in non-neutropenic critically ill patients. *Cochrane Database Syst Rev* 2006; **1**: CD004920.

92 Flynn JT, Kaiser BA, Long SS, Schulman SL, Deforest A, Polinsky MS *et al.* Intravenous immunoglobulin prophylaxis of cytomegalovirus infection in pediatric renal transplant recipients. *Am J Nephrol* 1997; **17(2)**: 146–152.

93 Bock GH, Sullivan EK, Miller D, Gimon D, Alexander S, Ellis E *et al.* Cytomegalovirus infections following renal transplantation–effects on antiviral prophylaxis: a report of the North American Pediatric Renal Transplant Cooperative Study. *Pediatr Nephrol* 1997; **11(6)**: 665–671.

94 Filler G, Lampe D, von Bredow MA, Lappenberg-Pelzer M, Rocher S, Strehlau J *et al.* Prophylactic oral ganciclovir after renal transplantation-dosing and pharmacokinetics. *Pediatr Nephrol* 1998; **12(1)**: 6–9.

95 Rubik J, Kozlowski K, Grenda R, Prokurat S. [Evaluation of pharmacokinetics and safety of valganciclovir oral suspension treatment in pediatric kidney graft recipients–preliminary report.] *Przegl Lek* 2006; **63(Suppl 3)**: 184–186.

96 Melgosa Hijosa M, Garcia Meseguer C, Pena Garcia P, Alonso Melgar A, Espinosa Roman L, Pena Carrion A *et al.* Preemptive treatment with oral ganciclovir for pediatric renal transplantation. *Clin Nephrol* 2004; **61(4)**: 246–252.

97 Srivastava T, Zwick DL, Rothberg PG, Warady BA. Posttransplant lymphoproliferative disorder in pediatric renal transplantation. *Pediatr Nephrol* 1999; **13(9)**: 748–754.

98 Shroff R, Trompeter R, Cubitt D, Thaker U, Rees L. Epstein-Barr virus monitoring in paediatric renal transplant recipients. *Pediatr Nephrol* 2002; **17(9)**: 770–775.

99 Playford EG, Webster AC, Sorell TC, Craig JC. Antifungal agents for preventing fungal infections in solid organ transplant recipients. *Cochrane Database Syst Rev* 2004; **3**: CD004291.

100 Cochat P, Fargue S, Liutkus A, Ranchin B. Récidive du syndrome néphrotique après transplantation rénale. *Courrier Transplant* 2006; **6**: 154–160.

101 Seikaly MG. Recurrence of primary disease in children after renal transplantation: an evidence-based update. *Pediatr Transplant* 2004; **8**(2): 113–119.

102 Burgess E. Management of focal segmental glomerulosclerosis: evidence-based recommendations. *Kidney Int Suppl* 1999; **70**: S26–S32.

103 Vincenti F, Ghiggeri GM. New insights into the pathogenesis and the therapy of recurrent focal glomerulosclerosis. *Am J Transplant* 2005; **5**(6): 1179–1185.

104 Gohh RY, Yango AF, Morrissey PE, Monaco AP, Gautam A, Sharma M *et al.* Preemptive plasmapheresis and recurrence of FSGS in high-risk renal transplant recipients. *Am J Transplant* 2005; **5**(12): 2907–2912.

105 Ohta T, Kawaguchi H, Hattori M, Komatsu Y, Akioka Y, Nagata M *et al.* Effect of pre-and postoperative plasmapheresis on posttransplant recurrence of focal segmental glomerulosclerosis in children. *Transplantation* 2001; **71**(5): 628–633.

106 Baum MA, Stablein DM, Panzarino VM, Tejani A, Harmon WE, Alexander SR. Loss of living donor renal allograft survival advantage in children with focal segmental glomerulosclerosis. *Kidney Int* 2001; **59**(1): 328–333.

107 Newstead CG. Recurrent disease in renal transplants. *Nephrol Dial Transplant* 2003; **18**(Suppl 6): vi68–vi74.

108 Dall'Amico R, Ghiggeri G, Carraro M, Artero M, Ghio L, Zamorani E *et al.* Prediction and treatment of recurrent focal segmental glomerulosclerosis after renal transplantation in children. *Am J Kidney Dis* 1999; **34**(6): 1048–1055.

109 Salomon R, Gagnadoux MF, Niaudet P. Intravenous cyclosporine therapy in recurrent nephrotic syndrome after renal transplantation in children. *Transplantation* 2003; **75**(6): 810–814.

110 Dantal J, Bigot E, Bogers W, Testa A, Kriaa F, Jacques Y *et al.* Effect of plasma protein adsorption on protein excretion in kidney-transplant recipients with recurrent nephrotic syndrome. *N Engl J Med* 1994; **330**(1): 7–14.

111 Quan A, Sullivan EK, Alexander SR. Recurrence of hemolytic uremic syndrome after renal transplantation in children: a report of the North American Pediatric Renal Transplant Cooperative Study. *Transplantation* 2001; **72**(4): 742–745.

112 Loirat C, Niaudet P. The risk of recurrence of hemolytic uremic syndrome after renal transplantation in children. *Pediatr Nephrol* 2003; **18**(11): 1095–1101.

113 Ponticelli C, Traversi L, Banfi G. Renal transplantation in patients with IgA mesangial glomerulonephritis. *Pediatr Transplant* 2004; **8**(4): 334–338.

114 Griffin KJ, Elkin TD. Non-adherence in pediatric transplantation: a review of the existing literature. *Pediatr Transplant* 2001; **5**(4): 246–249.

115 Ingulli E, Tejani A. Steroid withdrawal after renal transplantation. In: Tejani A, Fine R, editors. *Pediatric Renal Transplantation.* Wiley Liss, New York, 1994; 221–238.

116 Butani L. Investigation of pediatric renal transplant recipients with heavy proteinuria after sirolimus rescue. *Transplantation* 2004; **78**(9): 1362–1366.

117 Nagarajan S, Friedrich T, Garcia M, Kambham N, Sarwal MM. Gastrointestinal leukocytoclastic vasculitis: an adverse effect of sirolimus. *Pediatr Transplant* 2005; **9**(1): 97–100.

118 Falger JC, Mueller T, Arbeiter K, Boehm M, Regele H, Balzar E *et al.* Conversion from calcineurin inhibitor to sirolimus in pediatric chronic allograft nephropathy. *Pediatr Transplant* 2006; **10**(4): 474–478.

119 Shroff R, Rees L. The post-transplant lymphoproliferative disorder-a literature review. *Pediatr Nephrol* 2004; **19**(4): 369–377.

120 Webster AC, Playford EG, Higgins G, Chapman JR, Craig J. Interleukin 2 receptor antagonists for kidney transplant recipients. *Cochrane Database Syst Rev* 2004; **1**: CD003897.

121 Mulay AV, Cockfield S, Stryker R, Fergusson D, Knoll GA. Conversion from calcineurin inhibitors to sirolimus for chronic renal allograft dysfunction: a systematic review of the evidence. *Transplantation* 2006; **82**(9): 1153–1162.

122 Wang K, Zhang H, Li Y, Wei Q, Li H, Yang Y *et al.* Efficacy of mycophenolate mofetil versus azathioprine after renal transplantation: a systematic review. *Transplant Proc* 2004; **36**(7): 2071–2072.

123 Tan JY, Zhao N, Wu TX, Yang KH, Zhang JD, Tian JH *et al.* Steroid withdrawal increases risk of acute rejection but reduces infection: a meta-analysis of 1681 cases in renal transplantation. *Transplant Proc* 2006; **38**(7): 2054–2056.

63 Peritoneal Dialysis in Children

Jaap W. Groothoff & Maruschka P. Merkus

Department of Pediatric Nephrology, Emma Children's Hospital, Academic Medical Center, 1105AZ Amsterdam, The Netherlands.

Introduction

Soon after the introduction of continuous ambulatory peritoneal dialysis (CAPD) in 1978 [1], PD became the most popular mode of chronic dialysis for children in most countries. In comparison with hemodialysis (HD), PD has the social advantage of being a home treatment with relatively low cost [2]. Especially in small children, PD is technically more feasible and offers easier metabolic control, a more liberal diet, and less fluid restriction. Yet, no evidence exists on the advantage of PD over HD in children with respect to mortality or end-stage renal disease (ESRD)-related comorbidity, such as cardiovascular disease and metabolic bone disease. The apparent advantages of PD in the care of children have led to a preference for PD over HD for children in most countries, leaving HD for the more complicated patients. This has made unbiased comparison of the relative effects of PD and HD very difficult. Combined with a general policy to keep time on dialysis while waiting for transplantation to a minimum, this has meant a lack of studies on the outcome of chronic dialysis treatment in the pediatric population.

Searching for evidence

We searched the Renal Health Library 2005, produced by The Cochrane Renal Group for Systematic Reviews, randomized controlled trials (RCTs) on management of PD and, additionally, the Cochrane Central Register of Controlled Trials, DARE, MEDLINE, and EMbase for RCTs published more recently. In light of the available trial evidence, we critically reviewed the most recent guidelines on management of PD in children. In the absence of any RCT, important observational studies were reviewed. Data on mortality

and comorbidity were obtained from registries and cohort studies published after 1996. Studies published before 1990 were excluded, as they are not applicable to current practice. We also excluded studies on additive medication (phosphate binding, erythropoietin [EPO], etc.) in PD, as this is covered in other chapters.

Patient survival and causes of death

Most data were obtained from registry analyses and a few cohort studies [3–14], and they are summarized in Table 63.1. All studies suffer from lack of information on ESRD patients who were not accepted for chronic renal replacement therapy (RRT). Moreover, most reports concern chronic RRT and not chronic PD, because transplantation is the preferred RRT in children and, therefore, time on dialysis is usually kept to a minimum. Two comprehensive nationwide cohort studies both reported a 30-fold-increased overall mortality risk in children with ESRD [9,11]. Survival rates had increased over time, especially in very young children, until the mid 1980s, after which survival has not improved [9,11].

Determinants

Young age at onset of RRT and a prolonged dialysis period (beyond 2 years) are reported by all studies as the most important risk factors for death [9]. Over time, a trend towards improved survival is found predominantly among children under the age of 10 years, especially among the very young, but not in older children [9,11]. Yet, all these studies suffer from the lack of registration of those children with ESRD who were never accepted for therapy. Because there has been an increased acceptance of relatively sick children for RRT over time, these data probably underestimate the progress that has been made.

PD versus HD

Comparison between outcomes of PD and HD suffers from selection bias. Some studies found a higher mortality rate with PD than with HD (Italian Registry, patients ages 0–19 years, onset of RRT, 1989–2000: 17/295 deaths among PD group versus 2/163 in HD

Evidence-based Nephrology. Edited by Donald Molony and Jonathan Craig
© 2009 Blackwell Publishing, ISBN: 978-1-4051-3975-5.

Table 63.1 Studies on mortality in children on chronic dialysis.

Study and design [reference]	Patients	Outcome	Risk factor(s) for adverse outcome	Comments on study quality	Clinical implications
Italian Registry, 23 centers, PD & HD [3]	295 CPD 163 HD (1989–2000)	Overall 5-yr survival: HD 96.9%, PD 90.5% 17 PD pts died, 10 cardiovascular deaths	Young age (<5 yrs)	+ large study − incomplete data, registry study − no registration of untreated pts	Advocates more attention for prevention of cardiovascular disease
NAPRTCS, 150 centers [4]	584 HD (1992) & PD (1992–1998)	MR/100 pt-yrs: 0–2 mos, 15.7; 2–12 mos, 11.5; 1–2 yrs, 8.2; 2–5 yrs, 6.1; 6–12 yrs, 3.5; >12 yrs, 2.2	Young age	+ large study − incomplete data, registry study −no registration untreated pts	No conclusion for clinical practice
USRDS, 1991–1996 [5]	1454 ESRD, 0–19 yrs old	MR/100 pt-yrs: 3.84	Young age	+ large group − retrospective − incomplete data − no registration untreated pts	Advocates more attention for prevention of cardiovascular disease
USRDS, all patients, 1990–1996 [6]	1380 ESRD, 0–19 yrs old, deaths	23% cardiovascular deaths	Predictors of cardiac death: Black race (OR 1.56), dialysis status (Tx vs. dialysis, OR 0.22)	+ large group − no data on total cohort − incomplete data − no information on methodology registration cause of death	Advocates early transplantation
NAPRTCS Registry [7]	2971 PD, 1572 HD (1992–2001) 0–15 yrs old	Overall 3-yr survival : 85.7 ± 1.4%; 3-yr survival for 0–1 yr, 68.2 ± 3.9%; infection 24.3%, cardiovascular 21.5%	Young age	+ large study − incomplete data, registry study − no registration untreated pts − large group cause of death unknown'' (11.7%)	Advocates more attention for prevention of infections and cardiovascular disease
Turkish Registry, 12 centers, PD [8]	514 PD (1989–2002) CAPD	5-yr PD 70% survival, overall MR/100 pt-yrs 8.3	Young age RR vs >15 yrs old: <2 yrs old, 7.3 (CI 2.8–19.2) ; <1 yr, 9.7 (CI 3.5–26.5)	+ large study of children commencing RRT with PD -no completeness check	No conclusion for clinical practice
ANZDATA Registry [9]	1634 ESRD, 0–19 yrs old (1962–2002)	MR/100 pt-yrs: HD 4.8 (4.2–5.6), PD 5.9 (4.9–7.2); Tx 1.1 (0.9–1.3); SMR 30, cardiovascular cause of death 45% all pts, 43% PD pts	Young age, no transplantation, RRT onset before 1983; for PD vs. HD, delay to Tx <2 yrs not significant	+ large study + complete and comprehensive + methodology + long-term follow-up − retrospective − no registration untreated pts − no quality check death causes	Advocates transplantation within 2 yrs after onset RRT and attention for prevention of cardiovascular disease
Japanese Registry, 1981–1997 [10]	807 PD	87 deaths (10.8%) patient 3 y. survival 91%; 5 y.. 86% cardiovascular death 39.4% infection 36.6%	Young age	+ large study − registry study − incomplete data	Change from lethal infections to relatively more cardiovascular casualties over time advocates attention for prevention of cardiovascular disease
National Cohort study [11]	249 Dutch patients, <15 yrs, onset RRT 1972–1992, born before 1979	Overall survival, 87% 5-yr, 82% 10-yr, 78% 20-yr survival Overall SMR, 31 (1972–1999), 21 (1992–1999) Causes of death RRT: cardiovascular (41%), infection (21%), cessation of therapy (11%), malignancies (10%), complication of treatment (8%)	Predictors: young age (<6 yrs old), RRT onset <1982, hypertension, HD vs. PD, long duration dialysis	+ complete data of all Dutch pts <15 yrs old, no missing data + quality check cause of death + long follow-up − no registration for untreated pts − period/inclusion bias PD vs. HD − adolescents >14 yrs old not included	Advocates more attention for prevention of cardiovascular disease and treatment, hypertension, and early transplantation

(*Continued*)

Table 63.1 *(Continued)*

Study and design [reference]	Patients	Outcome	Risk factor(s) for adverse outcome	Comments on study quality	Clinical implications
EDTA registry [12]	3184, 0–19 yrs old (1980–2000)	Adjusted mortality HR (95% CI): Onset dialysis in 1995–2000 vs. 1980–1984, overall 0.64 (0.41–1.00), age 0–4 yrs 0.21 (0.09–0.51) Causes of death, PD pts: infection (23%), cardiovascular (10%)	Infection most important cause of death in PD, large "unknown" group	+ large population − registry study − incomplete data from several countries − unreliable data on cause of death	Advocates more attention for prevention of infections
1 centre [13]	98 (80 PD, 18 HD), 0–16 yrs old; (1984–2006)	17/98 deceased (7 PD, 3 HD, 7 Tx); survival at 1 yr 92%, 5 yrs 88%, 10 yrs 84%; cardiovascular deaths in 7/17	Young age Comorbid condition present in 76%	+ no missing patients + long-term follow-up −only retrospective chart data −small cohort	PD probably not superior to HD with respect to cardiovascular comorbidity
1 centre [14]	20 PD, age 32 wks (gest.)–1 yr, RRT 1986–1998	Duration PD 17.3 mos (1–59); 4 deceased, 11 successful transplant, 4 to HD followed by Tx, 1 continued PD, 14/16 survivors normal development milestones	Not determined	+ complete cohort + comprehensive + data on primary refusal RRT − small study	CPD feasible in (premature) infants
Japanese registry [21]	582 ESRD <20 yrs old, 1998	41.5% PD, 17.3% HD, 41.1% Tx Causes of death all patients: cardiovascular (56.9%), infection (42.9%)	Young age MR/100 pt-yrs, 0–4 yrs old, 2.22; 5–9 yrs, 3.39; 10–14 yrs, 1.48; 15–19 yrs, 0.10	+ large cohort + large PD population − registry study − very incomplete response (61.7%) −short-term follow-up	Cardiovascular disease most prominent

Abbreviations: Tx, transplantation; MR, mortality rate; SMR, standardized mortality rate; EDTA, European Dialysis and Transplant Association; USRDS = United States Renal Data System; ANZDATA = Australia & New Zealand and Transplant Registry.
Sources: References 3 to 14 and 21.

group) [15], but others have found no difference [9] or conflicting results (Dutch cohort, hazard ratio [HR] for HD versus PD, 2.1; 95% confidence interval [CI], 1.0–4.4) [11]. However, in the Italian study the PD patients were on average much younger than the HD patients (7.7 ± 4.8 versus 11.4 ± 3.1 years), and nearly all patients under the age of 5 years were on PD. Sixteen of the 17 deaths in PD patients occurred in those with onset of ESRD while they were children less than 5 years old, with six occurring in infancy [15]. No difference in survival was found between PD and HD patients in the age group 5–15 years. The Dutch analysis suffers from period and selection bias. During the period with the highest mortality (1972–1982), very few patients were treated with PD, and after 1982 most Dutch centers chose PD, leaving the more complicated patients to receive HD [11].

Adult studies have shown that preservation of residual kidney function is the most important determinant for survival in PD patients [16]. As in adults, PD is associated with better preservation of residual kidney function compared with HD [17], but there are no data that show a survival benefit in children with PD compared with HD.

Causes of death

Establishment of the exact cause of death in kidney disease patients can be troublesome. Apart from the Dutch study, no study defined the methodology used for cause of death assessment [11]. Cardiovascular disease is the most important cause of death in children on RRT in all studies, followed by infection [5,9–11,18–20]. Data on PD-associated causes of death are difficult to interpret, because most studies do not mention explicitly if patients had been treated only with PD during their RRT history. According to most studies, cardiovascular disease is also the most important cause of death in PD-treated children. Most comprehensive and reliable studies indicate a high burden of cardiovascular deaths in PD-treated children. In the Italian Registry study, 10 of 17 cardiovascular deaths occurred on PD. In the Japanese Registry study, cardiovascular disease was the cause of 56.9% of all deaths, 80% of which occurred on PD. In the Australian cohort study 43% of cardiovascular deaths occurred on PD, but there was no mention of the other causes of death in PD patients [9,15,21]. Two other registry studies with incomplete data have reported infection as the most important cause of death in PD patients [7,12].

Technique survival

Large European studies on PD in children reported catheter survival rates of 82–80% and 57–58% after 1 and 4 years, respectively [22,23]. The North American Pediatric Renal Transplant Cooperative Study (NAPRTCS) has reported a 20% transition (194 of 994 incident patients) from PD to HD [4]. The most common reasons were infection (43%), patient choice (7%), access failure (7%), and ultrafiltration failure (7%) [4,24].

Technique failure occurs more commonly with PD than HD (Italian Registry: 14.9% modality failure for PD, 7.4% for HD patients; patients aged 5–15 years; PD vs. HD technique failure rates of 40% vs. 5%; $P = 0.002$). Infection (peritonitis and/or exit site infection) accounted for 65.9% of all modality switches to HD [15]. Data on the association between age and technique failure are conflicting and often biased by unequally divided early cessations of PD in various age groups [15,24].

Comorbidity

Growth retardation, cardiovascular disease, metabolic bone disease causing pathological fractures, pain, impairment of movement, and cognitive impairment are the most important comorbidities in children and young adults with ESRD [5,18,25–30]. A prolonged period of dialysis is the most important risk factor for most of these complications, but the exact roles of PD versus HD remain to be elucidated. There is evidence that hypertension is an important determinant for cardiovascular disease, as in adults [11,31]. Observational studies in young adults with pediatric ESRD suggest that, among other factors, a high parathyroid hormone and high calcium–phosphate product might be responsible for early life-threatening vascular calcification [32]. After follow-up of 6–30 years, a 10-fold-increased incidence in malignancies was found among children with ESRD [19].

Hospitalization

In a multicenter Italian study, the hospitalization rates of a cohort of 149 PD and 111 HD patients in the period 1989–1994 were compared. Patients more than 5 years old on PD had a significantly higher hospitalization rate than age-matched HD children (days per dialysis month, 1.87 vs. 0.92; $P < 0.01$) [33].

Clinical implications with respect to choice of RRT

Early transplantation remains the ultimate goal in the treatment of children with ESRD. Currently there is no evidence in favor of PD over conventional HD treatment three times per week with respect to mortality or comorbidity. A recent small study by Fischbach *et al.* showed promising results of extended 5–6 times per week HD for the prevention of cardiovascular and metabolic bone disease, as well as improved a general well feeling [34]. This is in line with our own experience, but these data have to be confirmed in larger prospective studies.

Use and placement of PD catheter

Guidelines
An Ad Hoc Committee for elective chronic PD in pediatric patients that includes representatives of 12 European countries has formulated guidelines regarding the initiation of PD in children on behalf of the European Pediatric Peritoneal Dialysis Working Group. These guidelines are largely based on expert opinion [35]. The most important recommendations regarding the use and placement of the PD catheter are given in Table 63.2.

Available evidence
Most guidelines aim to prevent mechanical and, in particular, infectious complications. The recommendations for partial omentectomy and intraperitoneal heparin at PD catheter insertion to avoid catheter obstruction are not supported by evidence from pediatric RCTs. There are only data from retrospective observational studies to support the recommendation for partial omentectomy (no omentectomy versus omentectomy, 7/27 obstructions vs. 4/62 obstructions [Macchini], and 4/10 obstructions vs. 0/11 obstructions [Pumford]) [22,36]. Several studies in adults show evidence for anti-inflammatory, membrane-protective, and improved ultrafiltration properties of intraperitoneal heparin [37,38]. Yet, the protective effects of heparin against catheter obstruction by fibrin clot formation are based solely on clinical experience and have not been shown in studies.

In a nonrandomized prospective study in 42 children age 0.1–19 years, Daschner *et al.* found less leakage and similar rates of obstruction after laparoscopic implantation compared to conventional implantation of Tenckhoff catheters, despite the fact that patients with preexistent intra-abdominal adhesions were preferentially allocated to the laparoscopic procedure [39]. A retrospective study showed a favorable effect of delayed (>14 days) compared to early (<14 days) catheter use after placement on incidence of dialysate leakage but no effect on malfunction or infection rates [40]. In a single-center, open-label RCT of 45 CPD children with 52 catheter placements, application of fibrin glue to the peritoneal cuff suture resulted in a significantly lower incidence of leakage during the first 60 days after implantation compared to no sealant. No effect was seen on incidence of infection [41] (Table 63.3).

Table 63.2 Guidelines on inititation of PD and management of peritonitis.

Guideline

Implantation catheter
- Double-cuff, swan neck designed, curled Tenckhoff catheter
- Exit site downward; partial omentectomy
- Luer lock connections
- A disconnect "flush-before-fill" system
- Irrigation of catheter in-theater until dialysate is clear
- Heparin at 500 IU/L i.p. until clear effluent
- Immobilization of catheter and no application of keyhole dressing
- If possible, leave catheter for 2 weeks until patient returns for training, otherwise only use low volumes (10 mL/kg/cycle)
- Cephalosporin prophylactic antibiotic at time of catheter insertion.

Diagnosis of infection
- Peritonitis: cloudy effluent and effluent white blood cell count of $>100/mm^3$, $>50\%$ polymorphnuclear leukocytes
- Catheter exit site infection: purulent discharge from sinus tract or marked pericatheter swelling, redness, and/or tenderness, with or without pathogenic organism cultured from exit site

Treatment of peritonitis
- Empirical start with antibiotics as soon as peritonitis is suspected
- Fever and/or severe abdominal pain, recent methicillin-resistant *S. aureus* infection, recent or current exit site or tunnel infection or nasal exit site colonization with *S. aureus*, patients <2 years: glycopeptide (vancomycin or teicoplanin) and ceftazidime i.p.
- All other patients: cephalosporin and ceftazidime
- Modification according antibiogram (see Figure 63.1)
- 2 week treatment for all organisms, unless *S. aureus, Pseudomonas* or *Stenotrophomonas* species, multiple organisms, and/or anaerobes, then treatment for 3 weeks
- For fungal peritonitis, amphotericin B i.v. or a combination of imidazole–triazole and flucytosine; early catheter removal recommended; always if improvement does not occur with 3 days of treatment initiation; treatment duration following catheter removal for all patients should be at least 2 weeks

Indications for catheter removal and replacement
- Relapse of treated *S. aureus* or *Pseudomonas* peritonitis with an *S. aureus/Pseudomonas* catheter-related infection, fungal peritonitis, refractory (at 72–96 h) peritonitis, refractory (at 72–96 h) anaerobic peritonitis, refractory catheter exit site, tunnel infection.

Prophylactic antibiotic therapy
- *S. aureus* nasal carriage (single dose of antibiotics at time of catheter implantation), accidental intraluminal contamination, prior to dental procedures, and prior to procedures involving the gastrointestinal or urinary tract

Treatment of catheter exit site infection
- Treatment after culture results have been obtained, unless signs of severe infection
- Treatment duration 2–4 weeks

Sources: ISPD guidelines [35,47; www.peritonitis.org].

Clinical implications

There is weak evidence that omentectomy at implantation may reduce the risk for obstruction. Intraperitoneal heparin does no harm, but its benefit has not been proven. Laparoscopic catheter implantation might be advantageous over conventional implantation. Fibrin glue application on the peritoneal cuff at implantation may reduce the risk for leakage.

PD-associated infections

Epidemiology

Peritonitis and catheter-related infections are the major causes of morbidity and treatment failure of peritoneal dialysis in children. The control of infectious complications is particularly relevant to pediatric patients, because peritoneal adhesions and fibrosis caused by severe or recurrent peritonitis may prevent further use of the peritoneal membrane [42]. Exit site and tunnel infections occur in approximately one-third of pediatric PD patients after 1 year on PD and are the main reason for catheter removal [43]. Reported rates of peritonitis worldwide vary, with one episode every 13–70 patient PD months [7,15,24,43–45].

The incidence of peritonitis in pediatric patients is higher than that seen in adults and is highest in infants and younger children [7,43,44]. Data from NAPRTCS show an increasing frequency of exit site and tunnel infections and peritonitis with time on PD [43]. Exit site and tunnel infections increase the risk of peritonitis and access revision twofold and of hospitalization for access complications almost threefold [43]. Nasal carriage of *Staphylococcus aureus* in patients and caregivers is a risk factor for catheter-related

Table 63.3 Evidence ratings and recommendations for interventions to treat and prevent exit site and tunnel infections and peritonitis in pediatric PD patients.

Intervention	Evidence rating[a]			Comment [reference(s)]	Recommendation[c]			Comment
	SR	Moderate	Low		I	II	III	
Antibiotic treatment of peritonitis								
Intermittent vs continuous glycopeptide (vancomycin or teicoplanin)/ceftazidime, i.p.	—	•		1 RCT, relatively large sample size (152 pts, 168 episodes); suboptimal methodological quality [47]		•		Gram-positive peritonitis: Success rate (overall 95%) not different between intermittent and continuous or between vancomycin and teicoplanin treatment; 3 pts with vancomycin oversensitivity, 1 pt with ototoxicity vs. 0 pts teicoplanin side effects
								Gram-negative peritonitis: Intermittent treatment less effective than continuous according to clinical judgment (success rate, 3/11), but not according to DSS (10/14); no ceftazidime side effects
								More evidence needed for gram-negative peritonitis; teicoplanin has some advantages over vancomycin regarding side effects and reliability of blood levels after intermittent administration
Ceftazidime, cefazolin combination, i.p.	—		•	1 case series (27 pts, 50 episodes) [53]			•	Effective in 90% of episodes, no mention of adverse effects
								Advantage of this combination is that harms of aminoglucosides are avoided; disadvantage is that methicillin-resistant staphylococci are resistant to this combination
								Further evidence required.
Fluconazole and catheter removal for treatment of fungal peritonitis; adjunct amphotericin B in case of clinical sepsis	—		•	2 case series (6 and 12 pts) [54,55]			•	Success rate 4/6 and 9/12, respectively
								More data needed
Technique-related treatment of peritonitis								
Endoluminal brushing	—		•	1 case serie (3 pts) [56]			•	Peritonitis resolved in 2 of 3 cases; no adverse effects
								More data needed
Antimicrobial prophylactic interventions								
Mupirocin vs. placebo, intranasal in patients and caregivers with *S. aureus* carriage	—	•		1 RCT (92 families of CPD pts), double blind, placebo controlled; results not yet published [46]		•		Significant protective effect of mupirocin prophylaxis on ESI rate; *S. aureus* strains are shared among family members and transmission from parental noses to exit sites is common (Schaefer, pers. commun. 2006)
								Risk of resistance; trial not yet published; low likelihood that trial will show harm; evidence from adult studies shows benefit
Mupirocin intranasal in patients with *S. aureus* carriage	—		•	1 single-arm trial (47 pts) with historical controls (77 pts), 1 case series (13 pts); inconsistent results [65,66]			•	Both no benefit and benefit reported
								More data needed
								Prophylactic treatment of both patient and caregivers with *S. aureus* carriage suggested (see above)
Oral rifampin and topical bacitracin vs. no treatment in patients with *S. aureus* carriage	—		•	1 small RCT (15 pts), suboptimal quality [57]			•	Infection rate in treated vs no treatment group, 0/7 vs. 4/8; rate diff −50% (95% CI, −79 to −0.05)
								More data needed

(Continued)

Table 63.3 *(Continued)*

Intervention	Evidence rating[a]			Comment [reference(s)]	Recommendation[c]			Comment
	SR	Moderate	Low		I	II	III	
Perioperative antibiotics at surgical catheter placement vs. no treatment	—		•	1 retrospective cohort study (73 pts, 29 CPD pts) [58]	•			Postoperative peritonitis rate 6/61 in antibiotic group vs. 7/16 in no-treatment group
								Low likelihood that trials will show harm; evidence from SR of adult RCTs shows benefit for perioperative antibiotics
Povidone iodine (PI) vs. chlorhexidine (CH) exit site care	—		•	2 retrospective cohort studies (130 and 33 pts), inconsistent results [45,63]		•		Increases and no increases in ESI rates reported for PI vs. CH; no difference in peritonitis rates; adverse effects for PI reported; CH occasionally causes skin irritation
								Inconsistent evidence; more data needed
3% amuchina vs. 50% amuchina exit site care	—		•	1 single-arm trial (27 pts) (case series) with historical controls (18 pts) [64]		•		Similar ESI rates in both groups; no side effects
								More data needed
Technique-related prophylactic interventions								
Flush-before-fill APD	—	•		1 RCT (121 pts), suboptimal methodological quality [59]		•		Uncertain benefit; only benefit shown in women was peritonitis rate, flush vs no-flush group 1/44.7 vs. 1/12.4 pt-mos; no expected harm in men
								Further data needed
Fibrin glue vs. no sealant	—		•	1 RCT (45 pts, 52 catheters), small sample size, suboptimal methodological quality, one case series (8 pts) [41,60]	•			RCT: ESI (3/26) and peritonitis rates (1/26) similar; leakage with fibrin glue vs. no sealant, 3/26 vs. 14/26, rate diff −42% (95% CI, −61 to −17%); no side effects
								Use to prevent leakages suggested, more evidence needed regarding prevention of infections
Double vs. single cuff	—		•	NAPRTCS Registry (2971 pts), 1 retrospective cohort study (78 pts), 1 pseudo-controlled trial (two consecutive groups) (40 pts); inconsistent results [7,22,61]		•		Both increased and decreased infection rates of single vs. double cuff have been reported
								Inconsistent evidence, more data needed. No benefit of single or double cuff shown in SR of adults RCTs
Two disconnect vs. spike	—		•	One retrospective cohort study [67]	•			Peritonitis rate two-disconnect vs. spike, 1/58 vs. 1/10
								Superiority of two disconnect shown in SR of adult RCTs; low likelihood that trials will show harm
Exit sites pointing downward vs. upward or lateral	—		•	NAPRTCS Registry (2971 pts), one retrospective cohort study (130 pts). Inconsistent evidence [7,45]		•		Both decreased and similar infection rates of downward vs. upward and lateral reported
								Low and inconsistent evidence base, more data needed
Delayed vs. early catheter use postplacement	—		•	2 retrospective observational studies (90, 53 pts) [40,62]		•		No difference in infection rates (ESI, TI, peritonitis) between both groups; different definitions of early and delayed use (14 vs. 7 days)
								More data needed

Abbreviation: ESI, TI,

[a] Evidence rating based on study design, study quality, consistency, and directness of results. No intervention was rated with a high evidence rating.

[b] Recommendations based on trade-offs between benefits and harms, quality of evidence, translation into clinical pratice, uncertainty about the baseline risk of the disease in the population. I, recomend; II, suggest; III, no recommendation possible.

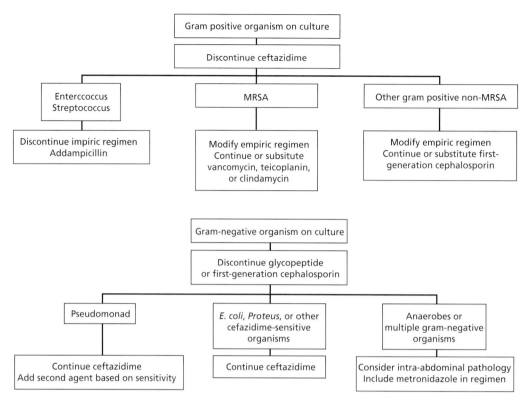

Figure 63.1 Proposed therapeutic strategy of peritonitis in gram-positive and gram-negative organisms on culture. From the ISPD Guidelines (www.ispd.org) published by Warady [48].

infections [46]. *S. aureus* peritonitis is responsible for the most serious episodes of infection [47].

Guidelines

The International Society for Peritoneal Dialysis (ISPD) guidelines, which are largely expert opinion-based, for the management of peritonitis in pediatric PD patients are currently the most specific, clinically useful guide to the appropriate treatment of these patients [48]. Recently, an International Pediatric Peritonitis Registry has been established among pediatric PD centers worldwide to evaluate the impact of these guidelines (www.peritonitis.org) [49]. The most important issues are summarized in Table 63.2 and Figure 63.1.

Available evidence

Our search identified three Cochrane systematic reviews of RCTs on antimicrobial and technique-related strategies to prevent PD-related infections that included both adult and pediatric patients [50–52]. However, pediatric data could not be separated from most individual trial data. Moreover, numbers were far too small to allow subgroup analyses. Only a few pediatric RCTs have been conducted, with most of them including a small number of patients and of suboptimal methodological quality to allow evidence-based treatment recommendations. Most pediatric studies are retrospective observational studies or case series. Table 63.3 summarizes the evidence on interventions to treat and prevent PD-associated in-

fections [7,22,40,41,45,46,47,53–67]. We have focused on only the most important studies.

Treatment of peritonitis and catheter-related infections

The best pediatric evidence has been provided by a multicenter RCT in a relatively large pediatric sample of 152 children with CPD-associated peritonitis that compared continuous versus intermittent intraperitoneal glycopeptide–ceftazidime treatment on treatment response [47]. This RCT showed that a combination of a glycopeptide with ceftazidime as first-line treatment is efficacious and safe. Intermittent and continuous treatment, either with vancomycin or teicoplanin, are equally efficacious and safe when measured by objective clinical criteria (DSS score). In gram-negative peritonitis, intermittent treatment was less successful than continuous treatment according to clinical judgment (27% vs. 73%) but not according to DSS (73% vs. 86%). Hence, more evidence is needed for this subgroup. These findings are in line with results in adults [68] and support the ISPD guidelines. Pediatric RCTs evaluating the efficacy of interventions to treat exit site and tunnel infections are lacking.

Preventive antibiotic interventions

S. aureus is the most frequent microorganism involved in catheter-related infections [69]. We identified two RCTs [46,57] on antibiotic preventive strategies in pediatric PD patients. In line with evidence from adult studies [52], a recently completed placebo-controlled RCT showed that the use of intranasal mupirocin in nasal *S. aureus* carrier families, that is, patients and caregivers, had a significant protective effect on|exit site|infection rate in the first treatment year (F. Schaefer, personal communication, 2006). It also showed that *S. aureus* strains are shared among family members and that transmission from parental noses|to exit sites is common. Up to 50% of patients and/or caregivers were colonized with *S. aureus* within 6 months [46]. These findings support ISPD recommendations to use prophylactic antibiotic therapy for *S. aureus* carriers. Widespread use of mupirocin carries the risk of emergence of mupirocin-resistant *S. aureus* strains (MuRSA). The emergence of high-level MuRSA was reported in 4 of 149 adult CPD patients of one dialysis unit after 4 years of prophylactic use of mupirocin at the exit site. Therefore, large PD centers using mupirocin in CPD patients should have periodic surveillance, at least yearly, to detect the emergence of MuRSA [70].

The recommendation by the Ad Hoc Committee [35] of prophylactic antibiotic treatment prior to PD catheter insertion is only supported by one retrospective analysis in pediatric CPD patients. This study showed a peritonitis rate, within 14 postoperative days, of 44% in untreated patients versus 10% in prophylactically treated patients [58]. A meta-analysis of RCTs in adult PD patients showed a significantly reduced risk of early peritonitis in patients who received perioperative antibiotics compared to no treatment. No effect was seen on exit site infections and peritonitis at 1 month after catheter insertion (RR, 0.15; 95% CI, 0.15–0.80) [52].

Technique-related preventive strategies

RCTs in pediatric PD patients to evaluate the effect of technique-related preventive strategies are scarce. We identified one RCT of 121 children on APD that evaluated the impact of the flush-before-fill technique on peritonitis frequency [59]. Overall, no difference in peritonitis rate was seen between patients in the flush and no-flush groups. Gender-stratified analysis showed a significant improvement in peritonitis rate in the flush compared to no-flush group in female patients but no difference in male patients. Because this subgroup analysis was not based on an *a priori* hypothesis and there is no biological plausibility for this finding, confirmation of this result is needed. Use of fibrin glue, compared with no sealant, prevented catheter leakage in an RCT of 45 CPD children. No effect was seen on incidence of catheter infections or peritonitis [41]. Studies evaluating the effect of catheter type (double- vs. single-cuffed catheters; downward- vs. upward- or lateral-pointing exit sites) in children have shown conflicting results [7,22,45,61]. Evidence from two systematic reviews of adult RCTs on technique-related preventive interventions showed that the only technique-related measure that reduced infection rate was the use of disconnect rather than conventional spike systems. Because many studies have been small and follow-up is often short, the possibility of a type 2 statistical error cannot be excluded [50,51].

Recommendations regarding proper training were supported by an ISPD survey [71]. This survey found that the peritonitis rate was significantly lower in programs with longer training time dedicated to theory and practical, technical skills [71]. Also, the low peritonitis rates reported by Japanese centers with long and rigorous training programs support these recommendations [45]. Observational studies in children report improvement of catheter survival over time, suggesting that routine and local skills with respect to the technical procedure might be of more importance than the specific type of catheter used [15,24].

Clinical implications

There is a lack of good-quality evidence from studies on the prevention and treatment of PD-related infections in children on which to base definitive treatment recommendations. There is a need for better-designed RCTs in this area.

The skills of the surgeons who place the catheters, and also the nurses and caregivers in achieving aseptic technique, may be of more importance in the prevention of PD-associated infections than the type of catheter or the several proposed prophylactic antibiotic strategies. There is no evidence supporting the superiority of any specific catheter design. Intravenous antibiotics at implantation may reduce the incidence of early peritonitis and can be recommended. The use of mupirocin may reduce the incidence of *S. aureus* infections, but possibly at the cost of an increase in resistance. A strategy to start mupirocin prophylactically after the first *S. aureus* infection is reasonable. Vancomycin or teicoplanin can be safely administered intermittently in case of peritonitis.

Adequacy of Dialysis

It is difficult to define outcomes of adequate dialysis in children, because most children remain on dialysis for a relatively short period and, although the death rate for children on RRT is high in relation to children without RRT, in absolute terms it is low. Only two observational studies have assessed the association between adequacy of PD treatment and clinical outcome. Höltta *et al.* compared the outcome of 10 PD patients less than 5 years old, who were treated between 1995 and 1999, with 27 age-matched patients who had been treated between 1989 and 1995 [72,73]. Peritoneal equilibration tests (PET), urea Kt/V, and creatinine clearance assessments were added to the program, and the optimal dialysis regimen was calculated using the PD ADEQUEST program (Baxter Healthcare). Targets for total weekly urea Kt/V and normalized creatinine clearance were >1.7 and >40 L/week, respectively, between 1995 and 1997 and >2.0 and >60 L/week, respectively, after 1997. Other treatment guidelines and the care team were unchanged. They found a 37% reduction in hospitalization, a 30% reduction in peritonitis rate, and a reduction from 41% to 0% of pulmonary edema in the 1995–1999 group compared to the 1989–1995 cohort. Metabolic control was significantly better in the 1995–1999 group with respect to serum mean phosphate levels (1.51 ± 0.48 vs. 2.01 ± 0.42; $P = 0.004$) with a lower calcium supplementation (836 ± 558 vs. 3641 ± 1717 mg/day; $P < 0.0001$). Schaefer *et al.* prospectively evaluated growth velocity, nutritional status, dialysis adequacy, and peritoneal membrane characteristics in a cohort of 51 CPD patients, ages 0.1–15.7 years, during an 18-month period [74]. A high transporter state appeared associated with poor growth velocity and a high creatinine clearance. Moreover, high transporters appeared to be at risk for obesity.

In 2002, the Ad Hoc committee published guidelines, based largely on clinical experience, on adequacy of PD prescription in children [75]. The committee identified 15 clinical studies that evaluated the effects of strategies aimed at increasing adequacy. Only surrogate outcomes were studied, such as metabolic control, ultrafiltration, Kt/V, and creatinine clearance [73,76–89]. Details of these studies are summarized in Table 63.4 and will briefly be discussed below in the context of the European Workgroup guidelines.

Bicarbonate-buffered versus lactate-buffered dialysate

Three trials comparing the effects of bicarbonate-buffered versus lactate-buffered dialysate in children on PD and that used surrogate outcomes have been carried out [76–78]. Two of these studies were of moderate quality [76,77]. Results of a randomized crossover trial in 28 children on APD showed that neutral pH bicarbonate-buffered PD provided more effective correction of metabolic acidosis than conventional lactate dialysate after 12 weeks of treatment. Younger age appeared to be associated with increasing pH towards alkalosis on bicarbonate dialysis. Additionally, a twofold increase in carcinogen antigen-125 appearance rate in the effluent during bicarbonate dialysis was seen, suggesting a higher mesothelial regeneration rate during bicarbonate-buffered sessions (Table 63.4). A crossover RCT compared peritoneal transport in one PET using bicarbonate dialysate versus one PET using lactate PD in 25 children on APD [77]. Creatinine and phosphate clearances were 10% lower with bicarbonate dialysate compared to lactate dialysate. No other differences in peritoneal transport kinetics were found [76–78].

A small crossover trial in six children on APD showed less intraperitoneal pressure at a given intraperitoneal volume with combined bicarbonate–lactate–buffered dialysis compared to pure lactate-buffered dialysis [78], but these findings were not confirmed by others [80]. None of the studies reported differences in adverse effects between the two fluids. To clarify the clinical significance of the buffer choice in biocompatible PD fluids, a multicenter European RCT in 60 CPD children (EPPS) comparing 10 months of use of bicarbonate- versus lactate-buffered dialysate on the preservation of the peritoneal membrane, metabolic control, and peritonitis rate, is ongoing [79]. No intervention studies are reported on the combination of bicarbonate dialysis and daytime icodextrin. One observational retrospective analysis reported a rise in mean blood bicarbonate from 23 ± 2 mmol/L up to 27 ± 2 mmol/L ($P < 0.05$) in 12 children 14 days after conversion from lactate-based dialysis to partly bicarbonate-buffered and partly lactate-buffered dialysate (Physioneal; Baxter) in combination with a daytime dwell with icodextrin [20].

Icodextrin

Five crossover trials have been performed in order to investigate the use of icodextrin dialysate on adequacy and safety aspects in children [80–82,84]. Although these studies were of insufficient methodological quality (small sample sizes, not randomized, short observation period), they support results of adult studies with respect to ultrafiltration and solute clearances [90], at least in children older than 2 years of age.

In a crossover study in eight children, 2–12 years old, undergoing nocturnal intermittent PD (NIPD), the addition of a daytime dwell with icodextrin increased weekly Kt/V from 1.99 to 2.54, phosphate clearance by 23%, and ultrafiltration by 44%. At the same time, a significant increase in peritoneal loss of essential amino acids was observed [83]. Although lower serum levels of amino acids were not found, the follow-up period was only 2 weeks, so studies with longer follow-up are necessary. Ultrafiltration was found to be much higher with daytime icodextrin than with a daytime 1.36% dextrose dwell and were comparable with a daytime 3.86% dextrose dwell in a crossover trial in 11 children ages 2.8–15.5 years [84].

Amino acid dialysate

Only three trials have been performed on the use of amino acid dialysis in children. In a randomized crossover study in seven children treated with CCPD for 3 months, amino acid dialysis appeared comparable to dextrose dialysis regarding peritoneal transport and metabolic control, except for higher urea levels. Improved appetite was the only benefit observed [86]. The amino acid dialysis was well-tolerated. No differences were found in growth velocity or nutritional status, although the follow-up was only 3 months. The same research group found similar results in a study of similar design in eight children on CAPD [85] treated with pure dextrose dialysate for 6 months and subsequently for 6–12 months with 1% amino acid dialysate substitution for one dwell per day. Correction of low blood levels of some essential amino acids (histidine, leucine, phenylalanine, valine, and isoleucine) was seen, but no change in anthropometric measures was found [87].

Fill volume, Kt/V, and creatinine clearance

In the previously discussed study by Schaefer et al. on adequacy in 52 CPD children, they found low fill volumes to be associated with low creatinine clearance and impaired growth and a hyperpermeable state to be associated with impaired growth [74]. RCTs are needed to confirm this association.

The area of the peritoneal membrane is twofold larger in infants than in adults if expressed per kg body weight (533 vs. 284 cm^2/kg) but independent of age if expressed per square meter of body surface. This implies that fill volumes should be prescribed per body surface and not by body weight. De Boer et al. compared the effect of dwell volume prescription by body weight (40 mL/kg) with prescription by body surface area (1,200 mL/m^2) on peritoneal transport within the same patients. An association was observed between age and net ultrafiltration when patients were treated with a dwell volume of 40 mL/kg body weight ($r = 0.68$; $P < 0.01$) but not when they were treated with a dwell volume of 1200 mL/m^2 body surface area [88]. The Ad Hoc Committee advises a maximal target of 1400 mL/m^2 fill volume in supine

Table 63.4 Evidence ratings and recommendations for interventions to enhance the adequacy of treatment in paediatric PD patients.

Intervention	SR	Moderate	Low	Comments [reference(s)]	I	II	III	Comments
Bicarbonate 34 m M vs. lactate 35 mM dialysate	—	•		3 multicenter RCTs (28, 25, and 60 pts); relatively large pt numbers, suboptimal methodological quality; consistent results; 1 trial ongoing [76,77,79]	•			*Favors bicarbonate dialysate* *Better treatment acidosis *Less mesothelial damage *Small children alkalosis (?) *Equal transport, lower phosphate clearance not of clinical relevance *Well-tolerated *Less acidotic dialysate No clinical outcomes; insufficient follow-up time; more data needed
Bicarbonate/lactate vs. lactate dialysate (Physioneal vs. Dianeal, [Baxter])	—		•	1 single-center RCT, crossover (6 pts); small study, suboptimal methodological quality [78]	•			*Favors bicarbonate dialysate* *Less inflow pain *Less intraperitoneal pressure, enhanced fill volume tolerance *Less capillary recruitment, better preservation membrane No clinical outcome, except dialysis comfort; more data needed
Icodextrin 7.5% vs. dextrose 3.86%	—		•	3 small open trials (9, 9, and 11 pts); suboptimal methodological quality; consistent results [80,82,84]	•			*Icodextrin can replace dextrose 3.86 and is safe* Icodextrin: long dwells needed for adequate UF Short follow-up; no small children; clinical implications maltose/icodextrin in serum not known; more data needed
Icodextrin 7.5% vs. dextrose 1.36%	—		•	2 open trials (5, 9 pts); very small studies, wide age range, insufficient methodological quality; consistent results [81,82]	•			*Icodextrin better UF and phosphate & clearance clear but caution because of protein loss* No small children; very short observation period; more data needed
Icodextrin 7.5% vs. no last bag	—		•	1 crossover trial (8 pts); small sample size; insufficient methodological quality; no information on serum AA levels at midterm (intervention stopped after 2 wks of increasing AA loss) [83]	•			*Increased loss of amino acids by icodextrin daytime dwell vs. no daytime dwell* More data needed; monitoring serum levels of essential amino acids, indicated especially in young children
Amino acid (AA) daytime dwell vs. dextrose daydwell in CCPD (1) & CAPD (2,3)	—		•	3 open trials (7, 7, and 8 pts); small studies; insufficient methodological quality; consistent results [85–87]	•			*Amino acid is probably safe and could enhance appetite in children on PD* No hard clinical outcome or apparent advantage; more data needed
Dwell volume 1200 m/m² vs. 40 mL/kg	—		•	1 open trial (4/4 pts.); small study; no mention of age of study group; insufficient methodological quality [88]	•			Dwell volumes scaled by kg body wt may lead to underdialysis with respect to UF in small children More data needed
Tidal vs. CCPD: 50% TD vs. CCPD, both overnight 1000 mL/m² fill volume & daytime dwell, 500 mL/m²	—	•		1 crossover trial (17 pts); suboptimal methodological quality [73]	•			Tidal higher dialysate flow rate and lower glucose concentration dialysate; both groups same Kt/V urea Tidal dialysis indicated in patients with high transport and reduced UF More data needed
Supine vs. upside posture	—		•	1 trial (6 pts); small study; insufficient methodological quality [89]	•			NIPD might be advantageous over CAPD as result of lower IPP and consequently superior solute transport. More data needed

[a] Evidence rating based on study design, study quality, consistency, and directness of results. No intervention was rated with a high evidence rating.

[b] Recommendations based on trade-offs between benefits and harms, quality of evidence, translation into clinical pratice, and uncertainty about the baseline risk of the disease in the population. I, recommend; II, suggest, III, no recommendation possible.

position and 1000–1200 mL/m^2 in the upright position [75]. This was suggested by the mass transfer area coefficient and ultrafiltration outcomes under various fill volumes in an observational study by Fischbach *et al.* in which fill volumes over 1400 mL/m^2 were associated with decreased phosphate clearance and clinical intolerance [91]. Apart from the prospective cohort study of Schaefer *et al.* [74], there are no pediatric data that support the adult recommendations of a weekly *Kt/V* of >2.0–2.2 or a weekly creatiine clearance of >60–66 L/1.73 m^2.

CCPD/NIPD CAPD tidal PD

Automatic PD is mostly prescribed for its obvious social advantages over CAPD in children. No studies exist that have compared the outcomes of CAPD and continuous cycling PD (CCPD) in children. Fischbach *et al.* studied the effects of supine versus upright position on peritoneal transport in six children. The use of the same dialysis prescription in the supine position compared to the upright position resulted in an approximately 17% higher equilibration of creatinine and phosphate as well as urea, lower loss of protein, a higher glucose absorption rate, and a lower intraperitoneal pressure. The net ultrafiltration was equal in both positions [89]. In theory, these outcomes favor the supine position, that is, NIPD over CAPD. However, the clinical significance of these outcomes is unclear, and the quality of the study is insufficient for clinical decision making. Höltta *et al.* compared tidal peritoneal dialysis and CCPD in a randomized, crossover trial in 17 children and found better clearances and lower glucose exposure in patients on tidal PD, especially in "high transporters" [73].

Clinical implications of the evidence on adequacy of PD in children

There is sufficient evidence that dialysate buffered with bicarbonate or combined bicarbonate–lactate is well-tolerated in children, at least in older children. In young children, at least in combination with an icodextrin daytime dwell, overt alkalosis may occur, which could lead to low ionized calcium levels. Phosphate clearances may be somewhat lower than with lactate-buffered dialysate, but not to an extent that has clinical implications. There is indirect evidence that, compared to lactate, pure bicarbonate-buffered or partly bicarbonate-buffered dialysate causes less mesothelial damage. Whether this will also lead to a more prolonged preservation of the peritoneal membrane still must be proven in long-term studies. There is sufficient evidence that icodextrin is as effective as 3.86% dextrose with respect to ultrafiltration and solute clearance. Because of the avoidance of high glucose exposure to the peritoneal membrane, icodextrin can be recommended in children over 2 years of age. Little data exist on its use in children less than 2 years of age.

Further studies are warranted to explore the possible harm of extensive loss of essential and nonessential amino acids, as well as the impact of high blood pH, that might occur in small children on icodextrin in combination with bicarbonate-buffered NIPD. A daytime dwell with amino acid dialysate might correct low blood levels of amino acids and enhance the appetite and caloric intake in undernourished children on PD, but more data are warranted to prove its real benefit in the long term. There is only very weak evidence that increasing creatinine clearance due to PD is associated with better clinical outcome in children; there is even more uncertainty with urea *Kt/V*. Optimal fill volumes are associated with optimal ultrafiltration and offer the possibility for use of dextrose concentrations as low as possible, which may enhance peritoneal membrane preservation. There is moderate evidence that tidal PD is advantageous over NIPD in high transporters. There is no evidence that NIPD is superior to CAPD.

References

1 Oreopoulos DG, Katirtzoglou A, Arbus G, Cordy P. Dialysis and transplantation in young children. *Br Med J* 1979; **1(6178)**: 1628–1629.

2 Coyte PC, Young LG, Tipper BL, Mitchell VM, Stoffman PR, Willumsen J et al. An economic evaluation of hospital-based hemodialysis and home-based peritoneal dialysis for pediatric patients. *Am J Kidney Dis* 1996; **27(4)**: 557–565.

3 Verrina E, Edefonti A, Gianoglio B, Rinaldi S, Sorino P, Zacchello G et al. A multicenter experience on patient and technique survival in children on chronic dialysis. *Pediatr Nephrol* 2004; **19(1)**: 82–90.

4 Leonard MB, Donaldson LA, Ho M, Geary DF. A prospective cohort study of incident maintenance dialysis in children: an NAPRTC study. *Kidney Int* 2003; **63(2)**: 744–755.

5 Chavers BM, Li S, Collins AJ, Herzog CA. Cardiovascular disease in pediatric chronic dialysis patients. *Kidney Int* 2002; **62(2)**: 648–653.

6 Parekh RS, Carroll CE, Wolfe RA, Port FK. Cardiovascular mortality in children and young adults with end-stage kidney disease. *J Pediatr* 2002; **141(2)**: 191–197.

7 Neu AM, Ho PL, McDonald RA, Warady BA. Chronic dialysis in children and adolescents. The 2001 NAPRTCS Annual Report. *Pediatr Nephrol* 2002; **17(8)**: 656–663.

8 Bakkaloglu SA, Ekim M, Sever L, Noyan A, Aksu N, Akman S et al. Chronic peritoneal dialysis in Turkish children: a multicenter study. *Pediatr Nephrol* 2005; **20(5)**: 644–651.

9 McDonald SP, Craig JC. Long-term survival of children with end-stage renal disease. *N Engl J Med* 2004; **350(26)**: 2654–2662.

10 Honda M. The 1997 report of the Japanese National Registry data on pediatric peritoneal dialysis patients. *Perit Dial Int* 1999; **19(Suppl 2)**: S473–S478.

11 Groothoff JW, Gruppen MP, Offringa M, Hutten J, Lilien MR, Van De Kar NJ et al. Mortality and causes of death of end-stage renal disease in children: a Dutch cohort study. *Kidney Int* 2002; **61(2)**: 621–629.

12 van der Heijden BJ, van Dijk PC, Verrier-Jones K, Jager KJ, Briggs JD. Renal replacement therapy in children: data from 12 registries in Europe. *Pediatr Nephrol* 2004; **19(2)**: 213–221.

13 Shroff R, Rees L, Trompeter R, Hutchinson C, Ledermann S. Long-term outcome of chronic dialysis in children. *Pediatr Nephrol* 2006; **21(2)**: 257–264.

14 Ledermann SE, Scanes ME, Fernando ON, Duffy PG, Madden SJ, Trompeter RS. Long-term outcome of peritoneal dialysis in infants. *J Pediatr* 2000; **136(1)**: 24–29.

15 Verrina E, Perfumo F, Zacchello G, Edefonti A, Bassi S, Capasso G et al. Chronic peritoneal dialysis catheters in pediatric patients: experience of

the Italian Registry of Pediatric Chronic Peritoneal Dialysis. *Perit Dial Int* 1993; **13(Suppl 2)**: S254–S256.

16 Termorshuizen F, Korevaar JC, Dekker FW, van Manen JG, Boeschoten EW, Krediet RT. The relative importance of residual renal function compared with peritoneal clearance for patient survival and quality of life: an analysis of the Netherlands Cooperative Study on the Adequacy of Dialysis (NECOSAD)-2. *Am J Kidney Dis* 2003; **41(6)**: 1293–1302.

17 Fischbach M, Terzic J, Menouer S, Soulami K, Dangelser C, Helmstetter A et al. Effects of automated peritoneal dialysis on residual daily urinary volume in children. *Adv Perit Dial* 2001; **17**: 269–273.

18 Oh J, Wunsch R, Turzer M, Bahner M, Raggi P, Querfeld U et al. Advanced coronary and carotid arteriopathy in young adults with childhood-onset chronic renal failure. *Circulation* 2002; **106(1)**: 100–105.

19 Coutinho HM, Groothoff JW, Offringa M, Gruppen MP, Heymans HS. De novo malignancy after paediatric renal replacement therapy. *Arch Dis Child* 2001; **85(6)**: 478–483.

20 Vande Walle JG, Raes AM, Dehoorne J, Mauel R. Use of bicarbonate/lactate-buffered dialysate with a nighttime cycler, associated with a daytime dwell with icodextrin, may result in alkalosis in children. *Adv Perit Dial* 2004; **20**: 222–225.

21 Hattori S, Yosioka K, Honda M, Ito H. The 1998 report of the Japanese National Registry data on pediatric end-stage renal disease patients. *Pediatr Nephrol* 2002; **17(6)**: 456–461.

22 Macchini F, Valade A, Ardissino G, Testa S, Edefonti A, Torricelli M et al. Chronic peritoneal dialysis in children: catheter related complications. A single centre experience. *Pediatr Surg Int* 2006; **22**: 524–528.

23 Schaefer F, Klaus G, Muller-Wiefel DE, Mehls O. Current practice of peritoneal dialysis in children: results of a longitudinal survey. Mid European Pediatric Peritoneal Dialysis Study Group (MEPPS). *Perit Dial Int* 1999; **19(Suppl 2)**: S445–S449.

24 Rinaldi S, Sera F, Verrina E, Edefonti A, Gianoglio B, Perfumo F et al. Chronic peritoneal dialysis catheters in children: a fifteen-year experience of the Italian Registry of Pediatric Chronic Peritoneal Dialysis. *Perit Dial Int* 2004; **24(5)**: 481–486.

25 Gruppen MP, Groothoff JW, Prins M, van der WP, Offringa M, Bos WJ et al. Cardiac disease in young adult patients with end-stage renal disease since childhood: a Dutch cohort study. *Kidney Int* 2003; **63(3)**: 1058–1065.

26 Groothoff JW, Gruppen MP, Offringa M, de GE, Stok W, Bos WJ et al. Increased arterial stiffness in young adults with end-stage renal disease since childhood. *J Am Soc Nephrol* 2002; **13(12)**: 2953–2961.

27 Groothoff JW, Offringa M, Van Eck-Smit BL, Gruppen MP, Van De Kar NJ, Wolff ED et al. Severe bone disease and low bone mineral density after juvenile renal failure. *Kidney Int* 2003; **63(1)**: 266–275.

28 Groothoff JW, Grootenhuis M, Dommerholt A, Gruppen MP, Offringa M, Heymans HS. Impaired cognition and schooling in adults with end stage renal disease since childhood. *Arch Dis Child* 2002; **87(5)**: 380–385.

29 Holtta T, Happonen JM, Ronnholm K, Fyhrquist F, Holmberg C. Hypertension, cardiac state, and the role of volume overload during peritoneal dialysis. *Pediatr Nephrol* 2001; **16(4)**: 324–331.

30 Mitsnefes MM, Daniels SR, Schwartz SM, Khoury P, Strife CF. Changes in left ventricular mass in children and adolescents during chronic dialysis. *Pediatr Nephrol* 2001; **16(4)**: 318–323.

31 Mitsnefes M, Stablein D. Hypertension in pediatric patients on long-term dialysis: a report of the North American Pediatric Renal Transplant Cooperative Study (NAPRTCS). *Am J Kidney Dis* 2005; **45(2)**: 309–315.

32 Mitsnefes MM, Kimball TR, Kartal J, Witt SA, Glascock BJ, Khoury PR et al. Cardiac and vascular adaptation in pediatric patients with chronic kidney disease: role of calcium-phosphorus metabolism. *J Am Soc Nephrol* 2005; **16(9)**: 2796–2803.

33 Verrina E, Perfumo F, Zacchello G, Sorino P, Edefonti A, Bassi S et al. Comparison of patient hospitalization in chronic peritoneal dialysis and hemodialysis: a pediatric multicenter study. *Perit Dial Int* 1996; **16(Suppl 1)**: S574–S577.

34 Fischbach M, Terzic J, Dangelser C, Schneider P, Roger ML, Geisert J. Improved dialysis dose by optimizing intraperitoneal volume prescription thanks to intraperitoneal pressure measurements in children. *Adv Perit Dial* 1997; **13**: 271–273.

35 Watson AR, Gartland C. Guidelines by an Ad Hoc European Committee for Elective Chronic Peritoneal Dialysis in Pediatric Patients. *Perit Dial Int* 2001; **21(3)**: 240–244.

36 Pumford N, Cassey J, Uttley WS. Omentectomy with peritoneal catheter placement in acute renal failure. *Nephron* 1994; **68(3)**: 327–328.

37 Sjoland JA, Pedersen RS, Jespersen J, Gram J. Intraperitoneal heparin ameliorates the systemic inflammatory response in PD patients. *Nephron Clin Pract* 2005; **100(4)**: c105–c110.

38 Sjoland JA, Smith PR, Jespersen J, Gram J. Intraperitoneal heparin reduces peritoneal permeability and increases ultrafiltration in peritoneal dialysis patients. *Nephrol Dial Transplant* 2004; **19(5)**: 1264–1268.

39 Daschner M, Gfrorer S, Zachariou Z, Mehls O, Schaefer F. Laparoscopic Tenckhoff catheter implantation in children. *Perit Dial Int* 2002; **22(1)**: 22–26.

40 Rahim KA, Seidel K, McDonald RA. Risk factors for catheter-related complications in pediatric peritoneal dialysis. *Pediatr Nephrol* 2004; **19(9)**: 1021–1028.

41 Sojo ET, Grosman MD, Monteverde ML, Bailez MM, Delgado N. Fibrin glue is useful in preventing early dialysate leakage in children on chronic peritoneal dialysis. *Perit Dial Int* 2004; **24(2)**: 186–190.

42 Andreoli SP, Langefeld CD, Stadler S, Smith P, Sears A, West K. Risks of peritoneal membrane failure in children undergoing long-term peritoneal dialysis. *Pediatr Nephrol* 1993; **7(5)**: 543–547.

43 Furth SL, Donaldson LA, Sullivan EK, Watkins SL. Peritoneal dialysis catheter infections and peritonitis in children: a report of the North American Pediatric Renal Transplant Cooperative Study. *Pediatr Nephrol* 2000; **15(3–4)**: 179–182.

44 Boehm M, Vecsei A, Aufricht C, Mueller T, Csaicsich D, Arbeiter K. Risk factors for peritonitis in pediatric peritoneal dialysis: a single-center study. *Pediatr Nephrol* 2005; **20(10)**: 1478–1483.

45 Hoshii S, Wada N, Honda M. A survey of peritonitis and exit-site and/or tunnel infections in Japanese children on PD. *Pediatr Nephrol* 2006; **21(6)**: 828–834.

46 Oh J, von Baum H, Klaus G, Schaefer F. Nasal carriage of Staphylococcus aureus in families of children on peritoneal dialysis. European Pediatric Peritoneal Dialysis Study Group (EPPS). *Adv Perit Dial* 2000; **16**: 324–327.

47 Schaefer F, Klaus G, Muller-Wiefel DE, Mehls O. Intermittent versus continuous intraperitoneal glycopeptide/ceftazidime treatment in children with peritoneal dialysis-associated peritonitis. The Mid-European Pediatric Peritoneal Dialysis Study Group (MEPPS). *J Am Soc Nephrol* 1999; **10(1)**: 136–145.

48 Warady BA. Guidelines for the treatment of peritonitis in children. *Perit Dial Int* 2000; **20(6)**: 607.

49 Feneberg R, Warady BA, Alexander SR, Schaefer F. The international pediatric peritonitis registry: a global internet-based initiative in pediatric dialysis. *Perit Dial Int* 2005; **25(Suppl 3)**: S130–S134.

50 Strippoli GF, Tong A, Johnson D, Schena FP, Craig JC. Catheter type, placement and insertion techniques for preventing peritonitis in peritoneal dialysis patients. *Cochrane Database Syst Rev* 2004; **4**: CD004680.

51 Daly CD, Campbell MK, MacLeod AM, Cody DJ, Vale LD, Grant AM et al. Do the Y-set and double-bag systems reduce the incidence of CAPD peritonitis? A systematic review of randomized controlled trials. *Nephrol Dial Transplant* 2001; **16(2)**: 341–347.

52 Strippoli GF, Tong A, Johnson D, Schena FP, Craig JC. Antimicrobial agents for preventing peritonitis in peritoneal dialysis patients. *Cochrane Database Syst Rev* 2004; **4**: CD004679.

53 Rusthoven E, Monnens LA, Schroder CH. Effective treatment of peritoneal dialysis-associated peritonitis with cefazolin and ceftazidime in children. *Perit Dial Int* 2001; **21(4)**: 386–389.

54 Montane BS, Mazza I, Abitbol C, Zilleruelo G, Strauss J, Coakley S et al. Fungal peritonitis in pediatric patients. *Adv Perit Dial* 1998; **14**: 251–254.

55 Chen CM, Ho MW, Yu WL, Wang JH. Fungal peritonitis in peritoneal dialysis patients: effect of fluconazole treatment and use of the twin-bag disconnect system. *J Microbiol Immunol Infect* 2004; **37(2)**: 115–120.

56 Aksu N, Yavascan O, Kara OD, Erdogan H, Kangin M. Does endoluminal brushing eliminate the need for catheter removal in peritoneal dialysis patients with persistent peritonitis? *Adv Perit Dial* 2003; **19**: 260–263.

57 Blowey DL, Warady BA, McFarland KS. The treatment of Staphylococcus aureus nasal carriage in pediatric peritoneal dialysis patients. *Adv Perit Dial* 1994; **10**: 297–299.

58 Sardegna KM, Beck AM, Strife CF. Evaluation of perioperative antibiotics at the time of dialysis catheter placement. *Pediatr Nephrol* 1998; **12(2)**: 149–152.

59 Warady BA, Ellis EN, Fivush BA, Lum GM, Alexander SR, Brewer ED et al. "Flush before fill" in children receiving automated peritoneal dialysis. *Perit Dial Int* 2003; **23(5)**: 493–498.

60 Rusthoven E, van de Kar NA, Monnens LA, Schroder CH. Fibrin glue used successfully in peritoneal dialysis catheter leakage in children. *Perit Dial Int* 2004; **24(3)**: 287–289.

61 Lewis MA, Smith T, Postlethwaite RJ, Webb NJ. A comparison of double-cuffed with single-cuffed Tenckhoff catheters in the prevention of infection in pediatric patients. *Adv Perit Dial* 1997; **13**: 274–276.

62 Donmez O, Durmaz O, Ediz B, Cigerdelen N, Kocak S. Catheter-related complications in children on chronic peritoneal dialysis. *Adv Perit Dial* 2005; **21**: 200–203.

63 Jones LL, Tweedy L, Warady BA. The impact of exit-site care and catheter design on the incidence of catheter-related infections. *Adv Perit Dial* 1995; **11**: 302–305.

64 Grosman MD, Mosquera VM, Hernandez MG, Agostini S, Adragna M, Sojo ET. 3% Amuchina is as effective as the 50% concentration in the prevention of exit-site infection in children on chronic peritoneal dialysis. *Adv Perit Dial* 2005; **21**: 148–150.

65 Araki H, Miyazaki R, Matsuda T, Gejyo F, Koni I. Significance of serum pepsinogens and their relationship to Helicobacter pylori infection and histological gastritis in dialysis patients. *Nephrol Dial Transplant* 1999; **14(11)**: 2669–2675.

66 Kingwatanakul P, Warady BA. Staphylococcus aureus nasal carriage in children receiving long-term peritoneal dialysis. *Adv Perit Dial* 1997; **13**: 281–284.

67 Garcia-Lopez E, Mendoza-Guevara L, Morales A, Guilar-Kitzu A, Vicencio LM, Hernandez-Fernandez M et al. Comparison of peritonitis rates in children on CAPD with spike connector versus two disconnect systems. *Adv Perit Dial* 1994; **10**: 300–303.

68 Boyce NW, Wood C, Thomson NM, Kerr P, Atkins RC. Intraperitoneal (IP) vancomycin therapy for CAPD peritonitis—a prospective, randomized comparison of intermittent v continuous therapy. *Am J Kidney Dis* 1988; **12(4)**: 304–306.

69 Klaus G. Prevention and treatment of peritoneal dialysis-associated peritonitis in pediatric patients. *Perit Dial Int* 2005; **25(Suppl 3)**: S117–S119.

70 Annigeri R, Conly J, Vas S, Dedier H, Prakashan KP, Bargman JM et al. Emergence of mupirocin-resistant Staphylococcus aureus in chronic peritoneal dialysis patients using mupirocin prophylaxis to prevent exit-site infection. *Perit Dial Int* 2001; **21(6)**: 554–559.

71 Holloway M, Mujais S, Kandert M, Warady BA. Pediatric peritoneal dialysis training: characteristics and impact on peritonitis rates. *Perit Dial Int* 2001; **21(4)**: 401–404.

72 Holtta TM, Ronnholm KA, Jalanko H, la-Houhala M, Antikainen M, Holmberg C. Peritoneal dialysis in children under 5 years of age. *Perit Dial Int* 1997; **17(6)**: 573–580.

73 Holtta T, Ronnholm K, Holmberg C. Adequacy of dialysis with tidal and continuous cycling peritoneal dialysis in children. *Nephrol Dial Transplant* 2000; **15(9)**: 1438–1442.

74 Schaefer F, Klaus G, Mehls O. Peritoneal transport properties and dialysis dose affect growth and nutritional status in children on chronic peritoneal dialysis. Mid-European Pediatric Peritoneal Dialysis Study Group. *J Am Soc Nephrol* 1999; **10(8)**: 1786–1792.

75 Fischbach M, Stefanidis CJ, Watson AR. Guidelines by an ad hoc European committee on adequacy of the paediatric peritoneal dialysis prescription. *Nephrol Dial Transplant* 2002; **17(3)**: 380–385.

76 Haas S, Schmitt CP, Arbeiter K, Bonzel KE, Fischbach M, John U et al. Improved acidosis correction and recovery of mesothelial cell mass with neutral-pH bicarbonate dialysis solution among children undergoing automated peritoneal dialysis. *J Am Soc Nephrol* 2003; **14(10)**: 2632–2638.

77 Schmitt CP, Haraldsson B, Doetschmann R, Zimmering M, Greiner C, Boswald M et al. Effects of pH-neutral, bicarbonate-buffered dialysis fluid on peritoneal transport kinetics in children. *Kidney Int* 2002; **61(4)**: 1527–1536.

78 Fischbach M, Terzic J, Chauve S, Laugel V, Muller A, Haraldsson B. Effect of peritoneal dialysis fluid composition on peritoneal area available for exchange in children. *Nephrol Dial Transplant* 2004; **19(4)**: 925–932.

79 Nau B, Schmitt CP, Almeida M, Arbeiter K, Ardissino G, Bonzel KE et al. BIOKID: randomized controlled trial comparing bicarbonate and lactate buffer in biocompatible peritoneal dialysis solutions in children (ISRCTN81137991). *BMC Nephrol* 2004; **5(1)**: 14.

80 Rusthoven E, van der Vlugt ME, van Lingen-van Bueren LJ, van Schaijk TC, Willems HL, Monnens LA et al. Evaluation of intraperitoneal pressure and the effect of different osmotic agents on intraperitoneal pressure in children. *Perit Dial Int* 2005; **25(4)**: 352–356.

81 Michallat AC, Dheu C, Loichot C, Danner S, Fischbach M. Long daytime exchange in children on continuous cycling peritoneal dialysis: preservation of drained volume because of icodextrin use. *Adv Perit Dial* 2005; **21**: 195–199.

82 Rusthoven E, Krediet RT, Willems HL, Monnens LA, Schroder CH. Peritoneal transport characteristics with glucose polymer-based dialysis fluid in children *J Am Soc Nephrol* 2004; **15(11)**: 2940–2947.

83 van Hoeck KJ, Rusthoven E, Vermeylen L, Vandesompel A, Marescau B, Lilien M *et al.* Nutritional effects of increasing dialysis dose by adding an icodextrin daytime dwell to nocturnal intermittent peritoneal dialysis (NIPD) in children. *Nephrol Dial Transplant* 2003; **18(7)**: 1383–1387.

84 de Boer AW, Schroder CH, van Vliet R, Willems JL, Monnens LA. Clinical experience with icodextrin in children: ultrafiltration profiles and metabolism. *Pediatr Nephrol* 2000; **15(1–2)**: 21–24.

85 Qamar IU, Levin L, Balfe JW, Balfe JA, Secker D, Zlotkin S. Effects of 3-month amino acid dialysis compared to dextrose dialysis in children on continuous ambulatory peritoneal dialysis. *Perit Dial Int* 1994; **14(1)**: 34–41.

86 Qamar IU, Secker D, Levin L, Balfe JA, Zlotkin S, Balfe JW. Effects of amino acid dialysis compared to dextrose dialysis in children on continuous cycling peritoneal dialysis *Perit Dial Int* 1999; **19(3)**: 237–247.

87 Canepa A, Perfumo F, Carrea A, Giallongo F, Verrina E, Cantaluppi A *et al.* Long-term effect of amino-acid dialysis solution in children on continuous ambulatory peritoneal dialysis. *Pediatr Nephrol* 1991; **5(2)**: 215–219.

88 de Boer AW, van Schaijk TC, Willems HL, Reddingius RE, Monnens LA, Schroder CH. The necessity of adjusting dialysate volume to body surface area in pediatric peritoneal equilibration tests. *Perit Dial Int* 1997; **17(2)**: 199–202.

89 Fischbach M, Terzic J, Dangelser C, Schneider P, Roger ML, Geisert J. Effect of posture on intraperitoneal pressure and peritoneal permeability in children. *Pediatr Nephrol* 1998; **12(4)**: 311–314.

90 Finkelstein F, Healy H, bu-Alfa A, Ahmad S, Brown F, Gehr T *et al.* Superiority of icodextrin compared with 4.25% dextrose for peritoneal ultrafiltration *J Am Soc Nephrol* 2005; **16(2)**: 546–554.

91 Fischbach M, Terzic J, Gaugler C, Bergere V, Munch K, Hamel G *et al.* Impact of increased intraperitoneal fill volume on tolerance and dialysis effectiveness in children. *Adv Perit Dial* 1998; **14**: 258–264.

64 Pediatric Hemodialysis

Stuart L. Goldstein

Renal Dialysis Unit and Pheresis Service, Baylor College of Medicine, Houston, USA

Introduction

Provision of evidence-based pediatric hemodialysis recommendations is hampered by a number of epidemiological issues. Kidney transplantation remains predominant and the preferred renal replacement therapy modality for children, peritoneal dialysis is a viable modality option for many pediatric patients [1], and children with end-stage renal disease (ESRD) exhibit significantly better survival rates compared to adult patients [2]. Thus, no long-term pediatric outcome study comparable to the HEMO study [3] or the National Cooperative Dialysis Study [4] would be adequately powered to detect an effect of delivered hemodialysis dose on pediatric patient outcome.

Technological advances and professional expertise specific for pediatric patients with kidney failure have developed relatively slowly. In the past 10 years, however, the hemodialysis procedure has become increasingly sophisticated, and many of the theoretical and technological advances studied previously in adult patients have been applied to children receiving hemodialysis. In fact, the most recent US Renal Data System report revealed that more children receive hemodialysis than peritoneal dialysis for their maintenance dialysis modality [1].

Data to support the recommendations cited in this chapter, therefore, are generally limited to reports from large, multicenter registries or government-sponsored databases and single-center reports. Specifically, pediatric data related to small-solute clearance measurement, vascular access placement and surveillance, ultrafiltration management, and nutrition provision will be reviewed. Recommendations and consensus guidelines from various working groups will be presented in each section, but they are collated together in a single table (Table 64.1).

Physiology of hemodialysis: pediatric issues

The factors that govern the physiology of hemodialysis, namely, diffusion and convection, are the same for pediatric and adult patients. Currently, most pediatric patients receive maintenance hemodialysis on a thrice-weekly in-center schedule, but recent data suggest that home nocturnal hemodialysis or more frequent hemodialysis may lead to improved blood pressure control and growth, a decreased need for dietary and fluid restrictions, and improved health-related quality of life [5,6]. Most pediatric-specific issues arise in hemodialysis provision to infants and small children, for whom the size of the extracorporeal circuit and blood pump flow rates can affect hemodynamic stability.

The hemodialysis circuit is comprised of the patient's blood compartment access in the form of an arteriovenous fistula (AVF) or graft (AVG) or a venous catheter, polyethylene tubing through which the patient's blood travels to and from the dialyzer, and the dialyzer itself. Blood tubing is produced in a variety of sizes and should be matched to allow for optimal blood flow while minimizing the volume of the extracorporeal circuit, which is the sum of the blood tubing volume and hollow fiber dialyzer volume. To prevent excessive repeated blood loss in the circuit and hemodynamic instability, the extracorporeal circuit should not exceed 10% of the patient's calculated blood volume [7]. Neonatal lines with a volume of 40 mL are available for use in children weighing less than 15 kg.

In order to prevent hypovolemia during initiation of dialysis treatment, the circuit should be primed with either saline or colloid. In some infants, for whom even the smallest blood tubing and dialyzer volumes would exceed 10% of patient blood volume, the circuit should be primed with colloid (5% albumin or packed red blood cells diluted with albumin to a measured hematocrit of 35%) instead of crystalloid. Weekly serum hematocrit values should be obtained to monitor for anemia resulting from excessive blood loss in the hemodialysis circuit for infants less than 10 kg maintained on chronic hemodialysis. The blood pump flow rate (Qb) should be prescribed to provide optimal clearance of solute safely. Use of

Evidence-based Nephrology. Edited by Donald Molony and Jonathan Craig
© 2009 Blackwell Publishing, ISBN: 978-1-4051-3975-5.

Table 64.1 Current guidelines and clinical practice recommendations for pediatric patients receiving maintenance hemodialysis.

Guideline	Country or Region	Year	Recommendations
Hemodialysis Adequacy			
K/DOQI	USA	2006	spKt/V, calculated either by formal UKM or by the second-generation natural logarithm formula should be used for month-to-month assessment of delivered hemodialysis dose.
			Pediatric patients should receive at least the delivered dialysis dose recommended for the adult population.
			For younger pediatric patients, prescription of higher dialysis doses and higher protein intake at 150% of the RNI for age may be important.
			Dialysis dose prescription should not only be a urea dialysis dose. Removal of the other uremic toxins should be considered, not only middle molecules but overall phosphate.
European Pediatric Dialysis Working Group	Europe	2005	Urea kinetic assessment enables not only urea dialysis dose calculation, i.e.Kt/V, but also estimation of protein intake by use of nPCR. Fasting to enable a short-duration three times/week dialysis schedule is inadequate care management.
Ultrafiltration Management			
K/DOQI	USA	2006	Accurate assessment of patient intravascular volume during hemodialysis treatment should be provided to optimize ultrafiltration.
Vascular Access Management			
K/DOQI	USA	2006	Permanent access in the form of an AVF or AVG is the preferred form of pediatric vascular access. Circumstances under which a central venous catheter may be acceptable for chronic access include lack of local surgical expertise to place permanent vascular access in small children, patient size too small to support a permanent vascular access, bridging hemodialysis for peritoneal training or peritoneal catheter removal and expectation of expeditious kidney transplantation.
			If surgical expertise to place permanent access does not exist in the patient's pediatric setting, efforts should be made to consult vascular access expertise among local adult-oriented surgeons to either supervise or place permanent vascular access in children.
			Serious consideration should be given to placing permanent vascular access in children >20 kg who are expected to wait more than 1 year for kidney transplant.

a maximum Qb of less than 400 mL/min/1.73 m² of patient body surface area minimizes the risk of cardiovascular compromise.

Hemodialysis adequacy

Definition and background

The term hemodialysis adequacy is derived from the National Co-operative Dialysis Study, which aimed to control dialysis treatment dosing in adult patients and correlate a particular dose with patient outcome [4]. Formal urea kinetic modeling (UKM) solves two unique, but interrelated, differential equations for two variables: patient total body water (V, in milliliters) and urea generation rate (G, in milligrams per minute). Values for V and G are then used to calculate normalized urea clearance during a dialysis treatment and the patient protein catabolic rate (PCR). The PCR is then divided by the postdialysis patient weight (in kilograms) to yield a normalized protein catabolic rate (nPCR). The fractional urea mass removed during hemodialysis is affected by the following factors: dialyzer urea clearance coefficient (K, in milliliters per minute), pre- and posttreatment blood urea nitrogen (BUN), treatment duration (t, in minutes), patient total body water (V, in milliliters), the amount of plasma water removed during dialysis

(ultrafiltrate), and the intradialytic G. Pre- and postdialysis measured BUN levels, the dialyzer K for urea at the delivered blood pump flow rate, time of treatment, and pre- and postdialysis patient weight are provided to the UKM algorithm. The difference between the pre- and postdialysis weights yields the ultrafiltration volume obtained during the treatment.

Pediatric-specific issues

Subsequent studies, such as the HEMO trial [3], which assessed the effect of small-solute clearance and increased convective clearance on mortality in adult maintenance hemodialysis patients, have not been performed in pediatric patients because relatively few children receive hemodialysis. Nevertheless, some recent pediatric data exist to describe the most accurate methods for quantifying urea removal, correlate delivered dose of dialysis with inflammation, and looking at other components of the dialysis prescription, including ultrafiltration and nutrition provision. These data can serve as a basis for clinical practice recommendations in caring for children receiving hemodialysis [8]. Although no current data exist to recommend a minimally acceptable hemodialysis dose for children, measurement of Kt/V is important in order to control for hemodialysis dose in outcome studies. For instance, Tom and colleagues demonstrated that improved growth could be achieved

Table 64.2 Pediatric hemodialysis adequacy studies.

Study ID	Assessment	No. of measurements
spKt/V		
Goldstein 1999	Comparison of Daugirdas II to UKM	21 patients, 103 measurements
Goldstein 2001	Comparison of Daugirdas II to UKM	39 patients, 367 measurements
eqKt/V		
Smye 1994	Mid-dialysis BUN sample to estimate eqBUN	14 patients, 14 measurements
Goldstein 1999	Logarithmic extrapolation of a 15-min post-BUN sample to estimate eqBUN	6 patients, 6 measurements
Sharma 2000	Use of a variable volume two-pool UKM to estimate eqKt/V	17 patients, 17 measurements
Goldstein 2000	Logarithmic extrapolation of a 15-min post-BUN sample to estimate eqBUN	21 patients, 21 measurements
Marsenic 2004	Linear regression equation	15 patients, 38 measurements
Goldstein[a] 2006	Comparison of eqKt/V and spKt/V to determine if 0.20 expected difference would lead to prescription changes	1513 measurements

[a] Conducted as part of the Center for Medicare and Medicaid Services Clinical Performance Measures (CMS CPM) project.

in patients with intensive hemodialysis (Kt/V of 2) and nutrition [9]. Goldstein showed that the proinflammatory cytokine concentrations were inversely proportional to Kt/V [10].

Current recommendations from the Kidney Disease Outcomes Quality Initiative (K/DOQI) suggest that children undergoing thrice-weekly maintenance hemodialysis receive at least the same minimum amount of urea clearance recommended for adults, namely, a single-pool Kt/V (spKt/V) of 1.2 [11]. No other guideline committee has offered pediatric-specific hemodialysis dose recommendations to date.

The K/DOQI recommendations are based on a number of single-center studies, which mostly focus upon urea clearance measurement methods. Substantial investigation has been performed to develop and validate Kt/V measurement methods more simple than UKM. Of these, only the natural logarithm formula of Daugirdas [12] garnered acceptance for spKt/V approximation in adults and children. The Daugirdas natural logarithm formula (Daugirdas II) is as follows: $Kt/V = -\ln(C_1/C_0 - 0.008 \times t) + [4 - 3.5 \times C_1/C_0)] \times UF/W$, where C_0 is the predialysis BUN, C_1 is the postdialysis BUN, t is the session duration (in hours), UF is the ultrafiltration volume (in milliliters), and W is the postdialysis weight (in kg). The accuracy of the Daugirdas II equation resides in the accounting for dialysis treatment duration and urea removed by ultrafiltration.

Goldstein demonstrated Daugirdas II to be a reliable and practical alternative to formal UKM for estimation of Kt/V in a large group of pediatric patients receiving hemodialysis [13,14]. A total of 367 dual Kt/V analyses comparing UKM Kt/V to Daugirdas II Kt/V demonstrated less than a 6% difference in every treatment, and the difference did not vary with patient size. K/DOQI guidelines recommend a prescription for Kt/V of 1.3 to ensure Kt/V delivery of 1.2 and allow for the use of Daugirdas II to calculate spKt/V [15].

The Kt/V calculation is based upon sampling the pre- and post-treatment BUN levels. In adults and children, the posthemodial-ysis BUN concentration rises in a logarithmic fashion until equilibration occurs 30 to 60 min after a hemodialysis treatment, a phenomenon termed urea rebound. As the BUN rises with equilibration posthemodialysis, the resultant calculation of Kt/V yields a lower value. Calculation of Kt/V by single-pool kinetics using the immediate, 30-s postdialysis BUN (BUN_{30s}) sample does not take urea rebound into account and leads to overestimation of the true urea mass removed during dialysis. Calculation of Kt/V by double-pool kinetics (eqKt/V) is based on a postdialysis BUN level actually drawn or estimated after the completion of urea rebound. Numerous studies in both children and adults have demonstrated that urea rebound ranges from 7.6% to 24% and accounts for a 12.3–16.8% difference between spKt/V and eqKt/V values [16–21]. It is impractical to wait 1 h after a treatment to obtain an equilibrated BUN (eqBUN) level for calculation of eqKt/V. Many formulas have been devised to estimate eqKt/V by applying a cofactor to spKt/V and relying solely on a pretreatment and 30-s posttreatment BUN levels. Smye and colleagues used a mid-dialysis BUN sample 80 min after treatment initiation and used the following approximation formula to estimate eqBUN: $C_{eq} = C_0 \times e^{-\lambda T}$, where $\lambda = (1/T - S)\ln(C_s/C_t)$ and C_0 is the pre-hemodialysis urea concentration, T is the duration of the dialysis session, S is the time into the hemodialysis session that the urea sample C_s was drawn, C_s is the BUN concentration at time S, and C_t is the BUN concentration at the end of hemodialysis [17]. In 14 patients, an average error in the calculation of Kt/V of 35% (range, 19–75%) by the single-pool UKM was reduced to 13% (range, 1–55%, but eight measurements were <7%) using the approximate technique. Marsenic has derived linear regression equations to describe a relationship between spKt/V and eqKt/V in children, demonstrating a mean difference of $0.26 + 0.18$ and an excellent correlation ($R^2 = 0.76$; $P < 0.0001$) [22]. However, this regression equation has not been validated in a different patient group.

Sharma developed a pediatric-specific variable volume double pool kinetic model with measurements from a cohort of

15 patients and then applied that model to predict measured eqKt/V in 17 different measurements [16]. Results from this study demonstrated a very low difference in measured versus estimated eqKt/V (0.06 + 0.07) and performed better than the Smye method, variable-volume, and fixed-volume single-pool methods. Because urea rebound is primarily characterized by a first-order logarithmic, concentration-dependent intercellular fluid (ICF)-to-extracellular fluid (ECF) urea movement, Goldstein evaluated a more recent method for estimating eqBUN by extrapolating the rise in BUN from 30 s to 15 min posttreatment (ΔBUN) [19]. Since urea rebound is 69% complete at 15 min postdialysis [21], eqBUN can be estimated (estBUN) using the following formula: estBUN = [(BUN$_{15min}$ − BUN$_{30s}$)/0.69] + BUN$_{30s.}$

The difference between eqKt/V based on a measured eqBUN and estimated eqKt/V based on estBUN by logarithmic extrapolation was less than that of other published eqKt/V estimation methods used in adult and pediatric patients.

A recent pediatric study evaluated potential differences in hemodialysis treatment prescription using the Center for Medicare and Medicaid Services Clinical Performance Measures data sets [23]. An expected difference in Kt/V (ΔKt/V = spKt/V − eqKt/V) of 0.20 was set based on results of the HEMO study [3]. Adequacy discordance was defined as a ΔKt/V of >0.20, because such a discordance could lead to an adequate spKt/V but an inadequate eqKt/V, thereby resulting in different clinical actions. A total of 1513 paired spKt/V and estimated eqKt/V results were available for comparison. Examination of the different spKt/V and estimated eqKt/V pairings revealed a greater adequacy discordance rate between a 0.20 difference in spKt/V and estimated eqKt/V at higher Kt/V values, but Kt/V discordance rates only varied from 0.3 to 5.5%, depending on the paired Kt/V values used. The authors suggested that these low discordance rates supported the use of spKt/V as acceptable for patient management.

The K/DOQI hemodialysis guidelines do not recommend eqKt/V as essential in the measurement of month-to-month patient hemodialysis adequacy, stating that spKt/V assessment of urea clearance is sufficient for patient management. However, the guidelines recommend use of eqKt/V to control for hemodialysis dose in outcome studies [11].

Target dry weight assessment and ultrafiltration management

Accurate determination of patient target weight is a challenging task when treating hemodialysis patients. Symptoms of hypovolemia may be difficult to assess, as the behavior of small children receiving dialysis is often difficult to interpret. Furthermore, children are growing and have variable appetites, so that real weight loss and weight gain may occur more frequently than in adults.

Accurate determination of pediatric target weight is critical, because an underestimation of dry weight can lead to hypovolemia with acute symptoms, whereas chronic overestimation of target weight can lead to chronic volume overload with resultant hypertension, pulmonary edema, congestive heart failure, and left ventricular hypertrophy. Ultrafiltration-associated symptoms may occur with an appropriately determined dry weight, especially in patients with large interdialytic weight gains. Approaches to minimize ultrafiltration-associated symptoms include sequential ultrafiltration and dialysis (or isolated ultrafiltration at the start of a treatment), sodium modeling, and noninvasive monitoring (NIVM) of hematocrit.

Sodium modeling

Sodium modeling is a machine-programmed algorithm that varies the dialysate sodium concentration during the treatment. Most modeling programs utilize hyperosmolar dialysate sodium concentrations at the beginning of treatment, which are designed to offset the decrease in serum osmolarity resulting from urea removal during dialysis. Sadowski demonstrated sodium modeling to be effective in decreasing both intra- and interdialytic symptoms in a prospective study of 16 adolescent and young adult patients [24].

NIVM of hematocrit

Because red blood cell volume remains constant during dialysis, changes in hematocrit will be inversely proportional to changes in intravascular volume. Continuous optical methods of NIVM for hematocrit take advantage of this relationship to demonstrate a real-time association between fluctuating hematocrit and intravascular volume during the hemodialysis treatment.

NIVM has been studied recently in pediatric patients receiving hemodialysis. Jain conducted a retrospective single-center review of ultrafiltration-associated event rates (hypotension, headache, or cramping that required a nursing intervention) in 200 matched treatments with and without NIVM. Event rates were lower, especially for patients less than 35 kg, when NIVM was performed, without a sacrifice in target weight achievement [25]. When NIVM was performed, symptom events in the first 90 min of a treatment occurred only with a blood volume change of greater than 8%/h. Seventy-one per cent of events occurring after 60 min of treatment initiation were associated with a blood volume change greater than 4%/h. Michael employed these treatment time and event observations to prospectively model ultrafiltration rates to lessen the need for antihypertensive medications and minimize intra- and interdialytic patient symptoms [26]. That model prescribes half of the total treatment ultrafiltration volume to be removed in the first 60 min of treatment with a maximum of a total 12% blood volume change as depicted on the NIVM. The remainder of the ultrafiltration volume is then removed during the final 2–3 h of treatment. Goldstein conducted a retrospective review before and after institution of this NIVM-guided UF algorithm and found a significant reduction in patient hospitalizations and additional treatments for fluid overload and hypertension [27]. The current K/DOQI guidelines now recommend NIVM for ultrafiltration modeling in children receiving maintenance hemodialysis [11].

Table 64.3 Semipermanent hemodialysis catheter and patient size guidelines.

Patient size (kg)	Catheter option(s)
<10	Made on case-by-case basis
10–20	8-French dual lumen
20–25	7 French twin Tesio®
25–40	10 French dual lumen
	10 French Ash Split®
	10 French twin Tesio®
>40	10 French twin Tesio®
	11.5 or 12.5 French dual lumen

Source: National Kidney Foundation [11].

Nutrition management

The important relationship between nutrition status and outcome for patients with ESRD prompted the K/DOQI to create guidelines to assess and treat malnutrition in both children and adults with ESRD [28]. The pediatric K/DOQI guidelines recommend measurement of serum albumin, height or length, dry weight, midarm circumference, skinfold thickness, fronto-occipital circumference, and height Z-score to monitor nutrition status and intensive enteral nutrition administration to treat protein energy malnutrition (PEM). There are also data on prealbumin being a more sensitive measure of current nutritional status than anthropomorphic indices. Although these measures may be important to monitor for and treat PEM, they may not be sufficient in all cases. Investigation into the validity of nPCR has been performed since the early 1980s and has demonstrated a positive correlation between dietary protein intake and nPCR [29]. These studies suggested that positive

nitrogen balance, which is essential for growth, can be achieved with moderate protein intake and without an increase in dialysis requirements. A recent investigation has shown nPCR to be more sensitive and specific than serum albumin as a marker for nutrition status in malnourished pediatric hemodialysis patients [30,31].

Provision of adequate nutrition is essential to delivering optimal dialysis. Tom performed a prospective study of 12 patients and showed that increased protein administration (150% of the recommended daily allowance for protein) and urea clearance (Kt/V, 2.0) led to improved growth in children receiving hemodialysis who did not receive growth hormone [9]. Krause [32], Goldstein [30], and Orellena [31] have used intradialytic parenteral nutrition to treat severe PEM in a total of 13 children receiving hemodialysis.

Vascular access

Adequate provision of hemodialysis depends upon a properly functioning vascular access. Current maintenance hemodialysis access options are divided into two categories: permanent access in the form of an AVF or AVG and semipermanent access in the form of catheters with a subcutaneous cuff.

Permanent vascular access in the form of an AVF or AVG can function for many years and is preferred over indwelling catheters for most children. The majority of children receiving maintenance hemodialysis in the USA are dialyzed via a catheter [33,34]. Reasons for high catheter use include small patient size, lack of local surgical experience of permanent access creation in smaller patients, anticipation of a short dialysis course prior to transplantation, or a dialysis unit philosophy to decrease painful procedures (i.e. repeated needle sticks for children with AVF or AVG). The 2006 K/DOQI Vascular Access update featured pediatric-specific

Table 64.4 Evidence ratings and recommendations for hemodialysis prescription to improve outcomes in pediatric patients.

Intervention	SR[a]	Evidence rating[a,b]		Comment	Recommendation[c]			Comment
		Moderate	Low		I	II	III	
eqKt/V and spKt/V vs UKM	—	•		8 studies (767 patients); generally consistent results	•			Simple, convenient, consistent measurements
Increased Kt/V (>1.2)	—		•	2 studies (12 patients for growth, 13 for inflammation)			•	Increased growth; reduced risk of inflammation, no separation of dialysis dose vs duration
Sodium modeling	—		•	1 study (16 patients)			•	Reduced intra- and interdialytic symptoms
NIVM	—		•	3 studies (74 patients); generally consistent results		•		Reduced hospitalization, hypertension, and intradialytic event rates
Ultrasound dilution to predict access stenosis	—		•	2 studies (22 patients); generally consistent results			•	Reduced flow predicts thrombosis

[a] Systematic review of randomized controlled trials.
[b] Evidence rating based on number of studies, study design, study quality, and consistency of results. No intervention was rated with a high evidence rating.
[c] Recommendations based on efficacy, trade-offs between benefits and harms, quality of evidence, and availability of intervention. I, recommend; II, suggest; III, no recommendation possible.

recommendations for the first time [11]. While the K/DOQI guidelines advocate permanent access placement in children >20 kg in size, Bourquelot has demonstrated successful AVF placement in children <10 kg in size by using microsurgical techniques [35,36]. The main drawback for AVF creation in such small children is an extended maturation time of up to 6 months.

Thrombosis of permanent access is a significant cause of morbidity for the hemodialysis patient population [37]. In many instances, thrombosis results from decreased access flow caused by a stenosis of the access venous outflow tract [38,39]. Many methods for assessing outflow stenosis in adult patients have significant drawbacks that preclude routine use. Ultrasound dilution is a practical, noninvasive, and reliable indicator of vascular access flow (QA, in milliliters per minute) and has been used effectively to identify venous stenosis in adult patients receiving hemodialysis [40–42]. The hemodialysis lines are temporarily reversed (to create recirculation), and a 20-mL bolus of saline is injected quickly into the venous line proximal to a sensor. The sensors are attached to a computer that interprets the changes in Doppler velocity within each line as the hematocrit changes in relation to dialyzer blood flow to report QA.

Goldstein has shown that a QA corrected for patient size (QA_{corr}) of <650 mL/min/1.73 m^2 is extremely sensitive and specific for predicting AVG and AVF stenosis in pediatric patients receiving hemodialysis [43]. Furthermore, when patients with a QA_{corr} of <650 mL/min/1.73 m^2 were referred for venography and balloon dilatation angioplasty within 48 h of ultrasound dilution measurement, a 90% reduction in the vascular access thrombosis rate was realized, compared to an aggressive surveillance venography protocol [44]. The reduction in thrombosis rate was associated with decreased patient hospitalization and a 40% reduction in unit cost per patient for vascular access management [27].

Chand assessed the ability of increased dynamic venous pressure to detect AVG venous stenosis and decrease thrombosis rates. She found increased venous pressures to be poorly predictive of stenosis and did not correlate with thrombotic events [45].

Sheth evaluated long-term AVG and AVF survival in pediatric patients [48]. One, 3-, and 5-year pediatric AVF survival was 90, 60, and 40%, respectively. One-, 3-, and 5-year pediatric AVG survival was 90, 50, and 40%, respectively [46]. These data demonstrated that although 5-year AVG and AVF survival rates are not significantly different, AVG rates do exhibit higher thrombosis and surgical intervention rates. However, this cohort was studied prior to institution of the ultrasound dilution venous stenosis surveillance protocol, so current AVG survival potential may be extended in the future.

Although catheters are not preferred for hemodialysis vascular access, a patient size of <20 kg and expectation of kidney transplantation in less than 1 year are acceptable reasons for provision of hemodialysis to children with catheters [11]. Table 64.3 lists some of the available cuffed hemodialysis catheter options and provides a guideline for matching catheter size and type with patient size [11].

A few pediatric cross-sectional descriptive studies have assessed the survival rates and complications for pediatric hemodialysis catheters [47–49]. The most common complications observed include infection (either tunnel infection or line sepsis), kinking of the catheter, and thrombosis. Gram-positive organisms, especially *Staphylococcus* species, are the most common causative organisms in hemodialysis catheter infections.

Pediatric studies have demonstrate a dual-lumen hemodialysis catheter median survival of 204–280 days. Sheth conducted a single-center comparison of Tesio catheters versus dual-lumen catheters and found Tesio catheters exhibited significantly longer survival and provided adequate hemodialysis more reliably than dual-lumen catheters of similar size [49].

Evidence table

An evidence table summarizing the research base for various aspects of hemodialysis prescription in children is provided at the end of the chapter (Table 64.4). The most extensive research has occurred in hemodialysis dose measurement and vascular access management. No randomized controlled trials have been conducted in the pediatric hemodialysis population, but moderate evidence exists to support the routine measurement of hemodialysis dose in terms of Kt/V, and more specifically as eqKt/V, to control for hemodialysis dose in interventional trials. Further study is warranted to determine if more frequent, shorter-duration hemodialysis would lead to improved outcomes in pediatric patients.

References

1 US Renal Data System. Excerpts from the USRDS Annual Report. *Am J Kidney Dis* 2006; **47**: S1–S286.

2 McDonald SP, Craig JC. Long-term survival of children with end-stage renal disease. *N Engl J Med* 2004; **350**: 2654–2662.

3 Eknoyan G, Beck GJ, Cheung AK, Daugirdas JT, Greene T, Kusek JW *et al.* Effect of dialysis dose and membrane flux in maintenance hemodialysis. *N Engl J Med* 2002; **347**: 2010–2019.

4 Gotch FA, Sargent JA. A mechanistic analysis of the National Cooperative Dialysis Study (NCDS). *Kidney Int* 1985; **28**: 526–534.

5 Geary DF, Piva E, Tyrrell J, Gajaria MJ, Picone G, Keating LE *et al.* Home nocturnal hemodialysis in children. *J Pediatr* 2005; **147**: 383–387.

6 Fischbach M, Terzic J, Menouer S, Dheu C, Soskin S, Helmstetter A *et al.* Intensified and daily hemodialysis in children might improve statural growth. *Pediatr Nephrol* 2006; **21**: 1746–1752.

7 Goldstein SL, Jabs K. Hemodialysis. In: Avner ED, Harmon WE, Niaudet P, editors, *Pediatric Nephrology*. Lippincott Williams & Wilkins, Philadelphia, 2004.

8 Goldstein SL. Adequacy of dialysis in children: does small solute clearance really matter? *Pediatr Nephrol* 2004; **19**: 1–5.

9 Tom A, McCauley L, Bell L, Rodd C, Espinosa P, Yu G *et al.* Growth during maintenance hemodialysis: impact of enhanced nutrition and clearance. *J Pediatr* 1999; **134**: 464–471.

10 Goldstein SL, Currier H, Watters L, Hempe JM, Sheth RD, Silverstein D. Acute and chronic inflammation in pediatric patients receiving hemodialysis. *J Pediatr* 2003; **143**: 653–657.

11 National Kidney Foundation. KDOQI clinical practice guidelines and clinical practice recommendations for 2006 updates: hemodiolysis adequacy, peritoneal dialysis adequacy, and vascular access. *Am J Kidney Dis* 2006; **48**: S1–S322.

12 Daugirdas JT. Second generation logarithmic estimates of single-pool variable volume Kt/V: an analysis of error. *J Am Soc Nephrol* 1993; **4**: 1205–1213.

13 Goldstein SL, Sorof JM, Brewer ED. Natural logarithmic estimates of Kt/V in the pediatric hemodialysis population. *Am J Kidney Dis* 1999; **33**: 518–522.

14 Goldstein SL. Hemodialysis in the pediatric patient: state of the art. *Adv Ren Replace Ther* 2001; **8**: 173–179.

15 NKF-DOQI clinical practice guidelines for hemodialysis adequacy. National Kidney Foundation. *Am J Kidney Dis* 1997; **30**: S15–S66.

16 Sharma A, Espinosa P, Bell L, Tom A, Rodd C. Multicompartment urea kinetics in well-dialyzed children. *Kidney Int* 2000; **58**: 2138–2146.

17 Smye SW, Evans JH, Will E, Brocklebank JT. Paediatric haemodialysis: estimation of treatment efficiency in the presence of urea rebound. *Clin Phys Physiol Meas* 1992; **13**: 51–62.

18 Marsenic O, Pavlicic D, Bigovic G, Peco-Antic A, Jovanovic O. Effects of postdialysis urea rebound on the quantification of pediatric hemodialysis. *Nephron* 2000; **84**: 124–129.

19 Goldstein SL, Brewer ED. Logarithmic extrapolation of a 15-minute postdialysis BUN to predict equilibrated BUN and calculate double-pool Kt/V in the pediatric hemodialysis population. *Am J Kidney Dis* 2000; **36**: 98–104.

20 Maduell F, Garcia-Valdecasas J, Garcia H, Hernandez-Jaras J, Siguenza F, del Pozo C *et al.* Validation of different methods to calculate Kt/V considering postdialysis rebound. *Nephrol Dial Transplant* 1997; **12**: 1928–1933.

21 Goldstein SL, Sorof JM, Brewer ED. Evaluation and prediction of urea rebound and equilibrated Kt/V in the pediatric hemodialysis population. *Am J Kidney Dis* 1999; **34**: 49–54.

22 Marsenic OD, Pavlicic D, Peco-Antic A, Bigovic G, Jovanovic O. Prediction of equilibrated urea in children on chronic hemodialysis. *ASAIO J* 2000; **46**: 283–287.

23 Goldstein SL, Brem A, Warady BA, Fivush B, Frankenfield D. Comparison of single-pool and equilibrated Kt/V values for pediatric hemodialysis prescription management: analysis from the Centers for Medicare & Medicaid Services Clinical Performance Measures Project. *Pediatr Nephrol* 2006; **21**: 1161–1166.

24 Sadowski RH, Allred EN, Jabs K. Sodium modeling ameliorates intradialytic and interdialytic symptoms in young hemodialysis patients. *J Am Soc Nephrol* 1993; **4**: 1192–1198.

25 Jain SR, Smith L, Brewer ED, Goldstein SL. Non-invasive intravascular monitoring in the pediatric hemodialysis population. *Pediatr Nephrol* 2001; **16**: 15–18.

26 Michael M, Brewer ED, Goldstein SL. Blood volume monitoring to achieve target weight in pediatric hemodialysis patients. *Pediatr Nephrol* 2004; **19**: 432–437.

27 Goldstein SL, Smith CM, Currier H. Noninvasive interventions to decrease hospitalization and associated costs for pediatric patients receiving hemodialysis. *J Am Soc Nephrol* 2003; **14**: 2127–2131.

28 NKF. K/DOQI clinical practice guidelines for nutrition in chronic renal failure. *Am J Kid Dis* 2000; **35(6 Suppl 2)**: S1–S140.

29 Grupe WE, Harmon WE, Spinozzi NS. Protein and energy requirements in children receiving chronic hemodialysis. *Kidney Int Suppl* 1983; **15**: S6–S10.

30 Goldstein SL, Baronette S, Gambrell TV, Currier H, Brewer ED. nPCR assessment and IDPN treatment of malnutrition in pediatric hemodialysis patients. *Pediatr Nephrol* 2002; **17**: 531–534.

31 Orellana P, Juarez-Congelosi M, Goldstein SL. Intradialytic parenteral nutrition treatment and biochemical marker assessment for malnutrition in adolescent maintenance hemodialysis patients. *J Ren Nutr* 2005; **15**: 312–317.

32 Krause I, Shamir R, Davidovits M, Frishman S, Cleper R, Gamzo Z *et al.* Intradialytic parenteral nutrition in malnourished children treated with hemodialysis. *J Ren Nutr* 2002; **12**: 55–59.

33 NAPRTCS. North American Pediatric Renal Transplant Cooperative Study: 2004 annual report. NAPRTCS, Boston, 2004.

34 Neu A, Goldstein S, Fivush B *et al.* Longitudinal analysis of clinical parameters in pediatric hemodialysis patients: results of the CMS ESRD CPM Project. *J Am Soc Nephrol* 2004; **15**: 400A (meeting abstract).

35 Bourquelot P, Cussenot O, Corbi P, Pillion G, Gagnadoux MF, Bensman A *et al.* Microsurgical creation and follow-up of arteriovenous fistulae for chronic haemodialysis in children. *Pediatr Nephrol* 1990; **4**: 156–159.

36 Bourquelot P, Raynaud F, Pirozzi N. Microsurgery in children for creation of arteriovenous fistulas in renal and non-renal diseases. *Ther Apher Dial* 2003; **7**: 498–503.

37 USRDS: the United States Renal Data System. *Am J Kidney Dis* 2003; **42**: 1–230.

38 Swedberg SH, Brown BG, Sigley R, Wight TN, Gordon D, Nicholls SC. Intimal fibromuscular hyperplasia at the venous anastomosis of PTFE grafts in hemodialysis patients. Clinical, immunocytochemical, light and electron microscopic assessment. *Circulation* 1989; **80**: 1726–1736.

39 Kanterman RY, Vesely TM, Pilgram TK, Guy BW, Windus DW, Picus D. Dialysis access grafts: anatomic location of venous stenosis and results of angioplasty. *Radiology* 1995; **195**: 135–139.

40 Krivitski NM. Theory and validation of access flow measurement by dilution technique during hemodialysis. *Kidney Int* 1995; **48**: 244–250.

41 Neyra NR, Ikizler TA, May RE, Himmelfarb J, Schulman G, Shyr Y *et al.* Change in access blood flow over time predicts vascular access thrombosis. *Kidney Int* 1998; **54**: 1714–1719.

42 May RE, Himmelfarb J, Yenicesu M, Knights S, Ikizler TA, Schulman G *et al.* Predictive measures of vascular access thrombosis: a prospective study. *Kidney Int* 1997; **52**: 1656–1662.

43 Goldstein SL, Allsteadt A. Ultrasound dilution evaluation of pediatric hemodialysis vascular access. *Kidney Int* 2001; **59**: 2357–2360.

44 Goldstein SL, Allsteadt A, Smith CM, Currier H. Proactive monitoring of pediatric hemodialysis vascular access: effects of ultrasound dilution on thrombosis rates. *Kidney Int* 2002; **62**: 272–275.

45 Chand DH, Poe SA, Strife CF. Venous pressure monitoring does not accurately predict access failure in children. *Pediatr Nephrol* 2002; **17**: 765–769.

46 Sheth RD, Brandt ML, Brewer ED, Nuchtern JG, Kale AS, Goldstein SL. Permanent hemodialysis vascular access survival in children and adolescents with end-stage renal disease. *Kidney Int* 2002; **62**: 1864–1869.

47 Goldstein SL, Macierowski CT, Jabs K. Hemodialysis catheter survival and complications in children and adolescents. *Pediatr Nephrol* 1997; **11**: 74–77.

48 Sharma A, Zilleruelo G, Abitbol C, Montane B, Strauss J. Survival and complications of cuffed catheters in children on chronic hemodialysis. *Pediatr Nephrol* 1999; **13**: 245–248.

49 Sheth RD, Kale AS, Brewer ED, Brandt ML, Nuchtern JG, Goldstein SL. Successful use of Tesio catheters in pediatric patients receiving chronic hemodialysis. *Am J Kidney Dis* 2001; **38**: 553–559.

Specific Pediatric Renal Disease

65 Urinary Tract Infection, Vesicoureteric Reflux, and Urinary Incontinence

Gabrielle Williams,[1,2] **Premala Sureshkumar,**[1] **Patrina Caldwell,**[1,3] **& Jonathan C. Craig**[1,2]

[1]Centre for Kidney Research, The Children's Hospital at Westmead, Westmead, Australia.
[2]School of Public Health, University of Sydney, Sydney, Australia.
[3]Discipline of Paediatrics and Child Health, University of Sydney, Sydney, Australia.

Introduction

Urinary tract infection (UTI), vesicoureteric reflux (VUR), and incontinence are the most commonly encountered problems in pediatric nephrology. The treatment of these conditions is important yet often controversial.

Urinary tract infection

Clinical presentation

UTIs can be grouped into asymptomatic bacteruria, cystitis, and acute pyelonephritis. Cystitis is most commonly seen in girls over 2 years of age and is an infection limited to the urethra and bladder. Patients usually present with localizing symptoms, which may include pain on urination (dysuria), frequency, urgency, cloudy urine, and lower abdominal discomfort.

A positive urine culture can be found in children without symptoms of illness (asymptomatic or covert bacteriuria), and antibiotics are not required because long-term outcomes appear similar in treated compared with untreated patients [1,2].

Pyelonephritis is the most severe form of UTI in children and is associated with systemic features such as high fever, vomiting, malaise, abdominal pain or tenderness, poor feeding, irritability in infants. Diagnosis may be assisted by imaging of the kidneys with a technetium 99[m]-labeled dimercaptosuccinic acid (DMSA) scan and assessment of inflammatory markers in the blood, for example, erythrocyte sedimentation rate and C-reactive protein.

Diagnosis

The diagnosis of UTI is based on the culture of a pure growth of bacteria in an uncontaminated sample of urine in the presence of symptoms of illness. Microbiological criteria for diagnosis of UTI are provided in Table 65.1.

Urine collection methods in children are important for the diagnosis, because of the problems with contamination and false-positive tests. The method least likely to involve contamination, the suprapubic bladder tap, may be impractical in some settings. Transurethral catheterization, the collection method second to a bladder tap for false positivity, also presents technical challenges, and both of these tests are invasive. Voided samples are more feasible but can be problematic. Some clinicians use a urine bag, but contamination rates are too high for this method to be recommended [3]. The clean catch method is reasonable but requires patience and cooperation from parents. Across health care settings, collection methods vary widely because time, skill, attitudes, and facilities, as well as contamination rates, are all influential.

The preferred method for urine collection in children who cannot void upon request is catheterization, after weighing criteria of contamination, technical feasibility, and invasiveness. For children above 2 years of age who are toilet trained, a midstream urine sample is recommended.

Urine culture requires a minimum of 18 h before a result is known, and this may be longer in some situations. Clinicians often use rapid tests to guide initial diagnosis and management decisions. Urinalysis, or dipsticks, and urine microscopy for white cells or visible bacteria are widely used. Dipsticks are quick, easy, and inexpensive and can be used in any setting. Microscopic examination usually requires specialized technical personnel. A systematic review of the literature [4] demonstrated that a dipstick result showing positive findings for both leukocyte esterase and nitrite is reasonably good for identifying UTI (LR+, 28.2). A dipstick negative for both generally rules out UTI (LR−, 0.20). The more common finding of a single positive result is considerably less helpful for guiding decisions (leukocyte esterase LR+, 5.5; nitrite LR+,15.9). When available, combined positive microscopy findings perform well at ruling in the diagnosis (LR+, 37.0), and two negative microscopy results also perform reasonably well at excluding UTI (LR, −0.21). A single positive microscopy result is less helpful in guiding management (pyuria LR+, 5.9; bacteriuria

Evidence-based Nephrology. Edited by Donald Molony and Jonathan Craig
© 2009 Blackwell Publishing, ISBN: 978-1-4051-3975-5.

Table 65.1 Microbiological criteria for diagnosis of UTI in children.

Collection method	Definite UTI[a]		Probable UTI[b]	
	No. of organisms (species)	CFU/L	No. of organisms (species)	CFU/L
Suprapubic bladder tap	1	Any	2	Any
Transurethral catheter	1	$\geq 10^7$	1	$\geq 10^6$
			2	$\geq 10^7$
Voided samples (clean catch, midstream, bag)	1	$\geq 10^8$	1	$\geq 10^7$
			2	$\geq 10^8$

CFU, colony-forming unit(s).
[a] Based on review of 85 studies comparing urine screening tests with urine culture for diagnosis of UTI in children.
[b] Based on consensus opinion of three senior staff specialists in infectious disease, general medicine and nephrology (Children's Hospital at Westmead).

LR+, 14.7). Urine culture is always needed to confirm the diagnosis.

Epidemiology

Precise estimates of rates of UTI are difficult to ascertain; however, a large population-based study, with a verified outcome of UTI, showed that 8% of girls and 2% of boys had at least one UTI by 7 years of age [5]. Rates of disease in subgroups of the population have been studied more readily, with one systematic review of 12 studies of febrile children showing that approximately 5% of febrile infants (0–2 months) had had a UTI [6]. A similar rate was found in studies that included older children (0–5 years) with fever [7,8].

Pathogenesis

UTIs are more common in girls after the first year of life, whereas boys are 5–10 times more susceptible to UTIs in the neonatal period. The increased rate in infant boys is highest in uncircumcised males [9,10].

Infection of the urinary tract is likely to be related to host and bacterial factors. Bacterial virulence factors that have been well-studied in UTI include adherence, growth factors, and features that allow the bacteria to avoid destruction by the human immune response [11]. Characteristics of bacteria only partly explain the differential colonization of the urinary tract, because healthy volunteers inoculated with virulent *Escherichia coli* rapidly eradicate the bacterium [12]. Characteristics of the human immune system are likely to contribute to disease risk. With so many components involved, any of which can vary with genetic and environmental factors, identifying attributable risk for each is difficult. Studies looking at some of these components have found inconsistent results [13–16]. Study design limitations are likely to explain the variability.

Children with lesions of the spinal cord and neurologic abnormalities have increased risk of UTI, but the management issues are different and thus are not discussed here.

Recurrence

Ten to 30% of children with UTI will have at least one more infection [17,18]. The majority occur within the first 12 months after the primary infection, and risks for recurrence include age less than 6 months at first UTI (odds ration [OR], 2.9; 95% confidence interval [CI], 1.4–6.2), presence of dilating VUR (OR, 3.6; CI, 1.5–8.3), and renal damage detected at primary UTI [18], which may be congenital in origin.

Acute treatment

Evidence on which to base specific treatment choices is limited in very young children, because they are often excluded from randomized controlled trials. However, clinical experience suggests infants aged 1 month or less with UTI require intravenous antibiotics, because there is an approximately 10% risk of concomitant bacteremia [19,20] and a significant chance of finding uropathology [21], such as posterior urethral valves or obstructed duplex systems. *E. coli* and *Enterococcus faecalis* are the most likely pathogens in this age group [22], indicating empirical treatment with a β-lactam antibiotic and an aminoglycoside. Intravenous treatment is usually continued until systemic signs have resolved (2–3 days), after which time an oral antibiotic is given for 7–10 days.

Evidence supporting treatment for children over the age of 1 month with pyelonephritis includes 18 randomized controlled trials and was summarized in a Cochrane review [23]. Two well-designed trials of 693 children compared oral antibiotics (cefixime, amoxicillin-clavulinic acid) with intravenous (IV) antibiotics for 3 days, or until defervescence, followed by oral antibiotics. No differences in time to fever resolution (weighted mean difference, 1.54 days; 95% CI, 1.67–4.76), recurrence of UTI (relative risk [RR], 0.67; 95% CI, 0.27–1.67), or frequency of renal parenchymal defect at 6–12 months (RR, 1.45; 95% CI, 0.63–3.03) were demonstrated (Figure 65.1). Four trials involving 480 children compared oral with IV administration of antibiotic after 3–4 days of IV treatment for both groups. Although antibiotic type varied, there was no difference in recurrence of UTI (Figure 65.1) or renal parenchymal defects between the long-duration IV antibiotics and the short-duration IV plus oral antibiotic groups. These findings provide good evidence that oral antibiotics are an effective treatment choice for children with a diagnosis of acute pyelonephritis (Table 65.2). Intravenous treatment can be reserved for children who present seriously ill or have persistent vomiting. Optimal

Oral vs IV for initial treatment of acute pyelonephritis

Review: Antibiotics for acute pyelonephritis in children
Comparison: 01 Pral (14 days) versus intravenous (3 days) followed by ora (11 days) therapy
Outcome: 01 Time to fever resolutioin (hours)

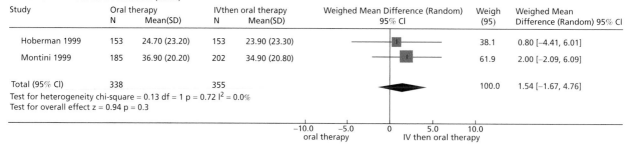

Study	Oral therapy		IVthen oral therapy		Weighed Mean Difference (Random) 95% CI	Weigh (95)	Weighed Mean Difference (Random) 95% CI
	N	Mean(SD)	N	Mean(SD)			
Hoberman 1999	153	24.70 (23.20)	153	23.90 (23.30)		38.1	0.80 [−4.41, 6.01]
Montini 1999	185	36.90 (20.20)	202	34.90 (20.80)		61.9	2.00 [−2.09, 6.09]
Total (95% CI)	338		355			100.0	1.54 [−1.67, 4.76]

Test for heterogeneity chi-square = 0.13 df = 1 p = 0.72 I^2 = 0.0%
Test for overall effect z = 0.94 p = 0.3

Short versus long initial IV treatment for acute pyelonephritis

Review: Antibiotics for acute pyelonephritis in children
Comparison: 02 short duration (3–4 days) versus long duration (7–14 days) intravenous therapy
Outcome: 02 Recurrent UTI within 6 months

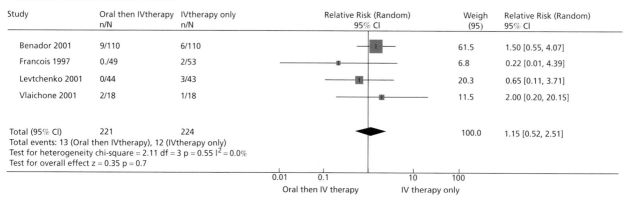

Study	Oral then IVtherapy n/N	IVtherapy only n/N	Relative Risk (Random) 95% CI	Weigh (95)	Relative Risk (Random) 95% CI
Benador 2001	9/110	6/110		61.5	1.50 [0.55, 4.07]
Francois 1997	0./49	2/53		6.8	0.22 [0.01, 4.39]
Levtchenko 2001	0/44	3/43		20.3	0.65 [0.11, 3.71]
Vlaichone 2001	2/18	1/18		11.5	2.00 [0.20, 20.15]
Total (95% CI)	221	224		100.0	1.15 [0.52, 2.51]

Total events: 13 (Oral then IVtherapy), 12 (IVtherapy only)
Test for heterogeneity chi-square = 2.11 df = 3 p = 0.55 I^2 = 0.0%
Test for overall effect z = 0.35 p = 0.7

Short (2-4 days) versus standard (7–10 days) duration of antibiotics for cystitis

Review: Short versus standard duration oral antibiotic therapy for acute urinary tract infection in children
Comparison: 01 Short duration versus standard duration
Outcome: 01 UTI at end of treatment

Study	Short duration n/N	Standard duration n/N	Relative Risk (Random) 95% CI	Weigh (95)	Relative Risk (Random) 95% CI
CSG 1991	18/96	18/78		57.9	0.81 [0.45, 1.46]
× Gaudreault 1992	0/20	0/20		0.0	Not estimable
× Helin 1981	0/23	0/20		0.0	Not estimable
Johnson 1993	9/20	3/17		18.3	2.55 [0.82, 7.94]
Komberg 1994	4/12	2/13		10.7	2.17 [0.48, 9.76]
Lohr 1981	2/26	2/23		7.0	0.88 [0.14, 5.79]
Zaki 1986	0/16	0/10		2.6	0.22 [0.01, 4.83]
Zaki 1986a	1/19	0/10		3.5	0.53 [0.04, 7.55]
Total (95% CI)	232	191		100.0	1.06 [0.64, 1.76]

Total events: 34 (Short duration), 27 (Standard duration)
(Test for heterogeneity chi-square = 5.27 df = 5 p = 0.38 I^2 = 5.1%
Test for overall effect z = 0.24 p = 0.8

Figure 65.1 Acute antibiotic treatment options for UTI in children.

Table 65.2 Evidence ratings and recommendations for acute treatment and prophylaxis of UTI in children.

Intervention	Treatment type	Evidence rating[a]	Comment	Recommendation[b]			Comments
				I	II	III	
Oral vs IV initial treatment	Acute	High	2 trials, 693 children, good design	• oral			Oral cefixime as effective as IV
Short (3–4 days) vs long (10–18 days) initial IV treatment	Acute	Moderate	4 trials, 480 children, reasonable design		• Short		3–4 days initial IV
Duration of antibiotic therapy for cystitis (lower tract UTI) 2–4 days vs 7–14 days Single dose vs 7–14 days	Acute	Moderate	3 systematic reviews 11 trials, 652 children 9 trials, 383 children, inconsistent quality		•	•	2–4 days sufficient; single dose less effective
Duration of antibiotic therapy for pyelonephritis	Acute	Low	1 trial 10 vs 42 days 2 trials 1dose vs 7–10 days			•	Suggest standard therapy 7–14 days
Renal tract imaging For localization of infection For detection of VUR For detection of renal scarring	Acute	Low	Included studies poorly reported; primarily cross-sectional design, no long-term follow-up			•	Suggest ultrasound after first UTI (inexpensive, noninvasive, readily available, will detect gross abnormalities); consider DMSA if recurrence
Prophylactic antibiotics vs no prophylaxis (<50% participants with VUR)	Prophylactic	Low	2 trials had outcome of symptomatic UTI, inconsistent results 4 trials had outcome of repeat positive urine culture, antibiotics were beneficial			•	Possible benefit, may elect to try after second infection
Prophylactic interventions for children with VUR Antibiotics vs no treatment Antibiotics vs surgery + antibiotics	Prophylactic	Moderate	2 trials, showed no difference in effect 7 trials, showed little difference in effect			•	Possible benefit, may elect to try antibiotics after second infection
Cranberries for prevention of recurrent UTI	Prophylactic	Moderate, but uncertain applicability	Most trials were adults, 2 trials in children with neuropathic bladder		•		Harmless intervention, possible benefit in children, uncertainty about dose
Circumcision for prevention of UTI	Prophylactic	Low	1 trial, 4 cohort studies, ORs concordant		• (restricted application)		Suggested for boys with recurrent UTI or high-grade (≥3) VUR

[a]Rating of systematic reviews: "high," included trials are good quality and applicable; "moderate," included trials are of moderate quality and applicability; "low," included trials are of low quality and are not directly applicable.

[b]I, recommend; II, suggest; III, evidence does not support a recommendation.

duration of antibiotic treatment for children with acute pyelonephritis is poorly supported by evidence because the existing trials have not compared short-course with standard therapy [23].

A large evidence base (22 trials and three systematic reviews) [24–26] (Table 65.2; Figure 65.1) supports the treatment options for children presenting with symptoms suggestive of cystitis. Findings show that short-duration therapy (2–4 days) is as effective as standard treatment (7–14 days) in eradicating urinary bacteria at 0–10 days posttreatment and 1–15 months posttreatment [25]. Further trials have demonstrated than single-dose therapy may be insufficient to successfully treat cystitis in children [26].

Prevention of recurrence

Good evidence exists to show that children who have had one UTI are at considerable risk (10–30%) for recurrence [17]. Without proper understanding of causality, it is not possible to reliably prescribe methods to prevent recurrence of UTI. However, many people recommend avoidance of constipation, complete bladder emptying, good intake of fluids, and avoidance of possible irritation from underclothing or bubble baths. These measures are supported by a weak evidence base.

A systematic review [27] of five trials, including one with a crossover design, that have compared prophylactic antibiotics with placebo or no treatment in a group of children where the majority did not have VUR is summarized in Table 65.2. One trial,

Review: Long-term antibiotics for preventing recurrent urinary tract infection in children
Comparison: 01 Antibiotic treatment versus placebo/no treatment
Outcome: 01 Recurrent of symptomatic UTI

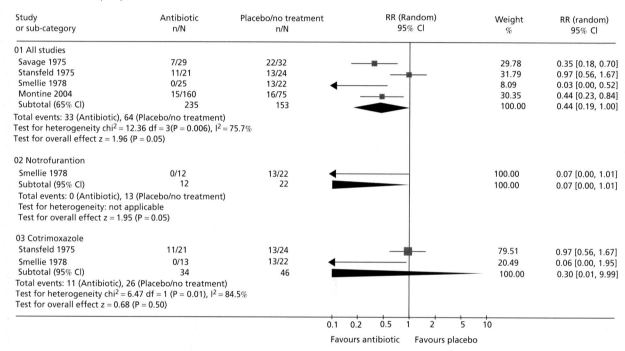

Figure 65.2 Antibiotic prophylaxis to prevent recurrent UTI in children, of whom the majority do not have VUR.

involving 61 children, in which repeat symptomatic UTI was the primary outcome, found that twice as many repeat infections occurred in the antibiotic arm compared to the placebo group [28] (Figure 65.2). In the crossover trial, 14 of 18 children had recurrent symptomatic infections, and all occurred during the placebo phase [29]. This rate of recurrence (78%) is large, very different from the findings of other studies, and suggests considerable selection bias in trial participants. The other four trials, which utilized repeat positive urine culture as the primary outcome, demonstrated a reduced risk of 0.44 (95% CI, 0.19–1.0) of repeat positive culture in the antibiotic prophylaxis group [28,30–32] (Figure 65.2). Three trials, including one with a crossover design, compared different antibiotic types [33–35]. Findings were variable, and without clear evidence that antibiotics are effective in preventing recurrent UTI,

it is potentially misleading to recommend one antibiotic over another. The evidence to support the use of prophylactic antibiotics to prevent recurrent UTI in children without reflux is weak and probably not generalizable to children experiencing their first UTI.

Other interventions for prevention that have been studied in randomized controlled trials include cranberry products [36], immuno-active agents (e.g. Uro-vaxom) [37], and probiotics [38]. Most trials demonstrating benefit have not focused on children, and thus the applicability of their results is questionable. Despite the absence of appropriate studies in children, cranberry products are harmless, readily available, beneficial in adults, and may prevent recurrent UTI in children (except in those with spina bifida).

Circumcision as a treatment for prevention of recurrent UTI has been evaluated in studies of various designs. A meta-analysis of randomized trials and observational studies [39] identified one randomized controlled trial, four cohort studies, and seven case–control studies that addressed this issue. Circumcision significantly reduced the risk of UTI (OR, 0.13; 95% CI, 0.08–0.20), but importantly, 111 circumcisions would need to be done to prevent 1 UTI. In boys with a considerably greater risk of recurrent UTI (high-grade VUR, recurrent UTIs), the number of circumcisions needed to prevent 1 UTI drops to less than 11 circumcisions. In summary, there is a net benefit of the intervention only in boys at greater risk than those presenting with first UTI.

Renal tract evaluation and imaging

Available guidelines [40,41] recommend renal tract imaging for very young children with UTI. However, a systematic review has shown that the evidence for improved outcomes for children is weak [42]. Renal ultrasound reveals anatomical information about the kidneys and urinary tract. It is noninvasive, inexpensive, and readily available, but results rarely change management. Micturating or voiding cystourethrogram (VCUG) is performed to detect VUR. VCUG is a traumatic imaging technique, and in the absence of good evidence for improved outcomes through better management of children with VUR, it is not justifiable in children presenting with a first UTI. A DMSA scan demonstrates renal focal abnormalities and determines differential renal function. Identification of renal focal abnormalities in many cases does not alter management.

Imaging by ultrasound can be justified where there is easy access to qualified sonographers, as it is a noninvasive procedure and it has a high sensitivity for renal tract obstruction. Strong observational evidence demonstrates that surgical treatment of children with obstructive uropathy improves outcome. Accordingly, almost all pediatricians report they recommend ultrasonography for all children with UTI [43]. Considerable variability in the use of DMSA and VCUG reflects the uncertainty about whether these tests do more good than harm in children with UTI.

Vesicoureteric reflux

Definition and diagnosis

VUR is the retrograde flow of urine from the bladder into the ureter and towards the kidney. Severity is graded using the five-grade International Reflux Study system, which includes domains such as height of retrograde flow and dilatation and tortuosity of the ureters [44]. The reference standard test for diagnosis of VUR is a VCUG.

Epidemiology

VUR is common in children with UTI. There have been numerous case series of children with UTI, and they have consistently shown that 25–30% of children with UTI have VUR [45–48]. Incidence in the wider population is less clear, although most review articles suggest a rate of less than 1% in "well" children [49–51].

Clinical spectrum

VUR may be an isolated finding, primary VUR, or it may be associated with other urological abnormalities, such as posterior urethral valves or a neurogenic bladder, in which case it is referred to as secondary VUR [52–55]. VUR may also occur as part of multiorgan malformation syndromes [56–59]. The appearance of VUR with other abnormalities of kidney and ureteric development within families has led to the collective classification of these as CAKUT (congenital abnormalities of the kidney and ureteric tract) [60–62]. Although most well-designed, prospective studies are small, follow-up of children with primary VUR suggests that the majority have resolution of the VUR without further morbidity. In follow-up studies VUR is a poor predictor of kidney damage and longer-term hypertension [63–66].

VUR as an inherited trait

Many groups have studied reflux in the context of an inherited disorder, because sibling recurrence, parent–child transmission, and twin concordance rates support this theory [67–73]. The majority of reported pedigrees have shown dominant inheritance patterns [73–77], but cases of recessive [75] and X-linked inheritance [78,79] have also been reported. Clinical characteristics of VUR cases can differ within families [80,81]; therefore, the same genetic change can result in different disease expression. This suggests other factors also influence expression of the VUR phenotype, and these may include other genes, environmental exposures, and the interaction of genes with environmental factors.

Screening

An antenatal ultrasound finding of renal dilatation of ≥ 4 mm is commonly suggested as an indication of VUR. It is, however, a nonspecific screening tool for VUR, as fewer than 10% of VUR cases are diagnosed by subsequent VCUG [82–84]. Some clinicians advocate testing asymptomatic siblings of children with VUR, because VUR can be familial [85]. However, given the insufficiency of evidence for the benefits of early treatment for VUR, early detection cannot be justified.

Prognosis

From a comparison of the frequency of VUR overall and end-stage kidney disease attributed to VUR [86], it is evident that the outcome for the vast majority of children with VUR is excellent. Assuming that about 3% of children (or 30,000 per million children) have reflux, only about 1 in 6,000 (or 5 per million) will ultimately develop end-stage kidney disease. VUR is a relatively common condition, and end-stage kidney failure due to reflux nephropathy is a very rare problem. For around 5–7% of people entering end-stage kidney failure programs, reflux nephropathy is nominated as the primary cause [86–90].

Management

Management of a child with VUR is controversial. The use of low-dose prophylactic antibiotics to prevent recurrent UTI and kidney damage has been the standard of care for many children

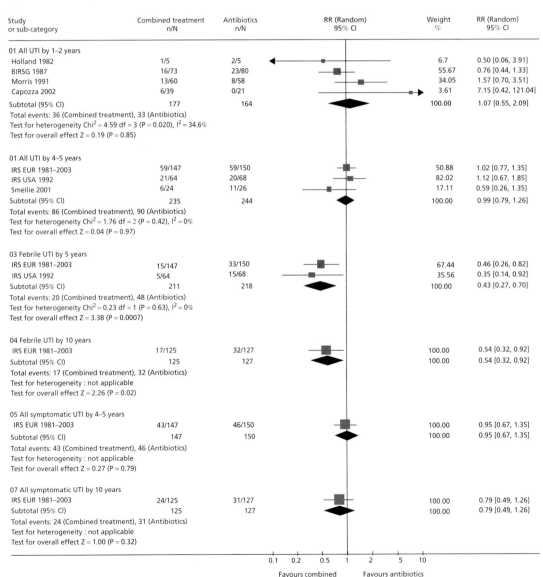

Figure 65.3 Interventions to prevent recurrent UTI in children with VUR.

with VUR. A recent systematic review highlighted the very weak basis for this practice [91]. Two trials, of 247 children, found no significant difference in risk of UTI or of renal parenchymal abnormality between the antibiotic group and the surveillance group [92,93] (Figure 65.3). Six trials compared ureteric reimplantation by open surgery plus antibiotic prophylaxis with antibiotic prophylaxis alone, and two trials compared subureteric injection plus antibiotics with antibiotics alone. Combining these studies demonstrates that the risks of UTI at 1–2 and 5 years (Figure 65.3) and of new or progressive renal parenchymal abnormality at 5 years are not significantly different between the surgery plus antibiotic groups compared to the antibiotics-alone group (RR of new renal parenchymal damage at 5 years, 1.09; 95% CI, 0.79–1.49; RR of progression of renal parenchymal damage at 5 years, 0.99; 95% CI, 0.69–1.42). The only difference was a lower risk (RR, 0.43; 95% CI, 0.27–0.70) of febrile UTI over 5 years in the surgery plus antibiotic group. This means that nine children would undergo surgery and take prophylactic antibiotics to prevent one febrile UTI over 5 years. In 2006, 10-year follow-up data on 252 of an original group of 306 trial participants were published [94]. These data showed that renal growth, UTI recurrence, somatic growth, and renal function did not differ between the antibiotic and the surgery plus antibiotic groups.

Two trials compared different subureteric injection substances, and numerous case series of this intervention have been published [91,95]. Common to most of these studies is the absence of the clinically relevant outcome, symptomatic UTI. Case series suggest subureteric injection frequently resolves the physical abnormality, VUR, but the effect on recurrence of UTI is not known. In summary, the trial data that support the use of prophylactic antibiotics, reimplantation surgery, and subureteric injection to prevent recurrent UTI in children with VUR is weak and inconclusive. Given that the risk of harm for no treatment is small, interventions to prevent recurrence of infection after first UTI are unjustifiable.

Urinary incontinence

Definition, clinical presentation, and diagnostic tests
Urinary incontinence may present as nocturnal enuresis, daytime incontinence, or both.

Nocturnal enuresis
Nocturnal enuresis is the involuntary loss of urine at night in the absence of organic disease by the developmental age of 5 years [96]. Nocturnal enuresis is classified as primary (no consistent night dryness) or secondary (bedwetting after a previous dry period of at least 6 months). It is also classified as monosymptomatic (with no daytime urinary symptoms) or non-monosymptomatic.

Epidemiology
Nocturnal enuresis occurs in up to 20% of school-aged children, with 2.4% wetting at least nightly [97]. The prevalence is approximately 20% in 5-year-olds, 10% in 10-year-olds, and 3%

in 15-year-olds [98]. Younger children tend to outgrow nocturnal enuresis, with a spontaneous remission rate of approximately 14% annually, while 3% remain enuretic as adults [98]. Nocturnal enuresis is more common in boys.

Risk factors
The etiology of nocturnal enuresis is a complex interaction of genetic and environmental factors. Secondary nocturnal enuresis is likely to be associated with recognizable psychological or organic causes. Non-monosymptomatic nocturnal enuresis (with daytime urinary symptoms) suggests an underlying bladder dysfunction [99,100].

Reported risk factors for primary nocturnal enuresis include nocturnal polyuria and a deranged circadian rhythm of antidiuretic hormone (ADH) [101], defects in sleep arousal [102], nocturnal detrusor overactivity with reduced functional bladder capacity [103], upper airway obstruction [104], and sleep apnea [105]. Nocturnal enuresis has also been linked to chromosomes 8, 12, 13, and 22 with an autosomal dominant inheritance [98]. Risk factors for secondary nocturnal enuresis include UTIs (which may cause temporary detrusor and/or urethral instability), diabetes mellitus and insipidus, stress, sexual abuse, and other psychopathology. Risk factors for both primary and secondary nocturnal enuresis include constipation [106], attention deficit hyperactivity disorder [107], and developmental delay and other neurological dysfunction [108]. Reported risk factors for non-monosymptomatic nocturnal enuresis are the same as those for daytime incontinence.

Assessment and investigation
Thorough history taking (from child and parents) and physical examination are essential for differentiating the type of nocturnal enuresis and directing management. Few investigations are required for children with monosymptomatic nocturnal enuresis. A urine culture to exclude UTI is recommended [109].

Management
Timing of when to seek treatment for bedwetting should be determined by the age of the child (at least 7 years), the severity of symptoms, and the child's level of concern. There are a number of Cochrane systematic reviews on the management of nocturnal enuresis (Table 65.3). First-line treatment for monosymptomatic nocturnal enuresis is the enuresis alarm, which is activated by micturition. Common alarm types include the bell and pad alarm (where a large mat is placed on the bed) and a personal alarm (which is clipped onto the child's underpants). There is insufficient evidence to draw conclusions on the relative effectiveness of the different types of alarms, but children generally prefer a personal alarm to a bell and pad alarm, and alarms using electric shock are unacceptable to children (Figure 65.4). Alarms are commonly used until 14 consecutive dry nights are achieved, with treatment beyond 16 weeks being unlikely to produce a cure [110]. Two-thirds of children become dry during alarm training (RR for failure, 0.38; 95% CI, 0.33–0.45), and one-half maintain dryness

Table 65.3 Evidence ratings and recommendations for treatment of nocturnal enuresis.

Intervention	Existing systematic reviews	Overall evidence rating			Recommendation[a]	Comments
		Moderate	Low	Comment		
Enuresis alarm vs no treatment	•	•			I	Alarms more effective than no treatment; insufficient evidence to compare different types of alarms (e.g. bed or personal alarms); alarms using electric shock not acceptable
Enuresis alarm vs desmopressin	•	•			I	Alarms and desmopressin equally effective; desmopressin more immediate effect than alarm, but alarm more prolonged effect compared with desmopressin
Overlearning with alarm training	•		•	Few studies, poor quality	II	Lower relapse rates after alarm training with overlearning
Desmopressin vs no treatment	•	•			II	Desmopressin more effective than no treatment
Tricyclics	•		•		Not recommended	Risk of significant side effects in children; treatment no longer recommended
Other drugs	•	•			III	Although some other drugs more effective than no treatment, there is insufficient evidence to recommend use of other drugs
Behavioral interventions	•		•	Few studies	II	Some simple methods such as rewards, lifting, and waking worked better than no treatment, but not as effective as alarm training; penalties reduced likelihood of success
Complementary therapies	•		•	Poor quality	III	Weak evidence to support hypnosis, psychotherapy, acupuncture, and chiropractic adjustment
Combination therapy	•		•	Few studies	II	Uncertainty whether combination therapy may be more effective than alarm alone

[a] I, recommend; II, suggest; III, evidence does not support a recommendation.

after completion of treatment compared with almost none after no treatment (RR of failure or relapse, 0.56; 95% CI, 0.46–0.68) [111]. Relapse can be halved, from about 50% to about 25%, with "overlearning" with extra bedtime fluids while continuing alarm training after initial success (RR, 1.92; 95% CI, 1.27–2.92) [112,113].

Desmopressin (an ADH analog) is a second-line therapy and is effective in 60% of children with monosymptomatic nocturnal enuresis. Desmopressin has a more immediate effect (RR, 0.71; 95% CI, 0.50–0.99) (Figure 65.5) and can be used for short-term overnight sleep-overs, but it has limited sustained effect compared with alarm training (RR, 0.27; 95% CI, 0.11–0.69) (Figure 65.6).

Although tricyclics and related drugs are effective in about 20% of cases, they are no longer recommended for the treatment of nocturnal enuresis because of their potentially serious cardiotoxic adverse effects [114,115]. In children with upper airway obstruction, treatment of the obstruction may improve nocturnal enuresis [116].

Although other therapies are often more effective than no treatment, studies comparing alarms to other therapies, including other pharmacological interventions [117], behavior interventions (such as reward systems, bladder training, lifting, and scheduled wakening) [118, 119], fluid deprivation, and complementary therapies such as hypnosis, psychotherapy, acupuncture, and chiropractic [111], were either inconclusive or showed alarm therapy to be superior. However, supplementing alarm therapy with other behavior interventions, such as dry bed training, reduced the relapse rate from 63% to 27% (RR, 2.0; 95% CI, 1.25–3.20), whereas penalties after wetting appear to reduce success [111].

For nonresponders to monotherapy with alarm or desmopressin, combination therapy with alarm and desmopressin can be tried [99]. Although combination therapy decreased the initial number of wet nights, success rates while on treatment or after treatment were not significantly different from alarm alone [111]. Antimuscarinics (oxybutynin) can be added to desmopressin in those who do not respond to monotherapy [120], although there is insufficient evidence to assess the effectiveness of this treatment.

Children with non-monosymptomatic enuresis should be treated for their daytime incontinence before addressing their nocturnal enuresis, as treatment failure rates for nocturnal enuresis

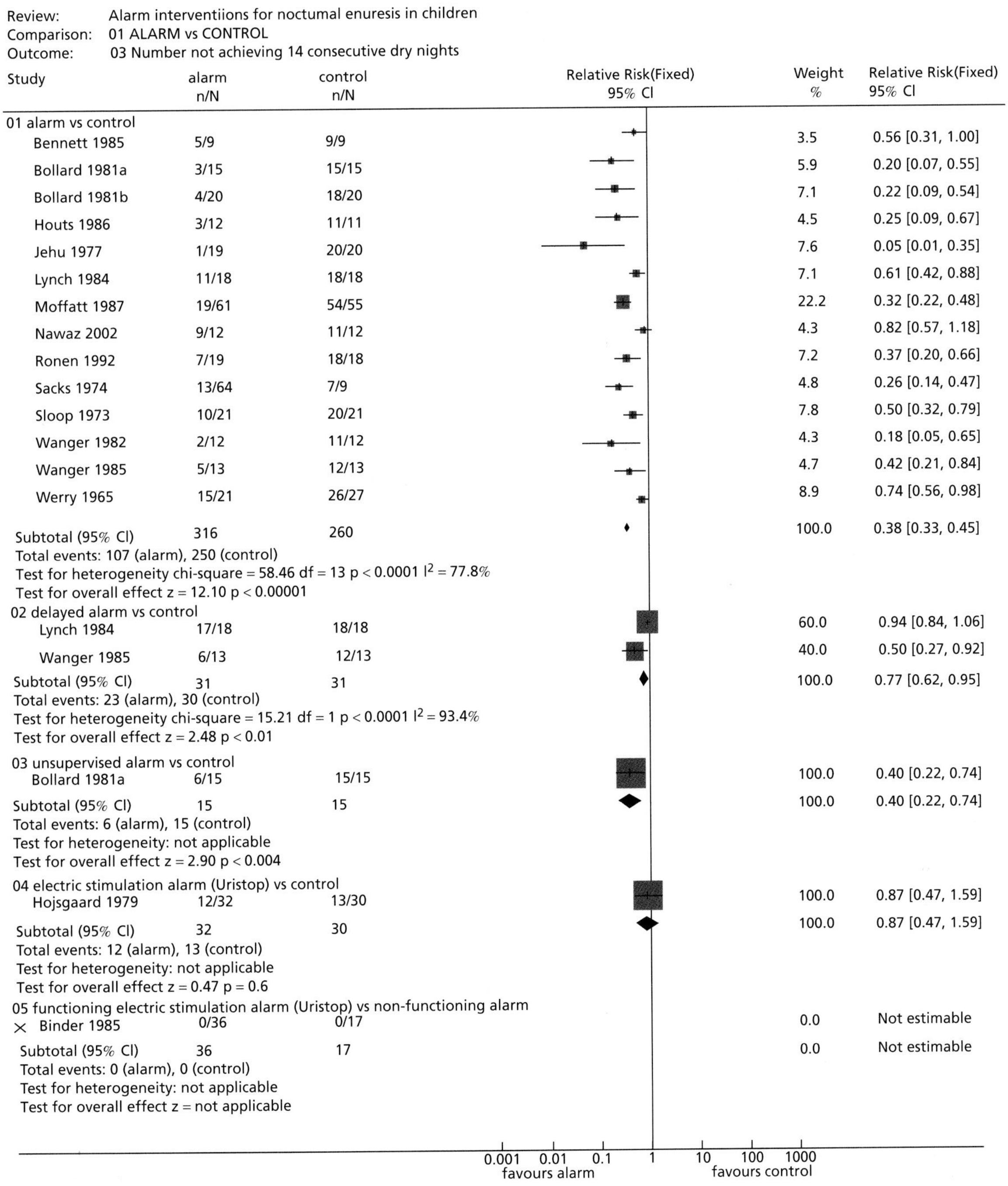

Review: Alarm interventiions for noctumal enuresis in children
Comparison: 01 ALARM vs CONTROL
Outcome: 03 Number not achieving 14 consecutive dry nights

Study	alarm n/N	control n/N	Relative Risk(Fixed) 95% CI	Weight %	Relative Risk(Fixed) 95% CI
01 alarm vs control					
Bennett 1985	5/9	9/9		3.5	0.56 [0.31, 1.00]
Bollard 1981a	3/15	15/15		5.9	0.20 [0.07, 0.55]
Bollard 1981b	4/20	18/20		7.1	0.22 [0.09, 0.54]
Houts 1986	3/12	11/11		4.5	0.25 [0.09, 0.67]
Jehu 1977	1/19	20/20		7.6	0.05 [0.01, 0.35]
Lynch 1984	11/18	18/18		7.1	0.61 [0.42, 0.88]
Moffatt 1987	19/61	54/55		22.2	0.32 [0.22, 0.48]
Nawaz 2002	9/12	11/12		4.3	0.82 [0.57, 1.18]
Ronen 1992	7/19	18/18		7.2	0.37 [0.20, 0.66]
Sacks 1974	13/64	7/9		4.8	0.26 [0.14, 0.47]
Sloop 1973	10/21	20/21		7.8	0.50 [0.32, 0.79]
Wanger 1982	2/12	11/12		4.3	0.18 [0.05, 0.65]
Wanger 1985	5/13	12/13		4.7	0.42 [0.21, 0.84]
Werry 1965	15/21	26/27		8.9	0.74 [0.56, 0.98]
Subtotal (95% CI)	316	260		100.0	0.38 [0.33, 0.45]

Total events: 107 (alarm), 250 (control)
Test for heterogeneity chi-square = 58.46 df = 13 p < 0.0001 I^2 = 77.8%
Test for overall effect z = 12.10 p < 0.00001

02 delayed alarm vs control					
Lynch 1984	17/18	18/18		60.0	0.94 [0.84, 1.06]
Wanger 1985	6/13	12/13		40.0	0.50 [0.27, 0.92]
Subtotal (95% CI)	31	31		100.0	0.77 [0.62, 0.95]

Total events: 23 (alarm), 30 (control)
Test for heterogeneity chi-square = 15.21 df = 1 p < 0.0001 I^2 = 93.4%
Test for overall effect z = 2.48 p < 0.01

03 unsupervised alarm vs control					
Bollard 1981a	6/15	15/15		100.0	0.40 [0.22, 0.74]
Subtotal (95% CI)	15	15		100.0	0.40 [0.22, 0.74]

Total events: 6 (alarm), 15 (control)
Test for heterogeneity: not applicable
Test for overall effect z = 2.90 p < 0.004

04 electric stimulation alarm (Uristop) vs control					
Hojsgaard 1979	12/32	13/30		100.0	0.87 [0.47, 1.59]
Subtotal (95% CI)	32	30		100.0	0.87 [0.47, 1.59]

Total events: 12 (alarm), 13 (control)
Test for heterogeneity: not applicable
Test for overall effect z = 0.47 p = 0.6

05 functioning electric stimuliion alarm (Uristop) vs non-functioning alarm					
✕ Binder 1985	0/36	0/17		0.0	Not estimable
Subtotal (95% CI)	36	17		0.0	Not estimable

Total events: 0 (alarm), 0 (control)
Test for heterogeneity: not applicable
Test for overall effect z = not applicable

0.001 0.01 0.1 1 10 100 1000
favours alarm   favours control

Figure 65.4 Alarm versus control for nocturnal enuresis in children.

are higher in the presence of daytime symptoms and nocturnal enuresis sometimes resolves with treatment of daytime symptoms alone [109].

Daytime urinary incontinence
Epidemiology
Daytime urinary incontinence is defined as any uncontrollable leakage of urine during the daytime [99]. Becoming continent

usually occurs between 2 and 3 years of age, with most children achieving full bladder control by the age of 4.

Prevalence
Daytime urinary incontinence is more common in girls than in boys [121–124]: 6% of girls compared to 4% of boys have at least one episode of wetting in the previous 3 months, and 2% of 7-year-old boys and 3% of 7-year-old girls wet every week [125].

Review: Desmopressin for nocturnal enuresis in children
Comparison: 01 DESMOPRESSIN VS PLACEBO
Outcome: 03 Number of wet nights per week during treatment

Study	Desmopressin N	Mean (SD)	Placebo N	Mean (SD)	Weighted Mean Difference (Fixed) 95% CI	Weight %	Weighted Mean Difference (Fixed) 95% CI
01 10 mcg vs placebo							
Aladjem 1982	15	1.52 (2.15)	17	4.40 (1.94)		62.1	−2.88 [−4.31, −1.45]
Kjoler 1984	13	2.49 (2.52)	12	3.84 (2.14)		37.9	−1.35 [−3.17, −0.47]
Subtotal (95A CI)	28		29			100.0	−2.30 [−3.42, −1.18]
Test for heterogeneity chi-square = 1.68 df = 0.20 I² = 40.4%							
Test for overall effect z = 4.01 p < 0.00006							
02 20 mcg vs placebo							
Folwell 1997#	31	3.24 (2.51)	31	4.86 (1.95)		4.3	−1.62 [−2.74, −0.50]
Janknegt 1990#	22	3.41 (2.50)	22	5.30 (1.80)		3.2	−1.90 [−3.19, −0.61]
Kjoller 1984	12	2.45 (1.84)	12	3.84 (2.13)		2.1	−1.39 [−2.98, −0.20]
Post 1983#	20	4.90 (1.92)	20	5.80 (1.14)		5.6	−0.90 [−1.88, −0.08]
Rushton 995	49	3.96 (2.37)	47	4.90 (1.64)		8.1	−0.94 [−1.75, −0.13]
Schulman 2001a	44	4.00 (1.33)	47	4.50 (1.37)		17.4	−0.50 [−1.05, −0.05]
Schulman 2001b	109	4.00 (1.57)	38	5.00 (1.54)		16.4	−1.00 [−1.57, −0.43]
Segni 1982	20	2.20 (1.34)	20	4.20 (1.79)		5.6	−2.00 [−2.98, −1.02]
Sener 1998	31	1.10 (1.39)	25	5.10 (2.00)		6.3	−4.00 [−4.92, −3.08]
Skoog 1997	33	4.00 (1.15)	36	5.00 (1.20)		17.5	−1.00 [−1.55, −0.45]
Terho 1984#	54	2.16 (2.00)	54	2.16 (1.83)		10.3	−1.86 [−2.58, −1.14]
Tuverno 1978#	18	1.60 (1.82)	18	3.97 (2.20)		3.1	−2.37 [−3.69, −1.05]
Subtotal (95% CI)	443		370			100.0	−1.34 [−1.57, −1.11]
Test for heterogeneity chi-square = 52 df = 11 p = <0.0001 I² = 78.9%							
Test for overall effect z = 11.35 p < 0.00001							
03 40 mcg vs placebo							
Janknegt 1990#	22	3.80 (2.20)	22	5.30 (1.80)		8.3	−1.50 [−2.69, −0.31]
Martin 1993	22	2.16 (2.25)	22	3.68 (2.25)		6.6	−1.52 [−2.85, −0.19]
Post 1983a#	52	3.90 (2.34)	52	5.00 (1.91)		17.3	−1.10 [−1.92, −0.28]
Schulman 2001a	48	3.50 (1.73)	47	4.50 (1.37)		29.6	−1.00 [−1.63, −0.37]
Skoog 1997	33	3.50 (1.44)	36	5.00 (1.20)		29.5	−1.50 [−2.13, −0.87]
Yap 1998#	34	2.50 (2.70)	34	4.50 (2.10)		8.8	−2.00 [−3.15, −0.85]
Subtotal (95% CI)	211		213			100.0	−1.33 [−1.67, −0.99]
Test for heterogeneity chi-square = 3.11 df = 5 p = 0.68 I² = 0.0%							
Test for overall effect z = 7.63 p < 0.00001							
04 60 mcg vs placebo							
Schulman 2001a	48	3.00 (1.73)	47	4.50 (1.37)		43.9	−1.50 [−2.13, −0.87]
Skoog 1997	33	3.50 (1.15)	36	5.00 (1.20)		56.1	−1.50 [−2.05, −0.95]
Subtotal (95% CI)	81		83			100.0	−1.50 [−1.92, −1.08]
Test for heterogeneity chi-square = 0.00 df = 1 p < 1.00 I² = 0.0%							
Test for overall effect z = 7.08 p < 0.00001							
05 combined close vs placebo							
Brikasova 1978#	22	2.10 (2.25)	22	5.50 (2.20)		100.0	−3.40 [−4.71, −2.09]
Subtotal (95% CI)	22		22			100.0	−3.40 [−4.71, −2.09]
Test for heterogeneity: not applicable							
Test for overall effect z = 5.07 p < 0.00001							
06 dose titration vs placebo							
Rushton 995	49	3.77 (2.52)	47	4.90 (1.82)		32.1	−1.13 [−2.01, −0.25]
Schulman 2001b	99	3.20 (1.69)	36	5.00 (1.54)		67.9	−1.80 [−2.40, −1.20]
Subtotal (95% CI)	148		83			100.0	−1.58 [−2.08, −1.09]
Test for heterogeneity chi-square = 1.52 df = 1 p = 0.22 I² = 34.3%							
Test for overall effect z = 6.25 p < 0.00001							

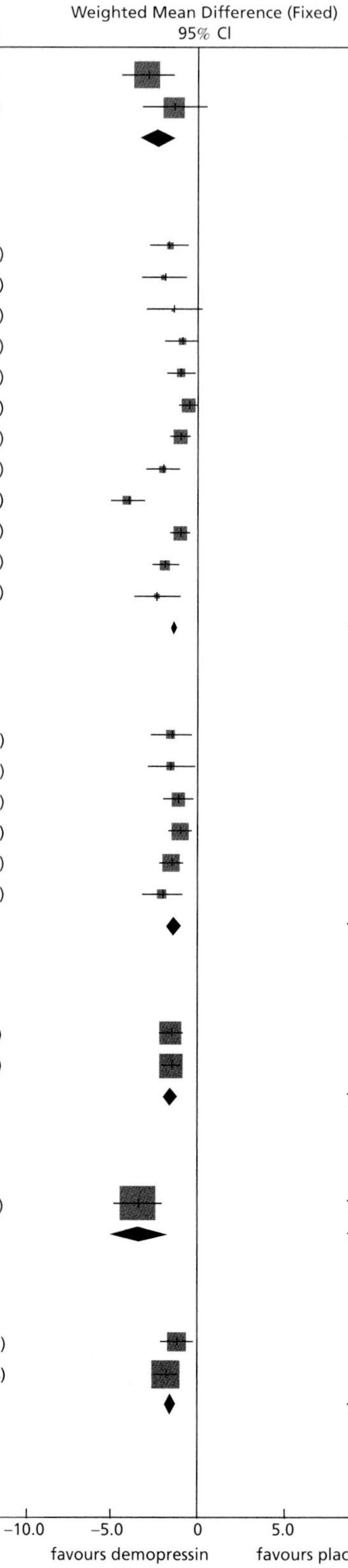

−10.0 −5.0 0 5.0 10.0
favours demopressin   favours placebo

Figure 65.5 Desmopressin versus placebo for nocturnal enuresis in children.

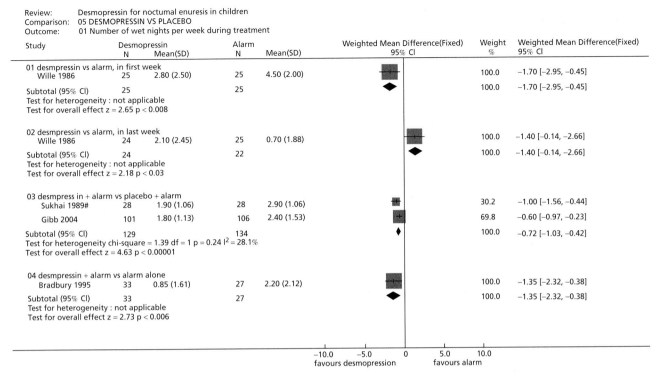

Review: Desmopressin for noctumal enuresis in children
Comparison: 05 DESMOPRESSIN VS PLACEBO
Outcome: 01 Number of wet nights per week during treatment

Figure 65.6 Alarm versus desmopressin for nocturnal enuresis in children.

Daytime urinary incontinence has been reported in 7% of boys and 17% of girls in the 11- to 12-years age group, a difference that is statistically significant [123]. The majority of these children wet occasionally.

Risk factors

In most children the cause(s) for their daytime urinary continence is unknown. Daytime urinary incontinence is commonly associated with other symptoms of bladder dysfunction (urgency, frequency, squatting to prevent incontinence, or incomplete bladder emptying), with constipation, fecal soiling, attention deficit hyperactivity disorder, and with UTI. From cross-sectional data, likely risk factors for daytime incontinence are family history of daytime incontinence, especially in the male lineage [126], low birth weight [127], developmental delay [127], a frightening or emotional stressful event [126], and psychiatric disorders [128]. One such study found that family history and emotional stressors accounted for up to 60% of the attributable risk for daytime incontinence in multivariate analysis [126]. None of these studies had a longitudinal component, so determining causality is difficult.

Natural history

Little is known about the natural history of daytime incontinence, and more prospective longitudinal studies are necessary. One study reported that daytime urinary incontinence decreased with age when children from 5 to 9 years of age were followed [129]. A study

of 1176 healthy adolescent school children assessed the prevalence of daytime urinary incontinence at two ages, 11–12 years and 15–16 years [130]. This study reported prevalence rates of daytime urinary incontinence of 12% at 11–12 years and 3% at 15–16 years. A Swedish cohort study reported that the point prevalence of daytime urinary incontinence decreased in girls from 6% at age 7 to 4% at age 17 [131].

Assessment

According to the recommendations of the International Children's Continence Society [99], initial assessment of daytime incontinence should include history taking, physical examination, and urinalysis to detect anatomical or neurological abnormalities, UTI, and diabetes mellitus. Noninvasive diagnostic investigations involve a frequency volume chart, which gives a detailed recording of fluid intake and urine output over a 24-h period, a 12-h pad test, which evaluates the quantity of urine lost, plain X-ray of the abdomen to quantify the grade of constipation, assessment of urinary flow patterns, and ultrasound of the upper and lower urinary tracts. Ultrasound of the urinary tract is an important noninvasive test to identify children who have renal tract abnormalities, residual urine, or thickening of the bladder wall. Based on the results of these tests, other invasive procedures, such as VCUG, urodynamics, renal scans, or intravenous urography or cystourethroscopy, may be required. Urodynamic investigations are invasive and usually performed on children who do not respond to conservative treatments, such as bladder training, education about how and

Table 65.4 Evidence rating and recommendations for treatment of daytime urinary incontinence.

Intervention	Existing systematic reviews	Overall evidence rating		Comment	Recommendation[a]	Comments
		Moderate	Low			
Bladder training	None	•		No available RCT	I	Noninvasive technique that offers effective first-line treatment and is less costly
Oxybutynin vs biofeedback	1	•		1 RCT	II	Adequately powered trial required to reveal effectiveness of intervention
Oxybutynin vs placebo	1	•		1 RCT	II	Adequately powered trial required to reveal effectiveness of intervention
Imipramine vs placebo	1	•		1 RCT	Not recommended	Historical interest only due to its side effects
Terodiline vs placebo	1	•		2 RCTs	Not recommended	Withdrawn due to serious cardiac side effects, hence historical interest only
Tolterodine vs placebo	None	•		2 large RCTs; limited evidence in children; reduction in wetting episodes and fewer side effects noted compared to oxybutynin	II	2 large RCTs did not show a difference in efficacy between the two treatment arms
Biofeedback vs standard therapy	1	•		1 RCT	II	Adequately powered trial required to reveal effectiveness of intervention
Electrical stimulation	None	•		Insufficient data available	II	Controlled trials needed to test efficacy of this treatment
Alarm treatment	1	•		1 RCT comparing contingent and with a noncontingent alarm	II	Adequately powered trial required; with current evidence does not appear useful for daytime incontinence

[a] I, recommend; II, suggest, III, evidence does not support a recommendation.

when to void, treatment of constipation, and management of UTI.

Management of daytime urinary incontinence

Bladder training is the first-line therapy for the management of daytime urinary incontinence, but the evidence about the efficacy of this treatment is variable [99]. Bladder training is a behavior therapy in which rehabilitation of the bladder and pelvic floor muscles is applied using different modalities, such as explanation and instructions for timed toileting [99]. When conservative treatment is not successful, more active treatments, including pharmacotherapy, pelvic floor muscle relaxation techniques, biofeedback, and electrical stimulation, are introduced.

Pharmacotherapy involves the use of antimuscarinics, which reduce detrusor overactivity. Oxybutynin has been shown to reduce daytime incontinence in uncontrolled studies. The randomized controlled study that compared oxybutynin with biofeedback and placebo did not show any decrease in the proportion of children with no improvement in the frequency of daytime incontinence after either biofeedback or oxybutynin treatment [132]. Side effects (headache, blurred vision, constipation, dry mouth, flushed cheeks, and incomplete bladder emptying) limit adherence. Other commonly used antimuscarinics include propantheline bromide and tolterodine. Recent studies, including two large randomized controlled studies, have shown that tolterodine is safe in children and has fewer side effects than oxybutynin [133,134]. Other drug therapies include imipramine and terodiline. The results of the imipramine trial showed that there was no significant increase in maximum functional bladder capacity [135]. Although the two terodiline trials [136,137] showed a small decrease (0.5–0.8) in the frequency of daily incontinent episodes compared with placebo, it is no longer used due to serious cardiac side effects. Table 65.4 summarizes the evidence for management of daytime urinary incontinence.

Several other interventions have been inadequately evaluated to allow recommendation. One randomized clinical trial evaluated the use of a contingent alarm (sounded when the children wet) versus a noncontingent alarm (sounded at intermittent intervals) and showed no difference in the proportion of children with persistent daytime wetting in the two alarm groups (RR, 0.67; 95% CI, 0.29–1.56) [138]. Many uncontrolled studies suggest that biofeedback using electromyograms may be a useful treatment for daytime urinary incontinence [139,140]. Similarly, oxybutynin with biofeedback may also be a useful intervention [141]. Neuromuscular electrical stimulation is an invasive, experimental treatment modality and can be used to stimulate the pelvic floor or the detrusor muscle [142,143].

Conclusions

UTI, VUR, nocturnal enuresis, and daytime incontinence are common problems in pediatric patients. Diagnosis and management can be controversial and difficult. Evidence supporting clinical practice is frequently suboptimal in quality or absent, and clinicians increasingly require critical appraisal skills to determine what evidence should be utilized and which should be ignored.

References

1 Verrier JK, Asscher AW, Verrier Jones ER, Mattholie K, Leach K, Thomson GM. Glomerular filtration rate in schoolgirls with covert bacteriuria. *Br Med J Clin Res Ed* 1982; **285**: 1307–1310.

2 Cardiff-Oxford Bacteriuria Study Group. Sequelae of covert bacteriuria in schoolgirls. *Lancet* 1978; **i**: 889–893.

3 Al-Orifi F, McGillivray D, Tange S, Kramer MS. Urine culture from bag specimens in young children: are the risks too high? *J Pediatr* 2000; **137**: 221–226.

4 Whiting P, Westwood M, Watt I, Cooper J, Kleijnen J. Rapid tests and urine sampling techniques for the diagnosis of urinary tract infection (UTI) in children under five years: a systematic review. *BMC Pediatr* 2005; **5**: 4.

5 Hellstrom A, Hanson E, Hansson S, Hjalmas K, Jodal U. Association between urinary symptoms at 7 years old and previous urinary tract infection. *Arch Dis Child* 1991; **66**: 232–234.

6 Slater M, Krug SE. Evaluation of the infant with fever without source: an evidence based approach. *Emergency Med Clin North Am* 1999; **17**: 97–126.

7 Trainor JL, Hampers LC, Krug SE, Listernick R. Children with first-time simple febrile seizures are at low risk of serious bacterial illness. *Acad Emergency Med* 2001; **8**: 781–787.

8 Hoberman A, Chao HP, Keller DM, Hickey R, Davis HW, Ellis D. Prevalence of urinary tract infection in febrile infants. *J Pediatr* 1993; **123**: 17–23.

9 Wiswell TE, Roscelli JD. Corroborative evidence for the decreased incidence of urinary tract infections in circumcised male infants. *Pediatrics* 1986; **78**: 96–99.

10 Fussell EN, Kaack MB, Cherry R, Roberts JA. Adherence of bacteria to human foreskins. *J Urol* 1988; **140**: 997–1001.

11 Roberts JA. Factors predisposing to urinary tract infections in children. *Pediatr Nephrol* 1996; **10**: 517–522.

12 Cox CE, Hinman EJ. Experiments with induced bacteriuria, vesical emptying and bacterial growth on the mechanism of bladder defense to infection. *J Urol* 1961; **86**: 739–748.

13 Lichodziejewska-Niemierko M, Topley N, Smith C, Verrier-Jones K, Williams JD. P1 blood group phenotype, secretor status in patients with urinary tract infections. *Clin Nephrol* 1995; **44**: 376–379.

14 Jantausch BA, Criss VR, O'Donnell R, Wiedermann BL, Majd M, Rushton *et al.* Association of Lewis blood group phenotypes with urinary tract infection in children. *J Pediatr* 1994; **124**: 863–868.

15 Albarus MH, Salzano FM, Goldraich NP. Genetic markers and acute febrile urinary tract infection in the 1st year of life. *Pediatr Nephrol* 1997; **11**: 691–694.

16 Winberg J, Bollgren I, Jacobson S, Kallenius G, Mollby R, Roberts JA *et al.* Host-bacteria interactions in the pathogenesis of urinary tract infections. *Acta Paediatr Jpn* 1986; **28**: 129–147.

17 Panaretto K, Craig JC, Knight JF, Howman-Giles R, Sureshkumar P, Roy LP. Risk factors for recurrent urinary tract infection in preschool children. *J Paediatr Child Health* 1999; **35**: 454–459.

18 Travis LB, Brouhard BH. *Infections of the urinary tract.* Prentice Hall International, Stamford, CT, 1996.

19 Hsiao AL, Chen L, Baker D. Incidence and predictors of serious bacterial infections among 57–180 day old infants. *Pediatrics* 2006; **117**: 1695.

20 Pantell RH, Newman TB, Bernzweig J, Bergman DA, Takayama JI, Segal M *et al.* Management and outcomes of care of fever in early infancy. *JAMA* 2004; **291**: 1203–1212.

21 Navarro M, Espinosa L, de las Heras JA, Garcia Meseguer MC, Pena MC, Larrauri M. Symptomatic urinary infection in infants less than 4 months old: outcome in 129 cases. *An Esp Peditr* 1984; **21**: 564–572.

22 Garcia FJ, Nager AL. Jaundice as an early diagnostic sign of urinary tract infection in infancy. *Pediatrics* 2002; **109**: 846–851.

23 Bloomfield P, Hodson EM, Craig JC. Antibiotics for acute pyelonephritis in children. *Cochrane Database Syst Rev* 2003; **3**: CD003772. (Updated in *Cochrane Database Syst Rev* 2005; **1**: CD003772.)

24 Keren R, Chan E. A meta-analysis of randomized, controlled trials comparing short- and long-course antibiotic therapy for urinary tract infections in children. *Pediatrics* 2002; **109**: E70.

25 Michael M, Hodson EM, Craig JC, Martin S, Moyer VA. Short versus standard duration oral antibiotic therapy for acute urinary tract infection in children. *Cochrane Database Syst Rev* 2003; **1**: CD003966.

26 Tran D, Muchant DG, Aronoff SC. Short-course versus conventional length antimicrobial therapy for uncomplicated lower urinary tract infections in children: a meta-analysis of 1279 patients. *J Pediatr* 2001; **139**: 93–99.

27 Williams GJ, Lee A, Craig JC. Long-term antibiotics for preventing recurrent urinary tract infection in children. *Cochrane Database Syst Rev* 2006; **3**: CD001534.

28 Savage DC, Howie G, Adler K, Wilson MI. Controlled trial of therapy in covert bacteriuria of childhood. *Lancet* 1975; **i**: 358–361.

29 Lohr JA, Nunley DH, Howards SS, Ford RF. Prevention of recurrent urinary tract infections in girls. *Pediatrics* 1977; **59**: 562–565.

30 Stansfeld JM. Duration of treatment for urinary tract infections in children. *Br Med J* 1975; **3**: 65–66.

31 Smellie JM, Katz G, Gruneberg RN. Controlled trial of prophylactic treatment in childhood urinary tract infection. *Lancet* 1978; **ii**: 175–178.

32 Montini G, Rigon L, Gobber D, Zucchetta P, Murer L, Calderan A *et al.* A randomised controlled trial of antibiotic prophylaxis in children with a previous documented pyelonephritis. *Pediatr Nephrol* 2004; **19(9)**: 70.

33 Carlsen NL, Hesselbjerg U, Glenting P. Comparison of long-term, low-dose pivmecillinam and nitrofurantoin in the control of recurrent urinary tract infection in children. An open, randomized, cross-over study. *J Antimicrob Chemother* 1985; **16**: 509–517.

34 Brendstrup L, Hjelt K, Petersen KE, Petersen S, Andersen EA, Daugbjerg PS *et al.* Nitrofurantoin versus trimethoprim prophylaxis in recurrent

urinary tract infection in children. A randomized, double-blind study. *Acta Paediatr Scand* 1990; **79**: 1225–1234.

35 Lettgen B, Troster K. Prophylaxis of recurrent urinary tract infections in children. Results of an open, controlled, randomised study about the efficacy and tolerance of cefixime compared to nitrofurantoin. *Klin Padiatrie* 2002; **214**: 353–358.

36 Jepson RG, Mihaljevic L, Craig J. Cranberries for preventing urinary tract infections. *Cochrane Database Syst Rev* 2004; **1**: CD001321. (update of *Cochrane Database Syst Rev* 2004; **1**: CD001321.)

37 Bauer HW, Rahlfs VW, Lauener PA, Blessmann GS. Prevention of recurrent urinary tract infections with immuno-active E. coli fractions: a meta-analysis of five placebo-controlled double-blind studies. *Int J Antimicrob Agents* 2002; **19**: 451–456.

38 Dani C, Biadaioli R, Bertini G, Martelli E, Rubaltelli FF. Probiotics feeding in prevention of urinary tract infection, bacterial sepsis and necrotizing enterocolitis in preterm infants: a prospective double-blind study. *Biol Neonate* 2002; **82(2)**: 103–108.

39 Singh-Grewal D, Macdessi J, Craig JC. Circumcision for the prevention of urinary tract infection in boys: a systematic review of randomised trials and observational studies. *Arch Dis Child* 2005; **90**: 853–858.

40 American Academy of Pediatrics, Committee on Quality Improvement, Subcommittee on Urinary Tract Infection. Practice parameter: the diagnosis, treatment, and evaluation of the initial urinary tract infection in febrile infants and young children *Pediatrics* 1999; **103(4)**: 843–852

41 Guidelines for the management of acute urinary tract infection in childhood. Report of a Working Group of the Research Unit, Royal College of Physicians. *J R Coll Physicians Lond* 1991; **25**: 36–42.

42 Westwood ME, Whiting PF, Cooper J, Watt IS, Kleijnen J. Further investigation of confirmed urinary tract infection (UTI) in children under five years: a systematic review. *BMC Pediatr* 2005; **5**: 2.

43 Williams G, Sureshkumar P, Chan S, Macaskill P, Craig JC. Ordering of renal tract imaging by pediatricians after urinary tract infection. *J Paediatr Child Health* 2007; **43**: 271–279.

44 Lebowitz RL, Olbing H, Parkkulainen KV, Smellie JM, Tamminen-Mobius TE. International system of radiographic grading of vesicoureteric reflux. International Reflux Study in Children. *Pediatr Radiol* 1985; **15(2)**: 105–109.

45 Craig JC, Irwig LM, Knight JF, Sureshkumar P, Roy LP. Symptomatic urinary tract infection in preschool Australian children. *J Paediatr Child Health* 1998; **34(2)**: 154–159.

46 Chand DH, Rhoades T, Poe SA, Kraus S, Strife CF. Incidence and severity of vesicoureteral reflux in children related to age, gender, race and diagnosis. *J Urol* 2003; **170**: 1548–1550.

47 Cleper R, Krause I, Eisenstein B, Davidovits M. Prevalence of vesicoureteral reflux in neonatal urinary tract infection. *Clin Pediatr* (Philadelphia) 2004; **43**: 619–625.

48 Siegel SR, Siegel B, Sokoloff BZ, Kanter MH. Urinary infection in infants and preschool children. Five-year follow-up. *Am J Dis Child* 1980; **134(4)**: 369–372.

49 Eccles MR, Jacobs GH. The genetics of primary vesico-ureteral reflux. *Ann Acad Med Singapore* 2000; **29(3)**: 337–345.

50 Mak RH, Kuo HJ. Primary ureteral reflux: emerging insights from molecular and genetic studies. *Curr Opin Pediat* 2003; **15**: 181–185.

51 Lama G, Russo M, De Rosa E, Mansi L, Piscitelli A, Luongo I *et al.* Primary vesicoureteric reflux and renal damage in the first year of life. *Pediatr Nephrol* 2000; **15**: 205–210.

52 Hassan JM, Pope JC, Brock JW, III, Adams MC. Vesicoureteral reflux in patients with posterior urethral valves. *J Urol* 2003; **170(4 Pt 2)**: 1677–1680.

53 Kass EJ, Koff SA. The management of vesicoureteral reflux in children with neurogenic bladders. *Zeitschrift Kinderchirurgie* 1981; **34(4)**: 379–383.

54 Puri P, Kumar R. Endoscopic correction of vesicoureteral reflux secondary to posterior urethral valves. *J Urol* 1996; **156(2 Pt 2)**: 680–682.

55 Upadhyay J, Bolduc S, Braga L, Farhat W, Bagli DJ, McLorie GA *et al.* Impact of prenatal diagnosis on the morbidity associated with ureterocele management. *J Urol* 2002; **167(6)**: 2560–2565.

56 Ahmed S. Vesico-ureteric reflux in Down's syndrome: poor prognosis. *Aust N Z J Surg* 1990; **60(2)**: 113–116.

57 Chou IC, Tsai FJ, Yu MT, Tsai CH. Smith-Magenis syndrome with bilateral vesicoureteral reflux: a case report. *J Formosan Med Assoc* 2002; **101(10)**: 726–728.

58 Grisaru S, Ramage IJ, Rosenblum ND. Vesicoureteric reflux associated with renal dysplasia in the Wolf-Hirschhorn syndrome. *Pediatr Nephrol* 2000; **14(2)**: 146–148.

59 Yildizdas D, Antmen B, Bayram I, Yapicioglu H. Klippel-Trenaunay-Weber syndrome with hydronephrosis and vesicoureteral reflux: an unusual association. *Turk J Pediatr* 2002; **44(2)**: 180–182.

60 Ichikawa I, Kuwayama F, Pope JC, Stephens FD, Miyazaki Y. Paradigm shift from classic anatomic theories to contemporary cell biological views of CAKUT. *Kidney Int* 2002; **61(3)**: 889–898.

61 Miyazaki Y, Ichikawa I. Ontogeny of congenital anomalies of the kidney and urinary tract, CAKUT. *Pediatr Int* 2003; **45**: 598–604.

62 Godley ML, Desai D, Yeung CK, Dhillon HK, Duffy PG, Ransley PG. The relationship between early renal status, and the resolution of vesicoureteric reflux and bladder function at 16 months. *BJU Int* 2001; **87(6)**: 457–462.

63 Smellie JM, Prescod NP, Shaw PJ, Risdon RA, Bryant TN. Childhood reflux and urinary infection: a follow-up of 10–41 years in 226 adults. *Pediatr Nephrol* 1998; **12(9)**: 727–736.

64 Goonasekera CD, Shah V, Wade AM, Barratt TM, Dillon MJ. 15-year follow-up of renin and blood pressure in reflux nephropathy. *Lancet* 1996; **347(9002)**: 640–643.

65 Gordon I, Barkovics M, Pindoria S, Cole TJ, Woolf AS. Primary vesicoureteric reflux as a predictor of renal damage in children hospitalized with urinary tract infection: a systematic review and meta-analysis. *J Am Soc Nephrol* 2003; **14(3)**: 739–744.

66 Hampel N, Levin DR, Gersh I. Bilateral vesico-ureteral reflux with pyelonephritis in identical twins. *Br J Urol* 1975; **47(5)**: 535–537.

67 Noe HN, Wyatt RJ, Peeden JN, Jr., Rivas ML. The transmission of vesicoureteral reflux from parent to child. *J Urol* 1992; **148**: 1869–1871.

68 Fried K, Yuval E, Eidelman A, Beer S. Familial primary vesicoureteral reflux. *Clin Genet* 1975; **7**: 144–147.

69 Connolly LP, Treves ST, Connolly SA, Zurakowski D, Share JC, Bar-Sever Z *et al.* Vesicoureteral reflux in children: incidence and severity in siblings. *J Urol* 1997; **157(6)**: 2287–2290.

70 Wan J, Greenfield SP, Ng M, Zerin M, Ritchey ML, Bloom D. Sibling reflux: a dual center retrospective study. *J Urol* 1996; **156(2 Pt 2)**: 677–679.

71 Kaefer M, Curran M, Treves ST, Bauer S, Hendren WH, Peters CA *et al.* Sibling vesicoureteral reflux in multiple gestation births. *Pediatrics* 2000; **105(4 Pt 1)**: 800–804.

72 Noe HN. The long-term results of prospective sibling reflux screening. *J Urol* 1992; **148**: 1739–1742.

73 Devriendt K, Groenen P, Van Esch H, van Dijck M, Van de Ven W, Fryns JP *et al.* Vesico-ureteral reflux: a genetic condition? *Eur J Pediatr* 1998; **157**: 265–271.

74 Chapman CJ, Bailey RR, Janus ED, Abbott GD, Lynn KL. Vesicoureteric reflux: segregation analysis. *Am J Med Genet* 1985; **20**: 577–584.

75 Malaga S, Santos F, Nuno F, Fernandez TJ, Matesanz JL, Crespo M. Familial vesicoureteral reflux. *An Esp Pediatr* 1979; **12**: 493–500.

76 Lewy PR, Belman AB. Familial occurrence of nonobstructive, noninfectious vesicoureteral reflux with renal scarring. *J Pediatr* 1975; **86**: 851–856.

77 Frye RN, Patel HR, Parsons V. Familial renal tract abnormalities and cortical scarring. *Nephron* 1974; **12(3)**: 188–196.

78 Middleton GW, Howards SS, Gillenwater JY. Sex-linked familial reflux. *J Urol* 1975; **114(1)**: 36–39.

79 Tobenkin MI. Hereditary vesicoureteric reflux. *South Med J* 1964; **57**: 139–147.

80 Feather SA, Malcolm S, Woolf AS, Wright V, Blaydon D, Reid CJ *et al.* Primary, nonsyndromic vesicoureteric reflux and its nephropathy is genetically heterogeneous, with a locus on chromosome 1. *Am J Hum Genet* 2000; **66(4)**: 1420–1425.

81 Heale WF. Hereditary vesicoureteric reflux: phenotypic variation and family screening. *Pediatr Nephrol* 1997; **11**: 504–507.

82 Ismaili K, Hall M, Piepsz A, Wissing KM, Collier F, Schulman C *et al.* Primary vesicoureteral reflux detected in neonates with a history of fetal renal pelvis dilatation: a prospective clinical and imaging study. *J Pediatr* 2006; **148**: 7.

83 Lim DM, Park J-Y, Kim JH, Paick SH, Oh S-J, Choi H. Clinical characteristics and outcomes of hydronephrosis detected by prenatal ultrasonography. *J Korean Med Sci* 2003; **18**: 859–862.

84 Hiraoka M, Kasuga K, Hori C, Sudo M. Ultrasonic indicators of ureteric reflux in the newborn. *Lancet* 1994; **343**: 519–520.

85 Chertin B, Puri P. Familial vesicoureteral reflux. *J Urol* 2003; **169**: 1804–1808.

86 Craig JC, Irwig LM, Knight JF, Roy LP. Does treatment of vesicoureteric reflux in childhood prevent end-stage renal disease attributable to reflux nephropathy? *Pediatrics* 2000; **105(6)**: 1236–1241.

87 Fenton S, Desmeules M, Copleston P, Arbus G, Froment D, Jeffery J *et al.* Renal replacement therapy in Canada: a report from the Canadian Organ Replacement Register. *Am J Kidney Dis* 1995; **25(1)**: 134–150.

88 Broyer M, Chantler C, Donckerwolcke R, Ehrich JH, Rizzoni G, Scharer K. The paediatric registry of the European Dialysis and Transplant Association: 20 years' experience. *Pediatr Nephrol* 1993; **7(6)**: 758–768.

89 Gusmano R, Perfumo F. Worldwide demographic aspects of chronic renal failure in children. *Kidney Int Suppl* 1993; **41**: S31–S35.

90 Incidence and prevalence of ESRD. *Am J Kidney Dis* 1999; **34(2 Suppl 1)**: S40–S50.

91 Wheeler D, Vimalachandra D, Hodson EM, Roy LP, Smith G, Craig JC. Antibiotics and surgery for vesicoureteric reflux: a meta-analysis of randomised controlled trials. *Arch Dis Child* 2003; **88**: 688–694.

92 Reddy PP, Evans MT, Hughes PA, Dangman B, Cooper J, Lepow ML *et al.* Antimicrobial prophylaxis in children with vesico-ureteral reflux: a randomized prospective study of continuous therapy vs intermittent therapy vs surveillance. *Pediatrics* 1997; **100(Suppl)**: 555–556.

93 Garin EH, Olavarria F, Garcia Nieto V, Valenciano B, Campos A, Young L. Clinical significance of primary vesicoureteralreflux and urinary antibiotic prophylaxis after acute pyelonephritis: a multicenter, randomized, controlled study. *Pediatrics* 2006; **117**: 626–632.

94 Jodal U, Smellie JM, Lax H, Hoyer PF. Ten-year results of randomised treatment of children with severe vesicoureteral reflux. Final report of the International Reflux Study in Children. *Pediatr Nephrol* 2006; **21**: 785–792.

95 Elder JS, Diaz M, Caldamone AA, Cendron M, Greenfield SP, Hurwitz R *et al.* Endoscopic therapy for vesicoureteral reflux: a meta-analysis. I. Reflux resolution and urinary tract infection. *J Urol* 2006; **175**: 716–722.

96 Pichot P. DSM-III: the 3rd edition of the Diagnostic and Statistical Manual of Mental Disorders from the American Psychiatric Association. *Rev Neurol* (Paris) 1986; **142(5)**: 489–499.

97 Bower WF, Moore KH, Shepherd RB, Adams RD. The epidemiology of childhood enuresis in Australia. *Br J Urol* 1996; **78(4)**: 602–606.

98 Hunskaar S, Burgio K, Diokno A, Herzog AR, Hjalmas K, Lapitan MC. Epidemiology and natural history of urinary incontinence in women. *Urology* 2003; **62(4 Suppl 1)**: 16–23.

99 Nijman RJM, Butler R, Van Gool J, Yeung CK, Bauer W, Hjalmas K. Conservative management of urinary incontinence in childhood. In: Abrams P, Cardozo L, Khoury S, Wein A, editors. *Incontinence.* Health Publication Ltd., Paris, 2002; 513–551.

100 Norgaard JP, van Gool JD, Hjalmas K, Djurhuus JC, Hellstrom AL. Standardization and definitions in lower urinary tract dysfunction in children. International Children's Continence Society. *Br J Urol* 1998; **81(Suppl 3)**: 1–16.

101 Rittig S, Knudsen UB, Norgaard JP, Pedersen EB, Djurhuus JC. Abnormal diurnal rhythm of plasma vasopressin and urinary output in patients with enuresis. *Am J Physiol* 1989; **256(4 Pt 2)**: F664–F671.

102 Kawauchi A, Imada N, Tanaka Y, Minami M, Watanabe H, Shirakawa S. Changes in the structure of sleep spindles and delta waves on electroencephalography in patients with nocturnal enuresis. *Br J Urol* 1998; **819(Suppl 3)**: 72–75.

103 Yeung CK, Sit FK, To LK, Chiu HN, Sihoe JD, Lee E *et al.* Reduction in nocturnal functional bladder capacity is a common factor in the pathogenesis of refractory nocturnal enuresis. *BJU Int* 2002; **90(3)**: 302–307.

104 Weider DJ, Hauri PJ. Nocturnal enuresis in children with upper airway obstruction. *Int J Pediatr Otorhinolaryngol* 1985; **9(2)**: 173–182.

105 Brooks LJ, Topol HI. Enuresis in children with sleep apnea. *J Pediatr* 2003; **142(5)**: 515–518.

106 O'Regan S, Yazbeck S, Hamberger B, Schick E. Constipation, a commonly unrecognized cause of enuresis. *Am J Dis Child* 1986; **140(3)**: 260–261.

107 Duel BP, Steinberg-Epstein R, Hill M, Lerner M. A survey of voiding dysfunction in children with attention deficit-hyperactivity disorder. *J Urol* 2003; **170(4 Pt 2)**: 1521–1523.

108 Jarvelin MR. Developmental history and neurological findings in enuretic children. *Dev Med Child Neurol* 1989; **31(6)**: 728–736.

109 Hjalmas K, Arnold T, Bower W, Caione P, Chiozza LM, von Gontard A *et al.* Nocturnal enuresis: an international evidence based management strategy. *J Urol* 2004; **171(6 Pt 2)**: 2545–2561.

110 Forsythe WI, Redmond A. Enuresis and the electric alarm: study of 200 cases. *Br Med J* 1970; **1(690)**: 211–213.

111 Glazener CM, Evans JH, Cheuk DK. Complementary and miscellaneous interventions for nocturnal enuresis in children. *Cochrane Database Syst Rev* 2005; **2**: CD005230.

112 Taylor PD, Turner RK. A clinical trial of continuous, intermittent and overlearning 'bell and pad' treatments for nocturnal enuresis. *Behav Res Ther* 1975; **13(4)**: 281–293.

113 Young GC, Morgan RT. Overlearning in the conditioning treatment of enuresis: a long-term follow-up study. *Behav Res Ther* 1972; **10(4)**: 419–420.

114 Moulden A. Management of bedwetting. *Aust Family Physician* 2002; **31(2)**: 161–163.

115 Glazener CM, Evans JH, Peto RE. Tricyclic and related drugs for nocturnal enuresis in children. *Cochrane Database Syst Rev* 2003; **3**: CD002117.

116 Weider DJ, Hauri PJ. Nocturnal enuresis in children with upper airway obstruction. *Int J Pediatr Otorhinolaryngol* 1985; **9(2)**: 173–182.

117 Glazener CM, Evans JH. Drugs for nocturnal enuresis in children (other than desmopressin and tricyclics). *Cochrane Database Syst Rev* 2000; **3**: CD002238. (Updated in *Cochrane Database Syst Rev* 2003; **4**: CD002238.)

118 Glazener CM, Evans JH. Simple behavioural and physical interventions for nocturnal enuresis in children. *Cochrane Database Syst Rev* 2002; **2**: CD003637.

119 Glazener CM, Evans JH, Peto RE. Complex behavioural and educational interventions for nocturnal enuresis in children. *Cochrane Database Syst Rev* 2004; **1**: CD004668.

120 Radvanska E, Kovacs L, Rittig S. The role of bladder capacity in antidiuretic and anticholinergic treatment for nocturnal enuresis. *J Urol* 2006; **176(2)**: 764–769.

121 Bakker E, van Sprundel M, van der Auwera JC, van Gool JD, Wyndaele JJ. Voiding habits and wetting in a population of 4,332 Belgian schoolchildren aged between 10 and 14 years. *Scand J Urol Nephrol* 2002; **36(5)**: 354–362.

122 Lee SD, Sohn DW, Lee JZ, Park NC, Chung MK. An epidemiological study of enuresis in Korean children. *BJU Int* 2000; **85(7)**: 869–873.

123 Swithinbank LV, Carr JC, Abrams PH. Longitudinal study of urinary symptoms in children. Longitudinal study of urinary symptoms and incontinence in local schoolchildren. *Scand J Urol Nephrol Suppl* 1994; **163**: 67–73.

124 Meadow SR. Day wetting. *Pediatr Nephrol* 1990; **4(2)**: 178–184.

125 Hellstrom A-L, Hanson E, Hansson S, Hjalmas K, Jodal U. Micturition habits and incontinence in 7-year-old Swedish school entrants. *Eur J Pediatr* 1990; **149(6)**: 437.

126 Sureshkumar P, Craig JC, Roy LP, Knight JF. Daytime urinary incontinence in primary school children: a population-based survey. *J Pediatr* 2000; **137(6)**: 814–818.

127 Jarvelin MR, Vikevainen-Tervonen I, Moilanen I, Hutteunen NP. Enuresis in seven-year-old children. *Acta Paediatr Scand* 1988; **77**: 148–153.

128 Kodman-Jones C, Hawkins L, Schulman SL. Behavioural characteristics of children with daytime wetting. *J Urol* 2001; **166**: 2392–2395.

129 McGee R, Makinson T, Williams S, Simpson A, Silva PA. A longitudinal study of enuresis from five to nine years. *Aust Paediatr J* 1984; **20(1)**: 39–42.

130 Swithinbank LV, Brookes ST, Shepherd AM, Abrams P. The natural history of urinary symptoms during adolescence. *Br J Urol Suppl* 1998; **81(3)**: 90–93.

131 Hellstrom A, Hanson E, Hansson S, Hjalmas K, Jodal U. Micturition habits and incontinence at age 17: reinvestigation of a cohort studied at age 7. *Br J Urol* 1995; **76(2)**: 231–234.

132 Sureshkumar P, Bower W, Craig JC, Knight JF. Treatment of daytime urinary incontinence in children: a systematic review of randomized controlled trials. *J Urol* 2003; **170(1)**: 196–200.

133 Ayan S, Kaya K, Topsakal K, Kilicarslan H, Gokce G, Gultekin Y. Efficacy of tolterodine as a first-line treatment for non-neurogenic voiding dysfunction in children. *BJU Int* 2005; **96(3)**: 411–414.

134 Bolduc S, Upadhyay J, Payton J, Bagli DJ, McLorie GA, Khoury AE *et al.* The use of tolterodine in children after oxybutynin failure. *BJU Int* 2003; **91(4)**: 398–401.

135 Meadow R, Berg I. Controlled trial of imipramine in diurnal enuresis. *Arch Dis Child* 1982; **57(9)**: 714–716.

136 Hellstrom AL, Hjalmas K, Jodal U. Terodiline in the treatment of children with unstable bladders. *Br J Urol* 1989; **63(4)**: 358–362.

137 Elmer M, Norgaard JP, Djurhuus JC, Adolfsson T. Terodiline in the treatment of diurnal enuresis in children. *Scand J Primary Health Care* 1988; **6(2)**: 119–124.

138 Halliday S, Meadow SR, Berg I. Successful management of daytime enuresis using alarm procedures: a randomly controlled trial. *Arch Dis Child* 1987; **62(2)**: 132–137.

139 Yamanishi T, Yasuda K, Murayama N, Sakakibara R, Uchiyama T, Ito H. Biofeedback training for detrusor overactivity in children. *J Urol* 2000; **164(5)**: 1686–1690.

140 Dolezal J, Zenisek J. The results of the treatment of voiding dysfunction by pelvic floor EMG biofeedback in children. *Br J Urol* 1997; **80(Suppl 2)**: 18.

141 van Gool JD, De Jong TPVM, Winkler-Seinstra P *et al.* A comparison of standard therapy, bladder rehabilitation with biofeedback, and pharmacotherapy in children with non-neuropathic bladder sphincter dysfunction. 2nd Annual Meeting of the International Children's Continence Society, Denver, CO, 1999; 89.

142 Hoebeke P, De Paepe H. Percutaneous electrical nerve stimulation in children with therapy resistant nonneuropathic bladder sphincter dysfunction: a pilot study. *J Urol* 2002; **168(6)**: 2605–2608.

143 Hoebeke P, Van Laecke E, Everaert K, Renson C, De Paepe H, Raes A *et al.* Transcutaneous neuromodulation for the urge syndrome in children: a pilot study. *J Urol* 2001; **166(6)**: 2416–2419.

66 Epidemiology and General Management of Childhood Idiopathic Nephrotic Syndrome

Nicholas J. A. Webb

Department of Nephrology, Royal Manchester Children's Hospital, Manchester M27 4HA, UK

Introduction

Nephrotic syndrome develops when an abnormality of glomerular permeability results in the development of heavy proteinuria, hypoalbuminemia, and generalized edema. The nephrotic syndrome can occur in the course of many different glomerular diseases. Nephrotic syndrome not associated with systemic disease is termed primary or idiopathic nephrotic syndrome, and where it occurs as part of a systemic disease or is related to a drug or other toxin it is termed secondary nephrotic syndrome. The list of causes of childhood nephrotic syndrome is extensive (Table 66.1), although the large majority of children have primary disease. Within this group, two histological subgroups predominate: minimal change disease (MCD) and focal segmental glomerulosclerosis (FSGS). There has been debate whether these should be considered distinct entities or whether they represent different ends of a single spectrum of disease, as there have been reports of transformation from MCD to FSGS histology [1]. In their typical presentation, they behave differently in their response to steroid therapy and the likelihood of progression to end-stage renal disease (ESRD). Furthermore, recent advances in genetics have revealed that a substantial proportion of children with FSGS have an underlying genetic basis for their disease.

Biopsy studies in the 1970s reported MCD to be the predominant cause of nephrotic syndrome, occurring in around 80% of cases [2,3]. This is in contrast to adult series, where MCD accounts for only around 25% of cases [4]. FSGS and mesangiocapillary glomerulonephritis (MCGN) were responsible for the majority of the remaining cases, along with a small number of cases of membranous nephropathy (MN) and a variety of other histological diagnoses [2,3]. Overall, 80% of children achieved remission with a standard 8-week course of corticosteroid (prednisone or prednisolone) therapy. Response varied according to histology, with

Evidence-based Nephrology. Edited by Donald Molony and Jonathan Craig
© 2009 Blackwell Publishing, ISBN: 978-1-4051-3975-5.

over 90% of children with MCD responding compared with only 17–30% of those with FSGS [3,5]. Of steroid-sensitive children, 91.8% had MCD and 8.2% had other histological diagnoses [5]. Consequently, the majority of children now receive an empiric course of steroid therapy, with biopsy being reserved for those with atypical presenting features (suggestive of non-MCD histology) or where the child is steroid unresponsive. As such, most children with nephrotic syndrome do not have a histological diagnosis but are classified according to their steroid responsiveness: so-called steroid-sensitive nephrotic syndrome (SSNS) and steroid-resistant nephrotic syndrome (SRNS).

Epidemiology

Incidence

The incidence of childhood idiopathic NS is reported to be around 2 cases/100,000 child population/year [6–10]. A recent study in Yorkshire, UK, reported an incidence of 2.3 cases/100,000 patient-years in children below 15 years of age [11]. Of these, 2.0 cases/100,000 had SSNS and 0.3 cases/100,000 had SRNS. Although the overall incidence of childhood nephrotic syndrome has been relatively stable, the incidence of FSGS appears to be increasing in children and adults [12–14], particularly in the African American and Hispanic populations in the USA.

Gender

Nephrotic syndrome is more common in boys, with a male/female ratio of 1.6:1 (1.7:1 for SSNS and 1.2:1 for SRNS) [11].

Age

The incidence of nephrotic syndrome and SSNS peaks in the 1- to 4-year-old age group (Table 66.2) [11]. In the International Study of Kidney Diseases in Children (ISKDC), the median ages at presentation with MCD, FSGS, and MCGN were 3, 6, and 10 years, respectively [2]. The age of the child at presentation is therefore a strong predictor of the likely underlying cause of the nephrotic syndrome. Children aged below 1 year generally have Finnish-type

Table 66.1 Causes of childhood nephrotic syndrome.

Primary (idiopathic) nephrotic syndromes
MCD
FSGS
McGN[a]
MN
Genetic causes of nephrotic syndromes
Congenital nephrotic syndrome of Finnish type
FSGS
Diffuse mesangial sclerosis
Denys Drash syndrome
Frasier syndrome
Schimke immuno-osseous dysplasia
Secondary nephrotic syndromes
Systemic disease
    Systemic lupus erythematosus
    Henoch-Schoenlein purpura
    Sickle cell disease
    IgA nephropathy
    Postinfectious glomerulonephritis
Infection
    Hepatitis B and C
    HIV/AIDS
    Malaria
    Syphilis
    Toxoplasmosis
Drugs
    Penicillamine
    Gold
    NSAIDs[b]
    Pamidronate
    Interferon
    Mercury
    Heroin
    Lithium
Immunologic or allergic disorders
    Castleman's disease
    Kimura's disease
    Bee sting
    Allergy
Malignancy
    Lymphoma
    Leukemia

[a]More commonly presents as an acute nephritic syndrome.
[b]NSAIDs, nonsteroidal anti-inflammatory agents.

congenital nephrotic syndrome, or variants thereof, congenital infections, and a variety of genetic disorders (Table 66.1). This group of disorders is outside the scope of this chapter.

Ethnic variation

The incidence of nephrotic syndrome and the underlying histological causes vary among ethnic groups. The incidence of SSNS in the UK South Asian population (Indian, Pakistani, and Bangladeshi) is four to six times higher than in the UK white population [9,11,15] (7.4 versus 1.6 per 100,000 children, respectively; $P < 0.01$). The

incidences in the Hungarian gypsy population, who migrated to Europe from the Indian subcontinent, and in the Arab population are also higher than in the white population [16,17]. The patterns of histological disease and steroid sensitivity in Indian children are similar to that seen in the ISKDC, and UK studies, and in white South Africans [18–20]. In black Africans, fewer cases of nephrotic syndrome are due to MCN [21–24]. Instead, the predominant causes are quartan malaria and MCGN in West Africa and MN (predominantly hepatitis B-associated) in South Africa. In the USA, African American and Hispanic children are more likely to have steroid-resistant FSGS than white children [25], with rates of FSGS as high as 69% in one series from Texas [13]. In this series the incidence of FSGS had risen in African Americans, Hispanics, and whites from 23% before 1990 to 47% after 1990. The differences in histological diagnoses between the different age and ethnic groups were further exemplified in a biopsy study in a predominantly African American group of adolescents, of whom only 20–30% had MCD histology [26].

Genetics

SSNS is more common in first-degree relatives of affected individuals. Of 1877 children with nephrotic syndrome (excluding congenital nephrotic syndrome), 63 (3.3%) had a positive family history [27]. Idiopathic nephrotic syndrome has been reported in identical twins [28]. Recent genetic family studies have identified a possible locus for the so-called SSNS1 gene at 2p12-p13.2 [29]. The congenital nephrotic syndromes are associated with mutations in the NPHS1 (nephrin), NPHS2 (podocin), and WT-1 genes. Familial and sporadic SRNS may be associated with NPHS2 mutations. Studies investigating children with SSNS have all failed to detect evidence of homozygous or compound heterozygous NPHS2 mutations [30,31].

SSNS

Definitions

Commonly used definitions in idiopathic nephrotic syndrome are shown in Table 66.3. These definitions are largely based upon those used in the ISKDC studies.

Indications for renal biopsy in childhood idiopathic nephrotic syndrome
Presenting episode

Because most children presenting with nephrotic syndrome will be steroid responsive, a therapeutic trial of steroids without prior biopsy is justified. Biopsy is generally restricted to those presenting with atypical clinical and laboratory features, who are more likely to have alternative histological diagnoses, such as MCGN or MN. Atypical presenting features include age of <12 months (congenital and infantile nephrotic syndrome), age of >16 years (adult pattern of disease), family history of nephrotic syndrome, impaired renal function unresponsive to volume correction, persistent hypertension, macroscopic hematuria, low C3, and evidence

Table 66.2 Nephrotic syndrome in Yorkshire, UK, 1987–1998.

Age group	SSNS		SRNS		All primary nephrotic syndromes	
	Incidence[a]	95% CI	Incidence	95% CI	Incidence	95% CI
0–<1	0.5	0.0–1.1	0.2	0.0–0.5	0.5	0.0–1.1
1–4	4.1	3.3–5.0	0.5	0.2–0.8	4.6	3.7–5.5
5–9	1.7	1.2–2.3	0.2	0.0–0.4	1.9	1.4–2.5
10–15	0.9	0.6–1.2	0.2	0.1–0.4	1.1	0.7–1.5
Total	2.0	1.7–2.3	0.3	0.2–0.4	2.3	2.0–2.6

Source: McKinney et al. [11].
[a] Incidence per 100,000 person.

of systemic disease (rash, arthropathy, etc). Isolated microscopic hematuria may be present in one-fourth of children with MCD histology [2] and is not an indication for biopsy. Steroid resistance is widely accepted as an absolute indication for renal biopsy before commencing alternative noncorticosteroid therapy, but there is no consistent definition of steroid resistance. Some define resistance as failure to respond to 4 weeks of daily steroid therapy, and others use the term after failure to respond to 4 weeks of daily and 4 weeks of alternate-day steroids. Although lacking in any evidence base,

Table 66.3 Definitions used in idiopathic nephrotic syndrome [2,5].

Classification	Definition
Nephrotic syndrome	Edema, proteinuria >40 mg/m^2/h or protein/creatinine ratio >0.2 g/mmol; hypoalbuminaemia <25 g/L
Remission	Urinary protein excretion ≤4 mg/m^2/h or 0-trace of protein on urine dipstick or protein/creatinine ratio <0.02 g/mmol for 3 consecutive days
Initial responder	Attainment of complete remission within initial 8 weeks of steroid therapy
Initial nonresponder/steroid resistance	Failure to achieve remission during initial 8 weeks of steroid therapy[a]
Relapse	Urinary protein >40 mg/m^2/h or protein/creatinine ratio >0.2 g/mmol or 2+ protein on urine dipstick for 3 consecutive days, having previously been in remission
Frequent relapse	Two or more relapses within 6 months of initial response or four or more relapses within any 12-month period
Steroid dependence	Two consecutive relapses during steroid therapy or within 14 days of ceasing therapy
Late nonresponder	Proteinuria for >8 weeks following one or more remissions

[a] There is a lack of a consistent definition of steroid resistance both in the literature and in clinical practice, with some using this term after failure to respond to 4 weeks of daily steroid therapy, but others using the term after failure to respond to 4 weeks of daily and 4 weeks of alternate-day steroids.

children in the UK resistant to 4 weeks of daily steroids are commonly given 3 days of intravenous methylprednisolone [32]. Those who respond appear to follow a typical course for steroid-sensitive patients. Biopsy is only performed in those who remain unresponsive to this additional therapy. There is evidence that prolonging oral steroid therapy beyond 8 weeks results in an additional 3.3% of children with MCD entering remission [33].

Frequently relapsing and steroid-dependent nephrotic syndrome

Biopsy of children with frequently relapsing and steroid-dependent disease was recommended previously, prior to giving an alkylating agent, because some studies suggested that the post-biopsy clinical course was strongly dependent upon histology. Permanent remission and long periods of remission occurred more frequently in those with MCD, compared with those with FSGS or a mesangioproliferative lesion [34–37]. Most children with SSNS have a favorable response to an alkylating agent irrespective of their histology [38–43]. Furthermore, response to therapy appears to correlate well with the prior pattern of relapses, as shorter post-alkylating agent remission periods occur in those with steroid dependency compared to those with non-steroid-dependent frequent relapses [44]. Among 75 children with steroid-dependent nephrotic syndrome treated with alkylating agents, the response to therapy did not differ between those who had or who had not undergone renal biopsy [45]. In Australia, the UK, and many other European countries, biopsy of the child with SSNS is no longer routine before alkylating agent therapy. Surveys of US and Spanish pediatric nephrologists indicate that about 60% would biopsy children with SSNS prior to alkylating agents [46–47]. It is the author's opinion that, given the good response to alkylating agents seen in the large majority of children with frequently relapsing or steroid-dependent disease, the inconvenience and risks of biopsy are not justified given the small amount of useful additional information that will be obtained by making a histological diagnosis.

Secondary steroid resistance

When steroid resistance occurs following relapse in a previously steroid-sensitive child, so-called secondary steroid resistance, biopsy is indicated. While most such cases will respond to further immunosuppressive therapy [42,48], a small number of children will remain steroid resistant, in association with the presence of FSGS on biopsy, and the rate of progression to ESRD is high.

Calcineurin inhibitor therapy

Chronic ciclosporin nephrotoxicity, characterized by arteriolar lesions (ciclosporin-associated arteriolopathy) and tubulointerstitial lesions, has been reported in some series in up to 50% of patients after 2 years of therapy [49,50]. Biopsy is therefore frequently recommended for children receiving calcineurin inhibitors for steroid-dependent nephrotic syndrome after 2 years of therapy. When the biopsy is normal, then treatment can be safely continued, although the biopsy should be repeated after a further 1–2 years.

Relapses of SSNS

At least 70% of children with SSNS will relapse following treatment of their first episode. The early ISKDC studies reported that after 8 weeks of corticosteroids, 45% of children were relapse-free at 6 months and 28% at 2 years [51]. Longer-term follow-up studies have shown the overall rate of relapse to be closer to 85% [52,53]. Of those children who experience relapses, approximately 50% will develop frequently relapsing or steroid-dependent disease [54].

Factors at presentation predicting subsequent pattern of relapse

The ISKDC reported that, among 218 steroid-responsive children, no correlation was found between the frequency of relapse following presentation and the different histological subtypes of MCD, baseline clinical and laboratory characteristics, time of initial response to corticosteroids, or the time to first relapse [51]. Similarly, no correlations were found with the presence of microscopic hematuria [52]. Young age at disease presentation was predictive for a higher number of relapses and longer disease duration [55–57]. Frequent relapses during the first 6 months after initial steroid therapy were predictive for frequent relapses over the subsequent 18 months [51,52]. In one study, time to remission of 9 or more days with steroid therapy was associated with an increased risk of steroid dependency [58]. There is emerging evidence that the rate of subsequent relapse can be reduced by the use of a longer initial corticosteroid regimen [59].

Triggers of relapses

Upper respiratory tract infections precede 71% of relapses; respiratory syncytial virus is the most commonly encountered pathogen [60]. In this same study, four children were exposed to varicella-zoster virus, all of whom developed relapses. Paradoxically, exposure to measles virus is known to induce permanent disease remission [61].

When to treat relapses

The ISKDC definition (Table 66.2) of relapse is 3 days of significant proteinuria. Exacerbation of proteinuria may be transient, with spontaneous remission occurring in 23% of frequently relapsing and 10% of steroid-dependent patients. Proteinuria resolves within 4–14 days in 79% of such cases [62]. It is generally accepted practice to defer commencement of corticosteroid therapy until after 5 days or so of proteinuria, although it is important to avoid the development of generalized edema. Although no definitive data exist on this subject, it is the author's observation that some individuals are more likely to consistently undergo spontaneous remission and others rapidly develop generalized edema and hypovolemia. With knowledge of the natural history of previous relapses, it is possible to individualize the timing of the commencement of relapse therapy.

Long-term outcome of SSNS

Early follow-up studies suggested that the long-term prognosis for children with SSNS was excellent, with all retaining normal renal function and over 90% achieving long-term remission at the end of puberty [53,57]. However, more recent follow-up studies have reported substantially higher rates of disease relapse occurring during adult life and have provided data on morbidity in adults treated for SSNS during childhood. In four studies from Finland [63], the UK [55], Switzerland [64], and France [65], the rate of relapse during adult life was reported to be 14%, 19%, 33%, and 42%, respectively. Of the 43 patients with disease continuing into adult life in the French series, 28 were receiving steroids, 3 were receiving cytotoxic agents, and 3 were receiving ciclosporin. These reports might imply that a change is occurring in the natural history of the disease, but it is more likely that these findings have arisen because of more complete follow-up [55,63] and tertiary center follow-up of a select group of patients with a more severe disease course [64,65].

Consistent risk factors for relapses continuing into adult life include very frequent relapses during childhood and adolescence and the use of either cytotoxic agents or ciclosporin. One study reported an increased risk with young age at presentation [65], although two other studies did not [55,64]. In patients in whom permanent remission was achieved during childhood, this appeared to occur in the majority at 13–16 years of age [65]. Renal function was preserved in almost all. Of the 309 patients followed in these four studies, only 2, who relapsed in adult life, developed abnormal renal function, 1 with ESRD [65] and the other with a creatinine clearance of 63 mL/min [63]. Other series have reported the incidence of renal failure in children with initial SSNS to be less than 1% and limited to those who develop secondary steroid resistance unresponsive to cytotoxic and other therapies in association with the presence of FSGS on biopsy [48,52].

The existing data on long-term follow-up of children with SSNS are insufficient to conclude that their outcome is universally good into adult life. Although sophisticated modern imaging modalities, such as electron beam computer tomography scanning, have not been used to identify early vascular changes, there is no evidence yet that this population has an increased rate of premature cardiovascular disease [64,66]. Similarly, the rate of malignancy in adult life does not appear to be increased [64,67].

A Finnish study reported an increased rate of diabetes mellitus, asthma, and ulcerative colitis compared with an age-matched population [63]. Hegarty *et al.* reported a decrease in forearm trabecular volumetric bone mineral density as measured by peripheral quantitative computed tomography in adult survivors at a median age of 35.5 years [68], although Leonard *et al.*, who used dual X-ray absorptiometry of the whole body and spine in 60 children with relapsing disease at a mean age of 9.0 years, did not detect any significant abnormalities during childhood [69]. Long-term side effects of corticosteroid therapy were present in 19 of 36 patients with proteinuria persisting into adulthood in the French series [65].

General management of nephrotic syndrome

Introduction and epidemiology

Children with nephrotic syndrome are at increased risk of bacterial infection because of edema, urinary losses of immunoglobulins and complement alternative pathway components factors B and D, impaired neutrophil function, immunosuppressive therapy, and other factors. Large follow-up series have reported an overall mortality rate for childhood SSNS of 1–7%, with deaths being largely due to sepsis and thrombosis [53,55,57]. Many of these deaths occurred in patients treated in the 1960s and 1970s, and current mortality rates are thought to be substantially lower, although there are no definitive data to support this view.

Peritonitis, bacteremia, and cellulitis remain the most common infections, and they are caused by bacteria with a polysaccharide capsule, particularly *Streptococcus pneumoniae* and gram-negative organisms, including *Escherichia coli*. There is a relatively high rate of bacteremia associated with peritonitis in children with nephrotic syndrome, in contrast to those on peritoneal dialysis [70]. Series from India have reported urinary tract infections and tuberculosis to be common [71,72]. Varicella is a highly contagious disease that is usually benign but may have serious and potentially fatal consequences in children with nephrotic syndrome receiving immunosuppressive agents.

Available evidence

No randomized controlled trials (RCTs) have investigated the use of prophylactic antibiotics or vaccination against pneumococcus or varicella-zoster virus. Five RCTs from China have investigated intravenous immunoglobulin (IVIG), thymosin, and Chinese herbs (Tiaojining).

Pneumococcal vaccination for prevention of infection

Two types of pneumococcal vaccine currently exist. The older 23-valent pneumococcal polysaccharide vaccine (23PS; Pneumovax), which was introduced in the early 1980s, is known to induce a good antibody response to *S. pneumoniae* serotypes 1, 2, 3, 4, 5, 6B, 7F, 8, 9N, 9V, 10A, 11A, 12F, 14, 15B, 17F, 18C, 19F, 19A, 20, 22F, 23F, and 33F in healthy adults and older children, but the

geometric mean antibody response is lower and of shorter duration in children with immunological impairment, including those with nephrotic syndrome [73–77]. The vaccine is not licensed for use in children less than 2 years of age, in whom the burden of the disease is highest, because it does not stimulate effective long-lasting immunity in this age group [78,79]. The newer heptavalent pneumococcal conjugate vaccine PCV7 (Prevnar in the US and Prevanar in the UK) contains polysaccharide from seven common capsular types (4, 6B, 9V, 14, 18C, 19F, and 23F) and is estimated to provide coverage against 82% of invasive infections in UK children under 5 years of age [80]. In the US, universal vaccination with PCV7 has been recommended in all children under 2 years of age at 2, 4, 6, and 12–15 months of age. The US guidelines for children at risk of invasive pneumococcal infection, including those with nephrotic syndrome, are shown in Table 66.4 [81,82]. The 23PS vaccine is administered after 2 years of age to boost the antibody concentrations of serotypes present in both PCV7 and 23PS vaccines and to broaden the serotype coverage. No efficacy data and limited safety and immunogenicity data are available regarding the use of PCV7 in children 5 years of age and older, and UK guidelines state that a single dose of 23PS should be administered. No RCTs of either vaccine have been performed specifically for this disease population to support these recommendations. In children with sickle cell disease, nine RCTs involving 547 children have compared a polysaccharide or conjugate pneumococcal vaccine regimen with a different regimen or no vaccination [83]. The risk of pneumococcal disease (reported in only one trial) was not significantly reduced by the polysaccharide pneumococcal vaccine PPV14 in children younger than 3 years [84]. Antibody responses were increased compared to control groups, including those in infants, in three trials of conjugate vaccines, but clinical outcomes were not measured.

Table 66.4 American Academy of Pediatrics recommendations for pneumococcal vaccination in children 24–59 months old with nephrotic syndrome [81].

Previous vaccination	Further vaccination
4 doses of PCV7	1 dose of 23PS at 24 months of age, at least 6–8 weeks after last dose of PCV7
1–3 doses of PCV7 before 24 months	1 dose of PCV7 at least 6–8 weeks after last dose of PCV7, then a dose of 23PS 6–8 weeks later; an additional dose of 23PS should be given no earlier than 3–5 years after the initial dose of 23PS
1 dose of 23PS	2 doses of PCV7 to be given at an interval of 6–8 weeks, commencing no earlier than 6–8 weeks after the last dose of 23PS; further dose of 23PS 3–5 years after first PS dose
No previous dose	2 doses of PCV7 at interval of 6–8 weeks, followed by single dose of 23PS no less than 6–8 weeks after the last dose of PCV7; an additional dose of 23PS is recommended 3–5 years after the last dose

Prophylactic antibiotics for prevention of infection

Many nephrologists routinely use prophylactic phenoxymethyl-penicillin when a child is edematous or has heavy proteinuria. No RCTs have been performed to evaluate the efficacy and safety of this therapy for this condition. Penicillin has been shown to reduce the risk of infection in children with sickle cell disease (three RCTs, 857 children; odds ratio, 0.37; 95% confidence interval [CI], 0.16–0.86) [85]. Adverse effects of therapy were rare and minor in nature. It has been estimated that 110 children with nephrotic syndrome would need to be treated with penicillin for 1 year to prevent one episode of pneumococcal infection [86].

IVIG for prevention of infection

Three RCTs (208 children) compared IVIG with no specific therapy in children with nephrotic syndrome [87–89]. The dosage and duration of IVIG varied considerably, and the quality of the studies was generally poor. There was a consistent positive effect of IVIG on preventing nosocomial infection or unspecified infection in children with nephrotic syndrome (relative risk [RR], 0.39; 95% CI, 0.18–0.82; $P = 0.01$) [90].

Thymosin for prevention of infection

Thymosin is an immunomodulating agent that can influence T-cell maturation and antigen recognition, the stimulation of interferon and cytokine production, and the activity of NK cell-mediated cytotoxicity [91]. Thymosin reduced the risk of infection compared to no specific therapy in children with nephrotic syndrome (one RCT, 40 patients; RR, 0.50; 95% CI, 0.26–0.97; $P = 0.04$) [92]. There was no significant difference in the types of infection observed in the treatment and control groups.

Chinese herbal preparations for prevention of infection

A single RCT showed a significant effect of Chinese herbs (Tiaojining) on preventing infections in children with nephrotic syndrome compared with no specific therapy (60 children; RR, 0.59; 95% CI, 0.43–0.81; $P = 0.001$) [93]. There was no significant difference in the range of infections between the two groups.

Strategies for the prevention of varicella-zoster infection

The current standard of care in the UK and Australia is that immunocompromised children should receive varicella-zoster immunoglobulin (VZIG) following exposure to varicella-zoster virus. VZIG significantly reduces morbidity and mortality, although breakthrough infection is well-recognized [94]. VZIG is no longer available in the USA. Postexposure acyclovir prophylaxis reduces the transmission rate of varicella in immunocompetent children [95]. In a RCT of eight patients (10 exposures) given acyclovir prophylaxis (10 mg/kg 6 hourly) and VZIG (12.5 U/kg of body weight; minimum of 125 U and maximum of 625 U), none developed varicella compared with one case in four controls given VZIG alone [96]. In two recent studies of varicella vaccines in children with SSNS, protective antibody levels developed in 85–100%. Three children developed mild varicella during the follow-up period. Thirteen children received alternate-day

steroids; none developed skin lesions secondary to replication of the vaccine strain. Studies were not powered to determine whether vaccination resulted in an increased risk of disease relapse [97,98]. Where vaccination is contraindicated because of the administration of high-dose steroids or other immunosuppressive agents, vaccination of household contacts is recommended.

Influenza vaccination for prevention of infection

UK guidelines recommend an annual influenza vaccination in children with nephrotic syndrome. This has been shown to be immunogenic [99,100], although no large-scale trials investigating efficacy and safety have been performed in this population. A single case report exists that describes an adult who developed MCD following the use of this vaccine [101].

Adverse effects of routine childhood vaccination

A single study has reported an association between the administration of the meningococcal C conjugate vaccine and relapse [102]. In the 12 months prior to the introduction of the vaccine in the UK, 63 relapses occurred in a population of 106 children with nephrotic syndrome compared with 96 relapses in the equivalent time period following the introduction of vaccination ($P = 0.009$). These findings have not been replicated elsewhere.

Thrombosis

Introduction and epidemiology

The reported incidence of symptomatic thromboembolic complications is as high as 50% in adults [103] and 2–4% in children [104–106]. The risk of thrombosis appears to be greater in children with SRNS who have persistent proteinuria, compared with children with SSNS who have intermittent proteinuria; 9 of 17 cases of thrombosis in two published series had SRNS [104,105]. Subclinical episodes of thrombosis are common. Of 26 children with nephrotic syndrome in remission who were examined via a ventilation perfusion scan, 7 had abnormal scans and 10 were found to have abnormal or suspicious changes [107].

Thromboembolic complications have been found to be more frequent in the venous rather than arterial system in some but not all series [104,105]. The deep leg veins are most frequently affected, except in congenital nephrotic syndrome, where renal vein thrombosis and thrombosis of the inferior vena cava predominate. Other reported sites of vascular thrombosis include the superior vena cava, the mesenteric artery, hepatic veins, the saggital sinus, and middle cerebral arteries. No single laboratory test can reliably predict thrombotic risk, although fibrinogen concentration has been proposed as a surrogate marker [108].

Prevention of thromboembolic complications

A number of general measures can be undertaken to reduce the risk of thromboembolic events. Bed rest should be avoided, sepsis prevented or adequately treated, and factors which cause

Table 66.5 Evidence ratings and recommendations for interventions to prevent infection and thromboembolic complications in childhood nephrotic syndrome.

Intervention	Evidence rating[a,b] SR[a]	Moderate	Low	Studies peformed	Recommendation[c] I	II	III	Comment
Prevention of bacterial infections								
Pneumococcal vaccination	—		●	No RCTs in NS patients; 9 RCTs (547 patients) in children with sickle cell disease	●			Benefit in well children; in children with sickle cell disease the conjugate vaccine has been shown to be immunogenic, although clinical outcomes were not measured; no significant harms.
Prophylactic antibiotics	—		●	No RCTs in NS patients; 3 RCTs (857 patients) in children with sickle cell disease		●		Odds of infection reduced (OR 0.37) with penicillin prophylaxis in children with sickle cell disease; adverse effects few and minor
IVIG	+	●		3 RCTs (208 patients); consistent results			●	Expensive medication; requires IV administration; dose unclear
Thymosin	+		●	1 RCT (40 patients)			●	Need more information on harms; not generally available
Chinese herbs	+		●	1 RCT (60 patients)			●	Need more information on harms; not generally available
Prevention of viral infections								
Varicella vaccination	—		●	No RCTs; 5 case series (238 patients) in NS patients	●			100% seroconverted with two-dose schedule; no significant harms; uncertain impact on disease relapses
VZIG + acyclovir	—		●	1 RCT (12 patients)			●	Uncertain benefit; no significant harms
Prevention of thromboembolic complications								
Anticoagulants	—		●	No RCTs			●	Risk of anticoagulant treatment likely to exceed benefit
Antiplatelet agents	—		●	No RCTs			●	Little value to prevent venous thrombosis

[a] Systematic reviews of RCTs;

[b] Evidence rating based on number of studies, study design, study quality, and consistency of results. No intervention was rated with a high evidence rating.

[c] Recommendations based on efficacy, trade-offs between benefits and harms, quality of evidence, and availability of medication. I, recommend; II, suggest; III, no recommendation possible.

hemoconcentration, such as dehydration from acute gastroenteritis and injudicious use of diuretic therapy, should also be avoided. Central venous catheters should not be used unless essential. Studies in adults have suggested that prophylactic oral anticoagulation may be of benefit in MN [109], but no RCTs or other studies have investigated the prophylactic use of any anticoagulant or antiplatelet agent to prevent thomboembolic complications in children with nephrotic syndrome. Possible approaches include the use of warfarin or subcutaneous low-molecular-weight heparin, although the latter is only likely to be effective where antithrombin III levels are adequate. Platelet function is consistently increased, and platelet aggregation inhibitors, such as low-dose aspirin and/or dipyridamole, are logical choices, although no data from controlled studies are available.

It is unclear how long prophylactic therapy should be continued following an episode of thrombosis: the use of prophylactic warfarin has been recommended for at least 6 months and perhaps during future relapses by some [110], but others have suggested that treatment with warfarin should continue for as long as nephrotic-range proteinuria is present [111].

Established thromboembolic complications

The treatment of thromboembolic complications in children with nephrotic syndrome has never been subjected to a RCT or other form of prospective clinical trial. Studies in adult patients have shown treatment with heparin and warfarin for renal vein thrombosis to be effective and safe, but this has not been assessed in RCTs [112]. In patients in whom thrombosis has been more extensive, involving both renal veins, the inferior vena cava, or where the vascular supply of other key organs is compromised, case reports describe successful therapy with anticoagulation and thrombolytic therapy with streptokinase [113] and tissue plasminogen activator

[114] therapy. This therapy is reserved for cases where critical organ function is compromised because of the risk of bleeding.

Edema

For some children, a modest fluid restriction alone may suffice, but in others oral diuretic therapy is necessary to induce diuresis. A combination of a loop diuretic such as furosemide, given two to three times daily, in combination with a potassium-sparing agent (spironolactone), is frequently used, particularly where there is significant ascites. The child should be regularly assessed for signs of intravascular volume depletion. The use of diuretic therapy in children with SSNS is controversial because of the risk of unrecognized hypovolemia once urine output increases.

Resistance to loop diuretics may occur because of a combination of hypoalbuminemia, which results in decreased delivery of protein-bound loop diuretic to the proximal tubules, increased volume of distribution, and intraluminal binding of secreted loop diuretics [115]. Increasing the dose of the diuretic may increase tubular delivery but may also increase the risk of toxicity. Where edema is unresponsive to diuretic therapy and there is risk of skin breakdown (the scrotum is a particularly vulnerable area), intravenous albumin given in conjunction with intravenous furosemide may be indicated. This intervention may cause acute pulmonary edema [116]. No studies have been performed to investigate the optimum dose and duration of intravenous 20% albumin, and some worldwide variation in practice exists. In the UK, a dose of 1 g/kg (5 mL/kg of 20% albumin) is generally given over 4 h, with furosemide given midway through the infusion. Elsewhere, others are more cautious, giving the same dose over 8 h, and others may use doses as large as 2 g/kg.

Evidence-based recommendations

On the basis of the available evidence, it is difficult to make strong evidence-based recommendations regarding the use of drug therapy, antibody therapy, or vaccination for the prevention of infection in children with nephrotic syndrome (Table 66.5). The routine use of IVIG for this indication is very infrequent in Western nations, and both thymosin and Chinese herbal preparations are unlicensed, making widespread adoption of their use unlikely. The evidence of efficacy of both pneumococcal and varicella vaccination based upon uncontrolled case series and RCTs in other disease groups suggests that their use should be recommended, although further studies are necessary to determine the optimal vaccine schedule. Following a similar rationale, the use of prophylactic phenoxymethylpenicillin for prevention of pneumococcal infection is suggested.

It is not possible to make any evidence-based recommendations for the use of anticoagulants or antiplatelet agents for the prevention or treatment of thrombosis.

References

1 Tejani A. Morphological transformation in minimal change nephrotic syndrome. *Nephron* 1985; **39**: 157–159.

2 International Study of Kidney Disease in Children. Nephrotic syndrome in children: prediction of histopathology from clinical and laboratory characteristics at time of diagnosis. *Kidney Int* 1978; **13**: 159–165.

3 White RHR, Glasgow EF, Mills RJ. Clinicopathologic study of nephrotic syndrome in childhood. *Lancet* 1970; **i**: 1353–1359.

4 Cameron JS, Turner DR, Ogg CS, Sharpstone R, Brown CB. The nephrotic syndrome in adults with minimal change glomerular lesions. *Q J Med* 1974; **43**: 461–488.

5 International Study of Kidney Disease in Children. The primary nephrotic syndrome in children. Identification of patients with minimal change nephrotic syndrome from initial response to prednisolone. *J Pediatr* 1981; **98**: 561–564.

6 Schlesinger ER, Sultz HA, Mosher WE, Feldman JG. The nephrotic syndrome: its incidence and implications for the community. *Am J Dis Child* 1968; **116**: 623–632.

7 Rothenburg MB, Heymann W. The incidence of the nephrotic syndrome in children. *Pediatrics* 1957; **19**: 446–452.

8 McEnery PT, Strife CF. Nephrotic syndrome in childhood. Management and treatment in patients with minimal change disease, mesangial proliferation or focal glomerulosclerosis. *Pediatr Clin North Am* 1982; **29**: 875–894.

9 Feehally J, Kendall NP, Swift PGF, Walls J. High incidence of minimal change nephrotic syndrome in Asians. *Arch Dis Child* 1985; **60**: 1018–1020.

10 Evans JHC, Long E. A national audit of steroid sensitive nephrotic syndrome. Presented at the Royal College of Paediatrics and Child Health Annual Meeting, York, April 1997.

11 McKinney PA, Feltblower RG, Brocklebank JT, Fitzpatrick MM. Time trends an ethnic patterns of childhood nephrotic syndrome in Yorkshire, UK. *Pediatr Nephrol* 2001; **15**: 1040–1044.

12 Gulati S, Sharma AP, Sharma RK, Gupta A. Changing trends of histopathology in childhood nephrotic syndrome. *Am J Kidney Dis* 1999; **34**: 646–650.

13 Bonilla-Felix M, Parra C, Danjani T, Ferris M, Swinford RD, Portman RJ *et al.* Changing patterns in the histopathology of idiopathic nephrotic syndrome in children. *Kidney Int* 1999; **55**: 1885–1890.

14 Filler G, Young E, Geier P, Carpenter B, Drukker A, Feber J. Is there really an increase in non-minimal change nephrotic syndrome in children? *Am J Kidney Dis* 2003; **42**: 1107–1113.

15 Sharples PM, Poulton J, White RHR. Steroid responsive nephrotic syndrome is more common in Asians. *Arch Dis Child* 1985; **60**: 1014–1017.

16 Horvath M, Sulyok E. Steroid responsive nephrotic syndrome in Asians (letter). *Arch Dis Child* 1986; **61**: 528.

17 Elzouki AY, Amin F, Jaiswal OP. Primary nephrotic syndrome in Arab children. *Arch Dis Child* 1984; **60**: 1014–1017.

18 Srivastava RN, Mayekar G, Anand R, Choudhry VP, Ghai OP, Tandon HD. Nephrotic syndrome in Indian children. *Arch Dis Child.* 1975; **50**: 626–630.

19 Adhikari M, Coovadia HM, Hammon MG. Associations between HLA antigens and nephrotic syndrome in African and Indian children in South Africa. *Nephron* 1985; **41**: 289–292.

20 Coovadia HM, Adhikari M, Morel-Maroger L. Clinicpathological feature of the nephrotic syndrome in South African children. *Q J Med* 1979; **189**: 77–91.

21 Hendrickse RG, Adeniyi A, Edington GM, Glasgow EF, White RHR, Houba V. Quartan malaria nephrotic syndrome collaborative clinicopathological study in Nigerian children. *Lancet* 1972; **i(7661)**: 1143–1149.

22 Abdurrahman MB, Aijhionbare HA, Babaoye FA, Sathiakumar N, Narayana PT. Clinicopathological features of childhood nephrotic syndrome in northern Nigeria. *Q J Med* 1990; **75**: 563–576.

23 Bhimma R, Coovadia HM, Adhikari M. Nephrotic syndrome in South African children: changing perspectives over 20 years. *Pediatr Nephrol* 1997; **11**: 429–434.

24 Asinobi AO, Gbadegesin RG, Adeyamo AA, Akang EE, Arowolo FA, Abiola OA *et al*. The predominance of membranoproliferative glomerulonephritis in childhood nephrotic syndrome in Ibadan, Nigeria. *West Afr J Med* 1999; **18**: 203–206.

25 Ingulli E, Tejani A. Racial differences in the incidence and renal outcome of idiopathic focal segmental glomerulosclerosis in children. *Pediatr Nephrol* 1991; **5**: 393–397.

26 Baqi N, Singh A, Balachandra S, Ahmad H, Nicastri A, Kytinski S *et al*. The paucity of minial change disease in primary nephrotic syndrome. *Pediatr Nephrol* 1998; **12**: 105–107.

27 White RHR. The familial nephrotic syndrome. A European survey. *Clin Nephrol* 1973; **1**: 215–219.

28 Roy S, Pitcock JA. Idiopathic nephrosis in identical twins. *Am J Dis Child* 1971; **121**: 428–439.

29 Ruf RG, Fuchshuber A, Karle SM, Lemainque A, Huck K, Wienker T *et al*. Identification of the first gene locus (SSNS1) for steroid sensitive nephrotic syndrome on chromosome 2p. *J Am Soc Nephrol* 2003; **14**: 1897–1900.

30 Ruf RG, Lichtenberger A, Karle SM, Haas JP, Anacletto FE, Schultheiss M *et al*. Patients with mutations in NPHS2 (podocin) do not respond to standard steroid treatment of nephrotic syndrome. *J Am Soc Nephrol* 2004; **1**: 722–732.

31 Caridi G, Bertelli R, Carrea A, Catarsi P, Artero M, Carraro M *et al*. Prevalence, genetics and clinical features of patients carrying podocin mutations in steroid resistant nonfamilial focal segmental glomerulosclerosis. *J Am Soc Nephrol* 2001; **12**: 2742–2746.

32 Haycock G. The child with idiopathic nephrotic syndrome. In: Webb NJA, Postlethwaite RJ, editors. *Clinical Paediatric Nephrology.* Oxford University Press, Oxford, UK, 2003.

33 International Study of Kidney Disease in Children. Primary nephrotic syndrome in children: clinical significance of histopathological variants of minimal change and of diffuse mesangial hypercellularity. *Kidney Int* 1981; **20**: 765–771.

34 Holliday MA, Barratt TM, Vernier R, editors. *Pediatric Nephrology*, 3rd edn. Williams & Wilkins, Baltimore, 1994.

35 Berns JS, Gaudio KM, Krassner LS, Anderson FP, Durante D, McDonald BM *et al*. Steroid responsive nephrotic syndrome of childhood: A long-term study of clinical course, histopathology, efficacy of cyclophosphamide therapy and effects on growth. *Am J Kidney Dis* 1987; **92**: 108–114.

36 Tejani A, Phadke K, Nicastri A, Adamson O, Chen CK, Trachtman H *et al*. Efficacy of cyclophosphamide in steroid sensitive childhood nephrotic syndrome with different morphological lesions. *Nephron* 1985; **41**: 170–173.

37 Siegel NJ, Gaudio KM, Krassner LS, McDonald BM, Anderson FP, Kasgarian M. Steroid-dependent nephrotic syndrome in children: histopathology and relapses after cyclophosphamide treatment. *Kidney Int* 1981; **19**: 454–459.

38 Gulati S, Sharma AP, Sharma RK, Gupta A, Gupta RK. Do current recommendations for kidney biopsy in nephrotic syndrome need modifications? *Pediatr Nephrol* 2002; **17**: 404–408.

39 Mattoo TJ. Kidney biopsy prior to cyclophosphamide therapy in primary nephrotic syndrome. *Pediatr Nephrol* 1991; **5**: 617–619 .

40 Schulman SL, Kaiser BA, Polinsky MS, Srinivasan R, Baluarte HJ. Predicting the response to cytotoxic therapy for childhood nephrotic syndrome: superiority of response to corticosteroid therapy over histopathologic patterns. *J Pediatr* 1988; **113**: 996–1001.

41 Garin EH, Pryor ND, Fennell RS, Richard GA. Pattern of response to prednisone in idiopathic minimal lesion nephrotic syndrome as a criterion for selecting patients for cyclophosphamide therapy. *J Pediatr* 1978; **92**: 304–308.

42 Webb NJ, Lewis MA, Iqbal J, Smart PJ, Lendon M, Postlethwaite RJ. Childhood steroid sensitive nephrotic syndrome: does the histology matter? *Am J Kidney Dis* 1994; **27**: 484–488.

43 Stadermann MB, Lilien MR, van de Kar NC, Monnenes LA, Schroder CH. Is biopsy required prior to cyclophosphamide in steroid-sensitive nephrotic syndrome? *Clin Nephrol* 2003; **60**: 315–317.

44 Durkan A, Hodson EM, Willis NS, Craig JC. Non-corticosteroid treatment for nephrotic syndrome in children. *Cochrane Database Syst Rev* 2005; **2**: CD002290.

45 Idczak-Nowicka E, Ksiazek J, Krynski J, Wyszynska T. Verification of indications for kidney biopsy in children with steroid-dependent nephrotic syndrome. *Pediatr Pol* 1996; **71**: 679–683.

46 Primack WA, Schulmann SL, Kaplan BS. An analysis of the approach to management of childhood nephrotic syndrome by pediatric nephrologists. *Am J Kidney Dis* 1994; **23**: 524–527.

47 Camacho Diaz JA. Indications for renal biopsy in idiopathic nephrotic syndrome in children. Results of a national survey. *An Esp Pediatr* 2000; **52**: 413–417.

48 Neuhaus TJ, Fay J, Dillon M, Trompeter RS, Barratt TM. Alternative treatment to corticosteroids in steroid sensitive nephrotic syndrome. *Arch Dis Child* 1994; **71**: 522–526.

49 Inoue Y, Iijima K, Nakamura H, Yoshikawa N. Two-year cyclosporine treatment in children with steroid dependent nephrotic syndrome. *Pediatr Nephrol* 1999; **13**: 33–38.

50 Yoshikawa N, Iijima K, Ito H. Cyclosporin treatment in children with steroid-dependent nephrotic syndrome. *Clin Exp Nephrol* 1999; **3(Suppl)**: S27–S33.

51 International Study of Kidney Disease in Children. Early identification of frequent relapsers among children with minimal change nephrotic syndrome. A report of the ISKDC. *J Pediatr* 1982; **101**: 514–518.

52 Tarshish P, Tobin JN, Bernstein J, Edelmann CM. Prognostic significance of the early course of minimal change nephrotic syndrome: report of the International Study of Kidney Disease in Children. *J Am Soc Nephrol* 1997; **8**: 769–776.

53 Koskimies O, Vilska J, Rapola J, Hallman N. Long-term outcome of primary nephrotic syndrome. *Arch Dis Child* 1982; **57**: 544–548.

54 Nephrotic syndrome in children: a randomized trial comparing two prednisone regimens in steroid-responsive patients who relapse early. Report of the International Study of Kidney Disease in Children. *J Pediatr* 1982; **95**: 239–243.

55 Lewis MA, Baildam EM, Houston IB, Postlethwaite RJ. Nephrotic syndrome: from toddlers to twenties. *Lancet* 1989; **i**: 255–259.

56 Kabuki N, Okugawa T, Hayakawa H, Tomizawa S, Kasahara T, Uchiyama M. Influence of age at onset on the outcome of steroid-sensitive nephrotic syndrome. *Pediatr Nephrol* 1998; **12**: 467–470.

57 Trompeter RS, Lloyd BW, Hicks J, Whie RH, Cameron JS. Long term outcome for children with minimal-change nephrotic syndrome. *Lancet* 1985; **i**: 368–370.

58 Yap H-K, Han EJ, Heng C-K, Gong W-K. Risk factors for steroid dependency in children with idiopathic nephrotic syndrome. *Pediatr Nephrol* 2001; **16**: 1049–1052.

59 Hodson EM, Knight JF, Willis NS, Craig JC. Corticosteroid therapy for nephrotic syndrome in children. *Cochrane Database Syst Rev* 2005; **1**: CD001533.

60 McDonald NE, Wolfish N, McLaine P, Phipps P, Rossier E. Role of respiratory viruses in exacerbation of primary nephrotic syndrome. *J Pediatr* 1986; **108**: 378–382.

61 Blumberg RW, Cassady HA. Effect of measles on the nephrotic syndrome. *Am J Dis Child* 1974; **73**: 151–166.

62 Wingen A-M, Muller-Wiefel DE, Scharer K. Spontaneous remissions in frequently relapsing and steroid dependent idiopathic nephrotic syndrome. *Clin Nephrol* 1985; **23**: 35–40.

63 Lahdenkari A-T, Suvanto M, Kajantie E, Koskimies O, Kestila M, Jalanko H. Clinical features and outcome of childhood minimal change nephrotic syndrome: is genetics involved. *Pediatr Nephrol* 2005; **20**: 1073–1080.

64 Ruth E-M, Kemper MJ, Leumann EP, Laube GF, Neuhaus TJ. Children with steroid sensitive nephrotic syndrome come of age: long-term outcome. *J Pediatr* 2005; **147**: 202–207.

65 Fakhouri F, Bocquet N, Taupin P, Presne C, Gagnadoux MF, Landais P et al. Steroid-sensitive nephrotic syndrome: from childhood to adulthood. *Am J Kidney Dis* 2003; **41**: 550–557.

66 Lechner BL, Bockenhauer D, Iragorri S, Kennedy TL, Siegel NJ. The risk of cardiovascular disease in adults who have had childhood nephrotic syndrome. *Pediatr Nephrol* 2004; **19**: 744–748.

67 Latta K, von Schnakenburg C, Ehrich JH. A meta-analysis of cytotoxic treatment for frequently relapsing nephrotic syndrome in children. *Pediatr Nephrol* 2001; **16**: 271–282.

68 Hegarty J, Mughal MZ, Adams J, Webb NJ. A reduced bone mineral density in adults treated with high-dose corticosteroids for childhood nephrotic syndrome. *Kidney Int* 2005; **68**: 2304–2309.

69 Leonard MB, Feldman HI, Shults J, Zemel BS, Foster BJ, Stallings VA. Long-term, high-dose glucocorticoids and bone mineral content in childhood glucocorticoid-sensitive nephrotic syndrome. *N Engl J Med* 2005; **351**: 868–875.

70 Krensky AM, Ingelfinger JR, Gorpe WE. Peritonitis in childhood nephrotic syndrome 1970–1980. *Am J Dis Child* 1982; **136**: 732–736.

71 Gulati S, Kher V, Alora P, Gupta S, Kole S. Urinary tract infection in nephrotic syndrome. *Pediatr Infect Dis J* 1966; **15**: 237–240.

72 Gulati S, Kher V, Gupta A, Arora P, Rai PK, Sharma RK. Spectrum of infections in Indian children with nephrotic syndrome. *Pediatr Nephrol* 1995; **9**: 431–434.

73 Butler JC, Breiman RF, Campbell JF, Lipman HB, Broome CV, Facklam RR. Pneumococcal polysaccharide vaccine efficacy: an evaluation of current recommendations. *JAMA* 1993; **270**: 1826–1831.

74 Wilkes JC, Nelson JD, Worthen HG, Morris M, Hogg RJ. Response to pneumococcal vaccination in children with nephrotic syndrome. *Am J Kidney Dis* 1982; **2**: 43–46.

75 Spika JS, Halsey NA, Fish AJ, Lum GM, Lauer BA, Schiffman G et al. Serum antibody response to pneumococcal vaccine in children with nephrotic syndrome. *Pediatrics* 1982; **69**: 219–223.

76 Fuchshuber A, Kuhnemund O, Keuth B, Lutticken R, Michalk D, Querfeld U. Pneumococcal vaccine in children and young adults with chronic renal failure. *Nephrol Dial Transplant* 1996; **11**: 468–473.

77 Guven AG, Akman S, Bahat E, Senyurt M, Yuzbey S, Uguz A et al. Rapid decline of anti-pneumococcal antibody levels in nephrotic children. *Pediatr Nephrol* 2004; **19**: 61–65.

78 Bogaert D, Hermans PW, Adrian PV, Rumke HC, de Groot R. Pneumococcal vaccines: an update on current strategies. *Vaccine* 2004; **22**: 2209–2220.

79 Fedson DS. The clinical effectiveness of pneumococcal vaccine: a brief review. *Vaccine* 1999; **17**: S85–S90.

80 George AC, Melegaro A. Invasive pneumococcal infection, England and Wales: *CDR weekly* **2003**: 3–9.

81 American Academy of Pediatrics Committee on Infectious Diseases. Policy statement: recommendations for the prevention of pneumococcal infections, including the use of pneumococcal conjugate vaccine (Prevnar), pneumococcal polysaccharide vaccine and antibiotic prophylaxis. *Pediatrics* 2000; **106**: 362–366.

82 Overturf GD. American Academy of Pediatrics, Committee on Infectious Diseases, technical report: prevention of pneumococcal infections, including the use of pneumococcal conjugate and polysaccharide vaccines and antibiotic prophylaxis. *Pediatrics* 2000; **106**: 367–376.

83 Davies EG, Riddington C, Lottenberg R, Dower N. Pneumococcal vaccines for sickle cell disease. *Cochrane Database Syst Rev* 2004; **1**: CD003885.

84 John AB, Ramlal A, Jackson H, Maude GH, Sharma AW, Serjeant GR. Prevention of pneumococcal infection in children with homozygous sickle cell disease. *Br Med J* 1984; **288**: 1567–1570.

85 Hirst C, Owusu-Ofori S. Prophylactic antibiotics for preventing pneumococcal infection in children with sickle cell disease. *Cochrane Database Syst Rev* 2002; **3**: CD003427.

86 McIntyre P, Craig JC. Prevention of serious bacterial infection in children with nephrotic syndrome. *J Paediatr Child Health* 1998; **34**: 314–317.

87 Dang X, Yi Z, Wang X, Wu X, Zhang X, He Q. Preventive efficacy of IVIgG on nosocomial infection in the children with nephrotic syndrome. *Bull Hunan Univ* 1999; **24**: 290–292.

88 Dou ZY, Wang JY, Liu YP. Preventative efficiency of low-dose IVIgG on infection in nephrotic syndrome. *Chin J Biol* 2000; **13**: 160.

89 Tong LZ, Mi LZ. Preventative efficiency of IVIgG on secondary nosocomial infection in nephrotic syndrome. *Mod Rehab* 1998; **2**: 236.

90 Wu HM, Tang JL, Sha ZH, Cao I, Li YP. Interventions for preventing infection in nephrotic syndrome (Cochrane review). *The Renal Health Library*, Update Software Ltd., Oxford, 2005.

91 Chan HL, Tang JL, Tam W, Sung JJ. The efficacy of thymosin in the treatment if hepatitis B virus infection: a meta-analysis. *Alim Pharmacol Ther* 2001; **15**: 1899–1905.

92 Zhang YJ, Wang Y, Yang ZW, Li XT. Clinical investigation of thymosin for preventing infection in children with primary nephrotic syndrome. *Chin J Contemp Pediatr* 2000; **2**: 197–198.

93 Li RH, Peng ZP, Wei YL, Liu CH. Clinical observation on Chinese medicinal herbs combined with prednisone for reducing the risks of infection in children with nephrotic syndrome. *Info J Chin Med* 2000; **7**: 60–61.

94 Zaia JA, Levin MJ, Preblud SR, Leszczynski J, Wright GG, Ellis RJ et al. Evaluation of varicella-zoster immune globulin: protection of

immunosuppressed children after household exposure to varicella. *J Infect Dis* 1983; **147**: 737–743.

95 Huang YC, Lin TY, Chiu CH. Acyclovir prophylaxis of varicella after household exposure. *Pediatr Infect Dis J* 1995; **14**: 152–154.

96 Goldstein SL, Somers MJG, Lande MB, Brewer ED, Jabs KL. Acyclovir prophylaxis of varicella in children with renal disease receiving steroids. *Pediatr Nephrol* 2000; **14**: 305–308.

97 Furth SL, Arbus GS, Hogg R, Tarver J, Chan C, Fivush BA *et al*. Varicella vaccination in children with nephrotic syndrome: a report of the Southwest Pediatric Nephrology Study Group. *J Pediatr* 2003; **142**: 145–148.

98 Alpay H, Yildiz N, Onar A, Temizer H, Ozcay S. Varicella vaccination in children with steroid sensitive nephrotic syndrome. *Pediatr Nephrol* 2002;**17**: 181–183.

99 Brydak LB, Rajkowski T, Machala M, Weglarska J, Sieniawska M. Humoral antibody response following influenza vaccination in patients with nephrotic syndrome. *Antiinfect Drugs Chemother* 1998; **16**: 151–155.

100 Poyrazoglu HM, Dusunsel R, Gunduz Z, Patiroglu T, Koklu S. Antibody response to influenza A vaccination in children with nephrotic syndrome. *Pediatr Nephrol* 2004; **19**: 57–60.

101 Kielstein JT, Termuhlen L, Sohn J, Kliem V. Minimal change nephrotic syndrome in a 65 year old patient following influenza vaccination. *Clin Nephrol* 2000; **54**: 246–248.

102 Abeyagunawardena AS, Goldblatt D, Andrews N, Trompeter RS. Risk of relapse after meningococcal C conjugate vaccine in nephrotic syndrome. *Lancet* 2003; **362**: 449–450.

103 Orth SR, Ritz E. The nephrotic syndrome. *N Engl J Med* 1998; **338**: 1202–1211.

104 Lilova MI, Velkovski IG, Topalov IB. Thromboembolic complications in children with nephrotic syndrome in Bulgaria (1974–1996). *Pediatr Nephrol* 2000;**15**: 74–78.

105 Mehls O, Andrassy K, Ritz E. Disseminated intravascular coagulation and platelet activation in the nephrotic syndrome. *Eur J Pediatr* 1984; **VOL**: 261–266.

106 Egli F, Elminger P, Stalder G. Thromboembolisms in nephrotic syndrome. Eur Soc Pediatr Nephrol, abstr. 42. *Pediatrics* 1974; **8**: 903.

107 Hoyer PF, Gonda S, Barthels M, Krohn HP, Brodehl J. Thromboembolic complications in children with nephrotic syndrome. Risk and incidence. *Acta Pediatr Scand* 1986; **75**: 804–810.

108 Eddy AA, Symons J. Nephrotic syndrome in childhood. *Lancet* 2003; **362**: 629–639.

109 Sarasin FP, Schifferli JA. Prophylactic oral anticoagulation in nephrotic patients with idiopathic membranous nephropathy. *Kidney Int* 1994; **45**: 578–585.

110 Andrew M, Michelson AD, Bovill E, Leaker M, Massicotte MP. Guidelines for antithrombotic therapy in pediatric patients. *J Pediatr* 1998; **132**: 577–588.

111 Cameron JS. Coagulation and thromboembolic complications in the nephrotic syndrome. *Adv Nephrol Necker Hosp* 1984; **13**: 75–114.

112 Singhal R, Brimble S. Thromboembolic complications in the nephrotic syndrome: pathophysiology and clinical management. *Thrombosis Res* 2006; **118**: 397–407.

113 Jones CL, Hébert D. Pulmonary thrombo-embolism in the nephrotic syndrome. *Pediatr Nephrol* 1991; **5**: 56–58.

114 Reid CJ, Segal T. Pulmonary thrombo-embolism in nephrotic syndrome treated with tissue plasminogen activator. *Eur J Pediatr* 1997; **156**: 647–649.

115 Brater DC. Diuretic therapy. *N Engl J Med* 1998; **339**: 387–395.

116 Reid CJ, Marsh MJ, Murdoch IM, Clark G. Nephrotic syndrome in childhood complicated by life-threatening pulmonary oedema. *Br Med J* 1996; **312**: 36–38.

67 Management of Steroid-Sensitive Nephrotic Syndrome

Elisabeth M. Hodson,[1,2] **Jonathan C. Craig,**[1,2] **& Narelle S. Willis**[1]

[1]Cochrane Renal Group, NHMRC Centre for Clinical Research Excellence in Renal Medicine, Centre for Kidney Research, The Children's Hospital at Westmead, Sydney, Australia.
[2]School of Public Health, University of Sydney, Sydney, Australia.

Introduction

The majority of children with idiopathic nephrotic syndrome have minimal change nephrotic syndrome, but 10% have mesangio-proliferative glomerulonephritis or focal and segmental glomerulonephritis [1]. The response to corticosteroids is highly predictive of histology, with 93% of children with minimal change nephrotic syndrome achieving remission following an 8-week course of prednisone [2]. Between 25 and 50% of children with mesangio-proliferative glomerulonephritis or focal and segmental glomerulonephritis on biopsy also responded to prednisone [2,3]. Children with idiopathic nephrotic syndrome are now classified according to their initial response to corticosteroids as having either steroid-sensitive nephrotic syndrome (SSNS) or steroid-resistant nephrotic syndrome, as the majority are steroid sensitive and do not undergo renal biopsy at diagnosis.

Of children with SSNS, 75–90% will have one or more relapses, and about half will relapse frequently or become steroid dependent [4,5]. The majority will continue to respond to corticosteroids throughout their subsequent disease course [4–6], and the long-term prognosis for complete resolution with normal renal function is good. In the International Study of Kidney Disease in Children (ISKDC), the proportion of children without relapse reached 80% by 8 years of follow-up [5]. About 10% of patients overall [7,8] and 30–40% of patients with steroid-dependent or frequently relapsing SSNS will continue to relapse as adults [6,9].

In children with SSNS, the aim of corticosteroid therapy is to induce and then maintain remission while minimizing adverse effects. Corticosteroid-sparing agents are used to achieve prolonged remissions in children with frequently relapsing or steroid-dependent disease who have significant adverse effects from prednisone therapy. In this chapter the current evidence base for cor-

ticosteroid therapy and corticosteroid-sparing agents in children with SSNS will be reviewed.

Treatment of the first episode of nephrotic syndrome with corticosteroids

Because of the clear benefits of corticosteroids compared with no treatment, no randomized controlled trials (RCTs) comparing prednisone with placebo have been performed in children with nephrotic syndrome. The ISKDC agreed on a standard corticosteroid regimen for the first episode of SSNS [10], and subsequently researchers have used this regimen or similar regimens as the standard comparator when testing other regimens. In the ISKDC regimen children received prednisone at 60 mg/m^2/day (maximum dose, 80 mg) in divided doses for 4 weeks followed by 40 mg/m^2/day (maximum, 60 mg/day) in divided doses on three consecutive days out of 7 days for 4 weeks. During the second month of therapy alternate-day prednisone is now preferred [11].

Table 67.1 lists the characteristics of study populations and interventions in relevant RCTs of prednisone in an initial episode of SSNS [12]. A single trial demonstrated that prednisone given for 8 weeks was more effective than a shorter duration of treatment (one trial, 60 patients; relative risk [RR], 1.46, 95% confidence interval [CI], 1.01–2.12) [13]. To investigate if longer courses of prednisone could reduce the 70% risk of relapse at 12–24 months seen in the control group after 2 months of therapy, six RCTs [14–19] compared 2 months of prednisone with periods of 3–7 months. A meta-analysis [12] of these trials demonstrated that the risk of relapse was reduced by 30% at 12–24 months (Figure 67.1a). In addition, there were significant reductions in the number of children who relapsed frequently (six trials; RR, 0.63; 95% CI, 0.46–0.84) and in the mean number of relapses per year (four trials; weighted mean difference [WMD], −0.65; 95% CI, −1.29 to 0.00). There was no significant difference in the cumulative prednisone dose (three trials; WMD, 0.71; 95% CI, −0.67 to 2.09), but significant heterogeneity between studies was found. In four trials [17,20–22], prednisone therapy for 6 months was

Evidence-based Nephrology. Edited by Donald Molony and Jonathan Craig
© 2009 Blackwell Publishing, ISBN: 978-1-4051-3975-5.

Table 67.1 Characteristics of populations and interventions in randomized trials of prednisone in the initial episode of SSNS.

Study ID [reference]	No. of patients	Experimental intervention	Control intervention	Follow-up (months)
1 month of prednisone vs 2 months				
APN 1988 [13]	61	60 mg/m^2/day to remission, 40 mg/m^2 alt days till albumin >35 g/L	60 mg/m^2/day for 4 weeks and 40 mg/m^2 alt days for 4 weeks	12
3–7 months of prednisone versus 2 months				
APN 1993 [14]	71	60 mg/m^2/day for 6 weeks and 40 mg/m^2 alt days for 6 weeks	60 mg/m^2/day for 4 weeks and 40 mg/m^2 alt days for 4 weeks	12
Bagga 1999 [15]	45	60 mg/m^2/day for 4 weeks, 40 mg/m^2/day for 4 weeks, 40 mg/m^2 alt days for 4 wks, and 30 mg/m^2 alt days for 4 wks	60 mg/m^2/day for 4 weeks and 40 mg/m^2 alt days for 4 weeks	12
Jayantha 2004a [16]	122	60 mg/m^2/day for 4 weeks, taper dose alt days for 6 months	60 mg/m^2/day for 4 weeks and 40 mg/m^2 alt days for 4 weeks	24
Ksiazek 1995* [17]	116	40–60 mg/m^2/day for 4 weeks, taper dose alt days for 5 months	40–60 mg/m^2/day for 4 wks and 30 mg/m^2 alt days for 4 weeks	24
Norero 1996 [18]	56	60 mg/m^2/day for 6 weeks and 40 mg/m^2 alt days for 6 weeks	60 mg/m^2/day for 4 weeks and 40 mg/m^2 alt days for 4 weeks	18
Ueda 1988 [19]	46	60 mg/m^2/day for 4 weeks, taper dose alt days for 6 months	60 mg/m^2/d for 4 weeks and 40 mg/m^2 on 3 of 7 days for 4 weeks	12
6 months of prednisone versus 3 months				
Hiraoka 2003 [20]	70	60 mg/m^2/day for 4 weeks, taper dose alt days for 5 months	60 mg/m^2/day for 6 weeks and 40 mg/m^2 alt days for 6 weeks	24
Ksiazek 1995* [17]	140	40–60 mg/m^2/day for 4 weeks, taper dose alt days for 5 months	40–60 mg/m^2/day for 4 weeks, taper dose alt days for 8 weeks	24
Pecoraro 2004* [21]	32	60 mg/m^2/day for 6 weeks, taper dose alt days for 4.5 months	60 mg/m^2/day for 4 weeks, taper dose alt days for 8 weeks	24
Sharma 2000 [22]	140	60 mg/m^2/day for 6 weeks, taper dose alt days for 4.5 months	60 mg/m^2/day for 6 weeks and 40 mg/m^2 alt days for 6 weeks	12
12 months of prednisone versus 5 months				
Kleinknecht 1992 [23]	58	60 mg/m^2/day for 4 weeks, taper dose alt days for 11 months	60 mg/m^2/day for 4 weeks, taper dose alt days for 4 months	15
High dose of prednisone compared with low dose given for same duration				
Hiraoka 2000 [24]	68	60 mg/m^2/day for 6 weeks and 40 mg/m^2 alt days for 6 weeks	40 mg/m^2/day for 6 weeks and 40 mg/m^2 alt days for 6 weeks	12
Pecoraro 2004* [21]	16	60 mg/m^2/day for 6 weeks, taper dose alt days for 4.5 months	IV MP 20 mg/kg for 3 days; 30 mg/m^2/day for 6 weeks, taper to alt days for 4.5 months	24
Other combinations of therapies				
APN 2006 [28]	104	Cyclosporine, 150 mg/m^2/day for 8 weeks Prednisone, 60 mg/m^2/day for 6 weeks and 40 mg/m^2 alt days for 6 wks	Prednisone, 60 mg/m^2/day for 6 weeks and 40 mg/m^2 alt days for 6 weeks	24

*Trials with three arms; only two of the three arms are included in each comparison.
Abbreviations: MP, methylprednisolone; IV, intravenous.

compared with 3 months of treatment. A meta-analysis [12] of these trials demonstrated that 6 months of therapy significantly reduced the risk for relapse compared with 3 months (Figure 67.1b). In addition, there were significant reductions in the number of children with frequent relapses (four trials; RR, 0.55; 95% CI, 0.39–0.80) and in the relapse rate per year (three trials; WMD, −0.44; 95% CI, −0.82 to −0.07). No additional benefit was demonstrated in one trial of treatment for 12 months compared with 5 months

[23]. In the six trials comparing 2 months of treatment with 3–7 months, the risk of individual prednisone-related adverse effects did not differ significantly between experimental and control groups of the RCTs [12], although there was heterogeneity between trials (Figure 67.2).

Increased duration of corticosteroid therapy results in an increased total dose of corticosteroid, making the effects of duration and dose difficult to separate. Compared with the standard

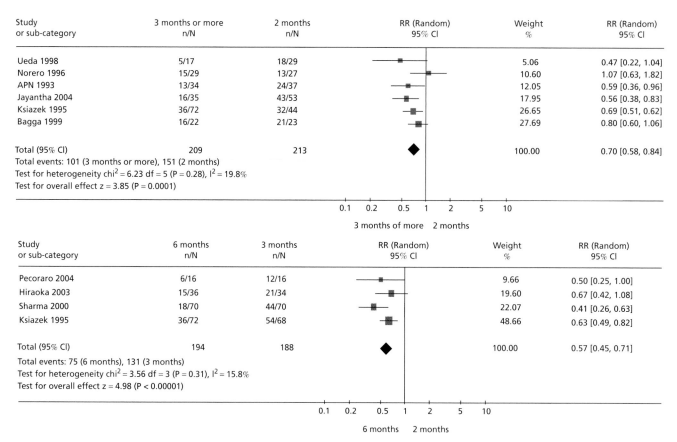

Study or sub-category	3 months or more n/N	2 months n/N	RR (Random) 95% CI	Weight %	RR (Random) 95% CI
Ueda 1998	5/17	18/29		5.06	0.47 [0.22, 1.04]
Norero 1996	15/29	13/27		10.60	1.07 [0.63, 1.82]
APN 1993	13/34	24/37		12.05	0.59 [0.36, 0.96]
Jayantha 2004	16/35	43/53		17.95	0.56 [0.38, 0.83]
Ksiazek 1995	36/72	32/44		26.65	0.69 [0.51, 0.62]
Bagga 1999	16/22	21/23		27.69	0.80 [0.60, 1.06]
Total (95% CI)	209	213		100.00	0.70 [0.58, 0.84]

Total events: 101 (3 months or more), 151 (2 months)
Test for heterogeneity chi^2 = 6.23 df = 5 (P = 0.28), I^2 = 19.8%
Test for overall effect z = 3.85 (P = 0.0001)

0.1 0.2 0.5 1 2 5 10
3 months of more   2 months

Study or sub-category	6 months n/N	3 months n/N	RR (Random) 95% CI	Weight %	RR (Random) 95% CI
Pecoraro 2004	6/16	12/16		9.66	0.50 [0.25, 1.00]
Hiraoka 2003	15/36	21/34		19.60	0.67 [0.42, 1.08]
Sharma 2000	18/70	44/70		22.07	0.41 [0.26, 0.63]
Ksiazek 1995	36/72	54/68		48.66	0.63 [0.49, 0.82]
Total (95% CI)	194	188		100.00	0.57 [0.45, 0.71]

Total events: 75 (6 months), 131 (3 months)
Test for heterogeneity chi^2 = 3.56 df = 3 (P = 0.31), I^2 = 15.8%
Test for overall effect z = 4.98 (P < 0.00001)

0.1 0.2 0.5 1 2 5 10
6 months   2 months

Figure 67.1 Meta-analyses of RR (95% CI) for relapse of nephrotic syndrome by 12–24 months after the initial episode of SSNS in (a) six trials comparing prolonged prednisone therapy (3–7 months) versus 2 months and in (b) four trials comparing 6 months versus 3 months of prednisone therapy in children. Results are shown ordered by trial weights. The test statistic *Z* indicates that an increased duration of prednisone was significantly more effective than 2 or 3 months of prednisone. (Reproduced from Hodson *et al.* [12] with permission from John Wiley and Sons.)

induction dose of prednisone of 2240 mg/m^2, administered doses of 2922–5235 mg/m^2 significantly reduced the risk for relapse at 12–24 months (seven trials [14–19,24], 481 children; RR, 0.69; 95% CI, 0.59–0.81). Plotting the RR for relapse against the dose/duration ratio suggested that duration was more important than dose [12]. Two trials [21,24] have now examined different total doses of prednisone administered for the same duration (3 or 6 months). A meta-analysis of these studies showed that the risk of relapse was reduced by 40% with higher doses of corticosteroids (two trials; RR, 0.59; 95% CI, 0.42–0.84), suggesting that both an increased dose and prolonged duration of corticosteroids are important determinants of the risk of relapse [12].

There is an inverse linear relationship between the risk for relapse and duration of induction therapy, suggesting an increase in benefit with treatment for up to 7 months (RR = 1.26 − 0.112 duration; $r^2 = 0.56$; $P = 0.03$) [12,25]. With each increase of 1 month of therapy beyond 2 months, the RR for relapse falls by 11%. With a relapse rate of 70% with treatment for 2 months, the calculated number of children relapsing by 12–24 months will fall by 8% for every increase by 1 month in the duration of therapy, so that treatment for 6 months would reduce the risk of relapse

by 32% (4 × 8%), to 38%. In populations with lower relapse rates following 2 months of therapy, the benefit of longer courses of prednisone will be smaller.

These data suggest that to reduce the risk of relapse following the first episode of SSNS, prednisone therapy should be given for 3 months or more, with increased benefit with up to 6 months of therapy. Despite the available data from RCTs, a survey of pediatric nephrologists in North America demonstrated considerable variation among respondents in their approach to the first episode of idiopathic nephrotic syndrome, although about 70% used durations of therapy exceeding the ISKDC's 8-week regimen [26]. Pediatric nephrologists may have been reluctant to increase the duration of prednisone therapy because data on benefits and harms have come from relatively small trials of varied methodological quality. Nevertheless, these trials have provided consistent results, demonstrating that increased duration and dose of corticosteroids reduces the risk for relapse without an increase in harm. The results of a well-designed adequately powered and placebo-controlled RCT comparing 2 months versus 4 months of prednisone therapy with an emphasis on adverse effects, which has recently commenced in the United Kingdom, are expected to help clarify this issue [27].

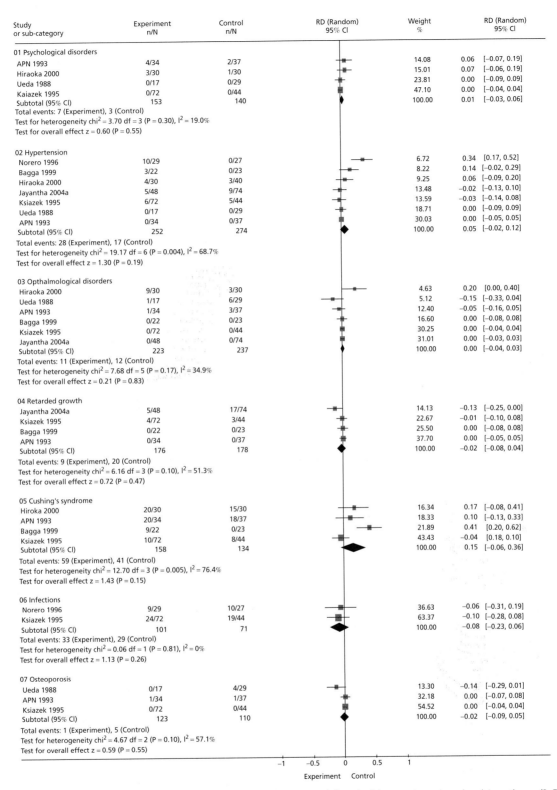

Figure 67.2 Meta-analyses of Risk Difference (RD) (95% CI) for adverse effects of corticosteroids from six trials comparing prolonged prednisone therapy (3–7 months) versus 2 months. Results are shown ordered by trial weights. The test statistic *Z* indicates that there were no significant differences in the risks of adverse effects with prolonged prednisone therapy (3–7 months) compared with 2 months. (Reproduced from Hodson *et al.* [12] with permission from John Wiley and Sons.)

Treatment of the first episode of nephrotic syndrome with corticosteroids and cyclosporine

Based on the hypothesis that increased immunosuppression reduces the risk for relapse further, but with physicians unwilling to use longer courses of corticosteroids because of the adverse effects, the Arbeitsgemeinschaft für Pädiatrische Nephrologie (APN) compared 12 weeks of prednisone alone with 12 weeks of prednisone plus 8 weeks of cyclosporine [28]. The risk of relapse was significantly lower in the cyclosporine group at 6 months (104 children; RR, 0.33; 95% CI, 0.13–0.83) but not at 12 or 24 months. The mean relapse rate per patient was significantly lower in the cyclosporine group at 6 and 12 months but not at 24 months. Blood pressure and renal function did not differ between groups. Psychological disturbances, hirsutism, and gum hypertrophy were more common during cyclosporine treatment but resolved when cyclosporine was ceased. The authors concluded that because of the attenuation of benefit after 1 year, the side effects of cyclosporine, and the need for monitoring of blood levels, this experimental protocol could not be recommended as a replacement for protocols using prednisone alone in the first episode of SSNS.

Treatment of relapsing SSNS with corticosteroids

There are few data from RCTs on corticosteroid regimens for children with relapsing SSNS, with individual trials addressing different questions. The trial populations and interventions are listed in Table 67.2. Alternate-day prednisone was more effective in maintaining remission than prednisone given on three consecutive days out of 7 days (48 children; RR, 0.60; 95% CI, 0.36–1.02) [11]. There were no significant differences in the time to remission (94 children; WMD, −0.30; 95% CI, −1.64 to −1.04) or risk for relapse (RR, 1.07; 95% CI, 0.77–1.50) between single daily doses and divided daily doses of prednisone. Prednisone can be administered as a single daily dose during daily therapy, which should improve adherence [29]. Deflazacort given for 12 months was significantly more effective than equivalent doses of prednisone in reducing the risk for relapse (40 children; RR, 0.44; 95% CI, 0.25–0.78) in children with steroid-dependent SSNS without differences in adverse effects [30], but deflazacort is not widely available. Prednisone given for 7 months reduced the risk of relapse by 1 year compared with 2 months of therapy (76 children; RR, 0.43; 95% CI, 0.29–0.65) [31]. No significant reduction in the risk of relapse at 1 year could be demonstrated with high-dose intravenous methylprednisolone followed by oral prednisone for 6 months compared with oral prednisone alone (64 children; RR, 1.06; 95% CI, 0.75–1.52) [32]. The total dose of oral prednisone administered was higher in the control group than in the group receiving intravenous prednisone. Children with steroid-dependent SSNS averaged three fewer relapses during 2 years of follow-up if they received daily rather than alternate-day therapy during intercurrent upper respiratory tract infections (38 children; WMD, −3.30; 95% CI, −4.03 to −2.57) [33].

Table 67.2 Characteristics of populations and interventions in randomized trials of corticosteroids in relapsing SSNS.

Trial ID [reference]	No. of patients	Experimental intervention	Control intervention	Follow-up (months)
Alternate-day prednisone versus intermittent therapy in frequently relapsing patients				
APN 1979 [11]	64	60 mg/m^2/day until remission, 35 mg/m^2 alt days for 6 months	60 mg/m^2/day till remission days, 40 mg/m^2 on 3 of 7 days for 6 months	12
Deflazacort versus prednisone in steroid-dependent patients				
Broyer 1997 [30]	40	Deflazacort equivalent to prednisone 60 mg/m^2/day until remission, tapering dose alt days for 12 months	Prednisone 60 mg/m^2/day until remission, tapering dose alt days for 12 months	12
Daily prednisone as single daily dose versus divided doses				
Ekka 1997 [29]	106	60 mg/m^2/day in single dose for 4 weeks, 40 mg/m^2 alt days for 4 weeks	60 mg/m^2/day in 3 doses for 4 weeks, 40 mg/m^2 alt days for 4 weeks	9
IV MP and oral prednisone versus oral prednisone alone in infrequently relapsing patients				
Imbasciati 1985 [32]	67	IV MP 20 mg/kg for 3 days, prednisone 20 mg/m^2/day for 4 weeks, tapering dose alt days for 5 month	Prednisone 60 mg/m^2/day for 4 weeks, tapering dose alt days for 5 months	24
Daily prednisone versus daily followed by alternate-day prednisone in patients relapsing <6 months after initial episode (7 months prednisone versus 2 months)				
Jayantha 2004b [31]	90	60 mg/m^2/day until remission, tapering dose alt days for 6 months	60 mg/m^2/day until remission and 60 mg/m^2 alt days for 4 weeks	24
Daily versus alternate-day prednisone during URTI in frequently relapsing patients				
Mattoo 2000 [33]	36	15 mg/m^2/day for 5 days in URTI and then 15 mg/m^2 alt days	15 mg/m^2 alt days continued in URTI	24

Abbreviations: IV, intravenous; MP, methylprednisolone; URTI, upper respiratory tract infection(s).

Table 67.3 Characteristics of populations and interventions in randomized trials of alkylating agents in SSNS.

Study ID [reference]	No. of patients	Experimental intervention	Control intervention	Follow-up (months)
Alkylating agents versus placebo or no treatment				
Barratt 1970 [34]	30	CPA 3 mg/kg/day for 8 weeks, prednisone for 16 weeks	Prednisone for 8 weeks	24
Chiu 1973 [35]	23	CPA 2.5 mg/kg/day for 16 weeks, prednisone for 16 weeks	Prednisone for 16 weeks	20
ISKDC 1974 [36]	53	CPA 5 mg/kg/day till leukopenia; 1–3 mg/kg/day; total 6 weeks	Prednisone for 26 weeks	6
Alatas 1978 [37]	20	CHL 0.3 mg/kg/day, prednisone for 8 weeks	Placebo. Prednisone for 8 weeks	12
Grupe 1976 [38]	21	CHL 0.1–0.2 mg/kg/day and increased till leukopenia (6–12 weeks); prednisone for 12 weeks	Prednisone for 12 weeks	12
Different durations or doses of alkylating agents				
Barratt 1973 [42]	32	CPA 3 mg/kg/day for 8 weeks, prednisone for 16 weeks	CPA 3 mg/kg/day for 2 weeks, prednisone for 16 weeks	12
Ueda 1990 [43]	73	CPA 2 mg/kg/day for 12 weeks	CPA 2 mg/kg/day for 8 weeks	24
IV versus oral cyclophosphamide				
Prasad 2004 [45]	47	IV CPA 500 mg/m^2 monthly for 6 doses, prednisone for 10–12 weeks	Oral CPA 2 mg/kg/day for 12 weeks, prednisone for 10–12 weeks	12
Cyclophosphamide versus chlorambucil				
APN 1982 [41]	50	CPA 2 mg/kg/day for 8 weeks, prednisone for 4 weeks	CHL 0.15 mg/kg/day for 8 weeks, prednisone for 4 weeks	24

Abbreviations: CPA, cyclophosphamide; CHL, chlorambucil; IV, intravenous.

Corticosteroid-sparing agents in frequently relapsing and steroid-dependent SSNS

Alkylating agents, cyclosporine, and levamisole have been demonstrated in RCTs to be effective in reducing the risk for relapse in frequently relapsing and steroid-dependent SSNS. There are no data demonstrating any differences in efficacy between alkylating agents, levamisole, and cyclosporine, so their use depends on availability and patient and physician preferences.

Alkylating agents

The characteristics of clinical trials with alkylating agents are shown in Table 67.3. A meta-analysis of five trials [34–38] demonstrated that cyclophosphamide or chlorambucil reduced the risk for relapse at 6–12 months by 70% in children with frequently relapsing SSNS compared with prednisone alone (Figure 67.3a) [39,40]. There was no significant difference in efficacy between cyclophosphamide and chlorambucil (50 children; RR, 1.15; 95% CI, 0.69–1.94) [41]. Cyclophosphamide therapy for 8 weeks was significantly more effective than administration for just 2 weeks in reducing the risk of relapse at 12 months (22 children; RR, 0.25; 95% CI, 0.07–0.92) [42]. There was no significant difference in the risk of relapse at 12 months between therapy lasting for 8 versus 12 weeks (73 children; RR, 1.04; 95% CI, 0.75–1.44) [43], although an APN study using historical controls had suggested that 12 weeks was superior [44]. Monthly intravenous cyclophosphamide given for 6 months reduced the risk of relapse at the end of therapy compared with oral cyclophosphamide given for 12 weeks (47 children; RR, 0.56; 95% CI, 0.33–0.92), but there was

no difference after 2 years [45]. To determine long-term outcomes, 26 studies of cyclophosphamide and chlorambucil usage in SSNS were analyzed [46]. Overall relapse-free survival after 5 years was below 40%. For frequently relapsing SSNS, relapse-free survivals were 72% and 36% after 2 and 5 years, respectively. For steroid-dependent children, relapse-free survival was 40% and 24% after 2 and 5 years, respectively.

Adverse effects with alkylating agents are frequent and may be severe. Latta and coworkers identified adverse effects from 38 reports on frequently relapsing SSNS that involved 866 children who received 906 courses of cyclophosphamide and 638 children who received 671 courses of chlorambucil [46]. With cyclophosphamide, 0.8% of children died, 1.5% suffered serious infections, 32% developed leukopenia, 2.2% had hemorrhagic cystitis, and 18% had hair loss. With chlorambucil therapy 1% of children died, 6.3% suffered serious infections, 33% developed leukopenia, and 5.9% had thrombocytopenia. Alkylating agents may cause gonadal dysfunction in men, but most reports observed little or no toxicity in women treated for SSNS [46]. With cyclophosphamide treatment in SSNS, there is a dose-dependent relationship between the number of men with sperm counts below 10^6/ml and the cumulative dose of cyclophosphamide. Some individuals have developed oligospermia at cumulative cyclophosphamide doses of 200 mg/kg, suggesting that single courses of cyclophosphamide at a dose of 2 mg/kg/day should not exceed 12 weeks (cumulative dose, 168 mg/kg) and that second courses should be avoided. There are few data on gonadal toxicity with chlorambucil in SSNS. However, in male patients treated for lymphoma, azoospermia occurred with cumulative doses of 10–17 mg/kg, which are equivalent to doses used in SSNS treatment [47].

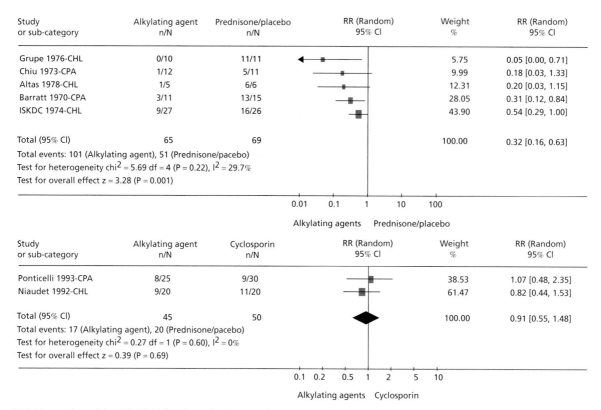

Study or sub-category	Alkylating agent n/N	Prednisone/placebo n/N	RR (Random) 95% CI	Weight %	RR (Random) 95% CI
Grupe 1976-CHL	0/10	11/11		5.75	0.05 [0.00, 0.71]
Chiu 1973-CPA	1/12	5/11		9.99	0.18 [0.03, 1.33]
Altas 1978-CHL	1/5	6/6		12.31	0.20 [0.03, 1.15]
Barratt 1970-CPA	3/11	13/15		28.05	0.31 [0.12, 0.84]
ISKDC 1974-CHL	9/27	16/26		43.90	0.54 [0.29, 1.00]
Total (95% CI)	65	69		100.00	0.32 [0.16, 0.63]

Total events: 101 (Alkylating agent), 51 (Prednisone/pacebo)
Test for heterogeneity chi^2 = 5.69 df = 4 (P = 0.22), I^2 = 29.7%
Test for overall effect z = 3.28 (P = 0.001)

0.01 0.1 1 10 100
Alkylating agents   Prednisone/placebo

Study or sub-category	Alkylating agent n/N	Cyclosporin n/N	RR (Random) 95% CI	Weight %	RR (Random) 95% CI
Ponticelli 1993-CPA	8/25	9/30		38.53	1.07 [0.48, 2.35]
Niaudet 1992-CHL	9/20	11/20		61.47	0.82 [0.44, 1.53]
Total (95% CI)	45	50		100.00	0.91 [0.55, 1.48]

Total events: 17 (Alkylating agent), 20 (Prednisone/pacebo)
Test for heterogeneity chi^2 = 0.27 df = 1 (P = 0.60), I^2 = 0%
Test for overall effect z = 0.39 (P = 0.69)

0.1 0.2 0.5 1 2 5 10
Alkylating agents   Cyclosporin

Figure 67.3 Meta-analyses of the RR (95% CI) for relapse of nephrotic syndrome at 6–12 months in children with frequently relapsing SSNS following (a) alkylating agents (cyclophosphamide [CPA] or chlorambucil [CHL]) compared with prednisone or placebo and (b) cyclosporin compared with alkylating agents. Results are shown ordered by trial weights. The test statistic *Z* indicates that alkylating agents are more effective than prednisone alone and that the efficacy of cyclosporine and alkylating agents is not significantly different. (Reproduced from Durkan *et al.* [40] with permission from John Wiley and Sons.)

Cyclosporine

Single trials [48,49] (Table 67.4) have demonstrated no significant difference in efficacy during treatment between cyclosporine (6 mg/kg/day in divided doses) and cyclophosphamide or chlorambucil (Figure 67.3b) [40]. The majority of children treated with cyclosporine relapse when therapy is ceased. Adverse effects are significant, with 4% of children developing hypertension, 9% reduced renal function, 28% gum hypertrophy, and 34% hirsutism [40]. In long-term studies remissions of 1 and 2 years are achieved in 60% and 40% of children, respectively. However, 40% of children require low-dose long-term alternate-day prednisone to maintain remission despite adequate blood levels of cyclosporine [50]. Cyclosporine is usually commenced at 5 mg/kg/day in two divided doses with subsequent dosing altered to achieve predose blood levels of 50–100 ng/mL (measured by fluorescence polarization immunoassay). The dose of cyclosporine required to maintain trough levels can be reduced by one-third by administering ketoconazole as a cyclosporine-sparing agent [51]. Glomerular filtration rate was significantly better in the group receiving ketoconazole. Recently, using a 2-h postdose level of 300–400 ng/mL to guide dosage, lower doses of cyclosporine could be used without changes in relapse rate [52].

Cyclosporine-induced tubulo-interstitial lesions on renal biopsy are reported in 30–40% of children who have received cyclosporine for 12 months or more [53, 54], with 80% having interstitial fibrosis when treated for 4 or more years. Cyclosporine-associated arteriopathy is uncommon. Risk factors for fibrosis are more than 3 years of cyclosporine therapy, age below 5 years at the start of therapy, and having heavy proteinuria for more than 30 days during therapy [53,55]. Arteriopathy, but not interstitial fibrosis, improves after cyclosporine has been ceased for 12 months or more [56]. Because of these histological changes, it is recommended that children with SSNS receive cyclosporine for periods of only 2–3 years [53,55] or undergo annual renal biopsies if cyclosporine is continued [53], particularly as interstitial changes may occur in the absence of renal impairment [57].

Levamisole

The efficacy of levamisole in SSNS has been demonstrated in many studies [58] and evaluated in four RCTs [59–62] (Table 67.4). Currently, levamisole is not available because its manufacturer ceased production [58]. Levamisole reduced the risk of relapse by 40% in comparison with prednisone alone in three trials (137 patients; RR, 0.60; 95% CI, 0.45–0.79) [40,59–61]. It was ineffective in a fourth trial [62] in which children with frequently relapsing

Table 67.4 Characteristics of populations and interventions in randomised trials of other corticosteroid sparing agents in relapsing steroid sensitive nephrotic syndrome

Study ID	Patient numbers	Experimental intervention	Control intervention	Follow up (months)
Cyclosporin compared with alkylating agents				
Niaudet 1992[48]	40	Cyclosporin 6 mg/kg/d × 3 mth, taper × 3 mth	Chlorambucil 0.2 mg/kg/d × 40 days	24
Ponticelli 1993[49]	55	Cyclosporin 6 mg/kg/d × 9 mth	Cyclophosphamide 2.5 mg/kg/d × 8 wk	24
Levamisole compared with placebo/no treatment				
BAPN* 1991[59]	61	Levamisole 2.5 mg/kg on alt days × 16wk	Placebo on alt days × 16wk	6
Dayal 1994[60]	37	Levamisole 2–3 mg/kg twice a week × 52 wk	No treatment × 52 wk	12
Rashid 1996[61]	40	Levamisole 2.5 mg/kg on alt days & prednisone × 26 wk	Prednisone × 26 wk	12
Weiss 1993[62]	49	Levamisole 2.5 mg/kg on 2 consecutive days/wk × 26 wk	Placebo on 2 consecutive days/wk × 26 wk	12
Levamisole compared with intravenous cyclophosphamide				
Donia 2005[63]	40	Levamisole 2.5 mg/kg on alt days × 26 wks	IV cyclophosphamide 500 mg/m^2 mthly × 26 wk	18
Azathioprine compared with placebo/no treatment				
Abramowicz 1970[67]	36	Azathioprine 60 mg/m^2/d × 26 wk, prednisone × 26 wk	Placebo × 26 wk, prednisone × 26 wk	6
Barratt 1977[68]	24	Azathioprine 2 mg/kg/d × 8 wk, prednisone × 16 wk	Prednisone × 16 wk	8
Mizoribine compared with placebo				
Yoshioka 2000[69]	197	Mizoribine 4 mg/kg/d × 48 wk, prednisone × 12 wk	Placebo × 48 wks, prednisone × 12 wk	18

*British Association for Paediatric Nephrology

and/or steroid-dependent SSNS received a total levamisole dose of 20 mg/kg/month, compared with the 35-mg/kg/month dose used in the other two trials [59,61] that enrolled children with frequently relapsing and/or steroid-dependent SSNS. In addition, levamisole was administered on two consecutive days of seven in the Weiss trial compared with alternate-day dosing in the other two trials. These data suggest that lack of efficacy in the Weiss trial [62] could have resulted from inadequate total dose and/or inappropriate dosing intervals. In an RCT comparing levamisole with intravenous cyclophosphamide, there was no significant difference in the risk of relapse at 12 months after the end of therapy (40 children; RR, 0.89; 95% CI, 0.68–1.16) [63]. Similarly, in a retrospective analysis of children with steroid-dependent SSNS treated with levamisole for 6 months or oral cyclophosphamide for 8–12 weeks, the proportion of children who were relapse-free after 1 year did not differ between treatment groups [64]. Adverse effects of levamisole are uncommon but include leukopenia, gastrointestinal effects, and occasionally vasculitis [65,66].

Other corticosteroid-sparing agents

In RCTs (Table 67.4), no significant reduction in the risk of relapse has been demonstrated with azathioprine compared with prednisone alone (two trials, 60 children; RR, 0.90; 95% CI, 0.59–1.38) [67,68]. There was no significant difference in relapse rates in an RCT comparing mizoribine with placebo (Table 67.4). The hazard ratio of cumulative remission rate was 0.79 (95% CI, 0.57–1.08) [69]. Sixteen percent of treated patients developed hyperuricemia.

Mycophenolate mofetil (MMF) is now widely used in children with SSNS as a corticosteroid-sparing agent, but to date no data on its efficacy are available from RCTs, although a crossover trial comparing MMF and cyclosporine is in progress through the APN [70]. Three prospective studies involving 76 children who were

treated with MMF for 6–12 months reported reductions in relapse rates of 50–75% during treatment [71–73]. Prednisone dose could be reduced in many patients, but most children relapsed when MMF was ceased. Studies have used 900–1200 mg/m^2/day in two divided doses. Trough levels of mycophenolic acid, measured by enzymatic immunoassay, below 2.5 μg/mL were associated with a slightly but not significantly greater risk of relapse, suggesting that dose regimens should be guided by therapeutic drug monitoring [73]. Kidney function improved on transfer from cyclosporine to MMF [73]. The main adverse effects of MMF in kidney transplant patients are abdominal pain, diarrhea, anemia, leukopenia, and thrombocytopenia, although to date MMF has been well-tolerated in children with SSNS, with only mild abdominal pain reported [71,73]. In children who relapse on MMF alone, a combination of cyclosporine and MMF may maintain remission with the potential for using lower cyclosporine doses [73].

There are few data on the use of tacrolimus, another calcineurin inhibitor, in children with steroid-dependent SSNS. A retrospective study reported data on 10 children who were transferred to tacrolimus because of a poor response to or adverse effects of cyclosporine, and it compared the therapy periods on cyclosporine versus tacrolimus therapy in these children [74]. There was no difference between the therapy periods in the rate of relapse per year, corticosteroid dose, glomerular filtration rate, need for antihypertensive agents, or calcineurin inhibitor toxicity on renal biopsy. One child on tacrolimus developed insulin-dependent diabetes mellitus. A second study of five children with steroid-dependent SSNS reported that only one patient improved substantially with tacrolimus and two children developed insulin-dependent diabetes mellitus [75]. Thus, to date there are no data suggesting that tacrolimus offers any additional benefits over cyclosporine in children with SSNS.

Table 67.5 Evidence rating and recommendations for corticosteroid therapy in steroid sensitive nephrotic syndrome.

Intervention	Evidence rating[a,b]			Recommendations[c]			
	Moderate	Low	Comment	I[d]	II[e]	III[f]	Comment
Corticosteroids in the initial episode of steroid sensitive nephrotic syndrome							
Prednisone 3–7 mths vs 2 mths	•		6 RCTs (422 patients), 3 trials of poor quality, consistent results	•			RD[g] −0.23 (95% CI −0.33 to −0.13). NNT[h] 4. Moderate evidence base, no excess harms documented.
Prednisone 6 mths vs 3 mths	•		4 RCTs (382 patients), 2 trials of poor quality, consistent results	•			RD −0.31 (95% CI −0.41 to −0.22). NNT 3. Moderate evidence base, no excess harms documented.
Prednisone high vs low dose		•	2 RCTs (91 patients), one trial of poor quality, consistent results			•	RD −0.32 (95% CI −0.51 to −0.13). Low evidence base. Need more data on harms.
Corticosteroids in relapsing steroid sensitive nephrotic syndrome							
Prednisone alt day vs 3/7 days	•		1 RCT (64 patients); wide 95% CI	•			RD −0.29 (95% CI −0.55 to −0.02). NNT 3.5. Moderate evidence base, no excess harms documented.
Prednisone daily vs divided dose	•		1 RCT (106 patients); wide 95% CI	•			No differences in efficacy or harms. Moderate evidence base. Could improve compliance.
Prednisone 7 mths vs 2 mths	•		1 RCT (90 patients); 20% lost to follow up		•		RD −0.50 (95% CI −0.68 to −0.32). NNT 2. Moderate evidence base. Further RCTs required.
Daily prednisone dose for URTI		•	1 small RCT (36 patients); poor quality			•	3 relapses fewer/yr. Low evidence base. Further RCTs required.
Deflazacort vs prednisone	•		1 small RCT (40 patients)			•	RD −0.50 (95% CI −0.75 to −0.25). NNT 2. Moderate evidence base. Further RCTs required. Deflazacort not generally available.

[a] Evidence rating based on study design, study quality, consistency and directness of results. All data from systematic reviews of randomized controlled trials.

[b] No intervention was rated with a high evidence rating.

[c] Recommendations based on trade-off between benefits and harms, quality of evidence, translation of evidence into practice in a specific setting including availability of medication and any uncertainty about the baseline risk of the disease in the population.

[d] Recommend, [e] Suggest, [f] No recommendation possible.

[g] Risk difference (95% confidence intervals).

[h] Number needed to treat.

Conclusions

The evidence ratings (based on numbers of trials, study design, study quality, and consistency of results) and recommendations (based on the trade-offs between benefits and harms, the quality of the evidence, and the ability to translate into clinical practice) for use of corticosteroids and corticosteroid-sparing agents in children with SSNS are listed in Tables 67.5 and 67.6.

For an initial episode of SSNS, the overall evidence rating is classified as moderate for the recommendation to use prednisone therapy for durations of 3–7 months compared with 2 months and for durations of 6 months compared with 3 months. Although the trials evaluating prolonged duration of prednisone are small

and of variable quality, the benefits are consistent across trials: the effect size is large (RR, 0.70; 95% CI, 0.58–0.84), and no significant differences in harm has been documented, although there is some heterogeneity among trials. The number needed to treat (NNT) is four, indicating that only four children need to be treated with prednisone for 3–7 months compared with 2 months to prevent one child from relapsing and avoiding the morbidity associated with relapse. The evidence rating for high total dose compared with lower total dose is low, so that no recommendation can be given for this medication schedule at present.

In relapsing SSNS, the evidence rating is classified as moderate for the recommendations to use single daily doses rather than divided doses to induce remission and to use alternate-day prednisone rather than three consecutive days out of seven to maintain

Table 67.6 Evidence ratings and recommendations for corticosteroid sparing agents in frequently relapsing steroid sensitive nephrotic syndrome

| Intervention | Evidence rating[a,b] | | | Recommendations[c] | | | |
	Moderate	Low	Comment	I[d]	II[e]	III[f]	Comment
Alkylating agents							
Alkylating agents for 8 wks vs prednisone	•		5 RCTs (134 patients), some of poor quality. Consistent results.	•			RD[g] −0.61 (95% CI −1.00 to −0.23). NNT[h] 2. Moderate evidence base for efficacy and safety.
Cyclophosphamide vs chlorambucil	•		1 RCT (50 patients).	•			No differences in efficacy or harms. Moderate evidence base.
Intravenous vs oral cyclophosphamide	•		1 RCT (47 patients).			•	No obvious difference in efficacy/harms by 2 yrs. Moderate evidence base.
Cyclosporin							
Cyclosporin vs alkylating agents	•		2 RCTs (95 patients). Consistent results.	•			No difference in efficacy between agents during treatment. Moderate evidence base.
Levamisole							
Levamisole for 4–12 mths vs prednisone	•		3 RCTs (137 patients) show benefit. Consistent results. 1 RCT (48 patients) using lower dose no effect.			•	RD −0.31 (95% CI −0.46 to −0.16) (3 RCTs). NNT 3. Moderate evidence base. No excess harms documented. Levamisole not currently available.
Levamisole vs cyclophosphamide		•	1 RCT (40 patients); poor quality			•	Sparse data; no obvious difference in efficacy. Levamisole not currently available.
Mycophenolate mofetil							
Mycophenolate mofetil		•	3 prospective studies (76 patients); consistent results			•	Poor evidence base. No RCTs. Apparent benefit in 50–75% patients.
Tacrolimus							
Tacrolimus		•	2 studies (15 patients); consistent results			•	Sparse data; no demonstrable benefit over cycloporin.

[a] Evidence rating based on study design, study quality, consistency and directness of results. All data from systematic reviews of randomized controlled trials.
[b] No intervention was rated with a high evidence rating.
[c] Recommendations based on trade-off between benefits and harms, quality of evidence, translation of evidence into practice in a specific setting including availability of medication and any uncertainty about the baseline risk of the disease in the population.
[d] Recommend, [e] Suggest, [f] No recommendation possible.
[g] Risk difference (95% confidence intervals). [h] Number needed to treat.

remission. There is no biological reason why these regimens should not be equally effective in the initial episode of SSNS, although this has not been evaluated in RCTs. It is suggested that prolonged duration of prednisone treatment can also be used for relapsing SSNS, but further RCTs are required to document the adverse effects of corticosteroids in children, who require multiple courses of prednisone. No recommendation can be made for deflazacort or for daily prednisone during upper respiratory infections without further RCTs to examine the benefits and harms.

In children with frequently relapsing or steroid-dependent SSNS, the evidence rating is classified as moderate for use of alkylating agents compared with prednisone or no treatment, with no difference demonstrated in efficacy between cyclophosphamide and chlorambucil. Alkylating agents can be recommended for children with frequently relapsing or steroid-dependent SSNS who

have serious adverse effects from corticosteroids. Significant harm is associated with alkylating agents, with about a 3% risk of serious infections and 1% risk of death. Alkylating agents reduce the risk of relapse by 70% (NNT, 2), so one can estimate that 3 serious infections and 1 death due to treatment will occur per 100 patients avoiding a relapse. The evidence rating for using intravenous compared with oral cyclophosphamide is moderate, but no recommendation for its routine use can be made because of the additional potential harm related to intravenous access and treatment costs, which were not considered in the study. The evidence rating for using cyclosporine is classified as moderate, and this agent can be recommended as an alternative to alkylating agents as no difference in efficacy between cyclosporine and these agents has been demonstrated. The evidence rating is classified as moderate for the efficacy of levamisole compared with prednisone or placebo, but no recommendation can be made for its use, as this medication is no longer manufactured. The evidence rating for MMF and tacrolimus is classified as low, and no recommendations can be made for their use.

Although the evidence base from randomized trials in the treatment of SSNS is relatively large, many of the trials performed have been small and/or of inadequate quality. Further information, particularly on potential harms, is required to determine the optimal duration and total dose of prednisone in the initial episode of SSNS, with clarification of the relative contributions of dose and duration. In frequently relapsing and steroid-dependent SSNS, more information is required on the relative efficacies of alkylating agents, cyclosporine, MMF, and levamisole (assuming that production of levamisole is resumed). In addition, information is needed on the relative efficacies of corticosteroid-sparing agents in children with steroid-dependent or frequently relapsing SSNS. These important questions can be answered with well-designed and adequately powered international multicenter trials.

References

1 Nephrotic syndrome in children: prediction of histopathology from clinical and laboratory characteristics at time of diagnosis. A report of the International Study of Kidney Disease in Children. *Kidney Int* 1978; **13**(2): 159–165.

2 The primary nephrotic syndrome in children. Identification of patients with minimal change nephrotic syndrome from initial response to prednisone. A report of the International Study of Kidney Disease in Children. *J Pediatr* 1981; **98**(4): 561–564 .

3 Childhood nephrotic syndrome associated with diffuse mesangial hypercellularity. A report of the Southwest Pediatric Nephrology Study Group. *Kidney Int* 1983; **24**(1): 87–94.

4 Koskimies O, Vilska J, Rapola J, Hallman N. Long-term outcome of primary nephrotic syndrome. *Arch Dis Child* 1982; **57**(7): 544–548.

5 Tarshish P, Tobin JN, Bernstein J, Edelmann CM, Jr. Prognostic significance of the early course of minimal change nephrotic syndrome: report of the International Study of Kidney Disease in Children. *J Am Soc Nephrol* 1997; **8**(5): 769–776.

6 Fakhouri F, Bocquet N, Taupin P, Presne C, Gagnadoux MF, Landais P *et al.* Steroid-sensitive nephrotic syndrome: from childhood to adulthood. *Am J Kidney Dis* 2003; **41**(3): 550–557.

7 Trompeter RS, Lloyd BW, Hicks J, White RH, Cameron JS. Long-term outcome for children with minimal-change nephrotic syndrome. *Lancet* 1985; **i**(8425): 368–370.

8 Lahdenkari AT, Suvanto M, Kajantie E, Koskimies O, Kestilä M, Jalanko H. Clinical features and outcome of childhood minimal change nephrotic syndrome: is genetics involved? *Pediatr Nephrol* 2005; **20**: 1073–1080.

9 Ruth EM, Kemper MJ, Leumann EP, Laube GF, Neuhaus TJ. Children with steroid-sensitive nephrotic syndrome come of age: long-term outcome. *J Pediatr* 2005; **147**(2): 202–207.

10 Arneil GC. The nephrotic syndrome. *Pediatr Clin North Am* 1971; **18**(2): 547–559.

11 Alternate-day versus intermittent prednisone in frequently relapsing nephrotic syndrome. A report of "Arbeitsgemeinschaft für Pädiatrische Nephrologie." *Lancet* 1979; **i**(8113): 401–403.

12 Hodson EM, Knight JF, Willis NS, Craig JC. Corticosteroid therapy for nephrotic syndrome in children. *Cochrane Database Syst Rev* 2005; **1**: CD001533.

13 Short versus standard prednisone therapy for initial treatment of idiopathic nephrotic syndrome in children. Arbeitsgemeinschaft für Pädiatrische Nephrologie. *Lancet* 1988; **i**(8582): 380–383.

14 Ehrich JH, Brodehl J. Long versus standard prednisone therapy for initial treatment of idiopathic nephrotic syndrome in children. Arbeitsgemeinschaft für Pädiatrische Nephrologie. *Eur J Pediatr* 1993; **152**(4): 357–361.

15 Bagga A, Hari P, Srivastava RN. Prolonged versus standard prednisolone therapy for initial episode of nephrotic syndrome. *Pediatr Nephrol* 1999; **13**(9): 824–827.

16 Jayantha UK. Comparison of ISKDC regime with a 7 months regime in the first attack of nephrotic syndrome. *Pediatr Nephrol* 2004; **19**: C81.

17 Ksiäžek J, Wyszyńska T. Short versus long initial prednisone treatment in steroid-sensitive nephrotic syndrome in children. *Acta Paediatr* 1995; **84**(8): 889–893.

18 Norero C, Delucchi A, Lagos E, Rosati P. [Initial therapy of primary nephrotic syndrome in children: evaluation in a period of 18 months of two prednisone treatment schedules. Chilean Co-operative Group of Study of Nephrotic Syndrome in Children]. [In Spanish]. *Rev Med Chile* 1996; **124**(5): 567–572.

19 Ueda N, Chihara M, Kawaguchi S, Niinomi Y, Nonoda T, Matsumoto J *et al.* Intermittent versus long-term tapering prednisolone for initial therapy in children with idiopathic nephrotic syndrome. *J Pediatr* 1988; **112**(1): 122–126.

20 Hiraoka M, Tsukahara H, Matsubara K, Tsurusawa M, Takeda N, Haruki S *et al.* A randomized study of two long-course prednisolone regimens for nephrotic syndrome in children. *Am J Kidney Dis* 2003; **41**(6): 1155–1162.

21 Pecoraro C, Caropreso MR, Malgieri G, Ferretti AVS, Raddi G, Piscitelli A *et al.* Therapy of first episode of steroid responsive nephrotic syndrome: a randomised controlled trial. *Pediatr Nephrol* 2004; **19**: C72.

22 Sharma RK, Ahmed M, Gupta A, Gulati S, Sharma AP. Comparison of abrupt withdrawal versus slow tapering regimens of prednisolone therapy in the management of first episode of steroid responsive childhood idiopathic nephrotic syndrome. *J Am Soc Nephrol* 2000; **11**: 97A.

23 Kleinknecht C, Broyer M, Parchoux B, Loriat C, Nivet H, Palcoux JB. Comparison of short and long treatment at onset of steroid sensitive nephrosis. *Int J Pediatr Nephrol* 1982; **3**: 45.

24 Hiraoka M, Tsukahara H, Haruki S, Hayashi S, Takeda N, Miyagawa K *et al.* Older boys benefit from higher initial prednisolone therapy for nephrotic syndrome. The West Japan Cooperative Study of Kidney Disease in Children. *Kidney Int.* 2000; **58**(3): 1247–1252.

25 Hodson EM, Craig JC, Willis NS. Evidence-based management of steroid-sensitive nephrotic syndrome. *Pediatr Nephrol* 2005; **20**: 1523–1530.

26 Lande MB, Leonard MB. Variability among pediatric nephrologists in the initial therapy of nephrotic syndrome. *Pediatr Nephrol* 2000; **14**(8–9): 766–769.

27 Webb NJ. Personal communication. 2006.

28 Hoyer PF, Brodehl J, *et al.* Initial treatment of idiopathic nephrotic syndrome in children: prednisone versus prednisone plus cyclosporine A: a prospective, randomized trial. *J Am Soc Nephrol* 2006; **17**: 1151–1157.

29 Ekka BK, Bagga A, Srivastava RN. Single- versus divided-dose prednisolone therapy for relapses of nephrotic syndrome. *Pediatr Nephrol* 1997; **11**(5): 597–599.

30 Broyer M, Terzi F, Lehnert A, Gagnadoux MF, Guest G, Niaudet P. A controlled study of deflazacort in the treatment of idiopathic nephrotic syndrome. *Pediatr Nephrol* 1997; **11**(4): 418–422.

31 Jayantha UK. Prolong versus standard steroid therapy for children with a relapsing course of nephrotic syndrome. *Pediatr Nephrol* 2004; **19**: C99.

32 Imbasciati E, Gusmano R, Edefonti A, Zucchelli P, Pozzi C, Grassi C *et al*. Controlled trial of methylprednisolone pulses and low dose oral prednisone for the minimal change nephrotic syndrome. *Br Med J Clin Res Ed* 1985; **291**: 1305–1308.

33 Mattoo TK, Mahmoud MA. Increased maintenance corticosteroids during upper respiratory infection decrease the risk of relapse in nephrotic syndrome. *Nephron* 2000; **85(4)**: 343–345.

34 Barratt TM, Soothill JF. Controlled trial of cyclophosphamide in steroid-sensitive relapsing nephrotic syndrome of childhood. *Lancet* 1970; **ii(7671)**: 479–482.

35 Chiu J, McLaine PN, Drummond KN. A controlled prospective study of cyclophosphamide in relapsing, corticosteroid-responsive, minimal-lesion nephrotic syndrome in childhood. *J Pediatr* 1973; **82(4)**: 607–613.

36 Prospective, controlled trial of cyclophosphamide therapy in children with nephrotic syndrome. Report of the International study of Kidney Disease in Children. *Lancet* 1974; **ii(7878)**: 423–427.

37 Alatas H, Wirya IG, Tambunan T, Himawan S. Controlled trial of chlorambucil in frequently relapsing nephrotic syndrome in children (a preliminary report). *J Med Assoc Thail* 1978; **61(Suppl 1)**: 222–228.

38 Grupe WE, Makker SP, Ingelfinger JR. Chlorambucil treatment of frequently relapsing nephrotic syndrome. *N Engl J Med* 1976; **295(14)**: 746–749.

39 Durkan AM, Hodson EM, Willis NS, Craig JC. Immunosuppressive agents in childhood nephrotic syndrome: a meta-analysis of randomized controlled trials. *Kidney Int* 2001; **59(5)**: 1919–1927.

40 Durkan A, Hodson EM, Willis NS, Craig JC. Non-corticosteroid treatment for nephrotic syndrome in children. *Cochrane Database Syst Rev* 2005; **2**: CD002290.

41 Effect of cytotoxic drugs in frequently relapsing nephrotic syndrome with and without steroid dependence. *N Engl J Med* 1982; **306(8)**: 451–454.

42 Barratt TM, Cameron JS, Chantler C, Ogg CS, Soothill JF. Comparative trial of 2 weeks and 8 weeks cyclophosphamide in steroid-sensitive relapsing nephrotic syndrome of childhood. *Arch Dis Child* 1973; **48(4)**: 286–290.

43 Ueda N, Kuno K, Ito S. Eight- and 12-week courses of cyclophosphamide in nephrotic syndrome. *Arch Dis Child* 1990; **65(10)**: 1147–1150.

44 Cyclophosphamide treatment of steroid dependent nephrotic syndrome: comparison of eight-week with 12-week course. Report of Arbeitsgemeinschaft für Pädiatrische Nephrologie. *Arch Dis Child* 1987; **62(11)**: 1102–1106.

45 Prasad N, Gulati S, Sharma RK, Singh U, Ahmed M. Pulse cyclophosphamide therapy in steroid-dependent nephrotic syndrome. *Pediatr Nephrol* 2004; **19**: 494–498.

46 Latta K, von Schnakenburg C, Ehrich JH. A meta-analysis of cytotoxic treatment for frequently relapsing nephrotic syndrome in children. *Pediatr Nephrol* 2001; **16(3)**: 271–282.

47 Miller DG. Alkylating agents and human spermatogenesis. *JAMA* 1971; **217(12)**: 1662–1665.

48 Niaudet P. Comparison of cyclosporin and chlorambucil in the treatment of steroid-dependent idiopathic nephrotic syndrome: a multicentre randomized controlled trial. The French Society of Paediatric Nephrology. *Pediatr Nephrol* 1992; **6(1)**: 1–3.

49 Ponticelli C, Edefonti A, Ghio L, Rizzoni G, Rinaldi S, Gusmano R *et al*. Cyclosporin versus cyclophosphamide for patients with steroid-dependent and frequently relapsing idiopathic nephrotic syndrome: a multicentre randomized controlled trial. *Nephrol Dial Transplant* 1993; **8(12)**: 1326–1332.

50 Hulton SA, Neuhaus TJ, Dillon MJ, Barratt TM. Long-term cyclosporin A treatment of minimal-change nephrotic syndrome of childhood. *Pediatr Nephrol* 1994; **8(4)**: 401–403.

51 El Husseini A, El Basuony F, Mahmoud I, Donia A, Hassan N, Sayed-Ahmad N *et al*. Co-administration of cyclosporine and ketoconazole in idiopathic childhood nephrosis. *Pediatr Nephrol* 2004; **19**: 976–981.

52 Fujinaga S, Kaneko K, Takada M, Ohtomo Y, Akashi S, Yamashiro Y. Preprandial C2 monitoring of cyclosporine treatment in children with nephrotic syndrome. *Pediatr Nephrol* 2005; **20**: 1359–1360.

53 Iijima K, Hamahira K, Tanaka R, Kobayashi A, Nozu K, Nakamura H *et al*. Risk factors for cyclosporine-induced tubulointerstitial lesions in children with minimal change nephrotic syndrome. *Kidney Int* 2002; **61(5)**: 1801–1805.

54 Niaudet P, Habib R, Tete MJ, Hinglais N, Broyer M. Cyclosporin in the treatment of idiopathic nephrotic syndrome in children. *Pediatr Nephrol* 1987; **1(4)**: 566–573.

55 Fujinaga S, Kaneko K, Muto T, Ohtomo Y, Murakami H, Yamashiro Y. Independent risk factors for chronic cyclosporine induced nephropathy in children with nephrotic syndrome. *Arch Dis Child* 2006; **91**: 666–670.

56 Hamahira K, Iijima K, Tanaka R, Nakamura H, Yoshikawa N. Recovery from cyclosporine-associated arteriolopathy in childhood nephrotic syndrome. *Pediatr Nephrol* 2001; **16(9)**: 723–727.

57 Niaudet P, Broyer M, Habib R. Treatment of idiopathic nephrotic syndrome with cyclosporin A in children. *Clin Nephrol* 1991; **35(Suppl 1)**: S31–S36.

58 Davin JC, Merkus MP. Levamisole in steroid-sensitive nephrotic syndrome of childhood: the lost paradise? *Pediatr Nephrol* 2005; **20**:10–14.

59 Levamisole for corticosteroid-dependent nephrotic syndrome in childhood. British Association for Paediatric Nephrology. *Lancet* 1991; **337(8757)**: 1555–1557.

60 Dayal U, Dayal AK, Shastry JC, Raghupathy P. Use of levamisole in maintaining remission in steroid-sensitive nephrotic syndrome in children. *Nephron* 1994; **66(4)**: 408–412. [Erratum, **67(4)**: 507.]

61 Rashid HU, Ahmed S, Fatima N, Khanam A. Levamisole in the treatment of steroid dependent or frequently relapsing nephrotic syndrome in children. *Bangladesh Ren J* 1996; **15(1)**: 6–8.

62 Weiss R. Randomized double-blind placebo controlled, multi-center trial of levamisole for children with frequently relapsing/steroid dependent nephrotic syndrome. *J Am Soc Nephrol* 1993; **4**: 289.

63 Donia AF, Ammar HM, El Agroudy A, Moustafa F, Sobh MA. Long-term results of two unconventional agents in steroid-dependent nephrotic children. *Pediatr Nephrol* 2005; **20**: 1420–1425.

64 Alsaran K, Grisaru S, Stephens D, Arbus G. Levamisole vs. cyclophosphamide for frequently-relapsing steroid-dependent nephrotic syndrome. *Clin Nephrol* 2001; **56(4)**: 289–294.

65 Palcoux JB, Niaudet P, Goumy P. Side effects of levamisole in children with nephrosis. *Pediatr Nephrol* 1994; **8(2)**: 263–264.

66 Barbano G, Ginevri F, Ghiggeri GM, Gusmano R. Disseminated autoimmune disease during levamisole treatment of nephrotic syndrome. *Pediatr Nephrol* 1999; **13(7)**: 602–603.

67 Abramowicz M, Barnett HL, Edelmann CM, Jr, Greifer I, Kobayashi O, Arneil GC *et al*. Controlled trial of azathioprine in children with nephrotic syndrome. A report for the international study of kidney disease in children. *Lancet* 1970; **i(7654)**: 959–961.

68 Barratt TM, Cameron JS, Chantler C, Counahan R, Ogg CS, Soothill JF. Controlled trial of azathioprine in treatment of steroid-responsive nephrotic syndrome of childhood. *Arch Dis Child* 1977; **52**: 462–463.

69 Yoshioka K, Ohashi Y, Sakai T, Ito H, Yoshikawa N, Nakamura H *et al*. A multicenter trial of mizoribine compared with placebo in children

with frequently relapsing nephrotic syndrome. *Kidney Int* 2000; **58**(**1**): 317–324.

70 Hoyer PF. Personal communication. 2006.

71 Bagga A, Hari P, Moudgil A, Jordan SC. Mycophenolate mofetil and prednisolone therapy in children with steroid-dependent nephrotic syndrome. *Am J Kidney Dis* 2003; **42**(**6**): 1114–1120.

72 Hogg RJ, Fitzgibbons L, Bruick J, Bunke M, Ault B, Baqi N *et al*. Clinical trial of mycophenolate mofetil (MMF) for frequent relapsing nephrotic syndrome in children. *Pediatr Nephrol* 2004; **19**: C18.

73 Mendizabal S, Zamora I, Berbel O, Sanahuja MJ, Fuentes J, Simon J. Mycophenolate mofetil in steroid/cyclosporine-dependent/resistant nephrotic syndrome. *Pediatr Nephrol* 2005; **20**: 914–919.

74 Sinha MD, MacLeod R, Rigby E, Clark AG. Treatment of severe steroid-dependent nephrotic syndrome (SDNS) in children with tacrolimus. *Nephrol Dial Transplant* 2006; **21**: 1848–1854.

75 Dotsch J, Dittrich K, Plank C, Rascher W. Is tacrolimus for childhood steroid-dependent nephrotic syndrome better than cyclosporin A? *Nephrol Dial Transplant* 2006; **21**: 1761–1763.

68 Steroid-Resistant Nephrotic Syndrome

Annabelle Chua[1] & Peter Yorgin[2]

[1] Section of Pediatric Nephrology, Texas Children's Hospital, Baylor College of Medicine, Houston, USA
[2] Section of Pediatric Nephrology, Loma Linda University, Loma Linda, CA, USA

Introduction

Steroid-resistant nephrotic syndrome (SRNS) is a heterogeneous disease characterized by the persistence of proteinuria after 4–8 weeks of corticosteroid therapy [1,2]. The incidence of new-onset childhood SRNS is about 0.3 cases/100,000 patient years [3]. Approximately 15% of children treated for new-onset nephrotic syndrome are steroid resistant [4–6]; some patients are corticosteroid resistant after the first corticosteroid course, whereas others become corticosteroid resistant after receiving two or more treatment courses. Steroid resistance is more common in South Asians [3], African Americans [4], older children [4], and those children who relapse more rapidly [4].

Most pediatric nephrologists perform a renal biopsy to determine the glomerular histology prior to initiating a non-corticosteroid-based therapy in SRNS [7]. The International Study of Kidney Diseases in Children (ISKDC) reported that focal segmental glomerulosclerosis (FSGS) was responsible for 7% of new-onset nephrotic syndrome cases [1]. A recent study suggested that the number of children with FSGS may be increasing to 0.5 cases/100,000 children/year [8]. A retrospective study of 42 children with SRNS at Stanford University reported 24% with minimal change disease (MCD), 17% with mesangial proliferative glomerulonephritis (MesPGN), 24% with FSGS, and 36% with FSGS and mesangial proliferation [9].

The treatment of SRNS can be directed toward abrogating the causes of the proteinuria through the use of additional corticosteroids, alkylating agents, and calcineurin inhibitors or by inhibiting the damaging effects of the proteinuria and nephrotic syndrome through the use of statins and angiotensin converting inhibitors. The stakes are high, as patients who respond to therapy regain a sense of well-being and are less likely to progress to end-stage renal disease (ESRD) [10,11]. Treatment failure, even after achieving an initial remission, correlates with poor long-term

outcome. Overall, children with MCD-associated SRNS tend to respond best to therapy, whereas those with FSGS comprise the majority of those who progress to ESRD [9,12]. Despite one case report of successful treatment of familial FSGS [13], patients with familial (genetic) forms of SRNS generally do not respond to therapy, and so this form of the disease will not be considered further in this chapter.

Treatment of SRNS: methods

A MEDLINE search was conducted to develop evidence-based treatment guidelines for children with SRNS. Pediatric studies were preferentially selected. However, if pediatric data could be extracted from a study population that also included adults, the information was added to the analysis. For consistency, the results reported reflect initial, not final or long-term, responses to therapy. Patients respond to therapy either completely, where urinary protein/creatinine (U_{Prot}/U_{Creat}) ratios return to normal (<0.20 mg/mg; <0.02 g/mmol), partially with at least a halving of the proteinuria (U_{Prot}/U_{Creat}, <2 mg/mg, or <0.2 g/mmol), or not at all (treatment failure).

There is controversy regarding the nomenclature of MesPGN, as some pathologists consider MesPGN to be an early form of FSGS. Because a significant number of the pediatric studies have characterized their patients as having MesPGN, the term MesPGN is used in the tables found in this chapter.

Calcineurin inhibitor therapy

Cyclosporine

There is more literature supporting calcineurin inhibitor therapy in SRNS than any other medication [14,15] (Table 68.1). Although both cyclosporine (CsA) and tacrolimus have been used to treat SRNS in children, there are substantially more data regarding the outcomes of patients treated with CsA. Twenty-four retrospective and prospective uncontrolled studies, with a total of 531 patients

Evidence-based Nephrology. Edited by Donald Molony and Jonathan Craig
© 2009 Blackwell Publishing, ISBN: 978-1-4051-3975-5.

Table 68.1 Evidence ratings and recommendations for interventions to achieve remission in SRNS.

Intervention	SR[a]	Evidence rating[b]		Studies conducted	Recommendation[c]			Benefit–risk trade-offs
		Moderate	Low		I	II	III	
Calcineurin inhibitors (vs standard care)	+	•		3 small RCTs (46 patients); 21 case series (507 patients); generally consistent results	•			Benefits exceed harms; RR −0.26 (95% CI −0.49 to −0.04); NNT 4
Oral steroids (vs oral alkylating agents)	+	•		2 RCTs (88 patients) with consistent results; 11 case series (104 patients) with inconsistent results		•		No evidence of benefit in FSGS in RCTs; significant harms
ACEi (vs standard care)	+	•		3 RCTs (87 patients) with consistent results; 6 case series (46 patients) with inconsistent results	•			Benefits exceed harms; proteinuria reduced by 0.95 g/day (95% CI −1.21 to −1.05) in 1 RCT; few harms reported
Pulse intravenous steroids	−		•	3 case series (94 patients), generally consistent results			•	Remission in 30–60%; need more data on harms
Intravenous alkylating agents	−		•	5 case series (71 patients), generally consistent results			•	Remission in 30–100%; need more data on harms
Combined therapy (PMT + CPA)	−		•	8 case series (204 patients), generally consistent results			•	Remission in 50–80%; need more data on harms

[a]SR, systematic review(s) available on RCT(s).

[b]Evidence rating based on study design, study quality, consistency, and directness of results. No intervention received a high evidence rating.

[c]Recommendation based on trade-off between benefits and harms, quality of evidence, and translation of evidence into practice in a specific setting, including availability of medication and any uncertainty about the baseline risk of the disease in the population. I, recommend to give or not to give; II, suggest to give or not to give; III, no recommendation possible; NNT, number needed to treat.

(497 treated with a calcineurin inhibitor) have been conducted to evaluate the effectiveness of CsA in the treatment of SRNS (Table 68.2) [13,16–33]. The response to CsA is variable, with complete remission rates that range from 7 to 100%. The recent Cochrane review of randomized controlled trials (RCTs) concluded that CsA, compared with placebo or no treatment, significantly increased the number of children who achieved complete remission (three RCTs, 49 children; relative risk [RR] for persistent nephrotic syndrome, 0.64; 95% confidence interval [CI], 0.47–0.88) [34].

The dosing regimen of CsA varies widely and has changed over time. Although lower-dose CsA therapy (100 mg/m²/day) has been advocated [25], most current treatment regimens empirically start with a dose of 5–7 mg/kg/day [22,24,31,32]. Inguilli *et al.* suggested that the CsA dose and trough level should be titrated upwards when patients have higher cholesterol levels [24]. Most regimens report twice-daily dosing; however, single-daily dosing of CsA has also been effective [16,21]. When starting with a higher dose, tapering of the CsA to 3–4 mg/kg is frequently undertaken after treatment response [31,35]. CsA trough levels effective in inducing remission have ranged from 50 to 300 ng/mL [22,24,28,32,36,37].

CsA-induced side effects include hirsutism [30,32], gingival hyperplasia [16,30,32,36], hypertension [16,22,32,33,36,38–40], and nephrotoxicity characterized by tubular atrophy and progressive interstitial fibrosis [16,22,25,28,29,36,41,42]. Investigators have reported that CsA reduces the glomerular filtration rate (GFR)

and causes significant nephrotoxicity [36,43]. Some children have reversible arteriopathy [42], with recovery of GFR when CsA is ceased [43], but about 15% have irreversible changes [22,28].

Relapses of nephrotic syndrome after withdrawal of CsA therapy are common, affecting approximately 50% of patients [16,18,23,25,28,29,32,36,44]. It is unclear how relapses impact long-term kidney function, how long patients can reasonably continue to receive therapy, whether resistance to treatment develops over time [45], and how frequently renal biopsies should be performed to monitor CsA nephrotoxicity.

Tacrolimus

Two pediatric case series have demonstrated that tacrolimus has an antiproteinuric effect similar to CsA and may be effective in achieving remission in CsA-resistant SRNS children [39,46]. Tacrolimus therapy does not induce hirsutism or gingival hyperplasia, which are common with CsA, but it dose cause insulin resistance and diabetes (in 2–3% of pediatric kidney transplant recipients) [47,48]. The lack of an RCT means that tacrolimus therapy cannot be recommended until further data are available.

Corticosteroid therapy

Oral corticosteroid therapy

Oral corticosteroid therapy remains a therapeutic "cornerstone" in the management of SRNS. Given that children with SRNS are,

Table 68.2 Evidence ratings and recommendations for calcineurin inhibitor therapy studies and SNRS[a].

Study ID [reference]	Study type[b]	No. of patients	Histology	Primary intervention	Other treatment	No. with complete/ partial response	Follow-up
Iyengar A/2006 [31]	P NR SC OL	12	2 MCD 4 MesPGN 3 MPGN[c] 3 FSGS	CsA, 6–7 mg/kg/day in two divided doses; dose titrated to target 100–200 ng/mL	Oral corticosteroids tapered over 1–2 months	5 (42%)/NR[d]	71 months
Garcia C/1998 [27]	P NR MC OL	19	2 MCD 17 FSGS	CsA, 6 mg/kg/day divided twice daily	PR[e] at 1 mg/kg/day for 1 month, 1 mg/kg on alternate days for 5 months, then tapered off	5 (26%)/5 (26%) MCD: 0/1 (50%) FSGS: 5 (29%)/4 (24%)	13 months
Kim PK/1997 [25]	P NR SC OL	7	7 MCD	CsA, 100 mg/m²/day	PR at 2 mg/kg every other day for 4 weeks then 1 mg/kg every other day	7 (100%)/ MCD: 7 (100%)/	36 months
Gregory MJ/1996 [22]	P NR SC OL	15	3 MCD 3 FSGS 9 MesPGN	CsA, 5–10 mg/kg/day divided twice daily, titrated to target 70–120 ng/mL	PR at 2 mg/kg on alternate days until complete remission;. PR slowly tapered over 3–6 months.	13 (87%)/2 (13%) MCD: 2 (67%)/1 (33%) FSGS: 3 (100%)/ MesPGN: 8 (89%)/1 (11%)	22 months
Lieberman KV/1996 [139]	P **RCT** MC B	25	FSGS	A: CsA, 3 mg/kg/day divided twice daily, titrated to target 300–500 ng/mL (12 patients) B: Placebo (13 patients)	None	**A:** 4 (33.3%)/8 (66.7%) **B:** 0 (0%)/2 (17%)	6 months
Ingulli E/1995 [24]	P NR SC OL	21	FSGS	CsA, 7–10 mg/kg/day, titrated to response, max 32 mg/kg/day	<6 years old, PR at 5 mg/day; 6–12 years PR at 10 mg/day; 12–18 years, PR at15 mg/day. In stable patients, PR was discontinued. Edematous patients received furosemide.	5 (24%)/12 (57%)	8.5 ± 4.7 years
Hymes LC/1995 [23]	P NR SC OL	18	7 MCD 4 FSGS 7 MesPGN	CsA, 5 mg/kg/day titrated to maintain whole blood trough levels 80–200 ng/mL	PR at 0.4–05 mg/kg on alternate days, except two children who received 5 mg/day	9 (50%)/5 (27.8%) MCD 5 (71%)/0 FSGS 1 (25%)/2 (50%) MesPGN 3 (43%)/ 3 (43%)	NR

(Continued)

Table 68.2 (Continued)

Study ID [reference]	Study type[b]	No. of patients	Histology	Primary intervention	Other treatment	No. with complete/ partial response	Follow-up
Niaudet P/1994 [18]	P MC NR OL	65	45 MCD 20 FSGS	CsA, 150 mg/m²/day adjusted to target 100–200 ng/mL	PR at 30 mg/m²/day for 1 month, then 30 mg/m² every other day for 5 months	27(42%)/4 (6%) MCD 21 (47%)/2 (9%) FSGS 6(30%)/2 (10%)	14–60 months
Ponticelli C/1993 [40]	P MC RCT OL	18	A: 6 MCD 5 FSGS B: 2 MCD 5 FSGS	A: CsA, 6 mg/kg/day (10 patients) B: Controls (7 patients)	Rescue treatment with PR if worsening kidney failure	A: 4 (40%)/ 2 (20%) MCD 3 (50%)/1 (17%) FSGS 1 (20%)/2 (40% B: 0/NR (16%, combined adults and children)	18 months
McCauley J/1993 [46]	P SC NR OL	4	4 FSGS	Tacrolimus, 0.15 mg/kg/day divided twice daily to achieve trough level of 0.5–2 ng/mL		2 (50%)/2 (50%)	3 months
Melocoton TL/1991 [17]	P SC NR OL	10	6 FSGS 4 MCD	CsA, 6 mg/kg/day in two divided doses to maintain trough levels 100–150 ng/mL	PR variable, tapered after 1– 3 months of remission.	1 (10%)/1 (10%)	NR
Niaudet P/1991 [19]	P SC NR OL	28	12 MCD 11 FSGS 1 Idiopathic 2 DMS[f]	A: CsA monotherapy (14 patients) B: CsA + PR (14 patients) (for both groups, CsA at 6 mg/kg/day divided twice daily; target trough levels 50–150 ng/mL)	B: PR at 30 mg/m²/day for 1 month then alternate days for 5 months	A: 1 (7%)/ 4 (29%) MCD 1 (20%)/0 FSGS 0/3 (50%) DMS 0/0 B: 8 (57%)/2 (14%) MCD 5 (63%)/0 FSGS 3 (50%)/2 (33%)	>180 days

(Continued)

Table 68.2 *Continued*

Study ID [reference]	Study type[b]	No. of patients	Histology	Primary intervention	Other treatment	No. with complete/ partial response	Follow-up
Garin EH/1988 [140]	P SC RCxT OL	8	4 MCD 4 FSGS	**A:** CsA at 5 mg/kg/day for 8 weeks then off for 1 month; patients became controls for 8 weeks **B:** Control group received no treatment for 1 month, then CsA at 5 mg/kg/day for 8 weeks	None	**A:** 0 (0%) **B:** 0 (0%) **A:** U_P/U_C 11.7 ± 2.3 **B:** U_P/U_C 15.1 ± 3.2 $P = 0.03$	5 months
Loeffler K/2004 [39]	R SC NR OL	16	13 FSGS 1 MCD 2 IgA	Tacrolimus 0.1 mg/kg divided twice daily dosing; adjusted to maintain trough level between 5-10	For patients on steroids at initiation of tacrolimus, steroid dose tapered once reduction in urine protein excretion; when complete remission achieved, steroids tapered over 1–3 months	13 (81%)/2 (12.5) MCD 1 (100%) FSGS 11 (85%)/1 (8%) IgA 1 (50%) /1 (50%)	NR
Other studies [16, 21, 28–30, 32, 37, 141–143]	R	264	72 MCD 171 FSGS 19 MesPGN 8 other	Various CsA-based regimens		168 (64%)/24 (%)	Various
Total		529 (494 treated with a calcineurin inhibitor)	167 MCD 298 FSGS 39 MesPGN 16 other	Various	**Cumulative remission** Remission: 259 (49%) Partial remission: 71 (13%) **Response by histology**[g] MCD: 79/166 (48%) FSGS: 86/153 (56%) MesPGN: 26/33 (79%)		

[a]Details are summarized for 14 of 24 studies, with the remaining studies grouped as "other studies."
[b]Study type abbreviations: XXXXX
[c]MPGN, membranoproliferative glomerulonephritis.
[d]NR, not reported.
[e]PR, prednisone.
[f]DMS, diffuse mesangial sclerosis.
*only pediatric data reported.
[o]pediatric and adult data (could not be separated).
[g]Data from Iyengar, Melocoton, Mamoud, El-Husseini, Frassinetti, and Kim studies were excluded.

by definition, resistant to steroid therapy, resuming or continuing oral corticosteroid therapy may seem counterintuitive. Yet, there is evidence that some patients with SRNS can respond to oral corticosteroids.

There have been two prospective RCTs in children with SRNS in which oral corticosteroid therapy was selected as the control treatment arm [49,50]. Children with MCD-induced SRNS may have higher remission rates [49] than those with FSGS [50]. Studies of children with FSGS have reported complete remission rates of 0–28% [49–51]. Yet, oral corticosteroid therapy alone may be insufficient to maintain remission, as 25% subsequently relapsed and progressed to ESRD [50,51].

Despite their well-known adverse effect profile, 3–6 months of oral corticosteroids has been recommended in the therapy of SRNS when combined or used in sequence with other therapies [52]. The current NIH-funded SRNS FSGS study is using alternate-day oral corticosteroid therapy at a dose of 0.5 mg/kg/day for 6 months.

Short course of high-dose (pulse) intravenous corticosteroid therapy

Early reports of successful treatment of glomerular diseases with pulse methylprednisolone therapy (PMT) [53,54] led to PMT studies in children with SRNS. Whereas some investigators used three consecutive doses or alternate-day doses [55–57], others used six doses of intravenous PMT ($1 g/1.73 m^2$ or 30 mg/kg with a maximum dose of 1 g) or dexamethasone (5 mg/kg) [54,58–60].

Ninety-four children were treated with intravenous corticosteroids in three prospective, nonrandomized studies [54,58,60] (Table 68.3). When intravenous PMT or dexamethasone therapy was used alone, 33–63% of patients achieved complete remission. Equivalent remission rates have been achieved using intravenous dexamethasone or methylprednisolone [59,60] ($P = 1.00$; RR, 0.958; 95% CI, 0.335–2.461). Although patients may go into remission, most require another agent to maintain remission [54,58,60].

The adverse effects of pulse intravenous methylprednisolone or dexamethasone therapy can include dysrhythmias [61], hyperglycemia (3%) [60], hypokalemia (48%) [60], nausea and vomiting (9%) [62], mood swings (18%) [62], and posterior lenticular cataracts (9%) [62]. Hypertension has been reported to occur in about 50% of children [60].

An RCT examining the efficacy of pulse intravenous corticosteroid therapy in the treatment of SRNS is needed.

Purine synthesis inhibitors

Azathioprine

Abramowicz *et al.* conducted an RCT comparing azathioprine (60 mg/m²/day) plus intermittent prednisone (40 mg/m²/day for three consecutive days per week) versus intermittent prednisone alone [2]. There was no difference in outcomes (12.5% achieved remission) between the azathioprine and prednisone alone groups ($P = 1.00$). White *et al.* reported the use of high-dose azathioprine therapy (4–14 mg/kg/day for 4–60 weeks) in combination

with steroid therapy to treat children with SRNS [63]. Although 38% of those treated with high-dose azathioprine improved, two patients died. The remission rate for azathioprine treatment is so low that it cannot be recommended in the treatment of SRNS.

Mycophenolate mofetil

No RCTs have evaluated the effect of mycophenolate mofetil (MMF) in childhood SRNS. A retrospective analysis of five pediatric patients with SRNS who were treated with MMF, with or without subsequent weaning of CsA, reported fewer relapses per year on treatment (1.4 ± 1.1) compared to the 12 months prior to MMF (2.8 ± 1.3) [64]. Only two patients were weaned off CsA, and two had the same number of relapses pre- and posttreatment with MMF. A cohort study of five patients with cyclophosphamide (CPA)-resistant and CsA-resistant SRNS reported only one MMF-induced remission [65]. A study conducted by Ulinski *et al.* evaluated treatment conversion from CsA to MMF in children with steroid-dependent nephrotic syndrome and SRNS [43]. Overall, the calculated GFR increased while the amount of corticosteroid therapy needed to retain the remission decreased.

The current NIH-sponsored FSGS study is comparing MMF (25–36 mg/kg/day) and dexamethasone in one group and CsA treatment in the other group [41]. An RCT of MMF is needed to determine its efficacy for this indication.

Mizoribine

The mechanism of action for mizoribine is similar to that of MMF. Although studies conducted in Japan reported that mizoribine was effective in the treatment of a limited number of children with SRNS [66,67], there have been no RCTs. In a study of patients with SRNS due to FSGS, 7 of the 15 (47%) children achieved remission [67]. Doses of 3–10 mg/kg have been used without significant adverse effects [66,68,69].

Alkylating agents

Oral CPA

Two RCTs concluded that children with SRNS respond poorly to alkylating agents, with only 17–25% of patients achieving remission [50,70]. The RCT performed by Tarshish *et al.* reported that there was no significant difference between the outcomes in children with FSGS treated with cyclophosphanide (CPA) ($P = 1.00$; RR, 1.050; 95% CI, 0.750–1.470) compared to oral prednisone alone. In addition, those study authors reported that 9/25 subjects receiving prednisone and 20/35 on CPA had kidney dysfunction ($P = 0.13$; RR, 1.59; 95% CI, 0.87–2.88). The ISKDC study, which included children with MCD or FSGS, reported a somewhat higher complete remission rate with CPA and intermittent prednisone (56%) than with intermittent prednisone alone (40%), but there was no significant difference in outcomes between the treatments ($P = 0.718$; RR, 0.714; 95% CI, 0.158–3.231) [49]. When the two RCTs are combined in a meta-analysis for the outcome of failure to achieve remission, results are no different ($P = 1.00$; RR, 1.01; 95% CI, 0.74–1.36). A large observational study by Martinelli *et al.*

Table 68.3 Evidence ratings and recommendations for pulse intravenous corticosteroid therapy and SNRS studies[a].

Study ID [reference]	Study type[b]	No. of patients	Histology	Primary intervention	Other treatment[b]	No. with complete/partial response of proteinuria	Follow-up
Hari P[c]/2004 [60]	P SC	NR OL	81	26 MCD 41 FSGS 14 MesPGN	**A:** Dexamethasone, 5 mg/kg; 6 alternate-day pulses (59 patients) **B:** Methylprednisolone, 30 mg/kg; 6 alternate-day pulse (22 patients)	Oral PR 2 mg/kg on days when not receiving PICT	**A:** 20 (35%)/7 (12%) **B:** 7 (33%)/3 (14%) **Total:** 29 (36%)/10 (12%) $P = 1.00$; RR 0.958; 95% CI 0.335–2.461	NR[d]
Murnaghan K/1984 [58]	P SC	NR OL	8	4 MCD 3 FSGS 1 MesPGN	Methylprednisolone 1g/1.73 m² for 6 pulses	None	5 (63%)/-	NR
Rose GM/1981 [54]	P SC	NR OL	5	3 MCD 2 FSGS	Methylprednisolone 30 mg/kg for 6 pulses over 2 weeks	None	MCD 3 (100%)/0 FSGS 0/1(50%) Total: 3 (60%)/1 (20%)	40.1 months 39 months 6.5 months
Total			94	All patients 33 MCD 46 FSGS 15 MesPGN	Dexamethasone (59 patients) Methylprednisolone (35 patients)	1 study added oral PR therapy	**Cumulative remission** Complete remission: 37 (39%) Partial remission: 8 (9%)	

[a]Three of three studies are shown.
[b]Treatment abbreviations: PR, prednisone; PICT, pulse intravenous corticosteroid therapy.
[c]There was an overlap of study patients in the two Hari reports (2001 and 2004) [59,60].
[d]NR, not reported.

[51] reported comparable outcomes for children treated with CPA compared to those treated with prednisone, but CPA-induced remission rates were still low (27%).

There may be a differential response to alkylating agents that depends on the underlying renal pathology in children with SRNS (Table 68.4). Oral CPA appears to be more effective in children with MCD-associated SRNS, with short-term remission rates of 50–100% [71–75].

Both chlorambucil and CPA have been successfully used to treat children with SRNS. Elzouki and Jaiswal [76] reported chlorambucil responsiveness despite CPA resistance in five SRNS patients. Because 4–8% of patients treated with chlorambucil develop seizures [77,78] and reported outcomes are similar, there appears to be no advantage to using chlorambucil compared with CPA.

Dosing for CPA in children has been based on studies performed by Barrett and Soothill. Patients who received 3 mg/kg/day for 8 weeks had longer remissions and fewer relapses [79]. Most of the current studies report using 2–3 mg/kg for 8–12 weeks [8,51,77,80,81]. Some investigators reported using a second, or even third, course of alkylating agent when the first course was not effective [75]. The study by Drummond et al. reported excellent results with longer-term therapy (up to 1 year) with CPA [82].

All patients receiving oral alkylating therapy should be advised of the risks of infertility [83–85], alopecia [86], leucopenia [77,87], and hemorrhagic cystitis [49]. Alkylating agent-induced infertility is particularly concerning. In the meta-analysis by Latta et al., there was no safe threshold CPA cumulative dose for men; greater cumulative doses correlated with a greater risk of infertility [77]. Conversely, women rarely develop oral alkylating agent-induced infertility [77]. A recent study by Ruth et al. reported that only 8 of 42 adults who had received CPA therapy for nephrotic syndrome as children had borne children, although it was uncertain whether CPA-induced fertility was the cause [84]. Etledorf et al. reported that four men who received CPA at 2–4 mg/kg/day for 49–60 days had normal semen, whereas four other men who received 2–5 mg/kg for 89–489 days were azoospermic [88]. Trompeter et al. found lower ejaculate volumes and sperm densities with a higher percentage of immotile and abnormal forms in 19 men who received CPA at 3 mg/kg for 8 weeks [83], but the abnormalities were not severe enough to suggest infertility. Sperm banking may be offered to older adolescent men as a hedge against the possibility of sterility.

Intravenous CPA

Reports of excellent outcomes in patients with lupus nephritis treated with intravenous CPA have encouraged some investigators to attempt intravenous pulse CPA therapy in children with SRNS. Intravenous CPA has been used by clinicians in settings where frequent visits for therapy are not feasible. There have been six studies (involving a total of 71 patients) in which children received monthly pulse CPA (in doses ranging from 500 to 750 mg/m^2 per dose) for 6 months with concurrent oral corticosteroid therapy (Table 68.5) [86,89–92]. One RCT was performed that compared intravenous versus oral CPA [91]. All of the subjects ($n = 7$) who

received intravenous CPA achieved remission, whereas only one (25%) of the subjects ($n = 4$) who received oral CPA responded to therapy. However, small numbers led to imprecision of results, so that the difference was not significant (RR, 0.09; 95% CI, 0.01–1.39), and further RCTs are required.

Intravenous pulse CPA therapy has been described as well-tolerated, safe, and effective, but with some increase in the risks of infection [90], alopecia [86,89,90], and transient vomiting [86,89]. Although not reported in any intravenous CPA SRNS studies, patients treated with intravenous CPA may develop hemorrhagic cystitis [93], which may recur with reintroduction of intravenous CPA [94]. The use of 2-mercaptoethane sodium sulfonate (Mesna) has been shown to reduce the risk of hemorrhagic cystitis due to intravenous CPA [94–98].

The long-term effects on fertility of intravenous pulse CPA are concerning. Women with systemic lupus erythematosus treated with intravenous pulse CPA are at risk of ovarian toxicity. In a study by Park et al., logistic regression analysis showed that older age, high damage index at initiation of therapy, and high cumulative dose were the independent risk factors of ovarian failure [85].

Because of small patient numbers, diverse histology, and extreme variability of treatment responses, it is not possible to make a recommendation regarding intravenous CPA.

Other antineoplastic and immunosuppressant medications

Nitrogen mustard therapy (mechlorethamine) and vincristine

There have been no RCTs of mechlorethamine. Mechlorethamine therapy with corticosteroids or adrenocorticotropic hormone was advocated as an effective treatment for SRNS from the 1950s to the 1980s. All patients achieved partial or complete remission in the study conducted by Fine et al. [99], in which mechlorethamine was infused intravenously for four consecutive days. A subsequent study by Armugan et al. [100] did not report encouraging results. None of the seven patients achieved a complete remission. Vomiting was a common adverse effect of mechlorethamine therapy [99,101].

Although primarily used as an antineoplastic drug in the treatment of malignancies, there have been two small cohort studies of vincristine treatment in children with SRNS [102,103]. Response rates to therapy, defined as combined complete and partial remissions, were 38% [102] and 43% [103]. Both studies concluded that vincristine was relatively ineffective in inducing remission. However, patient selection for both studies appeared to be biased towards unresponsiveness to any therapy. There is insufficient evidence to make a recommendation regarding vincristine therapy.

Combination therapy

The use of combination therapy, consisting of two or three different medications, has been advocated by many investigators

Table 68.4 Evidence ratings and recommendations for oral alkylating agent therapy and SNRS studies[a].

Study ID [reference]	Study type	No. of patients	Histology	Primary intervention	Other treatment	No. with complete/partial remission of proteinuria	Follow-up
Martinelli R/2004 [51]	P NR SC	84	FSGS	**A:** CPA, 2.0–3.0 mg/kg/day for 12 weeks + PR dose as below (30 patients) **B:** PR, 1.0–2.0 mg/kg/day for 4–6 weeks, then alternate-day PR for 4 weeks, taper over 2–3 months (54 patients)	None	**A:** 8 (27%)/6(20%) **B:** 11(20%)/8(15%)	**A:** 113.8 ± 88.6 months **B:** 51.5 ± 59.1 months
Tarshish P/1996 [50]	P RCT MC OL	60 (only 53 with proteinuria data)	FSGS	**A:** CPA, 2.5 mg/kg in a single AM dose for 90 days + PR dose as below (35 patients) **B:** PR, 40 mg/m² on alternate days in a single AM dose for 12 months (25 patients)	None	**A:** 8(25%)/8(25%) **B:** 6(28%)/6(28%) P = 1.00; RR 1.200; 95% CI 0.347–4.145	**A:** 42.4 months **B:** 44.5 months
Elzouki AY/1990 [76]	P NR MC	5	4 FSGS 1 MesPGN	Chlorambucil, 0.2 mg/kg/day for 8–16 weeks	PR 60 mg/m²/day	3(75%)/1(25%) for FSGS 1 (100%) for MesPGN	Not reported, but most >2 years
ISKDC/1974 [49]	P RCT MC OL	28	14 MCD 10 FSGS 2 MesPGN 2 Unknown	**A:** CPA, 5 mg/kg/day until WBC 3000–5000/mm³, then reduce dose to 1–3 mg/kg/day until 90 days of therapy completed + PR as below (16 patients) **B:** PR, 40 mg/m²/day, 3 days/week for 4 weeks (12 patients)	None	**A:** 9(56%)/ MCD: 5 (71%) FSGS: 3 (43%) MesPGN: 1 (50%) **B:** 5(41%) MCD: 4(57%) FSGS: 0(0%) Unknown: 1 (50%) P = 0.718; RR 0.714; 95% CI 0.158–3.231	Not reported
Other studies [63, 70, 72, 73, 80, 82, 144–146]	R	111	27 MCD 63 FSGS 11 MesPGN	Various CPA-based treatments	Various, many with prednisone	48 (43%)/9 (8%)	Various
TOTAL		282 (but only 192 received alkylating agent therapy)	**All patients** 41 MCD 225 FSGS 14 MesPGN 2 Unknown **Treated**[b] 34 MCD 143 FSGS 9 MesPGN	CPA Chlorambucil	Varied	**Cumulative Remission** Remission, 77 (40%) Partial remission, 24 (13%) **Response by histology**[c] MCD: 29 of 34 (85%) FSGS 42 of 143 (29%) MesPGN 3 of 9 (33%)	

[a]Details for 4 of the 13 studies are shown; the other 9 are summarized in the row "Other studies."
[b]Complete remission only.
[c]Data from Kari et al were excluded.

Table 68.5 Evidence ratings and recommendations for intravenous CPA therapy and SNRS studies[a].

Study ID [reference]	Study type	No. of patients	Histology	Primary intervention	Other treatment	No. with complete/partial remission of proteinuria	Follow-up
Alshaya HO/2003 [89]	P SC / NR OL	5	3 MesPGN 2 MCD	500 mg/m² q month for 6 months	PR 40 mg/m² on alternate days for 6 months Enalapril (0.1–0.5 mg/kg) for 6 months	0 (0%)/3 (60%) MCD 0/1 (50%) MesPGN 0/2 (66%)	2 months
Bajpai A/2003 [90]	P SC / NR OL	24	11 MCD 9 FSGS 4 MesPGN	750 mg/m² q month for 6 months	Alternate-day oral PR	7 (29%)/7(29%) MCD 4 (36%)/2 (18%) FSGS 3 (33%)/5 (55%) MesPGN 0/0	1.8 ± 0.4 years
Gulati S/2000 [86]	P SC / NR OL	20	20 FSGS	500 mg/m² q month for 3 months; if proteinuria persisted and CPA was well-tolerated the dose was increased to 750 mg/m² q month for 3 months	PR 60 mg/m²/day for 4 weeks, 40 mg/m²/alternate day for 4 weeks, tapered off over 4 weeks	13 (65%)/3 (15%)	21 months
Rennert WP/1999 [138]	P SC / NR OL	10	FSGS	500 mg/m² q month for 6 months	PR 60 mg/m²/day for 2 months, then 60 mg/m² alternate days for 4 months, 30 mg/m² alternate days for 6 months, then tapered by 10 mg/month until discontinued	7 (70%)/1 (10%)	26 months
Adhikari M/1997 [147]	P SC / NR OL	12	FSGS	A: Intravenous CPA monthly doses for 6 months (5 patients) B: Oral CPA for 18 months (7 patients)	Intravenous PMT for 3 consecutive daily doses and oral PR 2 mg/kg on alternate days	A: 2 (40%)/1 (20%) B: 0/6 (86%) P = 0.364; RR 0.75, 95% CI 0.426–1.321	38.1 ± 8.8 months
Elhence R/1994 [91]	P SC / **RCT** OL	13	MCD	A: Intravenous CPA 500 mg/m² per month for 6 months (7 patients) B: Oral CPA 2.5 mg/kg/day for 8 weeks (6 patients; 2 dropped out)	PR 60 mg/m²/day for 4 weeks, 40 mg/m² alternate days for 4 weeks, tapered off over next 4 weeks	A: 7 (100%) B: 1 (17%) P = 0.015; RR 0.143, 95% CI 0.023–0.877	A: 12 ± 1.4 months B: 13 ± 3.9 months
Total		84 (but only 71 received intravenous pulse CPA)	**All Patients** 25 MCD 51 FSGS 8 MesPGN **Treated** 20 MCD 44 FSGS 7 MesPGN	Various		**Cumulative remission** Remission: 36 (51%) Partial remission: 15 (21%) **Response by histology**[b] MCD 11/20 (55%) FGSG 22/44 (50%) MesPGN 0/7	

[a] Details on six of six studies are shown.
[b] Complete remission only.

[38,59,92,104–108] (Table 68.6). There have been at least 10 studies with a total of 204 patients treated with combination therapy, but no RCT has been conducted. The mean complete remission rate for all combination therapies is 58%. Nearly all patients with MCD respond to combination therapy, whereas only 47% of FSGS patients achieve a complete remission.

Triple therapy: PMT + alternate-day oral corticosteroids + CPA

One of the most common combinations, a triple therapy with a combination of intravenous PMT, oral CPA, and alternate-day prednisone therapy, was first described by Griswold et al. [104]. Large doses, 30 mg/kg methylprednisolone up to a maximum of 1 g, were infused intravenously three times per week for 2 weeks (six doses) and then weekly for at least 4–6 weeks. Decreasing the frequency of the PMT dose to every other week and monthly occurred when U_{Prot}/U_{Creat} levels decreased to near normal levels. For patients who did not respond to pulse intravenous corticosteroid therapy (PICT) alone, oral CPA at 2 mg/kg/day was prescribed for 75–90 days. Alternate-day oral corticosteroid dosing was decreased relative to the patient's response.

In the six triple therapy studies (150 patients), 50–75% of patients achieved a complete or partial remission [57,59]. African American patients may be less responsive to triple therapy than other ethnic groups [109], and outcomes in patients who have failed treatment with calcineurin inhibitors have been disappointing [57]. A long-term analysis of FSGS patients by Tune et al. reported that 9% of patients progressed to ESRD [107].

Adverse effects, including transient hypertension, vomiting, steroid-induced cataracts, and headaches, are reported to be self-limited [38,59,104–108]. RCTs are needed to determine the effectiveness and safety of this therapy.

Other combination therapies

Waldo et al. conducted a prospective cohort study in which PMT and CsA therapy was combined in 10 children with FSGS, 80% of whom achieved remission [38]. Four of the patients were African American, and all four responded to therapy. Yorgin et al. also reported the use of combined PMT, angiotensin converting enzyme inhibitor (ACEi), and CsA therapy in a subset of study subjects [13]. CsA therapy was used to maintain remission after it had been achieved by PMT.

Kano et al. reported the successful use of combination therapy with PMT, intravenous immunoglobulin and a statin [110], with 77% achieving a complete or partial remission.

The study by Mori et al. prospectively evaluated the use of heparin therapy and PMT administered for three consecutive days [57]. The combination therapy was given 14 times over 2 years. The patient group consisted of children who were expected to have a poor prognosis due to their resistance to CPA or CsA, and 60% achieved a partial or complete remission.

El-Reshaid et al. reported a 100% remission rate in 21 children with SRNS in a sequential protocol consisting of a calcineurin in-

hibitor followed by the addition of MMF and then by monthly intravenous CPA for three consecutive months [92]. All patients required antihypertensive therapy after starting calcineurin inhibitor therapy.

Nonimmunosuppressant therapy

ACEi therapy

A recent Cochrane review [34] concluded that ACEi significantly reduced proteinuria in children with SRNS (two RCT trials [111,112] with 70 children in total). The RCTs and a small number of prospective and retrospective uncontrolled studies [113–117] reported a 40–80% reduction of proteinuria (Table 68.7). In the RCT by Yi et al., children with SRNS were randomized to receive fosinopril and prednisone treatment for 12 weeks or to receive prednisone alone for the same duration [111]. Fosinopril-treated subjects consistently had lower 24-h urinary protein excretion. After 12 weeks of treatment, fosinopril reduced proteinuria by 0.95 g/24 h (95% CI, −1.21 to −0.69).

ACEi therapy appears to have a dose-dependent effect. In a randomized crossover trial evaluating low-dose versus high-dose enalapril [112], patients who received enalapril at a dose of 0.6 mg/kg/day had an almost twofold greater reduction in the $U_{albumin}/U_{creat}$ ratio compared with patients who received 0.2 mg/kg/day. Investigators had initiated enalapril at a low dose of 0.2 mg/kg/day and then gradually increased the dose to 0.5–0.6 mg/kg/day. Careful monitoring of GFR and serum potassium values is necessary when using ACEi therapy.

Statin therapy

Patients with nephrotic syndrome typically have apoB overproduction, with high levels of very-low-density lipoproteins and low-density lipoproteins (LDL) in plasma. HMG-CoA reductase inhibitors (statins) have been evaluated in both animal and adult studies to ameliorate hypercholesterolemia associated with nephrotic syndrome [118,119]. Two small uncontrolled trials evaluated the efficacy of statin therapy in children with SRNS. Coleman et al. evaluated the efficacy of simvastatin in seven pediatric patients with SRNS and reported that study participants who received a median simvastatin dose of 10 mg/day had 41% and 44% reductions in cholesterol and triglycerides, respectively [120]. One patient who was concurrently treated with prednisolone experienced complete remission.

Sanjad et al. reported that statin therapy significantly reduced plasma levels of total cholesterol, LDL cholesterol, and triglycerides [121]. Statin therapy did not result in a significant reduction in the level of proteinuria or increase serum albumin levels. The rate of progression to ESRD was not affected by statin therapy.

RCTs of statin therapy in a larger population of patients with SRNS are necessary to evaluate if statins have renoprotective and/or cardioprotective roles.

Table 68.6 Evidence ratings and recommendations for combined therapy and SNRS studies[a].

Study ID [reference]	Study type	No. of patients	Histology	Primary intervention	Other treatment	No. with complete/ partial remission	Follow-up
El-Reshaid K/2005 [92]	P NR SC OL	21	6 MCD 15 FSGS	Methylprednisolone q month for 3 months	Sequential and additive use of calcineurin inhibitor, MMF Intravenous pulse CPA Oral PR	21 (100%) MCD 6 (100%)/ FSGS 15 (100%)	41.4 ± 15.3 months
Mori K/2004 [57]	P NR SC OL	10	3 MCD 7 FSGS	Methylprednisolone 30 mg/kg 3 consecutive days, weekly for 2 weeks, monthly for 6 months, quarterly for 2 years	Heparin (10–15 U/kg/h) administered from day before PMT to day after PR 1 mg/kg every other day starting after 3 doses of PMT	4 (40%)/2 (20%) MCD 3 (100%)/ FSGS 1 (14%)/3 (43%)	Not reported
Hari P/2001[59]	P NR SC OL	65	65 FSGS	**A:** Dexamethasone 5 mg/kg 6 alternate-day pulses, 4 2/week pulses, 8 monthly pulses (54 patients) **B:** Methylprednisolone 30 mg/kg 6 alternate-day pulses, 4 2/week pulses, 8 monthly pulses (11 patients)	CPA for 12 weeks and tapering doses of PR for 52 weeks	34 (52%)/not reported **A:** Dexamethasone 28/48 (58%) **B:** Methylprednisolone 6/11 (54%)	25.6 months
Sa GA/1996 [106]	P NR SC OL	5	5 FSGS	Methylprednisolone 30 mg/kg 3 times/week for 2 weeks, once weekly for 8 weeks, once every other week for 8 weeks, once per month for 8 months	CPA 2–2.5 mg/kg/day for 8–12 weeks PR 2 mg/kg alternate-day therapy	4 (80%)/not reported	12–24 months
Waldo FB/1992 [109]	P NR SC OL	13	4 MCD 9 FSGS	Methylprednisolone 20 mg/kg 3 times/week for 2 weeks, once weekly for 8 weeks, once every other week for 8 weeks, once monthly for 8 months, once every other month for 8 months	Chlorambucil 0.2 mg/kg/day for 8 weeks PR 40 mg/m² alternate-day oral dose	5 (38%)/2 (15%) MCD 4 (100%)/ FSGS 1 (11%)/2 (22%)	32 months
Griswold WR/1987 [104]	P NR MC OL	7	7 FSGS	Methylprednisolone 30 mg/kg (max 1 g)	CPA 2 mg/kg/day for 8 weeks or chlorambucil 0.15–0.2 mg/kg/day for 8 weeks PR 2 mg/kg on alternate days	5 (71%)/2 (29%)	47 months
Other studies [62, 105, 107, 110]	R	75	11 Idiopathic 5 MCD 2 MesPGN 57 FSGS	Various combined therapies with PMT		46 (61%)/10 (13%)	Various
TOTAL		204	Histology[c]: 18 MCD 165 FSGS 2 MesPGN 11 Idiopathic	Various		**Cumulative total** Complete: 119 (58%) Partial: 16 (14%) **Response by histology**[b,c] MCD 13/13 (100%) FSGS 78/165 (47%)	

[a] Details for 6 of 10 studies are shown; the remaining 4 studies are summarized in the "Other studies" row.
[b] Complete remission only.
[c] Excluding data from studies by Yorgin and Kano.

Table 68.7 Evidence ratings and recommendations for ACE inhibitor and SNRS studies[a].

Study ID [reference]	Study type	No. of patients	Histology	Primary intervention	Other treatment	No. with complete/ partial response	Follow-up
Yi Z/2006	P SC	RCT OL	45	**A:** Only 17 biopsied 1 MCD 5 FSGS 2 Membranous 2MPGN 7 MesPGN **B:** Only 14 patients biopsied 2 MCD 5 FSGS 1 Membranous 2 MPGN 4 MesPGN	**A:** Fosinopril 5 mg/day for children >5 years, 7.5 mg/day for children 5–10 years, 10 mg for children >10 years; prednisone 2 mg/kg/day tapered to 1 mg/kg/day; treatment duration was 12 weeks **B:** Prednisone 2 mg/kg/day tapered to 1 mg/kg/day; treatment duration was 12 weeks	None	**A:** Urinary protein decreased from 3.94 ± 2.17 to 1.10 ± 0.41 g/24 h at 12 weeks **B:** Urinary protein decreased from 4.44 ± 3.06 to 2.05 ± 0.46 g/24 h at 12 weeks. $P < 0.05$ Complete and partial remission rates not reported	12 weeks
Bagga A/2004 [112]	P SC	RCxT OL	25	**A:** 1 MCD 4 FSGS 4 MPGN 2 MesPGN **B:** 3 MCD 5 FSGS 3 MPGN 3 MesPGN	**A:** Low-dose enalapril (range, 0.16–0.27 mg/kg/day) followed by high dose (range, 0.54–0.77 mg/kg/day) **B:** High-dose enalapril (range, 0.53–0.76 mg/kg/day) followed by low dose (range, 0.18–0.26 mg/kg/day)	Diuretic (furosemide) used for control of significant edema	**A*:** Low dose 34.8% High dose 37.2% **B*:** Low dose 33.3% High dose 62.9% High-dose enalapril associated with significant reduction in Ualb/Ucreat ratio in groups A and B ($P < 0.01$ and 0.001, respectively)	20 weeks (8 weeks per course of therapy)
Kumar NS/2004 [148]	P SC	RCT	17	**A:** 5 MCD 3 FSGS 1 MPGN **B:** 3 MCD 3 FSGS 2 MesPGN	**A:** Ramapril 2.5–5.0 mg/day initially, increased to max 10 mg/day as tolerated (9 patients) **B:** Verapamil 120 mg/day increased to max 240 mg/day as tolerated (8 patients)	None	**A:** 2 (22%)/4 (44%) 71% decrease in 24-h urine protein **B:** 1 (13%)/4 (50%) 48% decrease in 24-h urine protein	12 months
Delucci A/2000 [114]	P SC	NR OL	13	4 FSGS 3 MPGN 3 CresGN 2 MCD with IgM 1 DMS	Enalapril 0.2 mg/kg/day (max 30 mg/day), increased 0.1 mg/kg/day each month until 50% decrease in basal proteinuria reached	PR introduced 2 months later in 11 patients at 30 mg/m² on alternate days	4 (31%)/9 (69%) MCD 0/1 (50%) FSGS 0/4 (100%)	24–84 months (mean 48 months)
Lama G/2000 [149]	P SC	NR OL	7	2 MesPGN 2 FSGS 2 Membranous 1 Alport	Enalapril 0.5 mg/kg/day for nonadolescent patients; 5 mg/day titrated to 20 mg/day for adolescent patients	None	3 (43%)/3 (43%) FSGS 1 (50%)/1 (50%) MesPGN 0/2(100%) Membranous 2 (100%) Alport 0/	2 years

(Continued)

Table 68.7 (*Continued*)

Study ID [reference]	Study type	No. of patients	Histology	Primary intervention	Other treatment	No. with complete/partial response	Follow-up
Proesmans W/1996 [150]	P NR SC OL	6	1 Alport 1 MPGN 2 SR-MCD 2 SR-FSGS	Enalapril 0.5 mg/kg/day for nonadolescent patients; 5 mg/day titrated to 20 mg/day for adolescent patients	One patient received dypyridamole	2 (33%)/3 (50%)	24 months
Milliner DS/1991 [151]	P NR SC OL	6	4 FSGS 1 HSP 1 MCD	Enalapril titrated as tolerated to 10 mg divided twice/day or captopril 12.5 mg three times/day	None	0 / 6 (100%) Total urinary protein decreased by mean 52.4% (*P* < 0.05)	
Trachtman H/1988 [117]	P NR SC OL	8	4 SLE 2 FSGS 1 CGN 1 SDK	Captopril 0.33–1 mg/kg/dose three times a day to max of 1–2 mg/kg/dose		Not reported; 60–70% reduction in proteinuria noted	6.5 months
Adedoyin OT/2003 [113]	R NR SC OL	25	**A:** 2 MCD 2 FSGS 10 Unknown **B:** 2 SR-MCD 1 MesPGN 8 Unknown	**A:** Lisinopril 5 mg/day if <5 years old, 10 mg/day if > 5 years old **B:** No lisinopril	None	**A:** 2 (14.2%)/not reported **B:** 0/not reported	Not reported
Total		96 (88 received treatment)	**All patients:** 19 MCD 31 FSGS 12 MPGN 9 MesPGN 4 CGN 4 SLE 2 Alport 2 Membranous 1 DMS 1 HSP 1 SDK 10 unknown	Various		**Cumulative total** Total remission[b]: 14 (16%) Partial remission[b]: 19 (22%)	

[a]Details from nine of nine studies are shown.

[b]Studies by Yi, Bagga, and Trachtman were excluded because remissions rates were not reported.

*, percent reduction of U_{alb}/U_{creat} ratio.

Pheresis-based therapies

The efficacy of plasma exchange (TPE) in children is thought to be due to the removal of the focal segmental permeability factor described by Savin *et al.* [122–124] and other nephrotic syndrome-inducing permeability factors. The successful use of TPE in treatment-resistant FSGS in nontransplanted children has been reported in a limited number of patients [125–129]. The largest series conducted is the multicenter prospective study by Franke *et al.*, who treated seven children with FSGS using 2.5 volume TPE, PMT, CsA, and replacement intravenous immunoglobulin. Four of the seven patients (57%) achieved a remission. One patient developed *Streptococcus pneumonia* sepsis after two TPE sessions.

Hattori *et al.* were the first to report decreased proteinuria and improved renal function in FSGS with LDL apheresis (LDL-A) [130]. Lipoprotein pheresis systems use a dextran sulfate cellulose column, which binds LDL cholesterol. Brunton used LDL-A to treat 20 patients with nephrotic syndrome. Two patients experienced a remission while receiving the therapy, and LDL-A was effective in reducing LDL cholesterol and was deemed safe [131]. In a multicenter trial, 17 patients with SRNS due to FSGS were treated with corticosteroid therapy and LDL-A twice a week for 3 weeks and then weekly for 6 weeks [132]. In addition to a rapid improvement in hyperlipidemia, 71% achieved remission or partial remission. In a retrospective study, where LDL-A was compared to corticosteroid treatment alone in patients with FSGS, the LDL-A treatment group experienced a decrease in phospholipid, cholesterol, and proteinuria [133]. Hattori *et al.* conducted a prospective study of LDL-A in which 7 of 11 nephrotic children with steroid- and CsA-resistant primary FSGS achieved remission [134]. In a retrospective study by Muso *et al.*, patients in one group ($n = 17$) received LDL-A twice a week for 3 weeks and then weekly for 6 weeks, whereas the other group ($n = 10$) was only treated with corticosteroids. The length of time required to achieve a U_{Prot}/U_{Creat} ratio was shorter in the LDL-A group. Seven patients in the LDL-A group (41%) experienced remission of nephrotic syndrome.

Antibody therapy

Rituximab (anti-CD20)

There are two case reports of remission in response to rituximab therapy. Benz *et al.* reported a 16-year-old boy with SRNS due to FSGS who responded to CPA and CsA therapy but had relapses whenever therapy was withdrawn. After an episode of idiopathic thrombocytopenic purpura treated with rituximab, the patient no longer experienced relapses while on CsA therapy [135]. Nozu *et al.* reported the case of a 12-year-old kidney transplant recipient with recurrent FSGS who developed posttransplant lymphoproliferative disorder [136]. After treatment of the posttransplant lymphoproliferative disorder with rituximab, the patient's nephrotic syndrome completely resolved. Insufficient data exist to recommend this treatment.

Bone marrow transplantation

Shueng-Wai Chan *et al.* reported a case of a 13-year-old with membranous glomerulopathy, which on rebiopsy showed FSGS; the patient achieved remission after bone marrow transplantation [137].

Conclusions

Children with SRNS have access to reasonably effective empiric therapy. Calciuneurin inhibitor therapy and ACEi therapy are recommended therapies for the treatment of SRNS (Table 68.1). Oral CPA may be helpful in the treatment of SRNS due to MCD. Other therapies, including combination therapy, intravenous alkylating agents, MMF, statins, and a brief course of pulse methylprednisolone, may hold promise but due to their low evidence base cannot be recommended. Children with SRNS who experience a sustained remission have better outcomes.

A "one size fits all" approach to immunosuppressive medications has yielded a less-than-optimal record of treatment success. Children with primary steroid resistance due to FSGS are a challenging population, as treatment outcomes are generally inferior to those with MCD [138]. When treating a child who does not respond to a first-line and then second-line of therapy, consideration should be given to performing podocin gene (NPHS2) and the focal segmental permeability factor laboratory studies.

The pediatric nephrology community will need to cooperate to a far greater extent than in the past to effectively assess treatment strategies. Most articles reviewed for this chapter concluded with a statement that, "prospective randomized studies are needed." No single center or regional cooperative group has sufficient numbers to conduct a meaningful RCT. The current slow enrollment for the FSGS NIH study is concerning and indicates that either there are far fewer patients to be studied than originally thought or there is insufficient nephrologist "buy-in" to the multicenter investigative process or the specific treatment regimen offered. The pediatric nephrology community must work cooperatively to answer the pressing challenges of SRNS treatment.

References

1 Churg J, Habib R, White RH. Pathology of the nephrotic syndrome in children: a report for the International Study of Kidney Disease in Children. *Lancet* 1970; **760**: 1299–1302.

2 Abramowicz M, Barnett HL, Edlemann CM, Jr., Greifer L, Kobayashi O, Ameil GC *et al.* Controlled trial of azathioprine in children with nephrotic syndrome. A report for the International Study of Kidney Disease in Children. *Lancet* 1970; **i**: 959–961.

3 McKinney PA, Feltbower RG, Brocklebank, JT, Fitzpatrick MM. Time trends and ethnic patterns of childhood nephrotic syndrome in Yorkshire, UK. *Pediatr Nephrol* 2001; **16**: 1040–1044.

4 Kim JS, Bellew CA, Silverstein DM, Aviles DH, Boineau FG, Vehaskari VM. High incidence of initial and late steroid resistance in childhood nephrotic syndrome. *Kidney Int* 2005; **68**: 1275–1281.

5 Gulati S, Sengupta D, Sharma RK, Sharma A, Gupta RK, Singh U *et al.* Steroid resistant nephrotic syndrome: role of histopathology. *Indian Pediatr* 2006; **43**: 55–60.

6 Andenmatten F, Bianchetti MG, Gerber HA, Zimmerman A, Meregalli P, Luthy C *et al.* Outcome of idiopathic childhood nephrotic syndrome. A 20 year experience. *Scand J Urol Nephrol* 1995; **29**: 15–19.

7 Nammalwar BR, Vijayakumar M, Prahlad N. Experience of renal biopsy in children with nephrotic syndrome. *Pediatr Nephrol* 2006; **21**: 286–288.

8 Srivastava T, Simon SD, Alon US. High incidence of focal segmental glomerulosclerosis in nephrotic syndrome of childhood. *Pediatr Nephrol* 1999; **13**: 13–18.

9 Kirpekar R, Yorgin PD, Tune BM, Kim MK, Sibley RK. Clinicopathologic correlates predict the outcome in children with steroid-resistant idiopathic nephrotic syndrome treated with pulse methylprednisolone therapy. *Am J Kidney Dis* 2002; **39**: 1143–1152.

10 Seikaly MG, Ho PL, Emmett L, Fine RN, Tejani A. Chronic renal insufficiency in children: the 2001 Annual Report of the NAPRTCS. *Pediatr Nephrol* 2003; **18**: 796–804.

11 Benfield MR, McDonald R, Sullivan EK, Stablein DM, Tejani A. The 1997 Annual Renal Transplantation in Children Report of the North American Pediatric Renal Transplant Cooperative Study (NAPRTCS). *Pediatr Transplant* 1999; **3**: 152–167.

12 Andreoli SP. Racial and ethnic differences in the incidence and progression of focal segmental glomerulosclerosis in children. *Adv Ren Replace Ther* 2004; **11**: 105–109.

13 Yorgin PD, Belson A, Higgins J, Alexander SR. Pulse methylprednisolone, cyclosporine, and ACE inhibitor therapy decreases proteinuria in two siblings with familial focal segmental glomerulosclerosis. *Am J Kidney Dis* 2001; **37**: E44.

14 Habashy D, Hodson E, Craig J. Interventions for idiopathic steroid-resistant nephrotic syndrome in children. *Cochrane Database Syst Rev* 2004; **2**: CD003594.

15 Habashy D, Hodson EM, Craig JC. Interventions for steroid-resistant nephrotic syndrome: a systematic review. *Pediatr Nephrol* 2003; **18**: 906–912.

16 Chishti AS, Sorof JM, Brewer ED, Kale AS. Long-term treatment of focal segmental glomerulosclerosis in children with cyclosporine given as a single daily dose. *Am J Kidney Dis* 2001; **38**: 754–760.

17 Melocoton TL, Kamil ES, Cohen AH, Fine RN. Long-term cyclosporine A treatment of steroid-resistant and steroid-dependent nephrotic syndrome. *Am J Kidney Dis* 1991; **18**: 583–588

18 Niaudet P. Treatment of childhood steroid-resistant idiopathic nephrosis with a combination of cyclosporine and prednisone. French Society of Pediatric Nephrology. *J Pediatr* 1994; **125**: 981–986.

19 Niaudet P, Broyer M, Habib R. Treatment of idiopathic nephrotic syndrome with cyclosporin A in children. *Clin Nephrol* 1991; **35**(**Suppl 1**): S31–S36.

20 Niaudet P. Habib R. Cyclosporine in the treatment of idiopathic nephrosis. *J Am Soc Nephrol* 1994; **5**: 1049–1056.

21 Singh A, Tejani C, Tejani A. One-center experience with cyclosporine in refractory nephrotic syndrome in children. *Pediatr Nephrol* 1999; **13**: 26–32.

22 Gregory MJ, Smoyer WE, Sedman A, Kershaw DB, Valentini RP, Johnson K *et al.* Long-term cyclosporine therapy for pediatric nephrotic syndrome: a clinical and histologic analysis. *J Am Soc Nephrol* 1996; **7**: 543–549.

23 Hymes LC. Steroid-resistant, cyclosporine-responsive, relapsing nephrotic syndrome. *Pediatr Nephrol* 1995; **9**: 137–139.

24 Ingulli E, Singh A, Baqi N, Ahmad H, Moazami S, Tejani A. Aggressive, long-term cyclosporine therapy for steroid-resistant focal segmental glomerulosclerosis. *J Am Soc Nephrol* 1995; **5**: 1820–1825.

25 Kim PK, Kim KS, Pai KS, Kim JH, Choi, IJ. Long-term results of cyclosporine-induced remission of relapsing nephrotic syndrome in children. *Yonsei Med J* 1997; **38**: 307–318.

26 Nakamura T, Ushiyama C, Shimada N, Sekizuka K, Ebihara I, Hara M *et al.* Effect of cyclophosphamide or azathioprine on urinary podocytes in patients with diffuse proliferative lupus nephritis. *Nephron* 2001; **87**: 192–193.

27 Garcia C, Michelon T, Barros V, Mota D, Uhlmann A, Randon R *et al.* Cyclosporine in the treatment of steroid-dependent and steroid-resistant idiopathic nephrotic syndrome in children. *Transplant Proc* 1998; **30**: 4156–4157.

28 Hino S, Takemura T, Okada M, Murakami K, Yagi K, Fukushima K *et al.* Follow-up study of children with nephrotic syndrome treated with a long-term moderate dose of cyclosporine. *Am J Kidney Dis* 1998; **31**: 932–939.

29 Seikaly MG, Prashner H, Nolde-Hurlbert B, Browne R. Long-term clinical and pathological effects of cyclosporin in children with nephrosis. *Pediatr Nephrol* 2000; **14**: 214–217.

30 Fernandes P, Silva G, Jr., Barros FA, Oliveira CM, Kubrusly M, Evangelista JB, Jr. Treatment of steroid-resistant nephrotic syndrome with cyclosporine: study of 17 cases and a literature review. *J Nephrol* 2005; **18**: 711–720.

31 Iyengar A, Karthik S, Kumar A, Biswas S, Phadke K. Cyclosporine in steroid dependent and resistant childhood nephrotic syndrome. *Indian Pediatr* 2006; **43**: 14–19.

32 Mahmoud I, Basuni F, Sabry A, El-Husseini A, Hassan N, Ahmad NS *et al.* Single-centre experience with cyclosporin in 106 children with idiopathic focal segmental glomerulosclerosis. *Nephrol Dial Transplant* 2005; **20**: 735–742.

33 Ghiggeri GM, Catarsi P, Scolari F, Caridi G, Bertelli R, Carrea A *et al.* Cyclosporine in patients with steroid-resistant nephrotic syndrome: an open-label, nonrandomized, retrospective study. *Clin Ther* 2004; **26**: 1411–1418.

34 Hodson EM, Habashy D, Craig JC. Interventions for idiopathic steroid-resistant nephrotic syndrome in children. *Cochrane Database Syst Rev* 2006; **2**: CD003594.

35 Phadke K, Ballal S, Maiya V. Cyclosporine experience in nephrotic syndrome. *Indian Pediatr* 1998; **35**: 111–116.

36 El-Husseini A, El-Basuony F, Majmoud I, Sheashaa H, Sabry A, Hazzan R *et al.* Long-term effects of cyclosporine in children with idiopathic nephrotic syndrome: a single-centre experience. *Nephrol Dial Transplant* 2005; **20**: 2433–2438.

37 Waldo FB, Kohaut EC. Therapy of focal segmental glomerulosclerosis with cyclosporine A. *Pediatr Nephrol* 1987; **1**: 180–182.

38 Waldo FB, Benfield MR, Kohaut EC. Therapy of focal and segmental glomerulosclerosis with methylprednisolone, cyclosporine A, and prednisone. *Pediatr Nephrol* 1998; **12**: 397–400.

39 Loeffler K, Gowrishankar M, Yiu V. Tacrolimus therapy in pediatric patients with treatment-resistant nephrotic syndrome. *Pediatr Nephrol* 2004; **19**: 281–287.

40 Ponticelli C, Rizzoni G, Edefonti A, Altieri P, Rivolta E, Rinaldi S et al. A randomized trial of cyclosporine in steroid-resistant idiopathic nephrotic syndrome. *Kidney Int* 1993; **43**: 1377–1384.

41 Moudgil A, Bagga A, Jordan SC. Mycophenolate mofetil therapy in frequently relapsing steroid-dependent and steroid-resistant nephrotic syndrome of childhood: current status and future directions. *Pediatr Nephrol* 2005; **20**: 1376–1381.

42 Hamahira K, Iijima K, Tanaka R, Nakamura H, Yoshikawa N. Recovery from cyclosporine-associated arteriolopathy in childhood nephrotic syndrome. *Pediatr Nephrol* 2001; **16**: 723–727.

43 Ulinski T, Dubourg L, Said MH, Parchoux B, Ranchin B, Cochat P. Switch from cyclosporine A to mycophenolate mofetil in nephrotic children. *Pediatr Nephrol* 2005; **20**: 482–485.

44 McBryde KD, Kershaw DB, Smoyer WE. Pediatric steroid-resistant nephrotic syndrome. *Curr Probl Pediatr Adolesc Health Care* 2001; **31**: 280–307.

45 Sairam VK, Kalia A, Rajaraman S, Travis LB. Secondary resistance to cyclosporin A in children with nephrotic syndrome. *Pediatr Nephrol* 2002; **17**: 842–846.

46 McCauley J, Shapiro R, Ellis D, Igdal H, Tzakis A, Starzl TE. Pilot trial of FK 506 in the management of steroid-resistant nephrotic syndrome. *Nephrol Dial Transplant* 1993; **8**: 1286–1290.

47 Al-Uzri A, Stablein DM, Cohn R. Posttransplant diabetes mellitus in pediatric renal transplant recipients: a report of the North American Pediatric Renal Transplant Cooperative Study (NAPRTCS). *Transplantation* 2001; **72**: 1020–1024.

48 Shapiro R, Scantlebury V, Jordan ML, Vivas C, Ellis D, Lombardozzi-Lane S et al. Posttransplant diabetes in pediatric recipients on tacrolimus. *Transplantation* 1999; **67**: 771.

49 Prospective, controlled trial of cyclophosphamide therapy in children with nephrotic syndrome. Report of the International Study of Kidney Disease in Children. *Lancet* 1974; **ii**: 423–427.

50 Tarshish P, Tobin JN, Bernstein J, Edelmann CM, Jr. Cyclophosphamide does not benefit patients with focal segmental glomerulosclerosis. A report of the International Study of Kidney Disease in Children. *Pediatr Nephrol* 1996; **10**: 590–593.

51 Martinelli R, Pereira LJ, Silva OM, Okumura AS, Rocha H. Cyclophosphamide in the treatment of focal segmental glomerulosclerosis. *Braz J Med Biol Res* 2004; **37**: 1365–1372.

52 Burgess E. Management of focal segmental glomerulosclerosis: evidence-based recommendations. *Kidney Int Suppl* 1999; **70**: S26–S32.

53 Cole BR, Brocklebank JT, Kienstra RA, Kissane JM, Robson AM. "Pulse" methylprednisolone therapy in the treatment of severe glomerulonephritis. *J Pediatr* 1976; **88**: 307–314.

54 Rose GM, Cole BR, Robson AM. The treatment of severe glomerulopathies in children using high dose intravenous methylprednisolone pulses. *Am J Kidney Dis* 1981; **1**: 148–156.

55 Yeung CK, Wong KL, Ng WL. Intravenous methylprednisolone pulse therapy in minimal change nephrotic syndrome. *Aust N Z J Med* 1983; **13**: 349–351.

56 Hafeez F, Ahmad TM, Anwar S. Efficacy of steroids, cyclosporin and cyclophosphamide in steroid resistant idiopathic nephrotic syndrome. *J Coll Physicians Surg Pak* 2005; **15**: 329–332.

57 Mori K, Honda M, Ikeda M. Efficacy of methylprednisolone pulse therapy in steroid-resistant nephrotic syndrome. *Pediatr Nephrol* 2004; **19**: 1232–1236.

58 Murnaghan K, Vasmant D, Bensman A. Pulse methylprednisolone therapy in severe idiopathic childhood nephrotic syndrome. *Acta Paediatr Scand* 1984; **73**: 733–739.

59 Hari P, Bagga A, Jindal N, Srivastava RN. Treatment of focal glomerulosclerosis with pulse steroids and oral cyclophosphamide. *Pediatr Nephrol* 2001; **16**: 901–905.

60 Hari P, Bagga A, Mantan M. Short term efficacy of intravenous dexamethasone and methylprednisolone therapy in steroid resistant nephrotic syndrome. *Indian Pediatr* 2004; **41**: 993–1000.

61 Fujimoto S, Kondoh H, Yamamoto Y, Hisanaga S, Tanaka K. Holter electrocardiogram monitoring in nephrotic patients during methylprednisolone pulse therapy. *Am J Nephrol* 1990; **10**: 231–236.

62 Yorgin PD, Krasher J, Al-Uzri AY. Pulse methylprednisolone treatment of idiopathic steroid-resistant nephrotic syndrome. *Pediatr Nephrol* 2001; **16**: 245–250.

63 White RH, Cameron JS, Trounce JR. Immunosuppressive therapy in steroid-resistant proliferative glomerulonephritis accompanied by the nephrotic syndrome. *Br Med J* 1966; **2**: 853–860.

64 Barletta GM, Smoyer WE, Bunchman TE, Flynn JT, Kershaw DB. Use of mycophenolate mofetil in steroid-dependent and -resistant nephrotic syndrome. *Pediatr Nephrol* 2003; **18**: 833–837.

65 Mendizabal S, Zamora I, Berbel O, Sanahuja MJ, Fuentes J, Simon J. Mycophenolate mofetil in steroid/cyclosporine-dependent/resistant nephrotic syndrome. *Pediatr Nephrol* 2005; **20**: 914–919.

66 Kawasaki Y, Hosoya M, Kobayashi S, Ohara S, Onishi N, Takahashi A et al. Oral mizoribine pulse therapy for patients with steroid-resistant and frequently relapsing steroid-dependent nephrotic syndrome. *Nephrol Dial Transplant* 2005; **20**: 2243-2247.

67 Nakamura T, Ushiyama C, Suzuki S, Hara M, Shimada N, Ebihara I et al. The urinary podocyte as a marker for the differential diagnosis of idiopathic focal glomerulosclerosis and minimal-change nephrotic syndrome. *Am J Nephrol* 2000; **20**: 175–179.

68 Honda, M. Nephrotic syndrome and mizoribine in children. *Pediatr Int* 2002; **44**: 210–216

69 Tanaka H, Tsugawa K, Nakahata T, Kudo M, Onuma S, Kimura S et al. Mizoribine pulse therapy for a pediatric patient with steroid-resistant nephrotic syndrome. *Tohoku J Exp Med* 2005; **205**: 87–91.

70 Geary DF, Farine M, Thorner P, Baumal R. Response to cyclophosphamide in steroid-resistant focal segmental glomerulosclerosis: a reappraisal. *Clin Nephrol* 1984; **22**: 109–113.

71 Srivastava RN, Agarwal RK, Moudgil A, Bhuyan UN. Late resistance to corticosteroids in nephrotic syndrome. *J Pediatr* 1986; **108**: 66–70.

72 Trainin EB, Boichis H, Spitzer A, Edelmann CM, Jr, Greifer I. Late nonresponsiveness to steroids in children with the nephrotic syndrome. *J Pediatr* 1975; **87**: 519–523.

73 Bergstrand A, Bollgren I, Samuelsson A, Tornroth T, Wasserman J, Winberg J. Idiopathic nephrotic syndrome of childhood: cyclophosphamide induced conversion from steroid refractory to highly steroid sensitive disease. *Clin Nephrol* 1973; **1**: 302–306.

74 Durand P, De Toni E, Jr. Treatment of nephrotic syndrome in children. *Ann Paediatr* 1955; **185**: 225–235.

75 Grushkin CM, Fine RN, Heuser E, Lieberman E. Cyclophosphamide therapy of idiopathic nephrosis. *Calif Med* 1970; **113**: 1–5.

76 Elzouki AY, Jaiswal OP. Evaluation of chlorambucil therapy in steroid-dependent and cyclophosphamide-resistant children with nephrosis. *Pediatr Nephrol* 1990; **4**: 459–462.

77 Latta K, von Schnakenburg C, Ehrich JH. A meta-analysis of cytotoxic treatment for frequently relapsing nephrotic syndrome in children. *Pediatr Nephrol* 2001; **16**: 271–282.

78 Latta K, von Schnakenburg C, Ehrich JH. A meta-analysis of cytoxic treatment for frequently relapsing nephrotic syndrome in children. *Pediatr Nephrol* 2001; **16**: 271–282.

79 Barratt TM, Soothill JF. Controlled trial of cyclophosphamide in steroid-sensitive relapsing nephrotic syndrome of childhood. *Lancet* 1970; **ii:** 479–482.

80 Abrantes MM, Cardoso LS, Lima EM, Silva JM, Diniz JS, Bambirra EA *et al.* Clinical course of 110 children and adolescents with primary focal segmental glomerulosclerosis. *Pediatr Nephrol* 2006; **21:** 482–489.

81 Tarshish P, Tobin JN, Bernstein J, Edelmann CM, Jr. Prognostic significance of the early course of minimal change nephrotic syndrome: report of the International Study of Kidney Disease in Children. *J Am Soc Nephrol* 1997; **8:** 769–776.

82 Drummond KN, Hillman DA, Marchessault JH, Feldman W. Cyclophosphamide in the nephrotic syndrome of childhood: its use in two groups of patients defined by clinical, light microscopic and immunopathologic findings. *Can Med Assoc J* 1968; **98:** 524–531.

83 Trompeter RS, Evans PR, Barratt TM. Gonadal function in boys with steroid-responsive nephrotic syndrome treated with cyclophosphamide for short periods. *Lancet* 1981; **i:** 1177–1179.

84 Ruth EM, Kemper MJ, Leumann EP, Laube GF, Neuhaus TJ. Children with steroid-sensitive nephrotic syndrome come of age: long-term outcome. *J Pediatr* 2005; **147:** 202–207.

85 Park MC, Park YB, Jung SY, Chung IH, Choi KH, Lee SK. Risk of ovarian failure and pregnancy outcome in patients with lupus nephritis treated with intravenous cyclophosphamide pulse therapy. *Lupus* 2004; **13:** 569–574.

86 Gulati S, Kher V. Intravenous pulse cyclophosphamide—a new regimen for steroid resistant focal segmental glomerulosclerosis. *Indian Pediatr* 2000; **37:** 141–148.

87 du Buf-Vereijken PW, Wetzels JF. Efficacy of a second course of immunosuppressive therapy in patients with membranous nephropathy and persistent or relapsing disease activity. *Nephrol Dial Transplant* 2004; **19:** 2036–2043.

88 Etteldorf JN, West CD, Pitcock JA, Williams DL. Gonadal function, testicular histology, and meiosis following cyclophosphamide therapy in patients with nephrotic syndrome. *J Pediatr* 1976; **88:** 206–212.

89 Alshaya HO, Al-Maghrabi JA, Kari JA. Intravenous pulse cyclophosphamide—is it effective in children with steroid-resistant nephrotic syndrome? *Pediatr Nephrol* 2003; **18:** 1143–1146.

90 Bajpai A, Bagga A, Hari P, Dinda A, Srivastava RN. Intravenous cyclophosphamide in steroid-resistant nephrotic syndrome. *Pediatr Nephrol* 2003; **18:** 351–356.

91 Elhence R, Gulati S, Kher V, Gupta A, Sharma RK. Intravenous pulse cyclophosphamide—a new regimen for steroid-resistant minimal change nephrotic syndrome. *Pediatr Nephrol* 1994; **8:** 1–3.

92 El-Reshaid K, El-Reshaid W, Madda J. Combination of immunosuppressive agents in treatment of steroid-resistant minimal change disease and primary focal segmental glomerulosclerosis. *Ren Fail* 2005; **27:** 523–530.

93 Plotz PH, Klippel JH, Decker JL, Grauman D, Wolff B, Brown BC *et al.* Bladder complications in patients receiving cyclophosphamide for systemic lupus erythematosus or rheumatoid arthritis. *Ann Intern Med* 1979; **91:** 221–223.

94 Andriole GL, Sandlund JT, Miser JS, Arasi V, Linehan M, Magrath IT. The efficacy of mesna (2-mercaptoethane sodium sulfonate) as a uroprotectant in patients with hemorrhagic cystitis receiving further oxazaphosphorine chemotherapy. *J Clin Oncol* 1987; **5:** 799–803.

95 Scheef W, Klein HO, Brock N, Burkert H, Gunther U, Hoefer-Janker H *et al.* Controlled clinical studies with an antidote against the urotoxicity of oxazaphosphorines: preliminary results. *Cancer Treat Rep* 1979; **63:** 501–505.

96 Mace JR, Keohan ML, Bernardy H, Junge K, Niebch G, Romeis P *et al.* Crossover randomized comparison of intravenous versus intravenous/oral mesna in soft tissue sarcoma treated with high-dose ifosfamide. *Clin Cancer Res* 2003; **9:** 5829–5834.

97 Katz A, Epelman S, Anelli A, Gorender EF, Cruz SM, Oliveira RM *et al.* A prospective randomized evaluation of three schedules of mesna administration in patients receiving an ifosfamide-containing chemotherapy regimen: sustained efficiency and simplified administration. *J Cancer Res Clin Oncol* 1995; **121:** 128–131.

98 Vose JM, Reed EC, Pippert GC, Anderson JR, Bierman PJ, Kessinger A *et al.* Mesna compared with continuous bladder irrigation as uroprotection during high-dose chemotherapy and transplantation: a randomized trial. *J Clin Oncol* 1993; **11:** 1306–1310.

99 Fine BP, Munoz R, Uy CS, Ty A. Nitrogen mustard therapy in children with nephrotic syndrome unresponsive to corticosteroid therapy. *J Pediatr* 1976; **89:** 1014–1016.

100 Arumugam R, Watson AR. Nitrogen mustard therapy and nephrotic syndrome. *Pediatr Nephrol* 1996; **10:** 130–131.

101 Arumugan R, Watson, AR, *Nitrogen mustard therapy and nephrotic syndrome pediatric nephrology* 1996; **10**(1): 130–1.

102 Almeida MP, Almeida HA, Rosa FC. Vincristine in steroid-resistant nephrotic syndrome. *Pediatr Nephrol* 1994; **8:** 79–80.

103 Goonasekera CD, Koziell AB, Hulton SA, Dillon MJ. Vincristine and focal segmental sclerosis: do we need a multicentre trial? *Pediatr Nephrol* 1998; **12:** 284–289.

104 Griswold WR, Tune BM, Reznik VM, Vazquez M, Prime DH, Brock P *et al.* Treatment of childhood prednisone-resistant nephrotic syndrome and focal segmental glomerulosclerosis with intravenous methylprednisolone and oral alkylating agents. *Nephron* 1987; **46:** 73–77.

105 Mendoza SA, Reznik VM, Griswold WR, Krensky AM, Yorgin PD, Tune BM. Treatment of steroid-resistant focal segmental glomerulosclerosis with pulse methylprednisolone and alkylating agents. *Pediatr Nephrol* 1990; **4:** 303–307.

106 Sa GA, Luis JP, Mendonca E, Almeida M, Rosa FC. Treatment of childhood steroid-resistant nephrotic syndrome with pulse methylprednisolone and cyclophosphamide. *Pediatr Nephrol* 1996; **10:** 250.

107 Tune BM, Kirpekar R, Sibley RK, Reznik VM, Griswold WR, Mendoza SA. Intravenous methylprednisolone and oral alkylating agent therapy of prednisone-resistant pediatric focal segmental glomerulosclerosis: a long-term follow-up. *Clin Nephrol* 1995; **43:** 84–88.

108 Tune BM, Lieberman E, Mendoza SA. Steroid-resistant nephrotic focal segmental glomerulosclerosis: a treatable disease. *Pediatr Nephrol* 1996; **10:** 772–778.

109 Waldo FB, Benfield MR, Kohaut EC. Methylprednisolone treatment of patients with steroid-resistant nephrotic syndrome. *Pediatr Nephrol* 1992; **6:** 503–505.

110 Kano K, Hoshi E, Ito S, Kyo K, Yamada Y, Ando T *et al.* Effects of combination therapy consisting of moderate-dose intravenous immunoglobulin G, pulsed methylprednisolone and pravastatin in children with steroid-resistant nephrosis. *Nephron* 2000; **84:** 99–100.

111 Yi Z, Wu XC, He QN, Dan XQ, He XJ. Effect of fosinopril in children with steroid-resistant idiopathic nephrotic syndrome. *Pediatr Nephrol* 2006; **21:** 967–972.

112 Bagga A, Mudigoudar BD, Hari P, Vasudev V. Enalapril dosage in steroid-resistant nephrotic syndrome. *Pediatr Nephrol* 2004; **19:** 45–50.

113 Adedoyin OT, Ologe MO, Anigilaje EA, Adeniyi A. Effect of lisinopril on proteinuria in children with nephrotic syndrome in Ilorin, Nigeria. *Pediatr Nephrol* 2003; **18:** 727–728.

114 Delucchi A, Cano F, Rodriguez E, Wolff E, Gonzalez X, Cumsille MA. Enalapril and prednisone in children with nephrotic-range proteinuria. *Pediatr Nephrol* 2000; **14**: 1088–1091.

115 Heeg JE, de Jong PE, van der Hem, GK, de Zeeuw D. Reduction of proteinuria by angiotensin converting enzyme inhibition. *Kidney Int* 1987; **32**: 78–83.

116 Lama G, Luongo I, Tirino G, Borriello A, Carangio C, Salsano ME. T-lymphocyte populations and cytokines in childhood nephrotic syndrome. *Am J Kidney Dis* 2002; **39**: 958–965.

117 Trachtman H, Gauthier B. Effect of angiotensin-converting enzyme inhibitor therapy on proteinuria in children with renal disease. *J Pediatr* 1988; **112**: 295–298.

118 D'Amico G. Statins and renal diseases: from primary prevention to renal replacement therapy. *J Am Soc Nephrol* 2006; **17**: S148–S152.

119 Vaziri ND, Liang K. Effects of HMG-CoA reductase inhibition on hepatic expression of key cholesterol-regulatory enzymes and receptors in nephrotic syndrome. *Am J Nephrol* 2004; **24**: 606–613.

120 Coleman JE, Watson AR. Hyperlipidaemia, diet and simvastatin therapy in steroid-resistant nephrotic syndrome of childhood. *Pediatr Nephrol* 1996; **10**: 171–174.

121 Sanjad SA, al-Abbad A, al-Shorafa S. Management of hyperlipidemia in children with refractory nephrotic syndrome: the effect of statin therapy. *J Pediatr* 1997; **130**: 470–474.

122 Savin VJ, McCarthy ET, Sharma M. Permeability factors in focal segmental glomerulosclerosis. *Semin Nephrol* 2003; **23**: 147–160.

123 Sharma M, Sharma R, McCarthy ET, Savin VJ. "The FSGS factor:" enrichment and in vivo effect of activity from focal segmental glomerulosclerosis plasma. *J Am Soc Nephrol* 1999; **10**: 552–561.

124 Sharma M, Sharma R, Reddy SR, McCarthy ET, Savin VJ. Proteinuria after injection of human focal segmental glomerulosclerosis factor. *Transplantation* 2002; **73**: 366–372.

125 Vecsei AK, Muller T, Schratzberger EC, Kircher K, Regele H, Arbeiter K *et al.* Plasmapheresis-induced remission in otherwise therapy-resistant FSGS. *Pediatr Nephrol* 2001; **16**: 898–900.

126 Rao PS, Bakir AA. The role of plasmapheresis in the treatment of focal segmental glomerulosclerosis (FSGS). *Int J Artif Organs* 2000; **23**: 798–801.

127 Mitwalli AH. Adding plasmapheresis to corticosteroids and alkylating agents: does it benefit patients with focal segmental glomerulosclerosis? *Nephrol Dial Transplant* 1998; **13**: 1524–1528.

128 Feld SM, Figueroa P, Savin V, Nast CC, Sharma R, Sharma M *et al.* Plasmapheresis in the treatment of steroid-resistant focal segmental glomerulosclerosis in native kidneys. *Am J Kidney Dis* 1998; **32**: 230–237.

129 Ginsburg DS, Dau P. Plasmapheresis in the treatment of steroid-resistant focal segmental glomerulosclerosis. *Clin Nephrol* 1997; **48**: 282–287.

130 Hattori M, Ito K, Kawaguchi H, Tanaka T, Kuboto R, Khono M. Treatment with a combination of low-density lipoprotein aphaeresis and pravastatin of a patient with drug-resistant nephrotic syndrome due to focal segmental glomerulosclerosis. *Pediatr Nephrol* 1993; **7**: 196–198.

131 Brunton C, Varghese Z, Moorhead JF. Lipopheresis in the nephrotic syndrome. *Kidney Int Suppl* 1999; **71**: S6–S9.

132 Muso E, Mune M, Fujii Y, Imai E, Ueda N, Hatta K *et al.* Low density lipoprotein apheresis therapy for steroid-resistant nephrotic syndrome. Kansai-FGS-Apheresis Treatment (K-FLAT) Study Group. *Kidney Int Suppl* 1999; **71**: S122–S125.

133 Muso E, Mune M, Fujii Y, Imai E, Ueda N, Hatta K *et al.* Significantly rapid relief from steroid-resistant nephrotic syndrome by LDL apheresis compared with steroid monotherapy. *Nephron* 2001; **89**: 408–415.

134 Hattori M, Chikamoto H, Akioka Y, Nakakura H, Ogino D, Matsunaga A *et al.* A combined low-density lipoprotein apheresis and prednisone therapy for steroid-resistant primary focal segmental glomerulosclerosis in children. *Am J Kidney Dis* 2003; **42**: 1121–1130.

135 Benz K, Dotsch J, Rascher W, Stachel D. Change of the course of steroid-dependent nephrotic syndrome after rituximab therapy. *Pediatr Nephrol* 2004; **19**: 794–797.

136 Nozu K, Iijima K, Fujisawa M, Nakagawa A, Yoshikawa N, Matsuo M. Rituximab treatment for posttransplant lymphoproliferative disorder (PTLD) induces complete remission of recurrent nephrotic syndrome. *Pediatr Nephrol* 2005; **20**: 1660–1663.

137 Chan GS, Chim S, Fan YS, Chan KW. Focal segmental glomerulosclerosis after membranous glomerulonephritis in remission: temporal diversity of glomerulopathy after bone marrow transplantation. *Hum Pathol* 2006; **37**: 1607–1610.

138 Rennert WP, Kala UK, Jacobs D, Goetsch S, Verhaart S. Pulse cyclophosphamide for steroid-resistant focal segmental glomerulosclerosis. *Pediatr Nephrol* 1999; **13**: 113–116.

139 Lieberman KV, Tejani A. A randomized double-blind placebo-controlled trial of cyclosporine in steroid-resistant idiopathic focal segmental glomerulosclerosis in children. *J Am Soc Nephrol* 1996; **7**: 56–63.

140 Garin EH, Orak JK, Hiott KL, Sutherland SE. Cyclosporine therapy for steroid-resistant nephrotic syndrome. A controlled study. *Am J Dis Child* 1988; **142**: 985–988.

141 El-Husseini, A, El-Basuony F, Donia A, Mahmoud I, Hassan N, Sayed-Ahmed N *et al.* Co-administration of cyclosporine and ketoconazole in children with minimal change nephrotic syndrome. *Nephron Clin Pract* 2005; **100**: c27–c32.

142 El-Husseini A, El-Basuony F, Majmoud I, Donia A, Hassan N, Sayed-Ahmed N *et al.* Effect of concomitant administration of cyclosporine and ketoconazole in children with focal segmental glomerulosclerosis. *Am J Nephrol* 2004; **24**: 301–306.

143 O'Regan S, Murphy GF, Robitaille P, Russo P, Klassen J. Decreased hospitalization and increased height velocity in focal segmental glomerulosclerosis responsive to ciclosporin A. *Child Nephrol Urol* 1991; **11**: 185–189.

144 Grushkin CM, Fine RN, Heuser E, Lieberman E. Cyclophosphamide therapy of idiopathic nephrosis. *Calif Med* 1970; **113**: 1–5.

145 el-Reshaid K, Kapoor M, Nampoory N, Madda J, Jawad N, Johny K. Treatment of children with steroid refractory idiopathic nephrotic syndrome: the Kuwaiti experience. *Ren Fail* 1999; **21**: 487–494.

146 Kari JA, Alkushi A, Alshaya HO. Chlorambucil therapy in children with steroid-resistant nephrotic syndrome. *Saudi Med J* 2006; **27**: 558–559.

147 Adhikari M, Bhimma R, Coovadia HM. Intensive pulse therapies for focal glomerulosclerosis in South African children. *Pediatr Nephrol* 1997; **11**: 423–428.

148 Kumar NS, Singh AK, Mishra RN, Prakash J. Comparative study of angiotensin converting enzyme inhibitor and calcium channel blocker in the treatment of steroid-resistant idiopathic nephrotic syndrome. *J Assoc Physicians India* 2004; **52**: 454–458.

149 Lama G, Luongo I, Piscitelli A, Salsano ME. Enalapril: antiproteinuric effect in children with nephrotic syndrome. *Clin Nephrol* 2000; **53**: 432–436.

150 Proesmans W, Wambeke IV, Dyck MV. Long-term therapy with enalapril in patients with nephrotic-range proteinuria. *Pediatr Nephrol* 1996; **10**: 587–589.

151 Milliner DS, Morgenstern BZ. Angiotensin converting enzyme inhibitors for reduction of proteinuria in children with steroid-resistant nephrotic syndrome. *Pediatr Nephrol* 1991; **5**: 587–590.

Other Pediatric Renal Diseases

69 Henoch-Schonlein Nephritis and Membranoprolifertive Glomerulonephritis

Sharon Phillips Andreoli

Department of Pediatrics, James Whitcomb Riley Hospital for Children,
Indiana University Medical Center, Indianapolis, USA

Introduction

The clinical manifestions of Henoch-Schonlein purpura (HSP), including the typical rash, arthralgias, arthritis, gastrointestinal involvement, and renal involvement, have been well-described. Less common manifestations include testicular inflammation and pulmonary and central nervous system, as well as other organ, involvement [1–5]. The occurrence of kidney disease has been estimated to be as low as 20% in some studies and up to 50% in other studies [1–4]. The renal disease in HSP is quite variable, with the majority of patients demonstrating spontaneous resolution of the nephritis. Treatment strategies are based on the risk of progressive disease [2–5]. HSP is a very common disorder in pediatric patients and is less common in adults, but the development of HSP nephritis is more common and more severe in adolescent and adult patients [6–12]. Treatment strategies for HSP are based on very few randomized controlled trials (RCTs) with prednisone to prevent the development of renal disease in HSP, and there have been virtually no RCTs for therapy of severe HSP nephritis. Although there are no controlled trials of therapy for HSP nephritis, there are multiple case series and anecdotal reports of successful immunosuppressive therapy for HSP nephritis.

Membranoproliferative glomerulonephritis (MPGN) types I, II (also known as dense deposit disease), and III are also common forms of glomerulonephritis in pediatric and adult patients [5,13–15]. In contrast to HSP nephritis, the natural history of all types of MPGN is progression to chronic kidney disease in the majority of patients [5,13–15]. However, the natural history and rate of progression within and between types I, II, and III are quite variable. Treatment strategies in MPGN are also based on reports of series of patients treated with immunosuppressive therapy and very few controlled trials of therapy. This chapter reviews the etiology, epidemiology, natural history, and treatment strategies for HSP nephritis and idiopathic MPGN.

Etiology, epidemiology, and natural history of HSP nephritis

Etiology

Although the clinical manifestations of HSP are well-known, the specific pathogen(s) that triggers the clinical features of HSP is unknown. Associations with group A beta-hemolytic streptococcal infections, infections with viruses including hepatitis B, herpes simplex, human parovovirus B, and influenza viruses, other infections, and other agents have been reported by many investigators [16]. However, the large majority of the reports associating specific infectious agents, drugs, or immunizations with HSP are anecdotal reports, and despite extensive investigation, there is no clear pathogen that is accepted as a trigger for the clinical manifestations of HSP. Given the lack of a single etiological agent identified for HSP, it is likely that the disease is caused by multiple agents and that the immune responses to different agents are similar in individuals who develop HSP. Recent studies suggest genetic susceptibility to the development of HSP, and it is also likely that genetic and environmental factors play a role in the development of HSP and HSP nephritis.

HSP is a leukocytoclastic vasculitis that affects small vessels. The pathology demonstrates white blood cell infiltration, small vessel inflammation, and deposition of immunoglobulin A (IgA) in vessels obtained from skin biopsies and in kidney biopsies. Since infections, particularly respiratory infections, are associated with HSP, it has been suggested that abnormal mucosal IgA production following infection may precipitate the vasculitis. Reported findings of IgA-containing immune complexes in the kidney and extrarenal sites, of IgA rheumatoid factor in some patients, and of IgA fibronectin complexes and mesangial cell autoantigens support immune dysregulation as a cause of the vasculitis [17]. Abnormalities in the O-linked glycosylation of IgA1 may contribute to the abnormal IgA in HSP and in IgA nephropathy [16].

Evidence-based Nephrology. Edited by Donald Molony and Jonathan Craig
© 2009 Blackwell Publishing, ISBN: 978-1-4051-3975-5.

Epidemiology of HSP nephritis

Whereas HSP and HSP nephritis have been described in all age ranges, HSP is most common in children, with a peak incidence at ages 4–6 years. Age has a major influence on the development of HSP nephritis; multiple studies have demonstrated that the incidence of renal disease in HSP and the severity of the renal disease increase with age. The large majority of children with HSP in the first decade of life do not develop serious renal involvement, but significant renal disease occurs commonly in adolescents and adults with HSP [7–12].

The incidence of HSP has been reported in several population studies. In Taiwan, the annual incidence of HSP was 12.9/100,000 children less than 17 years of age [18]. In a study of 78 children in Spain, the incidence of HSP was also noted to be the highest in the fall and winter months. The median age at the onset of symptoms was 5.5 years, and the annual incidence was 10.45/100,000 children aged 14 and younger [19]. In a study of 150 Italian children, the male/female ratio was 1.8:1, the mean age was 6.1 years, and renal involvement occurred in 54%, with 7% of the children demonstrating severe nephritis and 2% with acute renal failure [20].

Several interesting studies have demonstrated that genetic polymorphisms may predispose individuals to the development of HSP and/or to the pathogenic evolution to HSP nephritis. In a study of 57 patients with HSP, no significant differences in the allele or genotype frequencies for two vascular endothelial cell growth factor polymorphisms between patients with HSP and control patients were found, but the high vascular endothelial growth factor producer allele was increased in patients with HSP nephritis compared to healthy controls [21]. Polymorphisms of the interleukin-1β gene were not different in patients with HSP compared to controls, but each of the 5 patients who developed severe nephropathy carried the rare T allele, compared with 16 of the remaining 44 patients [22]. Other interesting studies have demonstrated that the TT genotype of the C-509T polymorphism of the transforming growth factor β gene was significantly more common in children with HSP than in control children, and the TT genotype was more common in children with severe HSP [23]. Polymorphisms of the renin–angiotensin system have also been associated with the development of HSP and possibly the development of renal disease [24]. Patients with familial Mediterranean fever have a higher incidence of HSP, with approximately 5% of patients with familial Mediterranean fever developing HSP [25]. Other studies have demonstrated no association with uteroglobin gene polymorphism in childhood HSP [26]. Similarly, polymorphisms in thrombophilia genes, including methylenetetrahydrofolate reductase, prothrombin, and factor V genes, did not differ in patients with HSP and controls [27]. Although more studies need to be performed, these early studies suggest that there may be a genetically determined susceptibility to risk and increased severity of HSP nephritis.

Natural history of HSP nephritis

The majority of children with HSP have mild to no renal disease, and when renal disease occurs it usually resolves spontaneously without need for therapy [1–5]. Older children, adolescents, and adults with HSP have a higher incidence of renal disease, and when renal disease occurs it is more severe than in younger children [6–12]. Children with HSP nephritis who were followed for several years were found to have a high incidence of renal disease in adulthood compared to those that did not have initial renal disease, and there was a high incidence of complications during pregnancy even in the absence of active kidney disease [4,28].

The majority of patients with HSP who are destined to develop nephritis will demonstrate renal disease within a few months of the onset of HSP, but unusual cases of the late occurrence of HSP nephritis also have been described [29]. A systematic review of 12 studies of 1,133 patients found that 34.2% developed renal involvement, of whom 85% developed renal disease within 4 weeks, 91% within 6 weeks, and 97% within 6 months [30]. The most common manifestation is hematuria alone, which generally resolves spontaneously and does not require therapy. Some patients also develop proteinuria in addition to hematuria, and in the majority of such patients the nephritis will also resolve spontaneously. Proteinuria that is increasing in quantity and/or has evolved into nephrotic syndrome, and/or evidence of rapidly progressive glomerulonephritis, is highly suggestive of more severe pathology and a worse long-term prognosis. Although there are many notable exceptions, in general the severity of the clinical presentation, including laboratory values, correlates with the severity of the pathologic findings [5,31–34]. Among 1,133 children, persistent renal impairment did not occur in any child with a normal urinalysis. Persistent renal impairment developed in 1.6% of children with minor urine abnormalities, and 19.5% of children with nephritic and/or nephrotic syndrome developed renal impairment [30].

Evidence for the efficacy of therapies in HSP nephritis

In this section we review two aspects of therapy for HSP nephritis. First, we review evidence that therapy can alter the development of nephritis in patients with HSP; second, we review the evidence that therapy can alter established HSP nephritis.

Evidence that therapy can alter the development of HSP nephritis

Steroid therapy has been used to treat the abdominal symptoms and joint pain of HSP, and it has been suggested that steroid therapy may prevent the development of nephritis. Four trials and other retrospective studies have been performed to address this issue [35–39] (Table 69.1). Two well-designed randomized, double-blind, placebo-controlled trials did not demonstrate any benefit of prednisone over placebo in preventing renal disease at 6–12 months after diagnosis. In one RCT 40 children with HSP seen in an emergency room were randomized to receive placebo or oral prednisone at 2 mg/kg/day for 1 week with weaning of the prednisone over the next week. At 1 year, there was no difference in the incidence of renal involvement between the two groups [35]. In a larger RCT, 84 children were treated with 1 mg/kg/day prednisone for 2 weeks with a tapering dose of prednisone over the next 2 weeks, while 87 children received placebo [36]. The investigators

Table 69.1 Evidence for therapy to prevent the the development of HSP Nephritis.

Study	Therapy	Number of patients and patient characteristics	Outcome
Mollica, 1992 randomised controlled study	1mg/kg/day prednisone for two weeks	84 patients treated with prednisone 84 patients not treated with prednisone (age not reported)	No treated patient developed nephritis 10 (11.9%) control patients developed nephritis
Saulsbury, 1993 retrospective study	any prednisone therapy	50 children without nephritis	20% of patients who received predisone and 20% who did not receive prednisone developed nephritis
Islek, 1999 randomized controled trial	1 mg/kg/day for 10 days and weaning dose for one week	70 patients treated with prednisone and 50 not treated with prednisone aged 9.2 +/− 2.7 yrs	21% (15/70) of treated patients and 36% (18/50) control patients developed nephritis
Huber, 2004 randomized placebo controlled, double blind trial	2 mg/kg/day prednisone for one week and weaning dose for one week	21 treated patients and 19 placebo patients treated aged 2-15 years	No difference in rate of renal involvement; 3/21 treated and 2/19 placebo developed nephritis
Ronkainen, 2006 randomized placebo controled double blind trial	1 mg/kg/day prednisone for two weeks and weaning dose for two more weeks	84 treated patients and 87 placebo children ages 1.7 to 15.6 years	No difference in rate of renal symptoms 38/84 treated and 36/87 control patients had renal symptoms

concluded that prednisone did not prevent the development of renal symptoms, although prednisone may be effective in treating HSP nephritis. A retrospective study of 50 children with HSP without renal disease at the time of diagnosis demonstrated that prednisone therapy did not prevent the development of nephritis [38]. In contrast, two poorly designed controlled studies of early administration of prednisone in children with HSP and no signs of renal involvement demonstrated that, in the two studies, respectively, 0% and 21% of children treated with prednisone compared with 12% and 36% not treated developed nephropathy within 2–6 weeks after the acute episode of HSP [37,38].

Evidence for whether therapy can alter established HSP nephritis

There are very few trials of therapy for established HSP nephritis (Table 69.2). In the study described above, to determine if prednisone therapy prevented the development of HSP nephritis, the investigators found that in those who developed nephritis and were treated with prednisone, renal symptoms resolved significantly more rapidly in the patients in the prednisone group compared to the placebo group [36]. However, this finding was the result of a post hoc analysis, and further trials are needed to determine if steroids are beneficial for HSP nephritis.

In a randomized trial of cyclophosphamide and supportive therapy or supportive therapy alone, 28 children received supportive therapy and 28 received supportive therapy plus cyclophosphamide at 90 mg/m^2/day for 42 days [40]. The clinical status at last follow-up (mean, 6.93 years) demonstrated that there was no difference in outcome between the two groups. In a study (published as a meeting abstract) of 19 patients with severe HSP, 10 of 10 (100%) cyclosporine A-treated patients achieved remission compared with 5 of 9 (56%) patients who received pulse solumedrol [41].

Although there is a dearth of high-quality studies to provide evidence-based recommendations for therapy in HSP nephritis, there are numerous retrospective case studies of therapy for HSP nephritis (Table 69.2) [34,42–52]. A case series of prednisone treatment, with or without methylprednisolone, found improvement in the majority of the children [44]. Similar studies of prednisone and other immunosuppressive agents, including cyclophosphamide and azathioprine, have also described improvement in most children [34,42,43,45,46]. Finally, at least two retrospective case studies have demonstrated that therapy with cyclosporine in severe HSP nephritis is beneficial [47,48]. Additional therapies, including intravenous immunoglobulin therapy, plasmapheresis, and tonsillectomy, have been reported to improve a patient's response to immunosuppressive therapy [49–52].

Recommendations for therapy of HSP and HSP nephritis

Two randomized double-blind controlled trials and one retrospective study of therapy with prednisone in patients with HSP did not demonstrate a benefit of therapy in preventing the development of HSP nephritis, whereas two RCTs with poor methodological quality demonstrated a benefit of prednisone therapy in preventing HSP nephritis. Although these studies are not conclusive, the body of evidence suggests that prednisone therapy should not be used to prevent the development of HSP nephritis in patients with HSP (Table 69.3).

The study described above that was conducted to determine if prednisone therapy was beneficial for the prevention of HSP nephritis found, as a secondary outcome, that prednisone was beneficial for HSP nephritis, but this was determined from a post hoc analysis and so further studies are needed [36]. A controlled trial of cyclophosphamide therapy did not demonstrate a benefit of therapy, but these patients did not receive pulse solumedrol or prednisone therapy [40]. Other than a very small trial with short

Table 69.2 Evidence that therapy can alter established HSP nephritis.

Study	Therapy	Number of patients and patient characteristics	Outcome
Oner, 1995 case reports	pulse SM, cyclophosmaide, dipyridamole, oral prednisone	12 patients, 6-14 years of age	7 patients complete remission 4 patients partial remission 1 patient persisent nephrotic syndrome
Faedda, 1996 case reports	pulse SM, oral cyclophosmide, oral prednisone	8 patients, ages 13-61 years of age	7 patients complete remission
Niaudet, 1998 prospective uncontrolled study	pulse SM followed by oral prednisone	38 children ages 3 to 14 years of age with severe HSP nephritis	27 children recovered normally 7 children had residial abnormalities 4 children had ESRDI
Bergstein, 1998 retrospective study	pulse SM followed by oral prednisone and azathihoprine	21 children ages 1 to 16 years with severe HSP nephritis	19 children improved 2 progressed to ESRD
Iijima, 1998 retrospective study	prednisone, cyclophosphamide, heparin/warfarin, and dipyridamole	14 children ages 5 to 17 years with severe HSP	9 children were normal 3 had minor abnormalites, 1 heavy proteinuria no child had ESRD
Foster, 2000 retrospective study	prednisone 1-2 mg/kg/day and azathioprine 1-2 mg/kg//day	17 children ages 4 to 19 years with severe HSP	15 of 17 (88%) had a favorable outcome
Tanaka, 2003 retrospective study	prednisone 1.5 mg/kg/day and cyclophosphosmide 2mg/kg/day	9 children ages 6 to 16 years with severe HSP	At last folowup (78 months) 7 were normal and two had protieniura, no ESRD
Ronkainen, 2003 retrospective study	cyclosporin A	7 children ages 7 to 15 with severe HSP	4 in remission off cyclosporin, 3 in remission on cyclospirin and are dependent
Tarshish, 2004 prospective randomized trial	supportive therapy with or with out 90mg/m2/day cyclophosmide	56 children; 28 treated 28 control	No difference in renal outcome
Shin, 2005 retrospective study	cyclopsorin A	7 children ages 3.9 to 13.8 years with severe HSP	all patients improved with reduction in proteinuria
Shin, 2005 retrospective study	comparision of prednisone alone or prednisone and azathioprine	10 children in each group	children treated with prednisone and azathioprine did better than children treated with prednisone alone
Ronkainen, 2006 randomized placebo controled double	1 mg/kg/day prednisone for two weeks and weaning dose for two more weeks	84 treated patients and 87 placebo children ages 1.7 to 15.6 years	61% of prednisone treated renal symptoms resolved 34% of placebo treated renal symptoms resolved

follow-up that compared cyclosporine with methylprednisolone treatment, there are no other trials to guide evidence-based treatment recommendations. Although there are no other clinical trials on which to make treatment recommendations, there are several retrospective case series reports that have described a benefit of immunosuppressive therapy in established HSP nephritis. Given the well-described poor outcome of severe HSP nephritis, RCTs of therapy versus placebo are unlikely to be conducted, but trials to compare specific therapies are needed. Until such studies have been performed, evidence-based treatment recommendations cannot be formulated, but steroids (pulse solumedrol followed by oral prednisone or oral prednisone alone, depending upon the severity of the nephritis) with or without other immunosuppressive agents are reasonable therapies for severe disease. Since HSP nephritis is a variable disease, individual risk factors for progressive renal disease need to be taken into consideration when formulating therapy for patients with HSP.

Etiology, epidemiology, and natural history of MPGN

MPGN can be secondary to infections, such as hepatitis B or C virus or human immunodeficiency virus infection, or it may be secondary to collagen vascular diseases [53,54]. Idiopathic MPGN occurs in the absence of infections or other known causes of secondary MPGN. When MPGN is secondary to another infection or disease, therapy needs to be directed at the underlying cause of MPGN, such as interferon therapy for hepatitis or immunosuppressive therapy for collagen vascular diseases.

Etiology

The precise etiologies of the various types of MPGN are unknown. MPGN also has been called mesangiocapillary glomerulonephritis

Table 69.3 Evidence rating and recommendations for therapy in Henoch-Schonlein Purpura

Intervention	Evidence rating[a,b]		Comment	Recommendations[c]			Comment
	Moderate	Low		I[d]	II[e]	III[f]	
Corticosteroids in the prevention of nephritis							
Prednisone compared with placebo/no treatment		•	4 RCTs (499 patients), 2 trials of poor quality, inconsistent results			•	No significant benefit for preventing nephritis in 2 trials; 2 trials of poor quality suggested benefit
Corticosteroids in the treatment of nephritis							
Corticosteroids compared with placebo		•	1 RCT (171 children); Post hoc analysis		•		Among children with nephritis, reduction in symptoms more rapid with prednisone
Solumedrol and oral prednisone			1 Case series (38 children)				Normal recovery in the majority of children
Cyclophosphamide in the treatment of nephritis							
Cyclophosphamide compared with supportive treatment		•	1 RCT (56 patients); wide 95% CI			•	No significant benefit in reducing risk of any renal involvement or ESRD in RCT
Cyclophosphamide and prednisone with or without dipyridamole			4 Case series (43 children)				Majority of children improved and majority returned to normal in case series
Cyclosporin in the treatment of nephritis							
Cyclosporin compared with methylprednisolone		•	1 RCT (19 patients); small numbers			•	More patients on cyclosporine achieved remission in RCT.
Cyclosporin			2 Case series (14 patients)				Majority of children improved in case series
Prednisone and azathioprine in the treatment of nephritis							
Prednisone and azathioprine compared to prednisone alone		•	1 Retrospective study (20 children)			•	Combined therapy was better than prednisone alone
Prednisone and azathiopine		•	2 Case series (38 children)				Treated patients improved more than historic controls

[a] Evidence rating based on number of studies, study design, study quality and consistency of results.

[b] No intervention was rated with a high evidence rating

[c] Recommendations based on efficacy, trade off between benefits and harms and quality of evidence and availability of medication

[d] Recommend

[e] Suggest

[f] No recommendation possible

or peripheral lobular glomerulonephritis. Type II MPGN is also called dense deposit disease, due to the characteristic deposits seen on electron microscopy. Although there are three types of MPGN, types I and III share similar clinical and pathologic features; in contrast, type II MPGN (dense deposit disease) has distinct clinical and pathological features. The pathologic features of MPGN include an inflammatory infiltrate with increased mesangial cellularity and increased mesangial matrix leading to an accentuated lobular appearance of the glomerular tuft, hence, the name peripheral lobular glomerulonephritis. Immunofluorescence studies in type I and type III MPGN are usually positive for several complement components and immunoglobulins, whereas immunofluorescence findings in type II MPGN are remarkable for the absence

of immunoglobulin deposition but with intense complement deposition [13–15,54]. The electron microscopic findings are distinct for each type of MPGN, and these findings provide the basis for the division of MPGN into three subtypes. Type I MPGN is characterized by prominent subendothelial deposits, whereas type III MPGN has subendothelial and subepithelial deposits. Electron microscopy findings in type II MPGN include characteristic dense deposits within the lamina densa and the basement membranes [13–15,54].

In MPGN types I and III complement C3 and C4 levels are usually depressed, suggesting that the classical pathway is preferentially activated, whereas in type II MPGN the C3 level is depressed and the C4 level is normal, suggesting activation of the

Table 69.4 Evidence that therapy can alter MPGN - randomized controled trials.

Study	Therapy	Number of patients	Outcome
Mota-Hernandez, 1985 double blind controlled trial	Prednisone vs lactose	18 children, biopsies performed at diagnosis, 3 and 5 years	At 6.5 years, 4 patients in control group and none in treatment group developed ESRD; two in control and one in treated in remission; decreased activity and increased chronic changes on biopies in all patients.
Tarshish, 1992 randomized, double blind controlled trial RTC	Prednisone 40mg/m2 every other day vs lactose (47 treatment, 33 controls)	80 children ages 5.2 to 16.9 years 42 type I, 14 type II, 17 type III mean duration of therapy was 41 months	Treatment failure 55% in controls, 40% in treated group; of types I and III, treatment failure 58% in controls and 33% in treated group. eatd
Zimmerman, 1983 prospective trial	warfarin and dipyridamole	18 completed a control or treatment year 13 completed both a control and treatment year	Renal function stable during year of therapy, renal function declined with no therapy, proteinuria decreased during therapy
Donadio, 1984 RCT	Dipyridamole 225 mgs and aspirin 975 mg for 1 year	40 adult patients, 21 treated, 19 control	GFR better in treated group, rate of decline in treated 1.3 ml/min per 1.73m2 compared to 19.6 ml/min/1.73m2 in control, fewer treated pateints progressed to ESRD
Cattran, 1985 RCT	cyclophosphamide, coumadin and dipyradimole vs control	59 patients (27 treated, 32 control) with greater than 2gm/day proteinuria	At 6, 12, and 18 months no difference in renal function, serum creatinine, slop of creatinine clearance, or proteinuria
Zauner, 1994 randomized trial RCT	aspirin and dipyridamole vs supportive therapy	18 adults (15 type I, 3 type II) with nephrotic syndrome followed for 36 months	No change in renal function both groups, proteinujria decrease more in the treated group (8.3 ± 1.4 to 1.6 ± 0.7 treated vs 7.1 ± 1.6 to 4.3 ± 1.1 gm/day controls)
Giri, 2002 RCT	All patients received diuretics & beta-blockers, 1/3 treated with ACEI, 1/3 treated with CCB, 1/3 no additional therapy (control)	30 adults, 28 completed nine months of therapy	Serum creatinine and proteinuria significantly increased in controls, ACEI group had decrease in serum creatinine proteinuria, CCB group had decrease in serum creatinine and increase in proteinuria

alternative pathway. C3 nephritic factor is present in all types but is more common in type II MPGN [14]. Because a low serum level of C3 is the laboratory hallmark of MPGN, abnormal regulation of the complement system in particular is thought to be central to the pathogenesis of MPGN [13–15,54,55]. Aberrant complement regulation is due to the presence of C3 nephritic factor, an autoantibody directed against the C3 convertase of the alternative pathway [55]. The binding of this antibody protects C3bBb from enzymatic inactivation so that there is continued C3 breakdown [56,57]. Genetic mutations of the factor H genotype have been implicated in the pathogenesis of type II MPGN [58,59]. Factor H is a soluble complement regulatory protein that has a primary role in regulating the activity of alternative complement pathway MPGN [59]. Factor H gene mutations result in a lack of plasma factor H or in a functional defect in factor H proteins. Loss of factor H function can also be caused by inactivating factor H autoantibodies, C3 mutations preventing interaction between C3 and factor H, or autoantibodies against C3 [59].

Epidemiology

MPGN occurs more commonly in children and young adults than in adults. All types of MPGN can occur in pediatric patients and are usually idiopathic and rarely associated with hepatitis B or C

virus infections. In adults, types I and III of MPGN are more common, and MPGN is frequently associated with hepatitis infections and mixed cryoglobulinemia [53,54,60]. Type II MPGN can occur in patients with partial lipodystrophy and may be associated with retinal changes [61,62]. Types I and III reoccur in renal transplant patients in approximately 20–30% of renal transplant recipients [63]. Graft loss due to recurrent disease is approximately 30–40% [64]. Type II MPGN reoccurs in renal transplant patients in up to 100% of cases, but graft loss due to recurrent disease is quite variable, with reports ranging from 10 to 50% [64,65]. In a large retrospective study, 5-year graft survival for patients with type II MPGN was significantly worse than for those transplanted for other causes (50.0% ± 7.5% versus 74.3% ± 0.6%, respectively) [66].

Natural history of MPGN

Since MPGN was first described in 1965, it has been recognized to be a progressive glomerulonephritis, and the natural history is progression to end-stage renal disease in the majority of cases [13–15,54,67]. In a series of 105 children with MPGN, 67% presented with nephrotic syndrome, 88% had hematuria, 33% had renal insufficiency, and 25% had hypertension [68]. After 5.75 years of follow-up, 34 patients had kidney failure or were dead, 8 had chronic kidney failure, 7 had hypertension with normal renal

Table 69.5 Evidence that therapy can alter MPGN - uncontrolled trials and case series.

Study	Therapy	Number of patients and patient characteristics	Outcome
McEnery PT, 1990 uncontroled trail	Alternate day prednisone in 50 children additional agents in 21 children	71 children treated for a mean of 7.7 years and followed for a mean of 10.6 years	Cummulative renal survival 75% at 10 years and 59% at 20 years
Ford, 1992 uncontroled trial	oral predinisone in all, pulse methylprednisolone in those more severe	19 children with type I MPGN followqed up for a mean of 6.5 years	Biopsy at two years showed decreased activity in 88% of children, Eight children have normal urinalysis
Bergstein, 1995 uncontroled trial	Pulse methylprednisolone followed by alternate day prednisone	16 children ages 5 to 14 years mean follow up 52 months	Improvement in serum albumin and creatinine clearance, decrease in proteinuria and hematuria; repeat kidney biopsies decreased active disease increased chronic changes
Iitaka, 1995	Low dose alternate prednisone, low dose followed by high dose alternate day prednisone, or high dose alternate day prednisone	41 children ages 3 to 15 years identified by school screening	Remission of urinary abnormalities was highest in those treated with high dose alternate day prednisone
Arslan, 1997 uncontrolled trail	All received oral steroids; those who did not respond received pulse MP and/ or cyclophosphamide	96 children, ages 2 to 17 years	Renal survival was 81.9% and 61% at 5 and 10 years respectively
Braun, 1999 retrospective comparison studies	Comparison of alternate day prednisone therapy in type I and type III MPGN	21 children with type I and 25 children with type III MPGN	At last follow-up, type I patients had improved GFR, type III had decreased GRF; type I had hematuria in 38%, type III had hematuria in 72%, type I had proteinuria 0% type III had proteinuria 28%.
Yanagihara, 2005 Case series	Prednisone 2mg/kg/day after pulse solumedrol (n = 16) or cyclophosamide (n = 3)	19 children ages 7 to 16 followed for more than 10 years, mean 14.6 ± 4.6 years	At last observation, 15 had normal UA, normal renal function, normal C3 levels; 4 had residual proteinuria, no ESRD
Ronkainen, 2006 RCT	cyclosporine or pulse solumedrol	19 children ages , 10 treated with cyclosporine and 9 treated with pulse solumedrol followed for three months	10 od 10 (100%) cyclosporine treated patients achieved remission compared with 5 of 9 (56%) pulse solumedrol treated patients
Orlowski, 1988 uncontroled trial	prednisone, azathioprine, chlorambucil and/or cyclophosphamide	40 adults mean age at diagnosis 23.5 ± 1.6 years followed for an average of 10.6 years	Triple therapy was more effective in reducing proteinuria.
Jones, 2004 retrospective study	Comparison of oral prednisolone and mycophenolate with no therapy	5 adults received therapy and 6 received no therapy	Significant protein reduction in the treated group from 5.09 to 2.59 at 18 months while there was no reduction in the untreated group; serum creatinine increased in controls and did not in treated patients

function, 50 had residual proteinuria, and 6 were protein free [68]. Thus, 95% of children had evidence of disease and only 5% were normal. In another large series of 104 adults and children with MPGN, follow-up of 2–21 years with a mean of 8 years demonstrated that only 7 (6.5%) of the patients were in clinical remission whereas 38% of the patients with type I and 49% of type II patients required dialysis or had died [14].

In a study of 53 children with MPGN, the mean age of presentation was 8.8 years, and these children were followed for a median of 3.5 years; 31 children had type I disease, 14 had type II disease, and 2 had type III disease (the others could not be classified) [13]. Those with nephrotic syndrome at presentation had a mean renal survival of 8.9 years compared to 13.6 years in those with-

out nephrotic syndrome [13]. A review of 273 patients in Norway with a mean age of 40 ± 17 years with a diagnosis of MPGN (some of whom had IgA deposits possibly representing IgA nephropathy) showed that 3 years after diagnosis, 7% had developed kidney failure and 8% had died [69]. Similar to other studies, clinical and laboratory variables associated with progressive disease were increased serum creatinine, high-grade proteinuria, hypertension, depressed serum albumin, focal sclerosis on biopsy, and interstitial fibrosis [69].

Evidence for efficacy of therapies in MPGN

Because the natural history of idiopathic MPGN is usually progression to chronic kidney failure, several therapies have been proposed

Table 69.6 Evidence rating and recommendations for therapy in MPGN

Intervention	Evidence rating[a,b]			Recommendations[c]			Comment
	Moderate	Low	Comment	I[d]	II[e]	III[f]	
Corticosteroids in the treatment of MPGN							
Alternate day prednisone compared with placebo/no treatment	•		2 RCT (98 children) Uncontrolled trials, retrospective studies and case series (309 children)	•			Each RCT showed benefit of therapy, uncontrolled trials, retrospective studies and case series support therapy, perhaps benefit is best in MPGN type I
Pulse methylprednisolone followed by alternate day prednisone therapy		•	4 uncontrolled trials, retrospective studies or case series. Indications for pulse methylprednisolone variable			•	Children with more severe MPGN treated with pulse methylprednisolone
Corticosteroids with other immunosuppressive agents in the treatment of MPGN							
Prednisone, azathioprine, chlorambucil or cyclophosphamide		•	1 Uncontrolled trial (40 adults)			•	Triple therapy reduced proteinuria
Prednisone and mycophenolate		•	1 Retrospective study (5 adults), small numbers			•	Proteinuria decreased and creatinine remained stable
Antiplatelet therapy in the treatment of MPGN							
Warfarin and dipyridamole		•	1 RCT (31 adults) small numbers, poor quality study			•	Beneficial effect of therapy
Dipyridamole and aspirin		•	2 RCTs (58 adults), small numbers, inconsistent results			•	One trial supports therapy, one does not
Cyclophosphamide, coumadin and dipyridamole		•	1 RCT (adults) *All performed prior to the association of hepatitis C with MPGN			•	No benefit of therapy

[a] Evidence rating based on number of studies, study design, study quality and consistency of results.
[b] No intervention was rated with a high evidence rating
[c] Recommendations based on efficacy, trade off between benefits and harms and quality of evidence and availability of medication
[d] Recommend
[e] Suggest
[f] No recommendation possible

to alter the natural history of MPGN (Tables 69.4 and 69.5) [70–84]. Antiplatelet therapy and immunosuppressive therapy have been tested in RCTs (Table 69.4) and in several uncontrolled trials, retrospective studies, and cases series (Table 69.5). Unfortunately, several of these trials and studies were performed before MPGN was known to be strongly associated with hepatitis C in adult patients, and the relevance of these trials to recommendations for current therapy is problematic. Three controlled trials have tested antiplatelet therapy, and an additional trial has tested antiplatelet therapy in combination with cyclophosphamide therapy [70,71,73,75]. Two studies concluded that antiplatelet therapy was beneficial, and two did not demonstrate efficacy of antiplatelet therapy (Table 69.4), but all of these studies probably included some patients with hepatitis C. Two controlled trials of prednisone versus placebo in children concluded that prednisone

therapy was beneficial, and follow-up biopsies in one study demonstrated decreased active disease (Table 69.4) [72,74]. In a trial of three groups that received either angiotensin converting enzyme (ACE) inhibitor therapy, calcium channel blocker therapy, or no additional therapy, in the patients with MPGN (also treated with diuretic therapy and beta blocker therapy), proteinuria and serum creatinine decreased with ACE inhibitor therapy, only creatinine decreased with calcium channel blocker therapy, and creatinine and proteinuria increased in the group that received no additional therapy [76].

Seven uncontrolled trials, retrospective studies, and case series using alternate-day prednisone therapy concluded that therapy was beneficial (Table 69.5) [77–84]. Four of these trials also incorporated pulse methylprednisolone into the treatment regimen for many patients [79–81,84]. An uncontrolled trial of prednisone, azathioprine, chlorambucil, and/or cyclophosphamide concluded that triple therapy was more effective in reducing proteinuria [77]. A recent retrospective study that compared patients treated with oral prednisone and mycophenolate to patients that received no therapy reported that proteinuria decreased more in the treatment group [82]. A retrospective comparison of alternate-day prednisone therapy in children with type I or type III MPGN concluded that therapy was more effective in type I MPGN [84].

Recommendations for therapy of MPGN

Controlled trials, uncontrolled trials, retrospective studies, and case series have demonstrated that alternate-day prednisone therapy is beneficial in MPGN (Table 69.6). Thus, alternate-day prednisone therapy is indicated in children with MPGN and could be considered in adults with idiopathic MPGN. Because the studies to test the efficacy of antiplatelet therapy were performed before the association of MPGN with hepatitis C was known and because the results of these trials demonstrated mixed findings, recommendations for antiplatelet therapy are difficult to formulate, but antiplatelet therapy is probably not indicated in patients with MPGN. A previous review of evidence-based treatment recommendations concluded that a trial of antiplatelet therapy is indicated in adult patients [85]. Adequate control of blood pressure and therapy to decrease residual proteinuria with ACE inhibitors should be used in patients with MPGN when indicated.

References

1 White RHR. Henoch-Schonlein nephritis. *Nephron* 1994; **68**: 1–9.

2 Stewart M, Savage JM, Bell B, McCord B. Long term renal prognosis of Henoch-Schonlein purpura in an unselected childhood population. *Eur J Pediatr* 1988; **147**: 113–115.

3 Meadow SR. The prognosis of Henoch Schonlein nephritis. *Clin Nephrol* 1978; **9**: 87–90.

4 Goldstein AR, White RH, Akuse R, Chantler C. Long term follow-up of childhood Henoch-Schonlein nephritis. *Lancet* 1992; **339**: 280–282.

5 Andreoli SP. Chronic glomerulonephritis in childhood; membranoproliferative glomerulonephritis, Henoch-Schonlein purpura and IgA nephropathy. *Pediatr Clin North Am* 1995; **42**: 1487–1504.

6 Uppal SS, Hussain MAS, Al-Raqum HA, Nampoory MPN, Al-Saeid K, Sl-Assousi A *et al.* Henoch-Schonlein purpura in adults versus children/adolescents: a comparative study. *Clin Exp Rheumatol* 2006; **24**: S26–S30.

7 Garcia-Porrua C, Calvino MC, Llorca J, Couselo JM, Gonzalez-Gay MA. Henoch-Schonlein purpura in children and adults. *Semin Arthritis Rheum* 2002; **32**: 149–156.

8 Kellerman PS. Henoch-Schonlein purpura in adults. *Am J Kidney Dis* 2006; **48**: 1009–1016.

9 Pillebout E, Thervet E, Hill G, Alberti C, Vanhille P, Nochy D. Henoch-Schonlein purpura in adults: outcome and prognostic factors. *J Am Soc Nephrol* 2002; **13**: 1271–1278.

10 Coppo R, Andrulli S, Amore A, Gianoglio B, Conti G, Peruzzi L *et al.* Predictors of outcome in Henoch Schonlein nephritis in children and adults. *Am J Kidney Dis* 2006; **47**: 993–1003.

11 Tancrede-Bohin E, Ochonisky S, Vignon-Pennamen M, Flaheul B, Morel P, Rybojad M. Henoch-Schonlein purpura in adult patients. *Arch Dermatol* 1977; **133**: 1114–1121.

12 Blanco R, Martinez-Taboada VM, Rodriguez-Valverde V, Garcia-Fuentes M, Gonzalez-Gay MA. Henoch-Schonlein purpura in adulthood and childhood. *Arthritis Rheum* 1997; **40**: 859–864.

13 Canisk JC, Lennon R, Cummins CL, Howie AJ, McGraw ME, Saleem MA *et al.* Prognosis, treatment and outcome of childhood mesangiocapillary (membranoproliferative) glomerulonephritis. *Nephrol Dial Transplant* 2004; **19**: 2769–2777.

14 Cameron JS, Turner DR, Heaton J, Williams DG, Ogg CS, Chantler C *et al.* Idiopathic mesangiocapillary glomerulonephritis. Comparisons of types I and II in children and adults and long-term prognosis. *Am J Med* 1983; **74**: 175–192

15 Bennett WM, Fassett RG, Walker RG, Fairley KF, D'Apice AJ, Kincaid-Smith P. Mesaniocapillary glomerulonephritis type II (dense deposit disease): clinical features of progressive disease. *Am J Kidney Dis* 1989; **13**: 469–476.

16 Saulsbury FT. Henoch-Schonlein purpura in children: report of 100 patients and review of the literature. *Medicine* 1999; **78**: 395–409.

17 O'Konoghue DJ, Darvill A, Ballardie FW. Mesangial cell autoantigens on immunoglobulin nephropathy and Henoch-Schonlein purpura. *J Clin Invest* 1991; **88**: 1522–1530.

18 Yang YH, Hung CF, Hsu CR, Wang CL, Chauang YH, Lin YT *et al.* A nationwide survey on epidemiological characteristics of childhood Henoch-Schonlein purpura in Taiwan. *Rheumatology* 2005; **44**: 618–622.

19 Calvino MC, Llorca J, Garcia-Porrua C, Fernandez-Iglesias JL, Rodriguez-Dedo P, Gonzalez-Gay MA. Henoch-Schonlein purpura in children from northwest Spain. *Medicine* 2001; **80**: 279–290.

20 Trapani S, Micheli A, Grisolia F, Resti M, Chiappini E, Falcini F *et al.* Henoch Schonlein purpura in childhood: epidemiological and clinical analysis of 150 cases over a 5 year period and review of the literature. *Semin Arthritis Rheum* 2005; **35**: 143–153.

21 Rueda B, Perez-Armengol C, Lopez-Lopez S, Garcia-Porrua C, Javier M, Gonzalez-Gay M. Association between functional haplotypes of vascular endothelial cell growth factor and renal complications in HSP. *J Rheumatol* 2006; **33**: 69–73.

22 Amoli MM, Calvino MC, Garcia-Porua C, Llorca J, Ollier WE, Gonzalez-Gay MA. Interleukin-1β gene polymorphisms association with severe renal manifestations and renal sequelae in Henoch-Schonlein purpura. *J Rheumatol* 2004; **32**: 295–298.

23 Yang YH, Lai HJ, Lin YT, Chiang BL. The association between transforming growth factor-β gene promoter C-509T polymorphism and Chinese children with HSP. *Pediatr Nephrol* 2004; **19**: 972–975.

24 Ozkaya O, Soylemezoglu O, Gonen S, Misirhoglu M, Tuncer S, Kalman S *et al.* Renin-angiotensin system gene polymorphisms: association with susceptibility to Henoch-Schonlein purpura. *Clin Rheumatol* 2006; **25**: 861–965.

25 Gershoni-Baruch R, Broza Y, Brik R. Prevalence and significance of mutations in the familial Mediterranean fever gene in Henoch-Schonlein purpura. *J Pediatr* 2003; **143**: 658–661.

26 Eisenstein EM, Choi M. Analysis of an uteroglobin gene polymorphism in childhood Henoch-Schonlein purpura. *Pediatr Nephrol* 2006; **21**: 782–784.

27 Dagan E, Brik R, Broza Y, Gershoni-Baruch R. Henoch-Schonlein purpura: polymorphisms in thrombophilia genes. *Pediatric Nephrol* 2006; **21**: 1117–1121.

28 Ronkainen J, Nuutinen M, Koskimies O. The adult kidney 24 years after childhood Henoch-Schonlein purpura: a retrospective cohort study. *Lancet* 2002; **360**: 666–670.

29 Fujunga S, Ohtomo Y, Maurkami H, Takemoto M, Yamashiro Y, Kaneko K. Recurrence of Henoch-Schonlein purpura after long term remission in a 15 years old girl. *Pediatr Nephrol* 2006; **21**: 1215–1216.

30 Narchi H. Risk of long term renal impairment and duration of follow up recommended for Henoch-Schonlein purpura with normal or minimal urinary findings; a systematic review. *Arch Dis Child* 2005; **90**: 916–920.

31 Sano H, Izumida M, Shimizu H, Ogawa Y. Risk factors of renal involvement and significant proteinuria in Henoch-Schonlein purpura. *Eur J Pediatr* 2002; **161**: 196–201.

32 Scharer K, Krmar R, Quefeld U, Ruder H, Waldherr R, Schaefer F. Clinical outcome of Schonlein purpura nephritis in children. *Pediatr Nephrol* 1999; **13**: 816–823.

33 Halling SFE, Soderberg MP, Berg U. Henoch Schonlein nephritis: clinical findings related to renal function and morphology. *Pediatr Nephrol* 2005; **20**: 46–51.

34 Bergstein J, Leiser J, Andreoli SP. Response of crescentric Henoch-Schonlein purpura to corticosteroid and azathioprine therapy. *Clin Nephrol* 1998; **49**: 9–14.

35 Huber AM, King J, McLaine P, Klassen T, Pothos M. A randomized, placebo-controlled trial of prednisone in early Henoch Schonlein purpura. *BMC Med* 2004; **2**: 1–7.

36 Ronkainen J, Kosimies O, Ala-Houhala M, Antikainen M, Merenmies J, Rajantie J *et al.* Early prednisone therapy in Henoch-Schonlein purpura: a randomized, double-blind, placebo controlled trial. *J Pediatr* 2006; **149**: 241–247.

37 Mollica F, Li VS, Garozzo G. Effectiveness of early prednisone treatment in preventing the development of nephropathy in anaphylactoid purpura. *Eur J Pediatr* 1992; **151**: 140–144.

38 Islek I, Sezer T, Totan M, Cakir M, Kucukoduk S. The effect of prophylactic prednisone therapy on renal involvement in Henoch-Schonlein purpura. *Congress of the European Renal Association/European Dialysis and Transplant Association*, 1999; p. 103.

39 Saulsbury FT. Corticosteroid therapy does not prevent nephritis in Henoch-Schonlein purpura. *Pediatr Nephrol* 1993; **7**: 69–71.

40 Tarshish P, Bernstein J, Edelman CM. Henoch-Schonlein purpura nephritis: course of disease and efficacy of cyclophosphamide. *Pediatr Nephrol* 2004; **19**: 51–56.

41 Ronkainen J, Ala-Houhala M, Antikainen M, Jahnukainene T, Koskimies O, Meremmies J *et al.* Cyclosporine A versus MP pulses in the treatment of severe Henoch-Schonlein nephritis. *Pediatr Nephrol* 2006; **21**: 1531A.

42 Oner A, Tinaztepe K, Erdogan O. The effect of triple therapy on rapidly progressive type of Henoch-Schonlein purpura nephritis. *Pediatr Nephrol* 1995; **9**: 6–10.

43 Faedda R, Pirisi R, Satta A, Bosincu L, Bartoli E. Regression of Henoch-Schonlein purpura disease with intensive immunosuppressive treatment. *Clin Pharmacol Ther* 1996; **60**: 576–581.

44 Niaudet P, Habib R. Methylprednisolone pulse therapy in the treatment of severe forms of Schonlein-Henoch purpura nephritis. *Pediatr Nephrol* 1998; **12**: 238–243.

45 Foster BJ, Bernard C, Drummond KN, Sharma AK. Effective therapy for severe Henoch-Schonlein purpura nephritis with prednisone and azathioprine: a clinical and histopathological study. *J Pediatr* 2000; **136**: 370–375.

46 Tanaka H, Suzuki K, Nakahata T, Ito E, Waga S. Early therapy with oral immunosuppressants in severe proteinuric purpura nephritis. *Pediatr Nephrol* 2003; **18**: 347–350.

47 Ronkainen J, Autio-Harmainen H, Nuutinen M. Cyclosporine A for the treatment of severe Henoch-Schonlein glomerulonephritis. *Pediatr Nephrol* 2003; **18**: 1138–1142.

48 Shin JI, Park JM, Shin YH, Kim JH, Kim PK, Lee JS *et al.* Cyclosporine A therapy for severe Henoch-Schonlein nephritis with nephrotic syndrome. *Pediatr Nephrol* 2005; **20**: 1093–1097.

49 Shin JI, Park JM, Shin YH, Kim JH, Lee JS, Kim PK *et al.* Can azathioprine and steroids alter the progression of severe Henoch-Schonlein nephritis in children? *Pediatr Nephrol* 2005; **20**: 1087–1092.

50 Sugiyama H, Watanabe N, Onoda T, Kikumoto Y, Yamamoto M, Maeta M *et al.* Successful treatment of progressive Henoch-Schonlein purpura nephritis with tonsillectomy and steroid pulse therapy. *Intern Med* 2005; **44**: 611–615.

51 Rostoker G, Desvaux-Belghiti D, Pilatte Y, Petit-Phar M, Philippon C, Deforges L *et al.* High-dose immunoglobulin therapy for severe IgA nephropathy and Henoch-Schonlein purpura. *Ann Intern Med* 1994; **120**: 476–484.

52 Chen TC, Chung FR, Lee CH, Huang SC, Chen JB, Hsu KT. Successful treatment of crescentric glomerulonephritis associated with adult onset Henoch-Schonlein purpura by double filtration plasmapheresis. *Clin Nephrol* 2004; **61**: 213–216.

53 Johnson RJ, Willson R, Yamabe H. Renal manifestations of hepatitis C virus infections. *Kidney Int* 1994; **46**: 1255.

54 Nakopoulou L. Membranoproliferative glomerulonephritis. *Nephrol Dial Transplant* 2001; **16**: 71–73.

55 Smith KD, Alpers CE. Pathogenetic mechanisms in membranoproliferative glomerulonephritis. *Curr Opin Nephrol Hypertens* 2005; **14**: 396–403.

56 Daha MR, Austen KF, Fearon DT. Heterogeneity, polypeptide chain composition, and antigenic reactivity of C3 nephritic factor. *J Immunol* 1978; **120**: 1389–1393.

57 Bennett WM, Fassett RG, Walder RG, Fairley KF, d'Apice AJ, Kincaid-Smith P. Mesangiocapillary glomerulonephritis type II (dense deposit disease): clinical features of progressive disease. *Am J Kidney Dis* 1989; **13**: 469–476.

58 Goodship THJ. Factor H genotype-phenotype correlations: lessons from HUS, MPGN type II and ADM. *Kidney Int* 2006; **70**: 12–13.

59 Licht C, Scvholtzer-Schrehardt U, Kirschfink M, Zipfel PF, Hoppe B. MPGN II genetically determined by defective complement regulation. *Pediatr Nephrol* 2007; **22**: 22–29.

60 Meyers C, Seef LB, Stehman-Breen CO, Hoofnagle JH. Hepatitis C and renal disease: an update. *Am J Kidney Dis* 2003; **42**: 631–637.

61 Eisinger AJ, Shortland JR, Moorhead PJ. Renal disease and partial lipodystrophy. *Q J Med* 1972; **163**: 343–354.

62 Duvall-Young J, Short CD, Raines MF, Gokal R, Lawler W. Fundus changes in mesangiocapillary glomerulonephritis. *Br J Opthalmol* 1989; **73**: 900–906.

63 Floege J. Recurrent glomerulonephritis following renal transplantation: an update. *Nephrol Dial Transplant* 2003; **18**: 1260.

64 Habib R, Antignac C, Hinglais N, Gagnadoux MF, Broyer M. Glomerular lesions in the transplanted kidney in children. *Am J Kidney Dis* 1987; **10**: 198.

65 Eddy A, Sibley R, Mauer SM, Kim Y. Renal allograft failure due to recurrent dense intramembranous deposit disease. *Clin Nephrol* 1984; **21**: 305.

66 Braun MC, Stablein DM, Hamiwka LA, Bell L, Bartosh SM, Strife CF. Recurrence of membranoproliferative glomerulonephritis type II in renal allographs: the North American Pediatric Renal Transplant Cooperative study. *J Am Soc Nephrol* 2005; **16**: 2225–2233.

67 West CD, McAdams AJ, McConville JM, Davis NC, Holland NH. Hypocompletemia in normal complementemic persistent chronic glomerulonephritis: clinical and pathologic characteristics. *J Pediatr* 1965; **67**: 1089–1012.

68 Habib R, Kleinknecht C, Gubler MC, Levy M. Idiopathic membranoproliferative glomerulonephritis. Report of 105 cases. *Clin Nephrol* 1973; **1**: 194–214.

69 Vikse BE, Bostad L, Aasarod K, Lysebo DE, Iverson BM. Prognostic factors in mesangioproliferative glomerulonephritis. *Nephrol Dial Transplant* 2002; **17**: 1603–1613.

70 Zimmerman SW, Moorthy AV, Dreher WH, Friedman A, Varanasi U. Prospective trial of warfarin and dipyridamole in patients with membranoproliferative glomerulonephritis. *Am J Med* 1983; **75**: 920–927.

71 Donadio JV, Anderson CF, Mitchell JC, Holley KE, Ilstrup DM, Fuster V *et al.* Membranoproliferative glomerulonephritis: a prospective clinical trial of platelet-inhibitor therapy. *N Engl J Med* 1984; **310**: 1421–1426.

72 Mota-Hernandez F, Gordillo-Paianua G, Munoz-Arizpe JA, Madueno L. Prednisone versus placebo in membranoproliferative glomerulonephritis: long term clinicopathologic correlations. *Int J Pediatr Nephrol* 1985; **6**: 25–28.

73 Cattran DC, Cardella CJ, Roscoe JM, Charron RC, Rance PC, Ritchie SM *et al.* Results of a controlled drug trial in membranoproliferative glomerulonephritis. *Kidney Int* 1985; **27**: 436–441.

74 Tarshish P, Bernstein J, Tobin JN, Edelmann CM. Treatment of mesangiocapillary glomerulonephritis with alternate day prednisone: a report of the International Study of Kidney Disease in Children. *Pediatr Nephrol* 1992; **6**: 123–130.

75 Zauner I, Bohler J, Braun N, Grupp C, Heering P, Schollmeyer P. Effect of aspirin and dipyridamole on proteinuria in idiopathic membranoproliferative glomerulonephritis: a multicenter prospective clinical trial. *Nephrol Dial Transplant* 1994; **9**: 619–622.

76 Giri S, Mahajan SK, Sen R, Sharma A. Effects of angiotensin converting enzyme inhibitor on renal function in patients of membranoproliferative glomerulonephritis with mild to moderate renal insufficiency. *J Assoc Physicians India* 2002; **50**: 1245–1249.

77 Orlowski T, Rancewicz M, Lao M, Juskowa J, Klepacka J, Gradowska L *et al.* Long-term immunosuppressive therapy of idiopathic membranoproliferative glomerulonephritis. *Klin Wochenschr* 1988; **66**: 1019–1023.

78 McEnery PT. Membranoproliferative glomerulonephritis: the Cincinnati experience. Cumulative renal survival from 1957 to 1989. *J Pediatr* 1990; **116**: S109–S114.

79 Ford DM, Briscoe DM, Shanley PF, Lum GM. Childhood membranoproliferative glomerulonephritis type I: limited steroid therapy. *Kidney Int* 1992; **41**: 1606–1612.

80 Arslan S, Saatci U, Ozen S, Bakkaloglu A, Besbas N, Tinaztepe K *et al. Int Urol Nephrol* 1997; **29**: 711–716.

81 Bergstein JM, Andreoli SP. Response of type I membranoproliferative glomerulonephritis to pulse methylprednisolone and alternate day steroid therapy. *Pediatr Nephrol* 1995; **9**: 268–271.

82 Jones G, Juszczak M, Kingdon E, Harber M, Sweny P, Burns A. Treatment of idiopathic membranoproliferative glomerulonephritis with mycophenolate mofetil and steroids. *Nephrol Dial Transplant* 2004; **18**: 3160–3164.

83 Yanagihara T, Hayakawa M, Yoshida J, Tsuchiya M, Morita T, Murakami M *et al.* Long term follow up of diffuse membranoproliferative glomerulonephritis type I. *Pediatr Nephrol* 2005; **20**: 585–590.

84 Braun MC, West CD, Strife CF. Differences between membranoproliferative glomerulonephritis types I and types III in long term response to alternate day prednisone regimen. *Am J Kidney Dis* 1999; **34**: 1022–1032.

85 Levin A. Management of membranoproliferative glomerulonephritis: evidence based guidelines. *Kidney Int* 1999; **55**: S41–S46.

70 Cystinosis

William G. van't Hoff

Nephro-Urology Unit, Great Ormond Street Hospital for Children, London, United Kingdom

Introduction and clinical course

Cystinosis is a disorder characterized biochemically by excess accumulation of cystine due to defective lysosomal efflux and clinically as the most common inherited cause of generalized proximal tubular dysfunction (renal Fanconi syndrome) in young children [1]. It is inherited in an autosomal recessive manner and is due to defective or absent function of cystinosin, the lysosomal proton-dependent cystine transporter, secondary to mutations in the *CTNS* gene [2,3]. Cystinosis is a rare condition, averaging approximately 1/150,000 births in the UK, but the incidence varies according to geographic region and ethnicity, being more common in populations with increased consanguinity.

Children typically present with slow weight gain, poor feeding, recurrent vomiting, and features of dehydration and rickets. These features are not present at birth, possibly related to the normally low glomerular filtration rate in newborn babies, but develop progressively from 4 to 6 months of life. Rarely, patients can present in adolescence or adult life with proteinuria or chronic renal failure [1]. Laboratory findings include hypokalemia, hypophosphatemia, and a hyperchloremic metabolic acidosis. Urinary data include generalized aminoaciduria, proteinuria (characteristically including large amounts of low-molecular-weight proteins), phosphaturia, and bicarbonaturia [4]. The diagnosis can be confirmed clinically by demonstration of cystine crystals in the cornea via slit lamp examination; the fundus is often characteristically "blond." However, these ocular signs may be missed, and all suspected cases should have the leukocyte cystine concentration determined. This is a specialized assay, and careful coordination with accredited laboratories is necessary to provide an accurate result.

The effects of the Fanconi syndrome are profound. Children require huge volumes of water, electrolyte supplements, and medications to try to normalize their biochemical and volume status. Feeding difficulties and vomiting exacerbate the problem. Without specific treatment, children suffer progressive growth failure, bone deformity from rickets, and chronic kidney failure (the median age of renal replacement therapy for untreated children is between 9 and 10 years) [1]. Kidney transplantation is highly successful and cystinosis does not recur in the graft, although cystine may be seen in interstitial cells within graft biopsies as cystine continues to accumulate in the rest of the body. Virtually every body system is affected in the long term, and in untreated patients, death occurs in early adulthood, usually secondary to neurological involvement [1].

Treatment

The treatment of cystinosis can be divided into general and specific measures. The aims of general treatment are to replace the deficits and normalize the biochemical homeostasis. Specific therapies address the underlying metabolic disorder or its progress.

In the context of evidence-based therapy for conditions affecting many thousands of patients, many treatments used in cystinosis would be regarded as having "poor" evidence. Most importantly, the disorder is extremely rare, so that studies are difficult to undertake. This review will not address the use of replacement electrolyte supplements, such as sodium and/or potassium chloride, sodium bicarbonate, sodium and/or potassium citrate, and phosphate preparations. Administration of combinations of these are essential, often in large volumes, to make up for the severe urinary losses.

Cysteamine acts by undergoing disulfide exchange with cystine to form a mixed disulfide, which exits the lysosome via the lysine transporter [5]. This effect was discovered during an investigation of a range of sulfhydryl agents, and its mechanism of action confirmed its utility in cystinosis. It has not been subject to a randomized controlled trial (which, in addition to the rarity of cystinosis, would be hampered by the taste and smell of cysteamine), but there is other considerable evidence for its efficacy (Table 70.1). What remains unclear is whether the efficacy is purely related to

Evidence-based Nephrology. Edited by Donald Molony and Jonathan Craig
© 2009 Blackwell Publishing, ISBN: 978-1-4051-3975-5.

Table 70.1 Evidence ratings and recommendations for cystinosis studies.

Intervention	SR	Evidence rating High	Moderate	Low	Comments	Recommendation I	II	III	Comment
Cysteamine (Mercaptamine)	—		•		4 case series (approx 376 patients, some possible duplications); very consistent reduction in progression renal damage; small number case reports with inconsistent results	•			Only available treatment at present
Topical cysteamine eye drops	—	•			4 RCTs (64 patients, 34 vs. placebo, 30 vs. other agents); cysteamine improved symptoms and objective score of corneal cystine density	•			Only available treatment at present
Cysteamine for nonrenal tissues	—		•		3 case series (>100 patients; likely marked overlap) studying thyroid function, swallowing dysfunction, and neurological status; clear preservation of thyroid function, reduced score for swallowing dysfunction; Possible effect on neurological status	•			Only available treatment at present
Growth hormone	—			•	Case series in children with very severe growth reduction (78 patients: 52 CRF, 7 dialysis, 15 transplanted); increased height SDS in CRF prepubertal group	•			10 RCTs for other CKD show benefit, increased risk with impaired glucose intolerance
Indomethacin to reduce urinary losses	—			•	1 RCT and 2 case reports; RCT (39 patients) showed no significant effect on polyuria or growth (over 6 months); RCT underpowered; case reports indicated improved electrolyte status			•	Used in approximately 50% UK patients pretransplant
Carnitine replacement	—			•	2 case series, 11 and 6 patients; improved plasma (short term) and muscle levels (long term)			•	Low toxicity, unproven clinical benefit
ACE inhibitor for proteinuria	—			•	Case series (5 patients); 43% reduction in albuminuria, reduction in systolic BP			•	Effective for other CKD, increased risks of hypotension in cystinosis
Proton pump inhibitor (omperazole, esomeprazole)	—			•	2 case series (23 children); improved symptom score and reduced cysteamine-induced gastric acid hypersecretion		•		Vomiting and feeding symptoms often worse with cysteamine, proton pump inhibitors well-tolerated
Ineffectiveness of ascorbic acid	—	•			1 RCT (64 patients vs. placebo); stopped after 2 years, as no benefit and 8/11 deaths or ESRD on ascorbic acid, RR of adverse event 2.7, CI 0.8–11.5	•			No evidence of efficacy

* Systematic review of randomised controlled trials (RCT).

a Evidence rating based on number of studies, study design, study quality, and consistency of results. No intervention was rated with a high evidence rating.

c Recommendations based on efficacy, trade-offs between benefits and harms, quality of evidence, and availability of medication. I, recommend; II, suggest; III, no recommendation possible.

cystine depletion or to other mechanisms as well (cysteamine is a radio-protective agent, and it may affect free radical production and other thiols in cystinotic cells). Cysteamine (Cystagon) has been licensed for use in cystinosis.

Cystinosis is a multisystem disorder, so responses to drugs shown to be beneficial in other chronic kidney disease (CKD) cannot necessarily be extrapolated. For instance, the bone disease in cystinosis children is caused by a combination of profound hypophosphataemic rickets, renal osteodystrophy, endocrinopathy, and potentially a direct effect of cystine accumulation on bone.

The $ctns^{-/-}$ mouse manifests severe bone disease but has no evident renal tubulopathy. The multisystem dysfunction needs to be considered when assessing the risk–benefit ratio of a drug, such as growth hormone. Likewise, angiotensin converting enzyme (ACE) inhibition can have profoundly adverse effects in cystinosis due to the chronic intravascular volume depletion.

Cystinosis patients who develop end-stage renal failure receive dialysis or transplantation as with other noncystinosis conditions. Graft survival is good in cystinosis; the disease cannot recur in the graft, although cystine crystals may be detected in the interstitium of graft biopsies [5-7]. However, because cystine continues to accumulate in other nonrenal tissues, cysteamine therapy is generally advised in posttransplant patients [1].

Recommendations for optimal management

Optimal management should initially correct the biochemical and intravascular volume abnormalities evident at presentation. However, achieving stable biochemistry can take months, and cysteamine should be started as soon as the diagnosis is confirmed. Cysteamine should be given in four divided doses throughout 24 h; better cystine depletion occurs in those who can manage a strict 6-h regimen, but this may not be realistic for all families [8,9]. The recommended dose is 1.3 g/m^2/day, but new patients should be commenced at lower doses (e.g. one-fourth of the maintenance dose) with increases every week. Breath smell, nausea, and vomiting are frequent adverse effects, but tolerance can develop. A proton pump inhibitor can reduce the gastrointestinal effects [10,11]. The leukocyte cystine level is considered the best marker of tissue cystine depletion, and the aim is a level (taken 4–6 h after the last dose) of <1 nmol $^1/_2$ cystine/mg of protein [1]. The determination of leukocyte cystine is difficult. Careful discussion with a specialized metabolic laboratory is vital, as difficulties with the assay tend to cause artificially low results, which may lead to inadequate dosing [7]. After stabilization, the cystine level should be checked 3–4 times/year. The maximal dose is 1.95 g/m^2/day. For patients over 12 years old or over 50 kg, the recommended dose is 2 g/day. A small number of European patients (six so far, and mostly on high doses) have experienced an Ehlers Danlos-like skin reaction, in one case with fatal complications. Families should be asked to report immediately to their physician any unexpected circumscribed hemorrhagic or bruising rash.

Expert nutritional support is needed in view of the extreme fluid requirement, poor feeding, and vomiting that are so prevalent with cystinosis. In Europe, many physicians advocate indomethacin (2–3 mg/kg/day in divided doses) to reduce urinary losses and use of growth hormone in those who fail to respond to conventional treatments. Cysteamine eye drops are clearly beneficial and may even reverse corneal crystal deposition. After transplant, cysteamine therapy is logical to minimize the long-term sequelae of cystinosis.

Conflict of Interest

The author is contracted as a medical consultant to Orphan Europe, distributor of Cystagon (mercaptamine or cysteamine). Payment for this work (totalling £1150 to date) has been made to a research fund for cystinosis, held at the Institute of Child Health, University College London, for cystinosis research.

References

1 Gahl WA, Thoene JG, Schneider JA. Cystinosis: a disorder of lysosomal membrane transport. In: Scriver CR, Beaudet AL, Valle D, & Sly WS, eds. *The Metabolic and Molecular Basis of Inherited Disease*, 8th edn., vol. III. McGraw-Hill, New York, 2001: 5085–5108

2 Town M, Jean G, Cherqui S, Attard M, Forestier L, Whitmore SA *et al.* A novel gene encoding an integral membrane protein is mutated in nephropathic cystinosis. *Nat Genet* 1998; **18**: 319–324.

3 Kalatzis V, Cherqui S, Antignac C, Gasnier B. Cystinosin, the protein defective in cystinosis, is a H$^+$-driven lysosomal cystine transporter. *EMBO J* 2001; **21**: 5940–5949.

4 van't Hoff, W. Fanconi syndrome. In: Davison AM, Cameron S, Grunfeld J-P, Ponticelli C, Ritz E, Winearls C *et al.*, eds. *Oxford Textbook of Clinical Nephrology*, 3rd edn. Oxford University Press, New York, 2005: 961–973.

5 Gahl WA, Reed GF, Thoene JG, Schulman JD, Rizzo WB, Jonas AJ *et al.* Cysteamine therapy in nephropathic cystinosis. *N Engl J Med* 1987; **361**: 971–977.

6 Markello TC, Bernardini IM, Gahl WA. Improved renal function in children with cystinosis treated with cysteamine. *N Engl J Med* 1993; **328**:1157–1162.

7 van't Hoff, WG, Gretz, N. The treatment of cystinosis with cysteamine and phosphocysteamine in the UK and Eire. *Pediatr Nephrol* 1995; **9**: 685–689.

8 Belldina EB, Huang MY, Schneider JA, Brundage RC, Tracy TS. Steady-state pharmacokinetics and pharmacodynamics of cysteamine bitartrate in paediatric nephropathic cystinosis patients. *Br J Clin Pharmacol* 2003; **56(5)**: 520–525.

9 Levtchenko EN, van Dael CM, de Graaf-Hess AC, Wilmer MJ, van den Heuvel LP, Monnens LA *et al.* Strict cysteamine dose regimen is required to prevent nocturnal cystine accumulation in cystinosis. *Pediatr Nephrol* 2006; **21**: 110–113.

10 Dohil R, Newbury RO, Sellers ZM, Deutsch R, Schneider JA. The evaluation and treatment of gastrointestinal disease in children with cystinosis receiving cysteamine. *J Pediatr* 2003; **143(2)**: 224–230.

11 Dohil R, Fidler M, Barshop B, Newbury R, Sellers Z, Deutsch R *et al.* Esomeprazole therapy for gastric acid hypersecretion in children with cystinosis. *Pediatr Nephrol* 2005; **20(12)**: 1786–1793.

12 Proesmans W, Baten E, Hoogmartens J, Bruyneel P. Nephropathic cystinosis: effect of long-term cysteamine therapy. *Clin Nephrol* 1987; **27**: 309–312.

13 Kleta R, Gahl WA. Pharmacological treatment of nephropathic cystinosis with cysteamine. *Expert Opin Pharmacother* 2004; **5(11)**: 2255–2262.

14 Gahl WA, Thoene JG, Schneider JA, O'Regan S, Kaiser-Kupfer MI, Kuwabra T. NIH conference. Cystinosis: progress in a prototypic disease. *Ann Intern Med* 1988; **109(7)**: 557–569.

15 Kaiser-Kupfer MI, Gazzo MA, Datiles MB, Caruso RC, Kuehl EM, Gahl WA. A randomized placebo-controlled trial of cysteamine eye drops in nephropathic cystinosis. *Arch Ophthalmol* 1990; **108(5)**: 689–693.

16 Bradbury JA, Danjoux JP, Voller J, Spencer M, Brocklebank T. A randomised placebo-controlled trial of topical cysteamine therapy in patients with nephropathic cystinosis. *Eye* 1991; **5(6)**: 755–760.

17 Iwata F, Kuehl EM, Reed GF, McCain LM, Gahl WA, Kaiser-Kupfer MI. A randomized clinical trial of topical cysteamine disulfide (cystamine) versus free thiol (cysteamine) in the treatment of corneal cystine crystals in cystinosis. *Mol Genet Metab* 1998; **64(4)**: 237–242.

18 Tsilou ET, Thompson D, Lindblad AS, Reed GF, Rubin B, Gahl WA *et al.* A multicentre randomised double masked clinical trial of a new formulation of topical cysteamine for the treatment of corneal cystine crystals in cystinosis. *Br J Ophthalmol* 2003; **87(1)**: 28–31.

19 Dureau P, Broyer M, Dufier JL. Evolution of ocular manifestations in nephropathic cystinosis: a long-term study of a population treated with cysteamine. *J Pediatr Ophthalmol Strabismus* 2003; **40(3)**: 142–146.

20 Sonies BC, Almajid P, Kleta R, Bernadini I, Gahl WA. Swallowing dysfunction in 101 patients with nephropathic cystinosis: benefit of long-term cysteamine therapy. *Medicine* (Baltimore) 2005; **84(3)**: 137–146.

21 Kimonis VE, Troendle J, Rose SR, Yang ML, Markello TC, Gahl WA. Effects of early cysteamine therapy on thyroid function and growth in nephropathic cystinosis. *J Clin Endocrinol Metab* 1995; **80(11)**: 3257–3261.

22 Schneider JA, Schlesselman JJ, Mendoza SA, Orloff S, Thoene JG, Kroll WA *et al.* Ineffectiveness of ascorbic acid therapy in nephropathic cystinosis. *N Engl J Med* 1979; **300(14)**: 756–759.

23 Broyer M, Tete MJ, Guest G, Bertheleme JP, Labrousse F, Poisson M. Clinical polymorphism of cystinosis encephalopathy. Results of treatment with cysteamine. *J Inherit Metab Dis* 1996; **19(1)**: 65–75.

24 Levtchenko E, Blom H, Wilmer M, van der Heuvel L, Monnens L. ACE inhibitor enalapril diminishes albuminuria in patients with cystinosis. *Clin Nephrol* 2003; **60(6)**: 386–389.

25 Gahl WA, Bernadini I, Dalakas M, Rizzo WB, Harper GS, Hoeg JM *et al.* Oral carnitine therapy in children with cystinosis and renal Fanconi syndrome. *J Clin Invest* 1988; **81(2)**: 549–560.

26 Gahl WA, Bernadini I, Dalakas MC, Markello TC, Krasnewich DM, Charnas LR. Muscle carnitine repletion by long-term carnitine supplementation in nephropathic cystinosis. *Pediatr Res* 1993; **34(2)**: 115–119.

27 Clark KF, Slymen DJ, Schneider JA, Thoene J, Stetz S, Gahl WA *et al.* A comparative study of indomethacin for treatment of the Fanconi syndrome in cystinosis. *J Rare Dis* 1996; **11**: 5–12.

28 Lemire J, Kaplan BS. The various renal manifestations of the nephropathic form of cystinosis. *Am J Nephrol* 1984; **4(2)**: 81–85.

29 Haycock GB, Al-Dahhan J, Mak RH, Chantler C. Effect of indomethacin on clinical progress and renal function in cystinosis. *Arch Dis Child* 1982; **57(12)**: 934–939.

30 Andersson HC, Markello T, Schneider JA, Gahl WA. Effect of growth hormone treatment on serum creatinine concentration in patients with cystinosis and chronic renal disease. *J Pediatr* 1992; **120(5)**: 716–720.

31 Wuhl E, Haffner D, Offner G, Broyer M, van't Hoff W, Mehls O. Long-term treatment with growth hormone in short children with nephropathic cystinosis. Long-term treatment with growth hormone in short children with nephropathic cystinosis. *J Pediatr* 2001; **138(6)**: 880–887.

32 Langlois V, Geary D, Murray L, Chapoux S, Hebert D, Goodyer P. Polyuria and proteinuria in cystinosis have no impact on renal transplantation. A report of the North American Pediatric Renal Transplant Cooperative Study. *Pediatr Nephrol* 2000; **15(1–2)**: 7–10. (Erratum in *Pediatr Nephrol* 2001; **16(2)**: 201.)

33 Theodoropoulos DS, Krasnewich D, Kaiser-Kupfer MI, Gahl WA. Classic nephropathic cystinosis as an adult disease. *JAMA* 1993; **270(18)**: 2200–2204.

34 Gagnadoux MF, Charbit M, Guest G, Arsan A, Broyer M. Clinical evaluation of 70 pediatric renal transplants after 10 to 17 years. *Ann Pediatr* (Paris) 1991; **38(6)**: 413–417.

Index

Note: page numbers in *italics* refer to figures and page numbers in **bold** refer to tables.

Index

Index